DIAGNOSTIC IMAGING
EMERGENCY

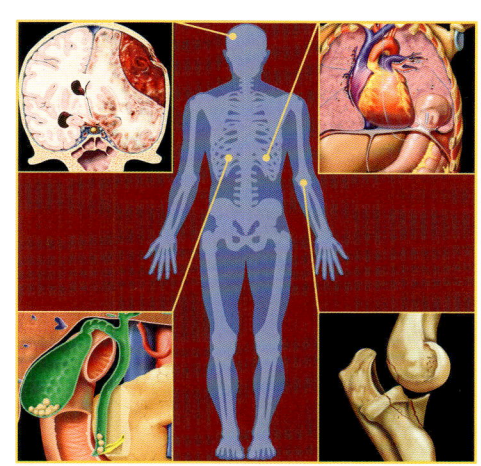

DIAGNOSTIC IMAGING
EMERGENCY

R. Brooke Jeffrey, MD
Professor of Radiology
Chief of Abdominal Imaging
Stanford University School of Medicine
Stanford, CA

B.J. Manaster, MD, PhD, FACR
Professor of Radiology
University of Utah
Salt Lake City, UT

Jud W. Gurney, MD, FACR
Charles A Dobry Professor of Radiology
University of Nebraska Medical Center
Omaha, NE

Robert D. Zimmerman, MD, FACR
Professor of Radiology
Executive Vice Chairman
Department of Radiology
Weill Medical College of Cornell University
Director of Diagnostic Imaging
New York Presbyterian Hospital
New York, NY

Joel K. Curé, MD
Associate Professor of Radiology
University of Alabama Medical Center
Birmingham, AL

Lane F. Donnelly, MD
Radiologist-in-Chief
Cincinnati Children's Hospital Medical Center
Professor of Radiology and Pediatrics
University of Cincinnati College of Medicine
Cincinnati, OH

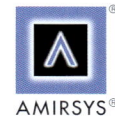

AMIRSYS®
Names you know, content you trust®

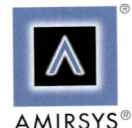

AMIRSYS®
Names you know, content you trust®

First Edition

Text and Radiologic Images - Copyright © 2007 Christopher G. Anton, MD, Corning Benton, MD, FACR, Miriam A. Bredella, MD, Russell W. Chapin, MD, Joel K. Curé, MD, Lane F. Donnelly, MD, Bradley R. Ferguson, MD, Jeffrey W. Grossman, MD, Jud W. Gurney, MD, FACR, H. Ric Harnsberger, MD, Keith D. Hentel, MD, R. Brooke Jeffrey, MD, Blaise V. Jones, MD, Steven J. Kraus, MD, B.J. Manaster, MD, PhD, FACR, Jay T. Morrow, MD, PhD, Misty Norman, MD, Anne G. Osborn, MD, FACR, Colin D. Strickland, MD, A. John Tsiouris, MD, Brant Wommack, MD, Robert D. Zimmerman, MD, FACR

Drawings - Copyright © 2007 Amirsys Inc.

Compilation - Copyright © 2007 Amirsys Inc.

All rights reserved. No part of this publication may be reproduced, stored in a retrieval system, or transmitted, in any form or media or by any means, electronic, mechanical, photocopying, recording, or otherwise, without prior written permission from Amirsys Inc.

Composition by Amirsys Inc, Salt Lake City, Utah

Printed in Canada by Friesens, Altona, Manitoba, Canada

ISBN-13: 978-1-4160-4934-0
ISBN-10: 1-4160-4934-7
ISBN-13: 978-0-8089-2397-8 (International English Edition)
ISBN-10: 0-8089-2397-8 (International English Edition)

Notice and Disclaimer

The information in this product ("Product") is provided as a reference for use by licensed medical professionals and no others. It does not and should not be construed as any form of medical diagnosis or professional medical advice on any matter. Receipt or use of this Product, in whole or in part, does not constitute or create a doctor-patient, therapist-patient, or other healthcare professional relationship between Amirsys Inc. ("Amirsys") and any recipient. This Product may not reflect the most current medical developments, and Amirsys makes no claims, promises, or guarantees about accuracy, completeness, or adequacy of the information contained in or linked to the Product. The Product is not a substitute for or replacement of professional medical judgment. Amirsys and its affiliates, authors, contributors, partners, and sponsors disclaim all liability or responsibility for any injury and/or damage to persons or property in respect to actions taken or not taken based on any and all Product information.

In the cases where drugs or other chemicals are prescribed, readers are advised to check the Product information currently provided by the manufacturer of each drug to be administered to verify the recommended dose, the method and duration of administration, and contraindications. It is the responsibility of the treating physician relying on experience and knowledge of the patient to determine dosages and the best treatment for the patient.

To the maximum extent permitted by applicable law, Amirsys provides the Product AS IS AND WITH ALL FAULTS, AND HEREBY DISCLAIMS ALL WARRANTIES AND CONDITIONS, WHETHER EXPRESS, IMPLIED OR STATUTORY, INCLUDING BUT NOT LIMITED TO, ANY (IF ANY) IMPLIED WARRANTIES OR CONDITIONS OF MERCHANTABILITY, OF FITNESS FOR A PARTICULAR PURPOSE, OF LACK OF VIRUSES, OR ACCURACY OR COMPLETENESS OF RESPONSES, OR RESULTS, AND OF LACK OF NEGLIGENCE OR LACK OF WORKMANLIKE EFFORT. ALSO, THERE IS NO WARRANTY OR CONDITION OF TITLE, QUIET ENJOYMENT, QUIET POSSESSION, CORRESPONDENCE TO DESCRIPTION OR NON-INFRINGEMENT, WITH REGARD TO THE PRODUCT. THE ENTIRE RISK AS TO THE QUALITY OF OR ARISING OUT OF USE OR PERFORMANCE OF THE PRODUCT

Library of Congress Cataloging-in-Publication Data

Diagnostic imaging : emergency / R. Brooke Jeffrey ... [et al.]. -- 1st ed.
   p. ; cm.
  Includes index.
  ISBN-13: 978-1-4160-4934-0
  ISBN-10: 1-4160-4934-7
  ISBN-13: 978-0-8089-2397-8 (international English ed.)
  ISBN-10: 0-8089-2397-8 (international English ed.)
  1. Medical emergencies--Imaging. 2. Emergency medicine--Diagnosis. 3. Wounds and injuries--Imaging. 4. Diagnostic imaging. I. Jeffrey, R. Brooke.
  [DNLM: 1. Diagnostic Imaging--methods--Handbooks. 2. Emergencies--Handbooks. 3. Wounds and Injuries--diagnosis--Handbooks. WN 39 D5357 2007]
RC86.7.D52 2007
616.02'5--dc22
                    2007029209

This book is dedicated to the memory of Jane P. Jeffrey.
RBJ

To all the residents, fellows, and colleagues I have so enjoyed teaching & learning from over the years. Their thirst for knowledge has contributed to a career of continued inquiry, which has been most satisfying.
BJM

To my wife, Mary, and my children Ian and Annie. There are many paths in life and you've made mine unbelievably gratifying. My children are just starting their journey, go where your heart takes you.
JWG

To my family Ellen, Max and Molly without whom none of this would be worthwhile.
RDZ

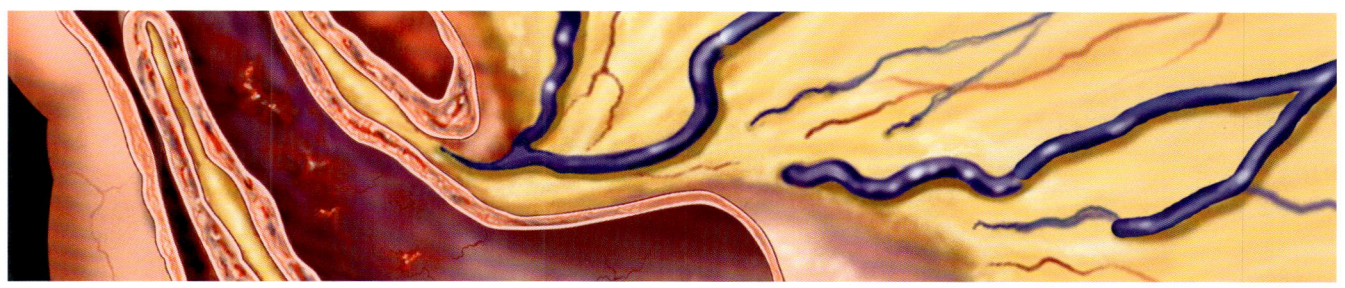

CONTRIBUTORS

Contributing Authors

Christopher G. Anton, MD
Assistant Professor, Radiology and Pediatrics
Section Chief of Abdominal Imaging
Cincinnati Children's Hospital Medical Center
Assistant Professor, Radiology
University of Cincinnati College of Medicine
Cincinnati, OH

Corning Benton, MD, FACR
Emeritus Staff Radiologist
Cincinnati Children's Hospital Medical Center
Emeritus Professor, Radiology and Pediatrics
University of Cincinnati College of Medicine
Cincinnati, OH

Anne G. Osborn, MD, FACR
University Distinguished Professor
William H. and Patricia W. Child
Presidential Endowed Chair in Radiology
University of Utah School of Medicine
Salt Lake City, Utah

Keith D. Hentel, MD
Chief, Section of Emergency/Musculoskeletal Radiology
Vice-chair, Department of Radiology
New York Presbyterian Hospital
Weill Cornell Medical Center
Assistant Professor
Weill Cornell Medical College
New York, NY

Steven J. Kraus, MD
Division Chief, Fluoroscopy and Radiography
Cincinnati Children's Hospital Medical Center
Associate Professor, Radiology and Pediatrics
University of Cincinnati College of Medicine
Cincinnati, OH

Blaise V. Jones, MD
Division Chief, Neuroradiology
Cincinnati Children's Hospital Medical Center
Associate Professor, Radiology and Pediatrics
University of Cincinnati College of Medicine
Cincinnati, OH

A. John Tsiouris, MD
Assistant Professor of Radiology
Weill Cornell Medical College
New York, NY

Miriam A. Bredella, MD
Assistant Radiologist
Massachusetts General Hospital
Assistant Professor
Harvard Medical School
Boston, MA

Russell W. Chapin, MD
Radiology Resident
University of Colorado Health Sciences Center
Denver, CO

Bradley R. Ferguson, MD
Radiology Resident
University of Colorado Health Sciences Center
Denver, CO

Jeffrey W. Grossman, MD
Radiology Resident
University of Colorado Health Sciences Center
Denver, CO

H. Ric Harnsberger, MD
Professor of Radiology/Neuroradiology
R.C. Willey Chair in Neuroradiology
University of Utah School of Medicine
Salt Lake City, Utah

Misty Norman, MD
Radiology Resident
University of Colorado Health Sciences Center
Denver, CO

Jay T. Morrow, MD, PhD
Radiology Resident
University of Colorado Health Sciences Center
Denver, CO

Colin D. Strickland, MD
Radiology Resident
University of Colorado Health Sciences Center
Denver, CO

Brant Wommack, MD
Radiology Resident
University of Colorado Health Sciences Center
Denver, CO

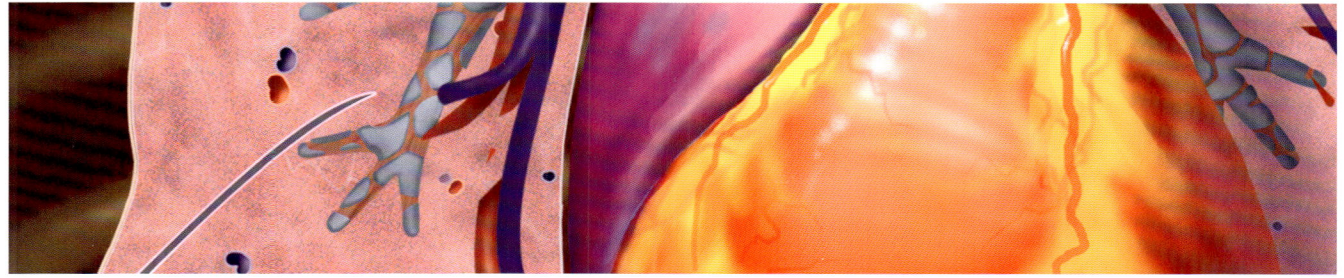

DIAGNOSTIC IMAGING: EMERGENCY

We at Amirsys and Elsevier are proud to present **Diagnostic Imaging: Emergency**, the twelfth volume in our acclaimed *Diagnostic Imaging (DI)* series. We began this precedent-setting, image- and graphic-rich series with David Stoller's Diagnostic Imaging: Orthopaedics. The next volumes, DI: Brain, DI: Head and Neck, DI: Abdomen, DI: Spine, DI: Pediatrics, DI: Obstetrics, DI: Chest, DI: Breast, DI: Ultrasound and DI: Pediatric Neuroradiology are now joined by Brooke Jeffrey's fabulous new textbook, DI: Emergency.

The pressure of handling an ever-increasing patient load is rising—relentlessly—at most emergency departments (EDs). EDs (or ERs, if you prefer) are no longer handling just acute medical emergencies such as trauma, heart attacks, and stroke but have become outpatient clinics for those without personal physicians. As patient numbers mount and waiting time in EDs everywhere increases, efficient handling of both emergent and nonemergent disease becomes paramount. In many institutions, patients may be sent to imaging by a triage nurse prior to seeing the ER physicians. Those that are sent to radiology get more studies than ever before—and, with the advent of multidetector-row CT, each study has more images (sometimes numbered in hundreds or even thousands). Some commentators have posited that radiology is rapidly becoming the "new triage officer." DI: Emergency shows you—whether radiologist or ED physician--just what to look for and includes both common and less common presentations of many diseases that can be quickly and accurately diagnosed with a variety of imaging techniques.

Again, the unique bulleted format of the DI series allows our authors to present approximately twice the information and four times the images per diagnosis compared to the old-fashioned traditional prose textbook. All the DI books follow the same format, which means that our many readers find the same information in the same place—every time! And in every body part! The innovative visual differential diagnosis "thumbnail" provides you with an at-a-glance look at entities that can mimic the diagnosis in question and has been highly popular (and much copied). "Key Facts" boxes provide a succinct summary for quick, easy review.

In summary, **Diagnostic Imaging: Emergency** is a product designed with you, the reader, in mind. Today's ERs and the radiologists who serve them demand efficiency in both image performance and interpretation. Many who find themselves covering literally everything that comes through the ER are sometimes faced with cases that require subspecialty expertise. Having **Diagnostic Imaging: Emergency** on your shelf is like having a group of subspecialty experts at your fingertips. We think you'll find this new volume a highly efficient and wonderfully rich resource that will significantly enhance your practice—and find a welcome place on your bookshelf. Enjoy!

Anne G. Osborn, MD
Executive Vice President & Editor-in-Chief, Amirsys, Inc.

H. Ric Harnsberger, MD
CEO & Chairman, Amirsys, Inc.

Paula J. Woodward, MD
Senior Vice President & Medical Director, Amirsys, Inc.

B.J. Manaster, MD
Vice President & Associate Medical Director, Amirsys, Inc.

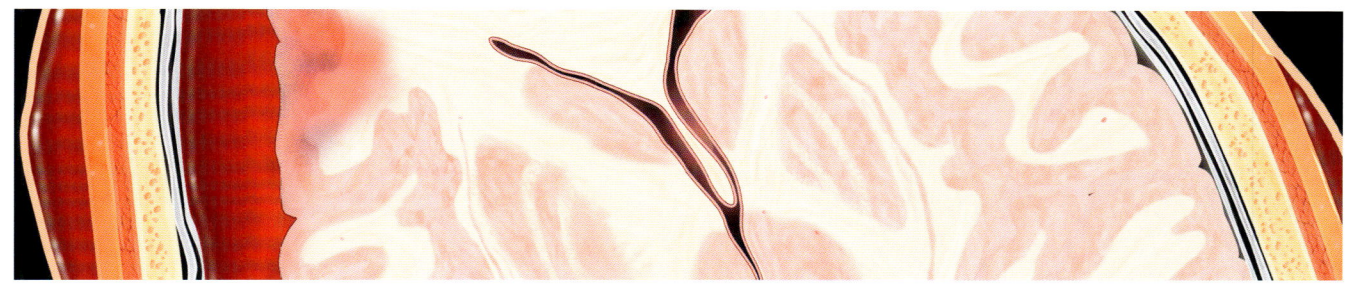

FOREWORD

The Diagnostic Imaging series of books has introduced an innovative, even revolutionary, alternative to traditional comprehensive reference texts, with the now familiar and very popular bulleted text, full color medical illustrations, and extensive high quality images. Each book in the series has quickly achieved "best seller" status, and DI: Emergency is destined to join the list. In this single text the reader will find the information necessary to handle all of the traumatic and non-traumatic conditions, in children and adults, that challenge radiologists and clinicians caring for patients in an emergency department setting.

Brooke Jeffrey has assembled an impressive and experienced group of co-authors, each of whom has written the majority of "chapters" in each section, assuring uniformity of style and substance. For each entity the reader will quickly find the essential diagnostic checklist, image interpretation pearls, differential diagnoses (illustrated), and clinical implications.

This book should be at the workstation of each radiologist and clinician who is evaluating acutely ill patients in the emergency department.

Michael P. Federle, MD
Professor of Radiology
Chief, Abdominal Imaging Section

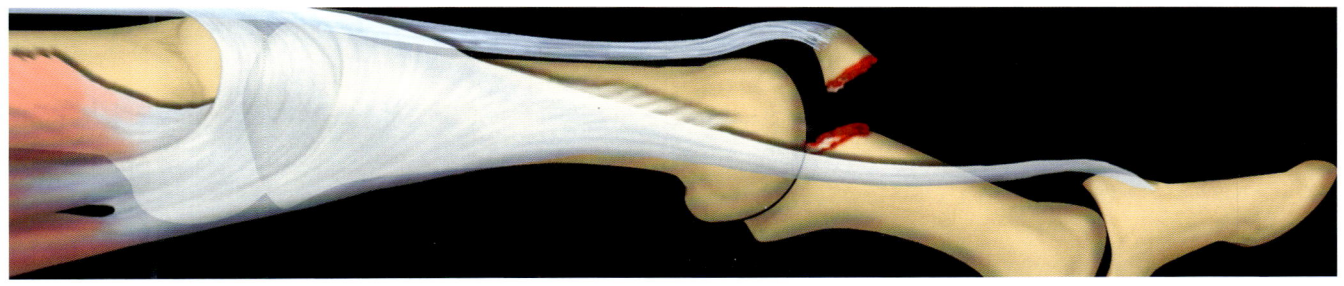

PREFACE

The evaluation of the acutely ill patient is one of the most challenging yet rewarding areas of all diagnostic imaging. Challenging, in the sense that time is of the essence in order to intervene and achieve an optimal clinical result, and rewarding when a precise diagnosis can be made expeditiously and prompt therapy can be initiated. Diagnostic imaging continues to evolve at a rapid pace, and in the past decade major hardware and software improvements to CT, MRI, and ultrasound have continued to improve our diagnostic abilities to evaluate all major organ systems in the acutely ill patient.

In my own professional lifetime, it is interesting to look back on the evolution of imaging in trauma. It was not that long ago that diagnostic peritoneal lavage and exploratory laparotomy were the only clinical tools used in the assessment of blunt abdominal trauma. Yet, through the pioneering efforts of individuals such as Mike Federle at San Francisco General Hospital, even early-generation CT scans proved their merit in the noninvasive evaluation of blunt abdominal trauma, and the entire concept of "nonoperative management" became a reality in the early 1990's. Today it would be unthinkable to have a state-of-the-art emergency room without a closely stationed multidetector CT scanner for global assessment of head and neck, vascular, abdominal, and musculoskeletal injuries.

This text is intended as a readable and approachable comprehensive reference for all major traumatic & non-traumatic illnesses that can be encountered in the acutely ill patient. Inevitably, some less common and indeed rare entitites will of necessity be excluded for consideration here, as the book evaluates multiple organ systems, including brain, spine, chest, abdomen, and pelvis in both adults and pediatric patients. It is intended that this book will not only be a resource for radiologists, but for all physicians caring for acutely ill patients, including emergency room physicians, surgeons, internists, and pediatricians.

As an abdominal radiologist, I am deeply indebted to my excellent co-authors for their significant contributions and superb illustrations dealing with CNS, spine, MSK, chest and pediatric diagnoses. Yet I am most indebted to Jeslyn Rumbold, my administrative assistant, whose phenomenal editorial and organizational skills kept me on track and focused. Indeed, without her assistance, this project would not have been possible.

I would also like to specifically thank Ric Harnsberger and the editorial staff at Amirsys, including Kaerli Main and Melissa Hoopes, for their expertise, support, and unfailing encouragement throughout this marathon of an academic exercise.

R. Brooke Jeffrey, MD
Professor of Radiology
Chief of Abdominal Imaging
Stanford University School of Medicine

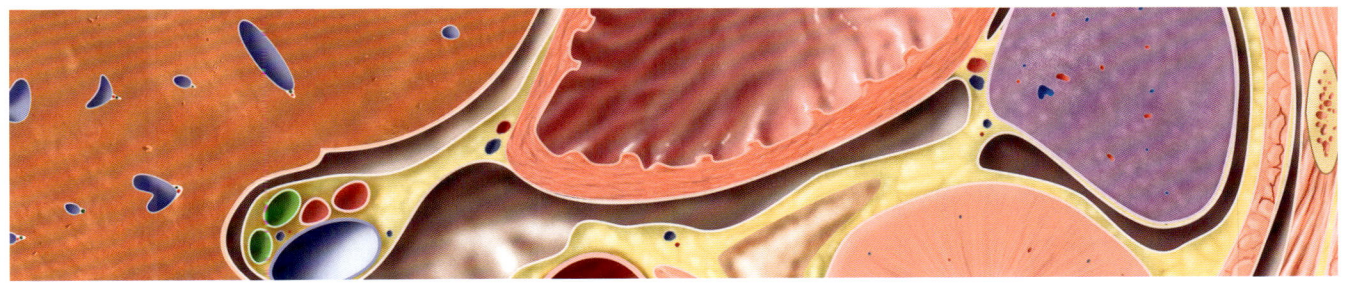

ACKNOWLEDGMENTS

Illustrations
Richard Coombs, MS
James A. Cooper, MD
Lane R. Bennion, MS

Image/Text Editing
Douglas Grant Jackson
Amanda Hurtado
Jeslyn Rumbold

Medical Text Editing
Henry J. Baskin, Jr., MD
Richard H. Wiggins III, MD

Case Management
Christopher Odekirk

Associate Editor
Kaerli Main

Production Lead
Melissa A. Hoopes

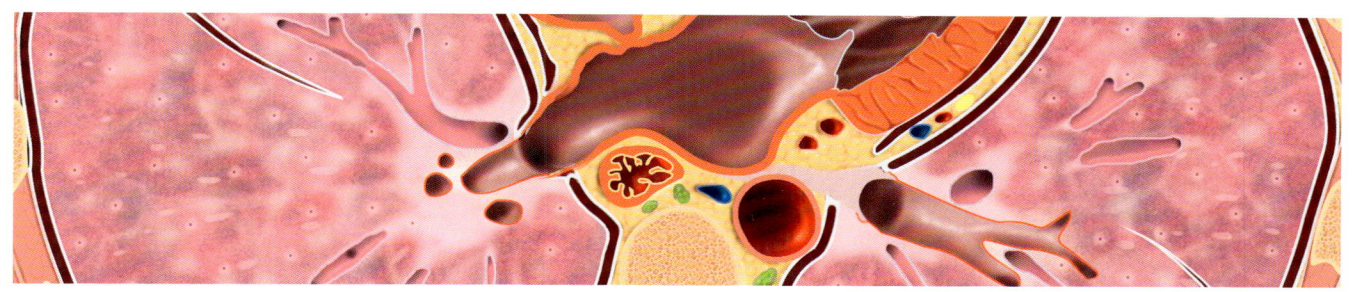

SECTIONS

PART I
Trauma

CNS 1

Chest/Cardiovascular 2

Abdomen/Pelvis 3

Musculoskeletal 4

PART II
Non-Trauma

CNS 1

Chest/Cardiovascular 2

Abdomen/Pelvis 3

Musculoskeletal 4

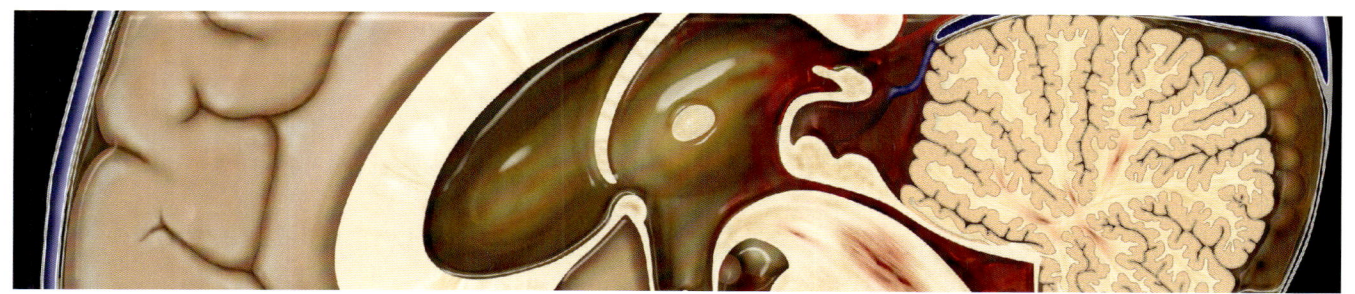

TABLE OF CONTENTS

PART I
Trauma

SECTION 1
CNS

Introduction and Overview

CNS Imaging Issues, Trauma I-1-2
Robert D. Zimmerman, MD, FACR

Brain

Epidural Hematoma I-1-4
Robert D. Zimmerman, MD, FACR

Acute Subdural Hematoma I-1-8
Robert D. Zimmerman, MD, FACR

Mixed Subdural Hematoma I-1-12
Robert D. Zimmerman, MD, FACR

Paratentorial Subdural Hematoma I-1-14
Robert D. Zimmerman, MD, FACR

Traumatic Subarachnoid Hemorrhage I-1-16
Robert D. Zimmerman, MD, FACR

Cerebral Contusion I-1-20
Robert D. Zimmerman, MD, FACR

Diffuse Axonal Injury (DAI) I-1-24
Robert D. Zimmerman, MD, FACR

Nonaccidental Trauma (Child Abuse) I-1-28
Robert D. Zimmerman, MD, FACR

Intracranial Herniation Syndromes I-1-32
Robert D. Zimmerman, MD, FACR

Intracranial Vascular Injury I-1-36
Robert D. Zimmerman, MD, FACR

Extracranial Vascular Injury I-1-40
Robert D. Zimmerman, MD, FACR

Carotid-Cavernous Fistula I-1-44
Robert D. Zimmerman, MD, FACR

Head & Neck

Temporal Bone Fractures I-1-46
Joel K. Curé, MD

CSF Leak I-1-50
Joel K. Curé, MD

Larynx Trauma I-1-52
Joel K. Curé, MD

LeFort Fractures I-III I-1-56
Joel K. Curé, MD

Spine

Atlanto-Occipital Dislocation I-1-60
Robert D. Zimmerman, MD, FACR

Jefferson C1 Fracture I-1-62
Robert D. Zimmerman, MD, FACR

Odontoid C2 Fracture I-1-66
Robert D. Zimmerman, MD, FACR

Hangman's C2 Fracture I-1-70
Robert D. Zimmerman, MD, FACR

Hyperflexion Injury, Cervical I-1-74
Robert D. Zimmerman, MD, FACR

Hyperextension Injury, Cervical I-1-76
Robert D. Zimmerman, MD, FACR

Hyperflexion-Rotation Injury, Cervical I-1-80
Robert D. Zimmerman, MD, FACR

Lateral Flexion Injury, Cervical I-1-84
Robert D. Zimmerman, MD, FACR

Posterior Column Injury, Cervical I-1-86
Robert D. Zimmerman, MD, FACR

Compression Fractures I-1-88
Robert D. Zimmerman, MD, FACR

Burst Thoracolumbar Fracture I-1-92
Robert D. Zimmerman, MD, FACR

Facet-Lamina Thoracolumbar Fracture I-1-94
Robert D. Zimmerman, MD, FACR

Chance Fracture I-1-98
Keith D. Hentel, MD

Sacral Traumatic Fracture I-1-102
Keith D. Hentel, MD

Traumatic Disc Herniation I-1-106
Keith D. Hentel, MD

Spinal Cord Injury I-1-110
Robert D. Zimmerman, MD, FACR

SECTION 2
Chest/Cardiovascular

Introduction and Overview

Chest Imaging Issues, Trauma I-2-2
Jud W. Gurney, MD, FACR

Chest/Cardiovascular

Pneumomediastinum I-2-4
Jud W. Gurney, MD, FACR

Pneumothorax I-2-8
Jud W. Gurney, MD, FACR

Tracheobronchial Tear I-2-12
Jud W. Gurney, MD, FACR

Rib Fractures and Flail Chest I-2-14
Jud W. Gurney, MD, FACR

Aortic Transection I-2-18
Jud W. Gurney, MD, FACR

Spinal Fracture, Thoracic I-2-22
Jud W. Gurney, MD, FACR

Sternal Fracture I-2-26
Jud W. Gurney, MD, FACR

Diaphragmatic Tear I-2-28
Jud W. Gurney, MD, FACR

Esophageal Tear I-2-32
Jud W. Gurney, MD, FACR

Lung Contusion I-2-36
Jud W. Gurney, MD, FACR

Neurogenic Pulmonary Edema I-2-40
Jud W. Gurney, MD, FACR

Negative Pressure Pulmonary Edema I-2-44
Jud W. Gurney, MD, FACR

SECTION 3
Abdomen/Pelvis

Introduction and Overview

Abdominal Imaging Issues, Trauma I-3-2
R. Brooke Jeffrey, MD

Abdomen/Pelvis

Splenic Trauma I-3-4
R. Brooke Jeffrey, MD

Hepatic Trauma I-3-8
R. Brooke Jeffrey, MD

Renal Trauma I-3-12
R. Brooke Jeffrey, MD

Pancreatic Trauma I-3-16
R. Brooke Jeffrey, MD

Duodenal Trauma/Hematoma I-3-20
R. Brooke Jeffrey, MD

Intestinal Trauma I-3-22
R. Brooke Jeffrey, MD

Testicular Trauma I-3-26
R. Brooke Jeffrey, MD

Hypoperfusion Complex I-3-28
Lane F. Donnelly, MD

SECTION 4
Musculoskeletal

Introduction and Overview

Musculoskeletal Imaging Issues, Trauma I-4-2
B.J. Manaster, MD, PhD, FACR

Fractures with other Contributing Etiolgies

Insufficiency Fractures, Sacrum I-4-4
B.J. Manaster, MD, PhD, FACR

Insufficiency Fractures, Appendicular I-4-8
B.J. Manaster, MD, PhD, FACR

Stress Fracture, Adult I-4-10
B.J. Manaster, MD, PhD, FACR

Pathologic Fracture I-4-14
B.J. Manaster, MD, PhD, FACR

Soft Tissue Trauma

Foreign Body I-4-18
Brant Wommack, MD

Compartment Syndrome I-4-22
B.J. Manaster, MD, PhD, FACR

Necrotizing Fasciitis I-4-26
Jeffrey W. Grossman, MD

Hematoma I-4-28
Brant Wommack, MD

Myositis Ossificans I-4-32
B.J. Manaster, MD, PhD, FACR

Fractures, Upper Extremity

Sternoclavicular Trauma I-4-36
Jay T. Morrow, MD, PhD

Clavicle Fracture I-4-40
Misty Norman, MD

Acromioclavicular Dislocation I-4-42
Misty Norman, MD

Scapular Trauma I-4-44
Colin D. Strickland, MD

Shoulder Dislocation I-4-48
B.J. Manaster, MD, PhD, FACR

Humeral Head/Neck Fracture I-4-52
Colin D. Strickland, MD

Humeral Shaft/Distal Humeral Fracture I-4-56
Colin D. Strickland, MD

Elbow Dislocation I-4-60
B.J. Manaster, MD, PhD, FACR

Olecranon Fracture/Triceps Tendon Rupture I-4-64
B.J. Manaster, MD, PhD, FACR

Radial Head/Neck Fracture I-4-68
B.J. Manaster, MD, PhD, FACR

Biceps Tendon Rupture I-4-72
B.J. Manaster, MD, PhD, FACR

Forearm Fractures — I-4-74
B.J. Manaster, MD, PhD, FACR

Distal Radius Fractures — I-4-76
B.J. Manaster, MD, PhD, FACR

Die Punch Fracture, Distal Radius — I-4-80
B.J. Manaster, MD, PhD, FACR

Scaphoid Fractures — I-4-82
B.J. Manaster, MD, PhD, FACR

Carpal Fractures, other than Scaphoid — I-4-86
B.J. Manaster, MD, PhD, FACR

Carpal Dislocations — I-4-90
B.J. Manaster, MD, PhD, FACR

Carpal Instabilities — I-4-94
B.J. Manaster, MD, PhD, FACR

Metacarpal Fractures and Dislocations — I-4-98
B.J. Manaster, MD, PhD, FACR

Ulnar Collateral Ligament Tear, Thumb — I-4-102
B.J. Manaster, MD, PhD, FACR

Flexor Annular Pulley Tears — I-4-106
B.J. Manaster, MD, PhD, FACR

Avulsion Fractures, Finger — I-4-110
B.J. Manaster, MD, PhD, FACR

Fractures, Lower Extremity

Avulsion Fractures, Pelvic — I-4-114
B.J. Manaster, MD, PhD, FACR

Pelvic Fractures, Stable — I-4-118
Bradley R. Ferguson, MD

Pelvic Fractures, Unstable — I-4-122
Bradley R. Ferguson, MD

Acetabular Fractures — I-4-126
Russell W. Chapin, MD

Hip Dislocation — I-4-130
B.J. Manaster, MD, PhD, FACR

Femoral Head Fractures — I-4-134
B.J. Manaster, MD, PhD, FACR

Femoral Neck Fractures — I-4-138
B.J. Manaster, MD, PhD, FACR

Knee Avulsion Fx: Internal Derangement — I-4-142
B.J. Manaster, MD, PhD, FACR

Patellar Fracture — I-4-146
Russell W. Chapin, MD

Patellar Tendon Tears & Tendinosis — I-4-150
B.J. Manaster, MD, PhD, FACR

Tibial Plateau Fracture — I-4-154
B.J. Manaster, MD, PhD, FACR

Ankle Fractures — I-4-158
Jeffrey W. Grossman, MD

Achilles Tendon Tear & Tendinopathy — I-4-162
B.J. Manaster, MD, PhD, FACR

Calcaneal Fractures — I-4-166
B.J. Manaster, MD, PhD, FACR

Talus Fractures — I-4-170
Jeffrey W. Grossman, MD

Navicular Fractures — I-4-174
Jay T. Morrow, MD, PhD

Lisfranc Fracture-Dislocation — I-4-178
B.J. Manaster, MD, PhD, FACR

Metatarsal Fractures — I-4-182
B.J. Manaster, MD, PhD, FACR

Pediatric Fractures

Physeal Fractures, Pediatric — I-4-186
Corning Benton, MD, FACR

Child Abuse, Metaphyseal Fracture — I-4-190
Corning Benton, MD, FACR

Incomplete Fractures, Pediatric — I-4-194
Corning Benton, MD, FACR

Supracondylar Fracture, Pediatric — I-4-198
Corning Benton, MD, FACR

Toddler's Fractures — I-4-202
Corning Benton, MD, FACR

Stress Fracture, Pediatric — I-4-206
Corning Benton, MD, FACR

Medial Epicondyle Avulsion, Pediatric — I-4-210
Christopher G. Anton, MD

PART II
Non-Trauma

SECTION 1
CNS

Introduction and Overview

CNS Imaging Issues, Non-Trauma — II-1-2
Robert D. Zimmerman, MD, FACR

Brain

Aneurysmal Subarachnoid Hemorrhage — II-1-4
Robert D. Zimmerman, MD, FACR

Nonaneurysmal Perimesencephalic SAH — II-1-6
Robert D. Zimmerman, MD, FACR

Saccular Aneurysm — II-1-8
A. John Tsiouris, MD

Fusiform Aneurysm — II-1-12
A. John Tsiouris, MD

Blood Blister-like Aneurysm — II-1-14
A. John Tsiouris, MD

Intracerebral Hematoma — II-1-16
Robert D. Zimmerman, MD, FACR

Spontaneous Intracranial Hemorrhage — II-1-20
Anne G. Osborn, MD, FACR

Hypertensive Intracranial Hemorrhage — II-1-24
Anne G. Osborn, MD, FACR

Acute Hypertensive Encephalopathy, PRES — II-1-28
Anne G. Osborn, MD, FACR

Acute Cerebral Ischemia-Infarction — II-1-32
A. John Tsiouris, MD

Dural Sinus Thrombosis — II-1-36
H. Ric Harnsberger, MD

Neonatal Meningitis — II-1-40
Blaise V. Jones, MD

Meningitis — II-1-44
Anne G. Osborn, MD, FACR

Abscess — II-1-48
Anne G. Osborn, MD, FACR

Extra-Axial Empyema — II-1-52
H. Ric Harnsberger, MD

Herpes Encephalitis — II-1-56
Anne G. Osborn, MD, FACR

Opportunistic Infection, AIDS — II-1-60
Robert D. Zimmerman, MD, FACR

Drug Abuse — II-1-64
Robert D. Zimmerman, MD, FACR

Hydrocephalus — II-1-68
Blaise V. Jones, MD

Inborn Errors of Metabolism — II-1-72
Blaise V. Jones, MD

Near-Drowning — II-1-76
Blaise V. Jones, MD

Carbon Monoxide Poisoning — II-1-78
Blaise V. Jones, MD

Head & Neck

Necrotizing External Otitis — II-1-80
Joel K. Curé, MD

Complicated Otitis Media — II-1-84
Joel K. Curé, MD

Idiopathic Orbital Inflammatory Disease — II-1-88
Joel K. Curé, MD

Subperiosteal Abscess, Orbit — II-1-92
Joel K. Curé, MD

Acute Rhinosinusitis — II-1-96
Joel K. Curé, MD

Fungal Sinusitis, Invasive — II-1-100
Joel K. Curé, MD

Parotitis, Acute — II-1-104
Joel K. Curé, MD

Retropharyngeal Space Abscess — II-1-108
Joel K. Curé, MD

Spine

Pyogenic Osteomyelitis, Spine — II-1-112
Keith D. Hentel, MD

Granulomatous Osteomyelitis, Spine — II-1-116
Keith D. Hentel, MD

Epidural Paravertebral Abscess — II-1-120
Keith D. Hentel, MD

Spinal Cord Infarction — II-1-124
Robert D. Zimmerman, MD, FACR

SECTION 2
Chest/Cardiovascular

Introduction and Overview

Chest Imaging Issues, Non-Trauma — II-2-2
Jud W. Gurney, MD, FACR

Chest/Cardiovascular

Cardiogenic Pulmonary Edema — II-2-4
Jud W. Gurney, MD, FACR

Mitral Regurgitation Pulmonary Edema — II-2-8
Jud W. Gurney, MD, FACR

Noncardiac Pulmonary Edema — II-2-12
Jud W. Gurney, MD, FACR

Smoke Inhalation — II-2-16
Jud W. Gurney, MD, FACR

Silo-Filler's Disease — II-2-20
Jud W. Gurney, MD, FACR

Community Acquired Pneumonia — II-2-24
Jud W. Gurney, MD, FACR

Immunocompromised Pneumonia — II-2-28
Jud W. Gurney, MD, FACR

Lung Abscess — II-2-32
Jud W. Gurney, MD, FACR

Viral Lung Infection, Pediatric — II-2-36
Lane F. Donnelly, MD

Round Pneumonia, Pediatric — II-2-40
Lane F. Donnelly, MD

Neonatal Pneumonia — II-2-44
Christopher G. Anton, MD

Exudative Tracheitis — II-2-48
Lane F. Donnelly, MD

Croup — II-2-52
Lane F. Donnelly, MD

Epiglottitis — II-2-56
Lane F. Donnelly, MD

Transient Tachypnea of the Newborn — II-2-60
Christopher G. Anton, MD

Pulmonary Interstitial Emphysema, Pediatric — II-2-64
Lane F. Donnelly, MD

Diffuse Alveolar Hemorrhage — II-2-68
Jud W. Gurney, MD, FACR

Vasculitis, Pulmonary — II-2-72
Jud W. Gurney, MD, FACR

Sickle Cell, Acute Chest Syndrome — II-2-76
Jud W. Gurney, MD, FACR

Eosinophilic Pneumonia — II-2-80
Jud W. Gurney, MD, FACR

Acute Interstitial Pneumonia — II-2-84
Jud W. Gurney, MD, FACR

Illicit Drug Abuse, Pulmonary — II-2-88
Jud W. Gurney, MD, FACR

Talcosis, Pulmonary — II-2-92
Jud W. Gurney, MD, FACR

Chronic Obstructive Pulmonary Disease — II-2-96
Jud W. Gurney, MD, FACR

Asthma — II-2-100
Jud W. Gurney, MD, FACR

Hypersensitivity Pneumonitis — II-2-104
Jud W. Gurney, MD, FACR

Aspiration — II-2-108
Jud W. Gurney, MD, FACR

Meconium Aspiration Syndrome — II-2-112
Christopher G. Anton, MD

Bronchial Foreign Body, Pediatric *Lane F. Donnelly, MD*	II-2-116
Pulmonary Emboli *Jud W. Gurney, MD, FACR*	II-2-120
Septic Emboli, Pulmonary *Jud W. Gurney, MD, FACR*	II-2-124
Aortic Dissection *Jud W. Gurney, MD, FACR*	II-2-128
SVC Syndrome *Jud W. Gurney, MD, FACR*	II-2-132
Pericardial Tamponade *Jud W. Gurney, MD, FACR*	II-2-136

SECTION 3
Abdomen/Pelvis

Introduction and Overview

Abdominal Imaging Issues, Non-Trauma *R. Brooke Jeffrey, MD*	II-3-2

Abdomen

Abdominal Abscess *R. Brooke Jeffrey, MD*	II-3-4
Peritonitis *R. Brooke Jeffrey, MD*	II-3-8
Inguinal Hernia *R. Brooke Jeffrey, MD*	II-3-12
Femoral Hernia *R. Brooke Jeffrey, MD*	II-3-16
Paraduodenal Hernia *R. Brooke Jeffrey, MD*	II-3-20
Transmesenteric Post-Operative Hernia *R. Brooke Jeffrey, MD*	II-3-24
Duodenal Ulcer *R. Brooke Jeffrey, MD*	II-3-28
Aorto-Enteric Fistula *R. Brooke Jeffrey, MD*	II-3-32
Crohn Disease *R. Brooke Jeffrey, MD*	II-3-34
Pneumatosis of the Intestine *R. Brooke Jeffrey, MD*	II-3-38
Acute Small Bowel Ischemia *R. Brooke Jeffrey, MD*	II-3-42
Vasculitis, Small Intestine *R. Brooke Jeffrey, MD*	II-3-46
Small Bowel Obstruction *R. Brooke Jeffrey, MD*	II-3-50
Gallstone Ileus *R. Brooke Jeffrey, MD*	II-3-54
Intussusception *R. Brooke Jeffrey, MD*	II-3-56
Infectious Colitis *R. Brooke Jeffrey, MD*	II-3-60
Pseudomembranous Colitis *R. Brooke Jeffrey, MD*	II-3-64
Typhlitis *R. Brooke Jeffrey, MD*	II-3-68
Ulcerative Colitis *R. Brooke Jeffrey, MD*	II-3-70
Toxic Megacolon *R. Brooke Jeffrey, MD*	II-3-74
Appendicitis *R. Brooke Jeffrey, MD*	II-3-76
Diverticulitis *R. Brooke Jeffrey, MD*	II-3-80
Epiploic Appendagitis *R. Brooke Jeffrey, MD*	II-3-84
Omental Infarct *R. Brooke Jeffrey, MD*	II-3-88
Ischemic Colitis *R. Brooke Jeffrey, MD*	II-3-92
Sigmoid Volvulus *R. Brooke Jeffrey, MD*	II-3-96
Cecal Volvulus *R. Brooke Jeffrey, MD*	II-3-100
Splenic Infection and Abscess *R. Brooke Jeffrey, MD*	II-3-102
Splenic Infarction *R. Brooke Jeffrey, MD*	II-3-106
Hepatic Candidiasis *R. Brooke Jeffrey, MD*	II-3-110
Hepatic Pyogenic Abscess *R. Brooke Jeffrey, MD*	II-3-114
Hepatic Amebic Abscess *R. Brooke Jeffrey, MD*	II-3-118
HELLP Syndrome *R. Brooke Jeffrey, MD*	II-3-122
Hepatic Infarction *R. Brooke Jeffrey, MD*	II-3-126
Portal Vein Occlusion *R. Brooke Jeffrey, MD*	II-3-130
Budd-Chiari Syndrome *R. Brooke Jeffrey, MD*	II-3-134
Ascending Cholangitis *R. Brooke Jeffrey, MD*	II-3-138
Recurrent Pyogenic Cholangitis *R. Brooke Jeffrey, MD*	II-3-140
Choledocholithiasis *R. Brooke Jeffrey, MD*	II-3-144
Cholecystitis *R. Brooke Jeffrey, MD*	II-3-148
Acute Pancreatitis *R. Brooke Jeffrey, MD*	II-3-152
Pyelonephritis *R. Brooke Jeffrey, MD*	II-3-156
Renal Abscess *R. Brooke Jeffrey, MD*	II-3-160
Xanthogranulomatous Pyelonephritis *R. Brooke Jeffrey, MD*	II-3-164
Emphysematous Pyelonephritis *R. Brooke Jeffrey, MD*	II-3-168
Renal Infarction *R. Brooke Jeffrey, MD*	II-3-170
Renal Vein Thrombosis *R. Brooke Jeffrey, MD*	II-3-174

Epididymo-Orchitis II-3-178
R. Brooke Jeffrey, MD

Testicular Torsion II-3-182
R. Brooke Jeffrey, MD

Midgut Volvulus II-3-186
Lane F. Donnelly, MD

Duodenal Atresia or Stenosis II-3-190
Steven J. Kraus, MD

Meconium Plug Syndrome II-3-194
Steven J. Kraus, MD

Meconium Ileus II-3-198
Steven J. Kraus, MD

Meconium Peritonitis II-3-202
Steven J. Kraus, MD

Necrotizing Enterocolitis II-3-206
Steven J. Kraus, MD

Hypertrophic Pyloric Stenosis II-3-210
Christopher G. Anton, MD

Gastric Volvulus II-3-214
Steven J. Kraus, MD

Ileocolic Intussusception (Idiopathic) II-3-218
Lane F. Donnelly, MD

Meckel Diverticulum II-3-222
Christopher G. Anton, MD

Mesenteric Adenitis II-3-226
Christopher G. Anton, MD

Small Bowel Intussusception, Pediatric II-3-230
Christopher G. Anton, MD

Pelvis

Uterine AVM II-3-234
R. Brooke Jeffrey, MD

Ovarian Torsion II-3-238
R. Brooke Jeffrey, MD

Ovarian Vein Thrombosis II-3-242
R. Brooke Jeffrey, MD

Ovarian Hemorrhage II-3-246
R. Brooke Jeffrey, MD

Pelvic Inflammatory Disease II-3-250
R. Brooke Jeffrey, MD

Ectopic Pregnancy, Tubal II-3-254
R. Brooke Jeffrey, MD

SECTION 4
Musculoskeletal

Introduction and Overview

Musculoskeletal Imaging Issues, Non-Trauma II-4-2
B.J. Manaster, MD, PhD, FACR

Infection

Soft Tissue Abscess II-4-4
B.J. Manaster, MD, PhD, FACR

Osteomyelitis, Adult II-4-6
B.J. Manaster, MD, PhD, FACR

Osteomyelitis, Pediatric II-4-10
Corning Benton, MD, FACR

Septic Joint II-4-14
B.J. Manaster, MD, PhD, FACR

Diabetes: MSK Complications II-4-18
B.J. Manaster, MD, PhD, FACR

Acute Arthritic Flares

Gout II-4-22
B.J. Manaster, MD, PhD, FACR

Pyrophosphate Arthropathy II-4-26
B.J. Manaster, MD, PhD, FACR

Calcific Periarthritis II-4-30
Miriam A. Bredella, MD

Joint Swelling

Pigmented Villonodular Synovitis (PVNS) II-4-34
B.J. Manaster, MD, PhD, FACR

Synovial Osteochondromatosis II-4-38
B.J. Manaster, MD, PhD, FACR

Charcot, Neuropathic II-4-42
B.J. Manaster, MD, PhD, FACR

Osteonecrosis

Transient Bone Marrow Edema II-4-46
B.J. Manaster, MD, PhD, FACR

Osteonecrosis, Hip II-4-48
B.J. Manaster, MD, PhD, FACR

Osteonecrosis, Wrist (Scaphoid & Lunate) II-4-52
B.J. Manaster, MD, PhD, FACR

Osteochondritis Dissecans II-4-54
B.J. Manaster, MD, PhD, FACR

Orthopedic Hardware Complications

Arthroplasty Loosening & Dislocation II-4-58
B.J. Manaster, MD, PhD, FACR

Arthroplasty Hardware/Periprosthetic Fx II-4-62
B.J. Manaster, MD, PhD, FACR

Arthroplasty Component Wear/Particle Disease II-4-66
B.J. Manaster, MD, PhD, FACR

Miscellaneous, Systemic Diseases

Sickle Cell Anemia: MSK Complications II-4-70
B.J. Manaster, MD, PhD, FACR

HIV-AIDS: MSK Complications II-4-74
Miriam A. Bredella, MD

Hemophilia: MSK Complications II-4-78
B.J. Manaster, MD, PhD, FACR

Diagnostic Imaging
EMERGENCY

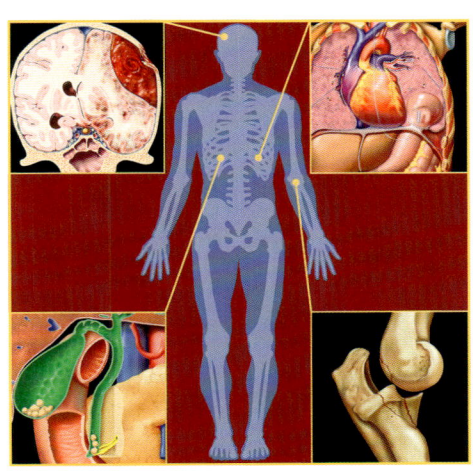

PART I
Trauma

CNS 1

Chest/Cardiovascular 2

Abdomen/Pelvis 3

Musculoskeletal 4

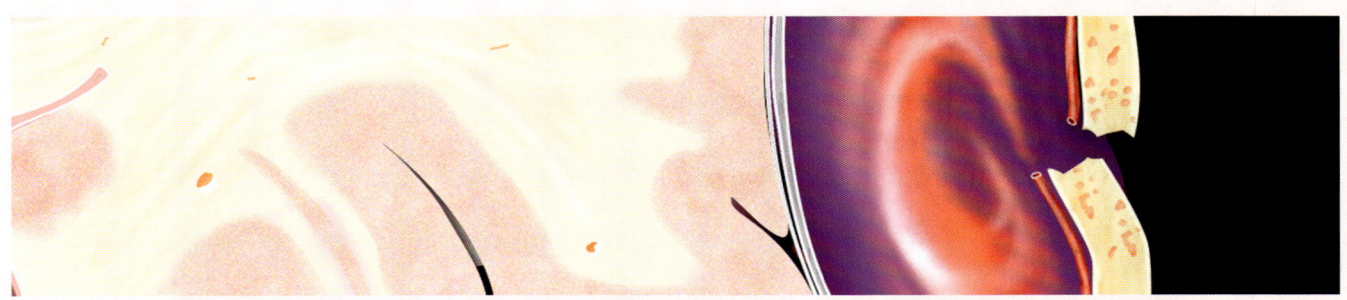

SECTION 1: CNS

Introduction and Overview
CNS Imaging Issues, Trauma   I-1-2

Brain
Epidural Hematoma   I-1-4
Acute Subdural Hematoma   I-1-8
Mixed Subdural Hematoma   I-1-12
Paratentorial Subdural Hematoma   I-1-14
Traumatic Subarachnoid Hemorrhage   I-1-16
Cerebral Contusion   I-1-20
Diffuse Axonal Injury (DAI)   I-1-24
Nonaccidental Trauma (Child Abuse)   I-1-28
Intracranial Herniation Syndromes   I-1-32
Intracranial Vascular Injury   I-1-36
Extracranial Vascular Injury   I-1-40
Carotid-Cavernous Fistula   I-1-44

Head & Neck
Temporal Bone Fractures   I-1-46
CSF Leak   I-1-50
Larynx Trauma   I-1-52
LeFort Fractures I-III   I-1-56

Spine
Atlanto-Occipital Dislocation   I-1-60
Jefferson C1 Fracture   I-1-62
Odontoid C2 Fracture   I-1-66
Hangman's C2 Fracture   I-1-70
Hyperflexion Injury, Cervical   I-1-74
Hyperextension Injury, Cervical   I-1-76
Hyperflexion-Rotation Injury, Cervical   I-1-80
Lateral Flexion Injury, Cervical   I-1-84
Posterior Column Injury, Cervical   I-1-86
Compression Fractures   I-1-88
Burst Thoracolumbar Fracture   I-1-92
Facet-Lamina Thoracolumbar Fracture   I-1-94
Chance Fracture   I-1-98
Sacral Traumatic Fracture   I-1-102
Traumatic Disc Herniation   I-1-106
Spinal Cord Injury   I-1-110

CNS IMAGING ISSUES, TRAUMA

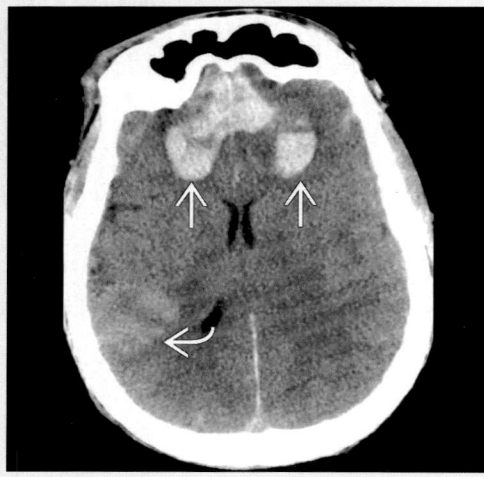

Axial NECT shows bifrontal hemorrhagic contusions ➔ and sylvian fissure subarachnoid hemorrhage ➔.

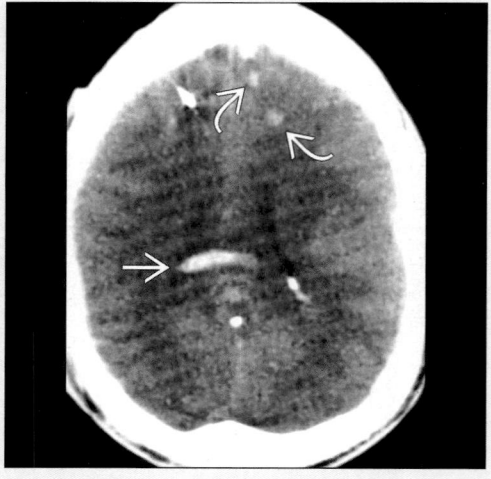

Axial NECT shows severe diffuse axonal injury with hemorrhage in the splenium of the corpus callosum ➔ and at the cortico-medullary junctions of the frontal lobes ➔.

TERMINOLOGY

Definitions
- Traumatic brain injury (TBI)
  - Injury of brain, vessels, cranial nerves, meninges, skull base & calvarium
- Spine trauma
  - Injury of vertebra, ligaments & spinal cord

IMAGING ANATOMY

General Anatomic Considerations
- TBI
  - Focal masses & diffuse brain swelling produce herniation of brain through confined openings → infarction
- Spina trauma
  - Disruption of osseous & ligamentous components of the spinal column → biomechanical instability → immediate or delayed cord injury

ANATOMY-BASED IMAGING ISSUES

Key Concepts or Questions
- Moving head lesions: Motor vehicle accidents (MVA) & falls
  - Cortical contusions
    - Superficial cortical bruises with variable hemorrhage
    - Most common in anterior medial, frontal & anterior temporal lobes
    - Deceleration injury: Frontal & temporal lobes abraded as slide across boney surfaces
  - Diffuse axonal injury (DAI)
    - Rotation & rapid deceleration shear axons
    - Most common mechanism of TBI
    - Occurs at regions of changes in brain density: Cortico-medullary junction, corpus callosum, deep gray matter & brain stem
    - Severe: Persistent vegetative state and/or death
    - Moderate: Initial coma or altered mental status with slow recovery (weeks to months)
    - Mild-acute: Loss of consciousness retrograde amnesia & headache
    - Mild-chronic: Post-concussive syndrome; headache memory loss, emotional lability & cognitive impairment lasting weeks to months
  - Subarachnoid hemorrhage (SAH)
    - Common: Typically in association with other injuries
    - Mild superficial SAH most common; self limiting
    - Basal SAH: Secondary to dissection/transection of major artery; mimics aneurysmal SAH
  - Subdural hematoma (SDH)
    - Rotational injury shears cortical veins as they cross from subarachnoid space to dural venous sinuses
    - Most common over convexities; may involve any dural surface - paratentorial, parafalcian, subfrontal and retroclival SDH
    - Young patients: Typically acute & associated with SAH, contusions & DAI
    - Older patients: Often isolated lesions resulting from repeated hemorrhage
  - Epidural hematoma (EDH)
    - Subperiosteal hemorrhage produced by fracture crossing major arterial (e.g., middle meningeal artery) or venous (dural sinus) structure
    - Most common in children and young adults where dura not tightly adherent to calvarium
- Stationary head injury (struck by object)
  - Depressed skull fracture
  - Epidural hematoma
  - Fracture contusion
    - Brain underlying impact is directly injured by displaced bone
- Vascular injuries
  - Dissection of extracranial carotid or vertebral artery with secondary embolic infarction
  - Dissection of intracranial vessels near skull base with extensive SAH - mimics aneurysmal SAH
- Herniations: Transfalcian, transtentorial, tonsillar

CNS IMAGING ISSUES, TRAUMA

Key Facts

- Detection of surgical treatable lesions (extra-axial hematomas, herniation, vascular injury) is critical on initial CT scan
- Arterial epidural hematomas may require emergent evacuation if large and near temporal lobe
- Herniation may result in secondary infarction of the occipital lobes due to compression of the posterior cerebral artery
- Routine CT & MR studies in minor TBI are typically normal
- If vascular injury suspected CTA or MR/MRA
- Assessment of spinal stability (CT) & detection of cord injury (MR) at time of initial exam critical in preserving function & prevention of further cord injury
- Plain radiographs are inadequate in individuals with moderate to high index of suspicion of cervical injury

- Mechanism of spinal injury
  - Flexion: Posterior ligament, laminar & facet fractures; facet joint disruption; cord initially spared; delayed cord injury due radiographically occult posterior ligamentous injury
  - Extension: Vertebral body fractures, traumatic disc herniations; spinal cord injury at time of trauma
  - Axial loading: Burst fractures, disc herniations, spinal cord contusions & hematoma
- Stable vs. unstable injuries (3 column approach of Denis)
  - Anterior column: Anterior longitudinal ligament to anterior vertebral body
  - Middle column: Posterior vertebral body annulus and posterior longitudinal ligament
  - Posterior column: Facet joints, lamina, spinous process and posterior ligaments
  - Injury is unstable when two columns involved

Imaging Approaches

- TBI
  - CT for evaluation of acute TBI
  - MR for extent of axonal injury or vascular injury
- Spine trauma
  - Plain radiographs extremely limited value
  - Thin section helical CT with multiplanar reformations required to identify or rule out significant spinal injury
  - MR for cord and/or ligamentous injury

Imaging Protocols

- Head
  - Routine non-contrast scan (5 mm)
  - Thin section scans of facial and temporal bones as warranted
  - Serial scans in first 48 hours
  - CT angiograms to assess for possible vascular injury if SAH extensive
  - MR: Gradient echo images for axonal injury
  - MRA for dissection if warranted
- Spine
  - Initial cross table lateral plain radiograph of cervical spine to assess for major injury
  - Thin section helical CT (< 2 mm) with reformations for cervical trauma
  - CT angiogram to evaluate for vascular injury - may use images from whole body trauma CT
  - MR for suspected cord or ligamentous injury

Imaging Pitfalls

- TBI: Anterior frontal contusions and DAI may be difficult to see on CT; basal SAH may mimic aneurysmal SAH
- Spine: Insensitivity of plain radiographs; no or poor quality reformations of spine CT

RELATED REFERENCES

1. Kelly AB et al: Head trauma: comparison of MR and CT--experience in 100 patients. AJNR Am J Neuroradiol. 9(4):699-708, 1988
2. Denis F: The three column spine and its significance in the classification of acute thoracolumbar spinal injuries. Spine. 8(8):817-31, 1983

IMAGE GALLERY

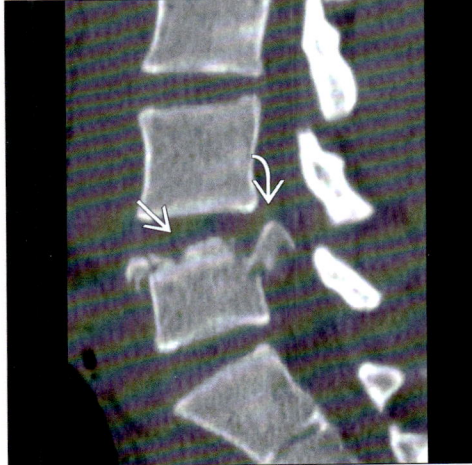
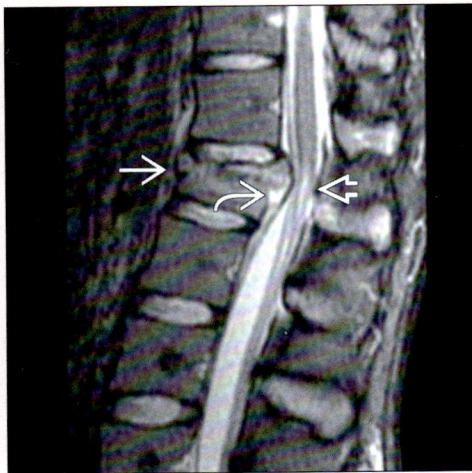

(Left) Sagittal bone CT shows fracture of the superior end plate of L4 ➡ with retropulsion of the posterior portion of the vertebral body ➡ into the spinal canal causing marked canal stenosis. (Right) Sagittal T2WI MR shows fracture of L1 ➡ with retropulsion of posterior portion of vertebral body into the spinal canal ➡ and secondary edema of the conus medullaris ➡.

EPIDURAL HEMATOMA

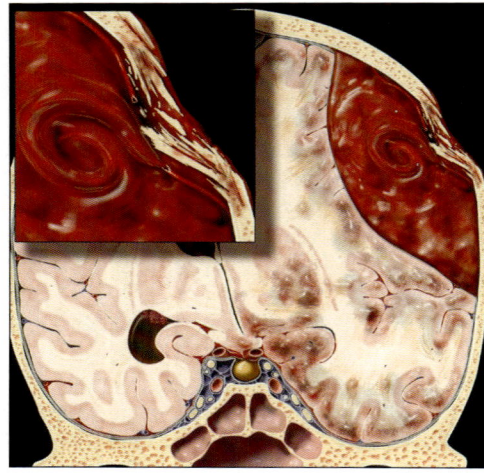

Coronal graphic illustrates swirling acute hemorrhage from laceration of middle meningeal artery by overlying skull fracture. Epidural hematoma displaces dura inward as it expands.

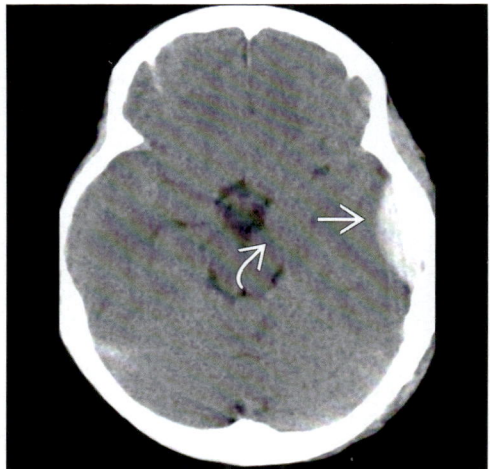

Axial NECT shows left temporal convexity EDH ➔. Note medial displacement of uncus ➔, indicative of early transtentorial herniation.

TERMINOLOGY

Abbreviations and Synonyms
- Epidural hematoma (EDH)

Definitions
- Blood collection within epidural space between skull inner table & dura mater

IMAGING FINDINGS

General Features
- Best diagnostic clue: Hyperdense biconvex extra-axial mass on NECT
- Location
  ○ Epidural space between skull & dura
  ○ Occurs at impact ("coup") site
  ○ 95% unilateral
    ▪ Bilateral EDH results from bilateral impacts
  ○ 90-95% supratentorial
    ▪ 66% temporoparietal
    ▪ 29% frontal, parietooccipital
  ○ 5-10% posterior fossa
  ○ Venous EDH adjacent to venous sinus
  ○ Rarely at vertex
- Size
  ○ Variable; rapidly expanding; attain maximum size within 36 hours
  ○ Slower accumulation of blood in venous EDH
- Morphology
  ○ Biconvex or lentiform extra-axial collection at impact site
  ○ Does not cross sutures unless sutural diastasis/fracture present
  ○ Venous EDH can cross falx & tentorium
  ○ Compresses & displaces underlying brain & subarachnoid space
  ○ Venous EDH
    ▪ Straddles multiple cranial compartments
    ▪ Sinus transgressed by fracture line
    ▪ Dural sinus displaced, usually not occluded
  ○ Skull fracture (> 95%)
  ○ One-third to one-half have other significant lesions
    ▪ Mass effect; secondary herniations common (subfalcine, transtentorial)
    ▪ "Contrecoup" subdural hematoma (SDH)

DDx: Epidural Hematoma

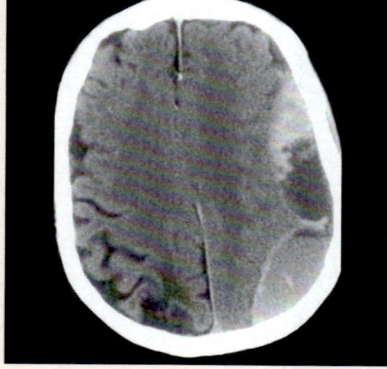
Loculated cSDH

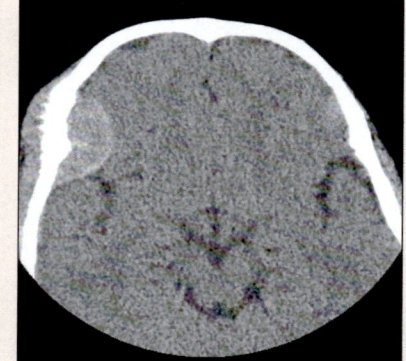
Neuroblastoma

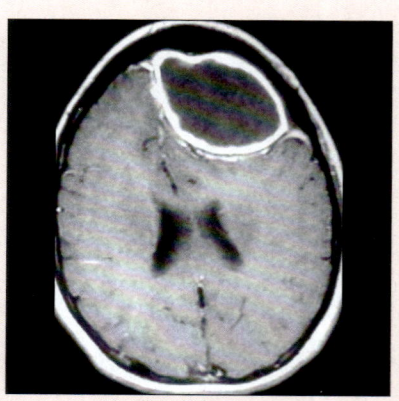
Epidural Empyema

EPIDURAL HEMATOMA

Key Facts

Terminology
- Blood collection within epidural space between skull inner table & dura mater

Imaging Findings
- Best diagnostic clue: Hyperdense biconvex extra-axial mass on NECT
- Biconvex or lentiform extra-axial collection at impact site
- Does not cross sutures unless sutural diastasis/fracture present
- Venous EDH can cross falx & tentorium
- Compresses & displaces underlying brain & subarachnoid space
- Acute: 2/3 Hyperdense, 1/3 mixed hyper-/hypodense

Top Differential Diagnoses
- Subdural Hematoma
- Neoplasm

Pathology
- 90% Arterial; 10% venous
- Arterial EDH with fracture often near MMA groove fracture
- Venous EDH usually related to fractures near dural sinus attachments

Clinical Issues
- Classic "lucid interval": Approximately 50% of cases
- More common in patients < 20 years; extremely rare in elderly
- Generally good outcome if promptly recognized & treated

- Cerebral contusions more common with venous EDH

Radiographic Findings
- Radiography: Skull fracture

CT Findings
- NECT
  - Acute: 2/3 Hyperdense, 1/3 mixed hyper-/hypodense
    - Low density "swirl sign": Active/rapid bleeding with unretracted clot
    - Acute extravasation: 30-50 HU; coagulated: 50-80 HU
    - Medial hyperdense margin: Displaced dura
  - Air within EDH (20%) suggests sinus or mastoid fracture
  - Vertex EDH easily overlooked
- CECT
  - Acute: Rarely contrast extravasation
  - Chronic: Peripheral dural enhancement

MR Findings
- T1WI
  - Acute: Isointense
  - Subacute/early chronic: Hyperintense
  - Black line between EDH & brain: Displaced dura
- T2WI
  - Acute: Variable hyper- to hypointense
  - Early subacute: Hypointense
  - Late subacute/early chronic: Hyperintense
  - Black line between EDH & brain: Displaced dura
- T1 C+
  - Venous EDH: Displaced dural sinus by hematoma
  - Spontaneous (non-traumatic) EDH: Enhancement of hemorrhagic epidural mass
- MRV
  - Assess for patency of venous sinus
  - Displaced venous sinus flow by hematoma

Angiographic Findings
- Conventional
  - Avascular mass effect; displaced cortical arteries
  - Laceration from middle meningeal artery (MMA)
  - "Tram-track" sign: Traumatic arteriovenous fistula? (AVF) between MMA and diploic veins
  - Displaced dural sinus (venous EDH)

Imaging Recommendations
- Best imaging tool: NECT for traumatic cases, MR if nontraumatic
- Protocol advice
  - Traumatic: Consider MR if EDH straddles dural compartments on NECT
  - Nontraumatic: Enhanced MR

DIFFERENTIAL DIAGNOSIS

Subdural Hematoma
- Usually crescentic, may also be biconvex
- Crosses sutures, does not cross falx
- No displaced dura

Neoplasm
- Meningioma
- Soft tissue component (subperiosteal) of osseous mass: Metastasis, lymphoma, primary sarcoma
- Dural-based mass: Metastases, lymphoma

Infection/Inflammation
- Subperiosteal extension of osseous inflammatory lesion
- Epidural empyema secondary to osteomyelitis
- Soft tissue component of granulomatous osseous lesion: Tuberculosis

Extramedullary Hematopoiesis
- History of blood dyscrasia

PATHOLOGY

General Features
- Etiology
  - Trauma most common
    - 90% Arterial; 10% venous

EPIDURAL HEMATOMA

- Arterial EDH with fracture often near MMA groove fracture
- Venous EDH usually related to fractures near dural sinus attachments
○ Nontraumatic
- Coagulopathy, thrombolysis, vascular malformation, neoplasm, epidural anesthesia, Paget disease of skull
• Epidemiology
○ 1-4% of imaged head trauma patients
○ 5-15% of patients with fatal head injuries
• Associated abnormalities
○ Skull fracture present in 95%, may cross MMA groove
○ Subdural hemorrhage, contusion

Gross Pathologic & Surgical Features

- Subperiosteal hematoma (outer layer of dura is periosteum of inner table of skull)
- May cross midline, dural attachments
- Hematoma collects between calvarium, outer dura
  ○ Rarely crosses sutures (exception: Large hematoma with diastatic fx)
- "Vertex" EDH (rare)
  ○ Usually venous: Linear or diastatic fracture crosses superior sagittal sinus
- At surgery or autopsy, 20% have blood in both epidural & subdural spaces
  ○ SDH usually not apparent on imaging

Microscopic Features
- Tear/laceration of adjacent vessel

Staging, Grading or Classification Criteria
- Type I: Acute EDH, arterial bleeding (58%)
- Type II: Subacute EDH (31%)
- Type III: Chronic EDH, venous bleeding (11%)

CLINICAL ISSUES

Presentation
- Most common signs/symptoms
  ○ Classic "lucid interval": Approximately 50% of cases
    - Initial brief loss of consciousness (LOC)
    - Subsequent asymptomatic time between LOC & symptom/coma onset
  ○ Headache, nausea, vomiting, seizures, focal neurological deficits (field cuts, aphasia, weakness)
  ○ Mass effect/herniation common
    - Pupil-involving CN3 palsy, somnolence, ↓ consciousness, coma
- Other signs/symptoms: Alcohol & other intoxications associated with ↑ incidence of EDH

Demographics
- Age
  ○ More common in patients < 20 years; extremely rare in elderly
  ○ Uncommon in infants
- Gender: M:F = 4:1

Natural History & Prognosis
- Factors affecting rate of growth
  ○ Arterial vs. venous flow rate, arterial spasm
  ○ Decompression through fracture into scalp
  ○ Tamponade
- Delayed development or enlargement common
  ○ 10-25% of cases
  ○ Usually occurs within first 36 hours
- Epidural abscess may develop if bacteria colonize EDH via fracture site
- Generally good outcome if promptly recognized & treated
  ○ Overall mortality approximately 5%
  ○ Bilateral EDH has 15-20% mortality rate
- Increased mortality in posterior fossa EDH (26%)
  ○ Can have delayed symptom onset 2° slower expansion from ↓ venous pressure

Treatment
- Prompt recognition, appropriate treatment essential
  ○ Poor outcome often related to delayed referral, diagnosis, or operation
- Nearly always requires surgical evacuation
  ○ Additional EDH may be unmasked post-procedure
- Small EDH sometimes followed without surgery
  ○ Repeat CT over 36 hrs to monitor for change
  ○ EDH ↑ during conservative management (23%)
    - Occurs within 36 hrs
    - Mean enlargement: 7 mm
- Complications: Mass effect causing herniations

DIAGNOSTIC CHECKLIST

Image Interpretation Pearls
- NECT highly sensitive
- If MR unavailable, coronal CT reconstructions to evaluate vertex EDH

SELECTED REFERENCES

1. Rochat P et al: Sequentially evolved bilateral epidural haematomas. Clin Neurol Neurosurg. 105(1):39-41, 2002
2. Server A et al: Vertex epidural hematoma - neuroradiological findings and management. Acta Radiol. 43(5):483-5, 2002
3. Al-Nakshabandi NA: The swirl sign. Radiology. 218(2):433, 2001
4. Khwaja HA et al: Posterior cranial fossa venous extradural haematoma: an uncommon form of intracranial injury. Emerg Med J. 18(6):496-7, 2001
5. Singleton SD et al: Lenticular lesions: not always an epidural hematoma. Pediatr Emerg Care. 17(4):252-4, 2001
6. Harbury OL et al: Vertex epidural hematomas: imaging findings and diagnostic pitfalls. Eur J Radiol. 36(3):150-7, 2000
7. Bozbuga M et al: Posterior fossa epidural hematomas: observations on a series of 73 cases. Neurosurg Rev. 22(1):34-40, 1999
8. Sullivan TP et al: Follow-up of conservatively managed epidural hematomas: implications for timing of repeat CT. AJNR Am J Neuroradiol. 20(1):107-13, 1999
9. Paterniti S et al: Is the size of an epidural haematoma related to outcome? Acta Neurochir (Wien). 140(9):953-5, 1998
10. Servadei F: Prognostic factors in severely head injured adult patients with epidural haematoma's. Acta Neurochir (Wien). 139(4):273-8, 1997

EPIDURAL HEMATOMA

IMAGE GALLERY

Typical

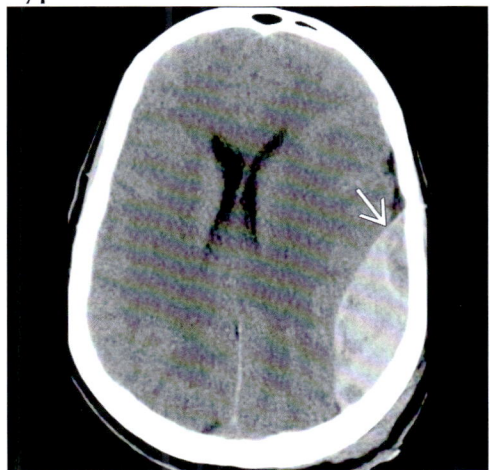
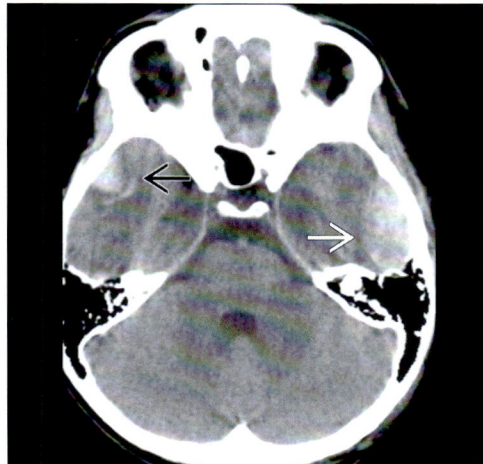

(Left) Axial NECT shows left parietal convexity EDH with dense medial margin ➡ representing displaced dura. *(Right)* Axial NECT shows lentiform acute EDH ➡ with contrecoup contusion in right temporal lobe ➡.

Variant

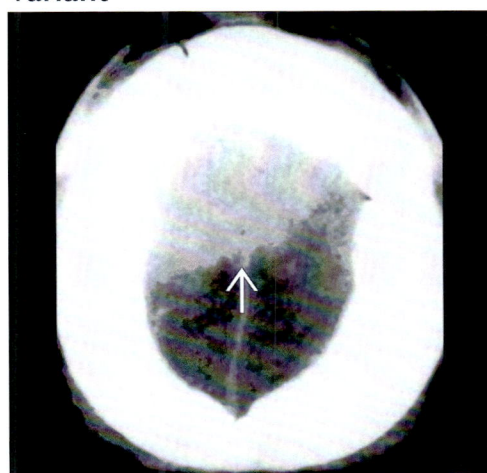
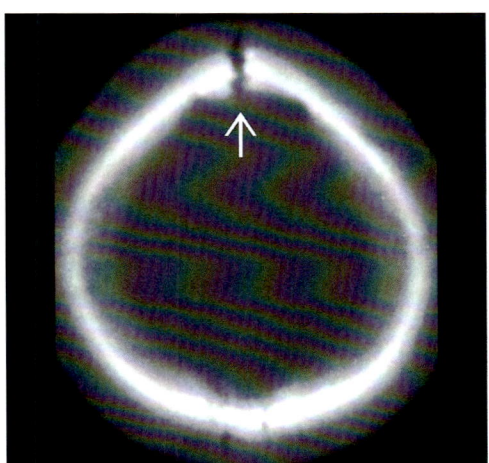

(Left) Axial NECT shows vertex EDH crossing midline ➡. *(Right)* Axial bone CT shows diastatic fracture of sagittal suture ➡ adjacent to superior sagittal sinus & EDH.

Variant

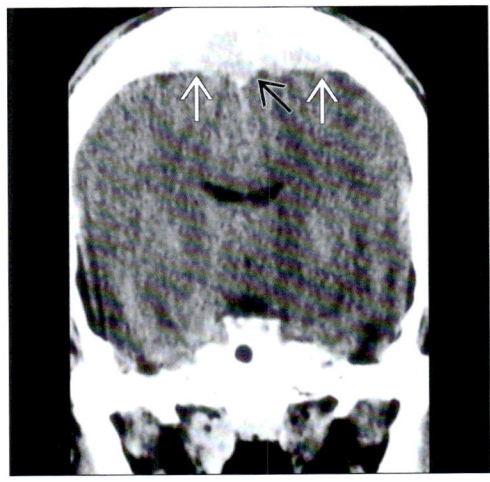
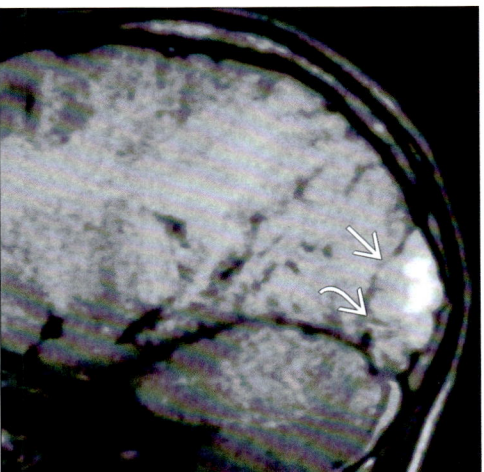

(Left) Coronal NECT shows vertex EDH ➡ crossing midline, displacing superior sagittal sinus inferiorly away from calvarium ➡. *(Right)* Sagittal T1WI MR shows venous EDH ➡ in occipital region, due to rupture of transverse sinus ➡.

ACUTE SUBDURAL HEMATOMA

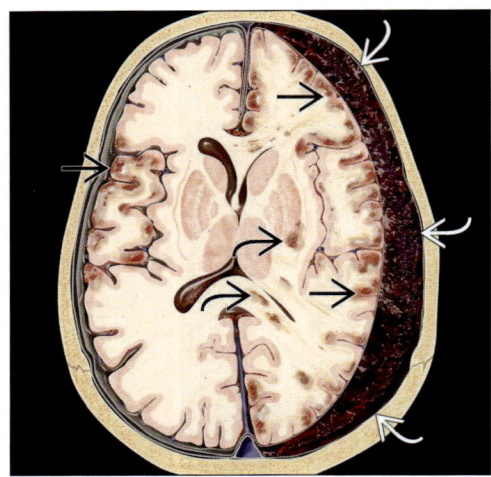

Axial graphic shows acute subdural hematoma ➡ compressing left hemisphere and lateral ventricle. Note contusions ➡ and axonal injuries ➡.

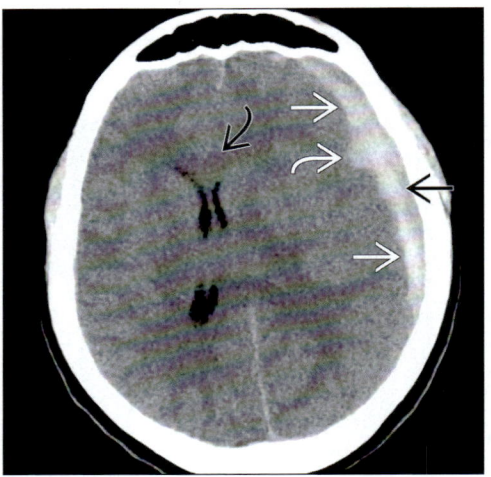

Axial NECT shows diffuse crescentic extra-axial hyperdense collection ➡, aSDH molding to brain surface ➡, & transfalcine herniation ➡. Lateral hypodense component is common ➡.

TERMINOLOGY

Abbreviations and Synonyms
- Acute subdural hematoma (aSDH)

Definitions
- Acute hemorrhagic collection in subdural space

IMAGING FINDINGS

General Features
- Best diagnostic clue: CT: Crescentic hyperdense extra-axial collection spread diffusely over convexity
- Location
  - Between arachnoid & inner layer of dura
  - Supratentorial convexity most common
- Morphology
  - Crescent-shaped extra-axial fluid collection
  - May cross sutures, not dural attachments
  - May extend along falx, tentorium & anterior and middle fossa floors

CT Findings
- NECT
  - Hyperacute SDH (≤ 6 hrs) may have heterogeneous density or hypodensity
  - aSDH (6 hours-3 days)
    - aSDH 60% homogeneously hyperdense
    - 40% mixed hyper-, hypodense with active bleeding ("swirl" sign), torn arachnoid with CSF accumulation, clot retraction
    - Rarely isodense → coagulopathy, anemia (Hgb < 8-10 g/dL)
    - Without recurrent hemorrhage density decreases ± 1.5 HU/day
- CECT
  - Inward displacement of cortical veins
  - Dura & membranes enhance when subacute, useful to visualize loculations

MR Findings
- T1WI
  - Hyperacute (< 12 hours): Iso- to mildly hyperintense
  - Acute: (12 hours-2 days) mildly hypointense
- T2WI
  - Hyperacute: Mildly hyperintense

DDx: Subdural Hematoma

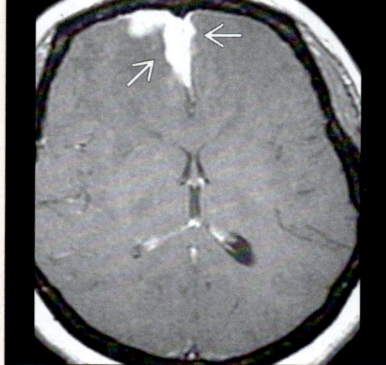
Sarcoidosis

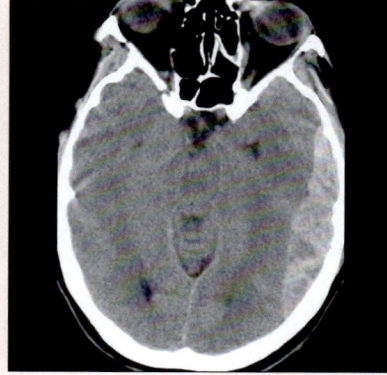
Epidural Hematoma

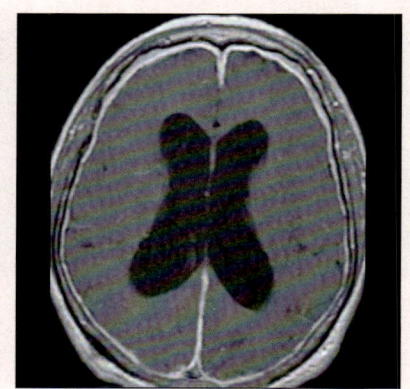
Intracranial Hypotension

ACUTE SUBDURAL HEMATOMA

Key Facts

Terminology
- Acute hemorrhagic collection in subdural space

Imaging Findings
- Best diagnostic clue: CT: Crescentic hyperdense extra-axial collection spread diffusely over convexity
- May extend along falx, tentorium & anterior and middle fossa floors
- aSDH (6 hours-3 days)
- aSDH 60% homogeneously hyperdense
- NECT as initial screen
- Protocol advice: Wide window settings (~ 150 HU)

Top Differential Diagnoses
- Other Subdural Collections
- Acute Epidural Hematoma
- Pachymeningopathies (Thickened Dura)
- Tumor

Pathology
- Tearing of bridging cortical veins as they cross subdural space to drain into dural sinus
- Associated abnormalities: > 70% have other significant associated traumatic lesions

Clinical Issues
- Coagulopathy or anticoagulation increase risk and extent of hemorrhage
- Recurrent, hemorrhage common; in children, raises suspicion of nonaccidental trauma

Diagnostic Checklist
- CT density & MR intensity vary with age & degree of recurrent hemorrhage

---

- Acute: Hypointense
- FLAIR
  - Intensity same as T2WI but conspicuity different because of contrast to CSF
    - Hyperacute hematomas highly conspicuous
    - Acute hematomas may be isointense to CSF: Difficult to identify when small
- T2* GRE: Hypointense
- DWI
  - Heterogeneous signal (nonspecific)
  - May differentiate extra-axial empyema (marked hyperintensity) from hemorrhage
- T1 C+
  - Enhancement of displaced bridging veins
  - Enhancement of subdural collection predictive of subsequent growth
- Recurrent hemorrhage common; mixtures of acute and chronic blood even at time of initial exam
  - Signal variable due to recurrent hemorrhage and therefore difficult to age hematoma

Angiographic Findings
- Conventional
  - Displacement, mass effect from extra-axial mass; veins displaced from inner table of skull
  - Perform only if suspect underlying vascular anomaly: Aneurysm or dural vascular malformation

Imaging Recommendations
- Best imaging tool
  - NECT as initial screen
  - MR more sensitive for extent of SDH & additional findings of traumatic brain injury
- Protocol advice: Wide window settings (~ 150 HU)

DIFFERENTIAL DIAGNOSIS

Other Subdural Collections
- Hygroma: Clear CSF, no encapsulating membranes
- Effusion: Xanthochromic fluid 2° extravasation of plasma from membrane; 1-3 days post-trauma; near CSF density/intensity
- Empyema: Peripheral enhancement, hyperintensity on FLAIR and DWI; restricted diffusion

Acute Epidural Hematoma
- Biconvex extra-axial collection
- Associated with fracture
- May cross dural attachments, limited by sutures

Pachymeningopathies (Thickened Dura)
- Chronic meningitis (may be indistinguishable); sarcoid "lumpy-bumpy"
- Post-surgical (e.g., shunt)
- Intracranial hypotension ("slumping" midbrain, tonsillar herniation)
- Thickened dura enhances intensely; MR > CT
- Calcified dural plaques hyperintense on T1WI due to yellow marrow; may mimic subacute SDH

Tumor
- Meningioma, lymphoma, leukemia, metastases
- Dural-based, enhancing mass
- ± Skull and extracranial soft tissue involved

Peripheral Infarct
- Cortex involved, not displaced
- Hyperintense DWI

Chemical Shift Artifact
- Marrow or subcutaneous fat may "shift", can appear intracranial, mimic T1 hyperintense SDH
  - Seen with ↑ field of view or ↓ bandwidth

PATHOLOGY

General Features
- Etiology
  - Trauma most common
    - Tearing of bridging cortical veins as they cross subdural space to drain into dural sinus
    - Nonimpact (falls) as well as direct injury
    - Trauma may be minor, particularly in elderly; often recurrent with initial episodes subclinical
  - Less common etiologies

ACUTE SUBDURAL HEMATOMA

- Dissection of intraparenchymal hematoma into subarachnoid, then subdural space
- Aneurysm rupture
- Vascular malformations: Dural arteriovenous fistula (AVF), arteriovenous malformation (AVM), cavernoma
- Dural invasion by tumor with secondary hemorrhage (prostate CA)
- Spontaneous hemorrhage with severe coagulopathy
  - Predisposing factors
    - Atrophy
    - Shunting (leads to increased traction on superior cortical veins)
    - Coagulopathy (e.g., alcohol abuse) & anticoagulation
- Epidemiology: Found in 30% of autopsy cases following craniocerebral trauma
- Associated abnormalities: > 70% have other significant associated traumatic lesions

Gross Pathologic & Surgical Features
- Hematoma
- Delayed development of membranes/granulation tissue

Microscopic Features
- Outer membrane of proliferating fibroblasts & capillaries
- Fragile capillaries hypothesized as source of recurrent hemorrhage (chronic SDH)
- Inner membrane of dural fibroblasts or border cells form fibrocollagenous sheet

CLINICAL ISSUES

Presentation
- Most common signs/symptoms
  - Most commonly following trauma
  - Varies from asymptomatic to loss of consciousness
    - "Lucid" interval in aSDH: Initially awake, alert patient who loses consciousness a few hours after trauma
    - Early symptomatic presentation (< 4 hours) and advanced age have poor prognosis
  - Other symptoms (focal deficit, seizure) from mass effect, diffuse brain injury, secondary ischemia
  - Coagulopathy or anticoagulation increase risk and extent of hemorrhage
- Other signs/symptoms: Other lesions (e.g., traumatic SAH) in > 70%

Demographics
- Age: Any age, more common in elderly
- Gender: No gender predilection

Natural History & Prognosis
- Can grow slowly with increased mass effect if untreated
- Compresses & displaces underlying brain
- Recurrent, hemorrhage common; in children, raises suspicion of nonaccidental trauma

Treatment
- Poor prognosis (35-90% mortality)
  - Emergency pre-operative high-dose mannitol may improve outcome
- Hematoma thickness, midline shift > 20 mm correlate with poor outcome
- Lethal if hematoma volume > 8-10% of intracranial volume

DIAGNOSTIC CHECKLIST

Consider
- NECT initial screen
- Consider MR if degree of mass effect and/or symptoms greater than expected for size of SDH
  - MR to identify extent of traumatic brain injury when patient is stable

Image Interpretation Pearls
- Wide window settings for CT increases conspicuity of subtle SDH
- FLAIR, T2* most sensitive sequences for SDH when isointense to CSF on T1 and T2
- CT density & MR intensity vary with age & degree of recurrent hemorrhage

SELECTED REFERENCES

1. Abe M et al: Analysis of ischemic brain damage in cases of acute subdural hematomas. Surg Neurol. 59(6):464-72; discussion 472, 2003
2. Tseng SH et al: Dural metastasis in patients with malignant neoplasm and chronic subdural hematoma. Acta Neurol Scand. 108(1):43-6, 2003
3. Burger PC et al: Surgical Pathology of the Nervous System & Its Coverings, 4th ed. New York, Churchill Livingstone, 2002
4. Lin DD et al: Detection of intracranial hemorrhage: comparison between gradient-echo images and b(0) images obtained from diffusion-weighted echo-planar sequences. AJNR Am J Neuroradiol. 22(7):1275-81, 2001
5. Matano S et al: Primary leptomeningeal lymphoma. J Neurooncol. 52(1):81-3, 2001
6. Mori K et al: Delayed magnetic resonance imaging with GdD-DTPA differentiates subdural hygroma and subdural effusion. Surg Neurol. 53(4):303-10; discussion 310-1, 2000
7. Campbell BG et al: Emergency magnetic resonance of the brain. Top Magn Reson Imaging. 9(4):208-27, 1998
8. Ashikaga R et al: MRI of head injury using FLAIR. Neuroradiology. 39(4):239-42, 1997
9. Cho SJ et al: Assumption of the age of subdural hematomas based on computed tomographic findings. Neurol Med Chir. 24:607-14, 1995
10. Oikawa A et al: Arteriovenous malformation presenting as acute subdural haematoma. Neurol Res. 15(5):353-5, 1993
11. Wilms G et al: Isodense subdural haematomas on CT:MRI findings. Neuroradiology. 34(6):497-9, 1992
12. Kelly AB et al: Head trauma: comparison of MR and CT--experience in 100 patients. AJNR Am J Neuroradiol. 9(4):699-708, 1988
13. Massaro F et al: One hundred and twenty-seven cases of acute subdural haematoma operated on. Correlation between CT scan findings and outcome.

ACUTE SUBDURAL HEMATOMA

IMAGE GALLERY

Other

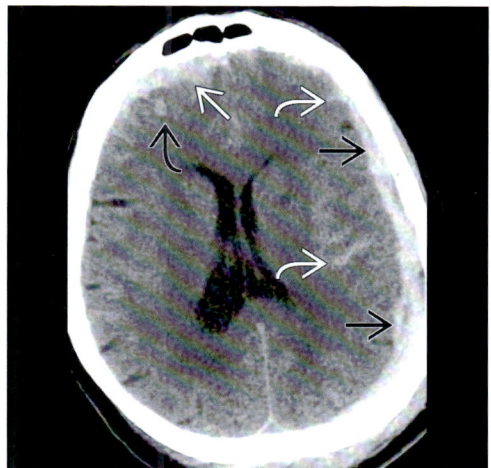 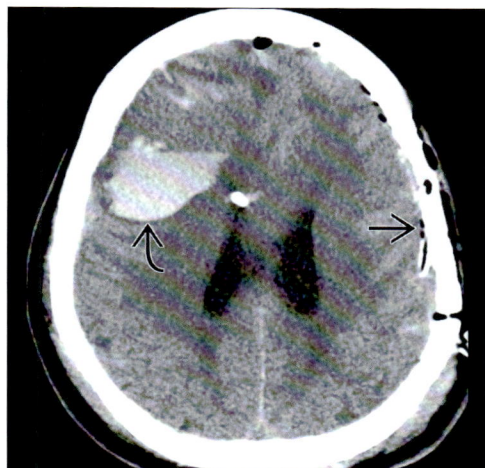

(Left) Axial NECT shows left convexity aSDH ➔, small right aSDH ➔, subarachnoid hemorrhage ➔ and left frontal contusion ➔. *(Right)* Axial NECT S/P evacuation of left aSDH ➔ in same patient as previous image shows blooming of left frontal contusion ➔ 6 hours after initial scan; patient expired 2 days later.

Other

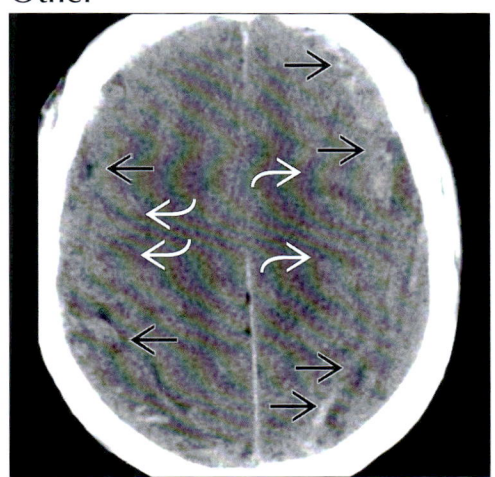 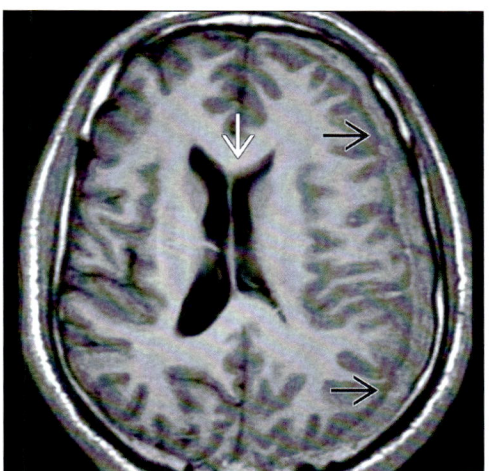

(Left) Axial NECT shows hyperacute SDH (< 3 hrs); bilateral mixed density SDHs ➔ predominantly isodense. Displaced cortico-medullary junctions ➔ are a sign of subdural location of lesions. *(Right)* Axial T1WI MR shows crescentic left convexity aSDH (24 hrs) ➔. Blood is isointense to white matter but well seen, due to ease of visualization of brain surface. Note transfalcine herniation ➔.

Typical

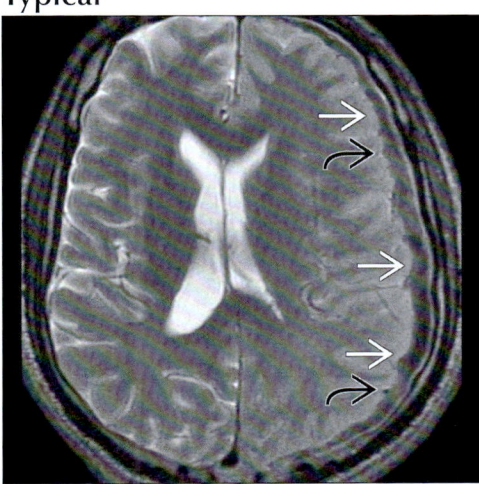 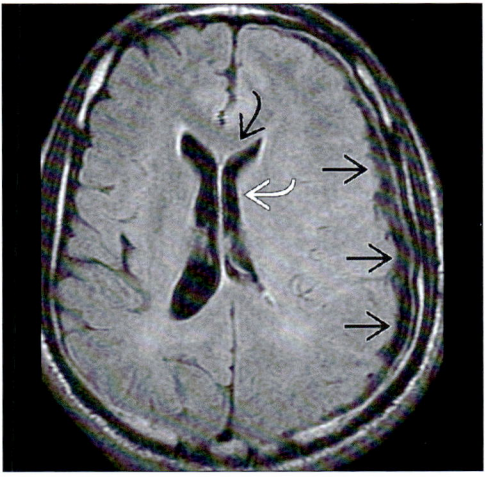

(Left) Axial T2WI MR in same patient as previous image shows hypodense left convexity aSDH (24 hrs) ➔. Medially displaced cortical veins are also visible ➔. *(Right)* Axial FLAIR MR in same patient as previous image shows hypointense aSDH ➔ difficult to differentiate from normal dark CSF & bone. Note lateral ventricular compression ➔ & transfalcine herniation ➔.

MIXED SUBDURAL HEMATOMA

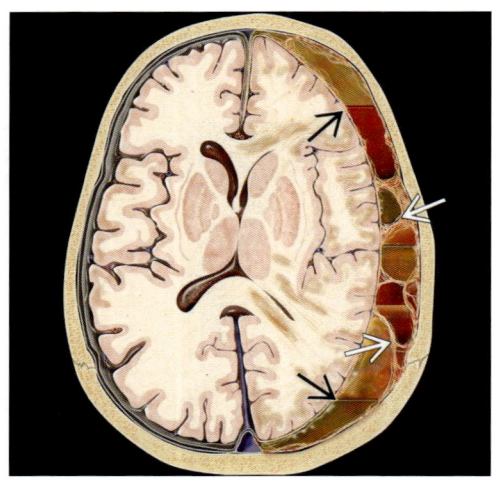

Axial graphic shows hemorrhage of multiple ages in subdural hematoma, with numerous loculations from membranes ➔; multiple fluid levels ➔.

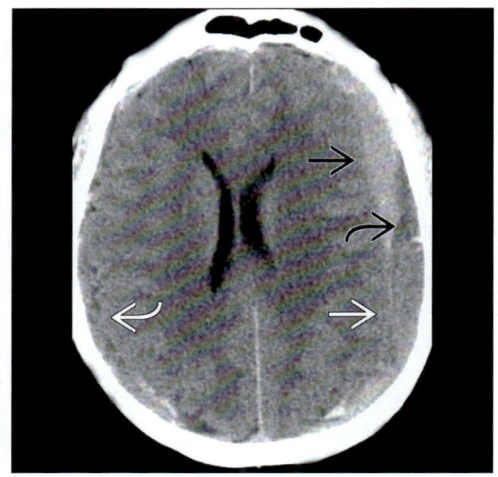

Axial NECT shows bilateral mixed-density SDHs. Left hematoma loculated with hyperdense ➔, isodense ➔ and hypodense ➔ components. Small right SDH ➔ is also present.

TERMINOLOGY

Abbreviations and Synonyms
- Subdural hematoma (SDH)

Definitions
- Hemorrhage of differing ages/evolution in subdural space

IMAGING FINDINGS

General Features
- Best diagnostic clue: Crescentic, mixed-density, signal intensity, and extra axial convexity collection
- Location
  ○ Potential space between inner layer of dura mater & arachnoid
  ○ Supratentorial convexity most common
- Morphology
  ○ Crescentic, extra-axial fluid collection
  ○ May cross sutures, but not dural attachments
  ○ Often septated, with internal membranes (biconvex)

CT Findings
- NECT
  ○ Variable heterogeneous density
    ▪ Dependent layering: Hyperdense posteriorly
    ▪ Loculated: Hypo- and hyperdense components
  ○ Bilateral isodense SDH: Medial displacement of corticomedullary junction
    ▪ Sulci & lateral ventricles small; ventricles parallel
    ▪ Central herniation: Non-visualization of suprasellar cistern; third ventricle posterior to sella
- CECT: Inward displacement of cortical veins

MR Findings
- T1WI: Mixed signal: Hyperintensity (hemorrhage > 3 days)
- T2WI: Mixed signal: Hypointensity (hemorrhage < 5 days)
- FLAIR: Mixed signal: Hyperintense to CSF
- Mixed signal due to recurrent bleed
- Loculations: Regions of different intensity (hemorrhage of different age)
- Dependent layering

DDx: Mixed Subdural Hematoma

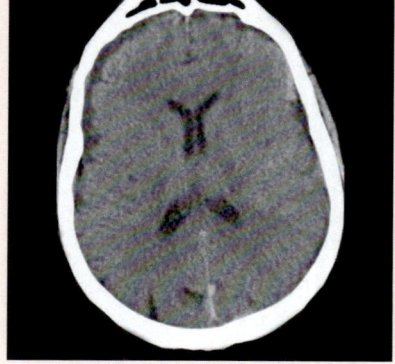

Traumatic Effusion

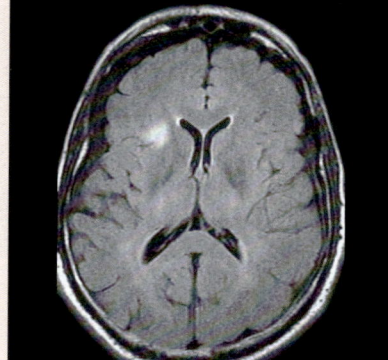

Traumatic Effusion

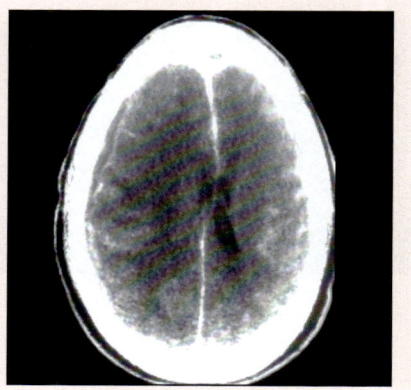

Subdural Empyema

MIXED SUBDURAL HEMATOMA

Key Facts

Terminology
- Hemorrhage of differing ages/evolution in subdural space

Imaging Findings
- Best diagnostic clue: Crescentic, mixed-density, signal intensity, and extra axial convexity collection
- Supratentorial convexity most common
- Often septated, with internal membranes (biconvex)
- Variable heterogeneous density

- Mixed signal due to recurrent bleed

Pathology
- Etiology: Re-hemorrhage into pre-existent SDH

Clinical Issues
- Age: Usually > 70 years of age; young children: Non-accidental trauma
- Surgical evacuation if symptomatic or growing

Imaging Recommendations
- Best imaging tool
  - NECT initial screen
  - MR more sensitive: Bleed age, extent of injuries
- Protocol advice: Wide window settings (150-200 HU)

DIFFERENTIAL DIAGNOSIS

Other Subdural Collections
- Acute traumatic effusion, empyema, hygroma

Acute Epidural Hematoma
- Hyperdense biconvex extra-axial mass on NECT

Pachymeningopathies (Thickened Dura)
- Chronic meningitis: Granulomatous
- Post-surgical (e.g., shunt)
- Intracranial hypotension

Tumor
- Meningioma, lymphoma, leukemia, metastases

PATHOLOGY

General Features
- Etiology: Re-hemorrhage into pre-existent SDH
- Epidemiology: 10-20% of imaged patients, 30% of autopsy cases following head trauma
- Associated abnormalities: > 70% of SDH: Significant associated traumatic lesions

CLINICAL ISSUES

Presentation
- Most common signs/symptoms: Asymptomatic, or headache, loss of consciousness

Demographics
- Age: Usually > 70 years of age; young children: Non-accidental trauma

Natural History & Prognosis
- Can spontaneously resolve or enlarge
- Onset 2 days to 2 weeks after trauma
  - Recurrent, mixed-age hemorrhages common; suspect non-accidental trauma in children
- Often bilateral

Treatment
- Surgical evacuation if symptomatic or growing

SELECTED REFERENCES
1. Nakaguchi H et al: Factors in the natural history of chronic subdural hematomas that influence their postoperative recurrence. J Neurosurg. 95(2):256-62, 2001
2. Kaminogo M et al: Characteristics of symptomatic chronic subdural haematomas on high-field MRI. Neuroradiology. 41(2):109-16, 1999
3. Wilms G et al: CT and MR in infants with pericerebral collections and macrocephaly: benign enlargement of the subarachnoid spaces versus subdural collections. AJNR Am J Neuroradiol. 14(4):855-60, 1993

IMAGE GALLERY

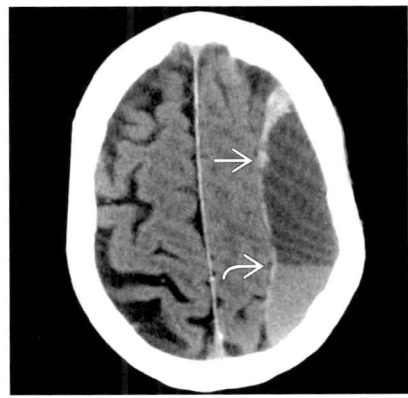 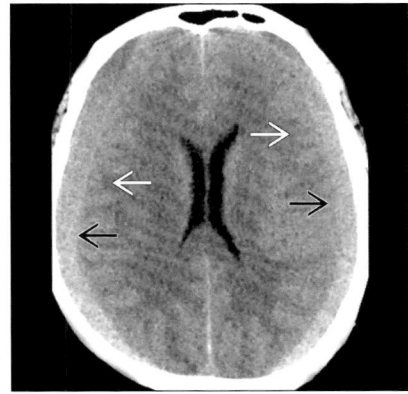 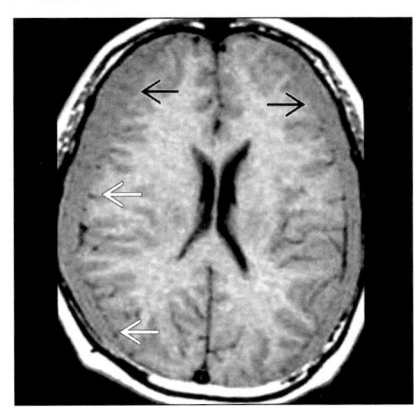

(Left) Axial NECT shows biconvex extra-axial collection with dense medial margin ➔ mimicking EDH. Dependent layering ➔ & age (83 y) favors SDH. (Center) Axial NECT shows bilateral isodense SDHs ➔. Medial displacement of cortico-medullary junction ➔, absent sulci and small, nearly parallel ventricles. (Right) Axial T1WI MR in same patient as previous image demonstrates SDHs ➔ mildly hypointense to cortex. Absence of bone artifacts improves visualization of cortex and displaced cortical veins ➔.

PARATENTORIAL SUBDURAL HEMATOMA

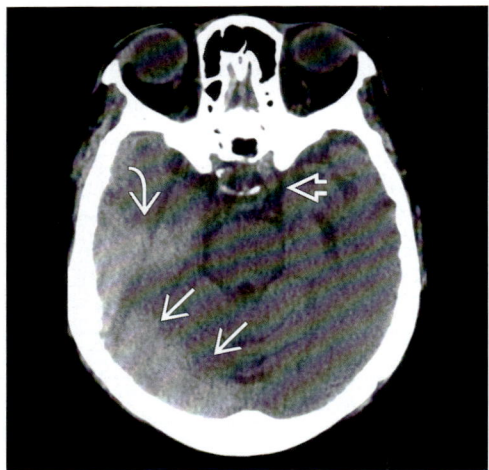 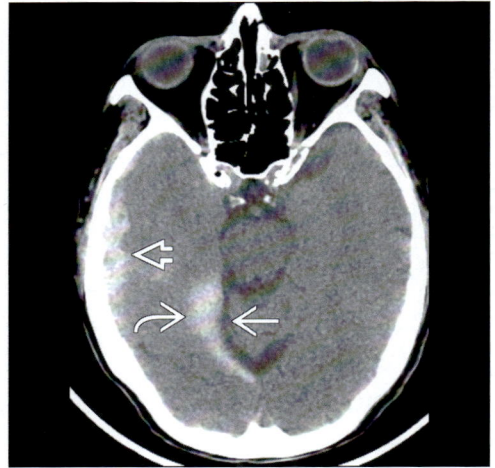

Axial NECT shows ill-defined hyperdensity along lateral margin of tentorium ➔ with subtemporal extension ➔. Despite size of SDH, there is no herniation ➔.

Axial NECT shows hyperdensity along lateral margin of tentorium with sharp medial margin ➔ and more ill-defined lateral border ➔. Right convexity SDH present ➔.

TERMINOLOGY

Abbreviations and Synonyms
- Supratentorial paratentorial (STPT) subdural hematoma (SDH)
- Infratentorial paratentorial (ITPT) SDH

Definitions
- Subdural hemorrhage along superior and/or inferior margin of tentorium (tent)

IMAGING FINDINGS

General Features
- Best diagnostic clue
  - STPT: Ill-defined hemorrhage along lateral margin of tent
  - ITPT: Discrete bilateral hemorrhage along medial margin of tent
- Location: Subdural space along superior and/or inferior margin of tent
- Size: Variable
- Morphology
  - Small: Thin layer of blood
  - Large: Bulbous mass bulging into brain

CT Findings
- NECT
  - Supratentorial
    - Linear or bulbous hyperdense lesion along lateral margin of tent if STPT
    - Sharp medial margin; ill-defined lateral margin
    - Usually unilateral
    - Interhemispheric fissure (IHF) & posterior convexity extension common in STPT
  - Infratentorial
    - Hyperdensity along medial margin of tent if ITPT
    - Bilateral but often asymmetric
    - Compresses quadrigeminal cistern & 4th ventricle
    - Secondary to hydrocephalus with larger lesions

MR Findings
- T1WI
  - Isointense if < 3 days, hyperintense if > 3 days
  - Coronal & sagittal views best for location & extent
- T2* GRE: Irregular "shaggy" hypointensity along tent

DDx: Mimics of Paratentorial SDH

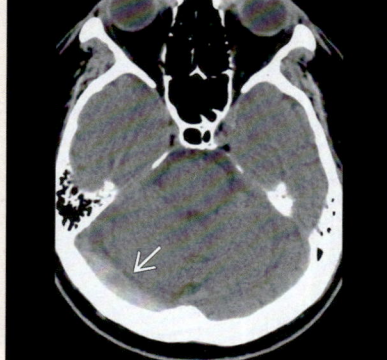 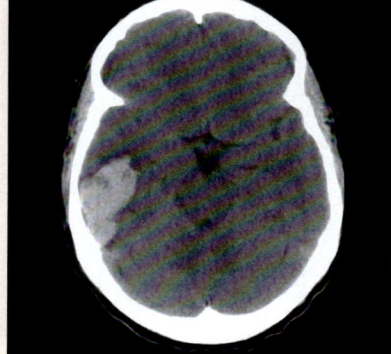 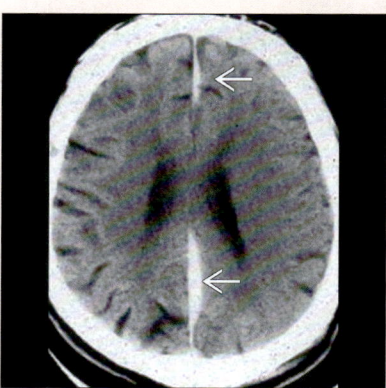

Transverse Sinus Thrombosis | Parenchymal Hematoma | Interhemispheric SDH

PARATENTORIAL SUBDURAL HEMATOMA

Key Facts

Terminology
- Supratentorial paratentorial (STPT) subdural hematoma (SDH)
- Infratentorial paratentorial (ITPT) SDH
- Subdural hemorrhage along superior and/or inferior margin of tentorium (tent)

Imaging Findings
- STPT: Ill-defined hemorrhage along lateral margin of tent
- ITPT: Discrete bilateral hemorrhage along medial margin of tent
- Linear or bulbous hyperdense lesion along lateral margin of tent if STPT
- Interhemispheric fissure (IHF) & posterior convexity extension common in STPT
- Hyperdensity along medial margin of tent if ITPT
- Coronal T1WI to confirm location, extent

Imaging Recommendations
- Best imaging tool
  - CT for initial screen
  - Coronal T1WI to confirm location, extent
- Protocol advice: MR to confirm diagnosis

DIFFERENTIAL DIAGNOSIS

IHF (Parafalcine) SDH
- Flat medial & convex lateral margin along falx

Parenchymal Hematoma
- No flat border along tent, more mass effect

Transverse Sinus Thrombosis
- Clot in sinus on CT or MR; confirm with MR or CT venography

PATHOLOGY

General Features
- Etiology
  - Closed head injury
  - Birth trauma
- Associated abnormalities
  - Other intracranial hemorrhage & edema
  - Hydrocephalus (infratentorial SDH)

Gross Pathologic & Surgical Features
- Acute/subacute hematoma along tent

CLINICAL ISSUES

Presentation
- Most common signs/symptoms: Altered mental status and/or focal deficit
- Other signs/symptoms: Signs of increased intracranial pressure 2° to infratentorial SDH & hydrocephalus

Demographics
- Age: Any

Natural History & Prognosis
- Small lesions: Spontaneous resolution
- Large lesions: Poor outcome without surgery

Treatment
- Surgery for large lesions

DIAGNOSTIC CHECKLIST

Image Interpretation Pearls
- Large STPT SDH bulges into brain
- Large ITPT SDH produces hydrocephalus

SELECTED REFERENCES
1. Young RJ et al: Imaging of traumatic intracranial hemorrhage. Neuroimaging Clin N Am. 12(2):189-204, 2002

IMAGE GALLERY

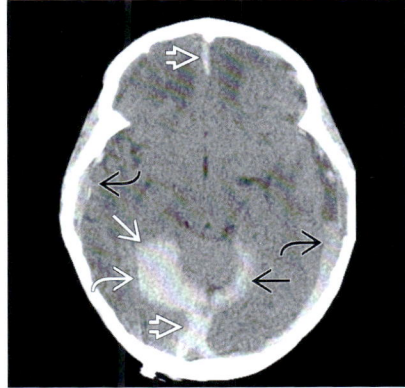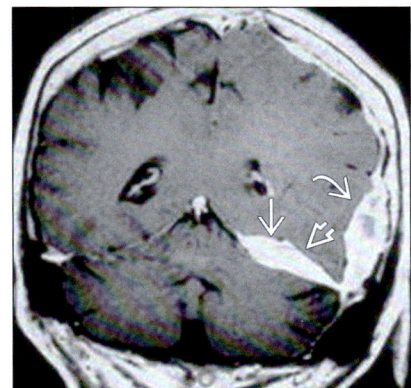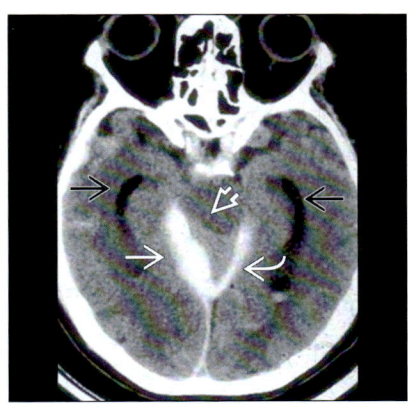

(Left) Axial NECT shows large right STPT SDH ➔ with bulbous anterior margin ➔ and extension into IHF ➔. Small left STPT SDH ➔ and bilateral convexity SDHs ➔ also present. (Center) Coronal T1WI MR shows SDH along superior margin of tent ➔ with extension over convexity ➔. Note upward convexity ➔ accounting for bulbous appearance on axial image. (Right) Axial NECT shows infratentorial bilateral SDH along medial margin of tent, larger on right ➔ than left ➔, with marked compression of quadrigeminal cistern ➔ & hydrocephalus ➔.

TRAUMATIC SUBARACHNOID HEMORRHAGE

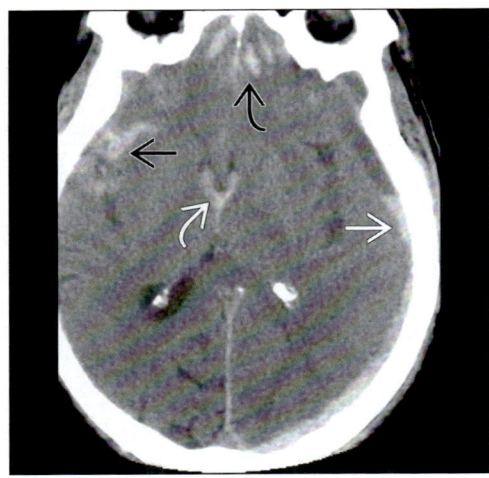

Axial NECT shows multi-compartment hemorrhage with subarachnoid hemorrhage in left sylvian fissure ➡, bifrontal contusions ➡, subdural ➡ and intraventricular hemorrhage ➡.

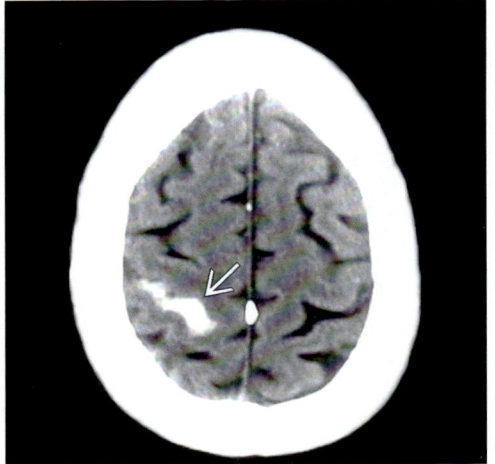

Axial NECT shows isolated superficial sulcal tSAH ➡.

TERMINOLOGY

Abbreviations and Synonyms
- Traumatic subarachnoid hemorrhage (tSAH)

Definitions
- Blood within subarachnoid spaces between pial & arachnoid membranes

IMAGING FINDINGS

General Features
- Best diagnostic clue: High density on CT, hyperintensity on FLAIR within sulci/cisterns in trauma patient
- Location
  - Focal adjacent to contusion, subdural hematoma (SDH), fracture, laceration
  - Diffusely throughout subarachnoid space &/or basal cisterns: Major arterial damage/dissection
  - Isolated focal superficial convexity sulci

CT Findings
- NECT
  - High density in subarachnoid space(s)/cisterns
  - Hyperdense blood in interpeduncular cistern may be only manifestation of subtle (benign) SAH
  - Identical to aneurysmal SAH except location
    - Adjacent to contusions, SDH
    - Convexity sulci > basal cisterns

MR Findings
- T1WI: Hyperintense to ventricular CSF ("dirty" CSF)
- T2WI: Hyperintense to brain, isointense to CSF (not detected)
- FLAIR: Hyperintense sulci/cisterns; more sensitive, less specific than CT
- T2* GRE: Occasionally hypointense; delayed or beneath SDH
- DWI
  - Evaluation of tSAH-induced spasm
    - Hyperintense restricted diffusion in areas of ischemia

Angiographic Findings
- Conventional

DDx: Traumatic Subarachnoid Hemorrhage

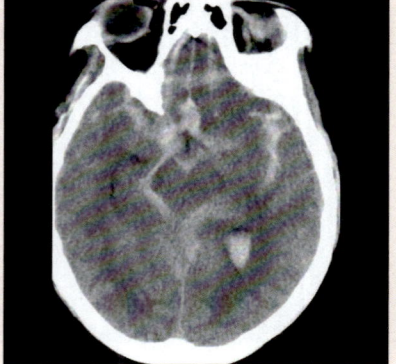
Aneurysmal SAH

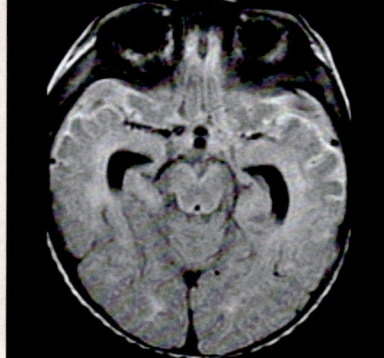
Meningitis

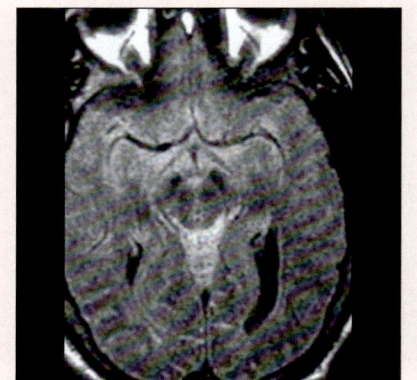
FLAIR: O₂ Therapy

TRAUMATIC SUBARACHNOID HEMORRHAGE

Key Facts

Terminology
- Blood within subarachnoid spaces between pial & arachnoid membranes

Imaging Findings
- Best diagnostic clue: High density on CT, hyperintensity on FLAIR within sulci/cisterns in trauma patient
- High density in subarachnoid space(s)/cisterns
- FLAIR: Hyperintense sulci/cisterns; more sensitive, less specific than CT
- Best imaging tool: NECT; FLAIR for subtle SAH

Top Differential Diagnoses
- Ruptured aneurysm
- Meningitis - Cellular & Proteinaceous Debris
- High Inspired Oxygen

Pathology
- Tearing of veins in subarachnoid space most likely etiology
- Evolutionary hemoglobin changes different than described for intracerebral hematoma

Clinical Issues
- Most common signs/symptoms: Headache, emesis, decreased consciousness
- Clinical Profile: Trauma most common cause of SAH, not ruptured aneurysm
- Amount of tSAH on initial CT correlates with delayed ischemia, poor outcome
- Supportive therapy is primary treatment

- DSA
  - Exclusion of aneurysm & evaluation of tSAH-induced spasm: CTA replaces DSA
  - "Beaded appearance" of spasm-involved vessels

Imaging Recommendations
- Best imaging tool: NECT; FLAIR for subtle SAH

DIFFERENTIAL DIAGNOSIS

Non-Traumatic SAH (ntSAH)
- Ruptured aneurysm
  - 80-90% ntSAH in North America
  - Aneurysm identified on DSA, CTA, MRA in > 90%
- Ruptured dissecting aneurysm
- Arteriovenous malformation (AVM)
  - 15% ntSAH
  - Identified on DSA, CTA, MRA
- Perimesencephalic venous hemorrhage
  - Limited to basal cisterns: Clot around basilar artery
  - Normal DSA, CTA, MRA
- Cerebral amyloid angiopathy
  - Recurrent cortical hemorrhages
- Cerebral infarction with reperfusion hemorrhage
  - Presence of known infarct
- Anticoagulation therapy
  - Long-term Coumadin therapy; usually unrecognized mild head trauma
  - Alcohol use/abuse also cause of abnormal coagulation
- Blood dyscrasia
  - Usually known pre-existing entity
- Eclampsia (pregnancy-induced hypertension)
  - Reported complication, eclampsia symptomatology
- Spinal vascular malformation
  - Spontaneous
  - Negative initial & repeat cerebral DSA
  - MR: Spinal SAH, cord edema
  - MRA and DSA to establish diagnosis

Meningitis - Cellular & Proteinaceous Debris
- Dirty CSF on CT
- Hyperintensity on FLAIR due to T1 shortening & failure of signal nulling

Carcinomatosis Meningitis
- Cellular CSF prevents FLAIR CSF nulling

Pseudo-Subarachnoid Hemorrhage
- Severe, diffuse cerebral edema → diffusely hypodense brain
- Dura & circulating blood appear hyperdense compared to adjacent brain

Gadolinium Administration
- IV contrast for routine enhanced MR may cause FLAIR hyperintensity
  - Stroke, high grade gliomas (neoplasm surfaces contact subarachnoid spaces/ventricles), meningiomas
  - CSF changes more evident close to pathology &/or hemisphere involved

High Inspired Oxygen
- Administration of 100% O_2 during general anesthesia
  - May cause incomplete nulling of subarachnoid CSF on FLAIR
  - Ventricular CSF not affected

PATHOLOGY

General Features
- Genetics: Less favorable outcome in patients with APOξ4 allele
- Etiology
  - Tearing of veins in subarachnoid space most likely etiology
  - Traumatic dissecting aneurysm causes basal cisternal SAH
    - Most often from vertebral artery dissection
    - Suspect with basilar skull fracture
    - Mimics aneurysmal SAH
- Epidemiology
  - 33% with moderate brain injury; nearly 100% at autopsy (typically mild)

TRAUMATIC SUBARACHNOID HEMORRHAGE

- tSAH-associated vasospasm in 2-10% of cases
- Associated abnormalities: Contusions, SDH or epidural hematoma, diffuse axonal injury

Gross Pathologic & Surgical Features
- Acute blood within sulci/cisterns

Microscopic Features
- Evolutionary hemoglobin changes different than described for intracerebral hematoma
  - Much slower progression, most likely 2° high ambient oxygen tension of subarachnoid CSF delaying degradation

Staging, Grading or Classification Criteria
- Grade 1: Thin tSAH ≤ 5 mm
- Grade 2: Thick tSAH > 5 mm
- Grade 3: Thin tSAH with mass lesion(s)
- Grade 4: Thick tSAH with mass lesion(s)
- Lower grades have better admission Glasgow coma scores & discharge Glasgow outcome scale scores

CLINICAL ISSUES

Presentation
- Most common signs/symptoms: Headache, emesis, decreased consciousness
- Clinical Profile: Trauma most common cause of SAH, not ruptured aneurysm

Demographics
- Age: Median age = 43 years (SD = 21.1 years)
- Gender: M:F = 2:1 for sustaining traumatic brain injury (TBI)
- Risk factors for TBI
  - Young age, low income, chronic alcohol abuse, substance abuse, prior episodes of TBI

Natural History & Prognosis
- Natural history: Breakdown & resorption from CSF
- Poor prognosis if associated with other intracranial injuries
  - Amount of tSAH on initial CT correlates with delayed ischemia, poor outcome
- Complications: Acute hydrocephalus, delayed hydrocephalus, vasospasm
- Acute hydrocephalus
  - Rare; usually obstruction of aqueduct or 4th ventricular outlet by clotted SAH
  - Obstructive, non-communicating hydrocephalus
    - Asymmetric ventricular dilatation
- Delayed hydrocephalus
  - Arachnoid granulation defect in CSF resorption
  - Obstructive communicating hydrocephalus
    - Symmetric ventricular dilatation
- Vasospasm
  - May develop quickly (2-3 days post-injury)
  - Peaks 7-10 days post-injury, threat remains up to 2 weeks
  - Uncommon cause of post-traumatic infarct

Treatment
- Supportive therapy is primary treatment
  - Intubation, supplemental oxygen, IV fluids, therapy of altered vital signs
  - Sedatives, medications for pain, nausea & vomiting
  - Anticonvulsants for seizures
- Nimodipine (calcium channel blocker) may prevent vasospasm & its complications

DIAGNOSTIC CHECKLIST

Image Interpretation Pearls
- Hyperdense blood in interpeduncular cistern may be only manifestation of subtle SAH
- Isolated supratentorial sulci common (benign)
- tSAH often accompanied by additional injuries

SELECTED REFERENCES

1. Prasad K et al: Traumatic subarachnoid hemorrhage. J Neurosurg. 100(4):739-40; author reply 740-1, 2004
2. Bozzao A et al: Cerebrospinal fluid changes after intravenous injection of gadolinium chelate: assessment by FLAIR MR imaging. Eur Radiol. 13(3):592-7, 2003
3. Given CA 2nd et al: Pseudo-subarachnoid hemorrhage: a potential imaging pitfall associated with diffuse cerebral edema. AJNR Am J Neuroradiol. 24(2):254-6, 2003
4. Kay A et al: Temporal alterations in cerebrospinal fluid amyloid beta-protein and apolipoprotein E after subarachnoid hemorrhage. Stroke. 34(12):e240-3, 2003
5. Mattioli C et al: Traumatic subarachnoid hemorrhage on the computerized tomography scan obtained at admission: a multicenter assessment of the accuracy of diagnosis and the potential impact on patient outcome. J Neurosurg. 98(1):37-42, 2003
6. Rumboldt Z et al: Hyperacute subarachnoid hemorrhage on T2-weighted MR images. AJNR Am J Neuroradiol. 24(3):472-5, 2003
7. Macmillan CS et al: Traumatic brain injury and subarachnoid hemorrhage: in vivo occult pathology demonstrated by magnetic resonance spectroscopy may not be "ischaemic". A primary study and review of the literature. Acta Neurochir (Wien). 144(9):853-62; discussion 862, 2002
8. Servadei F et al: Traumatic subarachnoid hemorrhage: demographic and clinical study of 750 patients from the European brain injury consortium survey of head injuries. Neurosurgery. 50(2):261-7; discussion 267-9, 2002
9. Filippi CG et al: Hyperintense signal abnormality in subarachnoid spaces and basal cisterns on MR images of children anesthetized with propofol: new fluid-attenuated inversion recovery finding. AJNR Am J Neuroradiol. 22(2):394-9, 2001
10. Server A et al: Post-traumatic cerebral infarction. Neuroimaging findings, etiology and outcome. Acta Radiol. 42(3):254-60, 2001
11. Taoka T et al: Sulcal hyperintensity on fluid-attenuated inversion recovery mr images in patients without apparent cerebrospinal fluid abnormality. AJR Am J Roentgenol. 176(2):519-24, 2001
12. Noguchi K et al: Comparison of fluid-attenuated inversion-recovery MR imaging with CT in a simulated model of acute subarachnoid hemorrhage. AJNR Am J Neuroradiol. 21(5):923-7, 2000
13. Noguchi K et al: Subacute and chronic subarachnoid hemorrhage: diagnosis with fluid-attenuated inversion-recovery MR imaging. Radiology. 203(1):257-62, 1997

TRAUMATIC SUBARACHNOID HEMORRHAGE

IMAGE GALLERY

Typical

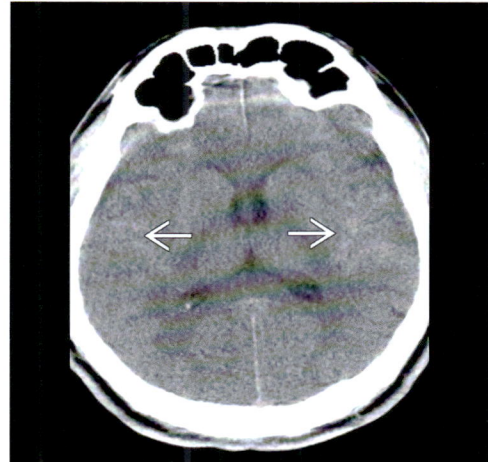
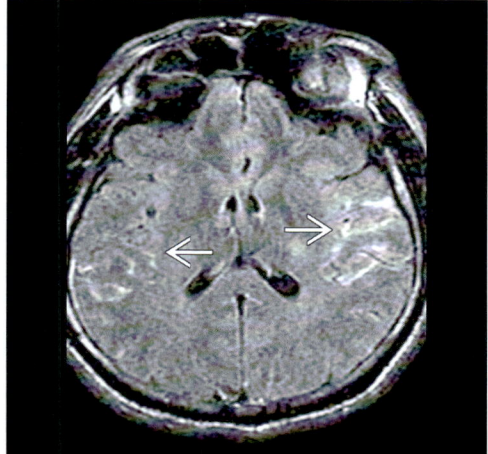

(Left) Axial NECT shows subtle hyperdensity in sylvian fissures ➡ not appreciated in prospect. *(Right)* Axial FLAIR MR one hour after CT in same patient as previous image shows obvious sulcal hyperintensity ➡, indicative of SAH.

Variant

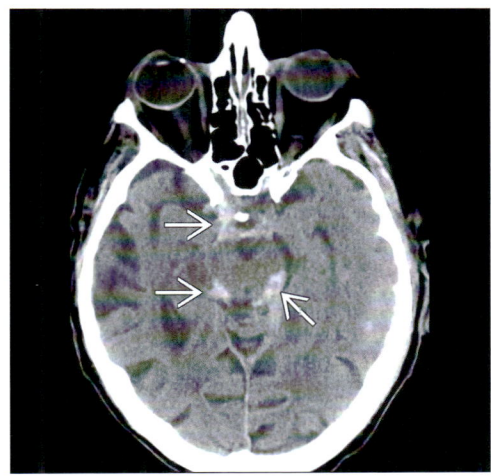
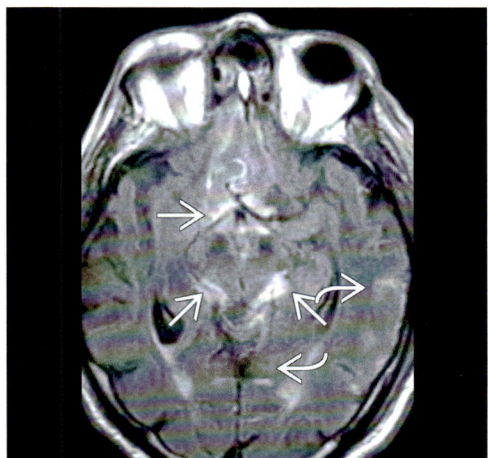

(Left) Axial NECT shows SAH secondary to pericallosal artery laceration ➡. *(Right)* Axial FLAIR MR in same patient as previous image shows basal subarachnoid hemorrhage ➡. Hemorrhage in posterior interhemispheric fissure and over convexity ➡ is better visualized than on CT.

Variant

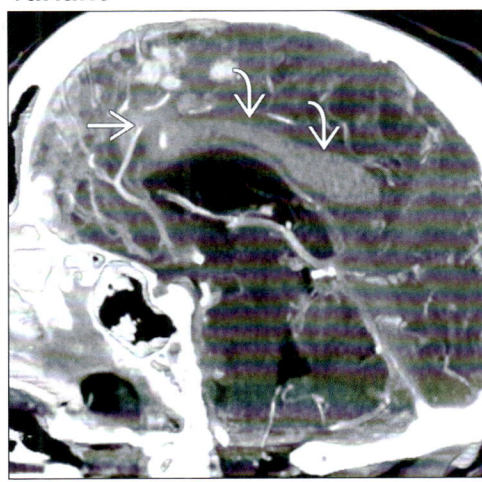
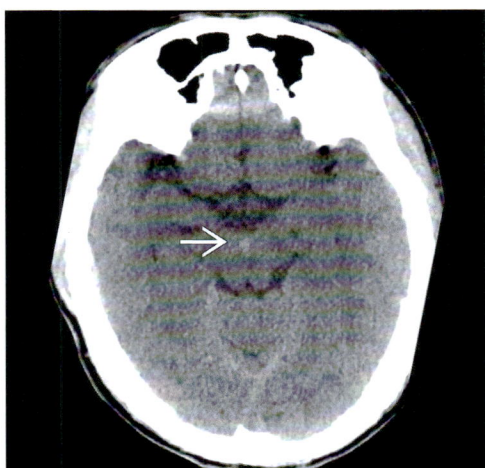

(Left) Sagittal CTA in same patient as previous two images shows focal occlusion of pericallosal artery ➡ and focal hematoma in pericallosal cistern ➡. *(Right)* Axial NECT shows focal interpeduncular cistern subarachnoid hemorrhage ➡.

CEREBRAL CONTUSION

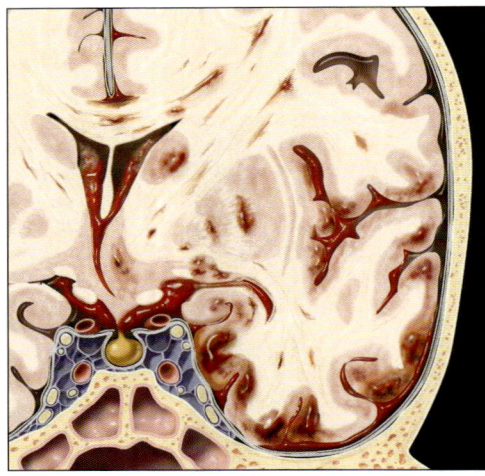
Coronal graphic illustrates hemorrhagic foci involving gray matter of several gyri as well as deeper white matter & gray nuclei. Mass effect is causing left to right shift.

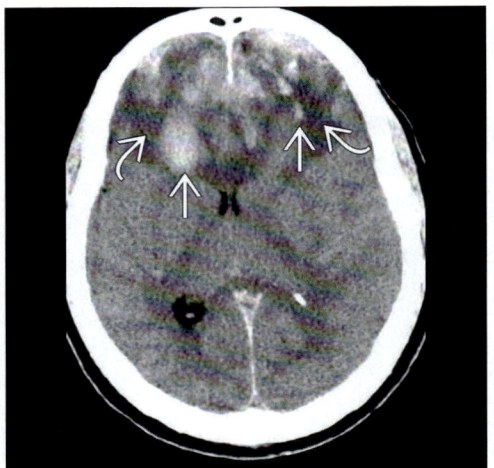
Axial NECT shows bifrontal mixture of hemorrhage ➡ and edema ➡.

TERMINOLOGY

Abbreviations and Synonyms
- Cerebral contusion (CC)

Definitions
- Brain surface injuries involving superficial gray matter (GM) and contiguous subcortical white matter

IMAGING FINDINGS

General Features
- Best diagnostic clue: Patchy superficial hemorrhages within edematous background
- Location
  - Characteristic locations: Adjacent to irregular bony protuberance or dural fold
    - Anterior inferior frontal lobes and anterior inferior temporal lobes most common
    - 25% parasagittal ("gliding" contusions)
  - Less common locations
    - Inferior cerebellar surfaces, parietal/occipital lobes, vermis, cerebellar tonsils
  - Focal contusions beneath site of depressed skull fracture ("fracture contusion")
- Size: Varies from barely discernible to large
- Morphology
  - Evolves over time
    - Early: Patchy, ill-defined superficial foci of punctate or linear hemorrhage along gyral crests
    - 24-48 hrs: Existing lesions enlarge and become more hemorrhagic; new lesions may appear
    - Chronic: Encephalomalacia with parenchymal volume loss
  - Multiple, bilateral lesions in 90% of cases

Radiographic Findings
- Radiography: Scalp hematomas, skull fractures

CT Findings
- NECT
  - Early: Patchy ill-defined, low-density edema with small foci of hyperdense hemorrhage
    - Rarely may be normal
  - 24-48 hrs
    - Edema hemorrhage and mass effect often increase
    - New foci of edema and hemorrhage
    - Delayed hemorrhage (~ 20%)

DDx: Contusion

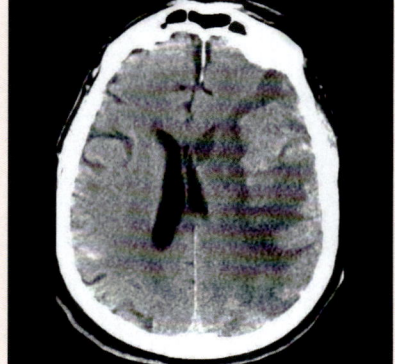
Hemorrhagic Infarct

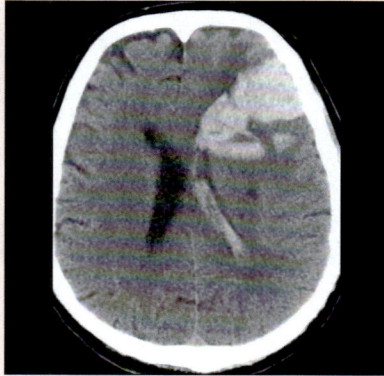
Amyloid Angiopathy

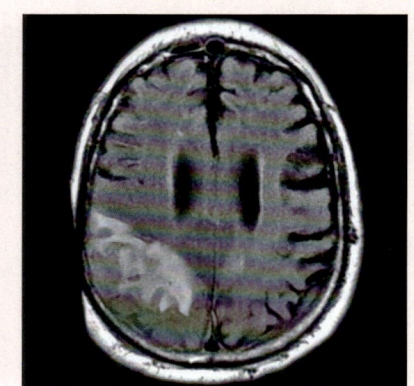
Venous Thrombosis

CEREBRAL CONTUSION

Key Facts

Terminology
- Brain surface injuries involving superficial gray matter (GM) and contiguous subcortical white matter

Imaging Findings
- Best diagnostic clue: Patchy superficial hemorrhages within edematous background
- Anterior inferior frontal lobes and anterior inferior temporal lobes most common
- MR to detect presence & delineate extent of lesions
- CT to detect acute hemorrhagic contusions, other intracranial lesions and herniations
- Protocol advice: FLAIR to evaluate edema & SAH, GRE for hemorrhagic foci

Top Differential Diagnoses
- Infarct
- Venous Sinus Thrombosis
- Cerebritis
- Low Grade Neoplasm
- Transient Post-Ictal Changes

Pathology
- Direct injury beneath impact site
- Contracoup: Deceleration injury opposite impact site
- Traumatic brain injury causes 6.5% of American deaths (32 per 100,000)

Diagnostic Checklist
- Repeat exam recommended if initial exam negative but symptoms persist 24-48 hours
- Inferior anterior frontal lobes most often injured
- Mixed-density contusions can be mistaken for common artifacts caused by orbital roof

---

- Petechial hemorrhage may coalesce to become frank hematomas
- Secondary lesions
  - Herniations/mass effect with secondary infarction
  - Hydrocephalus due to subarachnoid or intraventricular hemorrhage

MR Findings
- T1WI
  - Acute: Inhomogeneous relative isointensity (edema and hemorrhage) and mass effect
  - Chronic: Focal or diffuse atrophy
- FLAIR
  - Acute
    - Best for hyperintense cortical edema and subarachnoid hemorrhage (SAH)
  - Chronic
    - Hypointense hemosiderin "stains" in scarred parenchyma
    - Hyperintense demyelination & microglial scarring
    - Hypointense cavitation (cystic encephalomalacia)
- T2* GRE
  - Acute: Hypointense hemorrhagic foci "bloom" (often not detected on other sequences)
  - Chronic: Hemosiderin deposits; hypointense "stain" in scarred parenchyma
- DWI
  - Acute: Variable
    - Hyperintense in areas of cell death: Apparent diffusion coefficient (ADC) decreased
    - Isointense in regions of vasogenic edema: ADC increased
    - DTI can show white matter damage in minor head trauma when CT and routine MR normal

Imaging Recommendations
- Best imaging tool
  - MR to detect presence & delineate extent of lesions
  - CT to detect acute hemorrhagic contusions, other intracranial lesions and herniations
- Protocol advice: FLAIR to evaluate edema & SAH, GRE for hemorrhagic foci

DIFFERENTIAL DIAGNOSIS

Infarct
- No trauma history
- Characteristic acute onset focal neurologic deficit
- Vascular distribution: Spares frontal and temporal poles

Venous Sinus Thrombosis
- Subcortical edema and hemorrhage adjacent to occluded sinus

Cerebritis
- No trauma history
- Herpes typically involves medial temporal lobe & hippocampus

Low Grade Neoplasm
- No trauma history
- Solitary non-hemorrhagic lesion
- No predilection for anterior frontal and temporal lobes

Transient Post-Ictal Changes
- No trauma history
- Preceding or ongoing seizure activity
- May be hyperintense on DWI

PATHOLOGY

General Features
- Etiology
  - Stationary head (struck by object)
    - Direct injury beneath impact site
    - Contusion is rare without fracture
  - Moving head: Motor vehicle accident (MVA) and falls
    - Differential acceleration, deceleration and rotational forces on portions of brain with different densities
    - Coup: Direct injury to brain beneath impact site
    - Contracoup: Deceleration injury opposite impact site

CEREBRAL CONTUSION

- Contrecoup usually more severe than coup
- Gliding injury: Cortex anchored to dura by arachnoid granulations; subcortical tissue glides more than cortex
- Anterior inferior frontal lobes and temporal lobes most common location
• Epidemiology
  ○ 45% primary intra-axial traumatic lesions
  ○ Second most common primary traumatic neuronal injury (44%)
    - Diffuse axonal injury (DAI) is most common
  ○ 94% of non-missile head injuries in Glasgow postmortem series
  ○ Traumatic brain injury causes 6.5% of American deaths (32 per 100,000)
• Associated abnormalities
  ○ Soft tissue contusions (scalp, subgaleal) in 70% of patients
  ○ Subdural hematoma (SDH)
  ○ Traumatic SAH
  ○ Intraventricular hemorrhage (IVH)
  ○ Skull fracture

Gross Pathologic & Surgical Features
• Contusions
  ○ Coup lesions are associated with calvarial fractures
  ○ Contracoup lesions
  ○ Petechial hemorrhages (often more evident in first 24-48 hrs)
  ○ Edema along gyral crests
  ○ Small hemorrhages may coalesce
  ○ Large hematomas may occur within first 30-60 minutes
  ○ Delayed hematomas may develop 24-48 hrs later
• Lacerations
  ○ Intracerebral hematoma with "burst" lobe
  ○ SDH common
    - Communicates with hematoma via lacerated brain, torn pia-arachnoid
  ○ SAH and IVH common: Contusion tear

Microscopic Features
• Ultimately undergoes volume loss (atrophy) and cystic degeneration (encephalomalacia)
  ○ Whole brain atrophy may occur after moderate injury
• Capillary disruption
• Blood extravasation into tissue
  ○ Red blood cells account for visible hemorrhage
  ○ Plasma content leads to edema
  ○ Edema also result of inflammatory response to hemorrhage
• Liquefaction & encephalomalacia occur in chronic phase

CLINICAL ISSUES

Presentation
• Most common signs/symptoms
  ○ Initial symptom: Confusion - obtundation
  ○ Varied focal neurologic deficits
    - Focal cerebral dysfunction, seizures, personality changes
• Clinical Profile: Present in nearly half of moderate/severe closed head injury (CHI) cases

Demographics
• Age
  ○ Children:Adults = 2:1
  ○ Highest risk: 15-24 years
• Gender: M:F = 2:1

Natural History & Prognosis
• Varies
  ○ Extent of primary injury
  ○ Associated or secondary lesions (mass effect, herniations, perfusion alterations)
• Decreased CBF within first 24 hours associated with poor outcome
• Highest mortality rate: Elderly population
• 90% of patients survive injury
  ○ Approximately 25% have significant residual complaints

Treatment
• Mass effect and herniation may require surgical evacuation
  ○ Focal hematoma more amenable to surgery than hemorrhagic contusion
• Mitigate secondary effects of CHI (↑ intracranial pressure, perfusion disturbances)
  ○ Ventricular catheter to monitor and control intracranial pressure

DIAGNOSTIC CHECKLIST

Consider
• Repeat exam recommended if initial exam negative but symptoms persist 24-48 hours

Image Interpretation Pearls
• Inferior anterior frontal lobes most often injured
• Mixed-density contusions can be mistaken for common artifacts caused by orbital roof

SELECTED REFERENCES
1. MacKenzie JD et al: Brain atrophy in mild or moderate traumatic brain injury: a longitudinal quantitative analysis. AJNR Am J Neuroradiol. 23(9):1509-15, 2002
2. Hofman PA et al: MR imaging, single-photon emission CT, and neurocognitive performance after mild traumatic brain injury. AJNR Am J Neuroradiol. 22(3):441-9, 2001
3. Adams JH et al: The neuropathology of the vegetative state after an acute brain insult. Brain. 123 (Pt 7):1327-38, 2000
4. Laatsch L et al: Incorporation of SPECT imaging in a longitudinal cognitive rehabilitation therapy programme. Brain Inj. 13(8):555-70, 1999
5. Liu AY et al: Traumatic brain injury: diffusion-weighted MR imaging findings. AJNR Am J Neuroradiol. 20(9):1636-41, 1999
6. Friedman SD et al: Proton MR spectroscopic findings correspond to neuropsychological function in traumatic brain injury. AJNR Am J Neuroradiol. 19(10):1879-85, 1998

CEREBRAL CONTUSION

IMAGE GALLERY

Typical

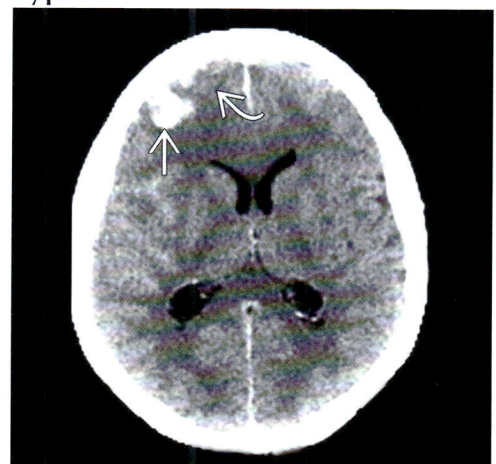
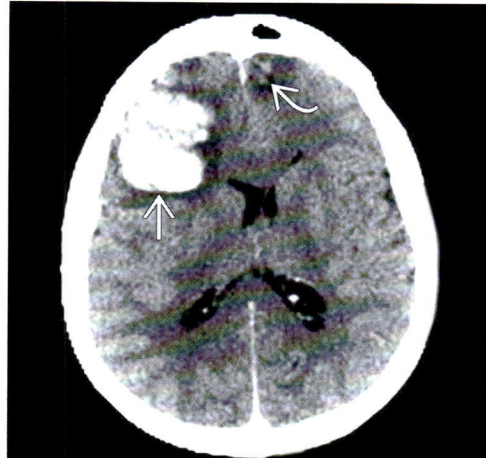

(Left) Axial NECT shows right frontal hemorrhagic contusion ➔ and edema ➔ at 4 hours. *(Right)* Axial NECT in same patient as previous image shows progressive enlargement and coalescence of hemorrhagic contusion ➔ at 24 hours. New contusion present in left frontal lobe ➔.

Typical

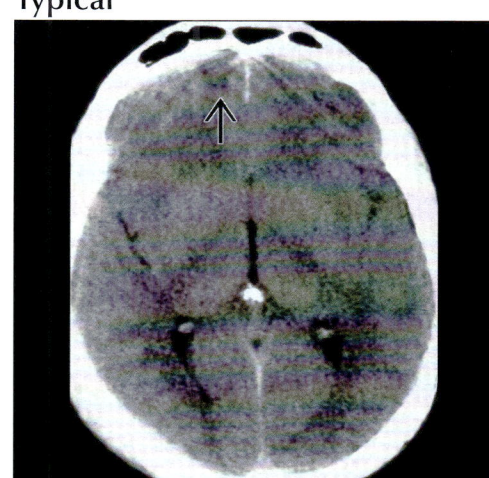
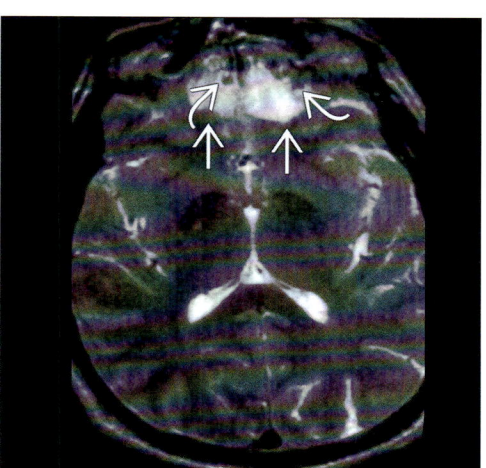

(Left) Axial NECT shows subtle hypodense edema ➔ in the frontal lobe. *(Right)* Axial T2WI FS MR in same patient as previous image shows bifrontal edema ➔ and mild petechial hemorrhage ➔.

Typical

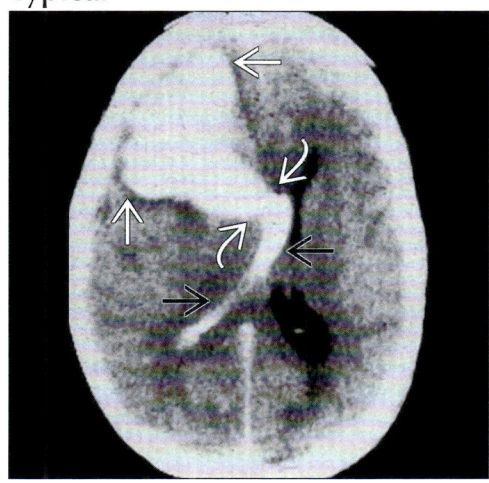
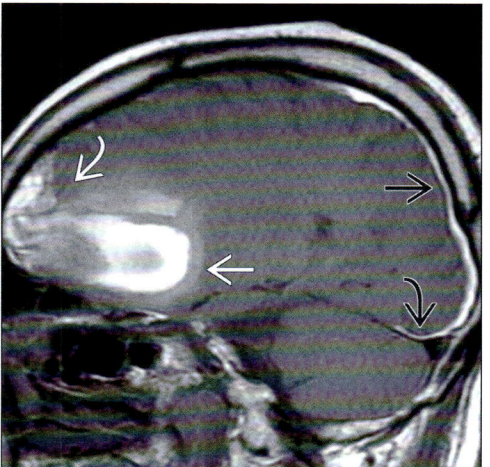

(Left) Axial NECT shows left frontal contusion tear. Homogeneous hematoma extends from the surface of the brain ➔ to the ventricle ➔ with rupture into the ventricle ➔. *(Right)* Sagittal T1WI MR shows inferior frontal ➔ and frontal polar ➔ hyperintense hemorrhagic contusion. Note convexity ➔ and paratentorial ➔ subdural hematoma.

DIFFUSE AXONAL INJURY (DAI)

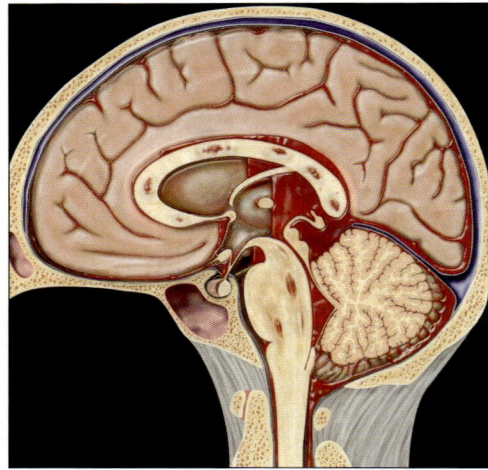

Sagittal graphic illustrates multiple hemorrhagic foci of diffuse axonal injury within the corpus callosum & brainstem.

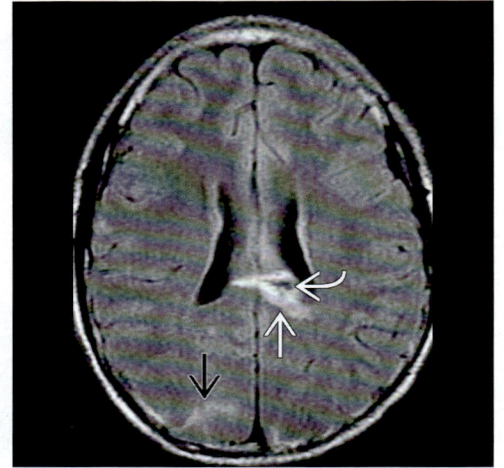

Axial FLAIR MR shows hyperintense edema of corpus callosum ➡ with central hypointense hemorrhage ➡ and edema in left parietal subcortical white matter ➡.

TERMINOLOGY

Abbreviations and Synonyms
- Diffuse axonal injury (DAI), traumatic brain injury (TBI)

Definitions
- Traumatic axonal stretch injury

IMAGING FINDINGS

General Features
- Best diagnostic clue: Punctate hemorrhages at corticomedullary junction, corpus callosum, deep gray matter & upper brainstem
- Location
  - Gray/white matter (GM/WM) interface (67%), especially frontotemporal lobes
  - Corpus callosum (20%); 3/4 involve splenium/undersurface of posterior body
  - Brainstem, especially dorsolateral midbrain & upper pons (poor prognosis)
  - Less common
    - Deep gray matter, internal/external capsule, tegmentum, fornix, corona radiata, cerebellar peduncles
- Size: Punctate to 15 mm
- Morphology
  - Punctate, round, ovoid or elliptical hemorrhagic foci
  - Nearly always multiple bilateral lesions

CT Findings
- NECT
  - Often normal (50-80%)
    - > 30% of patients with negative CT have positive MR
  - Small hypodense foci due to traumatic edema
  - Hyperdense petechial hemorrhage(s) (20-50%)
  - 10-20% evolve to focal mass lesion with hemorrhagic/edema admixture
  - Delayed scans may reveal "new" lesions

MR Findings
- T1WI
  - Usually normal
  - If > 1 cm and hemorrhagic, hyperintense (3-14 days)
- T2WI
  - Hyperintense foci at characteristic locations

DDx: Diffuse Axonal Injury

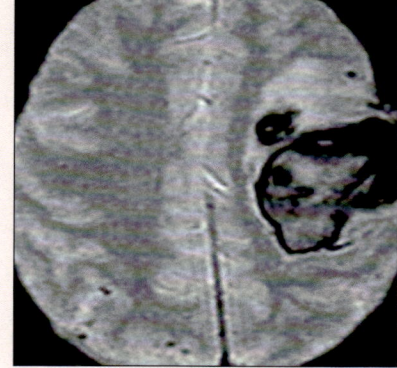
Cerebral Amyloid Angiopathy

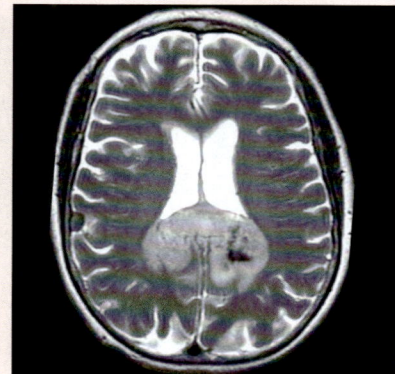
Hemorrhagic Glioma

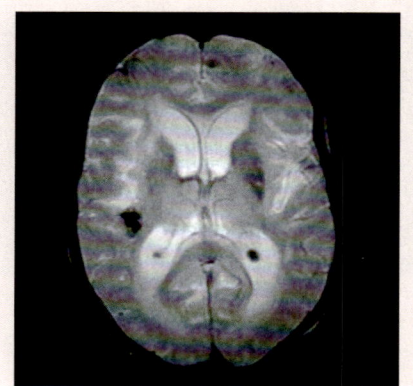
Hypertension

DIFFUSE AXONAL INJURY (DAI)

Key Facts

Terminology
- Traumatic axonal stretch injury

Imaging Findings
- Best diagnostic clue: Punctate hemorrhages at corticomedullary junction, corpus callosum, deep gray matter & upper brainstem
- Gray/white matter (GM/WM) interface (67%), especially frontotemporal lobes
- Corpus callosum (20%); 3/4 involve splenium/undersurface of posterior body
- Brainstem, especially dorsolateral midbrain & upper pons (poor prognosis)
- Most sensitive routine sequence; microbleeds may be visible only on GRE
- Best imaging tool: MR for detection
- GRE best routine sequence
- DTI and SWI may reveal lesions not seen on routine imaging in mTBI

Top Differential Diagnoses
- Multifocal Nonhemorrhagic Lesions
- Multifocal Hemorrhagic Lesions

Pathology
- Posterior falx indirectly contributes by preventing tissue displacement, allowing greater tensile stresses locally
- 80% of lesions are microscopic, nonhemorrhagic

Clinical Issues
- Transient loss of consciousness (LOC), retrograde amnesia in mTBI
- LOC at moment of impact: Moderate to severe TBI

  - Hypointense if hemorrhagic
  - Multifocal hypointense residua may remain for years
- FLAIR: Hyperintense and hypointense foci at characteristic locations
- T2* GRE
  - Hypointense foci 2° susceptibility from blood products at characteristic locations
  - Multifocal hypointense foci may remain for years
  - Most sensitive routine sequence; microbleeds may be visible only on GRE
  - Susceptibility-weighted imaging (SWI) may show more lesions than GRE
- DWI
  - May show hyperintense foci of restricted diffusion: ↓ Apparent diffusion coefficient (ADC)
  - Diffusion tensor imaging (DTI)
    - Fractional anisotropy (FA) maps document integrity & direction of white matter tracts
    - Damage to white matter reduces anisotropy: Visible on FA maps
    - DTI "tractograms" allow delineation of pattern of white matter tract disruption
    - Detects abnormalities when routine imaging, including GRE, normal
- MRS
  - In normal-appearing occipitoparietal WM & occipital GM
    - ↓ N-acetyl aspartate in WM 2° to neuronal injury
    - ↑ Choline in GM suggestive of inflammation
  - Decreased NAA/Cr correlates with poor outcome

Nuclear Medicine Findings
- SPECT and PET blood flow imaging
  - May show focal perfusion abnormalities in frontal lobes in patients with minor traumatic brain injury (mTBI)

Imaging Recommendations
- Best imaging tool: MR for detection
- Protocol advice
  - GRE best routine sequence
  - DTI and SWI may reveal lesions not seen on routine imaging in mTBI

DIFFERENTIAL DIAGNOSIS

Multifocal Nonhemorrhagic Lesions
- Aging: No trauma history; leukoariosis & lacunes
- Demyelinating disease: Ovoid, may enhance
- Marchiafava–Bignami syndrome: Splenium lesion in chronic alcoholism & poor nutrition
- Radiation therapy may cause focal lesions of splenium

Multifocal Hemorrhagic Lesions
- Cerebral amyloid angiopathy: Elderly, normotensive
- Chronic hypertension
- Cavernous malformations: Mixed-age hemorrhages
- Hemorrhagic tumors: Enhancing masses

PATHOLOGY

General Features
- General path comments: Overlying cortex moves at different speed in relation to underlying deep brain structures; results in axonal stretching, particularly where brain tissues of different density intersect
- Genetics
  - Significant genomic responses to brain trauma
    - Induction of "immediate early genes"
    - Activation of signal transduction pathways
    - Apolipoprotein E (apoE) genotype, amyloid deposition may influence clinical outcome
- Etiology
  - Trauma-induced forces of inertia
    - Differential acceleration/deceleration & rotational/angular forces
    - Head impact not required
  - Axons stretched, rarely disconnected or "sheared" (only in most severe injury)
  - Effect on non-disruptively injured axons
    - Traumatic depolarization, ion fluxes, spreading depression & excitatory amino acid release
    - Metabolic alterations with accelerated glycolysis, lactate accumulation
    - Cellular swelling & cytotoxic edema

DIFFUSE AXONAL INJURY (DAI)

- Corpus callosum injury
  - Believed due to rotational shear/strain forces
  - Posterior falx indirectly contributes by preventing tissue displacement, allowing greater tensile stresses locally
- Epidemiology
  - Spectrum of severity: mTBI to severe injuries, vegetative state and/or death
  - mTBI most common
  - Clinical abnormalities in mTBI may persist for months or longer
    - Headache, memory problems, mild cognitive impairment, personality change (post-concussive syndrome)
  - Subtle DAI likely substrate for mTBI
  - Approximately 50% of all primary intra-axial traumatic brain lesions in moderate and severe TBI
  - 80-100% autopsy prevalence in fatal injuries
- Associated abnormalities: Corpus callosal injury associated with intraventricular hemorrhage

Gross Pathologic & Surgical Features
- Multiple, small, round/ovoid/linear WM lesions
- Widely distributed: Parasagittal WM, corpus callosum, brainstem tracts

Microscopic Features
- 80% of lesions are microscopic, nonhemorrhagic
  - Visible lesions are "tip of the iceberg"
- Impaired axoplasmic transport, axonal swelling
- Axonal swelling 2° "axotomy", "retraction" balls
- Microglial clusters
- Macro-, microbleeds (torn penetrating vessels)
- Wallerian degeneration

Staging, Grading or Classification Criteria
- Adams & Gennarelli staging
  - Stage 1: Frontal & temporal lobe GM/WM interface (mTBI)
  - Stage 2: Lesions in lobar WM & corpus callosum (moderate TBI)
  - Stage 3: Lesions of dorsolateral midbrain & upper pons (severe TBI)
- Increasing severity of traumatic force correlates with deeper brain involvement

CLINICAL ISSUES

Presentation
- Most common signs/symptoms
  - Transient loss of consciousness (LOC), retrograde amnesia in mTBI
  - LOC at moment of impact: Moderate to severe TBI
  - Immediate coma typical
    - Persistent vegetative state in severe cases
    - Slow recovery in many cases
  - Greater impairment than with cerebral contusions, intracerebral hematoma, extra-axial hematomas
- Clinical Profile
  - Suggestive in patient with clinical symptoms disproportionate to imaging findings
  - Most common primary traumatic neuronal injury (48%)
  - Usually in setting of high velocity MVA
  - Admission Glasgow Coma Score may not correlate with outcome

Demographics
- Age: Any; may occur in utero if pregnant woman subjected to sufficient force

Natural History & Prognosis
- Severe DAI rarely causes death
  - > 90% remain in persistent vegetative state (brainstem spared)
  - Prognosis worsens as number of lesions increases
- 10% of patients who return to normal function do so within first year
  - May experience prolonged post-concussive symptoms
- Brainstem damage (pontomedullary rent) associated with immediate or early death

Treatment
- No real treatment; supportive therapy
- Treatment of associated abnormalities: Herniation, hematoma, hydrocephalus, seizures

DIAGNOSTIC CHECKLIST

Consider
- Consider DAI if symptoms disproportionate to imaging findings

Image Interpretation Pearls
- Lesions best detected by susceptibility-sensitive MR

SELECTED REFERENCES
1. Huisman TA et al: Diffusion tensor imaging as potential biomarker of white matter injury in diffuse axonal injury. AJNR Am J Neuroradiol. 25(3):370-6, 2004
2. Pekala JS et al: Focal lesion in the splenium of the corpus callosum on FLAIR MR images: a common finding with aging and after brain radiation therapy. AJNR Am J Neuroradiol. 24(5):855-61, 2003
3. Tong KA et al: Hemorrhagic shearing lesions in children and adolescents with posttraumatic diffuse axonal injury: improved detection and initial results. Radiology. 227(2):332-9, 2003
4. Arfanakis K et al: Diffusion tensor MR imaging in diffuse axonal injury. AJNR Am J Neuroradiol. 23(5):794-802, 2002
5. Hofman PA et al: MR imaging, single-photon emission CT, and neurocognitive performance after mild traumatic brain injury. AJNR Am J Neuroradiol. 22(3):441-9, 2001
6. Sinson G et al: Magnetization transfer imaging and proton MR spectroscopy in the evaluation of axonal injury: correlation with clinical outcome after traumatic brain injury. AJNR Am J Neuroradiol. 22(1):143-51, 2001
7. Kuzma BB et al: Improved identification of axonal shear injuries with gradient echo MR technique. Surg Neurol. 53(4):400-2, 2000

DIFFUSE AXONAL INJURY (DAI)

IMAGE GALLERY

Typical

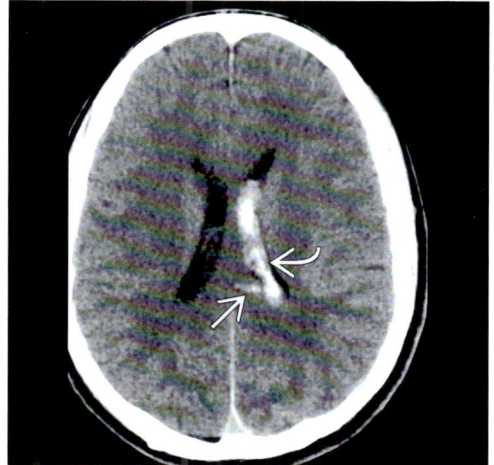 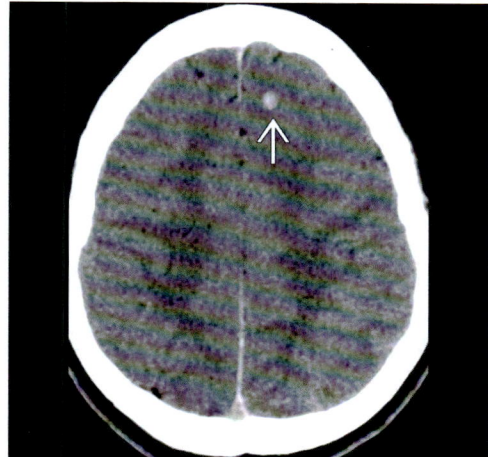

(Left) Axial NECT shows focal hemorrhage in splenium of corpus callosum ➡ with intraventricular spread ➡. *(Right)* Axial NECT in same patient as previous image reveals additional focus of hemorrhage in subcortical white matter of frontal lobe ➡.

Typical

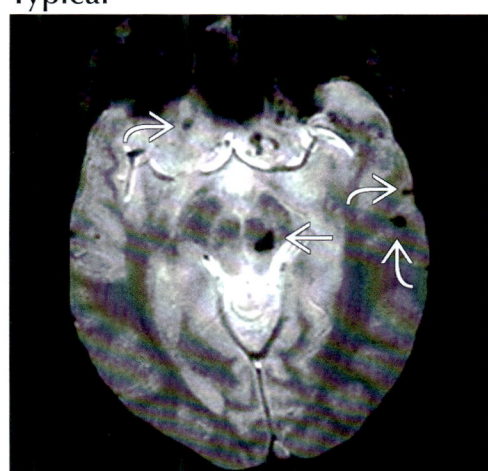 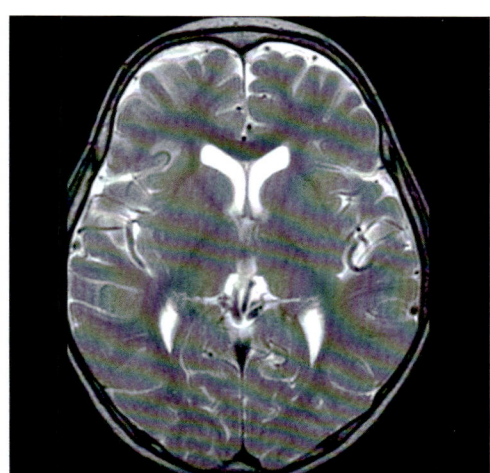

(Left) Axial T2* GRE MR shows focal hypointense hemorrhage in posterio-lateral mesencephalon ➡ & additional microbleeds in subcortical white matter of temporal & frontal lobes ➡. *(Right)* Axial T2WI MR at 3.0T is normal (head CT was also normal) in patient with severe post-traumatic headache and difficulty concentrating.

Typical

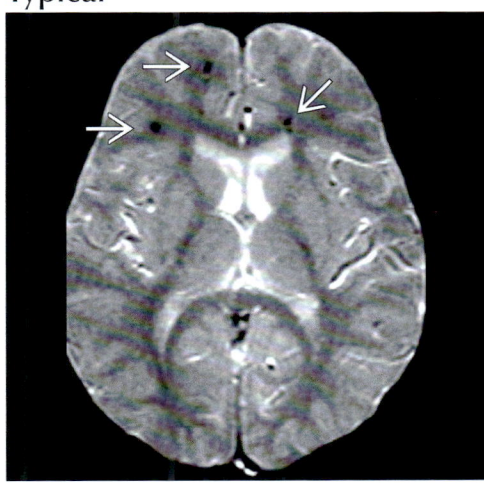 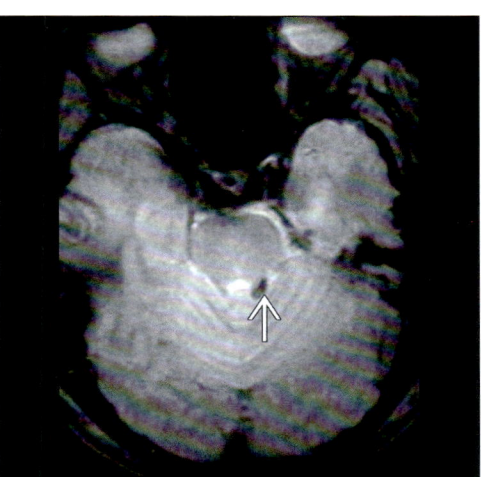

(Left) Axial T2* GRE MR at 3.0T in same patient as previous image shows foci of hypointensity in frontal white matter due to microbleeds ➡. *(Right)* Axial T2* GRE MR same patient as previous image reveals focal hemorrhage in left superior cerebellar peduncle ➡.

NONACCIDENTAL TRAUMA (CHILD ABUSE)

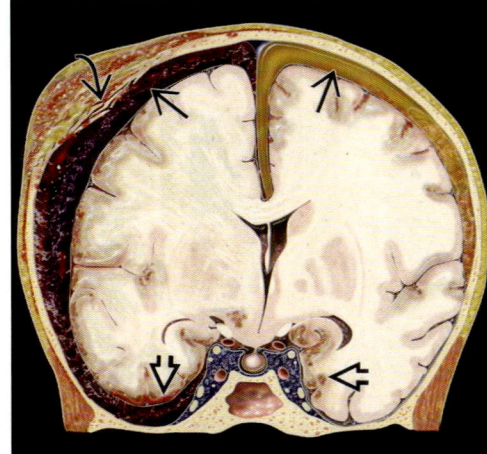

Coronal graphic shows features of NAT including subdurals of differing ages ➡, SAH, cortical contusions ➡, depressed skull fx ➡, scalp hematoma.

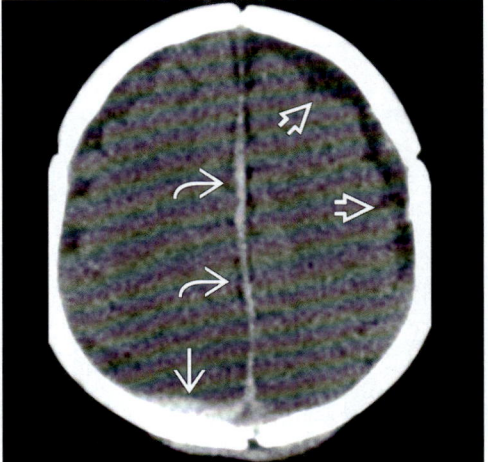

Axial NECT of small right high convexity ➡ & interhemispheric subdural hematoma ➡, hypodense left convexity subdural hematoma ➡; hemorrhage of different ages suspicious for NAT.

TERMINOLOGY

Abbreviations and Synonyms
- Nonaccidental trauma (NAT) or head injury (NAHI); child abuse; shaken-baby/infant syndrome; whiplash

Definitions
- Inflicted brain injury

IMAGING FINDINGS

General Features
- Best diagnostic clue: Multiple brain injuries at different stages of evolution
- Spectrum of findings: Scalp injuries, skull fractures (fxs), intracranial hemorrhages, cerebral contusions, shear injuries, ischemic brain injury
- Skull fxs
  ○ Linear: Low specificity NAT
  ○ Compound: Moderate specificity NAT
  ○ Multiple, depressed, diastatic (> 5 mm wide), non-parietal, growing fractures, crossing midline/sutures: High specificity NAT
- Intracranial hemorrhage
  ○ Subdural hemorrhage (SDH) is most common manifestation in NAT
    ▪ Multiple SDH in different locations, different ages
    ▪ Acute SDH typically small: High convexity & posterior interhemispheric fissure
  ○ Subarachnoid hemorrhage (SAH) ~ 50% of cases
  ○ Intraventricular hemorrhage
- Parenchymal features
  ○ Cortical contusions
    ▪ Typical locations: Surface of frontal & temporal lobes
    ▪ Mixture of hemorrhage and edema
  ○ Shear injuries
    ▪ Punctate focal hemorrhages
    ▪ Typical locations: Corticomedullary junction, centrum semiovale, corpus callosum
    ▪ Larger shearing injuries: Subcortical lacerations
  ○ Ischemic injury: Variable
    ▪ Global hypoxia 2° to strangulation
    ▪ Territorial infarction: Arterial dissection?
- Late sequelae
  ○ Subdural hygroma/chronic SDH
    ▪ Blood of different ages in subdural space

DDx: Nonaccidental Trauma Mimics

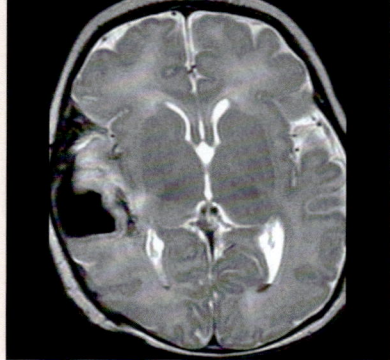
Coagulopathy

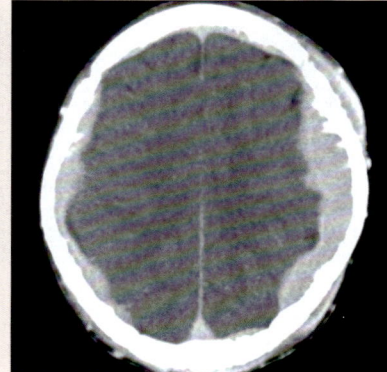
Leukemia

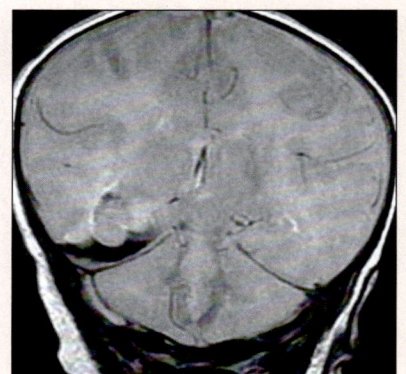
Dural Sinus Thrombosis

NONACCIDENTAL TRAUMA (CHILD ABUSE)

Key Facts

Terminology
- Nonaccidental trauma (NAT) or head injury (NAHI); child abuse; shaken-baby/infant syndrome; whiplash

Imaging Findings
- Best diagnostic clue: Multiple brain injuries at different stages of evolution
- Spectrum of findings: Scalp injuries, skull fractures (fxs), intracranial hemorrhages, cerebral contusions, shear injuries, ischemic brain injury
- Multiple, depressed, diastatic (> 5 mm wide), non-parietal, growing fractures, crossing midline/sutures: High specificity NAT
- Subdural hemorrhage (SDH) is most common manifestation in NAT
- Healing fxs of differing ages

Top Differential Diagnoses
- Accidental Trauma
- NAT Mimics
- Physiologic EVOH

Pathology
- 85% of non-survivors have evidence of head impact injury at postmortem examination
- Upper cervical cord stretching ⇒ apnea ⇒ ischemic brain injury
- Epidural hematoma (EDH) very rare in NAT
- Most common cause of traumatic death in infancy: 1,200 deaths per year in USA

Clinical Issues
- Notification to local Child Protection Agency mandated

- Hydrocephalus
- Encephalomalacia: Chronic infarction
- Atrophy
- Leptomeningeal cyst

Radiographic Findings
- Radiography: Best for skull fxs

CT Findings
- NECT
  - Primary tool in initial evaluation
  - High sensitivity for fxs, hemorrhage, edema & hypoxic-ischemic injury
    - Fxs oriented in axial plane may be missed
  - Age of hemorrhage (SDH) variable
    - Complex spectrum of appearances of intracranial hemorrhage on CT
    - General pattern: Hyperdense (< 7 days), isodense to brain (7-21 days), hypodense to brain (> 21 days)
  - Cortical contusions: Hypodense edema & focal hemorrhage
  - Shear injuries: Petechial hemorrhages
    - Corpus callosum, gray-white junction, basal ganglia, posterior brain stem
  - Ischemia
    - Basal ganglia hypodensity and/or diffuse edema: Hypoxia/anoxia
    - Hypodensity in vascular distribution: Infarction

MR Findings
- T1WI: Very sensitive to small acute SDH
- T2WI
  - Contusions: Hyperintense edema, hypointense hemorrhage
  - SDH: Intensity varies dependent upon age
- FLAIR: Same as T2WI
- T2* GRE: Petechial hemorrhages: Axonal injury
- DWI
  - Best for acute infarcts & global hypoxia/anoxia
    - Contusions hyperintense as well
- MR difficult to perform in acute setting
  - Overall increased sensitivity for most injuries (except fxs) outweigh difficulties of performing
    - T2* GRE most sensitive for depicting hemorrhage
    - DWI most sensitive for early ischemia in unmyelinated brain
    - DWI/FLAIR "mismatch" may confirm multiple or previous episodes of brain injury
    - Optimal method of cervical spine evaluation

Other Modality Findings
- Skeletal survey: Skeleton is most common site of inflicted injury
  - Healing fxs of differing ages
  - Metaphyseal corner, posterior rib, scapular, sternal fxs; T-L compression fxs; spinous process avulsion fxs

Imaging Recommendations
- Best imaging tool: NECT to start
- Protocol advice
  - NECT ± MR to document age of bleed; sequelae (first day of admission useful to confirm multiple ages of hemorrhages); evaluation of cervical spine
  - Skeletal survey ± scintigraphy (if > 2 yrs or if skeletal survey equivocal, clinical suspicion high)
  - Abdominal CT if multiple injuries, abnormal liver function test (LFT), or coma

DIFFERENTIAL DIAGNOSIS

Accidental Trauma
- Appropriate history of trauma
- Acute SDH 7% (70% in NAT)
- Retinal hemorrhage 0-2% (50-96% NAT)
- No evidence pre-existing brain injury (45% in NAT)
- Subsequent mental deficiency 5% (45% in NAT)

NAT Mimics
- Dural sinus thrombosis
- Brain: Coagulopathies (hemophilia, leukemia)
- Skeletal: Osteogenesis imperfecta, rickets, syphilis
- Metabolic: Glutaric aciduria type 1, Menkes

NONACCIDENTAL TRAUMA (CHILD ABUSE)

Physiologic EVOH
- Subarachnoid CSF prominence with traversing veins

PATHOLOGY

General Features
- General path comments
  - 85% of non-survivors have evidence of head impact injury at postmortem examination
  - 50% have significant extracranial injuries
  - Brain swelling (not hemorrhage) is cause of death in 80%
  - Upper cervical cord stretching ⇒ apnea ⇒ ischemic brain injury
    - Focal axonal damage to cranio-cervical junction of cervical cord
  - Severe hypoxic ischemic encephalopathy (HIE) 78% > classical diffuse axonal injury (DAI)
  - Retinal hemorrhage 70-96% (usually bilateral, always with SDH)
    - Non-ophthalmologists miss hemorrhages in 30%
  - 20-45% show evidence for prior brain injury
  - Epidural hematoma (EDH) very rare in NAT
- Etiology
  - Direct trauma, shaking injuries, strangulation, or combination thereof
  - Infants especially vulnerable
    - Large head:body ratio combined with weak neck muscles
    - Developing brain
  - Shaking/impact ⇒ torn bridging veins, retinal schisis
  - Minor falls do not typically cause rotational forces needed for spectrum of brain injuries seen in NAT
- Epidemiology
  - 17-25:100,000 annual incidence
  - Most common cause of traumatic death in infancy: 1,200 deaths per year in USA
  - Risk factors
    - < 1 year, prematurity, twin, male, physical handicap, stepchild
    - Young parents; ↓ socioeconomic status, 1/3 of perpetrators under influence of alcohol or drugs

Gross Pathologic & Surgical Features
- Acute (immediate)
  - Skull fxs, extra-axial hemorrhage, disrupted brain tissue, intra-ocular hemorrhages, brainstem dysfunction
- Early subacute (hours to days)
  - Impaired cerebral autoregulation/perfusion; chemically mediated cell death: Edema, HIE, infarction
- Late subacute or chronic
  - Hydrocephalus, atrophy, chronic SDH, gliosis, microcephaly, leptomeningeal cysts, delayed myelin maturation

CLINICAL ISSUES

Presentation
- Most common signs/symptoms
  - Discordance between stated history & injury on imaging (history of minimal or no trauma)
  - Presentation with "apnea" (33-45%), unexplained seizures, "unable to rouse"
  - Retinal hemorrhage in up to 96% of cases
- Clinical Profile: Poor feeding, vomiting, irritability, seizures, lethargy, coma, apnea

Demographics
- Age: Median age 2.2-4.6 months old
- Gender: Male > female (up to 2:1)

Natural History & Prognosis
- High mortality 15-38% (60% if coma at presentation)
- Neurologic deficits: Microcephaly (93%), early - seizures (79%), late - epilepsy (> 20%), poor visual outcome (20-65%)

Treatment
- Notification to local Child Protection Agency mandated
- Multidisciplinary child abuse & neglect team intervention

DIAGNOSTIC CHECKLIST

Consider
- Dural sinus thrombosis, inborn error of metabolism or bleeding dyscrasia may simulate NAT

Image Interpretation Pearls
- Look for combination of hemispheric brain swelling, HIE-like edema, bilateral or interhemispheric SDH

SELECTED REFERENCES

1. Jaspan T et al: Neuroimaging for non-accidental head injury in childhood: a proposed protocol. Clin Radiol. 58(1):44-53, 2003
2. Kemp AM et al: Apnoea and brain swelling in non-accidental head injury. Arch Dis Child. 88(6):472-6; discussion 472-6, 2003
3. Lo TY et al: Cerebral atrophy following shaken impact syndrome and other non-accidental head injury (NAHI). Pediatr Rehabil. 6(1):47-55, 2003
4. Wells RG et al: Intracranial hemorrhage in children younger than 3 years: prediction of intent. Arch Pediatr Adolesc Med. 156(3):252-7, 2002
5. Geddes JF et al: Neuropathology of inflicted head injury in children. I. Patterns of brain damage. Brain. 124(Pt 7):1290-8, 2001
6. Geddes JF et al: Neuropathology of inflicted head injury in children. II. Microscopic brain injury in infants. Brain. 124(Pt 7):1299-306, 2001
7. Suh DY et al: Nonaccidental pediatric head injury: diffusion-weighted imaging findings. Neurosurgery. 49(2):309-18; discussion 318-20, 2001
8. Ewing-Cobbs L et al: Acute neuroradiologic findings in young children with inflicted or noninflicted traumatic brain injury. Childs Nerv Syst. 16(1):25-33; discussion 34, 2000
9. Naidoo S: A profile of the oro-facial injuries in child physical abuse at a children's hospital. Child Abuse Negl. 24(4):521-34, 2000
10. Dashti SR et al: Current patterns of inflicted head injury in children. Pediatr Neurosurg. 31(6):302-6, 1999

NONACCIDENTAL TRAUMA (CHILD ABUSE)

IMAGE GALLERY

Typical

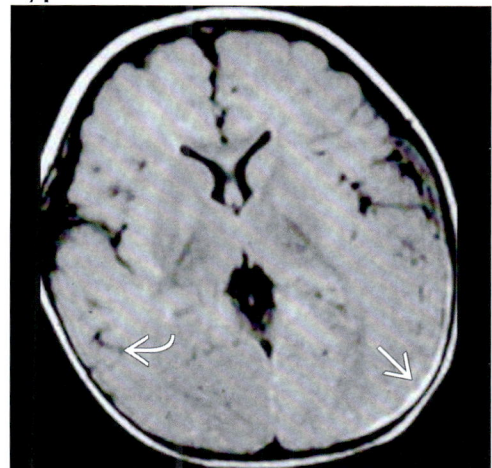 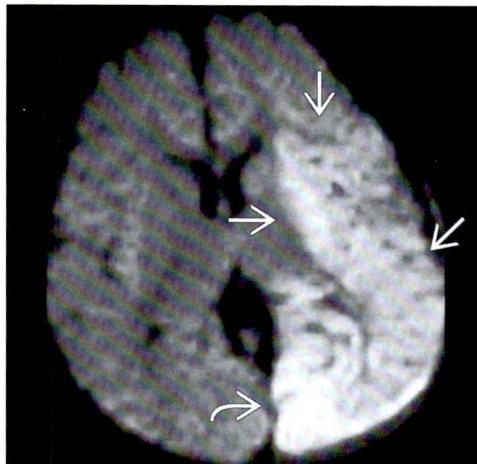

(Left) Axial FLAIR MR shows small left convexity subdural hematoma ➡. Sulci are more apparent in right parietal lobe than left ➡, but no apparent intensity abnormality on right. *(Right)* Axial DWI MR in same patient as left shows extensive hyperintensity in left middle ➡ and posterior cerebral artery ➡ distributions indicative of hyperacute infarction 2° to NAT.

Typical

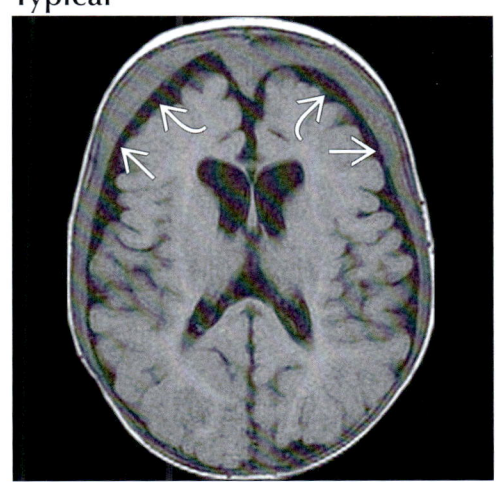 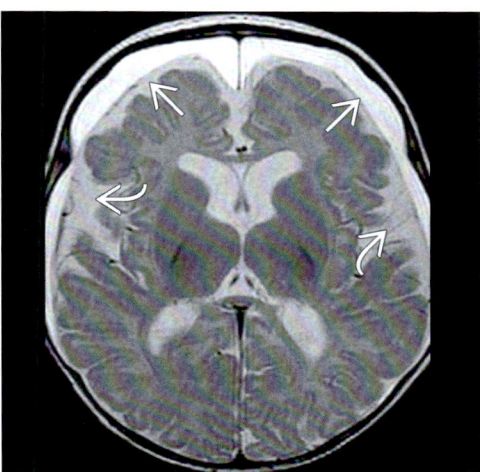

(Left) Axial T1WI MR shows large bilateral hyperintense chronic subdural hematomas ➡. Sulci ➡ and ventricles are dilated, indicative of atrophy due to recurrent NAT. *(Right)* Axial T2WI MR in same case as left shows bilateral hyperintense subdural hematomas ➡ & underlying atrophy with dilated sulci ➡ and ventricles.

Typical

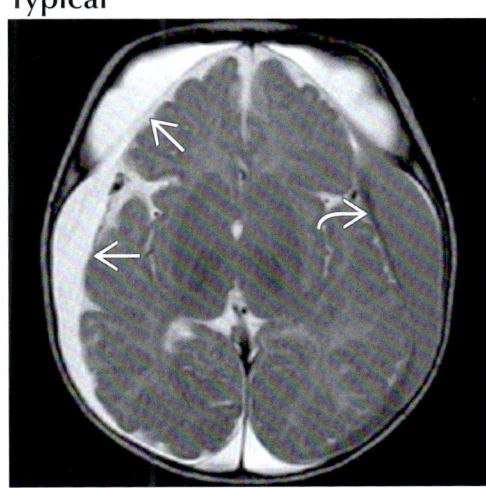 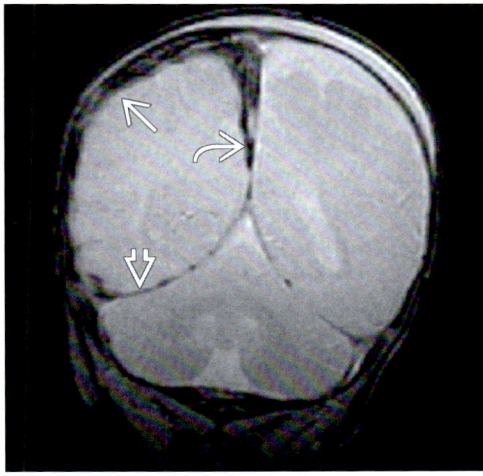

(Left) Axial T2WI MR shows bilateral chronic SDHs of different ages. Right SDH ➡ is hyperintense (chronic). Left SDH is hypointense ➡ (acute). *(Right)* Coronal T2* GRE MR shows small acute convexity ➡, interhemispheric ➡, and subtemporal ➡ SDHs.

INTRACRANIAL HERNIATION SYNDROMES

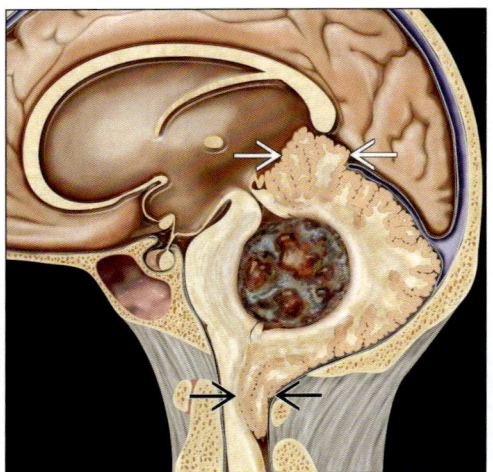

Sagittal graphic shows 4th ventricular mass resulting in superior transtentorial herniation ➡ and inferior tonsillar herniation ➡.

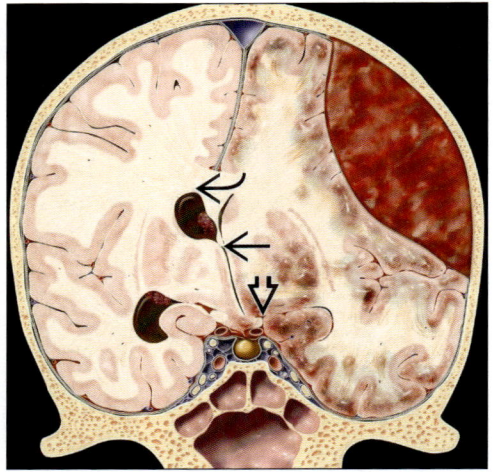

Coronal graphic shows acute epidural hematoma causing subfalcine ➡ and left uncal ➡ herniation. Note obstructed left foramen of Monro ➡.

TERMINOLOGY

Definitions
- Herniation of brain from one compartment (normally separated by calvarial &/or dural boundaries) to another

IMAGING FINDINGS

General Features
- Best diagnostic clue: CT and MR show same anatomic changes
- Subfalcine herniation: Herniation of cingulate gyrus under falx
  - Secondary to unilateral or asymmetric bilateral frontal lobe mass effect
  - Cingulate gyrus displaced under falx
  - Ipsilateral ventricle compressed and displaced across midline with midline shift
  - Contralateral ventricle obstructs & dilates at foramen of Monro
  - Anterior cerebral arteries (ACAs) displaced → compression on free edge of falx → occlusion
- Unilateral descending transtentorial herniation (DTH): Medial temporal lobe herniates inferiorly through incisura
  - Secondary to unilateral mass effect on temporal lobe
  - "Uncal" herniation: Type of early DTH, with uncus filling ipsilateral suprasellar cistern
- Unilateral DTH: Early (mild to moderate)
  - Ipsilateral suprasellar cistern partially effaced
  - Ipsilateral quadrigeminal plate cistern enlarged & contralateral narrowed → displaced stem
  - Contralateral temporal horn dilated 2° to obstruction caused by subfalcial herniation
- Unilateral DTH: Late (severe)
  - Suprasellar cistern completely obliterated
  - Medial temporal lobe and temporal horn displaced inferiorly into posterior fossa
  - Marked brainstem compression and displacement against tentorium: Kernohan notch
    - Duret hemorrhages in contralateral anterior stem
  - Posterior cerebral artery (PCA) displaced inferiorly over free edge of tentorium
    - Kinking of PCA leads to 2° occipital infarct
- Bilateral DTH ("central"): Bilateral downward herniation through incisura

DDx: Mimics of Intracranial Herniations

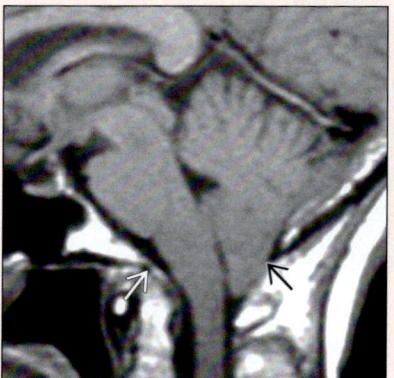

Chiari I/Low Tonsils

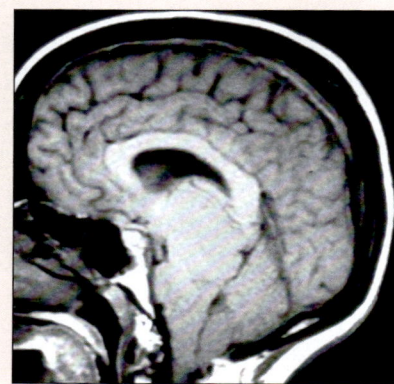

Intracranial Hypotension

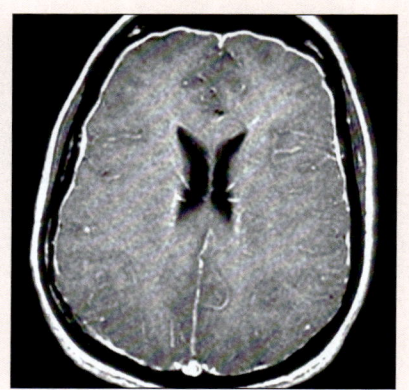

Intracranial Hypotension

INTRACRANIAL HERNIATION SYNDROMES

Key Facts

Terminology
- Herniation of brain from one compartment (normally separated by calvarial &/or dural boundaries) to another

Imaging Findings
- Subfalcine herniation: Herniation of cingulate gyrus under falx
- Unilateral descending transtentorial herniation (DTH): Medial temporal lobe herniates inferiorly through incisura
- Bilateral DTH ("central"): Bilateral downward herniation through incisura
- Ascending transtentorial herniation: Cerebellum & brainstem displaced up through incisura
- Tonsillar herniation into spinal canal
- Transalar herniation: Herniation across sphenoid wing
- T1WI: Sagittal and coronal images ideal for unilateral & bilateral DTH, tonsillar herniation

Top Differential Diagnoses
- Intracranial Hypotension Syndrome
- Chiari I Malformation

Pathology
- Herniations, ↑ ICP, altered cerebral hemodynamics → ischemia & infarction

Clinical Issues
- Decreased mental status or obtundation
- Brain death if ICP continues to rise & mass effect progresses unabated

---

- o Severe supratentorial mass effect
- o Both hemispheres, basal nuclei pushed downwards → diencephalon, midbrain displaced inferiorly
- o Suprasellar cistern obliterated
- o Both temporal lobes herniate into tentorial hiatus
- o Anterior inferior third ventricle displaced posteriorly behind dorsum sella
- o Angle between midbrain & pons becomes more acute
- o Optic chiasm/hypothalamus displaced downwards
- o Penetrating basal arteries often occlude → basal infarcts
- Ascending transtentorial herniation: Cerebellum & brainstem displaced up through incisura
  - o Secondary to cerebellar and dorsal posterior fossa extra-axial masses
  - o Quadrigeminal cistern compressed
  - o Midbrain displaced anteriorly
  - o May obstruct aqueduct → hydrocephalus
- Tonsillar herniation into spinal canal
  - o Secondary to posterior fossa mass effect or severe hydrocephalus
  - o Tonsils pushed inferiorly, impacted into foramen magnum
  - o Displacement > 5 mm below foramen magnum is abnormal, but morphology is more important
  - o Tonsil folia normally oriented horizontally → become vertically oriented when herniated
  - o Cisterna magna obliterated
  - o Fourth ventricle may obstruct → hydrocephalus
- Transalar herniation: Herniation across sphenoid wing
  - o Uncommon
  - o Few clinical symptoms
    - May compress middle cerebral artery (MCA) against sphenoid ridge → MCA infarct
  - o Can be ascending (middle cranial fossa or temporal lobe mass) or descending (frontal lobe mass)
  - o Displacement of temporal & frontal lobes, MCA across lesser sphenoid wing
- Transdural/transcranial herniation: Herniation through dural and/or skull defect
  - o Skull fracture & dural laceration; may also occur with craniotomy
  - o Elevated intracranial pressure (ICP)
  - o Brain extrudes through torn dura
  - o May extend under galea
- Secondary effects of herniation identified
  - o Hydrocephalus
  - o Duret hemorrhage in brain stem
  - o Infarcts 2° to vascular compression

CT Findings
- NECT: Hypodense acute infarcts and hyperdense hematomas
- CECT
  - o Variable causes of herniation demonstrated
    - Mass, leptomeningeal disease

MR Findings
- T1WI: Sagittal and coronal images ideal for unilateral & bilateral DTH, tonsillar herniation
- T2WI: Hyperintense infarcts
- T2* GRE: Hypointense hemorrhagic foci (e.g., Duret hemorrhages)
- DWI: Hyperintensity in secondary ischemic areas, due to vascular compression
- Variable causes of herniation demonstrated
  - o Mass, leptomeningeal disease

Imaging Recommendations
- Best imaging tool
  - o NECT best rapid screen
  - o Multiplanar ability of MR optimally demonstrates brain shift
- Protocol advice: Add DWI + GRE to imaging of post-trauma patients to identify infarcts & occult hemorrhagic foci

DIFFERENTIAL DIAGNOSIS

Intracranial Hypotension Syndrome
- Caused by brain "pulled" not "pushed" down
- Dural thickening, enhancement usually present

INTRACRANIAL HERNIATION SYNDROMES

Chiari I Malformation
- Congenital anomaly with low-lying tonsils
  - May be difficult to differentiate from tonsillar herniation in presence of posterior fossa mass

PATHOLOGY

General Features
- Etiology
  - Trauma most common clinical setting
  - Mass lesions, large infarcts and inflammatory lesions
  - Hemorrhage, extracellular fluid or added tissue accumulate within closed space
  - CSF spaces (cisterns, ventricles) initially compressed
  - Intracranial volume can't be accommodated
    - Gross mechanical displacement of brain, vessels → herniation
  - Secondary effects exacerbate severity of primary injuries
  - Herniations, ↑ ICP, altered cerebral hemodynamics → ischemia & infarction
    - PCA occlusion → occipital infarct most common
    - ACA occlusion → distal (cingulate gyrus) infarcts
    - Perforating vessels → basal ganglia, capsule infarcts
    - Midbrain Duret hemorrhage can occur from stretching/tearing of pontine perforators
- Associated abnormalities: Secondary hydrocephalus, ischemia, hemorrhage, necrosis

Gross Pathologic & Surgical Features
- Grossly swollen, edematous brain
- Gyri compressed, flattened against calvarium
- Sulci effaced

CLINICAL ISSUES

Presentation
- Decreased mental status or obtundation
- Focal neurologic deficit
  - Contralateral hemiparesis
  - Ipsilateral pupil-involving CN 3 palsy
  - Ipsilateral hemiplegia
    - Kernohan notch → compression of opposite cerebral peduncle against tentorium
    - "False localizing signs"
- Decreased brainstem blood flow, cardiovascular collapse
- Decerebrate posturing
- Chronic masses may produce anatomic herniation with few or no clinical signs & symptoms

Natural History & Prognosis
- Brain death if ICP continues to rise & mass effect progresses unabated

Treatment
- Treatment issues
  - Mitigate secondary effects of trauma
  - Removal of mass or decompressive craniectomy
  - Prolonged post-traumatic brain hypersensitivity
  - May offer potential "therapeutic window"
  - Possible use of neuroprotective agents

DIAGNOSTIC CHECKLIST

Consider
- DWI, GRE sequences in brain trauma, suspected herniation
- Intracranial hypotension syndrome can mimic DTH, tonsillar herniation caused by supratentorial mass

SELECTED REFERENCES

1. Cruz J et al: Successful use of the new high-dose mannitol treatment in patients with Glasgow Coma Scale scores of 3 and bilateral abnormal pupillary widening: a randomized trial. J Neurosurg. 100:376-83, 2004
2. Derakhshan I: Kernohan notch. J Neurosurg. 100(4):741-2; author reply 742, 2004
3. Stein SC et al: Association between Intravascular Microthrombosis and Cerebral Ischemia in Traumatic Brain Injury. Neurosurgery. 54(3):687-91, 2004
4. Parizel PM et al: Brainstem hemorrhage in descending transtentorial herniation (Duret hemorrhage). Intensive Care Med. 28(1):85-8, 2002
5. Server A et al: Post-traumatic cerebral infarction. Neuroimaging findings, etiology and outcome. Acta Radiol. 42(3):254-60, 2001
6. Juul N et al: Intracranial hypertension and cerebral perfusion pressure: influence on neurological deterioration and outcome in severe head injury. The Executive Committee of the International Selfotel Trial. J Neurosurg. 92(1):1-6, 2000
7. Sheehan JM et al: Resolution of tonsillar herniation and syringomyelia after supratentorial tumor resection: case report and review of the literature. Neurosurgery. 47(1):233-5, 2000
8. Mastronardi L et al: Magnetic resonance imaging findings of Kernohan-Woltman notch in acute subdural hematoma. Clin Neurol Neurosurg. 101(2):122-4, 1999
9. Laine FJ et al: Acquired intracranial herniations: MR imaging findings. AJR Am J Roentgenol. 165(4):967-73, 1995
10. Opeskin K: Traumatic pericallosal artery aneurysm. Am J Forensic Med Pathol. 16(1):11-6, 1995
11. Povlishock JT et al: Are the pathobiological changes evoked by traumatic brain injury immediate and irreversible? Brain Pathol. 5(4):415-26, 1995
12. Tachibana S et al: Syringomyelia secondary to tonsillar herniation caused by posterior fossa tumors. Surg Neurol. 43(5):470-5; discussion 475-7, 1995
13. Endo M et al: Capsular and thalamic infarction caused by tentorial herniation subsequent to head trauma. Neuroradiology. 33(4):296-9, 1991
14. Jones KM et al: Ipsilateral motor deficit resulting from a subdural hematoma and a Kernohan notch. AJNR Am J Neuroradiol. 12(6):1238-9, 1991
15. Osborn AG: Secondary effects of intracranial trauma. Neurosurg Clin N Amer. 1:461-74, 1991
16. Mirvis SE et al: Posttraumatic cerebral infarction diagnosed by CT: prevalence, origin, and outcome. AJNR Am J Neuroradiol. 11(2):355-60, 1990
17. Spiegelmann R et al: Upward transtentorial herniation: a complication of postoperative edema at the cervicomedullary junction. Neurosurgery. 24(2):284-8, 1989

INTRACRANIAL HERNIATION SYNDROMES

IMAGE GALLERY

Typical

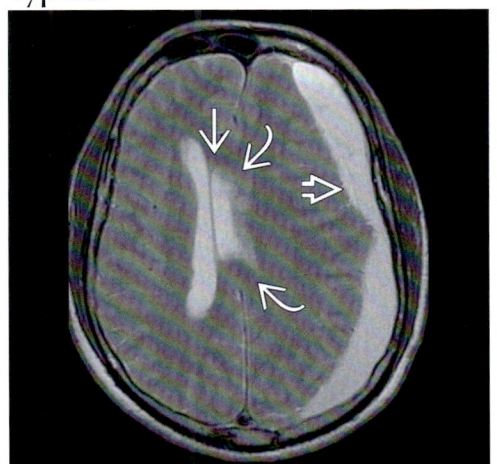 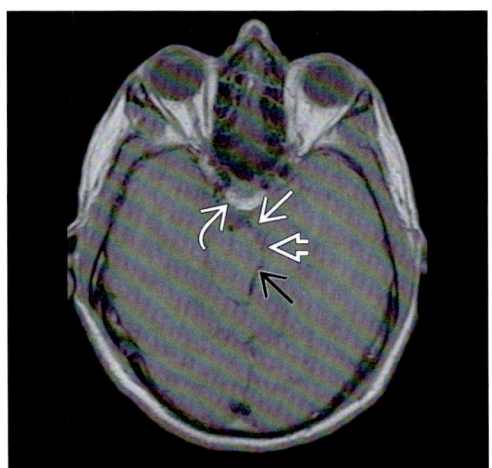

(Left) Axial T2WI FS MR shows subfalcial herniation with displacement across midline ➡ and compression of left lateral ventricle ➡ caused by subdural hematoma ➡. *(Right)* Axial T1WI MR shows unilateral descending transtentorial herniation. Uncus medially displaced ➡ narrowing suprasellar cistern ➡, compressing brain stem ➡ & widening ambient cistern ➡.

Typical

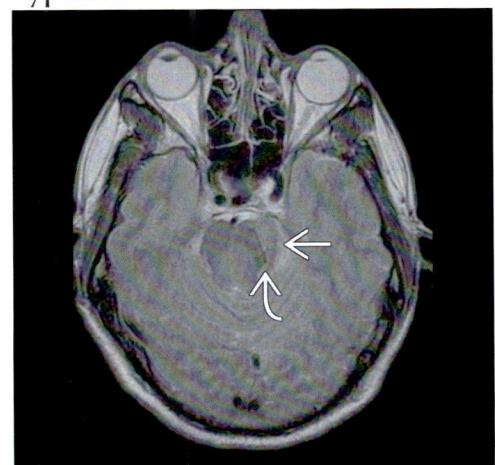 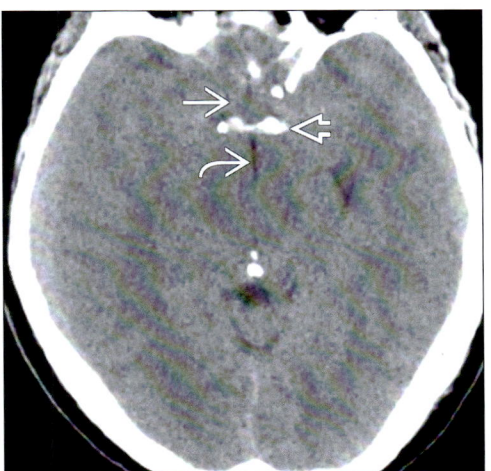

(Left) Axial T2WI MR in same patient as previous image shows temporal lobe herniated into posterior fossa ➡, where it compresses cerebral peduncle ➡. *(Right)* Axial NECT shows central herniation & obliteration of suprasellar cistern ➡. Inferior 3rd ventricle displaced posteriorly & inferiorly ➡ behind dorsum sellae ➡. No other cisterns visible.

Typical

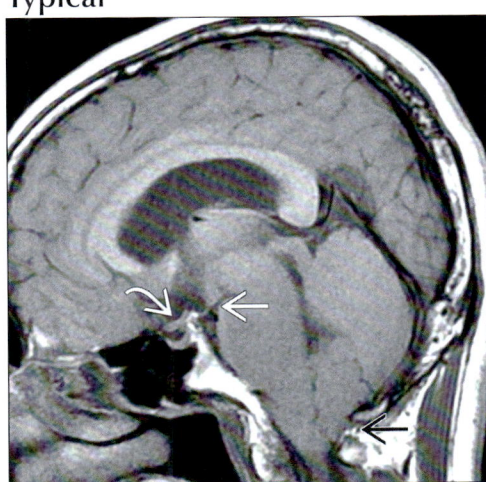 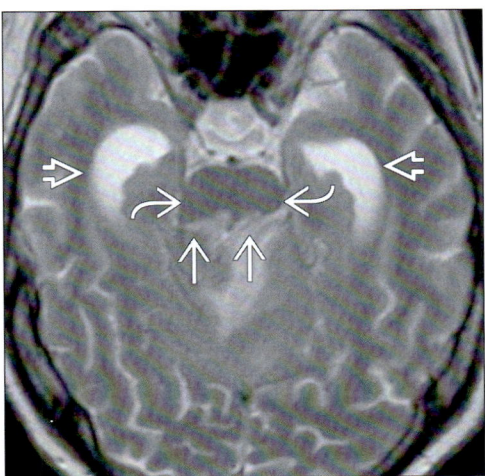

(Left) Sagittal T1WI MR shows central transtentorial & tonsillar herniation ➡ below foramen magnum. Chiasm ➡ & 3rd ventricle ➡ are inferiorly displaced, CSF spaces narrowed. *(Right)* Axial T2WI MR shows upward herniation. Mass obliterates quadrigeminal plate cistern ➡, brainstem compressed ➡, prepontine cistern narrowed. Hydrocephalus 2° to obstructed aqueduct ➡.

INTRACRANIAL VASCULAR INJURY

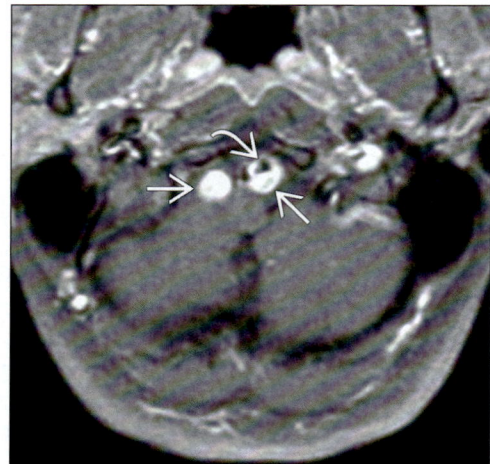

Axial T1 C+ FS MR shows hyperintensity within margins of both vertebral arteries, indicative of dissection ➡. Central hypointensity within left vertebral artery ➡ shows patent lumen.

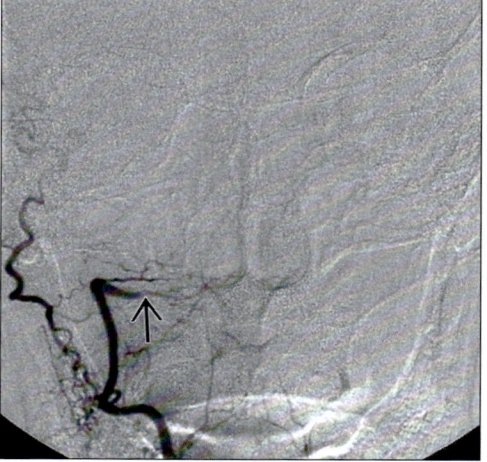

Anterior catheter angiography in same patient as previous image shows tapered occlusion of distal right vertebral artery ➡.

TERMINOLOGY

Abbreviations and Synonyms
- Traumatic dissection and pseudoaneurysm

Definitions
- Dissection: Intramural hematoma extends along vessel
- Intimal extension
  - Intimal flap
  - True and false lumen
- Arterial transection
  - Extension through adventitia
- Pseudoaneurysm: Focal collection of blood outside the vessel wall

IMAGING FINDINGS

General Features
- Best diagnostic clue
  - NECT: Basal subarachnoid hemorrhage (SAH) mimics aneurysmal SAH (aSAH)
  - MR: Hyperintense crescent in vessel wall with central flow void on axial T1WI & T2WI ("target sign")
    - Subarachnoid hyperintensity on FLAIR due to hemorrhage
  - MRA, CTA, conventional angiography
    - Long segment narrowing or tapered occlusion on MRA, CTA or conventional angiography
    - Intraluminal flap on MRA/CTA source images
- Location
  - Vertebral arteries most common (72%)
  - Basilar artery
  - Posterior inferior cerebellar artery (PICA)
  - Superior cerebral artery (SCA)
  - Posterior cerebral artery (PCA)
  - Anterior cerebral artery (ACA) (A2)
  - Middle cerebral artery (MCA)
- Morphology
  - Tapered stenosis with occlusion
  - Irregular vessel narrowing
  - Fusiform dilatation or focal pseudoaneurysm
  - Intimal flap and double (true and false) lumen
  - Intramural hematoma

DDx: Mimics of Intracranial Vascular Injury

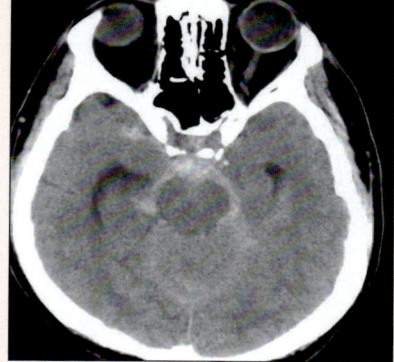

Spontaneous SAH

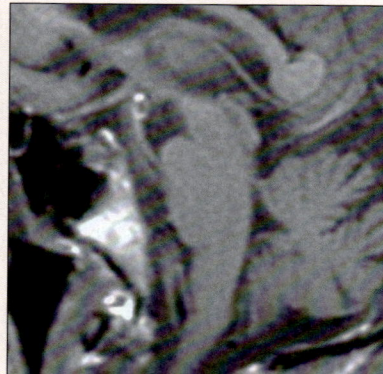

Atherosclerotic Dolichoectasia

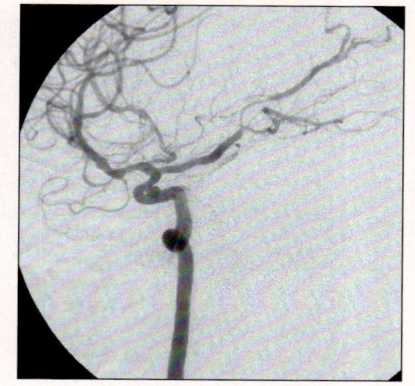

Primary Vasculitis

INTRACRANIAL VASCULAR INJURY

Key Facts

Imaging Findings
- NECT: Basal subarachnoid hemorrhage (SAH) mimics aneurysmal SAH (aSAH)
- MR: Hyperintense crescent in vessel wall with central flow void on axial T1WI & T2WI ("target sign")
- Long segment narrowing or tapered occlusion on MRA, CTA or conventional angiography
- Intraluminal flap on MRA/CTA source images
- Vertebral arteries most common (72%)
- Amorphous mild hyperintensity in wall of vessel (intramural hematoma) partially surrounds more marked flow-related hyperintensity
- Decreased flow may be manifested by decreased caliber and intensity of lumen of vessels distal to dissection
- MR and MRA are best imaging tools
- Initial NECT important to assess for SAH
- Conventional angiography indicated when clinical suspicion is high but MR/MRA negative, and/or for therapeutic intervention

Top Differential Diagnoses
- Atherosclerosis
- Vasospasm
- Vasculitis
- Fibromuscular Dysplasia (FMD)

Clinical Issues
- Most common signs/symptoms: Headache, obtundation, CN3 palsy
- If vessel patent may resolve spontaneously
- Acute emboli is a common complication in acute phase

CT Findings
- NECT
  - Basal extensive SAH mimics aSAH
  - Acute embolic infarct
    - Hypodensity in vascular distribution
    - Hemorrhagic conversion, gyral hyperdensity
  - Basal skull fracture in some cases
- CTA
  - Tapered narrowing and/or occlusion
  - False lumen and flap visible in minority of cases
  - CTA source images, intraluminal flap and vessel wall thickening

MR Findings
- T1WI
  - Hyperintense crescentic intramural hematoma within vessel wall
  - Absent or decreased flow void
- T2WI
  - Target sign: Central hypointense flow void surrounded by hyperintensity in vessel wall
  - Acute infarct hyperintense
  - Hemorrhagic conversion hypointense on T2WI and gradient echo
- FLAIR
  - Hyperintense CSF: SAH
  - Hyperintense acute infarct
- DWI: Hyperintensity in acute infarct
- MRA
  - Amorphous mild hyperintensity in wall of vessel (intramural hematoma) partially surrounds more marked flow-related hyperintensity
  - Decreased flow may be manifested by decreased caliber and intensity of lumen of vessels distal to dissection

Angiographic Findings
- Conventional
  - Tapered narrowing or occlusion
  - Irregular or spiral lumen of internal carotid artery
  - Focal aneurysmal dilatation
  - Embolic occlusion of distal branches

Imaging Recommendations
- Best imaging tool
  - MR and MRA are best imaging tools
  - CTA when MRA equivocal
- Protocol advice
  - Initial NECT important to assess for SAH
  - MR/MRA → CTA if MRA equivocal
  - Conventional angiography indicated when clinical suspicion is high but MR/MRA negative, and/or for therapeutic intervention

DIFFERENTIAL DIAGNOSIS

Atherosclerosis
- Luminal irregularity and stenosis most marked in cavernous carotid artery, vertebral, and basilar arteries
  - No aneurysmal dilatation
- Focal and eccentric when involves pial branches
- Mural calcification on NECT, CTA, or MRA source images

Vasospasm
- Smooth narrowing usually centered at vessel bifurcation
- Most severe where SAH is greatest
- No vasodilation

Vasculitis
- Short or long segment smooth narrowing not centered on vessel bifurcations
- Regions of narrowing alternate with normal vessel lumen or mild aneurysmal dilatation
- Isolated aneurysmal dilatation less common

Fibromuscular Dysplasia (FMD)
- Virtually always in association with extracranial involvement
  - Internal carotid artery opposite C2 in 2/3 of cases
- Alternating zones of focal narrowing and aneurysmal dilatation
  - Corrugated pipe appearance
- Long segment stenosis or aneurysmal dilatation

INTRACRANIAL VASCULAR INJURY

- May be the cause of spontaneous dissection
  - Visualization of vessel wall on MR needed to differentiate between FMD and dissection with or without FMD
  - FMD produces focal vessel wall thickening without hemorrhage or calcification

Spontaneous (Non-Traumatic) Basal SAH
- Ruptured aneurysm
- Benign perimesencephalic SAH

PATHOLOGY

General Features
- General path comments: Hematoma between media/adventitia
- Etiology
  - Skull base fracture: Clinically severe head injury
  - Rotation or flexion extension: Minor injury often overlooked in history
- Epidemiology: 1.5-10% of SAH
- Associated abnormalities
  - Fibromuscular dysplasia, arterial fenestrations
  - Collagen disorders, rheumatoid arthritis
  - Metabolic/genetic disorders: Angiolipomatosis, Marfan, Alpha-1-antitrypsin deficiency

CLINICAL ISSUES

Presentation
- Most common signs/symptoms: Headache, obtundation, CN3 palsy

Natural History & Prognosis
- If vessel patent may resolve spontaneously
- Acute emboli is a common complication in acute phase

Treatment
- Anticoagulation to prevent progressive thrombosis and embolization with distal infarction
- Endovascular occlusion or angioplasty and stenting
- Surgical occlusion, wrapping or bypass

DIAGNOSTIC CHECKLIST

Consider
- Dissection when young patient presents with acute "spontaneous" infarction
  - Inquire about chiropractic manipulation, neck torsion or blunt neck trauma in the 24 hours prior to onset of symptoms

Image Interpretation Pearls
- Look for "target sign" in internal carotid or vertebral artery on images at or just below skull base

SELECTED REFERENCES

1. Ahn JY et al: Endovascular treatment of intracranial vertebral artery dissections with stent placement or stent-assisted coiling. AJNR Am J Neuroradiol. 27(7):1514-20, 2006
2. Benninger DH et al: Mechanism of ischemic infarct in spontaneous carotid dissection. Stroke. 35(2):482-5, 2004
3. Chen CJ et al: Multisection CT angiography compared with catheter angiography in diagnosing vertebral artery dissection. AJNR Am J Neuroradiol. 25(5):769-74, 2004
4. Luo CB et al: Endovascular management of the traumatic cerebral aneurysms associated with traumatic carotid cavernous fistulas. AJNR Am J Neuroradiol. 25(3):501-5, 2004
5. Mizutani T et al: Healing process for cerebral dissecting aneurysms presenting with subarachnoid hemorrhage. Neurosurgery. 54(2):342-7; discussion 347-8, 2004
6. Anxionnat R et al: Treatment of hemorrhagic intracranial dissections. Neurosurgery. 53(2):289-300; discussion 300-1, 2003
7. Ohkuma H et al: Neuroradiologic and clinical features of arterial dissection of the anterior cerebral artery. AJNR Am J Neuroradiol. 24(4):691-9, 2003
8. Price RF et al: Traumatic vertebral arterial dissection and vertebrobasilar arterial thrombosis successfully treated with endovascular thrombolysis and stenting. AJNR Am J Neuroradiol. 19(9):1677-80, 1998
9. Quintana F et al: Traumatic aneurysm of the basilar artery. AJNR Am J Neuroradiol. 17(2):283-5, 1996

INTRACRANIAL VASCULAR INJURY

IMAGE GALLERY

Typical

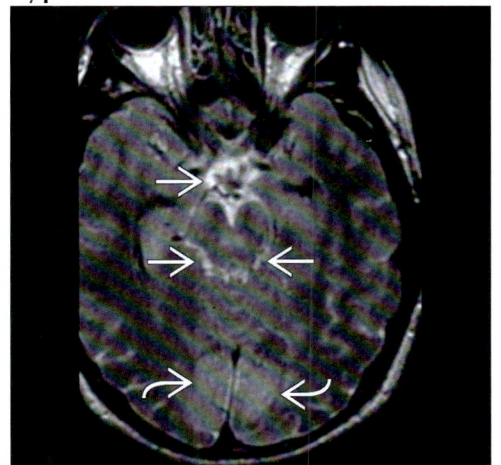
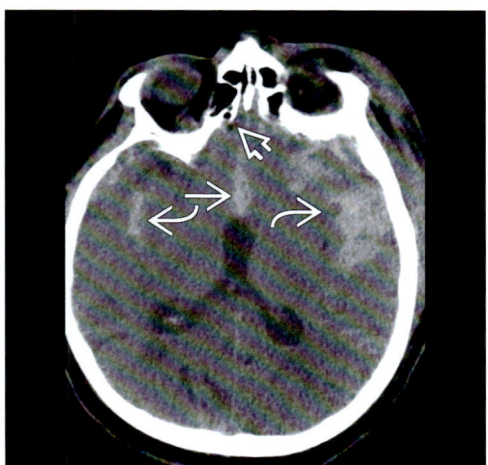

(Left) Axial FLAIR MR shows hyperintense SAH in basal cisterns ➔. Bioccipital cortical hyperintensity is present secondary to acute infarction ➔. *(Right)* Axial NECT shows extensive subarachnoid hemorrhage in interhemispheric fissure ➔ and left > right sylvian fissures ➔. Note pneumocephalus ➔ 2° to skull base fractures.

Typical

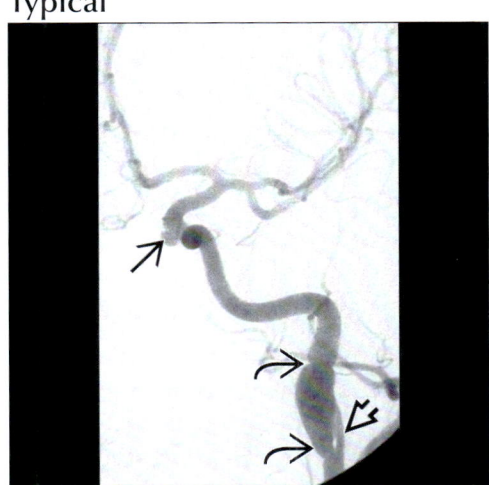
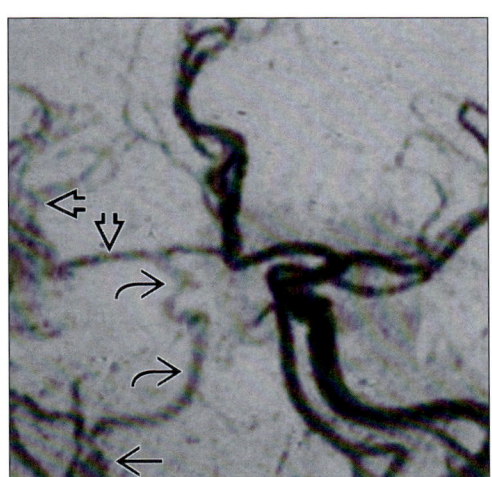

(Left) Anterior catheter angiography shows traumatic cavernous carotid artery pseudoaneurysm ➔ & dissection of internal carotid artery at skull base ➔. Note intimal flap ➔. *(Right)* Frontal MRA shows amorphous intramural hematoma ➔ in proximal internal carotid artery with decreased diameter and flow signal in remainder of ICA ➔ and MCA ➔.

Typical

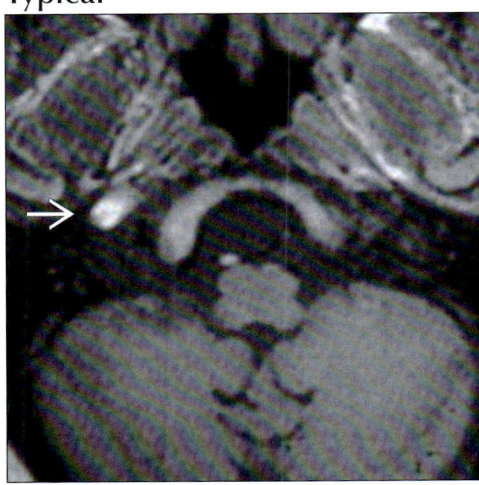
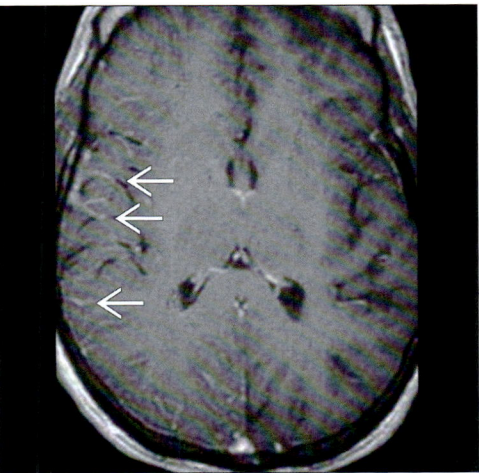

(Left) Axial T1WI MR in the same patient as previous image shows intramural hematoma ➔ in internal carotid artery at skull base. *(Right)* Axial T1 C+ MR in same patient as previous image shows arterial enhancement in right MCA branches ➔ due to slow flow. Patient presented with TIA 8 hours after being struck in neck by soccer ball.

EXTRACRANIAL VASCULAR INJURY

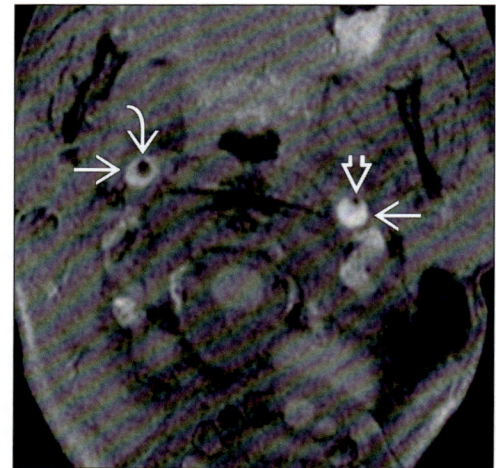
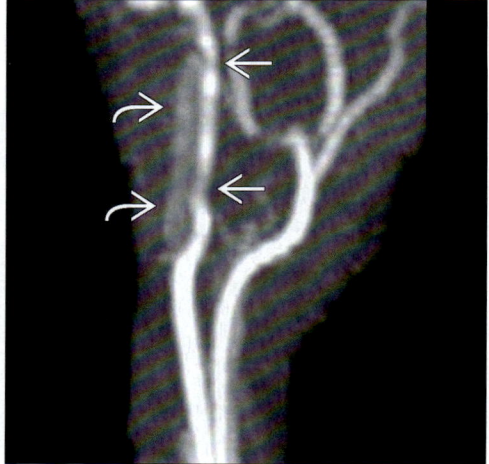

Axial T1WI FS MR shows bilateral mural hyperintensity in internal carotid arteries. Residual luminal flow voids present centrally on right and eccentrically on left.

Coronal MRA in same patient as previous image shows luminal narrowing of right ICA and amorphous hyperintensity within mural hematoma.

TERMINOLOGY

Abbreviations and Synonyms
- Cervicocephalic arterial dissection (CAD)

Definitions
- Traumatic intramural hemorrhage of internal carotid artery (ICA) or vertebral artery (VA)

IMAGING FINDINGS

General Features
- Best diagnostic clue
  - Tubular narrowing or focal dilatation in sites unusual for atherosclerosis
  - Crescentic, hyperintense intramural hematoma surrounding flow void on T1WI
    - "Target sign"
- Location
  - Between adventitia-media or between media-intima
  - Traumatic dissection: ICA > VA
  - ICA dissection: From few cm above carotid bifurcation to skull base or petrous segment
  - VA dissection most common at C1-C2 level
  - 15% involve multiple vessels
- Size: Intramural hematoma propagates distally for variable distance
- Morphology
  - Pseudoaneurysm or long stenosis
  - Secondary embolic infarct common

Radiographic Findings
- Radiography: ± Fracture of skull base or cervical spine

CT Findings
- NECT
  - Usually normal
  - Occasionally carotid space mass (dissecting aneurysm)
  - Brain may show arterial territorial low density 2° infarction
- CECT
  - Linear luminal filling defect: Intimal flap or false lumen
  - Thin rim of contrast-enhancement surrounding mural hematoma 2° vasa vasorum

DDx: Traumatic Extra-Cranial Dissection

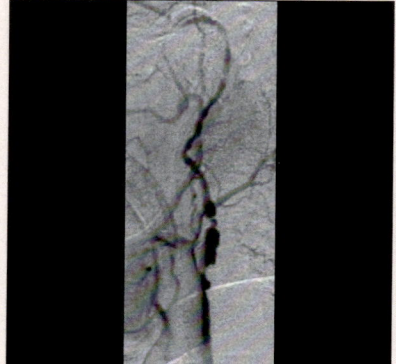
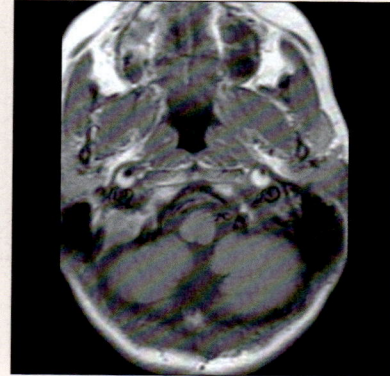
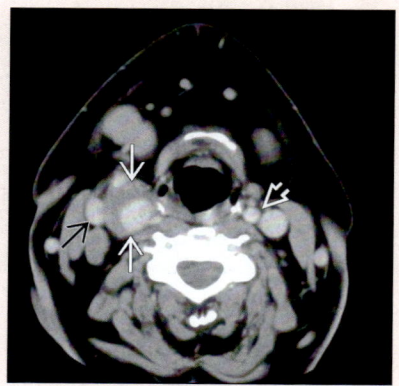

High-Grade Stenosis | Marfan ICA Dissections | Pseudoaneurysm ASCVD

EXTRACRANIAL VASCULAR INJURY

Key Facts

Terminology
- Traumatic intramural hemorrhage of internal carotid artery (ICA) or vertebral artery (VA)

Imaging Findings
- Tubular narrowing or focal dilatation in sites unusual for atherosclerosis
- Crescentic, hyperintense intramural hematoma surrounding flow void on T1WI
- ICA dissection: From few cm above carotid bifurcation to skull base or petrous segment
- VA dissection most common at C1-C2 level
- Segmental tapered narrowing ("string" sign)
- Segmental dilatation of vessel (pseudoaneurysm)
- Intimal flap at proximal margin of dissection
- MR with fat-suppressed T1WI, MRA
- CTA if MR/MRA negative or equivocal

Top Differential Diagnoses
- "Spontaneous" Dissection
- Arterial Thrombosis
- Atherosclerosis
- Proximal ICA Stenosis
- Vasospasm

Pathology
- Common cause of infarcts in patients < 40 y

Clinical Issues
- Unrelenting headache or neckache in young or middle-aged adults
- Delayed onset after relatively minor trauma or chiropractic treatment may obscure diagnosis

MR Findings
- Intramural hematoma ("target sign")
  - Curvilinear, crescentic, band-like or small focus adjacent to lumen
  - Usually circumferential & eccentric
  - Widens external diameter of artery
  - Surrounds normal/narrow flow void
  - Signal characteristics
    - Acute: Isointense/slightly hyperintense on T1WI, hypointense on T2WI
    - Subacute: Hyperintense on T1WI & T2WI
- Intimal flap
  - Thin curvilinear hypointense partition separating true & false lumen
- Flow void in residual lumen
  - Eccentrically narrowed
  - Absent flow void 2° to slow flow or occlusion

Ultrasonographic Findings
- Color Doppler
  - Echogenic intimal flap (most specific sign)
  - Echogenic thrombus
  - Abrupt smooth tapering of arterial lumen
  - False lumen occasionally seen with color Doppler

Angiographic Findings
- DSA/CTA/MRA
  - Segmental tapered narrowing ("string" sign)
  - MRA: Amorphous mild hyperintensity (intramural hematoma) partially engulfs hyperintense lumen (flow)
  - Segmental dilatation of vessel (pseudoaneurysm)
    - Oval, parallel to artery, variable size
    - Extraluminal pouch at midportion of stenotic segment
    - "Pearl & string" sign at distal margin of stenotic region
  - Intimal flap at proximal margin of dissection
    - Source MRA and CTA images, less commonly seen on DSA
  - Double lumen represents true lumen & intramural dissection
    - Uncommon, particularly in VA
  - True lumen may be completely occluded
  - Slow flow in parent artery
  - Distal branch occlusions due to embolization
  - CTA & MRA: Independent of flow phenomena
    - Shows small residual lumen & pseudoaneurysms

Imaging Recommendations
- Best imaging tool: MR & MRA of head and neck with overlapping imaging volumes
- Protocol advice
  - MR with fat-suppressed T1WI, MRA
  - CTA if MR/MRA negative or equivocal
  - DSA for equivocal cases and endovascular intervention

DIFFERENTIAL DIAGNOSIS

"Spontaneous" Dissection
- Underlying vasculopathy common
  - Fibromuscular dysplasia
    - "String of beads" appearance > long tubular stenosis
  - Marfan syndrome, type IV Ehlers-Danlos syndrome
- Familial ICA dissection
- Hypertension in 1/3 of patients
- Delayed presentation of undiagnosed blunt artery injury (occult CAD)

Arterial Thrombosis
- Often difficult to establish whether underlying dissection is present

Atherosclerosis
- Typically occurs at carotid bifurcation or VA origin
- Irregular > smooth tapered narrowing
- Ca++ often present

Proximal ICA Stenosis
- Severe extracranial arterial stenosis → slow flow in intracranial segment, simulating an intracranial dissection ("pseudodissection")

EXTRACRANIAL VASCULAR INJURY

- Can produce periarterial rim of abnormal signal that is not due to hematoma
- T1WI isointense, T2WI hyperintense; no marked T1WI hyperintensity or T2WI hyperintensity in wall

Vasospasm
- Catheter-placement induced
- Transient; resolves within minutes

PATHOLOGY

General Features
- General path comments
  - Intimal disruption or vasa vasorum hemorrhage
  - False lumen, true lumen stenosis ± occlusion, pseudoaneurysm, thrombosis & embolism
- Etiology
  - Penetrating injury (gunshot wound or stabbing) may injure common carotid, ICA, or VA
  - Blunt trauma may affect extracranial ICA
    - Motor vehicle accidents (high acceleration/hyperextension → whiplash injury)
    - Direct blow to neck; may be very mild and overlooked
    - Falls, strangulation digital carotid compression, iatrogenic (VA dissection in 5% of facet joint surgeries)
    - Rapid neck rotation or flexion; diving injuries
    - Chiropractic manipulation (stretching/torsion) affects VA > ICA
  - Potential mechanisms of injury
    - Sudden, severe stretch of artery over upper cervical spine in hyperextension & lateral flexion
    - Stretching of ICA over transverse processes of upper cervical vertebrae
    - Compression of ICA between angle of mandible & upper cervical vertebral bodies
    - Stretching of VA over C1-C2 vertebral bodies, primarily during head rotation
    - Combination of head, facial & cervical injuries
- Epidemiology
  - Incidence of ICA dissection in blunt trauma patients: 0.08-0.4%
  - CAD accounts for 0.4-2.5% of all infarcts
    - Common cause of infarcts in patients < 40 y
    - 20% of infarcts in young patients
- Associated abnormalities
  - Asymptomatic dissection of second artery (20%)
    - Usually accompanies symptomatic VA dissection
  - Severe trauma to cervical spine
  - Patients evaluated for blunt aortic trauma are 10 times more likely to have blunt carotid injury

Gross Pathologic & Surgical Features
- Hemorrhage between intima-media → luminal stenosis
- Hemorrhage between adventitia-media → pseudoaneurysm formation

CLINICAL ISSUES

Presentation
- Most common signs/symptoms
  - Headache, neck pain
    - 60-90% of patients with cervical ICA dissection
    - Onset often delayed, from hours to 3-4 weeks
  - Focal cerebral ischemic symptoms (TIA, infarct)
    - Often delayed hours to weeks post-injury
  - Horner syndrome
    - Stretching or injury of sympathetic nerves adjacent to ICA
    - May be incomplete (only miosis, ptosis)
- Other signs/symptoms
  - Uncommon
    - Cranial nerve palsy (CN 12 > 9, 10, 11)
    - Carotid bruits, pulsatile tinnitus
- Clinical profile
  - Unrelenting headache or neckache in young or middle-aged adults

Demographics
- Age
  - Spontaneous dissection → 70% between 35-50 y
  - Uncommon in children, adolescents (7% of cases)
- Gender
  - ICA dissection (all causes): M:F = 1.5:1
  - VA dissection (all causes): M:F = 1:3

Natural History & Prognosis
- Delayed diagnosis of blunt carotid injury common
- Traumatic CAD versus spontaneous CAD
  - Traumatic CAD less likely to spontaneously improve
  - Traumatic CAD more likely to lead to residual neurologic deficits
- More than 2/3 of patients have complete recovery

Treatment
- Anticoagulation with heparin followed by Coumadin
- Endovascular intervention: Occlusion, angioplasty, stenting
- Delayed onset after relatively minor trauma or chiropractic treatment may obscure diagnosis

DIAGNOSTIC CHECKLIST

Consider
- Early screening via MR/MRA of severely injured patients for detection of occult CAD
- CAD in any young or middle-aged patient with/unrelenting headache or neckache

SELECTED REFERENCES

1. Benninger DH et al: Mechanism of ischemic infarct in spontaneous carotid dissection. Stroke. 35(2):482-5, 2004
2. Mizutani T et al: Healing process for cerebral dissecting aneurysms presenting with subarachnoid hemorrhage. Neurosurgery. 54(2):342-7; discussion 347-8, 2004
3. Oelerich M et al: Craniocervical artery dissection: MR imaging and MR angiographic findings. Eur Radiol. 9(7):1385-91, 1999
4. Provenzale JM et al: Spontaneous vertebral dissection: clinical, conventional angiographic, CT, and MR findings. J Comput Assist Tomogr. 20(2):185-93, 1996
5. Provenzale JM: Dissection of the internal carotid and vertebral arteries: imaging features. AJR Am J Roentgenol. 165(5):1099-104, 1995

EXTRACRANIAL VASCULAR INJURY

IMAGE GALLERY

Variant

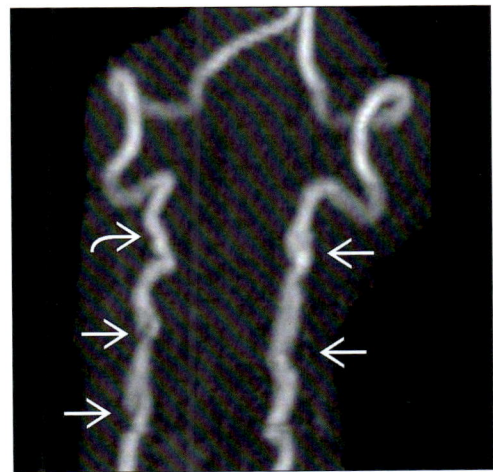
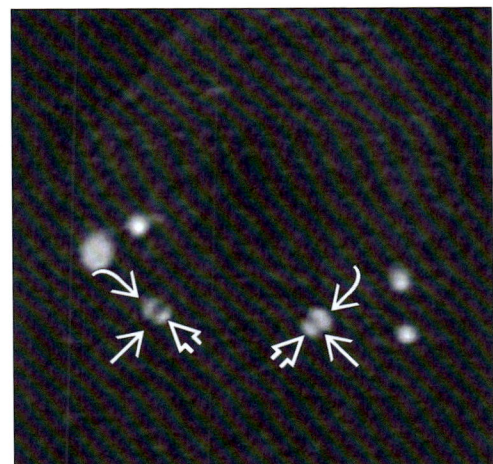

(Left) Coronal MRA shows bilateral spiral filling defects ➡ indicative of true & false lumens, and focal irregular narrowing of vertebral arteries ➡. *(Right)* Axial MRA in same patient as previous image shows intimal flaps ➡, true ➡ and false lumens ➡ on source MRA images.

Typical

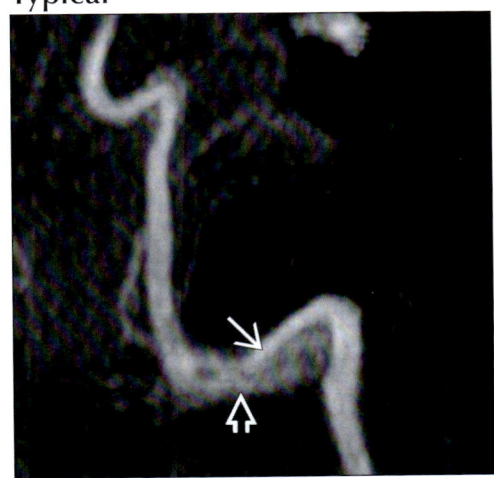
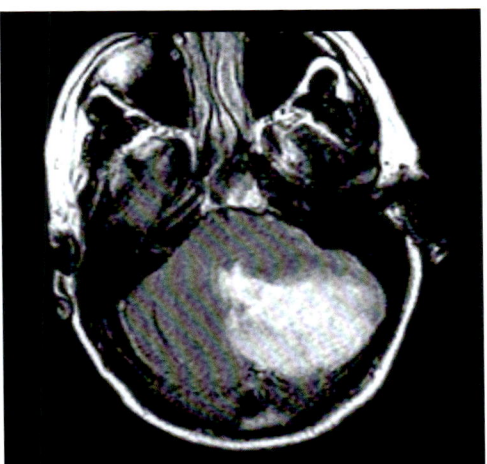

(Left) Coronal MRA shows true lumen ➡ and intramural hematoma ➡ in patient with acute onset neck pain & cerebellar findings 24 hrs after chiropractic manipulation. *(Right)* Axial FLAIR MR in same patient as previous image shows acute left cerebellar infarct 2° vertebral artery dissection from chiropractic manipulation.

Typical

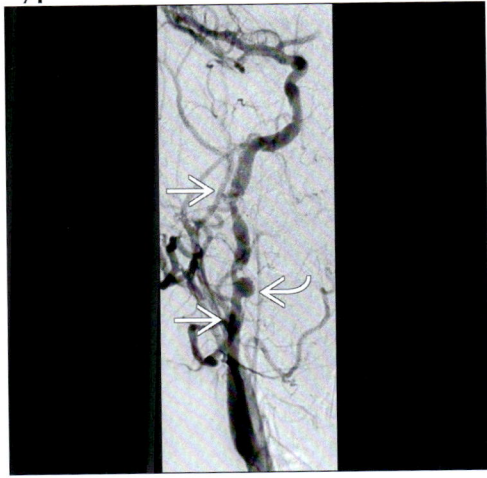
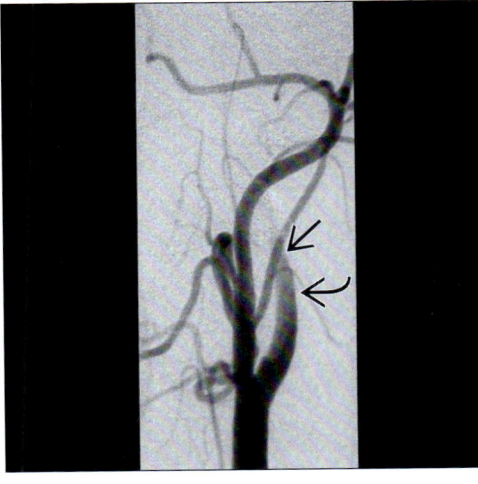

(Left) Anteroposterior catheter angiography shows long segment of irregular narrowing of extracranial ICA ➡ with focal pseudoaneurysm at site of maximal stenosis ➡. *(Right)* Lateral catheter angiography shows tapered narrowing of proximal ICA ➡ ending in occlusion ➡.

CAROTID-CAVERNOUS FISTULA

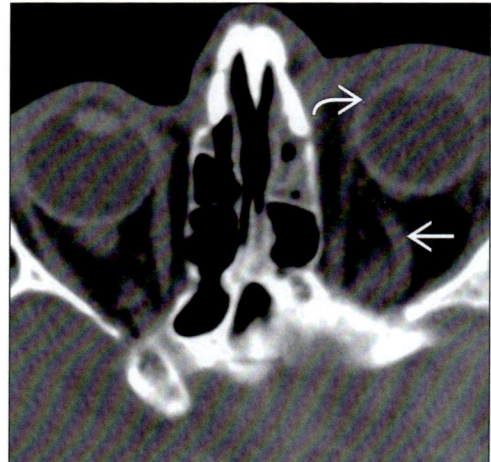

Axial NECT shows dilated SOV ➡ and mild proptosis ➡ two hours after head trauma.

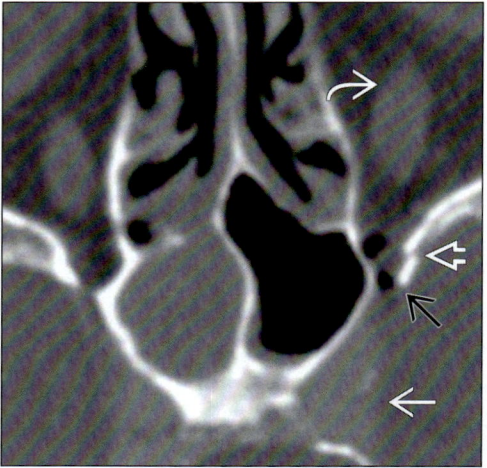

Axial NECT of the same patient as previous image shows enlarged cavernous sinus ➡, increased size of inferior rectus muscle ➡, sphenoid fracture ➡, & orbital emphysema ➡.

TERMINOLOGY

Abbreviations and Synonyms
- Carotid-cavernous fistula (CCF), direct or high-velocity

Definitions
- Direct fistula between cavernous internal carotid artery (ICA) & cavernous sinus (CS)

IMAGING FINDINGS

General Features
- Best diagnostic clue: Proptosis, large superior ophthalmic vein (SOV) & CS, extraocular muscle (EOM) enlargement

CT Findings
- NECT
  - Proptosis, enlarged SOV & EOMs
    - "Dirty" orbital fat 2° edema
  - Subarachnoid hemorrhage (SAH)
- CECT: Proptosis; prominent SOV & CS

MR Findings
- T1 C+: Same as CECT
- MRA
  - ↑ Flow-related signal in CS & SOV
  - Signal loss in ICA 2° turbulent flow

Ultrasonographic Findings
- Doppler: Reversal of flow in SOV

Angiographic Findings
- Conventional
  - Rapid filling of CS with retrograde filling of SOV
  - Opposite CS
  - Petrosal sinuses → internal jugular vein
  - Vein of Rosenthal → vein of Galen
  - Signs of danger: Filling of cortical veins, pseudoaneurysm, CS varices, thrombosis/obstruction of venous drainage

Imaging Recommendations
- Best imaging tool: CECT
- Protocol advice: Thin section scans with reformations

DDx: Traumatic Cavernous Carotid Fistula

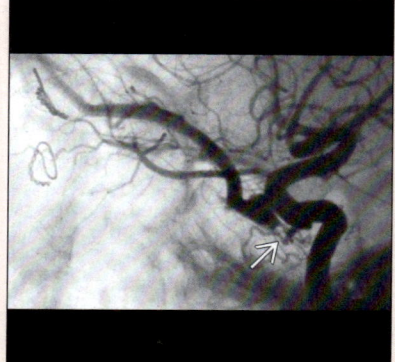

Spontaneous Low Flow Dural AVF

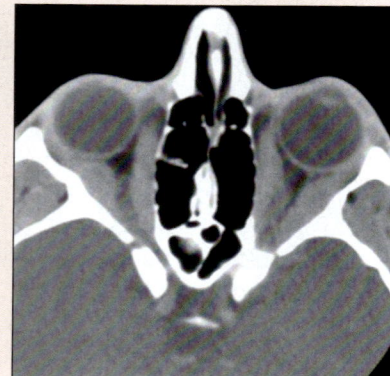

Orbital Myositis

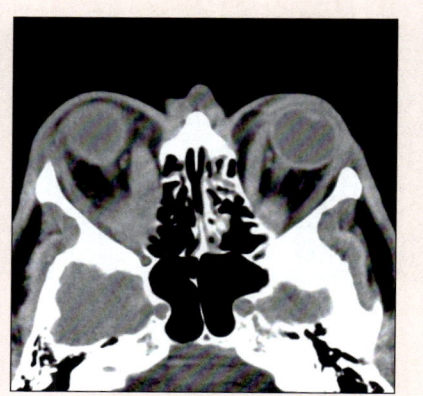

Graves Disease EOM Enlargement

CAROTID-CAVERNOUS FISTULA

Key Facts

Terminology
- Carotid-cavernous fistula (CCF), direct or high-velocity
- Direct fistula between cavernous internal carotid artery (ICA) & cavernous sinus (CS)

Imaging Findings
- Best diagnostic clue: Proptosis, large superior ophthalmic vein (SOV) & CS, extraocular muscle (EOM) enlargement
- Best imaging tool: CECT

Top Differential Diagnoses
- Spontaneous Slow Flow Dural AV Fistula
- SOV Enlargement
- EOM Enlargement

Pathology
- Etiology: Skull base fracture or ruptured intra-cavernous aneurysm

DIFFERENTIAL DIAGNOSIS

Spontaneous Slow Flow Dural AV Fistula
- Connection between dural artery and CS

SOV Enlargement
- CS thrombosis; orbital apex mass, varix

EOM Enlargement
- Graves disease; inflammatory pseudotumor; neoplasm

PATHOLOGY

General Features
- General path comments: Reflux into cortical veins when SOV/IOV & petrosal sinus cannot handle blood flow → ↑ risk SAH
- Etiology: Skull base fracture or ruptured intra-cavernous aneurysm
- Epidemiology: Spontaneous CCF in older patients

Gross Pathologic & Surgical Features
- Tears located at horizontal or vertical cavernous ICA

Staging, Grading or Classification Criteria
- Type A: Direct communication (traumatic)
- Types B-D: Indirect communications; meningeal branches of ICA and CS (usually non-traumatic)

CLINICAL ISSUES

Presentation
- Most common signs/symptoms
  - May develop days to weeks post-trauma
  - Bruit, pulsating exophthalmos, orbital edema/erythema, ↓ vision, glaucoma, headache
  - Severe/rapid vision loss, SAH → emergency
  - Focal deficits → CN 3-6

Natural History & Prognosis
- Progresses to blindness if untreated

Treatment
- Endovascular treatment: Transarterial or transvenous
- ICA/jugular vein compression for small indirect CCF

DIAGNOSTIC CHECKLIST

Image Interpretation Pearls
- Enlarged SOV & CS

SELECTED REFERENCES
1. Fattahi TT et al: Traumatic carotid-cavernous fistula: pathophysiology and treatment. J Craniofac Surg. 14(2):240-6, 2003
2. Chuman H et al: Spontaneous direct carotid-cavernous fistula in Ehlers-Danlos syndrome type IV: two case reports and a review of the literature. J Neuroophthalmol. 22(2):75-81, 2002

IMAGE GALLERY

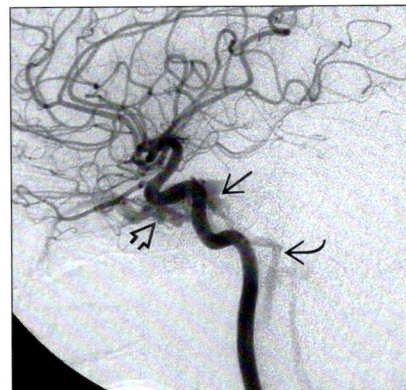 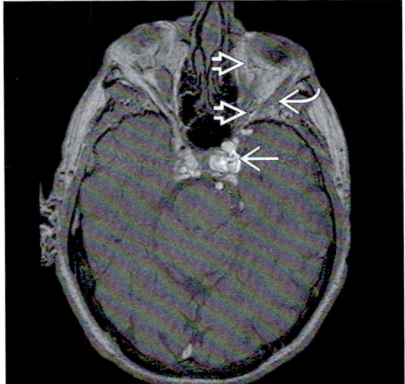 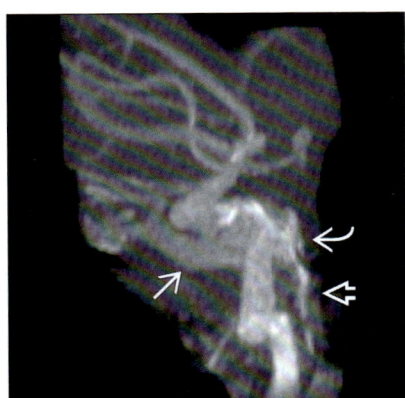

(Left) Lateral catheter angiography shows filling of the cavernous sinus ➡, SOV ➡, and pterygoid venous plexus ➡. *(Center)* Axial T1 C+ MR shows enlargement and increased flow signal in CS ➡, enlargement of the lateral rectus muscle ➡, & multiple dilated intraorbital veins ➡. *(Right)* Lateral MRA shows marked dilated SOV ➡, flow signal in CS ➡ and prominent dorsal venous plexus ➡.

TEMPORAL BONE FRACTURES

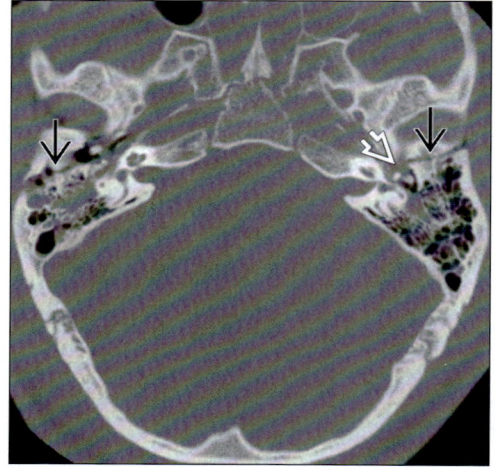

Axial bone CT shows bilateral otic capsule sparing fractures ➡ and left malleoincudal dislocation ➡. These previously would have been classified as longitudinal (R), transverse (L).

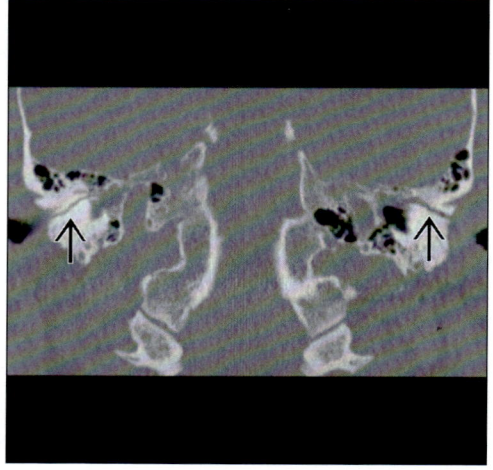

Coronal bone CT shows bilateral oblique fractures ➡. Note that fracture plane is horizontal.

TERMINOLOGY

Abbreviations and Synonyms
- T-bone fracture

Definitions
- Traumatic injury of temporal bone, ossicles

IMAGING FINDINGS

General Features
- Best diagnostic clue: Fracture line, hemotympanum
- Location: Petrous temporal bone (includes mastoid)
- Size: May be widely diastatic or subtle
- Morphology
  o Longitudinal fracture: Vertical plane parallels long axis of petrous ridge (PR)
  o Transverse fracture: Perpendicular to PR long axis
  o Oblique fracture: Most T-bone fractures, horizontal, parallels PR long axis
  o New classification as otic capsule (OC) violating vs. OC sparing better predicts complications

CT Findings
- NECT
  o Oblique T-bone fractures
    - Obliquely horizontal plane, crosses petrotympanic fissure, extends anteromedially along PR long axis
    - Involves EAC, middle ear, usually spares OC
  o Longitudinal T-bone fractures
    - Vertically oriented plane paralleling PR long axis, runs with (not across) petrotympanic fissure
    - EAC, middle ear involvement, hemotympanum & ossicular disruption common, usually spares OC
    - Facial nerve canal involvement less common than with transverse fracture
  o Transverse T-bone fractures
    - Perpendicular to PR, from foramen magnum or jugular foramen to middle fossa
    - Facial nerve canal involvement is common, often involves IAC or OC
    - Medial subtype: Posterior petrous surface through IAC to 1st genu of facial nerve
    - Lateral subtype: Posterior petrous surface through OC, pneumolabyrinth common

DDx: Temporal Bone Pseudofractures

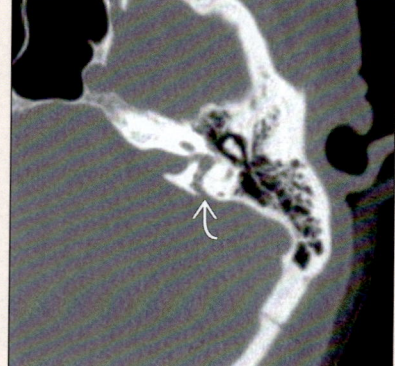

Enlarged Vestibular Aqueduct

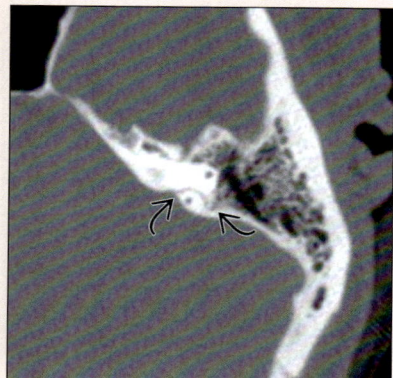

Petromastoid Canal

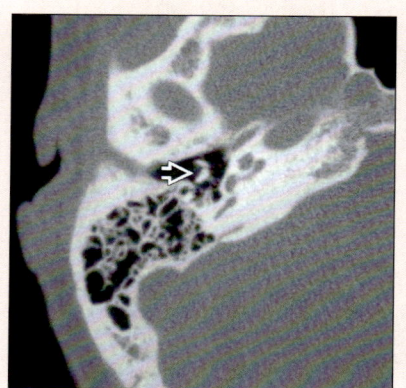

Incus Interposition

TEMPORAL BONE FRACTURES

Key Facts

Imaging Findings
- Longitudinal fracture: Vertical plane parallels long axis of petrous ridge (PR)
- Transverse fracture: Perpendicular to PR long axis
- Oblique fracture: Most T-bone fractures, horizontal, parallels PR long axis
- New classification as otic capsule (OC) violating vs. OC sparing better predicts complications
- Important to identify fractures with risk for CSF leak (e.g., tegmen)
- Best imaging tool: Computed tomography
- CTA or MRA if carotid canal involved, tinnitus, proptosis, or chemosis develop (suggesting AV fistula), or infarction (suggesting arterial occlusion or dissection with thromboembolism)

Pathology
- Most common fractures of skull base
- 20% of patients with skull fracture have T-bone fractures
- Only 2.5% of T-bone fractures involve OC

Clinical Issues
- Sensorineural hearing loss (SNHL), facial nerve injury, and intracranial complications more common with OC involvement
- Late CHL suggests ossicular dislocation
- Management of severe head injury is priority

Diagnostic Checklist
- Consider pseudofractures

- Middle ear & EAC involved less commonly than longitudinal
- All varieties: Facial nerve most commonly injured in perigeniculate region
- Important to identify fractures with risk for CSF leak (e.g., tegmen)
- Ossicular dislocation types
  - Incus dislocation most common (poor support): Incudostapedial > malleoincudal > complete incus dislocation
  - Stapediovestibular disruption
  - Malleus dislocation rare (supported by malleal ligaments, TM attachments)

MR Findings
- T1WI
  - Hemotympanum, hemolabyrinth (low signal acutely, high signal subacutely)
  - Fried egg sign (ICA dissection) or loss of ICA flow void in carotid injury
- T2WI
  - Middle ear & mastoid debris appears hyperintense
  - Look for hypointense line of intact dura over tegmen on coronal images if CSF leak suspected
- T1 C+
  - Most valuable for suspected intracranial complications (meningitis, abscess)
  - Facial nerve, membranous labyrinth may enhance when involved by fracture
- MRA: Carotid occlusion or dissection, carotid cavernous fistula
- MRV: Sigmoid sinus thrombosis = rare complication

Imaging Recommendations
- Best imaging tool: Computed tomography
- Protocol advice
  - Bone algorithm submillimeter axial helical CT, coronal reformats
    - 3D CT reconstructions helpful for clarifying fracture orientation, ossicular alignment
  - Routine brain CT or MR for intracranial complications (hemorrhage, CSF leak)
  - CTA or MRA if carotid canal involved, tinnitus, proptosis, or chemosis develop (suggesting AV fistula), or infarction (suggesting arterial occlusion or dissection with thromboembolism)

DIFFERENTIAL DIAGNOSIS

Pseudofractures
- Sutures-fissures
  - Occipitomastoid, petrooccipital, temporoparietal, petrotympanic, petrosquamosal, tympanosquamous, and tympanomastoid fissures
- Canaliculi
  - Mastoid, inferior tympanic, subarcuate (petromastoid canal), singular canaliculi
- Aqueducts
  - Cochlear, vestibular aqueducts

Incus Interposition Procedure (Mimics Incus Dislocation)
- Surgical remodeling/realignment of incus to bridge deficient ossicular chain, correct CHL

PATHOLOGY

General Features
- Etiology: Most common etiology is head injury during MVA
- Epidemiology
  - Most common fractures of skull base
  - 20% of patients with skull fracture have T-bone fractures
  - Only 2.5% of T-bone fractures involve OC
- Associated abnormalities: Pneumocephalus, temporal lobe contusion, CSF leak, ICA injury, traumatic arteriovenous fistula

TEMPORAL BONE FRACTURES

CLINICAL ISSUES

Presentation
- Most common signs/symptoms
  - Peri/postauricular swelling and ecchymosis (Battle sign), EAC hemorrhage, hemotympanum
  - Sensorineural hearing loss (SNHL), facial nerve injury, and intracranial complications more common with OC involvement
  - Longitudinal fracture
    - Lateral blow to temporal or parietal skull
    - High incidence of conductive hearing loss (CHL) due to ossicular injury
    - Typically spares OC, SNHL unusual
    - Facial nerve injury in up to 25%, often incomplete, delayed, tympanic segment
  - Transverse fractures
    - Frontal or occipital blow to the skull
    - Often involve OC, permanent complete SNHL common (medial type), perilymphatic fistula (lateral type)
    - Lower incidence of CHL
    - Facial nerve injury in 45-50%, with immediate, permanent facial paralysis more common than with longitudinal fractures
  - Chronic presentations
    - Late CHL suggests ossicular dislocation
    - Acquired cephalocele, delayed CSF leak
    - Acquired cholesteatoma (squamous invasion of fracture site)
    - EAC stenosis
- Other signs/symptoms
  - Dizziness, vertigo, imbalance, fluctuating SNHL (consider perilymph fistula)
  - CN VI injury
- Clinical Profile
  - Acute injury
    - Fracture usually incidentally discovered
  - Hearing loss, facial paralysis noted after stabilization from acute injuries
    - Occasionally history of trauma is remote

Demographics
- Age
  - All ages
  - Facial nerve paralysis less common in pediatric T-bone fractures
- Gender: M > F

Natural History & Prognosis
- Related to intracranial complications (intracranial pathology on CT in up to 84% of patients with T-bone fractures)
- Associated CSF leak common (15%)
  - Most resolve spontaneously within 7 days, surgery for persistent leak
  - 10% or less develop meningitis
- Perilymphatic fistula: Progressive dizziness and SNHL; early detection allows surgical repair, hearing preservation
- Most subacute cases of facial nerve paresis (due to swelling) resolve spontaneously, treated conservatively; surgical decompression or nerve repair for immediate paralysis

Treatment
- Management of severe head injury is priority
- Endovascular therapy for carotid injury
- Antibiotics if CSF leak is demonstrated

DIAGNOSTIC CHECKLIST

Consider
- Consider pseudofractures
- Consider postinflammatory or postsurgical ossicular changes

Image Interpretation Pearls
- Don't misdiagnose a pseudofracture!

SELECTED REFERENCES

1. Little SC et al: Radiographic classification of temporal bone fractures: clinical predictability using a new system. Arch Otolaryngol Head Neck Surg. 132(12):1300-4, 2006
2. Ishman SL et al: Temporal bone fractures: traditional classification and clinical relevance. Laryngoscope. 114(10):1734-41, 2004
3. Bergemalm PO: Progressive hearing loss after closed head injury: a predictable outcome? Acta Otolaryngol. 123(7):836-45, 2003
4. Exadaktylos AK et al: The clinical correlation of temporal bone fractures and spiral computed tomographic scan: a prospective and consecutive study at a level I trauma center. J Trauma. 55(4):704-6, 2003
5. Gross M et al: Cochlear involvement in a temporal bone fracture. Otol Neurotol. 24(6):958-9, 2003
6. Gross M et al: Pneumolabyrinth: an unusual finding in a temporal bone fracture. Int J Pediatr Otorhinolaryngol. 67(5):553-5, 2003
7. Sudhoff H et al: Temporal bone fracture and latent meningitis: temporal bone histopathology study of the month. Otol Neurotol. 24(3):521-2, 2003
8. Lin TF et al: Isolated transverse transcochlear temporal bone fracture. Otol Neurotol. 23(4):615-6, 2002
9. Singh S et al: Traumatic fracture of the stapes suprastructure following minor head injury. J Laryngol Otol. 116(6):457-9, 2002
10. Darrouzet V et al: Management of facial paralysis resulting from temporal bone fractures: Our experience in 115 cases. Otolaryngol Head Neck Surg. 125(1):77-84, 2001
11. Jager L et al: CT and MR imaging of the normal and pathologic conditions of the facial nerve. Eur J Radiol. 40(2):133-46, 2001
12. Swartz JD: Temporal bone trauma. Semin Ultrasound CT MR. 22(3):219-28, 2001
13. Cunningham CD 3rd et al: Neurotologic complications associated with deployment of airbags. Otolaryngol Head Neck Surg. 123(5):637-9, 2000
14. Dahiya R et al: Temporal bone fractures: otic capsule sparing versus otic capsule violating clinical and radiographic considerations. J Trauma. 47(6):1079-83, 1999
15. JD Swartz & HR Harnsberger: Imaging of the Temporal Bone, 3rd Edition, Thieme, Inc. Ch. 6, 1998
16. Brodie HA et al: Management of complications from 820 temporal bone fractures. Am J Otol. 18(2):188-97, 1997

TEMPORAL BONE FRACTURES

IMAGE GALLERY

Typical

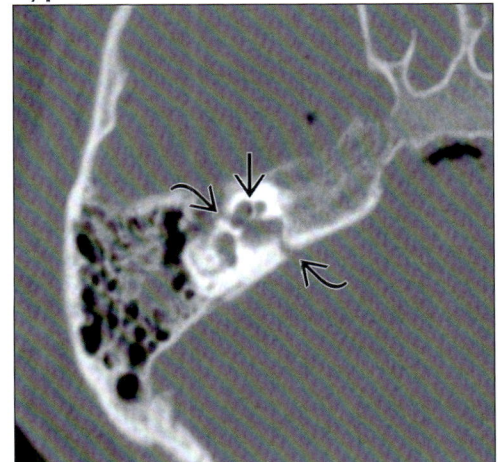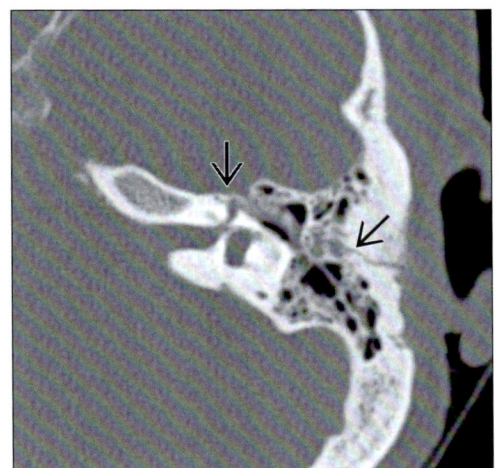

(Left) Axial bone CT shows transverse fracture crossing IAC and otic capsule ➔. Note tiny air bubble (pneumolabyrinth) ➔ in cochlea. *(Right)* Axial bone CT shows a longitudinal fracture ➔ crossing the region of the left geniculate ganglion in this patient with CN VII paralysis after a mountain bike riding injury.

Typical

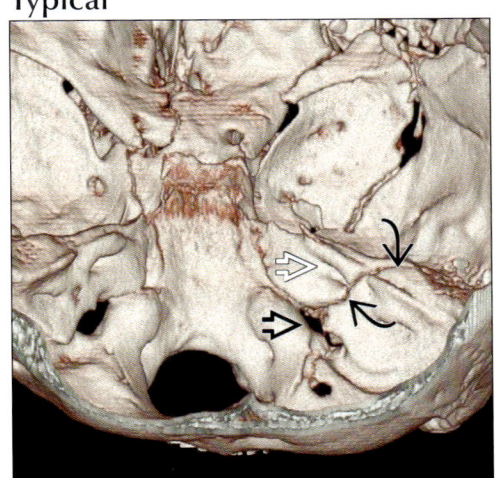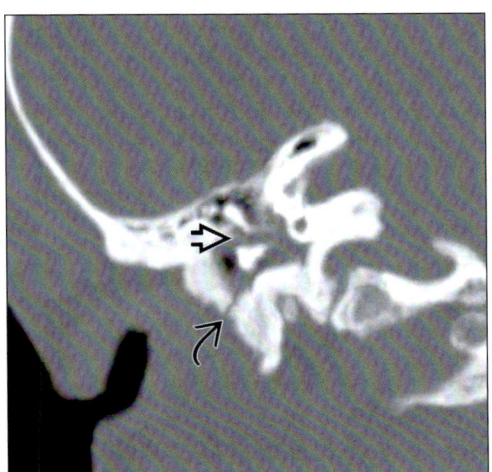

(Left) Oblique posterior projection of 3D volume rendered bone CT shows a transverse right temporal bone fracture ➔ traversing the jugular foramen ➔, IAC ➔, and petrous ridge. *(Right)* 3D coronal MIP reconstructed from axial helical bone CT clarifies the orientation of the dislocated malleoincudal joint ➔ in this oblique temporal bone fracture ➔.

Typical

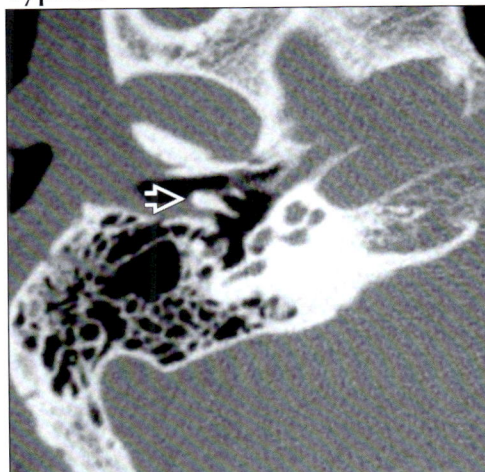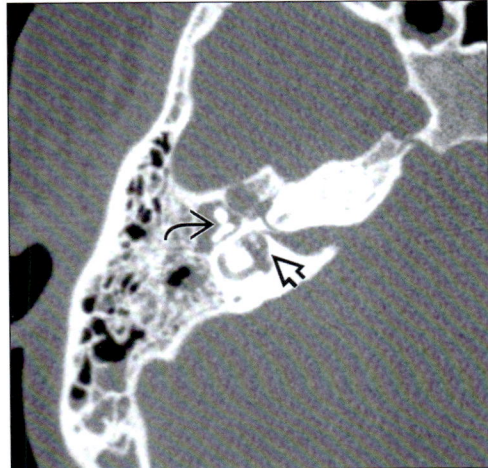

(Left) Axial NECT shows complete incus dislocation. The incus is laterally displaced into the EAC ➔ and rotated into the horizontal plane. Its articulations with the malleus and stapes are disrupted. *(Right)* Axial bone CT shows stapes displacement into vestibule ➔, malleoincudal dislocation ➔ due to airbag injury.

CSF LEAK

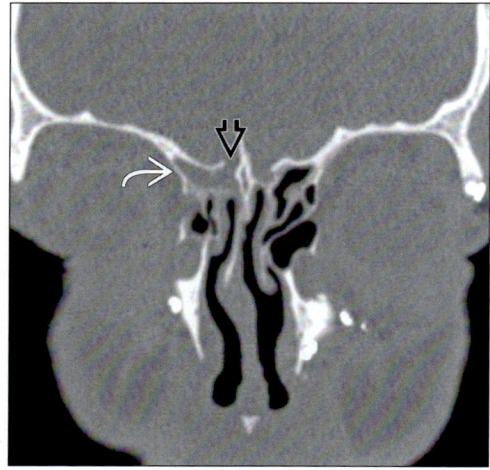

Coronal NECT shows bony defect between fovea ethmoidalis and olfactory groove ⇨, opacification of adjacent right frontal sinus ➡ in a patient with post-traumatic CSF rhinorrhea.

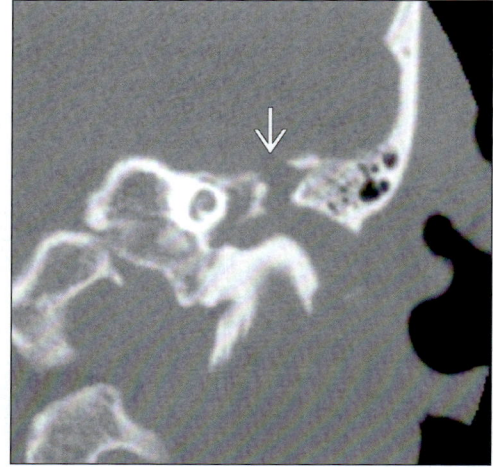

Coronal NECT shows left temporal bone fracture with large tegment defect ➡. Patient had left-sided CSF otorrhea.

TERMINOLOGY

Abbreviations and Synonyms
- Cerebrospinal fluid (CSF) otorhinorrhea, CSF fistula

Definitions
- Post-traumatic CSF leak into paranasal sinuses or temporal bone

IMAGING FINDINGS

General Features
- Best diagnostic clue: Fractures with fluid in adjacent paranasal sinuses, mastoid, or middle ear
- Location
  - Ethmoid (especially cribriform, fovea), frontal, sphenoid, or temporal bones; leaks may be multiple, intermittent
  - Post-traumatic leaks most common in anterior fossa

CT Findings
- NECT: Fracture with fluid in adjacent sinus or middle ear

MR Findings
- T2WI
  - Continuous fluid column from subarachnoid space to airspace
  - Distortion of adjacent sulcus or gyrus, cephalocele

Imaging Recommendations
- Best imaging tool: High resolution, non-contrast computed tomography (HRCT)
- Protocol advice
  - Axial helical HRCT, ≤ 1 mm thick, reformat coronals
  - Direct coronal images (after neck cleared) if necessary
  - Include all of paranasal sinuses, T-bones
  - MR cisternography (heavily T2WI)
  - CT or radionuclide cisternography if HRCT normal or multiple bone defects (usually not necessary)
  - Enhanced MR if cephalocele or meningitis suspected

DDx: Traumatic CSF Leak Mimics

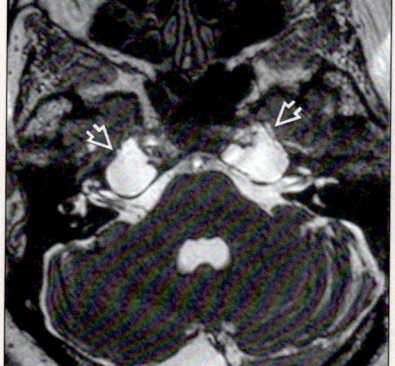

Petrous Apex Cephaloceles

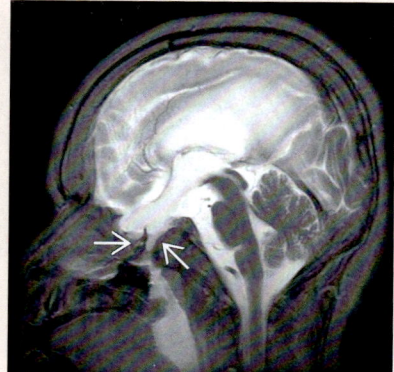

Sphenoidal Cephalocele

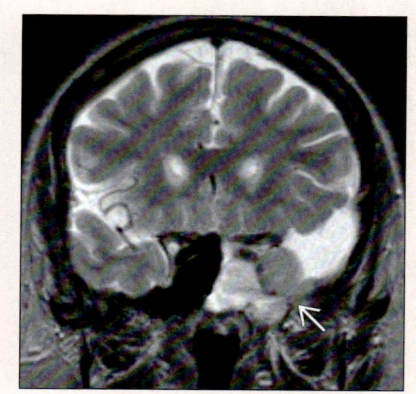

Transalar Cephalocele

CSF LEAK

Key Facts

Imaging Findings
- Ethmoid (especially cribriform, fovea), frontal, sphenoid, or temporal bones; leaks may be multiple, intermittent
- Post-traumatic leaks most common in anterior fossa
- NECT: Fracture with fluid in adjacent sinus or middle ear
- Axial helical HRCT, ≤ 1 mm thick, reformat coronals

Pathology
- Etiology: Most CSF leaks are traumatic (MVA, GSW, iatrogenic)

Clinical Issues
- Up to 85% resolve spontaneously within 7 days, almost all within 6 months

DIFFERENTIAL DIAGNOSIS

Rhinorrhea
- Vasomotor rhinitis, post-traumatic autonomic dysfunction

Otorrhea
- Otitis media with TM perforation, otitis externa, external auditory canal (EAC) foreign body

PATHOLOGY

General Features
- Etiology: Most CSF leaks are traumatic (MVA, GSW, iatrogenic)
- Epidemiology: Incidence: 2-9% of patients with head injury, 30% of patients with skull base fracture

CLINICAL ISSUES

Presentation
- Most common signs/symptoms: Watery fluid leaking from nose or EAC, usually within 48 hours of trauma
- Other signs/symptoms
  - Periorbital or mastoid ecchymosis, swelling
  - Optic neuropathy, oculomotor dysfunction (orbital injury), anosmia (olfactory bulb injury)
  - Conductive or sensorineural hearing loss, vertigo, CN VII paresis (temporal bone injuries)
- Laboratory tests for CSF: β2-transferrin = protein found in CSF, newer β trace protein test

Natural History & Prognosis
- Up to 85% resolve spontaneously within 7 days, almost all within 6 months
- Meningitis (up to 50% of persistent CSF fistulas)

Treatment
- Bedrest, lumbar drain
- Endonasal endoscopic repair for persistent sinonasal leaks vs. extracranial extradural or transcranial repair
- Middle fossa or mastoid approach for T-bone leaks

DIAGNOSTIC CHECKLIST

Consider
- T-bone as source of leak even if CSF rhinorrhea

SELECTED REFERENCES

1. Buchanan RJ et al: Traumatic cerebrospinal fluid fistulas. In: Winn HR, ed. Youmans Neurological Surgery. 5th ed. Philadelphia: W. B. Saunders Co. 5265-72, 2004
2. Stone JA et al: Evaluation of CSF leaks: high-resolution CT compared with contrast-enhanced CT and radionuclide cisternography. AJNR Am J Neuroradiol. 20(4):706-12, 1999
3. El Gammal T et al: Cerebrospinal fluid fistula: detection with MR cisternography. AJNR Am J Neuroradiol. 19(4):627-31, 1998

IMAGE GALLERY

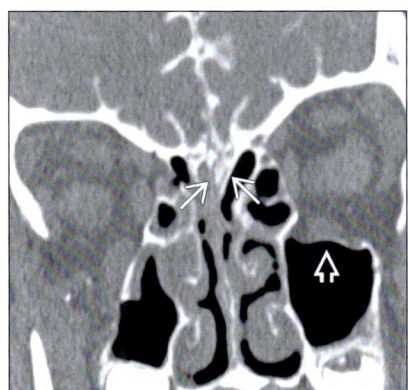 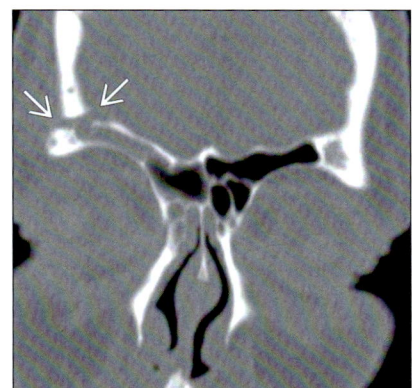 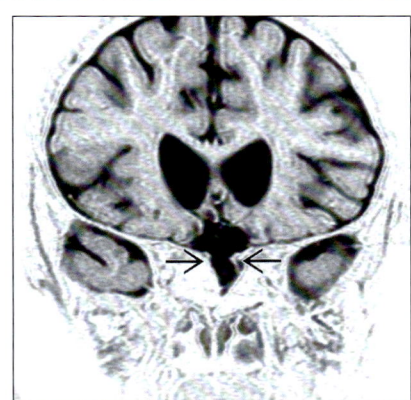

(Left) Coronal CT cisternogram shows contrast-opacified CSF traversing defect in left cribriform plate ➡. Also, note depressed left orbital floor fracture ➡. *(Center)* Coronal NECT shows iatrogenic CSF leak produced by craniotomy traversing apex of right frontal sinus ➡. *(Right)* Coronal heavily T2-weighted, video-inverted "MR cisternogram" shows post-traumatic defect in left planum sphenoidale ➡, responsible for CSF leak.

LARYNX TRAUMA

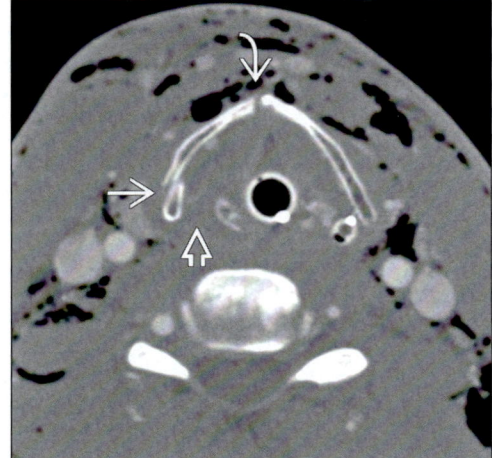

Axial CECT shows vertical fractures of thyroid ala ➡ and symphysis ⬆, with widening of right cricothyroid joint ➡.

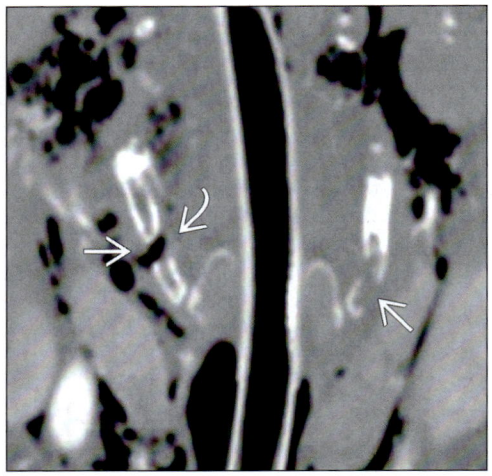

Coronal CECT shows bilateral horizontal thyroid alar fractures ➡. Note gas ➡ within right alar fracture, consistent with mucosal laceration.

TERMINOLOGY

Definitions
- Fracture of laryngeal cartilages or dislocation of laryngeal articulations by blunt or penetrating injury

IMAGING FINDINGS

General Features
- Best diagnostic clue: Airway narrowing and laryngeal cartilage deformity with vocal cord enlargement & extraluminal gas
- Location
  - Thyroid or cricoid cartilage fractures
  - Arytenoid cartilage, cricothyroid joint dislocation

Radiographic Findings
- Radiography
  - Deformity of larynx, narrowing of airway
  - Extraluminal gas (implies mucosal laceration)

CT Findings
- NECT
  - Laryngeal cartilage displacement
  - Vocal cord, paraglottic, subglottic swelling with airway narrowing
  - Extraluminal gas (mucosal laceration)
  - Thyroid cartilage fractures
    - Vertical: Midline or paramedian, alar splaying
    - Horizontal: Better depicted on coronal images
  - Cricothyroid joint dislocation, widening
  - Cricoid (ring) fractures typically bilateral
  - Arytenoid cartilage dislocation, typically anterior
  - Epiglottic injury with soft tissue swelling, posterior displacement of petiole, epiglottic tear

Imaging Recommendations
- Best imaging tool
  - CT demonstrates soft tissue and cartilage injury best
  - MR useful for epiglottic injuries
- Protocol advice
  - Thin (1-1.5 mm) axial helical CT slices
  - Review both bone and soft tissue windows
    - Soft tissue algorithm/window helpful for analyzing poorly ossified cartilage
  - Multiplanar & 3D reconstructions help define cartilage injury

DDx: Laryngeal Cartilage Deformity/Disruption

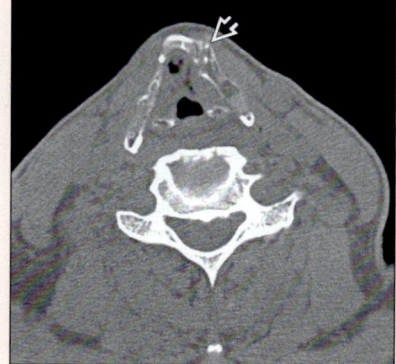

Chronic Fracture

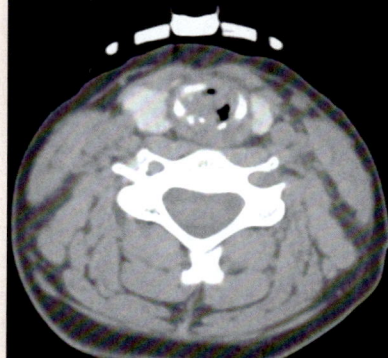

SLE Chondritis

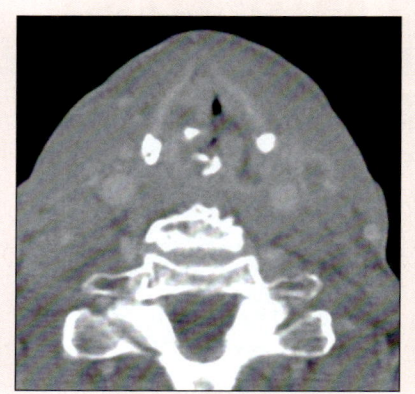

RT Cricoid Necrosis

LARYNX TRAUMA

Key Facts

Imaging Findings
- Best diagnostic clue: Airway narrowing and laryngeal cartilage deformity with vocal cord enlargement & extraluminal gas
- Laryngeal cartilage displacement
- Vocal cord, paraglottic, subglottic swelling with airway narrowing
- Extraluminal gas (mucosal laceration)
- CT demonstrates soft tissue and cartilage injury best

Top Differential Diagnoses
- Relapsing Polychondritis
- Anatomic/Rotational Deformity Related to Denervation
- Post-Radiation Chondronecrosis
- Vocal Cord Paralysis (VCP) Treatment

Pathology
- Blunt trauma, especially MVA (including airbag injury)
- Penetrating injury (GSW, knife)
- Arytenoid cartilage dislocation
- Cervical spine fractures, vascular, or esophageal injuries must be excluded

Clinical Issues
- Respiratory distress, stridor, cough, hemoptysis, anterior neck pain
- Hoarseness, dysphonia, vocal cord paralysis

Diagnostic Checklist
- Maintain low threshold for performing CTA in penetrating injuries
- View images in ST window!

- Non-penetrating injury: IV contrast not necessary
- Penetrating injuries: Conduct as cervical CT angiogram, evaluate larynx and cervical arteries

DIFFERENTIAL DIAGNOSIS

Relapsing Polychondritis
- Autoimmune cartilage destruction associated with collagen vascular diseases (especially SLE)
- Affects ear, nose, articular cartilage, larynx, tracheobronchial tree
- Laryngeal edema, sclerosis, enlargement or demineralization of cartilage

Anatomic/Rotational Deformity Related to Denervation
- Arytenoid displaced anteromedially
- Causative lesion often found along course of vagus or recurrent laryngeal nerve
- Atrophy of ipsilateral cricoarytenoid muscle

Post-Radiation Chondronecrosis
- Sclerosis, fragmentation of cartilage

Vocal Cord Paralysis (VCP) Treatment
- Teflon (hyperdense on CT) injected into paralyzed true vocal cord to improve voice quality

Old Fracture
- Thickening, deformity of affected cartilage, sclerosis of fracture margins

PATHOLOGY

General Features
- Etiology
  - Blunt trauma, especially MVA (including airbag injury)
    - Larynx compressed against cervical spine, splitting thyroid cartilage and crushing cricoid
    - Soft tissue injuries due to shearing forces
  - Penetrating injury (GSW, knife)
  - Clothesline injury (victim's neck collides with horizontal barrier)
    - Laryngeal fractures, laryngotracheal separation
    - High incidence of recurrent laryngeal nerve injury
  - Strangulation, hanging
    - Laryngeal fractures without mucosal lacerations
  - Iatrogenic injury 2° intubation
    - Mucosal injury: Abrasions or lacerations
    - Arytenoid cartilage dislocation
- Epidemiology
  - 1:30,000 ER visits
  - 1-6 patients per 15,000 to 42,500 trauma victims
  - Incidence decreasing in seat belt era (especially with shoulder harness, airbags)
- Associated abnormalities
  - Cervical spine fractures, vascular, or esophageal injuries must be excluded
  - Hyoid fractures rare (protective effect of mandible, hyoid mobility)
    - Direct blow or avulsion mechanisms (forced extension)
    - Managed conservatively unless airway compromise or pharyngeal perforation
  - Epiglottic injury
    - Blunt trauma or "clothesline" mechanisms
    - Include epiglottic tears, avulsion (at petiole)
    - Identification may be delayed
  - Arytenoid cartilage dislocation (usually anterior displacement)
    - More commonly due to traumatic intubation than blunt trauma
    - Important to identify early as delayed reduction is more difficult
  - Recurrent laryngeal nerve injury (self limited or permanent)

Gross Pathologic & Surgical Features
- Thyroid cartilage fractures tend to be horizontal and bilateral or vertical (midline or paramedian)
- Cricoid fractures usually multiple, disrupt ring, may lead to airway collapse

LARYNX TRAUMA

- Laryngotracheal separation involves horizontal tracheal tear, often acutely fatal

Staging, Grading or Classification Criteria
- Schaefer Group I: Minor hematoma, no fracture
- Schaefer Group II: Edema/hematoma, minor mucosal injury, no cartilage exposure, nondisplaced fracture
- Schaefer Group III: Massive edema, mucosal tear, exposed cartilage, VC immobility
- Schaefer Group IV: Group III + more than 2 fracture lines, massive mucosal trauma
- Schaefer Group V: Complete laryngotracheal separation

CLINICAL ISSUES

Presentation
- Most common signs/symptoms
  - Respiratory distress, stridor, cough, hemoptysis, anterior neck pain
  - Hoarseness, dysphonia, vocal cord paralysis
  - Subcutaneous emphysema, ecchymosis
  - Loss of tracheal protuberance ("Adam's apple"), tracheal deviation
- Clinical Profile: Patient with anterior neck trauma, stridor, change in voice, neck ecchymosis, subcutaneous emphysema

Demographics
- Age
  - Laryngeal injury less common in children (higher riding larynx sheltered by mandible)
  - Laryngeal soft tissue injuries more common in pediatric age group

Natural History & Prognosis
- Penetrating injuries more likely than blunt injuries to require open exploration/repair
- Severity of injury (especially to cricoid), adequacy of repair influence return to normal function
- Early definitive surgical treatment associated with better outcome
- Adverse outcomes from laryngeal trauma
  - Granulation tissue with airway compromise (early), laryngotracheal stenosis (late)
  - Vocal cord immobility with loss or alteration of voice (vocal cord paralysis or arytenoid dislocation)
  - Disordered swallowing ± aspiration

Treatment
- Stabilize airway: Intubation or tracheotomy for unstable airway
- Endoscopy and surgical exploration to assess for
  - Mucosal tears (predispose to infection), cartilage exposure (predisposes to chondronecrosis, fibrosis, granulation tissue formation)
  - Cricoid fractures, multiple or displaced fractures, displaced cricoarytenoid joint
  - Vocal cord immobility or laceration, hemorrhage
- Nonoperative management
  - Patients with only minor mucosal lacerations sparing free margin of vocal cord and anterior commissure
  - Single nondisplaced thyroid cartilage fracture, no exposed cartilage
- Displaced, comminuted laryngeal fractures treated with open reduction & internal fixation
- Airway stenting may be required for extensive laryngeal injuries
  - Helps prevent luminal stenosis, preserve normal shape of endolarynx
  - Stent should extend from level of false cord to level of first tracheal ring
- Treatment of epiglottic injuries may include primary repair with or without stenting or supraglottic hemilaryngectomy

DIAGNOSTIC CHECKLIST

Consider
- Maintain low threshold for performing CTA in penetrating injuries
- Arytenoid dislocation can mimic paralyzed vocal cord clinically and on imaging (look at cricoarytenoid muscles!)

Image Interpretation Pearls
- Fractures may be obscured or mimicked by incomplete ossification or artifacts from endotracheal tubes
- Aryepiglottic (AE) fold hematoma suggests cricoarytenoid joint disruption
- View images in ST window!

SELECTED REFERENCES
1. Bhojani RA et al: Contemporary assessment of laryngotracheal trauma. J Thorac Cardiovasc Surg. 130(2):426-32, 2005
2. Atkins BZ et al: Current management of laryngotracheal trauma: case report and literature review. J Trauma. 56(1):185-90, 2004
3. Hwang SY et al: Management dilemmas in laryngeal trauma. J Laryngol Otol. 118(5):325-8, 2004
4. Kuttenberger JJ et al: Diagnosis and initial management of laryngotracheal injuries associated with facial fractures. J Craniomaxillofac Surg. 32(2):80-4, 2004
5. de Mello-Filho FV et al: The management of laryngeal fractures using internal fixation. Laryngoscope. 110(12):2143-6, 2000
6. Perdikis G et al: Blunt laryngeal fracture: another airbag injury. J Trauma. 48(3):544-6, 2000
7. Brosch S et al: Clinical course of acute laryngeal trauma and associated effects on phonation. J Laryngol Otol. 113(1):58-61, 1999
8. Hoover CA et al: Vocal fold hemorrhage following laryngeal trauma. Ear Nose Throat J. 77(5):364-6, 1998
9. Cozzi S et al: Difficult diagnosis of laryngeal blunt trauma. J Trauma. 40(5):845-6, 1996
10. Duda JJ Jr et al: MR evaluation of epiglottic disruption. AJNR Am J Neuroradiol. 17(3):563-6, 1996
11. Bent JP 3rd et al: The management of blunt fractures of the thyroid cartilage. Otolaryngol Head Neck Surg. 110(2):195-202, 1994
12. Kadish H et al: Blunt pediatric laryngotracheal trauma: case reports and review of the literature. Am J Emerg Med. 12(2):207-11, 1994
13. Meglin AJ et al: Three-dimensional computerized tomography in the evaluation of laryngeal injury. Laryngoscope. 101(2):202-7, 1991

LARYNX TRAUMA

IMAGE GALLERY

Typical

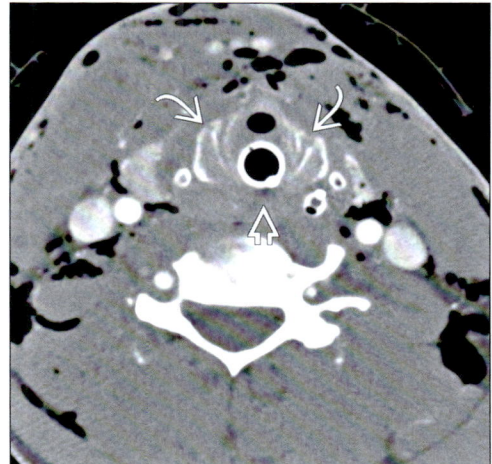
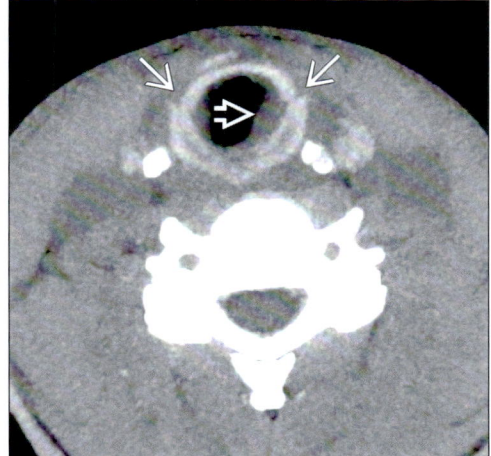

(Left) Axial CECT shows bilateral cricoid fractures ➔ with telescoped fragments. Endotracheal tube artifacts ➔ and poor cartilage ossification may complicate detection of laminar fractures. *(Right)* Axial NECT with slice averaging shows bilateral cricoid ring fractures ➔. Note mucosal edema on left side ➔.

Typical

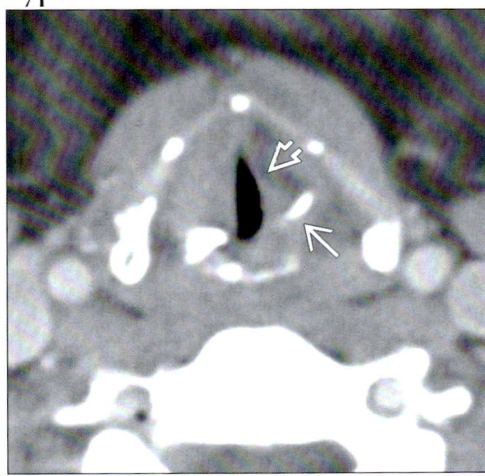
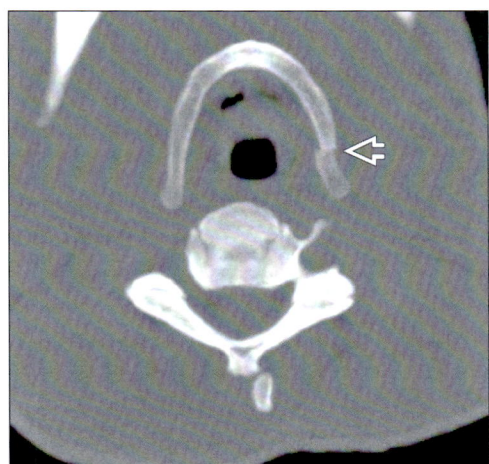

(Left) Axial CECT shows anteromedial left arytenoid cartilage dislocation ➔. Left true cord ➔ appears paretic, atrophic. *(Right)* Axial Bone CT shows mildly displaced left hyoid laminar fracture ➔ resulting from blow to lateral aspect of neck. These fractures are usually treated conservatively.

Typical

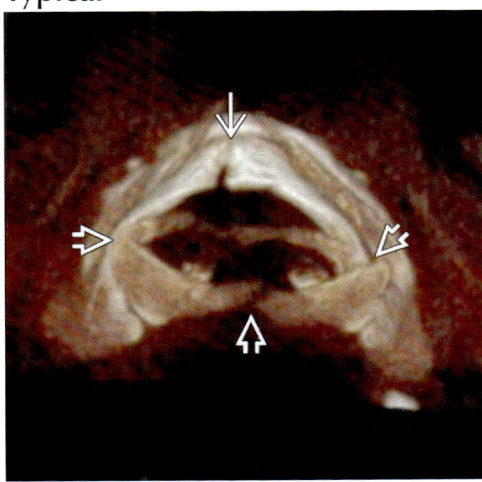
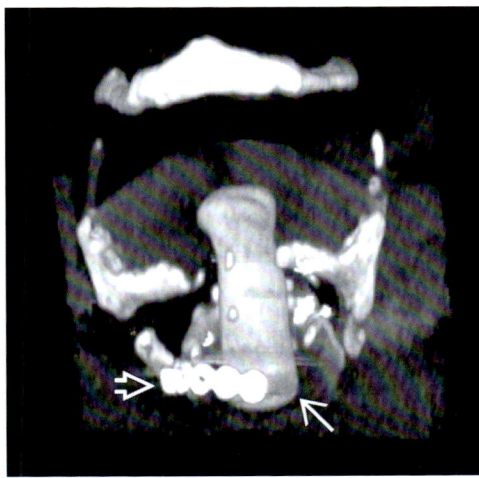

(Left) Axial oblique 3D volume-rendered CT shows laryngeal collapse due to blunt injury. Note vertical thyroid symphysis fracture ➔ and comminuted, collapsed cricoid ring ➔. *(Right)* Anterior 3D volume-rendered CT shows repaired laryngeal fractures with microplate ➔ and solid endoluminal stent ➔ in place.

LEFORT FRACTURES I-III

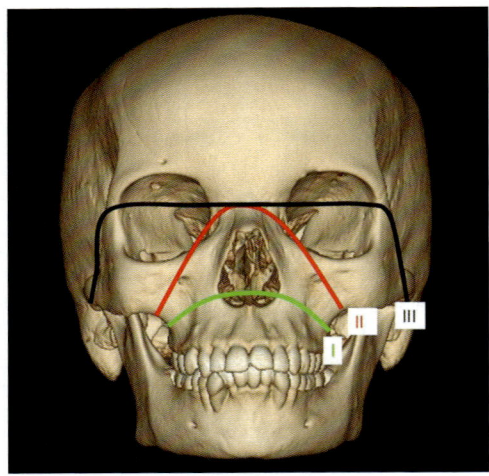

Coronal graphic shows lines defining the three types of LeFort fractures. LF I (green) involves the nasal aperture, LF II (red) the inferior orbital rim, and LF III (black) the zygomatic arch.

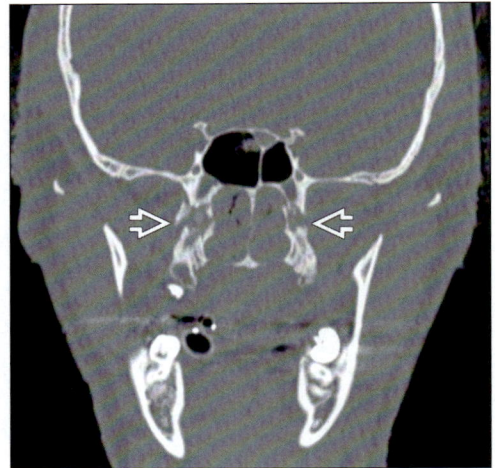

Coronal planar reconstruction from axial helical bone CT shows bilateral fractures ➡ through pterygoid processes, the sine qua non of LeFort fractures.

TERMINOLOGY

Abbreviations and Synonyms
- LF I-III; transfacial fractures

Definitions
- Fractures disrupting pterygomaxillary junction, fracturing pterygoid processes/plates & disjoining portions of face (maxilla) from skull
- Type I: Guerin fracture, "floating palate"
  - Separates palate & maxillary alveolus from remainder of the upper face and skull
  - Horizontal orientation, extends to anterolateral nasal fossa (pyriform aperture), involves medial and lateral walls of maxillary sinus and nasal septum
  - Result from blow to upper lip area
- Type II: Pyramidal fracture, separates midface from skull
  - Most common type of LeFort fracture
  - Involves inferomedial orbital rim, anteromedial orbital wall, frontonasal junction (or frontal process of maxilla)
  - May result from a descending impact to the nasal region or a broad blow to the midface
- Type III: Craniofacial disassociation
  - Rarest form, uncommon in isolation, associated with high energy injury, intracranial injuries
  - Separates entire face from skull
  - Involves frontonasal junction, medial & lateral orbital walls & zygomatic arch(es)
- Combinations of LeFort fracture types, unilateral/asymmetric LeFort fractures, and combinations of LeFort fractures with other facial fracture types (ZMC, nasoethmoid, smash) are all common

IMAGING FINDINGS

General Features
- Best diagnostic clue: Pterygoid process and pterygoid plate fractures in patients with clinically mobile facial skeleton
- Location: Central face
- Size: Variable
- Morphology: Facial features may be depressed or downwardly displaced and elongated

DDx: LeFort Fracture Mimics

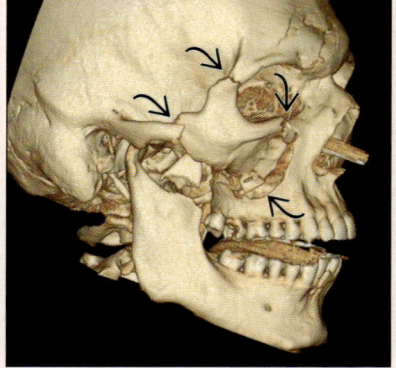

ZMC Fracture

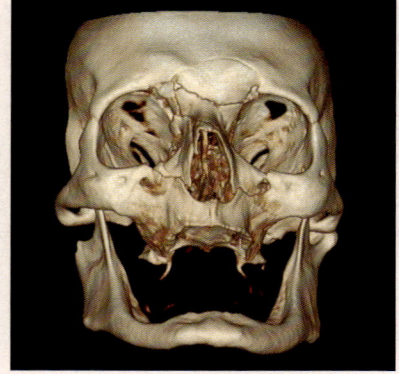

Nasoethmoid Fracture

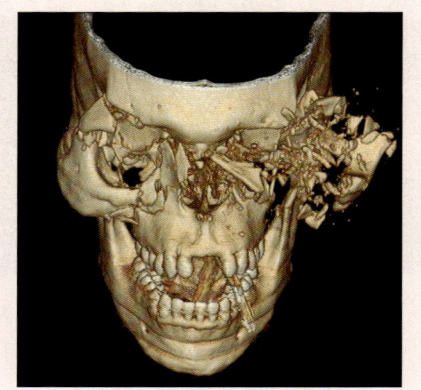

Smash Fracture

LEFORT FRACTURES I-III

Key Facts

Terminology
- Type I: Guerin fracture, "floating palate"
- Type II: Pyramidal fracture, separates midface from skull
- Type III: Craniofacial disassociation

Imaging Findings
- Non-contrast axial helical CT, slice thickness 1 mm or less, bone algorithm, coronal and 3D reconstructions
- Scan plane parallel to orbitomeatal (OM) line (from inferior orbital rim to top of external auditory meatus)
- Volume rendered 3D reconstructions from high resolution axial helical data sets greatly facilitate fracture analysis and assist in surgical planning

Diagnostic Checklist
- Remember the components that are unique to each LF fracture type
- Assess facial buttresses (transverse and vertical)
- Identify fractures or fracture fragments jeopardizing the optic nerve
- Be vigilant for fractures traversing central skull base/carotid canals; have a low threshold for performing conventional or CT angiography to exclude carotid injury
- Assess orbital volume, frontonasal duct integrity, floor and medial orbital wall, including bone at medial canthal ligament insertion
- Identify sagittal hard palate fractures (expected with displaced unilateral LeFort fractures) which must be addressed before repair of facial buttresses

Imaging Recommendations
- Best imaging tool
  - Computed tomography
  - CT cisternography for CSF leak
  - MRI for evaluation of posttraumatic optic neuropathy, diplopia unexplained by CT findings and possibly due to brainstem DAI
- Protocol advice
  - Non-contrast axial helical CT, slice thickness 1 mm or less, bone algorithm, coronal and 3D reconstructions
  - Precise patient positioning in center of gantry important for optimal analysis of symmetry for surgical planning
  - Scan plane parallel to orbitomeatal (OM) line (from inferior orbital rim to top of external auditory meatus)
  - Hard palate (or planum sphenoidale, if palate is displaced) may be used to optimally align axial slices from sagittal scanogram or sagittal planar reformation
  - Scan from above top of frontal sinuses to just below inferior mandibular margin
  - Reconstruct axials parallel to OM line when optimal positioning in scanner not possible
  - Volume rendered 3D reconstructions from high resolution axial helical data sets greatly facilitate fracture analysis and assist in surgical planning

DIFFERENTIAL DIAGNOSIS

Zygomaticomaxillary Complex Fractures
- Associated with blow to malar eminence
- Spares pterygoid process/plates
- Involves zygomaticofrontal, zygomaticomaxillary, zygomaticosphenoid, & zygomaticotemporal sutures
- Fragment often rotated or retracted by pull of masseter muscle on its zygomatic attachment
- May coexist with LeFort II fractures, but do not involve posteromedial wall of the orbit as "true" LeFort III fractures do

Nasoethmoid Fractures
- Spare pterygoid processes
- Associated with focal blow over nasal bridge
- Involve upper central midface, with accordioning of bone along lacrimal bone/lamina papyracea, depression of nasal pyramid
- Telecanthus due to displacement of medial canthal ligament attachment
- May be associated with cribriform plate injury/CSF leak, injuries of globe, optic nerve, lacrimal apparatus, nasofrontal ducts (with resultant frontal sinus mucocele formation)

Midface Smash Fracture
- Highly comminuted midface fracture
- Subdivided into nasoethmoid, frontal, central midface, & total craniofacial smash fractures
- In "pure form" spares pterygoid processes/plates, but frequently coexists with LF fractures
- Patients frequently clinically unstable, high incidence of intracranial injury

Pterygoid Plate Avulsion
- Associated with violent trauma to mandible, mandibular fractures
- Lateral pterygoid plate typically involved, pterygoid process usually spared

PATHOLOGY

General Features
- Etiology
  - Blunt facial trauma, fracturing along lines of weakness in facial skeleton
  - Most cases due to motor vehicle accidents, assaults, or falls
- Epidemiology
  - LeFort and maxillary fractures account for approximately 25.5% of facial fractures
  - LeFort II fracture is the most common type

LEFORT FRACTURES I-III

- LeFort III fracture least common type (in isolated form)
- Associated abnormalities: Intracranial and/or orbital injuries, CSF leak

CLINICAL ISSUES

Presentation
- Most common signs/symptoms
  - Mobile face (maxillary alveolus & hard palate, midface, or entire face)
  - Midface depression (retrusion), aka "dish face" deformity, facial elongation following craniofacial trauma, dental malocclusion
  - LeFort II and III fractures may present with periorbital ecchymosis and infraorbital nerve injury with resultant sensory loss, lacrimal apparatus injury with epiphora
- Other signs/symptoms: Enophthalmos, diplopia

Demographics
- Age
  - Children (up to age 16) account for only 15% of all types of facial fractures
  - Maxilla is least frequently fractured facial bone in pediatric population; mandible (especially condyle) is most frequently fractured facial bone in this group
- Gender: Male > female, but either may suffer LeFort fractures

Natural History & Prognosis
- May be complicated by long-term facial deformity, breathing difficulty, masticatory problems/malocclusion, telecanthus, visual loss, diplopia, anosmia, epiphora, facial numbness, and headaches

Treatment
- Surgical reduction and fixation of facial fractures usually starts with frontal bar (thickened frontal bone above frontonasal sutures & superior orbital rims)
- Other facial bones are "suspended" from frontal bar by open reduction/internal fixation with titanium plates & screws, fixing fractures in top-to-bottom fashion
- Zygomaticofrontal suture injuries usually repaired first, fixation of palatoalveolar complex last
- Associated orbital fractures are repaired after horizontal & vertical buttresses are surgically reconstituted

DIAGNOSTIC CHECKLIST

Image Interpretation Pearls
- Remember the components that are unique to each LF fracture type
  - I: Lateral margin of nasal aperture
  - II: Inferior orbital rim
  - III: Zygomatic arch
- Don't forget that more than one LF fracture type may coexist in the same patient
- Assess facial buttresses (transverse and vertical)
- Identify fractures or fracture fragments jeopardizing the optic nerve
- Be vigilant for fractures traversing central skull base/carotid canals; have a low threshold for performing conventional or CT angiography to exclude carotid injury
- Assess orbital volume, frontonasal duct integrity, floor and medial orbital wall, including bone at medial canthal ligament insertion
- Identify sagittal hard palate fractures (expected with displaced unilateral LeFort fractures) which must be addressed before repair of facial buttresses

SELECTED REFERENCES

1. Back CP et al: The conservative management of facial fractures: indications and outcomes. J Plast Reconstr Aesthet Surg. 60(2):146-51, 2007
2. Hopper RA et al: Diagnosis of midface fractures with CT: what the surgeon needs to know. Radiographics. 26(3):783-93, 2006
3. Zimmermann CE et al: Pediatric facial fractures: recent advances in prevention, diagnosis and management. Int J Oral Maxillofac Surg. 35(1):2-13, 2006
4. Connor SE et al: Computed tomography pseudofractures of the mid face and skull base. Clin Radiol. 60(12):1268-79, 2005
5. Rhea JT et al: How to simplify the CT diagnosis of Le Fort fractures. AJR Am J Roentgenol. 184(5):1700-5, 2005
6. Gassner R et al: Craniomaxillofacial trauma in children: a review of 3,385 cases with 6,060 injuries in 10 years. J Oral Maxillofac Surg. 62(4):399-407, 2004
7. Turner BG et al: Trends in the use of CT and radiography in the evaluation of facial trauma, 1992-2002: implications for current costs. AJR Am J Roentgenol. 183(3):751-4, 2004
8. Linnau KF et al: Imaging of high-energy midfacial trauma: what the surgeon needs to know. Eur J Radiol. 48(1):17-32, 2003
9. Linnau KF et al: Orbital apex injury: trauma at the junction between the face and the cranium. Eur J Radiol. 48(1):5-16, 2003
10. Salvolini U: Traumatic injuries: imaging of facial injuries. Eur Radiol. 12(6):1253-61, 2002
11. Sun JK et al: Imaging of facial trauma. Neuroimaging Clin N Am. 12(2):295-309, 2002
12. Girotto JA et al: Long-term physical impairment and functional outcomes after complex facial fractures. Plast Reconstr Surg. 108(2):312-27, 2001
13. Haug RH et al: Maxillofacial injuries in the pediatric patient. Oral Surg Oral Med Oral Pathol Oral Radiol Endod. 90(2):126-34, 2000
14. Rhea JT et al: Helical CT and three-dimensional CT of facial and orbital injury. Radiol Clin North Am. 37(3):489-513, 1999
15. Manson PN et al: Toward CT-based facial fracture treatment. Plast Reconstr Surg. 85(2):202-12; discussion 213-4, 1990

LEFORT FRACTURES I-III

IMAGE GALLERY

Typical

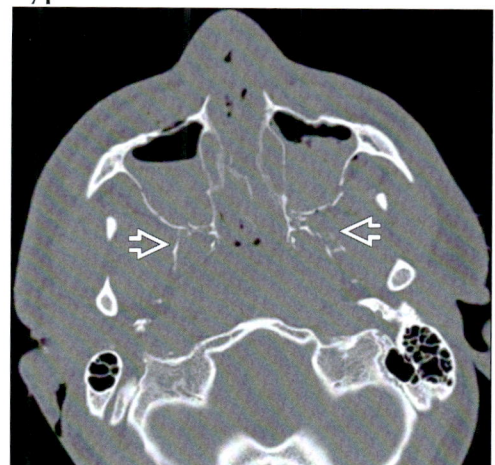
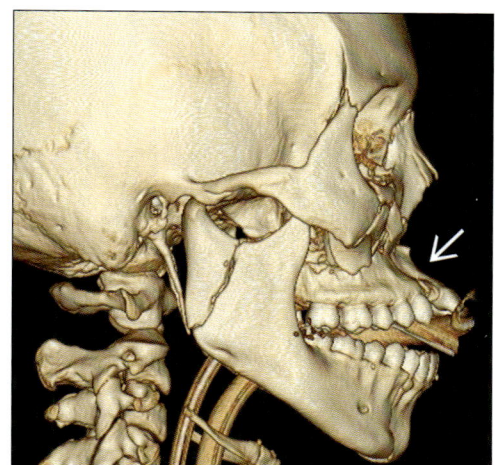

(Left) Axial bone CT shows bilateral pterygoid plate fractures ➔. *(Right)* Lateral 3D CT shows midface up-rotation and depression in patient with LeFort I, II, and III fractures. Note nearly horizontal orientation of premaxilla ➔.

Typical

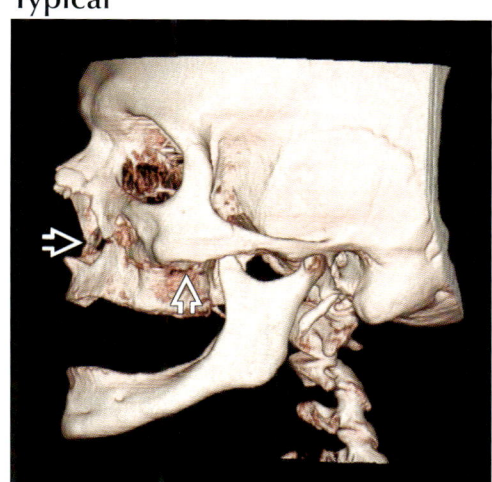
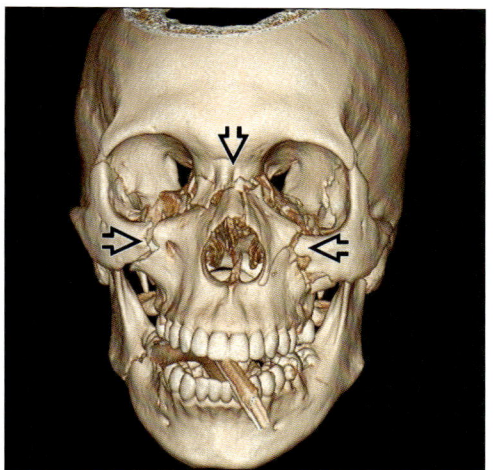

(Left) Oblique lateral 3D CT shows horizontal LeFort I fracture ➔ separating maxillary alveolus from midface. Note involvement of nasal aperture, but intact inferior orbital rim and zygomatic arch. *(Right)* Coronal 3D CT shows LeFort II fracture ➔ with subtle clockwise rotation of the midface and an asymmetric bite. Note bilateral inferior orbital rim involvement, sparing of nasal aperture.

Typical

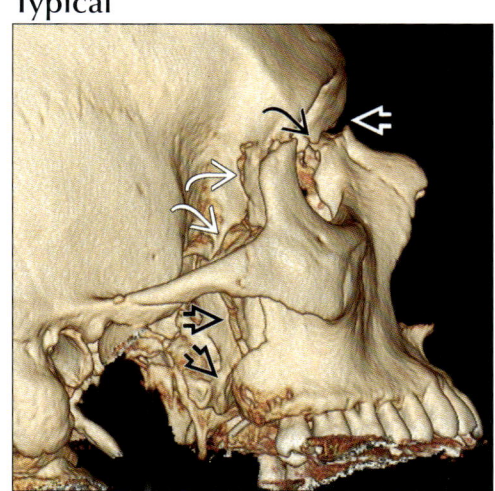
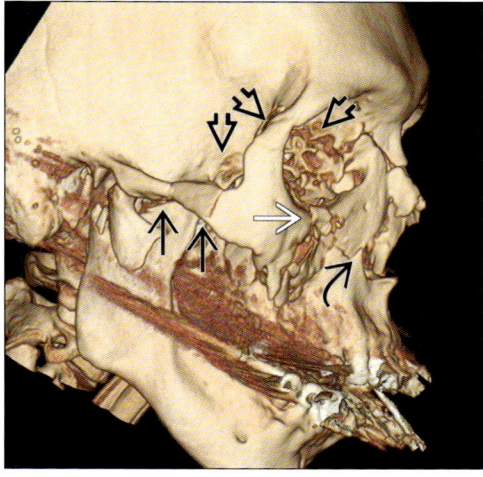

(Left) Lateral 3D CT (mandible removed) of right LeFort III fracture: Frontonasal diastasis ➔, medial ➔ and lateral ➔ orbital wall fractures, pterygoid plate fractures ➔; sparing of inferior orbital rim. *(Right)* Oblique 3D CT shows components of all LeFort fracture types including lateral, posteromedial orbit ➔ & zygomatic arch ➔ (LF III); nasal aperture ➔ (LF I); inferior orbital rim ➔ (LF II).

ATLANTO-OCCIPITAL DISLOCATION

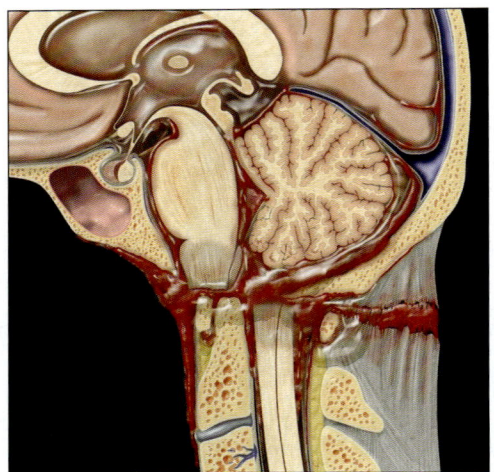

Sagittal graphic shows fatal AOD with cord transection. C1 is displaced posteriorly relative to skull base.

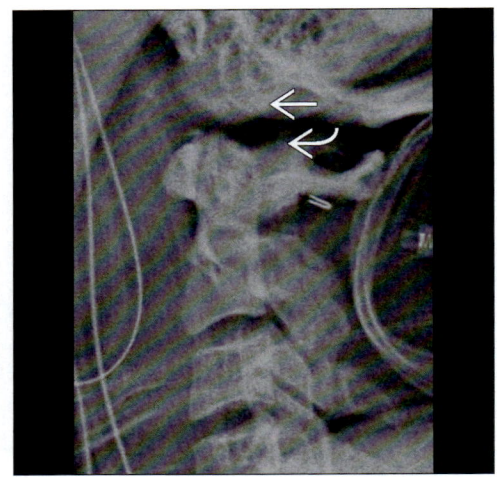

Lateral radiograph shows separation between occipital condyle ⇨ and C1 ⇨.

TERMINOLOGY

Abbreviations and Synonyms
- Craniocervical dissociation
- Atlanto-occipital dislocation (AOD)

Definitions
- Disruption of stabilizing ligaments occiput to C1

IMAGING FINDINGS

General Features
- Best diagnostic clue: Widening between occipital condyles and C1

Radiographic Findings
- Radiography
  - Increased distance from basion to odontoid
    - Normal < 4-5 mm; children < 10 mm
  - Powers ratio > 1.15 indicative of AOD
    - BC = distance from tip of clivus (basion) to anterior cortex of C1 posterior arch
    - AO = distance from C1 anterior arch to posterior margin foramen magnum (opisthion)
  - Odontoid view: ↑ Space between condyles & C1
  - Widened prevertebral soft tissues (nonspecific)

CT Findings
- Coronal & sagittal: Widened space between occipital condyles & C1
- Axial: May see portions of C1 on same image as occipital condyles

MR Findings
- Displacement seen on coronal, sagittal images
- STIR best shows ligamentous injury
- MRA for vertebral artery injury

Imaging Recommendations
- Best imaging tool: Thin section (~ 1 mm) helical CT with coronal & sagittal reformations

DIFFERENTIAL DIAGNOSIS

Occipital Condyle Fracture
- Best seen on CT; may be associated with AOD

DDx: Craniocervical Instability

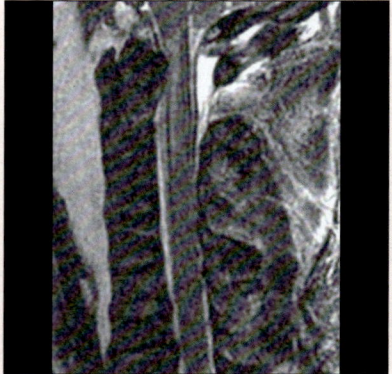

AOD Cord & Apical Ligament Edema

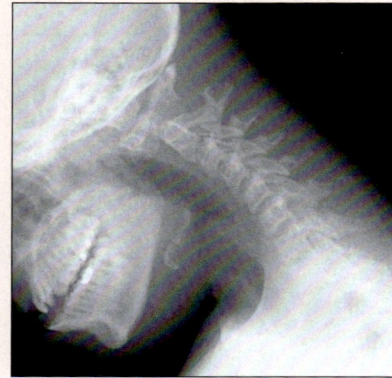

Down Syndrome

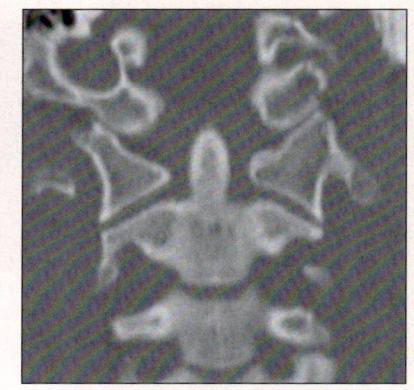

Occipital Condylar Fx

ATLANTO-OCCIPITAL DISLOCATION

Key Facts

Terminology
- Disruption of stabilizing ligaments occiput to C1

Imaging Findings
- Increased distance from basion to odontoid
- Powers ratio > 1.15 indicative of AOD
- Coronal & sagittal: Widened space between occipital condyles & C1
- Axial: May see portions of C1 on same image as occipital condyles

- Best imaging tool: Thin section (~ 1 mm) helical CT with coronal & sagittal reformations

Pathology
- Etiology: High speed motor vehicle accident

Clinical Issues
- Often immediately fatal with high incidence neurologic deficits in survivors

Down Syndrome
- Nontraumatic atlanto-occipital instability

PATHOLOGY

General Features
- Etiology: High speed motor vehicle accident
- Epidemiology: < 1% of acute cervical spine injuries
- Associated abnormalities: Brainstem, cranial nerve & multi-level cervical injuries

Gross Pathologic & Surgical Features
- Rupture of ligaments between C1 and skull, dens and skull
  - Tectorial membrane: Prime stabilizer occiput to C1
    - Continuation posterior longitudinal ligament; attaches to inner surface clivus
  - Alar ligaments
    - Tip of dens superolaterally to foramen magnum; rotational stability
  - Anterior atlanto-occipital ligament
    - Continuation anterior longitudinal ligament; C1 anterior arch to anterior cortex clivus
  - Posterior atlanto-occipital membrane
    - C1 posterior arch to opisthion
  - Apical ligament: Tip of dens to basion

Staging, Grading or Classification Criteria
- Distraction
- Anterior or posterior

CLINICAL ISSUES

Presentation
- Most common signs/symptoms: Cranial nerve injuries & motor deficit

Demographics
- Age: More common in children

Natural History & Prognosis
- Often immediately fatal with high incidence neurologic deficits in survivors

Treatment
- Occiput to C2 fusion required

DIAGNOSTIC CHECKLIST

Consider
- Separation between condyles & C1 key finding

SELECTED REFERENCES
1. Saeheng S et al: Traumatic occipitoatlantal dislocation. Surg Neurol. 55(1):35-40; discussion 40, 2001
2. Harris JH Jr et al: Radiologic diagnosis of traumatic occipitovertebral dissociation: 2. Comparison of three methods of detecting occipitovertebral relationships on lateral radiographs of supine subjects. AJR Am J Roentgenol. 162(4):887-92, 1994

IMAGE GALLERY

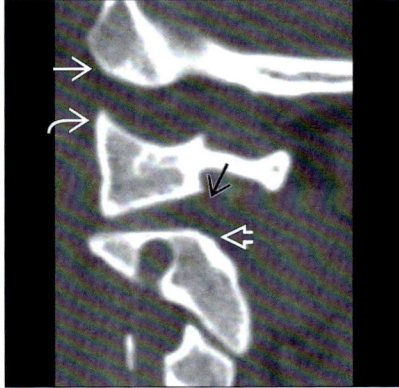
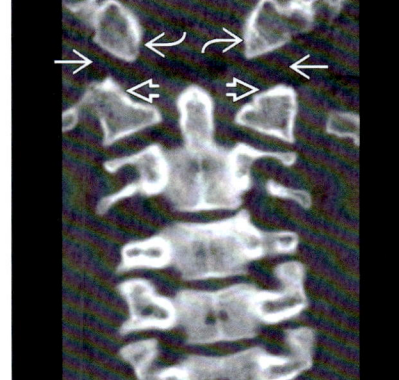
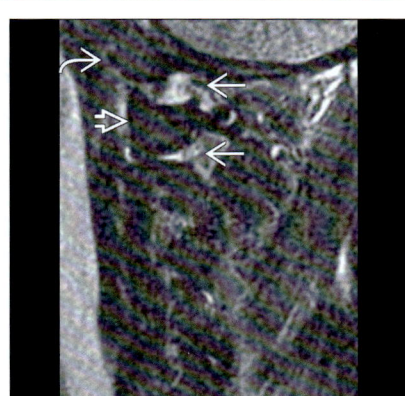

(Left) Sagittal HRCT in same patient as previous image shows marked separation between occipital condyle ➡ & lateral mass of C1 ➡. Abnormal angulation & widening between C1 ➡ & C2 ➡. *(Center)* Coronal HRCT in same case as previous image shows separation ➡ between occipital condyles & C1 lateral mass. Mild right displacement of condyles ➡ relative to C1 ➡. *(Right)* Sagittal STIR MR in same patient as previous image shows ligamentous edema ➡ & anterior superior displacement of occipital condyle ➡ relative to lateral mass of C1 ➡.

JEFFERSON C1 FRACTURE

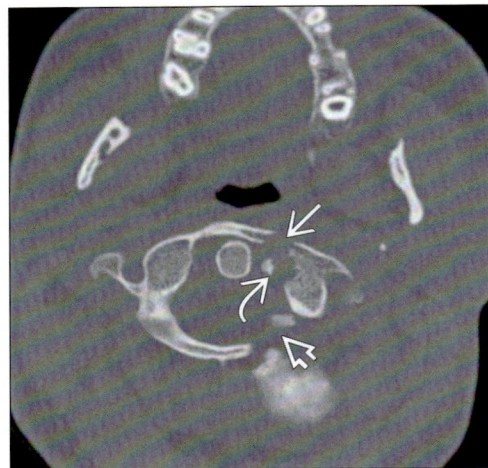

Axial bone CT shows fractures of the anterior ➡ and posterior ring ➡ of C1. Note avulsion of the odontoid ligamentous attachment ➡.

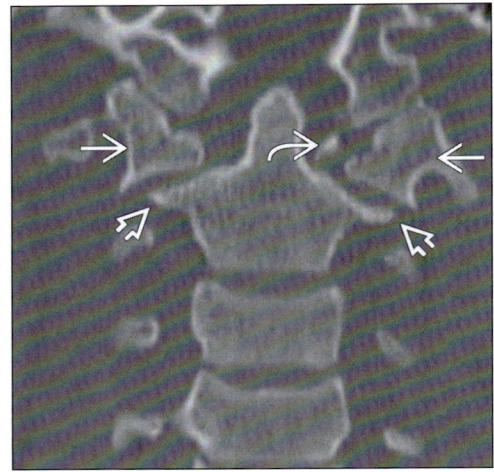

Coronal bone CT in the same patient as previous image shows lateral displacement of the C1 lateral masses ➡ relative to the C2 lateral masses ➡ as well as an avulsion fracture ➡.

TERMINOLOGY

Abbreviations and Synonyms
- Atlas burst fracture

Definitions
- Compression fracture of C1 arch

IMAGING FINDINGS

General Features
- Best diagnostic clue: Lateral displacement of both articular masses of C1 from those of C2 on open mouth radiograph

Radiographic Findings
- Radiography
  o Bony defects of C1 arch on lateral/oblique views
  o Both articular pillars of C1 offset laterally vs. C2 on open mouth view
    ▪ Normal rotation may produce apparent offset of pilar, simulating fracture
  o Separation between dens & C1 anterior arch
  o May demonstrate anterior subluxation of C1 vs. C2
    ▪ Unstable C1 fracture
    ▪ Associated C2 fracture, especially Hangman
  o Prevertebral soft tissue swelling at C1 level
  o Fractures at lower levels not uncommon

Fluoroscopic Findings
- Subluxation if unstable

CT Findings
- NECT
  o Axial CT defines components of fracture to best advantage
  o May demonstrate various patterns of arch disruption
  o May demonstrate hyperdensity in epidural space if bleeding occurs
- CTA: Loss of vertebral artery integrity if vertebrobasilar vascular syndrome present
- Bone CT
  o Disrupted ring of C1 arch
  o Multiple fractures of C1 arch
    ▪ Single site of arch fracture is rare
  o Posterior arch fracture more common than anterior
  o Both anterior and posterior arch fractures are seen in minority of cases

DDx: Jefferson Fracture

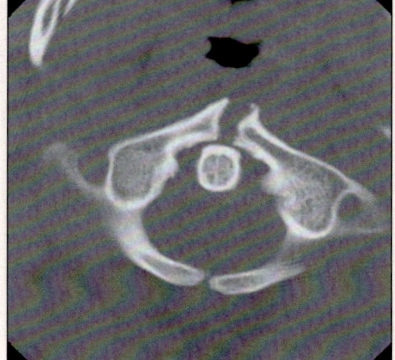

Congenital Fusion Anomaly

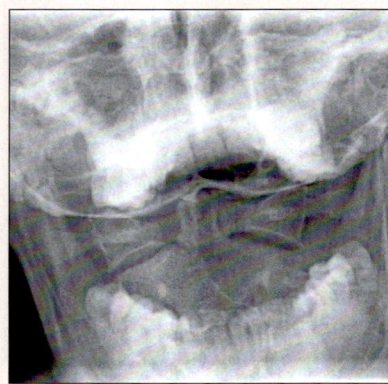

Congenital Fusion Anomaly

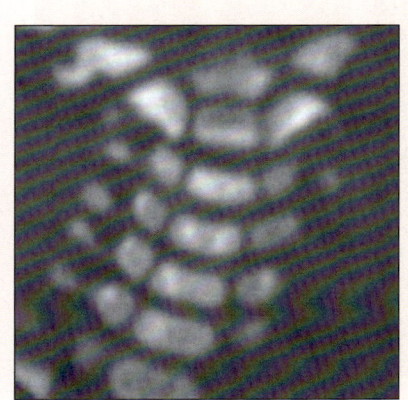

Pseudospread, 1 Year Old

JEFFERSON C1 FRACTURE

Key Facts

Terminology
- Atlas burst fracture
- Compression fracture of C1 arch

Imaging Findings
- Best diagnostic clue: Lateral displacement of both articular masses of C1 from those of C2 on open mouth radiograph
- Subluxation if unstable
- Axial CT defines components of fracture to best advantage
- May demonstrate various patterns of arch disruption
- Avulsion fragment off inner pillar at insertion of transverse ligament indicates instability
- Any lateral spread of C1 pillars on open mouth X-ray view requires CT
- Evaluate entire cervical spine as well as upper thoracic spine
- Associated fractures occur in 24-48% of cases

Top Differential Diagnoses
- Congenital Variants, Clefts, Malformations of Atlas
- Rotational Malalignment of Atlas, Axis Pillars
- Pseudospread of Atlas in Children

Diagnostic Checklist
- Routine CT of cervical spine in trauma victims with severe neck pain
- Evaluate lower levels for additional fractures
- 1-2 mm offset of C1 lateral masses vs. C2 on open mouth view in infants may be normal variant

---

- Lateral masses alone may be fractured
- Avulsion fragment off inner pillar at insertion of transverse ligament indicates instability
- Additional fractures may be present at lower levels

MR Findings
- T1WI: Prevertebral soft tissue swelling anterior to C1
- T2WI
  - High signal in soft tissue anterior to C1
  - Cord swelling
  - High or low signal if edema or hemorrhagic contusion present
- PD/Intermediate: Prevertebral soft tissue swelling
- MRA
  - Vertebral artery occlusion
  - MRA useful if delayed cerebellar or brainstem signs appear

Angiographic Findings
- Conventional
  - If CTA or MRA equivocal
  - Endovascular intervention

Imaging Recommendations
- Best imaging tool: Helical CT with reformations
- Protocol advice
  - Any lateral spread of C1 pillars on open mouth X-ray view requires CT
  - CT bone reconstruction algorithm details fracture sites
    - Distinguish well corticated margins of congenital clefts from jagged edges of fracture defect
  - Thin-section (1 mm) cuts mandatory, reformations very helpful
  - Evaluate integrity of vertebral basilar artery (VBA) foramina
  - Evaluate entire cervical spine as well as upper thoracic spine
    - Associated fractures occur in 24-48% of cases

DIFFERENTIAL DIAGNOSIS

Congenital Variants, Clefts, Malformations of Atlas
- May show 1-2 mm offset of C1 pillars from those of C2
- Clefts found in 4% of posterior arches, 0.1% of anterior arches
- 97% of posterior clefts are midline, 3% through sulcus of vertebral artery
- Various deficiencies of arch development can be seen
- Most are partial hemiaplasias of posterior arch
- Clefts, congenital defects show smooth or well-corticated edges

Rotational Malalignment of Atlas, Axis Pillars
- Generally seen unilaterally, with rotation and abduction of head

Pseudospread of Atlas in Children
- Common finding in children 3 months to four years of age evaluated for minor trauma
- Seen in 90% or more of two year olds
- Caused by disparity in growth rates of atlas and axis
- Jefferson fracture rare in young children, greater plasticity, synchondroses of C1 arch serve as "buffer"

PATHOLOGY

General Features
- General path comments
  - Rough-edge fragmentation of C1 arch at one or more sites
  - Typically stable fracture, unless transverse ligament avulsed
    - > 9 mm offset is clue to avulsion and instability
    - Unstable if transverse or posterior longitudinal ligaments disrupted or anterior arch severely comminuted
    - More often associated with severe neurological deficits, lower levels of injury

JEFFERSON C1 FRACTURE

- ○ Combined fractures occur (C2)
- Etiology
  - ○ Axial compressive force applied to skull vertex
  - ○ Force transmitted down through occipital condyles onto sloped C1 pillars with head & neck rigidly erect
    - Wedge effect
- Epidemiology
  - ○ C1 fractures represent 6% of all vertebral injuries
  - ○ One-third of C1 fractures conform to classic burst Jefferson fracture
  - ○ Rare in infants, young children
- Associated abnormalities
  - ○ Fractures at other levels
  - ○ VBA injury: Dissection or occlusion

CLINICAL ISSUES

Presentation
- Most common signs/symptoms: Upper neck pain after compression trauma (e.g., diving)
- Other signs/symptoms
  - ○ Neurologic signs uncommon unless unstable fracture or associated fractures present or VBA injured
  - ○ Fracture "blows" bone fragments away from cord
  - ○ Fracture can be missed on plain films
- Clinical Profile
  - ○ Trauma victim
  - ○ Upper neck pain

Natural History & Prognosis
- Stable fracture with healing in majority of isolated cases

Treatment
- Immobilization, fusion if gross instability

DIAGNOSTIC CHECKLIST

Consider
- Routine CT of cervical spine in trauma victims with severe neck pain
- Evaluate lower levels for additional fractures

Image Interpretation Pearls
- Well corticated edges of midline C1 arch defects are likely congenital clefts
- 1-2 mm offset of C1 lateral masses vs. C2 on open mouth view in infants may be normal variant

SELECTED REFERENCES

1. Lustrin ES et al: Pediatric cervical spine: normal anatomy, variants, and trauma. Radiographics. 23(3): 539-60, 2003
2. Torreggiani WC et al: Musculoskeletal case 20. Jefferson fracture (C1 burst fracture). Can J Surg. 45(1):16, 65-6, 2002
3. Connor SE et al: Congenital midline cleft of the posterior arch of atlas: a rare cause of symptomatic cervical canal stenosis. Eur Radiol. 11(9):1766-9, 2001
4. Harris J Jr: The cervicocranium: its radiographic assessment. Radiology. 218(2):337-51, 2001
5. Sharma A et al: Partial aplasia of the posterior arch of the atlas with an isolated posterior arch remnant: findings in three cases. AJNR Am J Neuroradiol. 21(6): 1167-71, 2000
6. Guiot B et al: Complex atlantoaxial fractures. J Neurosurg. 91(2 Suppl): 139-43, 1999
7. Haakonsen M et al: Midline anterior and posterior atlas clefts may simulate a Jefferson fracture. A report of 2 cases. Acta Orthop Scand. 66(4):369-71, 1995
8. Currarino G et al: Congenital defects of the posterior arch of the atlas: a report of seven cases including an affected mother and son. AJNR Am J Neuroradiol. 15(2):249-54, 1994
9. Kesterson L et al: Evaluation and treatment of atlas burst fractures (Jefferson fractures). J Neurosurg. 75(2):213-20, 1991
10. Lee C et al: Unstable Jefferson variant atlas fractures: an unrecognized cervical injury. AJNR Am J Neuroradiol. 12(6):1105-10, 1991
11. Gehweiler JA Jr et al: Malformations of the atlas vertebra simulating the Jefferson fracture. AJR Am J Roentgenol. 140(6):1083-6, 1983
12. Jefferson G: Fracture of the atlas vertebra. Report of four cases, and a review of those previously recorded. Br J Surg 7(27):407-22, 1919

JEFFERSON C1 FRACTURE

IMAGE GALLERY

Typical

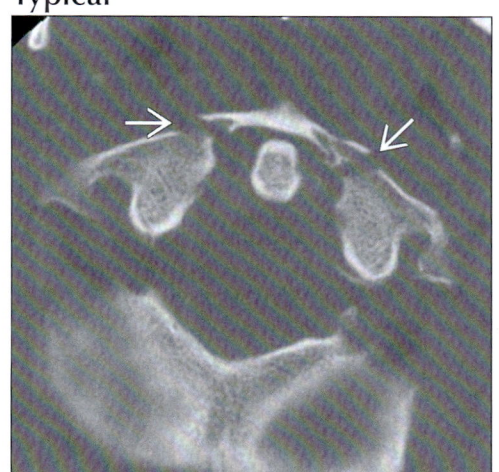
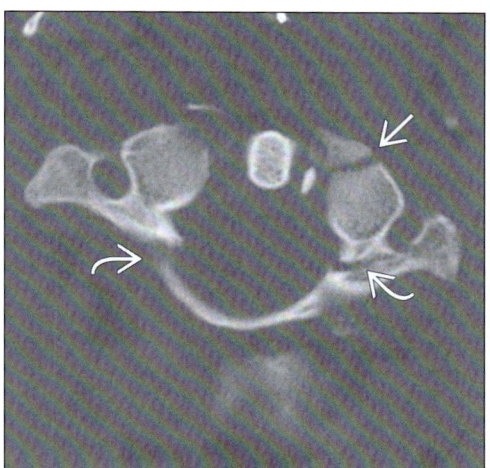

(Left) Axial NECT shows bilateral fractures of anterior ring of C1 ➡. (Right) Axial NECT in same patient as previous image shows anterior ➡ and posterior ➡ ring fractures.

Typical

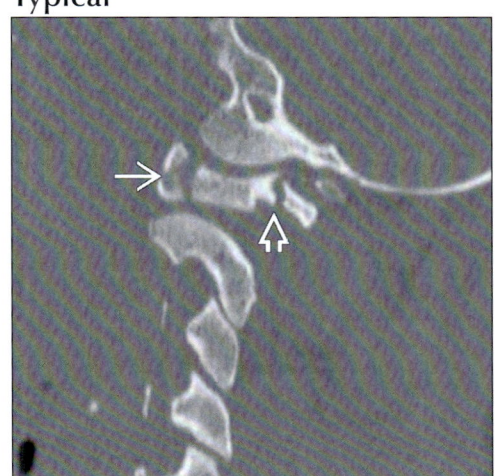
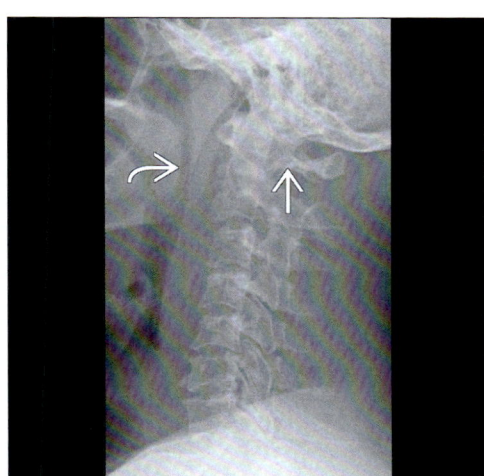

(Left) Sagittal NECT in same patient as previous image shows fractures of anterior ➡ and posterior ➡ portions of C1. (Right) Lateral radiograph shows prevertebral soft tissue swelling ➡ and fracture of posterior ➡ portion of C1 ring.

Typical

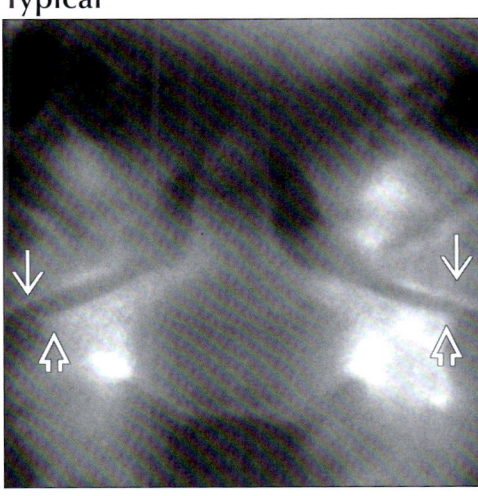
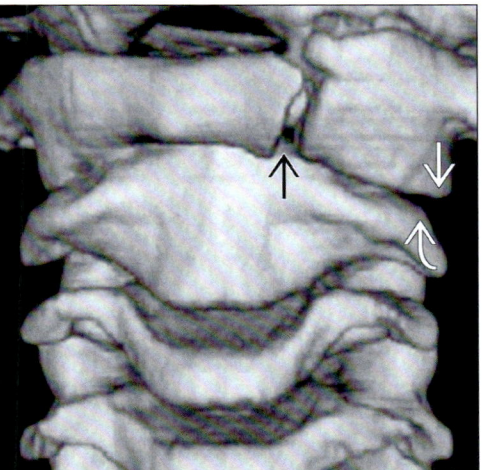

(Left) Frontal radiograph shows lateral displacement of C1 lateral masses ➡ relative to C2 lateral masses of ➡. (Right) Coronal bone CT 3D surface image reveals anterior C1 fracture ➡ with lateral displacement of C1 lateral mass ➡ on C2 ➡.

ODONTOID C2 FRACTURE

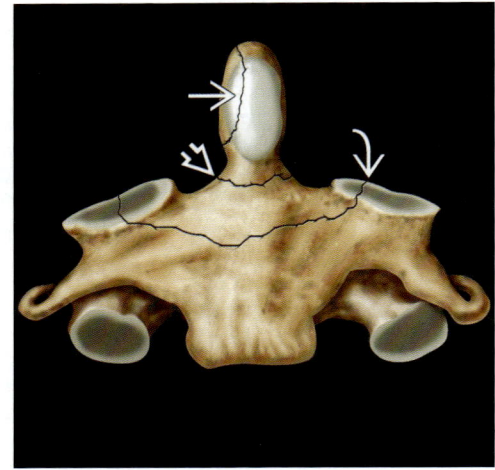

Anterior graphic shows three fractures through C2: Type I avulsion of the tip ➡; type II transverse fracture at base of dens ➡; and type III fracture extending through the body of C2 ➡.

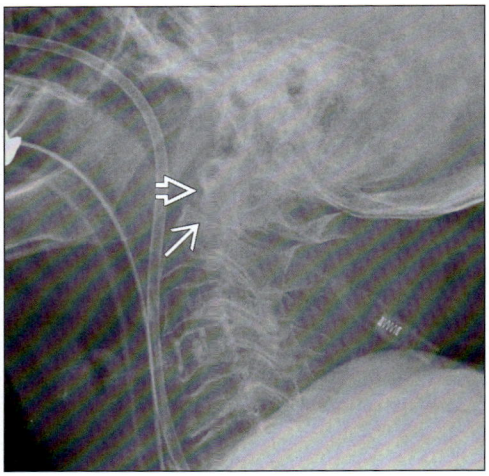

Lateral radiograph shows type II odontoid fracture ➡ with retrolisthesis of dens on C2 ➡.

TERMINOLOGY

Abbreviations and Synonyms
- Dens fracture

Definitions
- Traumatic bony disruption of odontoid process

IMAGING FINDINGS

General Features
- Best diagnostic clue
  - Lateral radiograph: Anterior or posterior displacement of C1 arch vs. C2, and prevertebral soft tissue swelling
  - Fracture visible on open mouth (dens) view

Radiographic Findings
- Radiography
  - Classic imaging appearance
    - Lucent linear defect through base of dens, posterior displacement of C1 dens arch relative to C2 body/arch
  - Open mouth frontal radiograph depicts transverse or oblique defect through dens
    - May be difficult to depict in elderly with osteoporosis
    - Overlying teeth may obscure/mimic fracture

Fluoroscopic Findings
- Evaluate stability of fusion

CT Findings
- NECT: Soft tissue swelling anterior to C2 in acute cases
- CTA: Use if vertebral artery injury is suspected
- Bone CT
  - Comminuted fracture at level of dens on axial views
  - Fracture line on reformations
  - Displacement at base of dens or tip of odontoid
  - Axial (source) images may miss or underestimate fracture if its plane parallels slice orientation
    - Use of thin section (1 mm) imaging with multi-detector scanners has made this a rare event
  - Coronal, sagittal reformations are mandatory

MR Findings
- T1WI
  - Loss of dens/C2 body contiguity

DDx: Odontoid Fracture

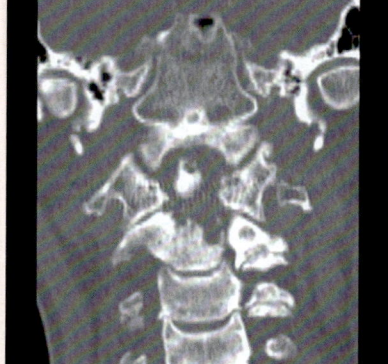

Rheumatoid Arthritis

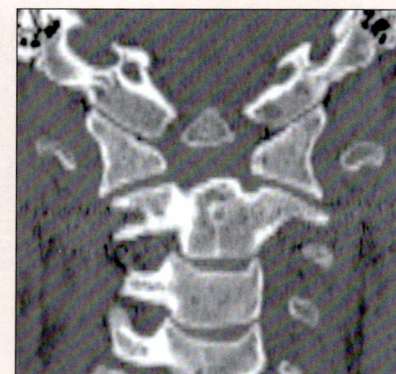

Os Odontoideum

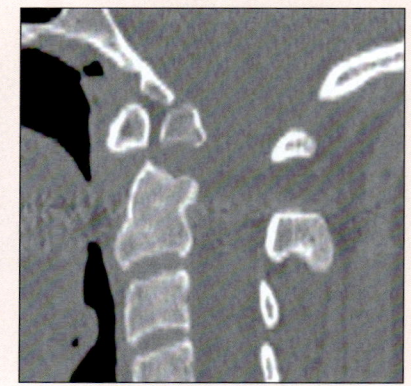

Os Odontoideum

ODONTOID C2 FRACTURE

Key Facts

Terminology
- Traumatic bony disruption of odontoid process

Imaging Findings
- Lateral radiograph: Anterior or posterior displacement of C1 arch vs. C2, and prevertebral soft tissue swelling
- Classic imaging appearance
- Open mouth frontal radiograph depicts transverse or oblique defect through dens
- May be difficult to depict in elderly with osteoporosis
- Axial (source) images may miss or underestimate fracture if its plane parallels slice orientation

Top Differential Diagnoses
- Congenital Nonunion of Odontoid Tip (Os Odontoideum)
- Congenital Variation: 3rd Occipital Condyle
- Rheumatoid Arthritis: C1/C2 Subluxation
- Pathologic C2 Fracture

Pathology
- Three ossification centers form C2
- Os odontoideum represents unfused ossification center atop dens C2
- Type III fracture follows embryologic line of union between dens and body of C2
- Sudden forward or backward movement of the head, neck rigidly erect & articulations locked
- Osteoporosis in elderly predisposes to Type II fracture and nonunion
- Type I: Avulsion of tip
- Type II: Transverse fracture at base of dens
- Type III: Fracture extending into body of C2

  - Replacement of normal marrow's high signal (fat) by low signal (edema)
  - Displacement of dens from C2 body, typically anterior subluxation
- T2WI
  - High signal of edema in marrow and prevertebral soft tissues
  - Hyperintense cord edema
  - Hypointense hemorrhage

Nuclear Medicine Findings
- Bone Scan: Used to detect old fracture with non-union

Imaging Recommendations
- Best imaging tool: Thin slice (1 mm or less) multidetector CT with reformations
- Protocol advice
  - Plain radiographs (especially lateral, open mouth views) initially suggest need for CT
  - Thin-section (1 mm) axial slices with bone reconstruction algorithm with fastest possible scan times for optimal reformation into sagittal and coronal planes
  - MR with T1WI in sagittal and coronal planes (3 mm slices), T2WI in sagittal plane to evaluate canal size, cord injury
  - GRE imaging to detect blood in cord if myelopathy is present

DIFFERENTIAL DIAGNOSIS

Congenital Nonunion of Odontoid Tip (Os Odontoideum)
- Well-corticated ossification center above rudimentary dens
- No soft tissue swelling
- No history of trauma, no pain

Congenital Variation: 3rd Occipital Condyle
- One of several anomalous bony structures which may form at foramen magnum as remnant of first sclerotome
- Midline bony peg off anterior lip of foramen magnum may articulate to dens, simulate odontoid fracture

Rheumatoid Arthritis: C1/C2 Subluxation
- Synovial proliferation erodes dens, leads to laxity & subluxation

Pathologic C2 Fracture
- Can produce pathologic odontoid fracture
- Metastases, infection, other inflammatory arthritidis

PATHOLOGY

General Features
- General path comments
  - Embryology: Anatomy
    - Three ossification centers form C2
    - Os odontoideum represents unfused ossification center atop dens C2
    - Type III fracture follows embryologic line of union between dens and body of C2
- Etiology
  - Sudden forward or backward movement of the head, neck rigidly erect & articulations locked
  - Osteoporosis in elderly predisposes to Type II fracture and nonunion

Staging, Grading or Classification Criteria
- Type I: Avulsion of tip
- Type II: Transverse fracture at base of dens
- Type III: Fracture extending into body of C2

CLINICAL ISSUES

Presentation
- Most common signs/symptoms: Neck pain
- Other signs/symptoms: Myelopathy
- Clinical Profile
  - Frequently elderly, osteoporotic patients

ODONTOID C2 FRACTURE

- Fluctuating long tract signs and spasticity may be only presentation in older patients with minor initial trauma; may be missed clinically

Natural History & Prognosis
- Chronic nonunion or fibrous union in elderly
- Nonunion common in elderly without primary fusion
  - May stabilize by fibrous union with prolonged immobilization
- Fusion produces stability

Treatment
- Fracture pattern dictates management
- Type I fracture
  - Considered stable
  - Treated with simple immobilization
- Type II fracture
  - Most likely to progress to nonunion
  - Primary fusion may be indicated to prevent myelopathy
- Type III fracture
  - Nonunion uncommon after treatment with traction followed by bracing

DIAGNOSTIC CHECKLIST

Consider
- T2WI to verify edematous marrow, better depict associated soft tissue edema in prevertebral space (missing in chronic nonunion)
- T1WI sagittal and coronal images to depict disruption of bone contiguity and degree of displacement
  - Marrow shows signal loss from edema in acute cases
  - Normal signal indicates chronic nonunion
- Flexion/extension films or fluoroscopy for evaluating stability

Image Interpretation Pearls
- Sclerotic margins of ununited dens indicate chronic nonunion of old fracture

SELECTED REFERENCES

1. Muller EJ et al: Non-rigid immobilisation of odontoid fractures. Eur Spine J. 12(5):522-5, 2003
2. Rao PV: Median (third) occipital condyle. Clin Anat. 15(2):148-51, 2002
3. Sanderson SP et al: Fracture through the C2 synchondrosis in a young child. Pediatr Neurosurg. 36(5):277-8, 2002
4. v Ludinghausen M et al: The third occipital condyle, a constituent part of a median occipito-atlanto-odontoid joint: a case report. Surg Radiol Anat. 24(1):71-6, 2002
5. Martin-Ferrer S: Odontoid fractures. J Neurosurg. 95(1 Suppl):158-9, 2001
6. Sasso RC: C2 dens fractures: treatment options. J Spinal Disord. 14(5):455-63, 2001
7. Teo EC et al: Biomechanical study of C2 (Axis) fracture: effect of restraint. Ann Acad Med Singapore. 30(6):582-7, 2001
8. Weisskopf M et al: CT scans versus conventional tomography in acute fractures of the odontoid process. Eur Spine J. 10(3):250-6, 2001
9. Govender S et al: Fractures of the odontoid process. J Bone Joint Surg Br. 82(8):1143-7, 2000
10. Swischuk LE et al: Is the open-mouth odontoid view necessary in children under 5 years? Pediatr Radiol. 30(3):186-9, 2000
11. Vaccaro AR et al: Contemporary management of adult cervical odontoid fractures. Orthopedics. 23(10):1109-13; quiz 1114-5, 2000
12. Ziai WC et al: A six year review of odontoid fractures: the emerging role of surgical intervention. Can J Neurol Sci. 27(4):297-301, 2000
13. Brant-Zawadzki M et al: CT in the evaluation of spine trauma. AJR Am J Roentgenol. 136(2):369-75, 1981
14. Charlton OP et al: Roentgenographic evaluation of cervical spine trauma. JAMA. 242(10):1073-5, 1979
15. Anderson LD et al: Fractures of the odontoid process of the axis. J Bone Joint Surg Am. 56(8):1663-74, 1974

ODONTOID C2 FRACTURE

IMAGE GALLERY

Typical

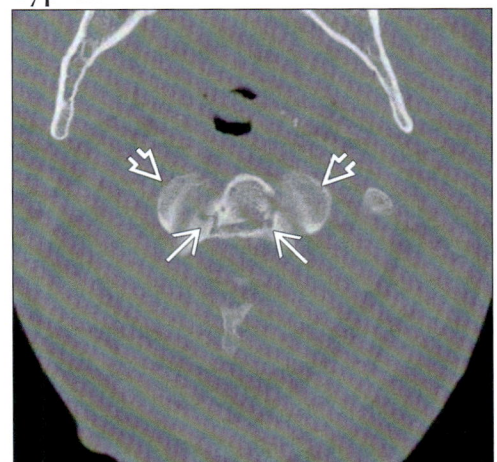
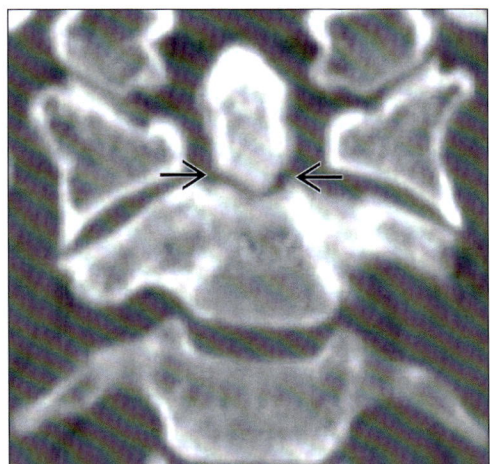

(Left) Axial bone CT shows complex fracture through base of dens ➡. Note anterior displacement of C1 arch relative to dens ➡. *(Right)* Coronal bone CT reformatted image shows type II fracture ➡ through base of dens.

Typical

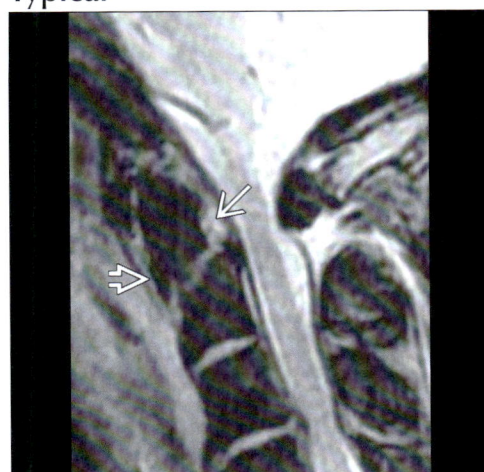
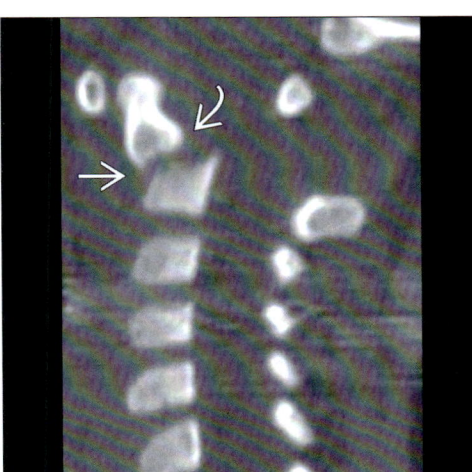

(Left) Sagittal STIR MR shows obliquely oriented type III fracture ➡ with hyperintensity within fracture and mild anterolisthesis of odontoid on C2 ➡. *(Right)* Sagittal bone CT shows type II fracture ➡ in a one year old with marked anterolisthesis and angulation ➡.

Typical

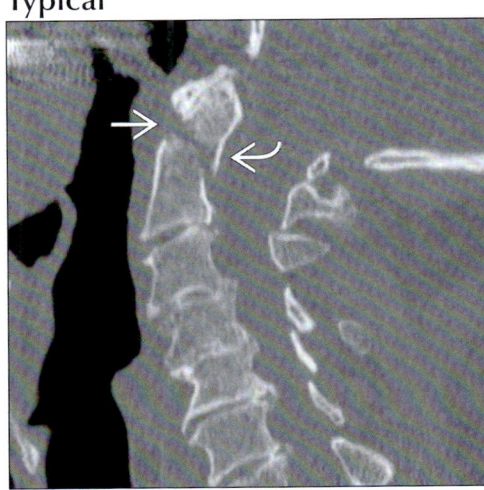
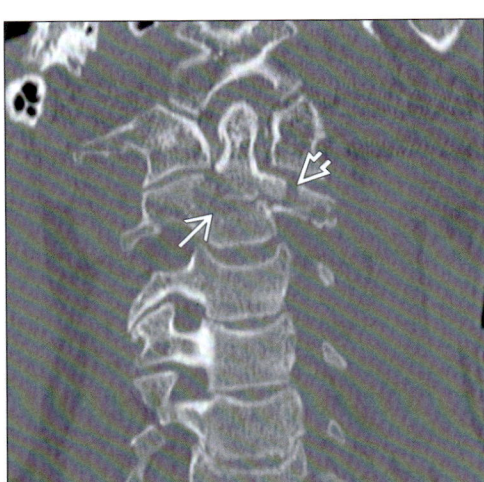

(Left) Sagittal bone CT shows type III obliquely oriented fracture ➡ with retrolisthesis of dens on C2 ➡. *(Right)* Coronal bone CT in the same patient as prior shows type III fracture extending into body ➡ and left lateral mass ➡ of C2.

HANGMAN'S C2 FRACTURE

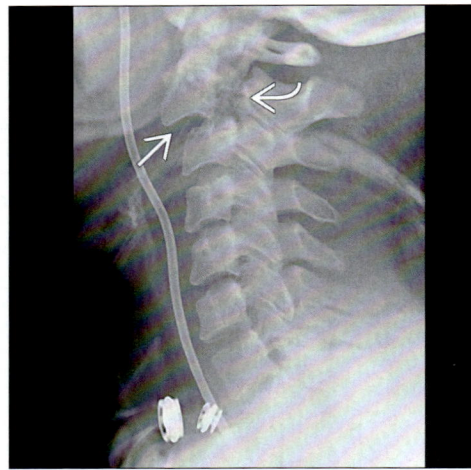

Lateral radiograph shows marked anterolisthesis of C2 on C3 ➔ and fracture disruption of pedicles of C2 ➔.

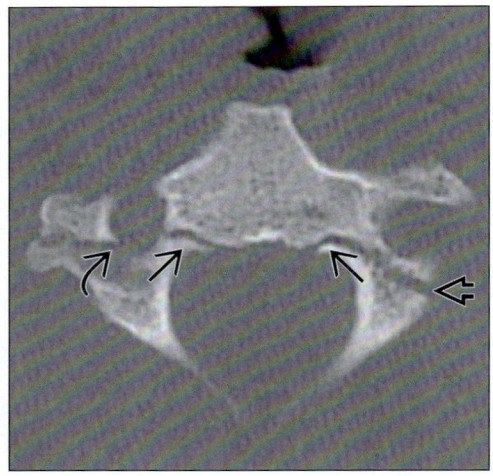

Axial bone CT shows fractures extending through posterior margin of C2 & bilateral pedicles ➔, with extension into foramen transversarium on right ➔ and lamina on left ➔.

TERMINOLOGY

Abbreviations and Synonyms
- Traumatic spondylolisthesis of axis (TSA)

Definitions
- Bilateral avulsion of C2 vertebral body (VB) from its arch

IMAGING FINDINGS

General Features
- Best diagnostic clue
  - Anterior displacement of C2 VB, C1, & skull vs. C3 on lateral X-ray
  - Classic imaging appearance: Defects through pedicles & C2 VB anterior to C3 VB; laminae aligned
    - CT defines components of fracture to best advantage
    - May see various patterns of arch, VB disruption
    - Soft tissue swelling anterior to VB common
    - May not see malalignment despite pedicle disruption
    - C1 & skull ride with anteriorly subluxed C2 VB
- Location: Both pedicles of C2

Radiographic Findings
- Radiography
  - C2 VB anteriorly subluxed vs. C3
  - Radiolucent gap in pedicles of C2
  - Prevertebral soft tissue swelling
  - C1 arch and skull ride forward with C2 VB
  - Posterior elements and laminal line of C2 and C3 remain aligned

Fluoroscopic Findings
- Flexion exaggerates C2-C3 subluxation
- Useful for verifying stability of therapeutic fusion

CT Findings
- NECT
  - Bone window CT
    - Multiple bilateral fractures of C2 arch, including pedicles
    - Axial slice shows disrupted ring of C2
    - Variation of fracture sites, including extension into body, not uncommon
    - Dens typically spared

DDx: Mimics of Hangman's Fracture

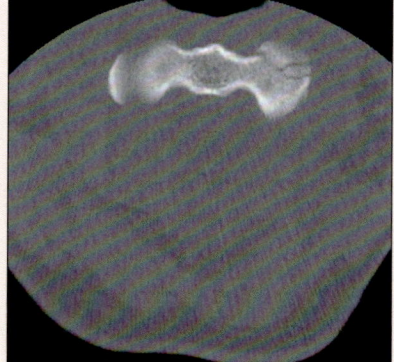

Unilateral Lateral Mass Fracture

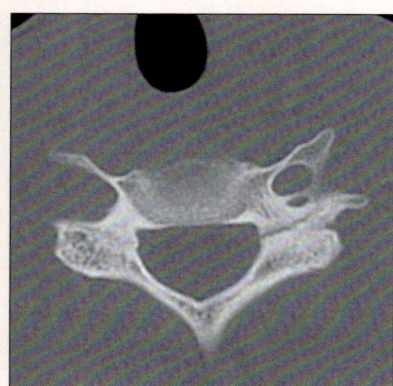

Chronic Unilateral Pedicle Fracture

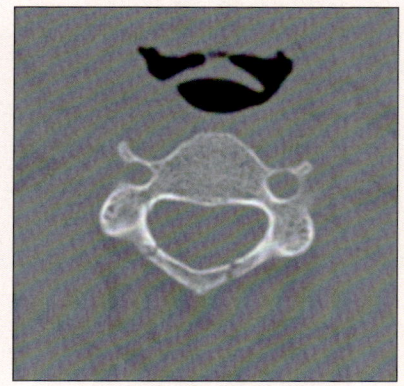

Posterior Arch Fractures

HANGMAN'S C2 FRACTURE

Key Facts

Terminology
- Traumatic spondylolisthesis of axis (TSA)

Imaging Findings
- Anterior displacement of C2 VB, C1, & skull vs. C3 on lateral X-ray
- Classic imaging appearance: Defects through pedicles & C2 VB anterior to C3 VB; laminae aligned
- Axial slice shows disrupted ring of C2
- Variation of fracture sites, including extension into body, not uncommon
- Dens typically spared
- Extension into vertebral artery foramen raises possibility of vertebral artery (VBA) damage
- Additional fracture levels seen in 33% of cases, C1 most commonly
- Canal at C2 enlarged
- Evaluate entire cervical spine (even upper thoracic): Associated fractures occur in 33% of cases
- Any anterior subluxation of C2 vs. C3 on lateral X-ray warrants CT
- MR if neurologic symptoms are present

Top Differential Diagnoses
- Pseudosubluxation
- Rotatory Subluxation of C2-C3
- Primary Spondylolysis

Diagnostic Checklist
- C2-C3 VB anterior subluxation with laminal line normally aligned requires CT even without fracture shown on X-ray

---

- Extension into vertebral artery foramen raises possibility of vertebral artery (VBA) damage
- Additional fracture levels seen in 33% of cases, C1 most commonly
- Canal at C2 enlarged
  - Soft tissue windows
    - Prevertebral soft tissue swelling
    - May show high density (blood) in spinal canal
- CTA: If VBA foramen fractured, CTA shows loss of VBA integrity

MR Findings
- T1WI: Low signal in pedicles of C2
- T2WI
  - High signal edema in thickened prevertebral soft tissue
  - Spinal cord injury - swelling and hyperintense edema in cord
  - Spinal cord hematoma - focal cord hypointensity
- STIR: High signal in pedicles of C2
- T2* GRE: Blood products in canal or cord produce marked hypointensity
- MRA: VBA signal loss if foramen fracture or significant subluxation occurred

Imaging Recommendations
- Protocol advice
  - Thin section (1 mm) helical CT with reformations
  - MR and MRA for cord and vascular injury when clinically warranted
  - Thin-section (1 mm) cuts & reformations mandatory to assess fractures, degree of subluxation, canal status
  - Evaluate entire cervical spine (even upper thoracic): Associated fractures occur in 33% of cases
  - Any anterior subluxation of C2 vs. C3 on lateral X-ray warrants CT
  - MR if neurologic symptoms are present
  - MRA or CTA if fracture line involves transverse foramen
  - Catheter angiography for endovascular intervention

DIFFERENTIAL DIAGNOSIS

Pseudosubluxation
- Seen in young children
- Affects multiple upper cervical levels
- Occurs on lateral X-ray view when mild flexion present
- No associated soft tissue swelling
- Due to ligamentous laxity of youth
- Laminal line remains aligned

Rotatory Subluxation of C2-C3
- Unilateral fracture(s) of C2 arch, pedicle

Primary Spondylolysis
- Rare anomaly
- Persistent embryonic synchondrosis

PATHOLOGY

General Features
- General path comments
  - Classical hanging with knot in submental position produces complete disruption of C2, C3 disc & ligaments
  - Sudden contusion or tearing of upper cord & brainstem by hyperextension and distraction
  - Traumatic TSA has different mechanism (e.g., chin vs. dashboard), similar results in bony spine
- Etiology: Traumatic TSA results from hyperextension with axial loading, or forced hyperflexion with compression in falls or MVA
- Epidemiology
  - Almost all modern cases represent sequelae of accidents rather than hanging
    - Only a minority of judicial hanging victims show C2 arch fracture
  - TSA represents 4-7% of all cervical fractures and/or dislocations
  - Isolated TSA represented 7% of all craniovertebral fractures in one series
- Associated abnormalities

HANGMAN'S C2 FRACTURE

- ○ Fractures at other levels, though not always contiguous
- ○ Associated C1 fracture is most common of other levels involved

Staging, Grading or Classification Criteria
- Type I: Non-displaced, no angulation
- Type II: Significant angulation and translation
- Type III: Type II plus unilateral or bilateral facet dislocations

CLINICAL ISSUES

Presentation
- Most common signs/symptoms: Acute neck pain
- Other signs/symptoms
  - ○ Neurological deficits
  - ○ Cerebellar findings suggest stroke due to vertebral artery dissection or occlusion
- Clinical Profile
  - ○ Upper neck pain after trauma
  - ○ Neurological sequelae occur in minority of traumatic cases (25%)
    - Canal wide here, further decompressed by fracture
  - ○ Vertebral artery injury may cause delayed neurological signs

Natural History & Prognosis
- Depends on presence of neurological damage
- Delayed stroke a possibility if vertebral artery damaged
- Accelerated degenerative changes

Treatment
- Immobilization
- Fusion

DIAGNOSTIC CHECKLIST

Consider
- Check VB alignment, soft tissue thickness (4 mm or less) on lateral X-ray and get CT if abnormal
- Evaluate transverse foramen for integrity; get MRA if any question to exclude vertebral artery injury

Image Interpretation Pearls
- C2-C3 VB anterior subluxation with laminal line normally aligned requires CT even without fracture shown on X-ray

SELECTED REFERENCES
1. No authors listed: Isolated fractures of the axis in adults. Neurosurgery. 50(3 Suppl):S125-39, 2002
2. No authors listed: Management of combination fractures of the atlas and axis in adults. Neurosurgery. 50(3 Suppl):S140-7, 2002
3. Ranjith RK et al: Hangman's fracture caused by suspected child abuse. A case report. J Pediatr Orthop B. 11(4):329-32, 2002
4. Harrop JS et al: Acute respiratory compromise associated with flexed cervical traction after C2 fractures. Spine. 26(4):E50-4, 2001
5. Samaha C et al: Hangman's fracture: the relationship between asymmetry and instability. J Bone Joint Surg Br. 82(7):1046-52, 2000
6. Agrillo U et al: Hangman's fracture. Spine. 24(22):2412, 1999
7. Guiot B et al: Complex atlantoaxial fractures. J Neurosurg. 91(2 Suppl):139-43, 1999
8. Williams JP 3rd et al: CT appearance of congenital defect resembling the Hangman's fracture. Pediatr Radiol. 29(7):549-50, 1999
9. Greene KA et al: Acute axis fractures. Analysis of management and outcome in 340 consecutive cases. Spine. 22(16):1843-52, 1997
10. Nunez DB Jr et al: Cervical spine trauma: how much more do we learn by routinely using helical CT? Radiographics. 16(6):1307-18; discussion 1318-21, 1996
11. Starr JK et al: Atypical hangman's fractures. Spine. 18(14):1954-7, 1993
12. James R et al: The occurrence of cervical fractures in victims of judicial hanging. Forensic Sci Int. 54(1):81-91, 1992
13. Parisi M et al: Hangman's fracture or primary spondylolysis: a patient and a brief review. Pediatr Radiol. 21(5):367-8, 1991
14. Burke JT et al: Acute injuries of the axis vertebra. Skeletal Radiol. 18(5):335-46, 1989
15. Fielding JW et al: Traumatic spondylolisthesis of the axis. Clin Orthop. (239):47-52, 1989
16. Mirvis SE et al: Hangman's fracture: radiologic assessment in 27 cases. Radiology. 163(3):713-7, 1987
17. Baumgarten M et al: Computed axial tomography in C1-C2 trauma. Spine. 10(3):187-92, 1985
18. Hadley MN et al: Axis fractures: a comprehensive review of management and treatment in 107 cases. Neurosurgery. 17(2):281-90, 1985
19. Sherk HH et al: Clinical and pathologic correlations in traumatic spondylolisthesis of the axis. Clin Orthop. (174):122-6, 1983
20. Bucholz RW: Unstable hangman's fractures. Clin Orthop. (154):119-24, 1981
21. Pepin JW et al: Traumatic spondylolisthesis of the axis: Hangman's fracture. Clin Orthop. (157):133-8, 1981
22. Seljeskog EL et al: Spectrum of the hangman's fracture. J Neurosurg. 45(1):3-8, 1976
23. Marar BC: Fracture of the axis arch. "Hangman's fracture" of the cervical spine. Clin Orthop. (106):155-65, 1975
24. Williams TG: Hangman's fracture. J Bone Joint Surg Br. 57(1):82-8, 1975

HANGMAN'S C2 FRACTURE

IMAGE GALLERY

Typical

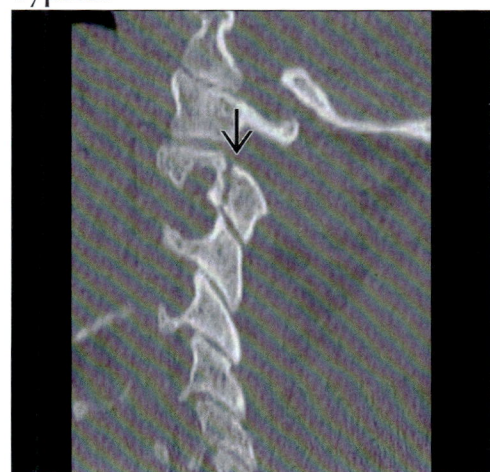
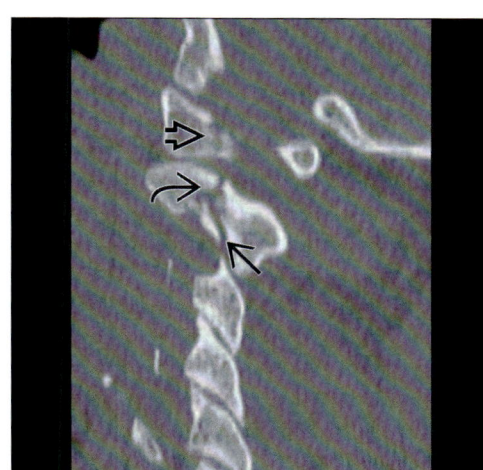

(Left) Sagittal bone CT shows fracture through right lateral mass extending into facet joint ➔ on sagittal reformation. *(Right)* Sagittal bone CT in same patient as previous image, shows complex fracture extending through left facet ➔ and pedicle ➔ of C2. Note additional fracture of lateral mass of C1 ➔.

Typical

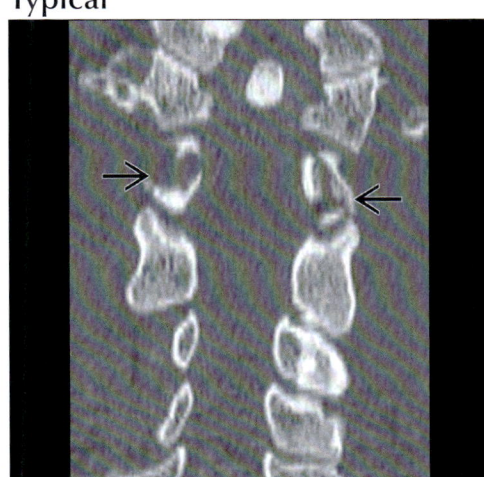
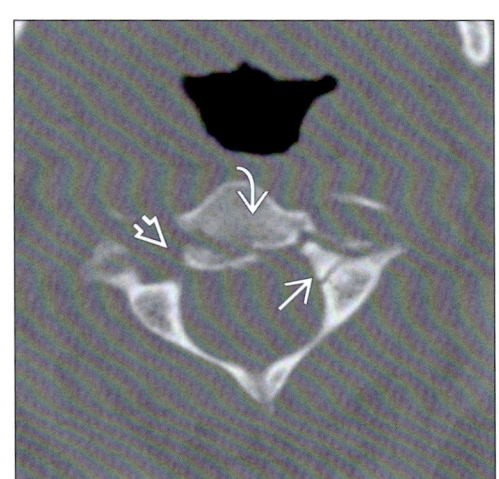

(Left) Coronal bone CT shows bilateral fractures ➔ through lateral masses and pedicles of C2. *(Right)* Axial bone CT shows fracture of left facet joint of C2 ➔. Fracture through posterior portion of vertebra on the right ➔ with anterior displacement and rotation of the body ➔.

Typical

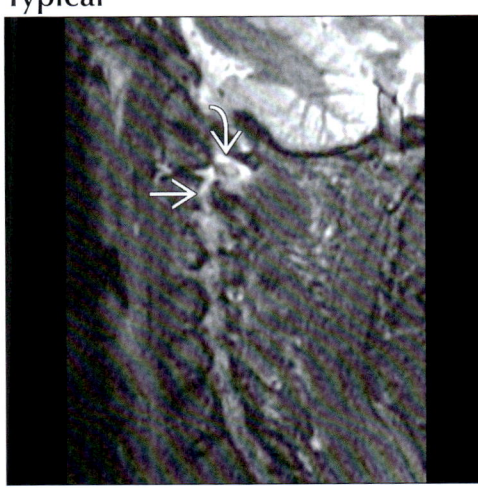
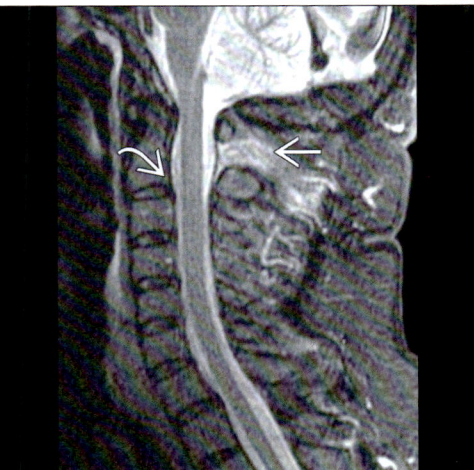

(Left) Sagittal STIR MR shows hyperintensity at site of the fracture of pedicle of C2 ➔ and adjacent ligamentous edema ➔. *(Right)* Sagittal STIR MR in same patient as previous image, shows edema of posterior ligaments and soft tissues ➔. Mild anterolisthesis ➔ is present but there is no cord injury.

HYPERFLEXION INJURY, CERVICAL

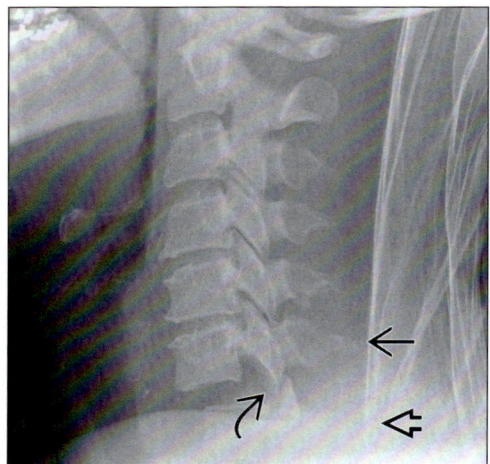

Lateral radiograph shows widening of space between the spinous process of C6 ➡ & C7 ➡. The inferior facet of C6 jumped anterior superior facet of C7 ➡.

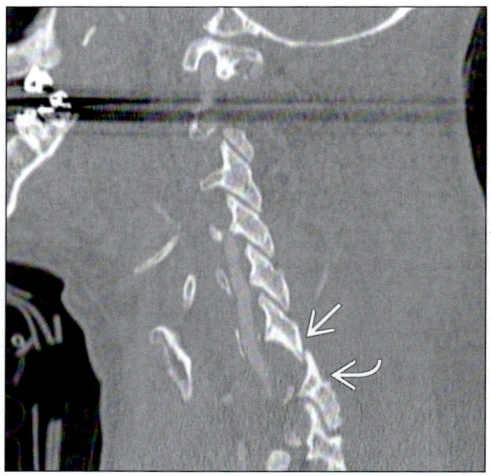

Sagittal CECT in same case as previous image shows inferior C6 facet ➡ anterior to superior facet of C7 ➡ ("jumped facet").

TERMINOLOGY

Abbreviations and Synonyms
- Traumatic anterior subluxation

Definitions
- Flexion force disrupts capsular & posterior ligaments, with anterior vertebral displacement/angulation

IMAGING FINDINGS

General Features
- Best diagnostic clue
  - Focal kyphosis, ↑ space between spinous processes
  - Widened, perched or jumped facets
- Location: Mid or lower cervical spine

Radiographic Findings
- Radiography: Focal kyphosis with ↑ space between adjacent facets, fanning of spinous processes

Fluoroscopic Findings
- ↑ Motion on flexion may confirm diagnosis

CT Findings
- Sagittal reformation: Separation between spinous processes, widened perched or jumped facets
- May see mild compression of superior end plate at involved interspace

MR Findings
- STIR
  - Hyperintensity in interspinous ligament & facet joints
  - Canal compromise, cord edema (sagittal view)

Imaging Recommendations
- Protocol advice
  - CT for facet relationships
  - MR to assess cord and ligaments

DIFFERENTIAL DIAGNOSIS

Burst Fracture
- Axial force is major component, flexion secondary

DDx: Hyperflexion Injury

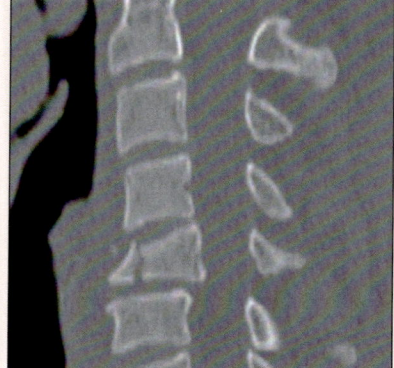

Cervical Burst Fracture

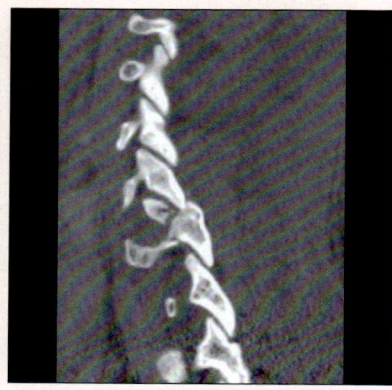

Hyperflexion Rotation Injury

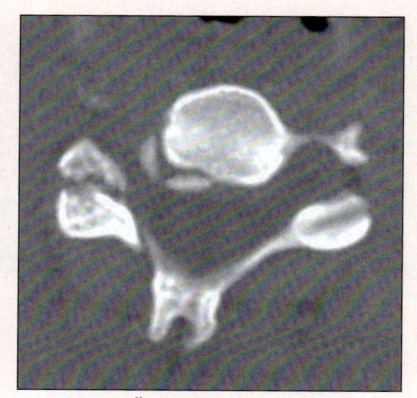

Hyperflexion Rotation Injury

HYPERFLEXION INJURY, CERVICAL

Key Facts

Terminology
- Flexion force disrupts capsular & posterior ligaments, with anterior vertebral displacement/angulation

Imaging Findings
- Focal kyphosis, ↑ space between spinous processes
- Widened, perched or jumped facets
- ↑ Motion on flexion may confirm diagnosis
- CT for facet relationships
- MR to assess cord and ligaments

Pathology
- Neurological compromise post-injury may occur if unstable fracture not recognized
- Ligamentous injury leads to instability

Diagnostic Checklist
- Evaluate other levels carefully; non-contiguous injury or fracture may occur

Flexion-Rotation Injury
- Unilateral facet subluxation; facet fracture common

Whiplash Fracture
- Extension → laminar fracture; flexion → vertebral body compression

PATHOLOGY

General Features
- General path comments
  - Disruption of middle column → mechanical instability
  - Neurological compromise post-injury may occur if unstable fracture not recognized
  - Disc displacement may contribute to cord compression
- Etiology
  - Small, flat, articular processes, horizontal articulation & little overlap of articular surfaces predisposes to flexion injury
  - Ligamentous injury leads to instability

CLINICAL ISSUES

Presentation
- Most common signs/symptoms
  - Trauma with flexion components (e.g., diving)
  - Acute neck pain with/without neurologic deficit

Natural History & Prognosis
- Good if no neurologic damage, & stabilization achieved
- Accelerated degenerative disease may be seen
- Fixed neurologic deficit if hemorrhagic cord contusion

Treatment
- Neurologically intact: Halo immobilization, deformity correction
- Neurologic signs & compression: Acute decompression
- Edematous cord: High dose steroids (< 1 day)

DIAGNOSTIC CHECKLIST

Image Interpretation Pearls
- Evaluate other levels carefully; non-contiguous injury or fracture may occur

SELECTED REFERENCES

1. Laporte C et al: Severe hyperflexion sprains of the lower cervical spine in adults. Clin Orthop. (363):126-34, 1999
2. Murakami H et al: Central cord syndrome secondary to hyperflexion injury of the cervical spine in a child. J Spinal Disord. 8(6):494-8, 1995
3. Fazl M et al: Posttraumatic ligamentous disruption of the cervical spine, an easily overlooked diagnosis: presentation of three cases. Neurosurgery. 26(4):674-8, 1990

IMAGE GALLERY

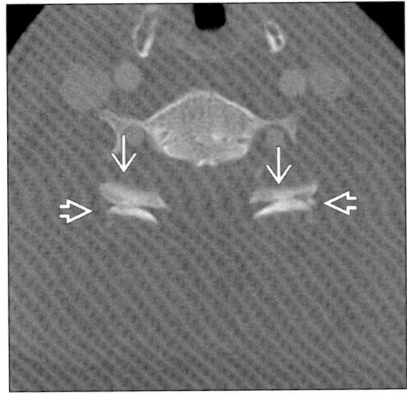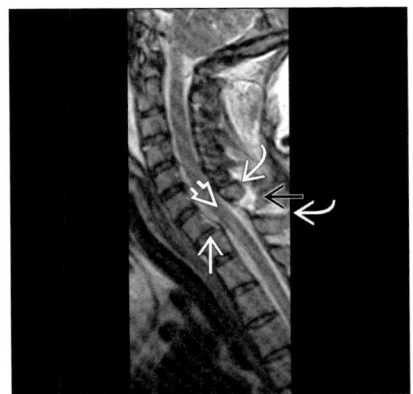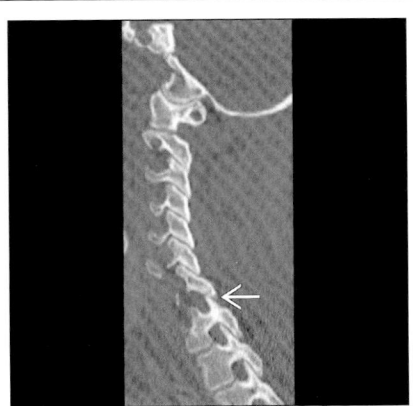

(Left) Axial CECT shows inferior facets of C6 ➔ anterior to superior facets of C7 ➔ ("naked facets"). *(Center)* Sagittal T2WI MR shows anterolisthesis of C7 on T1 ➔ with fanning of spinous processes ➔, edema of intraspinous ligament ➔, spinal cord edema ➔. *(Right)* Sagittal bone CT shows perching of inferior facet joint of C7 on superior facet joint of T1 ➔.

HYPEREXTENSION INJURY, CERVICAL

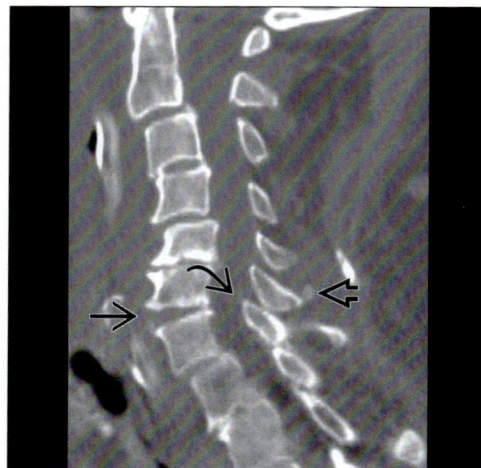

Sagittal bone CT shows widening of the anterior C6-C7 disc space ➡. The spinal laminar line is discontinuous 2° retrolisthesis ➡; note fracture of the spinous process ➡.

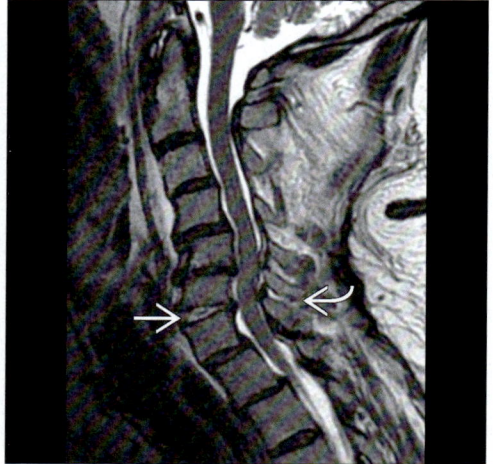

Sagittal T2WI MR in same case as previous image, shows widening of C6-C7 disc space, as well as edema of the intervertebral disc ➡ & interspinous ligament ➡.

TERMINOLOGY

Abbreviations and Synonyms
- Arch fracture (fx)
- Posterior element fx

Definitions
- Fracture of the laminae due to forceful posterior displacement of head and/or upper cervical spine

IMAGING FINDINGS

General Features
- Best diagnostic clue
  - Bony defect through posterior arch with posterior element malalignment
  - Widening of anterior portion of disc space with prevertebral soft tissue swelling
- Location: Typically mid or lower cervical spine
- Morphology: May see distraction or rotational malalignment

Radiographic Findings
- Radiography
  - Fx through posterior elements on lateral or oblique views
  - Malalignment of posterior spinal laminal line at level of fracture
  - Anterior widening of intervertebral disc space
  - Anterior vertebral avulsion fracture ("tear drop")
  - Fullness of prevertebral soft tissues

Fluoroscopic Findings
- Laxity at level of fracture
  - Performed only under controlled conditions

CT Findings
- NECT
  - High-resolution thin section (1 mm) algorithm best
  - Arch defect best shown on axial views of bone CT
  - Bone CT sagittal reformat: Listhesis, facet relationships, widening of disc space, anterior avulsion fracture
  - May show fractures at other levels
- CTA
  - Done when vertebral artery injury suspected

DDx: Cervical Hyperextension Injury

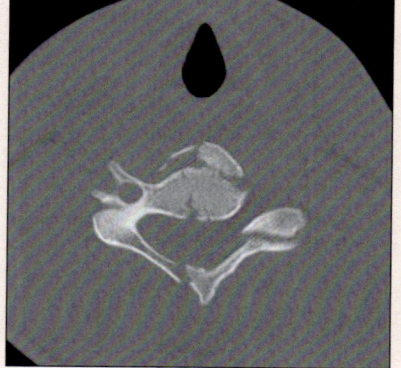
Whiplash Fracture

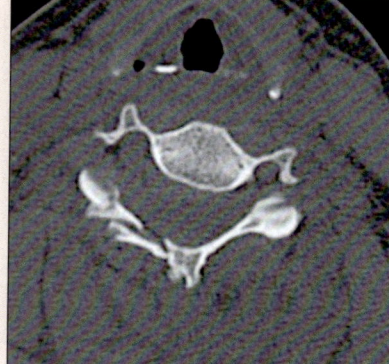
Rotational Fracture

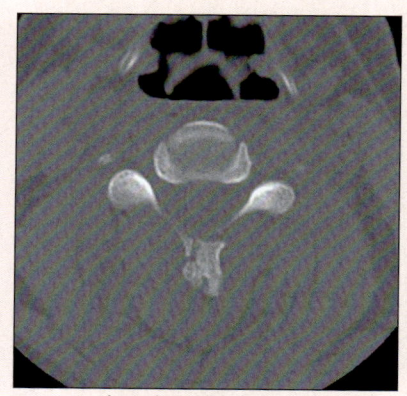
Clay Shoveler Fracture

HYPEREXTENSION INJURY, CERVICAL

Key Facts

Terminology
- Fracture of the laminae due to forceful posterior displacement of head and/or upper cervical spine

Imaging Findings
- Bony defect through posterior arch with posterior element malalignment
- Widening of anterior portion of disc space with prevertebral soft tissue swelling
- Arch defect best shown on axial views of bone CT
- Bone CT sagittal reformat: Listhesis, facet relationships, widening of disc space, anterior avulsion fracture
- T2WI shows cord edema if myelopathy present
- T2* GRE best depicts hemorrhagic cord contusion
- CT if high clinical level of suspicion of significant cervical injury regardless of plain film findings
- If neurologic signs present, MR vital to evaluate cord injury, compression

Top Differential Diagnoses
- Whiplash Fracture
- Rotational Fracture-Subluxation
- Clay Shoveler Fracture
- Congenital Cleft

Diagnostic Checklist
- CT in all cases with moderate to high clinical index of suspicion and when plain films inadequate
- CTA or MRA to exclude vertebral artery injury
- Subtle malalignment of spinal laminar line on lateral radiograph should prompt CT

- ○ Absence of enhancement within vertebral artery indicates injury

MR Findings
- T1WI: Difficult to see non-displaced fracture
- T2WI
  - ○ T2WI shows cord edema if myelopathy present
  - ○ May see soft tissue edema in retro-spinal tissues
  - ○ Hyperintense edema of anterior longitudinal ligament
  - ○ Hyperintense edema in disc
  - ○ Acute traumatic disc herniation
  - ○ Low sensitivity but high specificity for posterior element fracture
- STIR: Delineates soft tissue and disc edema
- T2* GRE
  - ○ T2* GRE best depicts hemorrhagic cord contusion
    - Hemorrhage in cord usually indicates irreversible damage
- MRA: Can show vertebral artery disruption

Angiographic Findings
- Conventional
  - ○ Done when endovascular therapy contemplated
    - Rarely required to confirm diagnosis of vertebral artery damage
  - ○ If arterial dissection is missed, risk of delayed neurologic damage

Imaging Recommendations
- Protocol advice
  - ○ CT if high clinical level of suspicion of significant cervical injury regardless of plain film findings
  - ○ CT mandatory if plain film findings suggest fracture
  - ○ Thin-section (1 mm maximum) cuts with reformations mandatory
  - ○ If neurologic signs present, MR vital to evaluate cord injury, compression
  - ○ Consider CTA, MRA to exclude dissection

DIFFERENTIAL DIAGNOSIS

Whiplash Fracture
- Associated vertebral body fracture
- Malalignment more common

Rotational Fracture-Subluxation
- May have associated laminar fracture

Clay Shoveler Fracture
- Spinous process avulsion from sudden severe force placed on ligamentum nuchae
- Laminae typically spared

Congenital Cleft
- Typically midline

PATHOLOGY

General Features
- General path comments
  - ○ Disruption of posterior spinal column causes mechanical instability
  - ○ Post-injury neurological compromise may occur if unstable nature of fracture not recognized
  - ○ Disc fragment displacement, though uncommon, can contribute to cord compression
- Etiology
  - ○ Hyperextension force during traumatic event
  - ○ Some degree of axial load usually present as well
  - ○ Disrupted ligaments (anterior, posterior longitudinal and capsular) add to considerable instability
- Epidemiology
  - ○ Sports are a common setting
  - ○ Increased incidence in individuals with limited spinal mobility
    - Ankylosing spondylitis & severe degenerative spine disease
- Associated abnormalities
  - ○ Cord contusion
  - ○ Traumatic disc herniation
  - ○ Vertebral artery dissection

HYPEREXTENSION INJURY, CERVICAL

- Additional fractures

Gross Pathologic & Surgical Features
- Typical traumatic bone disruption

CLINICAL ISSUES

Presentation
- Most common signs/symptoms
  - Severe neck pain with transient or lasting myelopathic signs
  - Midline cervical tenderness
- Clinical Profile: History of trauma with extension components and/or axial loading (e.g., diving)

Natural History & Prognosis
- Depends on presence/degree of neurologic compromise
- Good if no neurologic damage, and stabilization achieved
- Accelerated degenerative disease may occur if initial injury unrecognized
- Neurologic recovery can occur if only mild edema is seen in cord acutely
- Fixed neurologic deficit if cord shows hemorrhagic contusion
- Progression of fixed deficit superiorly if post-traumatic syrinx appears late

Treatment
- No neurological injury: Treatment aimed at halo immobilization & deformity correction
- Neurologic signs present with compression: Acute decompression
- Edematous cord: High dose steroids (first 24 hours) may help
- Cord hemorrhage or transection: Immobilization to prevent further deformity
- Endovascular treatment for associated vascular injury

DIAGNOSTIC CHECKLIST

Consider
- CT in all cases with moderate to high clinical index of suspicion and when plain films inadequate
- Evaluation of upper thoracic spine for associated fractures, as non-contiguous fractures can be present
- CTA or MRA to exclude vertebral artery injury

Image Interpretation Pearls
- Subtle malalignment of spinal laminar line on lateral radiograph should prompt CT
- Multiple, non-contiguous fractures may be seen

SELECTED REFERENCES

1. Ranger GS: "Radiographic clearance of blunt cervical spine injury: plain radiograph or computed tomography scan?", by Griffen MM, et al. J Trauma. 56(2):457; author reply 457, 2004
2. Berlin L: CT versus radiography for initial evaluation of cervical spine trauma: what is the standard of care? AJR Am J Roentgenol. 180(4):911-5, 2003
3. Cothren CC et al: Cervical spine fracture patterns predictive of blunt vertebral artery injury. J Trauma. 55(5):811-3, 2003
4. Hayes KC et al: Retropulsion of intervertebral discs associated with traumatic hyperextension of the cervical spine and absence of vertebral fracture: an uncommon mechanism of spinal cord injury. Spinal Cord. 40(10):544-7, 2002
5. Maiman DJ et al: Preinjury cervical alignment affecting spinal trauma. J Neurosurg. 97(1 Suppl):57-62, 2002
6. Biffl WL et al: The devastating potential of blunt vertebral arterial injuries. Ann Surg. 231(5):672-81, 2000
7. Hanson JA et al: Cervical spine injury: a clinical decision rule to identify high-risk patients for helical CT screening. AJR Am J Roentgenol. 174(3):713-7, 2000
8. Matar LD et al: "Spinolaminar breach": an important sign in cervical spinous process fractures. Skeletal Radiol. 29(2):75-80, 2000
9. Brady WJ et al: ED use of flexion-extension cervical spine radiography in the evaluation of blunt trauma. Am J Emerg Med. 17(6):504-8, 1999
10. Klein GR et al: Efficacy of magnetic resonance imaging in the evaluation of posterior cervical spine fractures. Spine. 24(8):771-4, 1999
11. Makan P: Neurologic compromise after an isolated laminar fracture of the cervical spine. Spine. 24(11):1144-6, 1999
12. Zhu Q et al: Traumatic instabilities of the cervical spine caused by high-speed axial compression in a human model. An in vitro biomechanical study. Spine. 24(5):440-4, 1999
13. Kinoshita H: Pathology of hyperextension injury of the cervical spine: a case report. Spinal Cord. 35(12):857-8, 1997
14. Kang JD et al: Sagittal measurements of the cervical spine in subaxial fractures and dislocations. An analysis of two hundred and eighty-eight patients with and without neurological deficits. J Bone Joint Surg Am. 76(11):1617-28, 1994
15. Kinoshita H: Pathology of hyperextension injuries of the cervical spine. Paraplegia. 32(6):367-74, 1994
16. Lukhele M: Fractures of the vertebral lamina associated with unifacet and bifacet cervical spine dislocations. S Afr J Surg. 32(3):112-4, 1994
17. Plezbert JA et al: Fracture of a lamina in the cervical spine. J Manipulative Physiol Ther. 17(8):552-7, 1994
18. Kiwerski J: Hyperextension-dislocation injuries of the cervical spine. Injury. 24(10):674-7, 1993
19. Silberstein M et al: Prevertebral swelling in cervical spine injury: identification of ligament injury with magnetic resonance imaging. Clin Radiol. 46(5):318-23, 1992
20. Goldberg AL et al: Hyperextension injuries of the cervical spine. Magnetic resonance findings. Skeletal Radiol. 18(4):283-8, 1989
21. Barquet A et al: An unusual extension injury to the cervical spine. A case report. J Bone Joint Surg Am. 70(9):1393-5, 1988
22. Edeiken-Monroe B et al: Hyperextension dislocation of the cervical spine. AJR Am J Roentgenol. 146(4):803-8, 1986
23. Coin CG et al: Diving-type injury of the cervical spine: contribution of computed tomography to management. J Comput Assist Tomogr. 3(3):362-72, 1979
24. Penning L: Functional pathology of the cervical spine. Baltimore, Williams and Wilkins, 1968

HYPEREXTENSION INJURY, CERVICAL

IMAGE GALLERY

Typical

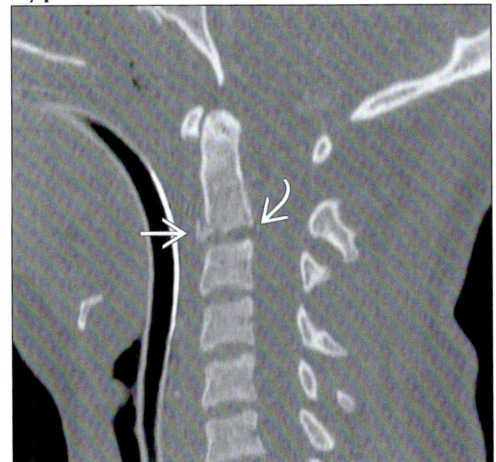
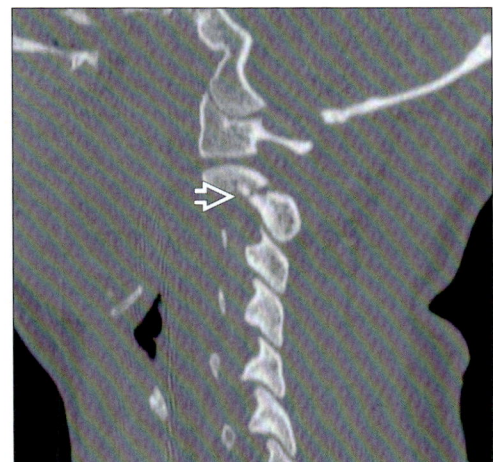

(Left) Sagittal bone CT shows anterior inferior fracture ("tear drop") of C2 ➡ with mild retrolisthesis of C2 on C3 ➡. (Right) Sagittal bone CT in same case as previous image, shows fracture through lamina of C2 ➡.

Typical

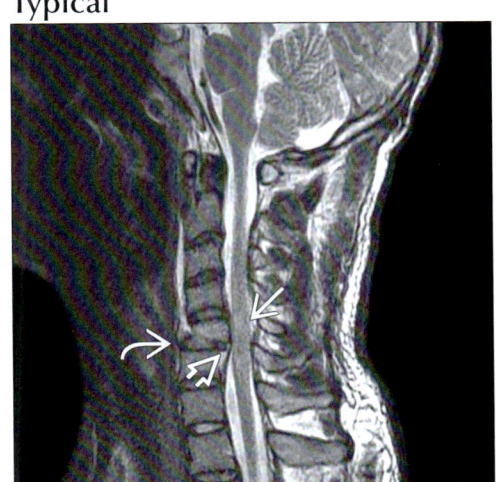
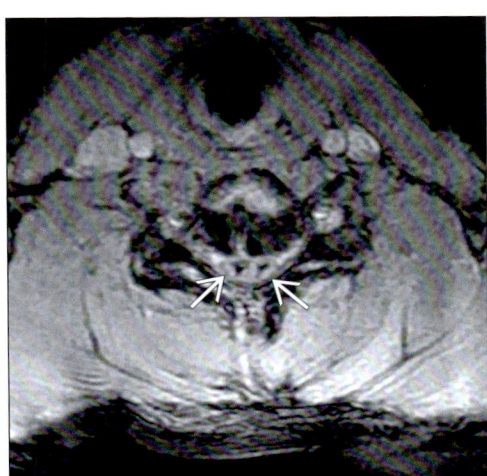

(Left) Sagittal T2WI MR shows widening of C5-C6 interspace and mild disc edema ➡. Note mild retrolisthesis with narrowing of the spinal canal ➡ & cord edema ➡. (Right) Axial T2* GRE MR in same case as previous image, shows focal hemorrhage within cord ➡ not visible on T2WI.

Typical

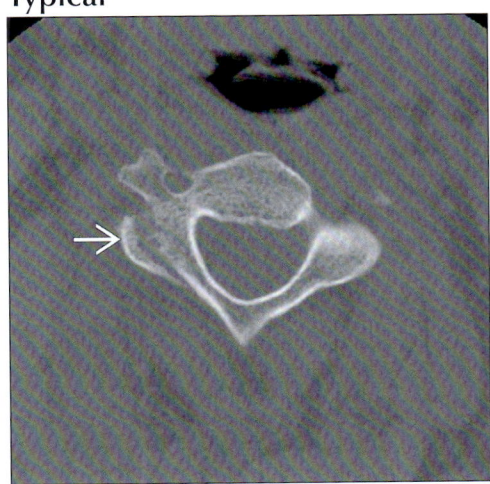
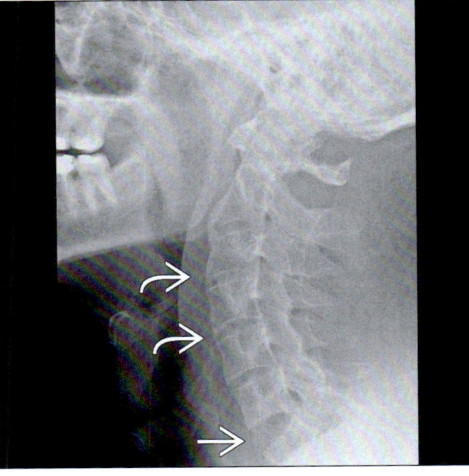

(Left) Axial NECT shows fracture through lamina ➡ of C5. (Right) Lateral radiograph shows anterior widening of disc space at C6-C7 ➡. Note anterior syndesmophytes at higher levels ➡, indicative of underlying ankylosing spondylitis.

HYPERFLEXION-ROTATION INJURY, CERVICAL

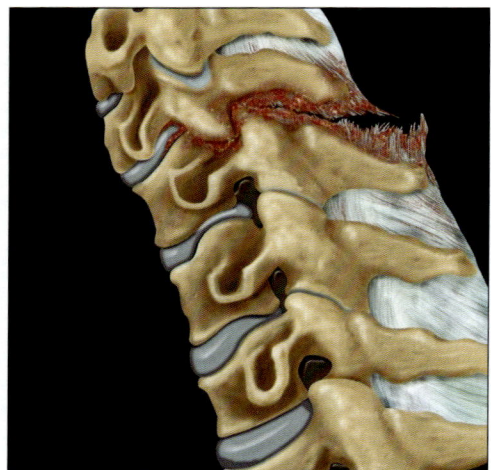

Lateral graphic shows disrupted facet and posterior ligaments with facet subluxation.

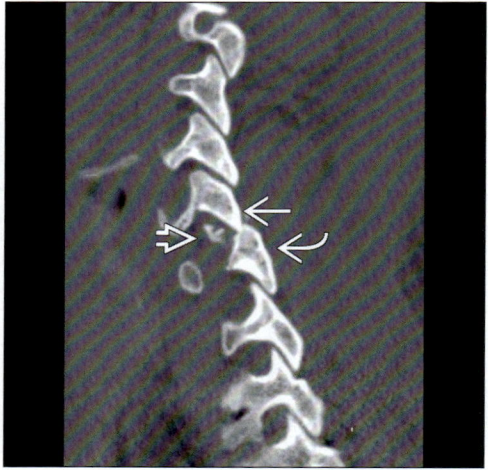

Sagittal bone CT shows inferior facet of C4 ➡ anterior to superior facet of C5 ➡ with fracture fragments of C5 facet ➡ (jumped and locked facet).

TERMINOLOGY

Abbreviations and Synonyms
- Jumped or locked facet(s)
- Rotatory subluxation of vertebral bodies (VB), posterior elements in the cervical spine

Definitions
- Traumatic disruption of cervical spine (ligaments alone or together with bony elements) causing facet subluxation

IMAGING FINDINGS

General Features
- Best diagnostic clue: Malalignment of adjacent facets with focal vertebral body angulation and rotation at site of injury
- Location: Typically mid or lower cervical spine

Radiographic Findings
- Radiography
  - Altered adjacent facet relationship on lateral radiograph
  - Focal VB kyphosis
  - Spinous process malalignment, especially vertical offset on anteroposterior view

CT Findings
- CTA: Detection of vertebral artery dissection or occlusion
- Bone CT
  - Normally, lower VB superior facet is anterior to upper neighbor's inferior facet
  - Axial: "Naked" inferior facet; subjacent neighbor, superior facet of lower VB, not seen at joint interface
  - Sagittal: Affected lateral mass "perched" on or jumped anterior to subjacent partner
  - May see fracture of facet tip
    - Fractures more common than previously thought due to improved CT detection
  - Axial views show rotated relationship between lower VB and upper neighbor

MR Findings
- T1WI: Demonstrates malalignment but insensitive to fracture

DDx: Hyperflexion Rotation

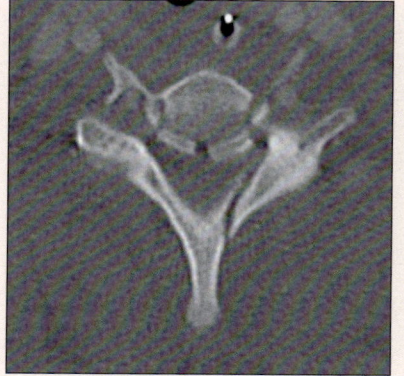

Burst Fracture

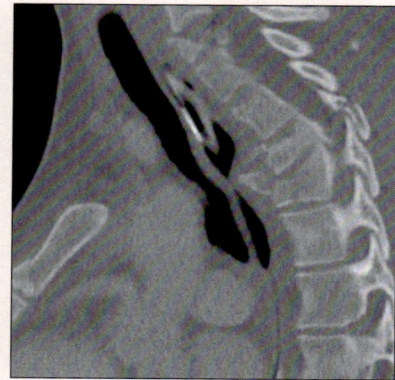

Burst Fracture

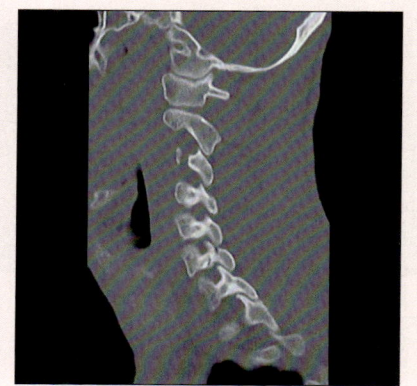

Hyperextension Rotation

HYPERFLEXION-ROTATION INJURY, CERVICAL

Key Facts

Terminology
- Jumped or locked facet(s)
- Rotatory subluxation of vertebral bodies (VB), posterior elements in the cervical spine

Imaging Findings
- Helical CT with 1 mm axial sections & mandatory reformations when diagnosis suspected clinically or on basis of plain radiographs
- Radiographs should include oblique views if initial images suggest diagnosis
- **Always evaluate the following relationships when examining C-spine trauma X-rays**
- Anterior VB edges should trace gentle C-like lordosis
- Posterior edges of VB should parallel anterior curve
- Facets should align on lateral and oblique views
- Posterior laminal line (point of junction of laminae) should show same gentle lordotic curve as anterior & posterior VB edges on lateral view
- Prevertebral soft tissue should show half thickness or less of AP VB diameter
- AP radiography should show regular spacing between spinous processes, all vertically aligned in midline
- Disc space height loss can be clue in absence of degenerative changes

Pathology
- Rotatory shear forces tear capsular, annular, longitudinal ligaments; allow even intact bony elements to sublux

---

- T2WI
  - Edema of disrupted ligaments and jumped facet
  - Cord compromise, contusion when present
- STIR
  - Best sequence for ligamentous and soft tissue injury
  - Most sensitive MR sequence for fracture; not as sensitive as CT
- T2* GRE: Most sensitive for cord hemorrhage
- MRA: Detect vertebral or carotid artery damage

Angiographic Findings
- Conventional: Verify suspected arterial damage and for endovascular treatment

Imaging Recommendations
- Best imaging tool: Helical CT with reformations
- Protocol advice
  - Helical CT with 1 mm axial sections & mandatory reformations when diagnosis suspected clinically or on basis of plain radiographs
  - Radiographs should include oblique views if initial images suggest diagnosis
- **Always evaluate the following relationships when examining C-spine trauma X-rays**
  - Anterior VB edges should trace gentle C-like lordosis
  - Posterior edges of VB should parallel anterior curve
  - Facets should align on lateral and oblique views
  - Posterior laminal line (point of junction of laminae) should show same gentle lordotic curve as anterior & posterior VB edges on lateral view
  - Prevertebral soft tissue should show half thickness or less of AP VB diameter
  - AP radiography should show regular spacing between spinous processes, all vertically aligned in midline
  - Disc space height loss can be clue in absence of degenerative changes

DIFFERENTIAL DIAGNOSIS

Whiplash Fracture
- No facet malalignment

- Some rotational component may be present

Burst or Tear-Drop Fracture
- May see slight separation of facet joints
- Less rotational malalignment

Rotatory Extension Fracture
- Similar, but greater disruption of posterior arch

PATHOLOGY

General Features
- General path comments
  - Capsular, other ligaments provide considerable support to relatively small facets of cervical VBs
  - Near-horizontal articulation of cervical facets predisposes to easy subluxation once ligaments are torn
  - Rotatory shear forces tear capsular, annular, longitudinal ligaments; allow even intact bony elements to sublux
    - Once facets "jump" each other and lock, fracture is stable
    - Considerable traction required to restore normal relationships
    - Neurological injury common
    - Facet fracture fragments often seen
- Etiology: Sudden, forceful rotational & flexion force on skull/spine
- Associated abnormalities
  - Spinal cord damage
  - Dissection of vertebral or carotid arteries

Gross Pathologic & Surgical Features
- Torn ligaments
- Displacement of inferior facet (articular pillar) on top of or anterior to inferior neighbor

Staging, Grading or Classification Criteria
- Facet subluxation may vary from mild (perched facets) with threat of further damage, to severe (locking) fixed injury

HYPERFLEXION-ROTATION INJURY, CERVICAL

- Fracture-subluxation combine to produce considerable instability

CLINICAL ISSUES

Presentation
- Most common signs/symptoms: Severe neck pain, often associated with neurological compromise
- Clinical Profile: Major trauma victim with neck pain, may have neurologic deficit

Natural History & Prognosis
- Dictated by type and degree of neurological deficit
- Mild cord contusion can regress
- Cord hematoma heralds grave prognosis

Treatment
- Traction
- Decompression and stabilization as necessary
- Fusion

DIAGNOSTIC CHECKLIST

Consider
- CT in any case of VB malalignment, facets on C spine radiographs or in presence of neurologic abnormality

Image Interpretation Pearls
- Check facet surface relationships on every lateral radiograph
- Sagittal reformations through both left & right lateral mass columns key to accurate diagnosis
- Look for associated vascular injury

SELECTED REFERENCES

1. Crawford NR et al: Unilateral cervical facet dislocation: injury mechanism and biomechanical consequences. Spine. 27(17):1858-64; discussion 1864, 2002
2. Hart RA: Cervical facet dislocation: when is magnetic resonance imaging indicated? Spine. 27(1):116-7, 2002
3. Vaccaro AR et al: Is magnetic resonance imaging indicated before reduction of a unilateral cervical facet dislocation? Spine. 27(1):117-8, 2002
4. Lingawi SS: The naked facet sign. Radiology. 219(2):366-7, 2001
5. Sim E et al: In vitro genesis of subaxial cervical unilateral facet dislocations through sequential soft tissue ablation. Spine. 26(12):1317-23, 2001
6. Argenson C et al: Traumatic rotatory displacement of the lower cervical spine. Bull Hosp Jt Dis. 59(1):52-60, 2000
7. Daffner RH et al: A new classification for cervical vertebral injuries: influence of CT. Skeletal Radiol. 29(3):125-32, 2000
8. Razack N et al: The management of traumatic cervical bilateral facet fracture-dislocations with unicortical anterior plates. J Spinal Disord. 13(5):374-81, 2000
9. An HS: Cervical spine trauma. Spine. 23(24):2713-29, 1998
10. Andreshak JL et al: Management of unilateral facet dislocations: a review of the literature. Orthopedics. 20(10):917-26, 1997
11. Halliday AL et al: The management of unilateral lateral mass/facet fractures of the subaxial cervical spine: the use of magnetic resonance imaging to predict instability. Spine. 22(22):2614-21, 1997
12. Korres DS et al: The significance of rotation in fracture-separation of the articular pillar of a lower cervical vertebra. A clinical and cadaveric study. Acta Orthop Scand Suppl. 275:17-20, 1997
13. Leite CC et al: MRI of cervical facet dislocation. Neuroradiology. 39(8):583-8, 1997
14. Sim E: Vertical facet splitting: a special variant of rotary dislocations of the cervical spine. J Neurosurg. 82(2):239-43, 1995
15. Shanmuganathan K et al: Rotational injury of cervical facets: CT analysis of fracture patterns with implications for management and neurologic outcome. AJR Am J Roentgenol. 163(5):1165-9, 1994
16. Willis BK et al: The incidence of vertebral artery injury after midcervical spine fracture or subluxation. Neurosurgery. 34(3):435-41; discussion 441-2, 1994
17. Shapiro SA: Management of unilateral locked facet of the cervical spine. Neurosurgery. 33(5):832-7; discussion 837, 1993
18. Beyer CA et al: Unilateral facet dislocations and fracture-dislocations of the cervical spine: a review. Orthopedics. 15(3):311-5, 1992
19. Hadley MN et al: Facet fracture-dislocation injuries of the cervical spine. Neurosurgery. 30(5):661-6, 1992
20. Roy-Camille R et al: Treatment of lower cervical spinal injuries--C3 to C7. Spine. 17(10 Suppl):S442-6, 1992
21. Myers BS et al: The role of torsion in cervical spine trauma. Spine. 16(8):870-4, 1991
22. Young JW et al: The laminar space in the diagnosis of rotational flexion injuries of the cervical spine. AJR Am J Roentgenol. 152(1):103-7, 1989
23. Rorabeck CH et al: Unilateral facet dislocation of the cervical spine. An analysis of the results of treatment in 26 patients. Spine. 12(1):23-7, 1987
24. Yetkin Z et al: Uncovertebral and facet joint dislocations in cervical articular pillar fractures: CT evaluation. AJNR Am J Neuroradiol. 6(4):633-7, 1985
25. Brant-Zawadzki M et al: Trauma, Computed Tomography of the Spine and Spinal Cord. Newton TH, Potts DG, Eds. Clavadel Press, 149-86, 1983
26. O'Callaghan JP et al: CT of facet distraction in flexion injuries of the thoracolumbar spine: the "naked" facet. AJR Am J Roentgenol. 134(3):563-8, 1980
27. Pick RY et al: C7--T1 bilateral facet dislocation: a rare lesion presenting with the syndrome of acute anterior spinal cord injury. Clin Orthop. (150):131-6, 1980
28. Ravichandran G: Traumatic single facet subluxation of cervical spine without neurological damage. A new clinical sign. Arch Orthop Trauma Surg. 92(2-3):221-4, 1978
29. Scher AT: Unilateral locked facet in cervical spine injuries. AJR Am J Roentgenol. 129(1):45-8, 1977
30. Babcock JL: Cervical spine injuries. Diagnosis and classification. Arch Surg. 111(6):646-51, 1976
31. Holdsworth FW et al: Fractures, dislocations and fracture-dislocations of the spine. J Bone Joint Surg Am. 45B: 6-20, 1963

HYPERFLEXION-ROTATION INJURY, CERVICAL

IMAGE GALLERY

Typical

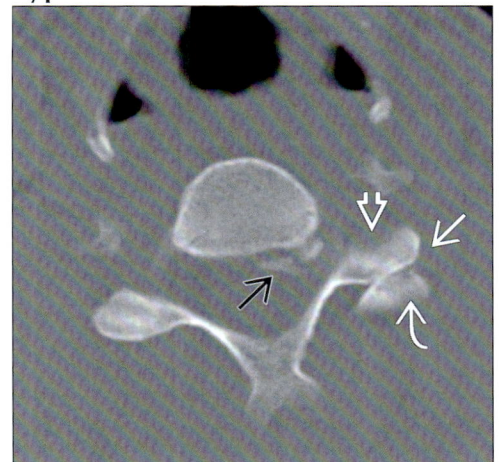
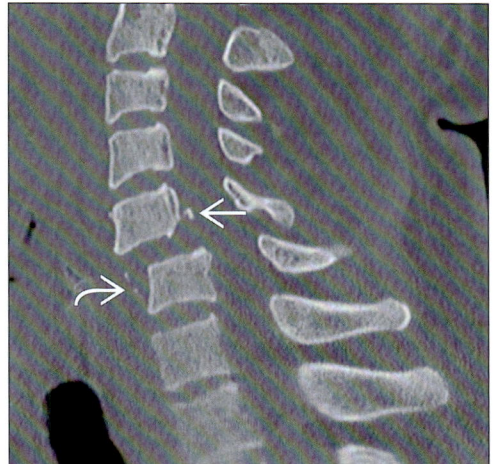

(Left) Axial bone CT shows left inferior facet ➡ anterior to superior facet ➡ (naked facet ➡). Note rotation of inferior body relative to superior body ➡. *(Right)* Sagittal bone CT shows anterolisthesis with fracture posterior margin of superior VB ➡ & avulsion anterior margin inferior VB ➡ 2° disruption of anterior & posterior longitudinal ligament.

Typical

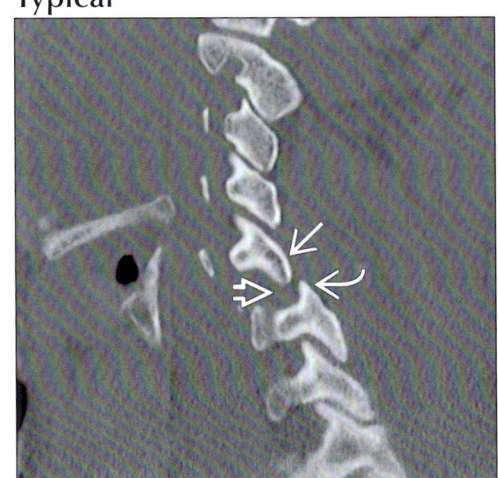
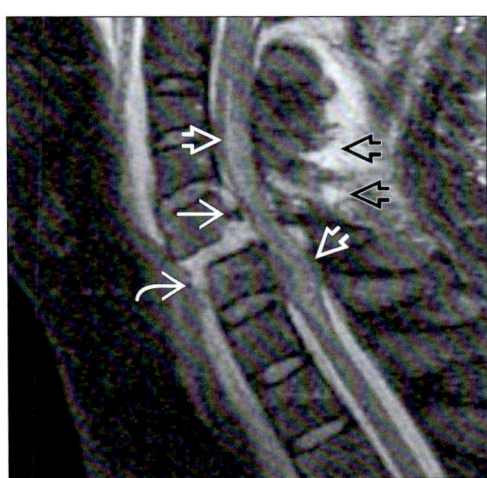

(Left) Sagittal bone CT in same patient as previous image. Anterior displacement of inferior facet of C5 ➡ relative to superior facet of C6 ➡, with separation and distraction of facet joint ➡. *(Right)* Sagittal STIR MR in same patient as left shows anterolisthesis with disruption of posterior ➡ & anterior ➡ longitudinal ligaments, cord edema ➡ and posterior soft tissue edema ➡.

Typical

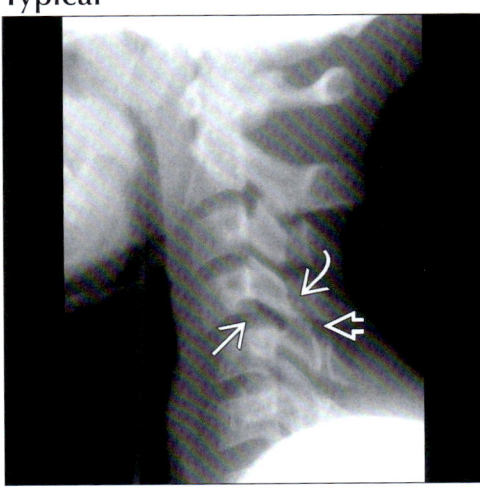
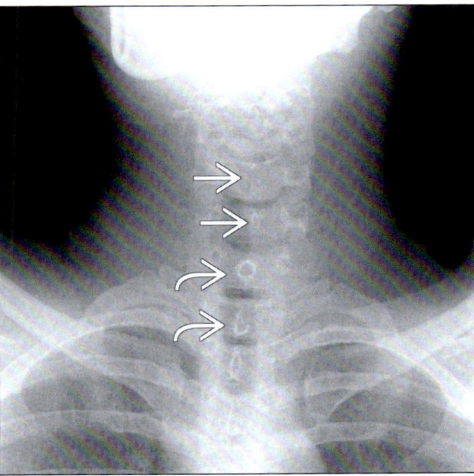

(Left) Lateral radiograph shows anterolisthesis of C4 on C5 ➡. Inferior facet of C4 ➡ is anterior to superior facet of C5 ➡. *(Right)* Anteroposterior radiograph shows spinous processes of C4 and C5 mildly displaced to right ➡ and obliquely oriented, compared to spinous processes of C7 and T1 ➡.

LATERAL FLEXION INJURY, CERVICAL

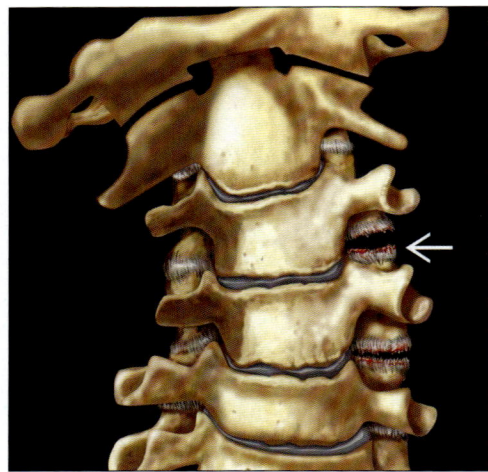

Anterior graphic shows disrupted facets and contralateral ligaments ➔ from lateral flexion injury.

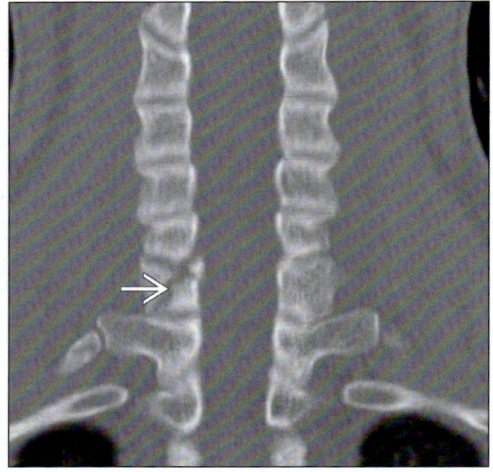

Coronal bone CT shows fracture lateral mass (pillar) of C7 ➔.

TERMINOLOGY

Abbreviations and Synonyms
- Articular mass fracture (fx), pillar fx

Definitions
- Fx of articular mass associated with fx of transverse, uncinate processes & vertebral body (vb)

IMAGING FINDINGS

General Features
- Best diagnostic clue: Articular pillar fx on AP view; widening uncovertebral joint
- Location: Mid-, lower cervical spine
- Morphology: Sagittal cleavage lateral mass

Radiographic Findings
- Radiography
  - Slight malalignment only clue on lateral view
  - Triangular appearance lateral mass on oblique view
  - Pillar view (cephalad angled AP): Articular mass fx

CT Findings
- NECT
  - Sagittal fx of pillar
  - Malaligned, impacted lateral mass on sagittal reformation
  - Associated transverse process or vb fx
- Bone CT
  - Thin section, bone algorithm with multiplanar reformations

MR Findings
- T1WI: Hypointense pillar fx
- T2WI: Hyperintense pillar fx, torn ligaments

Angiographic Findings
- Conventional: Confirm dissection and/or for endovascular treatment

Imaging Recommendations
- Best imaging tool: Bone algorithm CT with reformations
- Protocol advice: 1 mm or thinner slices

DDx: Lateral Flexion Injury Mimics

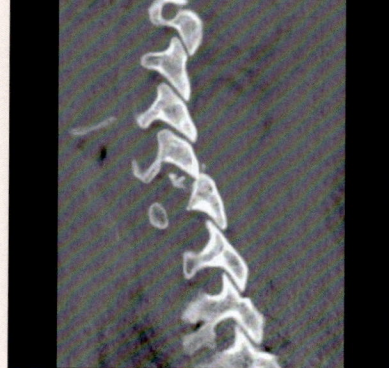

Unilateral Jumped Facet

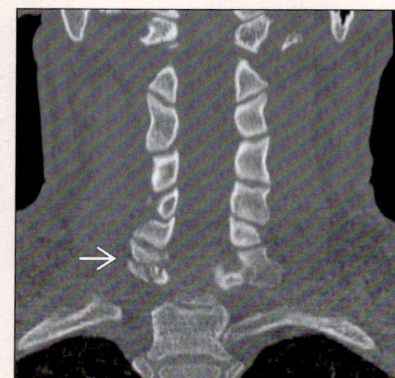

Flexion Rotation Injury

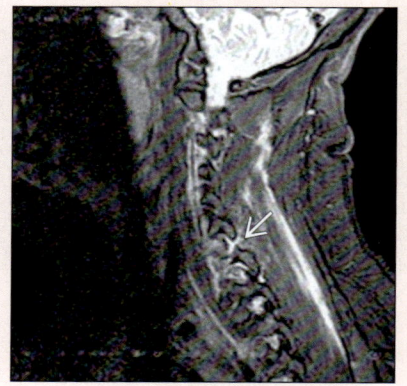

Flexion Rotation Injury

LATERAL FLEXION INJURY, CERVICAL

Key Facts

Terminology
- Articular mass fracture (fx), pillar fx

Imaging Findings
- Best diagnostic clue: Articular pillar fx on AP view; widening uncovertebral joint
- Sagittal fx of pillar
- Associated transverse process or vb fx

Top Differential Diagnoses
- Flexion/Rotation Fracture
- Fracture Isolation of Lateral Mass

Diagnostic Checklist
- CT if high clinical suspicion of fx
- Unilateral displacement of facet versus neighbor: Fx

DIFFERENTIAL DIAGNOSIS

Flexion/Rotation Fracture
- Different mechanism with rotational component
- Often see unilateral "jumped" facet

Fracture Isolation of Lateral Mass
- Separation of articular mass from vb & ipsilateral lamina ("floating" lateral mass)
- Produces three level instability

PATHOLOGY

General Features
- General path comments: Comminuted lateral mass, ipsilateral & contralateral capsular ligamentous injury
- Etiology: Lateral flexion forces during trauma
- Epidemiology: Sporadic traumatic injury
- Associated abnormalities: Neurological deficits (plegia, radiculopathy) in ~ 50%

Gross Pathologic & Surgical Features
- Fx instability

CLINICAL ISSUES

Presentation
- Most common signs/symptoms: Neck pain
- Other signs/symptoms: Plegia, radiculopathy

Natural History & Prognosis
- Depends on neurological damage

Treatment
- Options, risks, complications: Fusion for instability

DIAGNOSTIC CHECKLIST

Consider
- CT if high clinical suspicion of fx

Image Interpretation Pearls
- Unilateral displacement of facet versus neighbor: Fx

SELECTED REFERENCES

1. Halliday AL et al: The management of unilateral lateral mass/facet fractures of the subaxial cervical spine: the use of magnetic resonance imaging to predict instability. Spine. 22(22):2614-21, 1997
2. Shanmuganathan K et al: Traumatic isolation of the cervical articular pillar: imaging observations in 21 patients. AJR Am J Roentgenol. 166(4):897-902, 1996
3. Shanmuganathan K et al: Rotational injury of cervical facets: CT analysis of fracture patterns with implications for management and neurologic outcome. AJR Am J Roentgenol. 163(5):1165-9, 1994
4. Woodring JH et al: Fractures of the articular processes of the cervical spine. AJR Am J Roentgenol. 139(2):341-4, 1982

IMAGE GALLERY

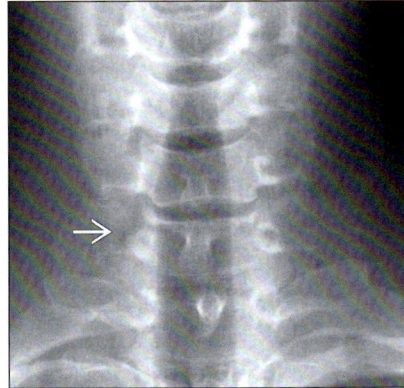 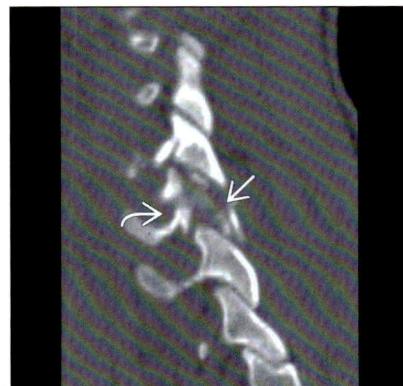 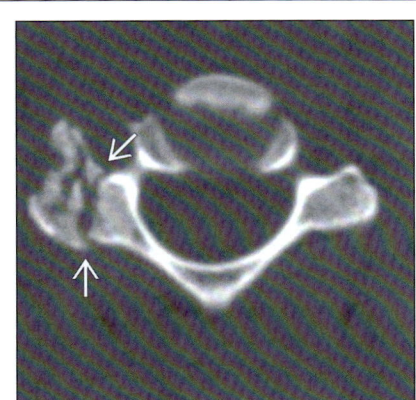

(Left) Anteroposterior radiograph in same case as previous image, shows ill defined hypodensity in lateral mass of C7 ➔. *(Center)* Sagittal bone CT shows fracture of lateral mass of facet ➔ and pedicle ➔. *(Right)* Axial bone CT in same case as previous image, shows fracture of lateral mass (pillar) ➔.

POSTERIOR COLUMN INJURY, CERVICAL

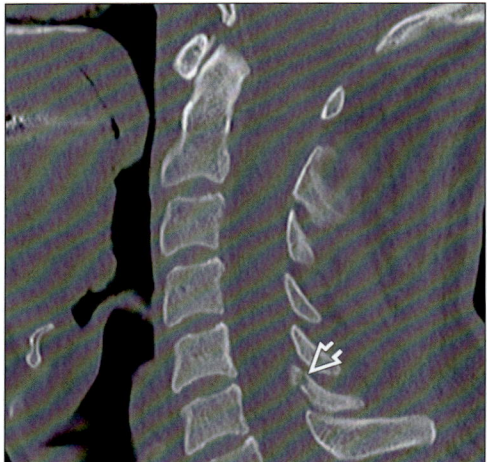

Sagittal bone CT shows fracture through spinous process of C6 ➡.

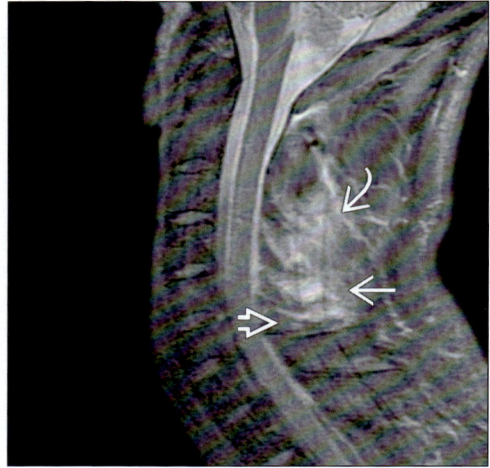

Sagittal STIR MR in same patient as previous image, reveals posterior spinal soft tissue edema from C4 ➡ through C6 ➡. Spinous process edema is visible ➡, but fracture cannot be seen.

TERMINOLOGY

Definitions
- Spinal structures beyond posterior longitudinal ligament (PLL) & posterior margin of vertebral body (VB)
  - Bones: Facets, laminae, spinous processes
  - Ligaments: Joint, interspinous & flavum

IMAGING FINDINGS

General Features
- Best diagnostic clue: Disrupted alignment, relation of posterior arch at adjacent vertebral levels

Radiographic Findings
- Radiography
  - Fracture through laminae, facets, or spinous process
  - Malaligned posterior elements

CT Findings
- NECT: Fracture of laminae or articular pillar, epidural hematoma
- Bone CT
  - High-resolution algorithm to detect non-displaced fracture

MR Findings
- T2WI
  - Increased signal in muscles, ligaments
  - Cord edema with contusion
- STIR: Best for soft tissue and marrow edema, fractured VB/arch

Imaging Recommendations
- Best imaging tool: CT with soft tissue & bone windows, reformations
- Protocol advice: 1 mm slice thickness, bone algorithm reconstruction of CT slices

DIFFERENTIAL DIAGNOSIS

Multicolumn Fractures with Element of Posterior Column Involvement
- Flexion or extension fracture
- Flexion or extension-rotation fracture

DDx: Posterior Column Injury

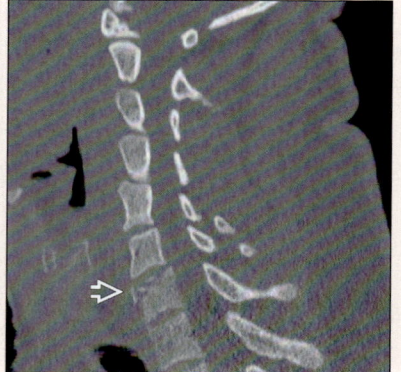

Flexion Rotation Fracture

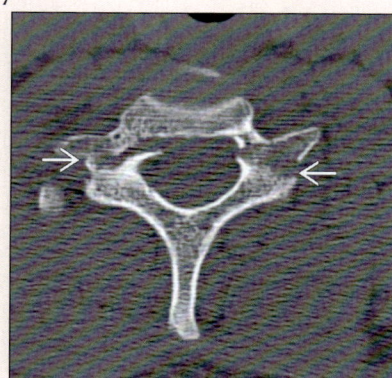

Extension Fracture

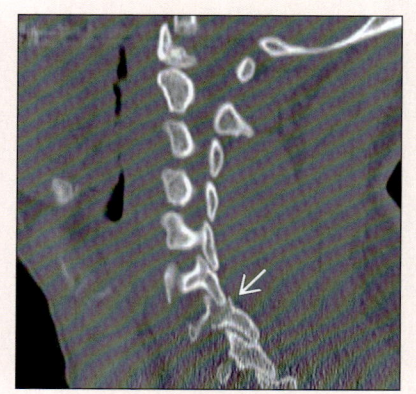

Extension Fracture

POSTERIOR COLUMN INJURY, CERVICAL

Terminology
- Spinal structures beyond posterior longitudinal ligament (PLL) & posterior margin of vertebral body (VB)

Pathology
- Tear of ligaments bridging spinous processes and laminae
- Fractures of laminae, facets, or spinous processes

Key Facts
- Posterior column fracture generally stable, as anterior/middle columns intact and prevent subluxation
- If capsular ligaments torn, facets and/or laminae both fractured, rotational instability may exist

Diagnostic Checklist
- Flexion extension films or fluoroscopy to assess for instability

- Jumped facets

PATHOLOGY

General Features
- General path comments
  - Tear of ligaments bridging spinous processes and laminae
  - Fractures of laminae, facets, or spinous processes
  - Posterior column fracture generally stable, as anterior/middle columns intact and prevent subluxation
    - If capsular ligaments torn, facets and/or laminae both fractured, rotational instability may exist
- Associated abnormalities: May have associated disruption of middle or anterior column, resulting in instability

CLINICAL ISSUES

Presentation
- Most common signs/symptoms: Neck pain, neurologic disturbance
- Clinical Profile: Neck pain, loss of mobility

Treatment
- Options, risks, complications
  - Immobilization
  - Surgical fusion

DIAGNOSTIC CHECKLIST

Consider
- Flexion extension films or fluoroscopy to assess for instability

Image Interpretation Pearls
- Minor malalignment → severe ligamentous disruption

SELECTED REFERENCES
1. Matar LD et al: "Spinolaminar breach": an important sign in cervical spinous process fractures. Skeletal Radiol. 29(2):75-80, 2000
2. Zhu Q et al: Traumatic instabilities of the cervical spine caused by high-speed axial compression in a human model. An in vitro biomechanical study. Spine. 24(5):440-4, 1999
3. Plezbert JA et al: Fracture of a lamina in the cervical spine. J Manipulative Physiol Ther. 17(8):552-7, 1994
4. Goldberg AL et al: Hyperextension injuries of the cervical spine. Magnetic resonance findings. Skeletal Radiol. 18(4):283-8, 1989

IMAGE GALLERY

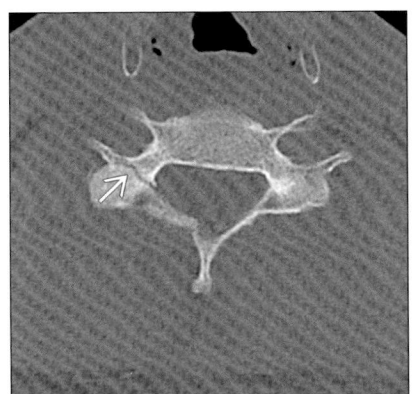
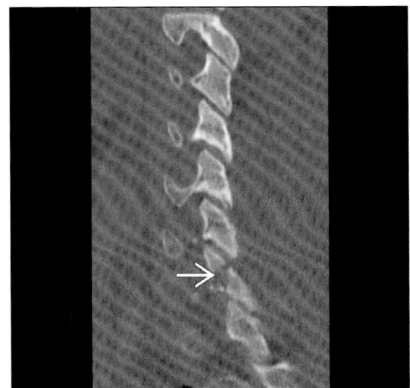
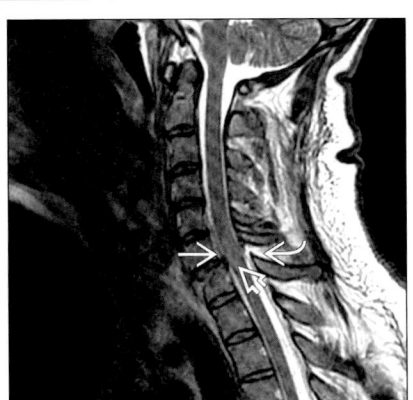

(Left) Axial bone CT shows fracture through the facet ➔. *(Center)* Sagittal bone CT in same patient as previous image, shows fractures through pars interarticularis and facets ➔. *(Right)* Sagittal T2WI MR shows anterolisthesis with disruption of PLL ➔ and spinal laminar ➔ line. Cord edema ➔ is also present.

COMPRESSION FRACTURES

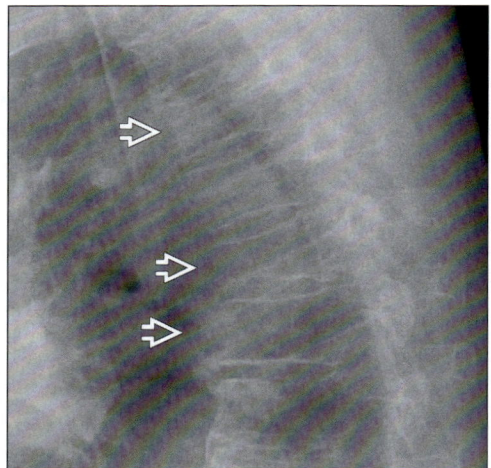

Lateral radiograph shows multiple mid-thoracic anterior compression fxs ➡.

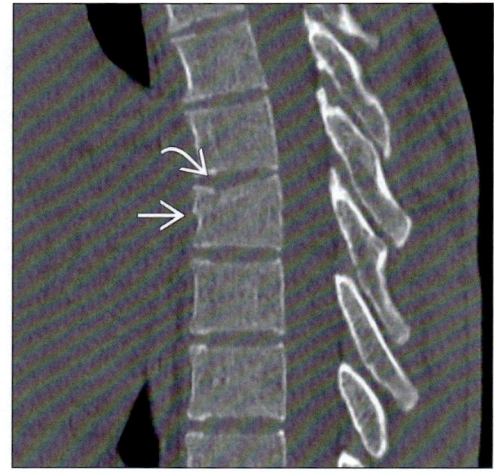

Sagittal bone CT shows compression fx in lower thoracic spine extending through superior endplate ➡ & anterior margin of vertebral body ➡.

TERMINOLOGY

Abbreviations and Synonyms
- Wedge compression

Definitions
- Vertebral body fracture (fx) compressing anterior cortex, sparing middle/posterior columns

IMAGING FINDINGS

General Features
- Best diagnostic clue: Wedge-shaped vertebral body
- Location
  - May occur at multiple levels, contiguous or noncontiguous
  - Mid- or lower thoracic most common; upper thoracic rare

Radiographic Findings
- Radiography
  - Diagnostic signs primarily visible on lateral radiography
    - Wedge-shaped vertebral body
    - Distinct fx line usually not visible
    - Kyphosis common
    - Most common: Superior endplate alone
    - May involve both endplates or inferior endplate (5%)
  - Anteroposterior radiography
    - Paraspinous hematoma apparent (acute)
    - Loss of vertebral height difficult to see
    - Endplate depression may be cup-like or angular
    - Angular deformity, stepoff anterior cortex
    - Normal posterior elements
  - < 40-50% loss of height in patients with normal density
    - If greater loss of height, probably Chance fracture
  - In osteoporotic patients, may develop vertebra plana

CT Findings
- Bone CT
  - Multiple fx
  - May extend to posterior cortex of vertebral body
  - Posterior cortical displacement absent
  - Fractures of posterior elements absent

DDx: Compression Fracture Mimics

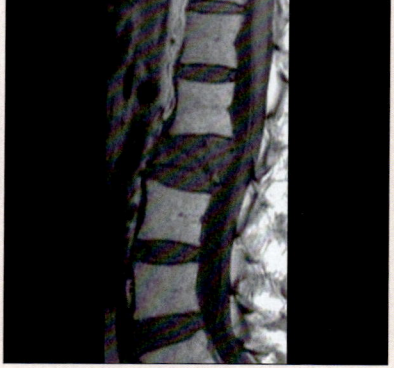

Pathologic Fracture (Mets)

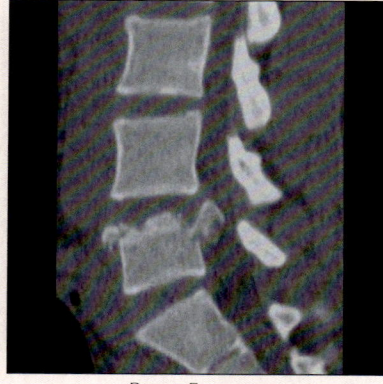

Burst Fracture

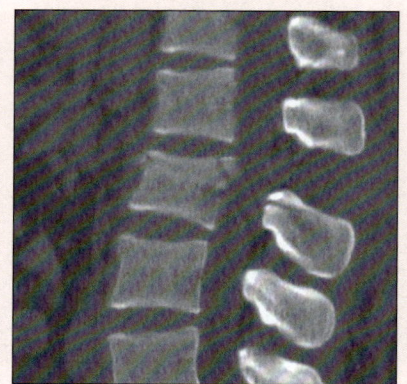

Chance Fracture

COMPRESSION FRACTURES

Key Facts

Terminology
- Vertebral body fracture (fx) compressing anterior cortex, sparing middle/posterior columns

Imaging Findings
- Best diagnostic clue: Wedge-shaped vertebral body
- May occur at multiple levels, contiguous or noncontiguous
- May extend to posterior cortex of vertebral body
- Fractures of posterior elements absent
- Best imaging tool: CT best to differentiate from Chance or burst fractures

Top Differential Diagnoses
- Compression-Distraction Injury (Chance Fx)
- Burst Fracture
- Pathologic Fracture Due to Tumor
- Scheuermann Kyphosis
- Physiologic Vertebral Wedging

Pathology
- Axial load ± flexion component
- Two distinct populations

Clinical Issues
- Patients with normal bone mineral density heal well with conservative management
- Osteoporotic patients may have progressive fx

Diagnostic Checklist
- Compression fx involving inferior endplate with normal superior endplate raises suspicion for pathologic fx

---

- Alignment of posterior elements normal on reformatted images

MR Findings
- T1WI
  - Low signal intensity fx visible in some cases
  - Band-like or triangular region of low signal parallel to endplate
  - Posterior cortex intact
  - Paraspinous hematoma may mimic tumor
- T2WI
  - High signal in vb
    - Parallels superior endplate
  - Ligaments intact
- STIR
  - Best sequence for marrow edema: Hyperintense
  - ± fx line
- T1 C+: May have diffuse or linear enhancement

Nuclear Medicine Findings
- Bone Scan
  - Positive in all three phases if acute
  - Nonspecific
    - Tumor, infection, degenerative disease

Imaging Recommendations
- Best imaging tool: CT best to differentiate from Chance or burst fractures
- Protocol advice
  - Thin section helical scans with multidetector unit
  - Sagittal/coronal reformations essential
  - If undergoing thoracic multidetector or whole body scan dedicated spine images not needed
    - Small field of view coronal/sagittal reformations obtained from original dataset
    - Bone algorithm applied retrospectively

DIFFERENTIAL DIAGNOSIS

Compression-Distraction Injury (Chance Fx)
- Involves middle, posterior columns
- If > 50% loss of vertebral body height & bone density normal, probably Chance fx
- Horizontally oriented posterior element fractures
- Disruption of facet joints, interspinous ligaments

Burst Fracture
- Loss of height anterior & posterior vertebral bodies
- Retropulsion of posterior vertebral cortex
- Less common in thoracic spine 2° stabilizing effect of ribs

Pathologic Fracture Due to Tumor
- Cortical destruction
- Trabecular destruction (best seen on CT)
- Hypointense on T1WI, hyperintense on STIR
  - Geographic distribution: Does not parallel endplate
  - Hyperintensity on DWI may differentiate malignant from benign fx
- More likely to involve inferior cortex of vertebral body & posterior elements
- Paraspinous mass may be 2° hematoma (benign compression fx) or tumor extension
- Often see tumor at other levels away from fx

Scheuermann Kyphosis
- Three contiguous levels
- Schmorl nodes
- Undulation of vertebral endplates

Physiologic Vertebral Wedging
- Seen at T12-L1
- Mild loss of height
- Usually involves both superior & inferior endplates

PATHOLOGY

General Features
- General path comments: Most common type of thoracic spine fx due to blunt trauma
- Etiology
  - Axial load ± flexion component

COMPRESSION FRACTURES

- Because of normal thoracic kyphosis, axial load affects anterior portion of vertebral body more than posterior
- Epidemiology
  - Two distinct populations
    - Young patients: Due to significant fall, major trauma
    - Elderly osteoporotic patients: Insufficiency fx
- Associated abnormalities
  - Other spine fx, contiguous or not contiguous
  - Fx of pelvis & lower extremities

CLINICAL ISSUES

Presentation
- Most common signs/symptoms
  - Acute trauma with focal back pain
  - Insidious back pain in elderly patients
- Other signs/symptoms
  - Radiculopathy
  - Kyphotic deformity

Demographics
- Age
  - Bimodal
  - Young trauma patients
  - Elderly osteoporotic patients

Natural History & Prognosis
- Patients with normal bone mineral density heal well with conservative management
- Increased risk of premature degenerative disc disease in young patients
- Osteoporotic patients may have progressive fx
  - Chronic pain
  - Kyphotic deformity often progressive
- Patients with one osteoporotic compression fx at increased risk for other fxs
- May have delayed onset of neurologic symptoms

Treatment
- Options, risks, complications: Conservative management usually successful
- Vertebroplasty & kyphoplasty used for chronic pain, kyphotic deformity
  - Usually affords immediate pain relief
  - May increase risk of compression fxs of adjacent vertebrae
- Bisphosphonates, calcitonin decrease pain & risk of further osteoporotic fx

DIAGNOSTIC CHECKLIST

Image Interpretation Pearls
- Compression fx involving inferior endplate with normal superior endplate raises suspicion for pathologic fx

SELECTED REFERENCES

1. Folman Y et al: Late outcome of nonoperative management of thoracolumbar vertebral wedge fractures. J Orthop Trauma. 17(3):190-2, 2003
2. Haba H et al: Diagnostic accuracy of magnetic resonance imaging for detecting posterior ligamentous complex injury associated with thoracic and lumbar fractures. J Neurosurg. 99(1 Suppl):20-6, 2003
3. Hiwatashi A et al: Increase in vertebral body height after vertebroplasty. AJNR Am J Neuroradiol. 24(2):185-9, 2003
4. Hsu JM et al: Thoracolumbar fracture in blunt trauma patients: guidelines for diagnosis and imaging. Injury. 34(6):426-33, 2003
5. Naves M et al: The effect of vertebral fracture as a risk factor for osteoporotic fracture and mortality in a Spanish population. Osteoporos Int. 14(6):520-4, 2003
6. Phillips FM: Minimally invasive treatments of osteoporotic vertebral compression fractures. Spine. 28(15):S45-53, 2003
7. Sapkas GS et al: Thoracic spinal injuries: operative treatments and neurologic outcomes. Am J Orthop. 32(2):85-8, 2003
8. Sheridan R et al: Reformatted visceral protocol helical computed tomographic scanning allows conventional radiographs of the thoracic and lumbar spine to be eliminated in the evaluation of blunt trauma patients. J Trauma. 55(4):665-9, 2003
9. Wintermark M et al: Thoracolumbar spine fractures in patients who have sustained severe trauma: depiction with multi-detector row CT. Radiology. 227(3):681-9, 2003
10. Baur A et al: Acute osteoporotic and neoplastic vertebral compression fractures: fluid sign at MR imaging. Radiology. 225(3):730-5, 2002
11. Lane JM et al: Minimally invasive options for the treatment of osteoporotic vertebral compression fractures. Orthop Clin North Am. 33(2):431-8, viii, 2002
12. O'Connor PA et al: Spinal cord injury following osteoporotic vertebral fracture: case report. Spine. 27(18):E413-5, 2002
13. Parisini P et al: Treatment of spinal fractures in children and adolescents: long-term results in 44 patients. Spine. 27(18):1989-94, 2002
14. Robertson A et al: Spinal injury patterns resulting from car and motorcycle accidents. Spine. 27(24):2825-30, 2002
15. Wittenberg RH et al: Noncontiguous unstable spine fractures. Spine. 27(3):254-7, 2002
16. Zhou XJ et al: Characterization of benign and metastatic vertebral compression fractures with quantitative diffusion MR imaging. AJNR Am J Neuroradiol. 23(1):165-70, 2002
17. Holmes JF et al: Epidemiology of thoracolumbar spine injury in blunt trauma. Acad Emerg Med. 8(9):866-72, 2001
18. Lindsay R et al: Risk of new vertebral fracture in the year following a fracture. JAMA. 285(3):320-3, 2001
19. Vaccaro AR et al: Post-traumatic spinal deformity. Spine. 26(24 Suppl):S111-8, 2001
20. Kerttula LI et al: Post-traumatic findings of the spine after earlier vertebral fracture in young patients: clinical and MRI study. Spine. 25(9):1104-8, 2000
21. van Beek EJ et al: Upper thoracic spinal fractures in trauma patients - a diagnostic pitfall. Injury. 31(4):219-23, 2000
22. Rechtine GR 2nd et al: Treatment of thoracolumbar trauma: comparison of complications of operative versus nonoperative treatment. J Spinal Disord. 12(5):406-9, 1999

COMPRESSION FRACTURES

IMAGE GALLERY

Typical

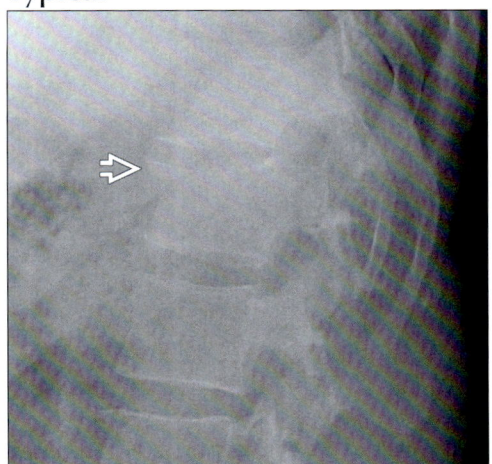
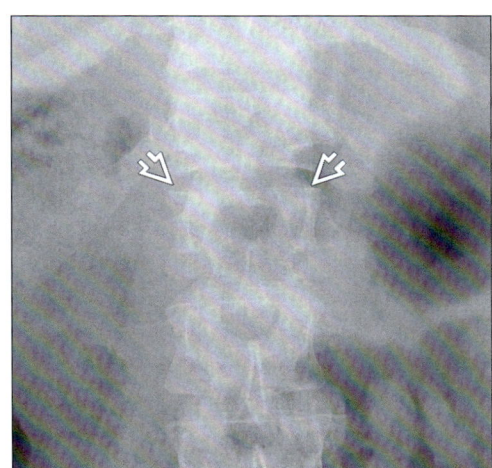

(Left) Lateral radiograph shows superior endplate fx of L1 ➡ with loss of height of anterior portion of vertebral body (wedge-shaped). *(Right)* Anteroposterior radiograph in same case as left shows subtle loss of height of L1 ➡; no fx visible.

Typical

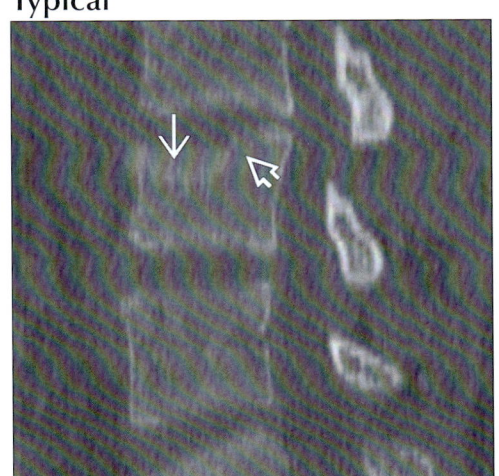
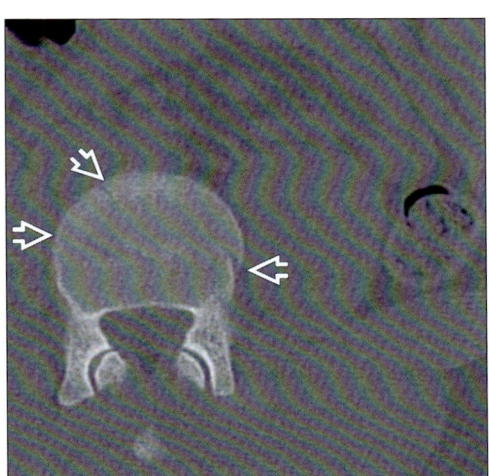

(Left) Sagittal bone CT in same patient as previous image, shows oval depression of superior endplate ➡ with acute angulation ➡ at posterior margin of fx. *(Right)* Axial bone CT in same case as left shows fx ➡ through anterior half of vertebral body; middle & posterior columns are spared.

Typical

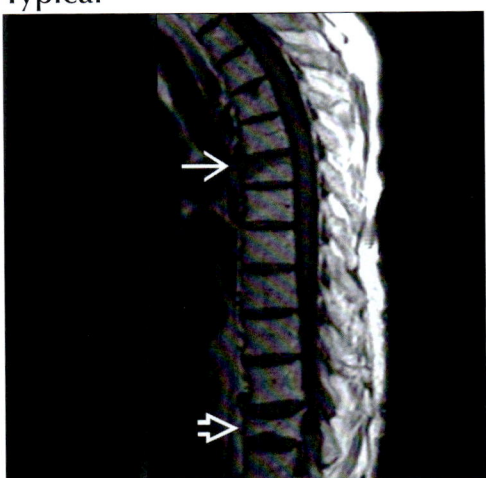
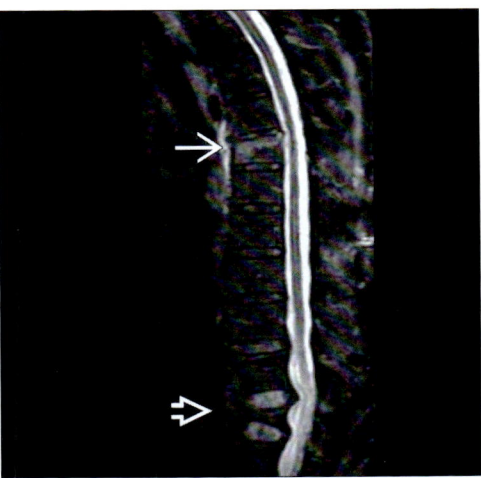

(Left) Sagittal T1WI MR shows two compression fxs: Acute superior fx ➡, with band of hypointense edema of vertebral body, and isointense chronic inferior fx involving both endplates ➡. *(Right)* Sagittal STIR MR in same case as left shows T2 hyperintense edema of superior acute fx ➡; chronic inferior fx is isointense ➡.

BURST THORACOLUMBAR FRACTURE

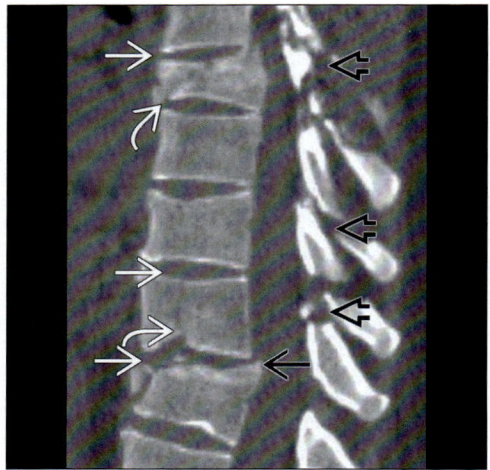

Sagittal bone CT shows multiple burst fx's with involvement of the superior ➔ & inferior end plates ➔ & spinous processes ➔. Note anterolisthesis & retropulsion of bone into spinal canal ➔.

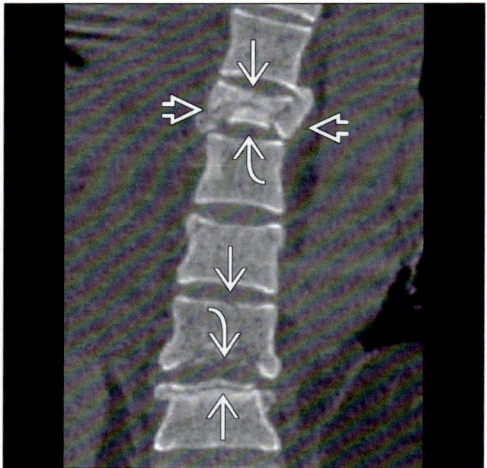

Coronal bone CT shows multiple burst fxs through the superior ➔ & inferior end plates ➔. Note lateral displacement of fracture fragments ➔.

TERMINOLOGY

Abbreviations and Synonyms
- Unstable compression fracture (fx)

Definitions
- Comminuted fx of vertebral body (VB) extending through superior & inferior endplates

IMAGING FINDINGS

General Features
- Best diagnostic clue: Compressed VB with endplate fxs, widened pedicles
- Location: Mid-thoracic to upper lumbar spine
- Morphology: Anterior wedging (lateral, sagittal views)

Radiographic Findings
- Radiography: Widened pedicles on anteroposterior & wedge VB on lateral view; malalignment

CT Findings
- NECT: Soft tissue swelling, blood in canal
- Bone CT
  - Comminuted fx on axial & reformatted views
  - Posterior displacement of bone into canal
  - Malalignment of VB and/or facets

MR Findings
- T1WI
  - Hypointensity in wedged VB; fx difficult to see
  - Soft tissue infiltration
- T2WI
  - Hyperintensity in VB & soft tissue
  - May see hyperintense cord contusion
- STIR: As with T2WI; better for bone edema
- T2* GRE: Hypointense hemorrhage in cord or canal

Imaging Recommendations
- Protocol advice
  - Thin-section axial slices; reformations, bone & soft tissue windows
  - MR for suspected cord injury or spinal hemorrhage

DIFFERENTIAL DIAGNOSIS

Benign Compression Fracture
- No retropulsion of fragments or pedicular widening

DDx: Fractures Resembling Burst Fracture

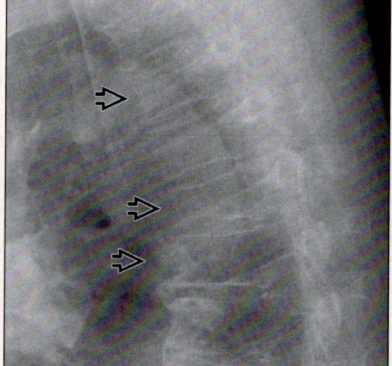

Benign Compression Fracture

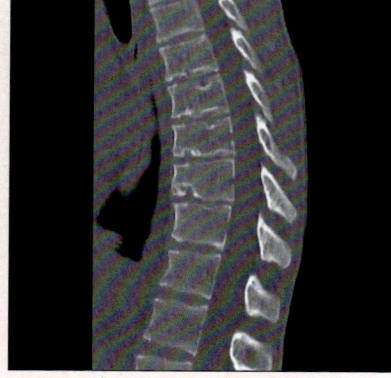

Scheuermann Syndrome

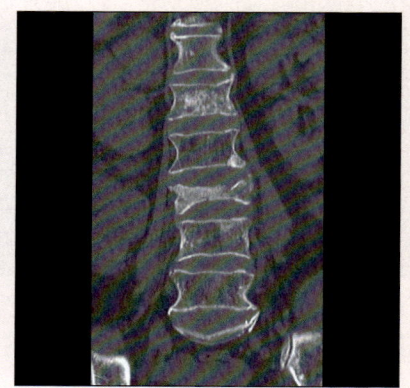

Pathologic Fracture

BURST THORACOLUMBAR FRACTURE

Key Facts

Terminology
- Unstable compression fracture (fx)
- Comminuted fx of vertebral body (VB) extending through superior & inferior endplates

Imaging Findings
- Location: Mid-thoracic to upper lumbar spine
- Radiography: Widened pedicles on anteroposterior & wedge VB on lateral view; malalignment
- Comminuted fx on axial & reformatted views

- Posterior displacement of bone into canal
- Hypointensity in wedged VB; fx difficult to see
- Hyperintensity in VB & soft tissue
- May see hyperintense cord contusion
- T2* GRE: Hypointense hemorrhage in cord or canal

Diagnostic Checklist
- If widened pedicles relative to superior VB, suspect burst fx, instability

Pathologic Compression Fracture
- Soft tissue mass replacing major portion of VB on MR

Scheuermann Syndrome
- Three contiguous wedged VBs

PATHOLOGY

General Features
- General path comments: Typically 2° to vertical force (jumping, landing on buttock)
- Etiology: Trauma
- Associated abnormalities
  - Spinal epidural hematoma
  - Cord contusion

Gross Pathologic & Surgical Features
- Disrupted VB
- Column instability

Microscopic Features
- Microtrabecular disruption, hemorrhage

CLINICAL ISSUES

Presentation
- Most common signs/symptoms
  - Acute local pain after trauma
  - Lower extremity weakness, +/- sphincter disruption
- Clinical Profile: Focal back pain with vertical force component injury; +/- neurologic deficit

Natural History & Prognosis
- Self-limited if no cord injury or spinal hematoma

Treatment
- Surgical stabilization ± canal decompression

DIAGNOSTIC CHECKLIST

Consider
- Neoplasm or osteoporosis if only minor trauma

Image Interpretation Pearls
- If widened pedicles relative to superior VB, suspect burst fx, instability

SELECTED REFERENCES

1. Verlaan JJ et al: Operative compared with nonoperative treatment of a thoracolumbar burst fracture without neurological deficit. J Bone Joint Surg Am. 86-A(3):649-50; author reply 650-1, 2004
2. Kim NH et al: Neurologic injury and recovery in patients with burst fracture of the thoracolumbar spine. Spine. 24(3):290-3; discussion 294, 1999
3. Saifuddin A et al: The role of imaging in the diagnosis and management of thoracolumbar burst fractures: current concepts and a review of the literature. Skeletal Radiol. 25(7):603-13, 1996

IMAGE GALLERY

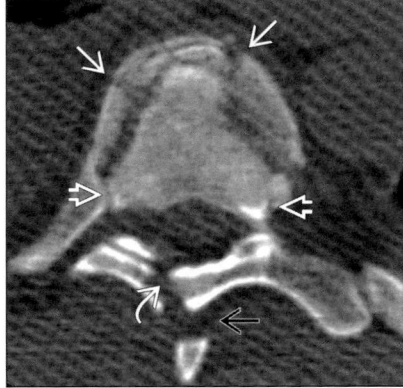 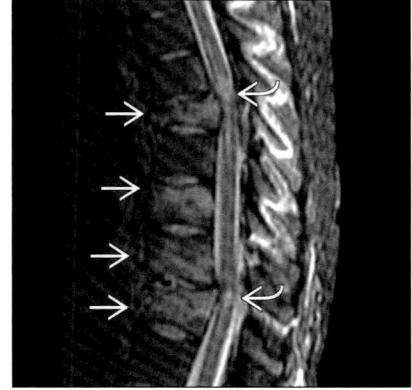 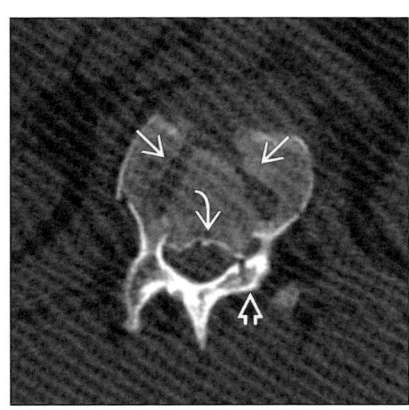

(Left) Axial bone CT shows fxs through the endplate anteriorly ➔ & the posterior margins of vertebral bodies ➔, as well as through lamina ➔ and spinous process ➔. *(Center)* Sagittal STIR MR shows edema ➔ within multiple burst fxs. Retropulsion of bone fragments produces cord edema ➔, which is indicative of contusions. *(Right)* Axial bone CT shows fxs through the end plate ➔ with retropulsion of the fragment into the spinal canal ➔, producing spinal stenosis. Posterior column fracture ➔ is also present.

FACET-LAMINA THORACOLUMBAR FRACTURE

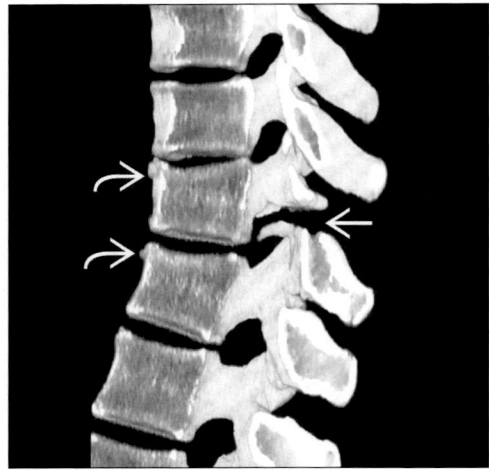

Sagittal bone CT 3D reformation shows fracture through pars intermedia ➔ with flexion distraction of fracture fragments & anterior compression fractures of adjacent vertebral bodies ➔.

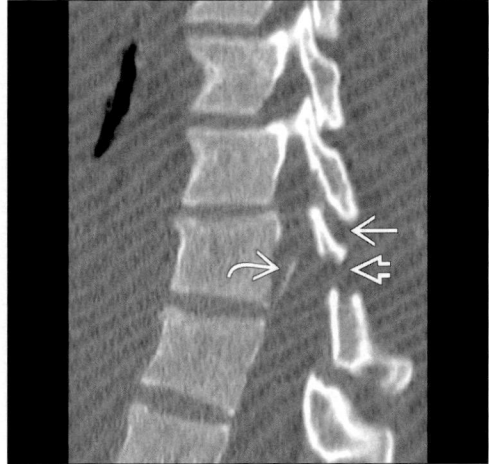

Sagittal bone CT in same case as previous image, shows pars fracture ➔ and widening of facet joint ➔. Note avulsion fracture of posterior vertebra 2° to PLL rupture ➔.

TERMINOLOGY

Abbreviations and Synonyms
- Neural (vertebral) arch fracture
- Posterior column fracture

Definitions
- Fracture through vertebral arch

IMAGING FINDINGS

General Features
- Best diagnostic clue: Cortical disruption/discontinuity through laminae, facet joints of thoracolumbar vertebrae
- Location
  ○ Uncommon in upper/mid-thoracic spine
    ▪ T1-T10 stabilized by ribs
    ▪ 60% of thoracolumbar fractures between T12-L2
    ▪ 90% of fractures between T11-L4
- Size: Multiple thoracic levels may be involved

Radiographic Findings
- Radiography
  ○ Widened paraspinal line
    ▪ Paraspinal hematoma
  ○ Vertebral height loss
    ▪ Posterior column usually not involved in compression fracture
  ○ Increased interpediculate distance
    ▪ Vertebral arch disrupted only in severe burst fractures
  ○ Facet dislocation/subluxation; vertebral dislocation; increased interspinous distance
    ▪ Indicates ruptured posterior ligamentous complex often with concomitant neural arch fractures

CT Findings
- NECT: Paraspinal hematoma on screening trauma CT
- CTA
  ○ Evaluation of aorta and major branches
    ▪ Especially in presence of upper thoracic and rib fractures
- Bone CT
  ○ Widened, comminuted neural arch
  ○ Fracture through facet joints

DDx: Facet-Lamina Thoracolumbar Fractures

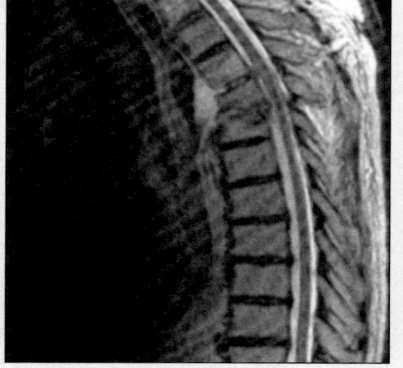

Osteomyelitis

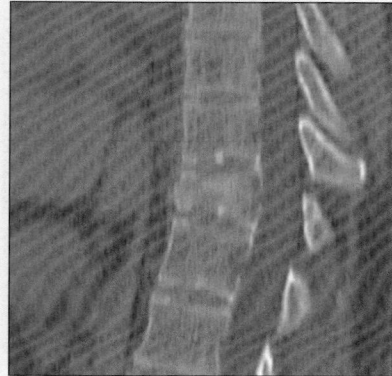

Compression Fracture

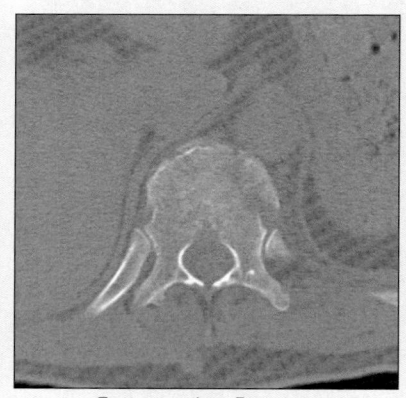

Compression Fracture

FACET-LAMINA THORACOLUMBAR FRACTURE

Key Facts

Terminology
- Neural (vertebral) arch fracture

Imaging Findings
- Best diagnostic clue: Cortical disruption/discontinuity through laminae, facet joints of thoracolumbar vertebrae
- 60% of thoracolumbar fractures between T12-L2
- Widened paraspinal line
- Increased interpediculate distance
- Facet subluxation/dislocation
- Vertebral body comminution
- Vertebral subluxation/dislocation
- Hyperintense marrow & soft tissue edema
- Hyperintense swollen cord: Edema
- Paraspinal & intraspinal hematoma

- Thin-section bone CT with reformation to characterize posterior column fracture
- MR when neurologic deficit to evaluate for cord injury
- Sagittal reformation from axial CT
- Sagittal STIR for posterior ligamentous injury

Top Differential Diagnoses
- Septic Facet Arthritis and Osteomyelitis
- Pathologic Fracture

Diagnostic Checklist
- Look for paraspinal soft tissue hematoma as clue to spinal fractures on CT

  - Facet subluxation/dislocation
    - "Naked facet" sign: Partially or completely uncovered articulating processes on axial imaging
    - Locked facets: Inferior facets of vertebra above anterior to superior facets of vertebra below
  - Vertebral body comminution
    - Retropulsed bony fragments within spinal canal
  - Vertebral subluxation/dislocation
    - "Double body" sign: Overlapping vertebrae on axial imaging

MR Findings
- T1WI
  - Hyperintense subacute intraspinal hemorrhage
  - Hypointense fracture lines
  - Separated osseous fragments
- T2WI
  - Hyperintense marrow & soft tissue edema
  - Hyperintense swollen cord: Edema
  - Hypointense swollen cord: Hematoma
- STIR: Hyperintense marrow & soft tissue edema accentuated
- T2* GRE
  - Hypointense cord hemorrhage
  - Herniated disc
  - Paraspinal & intraspinal hematoma

Non-Vascular Interventions
- Myelography: Evaluation for spinal cord swelling when MR not feasible

Imaging Recommendations
- Best imaging tool
  - Thin-section bone CT with reformation to characterize posterior column fracture
  - MR when neurologic deficit to evaluate for cord injury
- Protocol advice
  - Sagittal reformation from axial CT
    - Demonstrates extent of canal compromise
    - Shows horizontal fracture through posterior elements
  - Sagittal STIR for posterior ligamentous injury

DIFFERENTIAL DIAGNOSIS

Septic Facet Arthritis and Osteomyelitis
- Marrow edema in facet articular processes & adjacent laminae on MR
- Fluid intensity within facet joint
- Surrounding soft tissue edema, enhancement and abscess

Pathologic Fracture
- Underlying lytic or sclerotic lesion on CT
- Bony expansion
- Soft tissue mass
- More commonly associated with vertebral body

PATHOLOGY

General Features
- Etiology
  - Motor vehicle accidents
  - Falls
  - Sport-related injuries
  - Penetrating injuries
- Epidemiology
  - Prevalence of thoracolumbar injuries
    - 6% in blunt trauma patients
- Associated abnormalities
  - Intracranial hemorrhage
  - Visceral organ injuries
  - Other fractures
  - Vascular injury
- Anatomy
  - Neural (vertebral) arch
    - Pedicles, laminae, articular processes, base of spinous process
  - Posterior ligamentous complex
    - Ligamentum flavum, facet joint capsule, interspinous ligament, supraspinous ligament
  - Three-column concept of thoracic spine; two-column injury

FACET-LAMINA THORACOLUMBAR FRACTURE

- Anterior column: Anterior longitudinal ligament (ALL), anterior half of vertebral body & annulus fibrosis
- Middle column: Posterior longitudinal ligament (PLL), posterior half of vertebral body & annulus fibrosis
- Posterior column: Neural arch, facet joints, spinous process, transverse process, ligamentous complex
- Mechanism of injury
  - Neural arch fracture
    - Extension
    - Flexion-distraction: Horizontal fracture through vertebral body, PLL, posterior elements
    - Flexion-rotation: Ruptured posterior ligamentous complex, fractures, dislocation
    - Shear: All ligaments disrupted with listhesis in all three directions
  - If neural arch not involved
    - Flexion: Posterior ligaments may rupture
    - Compression: Neural arch involvement only in severe burst fractures
    - 75% of thoracolumbar fractures

Staging, Grading or Classification Criteria
- Mechanical stability depends on number of columns involved
  - Stable: One column injured
    - Anterior column: Compression fracture
    - Posterior column: Spinous process or unilateral laminar fracture
  - Unstable: Two or three columns involved
    - Burst and Chance fractures
    - All fracture dislocations

CLINICAL ISSUES

Presentation
- Most common signs/symptoms
  - Back pain
  - Neurologic deficits
- Other signs/symptoms: Multisystemic injury

Demographics
- Age: Mean age 25-40 years
- Gender
  - M:F ratio
    - 9:1 in motorcycle accidents
    - 3:2 in car accidents
- Ethnicity: No race predilection

Natural History & Prognosis
- Residual neurologic deficits in 15-20% of thoracolumbar trauma
  - Complete paraplegia at time of injury rarely improves despite therapy
  - Incomplete cord injury may achieve neurologic recovery

Treatment
- Initial IV high-dose steroids if cord injury present
- Conservative treatment if mechanically stable
  - Stabilization with bracing
  - Early mobilization
  - One- or two-column injuries
- Surgery to prevent instability and deformity, preserve neural function
  - Three-column injuries, kyphosis > 20°, progressive neurologic deficits
  - Anterior and/or posterior fusion
  - Spinal decompression may be indicated

DIAGNOSTIC CHECKLIST

Consider
- Bone windows to evaluate entire spine on screening trauma CT
  - Reconstruction to thinner collimation if spinal fractures detected
    - Sagittal and coronal reformation through area of interest
  - Evaluate spinal canal for hematoma, cord compromise

Image Interpretation Pearls
- Look for paraspinal soft tissue hematoma as clue to spinal fractures on CT

SELECTED REFERENCES

1. Haba H et al: Diagnostic accuracy of magnetic resonance imaging for detecting posterior ligamentous complex injury associated with thoracic and lumbar fractures. J Neurosurg. 99(1 Suppl):20-6, 2003
2. Sapkas GS et al: Thoracic spinal injuries: operative treatments and neurologic outcomes. Am J Orthop. 32(2):85-8, 2003
3. Sheridan R et al: Reformatted visceral protocol helical computed tomographic scanning allows conventional radiographs of the thoracic and lumbar spine to be eliminated in the evaluation of blunt trauma patients. J Trauma. 55(4):665-9, 2003
4. Wintermark M et al: Thoracolumbar spine fractures in patients who have sustained severe trauma: depiction with multi-detector row CT. Radiology. 227(3):681-9, 2003
5. Moon SH et al: Feasibility of ultrasound examination in posterior ligament complex injury of thoracolumbar spine fracture. Spine. 27(19):2154-8, 2002
6. Trivedi JM: Spinal trauma: therapy--options and outcomes. Eur J Radiol. 42(2):127-34, 2002
7. Holmes JF et al: Epidemiology of thoracolumbar spine injury in blunt trauma. Acad Emerg Med. 8(9):866-72, 2001
8. Denis F: Spinal instability as defined by the three-column spine concept in acute spinal trauma. Clin Orthop. (189):65-76, 1984
9. Denis F: The three column spine and its significance in the classification of acute thoracolumbar spinal injuries. Spine. 8(8):817-31, 1983

FACET-LAMINA THORACOLUMBAR FRACTURE

IMAGE GALLERY

Typical

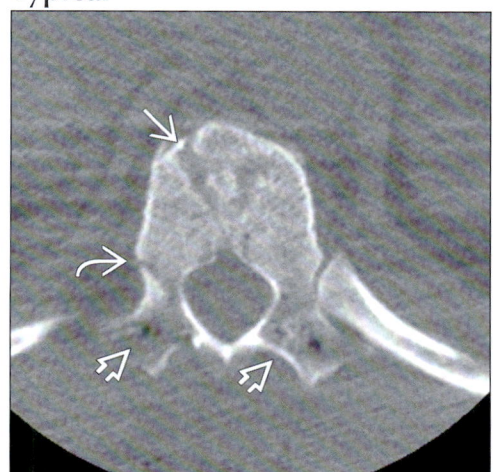
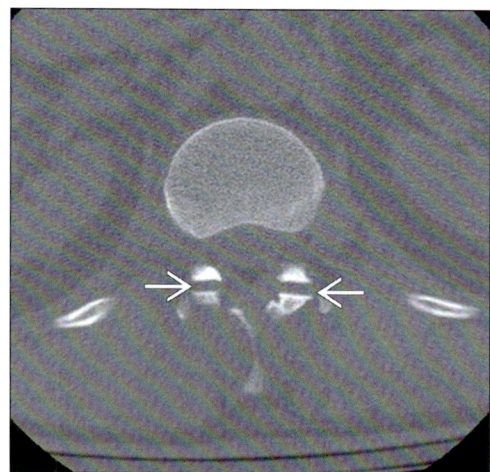

(Left) Axial bone CT in same case as previous image, shows anterior (vertebral body ➡), middle (posterior body ➡), and posterior (pedicle and facets ➡) column fractures. *(Right)* Axial bone CT shows widening of facet joints ➡.

Typical

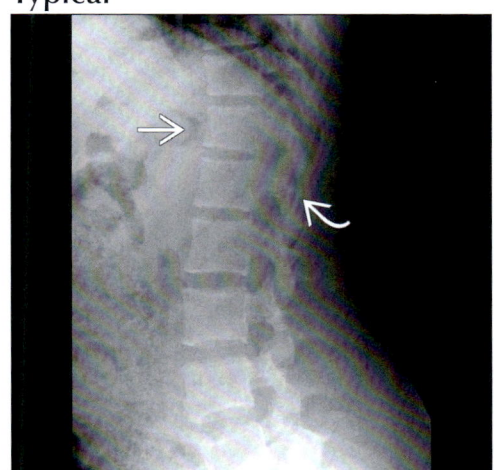
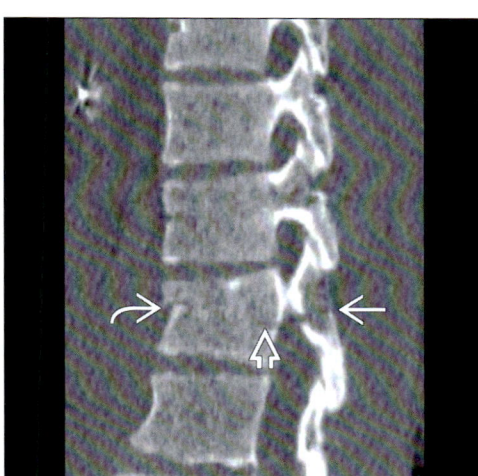

(Left) Lateral radiograph demonstrates anterior compression fracture ➡ and subtle widening of facet joint ➡. *(Right)* Sagittal bone CT of subtle unstable fracture through pars ➡ (posterior column), with extension through posterior ➡ (middle column) & anterior ➡ (anterior column) vertebral bodies.

Variant

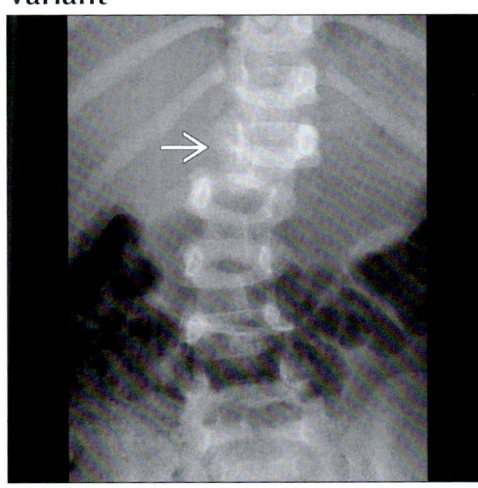
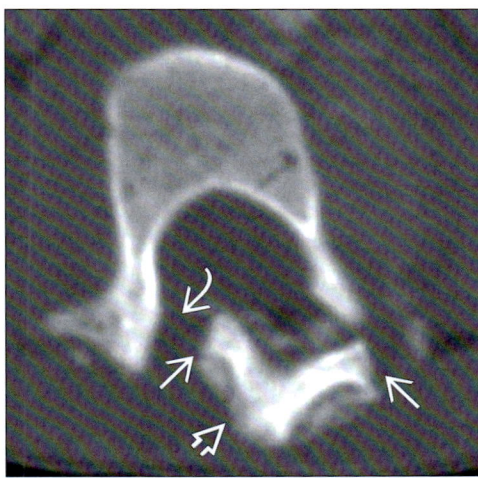

(Left) Frontal radiograph shows marked lateral displacement of L1 on L2 due to complete disruption and dissociation ➡. *(Right)* Axial bone CT shows marked lateral displacement and rotation of posterior elements ➡. There is marked widening of right facet joint ➡, and superior facets are "naked" ➡.

CHANCE FRACTURE

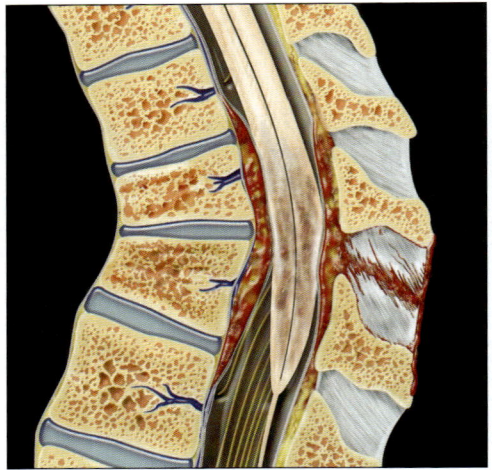
Sagittal graphic shows soft-tissue Chance injury through PLL, ligamentum flavum, facet joints, and interspinous ligaments with cord contusion.

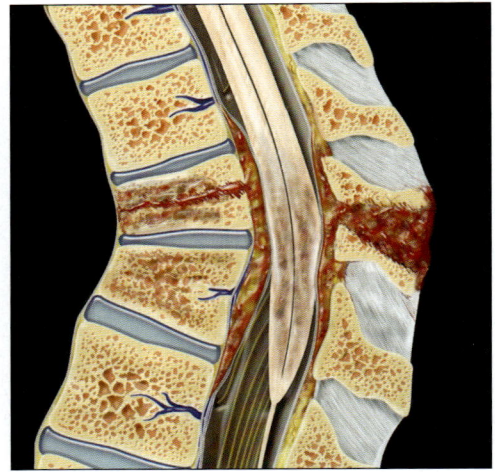
Sagittal graphic shows bony Chance injury through vertebral body, pedicles, and spinous process with cord contusion.

TERMINOLOGY

Abbreviations and Synonyms
- Flexion-distraction injury, seat-belt fracture (fx)

Definitions
- Compression injury of anterior column with distraction of middle & posterior columns
- Anterior column: Anterior longitudinal ligament (ALL), anterior 1/2 vertebral body, anterior annulus fibrosis
- Middle column: Posterior longitudinal ligament (PLL), posterior 1/2 vertebral body, posterior annulus fibrosis
- Posterior column: Posterior neural arch, facet joint capsular ligaments, ligamentum flavum, inter- & supraspinous ligaments
- Spine mechanical instability: 2 of 3 columns involved
- Spine neurologic instability: Neurologic injury, especially to spinal cord
- Transitional zone: T11 to L1 vertebrae, highly susceptible to fx

IMAGING FINDINGS

General Features
- Best diagnostic clue: Wedging anterior vertebral body + posterior element fx and/or increased intraspinous distance (ligamentous injury)
- Location
  - Usually occurs at T11-L3
    - 78% occur between T12 and L2
  - Occasionally at mid-thoracic spine
  - May occur at multiple levels

Radiographic Findings
- Radiography
  - Wedging anterior vertebral body
    - Usually more than 40-50% loss of vertebral body height
  - Focal kyphosis
  - Transversely oriented posterior element fx
  - Posterior ligamentous injury
    - Separation of facet joints
    - Increased interspinous distance
  - Listhesis of vertebral body absent

DDx: Chance Fracture Mimics

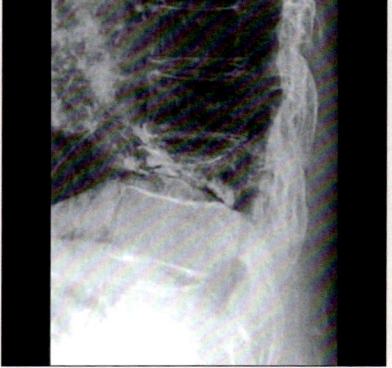
Osteoporotic Fracture

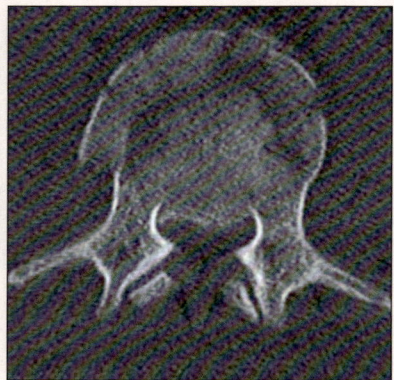
Burst Fracture

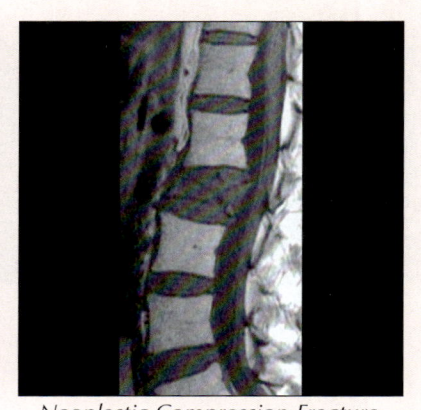
Neoplastic Compression Fracture

CHANCE FRACTURE

Key Facts

Terminology
- Flexion-distraction injury, seat-belt fracture (fx)
- Compression injury of anterior column with distraction of middle & posterior columns

Imaging Findings
- Best diagnostic clue: Wedging anterior vertebral body + posterior element fx and/or increased intraspinous distance (ligamentous injury)
- Usually occurs at T11-L3
- Occasionally at mid-thoracic spine
- Disruption of PLL, interspinous ligaments
- ALL usually intact

Top Differential Diagnoses
- Shear Injury
- Distraction Injury
- Burst Fracture
- Traumatic Compression Fracture
- Osteoporotic Compression Fracture
- Neoplastic Compression Fracture

Pathology
- 5-11% of thoracolumbar fxs
- 15-80% have significant abdominal injuries (bowel & mesentery most common)

Clinical Issues
- Options, risks, complications: Osteoligamentous & ligamentous injuries usually require spinal fusion

Diagnostic Checklist
- Always assess for posterior element fxs, widening of intraspinous distances in any patient with vertebral body compression & trauma history

---

- Increased radiolucency over affected vertebral body 2° displaced spinous processes: "Empty body sign"

CT Findings
- Vertebral body fx, often comminuted
- Transversely oriented posterior element fx
- Posterior ligamentous injury
  - Separation of facet joints: "Naked facet sign"
  - Increased interspinous distance
  - Focal kyphosis
- Gradual loss of pedicle definition on axial images: "Dissolving pedicle sign"
- May have mild buckling or retropulsion of posterior cortex

MR Findings
- T1WI: Discrete fxs as for CT or amorphous low signal in vertebral body
- T2WI
  - Disruption of PLL, interspinous ligaments
  - ALL usually intact
    - More likely to be disrupted in midthoracic injuries than lower thoracic
    - ALL may be stripped from vertebra inferior to fx
  - Bone marrow edema surrounding discrete fx line: "Sandwich sign"
  - May see T2 hyperintense cord contusion
    - Gradient echo best for hemorrhage
- STIR: More sensitive for acute bone marrow edema

Imaging Recommendations
- Best imaging tool
  - Thin section CT with reformations
    - Allows distinction between Chance, burst, compression fxs & assessment of stability
- Protocol advice
  - 1-3 mm overlapping helical MDCT
  - Coronal/sagittal reformations essential
  - MDCT of chest, abdomen & pelvis in trauma patient obviates need for dedicated spine CT
    - Reformatted images coned to spine
    - Expedites treatment of multitrauma patients

DIFFERENTIAL DIAGNOSIS

Shear Injury
- Cause: Transverse shearing force
- All three columns disrupted
- Anterior, posterior or lateral listhesis of vertebra

Distraction Injury
- Cause: Vertical distraction or hyperextension
- All three columns disrupted
- Distraction and/or listhesis of vertebra

Burst Fracture
- Cause: Axial load force
- Retropulsion of posterior vertebral cortex
- Vertically oriented fractures of posterior elements
- Normal interspinous distance

Traumatic Compression Fracture
- Cause: Axial load force ± flexion
- < 40% loss of vertebral body height
- No posterior element fx
- Normal interspinous distance

Osteoporotic Compression Fracture
- Cause: Normal weight-bearing stress or minor trauma
- May have complete loss of vertebral body height
- Pedicles may be involved
- Often at multiple levels
- Osteoporosis usually apparent on radiographs

Neoplastic Compression Fracture
- Cause: Normal weight-bearing stress or minor trauma
- May have complete loss of vertebral body height
- Trabecular destruction on CT
- Tumor may be difficult to see at fx site
- Often see marrow replacement at other levels on CT or MR (T1 STIR sequence)

CHANCE FRACTURE

PATHOLOGY

General Features
- General path comments
  - Fxs most common in transitional zone (T11-L1)
    - Ribs, sternum stabilize upper thoracic spine
    - Coronally oriented thoracic facet joints resist motion more than sagittally oriented lumbar facets
    - Usually see medial rib, transverse process fxs with mid-thoracic Chance
- Etiology
  - Motor vehicle accident or fall
  - Anterior compression, posterior distraction around fulcrum
  - Injury patterns depend on position of fulcrum
  - Classic pattern: Lap seat belt without shoulder strap
    - Seat belt fulcrum anterior to vertebral column
    - Compression of anterior column, distraction of posterior column
  - Midthoracic Chance fxs have fulcrum in middle column
    - Posterior column tension failure
    - Anterior column compression failure
  - ALL usually intact
    - In severe fxs, ALL may be stripped from vertebral body
- Epidemiology
  - 5-11% of thoracolumbar fxs
  - Decreased prevalence after institution of automobile shoulder belts
- Associated abnormalities
  - 15-80% have significant abdominal injuries (bowel & mesentery most common)
  - Retropulsion of posterior cortex has higher incidence of cord injury

Staging, Grading or Classification Criteria
- Osseous Chance fx
  - Vertebral body fx
  - Posterior element fxs: Pedicles, transverse processes, laminae, spinous process
- Ligamentous Chance injury (uncommon)
  - Intervertebral disc
  - Facet dislocation
  - Ruptured interspinous ligaments
- Osteoligamentous Chance injury
  - Variable combination of fracture & ligament injury

CLINICAL ISSUES

Presentation
- Most common signs/symptoms
  - Back pain following high-speed injury
  - Other signs/symptoms
    - Neurologic injury may be present

Natural History & Prognosis
- Long-term kyphotic deformity common without surgical fusion
- Osseous injury
  - Acutely unstable
  - May require fixation if reduction cannot be maintained
- Osteoligamentous, ligamentous injury
  - Poor prognosis for healing unless fusion performed

Treatment
- Options, risks, complications: Osteoligamentous & ligamentous injuries usually require spinal fusion

DIAGNOSTIC CHECKLIST

Image Interpretation Pearls
- Always assess for posterior element fxs, widening of intraspinous distances in any patient with vertebral body compression & trauma history

SELECTED REFERENCES

1. Bernstein MP et al: Chance-type fractures of the thoracolumbar spine: imaging analysis in 53 patients. AJR Am J Roentgenol. 187(4):859-68, 2006
2. Groves CJ et al: Chance-type flexion-distraction injuries in the thoracolumbar spine: MR imaging characteristics. Radiology. 236(2):601-8, 2005
3. Hsu JM et al: Thoracolumbar fracture in blunt trauma patients: guidelines for diagnosis and imaging. Injury. 34(6):426-33, 2003
4. Liu YJ et al: Flexion-distraction injury of the thoracolumbar spine. Injury. 34(12):920-3, 2003
5. Sapkas GS et al: Thoracic spinal injuries: operative treatments and neurologic outcomes. Am J Orthop. 32(2):85-8, 2003
6. Sheridan R et al: Reformatted visceral protocol helical computed tomographic scanning allows conventional radiographs of the thoracic and lumbar spine to be eliminated in the evaluation of blunt trauma patients. J Trauma. 55(4):665-9, 2003
7. Wintermark M et al: Thoracolumbar spine fractures in patients who have sustained severe trauma: depiction with multi-detector row CT. Radiology. 227(3):681-9, 2003
8. Beaunoyer M et al: Abdominal injuries associated with thoraco-lumbar fractures after motor vehicle collision. J Pediatr Surg. 36(5):760-2, 2001
9. Bouliane MJ et al: Instability resulting from a missed Chance fracture. Can J Surg. 44(1):61-2, 2001
10. Greenwald TA et al: Pediatric seatbelt injuries: diagnosis and treatment of lumbar flexion-distraction injuries. Paraplegia. 32(11):743-51, 1994
11. Anderson PA et al: Flexion distraction and chance injuries to the thoracolumbar spine. J Orthop Trauma. 5(2):153-60, 1991
12. Reid AB et al: Pediatric Chance fractures: association with intra-abdominal injuries and seatbelt use. J Trauma. 30(4):384-91, 1990
13. Rogers LF: The roentgenographic appearance of transverse or chance fractures of the spine: the seat belt fracture. Am J Roentgenol Radium Ther Nucl Med. 111(4):844-9, 1971
14. Chance GQ: Note on a type of flexion fracture of the spine. Br J Radiol. (21):452-3, 1948

CHANCE FRACTURE

IMAGE GALLERY

Typical

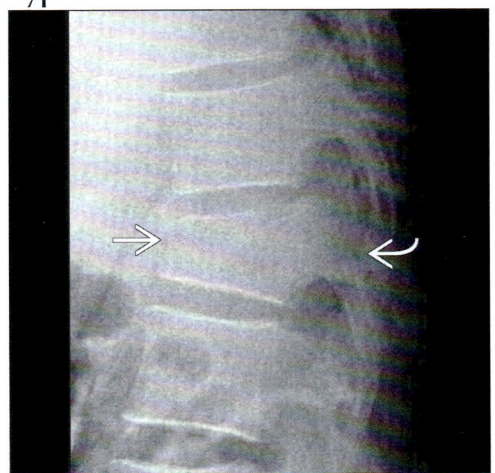
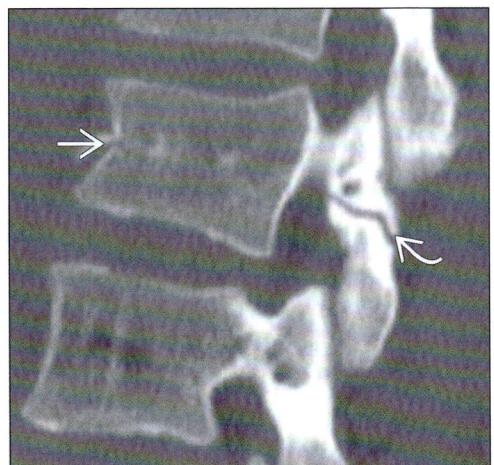

(Left) Lateral radiograph shows compression deformity of anterior aspect of T12 vertebral body ➡. Note faint linear lucency in posterior elements ➡. (Right) Sagittal bone CT shows fracture through midsection of vertebral body ➡ and facet ➡.

Typical

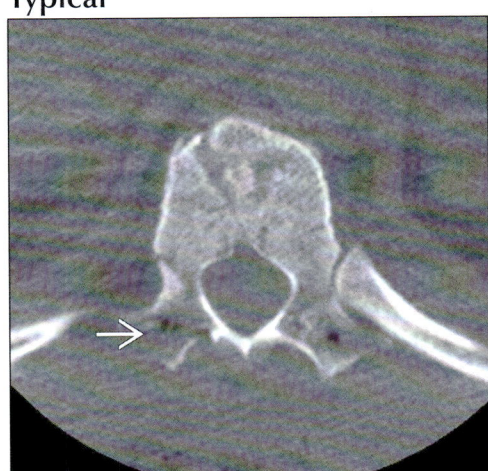
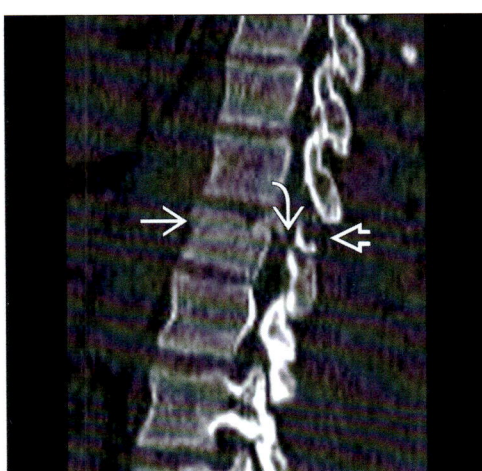

(Left) Axial bone CT shows vertebral body fracture. Right facet and pedicle are indistinct ➡ ("vanishing pedicle sign"), indicating posterior element fracture. (Right) Sagittal bone CT shows vertebral body fracture ➡, transverse fracture through posterior elements ➡, and increased distance between spinous processes ➡.

Typical

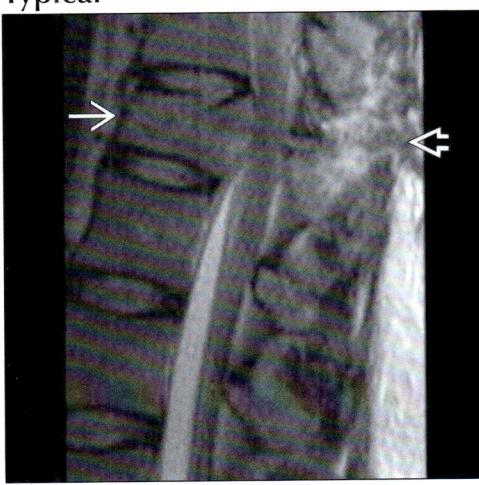
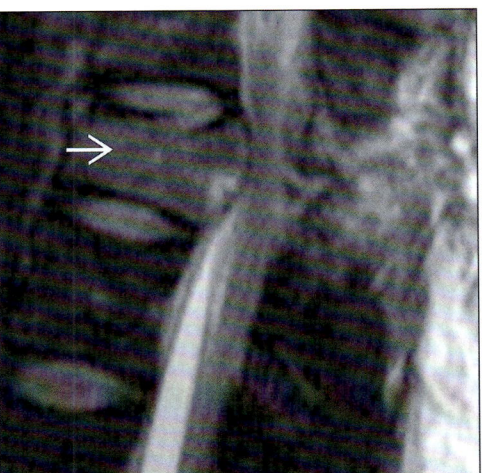

(Left) Sagittal T2WI MR shows compression and edema of vertebral body ➡. Bone marrow edema within posterior elements surrounds hypointense fracture line ➡ ("sandwich sign"). (Right) Sagittal STIR MR in the same patient as previous image, shows increased conspicuity of marrow edema ➡ when compared to non-fat-suppressed T2 image.

SACRAL TRAUMATIC FRACTURE

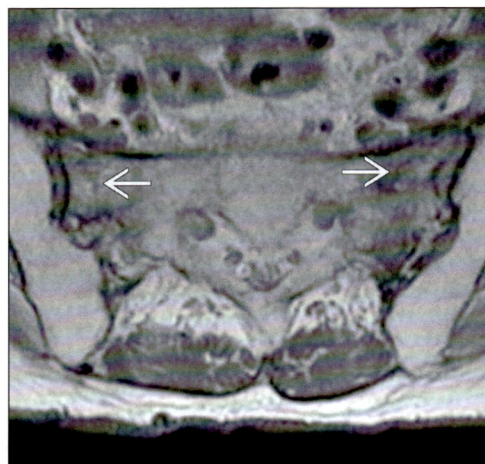

Axial T1WI MR shows decreased T1 signal (edema) bilaterally within the sacrum with linear low-intensity lines ➡ representing fractures.

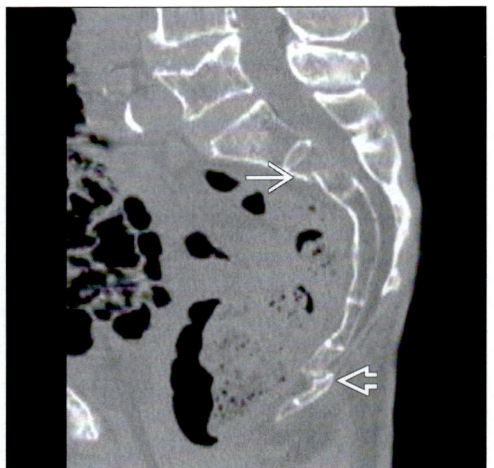

Sagittal bone CT shows transverse fracture of S2 ➡ with minimal posterior displacement. This was not clearly seen on axial images. Note old fracture deformity of coccyx ➡.

TERMINOLOGY

Definitions
- Pelvic ring: Pelvic bones form hollow, obliquely horizontal, ring-shaped structure around pelvic organs
- Pelvic ring disruption: Fractures and/or ligament injuries through anterior & posterior portions of pelvis
  - Posterior ring fracture: Behind ischial spine; usually sacrum or sacroiliac joint
  - Anterior ring fracture: Anterior to ischial spine, usually pubic rami

IMAGING FINDINGS

General Features
- Best diagnostic clue: Disruption of sacral arcuate lines
- Location: 95% vertical or oblique; 5% horizontal
- Morphology
  - Pelvic ring disruption: Vertically or obliquely oriented fracture
  - Isolated sacral fracture: Horizontally oriented fracture

Radiographic Findings
- Radiography
  - Difficult to see on routine radiography
    - Up to 60% reportedly missed prior to institution of CT scanning
  - Disruption of arcuate line of neural foramina
    - Normally see smooth curve above neural foramen
    - Angular contour of arcuate line indicates fracture
  - Lateral compression causes decreased width of sacrum on affected side
  - Displacement of fracture line uncommonly visible
  - Lateral radiography shows angular deformity of transverse fractures
  - Anteroposterior (AP) radiography
    - Inlet view of pelvis: 25° caudad angulation
    - Outlet view of pelvis: 25° cephalad angulation
    - Ferguson view sacrum: 15° cephalad angulation
  - Fracture best seen on outlet, Ferguson views
  - Paradoxical inlet view obtained with AP positioning suggestive of fracture
  - L5 transverse process fracture raises suspicion for sacral fracture
  - Children may have "greenstick" fracture of sacrum

DDx: Sacral Traumatic Fracture Mimics

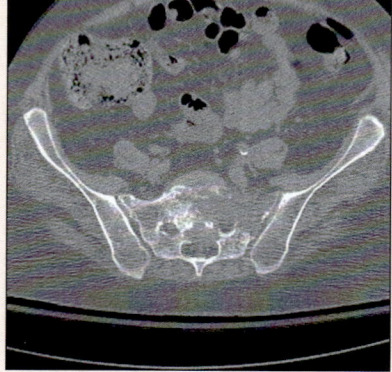

Sacral Metastasis

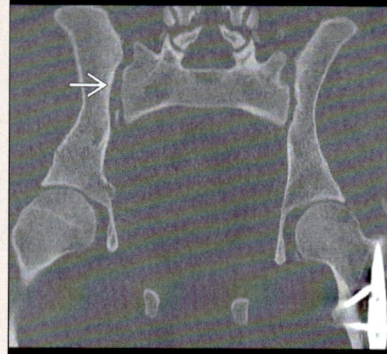

Diastasis Right Sacroiliac Joint

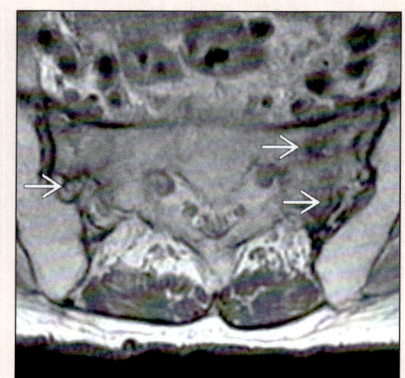

Insufficiency Fractures

SACRAL TRAUMATIC FRACTURE

Key Facts

Imaging Findings
- Best diagnostic clue: Disruption of sacral arcuate lines
- Pelvic ring disruption: Vertically or obliquely oriented fracture
- Isolated sacral fracture: Horizontally oriented fracture
- Difficult to see on routine radiography
- Best imaging tool: MDCT

Top Differential Diagnoses
- Sacroiliac Joint Disruption/Dislocation
- Stress Fracture
- Tumor
- Traumatic Lumbosacral Dislocation
- Accessory Centers of Ossification

Pathology
- 95% occur in association with pelvic fractures

- Neurologic injury may be masked by concurrent injuries at higher levels
- Neurologic injuries in 40% of displaced fractures
- **Denis classification (by zone)**
- Zone 1: Lateral to neural foramina
- Zone 2: Through neural foramina
- Zone 3: Through spinal canal

Clinical Issues
- Posterior pelvic pain or tenderness following high-velocity trauma
- Significant post-operative infection rate

Diagnostic Checklist
- If L5 transverse process fracture seen, suspect sacral fx
- If AP projection appears as paradoxical inlet view, suspect sacral fx

---

- Sacro-coccygeal junction fractures
  - Angular deformity at junction (but may be normal variant in this location)

CT Findings
- Bone CT
  - Shows displacement not apparent on radiography
  - Defines position of fracture relative to neural foramina, spinal canal
  - Most accurate for measurements
    - Axial images: AP displacement, horizontal displacement, canal occlusion
    - Coronal reconstructions: Vertical translation
    - Sagittal reconstructions: AP translation, angulation

MR Findings
- Because sacrum is thin & obliquely positioned, fracture may be missed or mistaken for tumor
  - Oblique coronal T1WI, STIR along plane of sacrum useful
- Evaluate for nerve root injury
  - Traumatic avulsion may be masked acutely by surrounding hematoma
  - Evaluate injury of sacral plexus on STIR sequences

Imaging Recommendations
- Best imaging tool: MDCT
- Protocol advice: 1-3 mm overlapping helical images; coronal & sagittal reformations

DIFFERENTIAL DIAGNOSIS

Sacroiliac Joint Disruption/Dislocation
- May require CT to differentiate from fracture

Stress Fracture
- Back pain of insidious onset & disabling severity
- No history of trauma
- Insufficiency fracture usually 2° osteoporosis
- Fatigue fracture in athletes
- Vertically oriented fracture through sacral ala
  - Unilateral or bilateral

- Horizontal component connecting two vertical fractures in < 50%
- Vacuum phenomenon often seen in anterior portion of fracture

Tumor
- Loss of arcuate lines on radiography
- Round or oval region of trabecular destruction on CT
- Round or oval region of high T2WI signal on MR

Traumatic Lumbosacral Dislocation
- Due to high speed injury, motor vehicle accident or fall
- Extremely rare
- Diagnosed with lateral radiograph or CT

Accessory Centers of Ossification
- Seen at lateral margins of sacrum in children
- Undulating contour, bilaterally symmetric

PATHOLOGY

General Features
- General path comments
  - 95% occur in association with pelvic fractures
  - Neurologic injury may be masked by concurrent injuries at higher levels
- Etiology
  - Sacral fractures without pelvic ring disruption
    - Often suicidal jumpers
    - Transverse fracture may occur if patient lands in seated or supine position
    - Fractures at sacro-coccygeal junction 2° minor falls
  - Three major mechanisms of pelvic ring disruption
  - Anteroposterior compression ("open book")
    - Vertically oriented sacral fracture, often slightly diastatic
  - Lateral compression ("T-bone injury")
    - Vertically oriented fracture
    - May see sclerotic rather than lucent line 2° impaction

SACRAL TRAUMATIC FRACTURE

- Impaction at sacral fracture causes decreased mediolateral dimension sacral ala
  - Vertical shear (fall from height)
    - Vertical displacement may be present, may have spontaneously reduced
    - ± Fractures of L5 transverse processes
- Epidemiology: Common injury
- Associated abnormalities
  - Lumbosacral junction injury
    - Seen in up to 1/3 of sacral fractures with pelvic ring involvement
    - Facet joint injury or L5-S1 disc injury
  - Fracture of L5 transverse process indicates unstable fracture
    - Fracture 2° avulsion of lumbosacral ligament
  - Anterior pelvic ring fractures
  - Lumbar spine fractures
    - Spine fracture with neurologic deficit may cause sacral fracture to be overlooked clinically
  - Neurologic injuries in 40% of displaced fractures
    - Nerve roots or sacral plexus
    - Transection or stretch injury
  - Vascular injuries
    - Therapeutic embolization may be needed
    - Active bleeding often seen on contrast-enhanced CT at time of trauma
  - Bladder or urethral injury
  - Lower extremity fractures
  - Degloving injury of posterior soft tissues

Staging, Grading or Classification Criteria
- **Denis classification (by zone)**
- Zone 1: Lateral to neural foramina
  - 50% of sacral fractures
  - Vertical or oblique orientation
  - Neurologic deficit in 6-24%
  - L5 nerve root may be entrapped in fracture
- Zone 2: Through neural foramina
  - 34% of sacral fractures
  - Vertical or oblique
  - Neurologic deficit in 28%
  - Traumatic "far-out syndrome"
    - L5 root caught between sacral alar fragment and transverse process
- Zone 3: Through spinal canal
  - 16% of sacral fractures
  - Transverse zone 3 fracture (fx)
    - 35% have associated avulsion of nerve roots
    - "Sacral burst fracture": Transverse fracture with retropulsion of bone into spinal canal
    - Fracture-dislocation may occur through rudimentary disc at S1-S2
    - Neurologic deficit in 57-60%
  - Vertical zone 3 fracture
    - Majority have neurologic deficit
    - Bowel, bladder, sexual dysfunction
  - Gibbons grading system for neurologic deficits
    - Grade 1: No neurologic deficit
    - Grade 2: Sensory changes only
    - Grade 3: Motor weakness
    - Grade 4: Loss of bowel/bladder control

CLINICAL ISSUES

Presentation
- Most common signs/symptoms
  - Posterior pelvic pain or tenderness following high-velocity trauma
  - Other signs/symptoms
    - Neurologic deficit
    - Bowel, bladder symptoms

Natural History & Prognosis
- Unstable injuries require open reduction internal fixation (ORIF)
- Neurologic injury
  - S1, S2 deficits tend to improve within 1 year regardless of treatment
    - If no improvement, consider nerve root avulsion
  - Dural laceration may lead to cerebrospinal fluid leak

Treatment
- Options, risks, complications
  - Bed rest, slow progression to weightbearing if stable
  - Stabilization of unstable fractures with trans-alar screws
  - Role of surgical decompression controversial
  - Significant post-operative infection rate

DIAGNOSTIC CHECKLIST

Image Interpretation Pearls
- High-velocity injuries in adults always involve anterior pelvic ring when sacrum fractured
- If L5 transverse process fracture seen, suspect sacral fx
- If AP projection appears as paradoxical inlet view, suspect sacral fx

SELECTED REFERENCES
1. Kuklo TR et al: Radiographic measurement techniques for sacral fractures consensus statement of the Spine Trauma Study Group. Spine. 31(9):1047-55, 2006
2. Bellabarba C et al: Midline sagittal sacral fractures in anterior-posterior compression pelvic ring injuries. J Orthop Trauma. 17(1):32-7, 2003
3. Kim MY et al: Transverse sacral fractures: case series and literature review. Can J Surg. 44(5):359-63, 2001
4. Rubel IF et al: Description of a rare type of posterior pelvis traumatic involvement: the green-stick fracture of the sarcum. Pediatr Radiol. 31(6):447-9, 2001
5. Leone A et al: Lumbosacral junction injury associated with unstable pelvic fracture: classification and diagnosis. Radiology. 205(1):253-9, 1997
6. Templeman D et al: Internal fixation of displaced fractures of the sacrum. Clin Orthop. (329):180-5, 1996
7. Albert TJ et al: Concomitant noncontiguous thoracolumbar and sacral fractures. Spine. 18(10):1285-91, 1993
8. Gibbons KJ et al: Neurological injury and patterns of sacral fractures. J Neurosurg. 72(6):889-93, 1990
9. Denis F et al: Sacral fractures: an important problem. Retrospective analysis of 236 cases. Clin Orthop. 227:67-81, 1988

SACRAL TRAUMATIC FRACTURE

IMAGE GALLERY

Typical

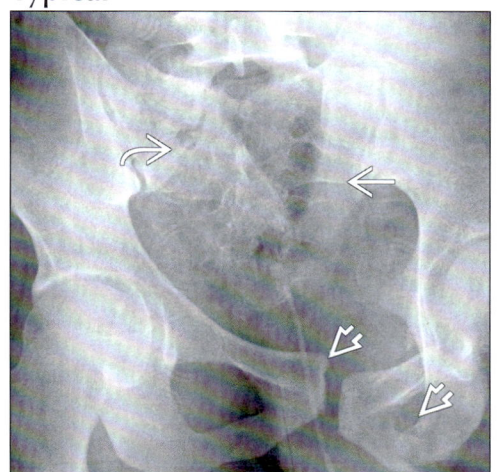
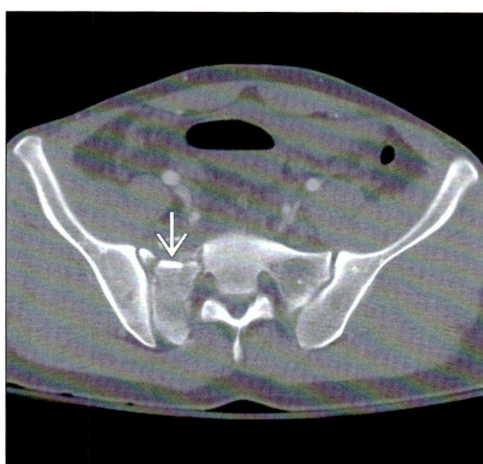

(Left) Anteroposterior radiograph shows normal left foraminal lines ➡. Right lines are disrupted and demonstrate acute angulation ➡. Note injury to symphysis pubis and left rami ➡. *(Right)* Axial bone CT of same patient as previous image shows Denis type II fracture involving sacral foramina. Note posterior displacement at fracture site ➡.

Typical

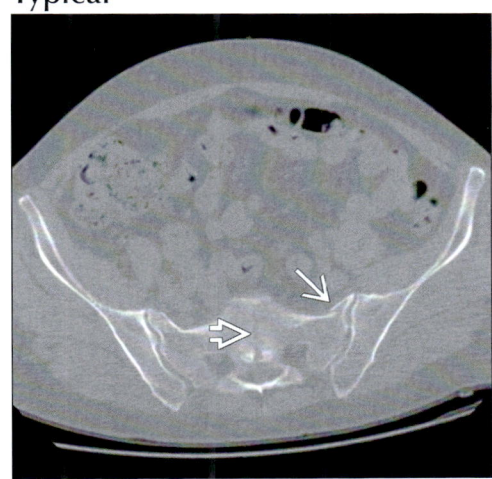
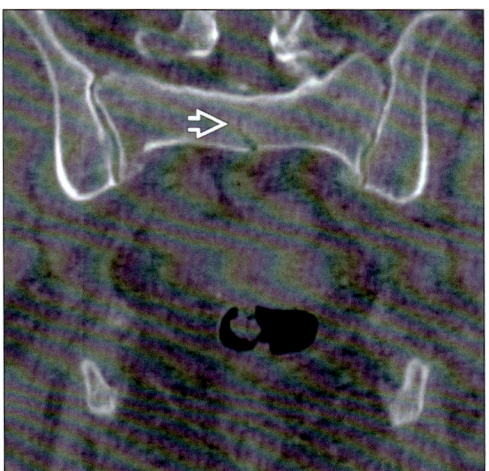

(Left) Axial bone CT shows Denis type I fracture on left ➡ and Denis type III fracture more centrally ➡. *(Right)* Coronal bone CT in the same patient as previous image, confirms a vertically oriented Denis type III fracture ➡. No AP translation noted. Multiplanar reformats are essential for evaluation of sacral fractures.

Typical

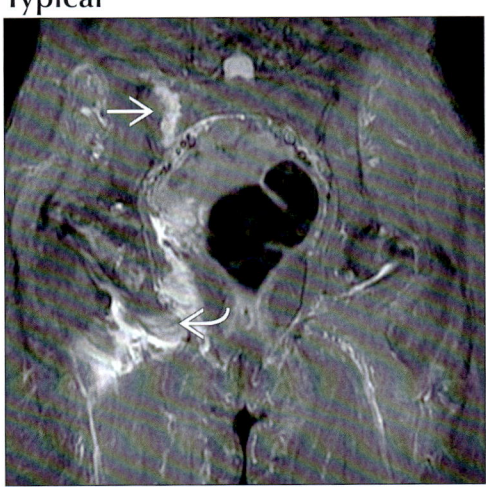
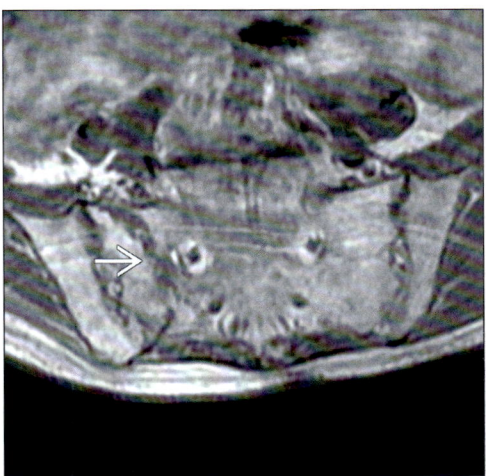

(Left) Coronal STIR MR shows linear hyperintense signal in right sacrum, indicating fracture ➡. Note edema within lower pelvis from associated pelvic injuries ➡. *(Right)* Axial T1WI MR shows linear T1 hypointense signal ➡, confirming fracture. Foramina are not involved, indicating a Denis type I fracture.

TRAUMATIC DISC HERNIATION

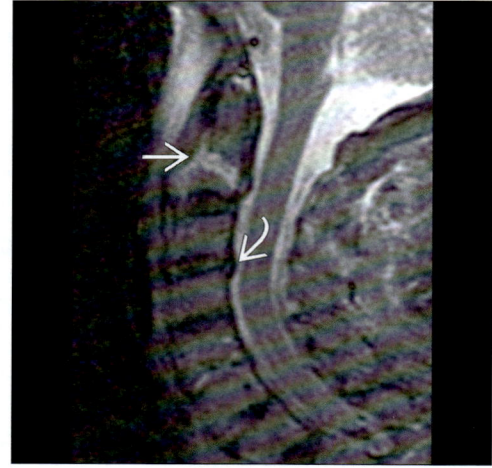

Sagittal T2WI MR shows fracture of C2 vertebral body ➔ with acute disc herniation at C3-4 level ➔.

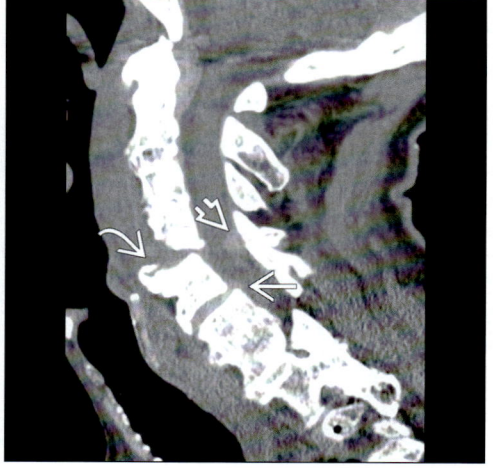

Sagittal bone CT shows fracture of C4 ➔. On narrow windows, disc herniation at C5-6 is apparent ➔. Soft tissue seen posteriorly at C4 level is epidural hematoma ➔.

TERMINOLOGY

Abbreviations and Synonyms
- Herniated nucleus pulposus (HNP)
  - Non-standard terminology
- Traumatic disc herniation (tHNP)
- Spinal cord injury (SCI)

Definitions
- Disc herniation induced by trauma

IMAGING FINDINGS

General Features
- Best diagnostic clue: Herniation of disc material most evident on T2WI
- Location
  - Cervical spine most frequent location
  - 50% of tHNP occur at level of injury or one level below/above fracture
- Size: Small to large
- Morphology: Same appearance as disc herniation unrelated to trauma

Radiographic Findings
- Radiography
  - Insensitive for disc pathology
  - Associated traumatic bone injuries

CT Findings
- NECT
  - Soft-tissue density projecting into spinal canal
    - Narrow windows helpful
  - Obliteration of adjacent epidural fat
  - Narrowing of disc space
- CTA: Quick screening for traumatic vascular injury
- Bone CT
  - THNP often obscured by associated fractures (fxs) epidural hematoma
  - May also see locked facets, joint subluxation, fxs

MR Findings
- T1WI
  - Disc material effacing anterior CSF, may compress cord or cauda equina
    - Young: Hydrated mid-intensity disc material
    - Older: Desiccated hypointense material
- T2WI

DDx: Traumatic Disc Herniation Mimics

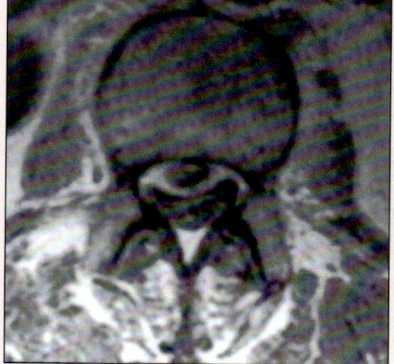

Epidural Abscess

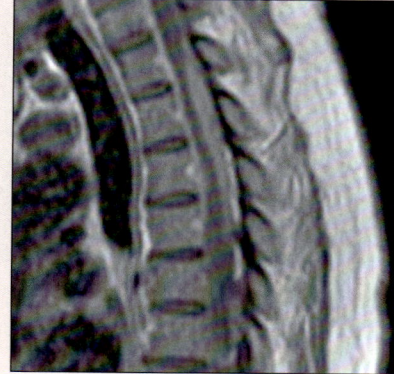

Epidural Tumor

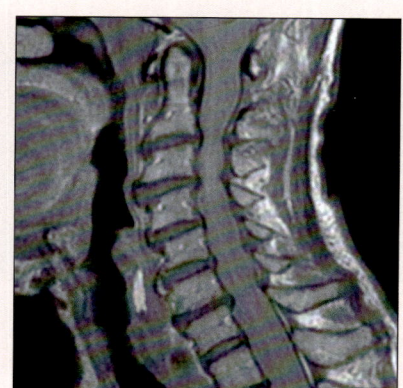

Degenerative Disc Disease

TRAUMATIC DISC HERNIATION

Key Facts

Terminology
- Disc herniation induced by trauma

Imaging Findings
- Best diagnostic clue: Herniation of disc material most evident on T2WI
- 50% of tHNP occur at level of injury or one level below/above fracture
- Morphology: Same appearance as disc herniation unrelated to trauma
- MR is modality of choice
- Bone CT better depicts associated osseous injuries

Top Differential Diagnoses
- Nontraumatic HNP
- Epidural Abscess, Phlegmon
- Epidural Tumor

Pathology
- Pre-existing disc degeneration likely
- Epidemiology: Seen in 3-9% of all SCI patients, 33-48% of unstable cervical spine injuries

Clinical Issues
- Radicular syndrome (pain & segmental neurologic deficit) (~ 65%)
- Myeloradiculopathy (~ 30%)
- Medullary symptoms (~ 7%)
- Anterior cord syndrome highly associated with traumatic disc herniation
- Good prognosis: Radiculopathy
- Poor prognosis: Myelopathy

Diagnostic Checklist
- tHNP in any patient who fails closed reduction

- Disc material effacing anterior CSF, may compress cord or cauda equina
  - Young: Hydrated hyperintense disc material, may be more hyperintense than normal
  - Older: Desiccated hypointense material
- Hyperintense cord contusion from compression
- Stripping of posterior longitudinal ligament
- STIR: Associated ligamentous or soft-tissue injury
- T2* GRE
  - Susceptibility from hemorrhage
  - Thin-section for cervical spine foraminal evaluation
- MRA: Quick screening for traumatic vascular injury

Angiographic Findings
- Conventional: Replaced by CTA, MRA

Non-Vascular Interventions
- Myelography
  - Extradural mass effacing anterior CSF-filled subarachnoid space
  - May see associated cord flattening
  - Distortion or obliteration of adjacent nerve root sleeve(s)

Imaging Recommendations
- Best imaging tool
  - MR is modality of choice
  - Bone CT better depicts associated osseous injuries
- Protocol advice
  - Best seen with sagittal T2WI
  - Add GRE to assess for cord hemorrhage
  - STIR for ligamentous & soft tissue injury

DIFFERENTIAL DIAGNOSIS

Nontraumatic HNP
- Disc herniation with little or no trauma
- Appears similar to tHNP on imaging

Epidural Abscess, Phlegmon
- Usually due to discitis
- Not as focal, may extend > 1 spinal segment
- Majority enhances, unlike disc material

Epidural Tumor
- Usually back pain without history of trauma
- Often diffuse enhancement
- Look for extension from adjacent bony metastasis

PATHOLOGY

General Features
- General path comments
  - Discs allow movement between vertebral bodies, transmit loads from one vertebral body to next
  - Annulus & nucleus disperse axial load pressure
  - Nucleus shortens & radially expands when axial load applied, exerting pressure on annulus
  - Annular resistance opposes outward pressure
  - Axial loads ≤ 40 kg cause only 1 mm of vertical compression, 0.5 mm of radial expansion
  - During movement, annulus acts as ligament restraining movement, partially stabilizing interbody joint
- Genetics
  - Collagen type II gene deficiency & vitamin D receptor intragenic polymorphism both map to same region on chromosome 12q13
    - Strong association with disc degeneration & herniation
    - Established for nontraumatic HNP
    - Most agree that pre-existing disc degeneration predisposes to tHNP
    - Same genes likely play some role in tHNP
- Etiology
  - Trauma-induced disruption of annulus → nucleus pulposus herniation
  - Pre-existing disc degeneration likely
- Epidemiology: Seen in 3-9% of all SCI patients, 33-48% of unstable cervical spine injuries
- Associated abnormalities
  - Bone fxs, subluxations, dislocations
  - Cord contusion, hemorrhage
  - Ligamentous, soft-tissue injury
  - Brain injury

TRAUMATIC DISC HERNIATION

Microscopic Features
- Fibrovascular tissue surrounds herniated disc material
- Vessels extend into annulus fibrosus but not endplate
- Scattered cartilage fragments & macrophages localize around disc margin
- Findings similar to degenerated herniated discs, suggest absorptive process

Staging, Grading or Classification Criteria
- Herniation: Presence of nuclear material within or beyond confines of annular tear
  - Protrusion: Focal or asymmetric disc extension beyond interspace with broader base than any other dimension of protrusion
  - Extrusion: Focal or asymmetric disc extension beyond interspace with base of origin narrower than diameter of extruding material
  - Free fragment: Herniation (extrusion) with no connection to original disc
- Modifiers
  - Contained: Restricted beneath intact posterior longitudinal ligament
  - Noncontained: Herniation extends through defective posterior longitudinal ligament

CLINICAL ISSUES

Presentation
- Most common signs/symptoms
  - Radicular syndrome (pain & segmental neurologic deficit) (~ 65%)
  - Myeloradiculopathy (~ 30%)
  - Medullary symptoms (~ 7%)
  - Anterior cord syndrome highly associated with traumatic disc herniation
    - Injury to anterior 2/3 of cord
    - Pain & temperature affected, touch & vibration intact
  - Brown-Sequard syndrome
    - Injury to 1/2 cord
    - Ipsilateral loss of touch & motor function
    - Contralateral loss of pain & temperature
    - Often superimposed on central cord syndrome
  - Central cord syndrome
    - Upper extremities involvement > lower
    - Older population, seen in spondylosis without fx
    - Historically associated with central hematoma, predominantly white-matter injury
  - Cauda equina syndrome: Pelvic & sacral pain 2° compression of cauda equina spinal nerve roots
- Clinical Profile: SCI patient, often with numerous injuries

Demographics
- Age: SCI: Mean age = 30.5 yrs, median = 26 yrs; 50% are 16-30
- Gender: SCI: > 80% male
- Ethnicity: SCI: More common in non-Caucasians
- Timing of SCI
  - Highest rate in July, lowest in February
  - 39% occur on Saturday or Sunday

Natural History & Prognosis
- Good prognosis: Radiculopathy
- Poor prognosis: Myelopathy

Treatment
- Number of large clinical series failed to establish relationship between tHNP & subsequent neurological deterioration with attempted closed traction-reduction in awake patients
  - No practice standard
- Surgical treatment often in association with repair of associated injuries

DIAGNOSTIC CHECKLIST

Consider
- tHNP in any patient who fails closed reduction

SELECTED REFERENCES
1. Martinez-Lage JF et al: Lumbar disc herniation in early childhood: case report and literature review. Childs Nerv Syst. 19(4):258-60, 2003
2. Tohme-Noun C et al: Imaging features of traumatic dislocation of the lumbosacral joint associated with disc herniation. Skeletal Radiol. 32(6):360-3, 2003
3. Hadley MN: Initial closed reduction of cervical spine fracture-dislocation injuries. Neurosurgery. 50(3 Suppl):S44-50, 2002
4. Hayes KC et al: Retropulsion of intervertebral discs associated with traumatic hyperextension of the cervical spine and absence of vertebral fracture: an uncommon mechanism of spinal cord injury. Spinal Cord. 40(10):544-7, 2002
5. Fuentes S et al: Traumatic thoracic disc herniation. Case illustration. J Neurosurg. 95(2 Suppl):276, 2001
6. Gray L et al: Thoracic and lumbar spine trauma. Semin Ultrasound CT MR. 22(2):125-34, 2001
7. Benedetti PF et al: MRI findings in spinal ligamentous injury. AJR Am J Roentgenol. 175(3):661-5, 2000
8. Dai L et al: Central cord injury complicating acute cervical disc herniation in trauma. Spine. 25(3):331-5; discussion 336, 2000
9. Lee JY et al: Histological study of lumbar intervertebral disc herniation in adolescents. Acta Neurochir (Wien). 142(10):1107-10, 2000
10. Katzberg RW et al: Acute cervical spine injuries: prospective MR imaging assessment at a level 1 trauma center. Radiology. 213(1):203-12, 1999
11. Vaccaro AR et al: Magnetic resonance evaluation of the intervertebral disc, spinal ligaments, and spinal cord before and after closed traction reduction of cervical spine dislocations. Spine. 24(12):1210-7, 1999
12. Bucciero A et al: Myeloradicular damage in traumatic cervical disc herniation. J Neurosurg Sci. 42(4):203-11, 1998
13. Carreon LY et al: Histologic changes in the disc after cervical spine trauma: evidence of disc absorption. J Spinal Disord. 9(4):313-6, 1996
14. Rumana CS et al: Brown-Sequard syndrome produced by cervical disc herniation: case report and literature review. Surg Neurol. 45(4):359-61, 1996
15. Doran SE et al: Magnetic resonance imaging documentation of coexistent traumatic locked facets of the cervical spine and disc herniation. J Neurosurg. 79(3):341-5, 1993

TRAUMATIC DISC HERNIATION

IMAGE GALLERY

Typical

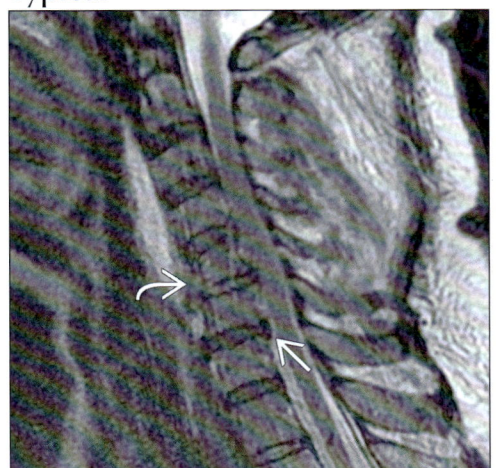
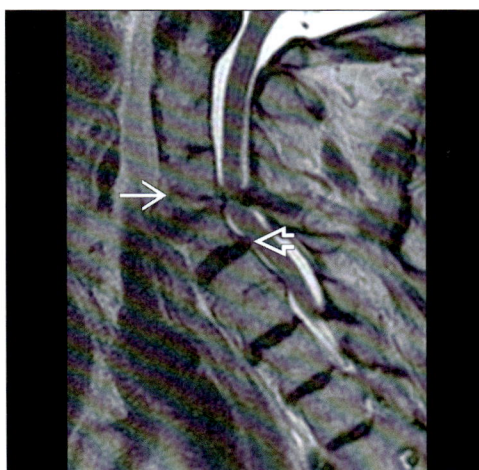

(Left) Sagittal T2WI MR shows traumatic disc protrusion at C6-7 ➡. Note flexion-type fracture of C5 ➡. *(Right)* Sagittal T2WI MR shows fracture of C4 vertebral body ➡. Traumatic disc herniation is noted at typical level inferior to fracture ➡.

Typical

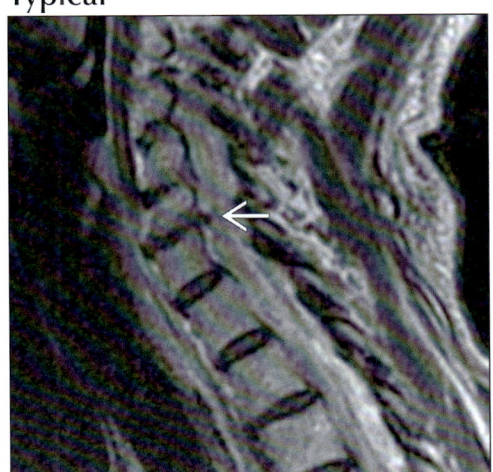
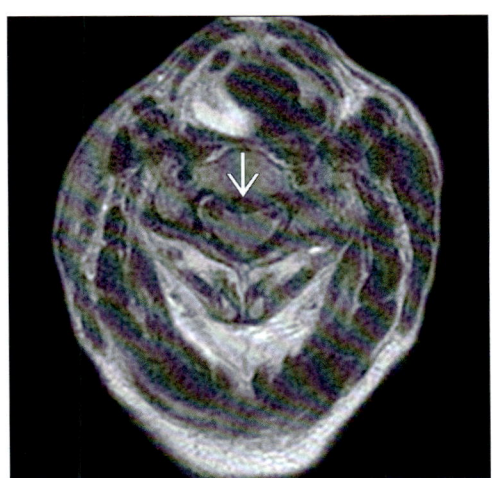

(Left) Sagittal T2WI FS MR shows disc protrusion in a patient following a motor vehicle accident ➡. Multiple fractures were present but not seen on this image. *(Right)* Axial T2WI MR in the same patient as previous image, demonstrates disc protrusion ➡ & resulting narrowing of thecal sac.

Typical

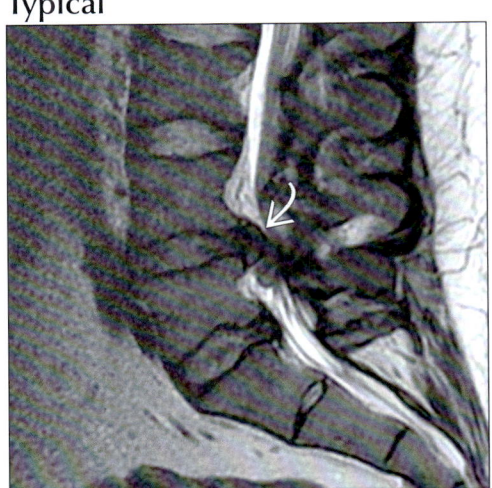
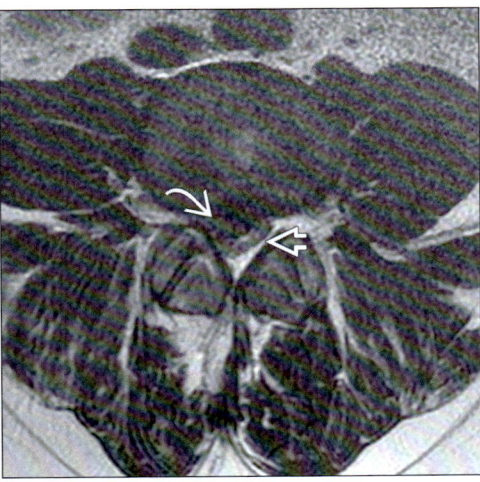

(Left) Sagittal T2WI MR shows a large disc protrusion ➡ following a fall in this 24 year old male. *(Right)* Axial T2WI MR in the same patient as previous image, shows a large disc protrusion ➡ and mass effect on the thecal sac ➡.

SPINAL CORD INJURY

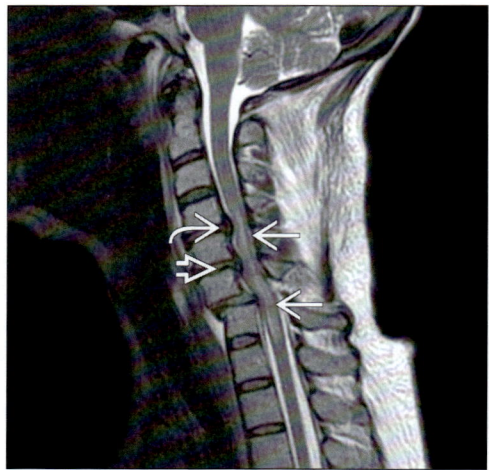

Sagittal T2WI MR shows acute traumatic subluxation at C6/C7 & extensive hyperintensity (contusion) ➡. Spinal stenosis at C4/C5 ➡ & C5/C6 ➡ contributed to extent of contusion.

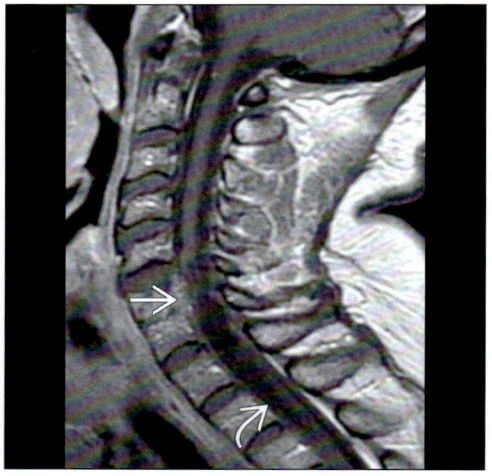

Sagittal T1WI MR shows cord transection secondary to gunshot wound. Note discontinuity of cord from C5 ➡ to T2 ➡.

TERMINOLOGY

Abbreviations and Synonyms
- Spinal cord injury (SCI)

Definitions
- Traumatic cord edema and/or hemorrhage

IMAGING FINDINGS

General Features
- Best diagnostic clue: Abnormal cord signal on MR
- Location
  - Most common level of SCI: C4-C6
  - With paraplegia, most common level is T10-L1

Radiographic Findings
- Radiography: Associated fracture (fx)/subluxation

CT Findings
- NECT
  - Hematoma: Cord hyperdensity
  - Contusion: Cord hypodensity (rare)
- CTA: Quick screening for associated vascular injury
- Bone CT
  - Associated fx, subluxation
  - Predisposing factors: Spondylosis, spinal stenosis

MR Findings
- T1WI
  - Acute contusion
    - Iso- to hypointense
    - Cord swelling
  - Hematoma: Hyperintense after 3 days
  - Transection: Sagittal T1WI best to show cord discontinuity
  - Chronic contusion: Atrophy ± cyst
- T2WI
  - Acute contusion (edema): Hyperintense
  - Hematoma: Follows typical temporal evolution
    - Acute: Hypointense
  - May see traumatic disc herniation
  - Chronic contusion: Hyperintense gliosis & atrophy
  - Chronic hematoma: Hypointense hemosiderin scar
    - Cystic change hyperintense
- T2* GRE: Hematoma: Hypointense (best for hemorrhage)
- MRA: Quick screening for associated vascular injury

DDx: Spinal Cord Injury Mimics

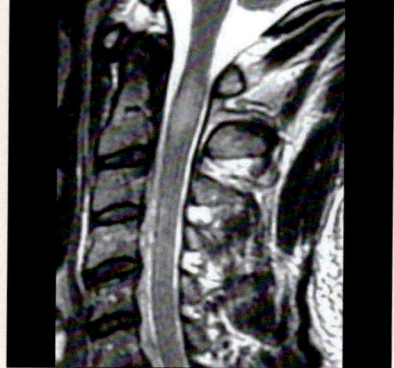

Multiple Sclerosis

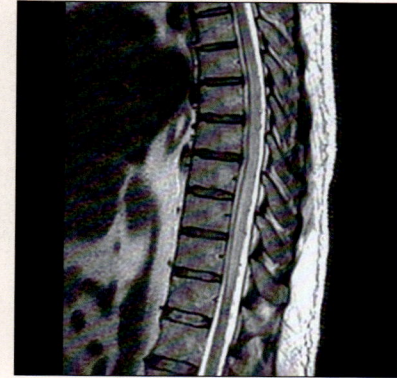

Dural AVF

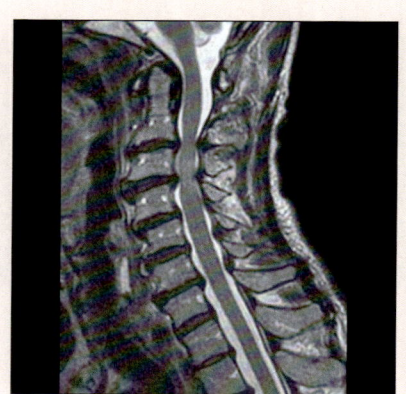

Cord Edema 2° Stenosis

SPINAL CORD INJURY

Key Facts

Terminology
- Traumatic cord edema and/or hemorrhage

Imaging Findings
- Best diagnostic clue: Abnormal cord signal on MR
- Acute contusion (edema): Hyperintense
- Hematoma: Follows typical temporal evolution
- May see traumatic disc herniation
- T2* GRE: Hematoma: Hypointense (best for hemorrhage)
- Best imaging tool: MR
- Protocol advice: Add STIR & GRE

Top Differential Diagnoses
- Degenerative Disease with Cord Compression
- Myelitis
- Myelomalacia

Pathology
- MVA (45%), falls (22%), acts of violence (16%), sports injury (13%)

Clinical Issues
- Mean age: 30.5 yrs; median age: 26 yrs
- Gender: Over 80% male
- Poor prognostic factors: C4, C5, C6 level injuries, age > 50 yrs
- Chronic care best approached from rehabilitation team approach

Diagnostic Checklist
- Screening MR for all symptomatic SCI
- Sagittal STIR is key to diagnosing marrow edema, ligamentous injury

---

Non-Vascular Interventions
- Myelography
  - Contusion: Focal cord enlargement effacing contrast
  - Hematoma: May mimic syrinx containing contrast
    - 140-300 Hounsfield units (HU)
  - Transection: No cord visible in affected axial slice

Imaging Recommendations
- Best imaging tool: MR
- Protocol advice: Add STIR & GRE

DIFFERENTIAL DIAGNOSIS

Degenerative Disease with Cord Compression
- Hyperintense cord compression on T2WI
- Severe spinal stenosis or large HNP
- Trauma superimposed on stenosis → edema

Myelitis
- Demyelinating disease (e.g., MS), ADEM, transverse myelitis
- All may enhance

Cavernous Malformation
- Best seen with GRE
- May be multiple
- May be asymptomatic

Dural Arteriovenous Fistula
- Cord edema: Swollen hyperintense cord on T2WI
- Flow voids posterior to cord: Dilated veins

Myelomalacia
- Cord volume loss, gliosis
- No CSF signal central cavitation seen on T1WI

PATHOLOGY

General Features
- Etiology
  - MVA (45%), falls (22%), acts of violence (16%), sports injury (13%)
    - Most common sports injury: Diving
    - If > 45 yrs, most likely due to fall
  - Spondylosis is significant risk factor for SCI
- Epidemiology
  - 14,000 SCI occur each year; 10,000 survive to reach treatment facility
  - Estimated societal cost ~ $2 billion annually

Gross Pathologic & Surgical Features
- Ranges in severity
  - Cord edema without hemorrhage
  - Cord petechial hemorrhage
  - Cord pulverization & bleeding
  - Complete transection

Microscopic Features
- Cord microcirculation alterations maximize in 24-48 hrs
- Intramedullary edema ± hemorrhage involving central gray matter
  - Edema peaks in 3-6 days, subsides by 1-2 weeks
- Extends outward with severity of trauma
- Hemorrhagic necrosis & liquefaction may occur
- Demyelination & cystic myelomalacia ensues

Staging, Grading or Classification Criteria
- American Spinal Injury Association (ASIA)
  - Grade A: No motor or sensory function preserved in sacral segments S4-S5
  - Grade B: Sensory, but no motor function preserved below neurologic level; sacral S4-S5 function preserved
  - Grade C: Motor function preserved below level, > 50% key muscles below have muscle grade < 3/5
  - Grade D: Motor function preserved below level, > 50% key muscles below have muscle grade > 3/5
  - Grade E: Normal
  - (Neurologic level of injury = most caudal cord segment with normal sensory & motor function on both sides of body)
- Kulkarni classification

SPINAL CORD INJURY

- Type 1: Cord hemorrhage evident acutely as T1 inhomogeneity; poorest prognosis
- Type 2 (most common): T2 hyperintense contusion & swelling with normal T1; good prognosis
- Type 3 (uncommon): T2 central hypointensity, thick peripheral hyperintensity at focal cord enlargement with normal T1; intermediate pattern & prognosis

CLINICAL ISSUES

Presentation
- Anterior cord syndrome
  - Injury to anterior 2/3 of cord
  - Pain & temperature affected
  - Touch & vibration intact
  - Highly associated with traumatic disc herniation
- Central cord syndrome
  - Upper extremity involvement more common than lower
  - Older population, seen with spondylosis without fx
  - Historically associated with central hematoma, predominantly a white-matter injury
- Posterior cord syndrome: Uncommon; loss of dorsal column function
- Brown-Sequard syndrome
  - Injury to half of cord
  - Ipsilateral loss of touch & motor function
  - Contralateral loss of pain & temperature
  - Often superimposed on central cord syndrome
- Autonomic hyperreflexia
  - Arise in SCI above T6
  - Paroxysmal hypertension with agonizing headache
  - May result in intracerebral hemorrhage, seizure, cardiac arrhythmias, death
- Contusion may be present in asymptomatic patients

Demographics
- Age
  - Mean age: 30.5 yrs; median age: 26 yrs
  - 50% are 16-30 yrs
- Gender: Over 80% male
- Ethnicity: More common in non-Caucasians
- Timing of injury
  - Highest rate in July, lowest in February
  - 39% occur on Saturday or Sunday

Natural History & Prognosis
- Contusion
  - Regresses over 1-2 weeks
  - Good prognosis for neurologic recovery
- Hematoma: Poor prognosis, often without recovery
- Poor prognostic factors: C4, C5, C6 level injuries, age > 50 yrs
- Anterior cord syndrome: 70% regain ambulation
- Central cord syndrome: < 50 yrs 70% ambulate, > 50 yrs 40%
- Posterior column syndrome: Ambulation usually possible unless proprioception involved, which then makes it difficult
- Brown-Sequard syndrome: 90% will ambulate
- Post-traumatic spinal cord syndrome (aka post-traumatic progressive myelopathy)
  - ≤ 2% post-traumatic SCI
  - Spinothalamic symptoms (i.e. pain, sensory loss)
  - Cysts may occur above or below original cord lesion
  - Cysts not related to site or severity of original lesion
  - May occur months to years following SCI

Treatment
- Surgical → stabilization
- Medical
  - Limit damaging processes → methylprednisolone bolus followed by infusion is standard
  - Respiratory support
  - Spinal shock
    - Loss of sympathetic tone below injury level
    - Unopposed vagal tone → asystole → atropine
  - Autonomic hyperreflexia
    - Occurs in 85% of patients with transection above T5
    - Lower blood pressure; sit patient upright to reduce intracranial pressures
    - Remove inciting factor; most often distended bladder, but also bowel distension, renal stones, sexual activity, numerous other stimuli
  - Neurogenic bladder: Intermittent catheter drainage to minimize potential complications
- Chronic care best approached from rehabilitation team approach
  - Rehab specialist, physical/occupational therapy, pain management, psychosocial support
- Vascular endothelial growth factor improves functional outcome, decreases secondary degeneration in experimental-rat SCI

DIAGNOSTIC CHECKLIST

Consider
- Screening MR for all symptomatic SCI

Image Interpretation Pearls
- Sagittal STIR is key to diagnosing marrow edema, ligamentous injury

SELECTED REFERENCES

1. Collignon F et al: Acute traumatic central cord syndrome: magnetic resonance imaging and clinical observations. J Neurosurg. 96(1 Suppl):29-33, 2002
2. Flanders AE et al: The relationship between the functional abilities of patients with cervical spinal cord injury and the severity of damage revealed by MR imaging. AJNR Am J Neuroradiol. 20(5):926-34, 1999
3. Katzberg RW et al: Acute cervical spine injuries: prospective MR imaging assessment at a level 1 trauma center. Radiology. 213(1):203-12, 1999
4. Lipper MH et al: Brown-Sequard syndrome of the cervical spinal cord after chiropractic manipulation. AJNR Am J Neuroradiol. 19(7):1349-52, 1998
5. Quencer RM et al: Acute traumatic central cord syndrome: MRI-pathological correlations. Neuroradiology. 34(2):85-94, 1992

SPINAL CORD INJURY

IMAGE GALLERY

Typical

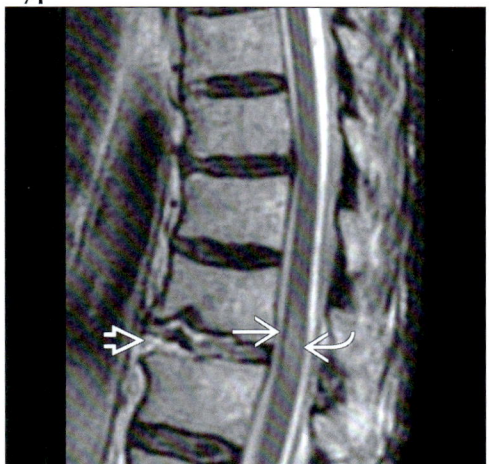
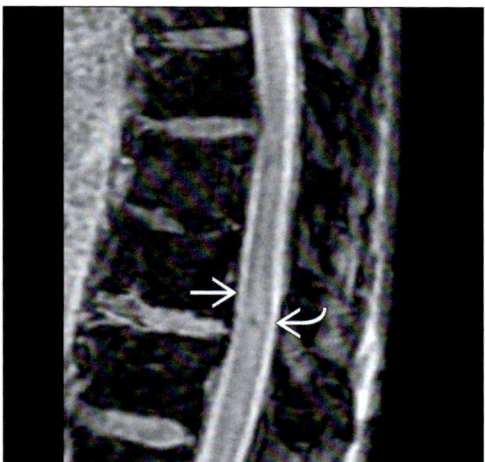

(Left) Sagittal T2WI MR shows focal hyperintense cord contusion ➡ with minimal central hemorrhage ➡. Disc edema is seen ➡ but superior vertebral fractures are not visible. (Right) Sagittal T2* GRE MR in the same case as previous image, better demonstrates focal hemorrhage ➡, though cord edema ➡ is not as apparent as on T2WI.

Typical

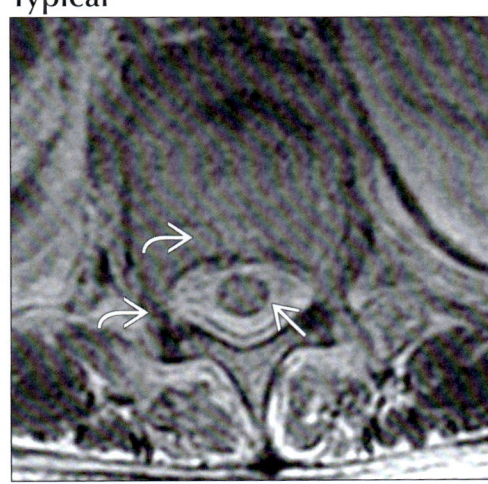
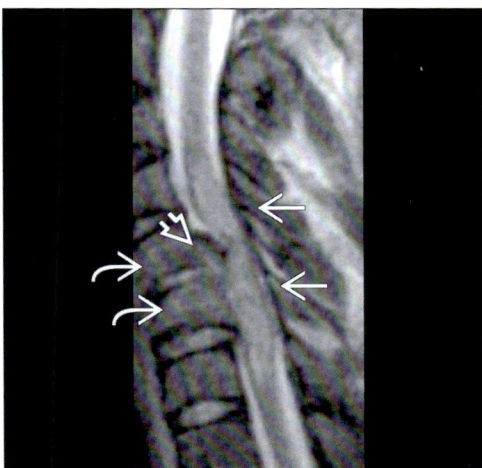

(Left) Axial T2WI MR in the same case as previous image, shows central cord edema ➡ indicative of contusion, as well as limited visualization of fractures ➡. (Right) Sagittal T2WI MR shows large area of swollen hyperintense edema ➡ indicative of contusion. Note edema of vertebral bodies ➡ & compression of cord by traumatic disc herniation ➡.

Typical

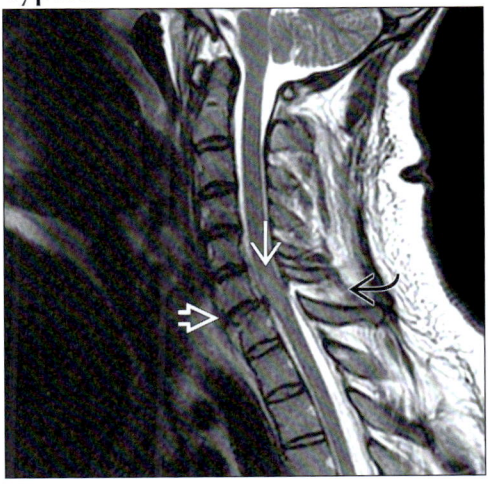
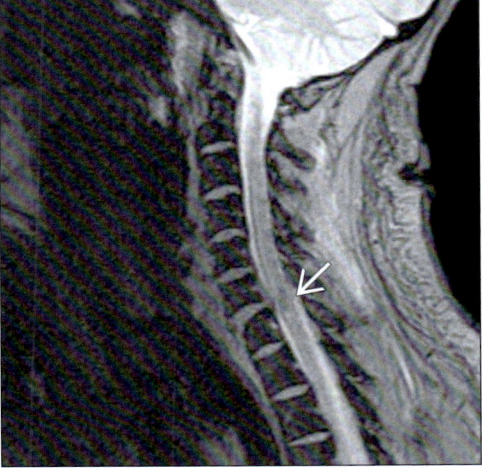

(Left) Sagittal T2WI MR shows focal hyperintense contusion ➡ with no evidence of hemorrhage. Note mild anterolisthesis ➡ & separation (flaring) of spinous processes ➡ due to flexion injury. (Right) Sagittal T2* GRE MR in the same same case as previous image shows hypointense susceptibility effect ➡ indicative of acute hemorrhage; not seen on T2WI.

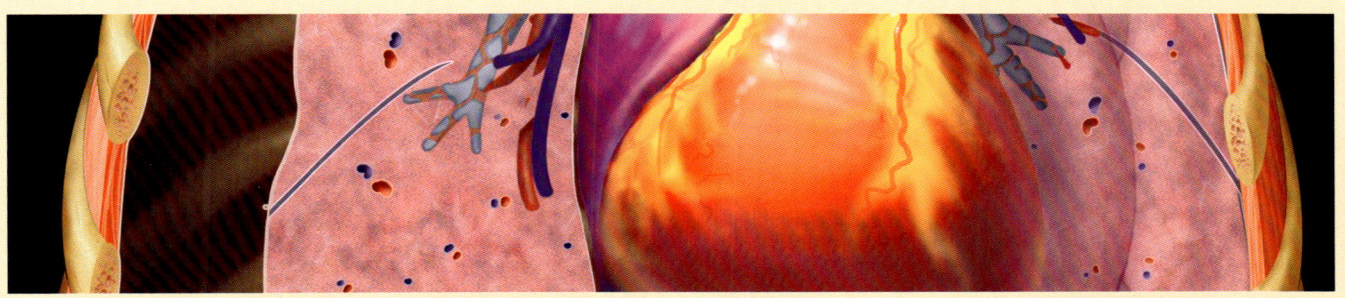

SECTION 2: Chest/Cardiovascular

Introduction and Overview
Chest Imaging Issues, Trauma   I-2-2

Chest/Cardiovascular
Pneumomediastinum   I-2-4
Pneumothorax   I-2-8
Tracheobronchial Tear   I-2-12
Rib Fractures and Flail Chest   I-2-14
Aortic Transection   I-2-18
Spinal Fracture, Thoracic   I-2-22
Sternal Fracture   I-2-26
Diaphragmatic Tear   I-2-28
Esophageal Tear   I-2-32
Lung Contusion   I-2-36
Neurogenic Pulmonary Edema   I-2-40
Negative Pressure Pulmonary Edema   I-2-44

CHEST IMAGING ISSUES, TRAUMA

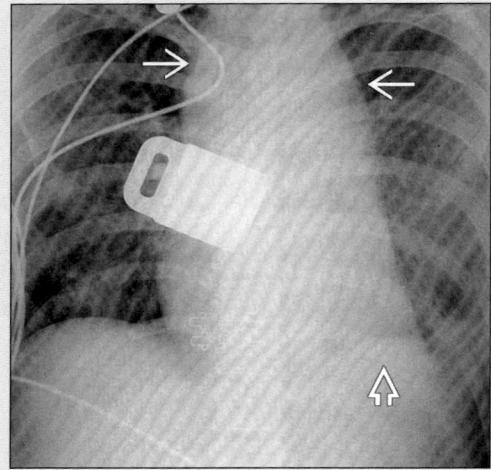

Anteroposterior radiograph shows widened mediastinum ➡, left hemidiaphragm is normal ➡. Patient made uneventful recovery.

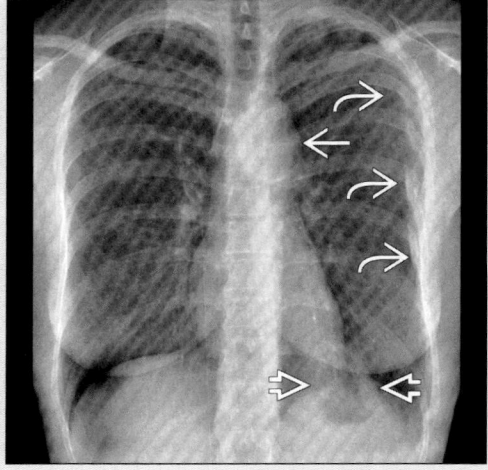

Frontal radiograph 4 years later shows abnormal aortic arch contour ➡ and abnormal left hemidiaphragm ➡. Multiple healed left rib fractures ➡.

TERMINOLOGY

Definitions
- Chest trauma is classified into blunt or penetrating

IMAGING ANATOMY

Critical Anatomic Structures
- Blunt chest trauma accounts for 20% of trauma-related deaths
  - Motor vehicle accidents account for 75% of blunt chest trauma
  - Most serious injury: Acute traumatic aortic injury
  - Most common injury: Rib fracture followed by pulmonary contusion

ANATOMY-BASED IMAGING ISSUES

Key Concepts or Questions
- Portable chest radiograph is a screening examination, sensitive but not specific for major intrathoracic injuries
  - Definitive diagnosis usually requires secondary examinations: CT, esophagram, MR
- MDCT rapidly replacing the portable chest radiograph as the initial examination in the traumatized patient
  - Chest radiograph sensitive (> 95%) for nearly all life-threatening injuries
  - However, stakes are too high, decision-making aided by MDCT evaluation

Imaging Approaches
- ABCs of blunt chest trauma
  - Sequential method to rapidly evaluate either chest radiograph or CT for major intrathoracic injuries
    - Starts with the most significant injury: Acute traumatic aortic injury
  - Mirrors the clinical approach to stabilizing seriously injured trauma patient ("ABCs": Airway, Breathing, Circulation)
  - Helps to obviate problem of satisfaction of search (SOS), recognizing the obvious non-life-threatening injury and missing the subtle life-threatening injury
  - Helps to obviate delayed diagnosis from overlooked injury
    - Delayed diagnosis > 30 days: 5% of aortic transections, 40% of bronchial tears, 60% of diaphragmatic tears
    - Of patients dying within 24 hours, 30% radiographs misinterpreted (missed injuries include aortic transection, diaphragmatic herniation, and flail segments)
- **A: Aortic transection**
  - Chest radiograph
    - Most common location at aortic isthmus
    - Radiograph will not show transection, rather shows the leakage of blood i.e., mediastinal widening, etc.
    - If suspected, CTA or aortography for diagnosis
- **B: Bronchial tear**
  - Chest radiograph
    - Most common location within 2.5 cm of carina
    - Radiograph usually will not show tear, rather shows the leakage of air
    - Persistent Progressive Pneumothorax or Pneumomediastinum ("P" sign)
    - If suspected, CT or bronchoscopy for diagnosis
- **C: Cord injury**
  - Chest radiograph
    - Most common location at the functional thoracolumbar junction (transition zone between thoracic facet and lumbar facet orientation) (T9-11)
    - Radiograph may not show spinal fracture, rather shows paraspinal mass or malalignment of spinous processes and pedicles
    - If suspected, CT or MR for diagnosis
- **D: Diaphragmatic tear**
  - Chest radiograph
    - Most common location through the posterolateral central tendon of the left hemidiaphragm

CHEST IMAGING ISSUES, TRAUMA

Differential Diagnosis

Pneumothorax
- Macklin effect
- Rib penetration
- Diaphragmatic tear
- Bronchial tear
- Esophageal tear

Pneumomediastinum
- Macklin effect
- Bronchial tear
- Esophageal tear

Increased Density Hemithorax
- Hemothorax
- Lung contusion
- Chest wall hematoma
- Aspiration
- Pulmonary edema
- Diaphragmatic hernia

- Herniation may be delayed, positive pressure ventilation may prevent abdominal contents from herniating into thorax
- If suspected, barium examinations remain useful but underutilized, CT or MR usually relied on
- Axial imaging less sensitive (90%) than coronal or sagittal reconstruction in diagnosing tear
- E: Esophageal tear
  - Chest radiograph
    - Most common location is the left posterolateral wall of the esophagogastric junction
    - Radiograph will not show tear, but will show signs from leakage of air and irritant fluids in the left costovertebral angle
    - If suspected, esophagram with nonionic contrast
- F: Flail chest & fractured ribs
  - Chest radiograph
    - Radiograph will not show paradoxical motion of chest wall
    - Radiograph insensitive for acute rib fractures
    - Suspect flail chest if more than 5 contiguous rib fractures or more than 3 contiguous segmental rib fractures (2 or more fractures in each rib)
    - 1st rib fracture signifies severity of trauma
- G: Gas collections
  - Chest radiograph
    - Supine portable radiograph less sensitive than upright radiograph for pneumothorax
    - Air collects in nondependent location, in supine position, inferior lateral hemithorax (deep sulcus)
    - Subtle air collections may be first hint of esophageal tears, bronchial tears, diaphragmatic tears
    - Simple pneumothorax can turn into tension pneumothorax, especially when patients ventilated
    - If suspected, CT, upright or decubitus radiographs
- H: Heart (cardiac) injury
  - Chest radiograph
    - Radiograph will not show cardiac injury, but may show signs related to cardiac dysfunction
    - Suspect with sudden development of pulmonary edema, especially in young
    - If suspected, echocardiography procedure of choice, CT or MR less useful
- I: Iatrogenic misplacement tubes & catheters
  - Chest radiograph
    - All lines and tubes must be accounted for
    - Hectic & harried environment of trauma bay may lead to more misplaced lines
    - Course of NG tube often useful as diagnostic aid in patients with aortic transection (displaced from aortic arch) or diaphragmatic tears (courses into abdomen and through herniated stomach)

RELATED REFERENCES

1. Euathrongchit J et al: Nonvascular mediastinal trauma. Radiol Clin North Am. 44(2):251-8, viii, 2006
2. Mirvis SE: Diagnostic imaging of acute thoracic injury. Semin Ultrasound CT MR. 25(2):156-79, 2004

IMAGE GALLERY

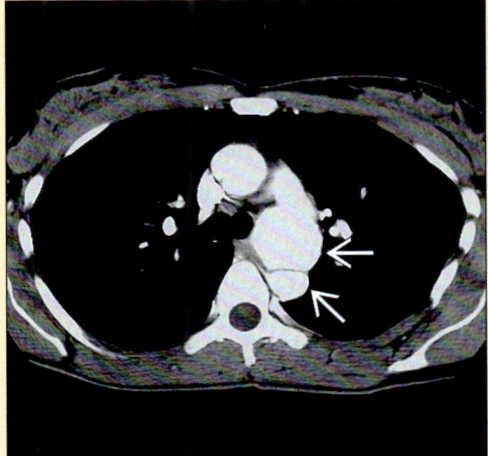
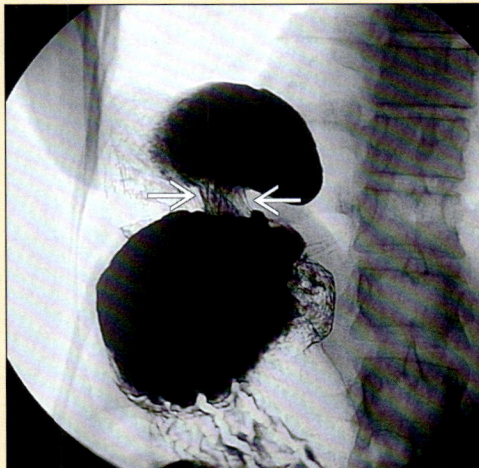

(Left) Axial CECT shows abnormal contour ➡ at aortic isthmus from chronic pseudoaneurysm. *(Right)* Tangential esophagram shows herniation of stomach through hemidiaphragm (collar sign, ➡). Both the aortic transection and the diaphragmatic rupture were missed during the first hospitalization.

PNEUMOMEDIASTINUM

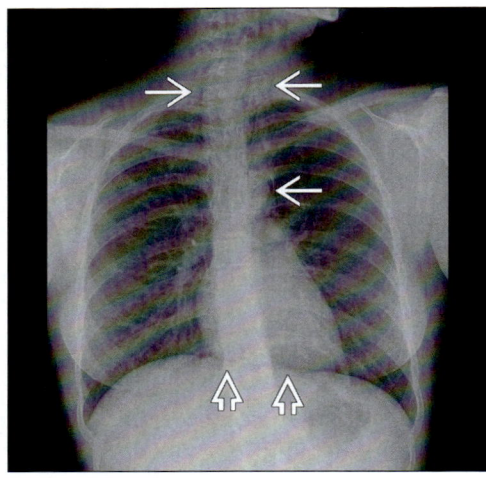
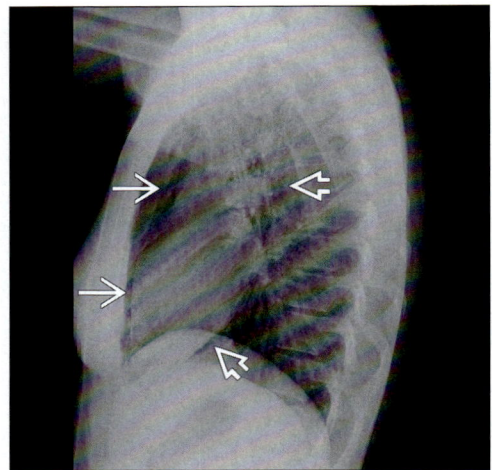

Frontal radiograph shows streaky lucencies outlining mediastinal structures and extending into the neck ➡. Majority of air above the carina. Continuous diaphragm sign ➡.

Lateral radiograph shows streaky lucencies anterior to the heart and great vessels ➡. Air also outlines posterior heart and hilar structures ➡. Spontaneous pneumomediastinum.

TERMINOLOGY

Abbreviations and Synonyms
- Pulmonary interstitial emphysema (PIE), Mediastinal emphysema, air block, pneumopericardium
- Barotrauma

Definitions
- Extra-alveolar air dissecting into pulmonary interstitium and mediastinum
  - Spontaneous: Usually secondary to Macklin effect
  - Traumatic includes tracheobronchial tear or esophageal tear

IMAGING FINDINGS

General Features
- Best diagnostic clue
  - Air outlining the heart borders and mediastinal vessels with subcutaneous emphysema
    - Usually more conspicuous on lateral view
- Location
  - Spontaneous: Air usually accumulates cephalad to carina
    - Esophageal tear: Air usually accumulates in paraesophageal location at level of diaphragm
  - On CT, look for air within the interlobular septa: Essentially, black Kerley B lines
    - Air can be followed, tracking medially around pulmonary arteries into mediastinum
- Size: Large especially if progressive should suggest visceral injury (trachea or esophagus)
- Morphology: Thin linear air streaks adjacent to mediastinal vessels and airways

Radiographic Findings
- Radiography: Air outlines normal mediastinal structures: Aorta and major arteries, lobar airways, anterior and posterior to heart
- Pulmonary interstitial emphysema (PIE)
  - Subtle, often unrecognized
  - Cysts: Small to large intrapulmonary cysts or subpleural location
  - Linear non-branching lucencies
  - Perivascular halos
  - Intraseptal air

DDx: Mediastinal Air Collections

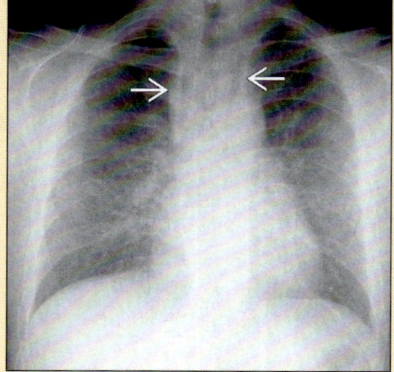
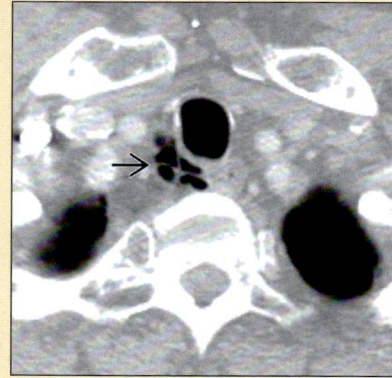
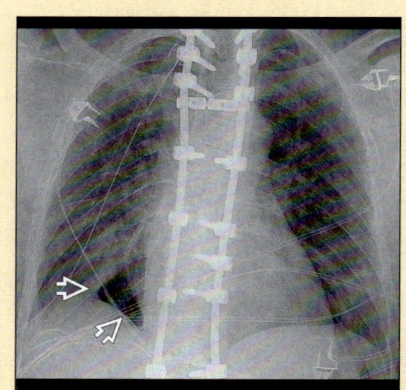

Achalasia | Paratracheal Cysts | Medial Pneumothorax

PNEUMOMEDIASTINUM

Terminology
- Extra-alveolar air dissecting into pulmonary interstitium and mediastinum

Imaging Findings
- Usually more conspicuous on lateral view
- Spontaneous: Air usually accumulates cephalad to carina
- Size: Large especially if progressive should suggest visceral injury (trachea or esophagus)
- Location: In esophageal tears air preferentially collects around esophagus at the level of the diaphragm

Top Differential Diagnoses
- Pneumothorax
- Pneumopericardium

Key Facts
- Mach Band
- Paratracheal Air Cyst

Pathology
- Macklin effect: Alveoli rupture along base, air then tracks through pulmonary interstitium and then decompresses into the mediastinum
- 10% incidence with blunt chest trauma

Clinical Issues
- Retrosternal chest pain (100%)
- Benign course usually resolves in 7 days (4-14 days)

Diagnostic Checklist
- Inhalational drug use in younger patients
- Asthma if pneumomediastinum associated with hyperinflated lungs

---

- Signs pneumomediastinum
  - Interstitial air
    - **Ring around the artery sign** or vein (vessel en face on radiograph)
    - Tubular artery sign (vessel in profile on radiograph)
    - Double bronchial wall (air on both sides of airway)
  - Subcutaneous emphysema (neck and chest wall)
  - **Continuous diaphragm sign**: Look for air between the pericardium and diaphragm
    - Can be similar to pneumoperitoneum
  - V sign of Naclerio
    - Costovertebral air adjacent to left hemidiaphragm and spine, raises question of esophageal tear
  - Thymic sail sign (pediatric patients)
- Signs suggestive of tracheobronchial tear or esophageal tear ("P" signs)
  - **P**rogressive enlargement **p**neumomediastinum
  - **P**ersistent (and or **p**rogressive) **p**neumothorax
    - Pneumothorax more common with visceral tears
  - **P**leural effusions (rare with spontaneous pneumomediastinum)
  - Location: In esophageal tears air preferentially collects around esophagus at the level of the diaphragm

CT Findings
- CECT
  - More sensitive than chest radiograph
  - Pulmonary interstitial emphysema
    - Interlobular septa (black Kerley B lines)
    - Air surrounding artery, veins, and/or airways
    - Lightning strikes or cracked lung: Air streaks not following normal bronchovascular structures
  - Pneumomediastinum
    - Streaky air collections within mediastinal fat and in connective tissue sheaths around tubular structures such as trachea and pulmonary arteries
    - Primarily paraesophageal at gastroesophageal junction suggests esophageal tear
  - Visceral injury
    - May not see tracheobronchial tears or esophageal tears, only the secondary affects of the tear (leakage of air or in the case of the esophagus air and/or oral contrast)
  - Tension pneumopericardium or pneumomediastinum
    - Compression superior vena cava, right ventricular cavity
    - Dilatation of inferior vena cava

Imaging Recommendations
- Best imaging tool
  - Chest radiograph usually suffices for diagnosis
    - Lateral view usually more sensitive than frontal view
  - CT more sensitive, may be useful in suspected tracheobronchial or esophageal tears
- Protocol advice
  - Consider using oral contrast when esophageal perforation suspected clinically
  - Decubitus views: In contrast to pneumothorax or pneumopericardium, air does not shift in pneumomediastinum

DIFFERENTIAL DIAGNOSIS

Pneumothorax
- Apical air cap
  - Pneumomediastinum may dissect extrapleurally over apex
  - Pneumothorax
    - Air will shift with decubitus position
    - Usually unilateral (apical air caps from pneumomediastinum may be bilateral)
    - Pleural line smooth (in pneumomediastinum pleural line irregular due to fascial tethering)

Pneumopericardium
- Less common but similar pathophysiology, air tracks along pulmonary veins into pericardium
- Etiology usually traumatic (penetrating, surgery, fistula from esophagus, or barotrauma)

PNEUMOMEDIASTINUM

- Air confined to pericardium key feature
  - Single gas collection outlining left ventricle, right atrium or if large both
  - Air does not extend above mid-ascending aorta
  - Air moves with decubitus position (pneumomediastinum will not shift)
  - Pericardial thickening or effusion (hydropneumopericardium)
  - Tension pneumopericardium
    - Heart size small (small heart sign)
  - Pneumomediastinum seldom completely surrounds heart

Mach Band
- Due to retinal inhibition, obscuring one edge with finger or hand will make Mach band disappear
- Convex soft tissue density into concave lung density = black Mach band, example heart border
- Convex lung density into concave soft tissue density = white Mach band, example paraesophageal stripe

Skin Fold
- Gradation of gray that fades medially, with a sharp Mach line laterally
- Follows non-anatomic course

Air Distended Esophagus
- Achalasia, can mimic extraluminal mediastinal air

Paratracheal Air Cyst
- Single or cluster of small rounded air-filled cysts in right paratracheal region at thoracic inlet

PATHOLOGY

General Features
- General path comments
  - Macklin effect: Alveoli rupture along base, air then tracks through pulmonary interstitium and then decompresses into the mediastinum
    - Mediastinal air communicates with retroperitoneum and fascial planes of the neck
    - In infants, pneumomediastinum may not decompress into neck or retroperitoneum leading to tension pneumomediastinum
  - PIE can lead to pneumothorax
    - Pneumothorax does not lead to PIE or pneumomediastinum
- Etiology
  - Spontaneous
    - Sustained Valsalva maneuver predisposes to alveolar rupture: Asthma, cough, weight lifting, straining, marijuana or inhalational drug use
  - Traumatic
    - Blunt chest trauma leads to pulmonary laceration and alveolar rupture
    - Bronchial or tracheal fracture
    - Esophageal tear
    - Mechanical ventilation: "Volutrauma" as opposed to barotrauma
  - Extrathoracic sources
    - Dental extraction, other head and neck operations
    - Sinus fracture
    - Duodenal ulcer or sigmoid diverticulitis
- Epidemiology
  - 10% incidence with blunt chest trauma
  - 1 in 30,000 ER visits

CLINICAL ISSUES

Presentation
- Most common signs/symptoms
  - Retrosternal chest pain (100%)
  - Subcutaneous emphysema (80%)
  - Neck pain (70%)
  - Dyspnea (70%)
  - Dysphagia (40%)
  - Hamman sign: Precordial crunching at auscultation
  - Mill wheel murmur (bruit de moulin): Succession splash with metallic tinkle from pneumopericardium
- Other signs/symptoms
  - Signs of pericardial tamponade
    - Consider pneumopericardium or tension pneumomediastinum (rare in adults)

Natural History & Prognosis
- Benign course usually resolves in 7 days (4-14 days)
- Morbidity and mortality related to etiology

Treatment
- None, observe for pneumothorax
- Treat underlying cause
- Bronchoscopy and esophagram useful for visceral injuries

DIAGNOSTIC CHECKLIST

Consider
- Inhalational drug use in younger patients
- Typically benign finding, so clinical history important to unearth more medically important disease

Image Interpretation Pearls
- Asthma if pneumomediastinum associated with hyperinflated lungs
- Lateral radiograph more sensitive than frontal radiograph

SELECTED REFERENCES

1. Sakai M et al: Frequent cause of the Macklin effect in spontaneous pneumomediastinum: demonstration by multidetector-row computed tomography. J Comput Assist Tomogr. 30(1):92-4, 2006
2. Newcomb AE et al: Spontaneous pneumomediastinum: a benign curiosity or a significant problem? Chest. 128(5):3298-302, 2005
3. Chapdelaine J et al: Spontaneous pneumomediastinum: are we overinvestigating? J Pediatr Surg. 39(5):681-4, 2004
4. Howton JC: Boerhaave's syndrome in a healthy adolescent male presenting with pneumomediastinum. Ann Emerg Med. 43(6):785, 2004

PNEUMOMEDIASTINUM

IMAGE GALLERY

Typical

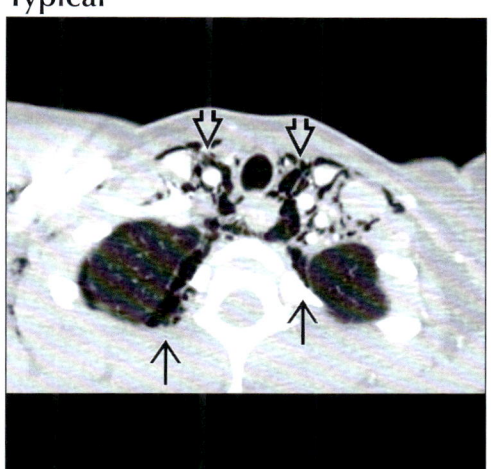
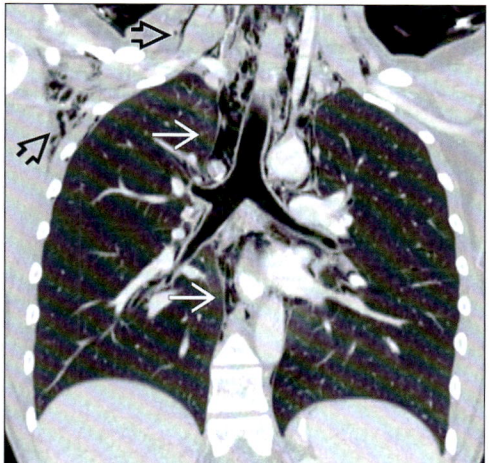

(Left) Axial CECT shows air extending into the neck ➡. Bilateral extrapleural extension ➡ produces apical air caps. Note the fascial tethering in the extrapleural space. *(Right)* Coronal CECT shows distribution of air throughout the mediastinum ➡ from spontaneous pneumomediastinum. Subcutaneous emphysema ➡.

Typical

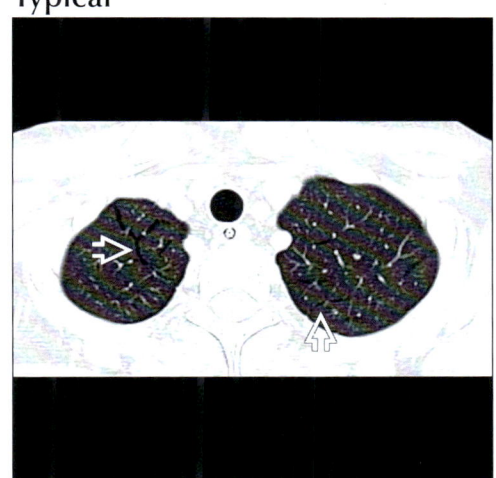
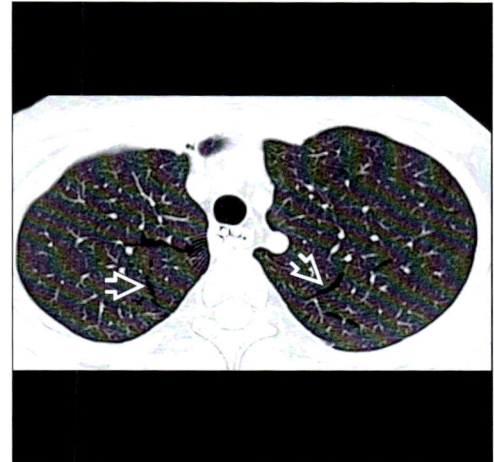

(Left) Axial HRCT shows air within interstitial space, "cracked lung" or "lightning strikes" ➡. Air does not follow airways or blood vessels. *(Right)* Axial HRCT shows air within interstitial space, short lines ➡ not following the airways or blood vessels. Note absence of mediastinal air.

Typical

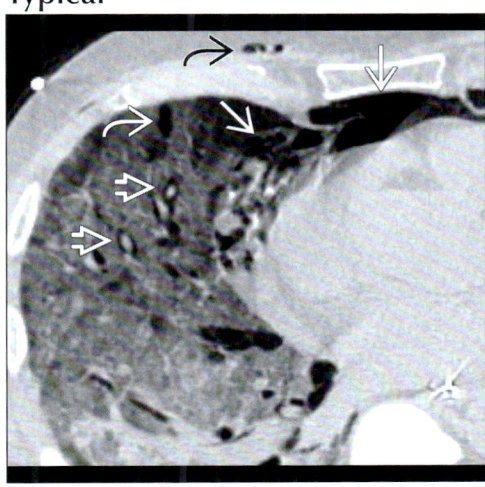
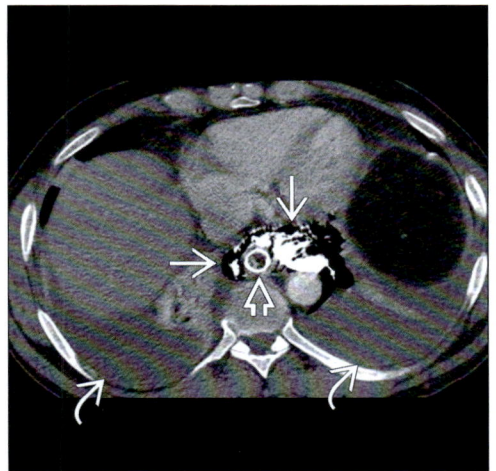

(Left) Axial CECT shows ring around the artery sign ➡ from interstitial emphysema in patient with Pneumocystis pneumonia. Black Kerley B line ➡. Pneumomediastinum ➡ and subcutaneous emphysema ➡. *(Right)* Axial CECT shows extravasation of air and contrast ➡ from esophageal rupture from ingested chicken bone ➡. Bilateral pleural effusion ➡.

PNEUMOTHORAX

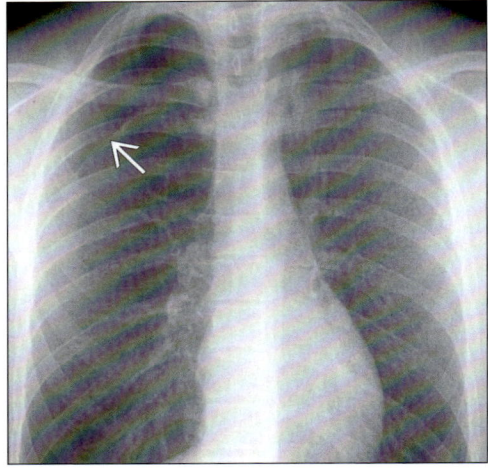

Frontal radiograph shows spontaneous right pneumothorax ➡ in young man.

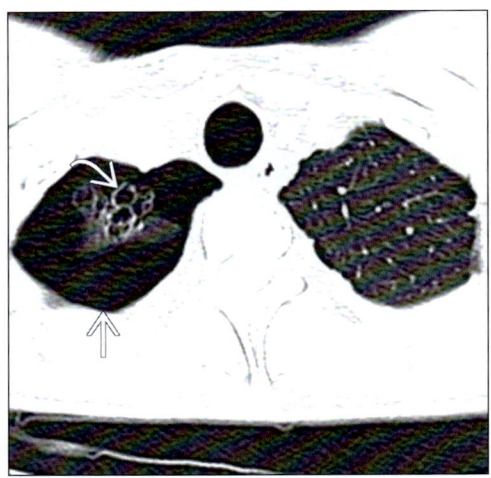

Axial HRCT shows right apical subpleural blebs ➡ surrounded by air in the pleural space ➡.

TERMINOLOGY

Abbreviations and Synonyms
- Pneumothorax (PTX)

Definitions
- Air in pleural space classified as spontaneous either primary (absence lung disease) or secondary (underlying interstitial or obstructive lung disease) or traumatic (includes iatrogenic)

IMAGING FINDINGS

General Features
- Best diagnostic clue: Observation of thin pleural line parallel to chest wall with no lung markings projecting beyond
- Location
  - Upright radiograph: Lung apex
  - Decubitus radiograph: Nondependent lung
  - Supine radiograph: Costophrenic sulcus
- Size: Small (< 2 cm maximal pleural separation), large (> 2 cm pleural separation)

Radiographic Findings
- Radiography
  - Visceral pleural line usually parallels chest wall
  - Size: Small or large
    - Based on maximum separation lung and chest wall: **Small < 2 cm; large > 2 cm**
    - Volume of PTX ~ lung diameter^3/hemithorax diameter^3
    - 1 cm PTX ~ 25% (if lung 9 cm diameter, hemithorax 10 cm: [10^3-9^3]/10^3 = 27%)
    - 2 cm PTX ~ 50%
  - Spontaneous pneumothorax
    - Bilateral 5%
    - Pleural effusion 10%, hemothorax 7%
    - Tension 1-3% of those with spontaneous pneumothorax
  - Supine, much less sensitive and underestimates size
    - **Deep sulcus**: Anterolateral inferior hemithorax most nondependent in supine position
    - Relative transradiancy hemithorax
    - Mediastinal contours, heart border, or hemidiaphragm sharper than uninvolved side

DDx: Pneumothorax

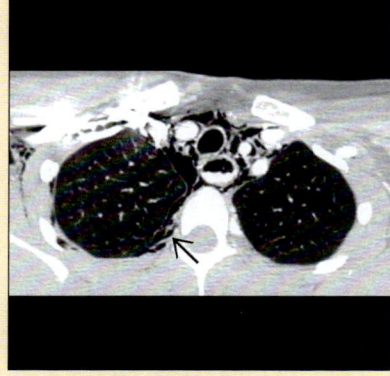

Pneumomediastinum

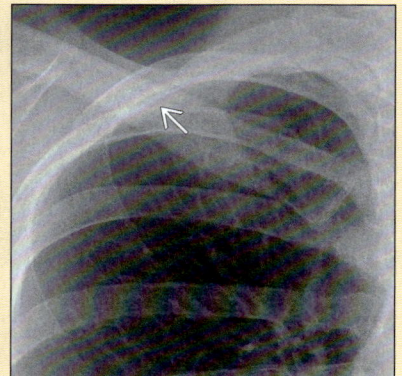

Companion Shadow

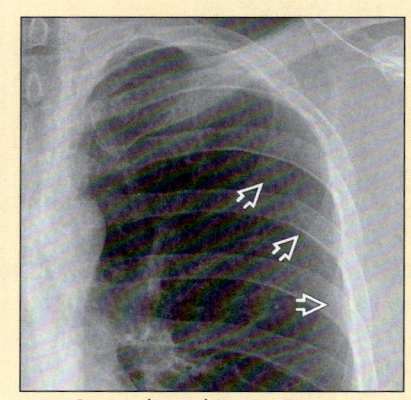

Superolateral Major Fissure

PNEUMOTHORAX

Key Facts

Terminology
- Air in pleural space classified as spontaneous either primary (absence lung disease) or secondary (underlying interstitial or obstructive lung disease) or traumatic (includes iatrogenic)

Imaging Findings
- Size: Small (< 2 cm maximal pleural separation), large (> 2 cm pleural separation)
- 2 cm PTX ~ 50%
- Tension pneumothorax: Radiographic findings + hemodynamic compromise
- Lateral or decubitus views recommended for equivocal cases (as sensitive as CT)
- Expiratory radiographs not recommended routinely

Top Differential Diagnoses
- Skin Fold, Scapula, Hair, Extraneous Monitoring or Support Lines
- Superolateral Major Fissure (SLMF), Companion Shadow
- Bullous Emphysema

Pathology
- **Buffalo chest**: Unilateral insult results in bilateral PTX, (buffalo have 1 common pleural space for both lungs)

Clinical Issues
- Absorption of air in pleural space: 1.5% per day on room air (50-75 ml/day)
- Persistent air leak: Air leak persisting > 10 days, usually due to bronchopleural fistula

---

- Visualization of pericardial tags or fat pads which become "mass-like"
- Air may accumulate in minor fissure
- Radiographic deep sulcus sign grossly underestimates true size of PTX
○ Expiratory exam
- Increases relative size of pleural space compared to overall lung volume
- Should aid detection but not shown to be more sensitive than full inspiratory examination
- Low lung volumes in expiratory exam often misinterpreted as interstitial lung disease or congestive heart failure
○ Tension pneumothorax: Radiographic findings + hemodynamic compromise
- Contralateral shift of mediastinum
- Ipsilateral hyperexpansion of ribs and flattening of hemidiaphragm
- Ipsilateral lung compressed
- With decreased lung compliance (stiff lungs like adult respiratory distress syndrome) PTX need not be large to compromise function
○ Pneumothorax ex vacuo
- Collection of air in pleural space adjacent to collapsed lobe
- Considered a vacuum phenomenon
- May resolve with reexpansion of lobe
- Conversely a large PTX may collapse an upper lobe due to bronchial kinking from weight of the lung, lobe will reexpand with chest tube drainage

CT Findings
- NECT
  ○ Very useful to distinguish pneumothorax from bullous emphysema or cystic lung disease
    - Important to distinguish prior to chest tube placement to avoid creating a bronchopleural fistula
  ○ More sensitive for PTX, distinguishing apical bulla, evaluating for underlying lung disease

Imaging Recommendations
- Best imaging tool: PA radiograph usually sufficient
- Protocol advice
  ○ Lateral or decubitus views recommended for equivocal cases (as sensitive as CT)
    - Expiratory radiographs not recommended routinely
  ○ CT for distinguishing bullous lung disease from PTX, to locate abnormal tube placement, or to evaluate for predisposing underlying lung disease
  ○ Immediate post-treatment radiograph necessary to ensure satisfactory chest tube position

DIFFERENTIAL DIAGNOSIS

Skin Fold, Scapula, Hair, Extraneous Monitoring or Support Lines
- Edge rather than a line, often extends outside chest wall
  ○ Skin fold: Gradation of grey with a black Mach line laterally that fades off medially, compared to distinct visceral pleural line of PTX

Superolateral Major Fissure (SLMF), Companion Shadow
- SLMF: Normally seen in 15%, edge rather than a line
  ○ Curved line does not parallel chest wall
    - Edge courses to the chest wall at the level of the posterior 5th or 6th rib
- Companion shadow: Extrapleural fat along subcostal groove
  ○ Most prominent along first or second rib
  ○ Usually confined to rib whereas visceral pleural line parallels the chest wall

Bullous Emphysema
- Air will not change location with position
- No visceral pleural line
- CT crucial to separate large bulla and PTX

Pneumomediastinum
- Can mimic medially loculated PTX
- Can also dissect parietal pleura away from thoracic fascia mimicking an apical PTX

PNEUMOTHORAX

PATHOLOGY

General Features
- General path comments
  - Spontaneous PTX associated with apical bulla or subpleural blebs (90%) (seen at CT 80%)
  - Apical bulla more common with connective tissue disorders: Marfan; Ehlers-Danlos, cutis laxa, pseudoxanthoma elasticum
- Etiology
  - Primary spontaneous pneumothorax
    - Height a risk factor; lungs of tall asthenic individuals may be subject to more gravitational stress
    - Gradient in pleural pressure increases from lung base to apex, alveoli at lung apex in tall lung subject to significantly greater distending pressure than those at the base
  - Most common predisposing conditions: Emphysema, pulmonary fibrosis, cystic fibrosis, cavities for any reason, cystic interstitial lung disease (e.g., Langerhans cell histiocytosis and lymphangiomyomatosis
  - Less common causes
    - Catamenial: Recurrent PTX associated with menses and pleural endometrial implants
    - Neoplastic: Osteosarcoma metastases
    - Rheumatoid arthritis: Necrobiotic nodules
    - Burt-Hogg-Dube syndrome: Cutaneous fibromas, renal cell carcinoma, spontaneous PTX
    - Post-infectious pneumatoceles: Pneumocystis jiroveci or Staphylococcus aureus pneumonia
  - Complication of intrathoracic interventional procedures such as lung biopsy and line placements

Gross Pathologic & Surgical Features
- Humans have separate pleural space for each lung
  - Transient communication (24 hours) immediately after median sternotomy, maybe long term (years) in heart-lung transplant patients
  - **Buffalo chest**: Unilateral insult results in bilateral PTX, (buffalo have 1 common pleural space for both lungs)
    - Single chest tube will drain both pleural spaces

Microscopic Features
- Air in pleural space can induce eosinophilia within pleural fluid

CLINICAL ISSUES

Presentation
- Most common signs/symptoms
  - Chest pain, sudden dyspnea
    - 50% wait more than 2 days before seeking medical attention
    - Re-expansion pulmonary edema directly related to length of time the lung has been collapsed
- Other signs/symptoms: Tension PTX: Severe dyspnea, cyanosis, sweating, and tachycardia

Demographics
- Gender: M:F = 2:1

Natural History & Prognosis
- Absorption of air in pleural space: 1.5% per day on room air (50-75 ml/day)
  - Full re-expansion usually takes a mean of 3 weeks
  - Daily radiographs often misleading as PTX may change little or not at all
    - Clinicians often get anxious and put in unnecessary chest tubes
  - Increased absorption with supplemental oxygen (increases reabsorption by a factor of 4)

Treatment
- Options, risks, complications
  - Chest tube drainage complications 20%
    - Aberrant tube placement
    - Pleural infection (1%)
  - Failure to expand lung may be due to chest tube malposition, underlying tracheal, bronchial, or esophageal tear, or due to trapped lung from visceral pleural thickening (usually metastases)
    - Persistent air leak: Air leak persisting > 10 days, usually due to bronchopleural fistula
  - Re-expansion pulmonary edema (< 1%)
    - Develops within hours of drainage of long-standing pneumothorax (or pleural effusion)
    - Transient, resolves over several days
- Stop smoking (lifetime risk smoking men 10% compared with 0.1% in nonsmoking men)
- Observation for small pneumothorax
  - Supplemental oxygen: Decreases inhaled Nitrogen concentration > decreases partial pressure nitrogen in blood > larger gradient between nitrogen concentration in pleura space and blood
  - Nitrogen limits the rate of absorption of gas from the pleural space
- Chest tube drainage common for large or symptomatic pneumothorax
  - **Size less important than patient's physiologic status**
  - Small pneumothorax can be problematic in patients with little reserve (COPD)
  - Large pneumothorax may not be clinically significant in young patient with large cardiopulmonary reserve
  - Small tubes work just as well as large tubes
- Pleurodesis or bullectomy for recurrent spontaneous pneumothorax or persistent pneumothorax
- Avoid air travel for 6 weeks, scuba diving avoided permanently

DIAGNOSTIC CHECKLIST

Image Interpretation Pearls
- Report size of pleural separation (small < 2 cm, large > 2 cm)

SELECTED REFERENCES
1. Henry M et al: BTS guidelines for the management of spontaneous pneumothorax. Thorax. 58 Suppl 2:ii39-52, 2003

PNEUMOTHORAX

IMAGE GALLERY

Typical

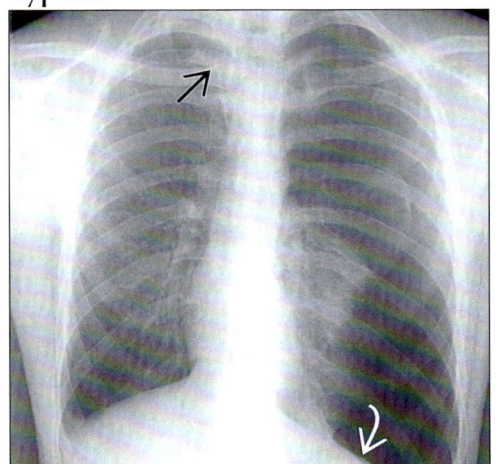
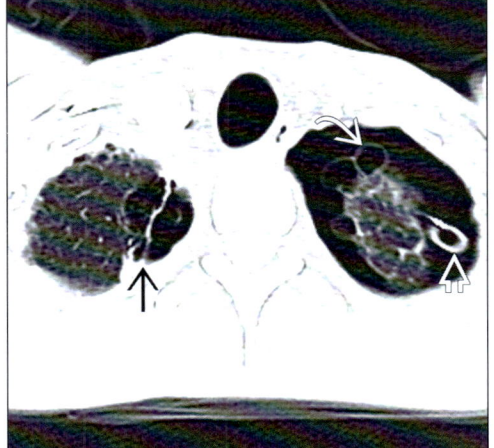

(Left) Frontal radiograph shows large left tension pneumothorax with depression of the left hemidiaphragm ➡. Surgical suture line from bleb repair ➡. Same patient as first page. *(Right)* Axial HRCT shows left chest tube ➡, subpleural blebs at lung apex ➡, and surgical suture line from previous repair of blebs right apex ➡.

Typical

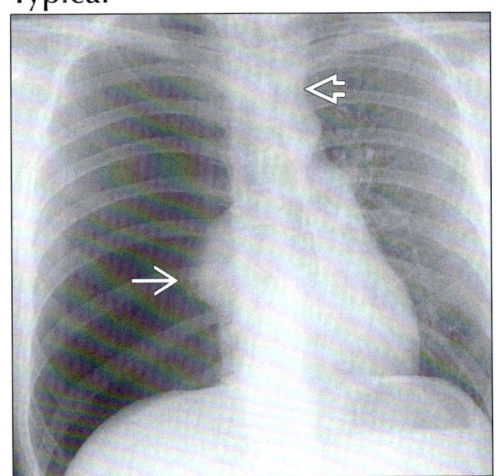
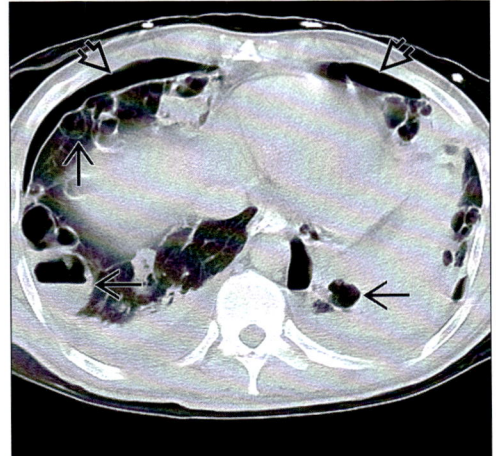

(Left) Frontal radiograph shows tension pneumothorax with lucent right hemithorax and collapsed right lung ➡ as well as mediastinum shift to the left ➡. Right hemidiaphragm is depressed and the right rib interspaces are larger than the left. *(Right)* Axial HRCT shows multiple bilateral cavitating lung nodules ➡ from staphylococcal pneumonia. Bilateral hydropneumothoraces ➡.

Typical

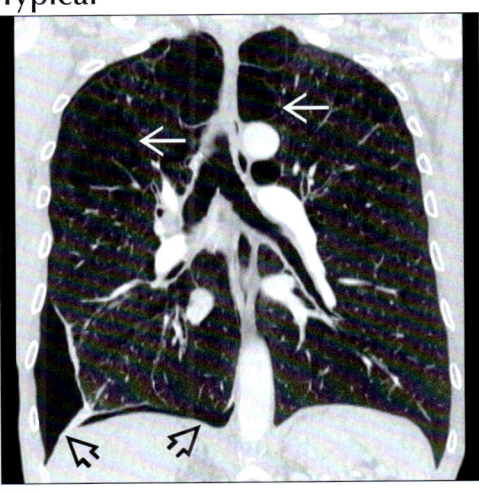
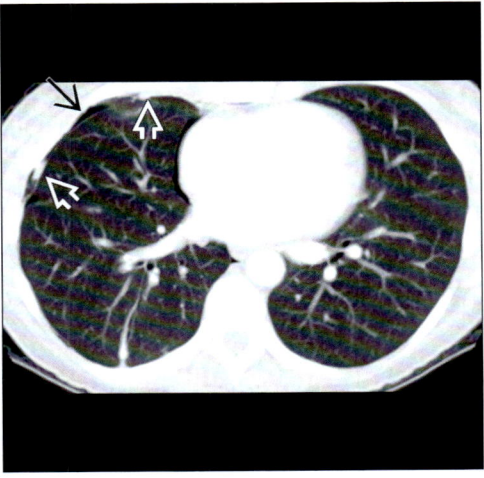

(Left) Coronal CECT shows extensive emphysema ➡ and right pneumothorax ➡. Basilar pneumothorax common in patients with emphysema. *(Right)* Axial CECT shows small pneumothorax ➡ and focal pleural thickening ➡ from endometriomas. Diagnosis: Catamenial pneumothorax.

TRACHEOBRONCHIAL TEAR

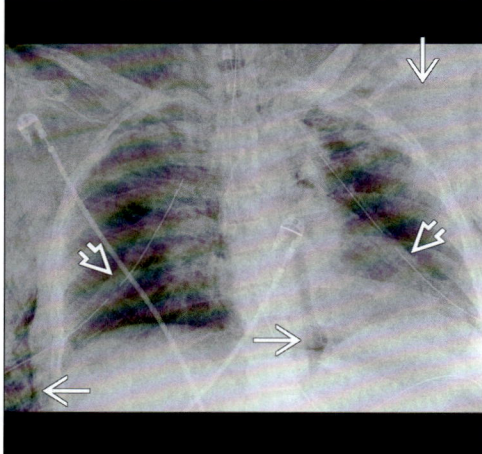 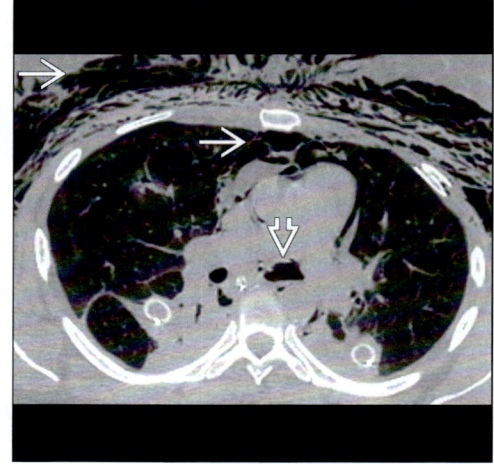

Anteroposterior radiograph shows massive pneumomediastinum and subcutaneous air ➔. Bilateral chest tubes ➔.

Axial CECT same patient as previous image shows extensive subcutaneous air and pneumomediastinum ➔. Left main bronchus interrupted ➔.

TERMINOLOGY

Abbreviations and Synonyms
- Fallen lung, bronchial fracture

IMAGING FINDINGS

General Features
- Best diagnostic clue: **P**ersistent or **p**rogressive **p**neumothorax or **p**neumomediastinum despite thoracostomy tube drainage (think **P**s)
- Location: Most within 2.5 cm of the tracheal carina, where airway fixed and subject to shearing
- Size: Partial thickness to complete disruption

Radiographic Findings
- Radiography
  - Rarely able to see tear
  - Subcutaneous emphysema, often massive and progressive
  - Pneumomediastinum, large and progressive
  - Pneumothorax (often tension)
  - Up to 80% have 1st rib fracture
  - "Fallen lung" sign
    - Lung falls away from hilum into a gravitationally dependent position
  - Endotracheal tube
    - Distended cuff beyond expected tracheal borders

CT Findings
- CTA
  - Look for associated injuries especially traumatic aortic rupture
  - 10% have no direct signs (tracheal defect, extensive air leak, or fractured cartilage)
  - Chronic: Airway stricture with volume loss affected lung

Imaging Recommendations
- Protocol advice: In severe blunt chest trauma, airways imaged along with aorta and great vessels

DIFFERENTIAL DIAGNOSIS

Pneumomediastinum
- Common with trauma, statistically unlikely from major airway injury

DDx: Bronchial Tear

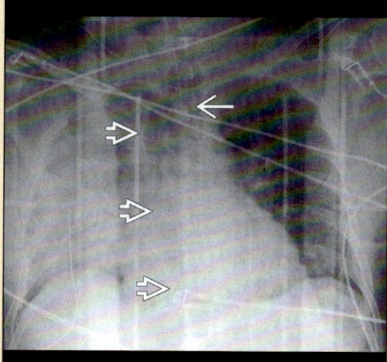 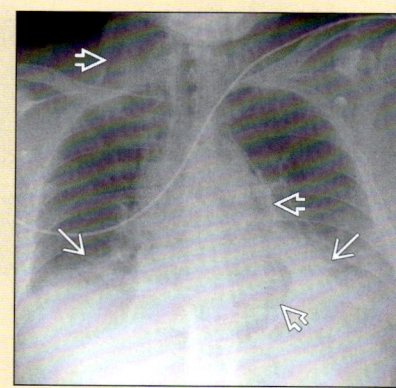 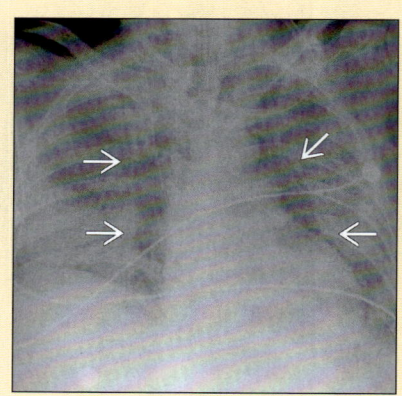

Esophageal Intubation | Esophageal Rupture | Pneumomediastinum

TRACHEOBRONCHIAL TEAR

Key Facts

Imaging Findings
- Best diagnostic clue: **P**ersistent or **p**rogressive **p**neumothorax or **p**neumomediastinum despite thoracostomy tube drainage (think **P**s)
- Location: Most within 2.5 cm of the tracheal carina, where airway fixed and subject to shearing
- Rarely able to see tear
- Pneumomediastinum, large and progressive
- Pneumothorax (often tension)

Top Differential Diagnoses
- Pneumomediastinum
- Pneumothorax
- Esophageal Rupture
- Esophageal Intubation

Clinical Issues
- Confirmation of diagnosis with bronchoscopy and prompt surgical repair

Pneumothorax
- Common with trauma, statistically unlikely from major airway injury

Esophageal Rupture
- From emetic injury, or blunt/penetrating trauma
- Also associated with pneumomediastinum (common) and pneumothorax (less common)

Esophageal Intubation
- Frontal radiograph shows balloon hyperinflation superimposed over the tracheal air column; lateral radiograph shows endotracheal tube posterior to trachea

PATHOLOGY

General Features
- Etiology
  - Direct compression between sternum and spine or
  - Sudden deceleration of lung with fixed trachea or
  - Forced expiration against closed glottis or
  - Penetrating trauma: Gunshot and stab wounds
- Epidemiology
  - Uncommon; 3% of patients who die from blunt chest trauma
  - Delayed diagnosis common: 70% not identified first 24 hours, 40% delayed more than 1 month

Gross Pathologic & Surgical Features
- Tears occur commonly at the attachment of the membranous posterior membrane with cartilage rings

CLINICAL ISSUES

Presentation
- Most common signs/symptoms
  - Respiratory distress
  - Continuous air leak despite chest tube drainage
  - Extensive subcutaneous emphysema

Natural History & Prognosis
- Delayed diagnosis leads to bronchostenosis

Treatment
- Confirmation of diagnosis with bronchoscopy and prompt surgical repair

DIAGNOSTIC CHECKLIST

Consider
- Don't overlook other life-threatening injuries

SELECTED REFERENCES
1. Tack D et al: The CT fallen-lung sign. Eur Radiol. 10(5):719-21, 2000

IMAGE GALLERY

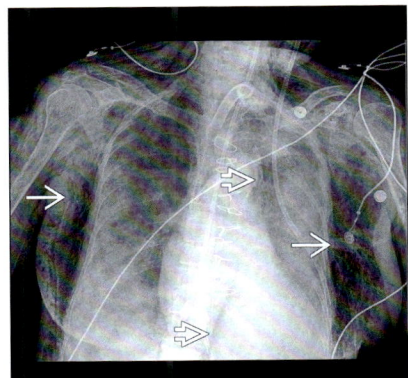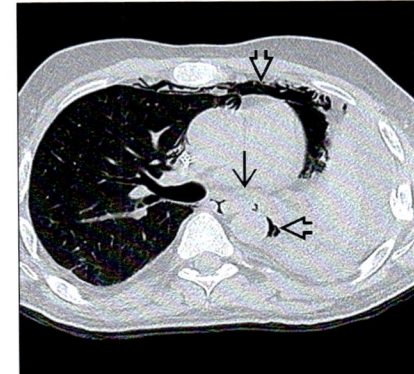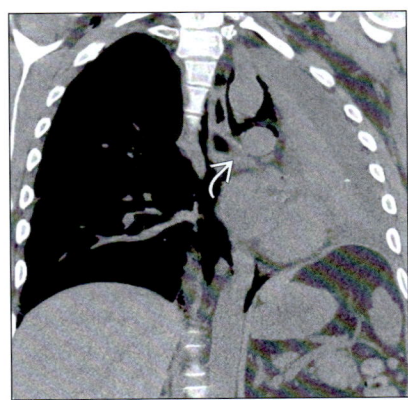

(Left) Anteroposterior radiograph 4 days after trauma shows massive subcutaneous emphysema ➡ and pneumomediastinum ➡. Left mainstem tear found at bronchoscopy. **(Center)** Axial NECT different patient shows pneumomediastinum ➡, but no pneumothorax. Left main bronchus is obliterated ➡. **(Right)** Coronal NECT in same patient as previous image shows a small fluid collection ➡ in the narrowed left main bronchus. Bronchoscopy showed fracture of the left main bronchus.

RIB FRACTURES AND FLAIL CHEST

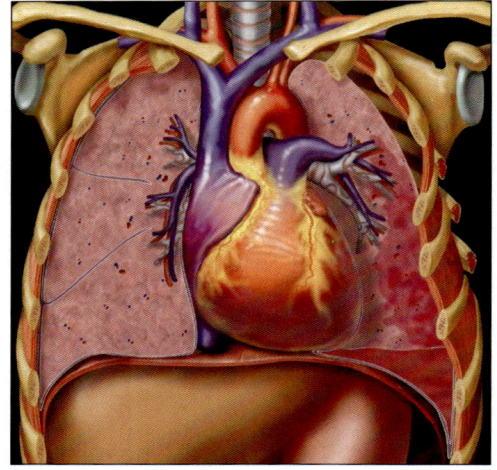

Graphic shows multiple, displaced, mid-left rib fractures, flail chest deformity with underlying pulmonary contusion, hemorrhage, and hemothorax/pneumothorax.

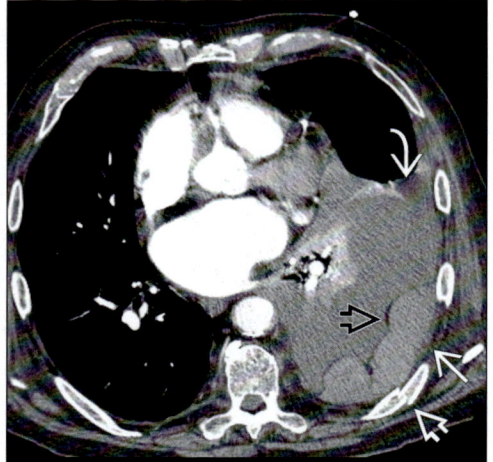

Axial CECT shows large pleural effusion ➡, displaced extrapleural fat ➡ and dense chest wall hematoma ➡. Rib fracture ➡.

TERMINOLOGY

Definitions
- Flail chest: 3 or more segmental rib fractures (more than 2 fractures within the same rib) or more than 5 adjacent rib fractures
  - Flail segment shows paradoxical motion with breathing

IMAGING FINDINGS

General Features
- Best diagnostic clue: Cortical break and step off
- Location: Dependent on site of energy absorption
- Morphology: Traumatic fractures are often multiple and in anatomic alignment

Radiographic Findings
- Radiography
  - Radiographs specific but not sensitive
    - 30% sensitivity for non-displaced fracture ("normal" to miss rib fractures)
    - Ribs 4-9 most commonly fractured
    - Fractures usually multiple
  - 1st rib fracture, in traumatic injury marker of high-energy chest trauma
    - 1st rib protected by clavicle, scapula
    - Statistically 2% have bronchial tear and 10% have aortic transection
    - Non-traumatic 1st rib fractures have a very low incidence of major vascular injury
  - Flail chest (up to 20% of patients with major trauma)
    - 3 or more adjacent ribs with segmental fractures or more than 5 adjacent rib fractures
    - Costal hook sign: Elephant trunk shaped ribs (due to rotation of segmental fractures)
  - Dedicated rib series occasionally helpful, especially when documentation of fracture important
    - Medical-legal cases
    - Should not substitute for a chest radiograph (may miss pneumothorax)
  - Fractures may only become evident after healing begins and callous forms
    - Initial radiographs often do not show fractures if they are not displaced

DDx: Chest Wall Deformity

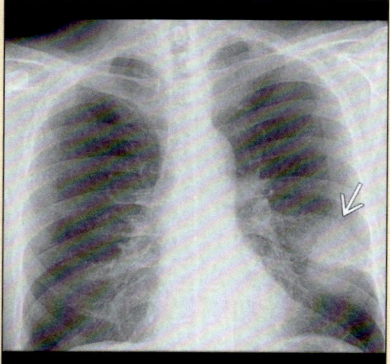

Rib Metastasis

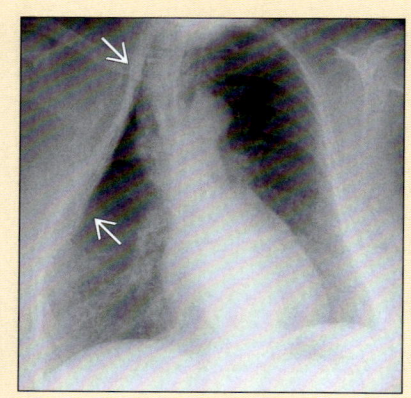

Thoracoplasty

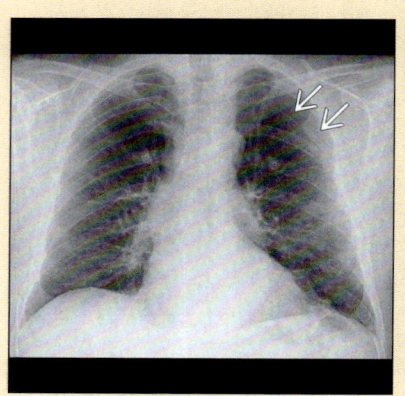

Old Thoracotomy

RIB FRACTURES AND FLAIL CHEST

Key Facts

Terminology
- Flail chest: 3 or more segmental rib fractures (more than 2 fractures within the same rib) or more than 5 adjacent rib fractures

Imaging Findings
- 30% sensitivity for non-displaced fracture ("normal" to miss rib fractures)
- Ribs 4-9 most commonly fractured
- 1st rib fracture, in traumatic injury marker of high-energy chest trauma
- Fractures may only become evident after healing begins and callous forms

Top Differential Diagnoses
- Pathologic Rib Fracture

Pathology
- Most common thoracic injury in blunt chest trauma (10%)
- Ribs difficult to fracture in children due to plasticity of ribs, therefore fractured ribs signify significant trauma

Clinical Issues
- Multiple bilateral healed rib fractures commonly seen in alcoholics
- Atelectasis a common sequela of rib fractures, predisposing to pneumonia

Diagnostic Checklist
- Dedicated rib radiographs only, without a chest radiograph, may miss associated pneumothorax

---

- Repeat radiographs taken 4 or more days after injury usually reveal fractures
- Early treatment for uncomplicated rib fracture is same as for bruised ribs; delay in diagnosis does not hinder treatment
  ○ Children with non-accidental trauma
    - 5-25% of all skeletal injuries in abused children
    - Typical location fractures costovertebral and costochondral junctions
    - Shaken baby injuries typically posterior near costovertebral junction
    - 1st rib fracture virtually diagnostic of abuse

CT Findings
- Primarily used for underlying visceral injuries
- More sensitive than chest radiographs
- Volume rendered images significantly reduce the time to interpret images for rib fractures

Ultrasonographic Findings
- Ultrasound can detect rib fractures
  ○ Does not significantly increase the detection rate
  ○ Too time-consuming to justify routine use

Nuclear Medicine Findings
- Bone scintigraphy useful and sensitive in detecting stress fractures, bone metastases, and detection of fractures in suspected child abuse

Imaging Recommendations
- Best imaging tool: Chest radiography usually sufficient for clinically important decisions
- Protocol advice: Routine radiographic follow-up for fractures not recommended

DIFFERENTIAL DIAGNOSIS

Pathologic Rib Fracture
- Typically not aligned
- Do not present with co-morbidities such as pneumothorax
- May present with minimal trauma only
- Lytic and expansile bone at fracture site

Thoracostomy Tube
- On CT, thoracostomy tubes can be confused with ribs and displaced fractures

PATHOLOGY

General Features
- Etiology
  ○ Rib stability
    - Area of maximal chest wall weakness found at 60° rotation from sternum where ribs flatter and less-supported
    - Anterior-posterior compression: Ribs fracture typically 2 places: 60° from sternum and posteriorly
  ○ Trauma: Direct blow from motor vehicle accidents, falls, assaults, contact sports
  ○ Severe coughing
  ○ Rib stress fractures uncommon
    - Typical locations: 1st anterolaterally, 4th-9th ribs laterally, and the posteromedial upper ribs
    - Occurs in golfers (Duffer fracture), canoeists, rowers, swimmers, weightlifters, ballet dancers
  ○ Isolated first rib fracture
    - In proper clinical setting, isolated first rib fracture can be avulsion injury, especially from throwing motion, rowing, or related to whiplash
    - Avulsion from scalene muscle attachment
- Epidemiology
  ○ Most common thoracic injury in blunt chest trauma (10%)
  ○ Rib fractures ominous in children and elderly
    - Ribs difficult to fracture in children due to plasticity of ribs, therefore fractured ribs signify significant trauma
    - Ribs fractures more common in elderly due to osteoporosis and decreased muscle mass: When present double the morbidity and mortality
  ○ Rib fractures common following cardiopulmonary resuscitation (CPR)
    - Fractures underreported, occur in up to 30%

RIB FRACTURES AND FLAIL CHEST

- Cough-induced rib fractures occur primarily in women with chronic cough
  - Middle ribs along the lateral aspect of the rib cage are affected most commonly
  - Also occurs in patients with Pertussis infection and post-nasal drip
- In proper clinical setting, isolated first rib fracture can be sports-related avulsion injury, especially from throwing motion or related to whiplash
- Flail chest: Level 1 trauma center 1-2 cases/month

Gross Pathologic & Surgical Features
- Flail segment moves paradoxically (Pendelluft breathing)
  - Segment moves inward with inspiration and outward with expiration

CLINICAL ISSUES

Presentation
- Most common signs/symptoms
  - Clinical examination sensitive but not specific
  - Chest wall pain or pain with deep breathing, sneezing, or coughing, accompanied by severe local rib tenderness, swelling, and/or crepitus
- Other signs/symptoms
  - Flail chest
    - May not be clinically evident in 1/3 of cases
    - Clinical findings masked by positive pressure ventilation resulting in delayed diagnosis
    - Traumatic extrathoracic intracostal lung herniation, a rare extraordinary associated injury

Demographics
- Age
  - More common with advancing age
    - Result in a longer duration of pain
    - Admission of elderly for observation and treatment, for isolated rib fractures, justified and beneficial
  - Overall trauma-related mortality higher in elderly patients with multiple rib fractures than younger patients
- Gender: Cough-induced rib fractures occur primarily in women with chronic cough

Natural History & Prognosis
- Typically heal with callous
  - Rarely non-union and pseudoarthrosis
- Multiple bilateral healed rib fractures commonly seen in alcoholics
- Greater number of fractured ribs = higher mortality and morbidity rates
- Location
  - Right-sided rib fractures below 8th rib: 20-50% probability of liver injury
  - Left-sided rib fractures below 8th rib: 25% probability of splenic injury
  - 1st and 2nd rib fractures not an indication for investigating aortic injury in absence of other findings for aortic transection
- Flail chest
  - Acutely, associated with mortality rates of 10-20%
  - Chronically, 25-50% have long term disability including chronic chest wall pain, and exertional dyspnea

Treatment
- Options, risks, complications
  - Atelectasis a common sequela of rib fractures, predisposing to pneumonia
  - Often complicated by lung contusion and laceration, pneumothorax, or hemothorax
  - Rarely, sharp edges of extremely displaced rib fractures can puncture or lacerate viscera such as the diaphragm, aorta, airway or heart
- Symptomatic pain management
  - Oral analgesia
  - Epidural analgesia, especially for flail chest, associated with decreased nosocomial pneumonia and shorter duration of mechanical ventilation
- Patients with rib fractures should be watched for development of delayed hemothorax
- Surgical fixation rarely necessary
- Intubation and mechanical ventilation
  - Need should be determined by underlying cardiopulmonary status, not the presence or absence of flail segments

DIAGNOSTIC CHECKLIST

Consider
- Pneumothorax and contusion more important than the rib fracture

Image Interpretation Pearls
- Lower rib fractures are marker for abdominal visceral injury
- Dedicated rib radiographs only, without a chest radiograph, may miss associated pneumothorax

SELECTED REFERENCES

1. Hanak V et al: Cough-induced rib fractures. Mayo Clin Proc. 80(7):879-82, 2005
2. Bulger EM et al: Epidural analgesia improves outcome after multiple rib fractures. Surgery. 136(2):426-30, 2004
3. Hurley ME et al: Is ultrasound really helpful in the detection of rib fractures? Injury. 35(6):562-6, 2004
4. Stawicki SP et al: Rib fractures in the elderly: a marker of injury severity. J Am Geriatr Soc. 52(5):805-8, 2004
5. Holcomb JB et al: Morbidity from rib fractures increases after age 45. J Am Coll Surg. 196(4):549-55, 2003
6. Sirmali M et al: A comprehensive analysis of traumatic rib fractures: morbidity, mortality and management. Eur J Cardiothorac Surg. 24(1):133-8, 2003
7. Barnea Y et al: Isolated rib fractures in elderly patients: mortality and morbidity. Can J Surg. 45(1):43-6, 2002
8. Velmahos GC et al: Influence of flail chest on outcome among patients with severe thoracic cage trauma. Int Surg. 87(4):240-4, 2002
9. Collins J: Chest wall trauma. J Thorac Imaging. 15(2):112-9, 2000
10. Westcott J et al: Rib fractures. American College of Radiology. ACR Appropriateness Criteria. Radiology. 215 Suppl:637-9, 2000

RIB FRACTURES AND FLAIL CHEST

IMAGE GALLERY

Typical

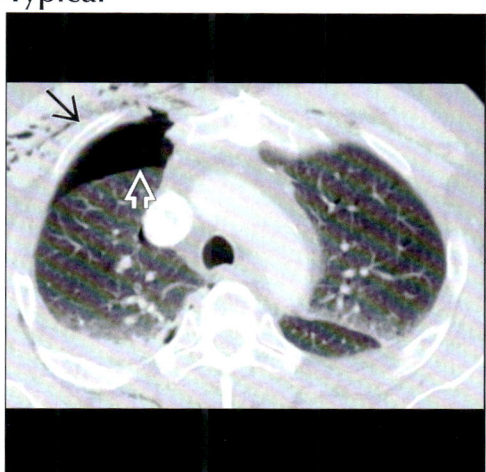
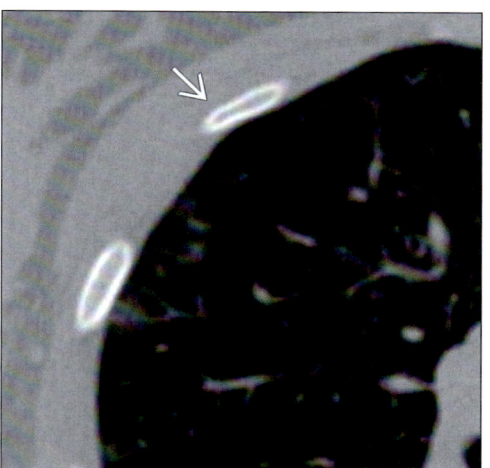

(Left) Axial CECT shows disruption of chest wall ➡ signifying flail chest deformity. Pneumothorax ➡. Subcutaneous emphysema right chest wall. (Right) Axial NECT shows subtle rib fracture ➡. Chest radiograph was normal. CT much more sensitive for rib fractures.

Typical

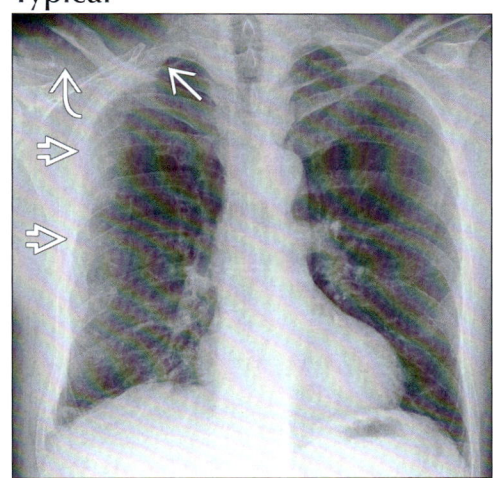
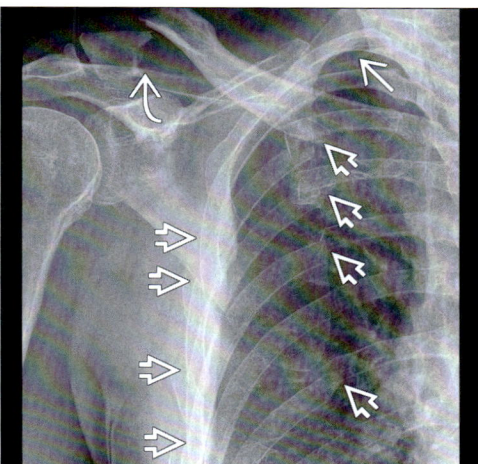

(Left) Frontal radiograph shows multiple rib fractures ➡, small pneumothorax ➡ and fractured clavicle ➡. Number of rib fractures suggests flail chest deformity. (Right) Dedicated rib radiograph better shows multiple segmental rib fractures ➡ consistent with flail segment, right clavicle fracture ➡ and pneumothorax ➡.

Typical

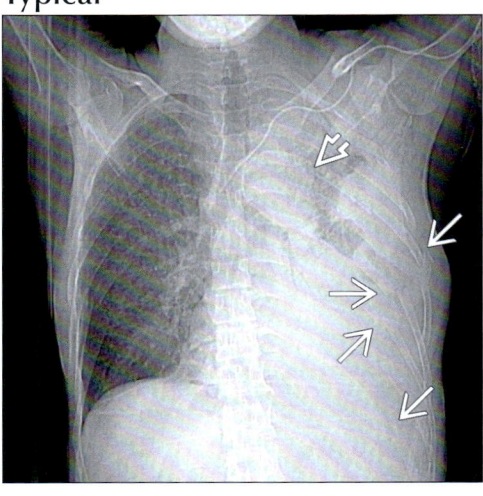
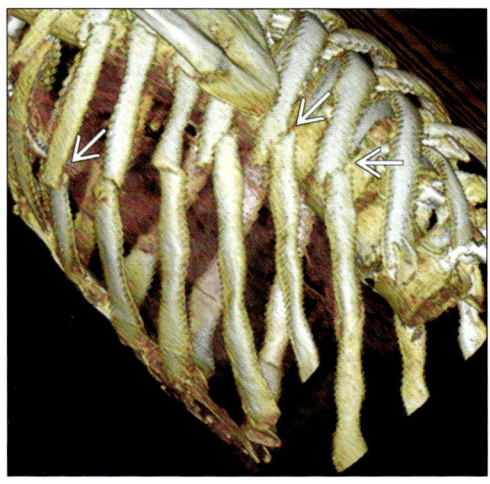

(Left) Frontal radiograph shows almost totally opacified left hemithorax from contusion and multiple rib fractures ➡. Aortic arch obscured ➡ requiring investigation for aortic injury. (Right) CECT VR reconstruction rapidly shows the number and location of rib fractures ➡.

AORTIC TRANSECTION

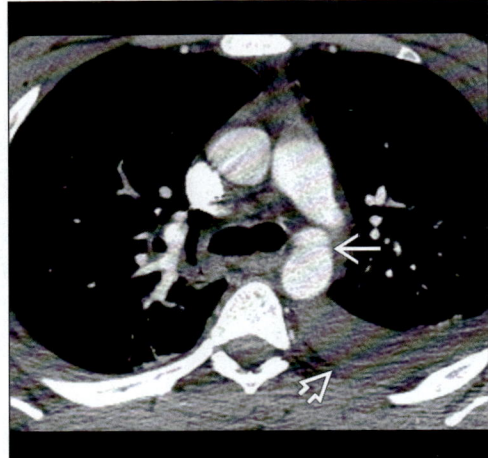

Axial CTA shows abnormal contour of distal aortic arch ➡ from pseudoaneurysm extending anteriorly from the aorta. Note left pleural effusion ➡.

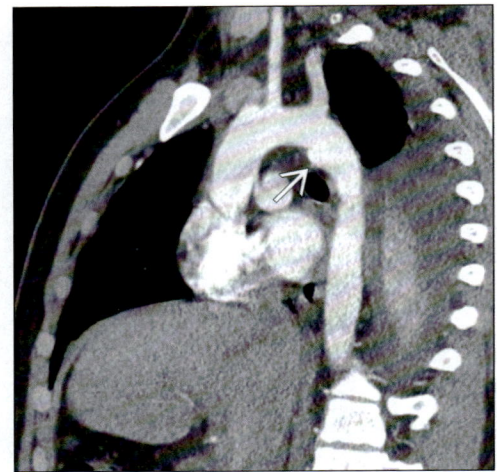

CTA sagittal oblique reconstruction in the same patient as previous image shows typical pseudoaneurysm ➡ in the aortic isthmus.

TERMINOLOGY

Abbreviations and Synonyms
- Traumatic aortic injury (TAI), acute traumatic aortic injury (ATAI), blunt traumatic aortic rupture (BTAR), blunt aortic trauma (BAT)

Definitions
- Tear of aortic wall, usually result of traumatic injury from motor vehicle accident (MVA) or serious fall
  - 80% complete tears: Rarely survive
  - 20% partial circumferential tear of intima or media: May survive

IMAGING FINDINGS

General Features
- Best diagnostic clue
  - Trauma chest radiograph: Widened mediastinum
  - CTA: Intimal flap, irregular contour aortic wall
- Location
  - 95% occur at aortic isthmus
  - 1% occur aortic root
  - 1% diaphragmatic aortic hiatus

Radiographic Findings
- Radiography
  - Normal chest radiograph once considered rare
    - Will be normal with little or no mediastinal hemorrhage
    - CTA has shown injures in up to 15% with normal chest radiographs
  - Chest radiograph: Usually abnormal (normal radiograph has 90-95% negative predictive value)
    - Will not see tear, only indirect signs from hemorrhage
    - Signs centered at aortic arch, most common location for transection
    - Erect positioning much superior to supine positioning
  - Signs of aortic transection
    - Widened superior mediastinum (70%)
    - Abnormal contour of aortic arch (40%)
    - Obscuration of AP window (55%)
    - Tracheal shift to right (65%)
    - Nasogastric (NG) tube shift to right (50%)
    - Widening of left paraspinal stripe (35%)

DDx: Aortic Transection

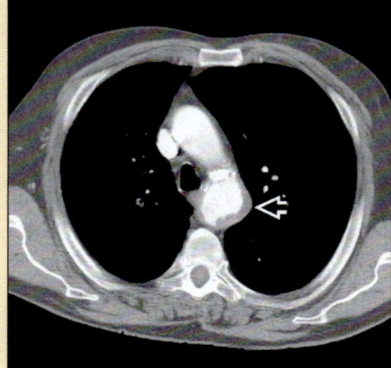

Aortic Atherosclerosis

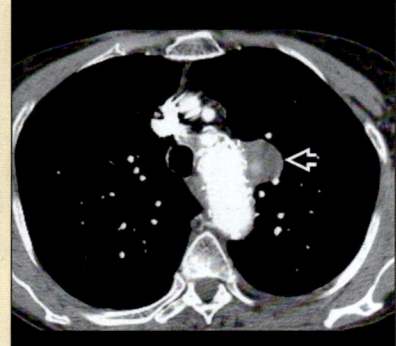

Atherosclerotic Aneurysm

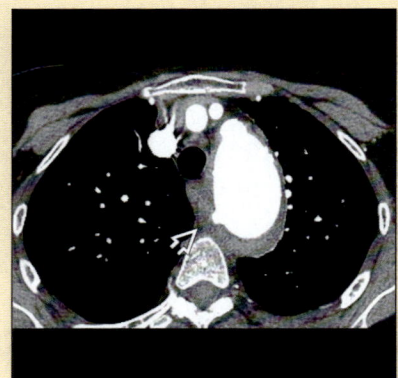

Aortic Ulcer

AORTIC TRANSECTION

Key Facts

Terminology
- Tear of aortic wall, usually result of traumatic injury from motor vehicle accident (MVA) or serious fall

Imaging Findings
- Trauma chest radiograph: Widened mediastinum
- CTA: Intimal flap, irregular contour aortic wall
- 95% occur at aortic isthmus
- CTA has shown injures in up to 15% with normal chest radiographs
- Chest radiograph: Usually abnormal (normal radiograph has 90-95% negative predictive value)
- Will not see tear, only indirect signs from hemorrhage
- Chronic aneurysm (2% survivors)
- CTA directly demonstrates aortic tear, markedly reducing need for aortography
- Accuracy: Sensitivity 85-100%, specificity 80%

Top Differential Diagnoses
- Widened Mediastinum
- Ductus Diverticulum (Type III Ductus)
- Normal Variant Fusiform Enlargement Proximal Descending Aorta
- Atherosclerosis
- Infundibulum of Bronchial-Intercostal Trunk

Pathology
- Multivariate causes likely: Combined shearing, torsion, stretching, and hydrostatic forces

Clinical Issues
- 15% of mortalities in MVA
- Delayed repair may be acceptable in many cases
- Endovascular stent grafts very promising

- Right paratracheal stripe thickening (50%)
- Left apical cap (65%)
- Depressed left mainstem bronchus (65%)
- Left pleural effusion (30%)
○ No combination of signs more specific for transection
○ Any above signs require further investigation to rule out transection
○ 1st rib fracture direct indicator of severity of trauma and likelihood of aortic transection
- Protected by clavicle and scapula, requires considerable force to break
- Frequency approximately 15% in those with transection
○ Chronic aneurysm (2% survivors)
- Calcified mass aorticopulmonary window

CT Findings
- NECT
  ○ May only visualize hematoma, will not obviate further testing
  ○ Initially used to reduce false-positive chest radiographs by demonstrating other causes of mediastinal widening, now replaced by CTA
- CTA
  ○ Now modality of choice
  ○ CTA directly demonstrates aortic tear, markedly reducing need for aortography
  ○ Direct signs
    - Periaortic hematoma
    - Pseudoaneurysm or irregular contour aortic wall
    - Intimal flap
    - Diminished caliber descending aorta (pseudocoarctation)
    - Extravasation of contrast material from aorta
    - Aortic occlusion (implies circumferential injury)
  ○ Indirect sign
    - Mediastinal hematoma
    - Absent in up to 10-15%
  ○ Accuracy: Sensitivity 85-100%, specificity 80%
  ○ Disadvantage: Requires intravenous contrast

MR Findings
- MR generally no role in evaluation of acute trauma
  ○ Limited transporting and monitoring critically injured patients

Echocardiographic Findings
- Transesophageal echocardiography
  ○ Demonstrate intimal tears and transection
- Downsides
  ○ More difficult in severely injured patients
  ○ Limited availability

Angiographic Findings
- Once considered gold standard for evaluating aorta and great vessels
  ○ Using chest radiograph as guide, perform 10 negative angiograms for each tear
- False negatives and false positives low
  ○ CTA shows 5% angiographic miss rate for aortic injury (tarnished gold)
- Small risk of rupture
- Rapidly being replaced by CTA

Imaging Recommendations
- Best imaging tool: CTA for direct evaluation of aorta
- Protocol advice: Thin-reconstructions and multiplanar reformations

---

DIFFERENTIAL DIAGNOSIS

Widened Mediastinum
- False positives from rotation, supine positioning, expiration
- Venous bleeding, sternal fracture, or spinal fracture

Ductus Diverticulum (Type III Ductus)
- Anteromedial outpouching of isthmus
- Smooth, gently sloping shoulders (obtuse angles with aorta)
- No intimal tear

AORTIC TRANSECTION

Normal Variant Fusiform Enlargement Proximal Descending Aorta
- Similar appearance, no intimal flap

Aortic Spindle
- Congenital narrowing ligamentum arteriosum

Atherosclerosis
- Ulcerated plaque or fusiform aneurysm
  - Often contain circumferential or eccentric thrombus
  - More common in older patients
  - Look for other aortic plaques

Infundibulum of Bronchial-Intercostal Trunk
- Take off may show bump in aortic contour

Technical Artifact
- Motion or streak artifact

PATHOLOGY

General Features
- General path comments
  - Etiology: Theories of pathogenesis
    - Deceleration injury: Stretching injury; aorta fixed at ligamentum arteriosum or
    - Osseous pinch: Manubrium and first ribs rotate and impact spine causing shear injury
    - Multivariate causes likely: Combined shearing, torsion, stretching, and hydrostatic forces
- Epidemiology: Accounts for 15% fatalities in MVAs

Gross Pathologic & Surgical Features
- 95% at aortic isthmus
  - From origin left subclavian artery to ligamentum arteriosum, often anteromedially
  - Transverse circumferential tear: Intima and media tear with intact adventitia (60%)
  - May involve layers to varying degrees
    - In survivors, pseudoaneurysm usually contained by adventitia or occasionally mediastinal structures
    - Complete tear through intima, media and adventitia usually leads to exsanguination
  - Noncircumferential tears more common posteriorly
- Other 1% ascending aorta or 1% descending aorta at diaphragmatic hiatus
- Ascending aorta location 20% coroner's cases, rarely survive to reach hospital

CLINICAL ISSUES

Presentation
- Most common signs/symptoms
  - Urgent diagnosis, 50% expire 24 hours if untreated
  - Majority have no signs or symptoms, nonspecific chest pain, dyspnea
- Other signs/symptoms
  - Acute coarctation syndrome rare
    - Upper extremity hypertension
    - Decreased femoral pulses
  - Multiple associated injuries: Diaphragm rupture, lung contusion, rib fractures, head injury

Natural History & Prognosis
- 15% of mortalities in MVA
- 85% mortality prior to reaching hospital
- Survival dependent on time from injury to intervention

Treatment
- Surgical repair
  - Delayed repair may be acceptable in many cases
  - Other injuries increase mortality of immediate repair
  - 70-85% surgical survival quoted (up to 20% surgical mortality)
  - Paraplegia 10% (directly related to cross-clamp time)
  - Circulatory assistance techniques decrease incidence of ischemia
- Beta-adrenergic blocking agents decrease wall stress
- Endovascular stent grafts very promising
  - Especially with multiple other associated injuries
  - Complete pseudoaneurysm resolution reported at 3 months
  - Long term follow-up not available
  - Complications
    - Stent-graft dislodgement
    - Migration
    - Stent fracture
    - Arterial wall injury may result in retrograde aortic dissection requiring surgical replacement aorta

DIAGNOSTIC CHECKLIST

Consider
- Look for signs of aortic transection in any blunt trauma chest radiograph or CTA

Image Interpretation Pearls
- Consider chronic pseudoaneurysm in any patient with vascular calcification in the aorticopulmonary window

SELECTED REFERENCES

1. Anakwe RE: Traumatic aortic transection. Eur J Emerg Med. 12(3):133-5, 2005
2. Pacini D et al: Traumatic rupture of the thoracic aorta: ten years of delayed management. J Thorac Cardiovasc Surg. 129(4):880-4, 2005
3. Takahashi K et al: Multidetector CT of the thoracic aorta. Int J Cardiovasc Imaging. 21(1):141-53, 2005
4. Alkadhi H et al: Vascular emergencies of the thorax after blunt and iatrogenic trauma: multi-detector row CT and three-dimensional imaging. Radiographics. 24(5):1239-55, 2004
5. Kondo N et al: Surgical repair for chronic traumatic thoracic aneurysm after 12-year follow-up. Jpn J Thorac Cardiovasc Surg. 52(12):586-8, 2004
6. Neuhauser B et al: Stent-graft repair for acute traumatic thoracic aortic rupture. Am Surg. 70(12):1039-44, 2004
7. Stamenkovic SA et al: Emergency endovascular stent grafting of a traumatic thoracic aortic dissection. Int J Clin Pract. 58(12):1165-7, 2004

AORTIC TRANSECTION

IMAGE GALLERY

Typical

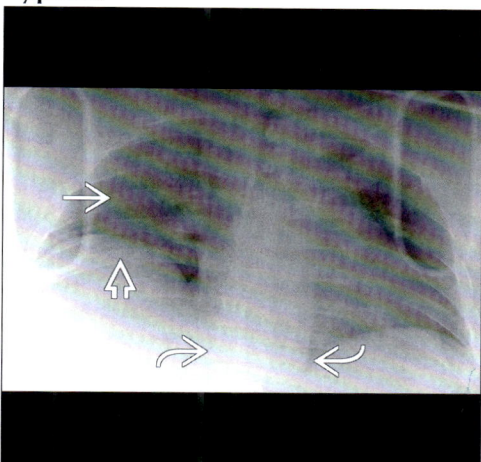
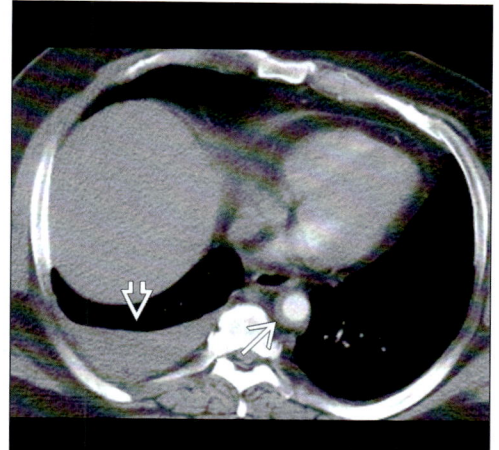

(Left) Anteroposterior radiograph shows elevation of right hemidiaphragm ➡, contusion of right lung ➡. Note paraspinal mediastinal widening ➡ inferiorly at the level of the diaphragm. *(Right)* Axial CECT shows right hemothorax ➡. Periaortic hematoma ➡. Rare aortic injury at the level of the aortic hiatus.

Typical

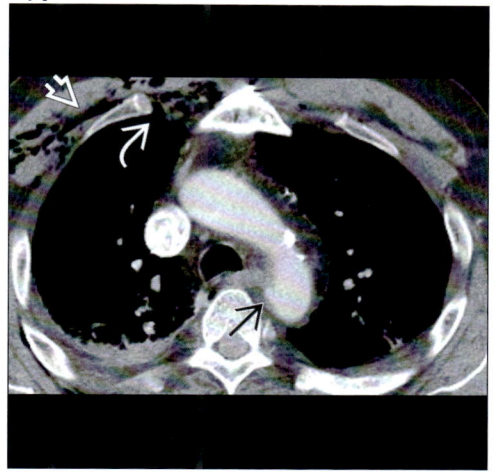
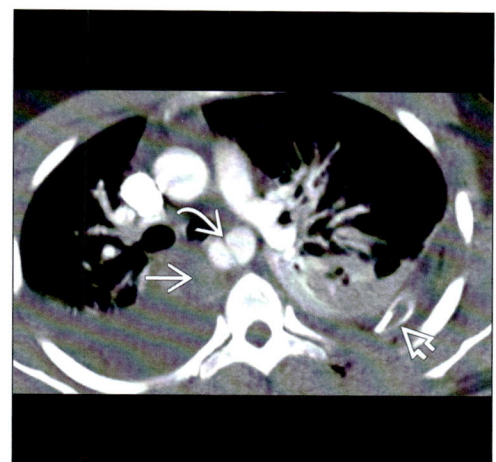

(Left) Axial CECT shows pseudoaneurysm ➡ of aortic arch. Subcutaneous emphysema ➡. Chest wall disruption ➡. Mediastinal hemorrhage is limited. *(Right)* Axial CECT shows mediastinal hematoma ➡ and aortic laceration ➡. Right pleural fluid is present. Left chest tube ➡. Aneurysm extends medially with hemorrhage into the opposite pleural space.

Typical

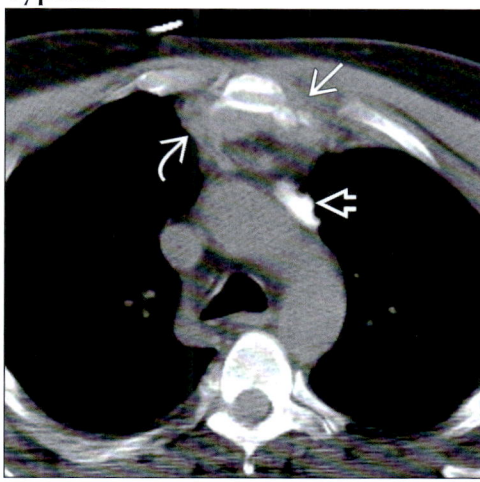
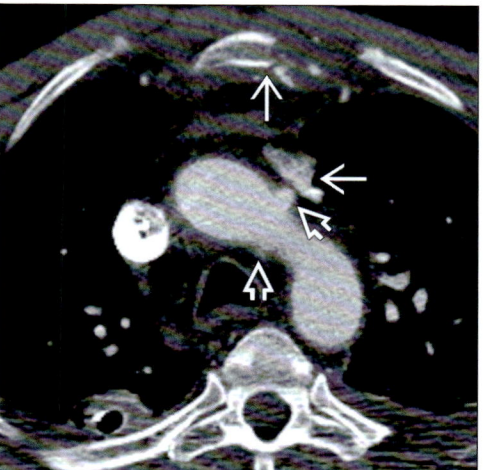

(Left) Axial NECT 5 mm collimation from outside hospital shows sternal fracture ➡ with displaced fragment adjacent to aortic arch ➡ & substernal hematoma ➡. Normal aorta. *(Right)* Axial CTA (same patient as previous image) 1.25 mm collimation the following day shows sternal fragment ➡ & pseudoaneurysm ➡. Combination of intravenous contrast & thin-sections required to evaluate aorta.

SPINAL FRACTURE, THORACIC

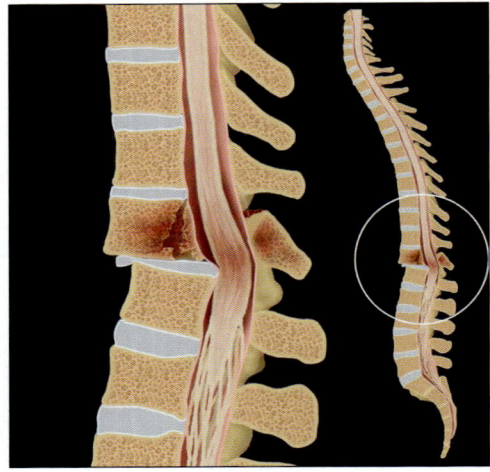 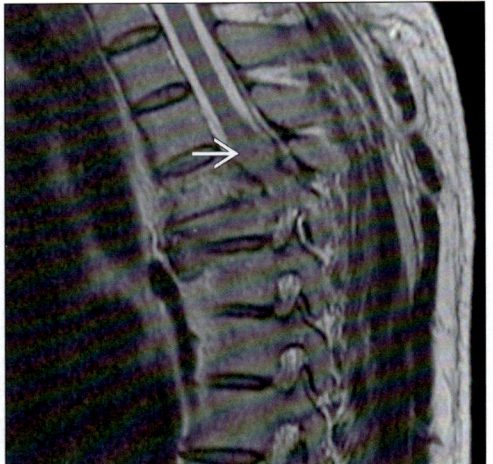

Sagittal graphic shows fracture dislocation in the thoracolumbar spine. In blunt chest trauma and flexion, the most common location for fractures is the thoracolumbar junction.

Sagittal T2WI MR shows fracture dislocation at thoracolumbar junction with retropulsed fragments causing cord compression ➡, patient was paraplegic.

TERMINOLOGY

Definitions
- Major injuries
  - Compression fracture
  - Burst fracture
  - Flexion-distraction fracture (Chance fracture)
  - Fracture-dislocation

IMAGING FINDINGS

General Features
- Best diagnostic clue
  - Compression fracture
    - Failure of anterior column from flexion force
    - Most common type of thoracic spine fracture due to blunt trauma
    - Wedge-shaped vertebral body, loss of body height > 50% suspicious for posterior injury
    - May occur at multiple levels, contiguous or noncontiguous
  - Burst fracture
    - Compression failure anterior and middle columns from axial load
    - Compressed thoracic vertebral body with fractured endplates, widened pedicles
  - Flexion-distraction (Chance) fracture
    - Injury involving compression of anterior column with distraction of middle and posterior columns
  - Fracture-dislocation
    - Failure of all 3 columns from combination flexion, rotation, and/or shearing
- Location
  - Thoracolumbar junction most vulnerable
    - Change in curvature from thoracic kyphosis to lumbar lordosis
    - Lack of rib cage support
    - Thoracic facets face in, lumbar facets face out: Transition zone (T9-T11) unstable with typical flexion injury

Radiographic Findings
- Radiography
  - Anterior compression fracture
    - Paraspinous hematoma
    - Distinct fracture line usually not visible

DDx: Thoracic Spine Fracture

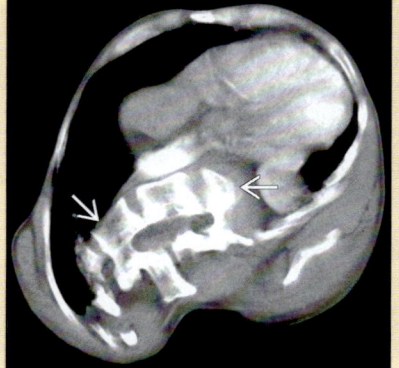 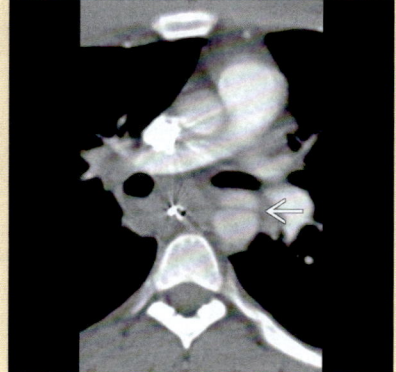 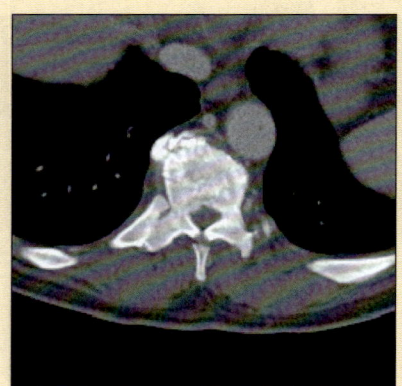

Kyphoscoliosis | Aortic Transection | Blastic Metastases

SPINAL FRACTURE, THORACIC

Key Facts

Imaging Findings
- Thoracolumbar junction most vulnerable
- Pedicle thinning with a slight increase in the interpediculate distance at the level of thinning normally seen at the thoracolumbar junction in 7%

Top Differential Diagnoses
- Spinal Abscess
- Spinal Metastasis
- Kyphoscoliosis
- Mediastinal Widening

Pathology
- Incidence 2% following blunt chest trauma
- 15% have fractures at multiple levels
- Spinal canal smallest in thoracic spine

Clinical Issues
- 20% with thoracic spine fractures have neurologic deficit

Diagnostic Checklist
- Widened pedicles relative to vertebral body above is strong clue to burst and instability of vertebral body
- Compression fracture involving inferior endplate with normal superior endplate raises suspicion for pathologic fracture
- Consider Chance fracture whenever radiography shows severe compression fracture in patient with normal bone density
- Look for paraspinal soft tissue hematoma as clue to spinal fractures on CT

- Kyphosis common
- Almost always involves superior endplate, < 5% involve inferior endplate only
- < 40-50% loss of height in patients with normal bone density; if greater loss of height, probably Chance fracture
- Osteoporotic patients may develop vertebra plana
○ Burst fracture
- Widened pedicles on AP view, wedge-shaped vertebral body on lateral view
- May see malalignment
○ Flexion-distraction (Chance) fracture
- Usually more than 40-50% loss of height of vertebral body
- Focal kyphosis
- Separation of facet joints
- **Increased interspinous distance**
- Listhesis and retropulsion of posterior vertebral body cortex absent
○ Fracture-dislocation
- Malalignment
- Thoracic spine
○ Pedicle thinning with a slight increase in the interpediculate distance at the level of thinning normally seen at the thoracolumbar junction in 7%
○ Rule of 2s: 2 mm is the normal upper limits for difference in
- Interspinous or interlaminar distance between adjacent vertebral bodies
- Interpedicular distance (transverse and vertical) between adjacent vertebral bodies
- Anterolisthesis or retrolisthesis with flexion and extension
- Facet joint width
- Difference in height between anterior and posterior vertebral bodies
○ Normal bone integrity
- Anterior height < posterior height: Ratio 0.80 males, 0.87 females
○ Instability if one of the following
- Displaced vertebra
- Widened interlaminar or interspinous distance
- Perched or dislocated facet joints
- Increased interpedicular distance
- Disrupted posterior vertebral body line

CT Findings
- Bone CT
  ○ Primarily used to investigate skeletal integrity
  ○ Anterior compression fracture
    - Multiple fracture lines often visible
    - Posterior cortical displacement and fractures of posterior elements absent
    - Alignment of posterior elements normal on reformatted images
  ○ Burst fracture
    - Soft tissue swelling surrounding vertebral body
    - May see blood in canal
    - Stellate pattern of fractures
  ○ Flexion-distraction (Chance) fracture
    - Fractured vertebral body, often comminuted
    - Separation of facet joints
    - Increased interspinous distance
    - Focal kyphosis
  ○ Fracture-dislocation
    - Widened, comminuted neural arch
    - Fracture through facet joints
    - "Naked facet" sign: Partially or completely uncovered articulating processes on axial imaging
    - Locked facets
    - Vertebral body comminution; retropulsed bony fragments within spinal canal
    - "Double body" sign: Overlapping vertebrae on axial imaging

MR Findings
- Primarily used to investigate spinal cord, disc, and ligaments
- Optimal timing for cord imaging: 24-72 hours following injury
- Anterior compression fracture
  ○ T1WI: Low signal intensity fracture line may not be seen
  ○ Posterior cortex intact
  ○ Paraspinous hematoma mimics tumor

SPINAL FRACTURE, THORACIC

- Burst fracture
  - May see cord contusion
- Flexion-distraction (Chance) fracture
  - T2WI: Disruption of posterior longitudinal ligament, interspinous ligaments
    - Anterior longitudinal ligament usually intact, may be stripped from vertebra inferior to fracture
    - May see cord contusion
  - Syringomyelia may develop chronically
- Fracture-dislocation
  - Cord edema, compression, distraction

Imaging Recommendations
- Best imaging tool
  - Anterior compression fracture
    - CT best to differentiate from Chance fracture, burst fractures
  - Burst fracture
    - MR vital if neurologic symptoms/signs present
  - Flexion-distraction (Chance) fracture
    - CT scan for surgical planning
  - Fracture-dislocation
    - Thin-section bone CT most effective in characterizing posterior column fractures
    - MR best for cord evaluation

DIFFERENTIAL DIAGNOSIS

Spinal Abscess
- Marrow edema in facet articular processes & adjacent laminae on MR
- Surrounding soft tissue edema, enhancement and abscess

Spinal Metastasis
- More likely to involve inferior cortex of vertebral body
- Metastases often involve posterior elements as well as vertebral body
- Cortical destruction

Kyphoscoliosis
- 3 contiguous levels
- Undulation of vertebral endplates

Mediastinal Widening
- Mimics aortic transection

PATHOLOGY

General Features
- General path comments
  - 3 column model of Davis
    - Anterior column: Anterior 2/3rds vertebral body
    - Middle column: Posterior 1/3rd vertebral body
    - Posterior column: Posterior elements
  - Spinal instability if more than 2 column failure
- Etiology
  - Thoracic spine flexion results in compression fractures (50% of all fractures)
  - Axial compression results in burst fracture (15% of all fractures)
  - Hyperflexion results in flexion-distraction (seat belt) fracture (15% of all fractures)
  - Shearing results in fracture-dislocation (5% of all fractures)
- Epidemiology
  - Incidence 2% following blunt chest trauma
  - 15% have fractures at multiple levels
- Associated abnormalities: < 5% have both aortic transection and cord injury

Gross Pathologic & Surgical Features
- Spinal canal smallest in thoracic spine
  - Limited leeway for fragments to cause cord injury

CLINICAL ISSUES

Presentation
- Most common signs/symptoms
  - Suggests spinal cord injury
    - Hypotension without tachycardia
    - Priapism
- Other signs/symptoms
  - Anterior cord syndrome
    - Injury anterior 2/3rds cord
    - Motor paralysis with sparring proprioception and vibration
  - Central cord syndrome
    - More effect on proximal function (arms > legs)
  - Brown-Sequard syndrome
    - Injury to 1/2 cord
    - Ipsilateral paralysis and loss of proprioception
    - Contralateral loss of pain and temperature

Natural History & Prognosis
- 20% with thoracic spine fractures have neurologic deficit

Treatment
- Surgical fixation thoracic spine fractures ± canal decompression

DIAGNOSTIC CHECKLIST

Image Interpretation Pearls
- Widened pedicles relative to vertebral body above is strong clue to burst and instability of vertebral body
- Compression fracture involving inferior endplate with normal superior endplate raises suspicion for pathologic fracture
- Consider Chance fracture whenever radiography shows severe compression fracture in patient with normal bone density
- Look for paraspinal soft tissue hematoma as clue to spinal fractures on CT

SELECTED REFERENCES
1. Vialle LR et al: Thoracic spine fractures. Injury. 36 Suppl 2(B65-72, 2005
2. Patel RV et al: Evaluation and treatment of spinal injuries in the patient with polytrauma. Clin Orthop Relat Res. 422):43-54, 2004

SPINAL FRACTURE, THORACIC

IMAGE GALLERY

Typical

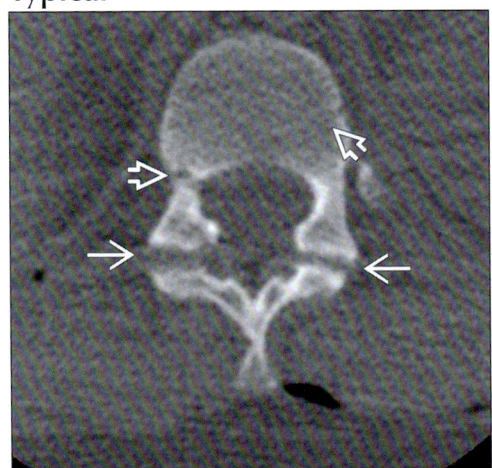 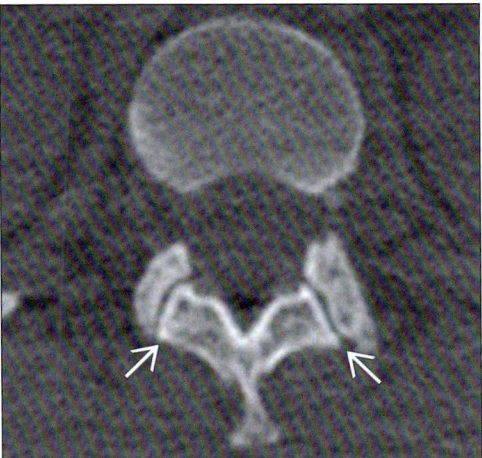

(Left) Axial NECT T11 thoracic spine shows thoracic facets face forward ➡. Fractured vertebral body ➡. (Right) Axial NECT shows T12 lumbar outward orientation spinal facets ➡. Transition between thoracic facet orientation and lumbar facet orientation often vulnerable in flexion injuries.

Typical

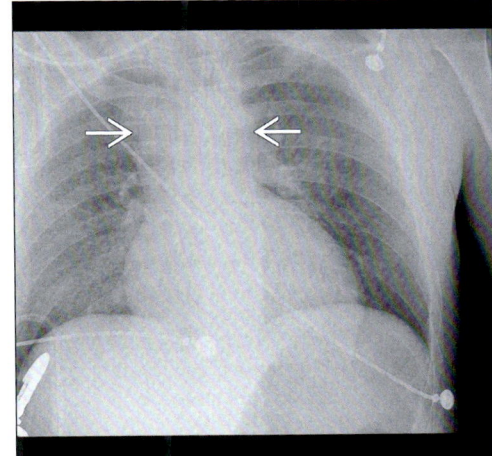 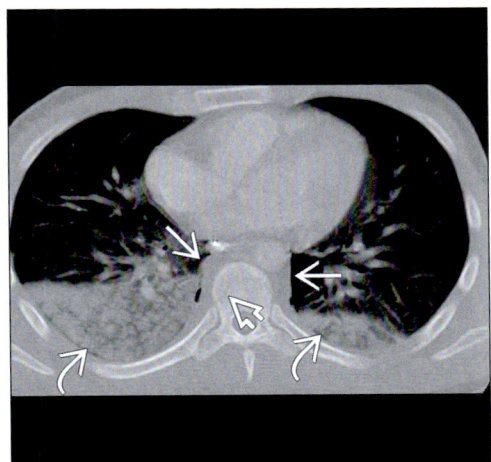

(Left) Anteroposterior radiograph shows mediastinal widening ➡ highly suspicious for aortic transection. (Right) Axial CECT shows paraspinal hematoma ➡ and nondisplaced fracture vertebral body ➡. Bilateral pulmonary contusions ➡.

Typical

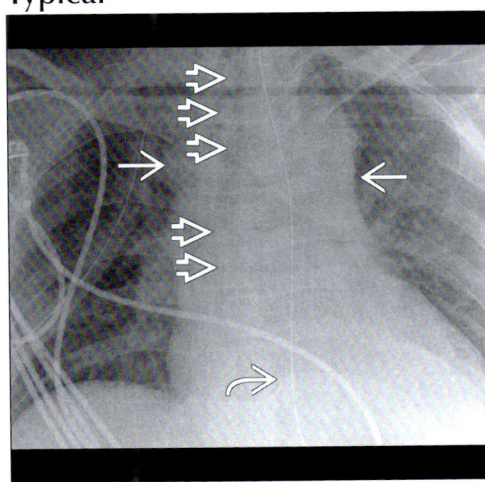 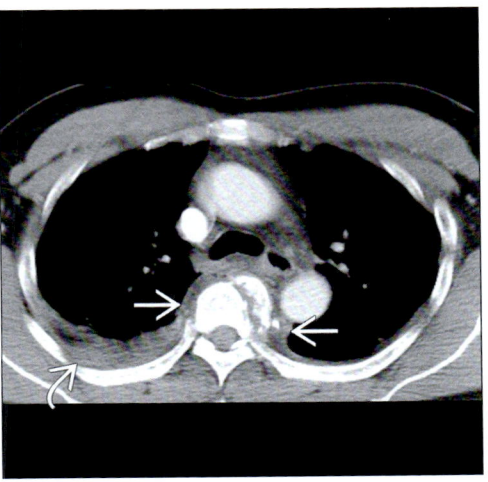

(Left) Anteroposterior radiograph shows mediastinal widening ➡. Spinal processes ➡ (maligned). Nasogastric tube ➡ is not deviated. Aortic injury must be excluded. (Right) Axial CECT at level of aortic arch shows fractured vertebral body and paraspinal hematoma ➡. Small right pleural effusion ➡. Aorta was normal.

STERNAL FRACTURE

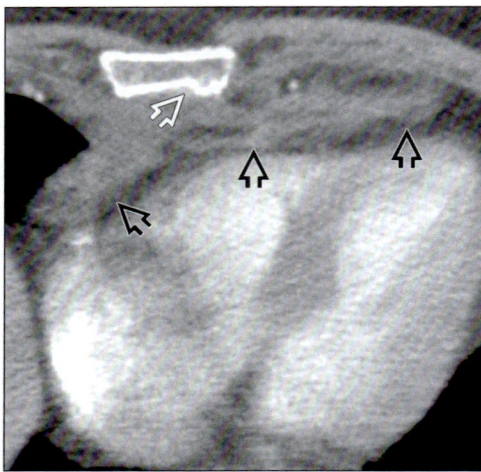
Axial CECT shows an anterior mediastinal hematoma ▷. Posterior step-off of the sternal fracture ▶.

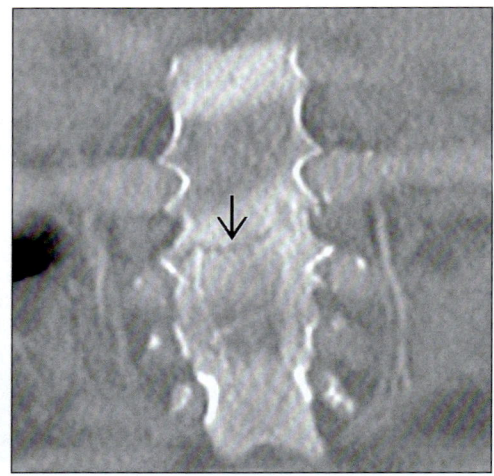
Coronal bone CT shows the nondisplaced fracture ➔ through the mid-body of the sternum.

TERMINOLOGY

Definitions
- Motor vehicle accidents account for 60-90% of sternal fractures

IMAGING FINDINGS

General Features
- Location: Transverse nondisplaced fracture through midbody most common

Radiographic Findings
- Radiography
  - Posteroanterior chest radiographs: Fractures usually not identified
    - Nonspecific findings: Mediastinal widening
  - Lateral radiograph
    - Transverse midbody fractures most common followed by fractured manubrium
    - 60% nondisplaced, 20% slightly displaced (1/4-1/2 sternal thickness), 15% moderately displaced (1/2-full sternal thickness), 5% completely displaced
  - Associated with compression fractures of the thoracic spine (10-15%) most frequently at the thoracolumbar junction or mid-thoracic spine

CT Findings
- MDCT with sagittal, coronal and 3D reconstructions improves the diagnostic accuracy for sternal injuries

MR Findings
- Useful in diagnosing insufficiency fractures
  - T1WI: Intermediate signal intensity; T2 weighted fat-suppressed images: High signal intensity

Imaging Recommendations
- Best imaging tool: Lateral radiograph key view

DIFFERENTIAL DIAGNOSIS

Pathologic Fractures
- Underlying neoplastic lesions with bone destruction

DDx: Parasternal Pathology

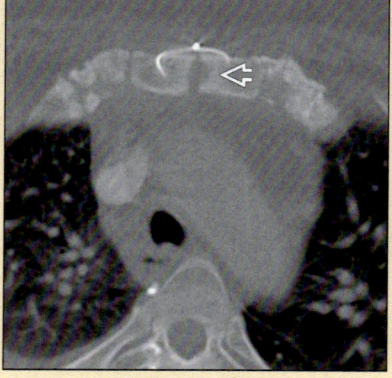
Osteomyelitis

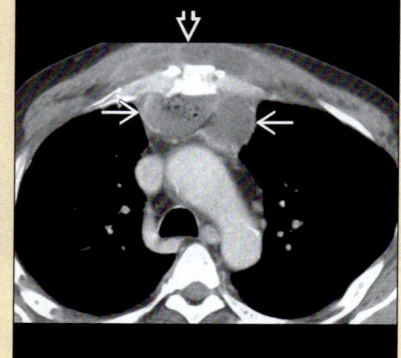
Mediastinal Abscess

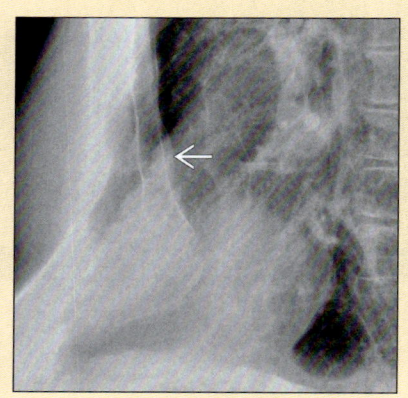
Pectus Excavatum

STERNAL FRACTURE

Key Facts

Imaging Findings
- Location: Transverse nondisplaced fracture through midbody most common
- Associated with compression fractures of the thoracic spine (10-15%) most frequently at the thoracolumbar junction or mid-thoracic spine
- Best imaging tool: Lateral radiograph key view

Top Differential Diagnoses
- Pathologic Fractures
- Osteomyelitis
- Pectus Excavatum
- Ossification Centers

Pathology
- Associated abnormalities: Cardiac contusion 10%

Clinical Issues
- Localized sternal pain (98%)
- Death and morbidity are related to associated injuries

- History of malignancy

Osteomyelitis
- Soft tissue mass usually prominent
- Constitutional symptoms: Fever, chills, malaise

Pectus Excavatum
- No cortical step off

Ossification Centers
- Nonunited ossification centers may simulate fracture

PATHOLOGY

General Features
- Etiology
  - Direct trauma: Motor vehicle accidents, especially common with seat belt injuries
  - Indirect trauma: Posterior displacement upper sternal fragment (spinal flexion "buckles" the sternum)
  - Osteoporosis: Often have associated thoracic compression fractures
  - After thoracic compression during cardiopulmonary resuscitation (CPR)
  - Stress fractures rare: Golfers, weight lifters
- Epidemiology: 5% of patients with blunt chest trauma have sternal fractures
- Associated abnormalities: Cardiac contusion 10%

CLINICAL ISSUES

Presentation
- Most common signs/symptoms
  - Localized sternal pain (98%)
  - Dyspnea in 15-20%
  - Palpitations (cardiac contusion)
  - 50% ecchymosis

Natural History & Prognosis
- Death and morbidity are related to associated injuries
  - Traumatic aortic rupture occurs in 2% of cases
  - Myocardial contusion in 10% (often clinically silent)

Treatment
- Directed toward associated injuries
- Monitor for cardiac injury
- Analgesia with appropriate opiates or nonsteroidal anti-inflammatory drugs

DIAGNOSTIC CHECKLIST

Consider
- Sternal fracture not an indication for aortography

SELECTED REFERENCES
1. von Garrel T et al: The sternal fracture: radiographic analysis of 200 fractures with special reference to concomitant injuries. J Trauma. 57(4):837-44, 2004

IMAGE GALLERY

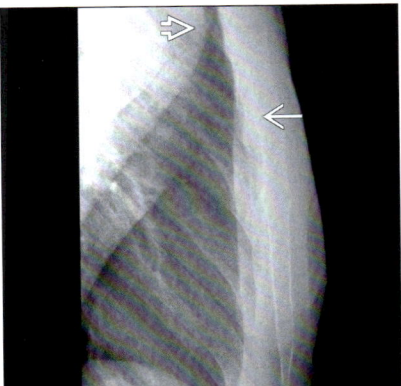 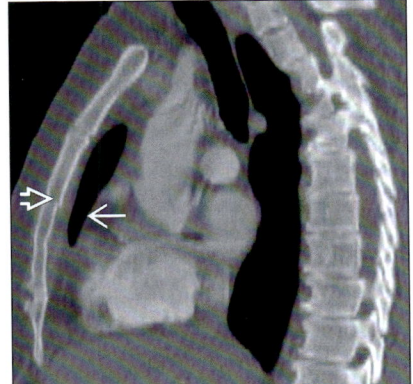 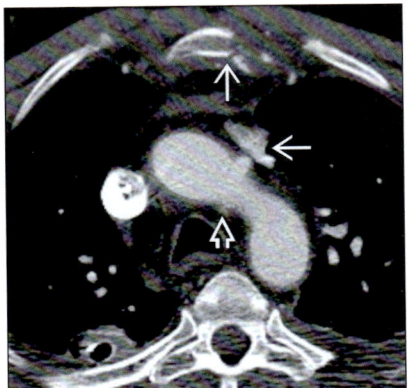

(Left) Lateral sternum shows nondisplaced fracture ➡. Manubriosternal junction ➡. *(Center)* Sagittal CECT shows slightly displaced fracture ➡ through mid-body of the sternum. Retrosternal hematoma ➡. *(Right)* Axial CTA shows comminuted sternal fracture and displaced fragment ➡ and aortic pseudoaneurysm ➡.

DIAPHRAGMATIC TEAR

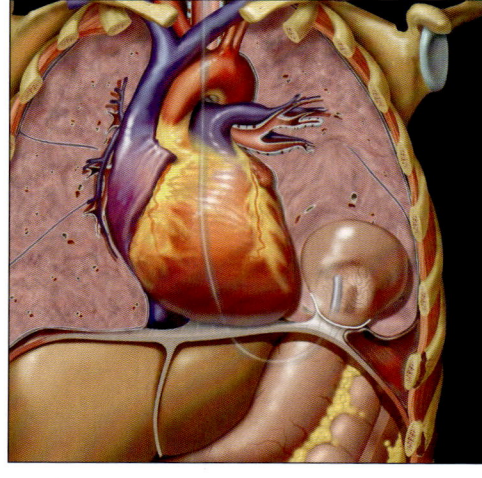

Graphic shows typical appearance of left hemidiaphragm rupture with herniation of portion of stomach into pleural space.

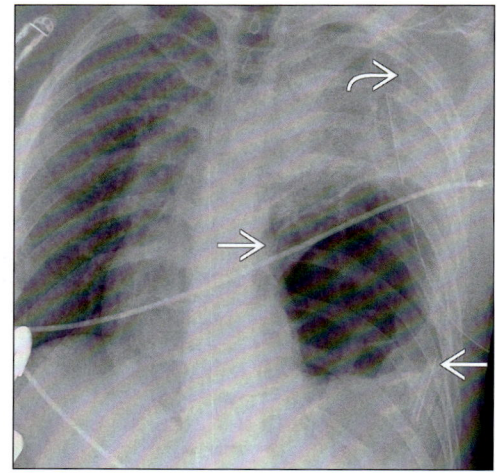

Anteroposterior radiograph shows intrathoracic bowel ➡, with mediastinal shift to the right. Left pleural effusion suggests strangulation ➡.

TERMINOLOGY

Abbreviations and Synonyms
- Hemidiaphragm rupture or laceration

Definitions
- Post-traumatic laceration of hemidiaphragm results in herniation of abdominal viscera into thorax
  - Blunt more common than penetrating trauma

IMAGING FINDINGS

General Features
- Best diagnostic clue
  - Air filled bowel above the hemidiaphragm
    - Even more accurate when nasogastric (NG) tube present above expected position of hemidiaphragm
- Location
  - Occur on right and left sides with equal frequency
    - Clinical manifestation (visceral herniation) much more common on left (70-90%)
    - Liver less likely to herniate through smaller right-sided lacerations
- Size
  - Tear in hemidiaphragm variable in size, small in penetrating trauma; large blunt trauma
    - Prevalence of visceral herniation increases with larger tears
- Morphology
  - Blunt: Linear or radial tears typically at dome of hemidiaphragm where tendon is thinnest
    - Most commonly extend posterolaterally along embryonic closure of pleuroperitoneal membrane

Radiographic Findings
- Radiography
  - Abnormal 90% but sensitivity in left-sided tears 50% and 20% for right-sided tears
    - Often nonspecific because of associated lower lobe atelectasis or contusion
  - Abnormal diaphragmatic contour
    - Elevated diaphragm > 7 cm
    - Diaphragmatic contour changes shape with change in position
  - Air filled bowel in hemithorax

DDx: Diaphragmatic Tear

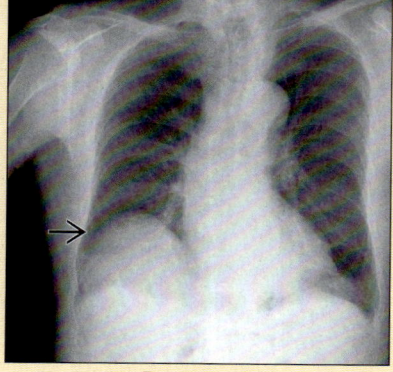
Eventration

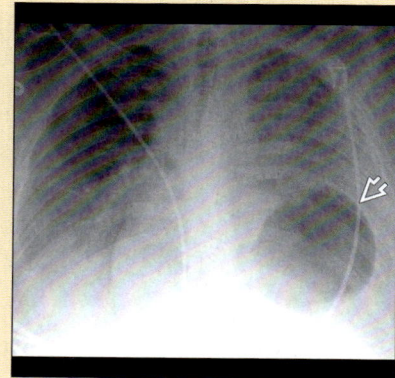
Esophageal Tear

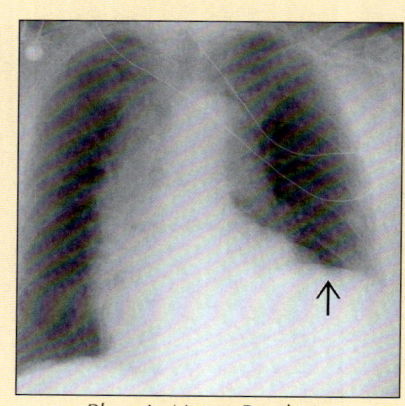
Phrenic Nerve Paralysis

DIAPHRAGMATIC TEAR

Key Facts

Terminology
- Post-traumatic laceration of hemidiaphragm results in herniation of abdominal viscera into thorax

Imaging Findings
- Air filled bowel above the hemidiaphragm
- Even more accurate when nasogastric (NG) tube present above expected position of hemidiaphragm
- Clinical manifestation (visceral herniation) much more common on left (70-90%)
- Blunt: Linear or radial tears typically at dome of hemidiaphragm where tendon is thinnest
- Contralateral mediastinal shift: Visceral herniation has mass effect
- **Dependent viscera sign**: In supine position: Herniated bowel or viscera no longer supported posteriorly by diaphragm
- **Collar sign**: Visceral herniation with focal constriction of bowel or liver at level of hemidiaphragm
- Protocol advice: Reformations increase sensitivity for diaphragmatic tears: Sagittal > coronal > axial

Top Differential Diagnoses
- Eventration of Diaphragm
- Diaphragm Paralysis
- Pleural Effusion
- Paraesophageal Hernia or Esophageal Tear

Clinical Issues
- Intubated patient on positive pressure may delay herniation until spontaneous respiration resumed
- New pleural effusion in patient with hernia heralds the onset of strangulation

---

  - Tip of NG tube in hemithorax
    - Tear usually spares esophageal hiatus
    - NG tube will course into abdomen and then traverse into hemithorax
  - Contralateral mediastinal shift: Visceral herniation has mass effect
  - Bowel strangulation
    - With open communication, pleural fluid should not accumulate in pleural space
    - Pleural effusion should suggest strangulation
    - Omental fat may simulate pleural effusion, including layering on decubitus examination

CT Findings
- **Dependent viscera sign**: In supine position: Herniated bowel or viscera no longer supported posteriorly by diaphragm
  - Right: Upper 1/3rd of liver in contact with ribs
  - Left: Stomach or bowel in contact with ribs or
    - Stomach or bowel posterior to spleen
  - Present in 90% of ruptures
- Diaphragmatic discontinuity
  - Segmental absence of hemidiaphragm
  - Present in 70%
  - Potential false positive: Posterolateral diaphragmatic defects present normally in 5%
    - Diagnosis should not be based on this sign alone
- **Collar sign**: Visceral herniation with focal constriction of bowel or liver at level of hemidiaphragm
  - Present in 30% (axial images) increased to 70% with sagittal or coronal reformations
- Diaphragmatic thickening
  - Either due to muscle retraction or muscular hematoma
  - Present in 30%
  - Very subjective with high proportion of false positives
    - Normal crura vary in thickness and crura vary in thickness with age and gender
- Blunt trauma
  - Left diaphragmatic tear: Sensitivity approaching 100%, specificity 100%
  - Right diaphragmatic tear: Sensitivity 70-80%, specificity 100%
  - Reformats in coronal and sagittal plane can increase diagnostic confidence
- Penetrating injury signs
  - Same as blunt trauma but includes
    - Trajectory of missile or penetrating instrument (sensitivity 35%, specificity 100%)
    - Active extravasation of contrast (sensitivity < 10%)

MR Findings
- Similar to CT, more difficult to perform in acute traumatic setting

Other Modality Findings
- Barium gastrointestinal findings
  - Approximation and narrowing of afferent and efferent bowel loops (pinched limbs) through the diaphragmatic defect (collar sign or kissing birds sign)
- Liver-spleen colloid scans have been used to diagnose right-sided diaphragmatic tears (collar sign)

Imaging Recommendations
- Best imaging tool: CT for global evaluation polytrauma
- Protocol advice: Reformations increase sensitivity for diaphragmatic tears: Sagittal > coronal > axial

DIFFERENTIAL DIAGNOSIS

Eventration of Diaphragm
- No dependent viscera sign
- Hemidiaphragm should appear intact
- No associated injuries
- Typically seen in elderly females without a history of recent trauma
- Bowel loops will not be approximated in eventration
- Can be difficult to distinguish if pre-existing condition is associated with recent blunt trauma

Diaphragm Paralysis
- Paradoxical motion at fluoroscopy (sniff test)

DIAPHRAGMATIC TEAR

- No recent history of trauma
  - Idiopathic or secondary to malignancy

Enlarged Liver
- No collar sign for liver

Pleural Effusion
- Subpulmonic or loculated
  - No abnormally positioned air-filled bowel
  - Crus intact

Paraesophageal Hernia or Esophageal Tear
- Tear rare at esophageal hiatus
- Extrathoracic air from tear may mimic bowel gas

Subphrenic Abscess
- Diaphragm intact, separate from bowel
- Clinical presentation of chronic infection, not trauma

PATHOLOGY

General Features
- General path comments
  - Kinetic energy absorption does not respect anatomic borders
    - Multiple simultaneous injuries above and below the hemidiaphragm frequent
  - Spontaneous healing uncommon, herniated abdominal contents prevent approximation of edges of tear
  - Most commonly herniated organs
    - Left: Stomach > colon > spleen
    - Right: Liver
  - Penetrating injuries usually smaller (< 1 cm diameter)
- Etiology
  - High-energy blunt torso trauma
    - Sudden rise in intraabdominal pressure ruptures diaphragm or
    - Lateral impact which distorts chest wall and shears diaphragm
  - Physiology
    - Diaphragm separates abdomen (Intraabdominal pressure positive) from thorax (intrapleural pressure negative)
    - Pressure gradient between abdomen and pleura 7-20 cm H_2O favors intrathoracic visceral herniation
- Epidemiology: Prevalence 5% blunt chest trauma
- Associated abnormalities
  - Rib fractures 90%
  - Liver or spleen laceration 60%
  - Pelvic fractures 50%
  - Aortic tear in 5%
  - Head injury commonly associated

Gross Pathologic & Surgical Features
- Blunt: Radial tear extends from central tendon posterolaterally
  - > 2 cm long, most > 10 cm long
- Penetrating: Any location, typically < 1 cm diameter
- CT normal diaphragmatic defects 5%
  - More common on the left
  - Normal process of aging
  - More common in women
  - More common with emphysema

CLINICAL ISSUES

Presentation
- Most common signs/symptoms: Nonspecific, consider in any patient with blunt torso injury
- Other signs/symptoms
  - Thoracic splenosis can rarely occur years after an injury
  - Rupture with intrapericardial herniation occurs rarely
- Latent: May present later in hospital course, especially after weaning from ventilator
  - In normal respiration there is a gradient for progressive herniation of abdominal contents
  - High index of suspicion important throughout the hospital course of trauma patients
- Obstructive
  - Strangulation of bowel
    - 85% strangulation within 3 years; however, cases have been undiagnosed for decades
    - Morbidity and mortality strangulation up to 50%
    - Obstructive symptoms, fever, chest pain

Demographics
- Age: Any age but young men most common

Natural History & Prognosis
- Diagnosis delayed 25%
  - Often other more compelling injuries such as aortic laceration
  - Nonspecific signs initially and injury not considered
  - Axial CT only may be overlooked
  - Gradient for herniation dependent on normal negative pleural pressure
    - Intubated patient on positive pressure may delay herniation until spontaneous respiration resumed
- Morbidity and mortality higher with strangulation
  - New pleural effusion in patient with hernia heralds the onset of strangulation

Treatment
- Surgical repair

DIAGNOSTIC CHECKLIST

Consider
- Must have a high index of clinical suspicion

SELECTED REFERENCES

1. Nchimi A et al: Helical CT of blunt diaphragmatic rupture. AJR Am J Roentgenol. 184(1):24-30, 2005
2. Karmy-Jones R et al: The impact of positive pressure ventilation on the diagnosis of traumatic diaphragmatic injury. Am Surg. 68(2):167-72, 2002
3. Bergin D et al: The "dependent viscera" sign in CT diagnosis of blunt traumatic diaphragmatic rupture. AJR Am J Roentgenol. 177(5):1137-40, 2001

DIAPHRAGMATIC TEAR

IMAGE GALLERY

Typical

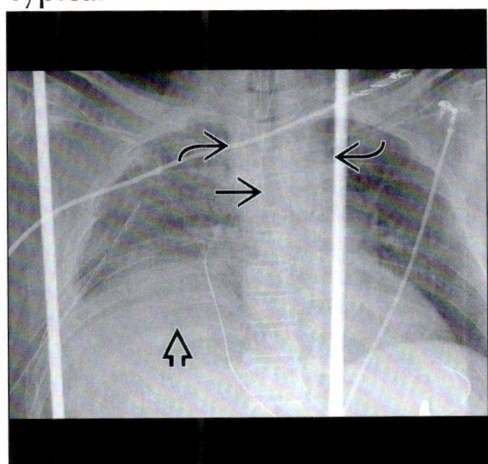
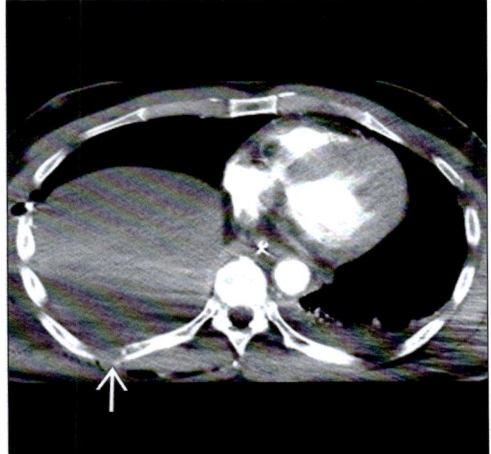

(Left) Anteroposterior radiograph shows elevation right hemidiaphragm ➡ and widened mediastinum ➡. NG tube ➡ is deviated. Right chest tube mid-hemithorax. *(Right)* Axial CECT shows liver adjacent to posterior fractured ribs ➡ "dependent viscera sign". Patient had ruptured right hemidiaphragm and pseudoaneurysm aorta (not shown).

Typical

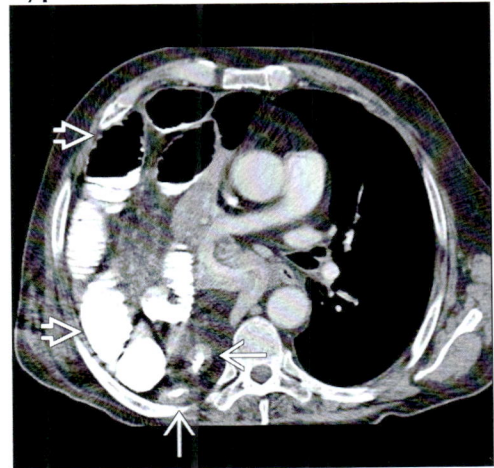
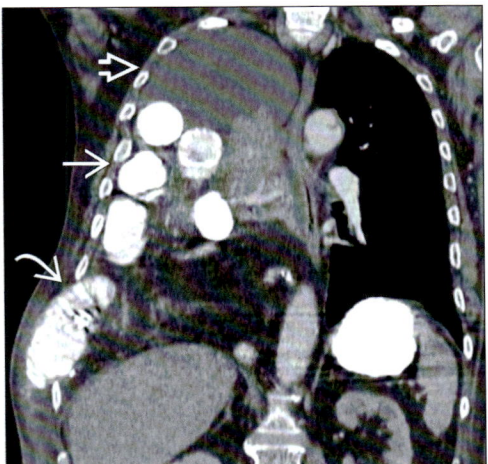

(Left) Axial CECT shows herniated small bowel loops ➡ and thickened small bowel loops ➡ from ischemic bowel. Small bowel loops contact ribs (dependent viscera sign). *(Right)* Coronal CECT reconstruction shows pleural fluid ➡ and herniated bowel ➡ through diaphragmatic defect. Chest wall hernia ➡. Diagnosis: Strangulated hernia.

Typical

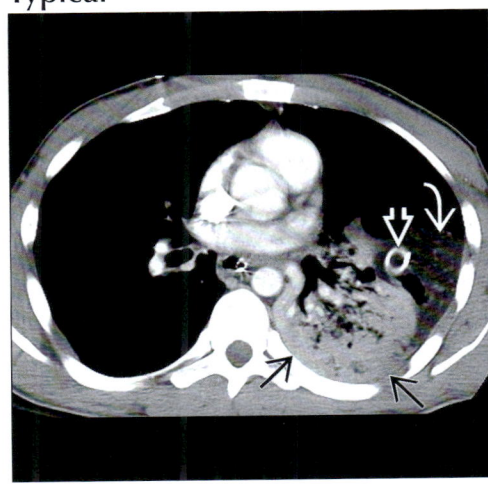
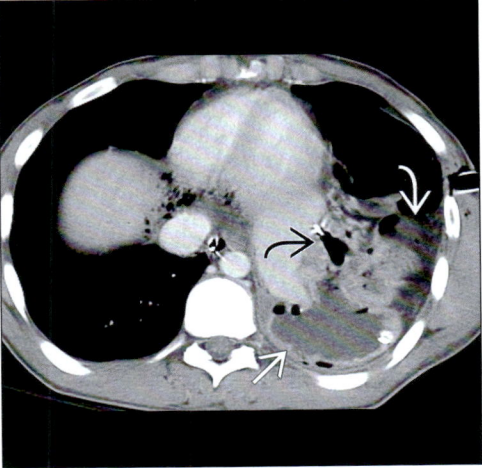

(Left) Axial CECT shows herniation of omentum ➡, chest tube ➡ and atelectatic lung ➡. CT corresponds to initial radiograph on first page. What was thought to be pleural effusion was omental fat. *(Right)* Axial CECT shows herniation of omentum ➡ and stomach ➡ and bowel loops ➡. Stomach ➡ contacts posterior ribs (dependent viscera sign).

ESOPHAGEAL TEAR

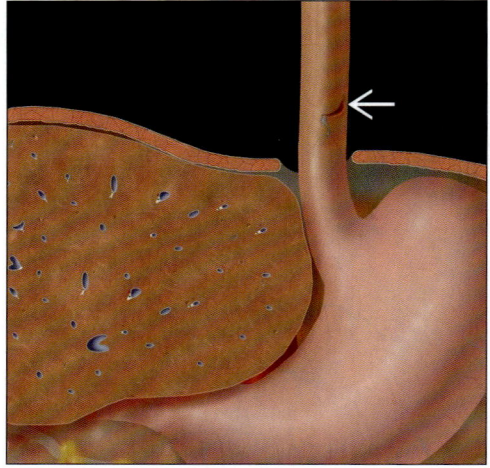

Graphic shows classic location of esophageal tear in Boerhaave syndrome. Small transverse laceration of the left lateral posterior wall of the distal esophagus ➡, 2-3 cm proximal to the gastroesophageal (GE) junction.

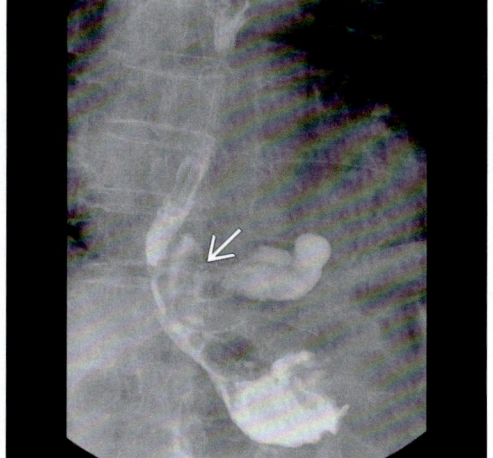

Frontal esophagram shows extravasation of contrast ➡ into the left costovertebral angle from an esophagus that was ruptured due to forced vomiting (Boerhaave syndrome).

TERMINOLOGY

Abbreviations and Synonyms
- Esophageal laceration, esophageal perforation, esophageal disruption

Definitions
- Transmural esophageal tear
- Boerhaave syndrome: Rupture of esophagus after forceful emesis
- Mallory-Weiss: Partial thickness tear after forceful emesis

IMAGING FINDINGS

General Features
- Best diagnostic clue
  - Diagnosis depends on high degree of suspicion and recognition of clinical features
  - Pneumomediastinum in the left costovertebral angle
- Location
  - Boerhaave syndrome or blunt chest trauma
    - Left lateral wall of distal esophagus 2-3 cm above gastroesophageal (GE) junction
  - Areas of anatomic narrowing
    - Site of extrinsic compression by aortic arch or left main bronchus
  - Post-surgical
    - At or above benign or malignant strictures, with biopsies or dilatation procedures
    - Anastomotic sites after esophageal surgery
- Morphology: Tear usually linear

Radiographic Findings
- Radiography
  - May be completely normal early (10%)
  - Diagnosis suspected in less than 20%
  - Pneumomediastinum & subcutaneous emphysema (60%)
    - Localized to left costovertebral angle (**V-sign of Naclerio**) (25%)
    - Pneumomediastinum, pleural effusion, and opacified lung usually occur together and although nonspecific should raise suspicion for esophageal tear

DDx: Esophageal Tear

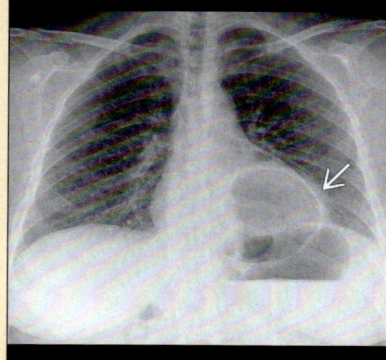

Paraesophageal Hernia

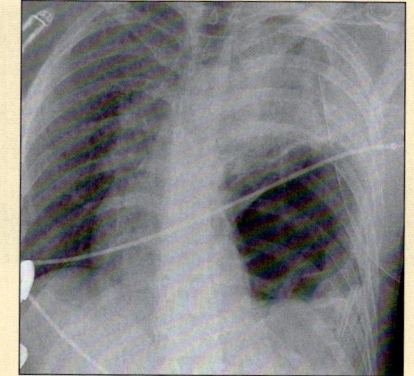

Diaphragmatic Tear

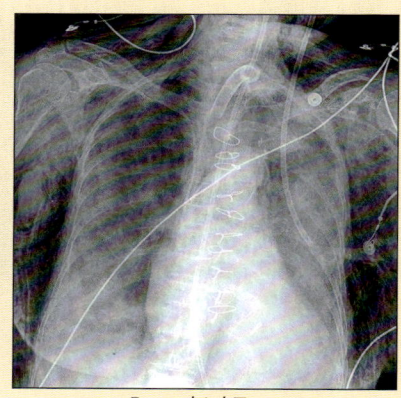

Bronchial Tear

ESOPHAGEAL TEAR

Key Facts

Terminology
- Transmural esophageal tear

Imaging Findings
- May be completely normal early (10%)
- Localized to left costovertebral angle (**V-sign of Naclerio**) (25%)
- Pneumomediastinum, pleural effusion, and opacified lung usually occur together and although nonspecific should raise suspicion for esophageal tear
- Water-soluble contrast agent may fail to detect 15-25% of esophageal tears

Top Differential Diagnoses
- Hiatal Hernia
- Diaphragmatic Rupture
- Paraesophageal Hernia

Clinical Issues
- Clinical diagnosis confused with acute myocardial infarction, aortic dissection, perforated peptic ulcer
- **Mackler triad**: Vomiting, severe chest pain, and subcutaneous emphysema (50%)
- Prognosis directly related to interval between perforation and initiation of treatment

Diagnostic Checklist
- Esophageal tear often overlooked, must have high index of suspicion
- Pneumomediastinum may be subtle, localization around esophagus (CT) or in left costovertebral angle (chest radiography) should raise suspicion for esophageal tear

---

- Due to caustic nature of gastric and ingested fluid, signs evolve rapidly within hours of perforation
  - Consolidation or atelectasis of the lung adjacent to tear (80%), nearly always associated with pleural effusion
  - Mediastinal widening usually delayed due to edema or accumulation of extraesophageal contents
  - Hydropneumothorax (50%)
    - Tear in mid or upper esophagus mainly right hemithorax (5%)
    - Tear in distal esophagus mainly left hemithorax (75%)
    - Bilateral pleural effusions (60%) > unilateral pleural effusion (40%): Left effusions usually larger than right effusions
    - Nearly always associated with pneumomediastinum
  - Pneumoperitoneum occasional with distal tears into the peritoneum

Fluoroscopic Findings
- Esophagram
  - Procedure of choice to determine site and extent of tear
  - Possible perforation should be evaluated with nonionic contrast
    - If nonionic contrast shows no tear, should be followed with barium contrast (20% tears will have falsely negative nonionic contrast esophagram)
  - Gastrografin should be avoided because of the risks of aspiration

CT Findings
- NECT
  - Pneumomediastinum centered on esophagus (90%)
  - Periesophageal fluid collections or extravasation of oral contrast
  - Esophageal thickening due to intramural hematoma or esophageal dissection
  - Pleural effusion or hydropneumothorax, usually small but enlarges with time
  - Mediastinal abscess, late
  - Does not show size of tear

Imaging Recommendations
- Best imaging tool: Esophagram to determine tear
- Protocol advice
  - Esophagography
    - Start with nonionic water-soluble contrast
    - If no leak, follow with barium
    - Water-soluble contrast agent may fail to detect 15-25% of esophageal tears
    - Barium may detect small leak not visible initially

DIFFERENTIAL DIAGNOSIS

Hiatal Hernia
- Pneumomediastinum absent
- Extravasation contrast absent

Diaphragmatic Rupture
- Also occurs in setting of blunt chest trauma
- Usually left-sided
- Stomach most common herniated organ
- Nasogastric (NG) tube may course through esophagogastric hiatus normally and then extend into hemithorax with herniated stomach
- No extra-alimentary air or pneumomediastinum
- No pleural effusion unless bowel strangulated

Paraesophageal Hernia
- Organoaxial gastric torsion most common
- Double air-fluid level, above and below diaphragm
- Usually no pleural effusion, unless bowel strangulated

Epiphrenic Diverticulum
- No free mediastinal gas or inflammation
- Extraluminal contrast, fluid + gas in mediastinal pocket may mimic diverticulum or even stomach

Esophageal Fistula
- Usually secondary to erosion from esophageal carcinoma
- Fistula may develop into trachea, mediastinum, aorta, pleura

ESOPHAGEAL TEAR

PATHOLOGY

General Features
- General path comments
  - Weakest part of esophageal wall: Left posterolateral wall just above gastroesophageal hiatus
    - Thinnest musculature, lack of serosa
    - Anterior angulation at diaphragmatic crus
- Etiology
  - Penetrating trauma (90%)
    - Iatrogenic following endoscopic procedures: Most common cause of esophageal tear (50%) especially with therapeutic procedures such as biopsy or dilatation
    - Post-surgical or knife/bullet wounds
    - Ingested foreign bodies (chicken and meat bones)
  - Spontaneous (15%)
    - Boerhaave syndrome: Increased intraluminal pressure due to retching against a closed glottis
    - Child abuse, in young children
  - Blunt chest trauma (10%)
    - Increased intraluminal pressure due to compression of esophagus against a closed glottis
  - Neoplasms: Esophageal carcinoma; lymphoma, rare
- Epidemiology
  - Esophagoscopy (50% of ruptures)
    - Pneumatic dilatation for achalasia: 2-6%
    - More common in those with pre-existing disease: Tumors, achalasia, strictures, or surgical anastomosis
    - Most common location: Pharynx or distal esophagus
  - Boerhaave syndrome: Incidence 1 in 6,000 (15% of ruptures)
  - < 1% in blunt chest trauma (10% of ruptures)
- Associated abnormalities: From blunt or penetrating trauma other injuries common: Aortic transection, bronchial fracture, spinal trauma

Gross Pathologic & Surgical Features
- Full-thickness linear tear of left lateral wall of distal esophagus just above GE junction
  - Range from 1-10 cm length
- Mallory-Weiss: Irregular linear tear or laceration in long axis of esophagus near GE junction involving mucosa only, does not penetrate the wall

CLINICAL ISSUES

Presentation
- Most common signs/symptoms
  - Sudden onset excruciating substernal or lower thoracic chest pain with vomiting
    - Clinical diagnosis confused with acute myocardial infarction, aortic dissection, perforated peptic ulcer
  - Dysphagia, hemoptysis or hematemesis (50%)
  - Subcutaneous crepitus neck (subcutaneous emphysema)
  - **Mackler triad**: Vomiting, severe chest pain, and subcutaneous emphysema (50%)
  - Hamman sign: Crunching sound on auscultation (20%)
  - Boerhaave syndrome typically occurs after drinking and eating binge
    - Classically vomiting but also straining during weight lifting, childbirth, severe coughing
- Other signs/symptoms
  - After instrumentation
    - May not have symptoms initially and present several hours after endoscopy

Demographics
- Gender: Boerhaave syndrome more common in males

Natural History & Prognosis
- Most serious and rapidly fatal type of perforation in gastrointestinal tract
- Life-threatening, associated with high morbidity and without intervention, high mortality 30-50%
- Prognosis directly related to interval between perforation and initiation of treatment
  - After 24 hours, 70% mortality rate
  - Untreated perforation, mortality rate nearly 100% due to fulminant mediastinitis

Treatment
- Drainage, antibiotics, surgical closure
- Conservative
  - For small tears especially in cervical esophagus contained leaks, or leaks draining back to esophagus
  - NG tube drainage, antibiotics, parenteral fluids
- Surgical
  - For large tears ideally performed within first 24 hours
  - Thoracotomy and primary closure, mediastinal drainage
  - For well-defined abscess or mediastinal fluid-collection: Percutaneous drainage and then primary closure
- Esophageal stents
  - Bridge the esophageal tear
  - May be useful in delayed diagnosis prior to definitive repair

DIAGNOSTIC CHECKLIST

Consider
- Esophageal tear often overlooked, must have high index of suspicion

Image Interpretation Pearls
- Pneumomediastinum may be subtle, localization around esophagus (CT) or in left costovertebral angle (chest radiography) should raise suspicion for esophageal tear
- CT does not necessarily substitute for esophagram

SELECTED REFERENCES
1. Fadoo F et al: Helical CT esophagography for the evaluation of suspected esophageal perforation or rupture. AJR Am J Roentgenol. 182(5):1177-9, 2004

ESOPHAGEAL TEAR

IMAGE GALLERY

Typical

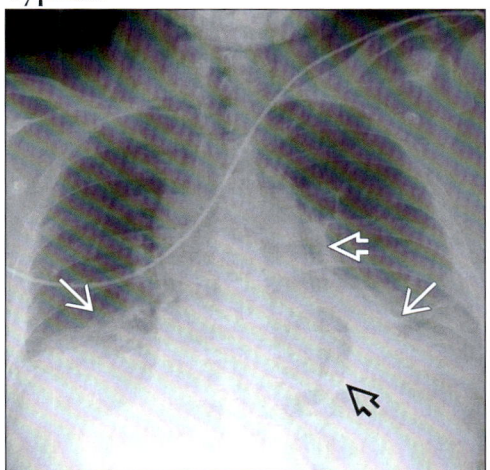 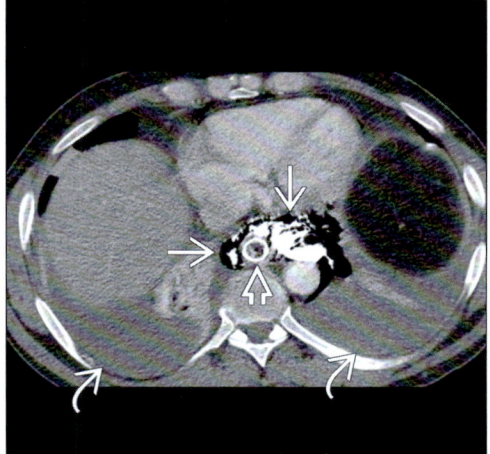

(Left) Anteroposterior radiograph shows massive pneumomediastinum ➡. Bibasilar atelectasis ➡. Note the large collection of air in the left costovertebral angle ➡. Sudden onset of pain after swallowing a chicken bone. *(Right)* Axial CECT shows extravasation of air and contrast ➡ surrounding a chicken bone in the esophagus ➡. Bilateral pleural effusion ➡.

Typical

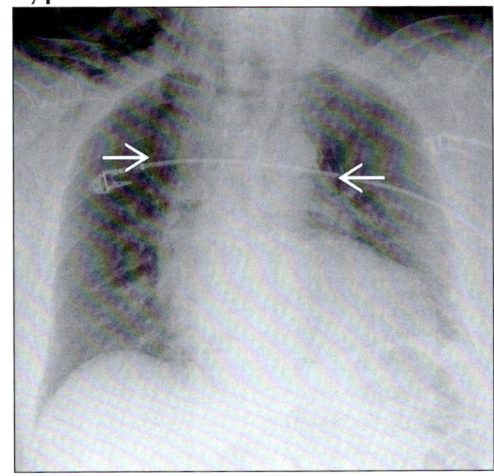 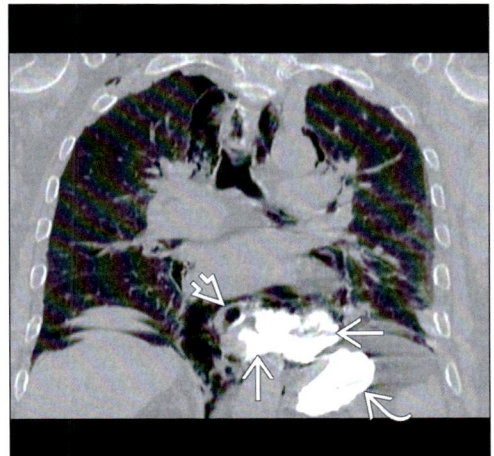

(Left) Anteroposterior radiograph shows massive pneumomediastinum ➡. Patient had just completed endoscopy and biopsy of distal esophagus. *(Right)* Coronal CECT shows collection of extravasated contrast ➡ adjacent to esophageal lumen ➡. Fundus of stomach ➡.

Typical

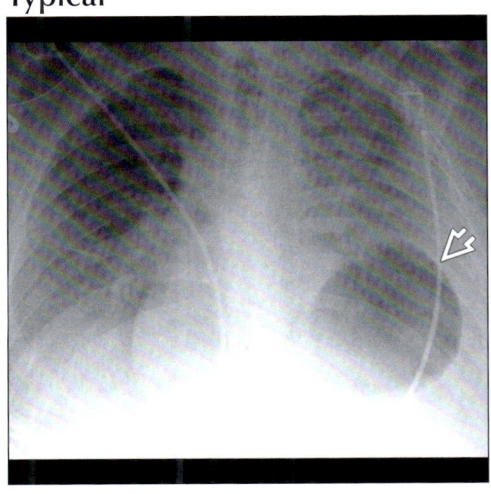 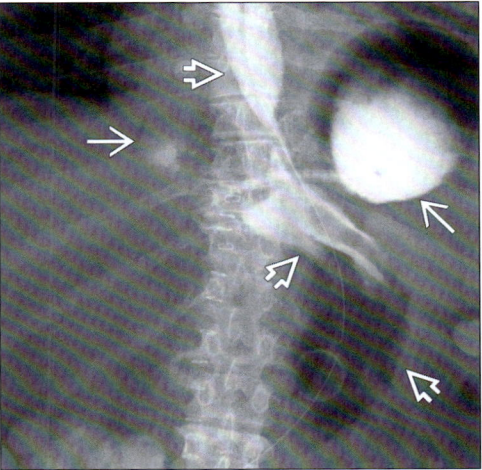

(Left) Anteroposterior radiograph following blunt chest trauma shows large air collection in lower left hemithorax ➡, thought to be ruptured diaphragm. *(Right)* Anteroposterior esophagram shows NG tube and contrast within stomach ➡. Other contrast collections are extravasation from ruptured esophagus ➡.

LUNG CONTUSION

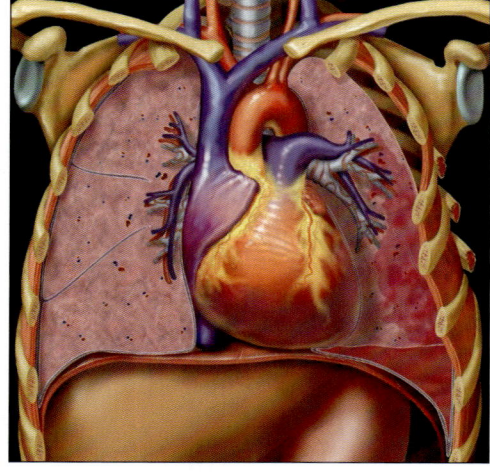

Graphic shows multiple left rib fractures, flail chest with pulmonary contusion and hemorrhage.

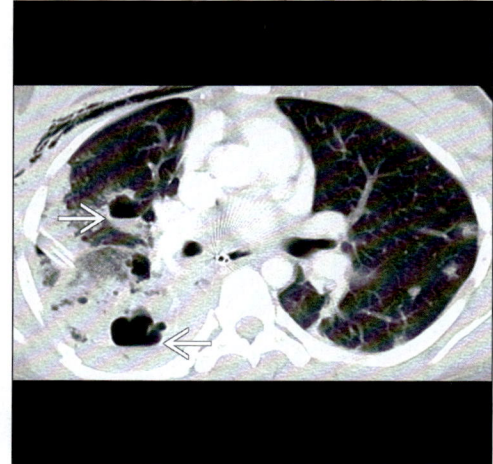

Axial CECT shows multiple post-traumatic lacerations with air/fluid levels ➡ surrounded by contused lung.

TERMINOLOGY

Abbreviations and Synonyms
- Lung bruise, pulmonary laceration, pneumatocele, pulmonary hematoma
- Adult respiratory distress syndrome (ARDS)

Definitions
- Contusion: Traumatic induced pulmonary hemorrhage filling airspaces from torn capillaries
  - Marker of rather severe kinetic energy absorption
- Laceration: Linear tear leading to radial retraction of parenchyma
  - Pulmonary hematoma: Blood-filled laceration
  - Pneumatocele: Air-filled laceration

IMAGING FINDINGS

General Features
- Best diagnostic clue
  - For contusion, posterior peripheral lung opacity following blunt chest trauma
  - For laceration, look for an air-fluid level or pneumatocele within consolidated lung
- Location
  - Contusions more common posteriorly (60%)
    - Typically peripheral lower lung, away from overlying chest wall musculature
    - Contusions do not respect anatomic boundaries such as fissures and do not follow bronchovascular distributions
    - Can occur as contrecoup injuries
  - Lacerations occur in four distinct locations, depending upon the mechanism of injury
    - Central pulmonary lacerations occur after forced chest compression (type 1 laceration)
    - Paravertebral lacerations occur as a shearing injury when the lung is compressed over the spine (type 2 laceration)
    - Small peripheral lacerations occur from rib fractures (type 3 laceration) or from preexisting pleural adhesions (type 4 laceration)
    - Lacerations will conform to the track of a penetrating object
- Size

DDx: Pulmonary Contusion

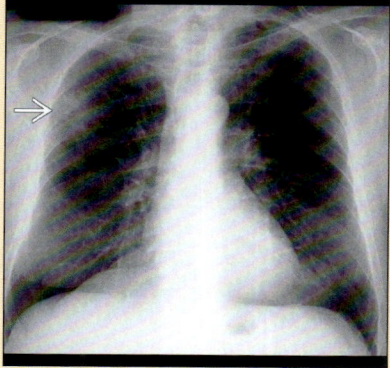
Aspiration

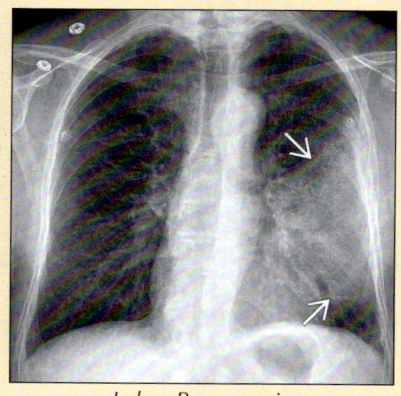
Lobar Pneumonia

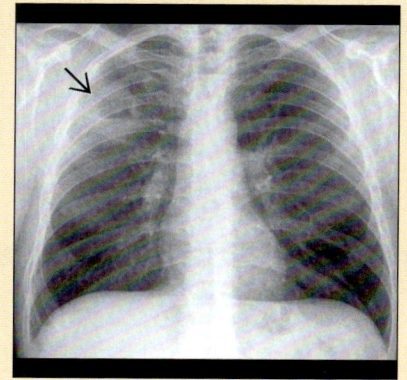
Lung Abscess

LUNG CONTUSION

Key Facts

Terminology
- Contusion: Traumatic induced pulmonary hemorrhage filling airspaces from torn capillaries
- Laceration: Linear tear leading to radial retraction of parenchyma

Imaging Findings
- Contusion volume > 28% of total lung volume usually requires intubation and may lead to ARDS
- Almost always apparent within 6 hours of trauma (rarely delayed appearance for up to 48 hours postinjury)
- Peripheral homogeneous consolidation of variable extent depending on extent of injury
- Posterior location (60%) often adjacent to ribs or vertebral bodies
- Resolution of contusion usually complete within 24-48 hours
- Worsening > 48 hours or persistence > 72 hours consider superimposed pneumonia or aspiration
- If develop diffuse interstitial thickening or consolidation consider development ARDS
- Type 1 laceration: Intraparenchymal pneumatocele or air-fluid level
- Type 2 laceration: Paravertebral pneumatocele or air-fluid level
- Type 3 laceration: Peripheral pneumatocele adjacent to rib fracture

Top Differential Diagnoses
- Aspiration
- Pneumonia
- Lung Abscess

- Contusions can be small (< 1 cm) to quite massive (whole lung) depending upon the extent of injury
  - Contusion volume > 28% of total lung volume usually requires intubation and may lead to ARDS
  - Contusion volume < 18% of total lung volume usually does not require intubation
- Lacerations from rib fractures usually small (< 2 cm)
- Morphology
  - Contusions typically present as peripheral homogeneous consolidation
  - Lacerations typically present spherical
    - In penetrating trauma, the laceration conforms to the path of the penetrating object

Radiographic Findings
- Radiography
  - Contusions
    - Almost always apparent within 6 hours of trauma (rarely delayed appearance for up to 48 hours postinjury)
    - May be normal initially
    - Peripheral homogeneous consolidation of variable extent depending on extent of injury
    - Posterior location (60%) often adjacent to ribs or vertebral bodies
  - Resolution of contusion usually complete within 24-48 hours
    - Worsening > 48 hours or persistence > 72 hours consider superimposed pneumonia or aspiration
    - If develop diffuse interstitial thickening or consolidation consider development ARDS
  - Associated injuries common: Pneumothorax, pneumomediastinum, and search for signs from visceral injuries to heart, aorta, diaphragm
  - Lacerations
    - May not become apparent for hours or even days after trauma, as can be obscured by surrounding contusion
    - Lacerations can change appearance over days to weeks, initially being air-filled but becoming blood-filled, or vice-versa
    - Lacerations heal over several weeks leaving only minimal scarring
    - Hematomas can appear as spiculated lung masses as they heal, mimicking malignancy, sometimes called "vanishing lung tumors"

CT Findings
- More sensitive than radiography for the initial detection of contusion and more accurate for the extent of contusion
  - Chest radiographs usually underestimate extent of contusion
- Contusion
  - Homogeneous or patchy peripheral consolidation in nonsegmental distribution
  - Subpleural lung (outer 1-2 mm) may be spared, especially in children
- Laceration
  - Type 1 laceration: Intraparenchymal pneumatocele or air-fluid level
    - From sudden compression of pliable chest wall and rupture of aerated lung
  - Type 2 laceration: Paravertebral pneumatocele or air-fluid level
    - From shearing of compressed lung across vertebral body
  - Type 3 laceration: Peripheral pneumatocele adjacent to rib fracture
    - From direct puncture from rib fracture
    - Associated hemopneumothorax common
  - Type 4 laceration: No specific abnormalities
    - Tear from tethering from preexisting pleural adhesions
  - Hematoma
    - Slight increased attenuation centrally
    - Contrast-enhancing rim
    - Nodule often results in work-up for lung cancer
  - Resolution pneumatoceles or hematomas
    - Pneumatocele: ↓ In size at rate of 1-2 cm/week
    - Hematoma: ↓ In size at rate of 0.5 cm/month

Imaging Recommendations
- Best imaging tool: CT more sensitive but usually not necessary for clinical decisions

LUNG CONTUSION

- Protocol advice: Chest radiographs usually sufficient to follow course of contusion

DIFFERENTIAL DIAGNOSIS

Aspiration
- In patients with loss of consciousness, aspiration may be superimposed
- Follows a bronchovascular distribution, perihilar predominant instead of peripheral
- Usually not acute

Pneumonia
- Can have similar radiographic findings, but develop later in hospital course
- If contusion fails to resolve in 72 hours or worsens after 48 hours consider superinfection
- Lacerations rarely become secondarily infected, and therefore should not be confused for a lung abscess

Lung Abscess
- Non-traumatic clinical scenario

PATHOLOGY

General Features
- General path comments
  - Linear laceration has spherical shape
    - Normal elasticity of lung pulls centrifugally on the tear
- Etiology
  - Types of blunt force
    - Compression of chest wall
    - Shearing from rapid acceleration or deceleration
    - Blast injury from pressure wave
  - Rib stability
    - Area of maximal chest wall weakness found at 60° rotation from sternum where ribs flatter and less-supported
    - AP compression: Ribs fracture typically 2 places: 60° and posteriorly
- Epidemiology
  - Rib fractures
    - Markers of injury, 4th-10th ribs most common, mean of 3 fractures/patient
    - Especially ominous in children and elderly
    - Ribs difficult to fracture in children due to plasticity, therefore signify significant trauma
    - Ribs fractures more common in elderly from osteoporosis and decreased muscle mass; when present double the morbidity and mortality
- Associated abnormalities
  - Common complications of contusion
    - Pneumonia up to 50%
    - ARDS in 5-20% (usually in those with contusion volumes that exceed 20%)

Microscopic Features
- Interstitial hemorrhage followed in 1-2 hours by interstitial edema, lung volumes usually maintained
- Lung architecture remains intact, airspaces filled with blood initially and then inflammatory cells

Staging, Grading or Classification Criteria
- Chest radiograph grade
  - Severe contusion: ≥ 20% of total lung volume
  - Moderate contusion: < 20% total lung volume
- CT staging of pulmonary lacerations
  - Type 1: From blunt trauma and sudden compression of pliable chest
  - Type 2: Lung compressed and sheared between chest wall and vertebra
  - Type 3: Punctured lung by fractured rib
  - Type 4: Preexisting pleural adhesions tear lung when chest wall compressed

CLINICAL ISSUES

Presentation
- Most common signs/symptoms
  - Nonspecific dyspnea and chest pain
  - Hemoptysis (50%)
  - Hypoxia marker of extent of contusion

Natural History & Prognosis
- Extent of pulmonary parenchymal injuries play a pivotal role in determining mortality
  - Most return to normal without long term sequela
  - > 20% pulmonary contusion at initial evaluation can be predicted to go on to develop ARDS with 90% specificity
- Long term dyspnea, decreased exercise tolerance and chest pain on side of injury in 50% of severe contusions associated with flail chest

Treatment
- Supportive therapy, surveillance for other major organ injuries, observe for complications
  - Prophylactic antibiotics and corticosteroid use unproven
- Severe lacerations with massive hemorrhage may require lobectomy
  - Pulmonary vein laceration, potential for systemic air embolism

DIAGNOSTIC CHECKLIST

Consider
- Pneumonia if contusion fails to resolve in 72 hours or increases in severity after 48 hours

Image Interpretation Pearls
- Lung hematoma may result in a solitary pulmonary nodule mimicking malignancy

SELECTED REFERENCES
1. Mirvis SE: Diagnostic imaging of acute thoracic injury. Semin Ultrasound CT MR. 25(2):156-79, 2004
2. Wanek S et al: Blunt thoracic trauma: flail chest, pulmonary contusion, and blast injury. Crit Care Clin. 20(1):71-81, 2004
3. Ullman EA et al: Pulmonary trauma emergency department evaluation and management. Emerg Med Clin North Am. 21(2):291-313, 2003

LUNG CONTUSION

IMAGE GALLERY

Typical

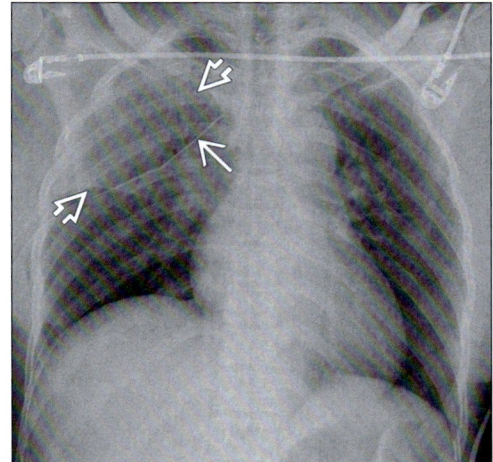
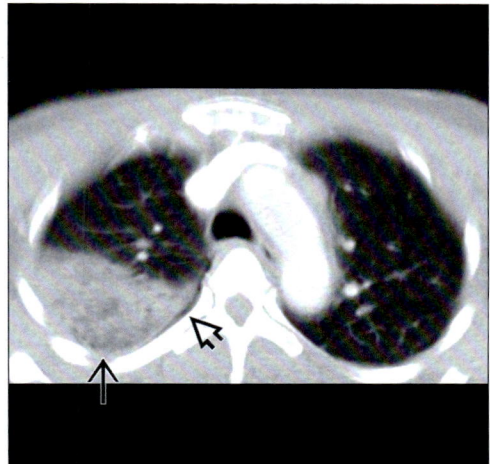

(Left) Anteroposterior radiograph shows homogeneous consolidation in the right upper lobe ➡ from lung contusion. Right chest tube ➡. *(Right)* Axial CECT shows posterior nonanatomic location of homogeneous consolidation from contusion ➡. No pneumothorax or laceration. Note subpleural sparing ➡.

Typical

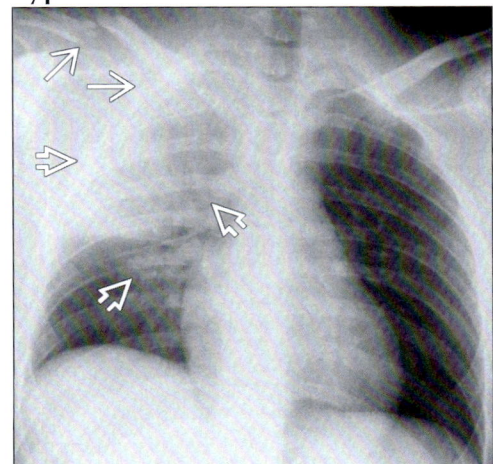
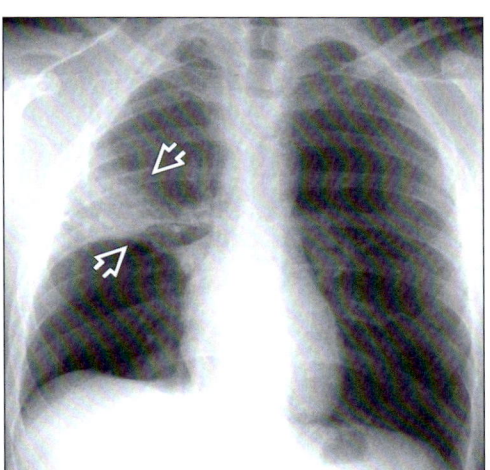

(Left) Anteroposterior radiograph shows homogeneous consolidation over the right upper lung ➡. Broken ribs and clavicle ➡. *(Right)* Anteroposterior radiograph next day shows marked reduction in area of consolidated lung ➡. Resolution of uncomplicated contusion usually rapid.

Typical

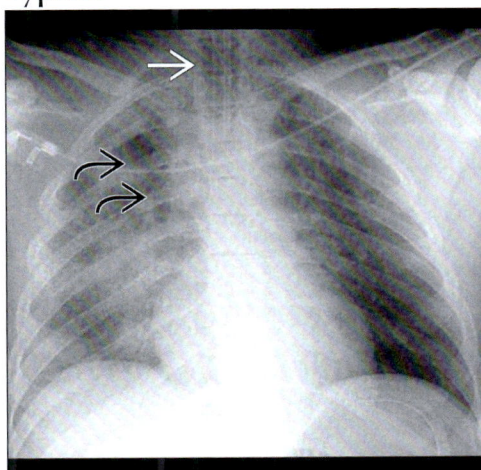
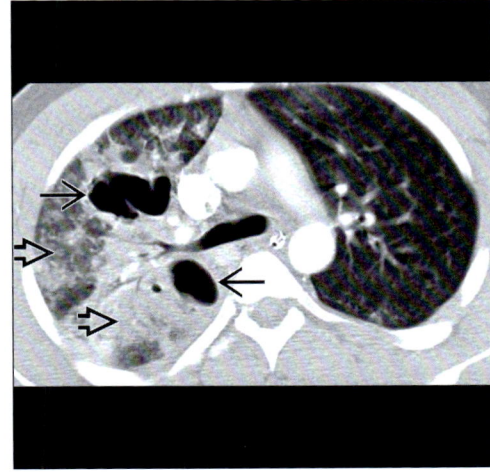

(Left) Anteroposterior radiograph shows extensive consolidation in the right lung from severe contusion, and an irregular cystic space in the right upper lung zone ➡. Patient intubated ➡. Note that the size of the contusion is > 20% total lung volume. *(Right)* Axial CECT shows traumatic lung cysts ➡ and variably consolidated lung consistent with hemorrhagic contusion ➡. Paravertebral laceration (type 2) ➡ anterior laceration (type 1) ➡.

NEUROGENIC PULMONARY EDEMA

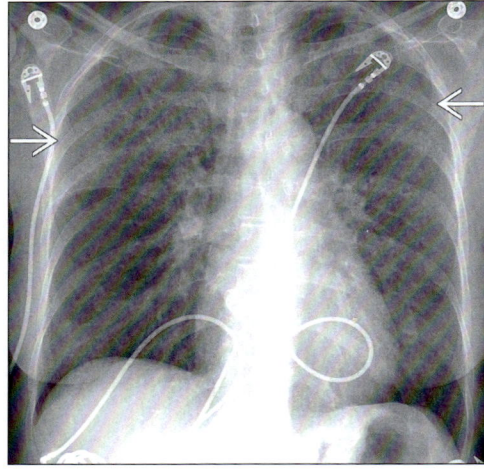

Frontal radiograph shows mild diffuse consolidation ➡ in the upper lobes, right more severely involved than the left. Heart size is normal.

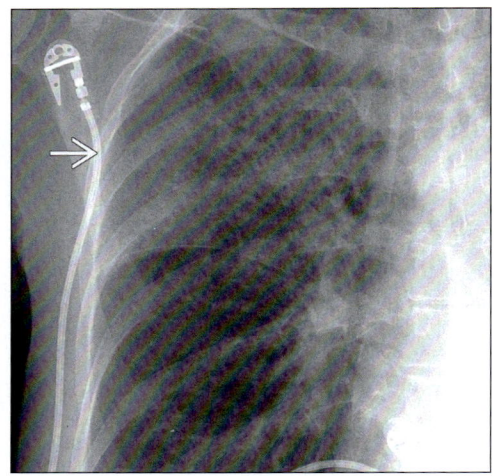

Frontal radiograph close-up shows edema ➡ in the right upper lobe. Radiograph obtained immediately following a ruptured intracranial aneurysm.

TERMINOLOGY

Abbreviations and Synonyms
- Neurogenic pulmonary edema (NPE)

Definitions
- Pulmonary edema due to a central nervous system (CNS) injury (including seizures) that causes a rapid increase in intracranial pressure (ICP)
- Pulmonary edema due to capillary stress failure: Edema based on both hydrostatic mechanisms and noncardiogenic (capillary) leak

IMAGING FINDINGS

General Features
- Best diagnostic clue: Rapid development pulmonary edema after CNS insult
- Location
  - Variable, often upper lung zone or unilateral
    - When unilateral usually right lung (pathophysiology unknown)
- Size: Variable extent dependent on extent of CNS injury

Radiographic Findings
- Radiography
  - Onset, acute (minutes), or subacute (12 hours), following CNS insult
  - Edema pattern often asymmetric
    - Upper lung predominant common finding
    - Usually bilateral but rare unilateral involvement (typically right lung)
  - Septal (Kerley) lines usually absent
  - Normal heart size
  - Pleural effusions absent
  - Resolves over 24-48 hours
    - Resolution usually rapid < 24 hours (33%)
    - Resolution between 24-72 hours (20%)
    - Resolution between 3-7 days (20%)
    - Rarely persists more than 7 days (5%)

Imaging Recommendations
- Best imaging tool: Chest radiographs usually sufficient for detection and monitoring
- Protocol advice: Cranial CT or MR useful to evaluate CNS etiology

DDx: Upper Lung Zone Consolidation

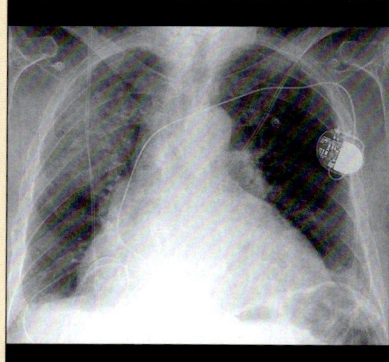

Mitral Regurgitation

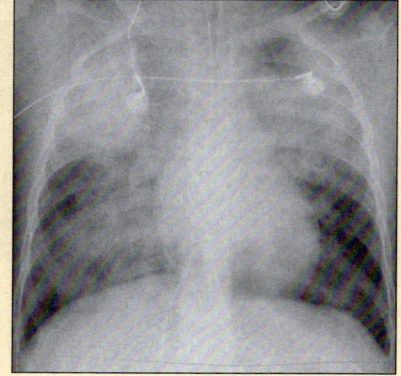

Smoke Inhalation

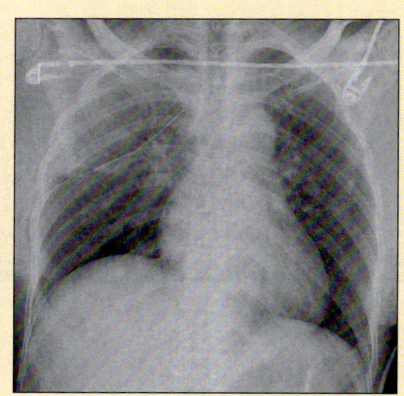

Contusion

NEUROGENIC PULMONARY EDEMA

Key Facts

Terminology
- Pulmonary edema due to a central nervous system (CNS) injury (including seizures) that causes a rapid increase in intracranial pressure (ICP)
- Pulmonary edema due to capillary stress failure: Edema based on both hydrostatic mechanisms and noncardiogenic (capillary) leak

Imaging Findings
- Best diagnostic clue: Rapid development pulmonary edema after CNS insult
- Variable, often upper lung zone or unilateral
- Onset, acute (minutes), or subacute (12 hours), following CNS insult
- Resolves over 24-48 hours

Top Differential Diagnoses
- Aspiration
- Cardiogenic Pulmonary Edema
- Pneumonia
- Contusion
- Smoke Inhalation

Pathology
- Underdiagnosed and unrecognized, NPE actually quite common

Diagnostic Checklist
- Upper lung zone predominance also seen with smoke inhalation, high altitude pulmonary edema, mitral regurgitant pulmonary edema, and negative pressure pulmonary edema: Many of which include CNS symptoms

DIFFERENTIAL DIAGNOSIS

Aspiration
- May be predominately upper lobes in supine comatose patient (gravitationally directed to posterior segments upper lobes)
- Aspiration extremely common with CNS insults
- Resolves more slowly than NPE
- Both associated with fever

Cardiogenic Pulmonary Edema
- Usually not predominately upper lobe
- Cardiomegaly and pleural effusions less likely with NPE
- Kerley B lines more common, rarely seen with NPE

Pneumonia
- Identical radiographic findings
- Like NPE, associated with fever
- Resolves more slowly than NPE

Contusion
- Immediately following trauma
- Motor vehicle accidents could give rise to both contusions and NPE
- Resolution similar
- Traumatic pneumatoceles not seen with NPE

High Altitude Pulmonary Edema
- Similar radiographic pattern
- Seen with ascent > 3,000 meters (10,000 feet)
- CNS insults from acute mountain sickness may result in high altitude pulmonary edema
- Also thought to be due to capillary stress failure

Smoke Inhalation
- Similar radiographic pattern
- May have subglottic edema
- May have carbonaceous particles in sputum and skin burns
- Develops within few hours of smoke inhalation

Mitral Regurgitant Pulmonary Edema
- Mitral regurgitant pulmonary edema predominant in right upper lobe
- Cardiomegaly
- Unilateral NPE usually involves the entire right lung

Negative Pressure Pulmonary Edema
- Develops acutely following relief of upper airway obstruction
- Most common following laryngospasm
- Victims often obtunded due to hypoxia
- Similar radiographic pattern

PATHOLOGY

General Features
- General path comments: Pulmonary edema with features of both hydrostatic edema and noncardiogenic (capillary) leak edema
- Etiology
  o Known features important in pathogenesis
    ▪ Acute elevation intracranial pressure: Common etiologies include subarachnoid or extra-axial hemorrhage, seizures, encephalitis
    ▪ Chronic slow onset of elevated intracranial pressure such as from intracranial tumors less likely to result in NPE
    ▪ Requires intact cervical spinal cord (NPE blocked with C7 cord transection)
    ▪ Release of catecholamines produces "sympathetic storm"
    ▪ Marked elevation of epinephrine and norepinephrine in blood
    ▪ NPE blocked by alpha-adrenergic blocking agents such as phentolamine
  o Pulmonary venoconstriction from catecholamines
    ▪ Markedly increases pulmonary capillary wedge pressure and may cause capillary stress failure or "blast injury"

NEUROGENIC PULMONARY EDEMA

- Edema has features of both hydrostatic (pulmonary venoconstriction) and noncardiogenic capillary leak (stress failure)
  - Initially, edema due to hydrostatic mechanisms and later, due to capillary leak
  - Stress failure
    - Pulmonary capillaries extremely thin
    - When subjected to high intravascular pressures, capillaries may fail (when pressures > 40 mm Hg)
    - Initially hydrostatic edema develops according to Starling's law
    - Disruption of capillary endothelium leads to noncardiogenic pulmonary edema
  - Stress failure differential diagnosis
    - Neurogenic pulmonary edema
    - High altitude pulmonary edema
    - Exercise-induced pulmonary hemorrhage in thoroughbred horses
  - CNS site responsible for NPE not fully established
    - Animal studies suggest hypothalamus or medulla
- Epidemiology
  - May result from any CNS injury that leads to rapid increase in intracranial pressure (ICP)
    - Most commonly trauma but can be seen with grand mal seizures and electroshock therapy
  - Underdiagnosed and unrecognized, NPE actually quite common
    - 70% incidence in fatal cases of subarachnoid hemorrhage
    - 50% incidence in head trauma
    - 33% incidence in status epilepticus
- Associated abnormalities
  - CNS injury usually obvious from subarachnoid hemorrhage, mass effect with herniation, subdural fluid collection
    - CT or MR may be normal with seizure induced NPE

Gross Pathologic & Surgical Features
- Increased lung weight from pulmonary edema

Microscopic Features
- Protein rich pulmonary edema with hyaline membrane formation
- Hemorrhage more common in severe cases

CLINICAL ISSUES

Presentation
- Most common signs/symptoms
  - Dyspnea
  - Nonspecific signs: Tachycardia, tachypnea
  - Rales and rhonchi
  - Mild leukocytosis common (leading to erroneous diagnosis of pneumonia)
  - Fever common (usually secondary to CNS insult)
  - Mild hemoptysis or pink frothy sputum
  - Hypoxia may require ventilatory support
  - Protein rich sputum (due to capillary leak)
- Other signs/symptoms
  - Swan Ganz catheterization
    - Usually pulmonary artery pressures and cardiac output normal
    - If pressure monitored at the time of CNS insult (subarachnoid hemorrhage in the ICU) there is a transient rise in pulmonary capillary wedge pressure
    - By the time patients reach hospital, pulmonary artery pressures have returned to normal

Demographics
- Age: Any age but more common in young adults (due to trauma related injuries and ruptured intracranial aneurysms)

Natural History & Prognosis
- Develops within minutes to hours of CNS insult
  - Characteristic rapid development of respiratory failure (< 4 hours)
- Outcome depends on successful treatment of CNS cause

Treatment
- Supportive
  - Supplemental oxygen
  - Often hyperventilated (to decrease CO_2) which decreases intracranial pressure
  - Mechanical ventilation including positive end-expiratory pressure (PEEP) may be necessary to maintain oxygenation
    - PEEP may increase intracranial pressure and should be used cautiously
- Alpha-adrenergic blocking agents early, benefit unproven but works in experimental animals
- Dilantin or other anticonvulsants for seizures

DIAGNOSTIC CHECKLIST

Consider
- Underdiagnosed, usually mistaken for aspiration, pneumonia, contusion, or cardiogenic edema

Image Interpretation Pearls
- Review neuroimaging studies
  - NPE a diagnosis of exclusion once contusion, aspiration, pneumonia excluded
- Upper lung zone predominance also seen with smoke inhalation, high altitude pulmonary edema, mitral regurgitant pulmonary edema, and negative pressure pulmonary edema: Many of which include CNS symptoms

SELECTED REFERENCES

1. Fontes RB et al: Acute neurogenic pulmonary edema: case reports and literature review. J Neurosurg Anesthesiol. 15(2):144-50, 2003
2. West JB: Invited review: pulmonary capillary stress failure. J Appl Physiol. 89(6):2483-9;discussion 2497, 2000
3. West JB: Invited review: pulmonary capillary stress failure. J Appl Physiol. 89(6):2483-9;discussion 97, 2000
4. Rogers FB et al: Neurogenic pulmonary edema in fatal and nonfatal head injuries. J Trauma. 39(5):860-6; discussion 66-8, 1995
5. Ell SR: Neurogenic pulmonary edema. A review of the literature and a perspective. Invest Radiol. 26(5):499-506, 1991

NEUROGENIC PULMONARY EDEMA

IMAGE GALLERY

Typical

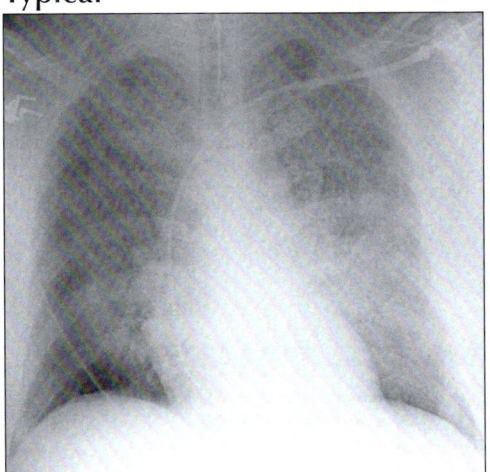
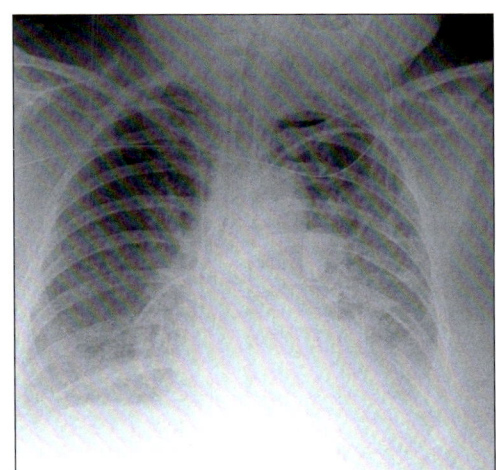

(Left) Anteroposterior radiograph shows moderately diffuse, dense consolidation with relative sparing of the costophrenic sulci and periphery of the right lung. Neurogenic pulmonary edema from subarachnoid hemorrhage. *(Right)* Anteroposterior radiograph shows diffuse consolidation (left > right) from neurogenic pulmonary edema manifesting 48 hours after cerebral angioplasty for vasospasm.

Typical

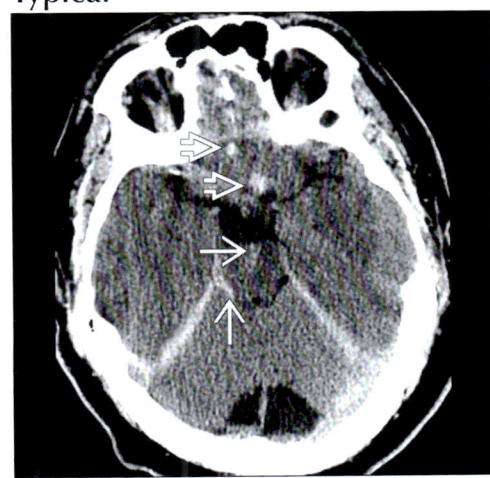
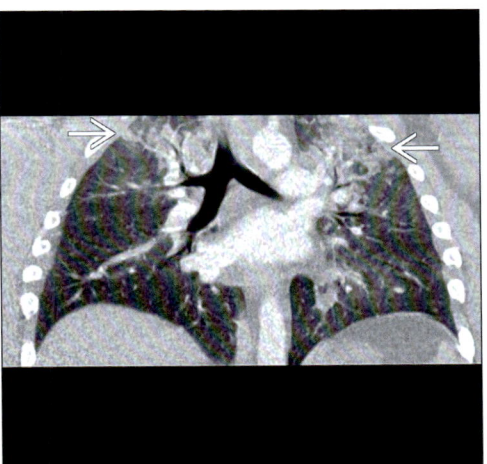

(Left) Axial CECT shows subarachnoid hemorrhage ➡ and intraparenchymal hemorrhage ➡. *(Right)* Coronal CECT shows ground-glass opacities and consolidation in both apices ➡. Neurogenic pulmonary edema.

Typical

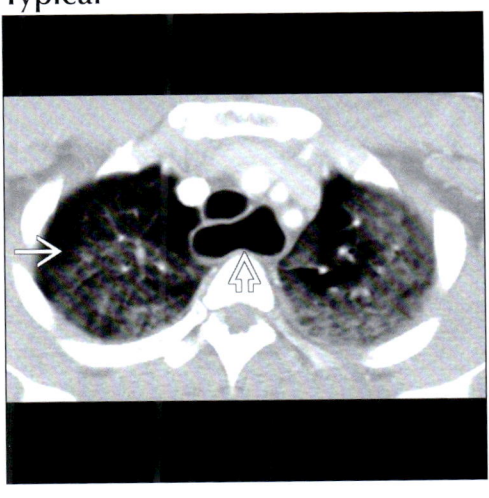
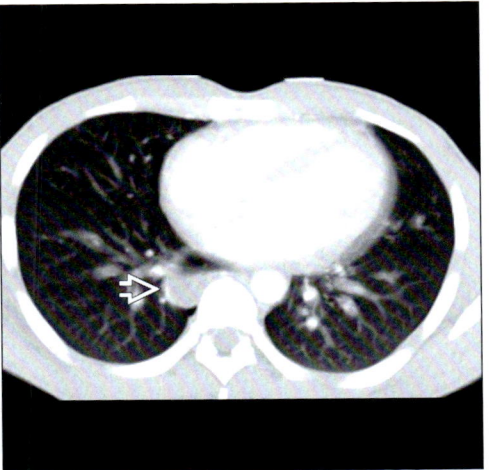

(Left) Axial CECT shows diffuse ground-glass opacities in the upper lobes ➡. Dilated esophagus ➡, etiology undetermined. Neurogenic pulmonary edema from epidural hematoma. *(Right)* Axial CECT shows lack of edema in the mid and lower lung. Dilated esophagus ➡.

NEGATIVE PRESSURE PULMONARY EDEMA

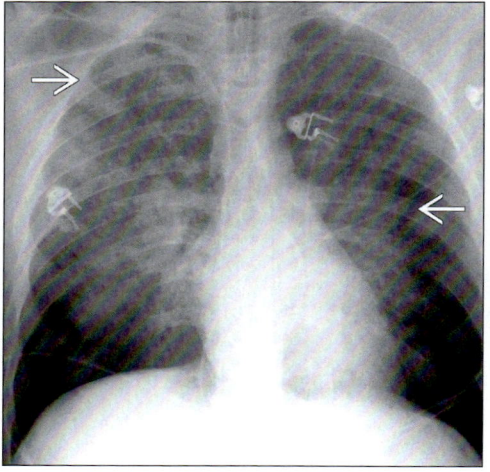

Anteroposterior radiograph shows central and upper lung zone consolidation ➡ which developed after intubation following failed suicidal hanging attempt.

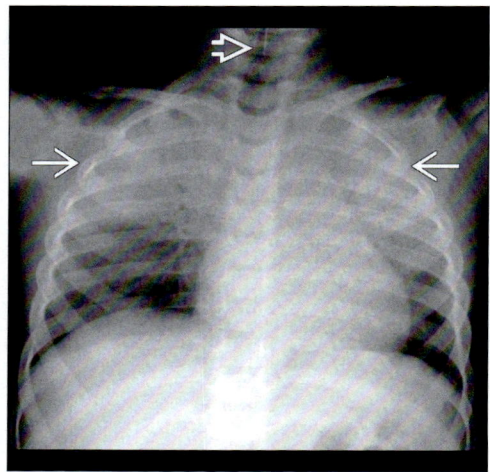

Anteroposterior radiograph following intubation ➡ for epiglottitis shows severe upper lung zone edema ➡.

TERMINOLOGY

Abbreviations and Synonyms
- Near-strangulation pulmonary edema, post-obstructive pulmonary edema, reexpansion pulmonary edema (RPE)
- Athletic pulmonary edema
- Negative pressure pulmonary edema (NPPE), adult respiratory distress syndrome (ARDS)

Definitions
- NPPE develops following relief of acute or chronic upper airway obstruction, most commonly post-extubation laryngospasm
- RPE develops following rapid expansion of a chronically collapsed lung after evacuation of a large amount of air or fluid from the pleural space

IMAGING FINDINGS

General Features
- Best diagnostic clue
  - NPPE: Recovery room radiograph showing pulmonary edema
  - RPE: Ipsilateral development of edema within few hours of removal of pleural air or fluid collections
- Location
  - NPPE: Central (bat-wing) pattern of pulmonary edema with relative sparing of the base
  - RPE: Ipsilateral to drainage of pleural space

Radiographic Findings
- Negative pressure pulmonary edema
  - Edema
    - Interstitial, alveolar pattern or mixed
    - Kerley lines uncommon
    - Most common central within lung (90%), symmetric 50%, asymmetric (right > left) 50%
    - Usually spares the costophrenic angles and basilar lung leaving the upper lung zones more severely involved
    - Unilateral (10%) right more common than left
  - Vascular pedicle width increased
  - Normal heart size
  - No pleural effusions

DDx: Atypical Edema

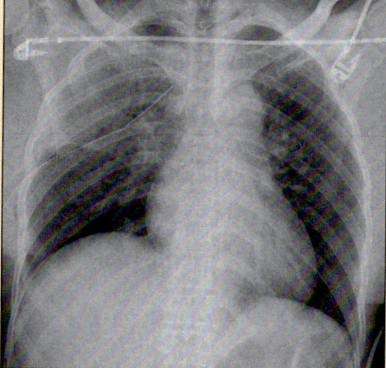

Lung Contusion

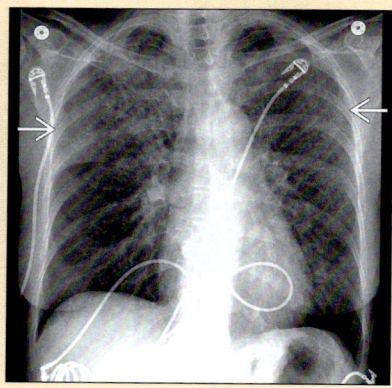

Neurogenic Edema

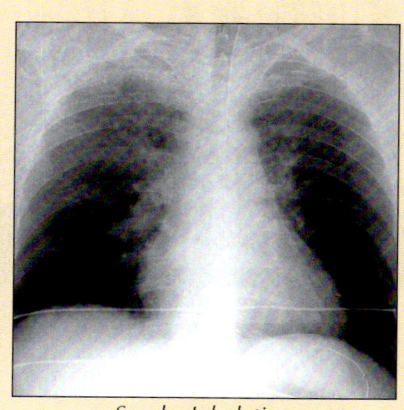

Smoke Inhalation

NEGATIVE PRESSURE PULMONARY EDEMA

Key Facts

Terminology
- NPPE develops following relief of acute or chronic upper airway obstruction, most commonly post-extubation laryngospasm
- RPE develops following rapid expansion of a chronically collapsed lung after evacuation of a large amount of air or fluid from the pleural space

Imaging Findings
- NPPE: Recovery room radiograph showing pulmonary edema
- RPE: Ipsilateral development of edema within few hours of removal of pleural air or fluid collections
- NPPE: Central (bat-wing) pattern of pulmonary edema with relative sparing of the base
- RPE: Ipsilateral to drainage of pleural space

Top Differential Diagnoses
- Contusion
- Aspiration
- IV Drug Abuse
- Cardiogenic Pulmonary Edema
- Neurogenic Pulmonary Edema

Clinical Issues
- Symptoms arise minutes to hours following relief of airway obstruction or drainage of pleural space

Diagnostic Checklist
- Suspect diagnosis when portable radiographs obtained in recovery room show pulmonary edema in young patient

---

  - Resolution usually rapid within hours or 2-3 days depending on severity of initial edema
- Reexpansion pulmonary edema
  - Pleural space occupying process usually chronic (average duration 14 days, minimum 3 days)
  - Pleural space occupying process usually large (more than 1/3rd of hemithorax)
  - Alveolar pattern ipsilateral to thoracentesis or chest tube drainage
    - Rarely limited to one lobe (perhaps due to torsion or asymmetric collapse)
    - Rarely also involves contralateral lung (probably reexpansion pulmonary edema incites ARDS)
  - Develops within 1 hour in 2/3rds
  - May progress for 24 hours
  - Resolution over 4-5 days

CT Findings
- Negative pressure pulmonary edema
  - Preferential central and nondependent distribution
    - Periphery typically spared
  - Nonspecific ground-glass opacities to consolidation
  - Near drowning
    - Central ground-glass opacities
    - Crazy-paving pattern
    - Ill-defined centrilobular nodules
    - May have interstitial pulmonary emphysema and pneumomediastinum
  - Neck CT in strangulation or hanging
    - Soft tissue edema or hemorrhage in neck
    - Fractured laryngeal skeleton (thyroid cartilage > hyoid bone > cricoid cartilage)

Imaging Recommendations
- Best imaging tool: Chest radiography usually suffices for diagnosis and follow-up

DIFFERENTIAL DIAGNOSIS

Contusion
- Follows trauma, usually motor vehicle accident
- Focal nonsegmental peripheral consolidation
- May have associated rib fractures

Aspiration
- Occurs in those obtunded and unable to protect airway
- Follows bronchovascular distribution in gravity dependent regions

IV Drug Abuse
- Consider in young adults with unexplained radiographic abnormalities, especially in ER
- Pulmonary hemorrhage most common with cocaine and crack
- Myocardial injury more common with cocaine
- Noncardiac pulmonary edema from crack and heroin

Cardiogenic Pulmonary Edema
- Kerley B lines common
- Pleural effusions
- Cardiomegaly and pulmonary venous hypertension

Smoke Inhalation
- Develops within hours of smoke inhalation
- Skin burns, carbonaceous sputum
- Edema more prominent in upper lung zones
- May have subglottic edema

Neurogenic Pulmonary Edema
- From intracranial hypertension
- Edema slightly more prominent upper lung zones

Mitral Regurgitant Pulmonary Edema
- Pulmonary edema due to heart failure in patient with incompetent mitral valve
- Edema diffuse but more severe in the right upper lobe due to directional back flow through the right superior pulmonary vein
- Cardiomegaly

Differential Unilateral Acute Consolidation
- Aspiration
- Pneumonia
- Contusion
- Edema

NEGATIVE PRESSURE PULMONARY EDEMA

- Neurogenic
- Cardiac (right lateral decubitus position)
- Acute rheumatic fever
- High altitude pulmonary edema (common with unilateral agenesis of pulmonary artery)
- Acute obstruction of pulmonary artery or pulmonary veins

PATHOLOGY

General Features
- Etiology
  - Relief of acute airway obstruction
    - **Post-extubation laryngospasm**
    - Epiglottitis or croup
    - Strangulation
    - Hanging
    - Choking or aspirated foreign body
    - Near drowning
    - Endotracheal tube obstruction
    - Asthma
  - Relief of chronic airway obstruction
    - Tonsillectomy
    - Substernal thyroid
    - Sleep apnea
    - Choanal stenosis
  - RPE: Drainage of large and usually chronic fluid or air collection in the pleural space
- Epidemiology
  - Incidence 10% in children with relief acute obstruction (typically epiglottitis or post-extubation laryngospasm)
  - Incidence 50% in children with relief chronic obstruction
  - Incidence 10% following removal large pleural effusion
  - NPPE & RPE may be clinically silent with radiographic evidence only suggesting the condition may be common
- Pathophysiology NPPE
  - Müller maneuver: Attempt to inhale against obstruction
  - Normal inspiratory pleural pressures: -2 to -5 cm of H_2O
    - May drop to -100 cm of H_2O with attempts to inspire past obstruction
  - Creates highly negative intrathoracic pressure
    - Increases venous return
    - Decreases cardiac output
    - Increased transmural pressure may rupture capillaries
  - During upper airway obstruction create more positive pressures during expiration (auto-PEEP)
- Pathophysiology RPE
  - Animal models: Incidence RPE 85% in which lung atelectatic for > 8 days
  - Exact pathophysiology unknown: Important factors
    - Rapid reexpansion using high negative intrapleural pressures
    - Rapid reperfusion of hypoxic lung
    - Chronically collapsed lung deficient in surfactant (surface tension lowering properties helps prevent fluid transudation)

Microscopic Features
- NPPE and RPE have increased capillary permeability
- NPPE common findings include
  - Admixture of alveolar collapse and alveolar hyperinflation
  - Alternating zones of bronchiolar constriction and bronchiolar dilatation

CLINICAL ISSUES

Presentation
- Most common signs/symptoms
  - Symptoms arise minutes to hours following relief of airway obstruction or drainage of pleural space
    - Agitation, cough, tachypnea, tachycardia, frothy secretions, rales, oxygen desaturation
  - Neck burns or bruises from strangulation or hanging
- Other signs/symptoms: Pulmonary capillary wedge pressure usually normal in NPPE and RPE

Demographics
- Age: Both more common in athletic young
- Gender: More common in men (probably from athleticism and ability to generate high intrathoracic pressures)

Natural History & Prognosis
- Both typically resolve over 3-5 days with no sequelae
- Rarely shock and death

Treatment
- Supportive, supplemental oxygen

DIAGNOSTIC CHECKLIST

Consider
- Suspect diagnosis when portable radiographs obtained in recovery room show pulmonary edema in young patient

SELECTED REFERENCES

1. Koh MS et al: Negative pressure pulmonary oedema in the medical intensive care unit. Intensive Care Med. 29(9):1601-4, 2003
2. Schwartz DR et al: Negative pressure pulmonary hemorrhage. Chest. 115(4):1194-7, 1999
3. Deepika K et al: Negative pressure pulmonary edema after acute upper airway obstruction. J Clin Anesth. 9(5):403-8, 1997
4. Tarver RD et al: Reexpansion pulmonary edema. J Thorac Imaging. 11(3):198-209, 1996
5. Cascade PN et al: Negative-pressure pulmonary edema after endotracheal intubation. Radiology. 186(3):671-5, 1993
6. Halow KD et al: Pulmonary edema following post-operative laryngospasm: a case report and review of the literature. Am Surg. 59(7):443-7, 1993

NEGATIVE PRESSURE PULMONARY EDEMA

IMAGE GALLERY

Typical

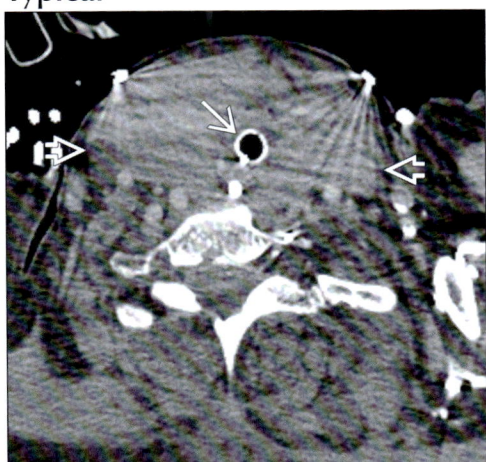
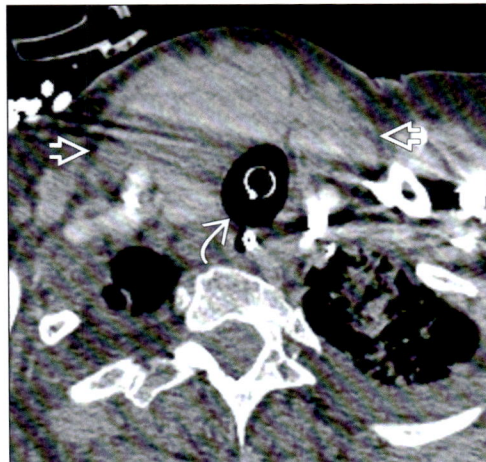

(Left) Axial CECT shows massive goiter ➡. Extrathoracic trachea narrowed around ET tube ➡. *(Right)* Axial CECT shows massive goiter ➡. Intrathoracic trachea normal size ➡.

Typical

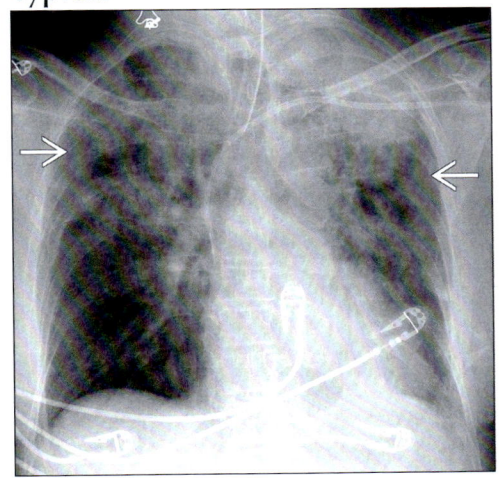
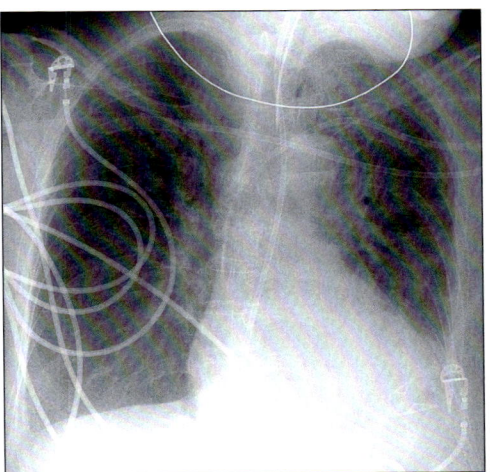

(Left) Anteroposterior radiograph post-intubation in the goiter patient shows diffuse consolidation in the upper lung zones ➡, from negative pressure pulmonary edema. *(Right)* Anteroposterior radiograph in same patient as previous image, 2 days later. Shows rapid resolution of upper lobe edema.

Typical

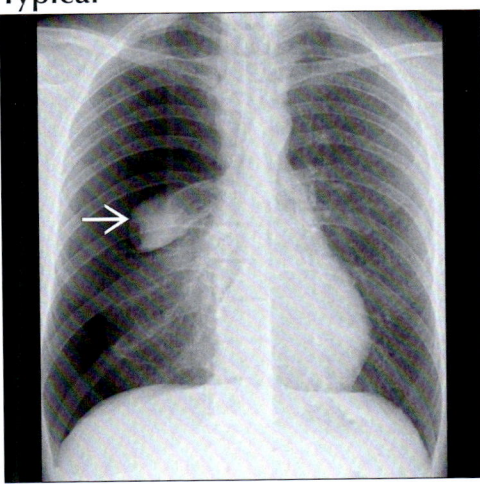
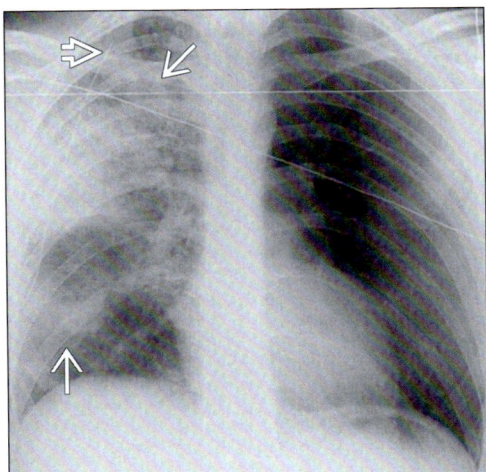

(Left) Frontal radiograph shows large pneumothorax with complete collapse (torsion) of right upper lobe ➡. *(Right)* Frontal radiograph in same patient as previous image, after insertion of chest tube ➡, few hours later. Dense consolidation in the right lung, especially in the right upper lobe ➡ from reexpansion edema.

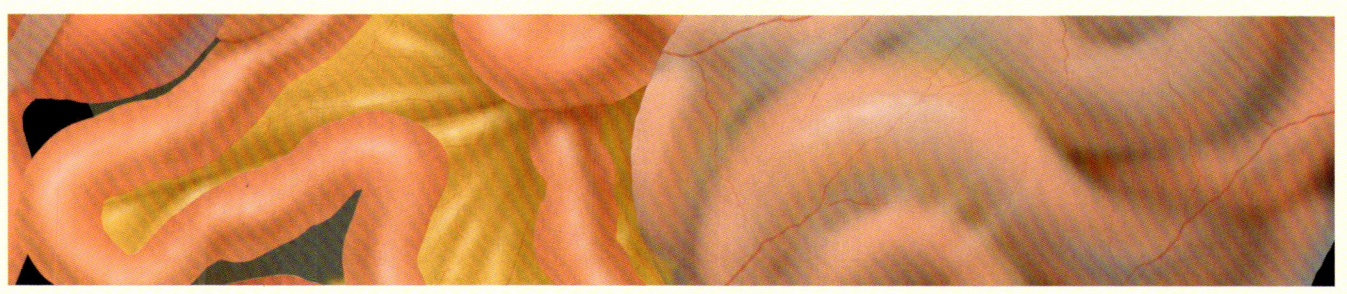

SECTION 3: Abdomen/Pelvis

Introduction and Overview
Abdominal Imaging Issues, Trauma   I-3-2

Abdomen/Pelvis
Splenic Trauma   I-3-4
Hepatic Trauma   I-3-8
Renal Trauma   I-3-12
Pancreatic Trauma   I-3-16
Duodenal Trauma/Hematoma   I-3-20
Intestinal Trauma   I-3-22
Testicular Trauma   I-3-26
Hypoperfusion Complex   I-3-28

ABDOMINAL IMAGING ISSUES, TRAUMA

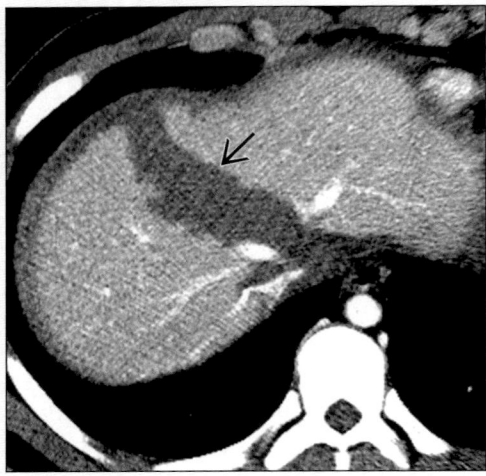

Axial CECT shows a hepatic fracture. Note linear low-attenuation laceration extending through entire substance of hepatic parenchyma ➔.

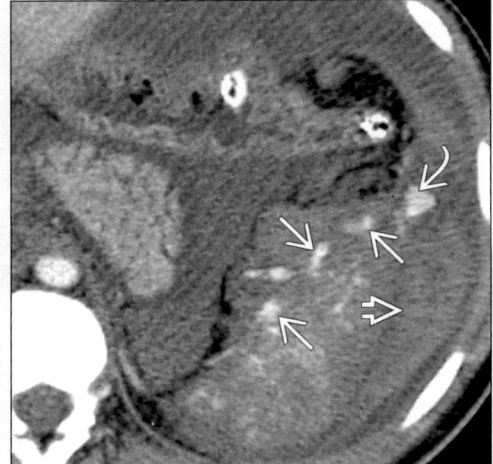

Axial CECT of high attenuation active extravasation ➔ lateral to spleen, massive surrounding hemoperitoneum ➔ & lack of splenic enhancement except for multiple high-attenuation pseudoaneurysms ➔.

ANATOMY-BASED IMAGING ISSUES

Clinical Overview
- Until recently, trauma not recognized as a "disease"
- New emphasis on government-designated trauma centers
  - Provide integrated & coordinated care with subspecialties, i.e., neurosurgery, orthopedics
- Survival depends on extent of injuries, length of time to resuscitation
  - "Golden hour" before hypovolemic shock
- Abdominal trauma often occurs in setting of multiple other injuries
  - Central nervous system (CNS), musculoskeletal (MSK), thoracic, vascular
    - With 16- & 64-slice MDCT, major CNS, thoracic, MSK & vascular injuries may be assessed concurrently in several minutes of scan time

Imaging Triage: Hemodynamically Unstable Patients
- Diagnostic peritoneal lavage (DPL) or US assessment of peritoneal fluid
  - DPL positive if RBC count > 100,000; WBC > 5,000; presence of bile, food material or fecal matter
  - 95% accurate, 1.2% false-negative rate
- Focused Assessment with Sonography for Trauma (FAST) exam
  - Positive if free fluid identified in peritoneal cavity
  - Increasing trend to replace DPL with FAST in hypotensive patients

Imaging Triage: Hemodynamically Stable Patients
- CT in patients with clinically moderate to high suspicion for intra-abdominal injury
- FAST exam or clinical observation for low clinical suspicion patients

Imaging Findings
- Global CT signs of abdominal trauma
  - Hemoperitoneum
    - Free lysed blood > 30 HU
    - Clotted blood > 45 HU
    - Active bleeding isodense with aorta (often > 150 HU)
  - "Caved in cava" sign
    - Flattened intra-abdominal inferior vena cava (IVC) due to decreased venous return & hypovolemia
  - "Sentinel clot" sign
    - Highest attenuation blood closest to anatomic site of injury
  - "Shock bowel" sign
    - Diffuse fold thickening of small bowel, reperfusion injury following volume replacement with submucosal edema
  - "Dependent viscera" sign
    - Lack of visualization of diaphragm between spleen & ribs
    - Indicates diaphragmatic rupture
  - "Collar sign"
    - Herniation of stomach through diaphragmatic defect causing tethering & narrowing of gastric folds
  - Periaortic blood at level of diaphragm
    - Aortic transsection, vertebral fracture, diaphragm rupture
  - Active arterial bleeding
    - Linear or irregularly shaped collection of extravasated contrast within hematoma or parenchymal laceration
    - Isodense with abdominal aorta
    - Diffuses on delayed images
  - Pseudoaneurysm
    - Rounded, contained area of contrast isodense with aorta
    - Does not diffuse on delayed images
- Parenchymal organ injuries
  - Contusion: Ill-defined area of decreased attenuation on CECT
  - Hematoma: Well-defined area of decreased attenuation on CECT
  - Subcapsular hematoma: Hematoma compresses lateral contour of organ, confined by capsule

ABDOMINAL IMAGING ISSUES, TRAUMA

Differential Diagnoses

Low Attenuation Intraperitoneal Fluid (< 15 HU)
- Trauma related: Intraperitoneal bladder rupture, bowel perforation (especially if intra-loop fluid), GB rupture
- Non-traumatic: Ascites, peritoneal dialysis fluid, peritonitis (especially TB), ruptured ovarian cyst

Low Attenuation Extraperitoneal Fluid
- Trauma related: Forniceal rupture and/or laceration of renal collecting system

High Attenuation Intraperitoneal Fluid (> 30 HU)
- Hemoperitoneum: Free lysed blood (30-45 HU); clotted blood (45-60 HU)
- Extravasated oral contrast (> 100 HU)
- Active arterial extravasation (> 150 HU)

- Laceration: Linear, jagged area of hematoma
- Fracture: Laceration extending through entire parenchyma
- Traumatic infarction: Vascular occlusion 2° intimal dissection causing complete lack of enhancement on CECT
- Bowel & mesenteric injury
  - Extraluminal air, extravasated oral contrast
  - Discontinuity of bowel wall, intramural air
  - Free intraperitoneal water-density fluid (< 15 HU)
    - Especially within intraloop compartment
  - Focal bowel wall thickening > 4 mm
  - High attenuation mesenteric hematoma (> 30 HU)
  - Active arterial extravasation
  - Secondary finding
    - Abnormal wall contusion 2° seat belt injury
- Pancreatic injury
  - Low-attenuation laceration or fracture in mid-body
  - Retropancreatic fluid adjacent to splenic vein
  - Post-traumatic pancreatitis with soft tissue stranding in anterior pararenal space

Visceral Injury Grading Systems
- American Association for the Surgery of Trauma (AAST) grading based on anatomic depiction of extent of injury
  - Splenic trauma Grade I
    - Hematoma: Subcapsular < 10% of surface area
    - Laceration: Capsular tear < 1 cm
  - Splenic trauma Grade II
    - Hematoma: Subcapsular hematoma 10-50% of surface
    - Laceration: 1-3 cm area
  - Splenic trauma Grade III
    - Hematoma: 75% of surface area, expanding or ruptured
    - Laceration: > 3 cm or involved trabecular vessel
  - Splenic trauma Grade IV
    - Laceration: Involves segmental or hilar vessel with > 25% devascularization
  - Splenic trauma Grade V
    - Laceration: Completely shattered spleen
    - Vascular: Hilar vascular injury, devascularized spleen
- CT-based splenic injury scale
  - Similar to AAST scale, except for grade IV A & IV B
  - Grade IV A
    - Active intraparenchymal and subcapsular splenic bleeding, pseudoaneurysm or arteriovenous fistula
  - Grade IV B
    - Active intraperitoneal bleeding

RELATED REFERENCES
1. Yao DC et al: Using contrast-enhanced helical CT to visualize arterial extravasation after blunt abdominal trauma: incidence and organ distribution. AJR Am J Roentgenol. 178(1):17-20, 2002

IMAGE GALLERY

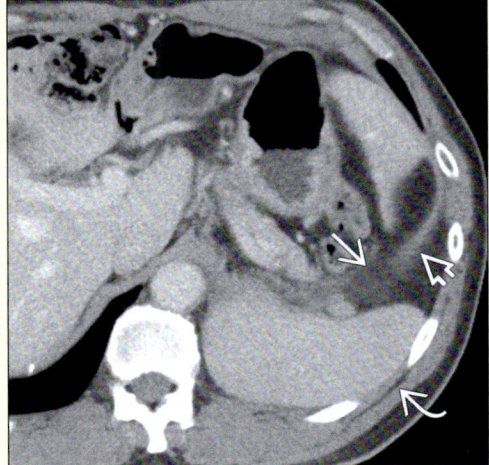
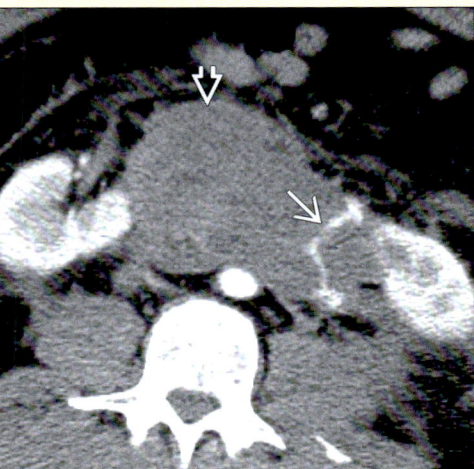

(Left) Axial CECT shows diaphragmatic rupture. Note focal interruption ➔ of diaphragm ➔ with non-visualization of diaphragm adjacent to spleen ➔ (dependent viscera sign). *(Right)* Axial CECT shows laceration of isthmus in horseshoe kidney. Note area of active arterial extravasation ➔ within large hematoma ➔ on isthmus.

SPLENIC TRAUMA

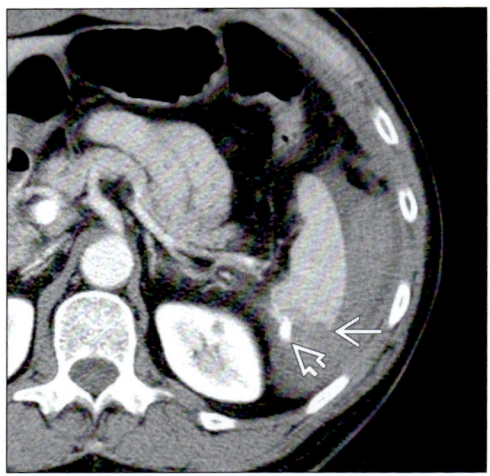

Axial CECT shows splenic fracture with active extravasation. Note fracture of lower pole ➡ with high attenuation area of arterial extravasation ➡.

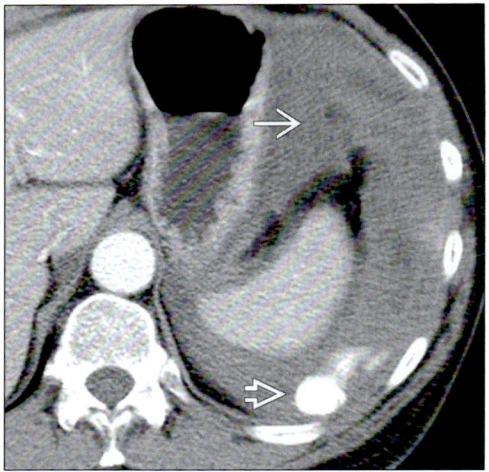

Axial CECT in same patient as left demonstrates large perisplenic hematoma ➡ and extensive arterial extravasation ➡.

TERMINOLOGY

Abbreviations and Synonyms
- Splenic laceration, splenic fracture, subcapsular hematoma of spleen

Definitions
- Splenic parenchymal injury with or without capsule disruption

IMAGING FINDINGS

General Features
- Best diagnostic clue: Low attenuation splenic laceration with high density active bleeding
- Morphology
  - Lacerations: Linear or jagged edges
  - Fracture: Laceration extending from outer cortex to hilum
  - Subcapsular hematoma: Flattened contour of splenic parenchyma

Radiographic Findings
- Radiography
  - Abdominal radiography
    - Left upper quadrant (LUQ) soft tissue mass
    - Signs of intraperitoneal fluid with widening of distance between flank strip and descending colon
    - Fluid in pelvis with prominent pelvic "dog ears"
  - Chest radiography
    - Left lower lobe atelectasis and/or consolidation
    - Left rib fractures
    - Left pneumothorax
    - Left pleural effusion

CT Findings
- NECT
  - High attenuation (> 30 HU) hemoperitoneum or perisplenic clot (> 45 HU)
  - Sentinel clot sign: Highest density blood adjacent to spleen
    - Indicates splenic injury even in absence of demonstrable laceration
  - Layered or lamellated clot when bleeding is intermittent
- CECT

DDx: Splenic Lesions Mimicking Trauma

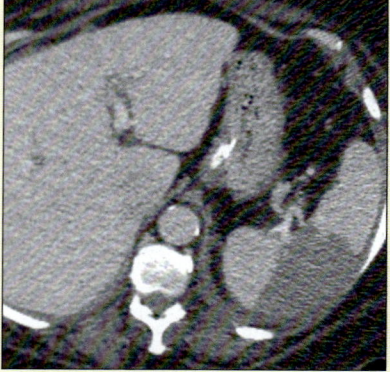

Splenic Infarct

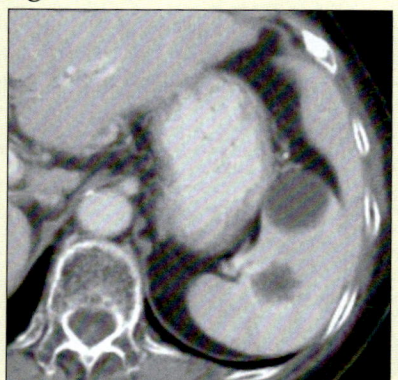

Splenic Cysts

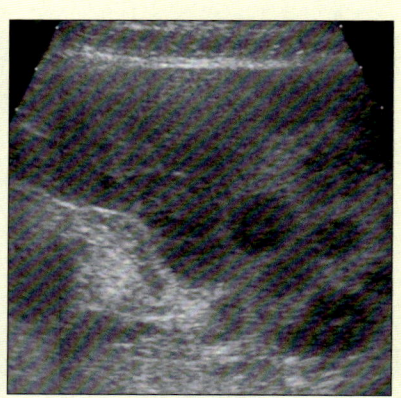

Splenic Lymphoma

SPLENIC TRAUMA

Key Facts

Terminology
- Splenic parenchymal injury with or without capsule disruption

Imaging Findings
- Best diagnostic clue: Low attenuation splenic laceration with high density active bleeding
- Sentinel clot sign: Highest density blood adjacent to spleen
- Best imaging tool: CECT
- 150 mL IV contrast at 2.5 mL/sec with 5 mm collimation

Top Differential Diagnoses
- Splenic Abscess
- Splenic Infarct
- Splenic Cyst
- Lymphoma

Pathology
- Etiology: Blunt trauma with blow to LUQ
- Most commonly injured solid abdominal organ in blunt trauma
- Associated abnormalities: Injuries to left thorax, tail of pancreas, left liver lobe and/or mesentery

Clinical Issues
- Prone to develop delayed hemorrhage, excellent prognosis with early intervention (surgery/embolization)

Diagnostic Checklist
- Congenital cleft if no hemoperitoneum
- Innocuous injury may lead to life-threatening delayed hemorrhage, especially with anticoagulation

---

  - Subcapsular hematoma: Compresses lateral margin of parenchyma
  - Parenchymal laceration: Jagged linear or stellate area of nonenhancement due to hematoma
  - Splenic fracture: Deep laceration extending from outer capsule through splenic hilum
  - Active arterial extravasation: High attenuation focus isodense with aorta, surrounded by lower attenuation clot or hematoma
    - High attenuation focus may be linear (spurting vessel) or rounded (pseudoaneurysm)

Ultrasonographic Findings
- Grayscale Ultrasound
  - Subtle laceration may be missed
  - Echogenic perisplenic clot
  - Hypo- or isoechoic hematoma or laceration
  - Free intraperitoneal fluid with low-level echoes representing hemoperitoneum
- Color Doppler
  - Color flow within round pseudoaneurysm
  - Hematomas are avascular

Angiographic Findings
- Avascular parenchymal laceration
- Flattened lateral contour due to subcapsular hematoma
- Rounded contrast collections (pseudoaneurysms)
- Amorphous parenchymal extravasation

Imaging Recommendations
- Best imaging tool: CECT
- Protocol advice
  - 150 mL IV contrast at 2.5 mL/sec with 5 mm collimation
  - Delayed images to confirm diffusion of active arterial extravasation

DIFFERENTIAL DIAGNOSIS

Splenic Abscess
- Rounded, irregular, low attenuation lesion
  - Clinical signs of infection
  - Associated with fever, ↑ white blood cell count, left pleural effusion

Splenic Infarct
- Wedge-shaped area of low attenuation
  - Associated with splenomegaly, systemic embolization
- Infarct may evolve into abscess

Splenic Cyst
- Rounded hypoechoic lesion on US
- Definable cyst wall
- No internal enhancement on CECT

Lymphoma
- Single or multiple hypodense lesions
  - Splenomegaly
- Hypoechoic on US with minimal color Doppler flow

PATHOLOGY

General Features
- General path comments: Laceration, fractures or subcapsular hematoma
- Etiology: Blunt trauma with blow to LUQ
- Epidemiology
  - Most commonly injured solid abdominal organ in blunt trauma
  - Most common abdominal organ injury requiring surgery
- Associated abnormalities: Injuries to left thorax, tail of pancreas, left liver lobe and/or mesentery

Gross Pathologic & Surgical Features
- Varies according to extent of injury

Microscopic Features
- Necrotic injured tissue with surrounding hematoma

Staging, Grading or Classification Criteria
- Grading may be misleading; minor injuries may go on to devastating delayed bleed

SPLENIC TRAUMA

- Current CT grading system emphasizes CECT appearance of active arterial bleed indicating need for intervention (surgery or embolization)
- Clinical grading system based on anatomic extent of injury at surgery (American Association for the Surgery of Trauma)
  - 1: Subcapsular hematoma or laceration < 1 cm
  - 2: Subcapsular hematoma or laceration 1-3 cm
  - 3: Capsular disruption, hematoma > 3 cm, parenchymal hematoma > 3 cm
  - 4A: Active parenchymal or subcapsular bleed, pseudoaneurysm or AV fistula, shattered spleen
  - 4B: Active intraperitoneal bleed

CLINICAL ISSUES

Presentation
- Most common signs/symptoms
  - Blunt abdominal trauma, LUQ pain, hypotension
    - Often associated with left chest pain 2° rib fractures, left lower lobe consolidation or left hemothorax

Natural History & Prognosis
- Prone to develop delayed hemorrhage, excellent prognosis with early intervention (surgery/embolization)
- Identification of active arterial extravasation or pseudoaneurysm is most predictive of need for surgery and failure of non-operative management

Treatment
- Non-operative management for minor injuries
  - Preserves splenic immune function
- Angiographic embolization if active arterial extravasation on CT
- Splenectomy or splenorrhaphy when surgery required

DIAGNOSTIC CHECKLIST

Consider
- Congenital cleft if no hemoperitoneum

Image Interpretation Pearls
- Innocuous injury may lead to life-threatening delayed hemorrhage, especially with anticoagulation

SELECTED REFERENCES

1. Becker CD et al: The trauma concept: the role of MDCT in the diagnosis and management of visceral injuries. Eur Radiol. 15 Suppl 4:D105-9, 2005
2. Chen LY et al: The role of diagnostic algorithms in the management of blunt splenic injury. J Chin Med Assoc. 68(8):373-8, 2005
3. Cooney R et al: Limitations of splenic angioembolization in treating blunt splenic injury. J Trauma. 59(4):926-32; discussion 932, 2005
4. Doody O et al: Blunt trauma to the spleen: ultrasonographic findings. Clin Radiol. 60(9):968-76, 2005
5. Fata P et al: A survey of EAST member practices in blunt splenic injury: a description of current trends and opportunities for improvement. J Trauma. 59(4):836-41; discussion 841-2, 2005
6. Haan JM et al: Nonoperative management of blunt splenic injury: a 5-year experience. J Trauma. 58(3):492-8, 2005
7. Harbrecht BG et al: Is outcome after blunt splenic injury in adults better in high-volume trauma centers? Am Surg. 71(11):942-8; discussion 948-9, 2005
8. Peitzman AB et al: Failure of observation of blunt splenic injury in adults: variability in practice and adverse consequences. J Am Coll Surg. 201(2):179-87, 2005
9. Rhodes CA et al: Clinical outcome of active extravasation in splenic trauma. Emerg Radiol. 11(6):348-52, 2005
10. Rozycki GS et al: Surgeon-performed bedside organ assessment with sonography after trauma (BOAST): a pilot study from the WTA Multicenter Group. J Trauma. 59(6):1356-64, 2005
11. Sharma OP et al: Assessment of nonoperative management of blunt spleen and liver trauma. Am Surg. 71(5):379-86, 2005
12. Shen HB et al: Clinical application of laparoscopic spleen-preserving operation in traumatic spleen rupture. Chin J Traumatol. 8(5):293-6, 2005
13. Smith J et al: Abdominal trauma: a disease in evolution. ANZ J Surg. 75(9):790-4, 2005
14. Shanmuganathan K: Multi-detector row CT imaging of blunt abdominal trauma. Semin Ultrasound CT MR. 25(2):180-204, 2004
15. Wahl WL et al: Blunt splenic injury: operation versus angiographic embolization. Surgery. 136(4):891-9, 2004
16. Katz S et al: Can ultrasonography replace computed tomography in the initial assessment of children with blunt abdominal trauma? J Pediatr Surg. 31(5):649-51, 1996
17. Black JJ et al: Subcapsular hematoma as a predictor of delayed splenic rupture. Am Surg. 58(12):732-5, 1992
18. Jeffrey RB Jr et al: Detection of active intraabdominal arterial hemorrhage: value of dynamic contrast-enhanced CT. AJR Am J Roentgenol. 156(4):725-9, 1991
19. Jeffrey RB Jr: CT diagnosis of blunt hepatic and splenic injuries: a look to the future. Radiology. 171(1):17-8, 1989
20. Orwig D et al: Localized clotted blood as evidence of visceral trauma on CT: the sentinel clot sign. AJR Am J Roentgenol. 153(4):747-9, 1989
21. Federle MP et al: Splenic trauma: evaluation with CT. Radiology. 162(1 Pt 1):69-71, 1987

SPLENIC TRAUMA

IMAGE GALLERY

Typical

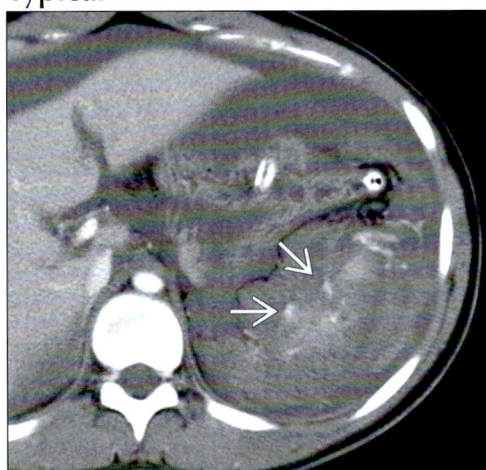
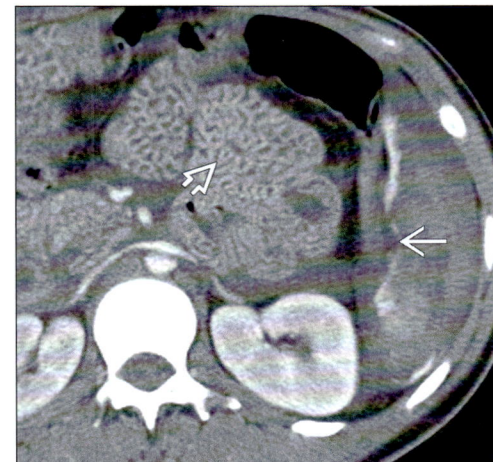

(Left) Axial CECT shows shattered spleen following blunt trauma. Note multiple areas of active arterial extravasation within poorly enhancing spleen ➡. *(Right)* Axial CECT at more caudal level (same patient as left): Note massive arterial extravasation into peritoneal cavity ➡. Thickened small bowel loops ➡, flattened IVC indicates hypoperfusion syndrome.

Typical

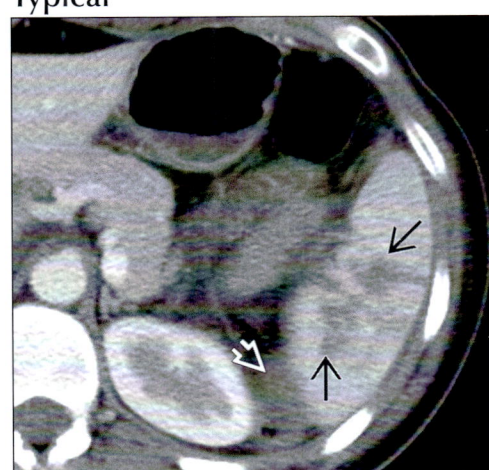
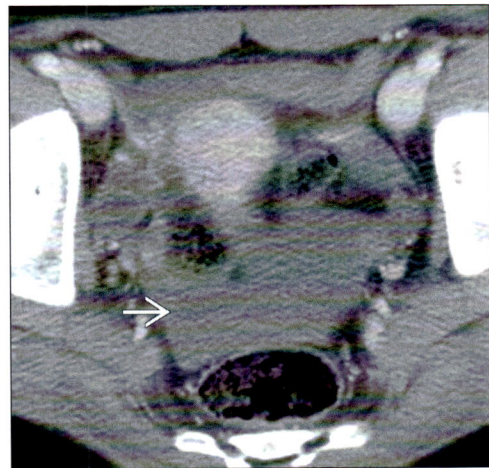

(Left) Axial CECT shows multiple deep splenic lacerations following blunt trauma ➡. Note small amount of perisplenic blood ➡. *(Right)* Axial CECT in same patient as left, shows moderate pelvic hemoperitoneum ➡. Despite hemodynamic stability during scan, patient had massive delayed bleed 24 hours later, requiring urgent surgery.

Variant

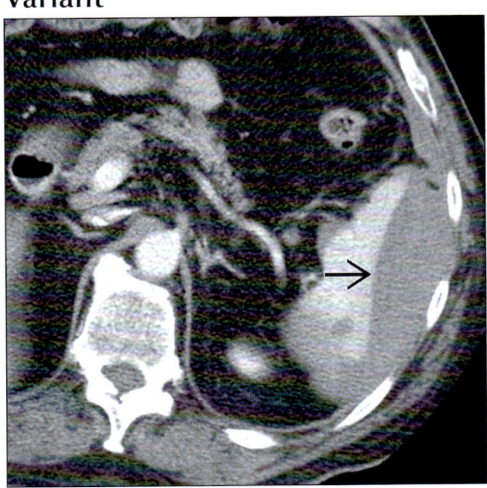
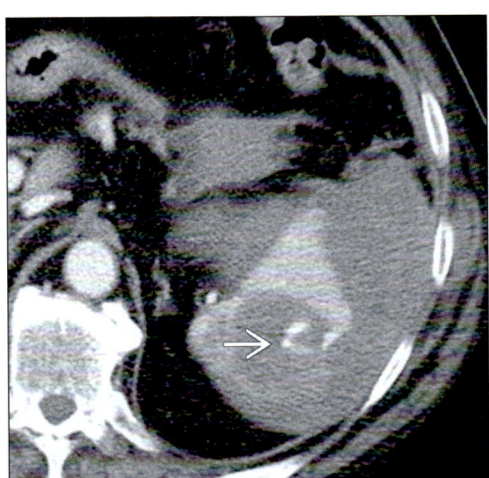

(Left) Axial CECT shows subcapsular hematoma with flattening of lateral contour of spleen ➡. *(Right)* Axial CECT at more caudal level in same patient as left demonstrates active arterial extravasation into subcapsular hematoma ➡.

HEPATIC TRAUMA

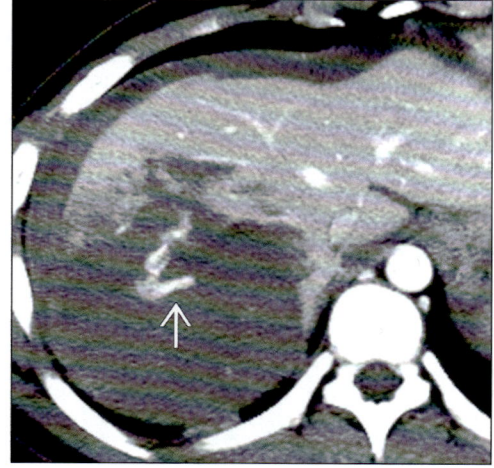

Axial CECT following blunt abdominal trauma. Note high attenuation area of active arterial extravasation ➡ within large avascular hematoma in right lobe.

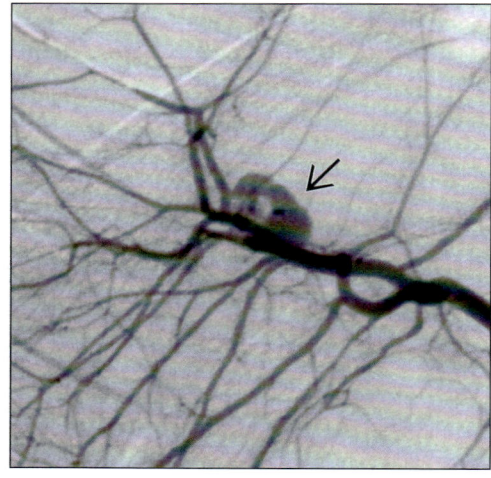

Selective hepatic arteriogram in same patient as left confirms arterial extravasation ➡. This was successfully treated with coil embolization.

TERMINOLOGY

Abbreviations and Synonyms
- Liver or hepatic injury

IMAGING FINDINGS

General Features
- Best diagnostic clue: CT evidence of irregular parenchymal lesions with intra- & perihepatic hemorrhage
- Location
  ○ Right lobe (75%), left lobe (25%)
    ▪ Intraparenchymal or subcapsular
- Key concepts
  ○ Liver 2nd most frequently injured solid intra-abdominal organ after spleen
    ▪ Due to anterior & partially subcostal location
  ○ Most common causes of hepatic trauma
    ▪ Blunt (more common), penetrating & iatrogenic injuries
  ○ Iatrogenic injury due to liver biopsy
    ▪ Most common cause of subcapsular hematoma in US
  ○ Abdominal trauma
    ▪ Leading cause of death in United States (< 40 yrs)

CT Findings
- Lacerations: Simple or stellate (parallel to portal/hepatic vein branches)
  ○ Simple: Hypodense solitary linear laceration
  ○ Stellate: Hypodense branching linear lacerations
- Parenchymal & subcapsular hematomas (lenticular configuration)
  ○ Unclotted blood (35-45 HU) soon after injury
    ▪ NECT: May be hyperdense relative to normal liver
    ▪ CECT: Hypodense compared to enhancing normal liver tissue
  ○ Clotted blood (60-90 HU)
    ▪ More dense than unclotted blood & normal liver
    ▪ May be more dense than unenhanced liver
- Active hemorrhage or pseudoaneurysm
  ○ CECT: Active hemorrhage
    ▪ Isodense to enhanced vessels
    ▪ Seen as contrast extravasation (85-350 HU)

DDx: Focal Liver Lesion with Hemorrhage

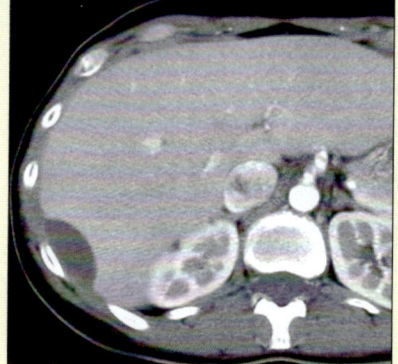

HELLP Syndrome

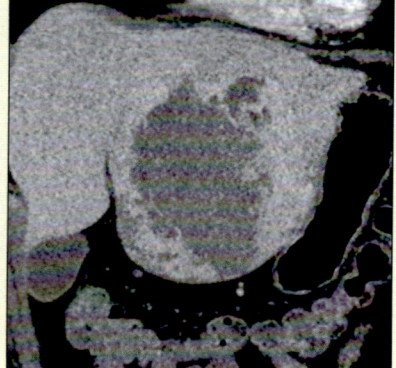

Bleeding Adenoma

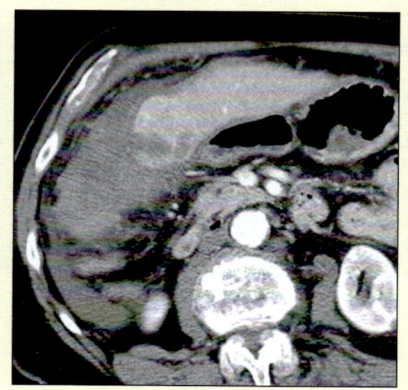

Ruptured HCC

HEPATIC TRAUMA

Key Facts

Imaging Findings
- Best diagnostic clue: CT evidence of irregular parenchymal lesions with intra- & perihepatic hemorrhage
- Right lobe (75%), left lobe (25%)
- Intraparenchymal or subcapsular

Top Differential Diagnoses
- HELLP Syndrome
- Spontaneous Hemorrhage (Coagulopathy)
- Bleeding Hepatic Tumor (e.g., HCC or Adenoma)

Pathology
- Blunt trauma (more common)

Clinical Issues
- Clinical Profile: Patient with history of MVA, RUQ tenderness, guarding & hypotension
- Mortality: 10-20%

Diagnostic Checklist
- Differentiate from HELLP syndrome, spontaneous hemorrhage (coagulopathy) & bleeding hepatic tumors such as HCC or adenoma
- CT evidence of active extravasation (intra- or extra-hepatic collection, isodense with vessels) usually indicates need for embolization or surgery regardless of "grade" of injury
- Laceration of left hepatic lobe often associated with bowel and pancreatic injury

---

- Extravasated contrast material & surrounding decreased attenuation clot
- Hemoperitoneum: Perihepatic and peritoneal recess collections of blood
- Periportal tracking: Linear, focal or diffuse periportal zones of decreased HU
  - Due to dissecting blood, bile or dilated periportal lymphatics
  - DDx: Overhydration (check for distended IVC)
    - Elevated venous pressure & transudation
- Areas of infarction
  - Small or large areas of low attenuation
  - Usually wedge-shaped; segmental or lobar
  - Intrahepatic/subcapsular gas (due to hepatic necrosis)
- CT diagnosis of liver trauma
  - Accuracy: 96%
  - Sensitivity: 100%
  - Specificity: 94%

MR Findings
- T1WI & T2WI
  - Varied signal intensity depending on degree/age of hemorrhage or infarct

Ultrasonographic Findings
- Grayscale Ultrasound
  - Subcapsular hematoma: Lentiform or curvilinear fluid collection
    - Initially: Anechoic
    - After 24 hrs: Echogenic
    - After 4-5 days: Hypoechoic
    - After 1-4 weeks: Internal echoes, septations develop within hematoma
  - Intraparenchymal hematoma
    - Rounded echogenic or hypoechoic foci
  - Bilomas
    - Rounded/ellipsoid, anechoic, loculated structures
    - Well-defined sharp margins, close to bile ducts
  - Parenchymal tears
    - Irregular defects
    - Abnormal echotexture relative to normal liver

Angiographic Findings
- Conventional
  - Active extravasation, pseudoaneurysm
  - A-V, arteriobiliary or portobiliary fistulas

Imaging Recommendations
- Best imaging tool
  - MDCT: In hemodynamically stable cases
  - Angiography: To localize active hemorrhage & embolization
- Protocol advice: MDCT: Include lung bases and pelvis

DIFFERENTIAL DIAGNOSIS

HELLP Syndrome
- Severe variant of preeclampsia
- HELLP: Hemolysis, elevated liver enzymes & low platelets
- Wedge-shaped areas of infarction
- Intrahepatic or subcapsular fluid collection (hematoma)
- Occasionally active extravasation

Spontaneous Hemorrhage (Coagulopathy)
- History of bleeding disorder
- Lab data: Abnormal hematologic coagulation values
- Subcapsular or intrahepatic blood collection
- Indistinguishable from hepatic trauma without history

Bleeding Hepatic Tumor (e.g., HCC or Adenoma)
- Spherical enhancing parenchymal masses
- Hepatocellular carcinoma (HCC)
  - Vascular, nodal & visceral invasion (common)

PATHOLOGY

General Features
- Etiology
  - Blunt trauma (more common)

HEPATIC TRAUMA

- Motor vehicle accidents (more common)
- Falls and assaults
  ○ Penetrating injuries
    - Gunshot and stab injuries
  ○ Iatrogenic
    - Liver biopsy, chest tubes, transhepatic cholangiography
- Epidemiology
  ○ 5-10% blunt abdominal trauma have liver injury
  ○ Mortality from hepatic trauma: 10-20%
- Associated abnormalities
  ○ Splenic injury (45%); bowel injury (5%); rib fractures
  ○ Left hepatic lobe laceration often associated with bowel or pancreatic injury

Gross Pathologic & Surgical Features
- Laceration or contusion
- Subcapsular or intraparenchymal hematoma

Staging, Grading or Classification Criteria
- Clinical classification based on American Association for the Surgery of Trauma (AAST)
  ○ Grade I
    - Subcapsular hematoma: < 10% surface area
    - Laceration: Capsular tear, < 1 cm parenchymal depth
  ○ Grade II
    - Subcapsular hematoma: 10-50% surface area
    - Intraparenchymal hematoma: < 10 cm diameter
    - Laceration: 1-3 cm parenchymal depth, < 10 cm length
  ○ Grade III
    - Subcapsular hematoma: > 50% surface area; expanding/ruptured subcapsular or parenchymal hematoma
    - Intraparenchymal hematoma: > 10 cm or expanding
    - Laceration: Parenchymal fracture > 3 cm deep
  ○ Grade IV
    - Laceration: Parenchymal disruption involving 25-75% of hepatic lobe or 1-3 Couinaud segments within a single lobe
  ○ Grade V
    - Laceration: Parenchymal disruption involving > 75% of hepatic lobe or > 3 Couinaud segments within a single lobe
    - Vascular: Juxtahepatic venous injuries (retrohepatic vena cava, major hepatic veins)
  ○ Grade VI
    - Vascular: Hepatic avulsion

CLINICAL ISSUES

Presentation
- Most common signs/symptoms
  ○ RUQ pain, tenderness, guarding, rebound tenderness
  ○ Hypotension, tachycardia, jaundice
  ○ Hematemesis or melena (due to hemobilia)
- Clinical Profile: Patient with history of MVA, RUQ tenderness, guarding & hypotension
- Lab data
  ○ Decreased hematocrit (not acutely)
  ○ Increased direct/indirect bilirubin
  ○ Increased alkaline phosphatase levels

Natural History & Prognosis
- Complications
  ○ Hemobilia, bilomas, A-V fistula, pseudoaneurysm
- Prognosis
  ○ Grade I, II & III: Good
  ○ Grade IV, V & VI: Poor
  ○ May not necessarily correlate with AAST grading
  ○ Mortality: 10-20%
    - 50% due to liver injury itself
    - Remainder due to associated injuries

Treatment
- Grade I, II, III
  ○ Conservative management for most injuries diagnosed on CT
- Grade IV, V, VI
  ○ Surgical intervention for shock & peritonitis
    - Control hemorrhage, drainage & repair
  ○ Embolization for active extravasation

DIAGNOSTIC CHECKLIST

Consider
- Differentiate from HELLP syndrome, spontaneous hemorrhage (coagulopathy) & bleeding hepatic tumors such as HCC or adenoma

Image Interpretation Pearls
- CT evidence of active extravasation (intra- or extra-hepatic collection, isodense with vessels) usually indicates need for embolization or surgery regardless of "grade" of injury
- Laceration of left hepatic lobe often associated with bowel and pancreatic injury

SELECTED REFERENCES

1. Cox JC et al: Routine follow-up imaging is unnecessary in the management of blunt hepatic injury. J Trauma. 59(5):1175-8; discussion 1178-80, 2005
2. Sharma OP et al: Assessment of nonoperative management of blunt spleen and liver trauma. Am Surg. 71(5):379-86, 2005
3. Yao DC et al: Using contrast-enhanced helical CT to visualize arterial extravasation after blunt abdominal trauma: incidence and organ distribution. AJR. 178(1):17-20, 2002
4. Patten RM et al: CT detection of hepatic and splenic injuries: usefulness of liver window settings. AJR. 175(4):1107-10, 2000
5. Poletti PA et al: CT criteria for management of blunt liver trauma: correlation with angiographic and surgical findings. Radiology. 216(2):418-27, 2000
6. Becker CD et al: Blunt hepatic trauma in adults: correlation of CT injury grading with outcome. Radiology. 201(1):215-20, 1996
7. Mirvis SE et al: Blunt hepatic trauma in adults: CT-based classification and correlation with prognosis and treatment. Radiology. 171(1):27-32, 1989

HEPATIC TRAUMA

IMAGE GALLERY

Typical

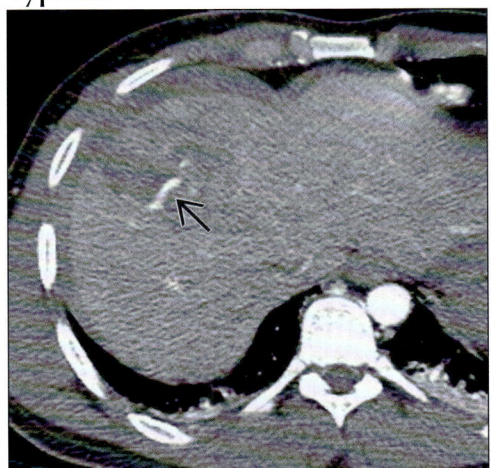
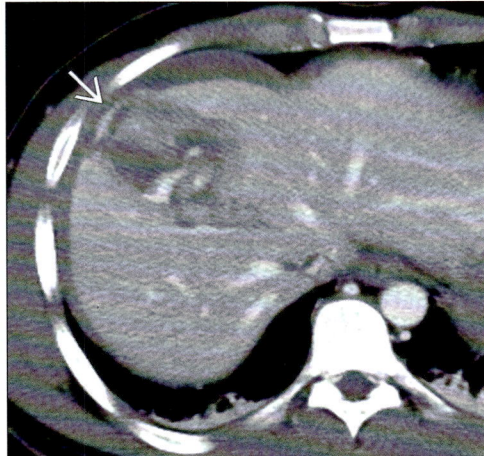

(Left) Axial arterial phase CECT following blunt abdominal trauma. Note high attenuation area of active arterial extravasation within right lobe hematoma ➡. *(Right)* Axial portal phase CECT image of same patient as left more clearly demonstrates extent of hepatic laceration & delineates extension of arterial leakage into adjacent peritoneal cavity ➡.

Typical

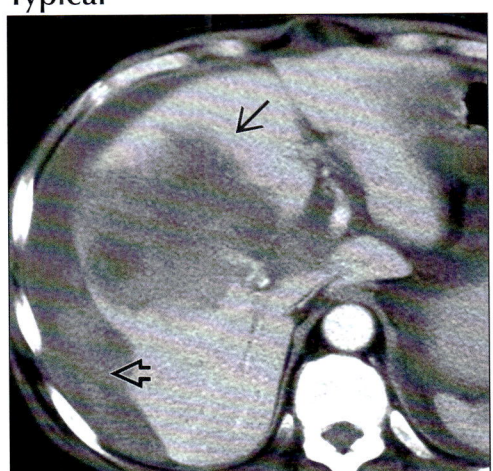
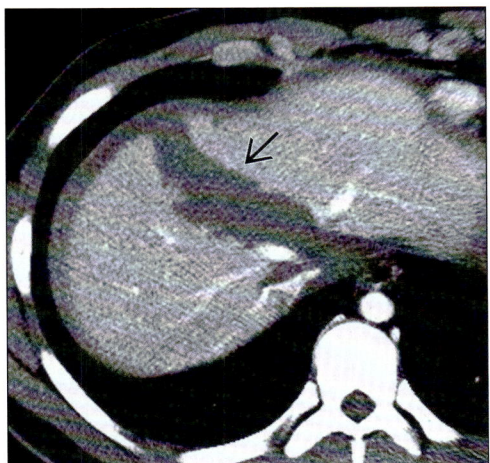

(Left) Axial CECT shows hepatic fracture following blunt trauma. Note large right lobe hematoma ➡ extending from peritoneal surface to liver hilum. Adjacent perihepatic clot is present ➡. *(Right)* Axial CECT shows hepatic fracture. Note fracture plane ➡ extending along middle hepatic vein. There is no arterial extravasation, and no surgery was required.

Variant

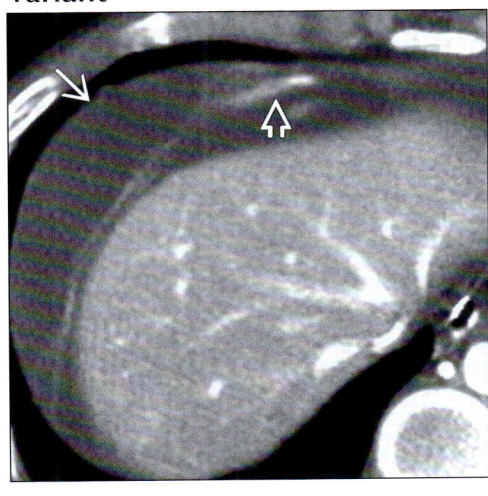
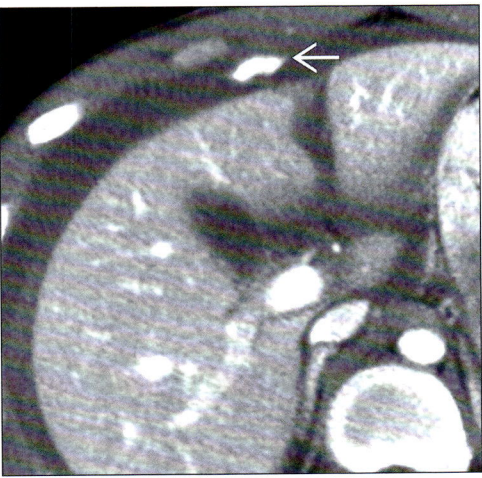

(Left) Axial CECT shows phrenic artery injury following blunt trauma. Note perihepatic hematoma ➡ and enhancing phrenic artery ➡. *(Right)* Axial CECT at lower plane of section in same patient as left demonstrates active arterial extravasation from phrenic artery ➡.

RENAL TRAUMA

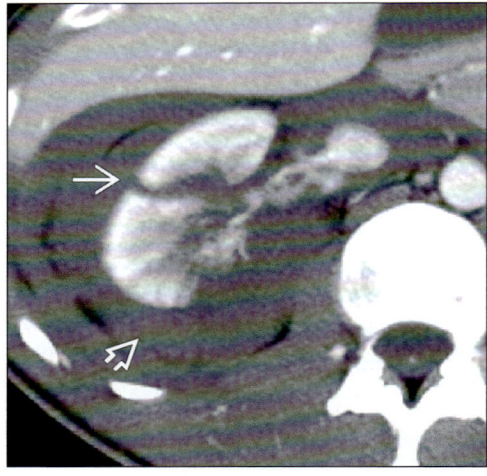

Axial CECT shows renal fracture following blunt trauma. Note linear fracture ➡ traversing renal parenchyma and large perinephric hematoma ⮫.

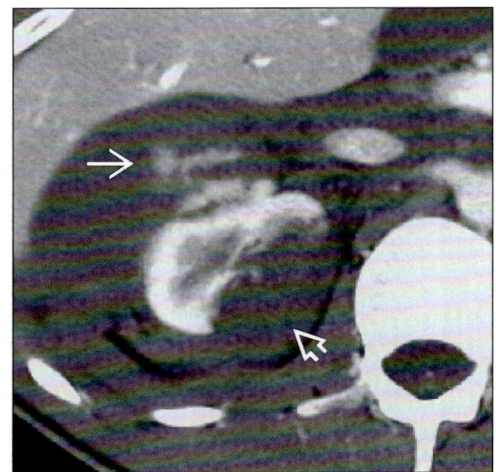

Axial CECT shows active extravasation into perinephric space ➡ & large avascular area in posterior half of kidney ⮫ due to intimal dissection and occlusion of segmental artery.

TERMINOLOGY

Definitions
- Injury to the kidney

IMAGING FINDINGS

General Features
- Best diagnostic clue: Renal parenchymal defect with perirenal hemorrhage ± extravasation of blood/urine
- Other general features
  o Seen in 8-10% of patients with blunt or penetrating abdominal injuries (80-90% are blunt)
  o Serious renal injuries usually associated with multi-organ involvement
    ▪ Due to penetrating trauma: 80% of cases
    ▪ Due to blunt trauma: 75% of cases
  o 98% of isolated renal injuries are minor & require no specific therapy

Radiographic Findings
- IVP
  o Grade I: Normal
  o Grade II-IV: Delayed, absent excretion or extravasation

CT Findings
- Grade I
  o Intrarenal hematoma or contusion
    ▪ Ill-defined, round or ovoid lesion
    ▪ Parenchymal phase: ↓ Enhancement relative to normal kidney
    ▪ Delayed phase: Hyperdense due to urine stasis + clot-filled tubules
  o Subcapsular hematoma
    ▪ Round or elliptical fluid collection (40-70 HU clotted blood)
  o Minor lacerations: Small linear hypodense areas in periphery
  o Limited perinephric hematoma adjacent to laceration
  o Subsegmental cortical infarct
    ▪ Small, sharply demarcated, wedge-shaped decreased attenuation area → scar
- Grade II
  o Major laceration through cortex extending to medulla

DDx: Parenchymal Lesion & Perirenal Fluid

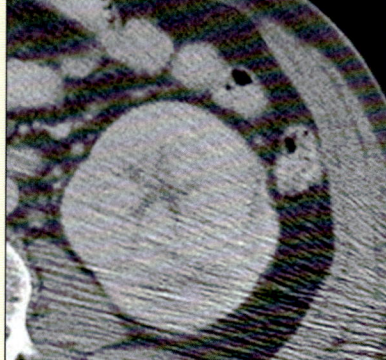

Renal Tumor

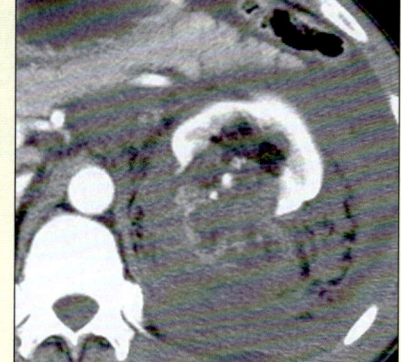

Bleeding Angiomyolipoma

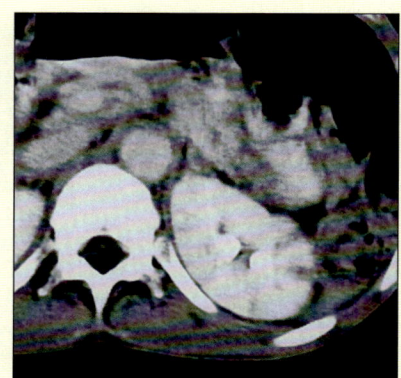

Polyarteritis

RENAL TRAUMA

Key Facts

Imaging Findings
- Best diagnostic clue: Renal parenchymal defect with perirenal hemorrhage ± extravasation of blood/urine
- Segmental renal infarct: Sharply demarcated, wedge-shaped area of decreased enhancement
- Global infarction (nonenhancement) + no perinephric hematoma: Renal artery thrombosis
- Global infarction (nonenhancement) + perinephric hematoma: Renal artery avulsion
- Protocol advice: For any renal laceration evident on CT, must obtain 8-10 minute delayed scans to evaluate for urinary extravasation

Top Differential Diagnoses
- Renal Tumor
- Vasculitis

Pathology
- Blunt, penetrating & deceleration injuries
- Other organ injuries in 75% of cases

Clinical Issues
- Flank pain, tenderness, ecchymosis
- Hematuria, anuria, uremia, shock
- Poor correlation between degree of hematuria & severity of renal injury

Diagnostic Checklist
- Possibility of underlying tumor if bleeding seems disproportionate to degree of trauma
- Arterial extravasation usually requires catheter embolization
- Urinary extravasation often requires ureteral stent ± catheter drainage of urinoma

---

    - Long irregular or linear hypodense area
  - Laceration may extend into collecting system
    - Nephrographic phase: Large, distracted renal fracture (hypodense)
    - Excretory phase: Contrast extravasation into perinephric space
    - ± Antegrade filling of ureter
  - Segmental renal infarct: Sharply demarcated, wedge-shaped area of decreased enhancement
- Grade III
  - Multiple renal lacerations & vascular injury
    - Nephrographic phase: Several irregular, linear or band-like interpolar hypodense areas ± areas of active arterial contrast extravasation
  - Subacute infarction
    - "Cortical rim" sign: Preserved capsular or subcapsular enhancement 6-8 hrs post-infarction
  - "Shattered kidney"
    - Segmental infarction: Nonenhancing wedge-shaped area (devitalized upper or lower renal pole branch)
    - Global infarction (nonenhancement) + no perinephric hematoma: Renal artery thrombosis
    - Global infarction (nonenhancement) + perinephric hematoma: Renal artery avulsion
- Grade IV
  - Ureteropelvic junction: Complete transection (avulsion) or laceration
    - Good excretion of contrast, medial perinephric extravasation
    - Circumferential urinoma may be seen around affected kidney

Imaging Recommendations
- Protocol advice: For any renal laceration evident on CT, must obtain 8-10 minute delayed scans to evaluate for urinary extravasation
- CECT: Gold standard imaging
- IVU: Limited urography (to evaluate hemodynamically unstable patient)
  - Plain film abdomen, 100-150 ml of 60% IV contrast, immediate "cone down" nephrogram film, full film after 8 minutes
  - "One-shot IVU": Assessment of normal kidney, not evaluation of injured kidney
- Retrograde pyelography: Assess ureteral & renal pelvic injuries
- US: Assess hemoperitoneum in hemodynamically unstable patient

DIFFERENTIAL DIAGNOSIS

Renal Tumor
- Spontaneous bleed/rupture may be seen
- Perinephric fluid collection of blood density
- Underlying renal mass lesion
  - Renal cell carcinoma (RCC)
    - Solid renal mass, usually hypervascular
    - Renal vein/IVC extension possible
    - Hypervascular metastatic foci common
  - Angiomyolipoma (AML)
    - Vascular, smooth muscle & fat components
    - Renal mass with variable amounts of fat is diagnostic
    - May significantly enhance with contrast

Vasculitis
- Polyarteritis nodosa, SLE, scleroderma, drug abuse
- Wedge-shaped or striated nephrogram
- Capsular retraction over parenchymal lesions
- Microaneurysms of small vessels

PATHOLOGY

General Features
- Etiology
  - Motor vehicle accidents (MVA), falls, assault
    - Blunt, penetrating & deceleration injuries
  - Children: Kidneys relatively large, more mobile, more vulnerable to trauma
- Epidemiology: Renal trauma accounts for 8-10% of all blunt abdominal trauma injuries
- Associated abnormalities
  - Other organ injuries in 75% of cases

RENAL TRAUMA

- Liver, spleen, bowel, pancreas

Gross Pathologic & Surgical Features
- Contusion, laceration, hematoma, infarction, vascular or ureteropelvic injury

Microscopic Features
- Contusion, laceration, ischemia of cortico-medullary or collecting system

Staging, Grading or Classification Criteria
- Grade I
  - 75-85% of all renal injuries
  - Minor injury (contusion, intrarenal/subcapsular hematoma)
  - Minor laceration, limited perinephric hematoma
  - No extension to collecting system or medulla
  - Small subsegmental cortical infarct
- Grade II
  - 10% of all renal injuries
  - Major injury (major cortical laceration, extension to medulla & collecting system
  - With or without urine extravasation or segmental renal infarct
- Grade III
  - 5% of cases
  - Catastrophic injury (multiple renal lacerations, vascular injury involving renal pedicle)
- Grade IV
  - Rare consequence
  - Ureteropelvic junction injury: Complete transection or laceration

CLINICAL ISSUES

Presentation
- Most common signs/symptoms
  - Flank pain, tenderness, ecchymosis
  - Hematuria, anuria, uremia, shock
  - Poor correlation between degree of hematuria & severity of renal injury
    - 14% of major, 10% of minor injuries may not have hematuria
- Clinical Profile: History of MVA, flank pain, hematuria or anuria
- Lab data: Hematuria (> 5 RBCs per high power field)
- Diagnosis: Clinical/classic imaging features diagnostic of renal trauma

Demographics
- Age: Any age group (children more vulnerable than adults)
- Gender: M = F

Natural History & Prognosis
- Complications
  - Early: Urinoma, perinephric abscess, sepsis, AV fistula, pseudoaneurysm
  - Late: Hydronephrosis, HTN, calculus formation, chronic pyelonephritis, renal failure & atrophy
- Prognosis
  - Grade I & II: Good
  - Grade III & IV
    - Unilateral after treatment: Good
    - Bilateral: Poor

Treatment
- Grade I & II: Conservative therapy
- Grade III & IV
  - Active bleeding: Angioembolization
  - Renal artery thrombosis: Anticoagulants, stent placement
  - Active urinary extravasation: Consider ureteral stent & catheter drainage
  - Indications for surgery
    - Vascular (renal pedicle) injury
    - Shattered kidney
    - Expanding or pulsatile hematoma
    - Shocked polytrauma patient
  - Severely damaged kidney: Surgical nephrectomy

DIAGNOSTIC CHECKLIST

Consider
- Possibility of underlying tumor if bleeding seems disproportionate to degree of trauma

Image Interpretation Pearls
- Arterial extravasation usually requires catheter embolization
- Urinary extravasation often requires ureteral stent ± catheter drainage of urinoma

SELECTED REFERENCES
1. Smith JK et al: Imaging of renal trauma. Radiol Clin North Am. 41(5):1019-35, 2003
2. Kawashima A et al: Imaging evaluation of posttraumatic renal injuries. Abdom Imaging. 27(2):199-213, 2002
3. Yao DC et al: Using contrast-enhanced helical CT to visualize arterial extravasation after blunt abdominal trauma: incidence and organ distribution. AJR Am J Roentgenol. 178(1):17-20, 2002
4. Harris AC et al: Ct findings in blunt renal trauma. Radiographics. 21 Spec No:S201-14, 2001
5. Kawashima A et al: Imaging of renal trauma: a comprehensive review. Radiographics. 21(3):557-74, 2001
6. Mizobata Y et al: Successful evaluation of pseudoaneurysm formation after blunt renal injury with dual-phase contrast-enhanced helical CT. AJR Am J Roentgenol. 177(1):136-8, 2001
7. Morey AF et al: Single shot intraoperative excretory urography for the immediate evaluation of renal trauma. J Urol. 161(4):1088-92, 1999
8. Kawashima A et al: Ureteropelvic junction injuries secondary to blunt abdominal trauma. Radiology. 205(2):487-92, 1997
9. Mirvis SE: Trauma. Radiol Clin North Am. 34(6):1225-57, 1996
10. Pollack HM et al: Imaging of renal trauma. Radiology. 172(2):297-308, 1989
11. Federle MP et al: Penetrating renal trauma: CT evaluation. J Comput Assist Tomogr. 11(6):1026-30, 1987
12. Lang EK et al: Renal trauma: radiological studies. Comparison of urography, computed tomography, angiography, and radionuclide studies. Radiology. 154(1):1-6, 1985
13. Federle MP et al: The role of computed tomography in renal trauma. Radiology. 141(2):455-60, 1981

RENAL TRAUMA

IMAGE GALLERY

Typical

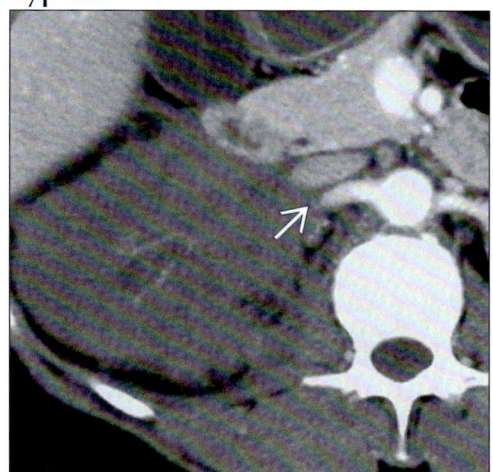
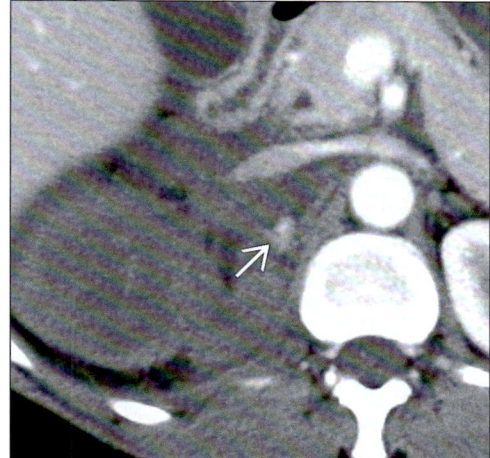

(Left) Axial CECT shows traumatic renal artery occlusion. Note abrupt cut-off of right renal artery ➔ and global lack of enhancement of right kidney. *(Right)* Axial CECT lower plane of section in same patient as previous image demonstrates paralumbar active extravasation from lumbar artery injury ➔.

Typical

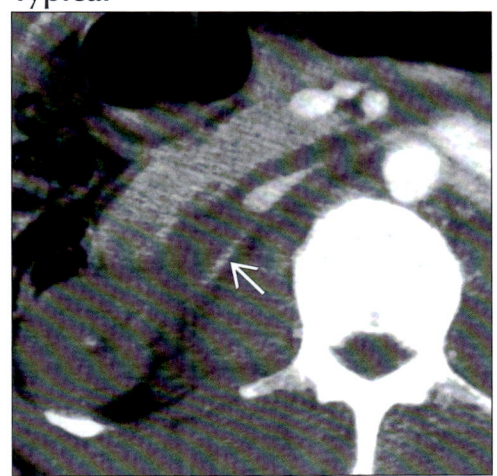
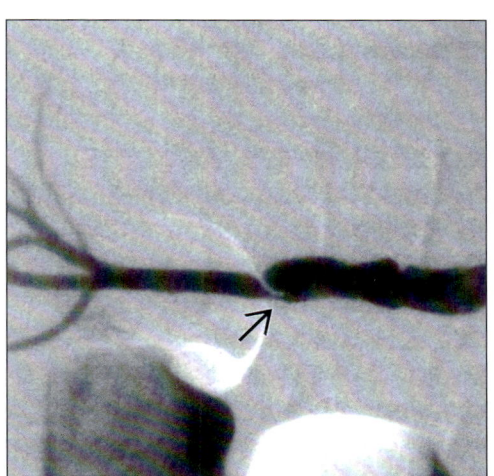

(Left) Axial CECT shows intimal dissection of main renal artery following blunt trauma. Note markedly decreased enhancement of right kidney with only minimal flow identified in right renal artery ➔. *(Right)* Selective right renal arteriogram confirms renal artery dissection with high grade obstruction ➔.

Variant

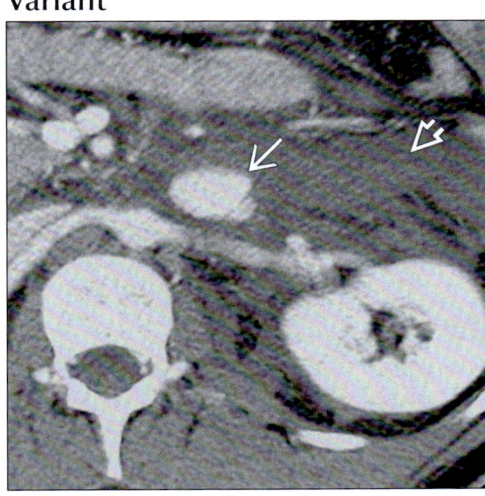
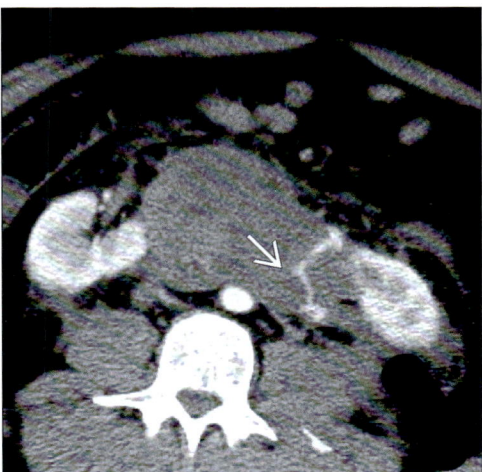

(Left) Axial CECT shows renal vein injury following blunt trauma. Note active extravasation from left renal vein ➔ & large perirenal hematoma ➔. Renal parenchyma was not injured. *(Right)* Axial CECT shows injury to isthmus of horseshoe kidney. Note midline hematoma containing high attenuation area of active arterial extravasation from isthmus ➔.

PANCREATIC TRAUMA

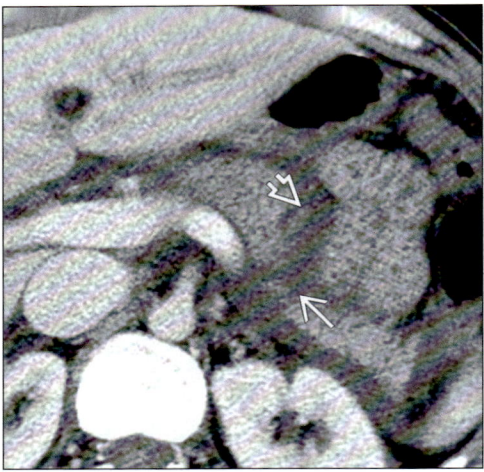

Axial CECT shows pancreatic fracture following blunt trauma. Note fracture in mid-body of pancreas ➡ and adjacent fluid in lesser sac ➡.

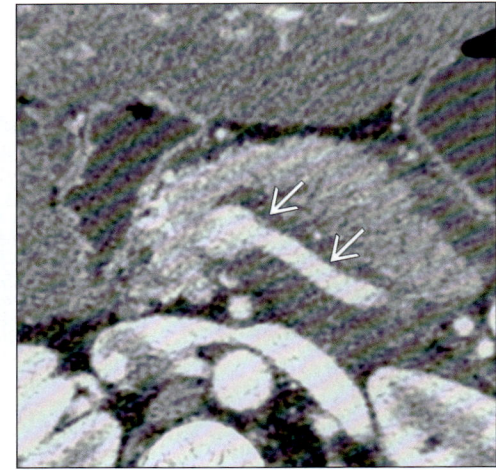

Axial CECT at lower plane of section (in same patient as previous image) demonstrates fluid dissection posterior to the pancreas anterior to splenic vein ➡.

TERMINOLOGY

Abbreviations and Synonyms
- Traumatic pancreatic injury

Definitions
- Inflammatory disease of pancreas secondary to trauma

IMAGING FINDINGS

General Features
- Best diagnostic clue: Enlargement of gland, heterogeneous parenchyma, peripancreatic fluid collections, history of trauma
- Morphology: Spectrum of injury: Acute pancreatitis, contusions, deep lacerations, fractures with ductal disruption

Radiographic Findings
- ERCP
  - Normal in cases of pancreatic "contusion"
  - Transection of pancreatic duct: Abrupt duct termination or contrast extravasation
  - Communication of pseudocyst with pancreatic duct
  - May cause pancreatitis

CT Findings
- Focal/diffuse pancreatic enlargement
- Irregularity of pancreatic contour
- Edema/fluid in peripancreatic fat
  - Loss of normal fat plane: Peripancreatic infiltration
- Heterogeneous parenchymal attenuation
- Thickening of anterior renal fascia
- Peripancreatic soft tissue changes of traumatic pancreatitis are often subtle; becoming more evident within 24-48 hours
- Laceration
  - Area of low attenuation (actual size of laceration difficult to visualize)
  - Linear cleft, usually oriented anteroposteriorly
- Pancreatic fracture or transection
  - Ill-defined low density area
  - Results in clear separation of two ends of gland
  - Nearly always extends through pancreatic neck
  - Retropancreatic fluid anterior to splenic vein
- Lacerations/fractures may produce subtle parenchymal density changes; may be undetectable on CT

DDx: Lesions Mimicking Pancreatic Trauma

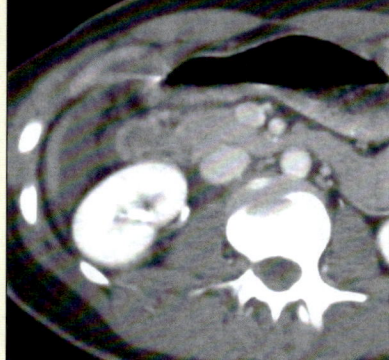

Duodenal Rupture

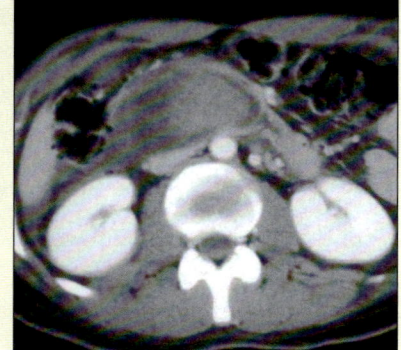

Duodenal Hematoma

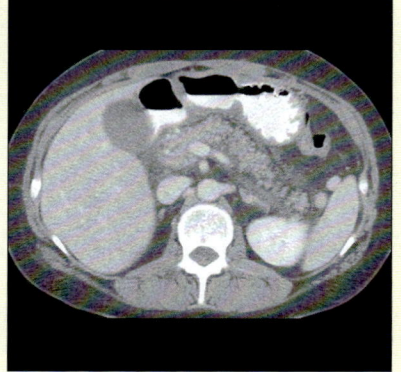

Pancreatitis

PANCREATIC TRAUMA

Key Facts

Imaging Findings
- Best diagnostic clue: Enlargement of gland, heterogeneous parenchyma, peripancreatic fluid collections, history of trauma
- Morphology: Spectrum of injury: Acute pancreatitis, contusions, deep lacerations, fractures with ductal disruption
- Irregularity of pancreatic contour
- Edema/fluid in peripancreatic fat
- Rupture of main pancreatic duct (MPD) (23%)
- Protocol advice: 24-48 hours delayed scans may uncover findings not present earlier

Top Differential Diagnoses
- "Shock" Pancreas
- Intramural Duodenal Hematoma ± Duodenal Rupture
- Pancreatitis

Pathology
- Penetrating/blunt trauma
- Pancreatic trauma uncommon, 3-12% of all abdominal injuries

Clinical Issues
- Complications: Recurrent pancreatitis, pseudocyst, hemorrhage, pseudoaneurysm, fistula, abscess
- Mortality from pancreatic injuries is nearly 20%

Diagnostic Checklist
- CT diagnosis of pancreatic trauma may be difficult in patients scanned soon after injury
- CT signs of traumatic pancreatitis become more evident after 24-48 hours

---

- Extrapancreatic fluid collections: Perivascular, transverse mesocolon, pararenal space, lesser sac, juxtasplenic, mesenteric root
- Pancreatic contusion/hematoma: Range from apparent contour deformity of pancreas to rounded mass several centimeters in diameter
  - Peripancreatic hematoma may mimic fluid-filled proximal small bowel loop
  - Frequently concomitant injury to liver (left lobe) and bowel
- Pancreatitis caused by ERCP (+/- papillotomy, etc.) usually more severe in & around pancreatic head

MR Findings
- T1WI: Variable decreased signal intensity
- T2WI: Fluid collections & pseudocyst: Hyperintense on fat-suppressed T2WI
- T1 C+
  - Heterogeneous enhancement pattern
  - Nonenhancing hypointense areas (fluid collection, pseudocyst, necrosis)
- MRCP
  - Rupture of main pancreatic duct (MPD) (23%)
  - Pseudocyst contiguous with MPD

Ultrasonographic Findings
- US (& CT) findings in traumatic pancreatitis may be similar to nontraumatic pancreatitis
- Not as sensitive as CT in diagnosing acute injury

Imaging Recommendations
- Best imaging tool
  - CT is more accurate for detecting extrapancreatic fluid collections, pancreatic lacerations or fractures
  - Emergency ERCP: Investigate pancreatic injuries when CT positive but status of pancreatic duct is uncertain
- Protocol advice: 24-48 hours delayed scans may uncover findings not present earlier

DIFFERENTIAL DIAGNOSIS

"Shock" Pancreas
- "Hypoperfusion complex" in severe injuries
- Abnormally intense enhancement of pancreas, bowel wall & kidneys
- Moderate to large peritoneal fluid collections
- Decreased caliber of aorta & inferior vena cava
- Diffuse dilatation of intestine with fluid
- Mesenteric & peripancreatic fat planes infiltrated
- Findings resolve spontaneously within 24 hours of fluid resuscitation

Intramural Duodenal Hematoma ± Duodenal Rupture
- Hematoma
  - Focal high attenuation thickening of duodenal wall
  - "Picket-fence appearance" from hemorrhage
  - Smooth intramural mass causing incomplete bowel obstruction
- Rupture
  - Air-fluid level in adjacent extraperitoneal space
  - Gas or fluid tracking into anterior pararenal space
  - Extravasation of oral contrast into anterior pararenal space
- May simulate or coexist with pancreatic injury

Pancreatitis
- Diffuse or focal pancreatic enlargement
- Low attenuation areas of nonenhancement (necrosis)
- Peripancreatic fluid in lesser sac and/or anterior pararenal space

PATHOLOGY

General Features
- Etiology
  - Penetrating/blunt trauma
    - Gunshot (45%), blunt (37%), stab wound (18%)
  - Mechanism in blunt trauma

PANCREATIC TRAUMA

- Compression against vertebral column with shear across pancreatic neck
- Relatively fixed position of pancreas anterior to spine
- Children: Trauma from bicycle handlebar, motor vehicle accident, child abuse
- Lacerations usually accompany midline compression injury, may involve left hepatic lobe, duodenum, central renal vascular pedicle
- Endoscopic procedures
  - ERCP, especially with papillotomy, stone extraction, stent placement
- Surgery: Billroth II resections, splenectomy, biliary surgery, aortic graft surgery
- Epidemiology
  - Pancreatic trauma uncommon, 3-12% of all abdominal injuries
  - Acute post-traumatic pancreatitis is infrequent disease, representing 0.4% of acute pancreatitis with pseudocyst formation
  - Penetrating injuries more common than blunt trauma
  - Combined injury of other organs seen in 80% of patients
  - Accounts for about 5% of all abdominal injuries in children
  - Trauma is most common cause of pseudocyst in children (often related to child abuse)

Staging, Grading or Classification Criteria

- Grade 1: Contusion/hematoma, pancreatic duct intact
- Grade 2: Parenchymal injury, pancreatic duct intact
- Grade 3: Major ductal injury
- Grade 4: Severe crush injury
- Grade of pancreatic injury is independent predictor of pancreatic complications & mortality

CLINICAL ISSUES

Presentation

- Most common signs/symptoms
  - History of traumatic injury
  - Upper abdominal pain
  - Postprandial vomiting, abdominal distention
- Clinical Profile
  - Serum amylase/lipase levels: Elevated in 90% of patients, may be normal immediately after trauma
  - Leukocytosis, hyperamylasemia
  - Diagnosis: Exploratory laparotomy
  - Blunt injuries to pancreas may be clinically occult & may go unrecognized on initial evaluation

Demographics

- Gender: More frequently seen in males (69%)

Natural History & Prognosis

- Complications: Recurrent pancreatitis, pseudocyst, hemorrhage, pseudoaneurysm, fistula, abscess
- Subcutaneous fat necrosis/polyarthritis secondary to post-traumatic pancreatitis reported in < 1% of patients with pancreatic disease
- Cerebral fat embolism is a rare possible complication of traumatic pancreatitis

- Mortality from pancreatic injuries is nearly 20%
- Morbidity (42%)
  - Pancreatic fistula (11%)
  - Pancreatitis (7%)
  - Pancreatic pseudocyst (3%)
  - Intra-abdominal abscesses (8%)
  - Associated liver or intestinal injuries (> 80%)
- Morbidity higher with external drainage compared to exploration without drainage

Treatment

- Grades 1 & 2: Conservative management
  - Total parenteral nutrition
  - Somatostatin or octreotide
  - More recently, endoscopy with pancreatic stenting
  - Superficial lesions not affecting major pancreatic duct can be managed nonoperatively
- Grades 3 & 4: Require surgery within 24 hours
  - Penetrating trauma generally requires immediate laparotomy
  - Surgical drainage
  - Partial pancreatectomy
  - Persistently elevated serum amylase levels, increasing cyst size are indications for surgery

DIAGNOSTIC CHECKLIST

Consider

- CT diagnosis of pancreatic trauma may be difficult in patients scanned soon after injury
- Thickening of anterior renal fascia on CT of trauma patient should prompt critical evaluation of pancreas
- CT signs of traumatic pancreatitis become more evident after 24-48 hours

SELECTED REFERENCES

1. Buccimazza I et al: Isolated main pancreatic duct injuries spectrum and management. Am J Surg. 191(4):448-52, 2006
2. Fang JF et al: Usefulness of multidetector computed tomography for the initial assessment of blunt abdominal trauma patients. World J Surg. 30(2):176-82, 2006
3. Cay A et al: Nonoperative treatment of traumatic pancreatic duct disruption in children with an endoscopically placed stent. J Pediatr Surg. 40(12):e9-12, 2005
4. Krige JE et al: The management of complex pancreatic injuries. S Afr J Surg. 43(3):92-102, 2005
5. Stringer MD: Pancreatitis and pancreatic trauma. Semin Pediatr Surg. 14(4):239-46, 2005
6. Kao LS et al: Predictors of morbidity after traumatic pancreatic injury. J Trauma. 55(5):898-905, 2003
7. Mayer JM et al: Pancreatic injury in severe trauma: early diagnosis and therapy improve the outcome. Dig Surg. 19(4):291-7; discussion 297-9, 2002
8. Akhrass R et al: Pancreatic trauma: a ten-year multi-institutional experience. Am Surg. 63(7):598-604, 1997
9. Lewis G et al: Traumatic pancreatic pseudocysts. Br J Surg. 80(1):89-93, 1993
10. Jeffrey RB Jr et al: Computed tomography of pancreatic trauma. Radiology. 147(2):491-4, 1983

PANCREATIC TRAUMA

IMAGE GALLERY

Typical

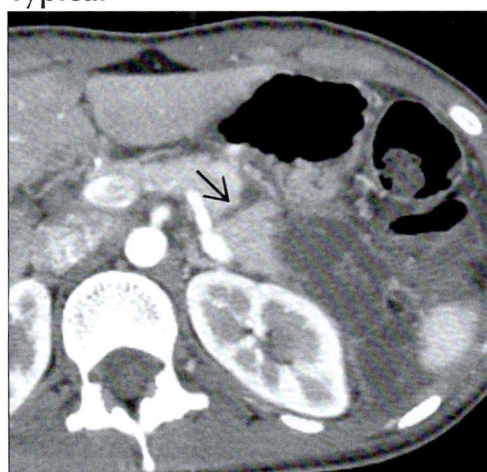
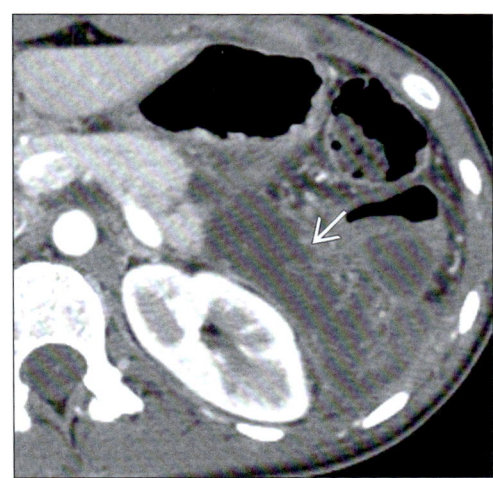

(Left) Axial CECT of missed pancreatic fracture. Scan performed 48 hours after blunt trauma reveals linear fracture in mid-body of pancreas ➡. *(Right)* Axial CECT (in same patient as previous image) at more caudal plane of section demonstrates acute fluid collection in anterior pararenal space ➡.

Typical

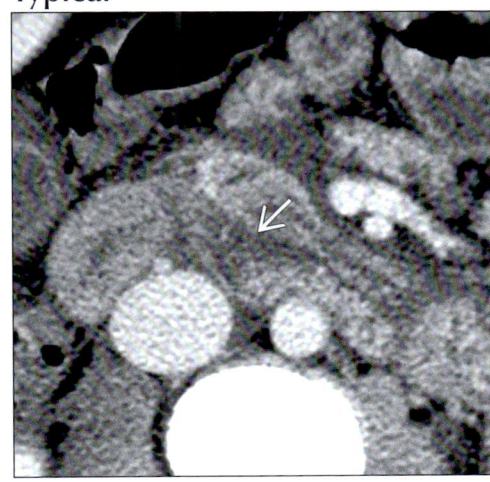
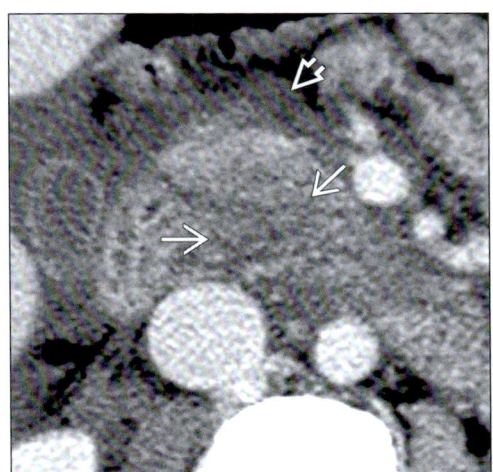

(Left) Axial CECT shows laceration to pancreatic head following blunt trauma. Note fracture plane in head of pancreas ➡. *(Right)* Plane of section through uncinate process demonstrates hematoma with ill-defined low attenuation mass ➡. Note surrounding peripancreatic fluid and blood ➡.

Variant

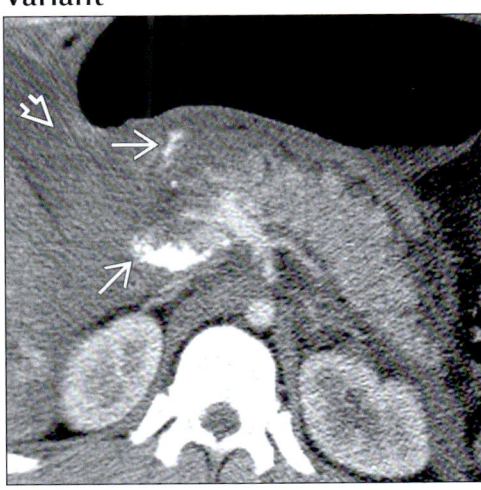
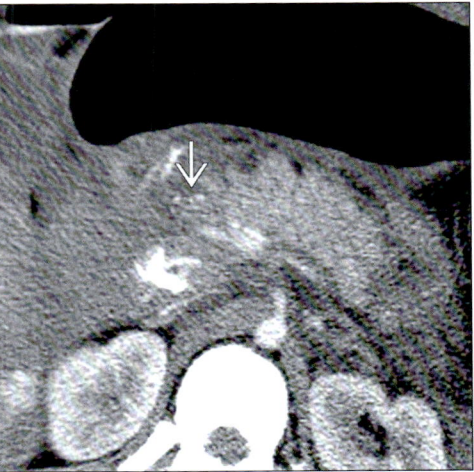

(Left) Axial CECT of combined duodenal and pancreatic trauma from blunt injury. Multiple high attenuation areas of peri-pancreatic active arterial bleed ➡ & large surrounding hematoma ➡. *(Right)* Axial CECT (in same patient as previous image) at lower plane of section. Note fracture plane through neck and body of pancreas ➡.

DUODENAL TRAUMA/HEMATOMA

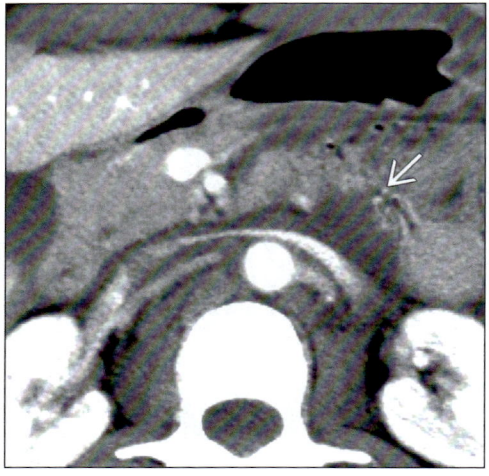

Axial CECT shows rupture of 3rd portion of duodenum following blunt trauma. Note water density fluid posterior to third portion of duodenum ➔.

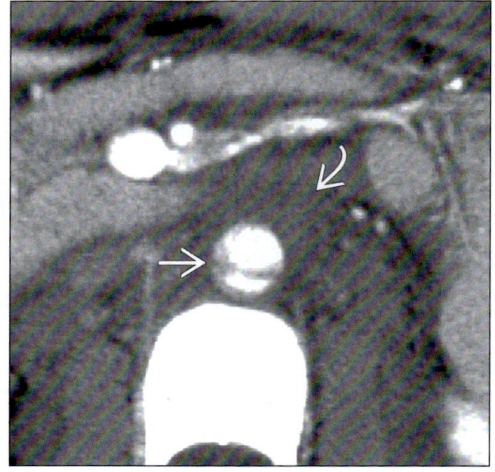

Axial CECT in same patient as left demonstrates traumatic aortic dissection with intimal flap ➔ in abdominal aorta. There is also associated retroperitoneal hemorrhage ➔.

TERMINOLOGY

Definitions
- Trauma to duodenum resulting in intramural hematoma or laceration

IMAGING FINDINGS

General Features
- Best diagnostic clue: High density intramural hematoma, pneumoperitoneum, anterior pararenal space fluid/air

Radiographic Findings
- Radiography: Pneumoperitoneum, ectopic retroperitoneal gas
- GI series: Duodenal lumen narrowing by hematoma, contrast extravasation (peritoneal cavity, retroperitoneum)

CT Findings
- NECT: High density intramural hematoma, pneumoperitoneum, anterior pararenal space fluid/air
- CECT: Nonenhancing intramural hematoma, active extravasation (gastroduodenal artery), interruption of duodenal wall, ectopic gas/fluid, periduodenal stranding

MR Findings
- T1WI: High signal intramural hematoma
- T2WI: High signal free fluid, high signal hematoma
- T1 C+: Thick duodenal wall, nonenhancing hematoma

Ultrasonographic Findings
- Echogenic intramural mass representing hematoma

Angiographic Findings
- Gastroduodenal artery bleed

Imaging Recommendations
- Best imaging tool: CECT, UGI

DIFFERENTIAL DIAGNOSIS

Perforated Duodenal Ulcer
- Pneumoperitoneum, anterior pararenal space fluid/air
- Periduodenal inflammatory changes

DDx: Duodenal Trauma/Hematoma

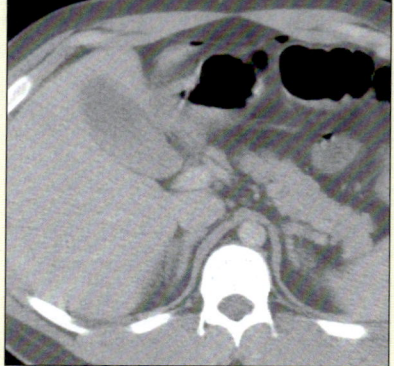

Perforated Ulcer

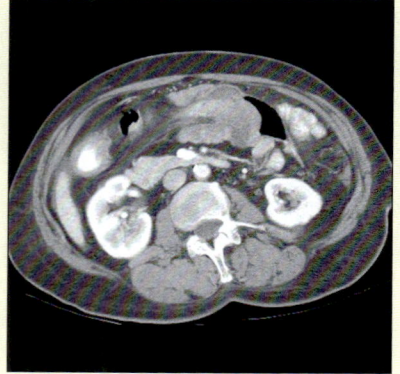

Villous Adenoma

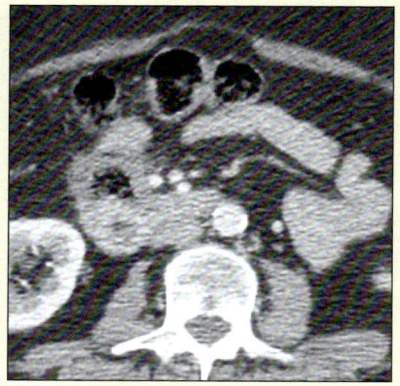

Duodenal Lymphoma

DUODENAL TRAUMA/HEMATOMA

Key Facts

Imaging Findings
- Best diagnostic clue: High density intramural hematoma, pneumoperitoneum, anterior pararenal space fluid/air
- Best imaging tool: CECT, UGI

Pathology
- Epidemiology: 4th most common organ injury in children, 2-10% of all blunt injuries

Clinical Issues
- Clinical Profile: Child with midepigastric blunt trauma, adult with high speed MVA injuries
- Non-operative management: Isolated hematoma without perforation
- Surgery for duodenal perforation & head of pancreas injury

Diagnostic Checklist
- Perforated duodenal ulcer

- Mural thickening of duodenum

Villous Adenoma
- Polypoid mucosal mass 3-9 cm

Duodenal Lymphoma
- Bulky submucosal mass

PATHOLOGY

General Features
- General path comments: Intramural hematoma
- Epidemiology: 4th most common organ injury in children, 2-10% of all blunt injuries
- Associated abnormalities: Pancreatic laceration/fracture (47%), liver or splenic laceration

Staging, Grading or Classification Criteria
- Isolated intramural hematoma; perforated duodenum; head of pancreas and duodenal injury

CLINICAL ISSUES

Presentation
- Most common signs/symptoms: Nausea, vomiting, abdominal pain/tenderness
- Clinical Profile: Child with midepigastric blunt trauma, adult with high speed MVA injuries

Natural History & Prognosis
- Isolated hematoma: Excellent prognosis with non-operative management
- Combined duodenal perforation with head of pancreas laceration: Morbidity 26%

Treatment
- Options, risks, complications
  - Non-operative management: Isolated hematoma without perforation
  - Surgery for duodenal perforation & head of pancreas injury

DIAGNOSTIC CHECKLIST

Consider
- Perforated duodenal ulcer

Image Interpretation Pearls
- Ectopic gas/fluid in pararenal space

SELECTED REFERENCES
1. Desai KM et al: Blunt duodenal injuries in children. J Trauma. 54(4):640-5; discussion 645-6, 2003
2. Zissin R et al: Pictorial review. CT of duodenal pathology. Br J Radiol. 75(889):78-84, 2002
3. Degiannis E et al: Duodenal injuries. Br J Surg. 87(11):1473-9, 2000

IMAGE GALLERY

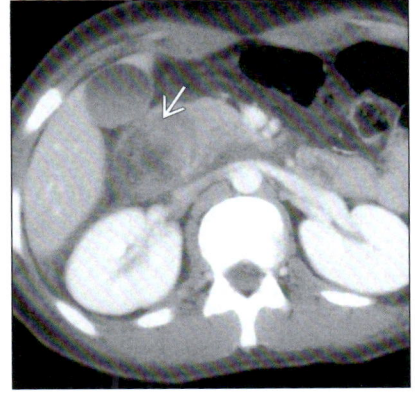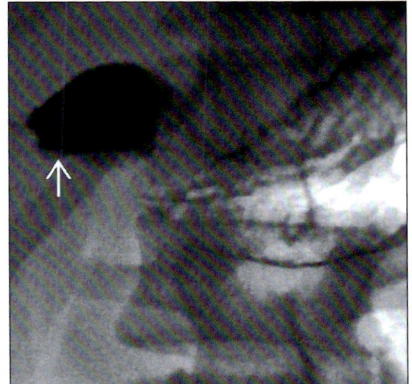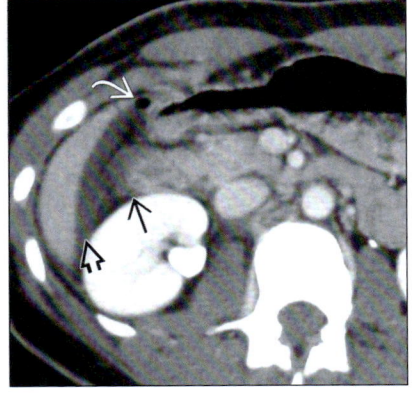

(Left) Axial CECT shows high attenuation hematoma ➔ within lumen of 2nd & 3rd portions of duodenum. *(Center)* UGI series in same patient as previous image shows obstructed post-bulbar duodenum ➔ but no evidence of perforation. *(Right)* Axial CECT of duodenal laceration from blunt trauma. Free intraperitoneal fluid ➔ and air ➔, as well as extraluminal fluid, adjacent to 2nd portion of duodenum ➔.

INTESTINAL TRAUMA

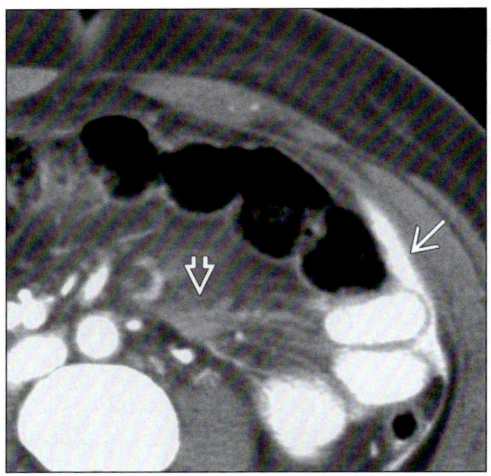

Axial CECT shows small bowel perforation following seat belt injury from MVA. Note extravasated oral contrast in left paracolic gutter ➡ associated with mesenteric hematoma ➡.

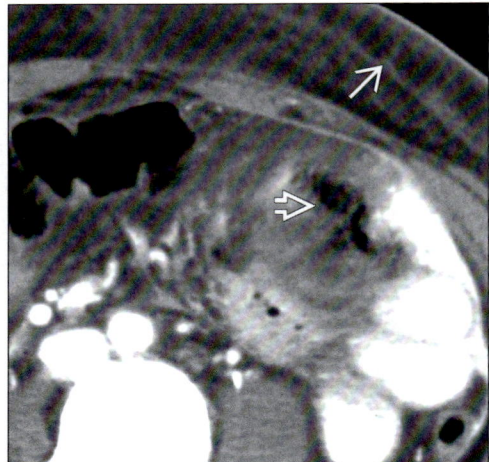

Axial CECT at more cranial plane of section in same patient as previous image demonstrates abdominal wall contusion ➡ from seat belt injury and pneumoperitoneum ➡.

TERMINOLOGY

Definitions
- Injury to bowel (duodenum, small bowel, colon)

IMAGING FINDINGS

General Features
- Best diagnostic clue: Bowel wall thickening, mesenteric infiltration ± extravasation of enteric or vascular contrast medium
- Location: Duodenum, proximal jejunum most common
- Other general features
  o Gastric injury
    ▪ More common in children than adults
    ▪ ↑ Risk: Distended stomach after eating
    ▪ Associated injuries: Rupture of spleen, left-sided thoracic injury
  o Duodenal injury
    ▪ Hematoma, ectopic air or contrast (perforation)
    ▪ Location: Descending 2nd & horizontal 3rd part
    ▪ 3rd part compressed against spine by direct blow
    ▪ Associated injuries: Pancreatic head, L lobe of liver
  o Jejunal & ileal injury
    ▪ Hematoma, bowel wall discontinuity, thickening
    ▪ At or near ligament of Treitz & ileocecal valve
    ▪ Symptoms & signs develop slowly (due to neutral pH & relative absence of bacteria)
  o Colon injury
    ▪ Compression of upper abdomen (steering wheel & seat belts)
    ▪ Location: Transverse colon, sigmoid colon, cecum
    ▪ Transverse: Intramural hematoma or serosal tear
    ▪ Ascending or descending: Mesenteric avulsion, full-thickness laceration, transection, ischemia
    ▪ Complications: Ischemic stricture or perforation
  o Mesenteric injury
    ▪ Hematoma: Most common GI injury seen on CT
    ▪ Complications: Disruption of mesenteric vasculature, hemorrhage, GI tract perforation
    ▪ Active mesenteric bleeding requires surgery

Radiographic Findings
- Radiography

DDx: Hemorrhage or Edema in Bowel Wall

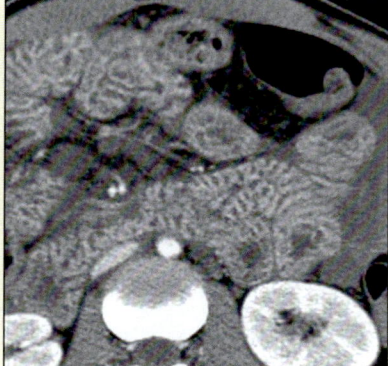

Shock Bowel

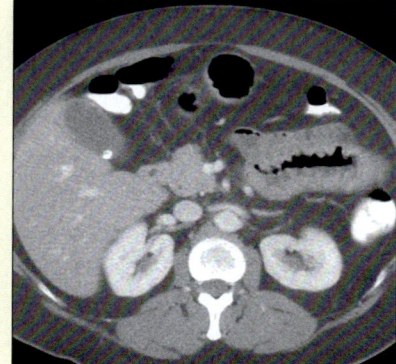

Intestinal Vasculitis

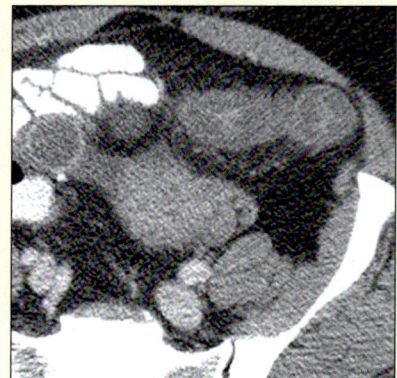

Ischemic Enteritis

INTESTINAL TRAUMA

Key Facts

Terminology
- Injury to bowel (duodenum, small bowel, colon)

Imaging Findings
- Best diagnostic clue: Bowel wall thickening, mesenteric infiltration ± extravasation of enteric or vascular contrast medium
- Intramural air, extraluminal air, interloop free fluid
- Bowel wall thickening: > 3 mm (seen in 75% of transmural injuries)
- Mesenteric infiltration or "stranding"
- Intra-/retroperitoneal free fluid: Hemoperitoneum or bowel contents
- Protocol advice: Helical CECT ± oral contrast; IV contrast @ 3 mL/sec

Top Differential Diagnoses
- Shock Bowel
- Coagulopathy
- Vasculitis
- Ischemic Enteritis

Clinical Issues
- Clinical Profile: History of MVA, abdominal pain, distension, tenderness & guarding
- Diagnostic peritoneal lavage (DPL): Severe injury if positive

Diagnostic Checklist
- Check for MVA history or other abdominal injury
- CT evidence of extraluminal air/contrast, bowel wall thickening, free fluids & mesenteric "stranding"

- "Flank-stripe" sign: ↑ Density zone (> 800 mL abdominal fluid) separates vertical colon segments from properitoneal fat & peritoneal reflection
- "Dog's-ear" sign: Pelvic fluid collections displace bowel from urinary bladder

Fluoroscopic Findings
- Water soluble contrast study
  - Fold thickening, luminal narrowing, extravasation
  - Mainly for duodenal hematoma/laceration

CT Findings
- Must view at abdominal & lung windows
- Extraluminal air: Intra- or retroperitoneal air
- Extraluminal gas not diagnostic of bowel perforation (also seen in barotrauma & mechanical ventilation)
  - Location
    - Perihepatic, perisplenic regions
    - Trapped in leaves of mesentery, omental interstices
    - Trapped by adhesions or ligaments (e.g., falciform)
- Intramural air, extraluminal air, interloop free fluid
  - Indicates full-thickness tear
- Bowel wall thickening: > 3 mm (seen in 75% of transmural injuries)
  - Circumferential or eccentric thickening in intramural hematoma, mesenteric trauma (arterial or venous injury)
- Bowel wall enhancement: > HU of psoas muscle or HU = blood vessels
  - Enhancement + thickening + free fluid: Strongly suggests perforation
- Mesenteric infiltration or "stranding"
  - Small hemorrhages: Streaky soft tissue infiltration of mesenteric fat
  - "Sentinel clot" sign: Localized > 60 HU mesenteric hematoma at site of bleeding
- Intra-/retroperitoneal free fluid: Hemoperitoneum or bowel contents
  - Polygonal fluid collections between folds of mesentery, bowel loops
  - Hematoma (> 60 HU), liquefied blood (35-50 HU)
  - Bowel content, extravasated enteric contrast
  - Free intraperitoneal fluids
  - Hemoperitoneum: Common in intraperitoneal bowel or mesenteric injury
  - Active bleeding isodense with enhanced vessels
  - Bowel rupture at sites of oral contrast extravasation
- Bowel discontinuity: Injury primary finding, unusual
- Extraluminal oral contrast material: 100% specific for bowel perforation, but uncommon

Ultrasonographic Findings
- Grayscale Ultrasound: Free fluid in abdomen & pelvis

Angiographic Findings
- Conventional: Vascular transection, laceration, pseudoaneurysm, arteriovenous fistula

Imaging Recommendations
- Best imaging tool: CECT
- Protocol advice: Helical CECT ± oral contrast; IV contrast @ 3 mL/sec

DIFFERENTIAL DIAGNOSIS

Shock Bowel
- Intense mucosal enhancement, submucosal edema (not blood)
- Often diffuse mesenteric edema & hypovolemia signs
  - Collapsed IVC & renal veins
- Reversible sign of recent hypotension
- Resolves quickly with fluid resuscitation

Coagulopathy
- Spontaneous, or due to anticoagulant treatment
- Spontaneous: Idiopathic thrombocytopenic purpura, leukemia, hemophilia
- Abdominal pain, melena, intestinal obstruction
- Barium studies or CT of small bowel
  - Segmental, extensive, or localized changes
  - Uniform, regular thickening of valvulae conniventes with symmetric, spike-like configuration, reduced luminal diameter simulating stack of coins
  - Localized bleeding may be seen as intramural mass

INTESTINAL TRAUMA

Vasculitis
- Polyarteritis nodosa
  - Bowel: Diffuse or segmental ischemia/hemorrhage
  - Frequent renal & liver involvement
  - Angiography: Small aneurysms of SMA branches
- Systemic lupus erythematosus
  - Small vessel arteritis in 10-60% of cases
  - Segmental bowel lesions → necrosis & perforation
- Henoch-Schönlein purpura
  - Children, young & middle-aged; GI tract (> 50%)
  - Present with clinical triad: Palpable purpura, arthritis, abdominal pain
- Barium studies or CT of small bowel in vasculitis
  - Extensive fold thickening + luminal narrowing
  - May show thumbprinting on mesenteric border
  - Intussusceptions may be seen in childhood purpura

Ischemic Enteritis
- Superior mesenteric vein (SMV) clot or narrowing
- Barium studies of small bowel
  - Markedly thickened valvulae conniventes
  - Thumbprinting along mesenteric border
- CT findings
  - Clot or reduced lumen in SMA or SMV
  - Segmental bowel wall thickening (> 3 mm)
  - Later phase: Focal or diffuse pneumatosis, gas within small bowel wall, venous radicles

PATHOLOGY

General Features
- Etiology
  - Most common causes
    - Motor vehicle accidents (MVA), falls, assault
  - Impact injuries
    - Crushing of bowel against spine
    - Location: Small bowel of limited mobility (duodenum, near ligament of Treitz & ileocecal valve)
    - Transverse tears of mesentery → hematoma → bowel infarction
  - Rapid deceleration injuries
    - Abrupt forward movement of proximal jejunum from its fixation by ligament of Treitz
    - Shearing force between restricted & mobile bowel: Transection at duodenojejunal flexure
- Epidemiology
  - Abdominal trauma: Leading cause of death in United States in patients < 40 yrs of age
  - Children: ↑ Incidence of intramural hematoma
  - Adults: ↑ Incidence of bowel wall transection
  - Bowel & mesenteric injuries seen in 5% of blunt trauma at laparotomy
- Associated abnormalities: Hepatic, splenic, renal & pancreatic injuries

Gross Pathologic & Surgical Features
- Contusion, laceration, bowel discontinuity
- Wall thickening, blood clot, rupture

CLINICAL ISSUES

Presentation
- Most common signs/symptoms
  - Abdominal pain, distension, tenderness, guarding
  - Hypotension, tachycardia
  - Loss of consciousness, shock due to ↑ blood loss
- Clinical Profile: History of MVA, abdominal pain, distension, tenderness & guarding
- Lab-data
  - Altered CBC, electrolytes, BUN, creatinine, amylase, PT, PTT & hematocrit
- Diagnostic peritoneal lavage (DPL): Severe injury if positive
  - RBC > 150,000/mm³; WBC > 500/mm³
  - Food, bile or bacteria on Gram stain from aspirate

Demographics
- Age: Any age group
- Gender: M = F

Natural History & Prognosis
- Complications
  - Perforation → sepsis → abdominal abscess → peritonitis → shock → death
- Prognosis
  - Good in early diagnosis & treatment
  - Poor in delayed diagnosis & treatment
    - Increased morbidity & mortality up to 65%

Treatment
- Minor: Airway, IV fluids, monitor vital signs, blood transfusion, antibiotics
- Major: Surgery for perforation or active bleed

DIAGNOSTIC CHECKLIST

Consider
- Check for MVA history or other abdominal injury

Image Interpretation Pearls
- CT evidence of extraluminal air/contrast, bowel wall thickening, free fluids & mesenteric "stranding"

SELECTED REFERENCES

1. Hanks PW et al: Blunt injury to mesentery and small bowel: CT evaluation. Radiol Clin North Am. 41(6):1171-82, 2003
2. Hawkins AE et al: Evaluation of bowel and mesenteric injury: role of multidetector CT. Abdom Imaging. 28(4):505-14, 2003
3. Butela ST et al: Performance of CT in detection of bowel injury. AJR Am J Roentgenol. 176(1):129-35, 2001
4. Brody JM et al: CT of blunt trauma bowel and mesenteric injury: typical findings and pitfalls in diagnosis. Radiographics. 20(6):1525-36; discussion 1536-7, 2000
5. Federle MP: Diagnosis of intestinal injuries by computed tomography and the use of oral contrast medium. Ann Emerg Med. 31(6):769-71, 1998
6. Levine CD et al: CT findings of bowel and mesenteric injury. J Comput Assist Tomogr. 21(6):974-9, 1997
7. Nghiem HV et al: CT of blunt trauma to the bowel and mesentery. AJR Am J Roentgenol. 160(1):53-8, 1993

INTESTINAL TRAUMA

IMAGE GALLERY

Typical

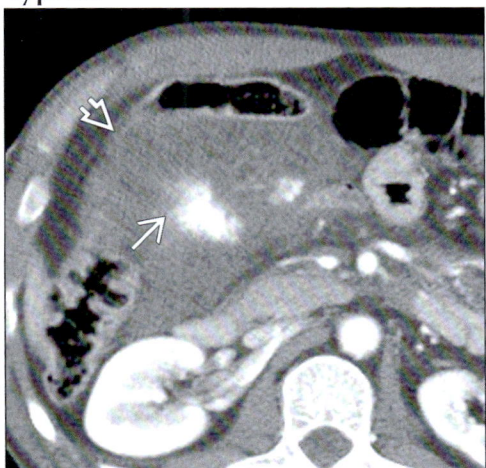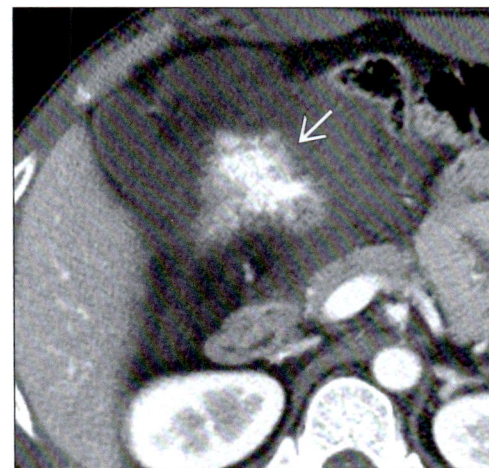

(Left) Axial CECT shows active arterial extravasation into mesentery of right colon following blunt trauma. Note high attenuation focus of arterial bleed ➡ surrounded by large hematoma ➡. *(Right)* Axial CECT in same patient as left shows diffusion of extravasated contrast into mesentery ➡. At surgery, a right hemicolectomy was required to stop bleeding.

Typical

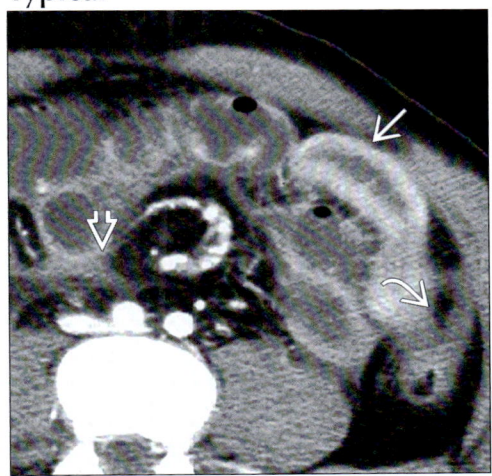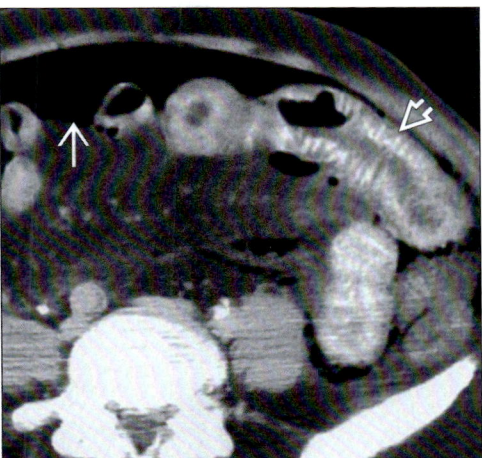

(Left) Axial CECT of bowel perforation. Note hyperdense small bowel from reperfusion injury ➡, water density in left paracolic gutter ➡ & intraloop compartment ➡. *(Right)* Axial CECT of bowel perforation with massive pneumoperitoneum ➡. Note hyperdense small bowel with visualization of vasa recta in thickened bowel wall from reperfusion injury ➡.

Typical

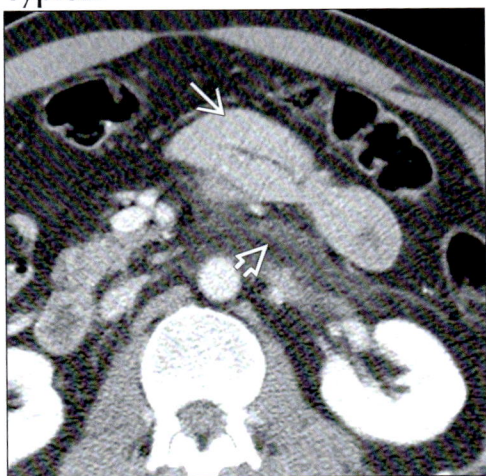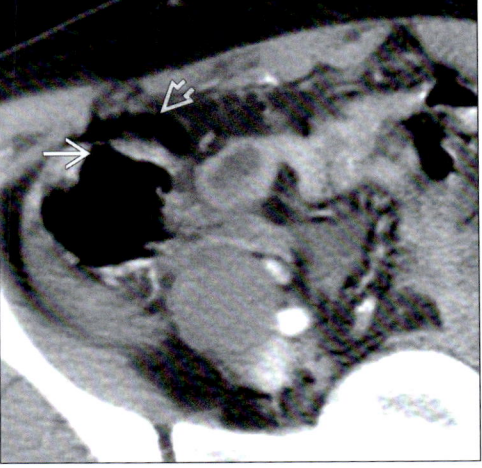

(Left) Axial CECT shows jejunal hematoma treated non-operatively following blunt trauma. Note marked thickening of proximal jejunum ➡ with adjacent mesenteric hematoma ➡. *(Right)* Axial CECT shows cecal perforation. Note mural thickening and focal interruption of cecal wall ➡. Adjacent ectopic gas is present ➡, confirming perforation.

TESTICULAR TRAUMA

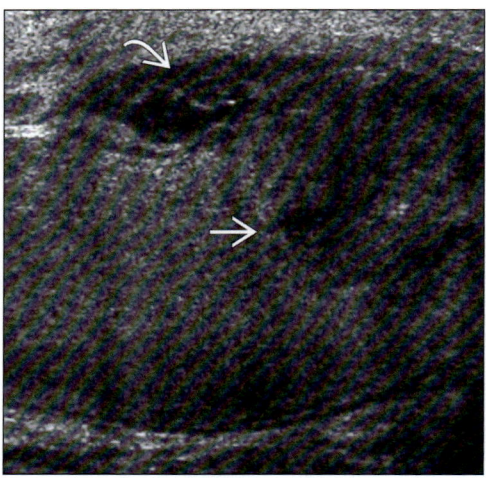

Sagittal grayscale sonogram shows testicular fracture following blunt trauma. Note hypoechoic parenchymal hematoma ➡ with adjacent hematocele ➢.

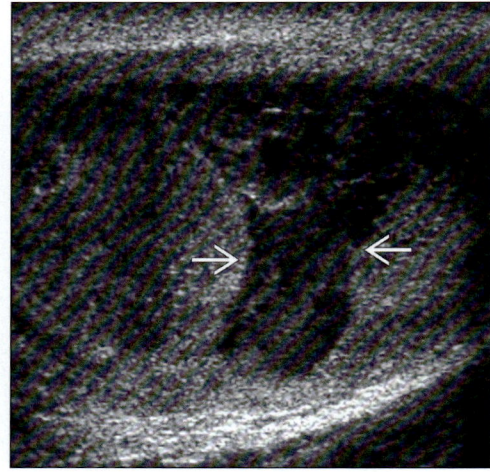

More medial sagittal scan in same patient as previous image reveals well-defined fracture plane within testis ➡.

TERMINOLOGY

Abbreviations and Synonyms
- Testicular rupture, fracture of testis

Definitions
- Laceration of tunica albuginea

IMAGING FINDINGS

General Features
- Best diagnostic clue: US: Heterogeneous parenchymal echogenicity of testis
- Morphology: Irregular testicular contour

MR Findings
- T1WI: High signal acute hematoma
- T2WI: High signal hematoma
- T1 C+: Avascular areas of injury post-contrast

Ultrasonographic Findings
- Grayscale Ultrasound
  - Hematocele & echogenic fluid, linear stranding in tunica vaginalis
  - Abnormal echogenicity of testicular parenchyma
  - Epididymal enlargement
  - Discrete linear/irregular fracture plane within testis
  - Focal intraparenchymal hematoma
- Color Doppler
  - Distorted intraparenchymal vascularity & interruption of vessels
  - Avascular intraparenchymal hematoma
  - Enlarged epididymis, ↑ flow

Imaging Recommendations
- Best imaging tool: High-resolution US (≥ 7.5 MHz)

DIFFERENTIAL DIAGNOSIS

Testicular Tumor
- Mild/moderate pain, palpable mass, no trauma history
- Focal grayscale abnormality, abnormal interval vascularity, vascular displacement

Epididymo-Orchitis
- Acute or chronic pain, no trauma history
- Enlarged hypoechoic epididymis, ↑ vascularity to epididymis & testis

DDx: Lesions Mimicking Testicular Trauma

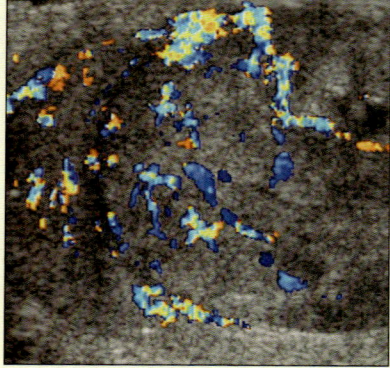

Testicular Tumor

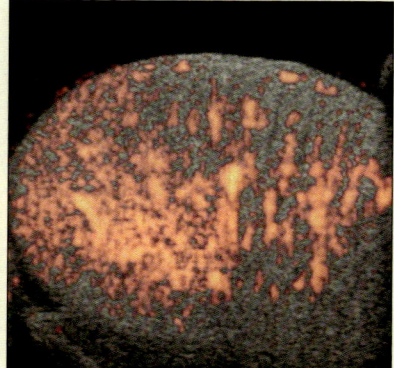

Orchitis

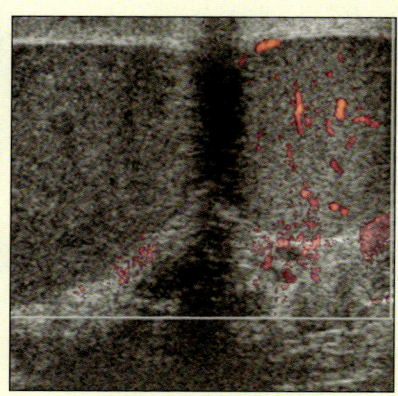

Testicular Torsion

TESTICULAR TRAUMA

Key Facts

Imaging Findings
- Best diagnostic clue: US: Heterogeneous parenchymal echogenicity of testis
- Hematocele & echogenic fluid, linear stranding in tunica vaginalis
- Abnormal echogenicity of testicular parenchyma
- Discrete linear/irregular fracture plane within testis
- Focal intraparenchymal hematoma
- Best imaging tool: High-resolution US (≥ 7.5 MHz)

Clinical Issues
- Salvage rate 45% if not repaired within 72 hours
- Options, risks, complications: Surgery mandatory

Diagnostic Checklist
- Isolated hematocele without rupture
- Irregular testicular contour, heterogeneous testicular parenchyma

Testicular Torsion
- ↓ Vascularity compared to normal testis

Segmental Infarct
- Acute pain, no trauma history
- Focal avascular hypoechoic area
- ↑ Incidence in hypercoagulable states, atherosclerosis

PATHOLOGY

General Features
- General path comments
  - Capsular disruption, hematocele
  - Necrotic testicular parenchyma within tunica vaginalis
- Etiology: Blunt trauma impales scrotal contents to symphysis pubis, pubic rami
- Associated abnormalities: Pelvic fractures

Microscopic Features
- Intraparenchymal bleed, necrotic lacerated tissue

Staging, Grading or Classification Criteria
- Extratesticular: Scrotal wall, tunica vaginalis, tunical & testicular parenchyma
- Intratesticular: Tunical and testicular parenchyma

CLINICAL ISSUES

Presentation
- Most common signs: Scrotal hematoma 2° trauma

Demographics
- Age: < 50 yrs

Natural History & Prognosis
- Salvage rate 45% if not repaired within 72 hours

Treatment
- Options, risks, complications: Surgery mandatory

DIAGNOSTIC CHECKLIST

Consider
- Isolated hematocele without rupture

Image Interpretation Pearls
- Irregular testicular contour, heterogeneous testicular parenchyma

SELECTED REFERENCES
1. Micallef M et al: Ultrasound features of blunt testicular injury. Injury. 32(1):23-6, 2001
2. Wessells H et al: Testicular trauma. Urology. 47(5):750, 1996
3. Altarac S: Management of 53 cases of testicular trauma. Eur Urol. 25(2):119-23, 1994

IMAGE GALLERY

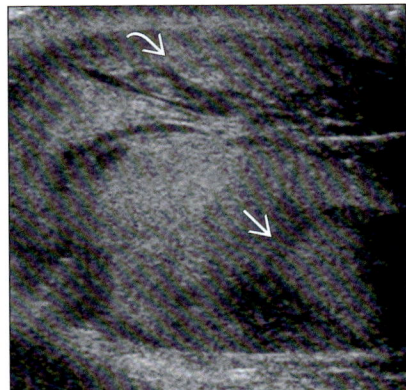 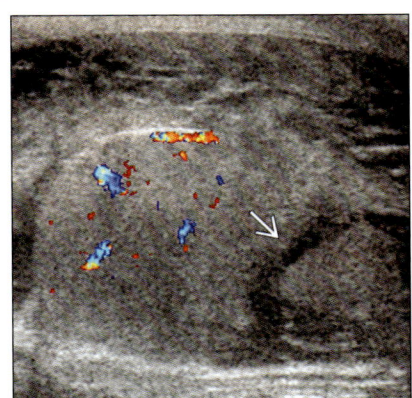 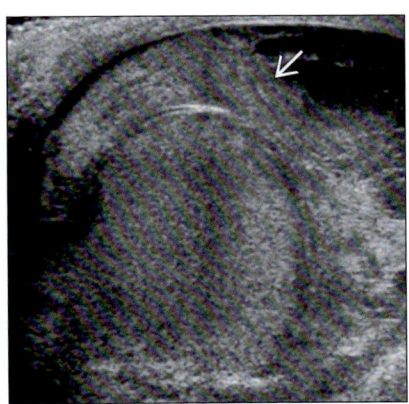

(Left) Grayscale sagittal sonogram of testicular fracture. Note marked heterogeneity of testicular parenchyma with hypoechoic laceration ➔ and surrounding hematocele ➔. *(Center)* Sagittal color Doppler sonogram in same patient as previous image reveals small amount of flow to normal testicle. Fracture plane is clearly identified ➔. *(Right)* Transverse grayscale sonogram in same patient as previous image reveals echogenic clotted blood ➔.

HYPOPERFUSION COMPLEX

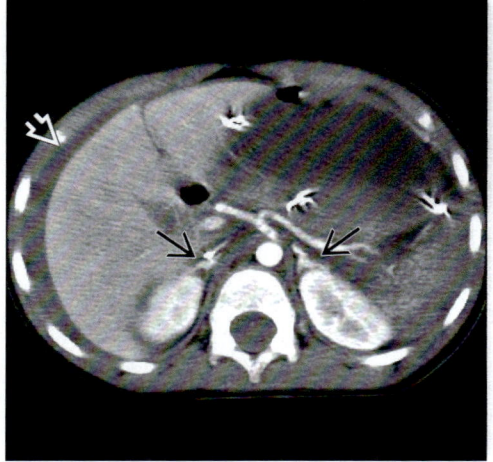

Axial CECT shows dramatic adrenal enhancement ➔, with small sized aorta and IVC. There is free fluid ➔ and a splenic laceration.

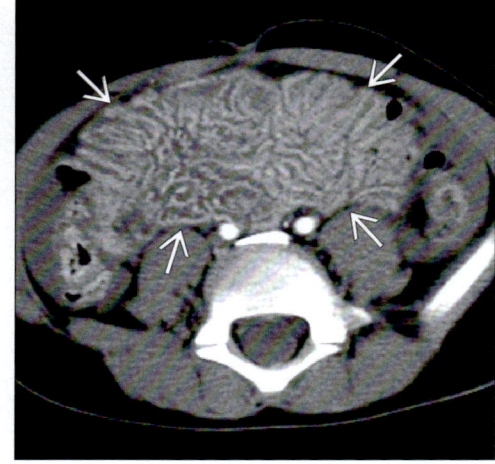

Axial CECT in same patient as previous image, shows dramatic small bowel wall enhancement and thickening ➔.

TERMINOLOGY

Abbreviations and Synonyms
- Shock bowel
- Shock abdomen
- Hypoperfusion complex (HC)

Definitions
- Hypoperfusion complex: A combination of CT findings seen in the abdomen of children with compensated shock
  - Most commonly encountered in young children who have significant hemorrhage after trauma
  - Associated with tenuous hemodynamic state and poor prognosis

IMAGING FINDINGS

General Features
- Best diagnostic clue: Diffuse bowel wall enhancement and thickening associated with abnormal enhancement of solid organs and abnormal enhancement and small caliber of vessels

CT Findings
- Best imaging clue: Diffuse bowel wall enhancement and thickening associated with abnormal enhancement of solid organs and abnormal enhancement and small caliber of vessels
- **Abnormal intense enhancement of:**
  - Bowel wall
    - Diffuse bowel wall enhancement involving large portions of bowel
    - In contrast to focal bowel wall enhancement seen with bowel injury
  - Mesentery
  - Adrenal glands
    - Adrenal glands normally soft tissue attenuation similar to muscle
    - With shock, adrenal glands enhance similar in attenuation to aorta
  - Liver
  - Kidneys
  - Pancreas
- **Intense enhancement and decreased caliber:**
  - Inferior vena cava

DDx: Bowel Wall Thickening/Enhancement

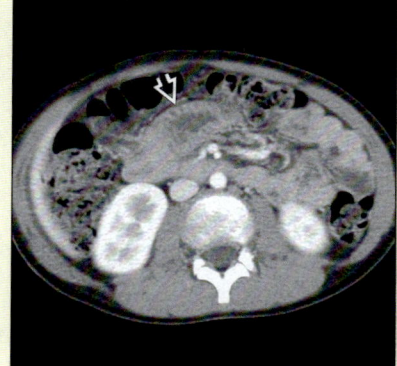
Bowel Injury

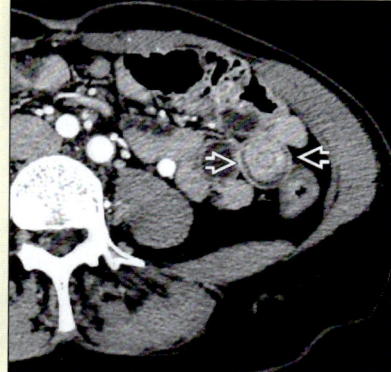
Small Bowel Intussusception

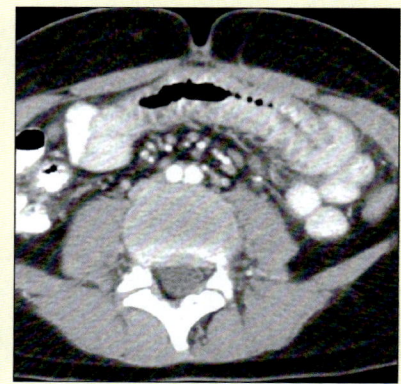
Henoch-Schönlein Purpura

HYPOPERFUSION COMPLEX

Key Facts

Imaging Findings
- Best imaging clue: Diffuse bowel wall enhancement and thickening associated with abnormal enhancement of solid organs and abnormal enhancement and small caliber of vessels
- **Abnormal intense enhancement of:**
- Bowel wall
- Mesentery
- Adrenal glands
- Liver
- Kidneys
- Pancreas
- **Intense enhancement and decreased caliber:**
- Inferior vena cava
- Aorta
- Diffuse bowel wall thickening
- Diffuse bowel dilatation
- Unexplained ascites
- CT findings may be apparent before clinical findings of shock

Clinical Issues
- In one series, progressive hypotension developed within 10 minutes of CT in 19% of children
- In same series, mortality rate associated with presence of hypoperfusion complex was 85%, compared with 2% of all children who suffered blunt trauma
- Immediately transfer child from CT to more supportive area or operating room
- Intense monitoring
- Fluid/blood volume replacement

  - Inferior vena cava will have a flat, "pancake" appearance
  ○ Aorta
- Diffuse bowel wall thickening
  ○ Involving large portions of small and occasionally large bowel
  ○ In contrast to bowel injury, in which thickening will often involve only a focal area of bowel
- Diffuse bowel dilatation
- Unexplained ascites
- CT findings may be apparent before clinical findings of shock

Ultrasonographic Findings
- Ultrasound may be used in "FAST" scanning of the abdomen for potential abdominal trauma screening
- May show peritoneal fluid
- Diffuse fluid-filled and dilated bowel
- Bowel wall thickening

Imaging Recommendations
- Immediate removal of child from CT scanner and transfer to intensive care area or operating room

DIFFERENTIAL DIAGNOSIS

Bowel Trauma
- Trauma to bowel associated with focal bowel wall thickening, wall enhancement, and dilatation
- Diffuse bowel involvement favors hypoperfusion complex
- Extra-bowel findings such as adrenal enhancement and small inferior vena cava (IVC) caliber favor shock bowel over direct bowel trauma
- Unexplained peritoneal fluid
- Mesenteric soft tissue stranding adjacent to involved bowel
- Both may coexist

Transient Small Bowel (SB) Intussusception
- With increased use of CT, transient small bowel intussusceptions are being visualized at increased frequency
- Believed to be incidental "normal" findings that resolve spontaneously and have no clinical relevance
- Seen with higher frequency in trauma patients than in patients with CT performed for other indications
- CT shows area of small bowel with alternating rings of high and low attenuation
- Bowel not diffusely abnormal

Henoch-Schönlein Purpura (HSP)
- Small vessel vasculitis of unknown origin
- Purpuric rash, abdominal pain, may have arthritis and nephritis
- 3-7 years old, boys more commonly affected
- Typically resolves spontaneously
- Edema and hemorrhage of bowel wall
  ○ CT shows multiple areas of bowel wall thickening, increased attenuation, and enhancement
- May also be areas of small bowel intussusception

Graft vs. Host Disease (GVHD)
- GVHD may have similar bowel findings as compared to hypoperfusion complex
  ○ Diffuse bowel wall enhancement and mild bowel wall thickening
  ○ Small bowel more often involved than large bowel
  ○ Increased soft tissue attenuation within mesenteric fat
  ○ Peritoneal fluid
- Clinical history of bone marrow transplant and absent history of trauma is obviously essential

Other Bowel Inflammatory Processes
- Pre-existing conditions may be present in setting of trauma
- Other inflammatory causes of bowel wall thickening and enhancement

HYPOPERFUSION COMPLEX

- Pseudomembranous colitis: Diffuse pancolitis, severe bowel wall thickening with disproportionately small amount of pericolonic inflammatory change, related to antibiotic use
- Crohn disease: Marked thickening typically of terminal ileum and cecum, "creeping fat"
- Infectious enterocolitis: Shigella, E. coli, etc., abnormal bowel wall thickening, dilatation, and wall enhancement

PATHOLOGY

General Features
- General path comments
  - Unlike in adults, in children with hypovolemic shock, compensation can occur in which increased sympathetic stimulation maintains adequate blood pressure and cardiac output
    - Differential vasospasm causes perfusion of vital organs
  - Child with hypovolemic shock may have normal blood pressures despite significant reductions in circulating blood volume
    - This may lead to patient appearing stable and having CT imaging
    - However, in children, transition from stable shock to decompensation is abrupt, not gradual
  - Increased sympathetic activity and resultant altered pathways of arterial flow result in findings seen at CT with hypoperfusion complex
    - Small caliber aorta and inferior vena cava are related to vasospasm and hypovolemia
    - Bowel dilatation and enhancement related to mesenteric vasoconstriction
    - Intense enhancement of adrenal glands related to central role of adrenal in generating sympathetic response to hypovolemic shock
- Epidemiology
  - Findings of hypoperfusion complex can be seen in compensated shock at any age
  - However, CT findings more common and more striking in young children
- Associated abnormalities
  - Findings of parenchymal organ hemorrhage - from liver, spleen, or kidney
  - Active extravasation from parenchymal organ
    - High attenuation material (similar in attenuation to aorta) surrounding an injured organ
  - Bowel injury may also be present

CLINICAL ISSUES

Presentation
- Most common signs/symptoms
  - Clinical findings of compensated shock
  - Children may be normotensive but often are tachycardic in an attempt to maintain adequate blood pressure
- Other signs/symptoms
  - CT findings seen most commonly in trauma patient but can occur with shock of any cause
  - CT findings often recognized prior to clinical recognition of severity of shock

Demographics
- Age
  - CT findings more common and more striking with shock seen in young children
  - CT findings, however, can be seen at any age

Natural History & Prognosis
- In one series, progressive hypotension developed within 10 minutes of CT in 19% of children
- In same series, mortality rate associated with presence of hypoperfusion complex was 85%, compared with 2% of all children who suffered blunt trauma
  - In other series, the mortality has been as low as 17%

Treatment
- Immediately transfer child from CT to more supportive area or operating room
- Intense monitoring
- Fluid/blood volume replacement
- Surgical management when necessary for underlying injuries

DIAGNOSTIC CHECKLIST

Consider
- When diffuse bowel wall enhancement, dilatation, and thickening: Think hypoperfusion complex
  - Look for supporting signs of intense enhancement of other organs and small caliber and intense enhancement of IVC and aorta

SELECTED REFERENCES

1. O'Hara SM et al: Intense contrast enhancement of the adrenal glands: another abdominal CT finding associated with hypoperfusion complex in children. AJR Am J Roentgenol. 173(4):995-7, 1999
2. Strouse PJ et al: CT of bowel and mesenteric trauma in children. Radiographics. 19(5):1237-50, 1999
3. Levine CD et al: CT in patients with blunt abdominal trauma: clinical significance of intraperitoneal fluid detected on a scan with otherwise normal findings. AJR Am J Roentgenol. 164(6):1381-5, 1995
4. Mirvis SE et al: Diffuse small-bowel ischemia in hypotensive adults after blunt trauma (shock bowel): CT findings and clinical significance. AJR Am J Roentgenol. 163(6):1375-9, 1994
5. Sivit CJ et al: CT in children with rupture of the bowel caused by blunt trauma: diagnostic efficacy and comparison with hypoperfusion complex. AJR Am J Roentgenol. 163(5):1195-8, 1994
6. Hara H et al: Significance of bowel wall enhancement on CT following blunt abdominal trauma in childhood. J Comput Assist Tomogr. 16(1):94-8, 1992
7. Sivit CJ et al: Posttraumatic shock in children: CT findings associated with hemodynamic instability. Radiology. 182(3):723-6, 1992
8. Jeffrey RB Jr et al: The collapsed inferior vena cava: CT evidence of hypovolemia. AJR Am J Roentgenol. 150(2):431-2, 1988
9. Taylor GA et al: Hypovolemic shock in children: abdominal CT manifestations. Radiology. 164(2):479-81, 1987

HYPOPERFUSION COMPLEX

IMAGE GALLERY

Typical

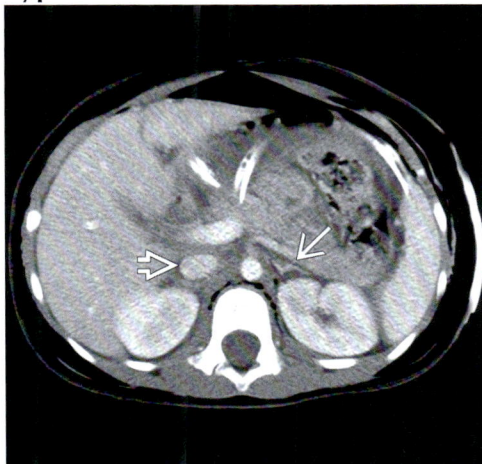
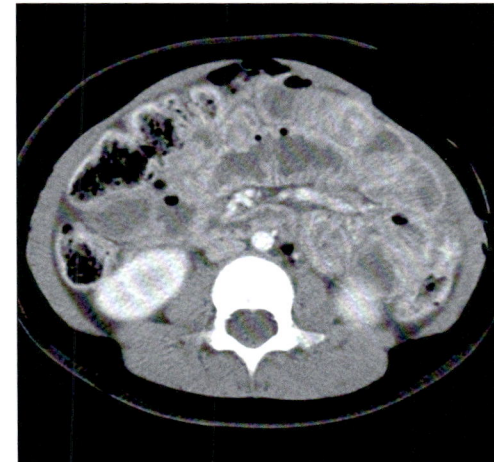

(Left) Axial CECT shows increased enhancement of adrenal gland ⇨ and mesenteric edema. An atypical characteristic for hypoperfusion complex is the normal appearing caliber of the IVC ⇨. *(Right)* Axial CECT in same patient as on left shows multiple loops of fluid-filled, slightly dilated bowel with abnormally enhancing walls.

Typical

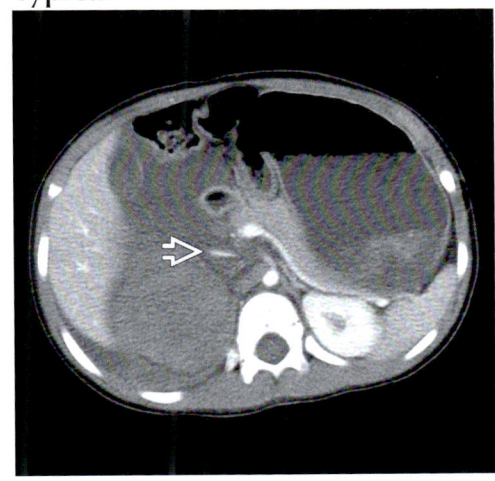
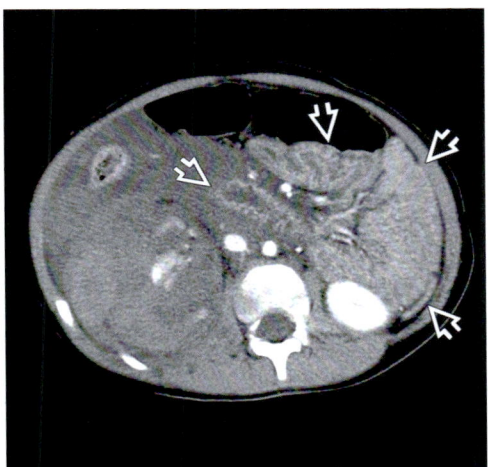

(Left) Axial CECT shows hypoperfusion complex in a patient with a right renal injury. Note small caliber of IVC ⇨ and right renal hematoma. *(Right)* Axial CECT in same patient as on left shows lacerated right kidney and surrounding fluid. Note densely enhancing bowel wall ⇨ and dense IVC and aorta.

Typical

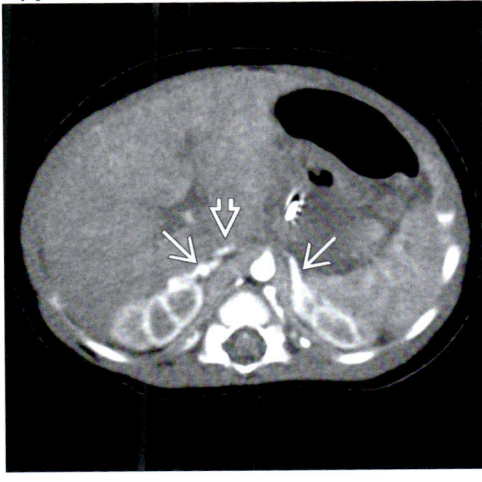
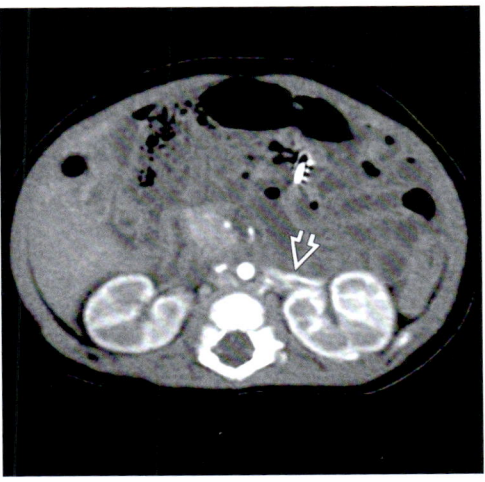

(Left) Axial CECT shows densely enhancing adrenal glands ⇨ and small caliber and densely enhancing IVC ⇨. There are also dense cortical nephrograms. *(Right)* Axial CECT in same patient as on left shows densely enhancing adrenal gland ⇨ and multiple loops of fluid-filled dilated bowel.

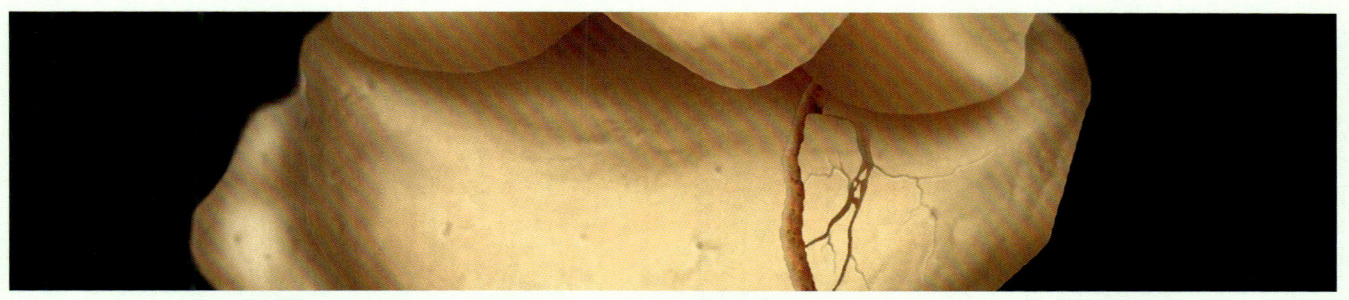

SECTION 4: Musculoskeletal

Introduction and Overview

Musculoskeletal Imaging Issues, Trauma	I-4-2

Fractures with other Contributing Etiolgies

Insufficiency Fractures, Sacrum	I-4-4
Insufficiency Fractures, Appendicular	I-4-8
Stress Fracture, Adult	I-4-10
Pathologic Fracture	I-4-14

Soft Tissue Trauma

Foreign Body	I-4-18
Compartment Syndrome	I-4-22
Necrotizing Fasciitis	I-4-26
Hematoma	I-4-28
Myositis Ossificans	I-4-32

Fractures, Upper Extremity

Sternoclavicular Trauma	I-4-36
Clavicle Fracture	I-4-40
Acromioclavicular Dislocation	I-4-42
Scapular Trauma	I-4-44
Shoulder Dislocation	I-4-48
Humeral Head/Neck Fracture	I-4-52
Humeral Shaft/Distal Humeral Fracture	I-4-56
Elbow Dislocation	I-4-60
Olecranon Fracture/Triceps Tendon Rupture	I-4-64
Radial Head/Neck Fracture	I-4-68
Biceps Tendon Rupture	I-4-72
Forearm Fractures	I-4-74
Distal Radius Fractures	I-4-76
Die Punch Fracture, Distal Radius	I-4-80
Scaphoid Fractures	I-4-82
Carpal Fractures, other than Scaphoid	I-4-86
Carpal Dislocations	I-4-90
Carpal Instabilities	I-4-94
Metacarpal Fractures and Dislocations	I-4-98
Ulnar Collateral Ligament Tear, Thumb	I-4-102
Flexor Annular Pulley Tears	I-4-106
Avulsion Fractures, Finger	I-4-110

Fractures, Lower Extremity

Avulsion Fractures, Pelvic	I-4-114
Pelvic Fractures, Stable	I-4-118
Pelvic Fractures, Unstable	I-4-122
Acetabular Fractures	I-4-126
Hip Dislocation	I-4-130
Femoral Head Fractures	I-4-134
Femoral Neck Fractures	I-4-138
Knee Avulsion Fx: Internal Derangement	I-4-142
Patellar Fracture	I-4-146
Patellar Tendon Tears & Tendinosis	I-4-150
Tibial Plateau Fracture	I-4-154
Ankle Fractures	I-4-158
Achilles Tendon Tear & Tendinopathy	I-4-162
Calcaneal Fractures	I-4-166
Talus Fractures	I-4-170
Navicular Fractures	I-4-174
Lisfranc Fracture-Dislocation	I-4-178
Metatarsal Fractures	I-4-182

Pediatric Fractures

Physeal Fractures, Pediatric	I-4-186
Child Abuse, Metaphyseal Fracture	I-4-190
Incomplete Fractures, Pediatric	I-4-194
Supracondylar Fracture, Pediatric	I-4-198
Toddler's Fractures	I-4-202
Stress Fracture, Pediatric	I-4-206
Medial Epicondyle Avulsion, Pediatric	I-4-210

MUSCULOSKELETAL IMAGING ISSUES, TRAUMA

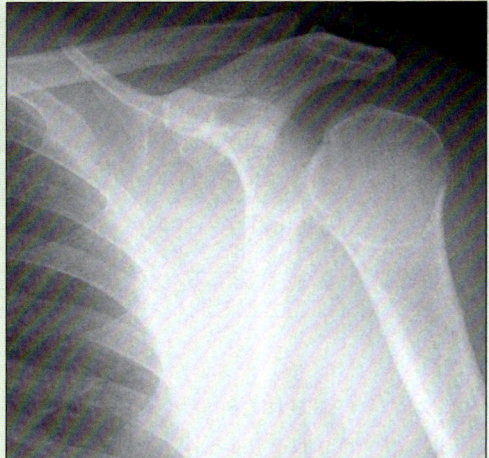

Anteroposterior, internal rotation radiograph shows apparently normal congruence of the humeral head & glenoid. Scapular "Y" view was initially obtained to check for dislocation, & appeared normal (not shown).

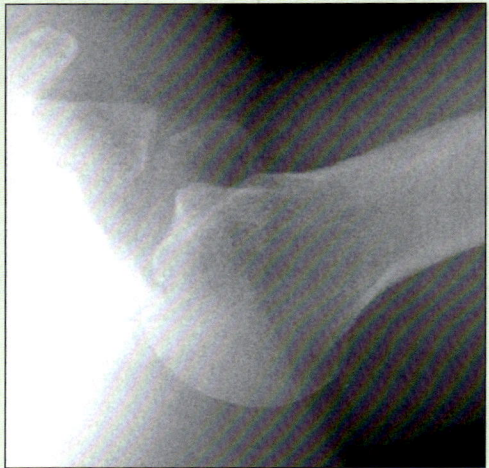

Axillary lateral radiograph however, confirms the posterior dislocation. This case is an example of the importance of obtaining true orthogonal views in trauma situations. Fractures can be missed easily as well.

ANATOMY-BASED IMAGING ISSUES

Key Concepts or Questions
- **Orthogonal imaging: The cornerstone of musculoskeletal trauma imaging**
  - Fx may be entirely obscured on one view but seen on a view 90° to that; orthogonal views required
  - Fx angulation must be assessed in both AP and lateral planes
  - A minority of orthogonal images may be difficult
    - Shoulder: Axillary lateral is the only true lateral; transthoracic or scapular "Y" views may not show a dislocation
    - Pelvis: In a trauma situation, oblique (Judet) views substitute for a true lateral view; they show both pelvic columns and acetabular rims
    - Hip: True lateral is the groin lateral view; frog lateral may be substituted, but does not show the true lateral femoral head/neck angle or the true acetabular anteversion
  - Thumb: If clinical concern is with the thumb, order thumb rather than hand views
    - Only thumb views give a true AP and lateral view
    - 3 views of hand all show the thumb in relatively the same obliquity
- **Quality filming with careful positioning is mandatory**
  - Portable technique: May be adequate if carefully done, but fractures can be missed in obese patients
  - Overlying material & backboard may obscure fx lines
  - Tech can "hide" any injury by poor positioning; examples that are especially prone to tech error
    - Wrist: PA view with wrist in radial deviation obscures waist of scaphoid fx
    - Wrist: Supinated lateral foreshortens scaphoid & makes colinear relationship of radius-lunate-capitate difficult to see
    - Elbow: Poor lateral obscures fat pads
    - Hip: External rotation on AP foreshortens neck and obscures usual fx site by greater trochanter
    - Lateral foot/ankle: Pronation and rotation obscure base of 5th metatarsal (MT)
- **Fracture description terminology: Consistent use of precise language required**
  - Open (gas in soft tissues or air in joint) vs. closed
  - Complete vs. incomplete (buckle, greenstick, plastic)
  - Comminution if present
    - Segmental: Fx at two sites of long bone, with an intact segment of bone between the fx sites: Affects blood supply
    - Butterfly: Wedge-shaped "butterfly fragment" involves a substantial portion of cortex: Often requires internal fixation
  - Location: Generally divide long bone into thirds for description; describe joint involvement if present
  - Displacement: Describe direction and amount
    - By convention, distal fragment is described as displaced relative to proximal fragment
    - Amount is described as % of cross sectional diameter of shaft
    - Describe any distraction by # mm; same for overlap (bayonet apposition)
  - Angulation: Described in one of two ways
    - Direction of the apex of the angle formed by the fx fragments (i.e. "apex lateral" or "apex varus" if the fracture angle points laterally)
    - Orientation of the distal fx fragment relative to the proximal (i.e. "medial angulation of the distal fx fragment" describes the same position as above)
  - Rotation: Generally need both joints on same image
- **How do you know where to look?**
  - Clinical site of pain
  - Knowledge of statistical likelihood of injury
  - Knowledge of "hidden" fractures and most frequently missed fx
  - Soft tissue swelling often points to injury
    - Distal to malleoli: Ligament injury more likely than fx
    - Fat pad signs: Distension around elbow or hip points to effusion & possible associated fx
    - Lipohemarthrosis: Fat blood level indicates intraarticular fx

MUSCULOSKELETAL IMAGING ISSUES, TRAUMA

Key Facts

- Orthogonal imaging is required in all trauma cases
- Quality filming with careful positioning is required
- Consistent use of precise descriptive language is mandatory in fx description
- Knowledge of statistical likelihood ↑'s sensitivity
- Knowledge of "hidden" or most frequently missed fractures improves sensitivity
- Normal variants can be confusing: Make liberal use of reference material
- Normal growth centers, particularly around the shoulder girdle & pelvis, are confusing in adolescents
- Width of AC joint, SI joint, and symphysis pubis is greater in adolescents than adults
- Although radiograph is usually the first imaging modality for trauma, there are circumstances (usually urgency) where CT is the appropriate first choice
- Rarely, MR may be a more appropriate choice than CT in an emergent setting (necrotizing fasciitis, femoral neck fx)

Imaging Approaches

- Imaging triage: Hemodynamically unstable patients will go straight to CT
- When is it not worthwhile to start with or pursue a radiograph?
  - High level trauma: C spine, pelvic CT
  - If abdominal CT is obtained as part of triage, may have to repeat with bone algorithm & submillimeter thickness to characterize an acetabular or pelvic fx
  - Sternoclavicular joint: Very difficult to characterize by radiograph; CT is study of choice
- When is CT not likely to provide the definitive answer and MR be required?
  - Understanding that MR availability may be limited in off-hours, CT is sometimes obtained initially in these cases; however it is not optimal
    - Necrotizing fasciitis: CT shows soft tissue gas, but will not define fascial fluid; thus it is often falsely negative & MR makes the correct diagnosis
    - Hip fx: Osteoporotic hip fx are not infrequently missed by CT; MR is the preferred modality; if CT is performed and is negative & clinical suspicion remains high, MR must be done
- When might US be a good place to start? search for FB
- Injuries that suggest other sites to be evaluated?
  - High rib fx: Consider aortic injury
  - Low transverse process fx: Consider sacral fx or SI joint dislocation
  - Pelvic fx: Bladder/urethral rupture, intrapelvic bleed
  - Dislocation finger: Volar plate fx
  - Calcaneus: Thoracolumbar fx
  - Acetabulum: Femoral head fx/intraarticular pieces

Imaging Protocols

- MR: Fluid sensitive sequences are most useful, but MUST include a non-fat-saturated T1 or T2 sequence
- CT: Increase kVp if metal present; < 1 mm slice thickness with reformats; principle of obliquity through thin bones

Imaging Pitfalls

- Use bone density in assessment; osteoporosis should lead to search for subtle insufficiency fx
- Watch for associated abnormalities: RA, ESRD
- Watch for destructive process mimicking trauma: Infection, tumor
- Normal variants: Many variants of ossification exist
  - Distinguish accessory ossicle from fx by sclerosis & rounded appearance
  - Reference material available: Make good use of Keats
- Normal growth centers: Apophyses around shoulder & pelvis are complex and may be confusing

Normal Measurements

- Different in children and adults: AC, SIJ, pubic symphysis all appear wider in children

RELATED REFERENCES

1. Keats TE et al: An atlas of normal roentgen variants that may simulate disease. 8th ed. Philadelphia PA, Elsevier, 2006

IMAGE GALLERY

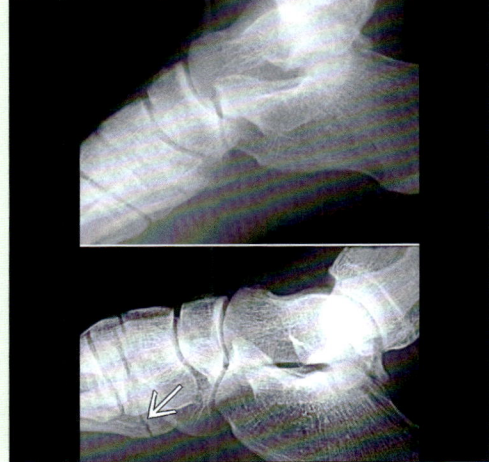
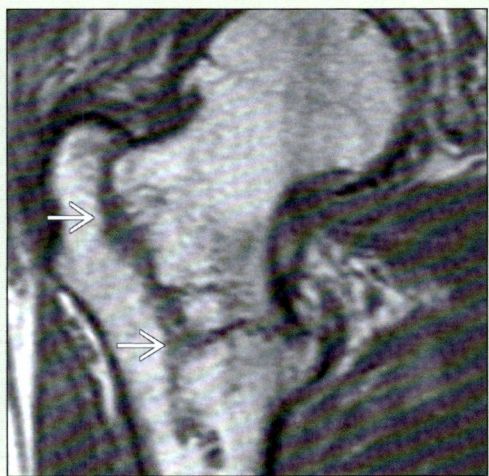

(Left) Two images of the same foot obtained at the same ER visit. The upper lateral is malpositioned, and completely obscures the fx at the base of the 5th MT seen easily in the well-positioned lower image ➡. Proper patient positioning is crucial to making diagnoses. *(Right)* Coronal T1WI MR shows incomplete, non-displaced intertrochanteric femoral neck fx ➡. The radiograph & CT obtained at the same setting were normal. MR is far more sensitive than other imaging for femoral neck fx in the osteoporotic patient.

INSUFFICIENCY FRACTURES, SACRUM

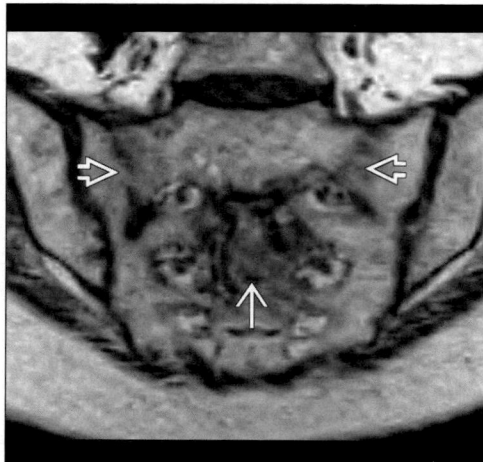

Coronal T1WI MR oriented along the long axis of the sacrum, demonstrates vertically oriented lines within both sacral ala ➔ with horizontally oriented edema ➔ which connects the vertically oriented abnormalities.

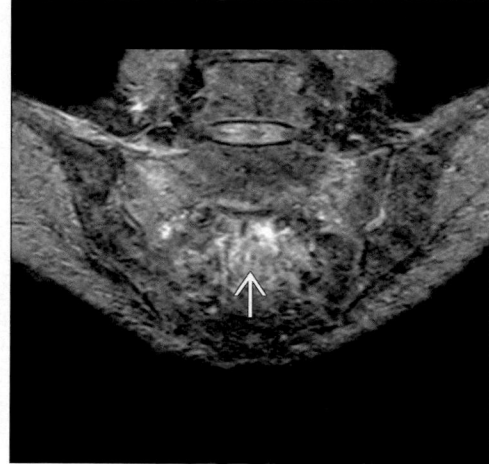

Coronal STIR MR shows edema along the bilateral sacral alar fracture lines, as well as in a transverse pattern ➔, crossing the sacral body to join the vertical fractures, forming the "Honda" sign.

TERMINOLOGY

Definitions
- Fracture crossing sacral ala vertically, related to normal stresses on abnormal bone
- "Stress fracture" is occasionally used synonymously, but is incorrect
  - Stress fracture refers to fracture resulting from abnormal stresses applied to normal bone

IMAGING FINDINGS

General Features
- Best diagnostic clue
  - Vertical fracture line through sacral ala seen on CT
  - Vertical fracture line through sacral ala seen on T1WI MR with surrounding edema seen on fluid sensitive sequences
- Location: Sacral ala, unilateral or bilateral
- Size
  - May be small & subtle initially
  - Eventually, may develop bilateral complete vertical fractures, with transverse bridge ("H" sign)

Radiographic Findings
- Radiograph is not sensitive
  - Osteopenic, so nondisplaced fx line not seen
  - Stool, gas overlying sacrum
- Late, in healing phase, may see "smudgy" vertical regions in the sacral ala (rare)

CT Findings
- Bone CT
  - CT provides direct visualization of vertical fracture lines, parallel to SI joints
  - Axial or reformatted angled coronal images
  - Sensitivity similar to MR
  - Has the advantage of identifying surrounding normal trabeculae and dispelling any concern for tumor

MR Findings
- T1WI
  - T1 MR: Vertical hypointense linear fracture line
  - Parallel to SI joints
  - No additional osseous destruction to suggest tumor
- T2WI FS
  - T2 MR: Hyperintense sacral ala marrow edema

Sacral Insufficiency Fractures: Other Imaging Modalities

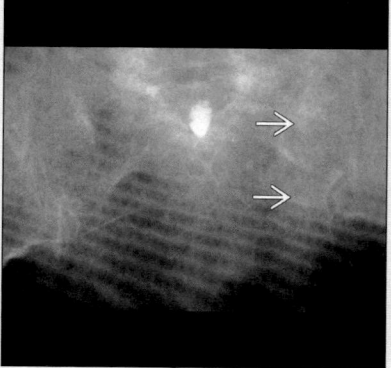

Radiograph: Smudgy Fracture Line

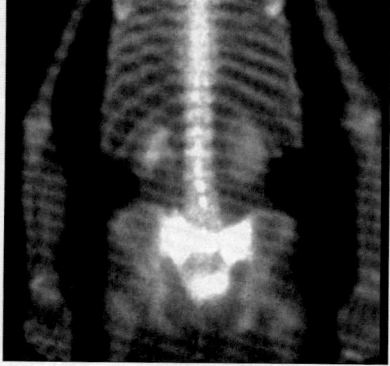

Bone Scan: Honda Sign

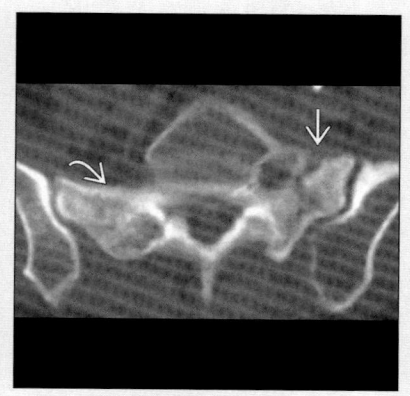

CT Bilateral Fractures

INSUFFICIENCY FRACTURES, SACRUM

Key Facts

Terminology
- Fracture crossing sacral ala vertically, related to normal stresses on abnormal bone

Imaging Findings
- Radiograph is not sensitive
- CT provides direct visualization of vertical fracture lines, parallel to SI joints
- T1 MR: Vertical hypointense linear fracture line
- T2 MR: Hyperintense sacral ala marrow edema
- Fracture line may be obscured by intense edema, do not misinterpret this as tumor
- Bone scan classic "Honda" sign with transverse component connecting 2 vertical fractures
- Bone scan highly sensitive, but nonspecific if pattern of uptake is not clearly vertical
- Angle to coronal oblique plane to best visualize entire sacrum

Clinical Issues
- Pain may not be localized in sacrum
- No history of trauma, or minimal to low velocity
- Symptoms may outweigh physical signs
- Majority heal with conservative treatment

Diagnostic Checklist
- Clinically, these patients may present with signs/symptoms suggesting hip insufficiency fracture
- Protocol for hip fracture MR should include one fluid sensitive sequence of full pelvis; this will demonstrate a sacral insufficiency fracture which is not more precisely localized by clinical exam

---

- ○ Hypointense fracture line
- ○ Fracture line may be obscured by intense edema, do not misinterpret this as tumor
- ○ May have adjacent soft tissue edema, but no mass
- ○ Often have concomitant pubic arch insufficiency fracture
- ○ Other fluid sensitive sequences (STIR, etc.) have identical findings
- ○ Extremely sensitive

Nuclear Medicine Findings
- Bone Scan
  - ○ Bone scan classic "Honda" sign with transverse component connecting 2 vertical fractures
  - ○ Incomplete Honda sign in unilateral fracture
  - ○ Bone scan highly sensitive, but nonspecific if pattern of uptake is not clearly vertical
  - ○ Nonspecific pattern often misinterpreted as metastatic disease
  - ○ Presence of pubic bone uptake in addition to sacral ala uptake improves specificity

Imaging Recommendations
- Best imaging tool
  - ○ MR identifies fracture line & should dispel other concerns (tumor)
  - ○ CT is similarly accurate and may be more available in an ER setting
- Protocol advice
  - ○ MR
    - ▪ T1WI and fluid sensitive sequences both required
    - ▪ Angle to coronal oblique plane to best visualize entire sacrum
  - ○ CT
    - ▪ Thin section (0.75 mm) bone algorithm
    - ▪ Angled coronal oblique reformatted images

DIFFERENTIAL DIAGNOSIS

Clinical Differential
- Lumbar radiculopathy
- Muscle strain/tear
- Other reasons for groin pain
  - ○ Pubic rami insufficiency fractures
  - ○ Hip pathology
    - ▪ Insufficiency fracture of femoral head or neck
    - ▪ Avascular necrosis

Radiographic Differential
- Tumor or metastatic disease
  - ○ Should have more significant osseous destruction
  - ○ Generally not vertically oriented or discrete fx line
  - ○ May have associated soft tissue mass
- Osteitis condensans ilii
  - ○ Mechanical stress induced osteosclerosis in the ilium
  - ○ Abnormality located in medial inferior iliac wing, adjacent to inferior aspect of SI joint
  - ○ Sacral ala is not involved
  - ○ Abnormality is triangular in shape
  - ○ Hypointense on all MR sequences
  - ○ Diagnosis confirmed on radiograph
- Sacroiliitis
  - ○ Abnormality centered in SI joint rather than sacral ala
  - ○ Osseous destruction on both sides of SI joint
  - ○ Hypointense on T1 MR, hyperintense on fluid sensitive sequences

PATHOLOGY

General Features
- General path comments
  - ○ Relevant anatomy
    - ▪ Sacrum transfers body weight to pelvic ring & hips
    - ▪ This constant transfer of weight puts an osteoporotic sacrum particularly at risk for fracture
    - ▪ Because of pelvic ring structure, associated pubic ring fractures frequently seen
- Etiology
  - ○ Insufficiency fracture: Normal forces of weight-bearing applied to abnormal bone
    - ▪ Osteoporosis
    - ▪ Rheumatoid arthritis
    - ▪ Pelvic irradiation

INSUFFICIENCY FRACTURES, SACRUM

- Corticosteroid use
- Metabolic bone disease (for example, renal osteodystrophy)
- Epidemiology
  - Occurs in 1% of females > 55 years
  - Occurs more frequently with other risk factors for osteoporosis
  - Occurs less frequently than pubic ramus insufficiency fractures

Gross Pathologic & Surgical Features
- Fracture sacral ala
- Vertical orientation of fracture
- Parallel to, but not involving SI joints
- May have transverse component if bilateral
- Associated pubic bone vertical fractures

Microscopic Features
- Microfractures
- Osteoclastic resorption prominent, with some osteoblastic activity
- Osteoporosis

CLINICAL ISSUES

Presentation
- Most common signs/symptoms
  - Pain with weight-bearing or ambulation
  - May present acutely, or with chronic symptoms
  - Pain may not be localized in sacrum
    - Groin pain is common presentation
    - Gluteal pain
    - Pain may even be referred to hip
- Clinical Profile
  - No history of trauma, or minimal to low velocity
  - Site of pain
    - May be point tender over sacrum
    - May be referred to other sites: Hip, groin, buttock
  - May be non-ambulatory or have gait abnormality
  - Limited range of motion
  - Symptoms may outweigh physical signs

Demographics
- Age
  - > 55 years
  - If at risk for osteoporosis, may present at earlier age
- Gender: M < F

Natural History & Prognosis
- Majority heal with conservative treatment
- May progress to complete fracture
- Healing is slow process (2-5 months) but does not require follow-up imaging
- Complications: Related to prolonged immobilization
  - Deep venous thrombosis
  - Pulmonary embolus
  - Decubitus ulcers

Treatment
- Conservative: Far most common
  - Analgesics
  - Bed rest
  - Reduced weight-bearing
  - Physical therapy (range of motion, gait training, muscle strengthening/stretching)
- Surgical (sacroplasty)
  - Interventional radiologic technique
  - Similar to vertebroplasty
  - Percutaneous injection of polymethylmethacrylate
  - When successful, nearly instantaneous relief of pain

DIAGNOSTIC CHECKLIST

Consider
- Clinically, these patients may present with signs/symptoms suggesting hip insufficiency fracture
  - If radiograph of hip is normal, MR is the next appropriate examination
  - Protocol for hip fracture MR should include one fluid sensitive sequence of full pelvis; this will demonstrate a sacral insufficiency fracture which is not more precisely localized by clinical exam
- Always identify hypointense fracture line; if obscured by edema, supplement MR with CT to assess trabecular integrity
- Associated pubic ramus fractures can be seen on all MR sequences or CT
- Coronal oblique and axial planes most useful
- Do not confuse sacral insufficiency fracture with osteitis condensans ilii or sacroiliitis; location of fracture line is distinctly different

Image Interpretation Pearls
- Do not mistake the intense high signal edema on fluid sensitive sequences for tumor
  - If there is any question of tumor versus insufficiency fracture, T1 MR or CT should show the fracture line more distinctly
- Sacral insufficiency fractures may be encountered following pelvic irradiation for adenocarcinoma
  - Do not misinterpret as metastatic site
  - Remember that radiation osteonecrosis weakens bone, putting it at risk for fracture
  - Timing for radiation osteonecrosis and fracture is many years earlier than timing for risk of radiation-induced sarcoma

SELECTED REFERENCES

1. Ikushima H et al: Pelvic bone complications following radiation therapy of gynecologic malignancies: clinical evaluation of radiation-induced pelvic insufficiency fractures. Gynecol Oncol. 103(3):1100-4, 2006
2. Tsiridis E et al: Treatment of sacral insufficiency fractures. AJR Am J Roentgenol. 186(6):E21; author reply E21, 2006
3. Zaman FM et al: Sacral stress fractures. Curr Sports Med Rep. 5(1):37-43, 2006
4. Blake SP et al: Sacral insufficiency fracture. Br J Radiol. 77(922):891-6, 2004
5. White JH et al: Imaging of sacral fractures. Clin Radiol. 58(12):914-21, 2003
6. Wild A et al: Sacral insufficiency fracture, an unsuspected cause of low-back pain in elderly women. Arch Orthop Trauma Surg. 122(1):58-60, 2002
7. Peh WC: Clinics in diagnostic imaging (60). Insufficiency fractures of the pelvis. Singapore Med J. 42(4):183-6, 2001

INSUFFICIENCY FRACTURES, SACRUM

IMAGE GALLERY

Typical

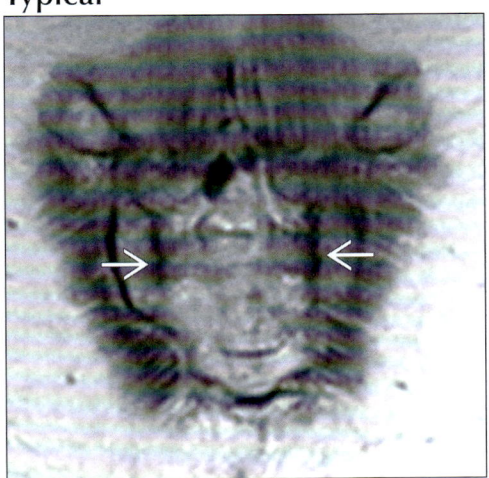
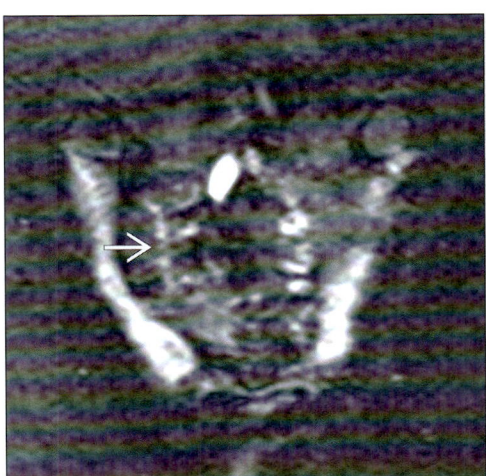

(Left) Coronal T1WI MR shows vertical low signal intensity fracture lines through each sacral ala ➡. This case shows use of obliquely oriented coronal images to display entire course of sacrum, facilitating delineation of subtle abnormalities such as these fractures. *(Right)* Coronal STIR MR shows faint bright line present along right sided fracture ➡. No edema is associated with fracture on left. Relative paucity of edema suggests that these fractures may be healing.

Typical

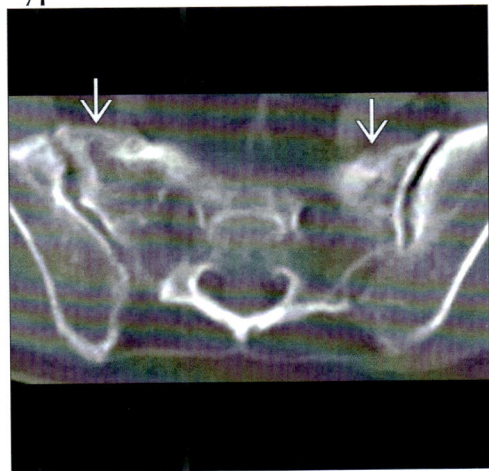
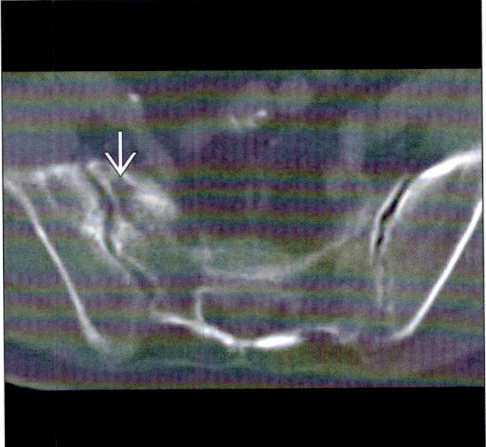

(Left) Axial NECT shows smudgy, fairly linear densities in both sacral wings, which should only be diagnosed as insufficiency fractures ➡. However, the fractures are not as distinctly seen as in some cases since the entire sacrum is abnormal in density, due to radiation osteonecrosis. *(Right)* Axial NECT located slightly more distally than the previous image shows the fracture line more distinctly ➡. This patient had pelvic irradiation one year earlier for adenocarcinoma.

Typical

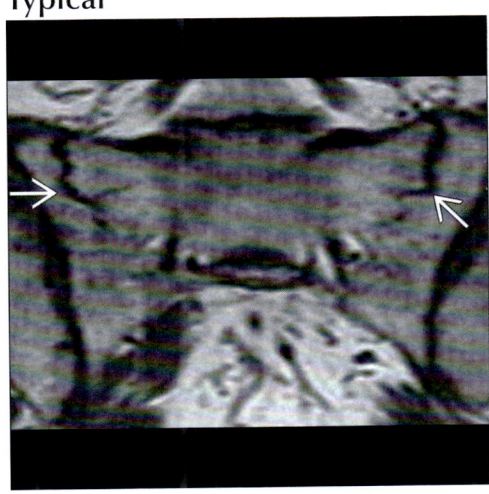
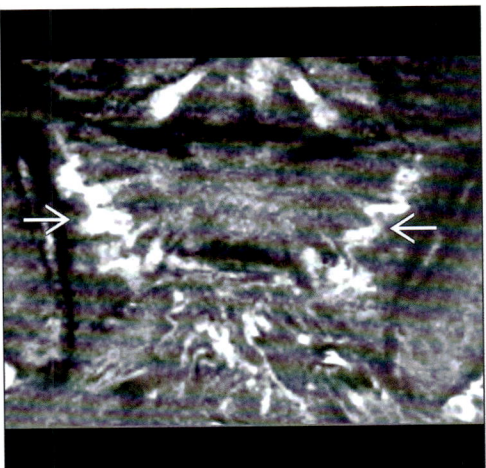

(Left) Coronal T1WI MR of the same case as previous two images shows the fracture lines ➡ much more distinctly. *(Right)* Coronal STIR MR obscures the actual fracture lines, but the linear nature of the edema ➡ makes the diagnosis easy. Occasionally, the edema appears less linear and can potentially be confusing.

INSUFFICIENCY FRACTURES, APPENDICULAR

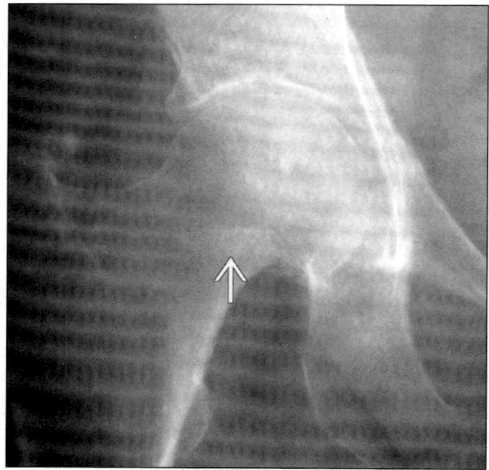

Anteroposterior radiograph shows underlying osteoporosis in this patient with RA; the linear sclerosis at the medial subcapital site ➡ is typical of an incomplete insufficiency fracture.

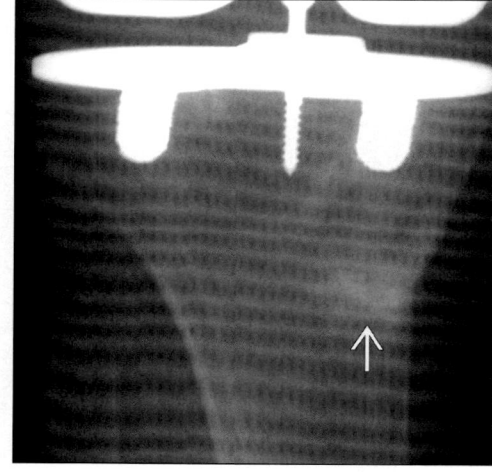

Anteroposterior radiograph shows a periprosthetic insufficiency fracture ➡ in the same patient, with linear sclerosis. This location is typical in osteoporotic patients following knee arthroplasty.

TERMINOLOGY

Abbreviations and Synonyms
- Occasionally considered a subset of pathologic fracture

Definitions
- Fracture resulting from normal stress applied to abnormal bone (excluding tumor)

IMAGING FINDINGS

General Features
- Best diagnostic clue
  - Radiograph: Linear sclerosis
  - MR: Fx line confirmed, with surrounding edema
- Location
  - Sacrum; pubic rami
  - Femoral neck: Subcapital, basicervical, intertrochanteric
  - Medial femoral condyle knee [formerly called spontaneous osteonecrosis of knee (SONK)]
  - Proximal tibia, distal fibula, calcaneus

Radiographic Findings
- Insensitive initially
- Linear sclerosis, often orthogonal to direction of major trabeculae
- Occasional focal periosteal reaction

MR Findings
- T1 weighted: Low signal linear fracture seen
- Fluid sensitive sequences: Marrow edema may obscure fx line; small amount of surrounding soft tissue edema

Nuclear Medicine Findings
- Bone scan sensitive but not specific
- Sensitivity ↓ in first 72 hours because of osteoporosis

Imaging Recommendations
- Best imaging tool: Radiograph; if negative & clinical suspicion is high, MR

PATHOLOGY

General Features
- Etiology

Osteoporotic Stress Fracture

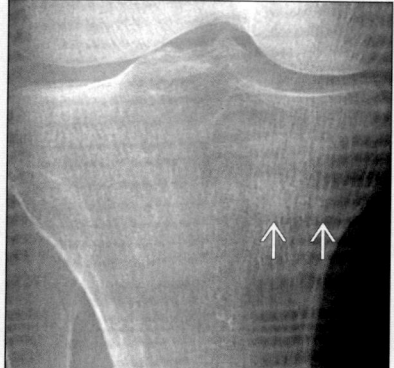

Linear Sclerosis

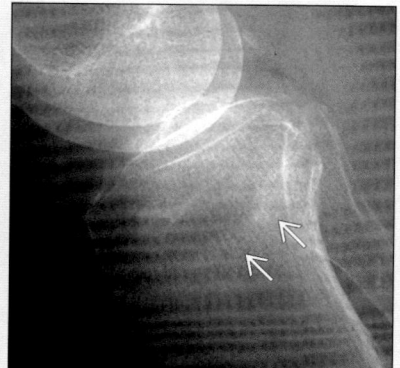

Linear on Lateral

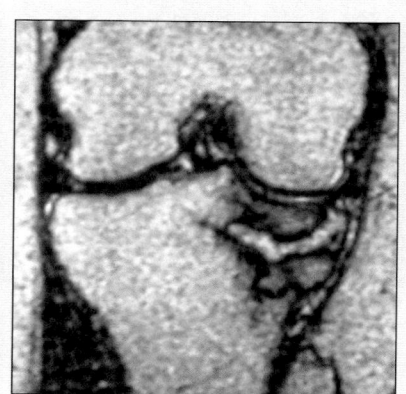

T2 MR Confirms Fracture

INSUFFICIENCY FRACTURES, APPENDICULAR

Key Facts

Terminology
- Fracture resulting from normal stress applied to abnormal bone (excluding tumor)

Imaging Findings
- Radiograph: Linear sclerosis
- MR: Fx line confirmed, with surrounding edema
- Best imaging tool: Radiograph; if negative & clinical suspicion is high, MR

Clinical Issues
- Discordance between severe pain & mild physical symptoms in an osteoporotic person is suggestive

Diagnostic Checklist
- Suggesting malignancy on the basis of non-specific bone scan or MR edema pattern is a pitfall; biopsy may lead to incorrect diagnosis since the attempts at healing give a histologically aggressive appearance

---

- Stress occurs beyond the bone's elastic range
  - Causes microfx & persistent plastic deformity
  - Osteoclastic resorption > osteoblastic activity
- Osteoporosis (↓ volume of otherwise normal bone)
  - Post-menopausal or senile osteoporosis
  - Rheumatoid arthritis (RA)
  - Steroids, smoking, alcohol
  - Diabetic/renal osteodystrophy
  - Anorexia
  - Radiation
  - Periprosthetic fx, particularly knee arthroplasty
- Epidemiology: In US, 1% of women older than 55 years have insufficiency fx

CLINICAL ISSUES

Presentation
- Most common signs/symptoms
  - Local pain without significant trauma; nonspecific
  - Discordance between severe pain & mild physical symptoms in an osteoporotic person is suggestive

Demographics
- Age: Usually > 60 years, unless patient has other predisposing conditions for osteoporosis
- Gender: Male < Female

Natural History & Prognosis
- If untreated, may progress to complete fracture
- Treated insufficiency fx resolve or improve significantly

Treatment
- Conservative: Reduced weight-bearing, analgesics for pain, then graded exercise
- Internal fixation for complete/near complete fx

DIAGNOSTIC CHECKLIST

Image Interpretation Pearls
- Strongly consider the diagnosis of insufficiency fracture particularly in these locations in an osteoporotic individual
  - At initial presentation, radiograph may be negative
  - At later presentation, radiograph will show sclerosis; watch for the pattern of linearity
  - Suggesting malignancy on the basis of non-specific bone scan or MR edema pattern is a pitfall; biopsy may lead to incorrect diagnosis since the attempts at healing give a histologically aggressive appearance

SELECTED REFERENCES

1. Prasad N et al: Insufficiency fracture of the tibial plateau: an often missed diagnosis. Acta Orthop Belg. 72(5):587-91, 2006
2. Guggenbuhl P et al: Osteoporotic fractures of the proximal humerus, pelvis, and ankle: epidemiology and diagnosis. Joint Bone Spine. 72(5):372-5, 2005
3. Ramnath RR et al: MR appearance of SONK-like subchondral abnormalities in the adult knee: SONK redefined. Skeletal Radiol. 33(10):575-81, 2004

IMAGE GALLERY

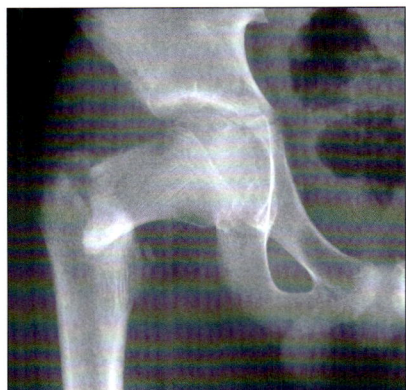 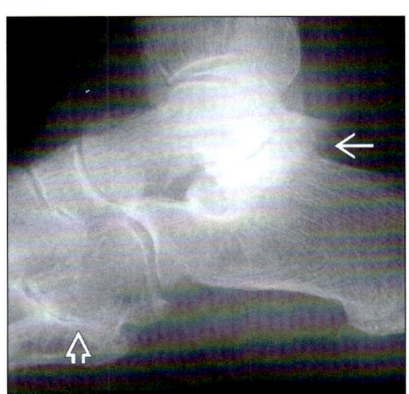 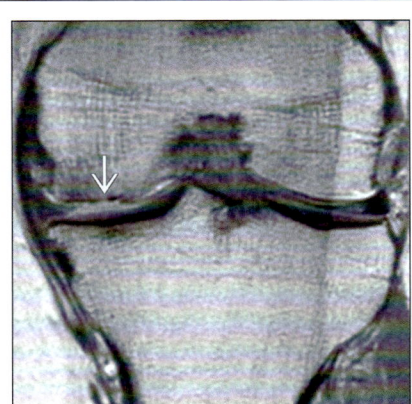

(Left) AP radiograph shows a basicervical fx in a patient who had low-level trauma. One must suspect insufficiency fx; patient proved to have transient juvenile osteoporosis. *(Center)* Lateral radiograph shows insufficiency fx of the calcaneal lateral facet ➡. Offset & sclerosis make the dx in this unusual location. T-MT erosions ➡ help confirm underlying dx of RA. *(Right)* Coronal T1WI MR shows a subchondral insufficiency fx in the weight-bearing region of the medial femoral condyle ➡. Lesion, seen mostly in elderly osteoporotic women, was formerly called SONK.

STRESS FRACTURE, ADULT

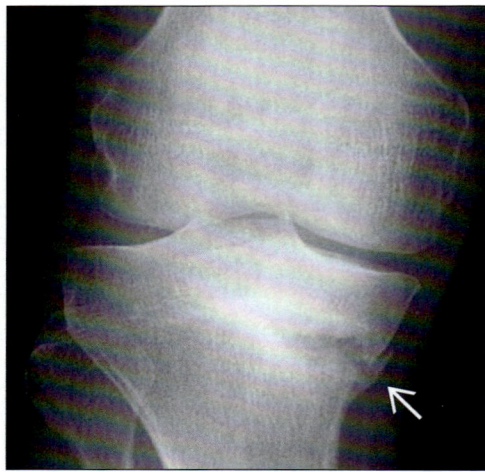

Anteroposterior radiograph shows obvious stress fracture. The fracture is subacute, with the lucent line easily seen, along with sclerosis surrounding it. Periosteal reaction is present ➡ as well.

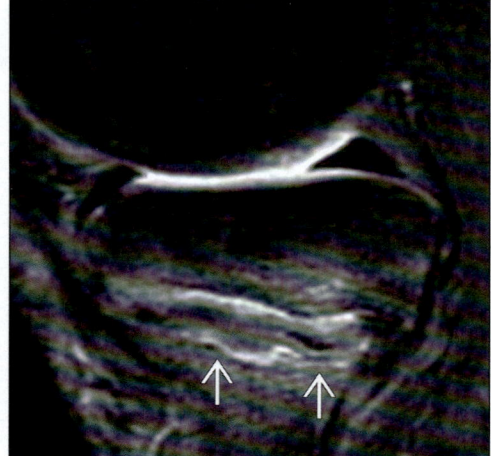

Sagittal STIR MR shows the fracture line which is so wide that fluid enters it ➡. It is unusual that a stress fracture is neglected long enough to have this prominent an appearance.

TERMINOLOGY

Abbreviations and Synonyms
- Fatigue fracture

Definitions
- Fracture resulting from abnormal stress on normal bone
  - Individual loads not enough to cause injury, but cyclical loading results in fracture

IMAGING FINDINGS

General Features
- Best diagnostic clue
  - Radiograph: Linear sclerosis, periosteal reaction
  - MR: Low signal fracture line with surrounding marrow and circumferential soft tissue edema
- Location
  - Pelvis
    - Sacrum
    - Pubic rami (inferior > superior)
  - Femur
    - Basicervical
    - Medial cortex in proximal & midshaft; proximal 1/3, including subtrochanteric region most common
    - Posterior cortex in distal shaft
  - Long bone longitudinal
    - Femur
    - Tibia
    - Fibula
  - Tibia
    - Posterior cortex proximal 1/3 (most frequent)
    - Distal 1/3; next most frequent
    - Mid 1/3; least common
  - Fibula
    - Distal 1/3, proximal to lateral malleolus most common
    - Proximal 1/3 less common
  - Ankle
    - Calcaneus
    - Navicular
  - Foot
    - Metatarsals (90% 2nd & 3rd; 4th next most common)
    - Sesamoid

Other Stress Fractures

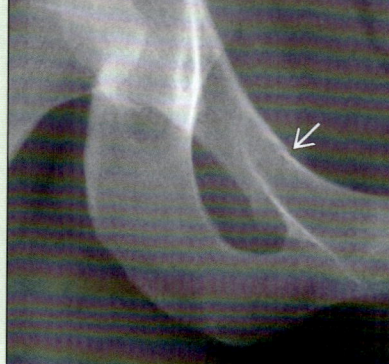

Pubic Ramus, Jogger

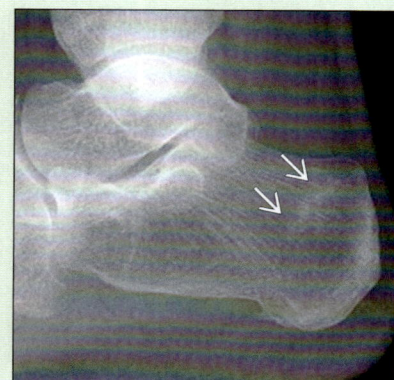

Calcaneal Stress Fracture

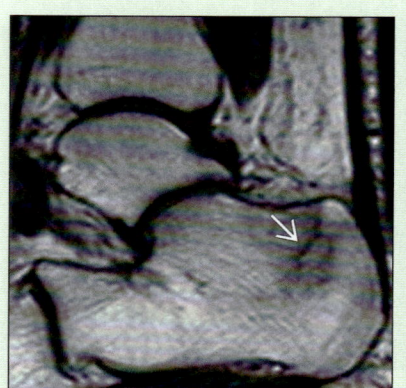

T1 MR Confirmation

STRESS FRACTURE, ADULT

Key Facts

Terminology
- Fracture resulting from abnormal stress on normal bone
- Individual loads not enough to cause injury, but cyclical loading results in fracture

Imaging Findings
- Linear sclerosis on radiograph, focal periosteal reaction
- Sclerosis usually perpendicular to major trabeculae
- CT with reformats is optimal imaging for longitudinal stress fracture
- MR: T1 shows linear fracture line
- MR: Fluid sensitive sequences show fracture line, surrounding marrow edema, & circumferential soft tissue signal
- MR: Highly specific

Top Differential Diagnoses
- Cortically based osteoid osteoma in long bones elicits prominent reactive bone formation & marrow edema which may mimic the sclerosis of a stress fx
- Brodie Abscess (Chronic Osteomyelitis)
- If the reactive bone formation is particularly prominent at one aspect of the cortex in a stress fx, it could mimic the osteoid of a surface osteosarcoma

Diagnostic Checklist
- It is extremely important to differentiate stress fx from considerations of tumor by means of imaging
- Biopsy of a stress fracture should be avoided
- Biopsy of fracture may be confusing histologically, with the healing osteoid giving the appearance of an aggressive bone tumor

---

　　o Upper extremity, ribs very uncommon

Radiographic Findings
- Early stress fracture
  - Radiograph identifies only 28%
  - Distributed over a long segment of cortex; radiographs normal or show faint cortical resorption or periosteal reaction
  - Termed stress reaction (shin splints in tibia)
- Subacute or chronic stress fracture
  - Radiographs more specific
  - Linear sclerosis on radiograph, focal periosteal reaction
  - Sclerosis usually perpendicular to major trabeculae

CT Findings
- Linear lucency of fracture line seen
- Adjacent sclerosis and reaction, depending on age of fracture
- Often requires reformats in a plane orthogonal to the fracture line
- CT with reformats is optimal imaging for longitudinal stress fracture

MR Findings
- Early stress fracture
  - Findings on fluid sensitive sequences
  - Periosteal reaction over long extent of cortex
  - Mild marrow edema
  - Surrounding circumferential soft tissue edema
- Subacute or chronic stress fracture
  - MR: T1 shows linear fracture line
  - MR: Fluid sensitive sequences show fracture line, surrounding marrow edema, & circumferential soft tissue signal
  - MR: Highly specific
- If negative for stress fx, MR may show nearby muscle strain which mimics fx clinically
- Longitudinal stress fracture may present a confusing picture on MR due to nonspecific edema

Nuclear Medicine Findings
- Early stress fracture: Tc-99m bone scan shows uptake along long extent of cortex
- Subacute or chronic stress fracture: Tc-99m bone scan shows more focal uptake
- Highly sensitive; less specific than MR
- High negative predictive value

Imaging Recommendations
- Best imaging tool
  - Radiograph is first modality
  - If radiograph negative, MR
  - If suspect longitudinal stress fracture, CT is best imaging tool

DIFFERENTIAL DIAGNOSIS

Osteoid Osteoma
- Cortically based osteoid osteoma in long bones elicits prominent reactive bone formation & marrow edema which may mimic the sclerosis of a stress fx
- Lytic central nidus is a differentiating factor when present
- Sclerotic reaction is not in a linear pattern as for stress fx

Brodie Abscess (Chronic Osteomyelitis)
- Osseous destruction may not be prominent in a slowly progressing infection
- Reactive bone formation is prominent, mimicking the sclerosis of stress fx

Surface Osteosarcoma
- If the reactive bone formation is particularly prominent at one aspect of the cortex in a stress fx, it could mimic the osteoid of a surface osteosarcoma

PATHOLOGY

General Features
- Etiology

STRESS FRACTURE, ADULT

- Bone responds to repetitive loading by remodeling
  - Cortical bone remodels first by resorption, then replacement
  - Stress fx occurs in the vulnerable period when bone is weakened by resorption & not yet strengthened by replacement
- Stress fractures evolve over time
  - Early, injury is distributed over a long segment of cortex (termed stress reaction)
  - With ongoing microfractures, a focal segment may weaken more rapidly
  - This segment becomes a focal point for bone deformation during repeated loading
  - Microfractures progress at this site
  - Reparative process becomes more focal, related to microfracture site
- Muscle fatigue may also contribute to the injury
  - If muscle is close to exhaustion, it provides less stress shielding & may increase load on bone
- Epidemiology
  - Up to 10% of patients seen in sports medicine clinics have stress fracture
  - Most common stress fx are in runners; of 1000 consecutive stress fx
    - 22% foot & ankle (20% metatarsals, 2% elsewhere in foot/ankle)
    - 14% femur (7% neck, 7% shaft)
    - 50% lower leg (34% tibia, 24% fibula)
    - 1-6% pelvis (inferior pubic ramus > superior)
  - Site usually relates to type of repetitive activity
    - Runners: Pubic rami (M < F), basicervical femoral neck, tibial shaft, fibula, metatarsal shaft, sesamoid
    - Backpacking (& heavy bookbags): Upper ribs, clavicle
    - Tennis: Humerus, ulna, metacarpal
    - Baseball pitching: Humerus, scapula, 1st rib, ulna
    - Baseball batting: Rib
    - Baseball catching: Patella
    - Basketball: Patella, tibia (anterior mid shaft, may heal poorly), calcaneus, sacrum, navicular
    - Javelin throwing: Ulna, humerus
    - Soccer: Tibia, pubis
    - Swimming: Tibia, metatarsals
    - Skating: Fibula, tibia, metatarsals
    - Curling: Ulna
    - Aerobics: Tibia, fibula
    - Ballet dancers: Spine (pars interarticularis), tibia, fibula, metatarsals, sesamoid
    - Cricket: Humerus, spine
    - Golf: Lower ribs, ulna, sternum, tibia, hook of hamate
    - Fencing: Pubis
    - Handball: Metacarpals
    - Water-skiing: Pars interarticularis
    - Rowing: Lower ribs
    - Trap shooting: Coracoid process
    - Volleyball: Pisiform
    - Gymnast: Fibula, pars intraarticularis, humerus (periostitis at pectoralis insertion, from iron ring performance)
    - Wrestlers: Sternum
    - Weight lifters: Humerus (periostitis at pectoralis insertion, from repeated lateral curls)

CLINICAL ISSUES

Presentation
- Most common signs/symptoms: Focal pain at the site, reproducible with the associated activity

Demographics
- Age: Generally young, athletic individuals
- Gender: Smaller bone structure may put female athletes more at risk

Natural History & Prognosis
- If protected, will heal without consequence
- If protection is not instituted or adhered to, may progress to complete fracture

Treatment
- Protect from weight bearing; if advanced, immobilization

DIAGNOSTIC CHECKLIST

Image Interpretation Pearls
- It is extremely important to differentiate stress fx from considerations of tumor by means of imaging
- Biopsy of a stress fracture should be avoided
  - Biopsy further weakens the bone, requiring longer protection from full weight bearing
  - Biopsy of fracture may be confusing histologically, with the healing osteoid giving the appearance of an aggressive bone tumor

SELECTED REFERENCES

1. Anderson MW: Imaging of upper extremity stress fractures in the athlete. Clin Sports Med. 25(3):489-504, vii, 2006
2. Chen RC et al: Troublesome stress fractures of the foot and ankle. Sports Med Arthrosc. 14(4):246-51, 2006
3. DeFranco MJ et al: Stress fractures of the femur in athletes. Clin Sports Med. 25(1):89-103, ix, 2006
4. Gaeta M et al: High-resolution CT grading of tibial stress reactions in distance runners. AJR Am J Roentgenol. 187(3):789-93, 2006
5. Gehrmann RM et al: Current concepts review: Stress fractures of the foot. Foot Ankle Int. 27(9):750-7, 2006
6. Pepper M et al: The pathophysiology of stress fractures. Clin Sports Med. 25(1):1-16, vii, 2006
7. Ruohola JP et al: Fatigue bone injuries causing anterior lower leg pain. Clin Orthop Relat Res. 444:216-23, 2006
8. Snyder RA et al: Epidemiology of stress fractures. Clin Sports Med. 25(1):37-52, viii, 2006
9. Umans HR: Imaging sports medicine injuries of the foot and toes. Clin Sports Med. 25(4):763-80, 2006
10. Wall J et al: Imaging of stress fractures in runners. Clin Sports Med. 25(4):781-802, 2006
11. Bolin D et al: Current concepts in the evaluation and management of stress fractures. Curr Sports Med Rep. 4(6):295-300, 2005
12. Joy EA et al: Stress fractures in the female athlete. Curr Sports Med Rep. 4(6):323-8, 2005
13. Knapp TP et al: Stress fractures: general concepts. Clin Sports Med. 16(2):339-56, 1997

STRESS FRACTURE, ADULT

IMAGE GALLERY

Typical

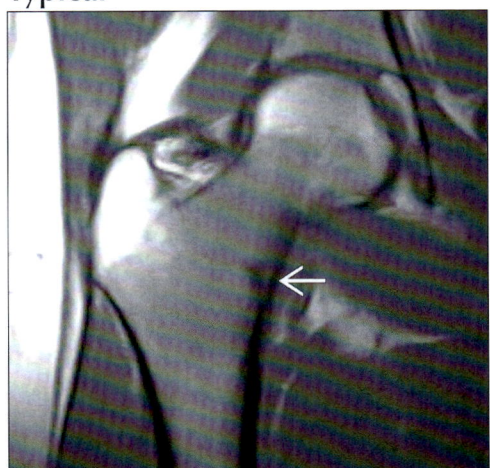
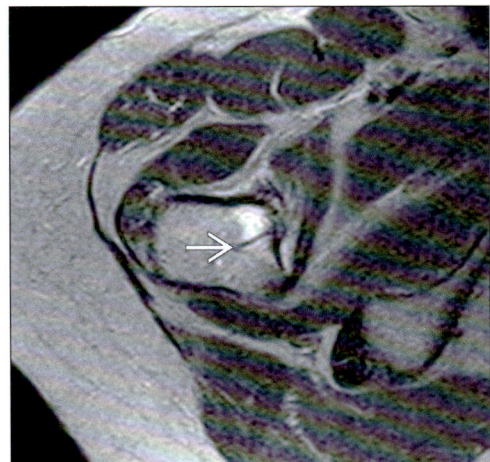

(Left) Coronal T1WI MR shows a low signal line ➡, representing early fatigue fracture in the medial proximal femur. Note the marrow pattern which is otherwise normal in this 18 year old female who runs 20 miles per week. *(Right)* Axial T2WI FS MR confirms the low signal fracture ➡, with surrounding edema. The radiograph was normal in this case of very early stress fracture.

Typical

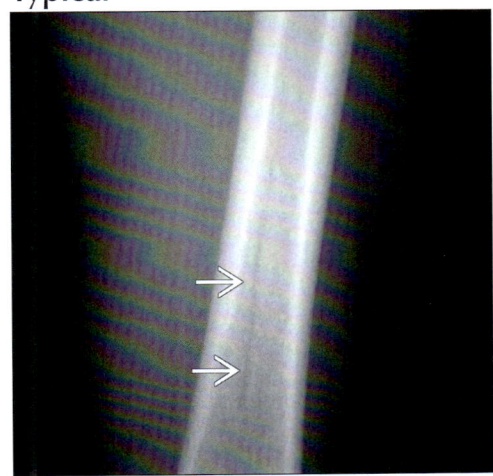
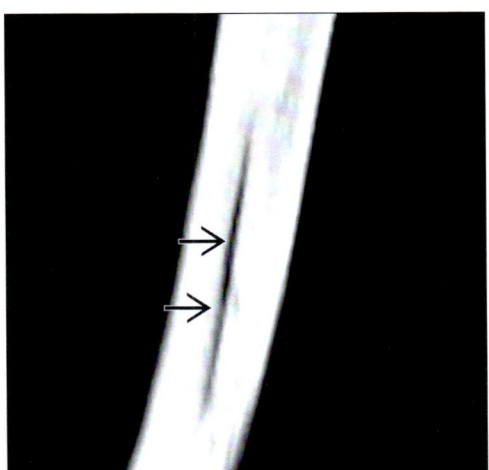

(Left) Anteroposterior radiograph shows a linear lucency which could be mistaken for a nutrient vessel ➡. However, the line is quite crisp, without the adjacent mild sclerosis seen with nutrient vessels. With high clinical suspicion, CT should be performed. *(Right)* Coronal bone CT reformat confirms that the lucency seen on radiograph is indeed a longitudinal stress fx ➡. MR (not shown) was confusing, with nonspecific edema & no definite fracture line.

Typical

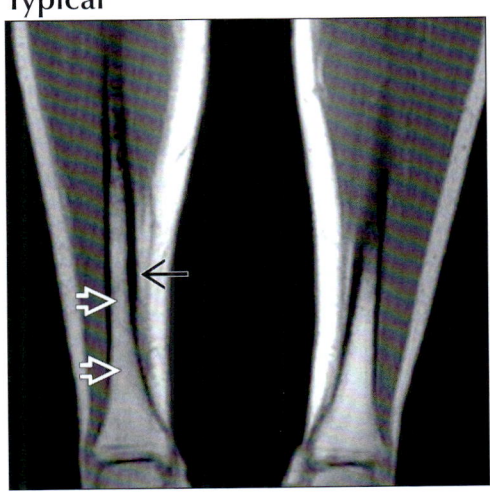
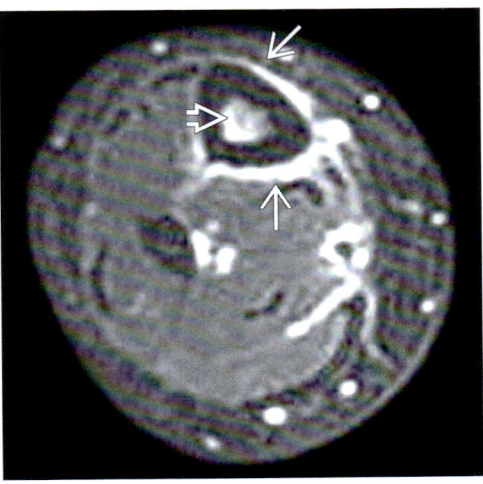

(Left) Coronal T1WI MR shows findings of medial tibial stress syndrome, with marrow edema ➡ and thickened periosteum ➡. *(Right)* Axial STIR MR confirms the marrow edema ➡. There is circumferential soft tissue edema as well ➡. No actual fracture line is seen. This stress reaction represents the earliest phase of stress injury.

PATHOLOGIC FRACTURE

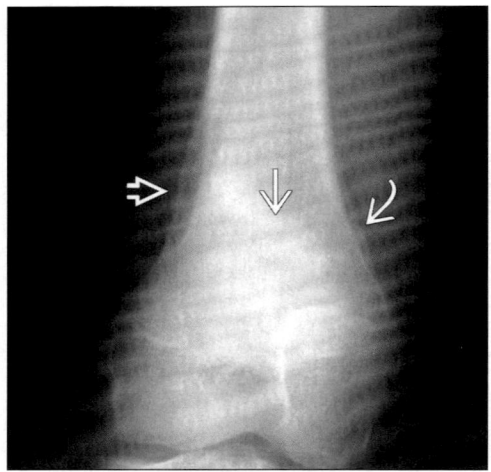

Anteroposterior radiograph shows a linear sclerotic fracture line ➡ extending from a non-ossifying fibroma ➡. This is subacute, as there is dense periosteal reaction ➡ seen as well.

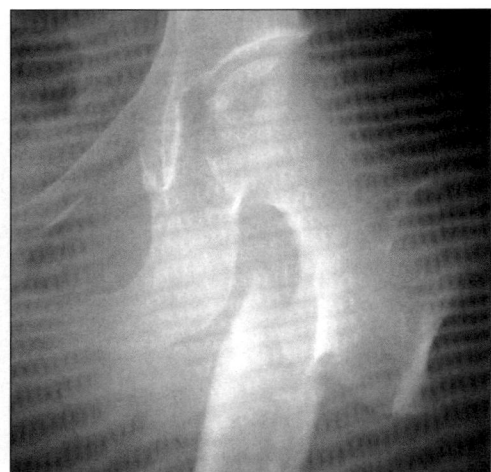

Anteroposterior radiograph shows a subtrochanteric transverse fx which occurred in the absence of significant trauma. This history & appearance leads one to suspect underlying pathology (metastatic breast).

TERMINOLOGY

Abbreviations and Synonyms
- Insufficiency fx (could be considered a subset of pathologic fx, but generally not)
- Stress fracture: Incorrect usage of this term since stress fracture refers to abnormal stresses applied to normal bone

Definitions
- Pathologic fracture results from normal stress on abnormal bone
- Several etiologies of abnormal bone may apply
  o Tumor (benign or malignant)
  o Insufficiency from osteopenia
    ▪ Radiation osteonecrosis
    ▪ Senile osteoporosis
    ▪ Corticosteroids, smoking, alcohol
    ▪ Metabolic bone disease
    ▪ Rheumatoid arthritis
    ▪ Diabetes
    ▪ Other arthritides with large subchondral cysts (pyrophosphate arthropathy & gout)

IMAGING FINDINGS

General Features
- Best diagnostic clue
  o Watch for underlying lesion, which weakens bone & may result in fx; these may be subtle
  o Watch for fractures in weight-bearing bones which are atypical in pattern or do not match the amount of force reported
    ▪ Transverse fractures in long weight-bearing bones are rare in the absence of significant trauma
    ▪ Basicervical femoral neck fractures are rare in the absence of either significant trauma or abnormal repetitive stress (serious runner)
    ▪ Though fractures in phalanges (hand or foot) are common, watch for an underlying enchondroma since this lesion is so common in these bones
- Location
  o Any bone may develop an underlying lesion
  o Those most likely to fracture are the long weight-bearing bones & phalanges
- Morphology

Other Fractures

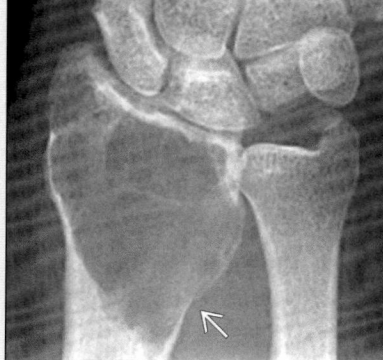

Pathologic Fx, Solitary Bone Cyst

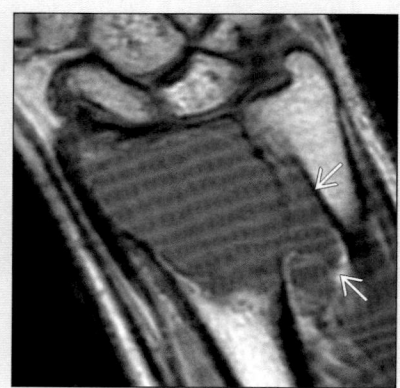

Hematoma from Fracture, not Tumor

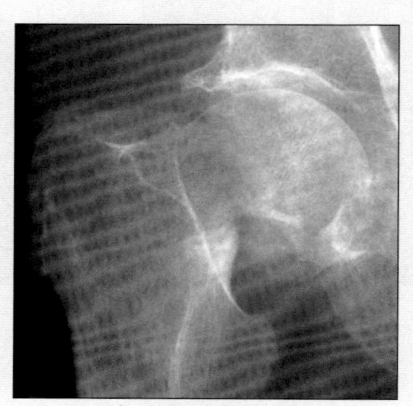

Garden IV, not Pathologic

PATHOLOGIC FRACTURE

Key Facts

Terminology
- Pathologic fracture results from normal stress on abnormal bone

Imaging Findings
- Watch for underlying lesion, which weakens bone & may result in fx; these may be subtle
- Watch for fractures in weight-bearing bones which are atypical in pattern or do not match the amount of force reported
- Transverse fractures in long weight-bearing bones are rare in the absence of significant trauma
- Basicervical femoral neck fractures are rare in the absence of either significant trauma or abnormal repetitive stress (serious runner)
- Though fractures in phalanges (hand or foot) are common, watch for an underlying enchondroma since this lesion is so common in these bones

Diagnostic Checklist
- Do not overcall a Garden III or IV subcapital fx as pathologic
- Pathologic fx may have soft tissue mass seen on MR
- This mass may be hematoma rather than tumor
- Subchondral pathologic fracture into a lytic lesion
- May not be tumor, but a subchondral cyst
- Look for other reasons to consider a diagnosis such as gout or pseudogout arthropathy
- Pathologic fracture of enchondroma in a phalanx does not imply malignant transformation, even when associated with cortical thinning

---

  ○ Transverse fracture is particularly common in pathologic fractures, as opposed to oblique or spiral patterns in trauma-induced fractures
  ○ It is difficult to predict likelihood of a lesion developing pathologic fx: Traditional criteria (not scientifically validated) include
    ▪ Endosteal scalloping over a "significant" distance
    ▪ Large size of lesion
    ▪ Location in a weight-bearing region (along the calcar, within the femoral neck, as examples)

Radiographic Findings
- Features which help differentiate pathologic from stress fracture in long bone
  ○ Surrounding permeative change in bone
  ○ Chondroid or osteoid matrix
  ○ Endosteal scalloping

CT Findings
- Features which help differentiate pathologic from stress fracture in long bone
  ○ Marrow abnormality
  ○ Endosteal scalloping
  ○ Aggressive periosteal reaction
  ○ Matrix

MR Findings
- Features which help differentiate pathologic from stress fracture in long bone
  ○ Well-defined T1 marrow signal in pathologic fracture (83% vs. 7%)
  ○ Endosteal scalloping in pathologic fracture (58% vs. 0%)
  ○ Abnormal muscle signal in pathologic fracture (83% vs. 48%)
  ○ Soft tissue mass in pathologic fracture (67% vs. 0%)

Imaging Recommendations
- Best imaging tool
  ○ Radiograph & high level of suspicion
  ○ MR may help to differentiate pathologic from stress fracture
    ▪ In-phase/opposed phase MR imaging shows a significant difference in signal intensity between benign vertebral compression fx & malignancy
    ▪ MR more accurate than radiograph (in turn more accurate than CT) in differentiating long bone pathologic from stress fracture
  ○ Quantitative CT may help predict likelihood of developing pathologic fracture through a known lesion
    ▪ Uses combination of bending & torsional rigidity measurements
    ▪ Reported to be 97% accurate for predicting pathologic fracture likelihood in benign bone lesions
    ▪ Standard radiographic criteria 42-61% accurate for similar prediction
- Protocol advice
  ○ Diffusion-weighted spin echo, fat-suppressed spin echo, & stimulated-echo sequences equally differentiate benign from malignant vertebral body fx
  ○ Consider in-phase/opposed phase imaging to differentiate benign from malignant

DIFFERENTIAL DIAGNOSIS

Pseudopathologic Subcapital Fracture
- Garden III-IV subcapital fracture results in external rotation of femoral shaft
  ○ Garden III: 32% have radiographic appearance simulating pathologic fx
  ○ Garden IV: 24% have radiologic appearance simulating pathologic fx
- Position of shaft in external rotation & distraction, compounded by osteoporosis, gives the impression of lytic lesion
- Do not overcall these as pathologic (tumor)

Stress Fracture
- May develop aggressive-appearing periosteal bone formation in the healing phase

PATHOLOGIC FRACTURE

- Marrow & adjacent tissue may have significant reactive change
- Generally, fracture line is seen in a long bone with careful attention to radiograph & MR
- Occasionally may need specialized MR to help differentiate between pathologic & stress fracture

PATHOLOGY

General Features
- Etiology: Mild trauma in weakened bone
- Epidemiology: Older patients most frequent, relating to ↑ probability of underlying osteopenia, tumor, etc.

Gross Pathologic & Surgical Features
- Fx + underlying pathology (osteopenia, tumor, etc.)

CLINICAL ISSUES

Presentation
- Most common signs/symptoms
  - Acute pain, without significant trauma
  - Remember that most tumors do not present with acute pain, but rather low-grade pain; with acute pain presentation, look for pathologic fx
- Clinical Profile
  - Statistically, most common patient will be
    - Adult with multiple myeloma
    - Adult with enchondroma involving phalanx
    - Adult with known primary tumor
  - Tumors most frequently metastatic to bone in adults
    - Breast
    - Prostate
    - Lung

Demographics
- Age: Any, but older adults are more likely to have osseous metastatic disease
- Gender: No predilection

Natural History & Prognosis
- Relates to the pathology

Treatment
- Relates to the pathology
  - Benign lesion
    - Curettage
    - Bone graft or cement
    - Hardware for support as necessary
    - Some benign lesions react to fracture with a healing response: Solitary (unicameral) bone cyst & nonossifying fibroma (fibroxanthoma) may heal with only external support (casting)
    - Fibrous dysplasia, though benign, generally is not cured by curettage; only complications of this disease are treated
  - Malignant lesion (primary)
    - Reduction & support of fx for patient comfort
    - Needs entire work-up, in appropriate order, usually in an outpatient setting
    - This generally includes MR of the site of the lesion
    - Biopsy
    - Consideration of metastatic sites: May use CT, MR, bone scan, PET/CT
  - Malignant lesion (metastatic)
    - For a weight-bearing long bone, IM rodding considered superior to ORIF
    - Radiation may be considered if lesion is responsive; may help alleviate pain, but may retard osseous healing
    - Cement or bone graft may be used to fill a significant defect
    - Radiofrequency ablation may be used in selected lesions for pain control (currently not FDA approved; undergoing clinical trials)

DIAGNOSTIC CHECKLIST

Consider
- Look for hints as to underlying diagnosis
  - Matrix within lesion
  - Aggressive versus nonaggressive features of lesion
  - Polyostotic lesion

Image Interpretation Pearls
- Do not overcall a Garden III or IV subcapital fx as pathologic
- Pathologic fx may have soft tissue mass seen on MR
  - This mass may be hematoma rather than tumor
  - If the osseous lesion otherwise does not appear aggressive, do not let this focal mass lead to an overcall of a malignant lesion
- Subchondral pathologic fracture into a lytic lesion
  - May not be tumor, but a subchondral cyst
  - Look for other reasons to consider a diagnosis such as gout or pseudogout arthropathy
- Pathologic fracture of enchondroma in a phalanx does not imply malignant transformation, even when associated with cortical thinning
  - Phalangeal enchondromas have a lower rate of malignant transformation to chondrosarcoma than more proximal enchondroma
  - Phalangeal enchondromas may show cortical thinning & expansion without being considered aggressive lesions

SELECTED REFERENCES

1. Erly WK et al: The utility of in-phase/opposed-phase imaging in differentiating malignancy from acute benign compression fractures of the spine. AJNR Am J Neuroradiol. 27(6):1183-8, 2006
2. Papagelopoulos PJ et al: Advances and challenges in diagnosis and management of skeletal metastases. Orthopedics. 29(7):609-20; quiz 621-2, 2006
3. Snyder BD et al: Predicting fracture through benign skeletal lesions with quantitative computed tomography. J Bone Joint Surg Am. 88(1):55-70, 2006
4. Fayad LM et al: Distinction of long bone stress fractures from pathologic fractures on cross-sectional imaging: how successful are we? AJR Am J Roentgenol. 185(4):915-24, 2005
5. Spuentrup E et al: Diffusion-weighted MR imaging for differentiation of benign fracture edema and tumor infiltration of the vertebral body. AJR Am J Roentgenol. 176(2):351-8, 2001

PATHOLOGIC FRACTURE

IMAGE GALLERY

Typical

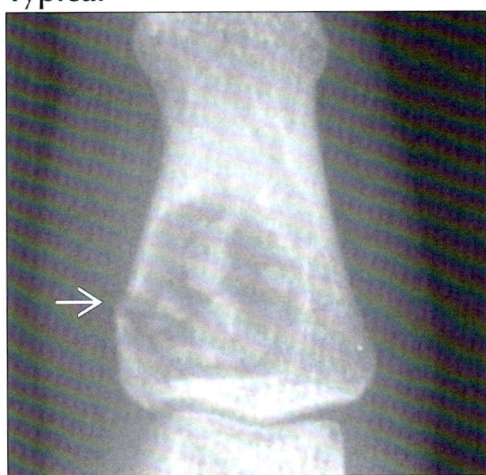
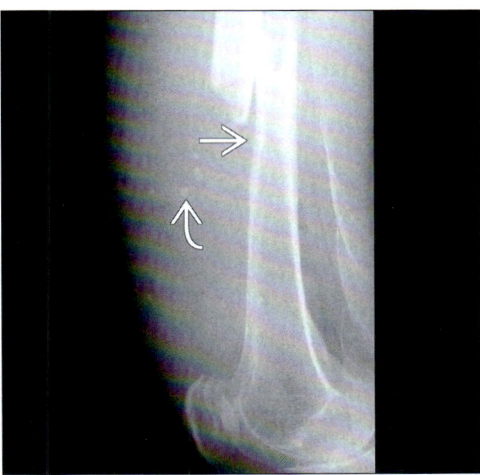

(Left) Anteroposterior radiograph shows a pathologic fx ➔ through a lytic lesion which contains chondroid matrix. This is a typical enchondroma (very common in phalanges). The underlying lesion is not always as distinctly seen. *(Right)* Lateral radiograph shows a pathologic fx in the mid femur. Note the transverse nature of the fx, as well as the extrinsic scalloping of the anterior cortex ➔. Phleboliths in a soft tissue mass ➔ make the diagnosis of hemangioma.

Typical

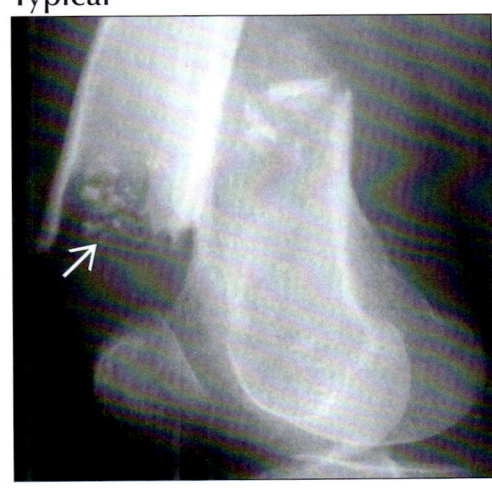
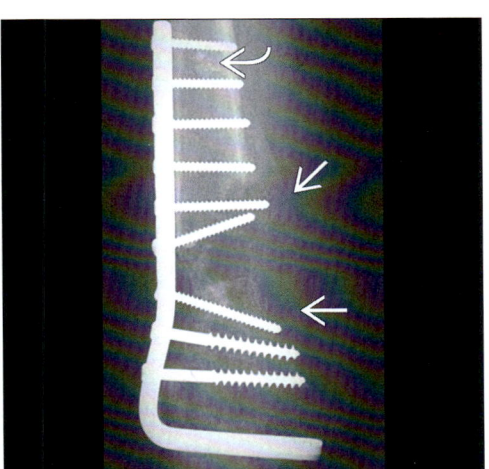

(Left) Lateral radiograph shows a transverse pathologic fx through the distal femur. There is chondroid matrix ➔ which should lead to a diagnosis of cartilage tumor. *(Right)* Anteroposterior radiograph shows fixation performed without regard to the underlying lesion seen in the prior image. There is now a soft tissue mass ➔, osseous destruction, & matrix seen proximally ➔. This is a chondrosarcoma.

Typical

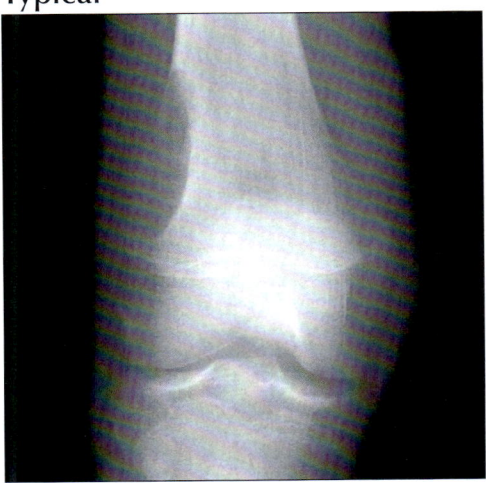
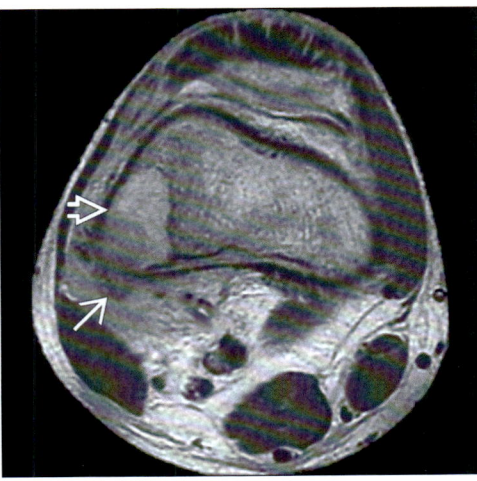

(Left) Anteroposterior radiograph shows nonaggressive appearing lesion. Patient had acute onset of pain, which would not be typical of this lesion & therefore suggests pathologic fx; fx is not seen. *(Right)* Axial T2WI MR shows underlying lesion ➔ as well as small soft tissue mass ➔. Given acute onset of pain as well as nonaggressive appearance by radiograph, mass should be diagnosed as hematoma from pathologic fracture rather than something more ominous.

FOREIGN BODY

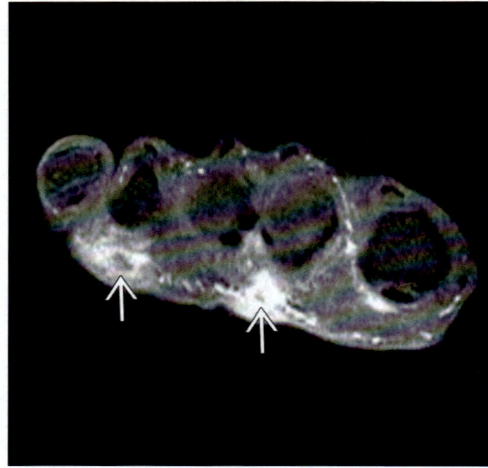

Coronal T1 C+ FS MR shows two pieces of glass in the subcutaneous plantar aspect of the foot ➡, with surrounding enhancing tissue. The foreign bodies were not apparent on radiograph, but suspected on US.

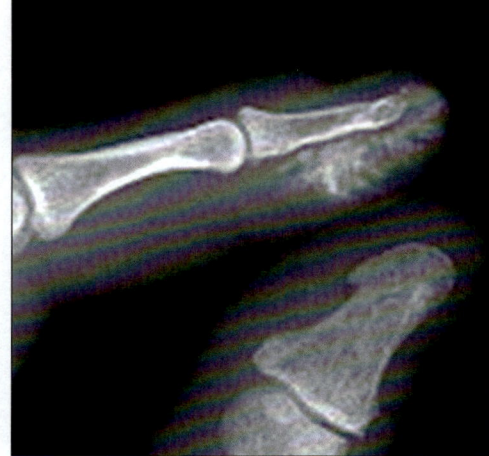

Lateral radiograph shows a radiodense foreign material in the soft tissues of the index finger. Paint gun injuries in which there is skin penetration have this typical appearance due to the lead in the paint.

TERMINOLOGY

Definitions
- Object of external origin that is retained within the tissues of the body
  - While foreign bodies within the trunk may also be from ingestion, those within extremities are almost exclusively from penetrating trauma

IMAGING FINDINGS

General Features
- Best diagnostic clue
  - Radiodensity on plain film with contours more characteristic of artificial than of natural material
    - Sometimes the object (e.g., bullet, nail, staple) may actually be recognizable
- Location: Most common in the hands, but can present anywhere
- Size: Variable
- Morphology: Variable

Radiographic Findings
- Radiographs will detect 80% of all foreign bodies
- Metal and glass (even non-leaded) are radiopaque relative to soft tissues
  - It is a myth that only leaded glass can be detected by radiography
- Wood and plastic are often isodense to muscle/water and not detected by plain film
  - Only 15% of wooden foreign bodies are visible on radiography
  - A large piece of porous wood may contain sufficient air to create a lucent defect in soft tissues
- Paint and grease guns cause numerous digital injuries annually
  - Index finger is most commonly involved since it is placed over the nozzle opening
  - Pressure injected contents dissect a path through tissue planes
    - Path commonly follows flexor tendon sheaths into palm
  - Oil or paint thinner causes a radiolucent stripe
  - Paint is radiopaque if it contains lead or other heavy metals

Other Foreign Bodies

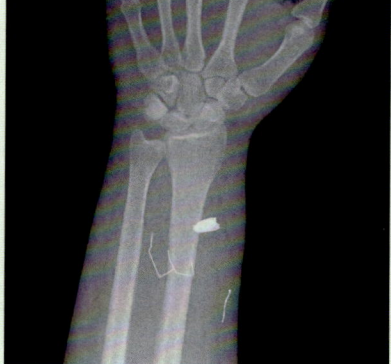

Wire

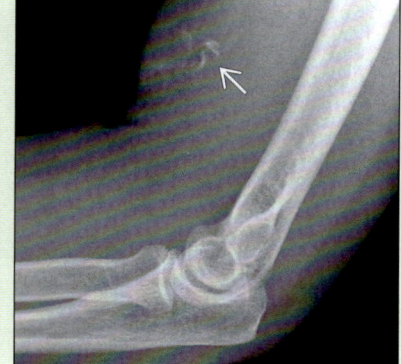

Gauze

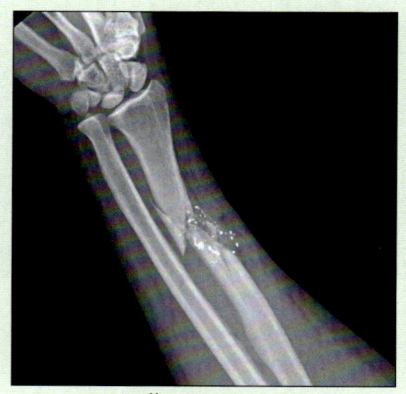

Bullet Fragments

FOREIGN BODY

Key Facts

Terminology
- Object of external origin that is retained within the tissues of the body

Imaging Findings
- Radiographs will detect 80% of all foreign bodies
- Metal and glass (even non-leaded) are radiopaque relative to soft tissues
- Wood and plastic are often isodense to muscle/water and not detected by plain film
- CT may be useful when other studies have failed to detect a suspected foreign body (i.e., wood or wood-like fragment)
- MR with gadolinium enhancement is useful in evaluating foreign body complications
- All foreign bodies are initially hyperechoic
- Ultrasound is the study of choice in the case of suspected foreign body with negative radiograph
- Best imaging tool: Plain radiographs in multiple views to cast the foreign body away from the underlying bone

Pathology
- Etiology: Extremity foreign bodies are almost exclusively due to penetrating trauma

Clinical Issues
- Pain and/or mass
- 38% are missed by the initial treating physician
- Complications include infection, granuloma formation, and nerve/tendon injury due to local inflammatory reaction

CT Findings
- NECT
  - Has the greatest advantage of distinguishing subtle differences in density
  - CT may be useful when other studies have failed to detect a suspected foreign body (i.e., wood or wood-like fragment)
  - Metal and glass are hyperdense
    - Metal may cause significant streak artifacts
  - Wood is initially low density due to air content
    - Chronically retained wood becomes hyperdense due to absorption of blood products and exudate
  - Limitations include cost, availability, and radiation exposure
- CECT
  - Usually only necessary if an abscess is suspected
  - May also be useful in evaluating for other complications, or in surgical planning

MR Findings
- Usually not necessary in the acute setting
  - Useful for planning surgical approach
    - Especially when foreign material is in a critical area
  - MR with gadolinium enhancement is useful in evaluating foreign body complications
    - Inflammatory reaction
    - Abscess
    - Osteomyelitis
    - Granuloma
    - Scar formation
- Superior to CT in soft tissue contrast resolution
- Metal will create local susceptibility artifact obscuring the soft tissue anatomic detail
- Wood and glass will create geometric areas of signal void (black), but no susceptibility artifact
  - Wood is hypointense to skeletal muscle on both T1WI and T2WI sequences
  - Surrounding inflammatory response is hypointense on T1WI but iso- to hyperintense on T2WI
- Should NOT be used in evaluating metallic foreign bodies in critical locations such as the eye or CNS
  - Ferromagnetic materials may be displaced by the magnetic field with catastrophic results

Ultrasonographic Findings
- All foreign bodies are initially hyperechoic
- Conspicuity is increased by hypoechoic halo of granulation tissue, edema, or hemorrhage
  - Halo usually develops by around 24 hours
- Sonographic artifacts can aid in identification
  - Objects with a rough surface (i.e., wood) have "clean" posterior acoustic shadowing
  - Objects with a smooth surface (i.e., glass, metal) have "dirty" shadowing and reverberation artifacts
- Plastic foreign bodies are less echogenic but have marked posterior shadowing
- Wooden foreign bodies become less echogenic over time
- 87% sensitivity and 97% specificity for wooden foreign bodies as small as 2.5 mm
  - Operator competence is a limiting factor in the clinical setting
  - High frequency transducers (↑ resolution, ↓ penetration) are more sensitive than those of lower frequency
- Ultrasound is the study of choice in the case of suspected foreign body with negative radiograph
- Intraoperative sonographic guidance can also be used during surgical removal

Angiographic Findings
- Contrast extravasation would suggest vascular damage

Other Modality Findings
- New techniques such as diffraction-enhanced imaging and multiple-image radiography show promise for future clinical use

Imaging Recommendations
- Best imaging tool: Plain radiographs in multiple views to cast the foreign body away from the underlying bone
- Protocol advice

FOREIGN BODY

- "Soft tissue" technique radiographs (i.e., lower kV and higher mA) may be more sensitive
  - Decreasing X-ray tube voltage lightens the film and enhances contrast between some materials and surrounding tissue

DIFFERENTIAL DIAGNOSIS

None
- Acute foreign bodies have no differential diagnosis
- Differential diagnosis of a chronic foreign body would be that of its complications (inflammation, abscess, granuloma, etc.)

PATHOLOGY

General Features
- Etiology: Extremity foreign bodies are almost exclusively due to penetrating trauma
- Epidemiology: 40% of foreign bodies in the hand (most common site) are work-related
- Associated abnormalities: May have fractures, vascular injury/hemorrhage, or nerve injury from the inciting trauma

Gross Pathologic & Surgical Features
- Wood comprises 36%
  - Glass 23%
  - Metal 20%
  - Other (plastic, gravel, etc.) 21%

CLINICAL ISSUES

Presentation
- Most common signs/symptoms
  - Pain and/or mass
  - Occasionally asymptomatic
    - Incidental finding on a study performed for another reason
- Other signs/symptoms
  - Patient may or may not give history of penetrating trauma
  - 13% present with a complication
- 38% are missed by the initial treating physician
- Missed foreign bodies are one of the leading causes of malpractice claims against ED physicians
- Average time for foreign body retention is 7 months
  - 43% removed within 1 week
  - 11% retained longer than 1 year

Demographics
- Age: Mean age = 35, but can affect any age
- Gender: M:F = 7:3

Natural History & Prognosis
- Complications include infection, granuloma formation, and nerve/tendon injury due to local inflammatory reaction
- Can wander locally, and may even work their way into circulation and travel to the heart

Treatment
- A foreign body may be left in place if it is inert, asymptomatic, not a threat to function, difficult to remove due to small size
- Should be removed if reactive, large, concerning to the patient, or near tendons/nerves/vessels
  - After removal, wound is loosely closed and extremity immobilized

DIAGNOSTIC CHECKLIST

Consider
- Plain radiographs are the mainstay in screening for foreign bodies
- If available, ultrasound should be considered in the case of a suspected foreign body with negative radiographs

SELECTED REFERENCES

1. Muehleman C et al: Multiple-image radiography for human soft tissue. J Anat. 208(1):115-24, 2006
2. Turkcuer I et al: Do we really need plain and soft-tissue radiographies to detect radiolucent foreign bodies in the ED? Am J Emerg Med. 24(7):763-8, 2006
3. Graham DD Jr: Ultrasound in the emergency department: detection of wooden foreign bodies in the soft tissues. J Emerg Med. 22(1):75-9, 2002
4. Manaster BJ et al: Musculoskeletal Imaging: The Requisites. 2nd ed. St. Louis, Mosby. 520-1, 2002
5. Peterson JJ et al: Wooden foreign bodies: imaging appearance. AJR Am J Roentgenol. 178(3):557-62, 2002
6. Horton LK et al: Sonography and radiography of soft-tissue foreign bodies. AJR Am J Roentgenol. 176(5):1155-9, 2001
7. Kornreich L et al: Preoperative localization of a foreign body by magnetic resonance imaging. Eur J Radiol. 26(3):309-11, 1998
8. Grechenig W et al: [Ultrasound imaging of foreign bodies--an experimental study] Biomed Tech (Berl). 41(11):308-15, 1996
9. Donaldson JS: Radiographic imaging of foreign bodies in the hand. Hand Clin. 7(1):125-34, 1991
10. Bodne D et al: Imaging foreign glass and wooden bodies of the extremities with CT and MR. J Comput Assist Tomogr. 12(4):608-11, 1988
11. Anderson MA et al: Diagnosis and treatment of retained foreign bodies in the hand. Am J Surg. 144(1):63-7, 1982

FOREIGN BODY

IMAGE GALLERY

Typical

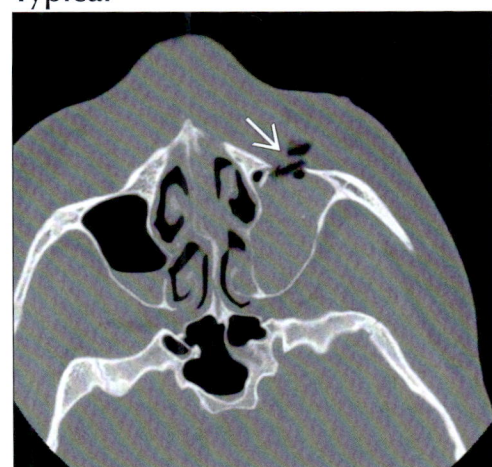
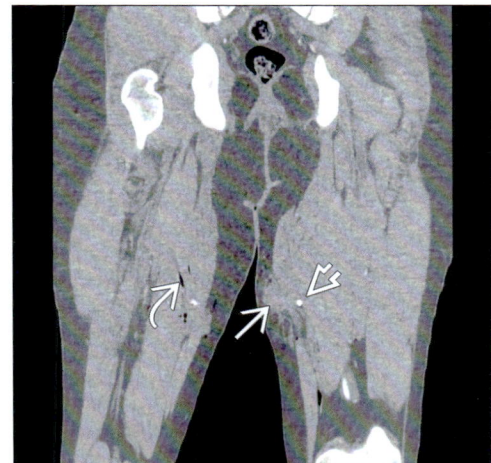

(Left) Axial NECT through the face of a patient assaulted with a tree branch shows a sliver of wood ➡ penetrating into the left maxillary sinus. Special windowing is necessary to distinguish the lucent wood from air. *(Right)* Coronal CECT of a gunshot victim shows multiple pellets ➡, as well as hemorrhage ➡ and gas ➡ secondary to the penetrating trauma.

Typical

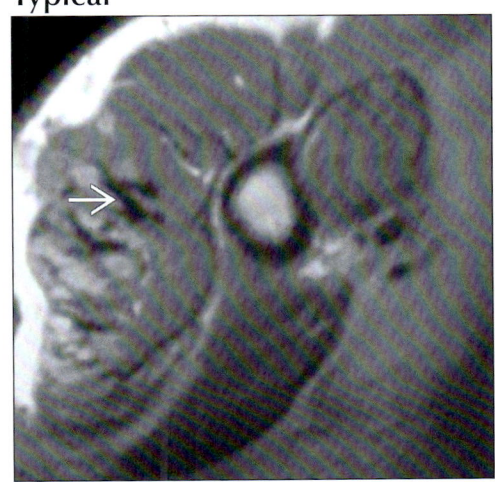
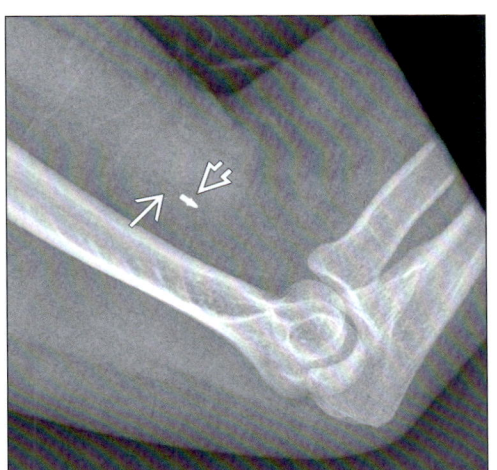

(Left) Axial T1 C+ MR shows hypointense foreign body reaction ➡ which was low signal on all sequences, surrounded by hyperintense edema. This patient had multiple injections of antibiotics over a several month period. *(Right)* Lateral radiograph of the elbow of a psychiatric patient shows the radiolucent plastic ➡ and radiopaque metal ➡ portions of a pen tip she stuck in her own arm.

Typical

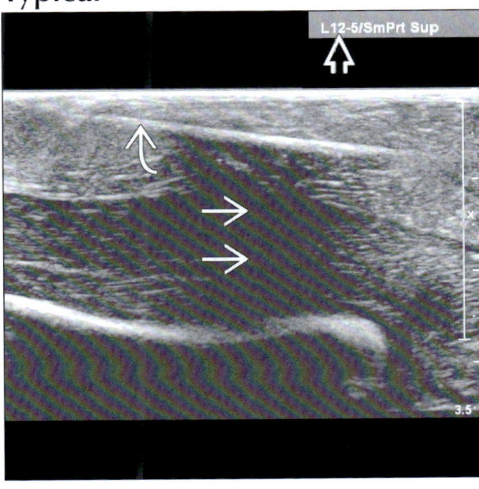
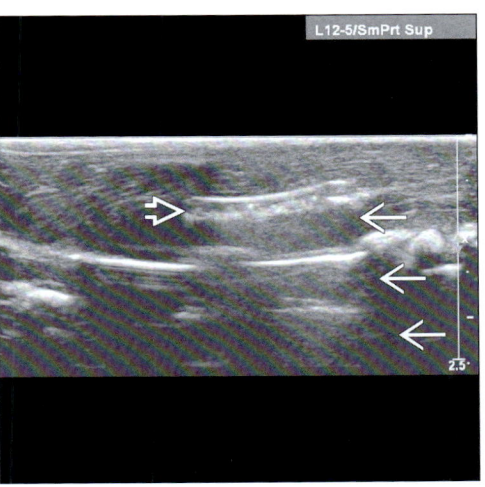

(Left) Ultrasound shows a wooden toothpick embedded in the muscle as a hyperechoic focus ➡ with complete posterior shadowing ➡. Note that a linear, high frequency (12 MHz) transducer was used ➡. *(Right)* Ultrasound shows a subcutaneous, hyperechoic focus ➡ representing a glass foreign body from a beer bottle. Note the classic posterior reverberation artifacts ➡.

COMPARTMENT SYNDROME

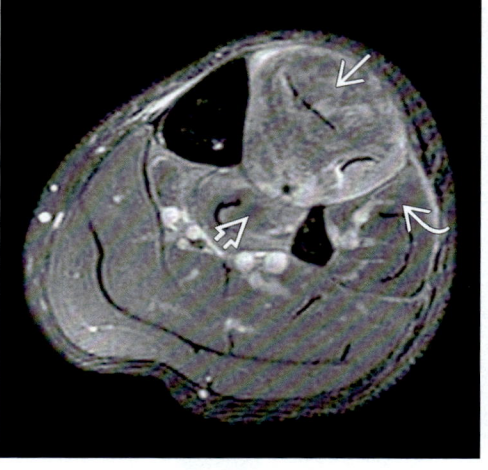

Axial T2WI FS MR reveals marked swelling of the anterior tibialis muscle ➡ with edema (hyperintensity) in the adjacent extensor hallucis longus ➡ as well as the posterior tibialis ➡.

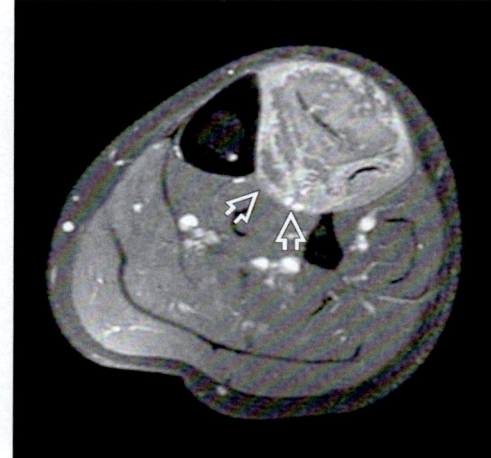

Axial T1 C+ FS MR demonstrates patchy diffuse enhancement of the swollen anterior tibialis. Note the bowing of the interosseous membrane ➡ which results in compromise of the adjacent neurovascular structures.

TERMINOLOGY

Abbreviations and Synonyms
- Acute compartment syndrome; chronic (exertional) compartment syndrome

Definitions
- Damage to soft tissues within anatomically confined space, resulting from elevated pressure

IMAGING FINDINGS

General Features
- Best diagnostic clue: Diffuse hyperintensity on fluid sensitive MR sequences within affected compartment muscle(s)
- Location
  - Most common: Anterior, lateral, superficial, deep posterior compartments of leg
  - Medial, central, lateral, interosseous, calcaneal compartments of foot
  - Flexor, extensor compartments of forearm
  - Thigh (exertional compartment syndrome)
  - Less frequent, often related to prolonged surgical positioning: Gluteal, deltoid
- Size: Variable along length of muscle or among more than one muscle of compartment
- Morphology
  - MR signal abnormality is elongated, along length of muscle or muscles in compartment
  - Combined leg & foot compartment syndromes may occur

MR Findings
- T1 WI
  - Intermediate signal intensity within edematous muscle
  - Loss of normal muscle striations
  - ± Increased signal in subacute hemorrhage
  - Hypointense hemosiderin foci
  - Enlargement of affected muscle group, ± peripheral bowing
  - Hypointense calcification in chronic compartment syndrome
  - Hyperintense fat in chronic muscle atrophy
  - Hypointense in chronic fibrous replacement
  - Calcific myonecrosis

DDx: Compartment Syndrome

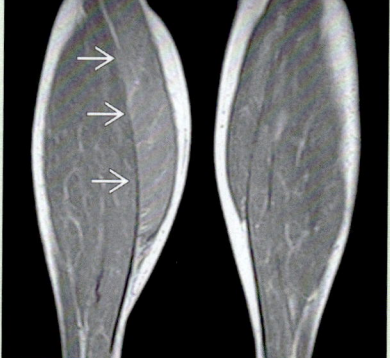

Denervation Hypertrophy

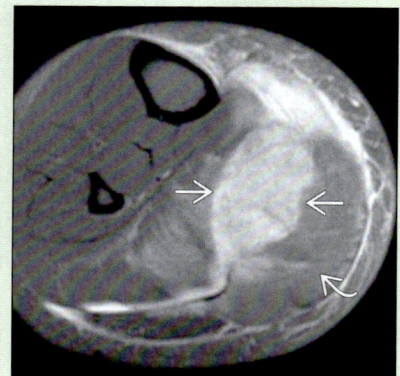

Hematoma; Muscle Strain

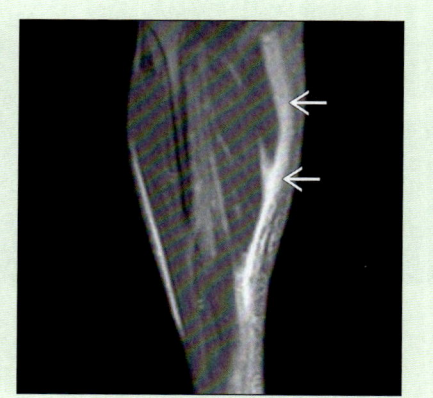

Necrotizing Fasciitis

COMPARTMENT SYNDROME

Key Facts

Terminology
- Damage to soft tissues within anatomically confined space, resulting from elevated pressure

Imaging Findings
- Best diagnostic clue: Diffuse hyperintensity on fluid sensitive MR sequences within affected compartment muscle(s)
- Most common: Anterior, lateral, superficial, deep posterior compartments of leg
- Medial, central, lateral, interosseous, calcaneal compartments of foot
- Flexor, extensor compartments of forearm
- Thigh (exertional compartment syndrome)
- Less frequent, often related to prolonged surgical positioning: Gluteal, deltoid
- MR signal abnormality is elongated, along length of muscle or muscles in compartment
- If acute syndrome is clinically suspected, direct measurement of intracompartmental pressure should not be delayed
- MR superior to bone scan, radiography, or CT
- Protocol advice: Axial plane required for identifying cross-sectional muscle compartment & neurovascular relationship

Clinical Issues
- Most common signs/symptoms: Disproportionate pain relative to injury
- Nerve/muscle ischemia > 12 hr → permanent injury
- Conservative treatment: Not an option

- Fluid sensitive sequences
  - Hyperintense diffusely within cross sectional anatomic boundaries of affected muscle
  - Hyperintense along variable proximal/distal extent of muscle
  - Hyperintense fluid/hemorrhage/edema also between muscles in fascial planes
  - Hyperintensity associated with both edema & rhabdomyolysis
  - Atrophied muscle suppresses without associated hyperintensity
  - ± Subcutaneous tissue hyperintense edema
  - Intermediate to increased signal of muscle in exertional compartment syndrome
  - Calcification & fibrosis (chronic) remain hypointense
- May have associated muscle herniation on any sequence

Imaging Recommendations
- Best imaging tool
  - If acute syndrome is clinically suspected, direct measurement of intracompartmental pressure should not be delayed
  - MR superior to bone scan, radiography, or CT
  - Edema, fibrosis, & fatty infiltration best visualized on MR
  - Conventional radiography & CT limited to ruling out associated injuries
- Protocol advice: Axial plane required for identifying cross-sectional muscle compartment & neurovascular relationship

DIFFERENTIAL DIAGNOSIS

Deep Vein Thrombosis
- Neurovascular bundle perivascular edema
- Edema in watershed distribution
- ± Enlarged popliteal vein with thrombus occlusion, ± collateral venous structures

Muscle Strain
- Partial tear muscle/musculotendinous unit
- Feathery/diffuse edema on fluid sensitive sequences

Cellulitis
- Reticular to circumscribed subcutaneous (superficial & deep) edema
- No muscle compartment involvement or fascial extension

Myositis Ossificans/Rhabdomyolysis
- Earliest stages of these may appear as muscle edema
- Both usually progress to mass pattern
- Myositis progresses to form calcifications by 4-8 weeks

Denervation Hypertrophy
- Enlarged & edematous muscle
- Fatty atrophy within muscle
- Onset more insidious; painless
- MR abnormality seen 2-4 weeks post denervation

Diabetic Muscle Infarct
- Edema, bulging of muscle similar
- May see decreased vascularity
- Generally end stage diabetes
- Extremely painful

Longitudinal Stress Fracture
- May have edema & swelling around fracture site
- Subtle fractures seen with careful imaging; CT with reformats useful

PATHOLOGY

General Features
- General path comments
  - Relevant anatomy
    - Anterior compartment (leg) muscles: Tibialis anterior, extensor hallucis longus, extensor digitorum longus, peroneus tertius
    - Anterior compartment neurovascular bundle: Deep peroneal nerve & anterior tibial artery

COMPARTMENT SYNDROME

- Posterior compartment divided by deep transverse fascia into superficial & deep sections
  - Superficial posterior compartment muscles: Gastrocnemius, plantaris, soleus
  - Deep posterior compartment muscles: Popliteus, flexor digitorum longus, flexor hallucis longus, tibialis posterior
  - Posterior compartment neurovascular bundle: Tibial nerve & posterior tibial artery
  - Anterolateral compartment muscles: Peroneus longus, peroneus brevis
  - Anterolateral compartment neurovascular bundle: Superficial peroneal nerve & peroneal artery
- Etiology
  - Arteriovenous gradient theory
    - Compromised blood flow → hypotension, increased vascular resistance → increased tissue pressure (extravasated blood)
  - Ischemia-reperfusion theory
    - Compromised blood flow → ischemia → impaired cellular metabolism → interstitial edema → increased compartmental pressure
  - Acute compartment syndrome etiologies
    - Fracture (especially tibia, forearm, & calcaneus)
    - Muscle rupture or hemorrhage
    - Crush injuries
    - Burns
    - Extrinsic pressure: From lying motionless on hard surface (drug or alcoholic stupor) or certain positions on OR table (deltoids or glutei)
    - Peripheral vasospasm from cocaine use
    - Axillary arteriography: Medial brachial fascial compartment syndrome
  - Chronic compartment syndrome
    - Exercise-induced
    - Pain during exercise that subsides with rest
- Epidemiology
  - Open tibial fractures: 20% complicated by compartment syndrome
  - Acute leg compartment syndrome most commonly related to tibial fracture
  - Muscle hernias in 40% of chronic compartment syndrome
  - 5% calcaneal fractures develop compartment syndrome of the foot
  - Bivalving a cast results in 85% reduction in intracompartmental pressure

Staging, Grading or Classification Criteria

- Acute: Resting intracompartment pressures > 30 mm Hg
- Chronic
  - Resting intramuscular pressure > 10 mm Hg
  - Pressure of 15 mm Hg at 15 minutes post exercise

CLINICAL ISSUES

Presentation

- Most common signs/symptoms: Disproportionate pain relative to injury
- Clinical Profile
  - Palpable swelling (± tense skin), pain, pallor, paralysis, paresthesias
  - Distal pulses usually intact
  - Chronic
    - Exercise related; usually runners
    - Resolves when exercise is stopped
  - Acute
    - Uncommon in athletic population
    - Most frequently related to fractures & casting
    - May have history of recent surgery, especially if in prolonged lithotomy position
    - Prolonged lying on hard surface (drug/alcoholic)

Demographics

- Age: Nonspecific
- Gender: No gender bias

Natural History & Prognosis

- Nerve/muscle ischemia > 12 hr → permanent injury
- Muscle necrosis
- Volkmann contracture (fibrous contracture & neurologic damage)
- Complication: Reperfusion injury (cellular activity restored → worsening of preexisting cellular damage)

Treatment

- Conservative treatment: Not an option
- Surgical
  - Acute: Fasciotomy
  - Chronic: Surgical decompression/fasciotomy

DIAGNOSTIC CHECKLIST

Consider

- Use axial images to identify diffuse muscle edema & muscle herniation
- Compartment syndrome should be strongly considered in case of casted tibial fracture with disproportionate pain

SELECTED REFERENCES

1. Dhawan SS et al: Four-extremity gangrene associated with crack cocaine abuse. Ann Emerg Med. 49(2):186-9, 2007
2. Armfield DR et al: Sports-related muscle injury in the lower extremity. Clin Sports Med. 25(4):803-42, 2006
3. Beraldo S et al: Lower limb acute compartment syndrome after colorectal surgery in prolonged lithotomy position. Dis Colon Rectum. 49(11):1772-80, 2006
4. Woolley SL et al: Acute compartment syndrome secondary to diabetic muscle infarction: case report and literature review. Eur J Emerg Med. 13(2):113-6, 2006
5. Bong MR et al: Chronic exertional compartment syndrome: diagnosis and management. Bull Hosp Jt Dis. 62(3-4):77-84, 2005
6. Olson SA et al: Acute compartment syndrome in lower extremity musculoskeletal trauma. J Am Acad Orthop Surg. 13(7):436-44, 2005
7. Kostler W et al: Acute compartment syndrome of the limb. Injury. 35(12):1221-7, 2004
8. Pell RF 4th et al: Leg pain in the running athlete. J Am Acad Orthop Surg. 12(6):396-404, 2004
9. Rominger MB et al: MR imaging of compartment syndrome of the lower leg: a case control study. Eur Radiol. 14(8):1432-9, 2004

COMPARTMENT SYNDROME

IMAGE GALLERY

Typical

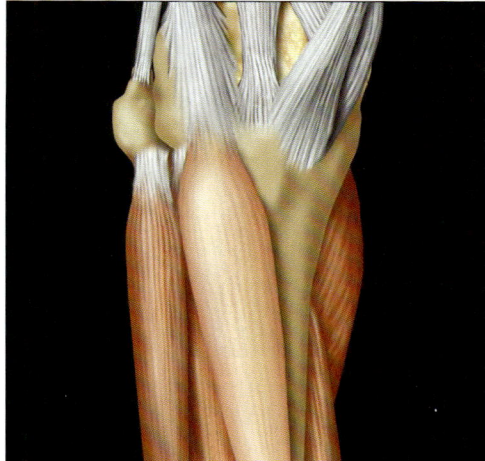
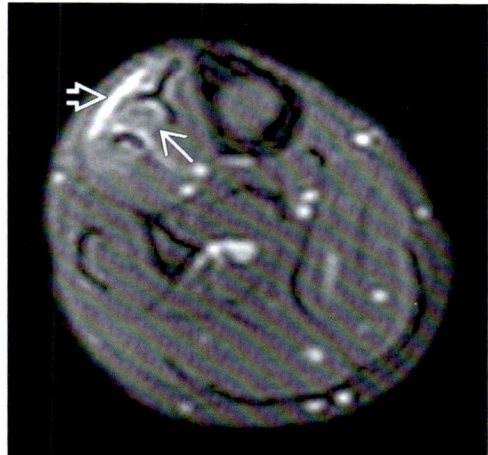

(Left) Frontal graphic depicts edema and swelling in tibialis anterior, as is seen in anterior compartment syndrome. *(Right)* Axial T2WI FS MR reveals diffuse high signal intensity throughout the anterior compartment ➡. The focal area of high signal just deep to the superficial fascia of the anterior tibial muscle represents fascial plane edema ➡.

Typical

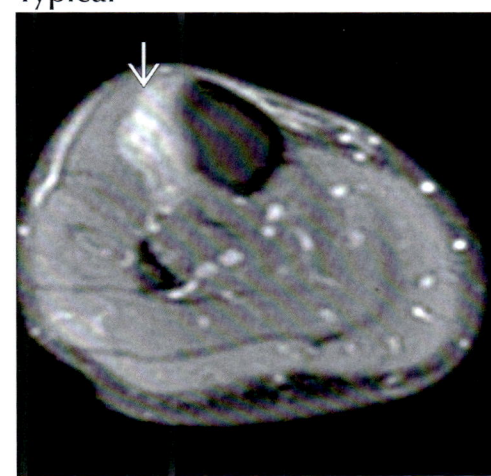
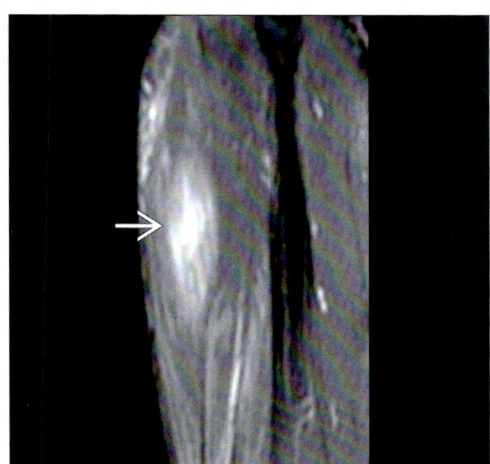

(Left) Axial T2WI FS MR reveals diffuse high signal intensity throughout the anterior tibialis muscle ➡. There is no evidence of muscle volume loss to suggest atrophy. *(Right)* Sagittal STIR MR emphasizes the elongate, diffuse nature of the edema ➡ within the muscle belly.

Other

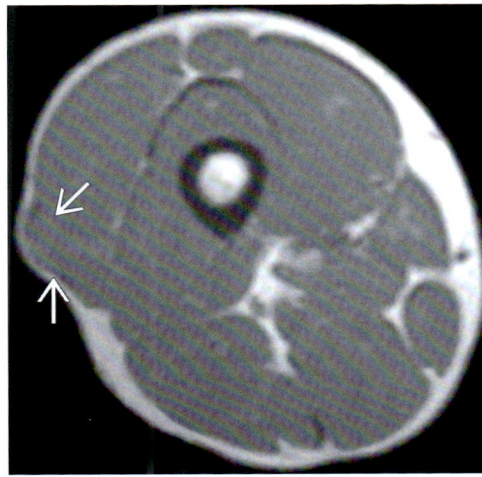
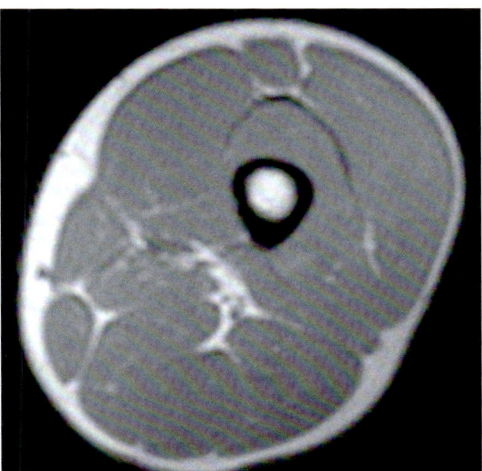

(Left) Axial T1WI MR of the right thigh in a patient with exercise-induced pain demonstrates herniation of vastus lateralis ➡. It is not uncommon to see muscle herniation in patients with chronic (exercise induced) compartment syndrome. *(Right)* Axial T1WI MR of the patient's asymptomatic left thigh at the same level shows no evidence of a similar herniation.

NECROTIZING FASCIITIS

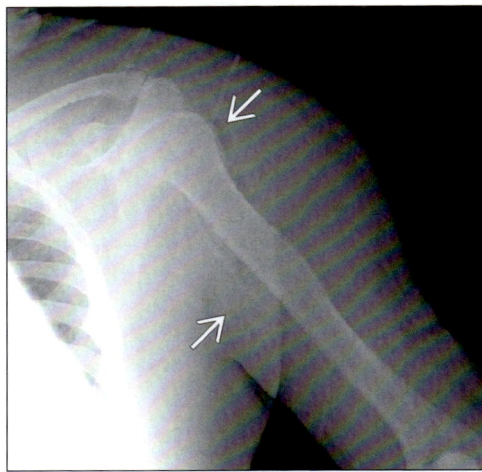

Frontal radiograph shows gas tracking along fascial planes ➡. In the absence of penetrating trauma, this is virtually pathognomonic of necrotizing fasciitis, confirmed in this patient.

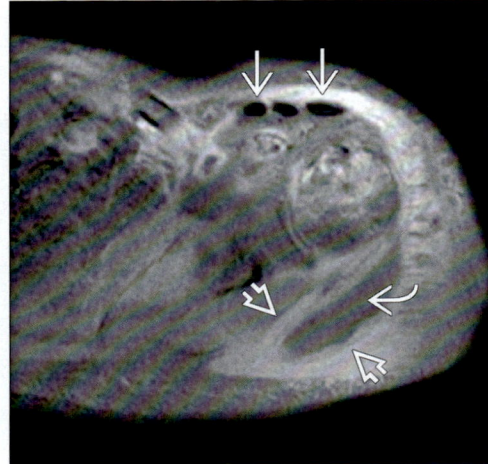

Axial T1WI FS C+ MR shows fascial gas anteriorly ➡ and fascial necrosis ➡ within abnormally enhancing fascia ➡ posteriorly.

TERMINOLOGY

Definitions
- Necrotizing fasciitis (NF): Aggressive, rapidly progressive soft tissue infection that tracks along both superficial (early) and deep fascial planes causing necrosis by microvascular occlusion

IMAGING FINDINGS

General Features
- Best diagnostic clue: In absence of penetrating trauma (including iatrogenic causes such as surgery or a chest tube), gas tracking along fascial planes is virtually pathognomonic
- **Necrotizing fasciitis is a clinical diagnosis;** if there is real clinical suspicion of NF, surgical biopsy is necessary, **regardless of imaging findings**
- Main utility of imaging in cases of suspected NF is to aid surgical planning
  - Rarely, **ENTIRELY** normal fascia can rule out NF
- If there is real clinical suspicion for necrotizing fasciitis, **imaging should not delay surgical biopsy**

MR Findings
- Fascial thickening with increased T2 (fluid) signal is invariably present, but not specific
- Areas of abnormal fascia often enhance
  - Enhancement may be uniform or patchy
  - Non-enhancing islands within & surrounded by enhancing abnormal fascia suggests necrosis & is the most suggestive MR feature (outside of fascial gas)
- In cellulitis, superficial fascia may be thickened, but deep fascia is not involved
- In NF, fascial thickening almost always involves **both** the superficial and deep fascia
  - NF begins in the superficial fascia, so in very early NF, differentiation from cellulitis may be difficult
    - If **only** superficial fascia is abnormal, cellulitis is statistically more likely, but **long** segment involvement, smooth fusiform thickening, necrosis, fascial gas, & marked thickening should raise the possibility of NF

Imaging Recommendations
- Best imaging tool: Contrast-enhanced MR

DDx: Necrotizing Fasciitis Mimics

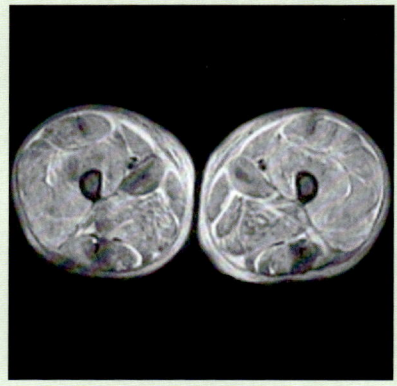

Dermatomyositis

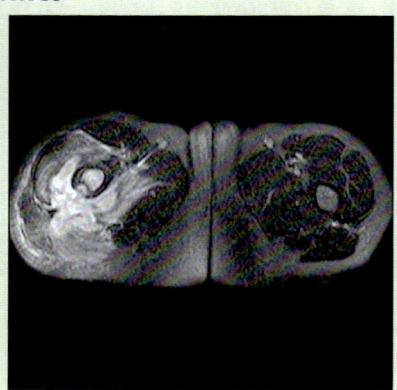

Osteomyelitis, Soft Tissue Extension

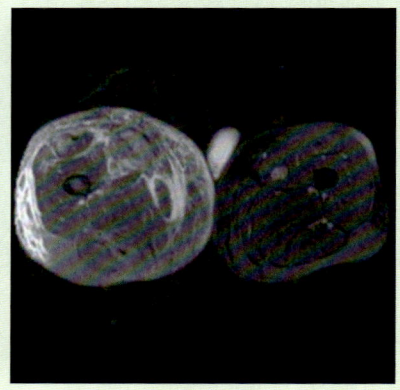

DVT

NECROTIZING FASCIITIS

Key Facts

Imaging Findings
- Best diagnostic clue: In absence of penetrating trauma (including iatrogenic causes such as surgery or a chest tube), gas tracking along fascial planes is virtually pathognomonic
- **Necrotizing fasciitis is a clinical diagnosis;** if there is real clinical suspicion of NF, surgical biopsy is necessary, **regardless of imaging findings**
- Non-enhancing islands within & surrounded by enhancing abnormal fascia suggests necrosis & is the most suggestive MR feature (outside of fascial gas)
- In NF, fascial thickening almost always involves **both** the superficial and deep fascia

Clinical Issues
- Morbidity and mortality is as high as 70-80%

DIFFERENTIAL DIAGNOSIS

Radiologic
- Trauma, myositis, non-necrotizing fasciitis & DVT can all produce deep fascial thickening with enhancement, but necrosis will not be present

Clinical
- Cellulitis: Deep fascial thickening is not present

PATHOLOGY

General Features
- Etiology
  - Predisposing factors: Immunocompromise, vascular insufficiency & recent trauma or surgery
    - Diabetics are at particular risk owing to both immunocompromise & vascular insufficiency

CLINICAL ISSUES

Presentation
- Most common signs/symptoms
  - Sudden onset of pain, swelling, and often erythema
    - Early on, can be very difficult to differentiate from cellulitis, but pain is often much more severe
- Other signs/symptoms
  - As the infection progresses, the pain may disappear and the area may become anesthetic
  - Skin may demonstrate patchy areas of bluish-purple discoloration and/or hemorrhagic bullae
  - Although patients may present in florid sepsis, many may appear remarkably well owing to a blunted immune response

Demographics
- Age: Any, but most are late middle-age to elderly

Natural History & Prognosis
- Extensive & rapid progression of soft tissue infection to sepsis & multi-organ system failure
  - Morbidity and mortality is as high as 70-80%

Treatment
- Broad spectrum antibiotics, general supportive measures, and early, extensive surgical debridement
  - 90% polymicrobial with aerobes & anaerobes
  - Only about 10% are due to isolated group A strep
- Hyperbaric oxygen therapy may reduce mortality

SELECTED REFERENCES

1. Arslan A et al: Necrotizing fasciitis: unreliable MRI findings in the preoperative diagnosis. Eur J Radiol. 36(3):139-43, 2000
2. Brothers TE et al: Magnetic resonance imaging differentiates between necrotizing and non-necrotizing fasciitis of the lower extremity. J Am Coll Surg. 187(4):416-21, 1998
3. Schmid MR et al: Differentiation of necrotizing fasciitis and cellulitis using MR imaging. AJR Am J Roentgenol. 170(3):615-20, 1998

IMAGE GALLERY

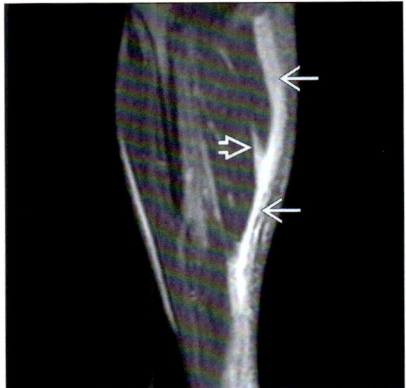 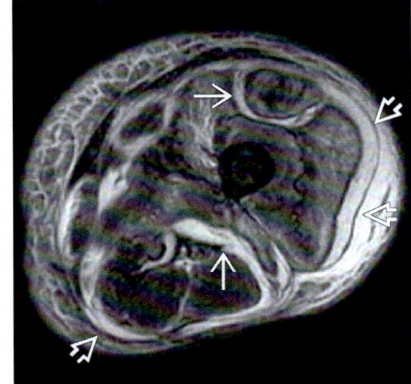 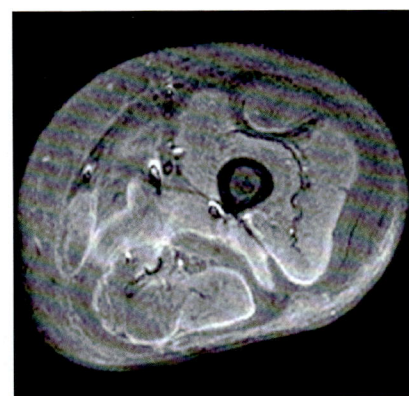

(Left) Coronal T2WI FS MR shows T2 thickening of superficial ➔ & deep ➔ fascia. Deep involvement & the magnitude & length of superficial thickening is not consistent with cellulitis. *(Center)* Axial T2WI FS MR shows extensive deep ➔ & superficial ➔ fascial thickening as well as subcutaneous and muscle edema. *(Right)* Axial T1 C+ FS MR shows that the abnormally thickened fascia (from previous image) enhances only peripherally, suggesting necrosis. This patient required amputation.

HEMATOMA

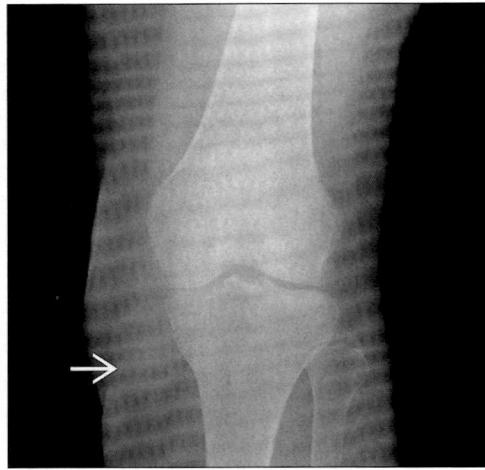

Frontal radiograph in a patient with blunt trauma to the knee shows focal area of soft tissue swelling medial to the tibial plateau ➔.

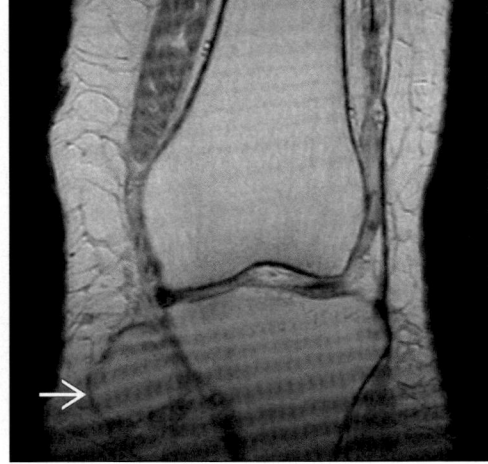

Coronal PD/Intermediate MR of the same patient as previous image, shows a hematoma in the subcutaneous tissue that is slightly hyperintense to muscle ➔.

TERMINOLOGY

Definitions
- A localized collection of blood (usually clotted) outside a blood vessel, but contained within a space
- In contrast, intraparenchymal hemorrhage = blood interspersed within an organ
- Either condition possible within muscles of the extremities

IMAGING FINDINGS

General Features
- Best diagnostic clue: Soft tissue mass highly variable on MR, but most often hyperintense to muscle on T2WI
- Location: Intra- or extra-muscular, depending on mechanism
- Size: Variable
- Morphology: Often extends longitudinally within fascial planes

Radiographic Findings
- Radiographs may only show focal soft tissue swelling
- Other evidence of trauma (e.g., joint effusion)

CT Findings
- NECT
  - CT shows asymmetric enlargement of the involved muscle or tissue plane
  - Usually isodense to muscle, but can be higher density in case of acute hemorrhage
  - Evolution to seroma will appear hypodense
- CECT: Focal areas of contrast extravasation into the hematoma suggest active bleeding

MR Findings
- T1WI
  - Initially iso/hypointense to muscle (deoxyhemoglobin)
  - Then hyperintense (methemoglobin)
  - Eventually hypointense (hemosiderin)
  - Residual seroma would appear hypointense
  - Development of fibrosis would cause foci of low signal

DDx: Hematoma

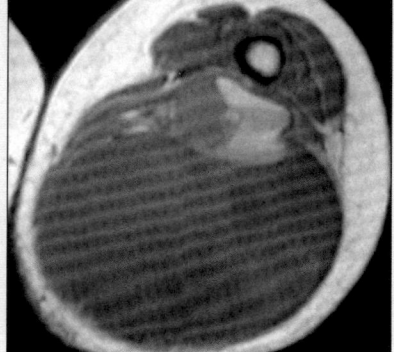

T1: Hematoma within Liposarcoma

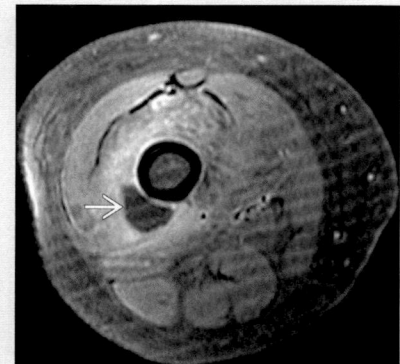

T1 C+: Abscess

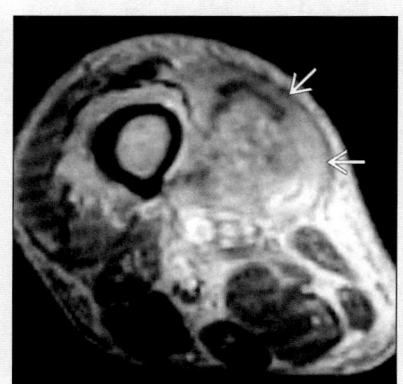

Chronic Hematoma Mimics Tumor

HEMATOMA

Key Facts

Terminology
- A localized collection of blood (usually clotted) outside a blood vessel, but contained within a space

Imaging Findings
- Best diagnostic clue: Soft tissue mass highly variable on MR, but most often hyperintense to muscle on T2WI
- Morphology: Often extends longitudinally within fascial planes
- Radiographs may only show focal soft tissue swelling
- CT shows asymmetric enlargement of the involved muscle or tissue plane
- Chronic hematomas often incite tremendous adjacent soft tissue reaction
- MR appearance is highly complex and variable
- US acutely anechoic, with irregular echoic areas developing later

Pathology
- **Exertional/sports related extremity hematomas:**
- Usually associated with a muscle tear (strain), often at myotendinous junction
- **Traumatic (non-exertional) hematomas:**
- Result from blunt or penetrating trauma causing sufficient vascular damage to generate intra/extramuscular bleeding

Diagnostic Checklist
- A hematoma with surrounding inflammation can be indistinguishable on MR from an aggressive tumor such as high grade sarcoma; any doubt should be resolved with a biopsy!

- Associated areas of intraparenchymal muscle hemorrhage would show high signal on both T1WI and T2WI
- T2WI
  - Initially hyperintense to muscle (oxyhemoglobin)
  - Then iso/hypointense (deoxyhemoglobin)
  - Then hyperintense (as intracellular methemoglobin becomes extracellular with RBC breakdown)
  - Eventually hypointense (hemosiderin)
  - Residual seroma would remain hyperintense
  - Reactive edema (high T2 signal) in the surrounding muscles may be seen at any stage
  - Occasionally a fluid-cellular layer (aka hematocrit level) is visible
    - Usually in patients who are anticoagulated or have intratumoral bleeding
- T1 C+
  - Typically no abnormal enhancement in acute stage
  - Chronic hematomas often incite tremendous adjacent soft tissue reaction
    - Causes inhomogeneous enhancement in multiple muscle groups and/or neurovascular bundles
    - Infiltrative appearance can make a chronic hematoma indistinguishable from an aggressive tumor on MR
- MR appearance is highly complex and variable
  - Varies by differences in individual MR unit field strengths and different patterns of blood breakdown
  - Much less predictable than intracranial hematomas due to larger and more complex/loculated nature

Ultrasonographic Findings
- Asymmetrical muscle enlargement
  - US acutely anechoic, with irregular echoic areas developing later

Angiographic Findings
- Hematomas will not show internal vascularization; a highly vascularized mass suggests malignancy

Imaging Recommendations
- Best imaging tool: MR

DIFFERENTIAL DIAGNOSIS

Depends on the Stage of the Hematoma
- **Acute hematoma** (low/intermediate signal on T1, low signal on T2)
  - Desmoid or other fibromatosis
  - Pigmented villonodular synovitis (PVNS)
  - Morton neuroma, fibrolipohamartoma, or xanthoma
  - High-flow arteriovenous malformation (AVM)
  - Scar tissue, mineralized mass, or amyloidosis
  - Granuloma annulare
- **Early subacute hematoma** (low signal on T1, high signal on T2)
  - Cyst, seroma, or abscess
  - Myxoma or myxoid liposarcoma
  - Sarcoma
    - Rhabdomyosarcoma
    - Leiomyosarcoma
    - Synovial cell sarcoma
- **Late subacute hematoma** (high signal on T1, high signal on T2)
  - Hemangioma or lymphangioma
  - Small AVM
  - Liposarcoma
- **Chronic hematoma** (low signal on T1, low signal on T2)
  - Similar differential to acute hematoma

PATHOLOGY

General Features
- Etiology
  - **Exertional/sports related extremity hematomas:**
    - Usually associated with a muscle tear (strain), often at myotendinous junction
    - If weakness is still present at 2-3 days post muscle strain, MR often ordered to rule out total muscular rupture or hematoma
  - **Traumatic (non-exertional) hematomas:**

HEMATOMA

- Result from blunt or penetrating trauma causing sufficient vascular damage to generate intra/extramuscular bleeding
- Epidemiology
  - Predisposing conditions (after little or no trauma)
    - Hemophilia (hematoma = "hemophilic pseudotumor")
    - Anticoagulation, Henoch-Schönlein purpura, Von Willebrand disease, and other bleeding diatheses
- Associated abnormalities
  - Intraparenchymal muscular hemorrhage
  - Muscle tear or rupture
  - Surrounding muscular edema/inflammation

Gross Pathologic & Surgical Features

- Hematomas progress through various stages of blood breakdown: Oxyhemoglobin, deoxyhemoglobin, intracellular methemoglobin, extracellular methemoglobin, hemosiderin
- Will often be heterogeneous, containing blood products at multiple stages
- Internal fibrotic clots often found at surgery

CLINICAL ISSUES

Presentation

- Most common signs/symptoms
  - Sports related muscular hematoma ⇒ sudden onset of pain/weakness during an explosive movement such as jumping (calf) or accelerating (hamstring)
  - Traumatic (non-exertional) hematomas ⇒ signs/symptoms related to blunt or penetrating trauma
- Other signs/symptoms: Swelling, ecchymoses, or other evidence of trauma

Demographics

- Age
  - Exertional/sports related hematomas are more prevalent in young athletes, M > F
  - Traumatic hematomas have no age/sex predilection

Natural History & Prognosis

- Without treatment (conservative or surgical), rebleeding will often occur
- Can lead to compartment syndrome
  - Venous congestion ⇒ neurovascular compromise ⇒ muscle degeneration/necrosis

Treatment

- Conservative treatment (i.e., activity restriction) if asymptomatic
- Surgical evacuation if symptomatic (weakness, hyperesthesia, pain on passive flexion)

DIAGNOSTIC CHECKLIST

Consider

- A hematoma with surrounding inflammation can be indistinguishable on MR from an aggressive tumor such as high grade sarcoma; any doubt should be resolved with a biopsy!

SELECTED REFERENCES

1. Mann HA et al: Synovial Sarcoma Mimicking Haemophilic Pseudotumour. Sarcoma. 2006
2. Suzuki T et al: Arterial injury associated with acute compartment syndrome of the thigh following blunt trauma. Injury. 36(1):151-9, 2005
3. Connell DA et al: Longitudinal study comparing sonographic and MRI assessments of acute and healing hamstring injuries. AJR Am J Roentgenol. 183(4):975-84, 2004
4. Gomez P et al: High-grade sarcomas mimicking traumatic intramuscular hematomas: a report of three cases. Iowa Orthop J. 24:106-10, 2004
5. Mahevas M et al: [Muscular haematoma in Henoch-Schonlein purpura] Rev Med Interne. 25(12):927-30, 2004
6. Saotome K et al: Enlarging intramuscular hematoma and fibrinolytic parameters. J Orthop Sci. 8(2):132-6, 2003
7. Krebs M et al: Massive postoperative intramuscular bleeding in acquired von Willebrand's disease. Ann Hematol. 81(7):394-6, 2002
8. Manaster BJ et al: Musculoskeletal Imaging: The Requisites. 2nd ed. St. Louis, Mosby. 9-12, 2002
9. Clanton TO et al: Hamstring strains in athletes: diagnosis and treatment. J Am Acad Orthop Surg. 6(4):237-48, 1998
10. Jaovisidha S et al: Hemophilic pseudotumor: spectrum of MR findings. Skeletal Radiol. 26(8):468-74, 1997
11. Manaster BJ: Handbook of Skeletal Radiology. 2nd ed. St. Louis, Mosby. 10-12, 1997
12. Bradley WG Jr: MR appearance of hemorrhage in the brain. Radiology. 189(1):15-26, 1993
13. De Smet AA et al: Magnetic resonance imaging of muscle tears. Skeletal Radiol. 19(4):283-6, 1990
14. Niemi P et al: MR imaging of experimental intramuscular hemorrhage at 0.02 T. Contrast enhancement with Gd-DOTA. Acta Radiol. 31(5):455-8, 1990
15. Pakter RL et al: Calf hematoma--computed tomographic and magnetic resonance findings. Skeletal Radiol. 16(5):393-6, 1987
16. Rubin JI et al: High-field MR imaging of extracranial hematomas. AJR Am J Roentgenol. 148(4):813-7, 1987
17. Dooms GC et al: MR imaging of intramuscular hemorrhage. J Comput Assist Tomogr. 9(5):908-13, 1985

HEMATOMA

IMAGE GALLERY

Typical

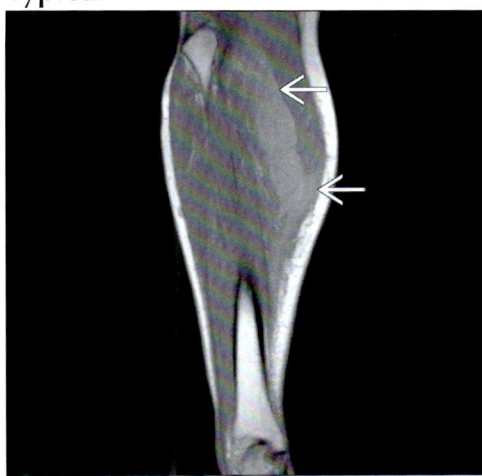
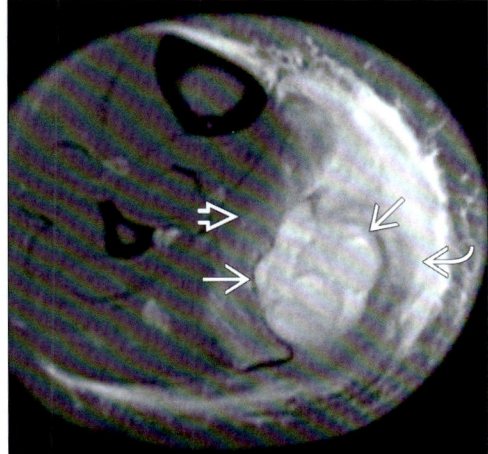

(Left) Coronal T1WI MR shows a longitudinal plane of tissue ➔ which is higher signal intensity than adjacent muscle. A hematoma often extends longitudinally within muscle or fascial planes. *(Right)* Axial T2WI FS MR shows an inhomogeneous collection that is high signal intensity ➔, located between the edematous soleus ➔ and gastrocnemius ➔. This collection is a hematoma which formed acutely when the medial head of gastrocnemius ruptured.

Typical

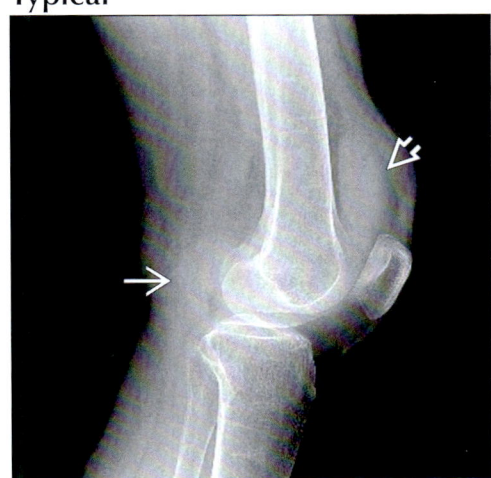
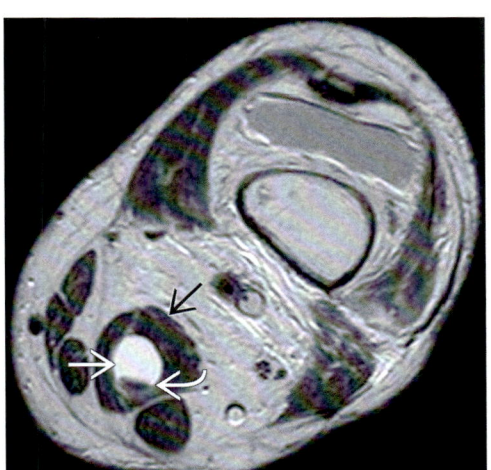

(Left) Lateral radiograph shows a focal round area of soft tissue prominence posterior to the distal femur ➔. Large joint effusion is also visible ➔. *(Right)* Axial T2WI MR of the same patient as previous image, shows a predominantly hyperintense hematoma ➔ within the semimembranosus muscle ➔. A hematocrit level is visible within the hematoma ➔.

Typical

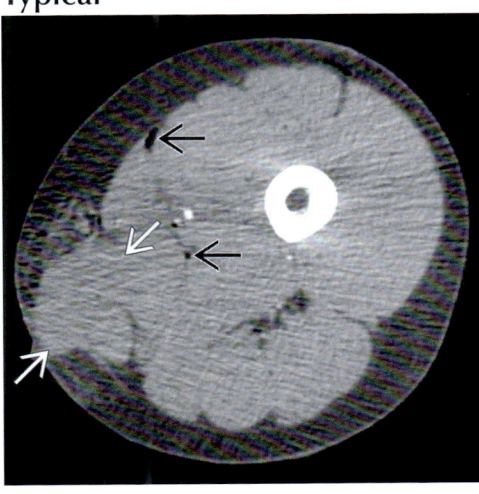
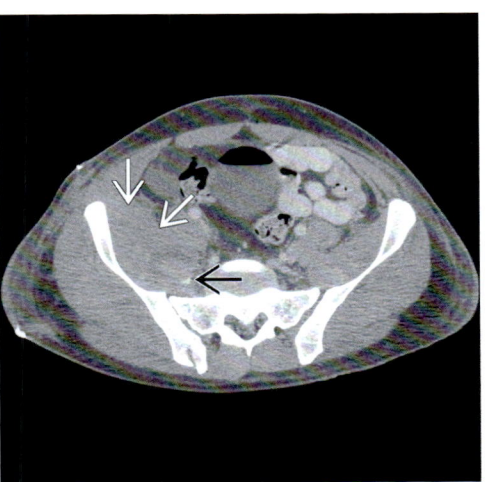

(Left) Axial NECT of a patient with penetrating trauma (gun shot wound) shows a hematoma ➔ in the medial thigh that is isodense to muscle. Several small gas pockets are also visible ➔. *(Right)* Axial CECT in a hemophilic patient shows a large isodense hematoma in the right iliopsoas muscle ➔. A focal area of active contrast extravasation is also visible ➔.

MYOSITIS OSSIFICANS

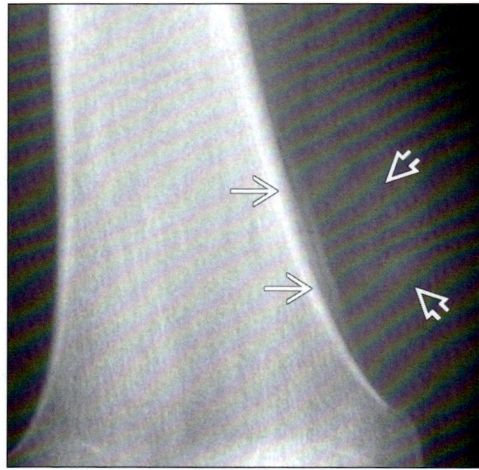

AP radiograph shows prominent periosteal reaction ➡ & amorphous bone formation in the adjacent soft tissues ➡. Differential is MO vs. surface osteosarcoma. The bone mass is not mature enough to show zoning.

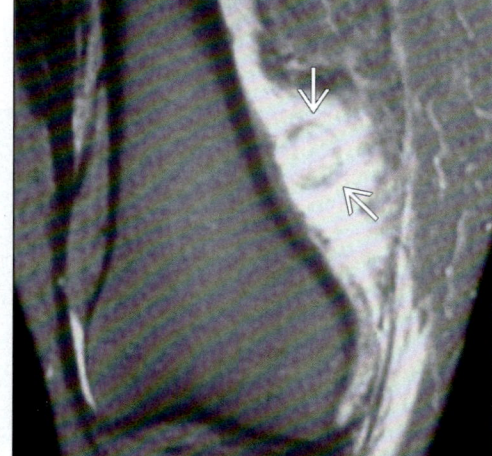

Coronal T2WI MR shows a halo of low signal with central & surrounding high signal at the site of the mass ➡. This is an early representation of the zoning phenomenon with peripheral maturity in MO.

TERMINOLOGY

Abbreviations and Synonyms
- Myositis ossificans (MO)
- Heterotopic ossification (HO)

Definitions
- Heterotopic formation of bone and cartilage in soft tissue: Benign, solitary, self-limiting
- Term "myositis" is misleading
  - Most frequently occurs in muscle
  - May also be found in fascia, tendons, & fat
  - "Heterotopic ossification" is a more correct term; however, "myositis ossificans" continues to be in popular usage at this time

IMAGING FINDINGS

General Features
- Best diagnostic clue
  - Mature bone formation within soft tissues, seen in later stages of the disease
  - Earlier stages are confusing: The bone is amorphous & appears similar to tumor bone formation
- Location
  - Common in areas prone to trauma
    - Antecubital fossa following elbow dislocation
    - Anterolateral thigh in football players
    - Fat adjacent to adductors in horseback riders
  - Shoulder & elbows in burn patients
  - Formed about the pelvis & hips in spinal cord or brain injured patients
- Size: May be several centimeters in length or diameter
- Morphology
  - Distinctive & related to time following trauma
  - All imaging modalities reflect progressive changes

Radiographic Findings
- Distinctive related to time following trauma
- 0-2 weeks: Soft tissue mass with indistinct surrounding soft tissue planes
- 3-4 weeks: Amorphous osteoid forms within the mass; adjacent periosteal reaction may be seen
- 6-8 weeks: Sharper cortex begins to form about the lacy central osseous mass
- 5-6 months: Mature bone formation

DDx: Myositis Ossificans

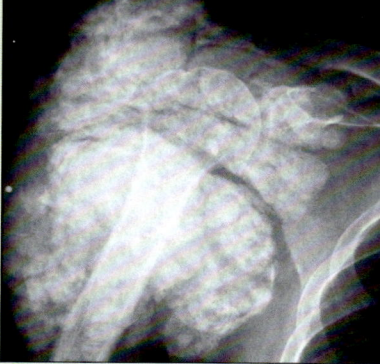

Tumoral Calcinosis

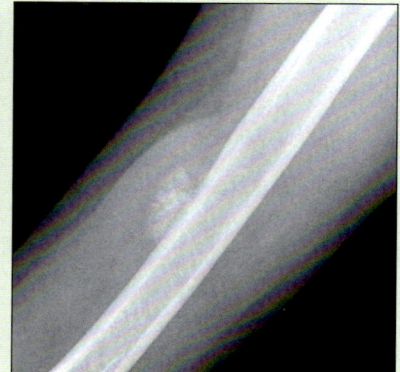

High Grade Surface Osteosarcoma

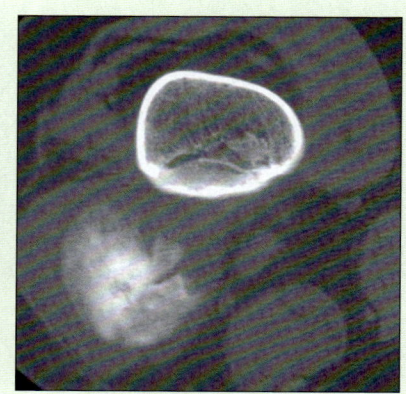

Parosteal Osteosarcoma

MYOSITIS OSSIFICANS

Key Facts

Imaging Findings
- Mature bone formation within soft tissues, seen in later stages of the disease
- Earlier stages are confusing: The bone is amorphous & appears similar to tumor bone formation
- Common in areas prone to trauma
- Shoulder & elbows in burn patients
- Formed about the pelvis & hips in spinal cord or brain injured patients
- Distinctive & related to time following trauma
- 0-2 weeks: Soft tissue mass with indistinct surrounding soft tissue planes
- 3-4 weeks: Amorphous osteoid forms within the mass; adjacent periosteal reaction may be seen
- 6-8 weeks: Sharper cortex begins to form about the lacy central osseous mass
- 5-6 months: Mature bone formation

Top Differential Diagnoses
- Tumoral Calcinosis
- Parosteal Osteosarcoma
- High Grade Surface or Soft Tissue Osteosarcoma

Diagnostic Checklist
- History of trauma & the timing relative to imaging is crucial to diagnosis, though trauma may be denied
- Must avoid biopsy during the early stages to avoid misdiagnosis of tumor
- Do not overinterpret early amorphous osteoid formation as tumor bone
- Watch for peripheral organization, either as organized bone on radiograph or CT, or as "halo" on MR

  - Note: During the 2-6 month period, the osseous maturation assumes the distinctive zoning pattern diagnostic of MO: Mature cortical bone peripherally, less mature bone centrally
  - Towards the end of this period, size may begin to ↓
- 7 + months: Mass may continue to decrease in size; trabeculae may be seen enclosed by mature cortex

CT Findings
- Appearance relates to age of lesion, paralleling histology and other imaging
- Earliest findings: Low-attenuation soft tissue mass
- Amorphous bone density seen by 3-4 weeks, more prominently than on radiograph
- Peripheral rim of more organized mineralization seen by 4-6 weeks, earlier than radiograph
- Mature lesions show peripheral cortical rim and central decreased attenuation (may contain trabeculae)

MR Findings
- Appearance relates to age of lesion, paralleling histology and other imaging
- May show marrow edema, periosteal reaction, & peripheral edema at any stage
- Early stages
  - T1: Signal intensity isointense to muscle
  - Fluid sensitive sequences: Hyperintense, markedly inhomogeneous
- Intermediate stages
  - T1: Normal, isointense to muscle, perhaps with local distortion of fat planes
  - Fluid sensitive sequences: Hyperintense mass, with curvilinear & irregular areas of decreased signal intensity surrounding lesion
    - This low signal "halo" may be incomplete & difficult to visualize, but serves to differentiate MO from tumor bone formation
    - It is the earliest equivalent to the well-organized cortical rim visualized on radiograph or CT
    - This curvilinear density occasionally seen in early lesions, but fairly reliably seen by 3-4 weeks
  - Marked enhancement with contrast
- Late stages
  - Well-defined inhomogeneous masses with signal approximating bone, without associated edema

Imaging Recommendations
- Best imaging tool: Depending on age of lesion, may need combination of radiograph + CT or MR

DIFFERENTIAL DIAGNOSIS

Tumoral Calcinosis
- Periarticular calcified (not ossified) soft tissue mass
- Separate from underlying bone

Parosteal Osteosarcoma
- Well-organized bone formation mostly in soft tissues, though there is usually an osseous attachment
- Opposite zoning pattern
  - Parosteal osteosarcoma has organized bone centrally, less mature bone peripherally

High Grade Surface or Soft Tissue Osteosarcoma
- Less well-organized tumor bone formation within soft tissues
- May have very similar appearance to MO in its early amorphous stages
- Opposite zoning pattern
  - More mature osteoid centrally, less mature bone peripherally, less organized overall

Osteochondroma (Exostosis)
- Normally organized bone arising from metaphyseal region of underlying bone
- "Stalk" of marrow, outlined by cortex, cartilage cap
- Careful evaluation shows there is no true similarity to MO

Fibrodysplasia Ossificans Progressiva (FOP)
- Also termed myositis ossificans progressiva or Munchmeyer disease
- Autosomal dominant mesodermal disorder with wide range of expressivity

MYOSITIS OSSIFICANS

- Target is interstitial tissues, with muscle involvement secondary to pressure atrophy
- Progressive ossification of striated muscle, tendons, ligaments, & fascial planes
- Often presents with acute torticollis, with painful ossified mass in sternocleidomastoid muscle
- Progresses to shoulder girdle, upper arms, spine, pelvis
- Bridges adjacent bones, eventually causing severe restriction of motion
- Progression to eventual loss of most range of motion; death may occur from recurrent respiratory infections due to chest wall restriction

PATHOLOGY

General Features
- Etiology
  - Progenitor stem cells for osteoid production exist within the affected soft tissues
  - With proper stimulus, stem cells differentiate into osteoblasts & form osteoid
  - Experiments suggest that bone morphogenic proteins (BMPs) can stimulate HO & may play a role
  - Overt stimulus is usually traumatic, though it may be inapparent or forgotten by patient
  - Avulsion fx, especially around pelvis, may result in heterotopic bone formation
    - Bone forms between donor site & avulsed bone
    - Follows same timing & zoning pattern as MO
    - Ages 14-25 particularly at risk: This ranges from the period of apophyseal ossification to fusion
    - Sites most frequently seen: Anterior superior iliac spine, anterior inferior iliac spine, ischial apophysis, adductor apophysis
  - Burn patients are at additional risk
  - Brain injury patients at additional risk
    - Extent & functional severity directly related to severity of intracranial injury
  - Spinal cord injury patients at risk
    - Strong propensity to recur following resection
  - Other causes of neurologic compromise may be associated: Tetanus, poliomyelitis, Guillain-Barre
  - Total hip arthroplasty patients at risk for local HO
- Epidemiology
  - 20-30% patients with neurologic deficits develop HO
  - 33-49% of paraplegics show HO
  - 5% total hip patients develop HO; 1% severe

Microscopic Features
- Histologic evolution of MO parallels that of imaging, with progression and a similar zoning phenomenon
  - Weeks 1-4: Pseudosarcomatous appearance in the central zone, giving the appearance of tumor bone
  - Weeks 4-8: Centrifugal pattern, with periphery of amorphous osteoid, surrounding a cellular center
  - Following week 8: Gradual organization into mature peripheral bone surrounding a cellular center

CLINICAL ISSUES

Presentation
- Most common signs/symptoms
  - First 2 weeks: Painful soft tissue mass
    - Warm, doughy
    - Patient may not recall episode of trauma (particularly if child or teenager)

Demographics
- Age
  - Any age
  - In FOP, disease usually manifests by age 5 & becomes severe by end of second decade
- Gender: M > F, particularly in spinal cord injury patients

Natural History & Prognosis
- Single traumatic lesion may stabilize & regress
  - Residual: Symptomatic based on size/location
- Brain/spinal cord HO tend not to regress
  - May cause decreased range of motion
  - May develop ulceration if in weight-bearing area

Treatment
- Following maturation of lesion, surgical resection may be considered if lesion is symptomatic
- May prophylax total hip patients at high risk for HO with low dose radiation
- Long term oral etidronate may be useful for early HO

DIAGNOSTIC CHECKLIST

Consider
- History of trauma & the timing relative to imaging is crucial to diagnosis, though trauma may be denied
- Must avoid biopsy during the early stages to avoid misdiagnosis of tumor
- Radiologist, oncologic surgeon, & pathologist must work as a team to avoid misdiagnosis

Image Interpretation Pearls
- Do not overinterpret early amorphous osteoid formation as tumor bone
- Watch for peripheral organization, either as organized bone on radiograph or CT, or as "halo" on MR

SELECTED REFERENCES

1. Balboni TA et al: Heterotopic ossification: Pathophysiology, clinical features, and the role of radiotherapy for prophylaxis. Int J Radiat Oncol Biol Phys. 65(5):1289-99, 2006
2. Eid K et al: Systemic effects of severe trauma on the function and apoptosis of human skeletal cells. J Bone Joint Surg Br. 88(10):1394-400, 2006
3. Higo T et al: The incidence of heterotopic ossification after cementless total hip arthroplasty. J Arthroplasty. 21(6):852-6, 2006
4. Hudson SJ et al: Heterotopic ossification--a long-term consequence of prolonged immobility. Crit Care. 10(6):174, 2006
5. McCarthy EF et al: Heterotopic ossification: a review. Skeletal Radiol. 34(10):609-19, 2005

MYOSITIS OSSIFICANS

IMAGE GALLERY

Typical

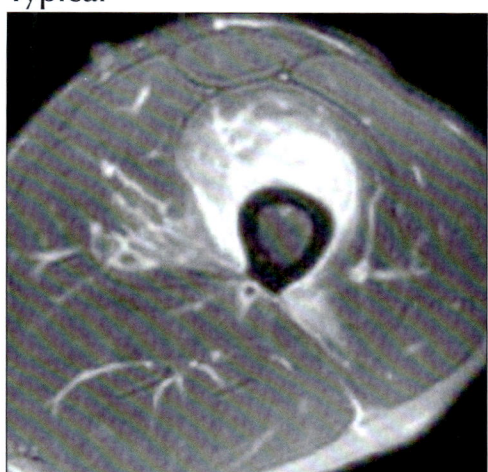
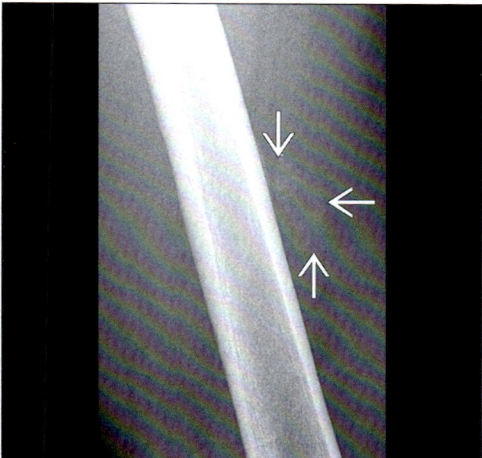

(Left) Axial T2WI FS MR shows signal abnormality involving much of the vastus intermedius, with surrounding edema. The MR does not add further specificity for the diagnosis. *(Right)* Lateral radiograph shows faintly ossified mass anterior to the thigh ➡, corresponding to the region seen on MR. There is a suggestion of greater maturation in the periphery; this zoning suggests the diagnosis is myositis ossificans.

Typical

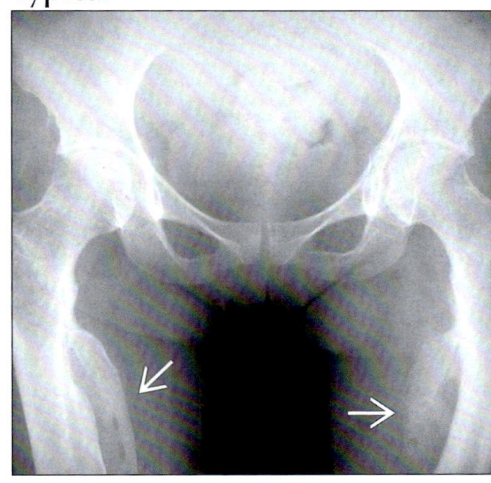
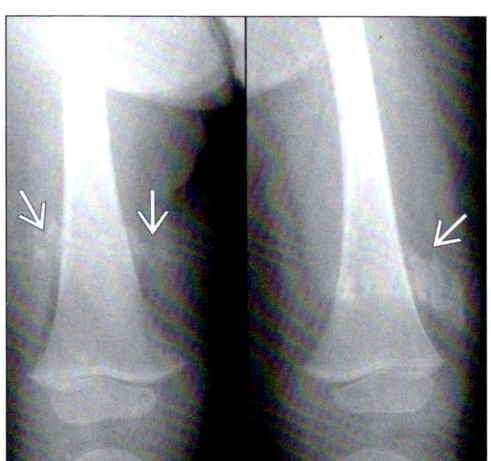

(Left) Anteroposterior radiograph shows mature MO within the adductors bilaterally ➡. Maturity is judged by the development of peripheral cortex & central trabeculae. This patient is an avid horseback rider. *(Right)* Anteroposterior radiograph of both thighs in a burn patient shows pin tracts & moderately early MO in the adjacent soft tissues ➡. This patient was severely burned & placed in traction; burn patients are at ↑ risk for development of MO.

Typical

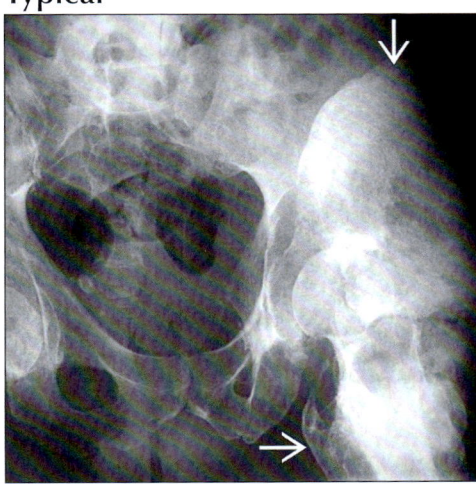
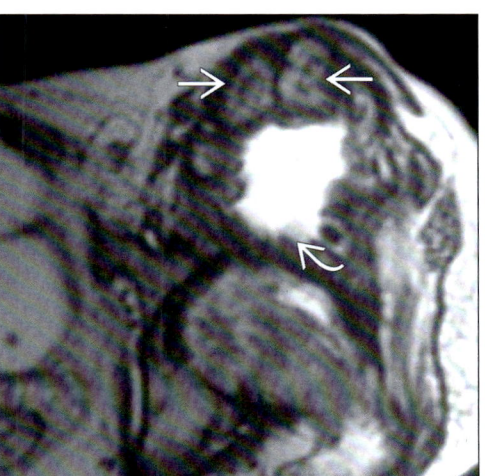

(Left) Anteroposterior radiograph in a paraplegic patient shows abundant mature MO adjacent to the entire left hemipelvis ➡. There was clinical concern for a mass, but the diagnosis is clear from this image. *(Right)* Axial T2WI MR confirms the diagnosis of MO. There is peripheral mature bone (note the signal which matches that of the femur ➡). There is central necrosis with liquefaction ➡. MO is frequently seen in the pelvic region in paraplegics.

STERNOCLAVICULAR TRAUMA

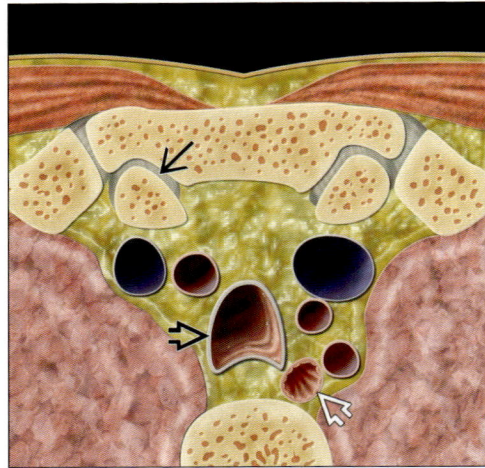

Graphic shows normal SC joint ➡ & structures at risk with posterior dislocation: Veins (blue): R subclavian, L innominate; arteries (red): R innominate, L common carotid, L subclavian; trachea ➡; esophagus ➡.

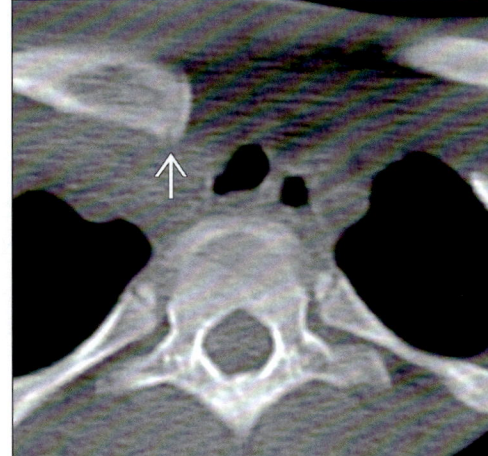

Axial CT shows a right posterior SC dislocation ➡. The open epiphysis remains in normal position relative to the clavicular shaft, making this is a true dislocation rather than a Salter fx as is often seen in this patient age group.

TERMINOLOGY

Abbreviations and Synonyms
- Sternoclavicular (SC) dislocation, subluxation, sprain

Definitions
- SC ligament injury with various degrees/directions of medial clavicle displacement from SC joint

IMAGING FINDINGS

General Features
- Best diagnostic clue: Abnormal position of medial clavicle in relation to manubrium
- Location
  - Anterior (presternal) dislocation (AD): Medial clavicle anterior or anterosuperior to manubrium
  - Posterior (retrosternal) dislocation (PD): Medial clavicle posterior or posterosuperior to manubrium
- Size: Symptomatic sprain to complete SC dislocation

Radiographic Findings
- Often misleadingly normal
  - Oblique SC joint normally appears subluxed
  - Overlapping thoracic structures obscure the joint
- Routine: PA, oblique, lateral views of SC joints
  - PA: Difference in relative craniocaudal positions of medial clavicles > 50% the width of clavicle head
- Special views
  - Rockwood (serendipity) view: Beam directed cephalad through manubrium in supine patient
    - AD: Medial clavicle above horizontal plane
    - PD: Medial clavicle below horizontal plane
  - Hobbs view: Patient seated, leaning over table with beam aimed through cervical spine
    - Approximates 90° lateral view of SC joint
- Stress maneuver
  - Classic: Ipsilateral arm across chest and pulling against contralateral elbow
  - Can also use with CT

CT Findings
- CECT
  - Identifies vascular and soft tissue injury
  - Easily distinguishes direction of dislocation
  - Useful for surgical planning
  - Can obtain quickly in trauma setting

DDx: Sternoclavicular Osteomyelitis and Abscess

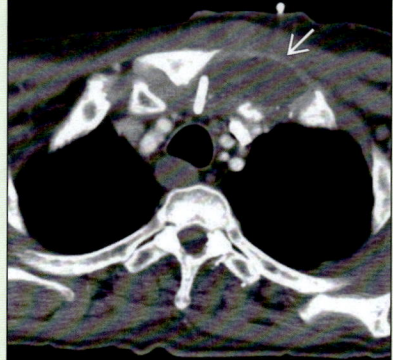

Axial CT with Contrast

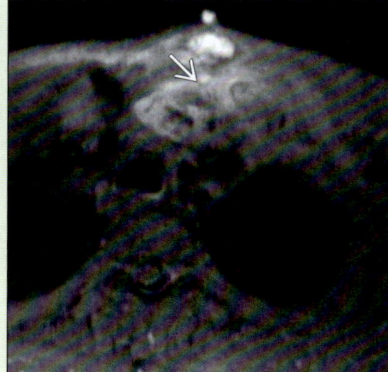

Axial MR STIR

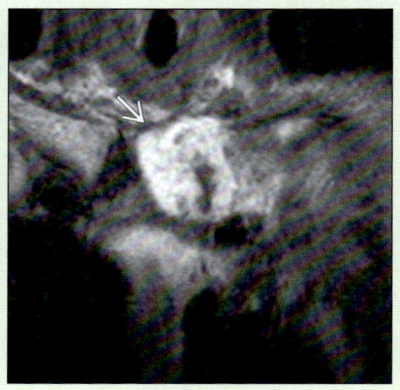

Coronal MR T2

STERNOCLAVICULAR TRAUMA

Key Facts

Terminology
- Sternoclavicular (SC) dislocation, subluxation, sprain

Imaging Findings
- Best diagnostic clue: Abnormal position of medial clavicle in relation to manubrium
- Anterior (presternal) dislocation (AD): Medial clavicle anterior or anterosuperior to manubrium
- Posterior (retrosternal) dislocation (PD): Medial clavicle posterior or posterosuperior to manubrium

Top Differential Diagnoses
- Physeal Fractures
- Osteomyelitis
- Neoplasia
- Arthritis

Pathology
- Usually result of profound direct or indirect force
- Most result from motor vehicle accident (40%) or sports-related trauma (21%)
- SC dislocations are rare

Clinical Issues
- Most common signs/symptoms: Pain, swelling, and deformity at SC joint
- Most regain adequate upper extremity function

Diagnostic Checklist
- AD are far more common than PD
- PD can result in damage to superior mediastinal structures that can be life-threatening
- CT is preferred diagnostic modality

MR Findings
- T1WI
  - Identify ligament disruption
  - Low signal joint effusion
- T2WI
  - Increased signal ligament tears
  - Increased signal joint effusion
- MRA: Identify vascular injury with PD
- Superior to CT in identifying articular cartilage and disc injury, joint effusions, ligament injury

Ultrasonographic Findings
- Quick pre-operative screen for dislocation
- Color Doppler allows quick assessment of vessels
- Helpful intraoperatively to guide relocation
- Confirm reduction before leaving operating room
- Correct state of SC joint found 89% time for US vs. 13% for radiographs
- Limited number of individuals with expertise in use

Imaging Recommendations
- Best imaging tool: CT best at revealing position of medial clavicle and associated injuries
- Protocol advice
  - Radiographs: Special views ± stress maneuvers
  - CT
    - Thin slices (≤ 1 mm) to include both SC joints + medial half of both clavicles
    - Coronal reformats useful; angle to plane of joint
    - Neutral position or with stress maneuver
    - Intravenous contrast: ↑ Conspicuity of vessels
  - MR
    - Coronal, sagittal, axial, and oblique axial planes
    - T1, T2, and STIR or T2 fat-suppressed

DIFFERENTIAL DIAGNOSIS

Physeal Fractures
- Medial clavicle physis closes between 22 and 26 years
- If < 22 years, displaced clavicle is usually a physeal fracture and not a true dislocation
- Ligaments remain intact

Osteomyelitis
- Uncommon: Usually occurs after surgery or radiation
- Seen in IV drug abusers, patients with infective endocarditis, with adjacent mediastinal infections
- Abscess & destruction differentiate from dislocation

Neoplasia
- Metastatic disease or primary neoplasm (multiple myeloma, lymphoma, or chondrosarcoma)
- Differentiate from dislocation by bone destruction, associated soft tissue mass, and tumor matrix

Arthritis
- Frequently involved with rheumatoid arthritis, scleroderma, ankylosing spondylitis, SAPHO syndrome and other collagen-vascular diseases
- Differentiate by joint space narrowing, erosions, osteophyte formation, sclerosis, & capsular thickening

PATHOLOGY

General Features
- Etiology
  - Usually result of profound direct or indirect force
  - Anterior dislocation
    - Atraumatic: Ligamentous laxity in young adults and teenagers when arm raised over head
    - Traumatic: Indirect; anterior force applied to shoulder that is posterior to the SC joint
  - Posterior dislocation
    - Direct: Blow to medial clavicle
    - Indirect: Posterolaterally applied force to shoulder that is anterior to the SC joint
  - Most result from motor vehicle accident (40%) or sports-related trauma (21%)
- Epidemiology
  - SC dislocations are rare
    - 3% of shoulder girdle injuries
    - < 1% of total dislocations
    - 0.6% of trauma patients

STERNOCLAVICULAR TRAUMA

- 90-95% of SC dislocations are anterior
- Often associated with significant injuries
  - \> 2/3 of AD associated with serious injuries
  - 25% of PD have superior mediastinal injury
  - Associated injuries not as serious for AD as PD
- Associated abnormalities
  - AD: Pneumothorax, hemothorax, pulmonary contusion, rib fractures if due to significant trauma
  - PD: Trachea, esophagus, nerves, and great vessel injury of superior mediastinum

Gross Pathologic & Surgical Features
- Anterior
  - Disruption of anterior SC ligament
  - Joint capsule disruption
- Posterior
  - Disruption of posterior SC ligament
  - Joint capsule disruption
- Anterior SC ligament is much weaker than posterior

Staging, Grading or Classification Criteria
- Severity grades of SC joint injury
  - Grade I: Sprain - incomplete tear or stretching of SC and costoclavicular ligaments
  - Grade II: SC joint subluxation - complete tear of SC ligament + partial tear of capsule
  - Grade III: SC dislocation - complete tear of SC and costoclavicular ligaments + complete tear of capsule

CLINICAL ISSUES

Presentation
- Most common signs/symptoms: Pain, swelling, and deformity at SC joint
- Other signs/symptoms
  - Chest + shoulder pain exacerbated by arm movement or assuming a supine position
  - Affected arm supported across chest by opposite arm
  - Head tilted toward affected side
  - Affected shoulder: Shortened + thrust forward
- Clinical Profile
  - Anterior dislocation
    - Less painful than PD
    - Prominent medial clavicle accentuated by shoulder motion
  - Posterior dislocation
    - Potential life threatening emergency
    - Dyspnea, dysphagia, venous congestion, paresthesias
    - Sulcus-type deformity near sternum: Soft tissue swelling can obscure → false appearance of AD
    - Physical findings more subtle than with AD
  - Atraumatic dislocation: Only mild symptoms

Demographics
- Age
  - Young adults
  - Older patients may develop AD without clear history of trauma → painless mass over medial clavicle
- Gender
  - M > F
  - Atraumatic more common in young girls

Natural History & Prognosis
- Most regain adequate upper extremity function
- AD: Symptoms usually subside rapidly
- PD: Significant disability & death (rarely) ↑ than in AD

Treatment
- Grade I: Ice for 12-24 h, heat, + immobilize for 3-4 d
- Grade II: Ice for 12 h, heat for 12-24 h, reduce subluxation, + immobilize for 3-6 weeks
- Anterior dislocation (grade III)
  - Usually closed reduction under conscious sedation
  - Immobilization for 4-6 weeks following reduction
  - Recurrent painful dislocations may require surgery
  - May leave unreduced in geriatric + less active pts
- Posterior dislocation (grade III)
  - Closed reduction preferred < 24 h after injury; often done in OR under general anesthesia
  - Surgery if closed reduction fails or joint unstable
  - Immobilization for 4-6 weeks following reduction
  - Should have cardiothoracic surgery available
  - Most require hospital admission
- Atraumatic: Benign course → treatment not required
- Complications (nonoperative management)
  - AD: Cosmetic deformity, degenerative changes, persistent pain, weakness, instability with activity
  - PD: Great vessel, tracheal, esophageal, or brachial plexus injury
- Complications (operative management)
  - Migration of fixation pins
  - SC joint infection
  - Recurrent pain, impaired shoulder mobility, fatigue, neurologic symptoms, thoracic outlet syndrome

DIAGNOSTIC CHECKLIST

Consider
- SC dislocations are rare
- AD are far more common than PD
- PD can result in damage to superior mediastinal structures that can be life-threatening

Image Interpretation Pearls
- CT is preferred diagnostic modality
- Radiographs unreliable for dislocation direction

SELECTED REFERENCES

1. Ernberg LA et al: Radiographic evaluation of the acromioclavicular and sternoclavicular joints. Clin Sports Med. 22(2):255-75, 2003
2. Aslam M et al: Pictorial review: MRI of the sternum and sternoclavicular joints. Br J Radiol. 75(895):627-34, 2002
3. Salgado RA et al: Post-traumatic posterior sternoclavicular dislocation: case report and review of the literature. Emerg Radiol. 9(6):323-5, 2002
4. McCulloch P et al: Radiographic clues for high-energy trauma: three cases of sternoclavicular dislocation. AJR Am J Roentgenol. 176(6):1534, 2001
5. Ferrera PC et al: Sternoclavicular joint injuries. Am J Emerg Med. 18(1):58-61, 2000
6. Destouet JM et al: Computed tomography of the sternoclavicular joint and sternum. Radiology. 138(1):123-8, 1981

STERNOCLAVICULAR TRAUMA

IMAGE GALLERY

Typical

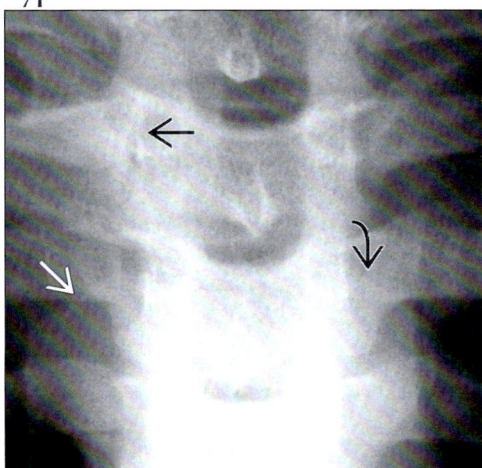 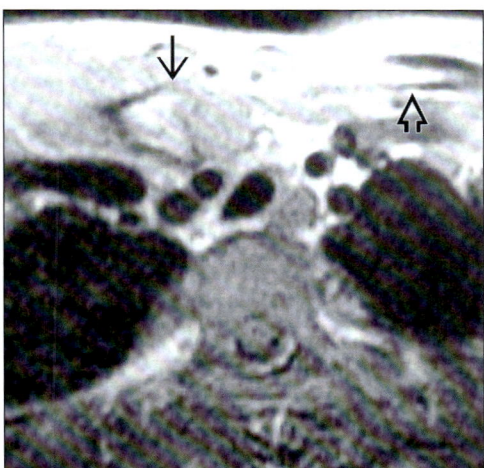

(**Left**) Anteroposterior radiograph shows a superior dislocation of the right clavicle ➔ relative to its site of articulation on the manubrium ➔. The contralateral normal SC joint is seen ➔. (**Right**) Axial T1WI MR shows the posterior & superior dislocation of the right clavicle ➔ relative to the left ➔. The superiorly displaced head of the right clavicle is seen in the same plane as the left midclavicle. There is no significant compression of major vessels.

Typical

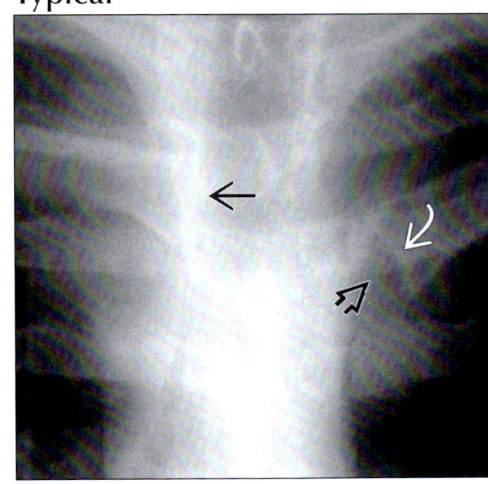 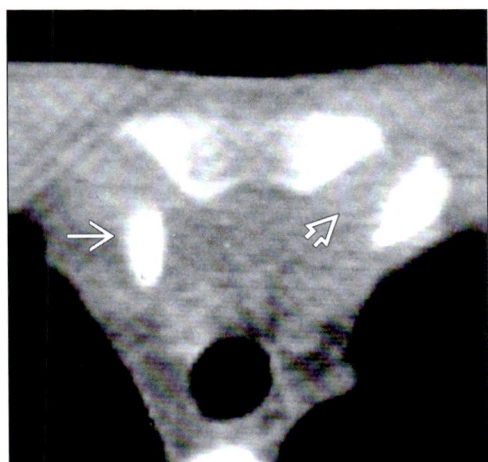

(**Left**) Anteroposterior radiograph shows normal mild offset of the left clavicle ➔ relative to the manubrium ➔. The right clavicle is superiorly displaced ➔. One cannot determine the direction of SC joint dislocation. (**Right**) Axial bone CT shows the normal left SC joint ➔; note that there is normally an incongruency because of the presence of the disc. The right SC joint is posteriorly dislocated ➔, putting the major vascular structures at risk.

Typical

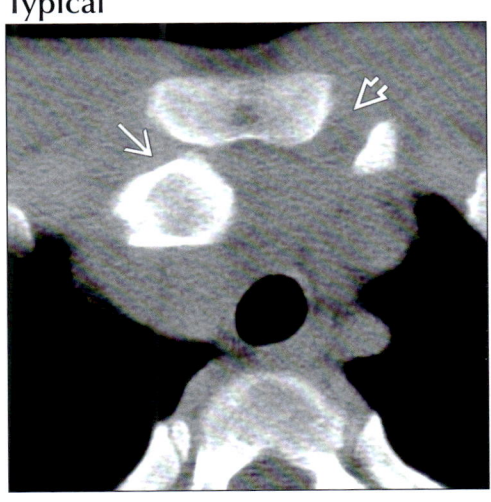 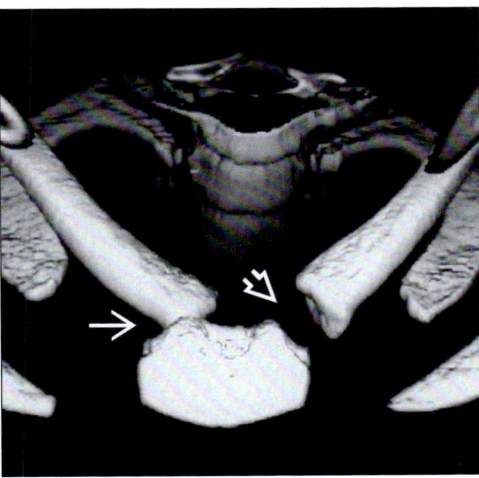

(**Left**) Axial bone CT shows a posterior dislocation of the right clavicle ➔. Compare the normal SC joint on the left ➔. The vessels are compressed & at risk with this dislocation. (**Right**) Frontal bone CT 3D reformat shows the right posterior SC joint dislocation ➔. This image shows nicely the normal arrangement of the left SC joint ➔. The clavicle is normally slightly superiorly placed relative to the manubrium because of the interposed triangular-shaped disc.

CLAVICLE FRACTURE

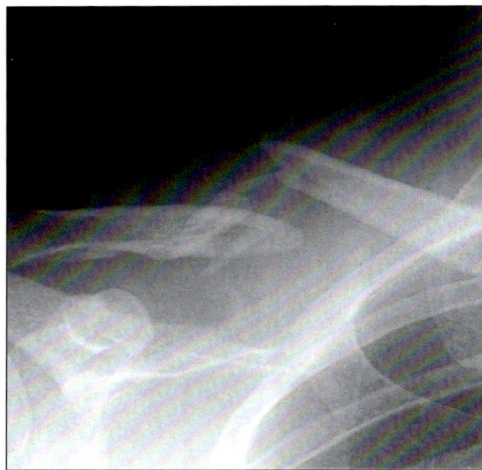

Anteroposterior radiograph shows a comminuted mid-clavicular fracture with superior displacement of the proximal fracture fragment.

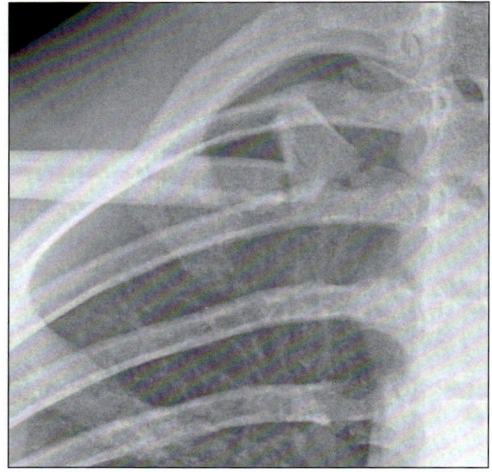

Anteroposterior radiograph shows a medial clavicular fracture in a child. In addition to the displaced fx, one must consider whether there is a dislocation or Salter I fx at the sternoclavicular joint.

TERMINOLOGY

Definitions
- Displaced and non-displaced fractures of the clavicle

IMAGING FINDINGS

General Features
- Best diagnostic clue: Linear fx line ± displacement
- Location: Allman classification: Group 1: Middle third (80%); group 2: Distal third (15%); group 3: Medial third (5%)
- Size: Varies from non-displaced cortical break to displaced and/or comminuted fracture

Radiographic Findings
- Linear lucency fracture line ± displacement

CT Findings
- Bone CT: Can aid in identifying intra-articular involvement and non-displaced medial fractures

MR Findings
- T1WI: Decreased marrow signal indicating edema with low signal fracture line; gross ligamentous disruption may be seen in distal and medial fractures
- Fluid sensitive sequences: Increased marrow signal indicating edema; subtle marrow and soft tissue findings are more easily seen with FS sequences

Imaging Recommendations
- Best imaging tool: Radiographs: Anteroposterior and 45° cephalic tilt anteroposterior view

DIFFERENTIAL DIAGNOSIS

Clinical
- AC dislocation: Pain & point tenderness over AC joint following direct trauma onto point of the shoulder
- Post-traumatic osteolysis of the distal clavicle: Shoulder pain within a variable time period (weeks to years) following episode of often minor trauma or repetitive trauma in weight lifters

DDx: Clavicle Injuries

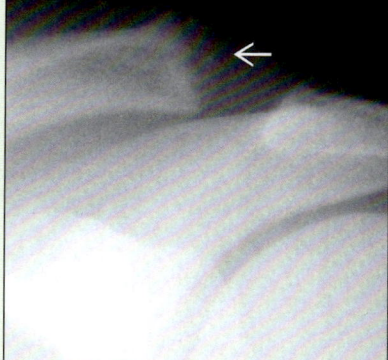

Distal Clavicle Osteolysis

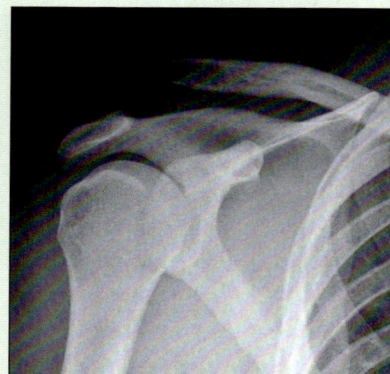

Type III AC Dislocation

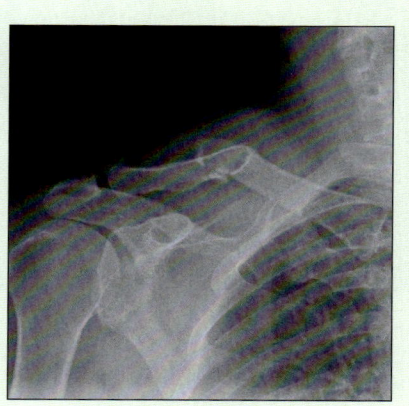

Mid-Clavicle Fracture

CLAVICLE FRACTURE

Key Facts

Imaging Findings
- Best imaging tool: Radiographs: Anteroposterior and 45° cephalic tilt anteroposterior view

Pathology
- Etiology: Direct fall onto shoulder (most common), direct blow to clavicle, or fall on outstretched hand

Clinical Issues
- Nonunion is rare (1-4% of cases); more likely to occur with unstable distal clavicle or poorly immobilized fx
- Post-traumatic osteoarthritis is common in type III distal clavicle fractures

Diagnostic Checklist
- Associated injuries, especially with high mechanism trauma

PATHOLOGY

General Features
- Etiology: Direct fall onto shoulder (most common), direct blow to clavicle, or fall on outstretched hand
- Epidemiology
  o Common fracture accounting for 5% of all fractures
  o Incidence: 64 per 100,000 people per year
  o 50% occur in children under the age of 10
  o M:F = 2.1:1
- Associated abnormalities
  o Rib fractures
  o Pneumothorax or hemothorax
  o Acromioclavicular disruptions

Staging, Grading or Classification Criteria
- Allman classification: Based on location
- Neer classification of distal clavicle fractures
  o Type I: Between AC joint & CC ligament attachment, minimal displacement and intact ligaments
  o Type II: At level of CC ligament, displaced with detachment of ligaments from proximal fragment
  o Type III: At the articular surface of the AC joint

CLINICAL ISSUES

Presentation
- Most common signs/symptoms: Pain, swelling and palpable deformity

Natural History & Prognosis
- Majority of fractures heal without difficulty
- Nonunion is rare (1-4% of cases); more likely to occur with unstable distal clavicle or poorly immobilized fx
- Post-traumatic osteoarthritis is common in type III distal clavicle fractures

Treatment
- Conservative: Protected immobilization
- Surgical: Open reduction and internal fixation may involve plate/screw or intramedullary rod placement
- Complications: Neurovascular symptoms from compression of subclavian vessels or brachial plexus; malunion with shortening may produce aesthetically unappealing deformity

DIAGNOSTIC CHECKLIST

Consider
- Associated injuries, especially with high mechanism trauma
- Nerve or vascular damage

SELECTED REFERENCES
1. Throckmorton T et al: Fractures of the medial end of the clavicle. J Shoulder Elbow Surg. 16(1):49-54, 2007
2. Jackson WF et al: Fractures of the lateral third of the clavicle: an anatomic approach to treatment. J Trauma. 61(1):222-5, 2006

IMAGE GALLERY

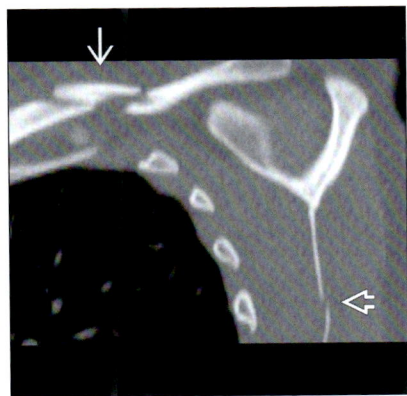 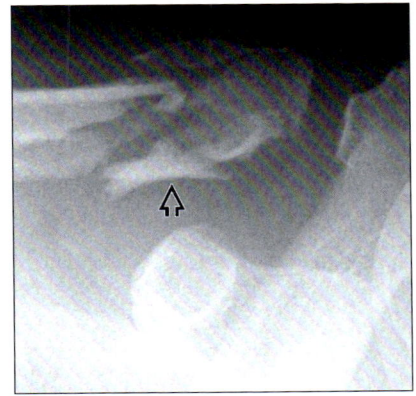 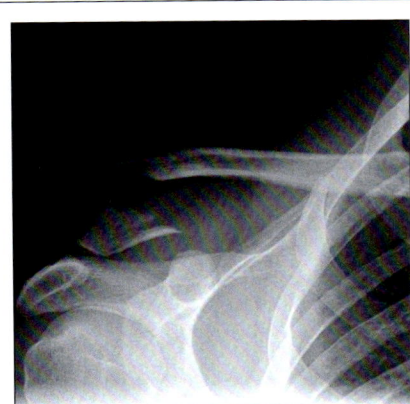

(Left) Oblique bone CT (reconstructed from axially acquired images) shows a comminuted mid-clavicle fracture ➡. There is also a minimally displaced fracture of the scapula ➡. *(Center)* Anteroposterior radiograph shows a comminuted type II distal clavicle fracture with an avulsion at the coracoclavicular insertion ➡. *(Right)* Anteroposterior radiograph shows a type II distal clavicular fracture with disruption of the coracoclavicular ligament and resulting superior displacement of the proximal fragment.

ACROMIOCLAVICULAR DISLOCATION

Anteroposterior radiograph shows a subtle type II AC dislocation with mild superior displacement of the clavicle. The AC distance is increased but the CC distance in normal.

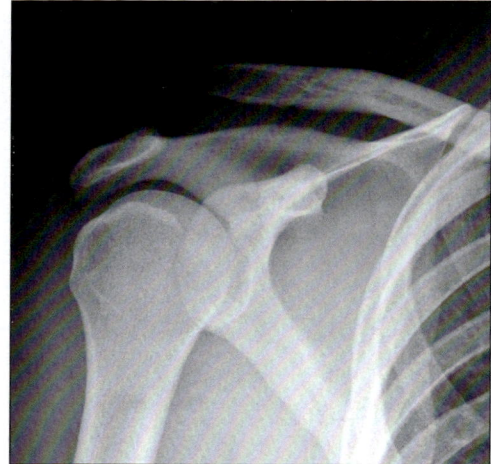

Anteroposterior radiograph shows a type III AC dislocation with moderate superior displacement of the clavicle and increased AC and CC distances.

TERMINOLOGY

Abbreviations and Synonyms
- Acromioclavicular (AC) separation

Definitions
- Distal clavicle dislocated relative to the acromion secondary to ligamentous injury

IMAGING FINDINGS

General Features
- Best diagnostic clue: Widening of the AC joint with variable displacement of the distal clavicle

Radiographic Findings
- Increased AC distance (normal: 3-6 mm) ± increased coracoclavicular (CC) distance (normal: 10-13 mm)
- Superior, posterior or inferior dislocation of the distal clavicle relative to the acromion

CT Findings
- Similar to radiographs, increased AC ± CC distances and variable distal clavicle displacement

MR Findings
- T1WI: Gross ligamentous disruption; low signal joint effusion; decreased marrow signal indicating edema
- T2WI, T2WI FS, PD/Intermediate FS, and STIR: High signal joint effusion; increased marrow signal indicating edema

Imaging Recommendations
- Best imaging tool: AP (with 15° cephalic angulation) and axillary lateral radiographs; normal side comparison useful; adding weights generally is not

DIFFERENTIAL DIAGNOSIS

Post-Traumatic Distal Clavicle Osteolysis
- Pain, weeks to years following episode of often minor trauma or repetitive trauma in weight lifters

Clavicle Fracture
- Pain and swelling following acute trauma

Normal Pediatric/Adolescent AC
- Distal clavicle epiphysis ossifies/fuses about 19 years

DDx: AC Dislocation

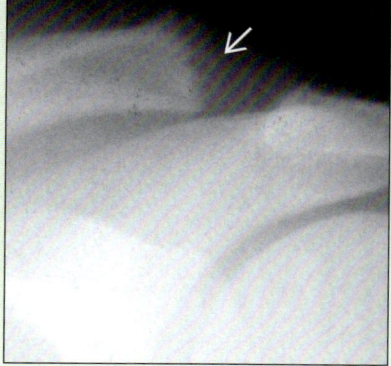
Distal Clavicle Osteolysis

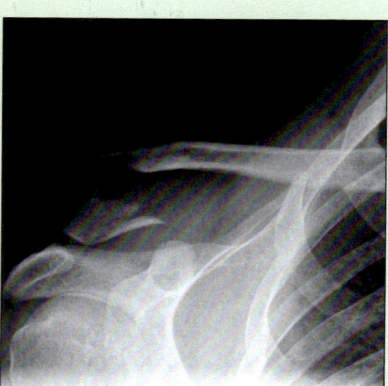
Distal Clavicle Fracture

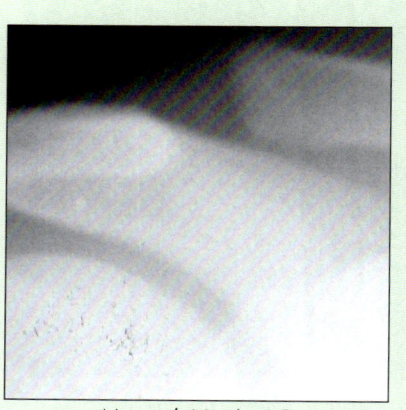
Normal 16 y/o AC

ACROMIOCLAVICULAR DISLOCATION

Key Facts

Terminology
- Distal clavicle dislocated relative to the acromion secondary to ligamentous injury

Imaging Findings
- Best diagnostic clue: Widening of the AC joint with variable displacement of the distal clavicle
- Increased AC distance (normal: 3-6 mm) ± increased coracoclavicular (CC) distance (normal: 10-13 mm)
- Superior, posterior or inferior dislocation of the distal clavicle relative to the acromion

Pathology
- Etiology: Direct force onto the point of the shoulder (most common) or indirect upward force/downward pull through the extremity

Clinical Issues
- Complications: Acromioclavicular osteoarthritis

- Compare to normal side; < 25% difference

PATHOLOGY

General Features
- Etiology: Direct force onto the point of the shoulder (most common) or indirect upward force/downward pull through the extremity
- Epidemiology: M > F; active patients between the ages of 15-44; rare < age 12
- Associated abnormalities: Acromion process, clavicle and rib fractures

Staging, Grading or Classification Criteria
- Type I: AC ligaments sprained but functionally intact; CC ligaments spared; normal radiograph
- Type II: AC ligaments completely disrupted; CC ligaments sprained but functionally intact
- Type III: AC and CC ligaments completely disrupted with mild to moderate superior displacement of clavicle
- Type IV: Similar to type III, complete AC and CC disruption with posterior displacement of clavicle into trapezius muscle
- Type V: Similar to type III, complete AC and CC disruption with severe superior displacement of clavicle into subcutaneous soft tissue
- Type VI: AC ligament disruption ± CC ligament disruption with inferior displacement of clavicle into a subacromial or subcoracoid location

CLINICAL ISSUES

Presentation
- Most common signs/symptoms: Pain, tenderness, deformity of the AC joint

Natural History & Prognosis
- High rate of persistent nuisance-type symptoms (pain and clicking)
- Residual weakness and instability are not uncommon

Treatment
- Conservative
  - Ice, analgesics and shoulder rest in sling (1-4 weeks)
  - Heavy lifting/sports restriction (6-12 weeks)
- Surgical: Repair of the AC and CC ligaments; distal clavicle excision; dynamic muscle transfers
- Complications: Acromioclavicular osteoarthritis

DIAGNOSTIC CHECKLIST

Consider
- Associated injuries, especially in high grade dislocations

SELECTED REFERENCES
1. Bishop JY et al: Treatment of the acute traumatic acromioclavicular separation. Sports Med Arthrosc. 14(4):237-45, 2006

IMAGE GALLERY

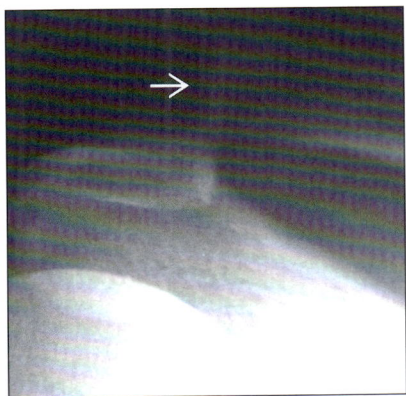 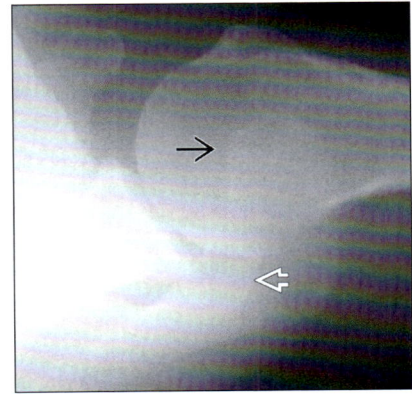 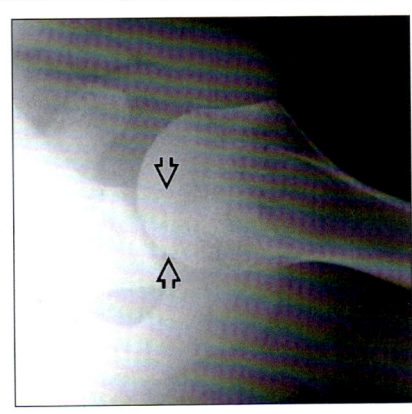

(Left) Anteroposterior radiograph shows an elevated clavicle relative to the acromion ➡. This might be considered a type III AC separation, but the axillary view changes it to a type IV. *(Center)* Axillary lateral radiograph shows type IV AC separation, with clavicle ➡ significantly posteriorly dislocated relative to the articular surface of the acromion ➡. *(Right)* Axillary lateral radiograph of a different (normal) patient, showing the normal acromioclavicular articulation ➡ superimposed over the humeral head.

SCAPULAR TRAUMA

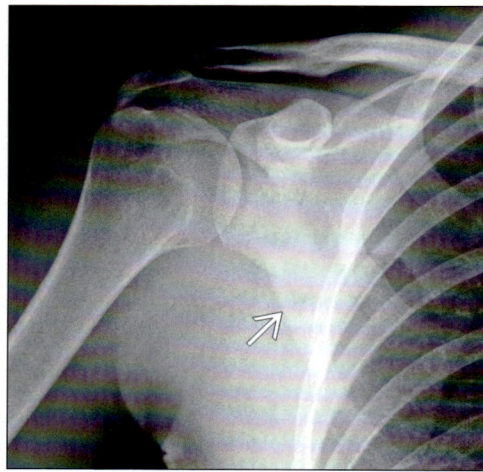

Anteroposterior radiograph shows a minimally displaced fracture of the scapular body ➡. The glenoid, coracoid, acromion, and adjacent clavicle are intact.

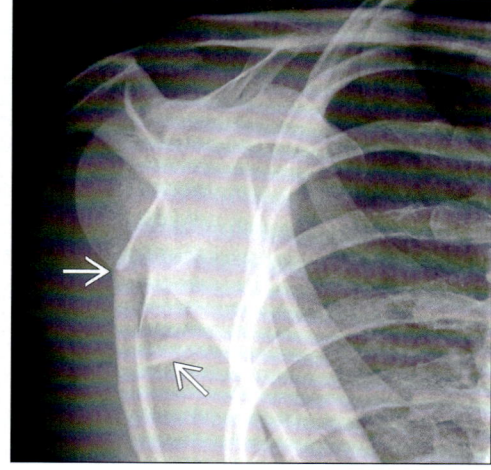

Lateral radiograph shows the same comminuted fracture of the scapular body ➡. In cases with isolated fractures of the scapular body, treatment is usually conservative.

TERMINOLOGY

Abbreviations and Synonyms
- Fracture may be termed according to involved structure such as: Glenoid fracture, acromion fracture, or coracoid fracture

Definitions
- Fracture of the scapula due to direct trauma, shoulder dislocation or avulsion

IMAGING FINDINGS

General Features
- Best diagnostic clue
  - Linear fracture line on AP, axillary, and scapula Y-view radiographs
  - Medialization of the glenohumeral joint on true AP radiograph (35° mediolateral AP projection)
  - Glenohumeral dislocation has associated glenoid rim fracture in approximately 20% of cases
- Location
  - Scapular body is most commonly fractured portion of the scapula and is often the result of direct trauma
  - Glenoid fracture may extend from body or may be isolated finding in relation to glenohumeral joint dislocation
  - Scapular neck fracture is usually the result of direct trauma and may be associated with inferior displacement of the distal fragment
  - Spinous process of scapula fracture is usually the result of direct trauma
- Size: Varies with mechanism and may involve one or more portions of the scapula ± severe comminution
- Morphology
  - Fracture may be difficult to detect if simple and without displacement
  - "Floating shoulder" may result from fracture of glenoid and ipsilateral clavicle with weight of arm pulling glenoid fragment anteromedially

Radiographic Findings
- Linear lucency through the scapula ± comminution of fragments

Assorted Scapular Fractures

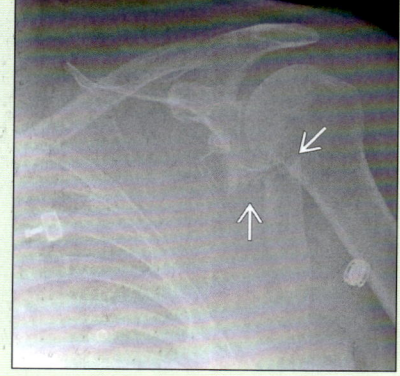

Infraglenoid Fracture

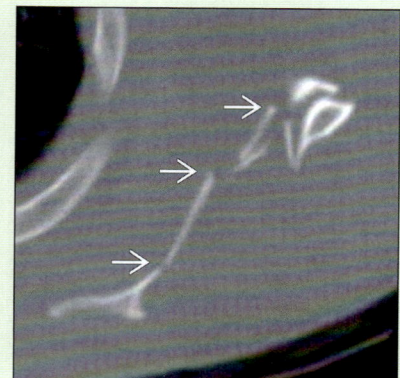

Scapular Body Fracture

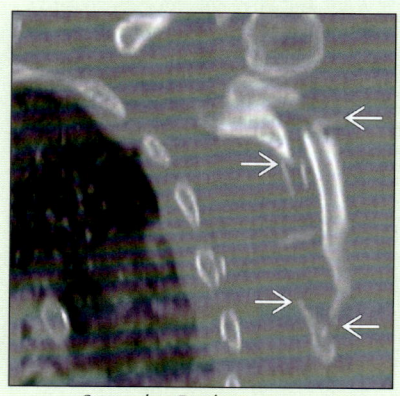

Scapular Body Fracture

SCAPULAR TRAUMA

Key Facts

Terminology
- Fracture may be termed according to involved structure such as: Glenoid fracture, acromion fracture, or coracoid fracture
- Fracture of the scapula due to direct trauma, shoulder dislocation or avulsion

Imaging Findings
- Glenohumeral dislocation has associated glenoid rim fracture in approximately 20% of cases
- Scapula fractures are frequently found in combination with other injuries including humerus, clavicle, and rib fractures
- True AP (Grashey) view to evaluate glenohumeral joint space, glenoid rim, and to detect medialization of the glenoid in cases of scapular neck fracture

Pathology
- High energy mechanism of injury usually responsible for fracture

Clinical Issues
- 90% of scapula fractures are minimally or nondisplaced and treatment is directed towards symptom relief and restoration of motion
- Displaced intra-articular fracture of glenoid is indication for surgical treatment
- Significantly displaced scapular spine, coracoid and acromial fractures may require surgical treatment
- Significant displacement or angulation of the scapular neck may require surgical treatment
- Associated injury such as clavicle fracture may result in "floating shoulder" and require surgical repair with aim of improving glenohumeral joint biomechanics

---

- May initially be identified on chest radiographs obtained during the evaluation of thoracic trauma
- Scapula fractures are frequently found in combination with other injuries including humerus, clavicle, and rib fractures
- Glenohumeral joint dislocation commonly associated with glenoid rim fracture

CT Findings
- Bone CT
  - Assists in detection and characterization of scapula fracture
  - Demonstrates whether there is intra-articular extension
  - Aids in surgical planning when necessary

MR Findings
- T1WI
  - Decreased signal intensity fracture line
  - Decreased signal intensity marrow edema
- T2WI
  - Decreased signal intensity fracture line
  - Increased signal intensity marrow edema
  - Increased signal intensity of surrounding musculature in regions of contusion
- PD/Intermediate FS: Evaluate for intra-articular extension and disruption of labrum, glenoid articular cartilage
- STIR
  - Increased signal intensity marrow edema
  - Increased signal intensity in surrounding musculature in regions of contusion
- May demonstrate associated ligamentous and muscular injury
- May demonstrate occult fracture not visible on plain radiographs

Imaging Recommendations
- Best imaging tool
  - AP, axillary, and scapula Y-views of the shoulder
    - True AP (Grashey) view to evaluate glenohumeral joint space, glenoid rim, and to detect medialization of the glenoid in cases of scapular neck fracture
    - Axillary view to evaluate glenoid, coracoid, acromion, and to detect glenohumeral dislocation
    - Scapula Y-view to detect angular deformity of body or neck of scapula and to detect glenohumeral dislocation
  - Bone CT
- Protocol advice
  - Bone CT with multiplanar reformatting including oblique coronal perpendicular to glenoid
    - Complicated fracture
    - Surgical planning

DIFFERENTIAL DIAGNOSIS

Os Acromiale
- Anatomic variant consisting of fibrocartilaginous union of the acromion to the scapular spine
- May contribute to shoulder impingement and rotator cuff tear

Osteochondral Injury
- Injury to articular cartilage ± underlying subchondral bone
- Typically gradual onset in physically active patient

Proximal Humerus/Humeral Head Fracture
- Overlapping mechanism of injury and presentation
- ± Glenohumeral dislocation

Glenohumeral Dislocation
- Commonly associated with glenoid rim fracture or labral injury

SCAPULAR TRAUMA

PATHOLOGY

General Features
- General path comments: 5-7% of fractures about the shoulder
- Etiology
  - Direct trauma
    - High energy mechanism of injury usually responsible for fracture
    - The scapula is surrounded by muscle and articulates with the clavicle and humerus, both of which are more likely to fracture before the scapula
  - Glenohumeral dislocation may lead to glenoid rim fracture
- Epidemiology
  - Approximately 1% of fractures
  - Mean age of patients with scapula fracture is 35-45 years
  - Motor vehicle accident most common etiology
- Associated abnormalities
  - Associated fracture in 80-90% of cases
    - Clavicle
    - Humerus
    - Ribs
  - Thoracic, spinal and cranial injuries may be present related to high energy mechanism
  - Vascular or neurologic injury may accompany scapula fracture
    - Suprascapular nerve at risk of injury with fracture extension into suprascapular notch or spinoglenoid notch

Microscopic Features
- Disruption of cortex and trabeculae

Staging, Grading or Classification Criteria
- Scapula fractures are described by the region and structures they involve
  - Ideberg classification of intra-articular glenoid fractures
    - Type I: Glenoid rim (type Ia: Anterior, type Ib: Posterior)
    - Type II: Glenoid fossa fracture with displacement of inferior glenoid fragment in same direction as humeral head
    - Type III: Glenoid fracture extending superiorly through the superior border of the scapula
    - Type IV: Horizontal fracture extending through the body to the medial edge of the scapular body
    - Type V: Horizontal fracture with additional fracture line separating inferior glenoid from the remaining scapula
    - Type VI: Severe comminution of the glenoid
  - Glenoid neck fractures
    - With associated clavicle fracture or AC joint separation
    - Without associated clavicle fracture or AC joint separation
  - Kuhn classification of acromion fractures
    - Type I: Minimally displaced
    - Type II: Displaced, but no loss of subacromial space
    - Type III: Displaced with associated loss of subacromial space
  - Coracoid fractures
    - Proximal to coracoclavicular ligaments
    - Distal to coracoclavicular ligaments

CLINICAL ISSUES

Presentation
- Most common signs/symptoms
  - Pain, inability to abduct arm, tenderness over shoulder and scapula
  - Shoulder may appear flattened
- Other signs/symptoms: Shoulder dislocation

Demographics
- Age: Young > old related to incidence of high energy mechanism trauma
- Gender: M > F related to incidence of high energy mechanism trauma

Natural History & Prognosis
- Treatment has historically been nonoperative

Treatment
- Overall goal of restoring function, avoiding/minimizing long-term stiffness
- Nondisplaced fracture may heal with conservative management
  - 90% of scapula fractures are minimally or nondisplaced and treatment is directed towards symptom relief and restoration of motion
- Certain features predict poor prognosis and may indicate surgical treatment
  - Intra-articular fracture
    - Displaced intra-articular fracture of glenoid is indication for surgical treatment
  - Extra-articular fracture
    - Significantly displaced scapular spine, coracoid and acromial fractures may require surgical treatment
    - Significant displacement or angulation of the scapular neck may require surgical treatment
    - Associated injury such as clavicle fracture may result in "floating shoulder" and require surgical repair with aim of improving glenohumeral joint biomechanics

SELECTED REFERENCES
1. Zlowodzki M et al: Treatment of scapula fractures: systematic review of 520 fractures in 22 case series. J Orthop Trauma. 20(3):230-3, 2006
2. Cole PA: Scapula fractures. Orthop Clin North Am. 33(1):1-18, vii, 2002
3. Resnick D: Diagnosis of Bone and Joint Disorders. vol 3. 4th ed. Philadelphia, W.B. Saunders Company. 2817-20, 2824-7, 2002
4. Bucholz RW et al: Rockwood and Green's Fractures in Adults. vol 1. 5th ed. Philadelphia, Lippincott Williams and Wilkins. 1079-92, 2001
5. Goss TP: The scapula: coracoid, acromial, and avulsion fractures. Am J Orthop. 25(2):106-15, 1996

SCAPULAR TRAUMA

IMAGE GALLERY

Typical

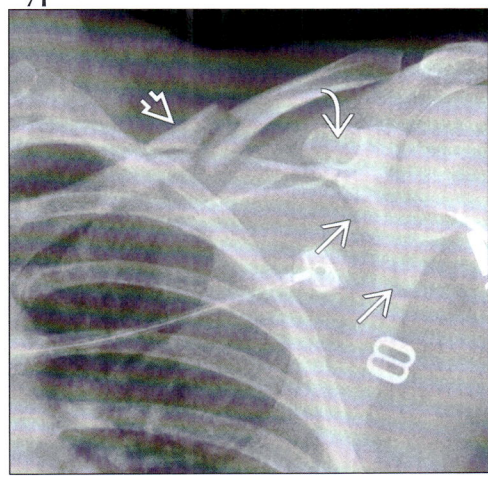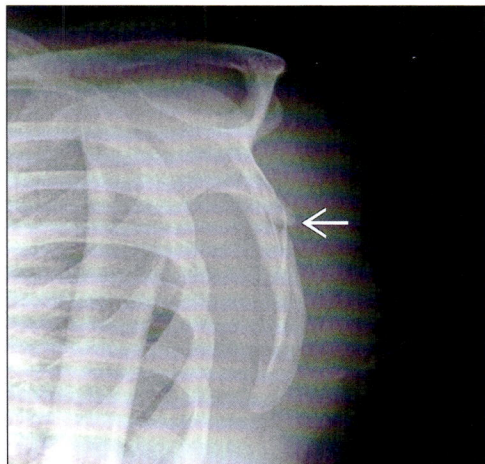

(Left) Anteroposterior radiograph shows a fracture ➡ extending from the suprascapular notch ➡ through the neck of the glenoid. Note the associated clavicle fracture ➡. *(Right)* Lateral radiograph shows a minimally displaced scapular body fracture ➡. Such fractures may be difficult to identify on anteroposterior views of the chest or shoulder.

Typical

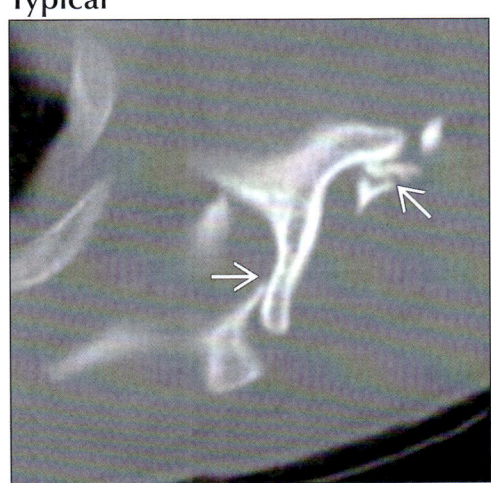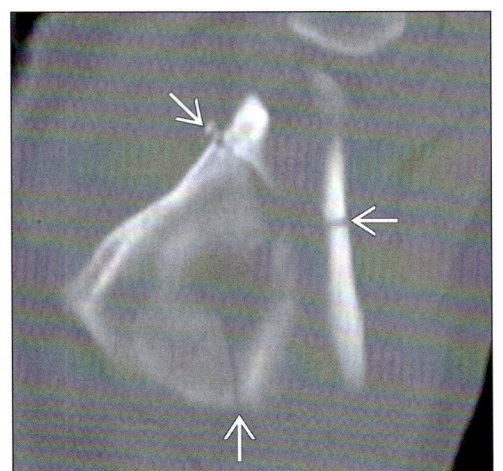

(Left) Axial bone CT shows a markedly comminuted scapular body fracture ➡ which extends through the scapular spine. *(Right)* Coronal bone CT shows a comminuted fracture of the scapular body ➡. Most of these fractures are treated without surgery unless there is significant displacement of the fragments.

Typical

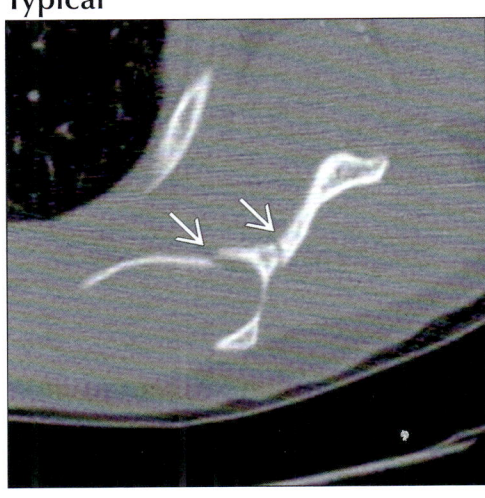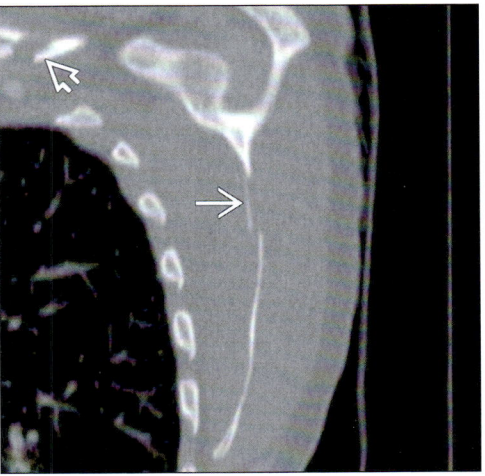

(Left) Axial bone CT shows a fracture ➡ involving the scapular body on both sides of the scapular spine. This nondisplaced fracture would be treated conservatively without surgery. *(Right)* Sagittal bone CT shows a minimally displaced scapular body fracture ➡. Note the associated clavicle fracture ➡. Scapular fractures are frequently associated with other fractures.

SHOULDER DISLOCATION

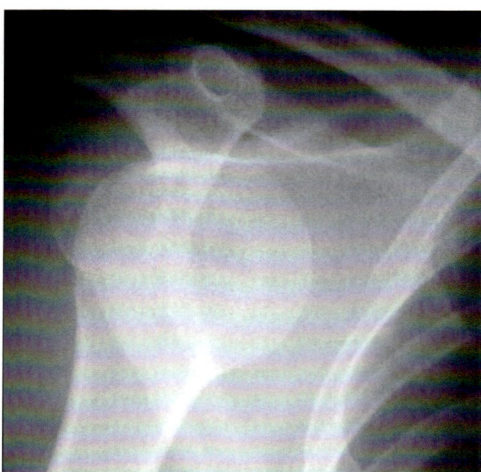

Anteroposterior radiograph shows an anterior glenohumeral dislocation, with the humeral head in the typical subcoracoid position.

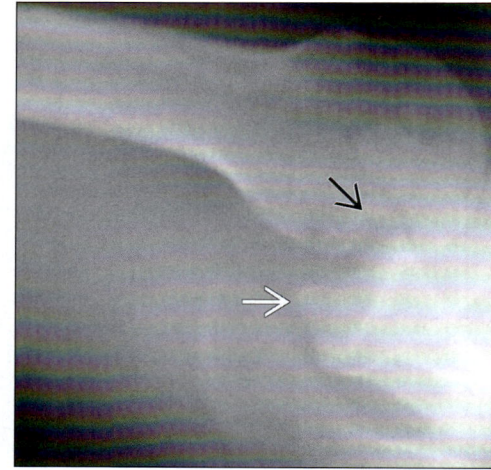

Lateral radiograph is confirmatory. The humeral head is anteriorly and medially dislocated relative to the glenoid, with impaction (Hill Sachs fracture) ➡ as well as Bankart fracture fragment ➡.

TERMINOLOGY

Definitions
- Complete loss of articulation between glenoid and humeral head

IMAGING FINDINGS

General Features
- Best diagnostic clue
  - Anterior dislocation: Usually dislocates anteriorly, inferiorly, & medially
  - Posterior dislocation: Usually dislocates directly posteriorly
    - Because there is usually not significant medial, lateral, superior, or inferior displacement, 50% of posterior dislocations are initially missed if only AP radiographs obtained
    - Axillary lateral radiograph confirms posterior dislocation, concurrent reverse Hill Sachs impaction, & glenoid rim fracture
  - Luxatio erecta: Dislocation of humeral head directly inferiorly
    - Loss of articulation, with humeral head located inferior to glenoid
    - Arm is in fixed abduction

Radiographic Findings
- Anterior dislocation
  - Subcoracoid position of humeral head shown on AP
  - Hill Sachs impaction fracture (located posterolaterally) best seen on AP internal rotation; may be more subtle or even entirely obscured on external rotation or axillary view
  - Bankart or subtle glenoid rim fractures best seen on axillary lateral
- Posterior dislocation
  - Direct posterior dislocation may result in apparent joint space being narrow, wide, or normal on AP
    - "Rim sign": Widened glenohumeral space on AP, indirect sign of posterior dislocation
  - Reverse Hill Sachs: Impaction fracture (located anteromedially) may be subtle
    - Humeral head locked in internal rotation
    - "Trough sign": Linear sclerosis seen in mid humeral head on internal rotation view; impacted bone of reverse Hill Sachs fracture is responsible

Other Shoulder Dislocations

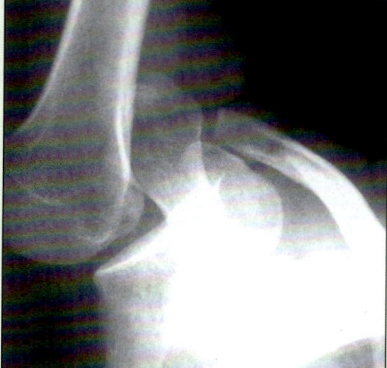

Luxatio Erecta

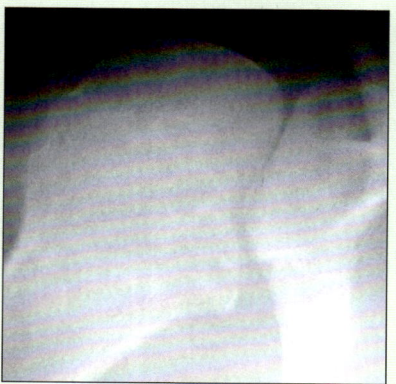

Chronic Posterior Dislocation

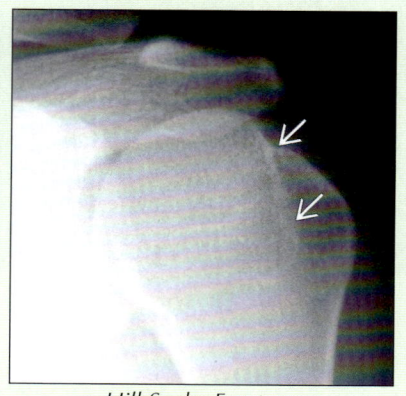

Hill Sachs Fracture

SHOULDER DISLOCATION

Key Facts

Terminology
- Complete loss of articulation between glenoid and humeral head

Imaging Findings
- Anterior dislocation: Usually dislocates anteriorly, inferiorly, & medially
- Posterior dislocation: Usually dislocates directly posteriorly
- Because there is usually not significant medial, lateral, superior, or inferior displacement, 50% of posterior dislocations are initially missed if only AP radiographs obtained
- Luxatio erecta: Dislocation of humeral head directly inferiorly
- Hill Sachs impaction fracture (located posterolaterally) best seen on AP internal rotation; may be more subtle or even entirely obscured on external rotation or axillary view
- Bankart or subtle glenoid rim fractures best seen on axillary lateral
- "Rim sign": Widened glenohumeral space on AP, indirect sign of posterior dislocation
- Reverse Hill Sachs: Impaction fracture (located anteromedially) may be subtle
- Humeral head locked in internal rotation
- "Trough sign": Linear sclerosis seen in mid humeral head on internal rotation view; impacted bone of reverse Hill Sachs fracture is responsible
- Posterior dislocation may be directly seen and diagnosed only with axillary lateral

---

- Posterior dislocation may be directly seen and diagnosed only with axillary lateral

MR Findings
- MR or MR arthrography may be performed subacutely if a reduced shoulder is unstable
- Demonstrates associated abnormalities which may lead to instability
  - Fracture: Impaction humeral head, bony glenoid, greater or lesser tuberosities
  - Rotator cuff tear
  - Capsular disruption or redundancy
  - Labral tear
  - Glenohumeral ligament disruption

Imaging Recommendations
- Best imaging tool: Radiograph: AP external & internal rotation, axillary lateral
- Protocol advice
  - Axillary lateral is preferable to transscapular or Y view; the latter two must be perfectly aligned, or a dislocation/significant subluxation will be missed
  - MR arthrogram: If it can be accomplished without re-dislocation, abduction external rotation view is extremely useful for evaluation of inferior glenohumeral ligament (IGHL) injury, frequently seen following anterior dislocation

DIFFERENTIAL DIAGNOSIS

Radiographic Differential: Inferior Humeral Head Subluxation
- Often seen following stroke or humeral head/neck fracture
- Due to muscle atony
- Note: Subluxation (some articulation remains) rather than dislocation

Clinical Differential: Multidirectional Instability
- Usually young female
- Usually bilateral
- Not frankly dislocated on radiograph
- MR excludes conventional causes of instability
  - No visible labral-ligamentous lesions
  - Capsule may be redundant
  - Labrum may be hypoplastic
  - May have early degenerative changes, with labral fraying/tear

PATHOLOGY

General Features
- Etiology
  - Glenohumeral is ball-and-socket joint
    - Hemispherical head & shallow scapular glenoid result in 4:1 disproportion in articular surface areas of head & glenoid
    - Allows wide range of motion
    - Puts structure at risk for dislocation
  - Anterior shoulder dislocation etiology
    - Abduction, external rotation; acromion contacts surgical neck of humerus & head is levered out of glenoid fossa
    - Direct blow to back of shoulder
    - Traction on limb
  - Posterior shoulder dislocation etiology
    - Fall on outstretched hand with arm flexed & abducted
    - Direct trauma
    - Violent muscle contractions: Electric shock or seizures
    - Hypoplastic or retroverted glenoid adds to risk
  - Luxatio erecta dislocation etiology
    - Direct axial force applied to fully abducted arm
    - Hyperabduction leading to leverage of humeral head across acromion
- Epidemiology
  - Shoulder is inherently unstable & is one of the most frequently dislocated joints
  - 96% dislocate anteriorly
  - 2-4% dislocate posteriorly
  - 1-2% dislocate inferiorly (luxatio erecta)

SHOULDER DISLOCATION

- ○ < 1% dislocate superiorly
- Associated abnormalities
  - ○ Anterior shoulder dislocation
    - Hill Sachs (posterolateral impaction fx): 50-75%
    - Anterior band IGHL is most important stabilizing structure at end of range of motion in the ABER direction; IGHL fails at capsular insertion site (40%), intrasubstance (35%), or humeral insertion site (25%)
    - Labral lesions (Bankart & its subsets)
    - Capsular separation from anterior glenoid rim (85%)
    - Bony glenoid fracture
    - Greater tuberosity fracture
    - Rotator cuff tear (supraspinatus or subscapularis): 25%
  - ○ Posterior shoulder dislocation
    - Reverse Hill Sachs (anteromedial impaction fx)
    - Posterior band of IGHL is primary capsuloligamentous restraint & most at risk
    - Labrum (posterior; reverse Bankart)
    - Capsular tear or laxity
    - Fracture or ectopic calcification of posterior glenoid rim
    - Fracture lesser tuberosity
    - Teres minor lesion (partial tear/edema)
  - ○ Luxatio erecta
    - Inferior capsule usually torn
    - May fracture greater tuberosity, acromion, clavicle, coracoid, glenoid rim
    - May have brachial plexus or axillary artery injury

Staging, Grading or Classification Criteria
- Classification of glenoid lesions: Aids surgical planning
  - ○ Type 1: Partial Bankart lesion without stripping of capsule from glenoid labrum
  - ○ Type 2: Moderate detachment of labrum & capsule from glenoid, with preservation of labral shape
  - ○ Type 3: Severe detachment of capsulolabral complex, with attenuation of glenoid labrum
  - ○ Type 4: Includes a fracture of glenoid

CLINICAL ISSUES

Presentation
- Most common signs/symptoms
  - ○ Trauma, with "popping" sensation and severe pain
  - ○ Anterior dislocation: Prominence of humeral head anteriorly & a hollow below acromion
  - ○ Posterior dislocation: Loss of the normal rounded appearance anteriorly; shoulder fixed in internal rotation & adduction
  - ○ May have axillary nerve damage
    - Loss of sensation on lateral aspect of shoulder (sergeant's stripe pattern)

Demographics
- Age
  - ○ Two age peaks for initial dislocation: 10-20 years, and 50-70 years
  - ○ Incidence of recurrence inversely related to age at initial dislocation

Natural History & Prognosis
- Following a single acute anterior dislocation, 40% become recurrent dislocators as a result of associated damage
- Young patients (teens through 3rd decade)
  - ○ Often have Bankart lesion (with subsets anterior ligamentous periosteal sleeve avulsion (ALPSA), Perthes, humeral avulsion glenohumeral ligament (HAGL), Bennett)
  - ○ Often need surgical reconstruction to regain stability
- Older patients
  - ○ Fewer Bankart lesions
  - ○ More frequent supraspinatus tears
  - ○ Fracture of greater tuberosity more frequent (30% of older patients)
  - ○ Avulsion of subscapularis & capsule from lesser tuberosity
  - ○ Usually treated conservatively, so may not need MR arthrography

Treatment
- Immediate reduction
- Repeated dislocations may require surgical treatment; MR demonstrates injuries associated with the instability
- Multidirectional instability usually treated with rehabilitative therapy for muscle strengthening; occasionally surgical treatment

DIAGNOSTIC CHECKLIST

Consider
- Look for associated fractures at initial dislocation
- Understand all stabilizing structures of shoulder in order to give a full interpretation of MR for instability

Image Interpretation Pearls
- Following anterior dislocation, do not dismiss the possibility of Hill Sachs impaction fracture if AP internal rotation radiograph not available
- Do not dismiss the possibility of dislocation if adequate lateral radiograph is not available; axillary lateral is preferred view

SELECTED REFERENCES

1. Robinson CM et al: Functional outcome and risk of recurrent instability after primary traumatic anterior shoulder dislocation in young patients. J Bone Joint Surg Am. 88(11):2326-36, 2006
2. Spatschil A et al: Posttraumatic anterior-inferior instability of the shoulder: arthroscopic findings and clinical correlations. Arch Orthop Trauma Surg. 126(4):217-22, 2006
3. Widjaja AB et al: Correlation between Bankart and Hill-Sachs lesions in anterior shoulder dislocation. ANZ J Surg. 76(6):436-8, 2006
4. Grimer RJ et al: The prognosis following acute primary glenohumeral dislocation. J Bone Joint Surg Br. 87(2):277; author reply 277, 2005
5. Takase K et al: Intraarticular lesions in traumatic anterior shoulder instability: a study based on the results of diagnostic imaging. Acta Orthop. 76(6):854-7, 2005

SHOULDER DISLOCATION

IMAGE GALLERY

Typical

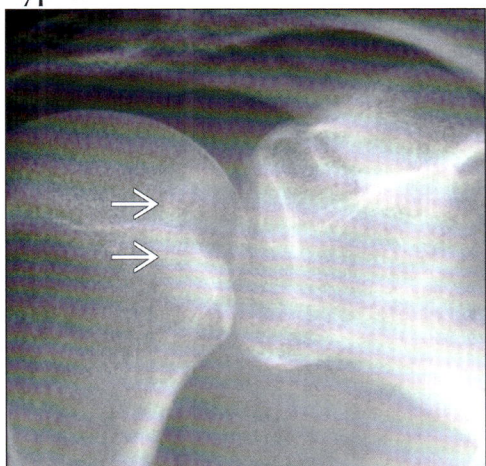
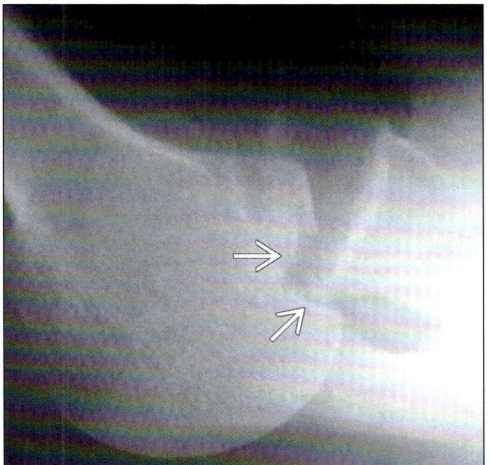

(Left) Anteroposterior radiograph shows a trough sign ➡, indicating a reverse Hill Sachs impaction fracture in a posterior dislocation. The humeral head is locked in internal rotation. *(Right)* Lateral radiograph confirms the posterior dislocation of the humeral head, with the large impaction fracture ➡ on the humeral head preventing easy relocation.

Typical

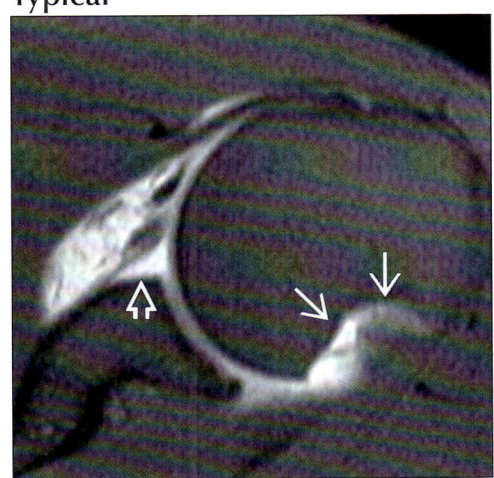
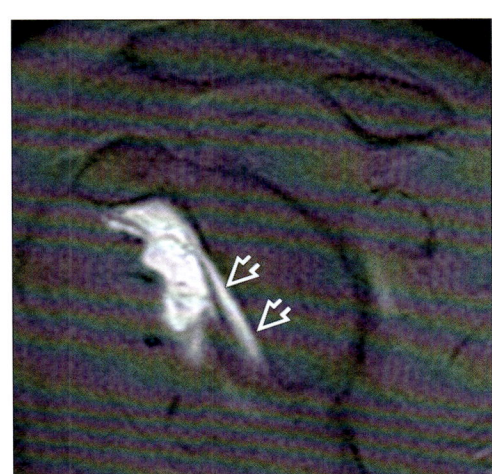

(Left) Axial T1WI FS MR following contrast injection shows a large Hill Sachs impaction fracture ➡ as well as a large osseous Bankart fracture ➡. *(Right)* Sagittal T1WI FS MR arthrogram at the level of the glenoid shows the large extent of the Bankart fracture ➡. This patient reported "over 200" dislocations and was severely unstable.

Typical

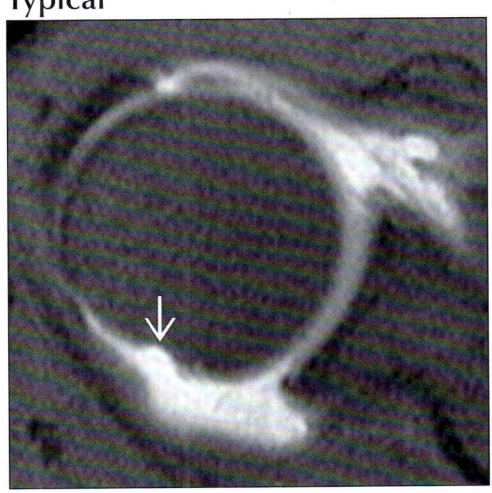
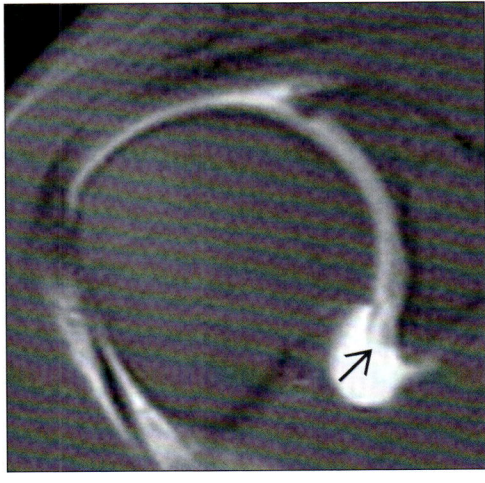

(Left) Axial T1WI FS MR arthrogram shows a small Hill Sachs impaction fracture ➡ in a patient with a single episode of anterior dislocation. *(Right)* Coronal T1WI FS MR arthrogram shows an anteroinferior labral tear, along with a glenolabral articular defect ➡. There is no capsular redundancy or other injury to contribute to instability.

HUMERAL HEAD/NECK FRACTURE

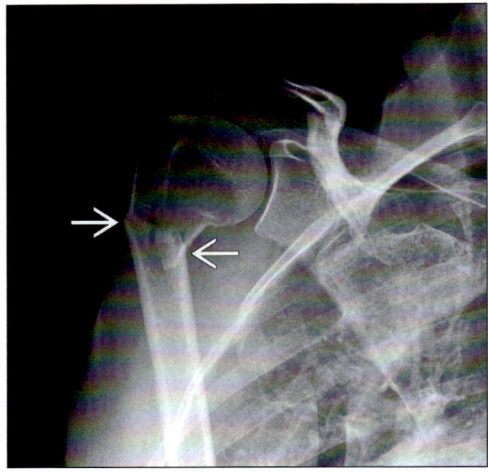

Anteroposterior radiograph shows a transverse fracture ➡ of the neck of the humerus. This appears to be a Neer 1-Part fracture as there is less than 45° of angulation and no apparent significant displacement.

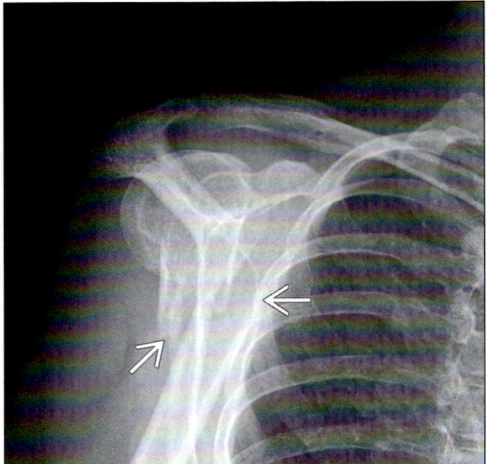

Lateral radiograph shows the same humeral neck fracture ➡ with mild angulation. However, anterior displacement of the shaft fragment is > 1 cm; this elevates the classification to Neer 2-Part.

TERMINOLOGY

Abbreviations and Synonyms
- Fracture may be termed according to involved structure including: Humeral head fracture or humeral neck fracture; surgical neck fx

Definitions
- Fracture of the proximal humerus due to fall on arm or direct trauma

IMAGING FINDINGS

General Features
- Best diagnostic clue
  - Oblique or transverse fracture line on radiographs
  - Discontinuity of the cortex of the proximal humerus
  - Separation of fragments
- Location
  - Humeral head
  - Surgical neck of the humerus
  - Greater tuberosity
  - Lesser tuberosity
- Size: Varies from nondisplaced fracture to severe comminution and displacement of fragments
- Morphology: Fractures described according to the separate fragments that are generated and the degree of displacement & angulation

Radiographic Findings
- Radiolucent fracture line extending through proximal humerus/humeral head or tuberosity
  - Fracture lines may be difficult to see due to osteopenia, obesity, overlapping fragments or nondisplacement
  - Impacted fractures may be seen as sclerotic lines
  - Fracture ± comminution of the humeral head may be difficult to distinguish from a tuberosity fracture
- Lipohemarthrosis may be demonstrated by upright or decubitus projections
- Degree of displacement and/or angulation of fragments may be difficult to appreciate with radiographs alone; axillary lateral helpful

CT Findings
- Bone CT
  - Assists in defining degree of displacement and/or angulation of fragments

Additional Humeral Head/Neck Fractures

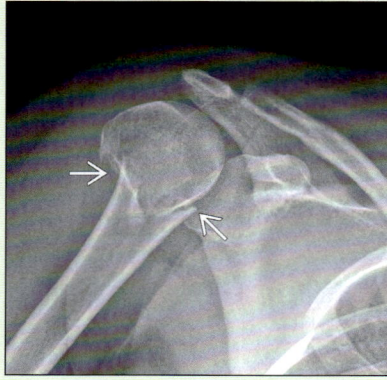

Neer 1-Part Humeral Neck Fracture

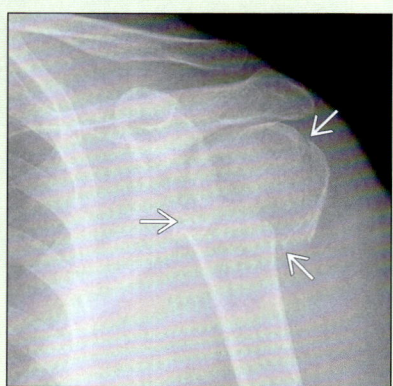

Neer 2-Part Head/Neck Fracture

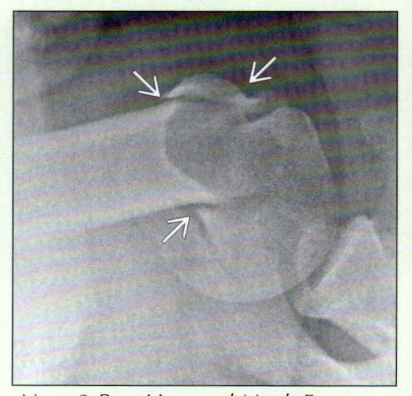

Neer 3-Part Humeral Neck Fracture

HUMERAL HEAD/NECK FRACTURE

Key Facts

Terminology
- Fracture may be termed according to involved structure including: Humeral head fracture or humeral neck fracture; surgical neck fx

Imaging Findings
- Size: Varies from nondisplaced fracture to severe comminution and displacement of fragments
- Degree of displacement and/or angulation of fragments may be difficult to appreciate with radiographs alone; axillary lateral helpful

Pathology
- Fragments considered displaced if there is > 1 cm of displacement or > 45° of angulation
- Neer Classification system most commonly used

- Approximately 80% of proximal humeral fractures are nondisplaced
- Hill-Sachs fracture (impaction fracture of humeral head) usually result of glenohumeral dislocation

Diagnostic Checklist
- Possible vascular injury to the axillary vessels
- Possible neurological injury to brachial plexus or axillary nerve
- Associated injury of the chest wall, neck, head or other site related to mechanism
- High-quality, well-positioned radiographs required for evaluation of proximal humerus fractures
- CT may be helpful in characterizing complex proximal humerus fractures

---

- Helpful in identifying dislocation
- May demonstrate associated glenoid fracture
- May show disorganized trabecular pattern of contusion or impaction
- May demonstrate lipohemarthrosis
- May aid in surgical planning

MR Findings
- T1WI
  - Decreased signal intensity fracture line
  - Decreased signal intensity of surrounding edema
  - High signal of intra-articular fat in lipohemarthrosis
- T2WI
  - Decreased signal intensity fracture line
  - Increased signal intensity of surrounding edema
  - Increased signal intensity of torn/injured ligaments and tendons

Imaging Recommendations
- Best imaging tool: AP, scapula Y-view, and axillary views of the shoulder
- Protocol advice: CT (< 1 mm slice, reformats) if fracture is not fully characterized by plain films

DIFFERENTIAL DIAGNOSIS

Glenohumeral Dislocation
- Loss of articulation of the humeral head with the glenoid
  - Glenohumeral dislocation may be seen in association with humeral head/neck fracture
- Pain, swelling, loss of function
- Pain with abduction of arm

Glenoid Fracture
- Fracture of the glenoid rim
  - Frequently associated with glenohumeral dislocation
  - Defect may be cartilaginous or osteocartilaginous

Unfused Growth Plate
- May mimic fracture in skeletally immature patient

PATHOLOGY

General Features
- Etiology
  - Fall on outstretched arm with severe abduction of the shoulder
  - Direct or indirect high-energy trauma
- Epidemiology
  - Approximately 2-3% of upper extremity fractures
  - Approximately 1% of all fractures
- Associated abnormalities
  - Risk of injury to axillary vessels and to brachial plexus
  - Tendon of long head of biceps brachii muscle may become entrapped between fracture fragments, preventing reduction
  - Isolation of the humeral articular segment puts the humeral head at risk for ischemia

Gross Pathologic & Surgical Features
- Fx fragments are displaced by tendinous insertions
  - Humeral shaft displaced medially by pectoralis major muscle
  - Greater tuberosity displaced superiorly by supraspinatus, infraspinatus and teres minor muscles
  - Lesser tuberosity displaced medially by the subscapularis muscle

Staging, Grading or Classification Criteria
- Classification scheme assesses four principle fragments (head, shaft, greater tuberosity and lesser tuberosity)
- Fx named by number of displaced or angulated parts and not by specific numbers or locations of fx lines
- Fragments considered displaced if there is > 1 cm of displacement or > 45° of angulation
- Neer Classification system most commonly used
  - 1-Part fracture: (e.g., Humeral neck fracture without significant displacement or angulation)
  - 2-Part fracture: (e.g., Humeral fracture with any one of the 4 possible parts significantly displaced or angulated from the others)

HUMERAL HEAD/NECK FRACTURE

- 3-Part fracture: (e.g., Humeral head, greater tuberosity and shaft as three separate parts, presuming 2 of them are significantly displaced or angulated)
- 4-Part fracture: (e.g., Significant displacement or angulation of the humeral head, shaft and both tuberosities)
  - "Classic" 4-Part fracture: Humeral head dislocated from glenohumeral joint
  - "Valgus-impacted" 4-Part fracture: Humeral head rotated to face superiorly
- Loss or disruption of the humeral head articular surface is an important fracture feature if present
  - Impaction fracture of humeral head
  - Split fracture of humeral head
- Approximately 80% of proximal humeral fractures are nondisplaced
- Hill-Sachs fracture (impaction fracture of humeral head) usually result of glenohumeral dislocation

CLINICAL ISSUES

Presentation
- Most common signs/symptoms
  - Pain, swelling
  - Swelling may worsen for several days
- Other signs/symptoms
  - Deformity if there is displacement of fragments
  - Inferior displacement of the humerus may be seen in association with intra-articular or extra-articular fractures; due to muscle atony

Demographics
- Age
  - Older patients, transverse humeral neck fracture related to osteopenia
  - Younger patients, wide range of fracture patterns related to high-energy trauma
- Gender: Humeral neck fractures more common in elderly women related to osteopenia

Natural History & Prognosis
- Nondisplaced fractures may heal with conservative management
  - Some degree of angulation may be tolerated due to compensation by range of motion at the shoulder
  - Bone contact necessary for healing to occur
- Fractures with significant displacement or rotation of fragments may require surgical management

Treatment
- Options, risks, complications
  - Osteonecrosis of the humeral head may result from fractures that interrupt the vascular supply (e.g., fractures at anatomic neck, muscular insertions or injury to arcuate branch of internal humeral circumflex artery)
  - Osteoarthritis may develop following intra-articular fracture
  - Heterotopic bone formation following proximal humerus fracture
  - Traumatic rotator cuff tear
- Immediate surgery for neurovascular compromise
- Minimally displaced fracture
  - Gradual mobilization and physical therapy
  - In elderly and sedentary patients, greater than 1 cm of displacement may occasionally be treated as "nondisplaced" as long as there is some bony contact of fragments
  - Surgery for neurovascular compromise, open fracture
- Humeral neck fracture
  - Closed reduction if sufficient to ensure stability
  - Surgery for displaced humeral neck fracture that is irreducible
- Greater tuberosity fracture
  - Surgery for > 5 mm of superior displacement or > 10 mm of posterior displacement
- Lesser tuberosity fracture
  - Surgery for > 5 mm of displacement
- Guidelines for surgical or conservative management are not absolute and multiple patient factors are considered when choosing the most appropriate treatment strategy

DIAGNOSTIC CHECKLIST

Consider
- Possible vascular injury to the axillary vessels
- Possible neurological injury to brachial plexus or axillary nerve
- Associated injury of the chest wall, neck, head or other site related to mechanism

Image Interpretation Pearls
- High-quality, well-positioned radiographs required for evaluation of proximal humerus fractures
  - Watch for overlapping fragments and impaction
  - Tuberosity fractures often missed or misdiagnosed on initial radiographs
- CT may be helpful in characterizing complex proximal humerus fractures
  - Tuberosity fractures typically well-demonstrated by CT
  - Rotation of fragments well-demonstrated by CT

SELECTED REFERENCES

1. Shrader MW et al: Understanding proximal humerus fractures: image analysis, classification, and treatment. J Shoulder Elbow Surg. 14(5):497-505, 2005
2. Bucholz RW et al: Rockwood and Green's Fractures in Adults. vol 1. 5th ed. Philadelphia, Lippincott Williams and Wilkins. 997-1023, 2001
3. Blake R et al: Emergency department evaluation and treatment of the shoulder and humerus. Emerg Med Clin North Am. 17(4):859-76, vi, 1999
4. Bernstein J et al: Evaluation of the Neer system of classification of proximal humeral fractures with computerized tomographic scans and plain radiographs. J Bone Joint Surg Am. 78(9):1371-5, 1996
5. Kilcoyne RF et al: The Neer classification of displaced proximal humeral fractures: spectrum of findings on plain radiographs and CT scans. AJR Am J Roentgenol. 154(5):1029-33, 1990

HUMERAL HEAD/NECK FRACTURE

IMAGE GALLERY

Typical

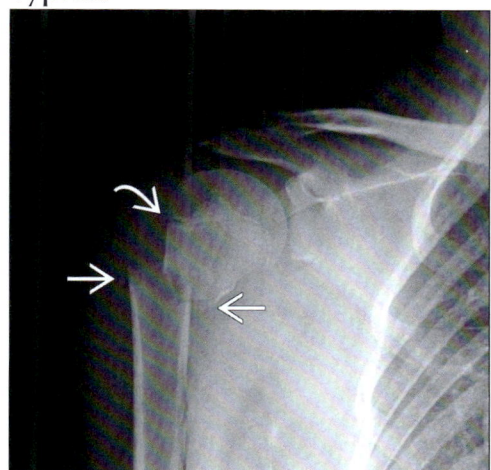
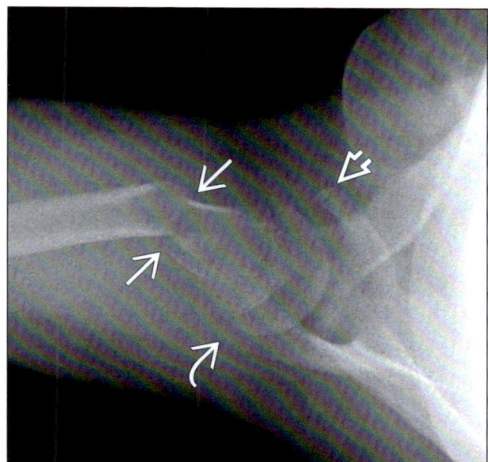

(Left) Anteroposterior radiograph shows a > 1 cm displaced transverse fracture ➔ of the humeral neck (Neer 2-Part). Note the normal humeral head growth plate ➔ in this skeletally immature patient. *(Right)* Lateral radiograph shows the same angulated humeral neck fracture ➔. Note the normal humeral head growth plate ➔ and coracoid process apophysis ➔ in this skeletally immature patient.

Typical

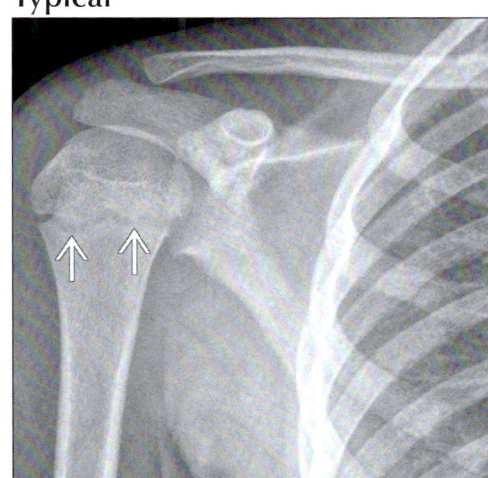
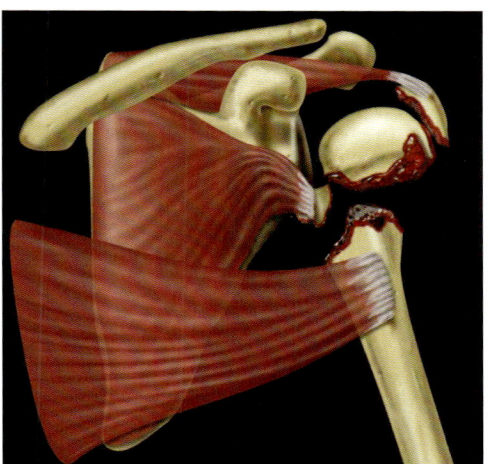

(Left) Anteroposterior radiograph shows the epiphyseal plate ➔ of the proximal humerus in a skeletally immature patient which may potentially mimic a fracture. *(Right)* Anterior graphic shows the 4 principle fragments of a Neer 4-part fracture. The greater and lesser tuberosities are displaced by the supraspinatus and subscapularis muscles, respectively. The humeral shaft is displaced by the pectoralis major muscle.

Other

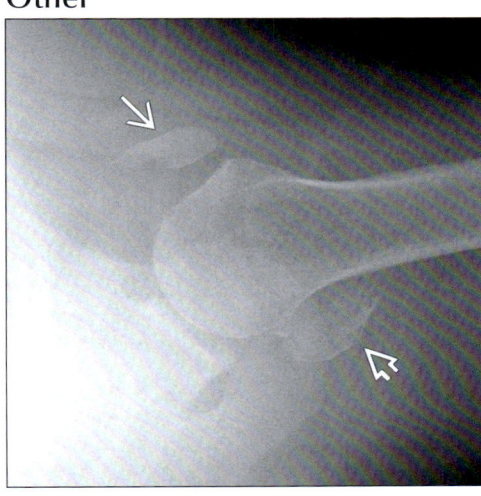
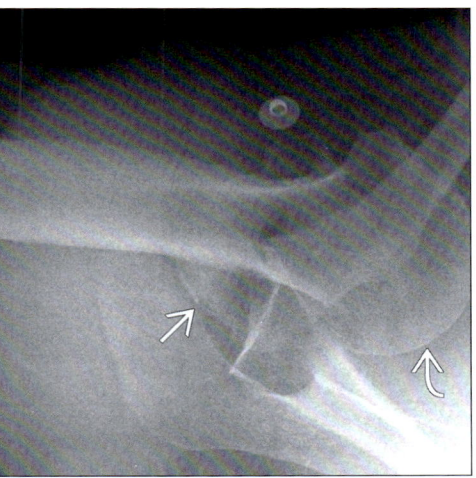

(Left) Lateral radiograph shows a Neer 3-Part fracture of the proximal humerus with displaced lesser tuberosity ➔ and greater tuberosity ➔ fractures. *(Right)* Lateral radiograph shows a Neer 2-Part fracture with a displaced greater tuberosity fracture ➔ and associated anterior glenohumeral dislocation ➔.

HUMERAL SHAFT/DISTAL HUMERAL FRACTURE

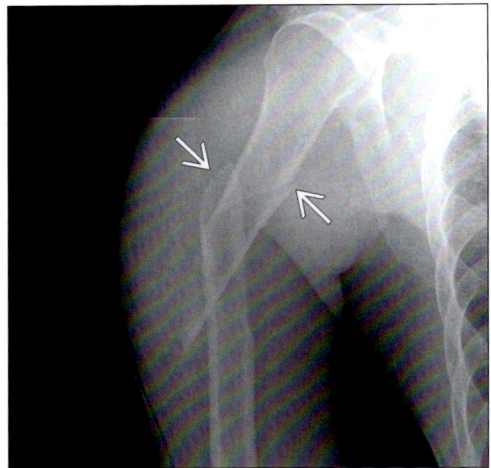

Anteroposterior radiograph shows a comminuted spiral fracture of the humeral shaft ➡. Note the abduction of the proximal fragment by the action of the deltoid with resultant deformity.

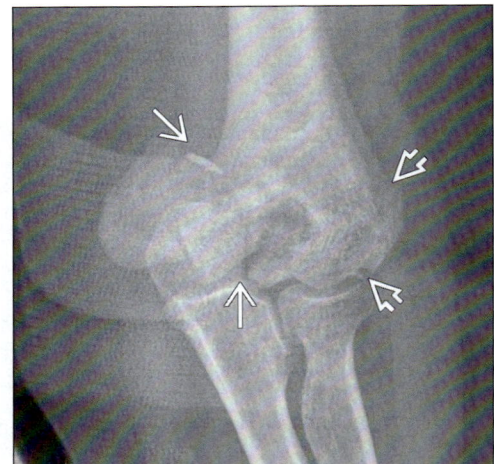

Anteroposterior radiograph shows a comminuted medial condylar fracture ➡ with intra-articular extension through the trochlea and a nondisplaced lateral condylar fracture ➡.

TERMINOLOGY

Abbreviations and Synonyms
- Fractures described according to involved structures including humeral shaft fx, lateral condylar fx, medial condylar fx, intercondylar fx, supracondylar fx, transcondylar fx and capitellum fx
- Capitellum fracture also called Hahn-Steinthal or Kocher-Lorenz fracture
- Supracondylar fracture also called Gartland fracture (See "Supracondylar Fracture")

Definitions
- Fracture of the shaft or distal humerus due to fall on elbow/arm, direct trauma, valgus/varus stress, hyperflexion/extension or torsional forces such as those generated when throwing a ball

IMAGING FINDINGS

General Features
- Best diagnostic clue
  - Transverse or oblique lucency on well-positioned radiograph
  - Positive fat pad sign in cases of intracapsular fracture
- Location
  - Humeral shaft
  - Supracondylar (extra-capsular) or transcondylar (intra-capsular) distal humeral metaphysis
  - Medial or lateral condyle
  - Medial or lateral epicondyle
  - Capitellum
- Size: Ranges from small epicondylar fracture to complex comminuted fracture of the entire distal humerus
- Morphology
  - Nondisplaced
  - Displaced or angulated by tendinous and ligamentous insertions

Radiographic Findings
- Radiography
  - Transverse or oblique lucency on AP and/or lateral radiographs
  - Positive fat pad sign on lateral radiograph from effusion is suggestive of intra-capsular fracture

DDx: Assorted Elbow Injuries

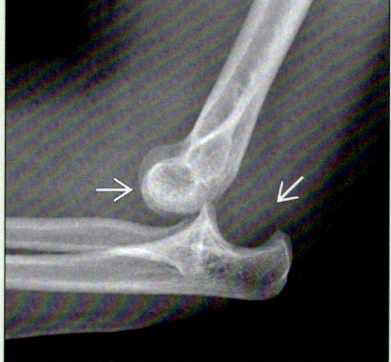

Elbow Dislocation

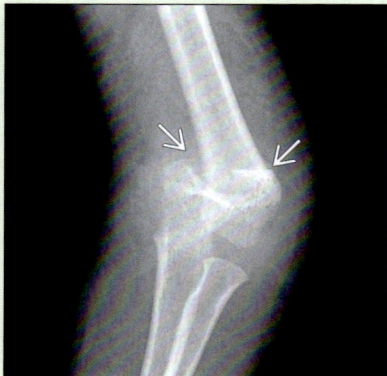

Supracondylar Fracture

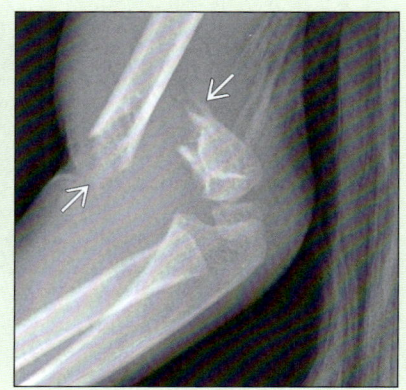

Supracondylar Fracture

HUMERAL SHAFT/DISTAL HUMERAL FRACTURE

Key Facts

Terminology
- Fractures described according to involved structures including humeral shaft fx, lateral condylar fx, medial condylar fx, intercondylar fx, supracondylar fx, transcondylar fx and capitellum fx

Imaging Findings
- Transverse or oblique lucency on AP and/or lateral radiographs
- Positive fat pad sign on lateral radiograph from effusion is suggestive of intra-capsular fracture
- Protocol advice: Image the elbow and shoulder joints to exclude adjacent injury

Pathology
- Radial nerve at risk for injury due to proximity to supracondylar humeral shaft
- Median nerve at risk from traction over angulated supracondylar fracture fragment
- Deformity of humeral shaft fractures depends on relative retraction from muscle insertions in relation to the fracture site

Clinical Issues
- Fracture patterns vary with age/mechanism

Diagnostic Checklist
- Evidence of neurovascular complications
- Presence of other injuries of wrist, elbow, or shoulder
- Positive fat pad sign on lateral radiograph suggestive of intra-capsular fracture

---

  - Anterior humeral line extends anterior to middle third of capitellum in supracondylar fracture

CT Findings
- Bone CT
  - Linear lucency through humeral shaft and/or distal humerus
  - Elbow effusion

MR Findings
- T1WI
  - Decreased signal intensity fracture line
  - Decreased signal intensity marrow edema
- T2WI
  - Decreased signal intensity fracture line
  - Increased signal intensity marrow edema
  - Hyperintense elbow effusion
- STIR: Increased signal intensity marrow edema along fracture line

Imaging Recommendations
- Best imaging tool
  - AP and lateral radiographs of the humerus or elbow (out of splint)
  - CT to assess degree of comminution
- Protocol advice: Image the elbow and shoulder joints to exclude adjacent injury

DIFFERENTIAL DIAGNOSIS

Elbow Dislocation
- Ulna and radius typically displaced posteriorly

Capitellum Osteochondritis Dissecans (Osteochondral Defect)
- Chronic valgus stress leading to microtrauma of the capitellum
- Commonly described in adolescent throwing athletes, especially baseball pitchers
- Subacute presentation

Radial Head Fracture
- Most common elbow fracture in adults; typically from fall on outstretched hand (FOOSH)
- 30% of adult elbow fractures

Olecranon Fracture
- Proximal displacement of olecranon fragment
- Fall on flexed supinated forearm
- 20% of adult elbow fractures

PATHOLOGY

General Features
- Etiology: Range of mechanisms including fall on outstretched hand, direct trauma, hyperflexion/extension, varus/valgus stress
- Epidemiology
  - Distal humerus fractures rare in adults (0.5% of all fractures)
  - Supracondylar fractures rare in adults (≤ 3%) but most common pediatric elbow fracture
  - Lateral and medial condylar fractures rare in adults; lateral condylar fracture peak age 6 years, medial condylar fracture peak age in adolescence
- Associated abnormalities
  - Radial nerve at risk for injury due to proximity to supracondylar humeral shaft
    - "Wrist drop" deformity
    - Transient radial nerve palsy common following humeral shaft fracture
  - Median nerve at risk from traction over angulated supracondylar fracture fragment
    - "Hand of benediction" deformity
  - Brachial artery at risk from traction over angulated supracondylar fracture fragment
  - Concomitant olecranon and distal radial fracture

Gross Pathologic & Surgical Features
- Deformity of humeral shaft fractures depends on relative retraction from muscle insertions in relation to the fracture site

HUMERAL SHAFT/DISTAL HUMERAL FRACTURE

- Above insertion of pectoralis major, proximal fragment is abducted by rotator cuff, distal fragment is retracted proximally by pectoralis major and deltoid
- Between pectoralis major and deltoid insertions, proximal fragment is displaced medially by pectoralis major, distal fragment is abducted by deltoid
- Below level of deltoid insertion, proximal fragment is abducted by deltoid
- Lateral condylar fracture fragment may be displaced/rotated by forearm supinators and extensors
- Medial condylar fracture fragment may be displaced/rotated by forearm flexors

Microscopic Features
- Disruption of cortex and trabeculae

Staging, Grading or Classification Criteria
- Orthopedic Trauma Association (OTA) classification of intercondylar humeral fractures
  - Type A: Nonarticular
  - Type B: Partially articular, with part of the articular surface contiguous with the remaining humeral shaft
  - Type C: Articular with no portion of the articular surface remaining in continuity with the humeral shaft
    - Classic "T" fracture
    - Classic "Y" fracture
- Specific classification systems based on involved structures
  - Capitellum fractures (involving only articular surface and not epicondyle or metaphysis)
    - Type I: Involves capitellum ± portion of trochlea
    - Type II: Involves capitellum articular cartilage and subchondral bone; associated injuries include ulnar collateral ligament disruption and radial head fracture
    - Type III: Comminuted
    - Type IV: Comminuted with extension into trochlea
  - Condylar fractures
    - Lateral condylar fracture more common
    - Type I: Lateral trochlear ridge not disrupted
    - Type II: Larger fracture fragment contains condyle and portion of trochlear ridge

CLINICAL ISSUES

Presentation
- Most common signs/symptoms
  - Localized pain and swelling
  - Arm carried at the side with the opposite hand
  - ± Gross deformity
- Other signs/symptoms: Possible neurovascular injury

Demographics
- Age
  - Fracture patterns vary with age/mechanism
    - Supracondylar and lateral condylar fractures more common in children than in adults

Natural History & Prognosis
- Degree of regained function depends on site of injury, success in restoring joint mechanics, bony union and avoidance of infection
- Complications may result from inadequate fixation at time of fracture

Treatment
- Options, risks, complications
  - Post-operative neuritis may complicate surgical repair
    - Ulnar nerve most frequently involved
  - Volkmann contracture may result from acute vascular injury or compartment syndrome
- Closed reduction is treatment of choice for most humeral shaft fractures
  - Hanging arm cast
  - Coaptation splint
- Surgical reduction of humeral shaft fractures in certain circumstances
  - Neurovascular compromise
  - Inability to achieve angulation ≤ 15° by closed reduction
  - Pathologic fracture
  - "Floating elbow" (radius and ulna fractures in addition to humeral shaft fracture)
  - Bilateral humeral fractures
  - Segmental fractures with free fragments
- Surgical repair for most displaced distal humerus fractures
  - ORIF for most fractures with goal of restoring painless elbow motion
  - Percutaneous pinning or traction and casting may be appropriate in some cases
- Capitellum fractures
  - ± Surgical fixation depending on degree of displacement
- Epicondylar fractures
  - Nonoperative treatment with splinting unless there is significant displacement

DIAGNOSTIC CHECKLIST

Consider
- Evidence of neurovascular complications
- Presence of other injuries of wrist, elbow, or shoulder

Image Interpretation Pearls
- Positive fat pad sign on lateral radiograph suggestive of intra-capsular fracture

SELECTED REFERENCES
1. McCarty LP et al: Management of distal humerus fractures. Am J Orthop. 34(9):430-8, 2005
2. O'Driscoll SW et al: Management of the smashed distal humerus. Orthop Clin North Am. 33(1):19-33, vii, 2002
3. Resnick D: Diagnosis of Bone and Joint Disorders. vol 3. 4th ed. Philadelphia, W.B. Saunders. 2817-20, 2824-7, 2002
4. Bucholz RW et al: Rockwood and Green's Fractures in Adults. vol 1. 5th ed. Philadelphia, Lippincott Williams and Wilkins. 953-96, 2001

HUMERAL SHAFT/DISTAL HUMERAL FRACTURE

IMAGE GALLERY

Typical

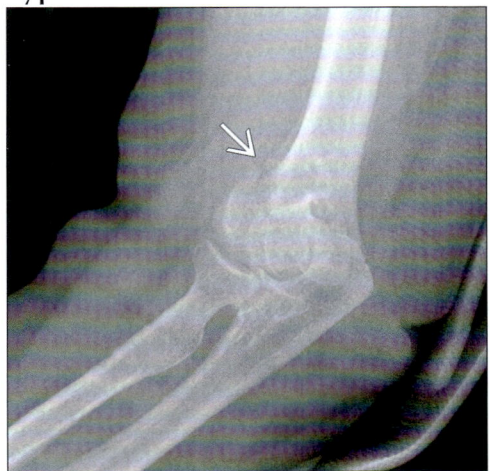 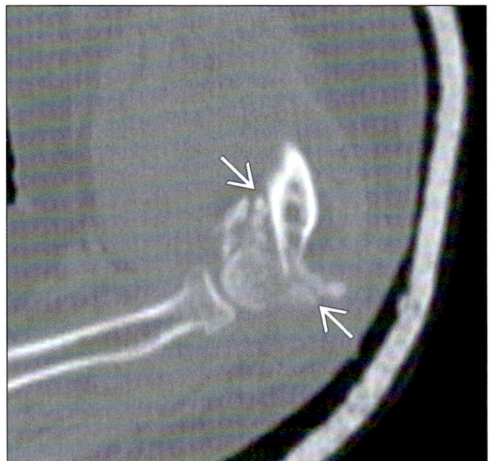

(Left) Oblique radiograph shows a complex fracture of the distal humerus ➔. The full extent of the fracture is difficult to characterize due to the splint and obliquity of the projection. *(Right)* Sagittal bone CT shows the same fracture ➔ and better demonstrates the degree of comminution involving the lateral condyle. CT is helpful in characterizing complex fractures.

Typical

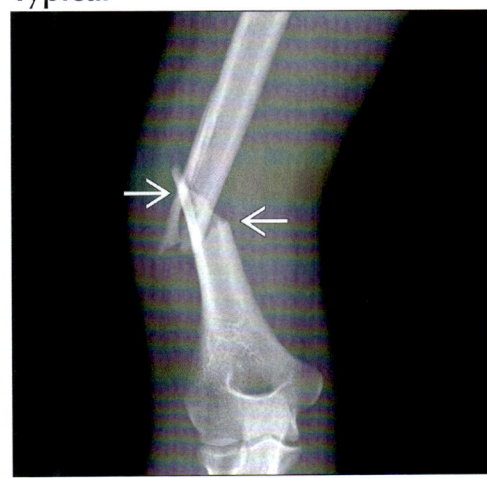 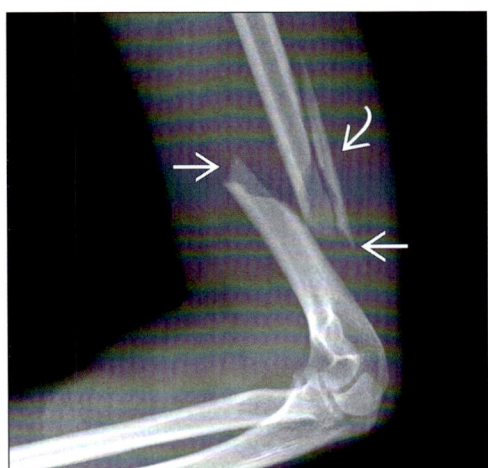

(Left) Anteroposterior radiograph shows a comminuted spiral fracture of the distal humeral shaft ➔. There is abduction of the proximal fragment related to contraction of the deltoid. *(Right)* Lateral radiograph shows the same comminuted, angulated, and displaced fracture of the humeral shaft ➔ with a prominent posterior butterfly fragment ➔.

Typical

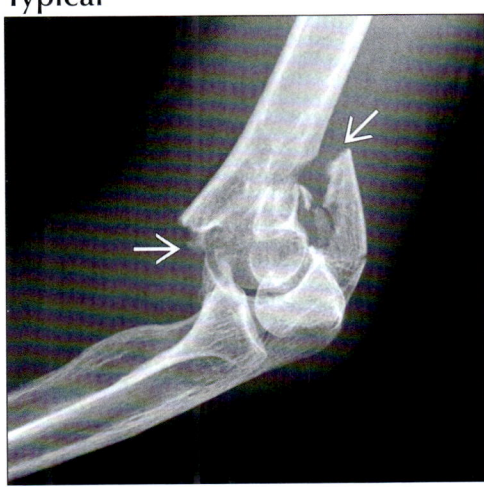 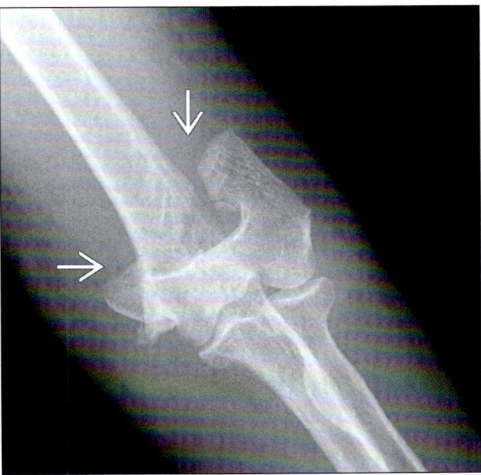

(Left) Lateral radiograph shows a comminuted supracondylar fracture ➔. There is proximal displacement of the distal fracture fragments. *(Right)* Anteroposterior radiograph shows the same supracondylar fracture ➔. There is no elbow dislocation and the articular surface of the distal humerus is intact.

ELBOW DISLOCATION

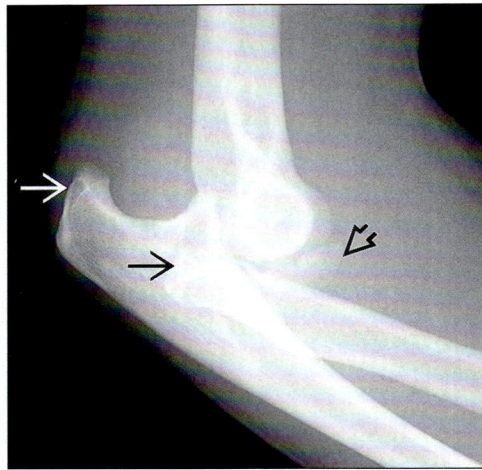

Lateral radiograph shows a posterior dislocation of the elbow, including olecranon ➡ and radial head ➡. A large radial head fragment remains located anterior to the capitellum ➡.

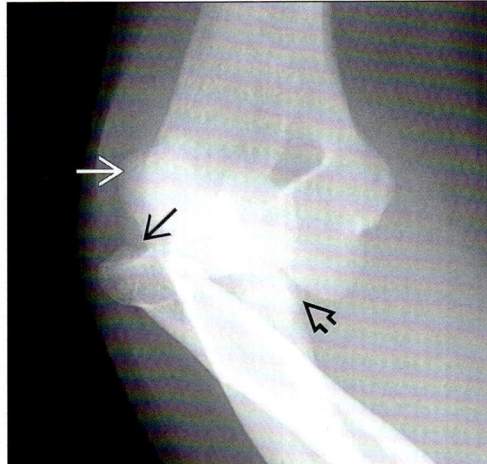

Anteroposterior radiograph shows the lateral direction of a typical dislocation. Dislocated radial head with large defect ➡, dislocated ulna ➡, and the radial head fracture fragment ➡ are seen.

TERMINOLOGY

Abbreviations and Synonyms
- Posterior elbow dislocation

Definitions
- Ulna dislocated relative to humerus
  - Ulna usually dislocates in posterior direction
  - Ulnar dislocation is usually associated with a radial head dislocation from capitellum
  - Dislocation may be directly posterior, but more often is posterolateral; posteromedial is uncommon

IMAGING FINDINGS

General Features
- Best diagnostic clue
  - Malalignment, with no articulation between ulna and trochlea
    - Often has associated lack of articulation between radius and capitellum
    - On lateral radiograph obtained in flexion, anterior humeral line extends through radial head or neck and through ulnar metaphysis
  - Empty semilunar notch of olecranon seen on lateral view
- Location: Humeroulnar joint, ± radiocapitellar joint and other injuries
- Size: Extent of injury is related to associated bony and ligamentous injuries
- Morphology
  - Posterior, posterolateral, or posteromedial dislocation of ulna relative to humerus
    - ± Impaction or avulsion fractures
    - ± Ligamentous disruptions

Radiographic Findings
- Complete loss of articulation between trochlea and ulna
- Often associated radial head dislocation
- Often associated fractures
  - Radial head
  - Coronoid process
  - Capitellum
  - Medial epicondylar apophysis in child (Salter I)

Elbow Dislocation, Other Cases

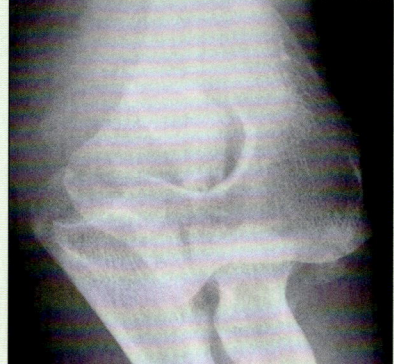

Posteromedial Dislocation

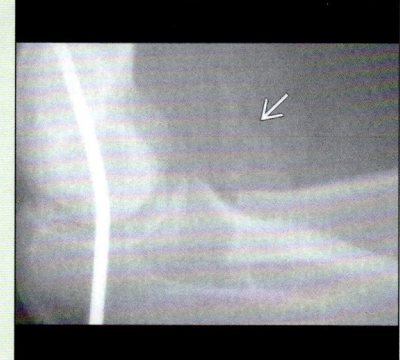

Myositis Following Dislocation

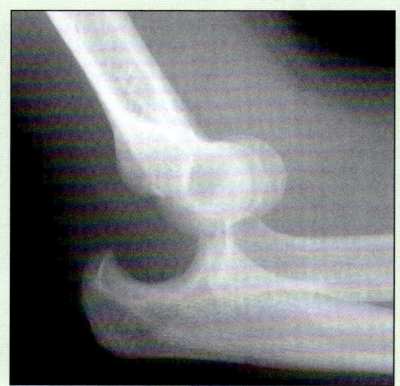

Perched Elbow

ELBOW DISLOCATION

Key Facts

Terminology
- Ulna dislocated relative to humerus
- Ulna usually dislocates in posterior direction
- Ulnar dislocation is usually associated with a radial head dislocation from capitellum
- Dislocation may be directly posterior, but more often is posterolateral; posteromedial is uncommon

Imaging Findings
- Radiographs: Anteroposterior, lateral, & oblique
- Re-image post reduction, to evaluate for displaced fracture fragments

Pathology
- Etiology: Fall on outstretched hand
- Fracture radial head
- Fracture coronoid process

- "Terrible triad" of coronoid process fracture, radial head fracture, and posterior dislocation has a poor prognosis
- In adolescents, avulsion of apophyses, particularly the medial epicondyle (Salter I)
- Medial collateral ligament tears
- Lateral ulnar collateral ligament tear
- Radial collateral ligament tear

Clinical Issues
- If uncomplicated, 60% have late symptoms of pain
- Fractures are associated with development of secondary osteoarthritis

Diagnostic Checklist
- Associated fractures, both pre and post reduction

CT Findings
- Bone CT
  - Axial imaging with reformats can be especially useful if standard radiographic positioning cannot be obtained
  - Fracture fragment location is best assessed by CT
  - Fracture fragment donor sites are located by CT
  - Post-reduction CT is useful if there is persistent pain, popping, or incomplete reduction
    - Search for entrapped fracture fragments
    - Small osseous fragments better seen on CT than MR

MR Findings
- T1WI
  - Decreased marrow signal indicating areas of bone edema
  - Fracture lines may be seen if fracture is incomplete
  - Low signal joint effusion
  - Displacement of high signal anterior and posterior fat pads
  - Gross ligamentous disruption may be seen, but subtle soft tissue disruption will not
- T2WI
  - Similar to T2WI FS and PD/Intermediate FS
  - Subtle marrow and soft tissue findings are more easily seen with fat saturated sequences
- T2WI FS
  - Increased marrow signal indicating edema
    - "Kissing" fractures or edema at sites of impaction, particularly radial head and capitellum
    - If fracture is nondisplaced, fracture line may be obscured by surrounding edema
    - Coronoid process fracture
  - High signal joint effusion ± periarticular leakage with capsular rupture
  - Disruption of medial collateral ligament anatomy with high signal tears
  - High signal stress lesions at bony attachments of torn ligaments
  - Edema/disruption of neurovascular structures
  - Disruption of lateral collateral ligament anatomy with high signal tears (radial collateral ligament, lateral ulnar collateral ligament)
  - ± Medial epicondylar avulsion in children or hyperintense edema at medial epicondyle
- PD/Intermediate FS: Same as T2WI FS
- STIR: Same as T2WI FS; sequence may be preferred on low field strength magnets

Imaging Recommendations
- Best imaging tool
  - Radiographs: Anteroposterior, lateral, & oblique
  - Re-image post reduction, to evaluate for displaced fracture fragments
- CT occasionally necessary
  - May be helpful if reduction cannot be achieved, to look for fracture fragments
  - Multichannel CT with 0.75 mm acquisition, reformats
- MR may be helpful in an outpatient setting to evaluate
  - Osteochondral injury
  - Ligament injury
    - Medial collateral ligament most frequent
    - Lateral ulnar collateral ligament
    - Radial collateral ligament

DIFFERENTIAL DIAGNOSIS

Radiographic
- No differential diagnosis
- Only degree of injury varies, including fracture fragments & ligament instability

Clinical
- Supracondylar fracture: Fall on outstretched hand
- Radial head/neck fracture: Fall on outstretched hand
- Lateral ulnar collateral ligament tear
  - Predisposes to posterior dislocation

ELBOW DISLOCATION

PATHOLOGY

General Features
- Etiology: Fall on outstretched hand
- Epidemiology
  - Incidence: 6/100,000 individuals
  - Second most common dislocation in adults
  - Most frequent dislocation in children
- Associated abnormalities
  - Fracture radial head
    - Most common associated injury
    - Found in 10% of elbow dislocations
  - Fracture coronoid process
    - Most frequent etiology of coronoid process fracture
    - "Terrible triad" of coronoid process fracture, radial head fracture, and posterior dislocation has a poor prognosis
  - Fracture distal humerus
    - Particularly capitellum
  - Osteochondral injury
  - In adolescents, avulsion of apophyses, particularly the medial epicondyle (Salter I)
  - Medial collateral ligament tears
  - Lateral ulnar collateral ligament tear
  - Radial collateral ligament tear

Staging, Grading or Classification Criteria
- Staging is generally not performed successfully in the ED setting due to pain and swelling & consequent inability to determine ligamentous injury
- Staging is based on instability
  - Stage I
    - Posterolateral subluxation of ulna & radius plus disruption of lateral ulnar collateral ligament
  - Stage II
    - Complete dislocation with coronoid perched on trochlea plus disruption of anterior and posterior joint capsule (perched elbow)
  - Stage III
    - Complete posterior dislocation plus disruption of medial collateral complex

CLINICAL ISSUES

Presentation
- Most common signs/symptoms: Pain, swelling, and deformity of elbow

Demographics
- Age: Active young patients; mean age 30 years
- Gender: M:F ratio 2-2.5:1

Natural History & Prognosis
- If uncomplicated, 60% have late symptoms of pain
  - Pain on valgus stress
  - Incomplete recovery more likely with
    - Fractures, especially coronoid
    - Delayed reduction
    - Rigid or prolonged immobilization
  - Fractures are associated with development of secondary osteoarthritis
  - Prolonged rigid immobilization associated with decreased range of motion and flexion contractures
  - Redislocation associated with poor outcome

Treatment
- Conservative
  - Reduction and bracing in pronation
  - Protected mobilization
- Surgical
  - Repair of medial collateral and other ligament or tendon avulsions
  - Preservation of radial head if possible; excessive comminution requires excision
  - Excision of interposed soft tissue or osteochondral fragments
  - Reconstruction of coronoid process
- Complications
  - Immediate
    - Failed reduction due to entrapped fragments
    - Failed reduction due to inverted cartilaginous flap
    - Failed reduction due to entrapped medial epicondylar avulsion in a child
    - Volkmann ischemic contracture: Rare
    - Brachial artery injury: Rare
  - Late
    - Medial collateral ligament laxity
    - Posterolateral instability; high association with coronoid process fracture
    - Myositis ossificans develops in the antecubital fossa relatively frequently
    - Flexion contracture
    - Neuropraxias may occur in up to 20% of cases: Ulnar nerve or else anterior interosseous branch of median nerve may be involved

DIAGNOSTIC CHECKLIST

Consider
- Associated fractures, both pre and post reduction
  - Evaluate coronoid process fractures carefully for size and type of fracture
  - CT may be helpful in locating these fragments if reduction is not satisfactory
- Instability
  - MR in an outpatient setting can identify disruption of ligaments and tendons
- Nerve or vascular damage

SELECTED REFERENCES

1. Doornberg JN et al: Coronoid fracture patterns. J Hand Surg [Am]. 31(1):45-52, 2006
2. Papandrea RF et al: Reconstruction for persistent instability of the elbow after coronoid fracture-dislocation. J Shoulder Elbow Surg. 2006
3. Tashjian RZ et al: Complex elbow instability. J Am Acad Orthop Surg. 14(5):278-86, 2006
4. Chung CB et al: Magnetic resonance imaging of elbow instability. Semin Musculoskelet Radiol. 9(1):67-76, 2005
5. Pacelli LL et al: Elbow instability: the orthopedic approach. Semin Musculoskelet Radiol. 9(1):56-66, 2005
6. Ring D et al: Posterior dislocation of the elbow with fractures of the radial head and coronoid. J Bone Joint Surg Am. 84-A(4):547-51, 2002

ELBOW DISLOCATION

IMAGE GALLERY

Typical

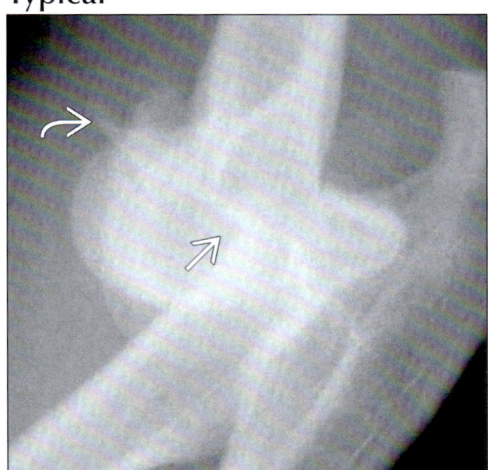
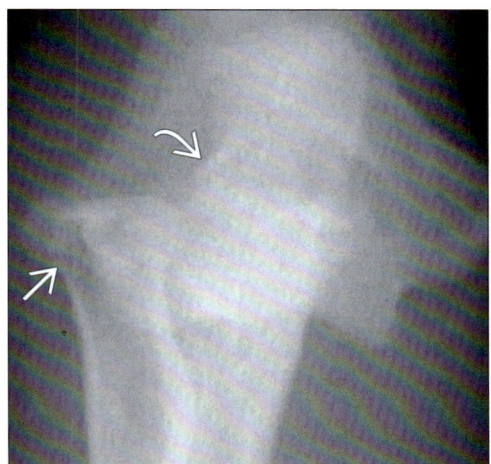

(Left) Lateral radiograph shows a classic appearance of dislocated elbow. Radius & ulna are dislocated posteriorly. Not surprisingly, there is often an associated radial head fx ➔ as well as coronoid process fx ➔. (Right) Anteroposterior radiograph shows that the radius and ulna simultaneously are displaced laterally. Radial head ➔ and coronoid process ➔ fractures are again noted.

Typical

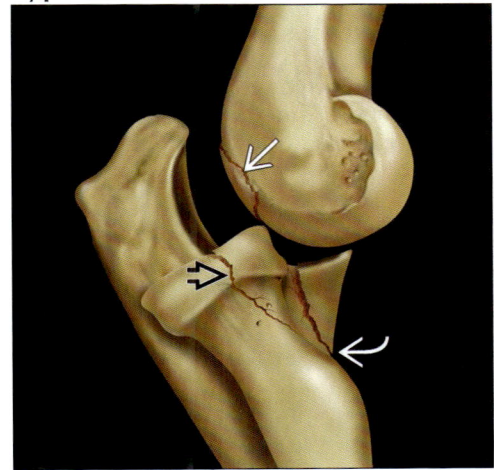
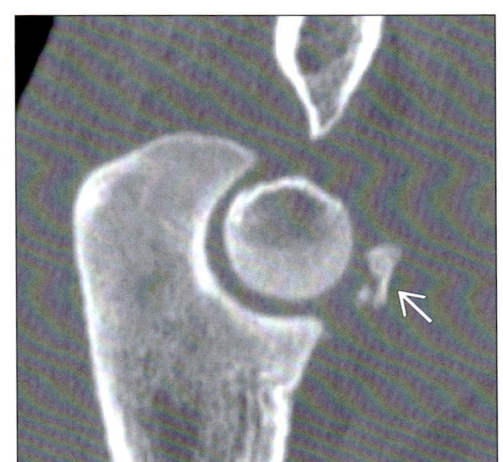

(Left) Lateral graphic of a posterior elbow dislocation shows the most typical associated fracture sites, including the coronoid process ➔, radial head ➔, and capitellum ➔. (Right) Sagittal bone CT shows reduced posterior elbow dislocation with displaced coronoid process fracture ➔.

Typical

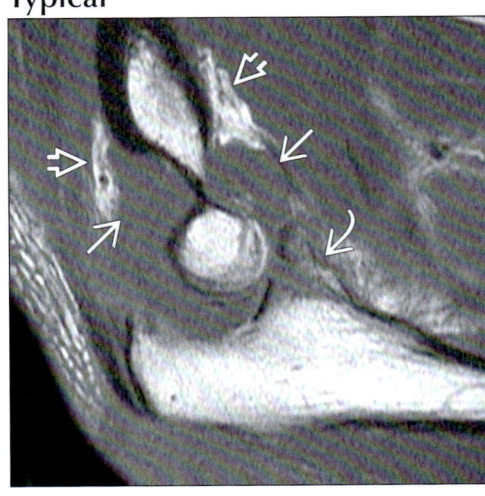
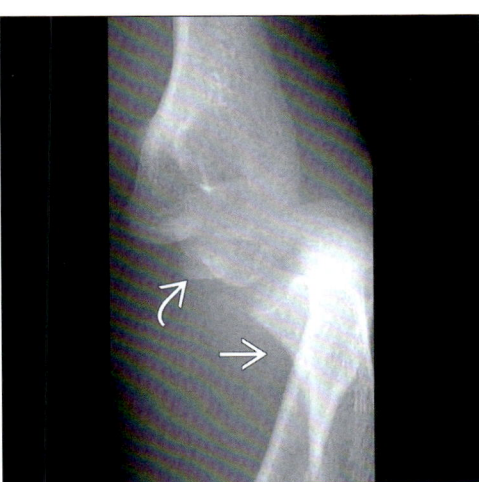

(Left) Sagittal T1WI MR shows a large elbow effusion ➔ elevating the anterior and posterior fat pads ➔. There is residual subluxation of the ulna and an associated fracture of the coronoid ➔. (Right) Oblique radiograph in a different patient shows a posterior elbow dislocation in a child ➔. There is an intraarticular fragment ➔; this proved to be an avulsion of the medial epicondylar apophysis.

OLECRANON FRACTURE/TRICEPS TENDON RUPTURE

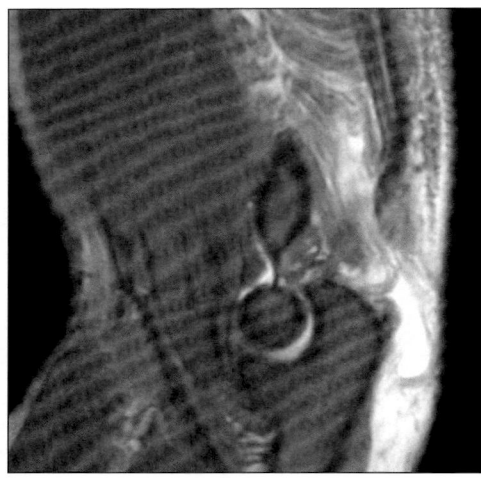

Sagittal T2WI FS MR shows a complete tear of the distal triceps tendon as well as retraction and surrounding hemorrhage. Note that there is no abnormal signal within the olecranon to suggest avulsion.

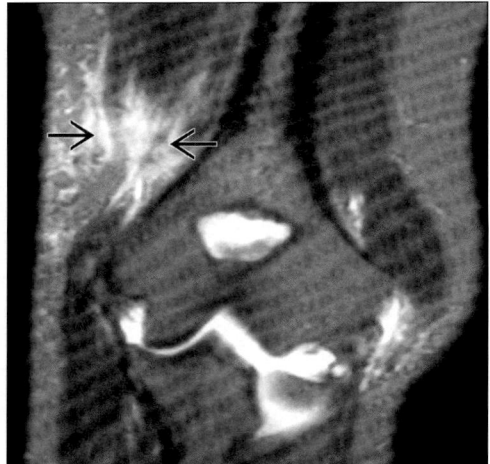

Coronal T2WI FS MR shows tear of the distal myotendinous junction of the medial triceps ➡ with surrounding edema. This type of triceps rupture is rare compared with a tear of the distal tendon.

TERMINOLOGY

Definitions
- Olecranon fracture
  - Distraction injury due to resisted triceps contraction
  - Direct impact injury
- Triceps rupture
  - Avulsion from site of insertion on olecranon
  - Intrasubstance triceps tendon rupture

IMAGING FINDINGS

General Features
- Best diagnostic clue
  - **Olecranon fracture**
    - Positive fat pad sign
    - If distracted, proximal displacement of olecranon fragment
    - If nondisplaced, linear fx line on MR with surrounding edema
  - **Triceps tendon rupture**
    - Tear or gap in tendon which can be filled with hemorrhage or granulation tissue
- Location
  - Ranges from musculotendinous junction to olecranon process
    - Musculotendinous rupture uncommon
    - Midtendon rupture uncommon
    - Injury usually occurs in distal triceps tendon or olecranon process
- Size
  - Fracture varies from an avulsed flake to complete olecranon process fragment
  - Triceps rupture varies from millimeter range to large (several centimeters)
- Morphology
  - Fracture varies from nondisplaced cortical disruption to wide distraction
  - Tendon rupture varies from partial disruption to complete, with irregular gap

Radiographic Findings
- Positive fat pad sign with intraarticular fx
  - Anterior displacement of anterior fat pad
  - Presence of posterior fat pad
- Linear lucency of fracture line; ranges from nondisplaced to widely displaced

Olecranon Fractures

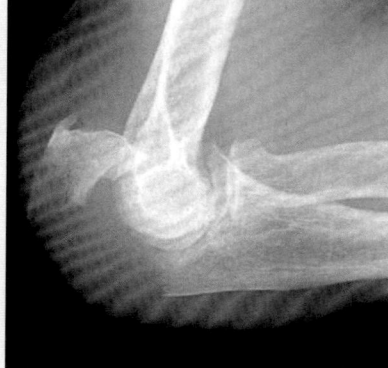

Widely Diastased

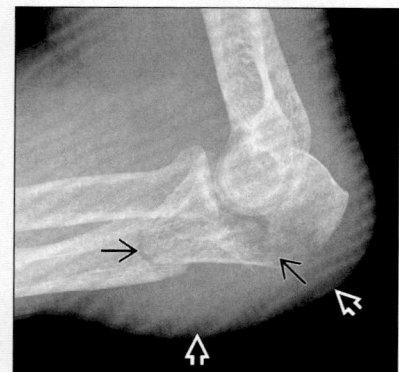

Comminuted/Hematoma

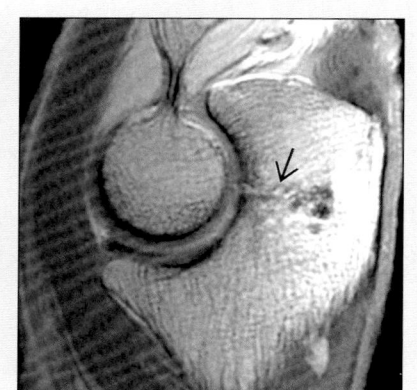

Nondisplaced Olecranon Fracture

OLECRANON FRACTURE/TRICEPS TENDON RUPTURE

Key Facts

Imaging Findings
- **Olecranon fracture**
- Positive fat pad sign
- If distracted, proximal displacement of olecranon fragment
- If nondisplaced, linear fx line on MR with surrounding edema
- **Triceps tendon rupture**
- Tear or gap in tendon which can be filled with hemorrhage or granulation tissue
- Best imaging tool: Radiograph, MR if radiograph is negative
- Protocol advice: Fracture or tear best seen on sagittal sequences

Top Differential Diagnoses
- **For Olecranon Fracture**
- Cortical notch
- Ulnar stress fracture
- Normal ossification center/variation
- **For Triceps Rupture**
- Olecranon bursitis
- Triceps muscle contusion/hematoma
- Fibroxanthoma

Pathology
- Olecranon apophysis fuses by 16-18 years
- Midpoint of trochlear notch of olecranon critical in determining stability of healing
- Previous bursectomy predisposes to triceps rupture
- Deceleration stress on a contracted triceps muscle
- Eccentric contraction against resistance: Sudden forced flexion of an extended forearm

CT Findings
- Fracture comminution & distraction can be assessed on sagittal reformats
- Soft tissue swelling/abnormal fat pads

MR Findings
- Fracture
  - T1WI: Decreased marrow signal & linear fracture line; low signal effusion elevating fat pads
  - Fluid sensitive sequence: Low signal fracture line could be obscured by edema; high signal joint effusion
- Triceps tendon tear
  - T1WI: Partial or complete disruption from olecranon; discontinuous decreased signal intensity tendon; hypointense fluid
  - Fluid sensitive sequence: Increased signal intensity
    - Complete tear: Fluid in gap
    - Partial tear: High signal defect within tendon
    - Tendinosis: Intermediate signal within a thickened tendon
    - +/- Reactive edema signal in olecranon
    - +/- Olecranon bursitis

Ultrasonographic Findings
- Tendon tear may be visualized & diastasis assessed

Imaging Recommendations
- Best imaging tool: Radiograph, MR if radiograph is negative
- Protocol advice: Fracture or tear best seen on sagittal sequences

DIFFERENTIAL DIAGNOSIS

For Olecranon Fracture
- Cortical notch
  - Normal variation at articular surface of mid olecranon
  - "Bare area" of olecranon
  - Mimics osteochondral defect
- Ulnar stress fracture
  - Proximal ulna; not olecranon
  - Abnormal stress on normal bone
- Normal ossification center/variation
  - Normal childhood apophysis at olecranon
  - May mimic fracture
  - Normally fuses at 16-18 years
  - Failure of fusion = os supratrochlear dorsale
  - Also termed bipartite olecranon or patella cubiti
  - Absent edema on MR

For Triceps Rupture
- Olecranon bursitis
  - Adult men, dominant arm; +/- sports activity
  - Tendon seen separate from fluid contained in bursa
- Triceps muscle contusion/hematoma
  - History of trauma more prominent
  - Contusion/hematoma more mass-like within muscle
  - True tear within triceps muscle rare
- Fibroxanthoma
  - Mass within dorsal tendons such as triceps
  - Related to hyperlipidemia
  - Low signal-intensity on all sequences

PATHOLOGY

General Features
- General path comments
  - Olecranon apophysis fuses by 16-18 years
  - Midpoint of trochlear notch of olecranon critical in determining stability of healing
  - Previous bursectomy predisposes to triceps rupture
  - Medial head of triceps has a separate tendinous insertion deep to common tendon of the lateral & long heads
    - Can rupture the medial head alone
    - Will lead to weakness of elbow extension with elbow flexed > 90°
- Etiology
  - Either fracture or triceps rupture from
    - Deceleration stress on a contracted triceps muscle
    - Eccentric contraction against resistance: Sudden forced flexion of an extended forearm

OLECRANON FRACTURE/TRICEPS TENDON RUPTURE

- Other etiologies of olecranon fracture
  - Fall on a flexed, supinated forearm
  - Direct blow to olecranon
  - Hyperextension
  - Throwing injury (pitchers; pain in acceleration phase of throwing)
- Other etiologies of triceps rupture
  - Direct trauma on tendon with muscle contracted & forearm extended
  - Systemic disease process: Hyperparathyroidism, rheumatoid arthritis
  - Steroid use
- Epidemiology
  - Olecranon fx 20% of all elbow fractures in adults, 6% in children
  - Triceps rupture uncommon; < 1% of all tendon tears at elbow

Gross Pathologic & Surgical Features

- Olecranon fracture pattern
  - Usually transverse
  - Intraarticular
  - Usually single fragment
  - Diastasis results from associated tearing of fibrous sheath formed from capsule, lateral ligaments, triceps tendon, and periosteum
  - 2-31% will be open fractures
- Triceps rupture pattern
  - Variable retraction
  - An intratendinous bursa may occur

Staging, Grading or Classification Criteria

- Olecranon fracture: Colton classification for displacement & pattern
  - Type I: Nondisplaced (< 2 mm) and stable
  - Type II: Displaced
    - A - avulsion
    - B - transverse
    - C - comminuted
    - D - fracture/dislocations
  - Number of fractures, displacement, & location will determine management
- Triceps rupture staging
  - Grade I - mild strain
  - Grade II - intermediate partial tear
  - Grade III - complete disruption

CLINICAL ISSUES

Presentation

- Most common signs/symptoms
  - Point tenderness over olecranon or distal triceps
  - Swelling and hemorrhagic effusion
  - May have inability to extend elbow against gravity
  - May rarely have ulnar neuropathy

Demographics

- Age
  - Fracture may be seen in children or adults
  - Triceps tear in middle-aged man who suffered forced flexion of an extended forearm
- Gender: M > F

Natural History & Prognosis

- Olecranon fracture
  - 80% will have little (< 2 mm) or no displacement; these have good outcomes
  - Degenerative changes seen in < 20%
  - Displacement of > 2 mm usually requires ORIF
  - Displacement of > 1.5 cm is unusual
- Triceps rupture
  - Complete ruptures need surgical repair
  - Partial tears may heal with conservative therapy

Treatment

- Olecranon fracture
  - Conservative
    - 3 weeks cast in 90 degrees flexion
    - For nondisplaced fractures
    - Acceptable for displaced fractures in elderly patients with concomitant illness
  - Surgical
    - Tension band wiring for fractures proximal to midpoint of trochlear notch
    - Plate fixation for fractures distal to midpoint
    - Locking nails and screws may also be used
    - Severe comminution or poor bone quality may require excision and triceps advancement
  - Complications
    - Loss of extension
    - Nonunion
    - Ulnar nerve palsies
    - Heterotopic bone formation
    - Ulna-humeral arthrosis
    - Painful hardware
- Triceps tendon rupture
  - Conservative
    - Rest, ice, temporary splinting
    - For partial tear
  - Surgical
    - Complete tear - repair
    - Acute tear - repair recommended
    - Delayed operative reconstruction: Periosteal flap, fascia flap, split triceps into reinforcing flap, rotation anconeus flap

DIAGNOSTIC CHECKLIST

Consider

- Presence of other fractures, especially coronoid
- Identify fx site relative to midpoint of trochlear notch

Image Interpretation Pearls

- Lateral radiograph, sagittal MR sequences most helpful

SELECTED REFERENCES

1. Madsen M et al: Surgical anatomy of the triceps brachii tendon: anatomical study and clinical correlation. Am J Sports Med. 34(11):1839-43, 2006
2. Kijowski R et al: Magnetic resonance imaging of the elbow. Part II: Abnormalities of the ligaments, tendons, and nerves. Skeletal Radiol. 34(1):1-18, 2005
3. Vidal AF et al: Biceps tendon and triceps tendon injuries. Clin Sports Med. 23(4):707-22, xi, 2004

OLECRANON FRACTURE/TRICEPS TENDON RUPTURE

IMAGE GALLERY

Typical

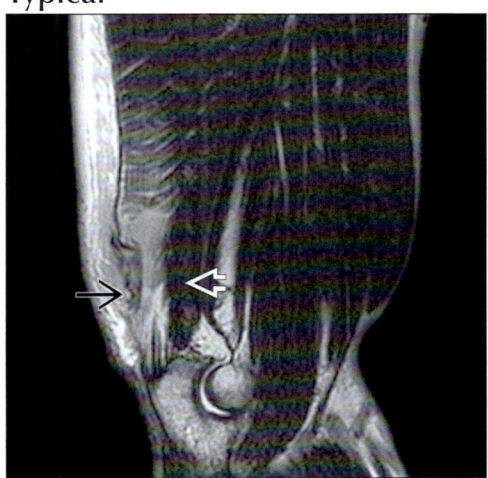
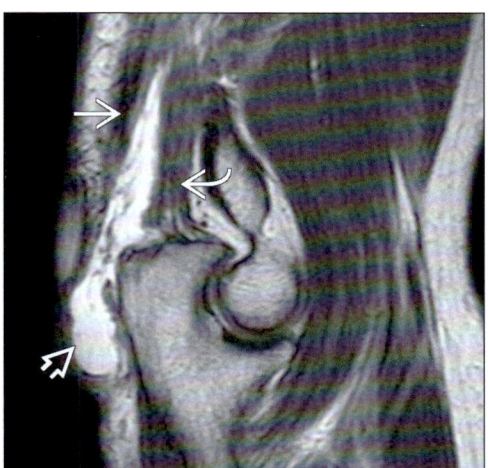

(Left) Sagittal T2WI MR shows partial triceps rupture in a patient with chronic renal failure. The ruptured and retracted superficial fibers are seen ➡ posteriorly, while the intact medial head fibers remain attached ➡. *(Right)* Sagittal T2WI MR shows partial tear of the distal triceps in a patient following a fall. The disrupted posterior tendon fibers ➡ (long and lateral heads) and deep fibers ➡ (medial head) are separated by interposed hematoma ➡.

Typical

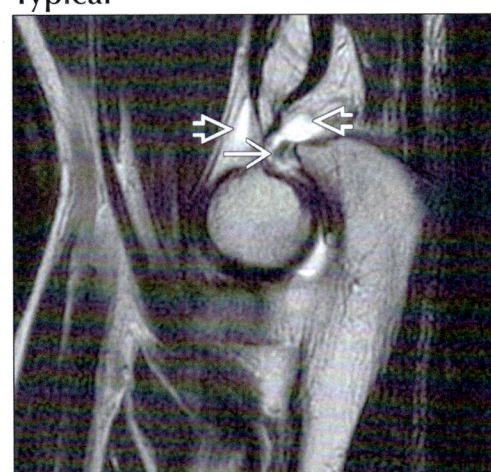
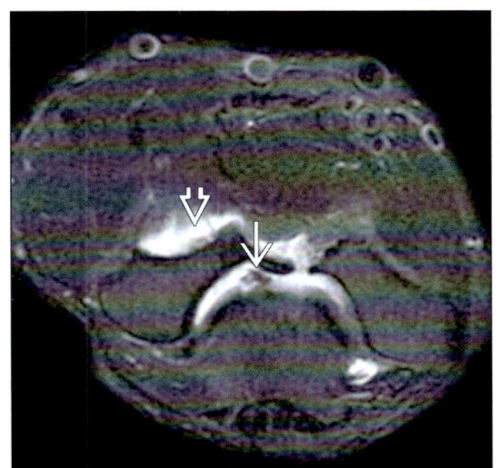

(Left) Sagittal T2WI MR shows a chondral flap tear of the proximal olecranon ➡. The cartilage fragment remains attached and bunched up, creating a mechanical impediment to complete elbow extension. A small joint effusion is present ➡. *(Right)* Axial T2WI FS MR also shows the chondral fragment ➡ in an obstructing position, as well as effusion ➡.

Typical

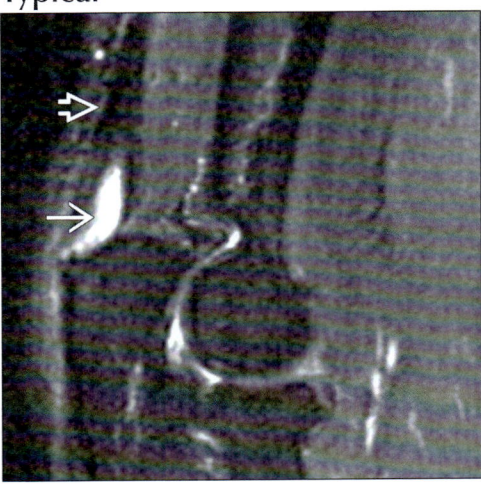
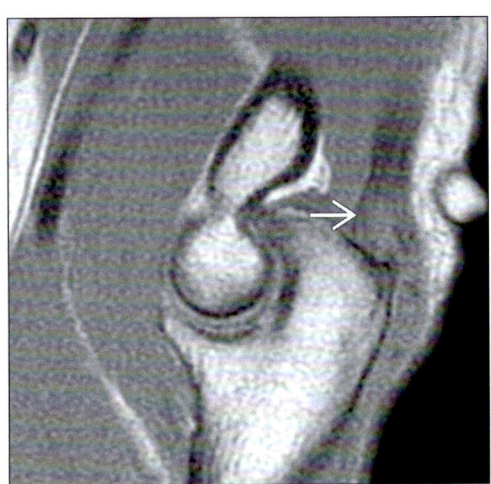

(Left) Sagittal T2WI FS MR shows high signal-intensity ➡ within the distal aspect of the triceps tendon ➡, indicating a large interstitial tear. *(Right)* Sagittal T1WI MR shows low grade triceps tendinopathy without rupture ➡, seen as an area of thickening and heterogeneous signal in the distal triceps. Fluid sensitive sequence showed no high signal to suggest tear.

RADIAL HEAD/NECK FRACTURE

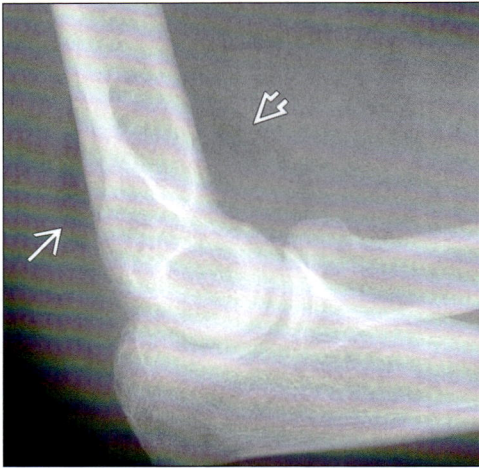

Lateral radiograph is suggestive of an occult radial head fx, owing to the presence of an elbow effusion, which is inferred by the presence of an elevated posterior fat pad ➡ as well as bowed anterior fat pad ➡.

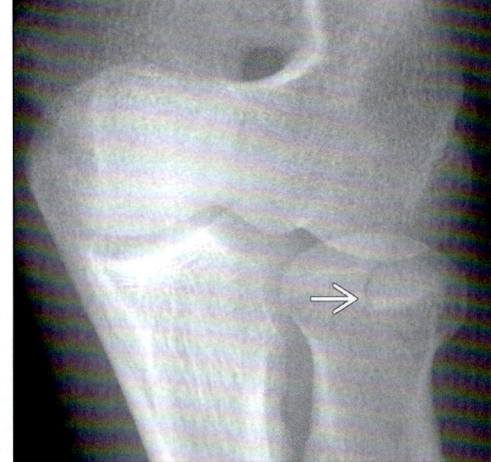

Oblique radiograph demonstrates the intraarticular radial head fx ➡, which was not seen on either AP or lateral views. It is not uncommon for a nondisplaced fx to be demonstrated on only a single view.

TERMINOLOGY

Abbreviations and Synonyms
- Essex-Lopresti fracture, terrible triad of the elbow, lateral column fracture

Definitions
- Impaction injury due to axial overloading in a fall on the outstretched hand (FOOSH)
- Essex-Lopresti: Constellation of significant injuries extending from radial head fx to forearm DRUJ
  ○ Radial head fx with comminution or significant displacement
  ○ ± Ligamentous injury at elbow
  ○ Force continues down forearm through interosseous membrane
  ○ Force exits through distal radioulnar joint (DRUJ), leaving it unstable

IMAGING FINDINGS

General Features
- Best diagnostic clue
  ○ Positive fat pad sign on lateral radiograph
  ○ Most radial head fx are nondisplaced and subtle
  ○ 3 routine elbow views plus radial head view may be necessary to identify fx
  ○ Essex-Lopresti
    ▪ Comminuted or displaced radial head fx
    ▪ May have opening of elbow joint suggesting instability
    ▪ Impaction may shorten radius
    ▪ Wrist shows signs of instability
- Location
  ○ Radial head/neck
  ○ Anterolateral aspect of head more vulnerable because of lack of subchondral bone
  ○ Essex-Lopresti involves DRUJ at wrist as well
- Size: Ranges from small nondisplaced to highly comminuted and significantly displaced
- Morphology
  ○ Elbow
    ▪ Low-energy injury: Nondisplaced intraarticular or radial neck fx
    ▪ High-energy injury: Comminuted/displaced radial head fx, often with impaction, other fxs, MCL tear
  ○ Wrist

Other Radial Head Fractures

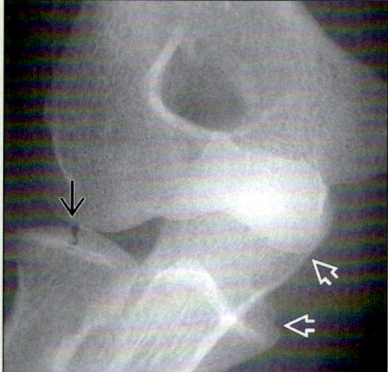

Fx With MCL Tear

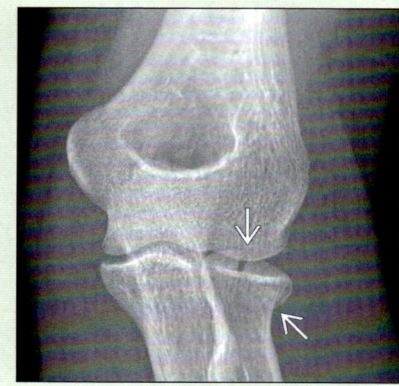

Minimally Impacted Head Fx

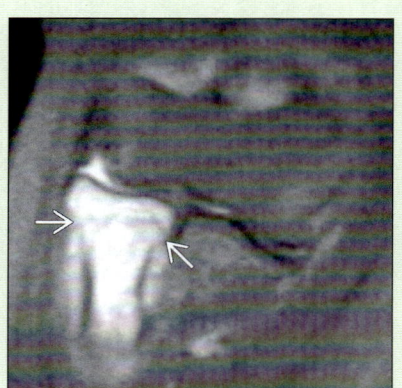

Nondisplaced, Occult on X-ray

RADIAL HEAD/NECK FRACTURE

Key Facts

Terminology
- Impaction injury due to axial overloading in a fall on the outstretched hand (FOOSH)
- Essex-Lopresti: Constellation of significant injuries extending from radial head fx to forearm DRUJ

Imaging Findings
- Positive fat pad sign on lateral radiograph
- Most radial head fx are nondisplaced and subtle
- CT useful to evaluate for stability of DRUJ
- MR used to evaluate for associated occult fx or ligament injury in high energy trauma
- Angled radial head view (isolates head from the usual overlap) may be useful additional view

Pathology
- 30% of adult elbow fractures
- Most common elbow fracture in adults

Clinical Issues
- Essex-Lopresti: Cascade of effects can occur which result in poor result if true extent of injury is not recognized and treated at outset

Diagnostic Checklist
- Presence of other fractures
- Presence of valgus instability
- Extent of comminution
- With either of the latter two in evidence, check for stability of DRUJ
- "Positive ulnar variance" in the setting of high energy radial head fx should suggest Essex-Lopresti: Check for stability of DRUJ

- If radial head is displaced or impacted, radius may be relatively short, leaving an ulnar + variance
- This combination of radial head fx & ulnar positive variance implies disruption of DRUJ
- Subluxation of DRUJ proves instability of wrist

Radiographic Findings
- Positive fat pad sign
  - Anterior bowing of anterior fat pad
  - Radiographic presence of posterior fat pad
- Linear fracture lines
- If highly comminuted or due to elbow dislocation, other fxs of adjacent bones (coronoid process, capitellum)
- Essex-Lopresti
  - Highly disrupted, often impacted radial head
  - Occasional relative ulnar positive variance
  - Disruption DRUJ: Diastasis on PA view of wrist & posterior subluxation ulna on lateral view
  - Occasional ulnar styloid fx

CT Findings
- Generally not necessary for radial head diagnosis
- CT useful to evaluate for stability of DRUJ

MR Findings
- Generally not necessary to diagnose radial head fx since most are subtle but not truly occult
- May be used to follow up unexplained and unimproved pain; evaluate for occult fracture, bone bruise, ligament injury
- MR used to evaluate for associated occult fx or ligament injury in high energy trauma
- T1 MR: Low signal fracture lines, ± displacement, with surrounding low signal edema
- Fluid sensitive sequences: Low signal fracture line surrounded by edema
- Ligament disruptions are hyperintense with possible associated stress lesions at bony attachments
- Effusion: Fat pads (high signal on all sequences unless fat-saturated) at anterior & posterior distal humerus bowed out by joint fluid (low signal T1/high signal on fluid sequences)

Imaging Recommendations
- Best imaging tool
  - Radiographs for initial diagnosis
  - CT/MR as above to answer specific questions
- Protocol advice
  - Angled radial head view (isolates head from the usual overlap) may be useful additional view
  - CT for DRUJ
    - Patient positioned prone with arms over head
    - Both wrists imaged simultaneously, axial cuts only
    - Position both wrists in neutral, then extreme pronation, then extreme supination
    - Comparison reveals extent of subluxation

DIFFERENTIAL DIAGNOSIS

Radial Neck Fx
- More frequently seen in children/adolescents
- Same mechanism and injury
- ± Cortical buckle

Osteoarthritis
- Ring osteophyte at neck can simulate impacted fx

PATHOLOGY

General Features
- Etiology
  - Nondisplaced fracture: Fall on outstretched arm
    - Relatively low energy trauma
  - Unstable elbow & Essex-Lopresti: Higher energy impaction
- Epidemiology
  - 30% of adult elbow fractures
  - Most common elbow fracture in adults
  - Proximal radial injuries are rare in children
    - When present, usually occur in radial neck
  - Essex-Lopresti rare, but also frequently missed
- Associated abnormalities
  - If associated with posterior elbow dislocation

RADIAL HEAD/NECK FRACTURE

- Capitellar fx
- Coronoid process fx
- Ligamentous disruption
  - If high energy trauma
    - Disruption of anterior band of medial collateral ligament (MCL)
    - Triceps tendon rupture
    - Scaphoid fracture
    - Dislocation of DRUJ (Essex-Lopresti)
    - Terrible triad: Radial head fx + coronoid fx + MCL

Gross Pathologic & Surgical Features
- Disruption of radial head with variable bone fragment size & number
- Osteochondral injury to adjacent capitellum
- Avulsion of insertion of anterior band of MCL

Staging, Grading or Classification Criteria
- Based on classification by Mason
  - Type I = displacement < 2 mm
  - Type II = displacement > 2 mm
  - Type III = comminuted
  - Type IV = comminution + dislocation

CLINICAL ISSUES

Presentation
- Most common signs/symptoms
  - Pain and loss of function
  - Swelling and discoloration
  - Point tenderness over radial head
  - Crepitus if fracture is displaced
  - ± Associated wrist tenderness
  - Loss of joint stability (late)

Demographics
- Age: Young to adult
- Gender: M > F

Natural History & Prognosis
- Minimally displaced radial head fx
  - Prognosis worsened by
    - Delayed recognition of fracture
    - Delayed mobilization
    - Presence of other fractures, especially coronoid
    - Deteriorates with increase in grade of fracture
    - Potentially worsened by radial head resection
  - Prognosis improved by
    - Early recognition
    - Early mobilization
    - Maintaining integrity of DRUJ
    - Repair of collateral ligaments
- Essex-Lopresti: Cascade of effects can occur which result in poor result if true extent of injury is not recognized and treated at outset
  - Radius may end up being effectively shortened
    - If highly comminuted, it may be resected
    - Impaction may shorten the radius
    - Severe instability may effectively shorten the radius
  - If radius is effectively shortened for any of the above reasons, ulna is relatively long
    - Effective ulnar positive variance & instability → pain
  - If wrist is diagnosed as ulnar positive variance without entire syndrome being recognized, distal ulna may be treated by a shortening procedure
  - Ulnar shortening, in turn, causes radius to impact capitellum
  - Impaction at either end of these forearm bones is aggravated by lack of stability usually provided by the interosseous membrane
  - Worse case scenario of unrecognized Essex-Lopresti
    - Sequential shortening procedures at both proximal radius and distal ulna, with no resolution of the instability

Treatment
- Nondisplaced radial head fracture
  - Conservative: NSAIDs & physical therapy
- Displaced radial head fracture
  - Surgical fixation of fracture
  - Repair of ligaments
- Essex-Lopresti
  - Internal fixation of radial head fracture
  - If severely comminuted, resection may be necessary
  - At the same time, stabilize DRUJ (usually percutaneous pinning)

DIAGNOSTIC CHECKLIST

Consider
- Presence of other fractures
- Presence of valgus instability
- Extent of comminution
- With either of the latter two in evidence, check for stability of DRUJ

Image Interpretation Pearls
- "Positive ulnar variance" in the setting of high energy radial head fx should suggest Essex-Lopresti: Check for stability of DRUJ

SELECTED REFERENCES

1. Auyeung J et al: The Essex-Lopresti lesion: a variant with a bony distal radioulnar joint injury. J Hand Surg [Br]. 31(2):206-7, 2006
2. Bano KY et al: Radial head fractures--advanced techniques in surgical management and rehabilitation. J Hand Ther. 19(2):114-35, 2006
3. Caputo AE et al: Articular cartilage injuries of the capitellum interposed in radial head fractures: a report of ten cases. J Shoulder Elbow Surg. 15(6):716-20, 2006
4. Doornberg JN et al: Coronoid fracture height in terrible-triad injuries. J Hand Surg [Am]. 31(5):794-7, 2006
5. Roidis NT et al: Current concepts and controversies in the management of radial head fractures. Orthopedics. 29(10):904-16; quiz 917-8, 2006
6. Tashjian RZ et al: Complex elbow instability. J Am Acad Orthop Surg. 14(5):278-86, 2006
7. Itamura J et al: Radial head fractures: MRI evaluation of associated injuries. J Shoulder Elbow Surg. 14(4):421-4, 2005
8. van Riet RP et al: Associated injuries complicating radial head fractures: a demographic study. Clin Orthop Relat Res. 441:351-5, 2005

RADIAL HEAD/NECK FRACTURE

IMAGE GALLERY

Typical

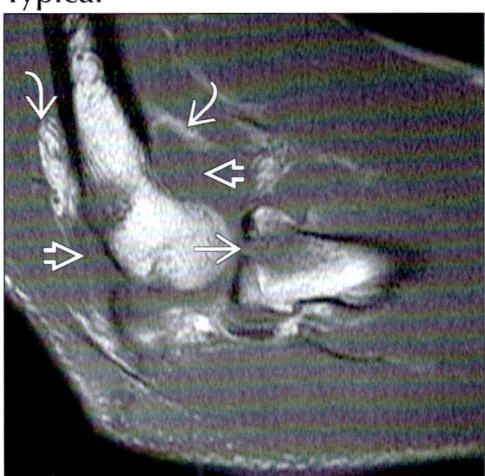 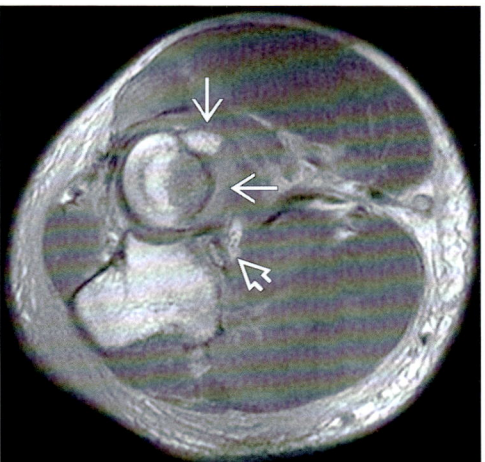

(Left) Sagittal T1WI MR shows a comminuted fracture of the radial head ➡. A large hemarthrosis is present ➡, with displacement of the periarticular fat pads ➡. *(Right)* Axial PD/Intermediate MR shows that, in addition to the comminuted radial head fx ➡, there is a coronoid process fx ➡. If there were also a tear of the MCL, this would represent the "terrible triad" of the elbow, which has a poor prognosis.

Typical

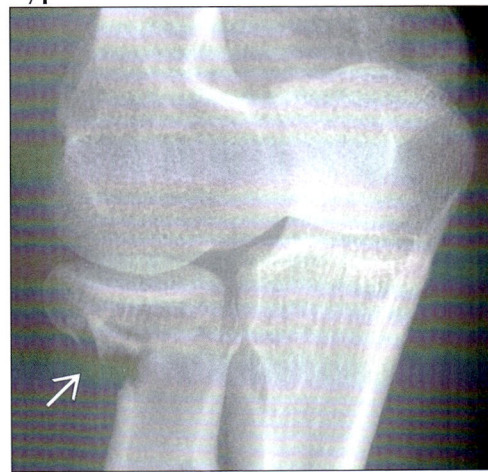 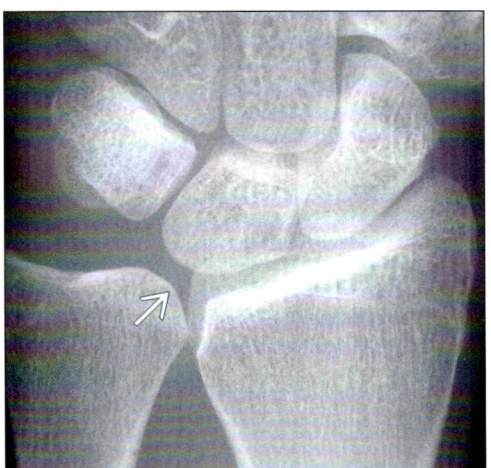

(Left) Oblique radiograph shows this patient had high-energy trauma, with a comminuted radial head/neck fracture showing displacement as well as some impaction ➡. This should alert the observer to search for a more substantial injury, such as MCL tear, coronoid process fx, or Essex-Lopresti. *(Right)* Posteroanterior radiograph confirms the latter diagnosis, showing relative ulnar positive variance ➡ and associated instability at the DRUJ.

Typical

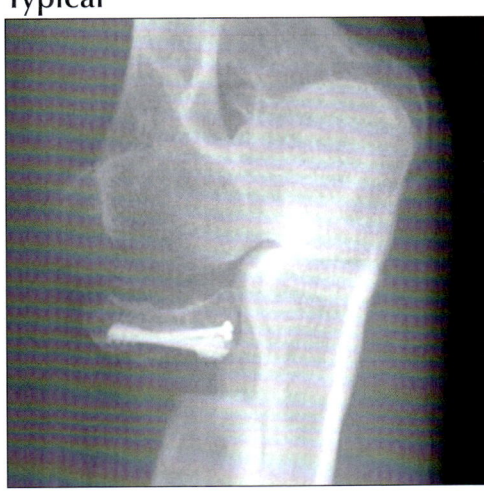 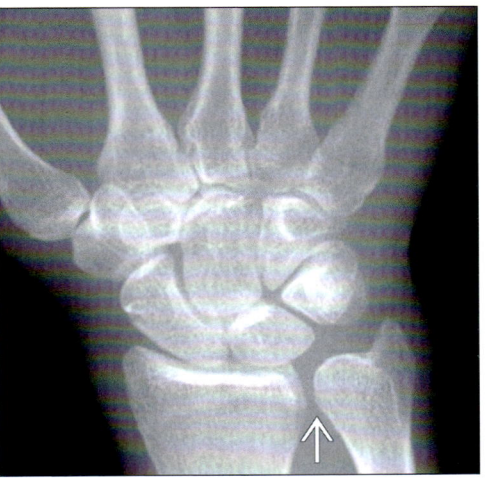

(Left) Oblique radiograph shows a surgically reduced comminuted radial head fx, with resection of the neck. This should lead to a concern about the possibility of interosseous membrane and DRUJ instability. *(Right)* Anteroposterior radiograph shows diastasis at the DRUJ ➡, confirming instability. This is a late finding in this case of Essex-Lopresti fracture-dislocation.

BICEPS TENDON RUPTURE

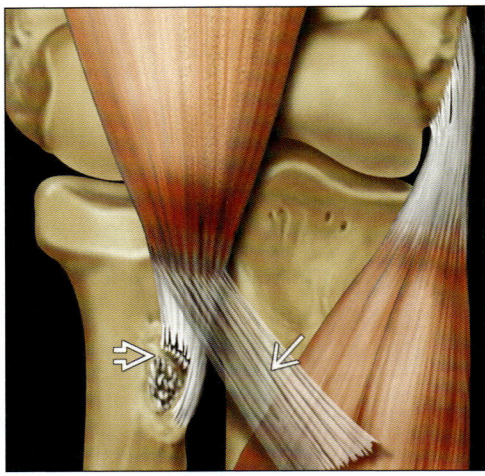

Coronal graphic shows a rupture of the biceps tendon from the radial tuberosity ⇨. Note the lacertus fibrosus ➡ which is intact, in this case preventing retraction of the tendon.

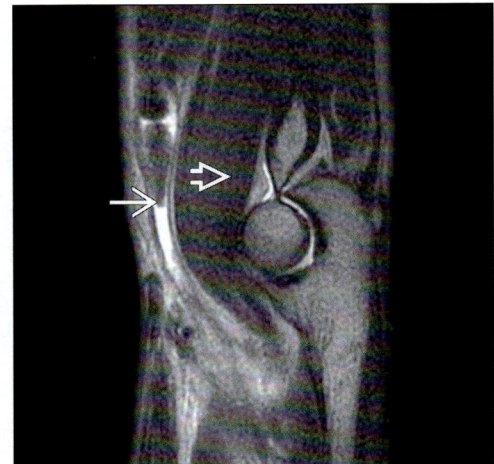

Sagittal T2WI MR shows the retracted ruptured biceps tendon ➡ surrounded by a small amount of fluid. The brachialis muscle ➡ lies deep to the biceps and should also not be mistaken for the biceps.

TERMINOLOGY

Definitions
- Rupture of distal biceps tendon, either in substance of tendon or from its insertion on radial tuberosity

IMAGING FINDINGS

General Features
- Best diagnostic clue: Disruption of distal biceps tendon
- Size: Partial or complete
- Morphology: Transverse or longitudinal tear

Radiographic Findings
- Generally negative; avulsion fracture extremely rare

MR Findings
- MR: Fluid within tendon sheath
- MR: Hypointense tendon may be thickened, thinned, absent/retracted
- Tendinosis: Increased signal intensity within a variably thickened tendon
- Edema in bicipital tuberosity

Ultrasonographic Findings
- Used to localize tendon within fluid-filled sheath

Imaging Recommendations
- Best imaging tool: MR
- Protocol advice
  - Axial most specifically identifies morphology & location of biceps tendon
  - Sagittal useful to measure retraction; do not confuse biceps tendon with adjacent vascular structures
  - **FABS positioning**
    - Patient prone, elbow **F**lexed, arm **AB**ducted, wrist **S**upinated (thumb up)
    - Slices parallel to coronal length of humerus; demonstrates biceps & brachialis tendons in their entire distal extent, to insertion sites

DIFFERENTIAL DIAGNOSIS

Bicipital Radial Bursitis
- Fluid within bursa of antecubital fossa; tendon intact

Biceps Tendon Rupture

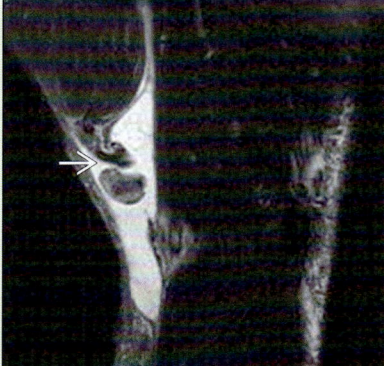

"Coat Hanger" Sign

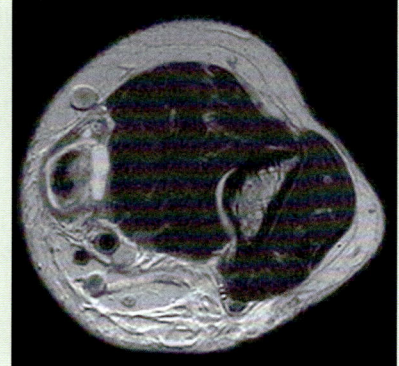

Myotendinous Junction Tear

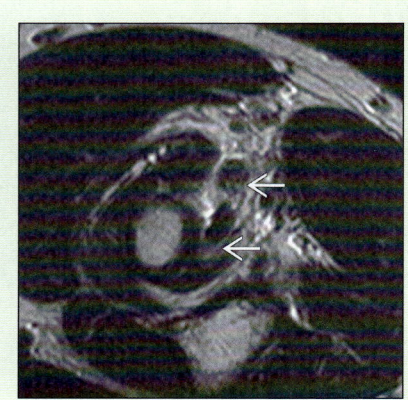

Longitudinal Split Biceps

BICEPS TENDON RUPTURE

Key Facts

Terminology
- Rupture of distal biceps tendon, either in substance of tendon or from its insertion on radial tuberosity

Imaging Findings
- MR: Fluid within tendon sheath
- MR: Hypointense tendon may be thickened, thinned, absent/retracted
- Axial most specifically identifies morphology & location of biceps tendon
- Sagittal useful to measure retraction; do not confuse biceps tendon with adjacent vascular structures
- **FABS positioning**
- Patient prone, elbow **F**lexed, arm **AB**ducted, wrist **S**upinated (thumb up)

Diagnostic Checklist
- Radial tuberosity is 5 cm distal to joint line; be sure to cover far enough distally to include entire structure

Brachialis Strain
- Similar mechanism; differentiate by anatomic location

PATHOLOGY

General Features
- General path comments
  - Lacertus fibrosus: Aponeurosis of biceps
    - Extends from musculotendinous junction to medial deep fascia of forearm
    - May prevent retraction of completely torn tendon
    - May preserve supination & forearm flexion
- Etiology
  - Eccentric contraction against resistance such as sudden forced extension of a flexed forearm
    - Heavy weightlifting; traumatic fall
- Epidemiology
  - Most common tendon rupture in elbow
  - Increasing frequency, especially in 40-60 year olds
  - Much less frequent than proximal biceps tendon ruptures (90-97% of all biceps tears)

Gross Pathologic & Surgical Features
- Disrupted tendon with variable degrees of retraction

CLINICAL ISSUES

Presentation
- Most common signs/symptoms
  - Forced extension of flexed forearm
  - Antecubital ecchymosis
  - Limited flexion; crepitus with supination/pronation
  - "Popeye" sign if retracted (limited by intact lacertus)

Demographics
- Age: Average 55 years of age
- Gender: M > F

Natural History & Prognosis
- Body builders & weight lifters may present earlier

Treatment
- Partial tear: Conservative: Rest, ice, immobilization, physical therapy
- Complete tear: Surgical repair, inserting tendon at apex of tuberosity, or tenodesis

DIAGNOSTIC CHECKLIST

Image Interpretation Pearls
- Radial tuberosity is 5 cm distal to joint line; be sure to cover far enough distally to include entire structure

SELECTED REFERENCES

1. Kijowski R et al: Magnetic resonance imaging of the elbow. Part II: Abnormalities of the ligaments, tendons, and nerves. Skeletal Radiol. 34(1):1-18, 2005
2. Vidal AF et al: Biceps tendon and triceps tendon injuries. Clin Sports Med. 23(4):707-22, xi, 2004

IMAGE GALLERY

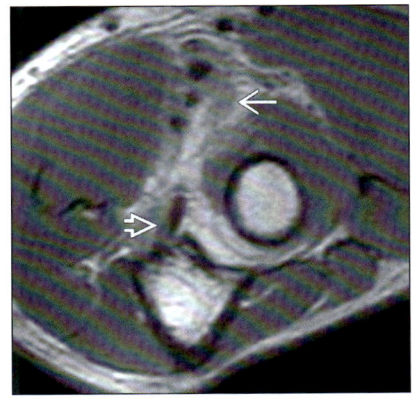 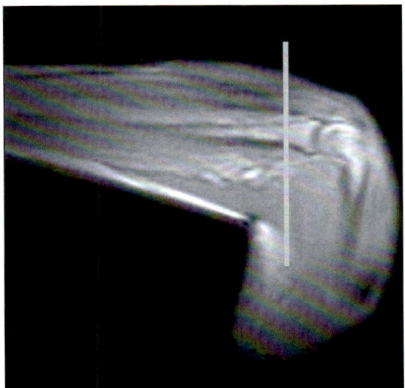 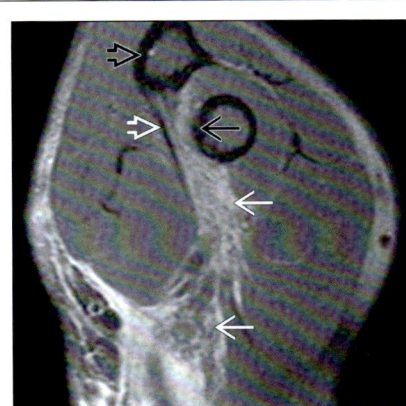

(Left) Axial T1WI MR at the coronoid process shows the brachialis tendon inserting normally ➡ while there is only intermediate signal where the biceps tendon should be ➡. This is a complete rupture of the biceps tendon, with retraction. *(Center)* FABS positioning localizer T2* GRE MR (flexed, abducted, supinated); the patient lies prone with the arm over the head. *(Right)* FABS T2WI MR shows a normal brachialis tendon ➡ inserting on the coronoid ➡. The biceps is torn ➡ and retracted; the expected site of insertion on the radial tuberosity is seen ➡.

FOREARM FRACTURES

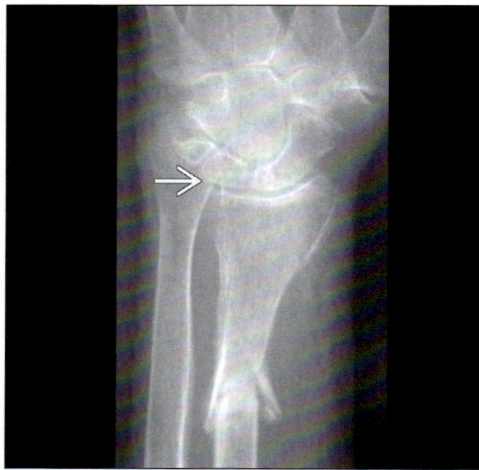

Posteroanterior radiograph shows a significantly impacted fracture of the radial shaft. This is associated with dislocation of the distal radioulnar joint; note the relationship of the distal ulna to the distal radius ➡.

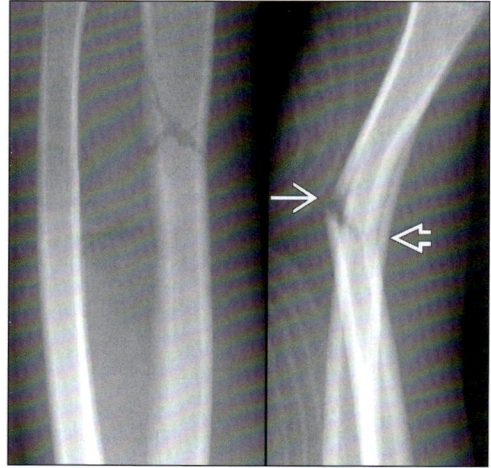

Anteroposterior & lateral radiographs show a both bone fracture of the forearm. The only complete fx is in the radius ➡. The ulna is bowed ➡; this is a plastic fx, which may be seen in long bones of narrow diameter.

TERMINOLOGY

Abbreviations and Synonyms
- Both bone fracture, nightstick fracture
- Forearm fracture dislocations: Galeazzi, Monteggia, Essex-Lopresti
- Incomplete fx: Torus (buckle), greenstick, plastic

Definitions
- Fx, complete or incomplete, of radius and/or ulna
- Fracture/dislocation: Generally fracture of one of the forearm bones, with associated dislocation of the other, either at elbow or wrist

IMAGING FINDINGS

General Features
- Best diagnostic clue: Fractures or dislocation
- Location: Anywhere along forearm, from radiocapitellar joint to distal radioulnar joint (DRUJ)
- Size: Ranges from complete, with displacement and angulation to incomplete & anatomic
- Morphology
  - Both bone fx: Generally middle to distal third of forearm
  - Nightstick fx: Isolated fx ulna, generally middle to distal third
  - Torus or greenstick fx: Generally distal metaphysis
  - Plastic fx: Ulna more common than radius; usually complete fx in the adjacent forearm bone
  - Galeazzi: Fracture radial shaft & dislocation DRUJ
  - Monteggia: Fracture ulnar shaft & dislocation radiocapitellar joint
  - Essex-Lopresti: Comminuted fx radial head (or simple fx & severe ligamentous disruption) & dislocation DRUJ

Radiographic Findings
- Fracture line in adults
- Focal disruption of cortex in incomplete fx
- Bowing of either bone (note: The radius has a normal bow in its midportion, in the lateral direction as seen on anteroposterior view)
- Radial head dislocation: Disruption of RC line
  - Radiocapitellar (RC) line: Bisects proximal 1/3 radius should intersect capitellum on any view of elbow
- Distal radioulnar joint (DRUJ) dislocation

Other Forearm Fractures

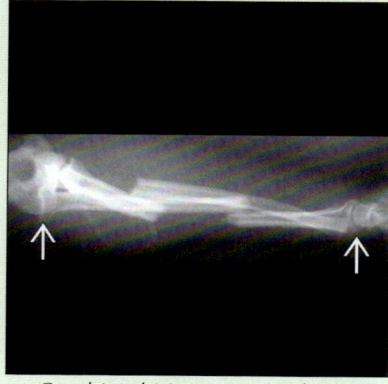
Combined Monteggia/Galeazzi

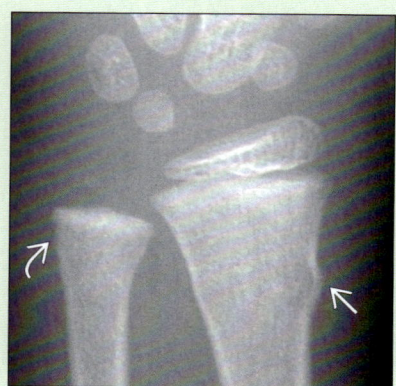
Buckle Fx, Both Bones

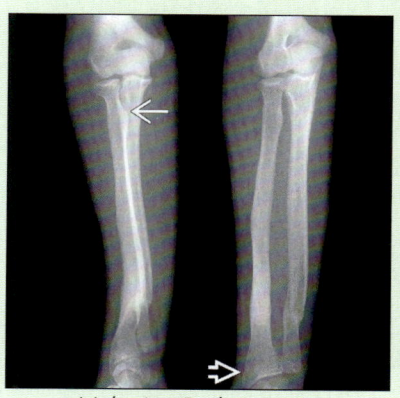
Malunion Both Bone Fx

FOREARM FRACTURES

Key Facts

Imaging Findings
- Both bone fx: Generally middle to distal third of forearm
- Nightstick fx: Isolated fx ulna, generally middle to distal third
- Torus or greenstick fx: Generally distal metaphysis
- Plastic fx: Ulna more common than radius; usually complete fx in the adjacent forearm bone
- Galeazzi: Fracture radial shaft & dislocation DRUJ
- Monteggia: Fracture ulnar shaft & dislocation radiocapitellar joint
- Essex-Lopresti: Comminuted fx radial head (or simple fx & severe ligamentous disruption) & dislocation DRUJ

Diagnostic Checklist
- Look for associated injuries if only single fx seen
- Compartment syndrome may be associated

- Anteroposterior view: Lack of the normal slight overlap of radius and ulna (diastasis of ulna)
- Lateral view: Slightly more dorsal placement of ulna

CT Findings
- May be used to confirm a subtle DRUJ dislocation

Imaging Recommendations
- Best imaging tool: Radiographs, orthogonal views
- Protocol advice: CT for DRUJ disruption: Axial cuts through both wrists (held over head), in neutral, full supination, & full pronation

PATHOLOGY

General Features
- General path comments
  - It is rare to have an isolated fracture of the shaft of one of the forearm bones
    - Exception: Nightstick fracture of ulna
    - Note: This "rule" applies to the shaft & does not include articular fx at either the elbow or wrist
- Etiology
  - Fall on outstretched hand (FOOSH)
  - Nightstick: Direct blow to ulna (often while forearm is held up to protect face)
- Epidemiology
  - Common: 23% of all fractures in children
  - Forearm fractures 10 times more frequent than carpal injuries in both adults & children

CLINICAL ISSUES

Presentation
- Most common signs/symptoms: Pain, possible deformity following FOOSH

Demographics
- Age: Children, age 1-10; adults
- Gender: No gender predilection

Natural History & Prognosis
- Incomplete fx heals in anatomic position
- Children's complete fx heals with remodeling
- Plastic fx does not remodel

Treatment
- Reduction; adult both bone fx generally require ORIF
- Reduction & stabilization of adjacent unstable joint

DIAGNOSTIC CHECKLIST

Consider
- Look for associated injuries if only single fx seen
- Compartment syndrome may be associated

SELECTED REFERENCES
1. Ward WT et al: The impact of trauma in an urban pediatric orthopaedic practice. J Bone Joint Surg Am. 88(12):2759-64, 2006

IMAGE GALLERY

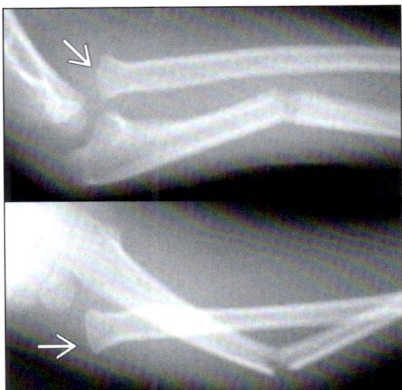 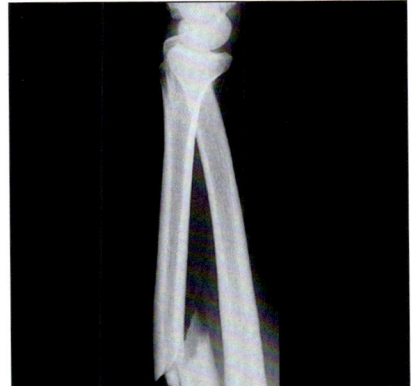 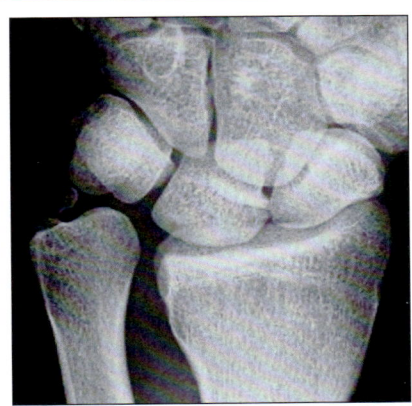

(Left) Lateral & anteroposterior radiographs show a midshaft ulnar fracture associated with a radial head dislocation ➡. This pattern of both-bone injury is termed a Monteggia fracture/dislocation. **(Center)** Lateral radiograph shows a fracture of the midshaft of the radius. There was no associated ulnar fracture. **(Right)** Posteroanterior radiograph of the wrist of the same patient as previous, shows dissociation of the distal radioulnar joint, as well as ulnar styloid fracture. The combined pattern is a Galeazzi fracture/dislocation.

DISTAL RADIUS FRACTURES

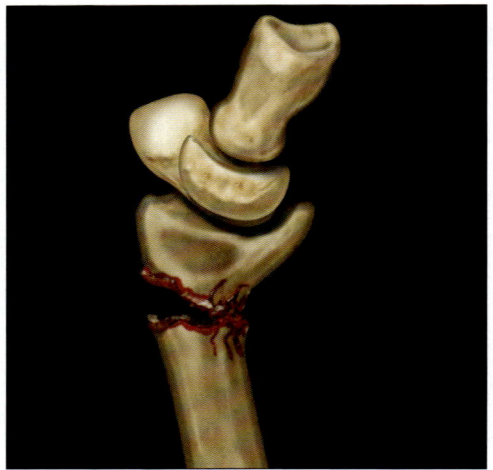

Lateral graphic shows the configuration of a typical Colles fx, with comminution at the dorsal fx line. This results in a volar angulation at the apex of the fx, & dorsal tilt of the radial articular surface.

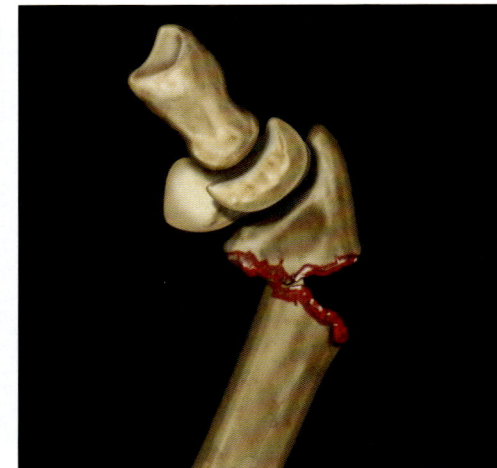

Lateral graphic demonstrates a reverse Colles (or Smith) fx pattern. It is also a transverse distal radial fx, but the apex of the fracture is directed dorsally. This results in exaggerated volar tilt of the distal radial surface.

TERMINOLOGY

Abbreviations and Synonyms
- Colles, Smith, Barton, reverse Barton, chauffeur (Hutchinson) are all types of distal radial fractures

Definitions
- Colles: Transverse fracture through distal radius which results in apex volar angulation of the fracture fragments
  - ± Intraarticular (most often)
  - ± Associated ulnar styloid fx
- Smith: Transverse fracture through distal radius which results in apex dorsal angulation of the fracture fragments (reverse Colles)
- Barton: Dorsal lip intraarticular fracture of distal radius
- Reverse Barton: Volar lip intraarticular fracture of distal radius
- Chauffeur (Hutchinson): Intraarticular fracture through the radial styloid
- Complex intraarticular fracture: Generally 3 intraarticular fragments, often with angulation
- Salter II fracture: Fx crosses physis, exiting through metaphysis
- Osteolysis of distal radial metaphysis: Irregular lysis of distal metaphysis adjacent to epiphyseal plate

IMAGING FINDINGS

Radiographic Findings
- Colles fracture
  - Usually osteoporotic
  - Transverse distal radial fx
  - On lateral, major fracture fragments are in apex volar angulation (reversal of the normal volar tilt of the distal radial articular surface)
    - This angulation relates to severe comminution of tiny osteoporotic bone fragments on dorsal aspect of radius
  - Intraarticular extension is common
    - Tends to occur near the ulnar aspect of the distal radius
    - When subtle, intraarticular extension easiest to see on pronated oblique image
  - Following reduction, watch for
    - Loss of length of radius relative to ulna
    - Loss of normal tilt of radial articular surface

Other Distal Radial Fractures

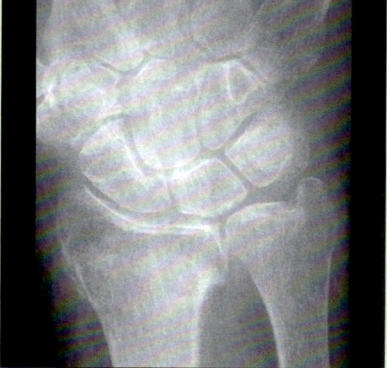

Colles, Loss of Length

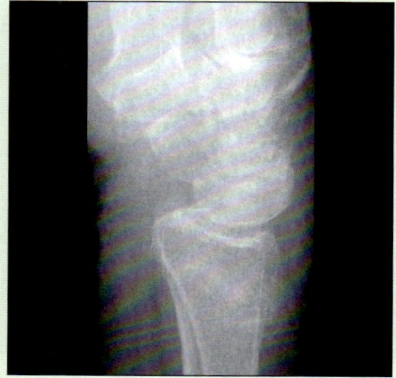

Colles, Loss of Volar Tilt

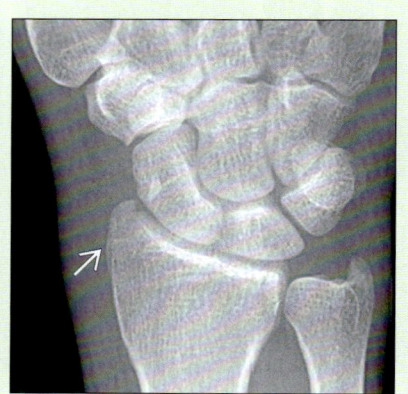

Chauffeur Fracture

DISTAL RADIUS FRACTURES

Key Facts

Terminology
- Colles: Transverse fracture through distal radius which results in apex volar angulation of the fracture fragments
- Smith: Transverse fracture through distal radius which results in apex dorsal angulation of the fracture fragments (reverse Colles)
- Barton: Dorsal lip intraarticular fracture of distal radius
- Reverse Barton: Volar lip intraarticular fracture of distal radius
- Chauffeur (Hutchinson): Intraarticular fracture through the radial styloid
- Complex intraarticular fracture: Generally 3 intraarticular fragments, often with angulation
- Salter II fracture: Fx crosses physis, exiting through metaphysis
- Osteolysis of distal radial metaphysis: Irregular lysis of distal metaphysis adjacent to epiphyseal plate

Diagnostic Checklist
- Not all distal radial fractures are Colles, and should not be identified as such!
- **All distal radial fractures should be specifically evaluated for:**
- Intraarticular extension
- Shortening of radius relative to ulna
- Severe comminution & angulation of fragments
- Loss of normal ulnar tilt of distal radial articular surface (normal approximates 30°)
- Loss of normal volar tilt of distal radial articular surface (normal approximates 10-15°)

- Smith fracture
  - Usually normal bone density
  - Transverse distal radial fx
  - May or may not have intraarticular extension
  - On lateral, major fracture fragments are in apex dorsal angulation (exaggeration of the normal volar tilt of the distal radial articular surface)
  - "Reverse Colles"
- Barton fracture
  - Dorsal lip fracture, intraarticular; this feature seen best on lateral
  - Carpus follows the diastased dorsal lip fragment
    - On lateral, lunate & remainder of carpus are dorsally displaced, along with the fragment, relative to the shaft of the radius
    - Unstable
- Reverse Barton fracture
  - Volar lip fracture, intraarticular; this feature seen best on lateral
  - Carpus follows the diastased dorsal lip fragment
    - On lateral, lunate & remainder of carpus are dorsally displaced, along with the fragment, relative to the shaft of the radius
    - Unstable
- Chauffeur fracture
  - PA & pronated oblique show avulsed radial styloid
  - Often associated with dislocation; check carpal arcs
- Complex intraarticular fracture
  - PA & pronated oblique show separate radial styloid fragment & generally dorsal and volar fragmentation of remaining medial distal radial fragments
  - Lateral shows dorsal or volar angulation of the fragments
- Salter II fracture
  - PA often appears normal since epiphyseal plate is dorsally displaced
  - Lateral view shows dorsal displacement of epiphysis, as well as the associated small dorsal metaphyseal fragment
- Osteolysis of distal radial metaphysis
  - Lysis of distal radial metaphysis, adjacent to epiphyseal plate
  - Repetitive trauma-related Salter I injury
  - Often bilateral

Imaging Recommendations
- Best imaging tool
  - 3 view radiograph of wrist: Posteroanterior (PA), lateral, pronated oblique
  - CT if further definition of fx displacement/angulation is required
  - MR if soft tissue evaluation is required

PATHOLOGY

General Features
- General path comments
  - Normal anatomy should be regained following reduction; watch for
    - PA radiograph, radius is normally 0-2 mm longer than ulna
    - PA radiograph, radial articular surface normally tilts 30° towards the ulna
    - Lateral radiograph, radial articular surface normally tilts 10-15° in a volar direction
    - Lateral radiograph, lunate should articulate concentrically with radial articular surface
    - Any articular diastasis ≥ 2 mm
- Etiology
  - Fall on outstretched hand (FOOSH) can result in many fracture and fx-dislocation patterns
  - Most frequent injury pattern for FOOSH relates to patient age
    - 4-10 years: Distal radius & ulna transverse metaphyseal, often incomplete
    - 11-16 years: Distal radius, usually Salter II (dorsal displacement best seen on lateral view)
    - 17-40 years: Scaphoid, occasionally triquetrum or both
    - > 40 years: Colles
  - Distal radial fracture patterns represent a spectrum of injuries based on four factors
    - Direction of 3-dimensional loading
    - Magnitude & duration of force

DISTAL RADIUS FRACTURES

- Position of hand & wrist at injury
- Biomechanical properties of affected ligaments & bones
  - Colles
    - Underlying osteoporosis makes bones vulnerable to fracture
    - Fall onto outstretched, dorsiflexed hand
    - Impact force aligned to long axis of radius
    - Tensile failure of cancellous metaphyseal bone on the volar side & compressive failure on the dorsal side
    - Ulnar styloid avulsed by TFCC in 60%
  - Complex distal radial fracture
    - High energy axial compression forces
    - Force transmitted through lunate to the medial half of the radial articular surface
    - Articular surface usually splits into three major fragments: Radial styloid & two medial fragments (dorsal and volar); these may be angulated
    - May have associated soft injuries & disrupted DRUJ
  - Osteolysis of distal radial metaphysis
    - Salter I injury due to repetitive stress at wrist, generally in a gymnast
- Epidemiology
  - Distal radius is among the most common fractures (1/6 of all fx seen in acute setting)
  - Colles fractures particularly common in elderly osteoporotic women
- Associated abnormalities: Colles fx: Because of osteoporosis, associated with humeral & femoral neck fractures

Staging, Grading or Classification Criteria
- Multiple published classifications: Melone is based on degree & direction of displaced articular fragments
  - 4 components: Radial shaft, radial styloid, dorsal-medial, volar-medial fragments
    - Type I: Minimally displaced
    - Type IIA: Dorsal (most common) or volar displacement
    - Type IIB: Die-punch fracture with lunate impaction (usually dorsal medial component)
    - Type III: Addition of spike fragment from volar metaphysis
    - Type IV: Separation or rotation of dorsal & volar medial fragments and disruption of distal radius articulations
    - Type V: Explosion with extensive comminution from articular surfaces to diaphysis

CLINICAL ISSUES

Presentation
- Most common signs/symptoms: Pain, swelling following fall on outstretched hand

Demographics
- Age
  - Colles: > 40 years
  - Salter II & stress osteolysis (Salter I): 11-16 years
- Gender: Colles: M < F; others not gender-specific

Natural History & Prognosis
- Stress osteolysis heals if activity ceased
- Fx heals; outcome depends on anatomic alignment
- Non-anatomic alignment may result in
  - Decreased grip strength
  - Decreased range of motion
  - Shortening of radius creates a relative ulnar positive variance & associated impaction on carpus
  - Osteoarthritis
- Any of these fractures may be complicated by reflex sympathetic dystrophy

Treatment
- Stress osteolysis: Stop activity
- Others: Reduce; cast immobilization if anatomic
- If reduction is nonanatomic, ORIF considered
  - Loss of radial length relative to ulna
  - Articular diastasis of fracture fragments (2 mm or more associated with osteoarthritis)
  - Loss of normal volar or ulnar tilt of distal radial articular surface

DIAGNOSTIC CHECKLIST

Consider
- Not all distal radial fractures are Colles, and should not be identified as such!
  - Differences relate to fracture line placement & angular deformity; these must be described accurately
  - Reduction technique & treatment is different for the different fx patterns

Image Interpretation Pearls
- **All distal radial fractures should be specifically evaluated for:**
  - Intraarticular extension
    - If intraarticular, determine whether fracture line interrupts scaphoid fossa, lunate fossa, or sigmoid notch at DRUJ
    - Amount of diastasis at intraarticular site
  - Shortening of radius relative to ulna
  - Severe comminution & angulation of fragments
  - Loss of normal ulnar tilt of distal radial articular surface (normal approximates 30°)
  - Loss of normal volar tilt of distal radial articular surface (normal approximates 10-15°)

SELECTED REFERENCES
1. Mackenney PJ et al: Prediction of instability in distal radial fractures. J Bone Joint Surg Am. 88(9):1944-51, 2006
2. Karnezis IA et al: Correlation between radiological parameters and patient-rated wrist dysfunction following fractures of the distal radius. Injury. 36(12):1435-9, 2005

DISTAL RADIUS FRACTURES

IMAGE GALLERY

Typical

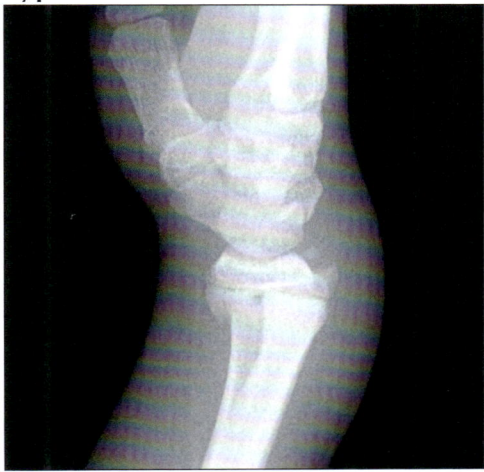 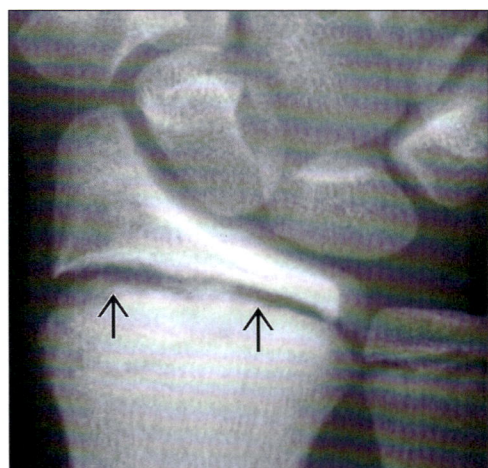

(Left) Lateral radiograph in a teenager shows a Salter II fx with volar displacement & apex dorsal angulation. This is a Smith-like fracture, with angulation opposite that of a Colles fx. It is not typical of a Salter II fx due to FOOSH injury (dorsal displacement of the physis). (Right) Posteroanterior radiograph shows resorption of the distal radial metaphysis in a teenaged gymnast ➡. The appearance suggests rickets, but this pattern is also seen as a Salter I injury, related to significant stress.

Typical

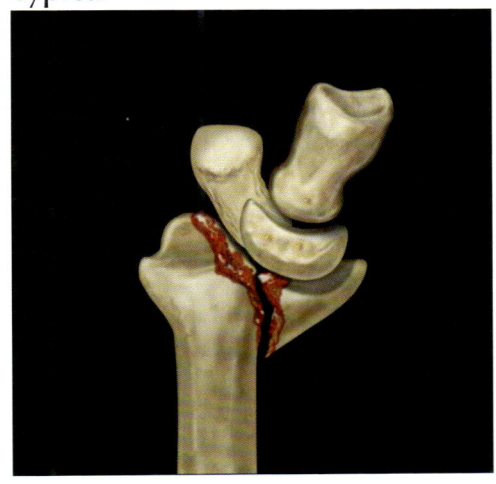 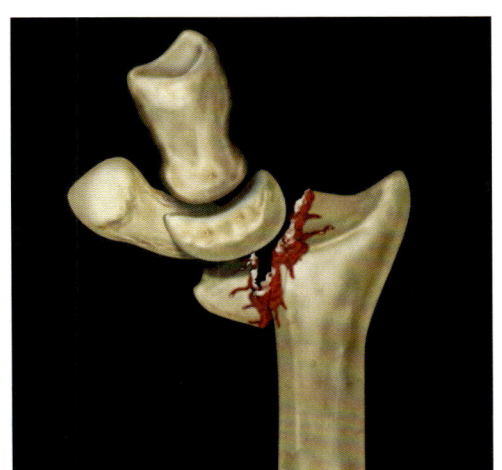

(Left) Lateral graphic shows an intraarticular dorsal lip (Barton) fx of the distal radius. Note that the carpus moves dorsally & proximally with the fracture fragment, & is no longer aligned with the radial shaft. (Right) Lateral graphic shows a reverse Barton (volar lip) fx. In this case, the intraarticular fx fragment is located volarly, & is displaced further volarly & inferiorly. As with the Barton fx, the carpus moves with the fragment, & the wrist is displaced from the radial shaft.

Typical

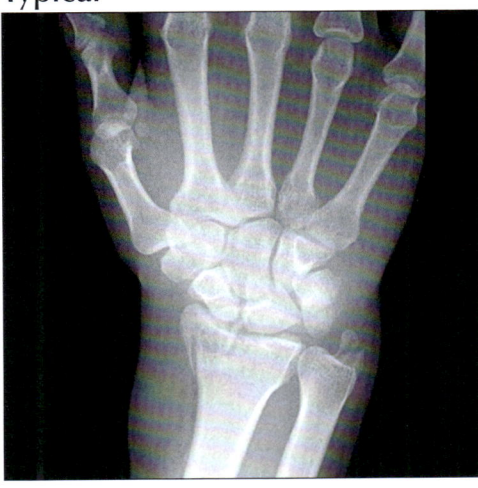 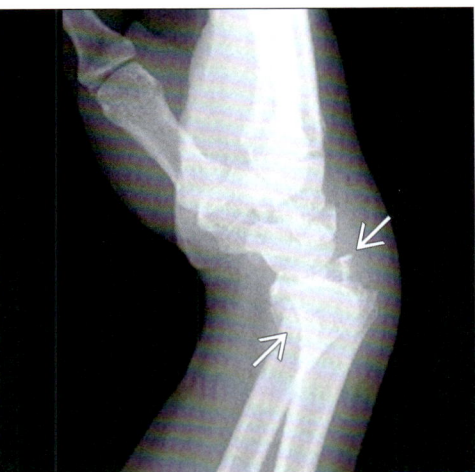

(Left) Posteroanterior radiograph shows a comminuted intraarticular fracture of the distal radius. This is a young adult, with normal bone density. (Right) Lateral radiograph of the same patient further defines the fracture as a volar lip (reverse Barton) fracture ➡. Note that the carpus moves with the volar lip fracture fragment. The lunate does not have its usual concentric articulation with the distal radius.

DIE PUNCH FRACTURE, DISTAL RADIUS

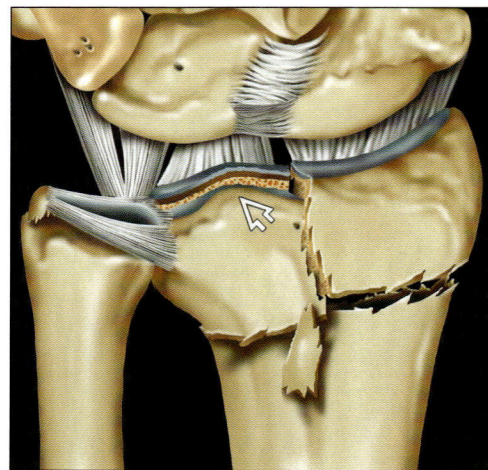

Posterior graphic shows a type II articular die punch fracture with dorsal displacement of the dorsal medial fragment ➔. This pattern matches that of the adjacent radiograph.

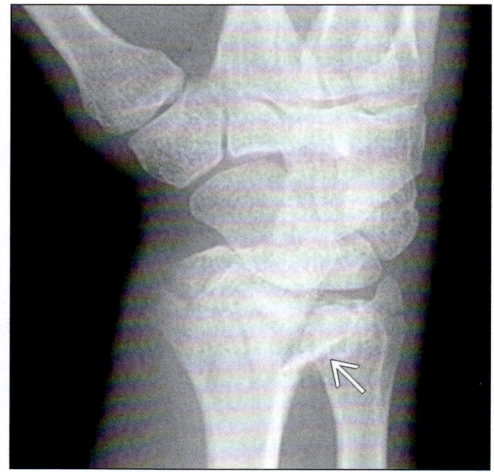

Oblique radiograph shows severe comminution of the articular surface typical of a die punch type II fx pattern. The major dorsal medial fragment is impacted & dorsally displaced ➔.

TERMINOLOGY

Abbreviations and Synonyms
- Lunate load fracture

Definitions
- Intraarticular comminuted distal radius fx occurring secondary to lunate impaction on distal radius, splitting it in both coronal & sagittal planes

IMAGING FINDINGS

General Features
- Best diagnostic clue: Fracture that extends to involve lunate fossa of distal radius
- Location: Lunate fossa (dorsal medial or volar medial fragments; these are split in the coronal plane)
- Size: Variable based on displacement of fragments
- Morphology
  - Dorsal or volar displacement of medial radial fragments
  - ± Metaphyseal spike fragment impaction

Radiographic Findings
- 3 views wrist identify fragments
- 4 main fragments identified: Metaphyseal, radial styloid, dorsal medial, volar medial
- Dorsal & volar medial fragments are those impacted by lunate & therefore the most likely to be displaced

CT Findings
- Bone CT with reformats best defines fx fragments

MR Findings
- T1 MR: Fx diastasis measured directly in all 3 planes
- Fluid sensitive sequences: Hyperintense edema seen in fx fragments as well as impacting lunate

Imaging Recommendations
- Best imaging tool: Radiographs; followed by CT/MR

DIFFERENTIAL DIAGNOSIS

Colles Fracture without Intraarticular Extension
- Major finding is apex volar angulation of distal radius

Die Punch Fx Distal Radius: CT

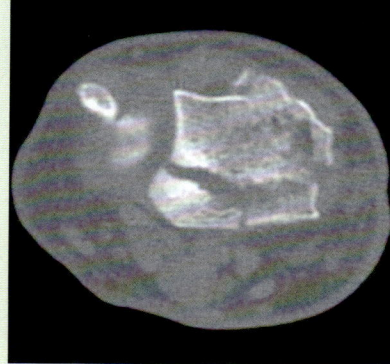

Axial: Diastasis Fragments

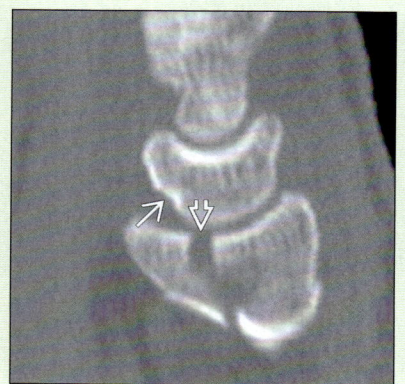

Sagittal: Lunate Impaction

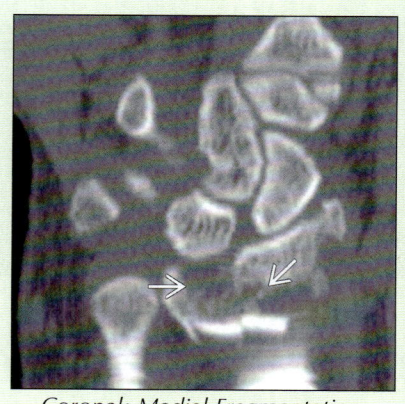

Coronal: Medial Fragmentation

DIE PUNCH FRACTURE, DISTAL RADIUS

Key Facts

Terminology
- Intraarticular comminuted distal radius fx occurring secondary to lunate impaction on distal radius, splitting it in both coronal & sagittal planes

Imaging Findings
- Location: Lunate fossa (dorsal medial or volar medial fragments; these are split in the coronal plane)
- 4 main fragments identified: Metaphyseal, radial styloid, dorsal medial, volar medial

- Dorsal & volar medial fragments are those impacted by lunate & therefore the most likely to be displaced
- Bone CT with reformats best defines fx fragments
- T1 MR: Fx diastasis measured directly in all 3 planes

Diagnostic Checklist
- Watch for associated fx of radial and/or ulnar styloid
- Characterize lunate fossa into dorsal medial & volar medial components on sagittal images

PATHOLOGY

General Features
- Etiology: Axial compression, lunate driven proximally, impacting dorsal medial aspect of radius
- Epidemiology: Distal radial fx common skeletal injury

Gross Pathologic & Surgical Features
- Lunate impaction on dorsal medial component of lunate fossa, with dorsal displacement

Staging, Grading or Classification Criteria
- Type I: No significant displacement or angulation
- Type IIa: Classic die punch fx; unstable fx with dorsal displacement & tilt of dorsal medial fragment
- Type IIb: Lunate impaction of volar medial component resulting in ↑ comminution & volar tilt
- Type III: Similar to type II fx with extra comminuted "spike" fragment displaced volarly
- Type IV: Wide diastasis dorsal & volar medial fragments
- Type V: Severe comminution ("exploded" wrist)

CLINICAL ISSUES

Presentation
- Most common signs/symptoms: Pain/FOOSH

Demographics
- Age: Adults (60-80 most common)
- Gender: F > M

Natural History & Prognosis
- Type I fx has best prognosis
- Complications
  - Chondral injury → eventual development of OA
  - TFCC, scapholunate, lunatetriquetral, extrinsic ligament, tendon tears
  - Arterial or nerve (ulnar, radial, median) injuries
  - Reflex sympathetic dystrophy

Treatment
- Conservative: Type I fx treated with closed reduction
- Surgical
  - Open reduction usually required for any fx > type 1, relating to articular diastasis, shortening, & tilt
  - May combine internal & external fixation

DIAGNOSTIC CHECKLIST

Consider
- Watch for associated fx of radial and/or ulnar styloid
- Characterize lunate fossa into dorsal medial & volar medial components on sagittal images

SELECTED REFERENCES
1. Anderson DD et al: A three-dimensional finite element model of the radiocarpal joint: distal radius fracture step-off and stress transfer. Iowa Orthop J. 25:108-17, 2005
2. Yamamoto K et al: Clinical results of external fixation for unstable Colles' fractures. Hand Surg. 8(2):193-200, 2003

IMAGE GALLERY

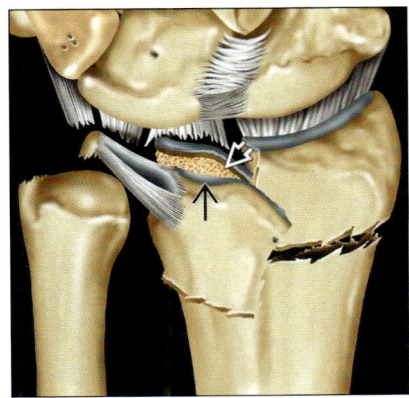 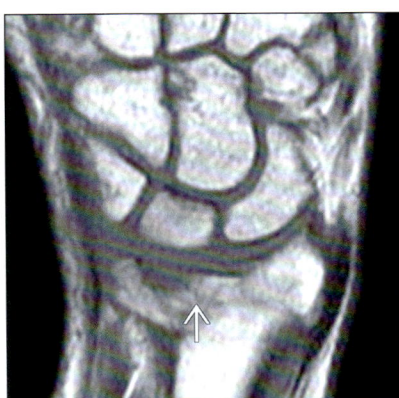 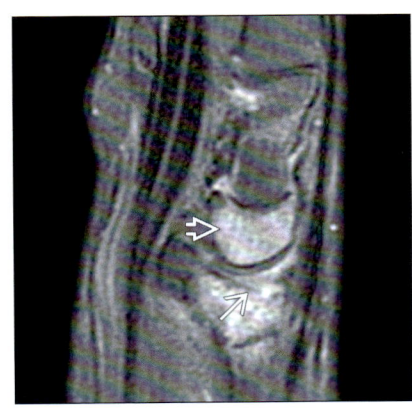

(Left) Posterior graphic shows an unstable type IV distal radius fx with wide separation of the dorsal ➔ & volar ➔ medial fragments. (Center) Coronal T1WI MR shows an impacted fx, with dorsal medial fragments driven into the subchondral bone ➔. (Right) Sagittal T2WI FS MR (same case) shows edema in the lunate related to its role in the impaction injury ➔. The impacted cortex of the volar medial fx fragment is seen ➔. With the diastasis & impaction of both dorsal & volar fragments, this constitutes a type IV injury, similar to that depicted in the graphic.

SCAPHOID FRACTURES

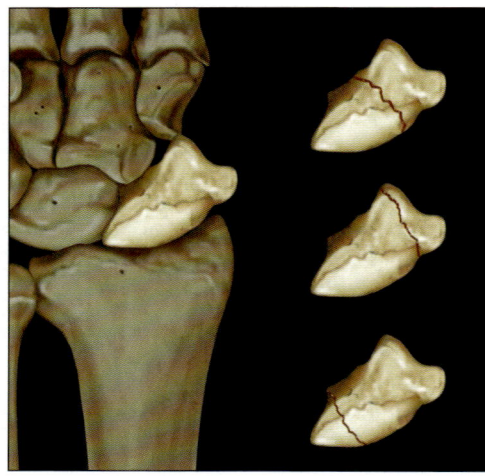

Graphic shows the 3 common types of scaphoid fx: Waist, distal pole, & proximal pole (top to bottom). Scaphoid waist fx is the most frequent (70%); proximal pole fx is the most likely to have a poor result.

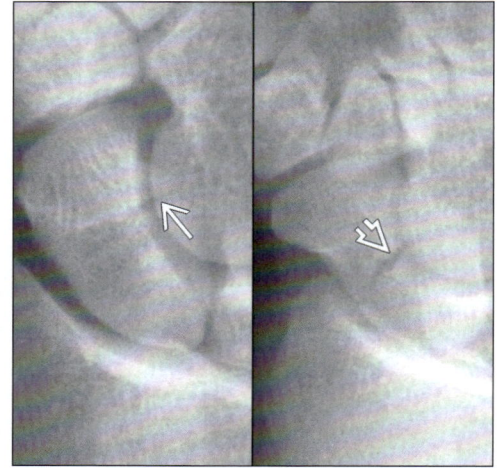

This scaphoid fx is extremely subtle on the PA ➡ but easily seen on the oblique ➡. It is not uncommon to be able to visualize a scaphoid fx on only a single view; occasionally a specialized navicular view is required.

TERMINOLOGY

Abbreviations and Synonyms
- Navicular fracture

Definitions
- Disruption of scaphoid trabecular and/or cortical bone

IMAGING FINDINGS

General Features
- Best diagnostic clue
  - Transverse fracture line most commonly in middle 1/3 of waist
  - Fracture is usually nondisplaced, so may be seen in only 1 view
- Location
  - Tubercle (distal volar prominence): 5%
  - Distal third: 10-20%
  - Waist (middle third): 70%
  - Proximal pole: 5-10%
- Size: Usually not comminuted or displaced
- Morphology: Transverse, or mildly oblique

Radiographic Findings
- Posteroanterior (PA), pronated oblique, lateral, navicular views
- Only 25% of scaphoid fxs are visible on all views
- 75% visible on PA & pronated oblique views
- 2-5% not visible on initial imaging
- Obliteration of scaphoid (navicular) fat stripe & dorsal soft tissue swelling are suggestive but nonspecific
- Beware of radial deviation on PA view; it obscures the waist of scaphoid
  - With radial deviation, scaphoid develops a volar tilt
  - Volar tilt is seen on PA view as a "target" or "ring" sign; it foreshortens the scaphoid and obscures the waist
  - Patients with wrist injuries tend to hold their hand in this position; must encourage neutral or ulnar deviation

CT Findings
- May be used to identify occult or chip fx
- Most frequently used to evaluate for healing & deformity

Other Scaphoid Fractures

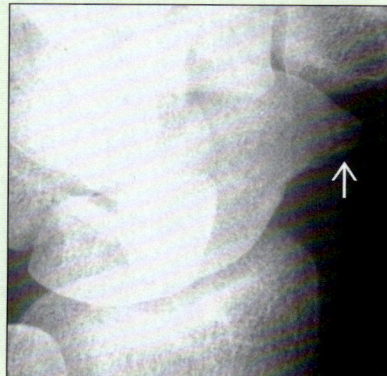

Scaphoid Tubercle Fx

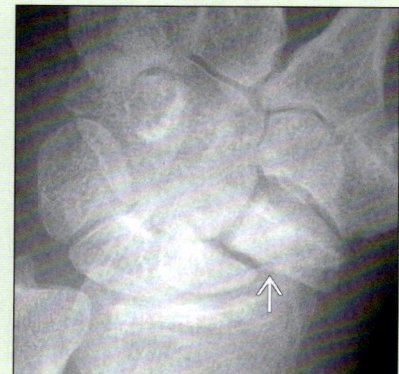

Scaphoid Nonunion

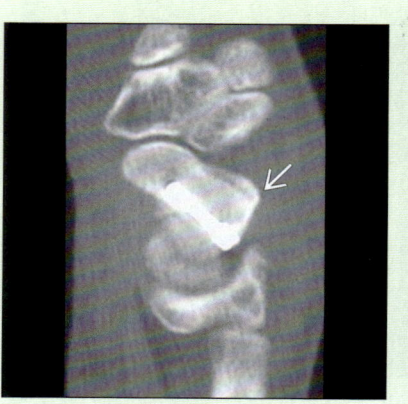

Humpback Deformity

SCAPHOID FRACTURES

Key Facts

Imaging Findings
- Transverse fracture line most commonly in middle 1/3 of waist

Clinical Issues
- Up to 90% of acute scaphoid fx heal if treated promptly
- **Complications**
- Most frequent malunion is the humpback angular deformity (apex dorsal angulation)
- Delayed union: Incomplete union after 4 months of cast immobilization
- Nonunion: 10-15% scaphoid fx do not unite
- 15-30% of all scaphoid fractures develop AVN, usually proximal pole

Diagnostic Checklist
- 2-5% scaphoid fx not visible on initial radiographs; with high clinical suspicion, may
- Splint and return for re-imaging in 7-10 days
- In many patients waiting for the diagnosis is not acceptable, for a variety of reasons; for these, MR
- Beware of PA view in radial deviation; fx line is obscured
- In follow-up CT for evaluation of union, perform direct sagittals through scaphoid
- Do not overinterpret resorption & cystic change at fx site as impending nonunion; it may be reversible
- Do not overinterpret density in proximal pole as AVN; this is often reversible
- MR, even with contrast, is not 100% accurate in determining viability of fragments

MR Findings
- For initial diagnosis if radiographs negative & waiting is not an option
  - Hypointense fracture line on T1
  - Hypo- to hyperintense fracture line with surrounding marrow edema on fluid sensitive sequences
  - Initial hypointensity of proximal pole on fluid sensitive sequences indicates ischemia of that segment; may or may not progress to avascular necrosis (AVN)
- MR not as specific for diagnosis of nonunion as CT
- Used to determine viability of proximal pole fragment
  - Not 100% sensitive or specific for vascularization status
  - Entire fragment may not be uniformly vascularized or avascular
  - Contrast-enhanced MR for viability of proximal pole
    - Sensitivity 66%, specificity 88%, accuracy 83%
    - Criteria: ↓ Signal intensity (SI) on both T1 & T2 → no healing with bone grafting
    - ↓ SI on T1 & slight hypointensity on T2 → 75% heal with bone graft
    - Slight hypointensity on T1 & isointensity on T2 → 92% healing with bone graft

Imaging Recommendations
- Best imaging tool
  - Radiographs initially; if negative, MR
  - CT for follow-up
  - MR for viability of fragment
- Protocol advice
  - Obtain navicular views if routine radiographs negative
  - CT: Use overhead positioning to obtain direct oblique sagittal along longitudinal axis of scaphoid; if reformatting from axials, reformat along scaphoid longitudinal axis rather than sagittal wrist
  - MR for viability requires use of contrast

DIFFERENTIAL DIAGNOSIS

Bone Bruise
- If edema present without fx line

PATHOLOGY

General Features
- General path comments
  - Relevant anatomy
    - Entire surface of scaphoid is covered with cartilage because of its extensive articulation with adjacent bones
    - Since there is no periosteum, vessels enter only at sites of ligamentous attachment
    - Primary blood supply to proximal pole is from the dorsal branch radial artery, which enters at waist & has branches coursing proximally and distally
    - Vascular supply to proximal pole is therefore at risk with proximal pole fractures or fractures of the waist, with degree of risk increasing as fracture line becomes more proximal
- Etiology
  - Dorsiflexion secondary to fall on outstretched hand
  - Forceful extension (hyperextension) + radial deviation maximizes forces across scaphoid
  - Tensile fractures: Transverse & begin in palmar cortex
- Epidemiology
  - 71% of all carpal bone fractures
  - 5-12% associated with other fractures
    - Radial styloid, triquetrum, fracture-dislocation
    - Usually due to higher-impact trauma

Gross Pathologic & Surgical Features
- Majority are in waist (70+%)
- Waist fractures stable if noncomminuted & perpendicular to long axis of scaphoid
- Increased obliquity, dorsal comminution & displacement result in instability

SCAPHOID FRACTURES

Staging, Grading or Classification Criteria
- Several classification systems
- Most important information from any of them is whether fracture is stable or unstable
  - Stable scaphoid fracture
    - Incomplete
    - If complete, no fracture motion with wrist motion (overlying cartilage likely intact)
  - Unstable scaphoid fracture
    - Motion about fracture site
    - Cortical offset > 1 mm
    - Fracture angulation
    - Associated ligamentous instability (scapholunate dissociation or DISI (dorsal intercalated segmental instability)
    - Motion with radial or ulnar deviation
    - Requires surgery; cast immobilization alone will not maintain reduction

CLINICAL ISSUES

Presentation
- Most common signs/symptoms: Pain over anatomic snuffbox following trauma

Demographics
- Age
  - 15-60 years
  - Most common in adolescents & young athletes
- Gender: M > F

Natural History & Prognosis
- Up to 90% of acute scaphoid fx heal if treated promptly
- Complications
  - Malunion
    - Most frequent malunion is the humpback angular deformity (apex dorsal angulation)
    - Evaluation: In sagittal plane, measure angle of lines bisecting proximal & distal scaphoid fragments; > 35° abnormal, > 45°, poor outcome
  - Delayed union
    - Delayed union: Incomplete union after 4 months of cast immobilization
    - Related to improper or incomplete immobilization or failure to diagnose & treat promptly
    - Some degree of delayed or nonunion occurs in nearly all proximal pole & 30% scaphoid waist fx
    - Often see resorption of bone & cyst formation at fx site; may still heal with ingrowth of granulation tissue & eventual bony bridging
  - Nonunion
    - Nonunion: 10-15% scaphoid fx do not unite
    - Rounded, sclerotic fracture edges with diastasis & movement of fragments
  - Avascular necrosis (AVN)
    - 15-30% of all scaphoid fractures develop AVN, usually proximal pole
    - Incidence increases with more proximal location of fracture line
    - Diagnosed by fragmentation & collapse
    - Early diagnosis of viability of fragment by contrast-enhanced MR is moderately accurate, but not definitive
    - 30% of scaphoid fx develop ↑ density of proximal pole (by radiograph or CT); this is a relative ischemia, but is frequently reversible; not a reliable sign of impending nonunion or AVN
- Complications result in
  - Limited range of motion & pain
  - Decreased grip strength
  - Osteoarthritis
    - Radioscaphoid joint
    - SNAC (scaphoid nonunion advanced collapse): Appears similar to SLAC (scapholunate advanced collapse), often with DISI as well
- Associated injuries
  - Ligamentous: Scapholunate dissociation & DISI
  - Capitate head shear fracture, triquetral fracture
  - Carpal dislocation

Treatment
- Conservative: Immobilization & casting
  - Stable fx
- Surgical
  - Unstable fx, delayed union, symptomatic nonunion
  - Some treat all nonunions, regardless of symptoms, because of association with secondary osteoarthritis
  - Surgical treatment: Bone graft & internal fixation
  - 82% success rate eventually for nonunions
  - If graft fails & patient in severe pain, intercarpal fusion with resection of proximal pole scaphoid

DIAGNOSTIC CHECKLIST

Consider
- 2-5% scaphoid fx not visible on initial radiographs; with high clinical suspicion, may
  - Splint and return for re-imaging in 7-10 days
  - In many patients waiting for the diagnosis is not acceptable, for a variety of reasons; for these, MR

Image Interpretation Pearls
- Do not expect to see fracture line on all, or even most, of initial radiographs
- Beware of PA view in radial deviation; fx line is obscured
- In follow-up CT for evaluation of union, perform direct sagittals through scaphoid
- Do not overinterpret resorption & cystic change at fx site as impending nonunion; it may be reversible
- Do not overinterpret density in proximal pole as AVN; this is often reversible
- MR, even with contrast, is not 100% accurate in determining viability of fragments

SELECTED REFERENCES
1. Brydie A et al: Early MRI in the management of clinical scaphoid fracture. Br J Radiol. 76(905):296-300, 2003
2. Rennie WJ et al: Posttraumatic cystlike defects of the scaphoid: late sign of occult microfracture and useful indicator of delayed union. AJR Am J Roentgenol. 180(3):655-8, 2003

SCAPHOID FRACTURES

IMAGE GALLERY

Typical

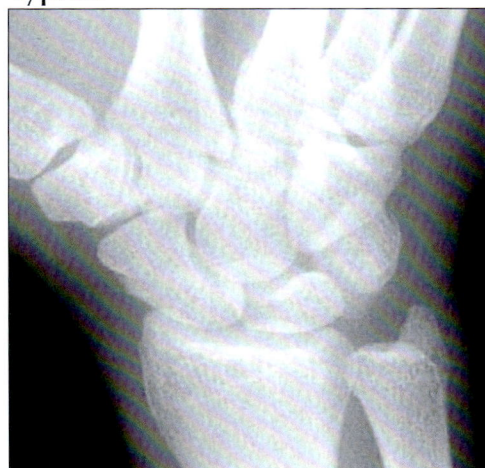 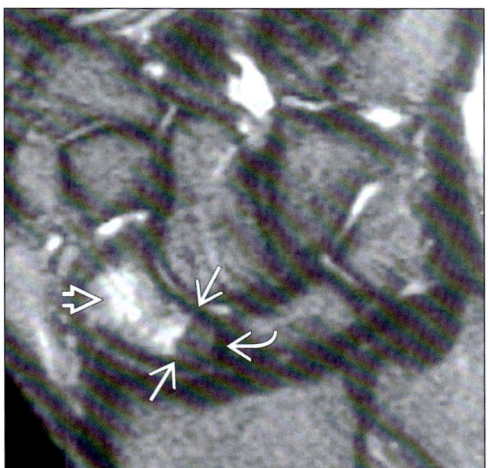

(Left) Oblique radiograph obtained in the ER following FOOSH injury is normal; no scaphoid fx could be seen on any view. *(Right)* Coronal T2WI FS MR (same patient as previous) obtained 20 minutes later, shows nondisplaced proximal scaphoid fx ➡ with marrow edema in the distal fragment ➡, but not in the proximal ➡. Absence of edema in the proximal pole, particularly in the setting of an acute injury, is highly suggestive of ischemia of that fragment, & may lead to osteonecrosis.

Typical

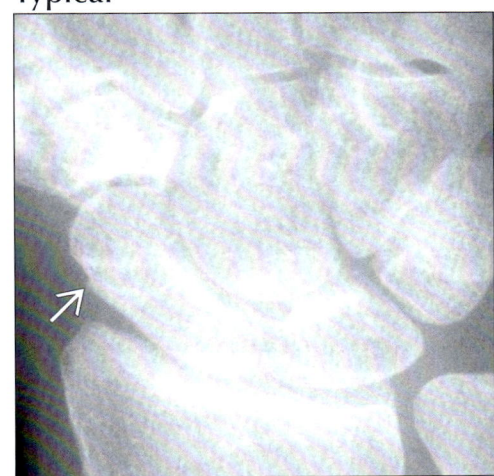 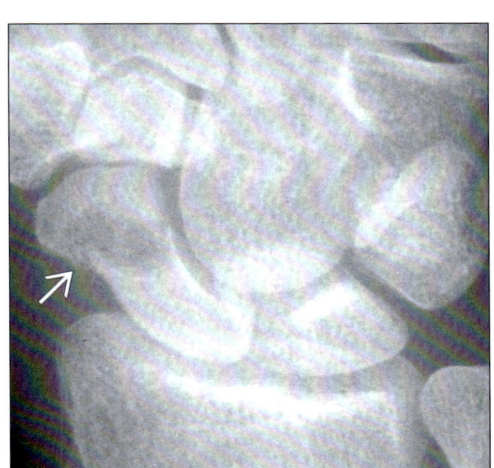

(Left) Posteroanterior radiograph obtained at time of injury does not convincingly show fx. Cortical irregularity at waist of scaphoid ➡ is normal. *(Right)* Posteroanterior radiograph (same patient as previous) obtained 2 months later, shows the missed fx of the distal pole. Resorption & cystic change have occurred at fx site ➡. However, since this is a distal pole fx, it will likely heal with proper immobilization. Granulation tissue forms, with eventual bony bridging.

Typical

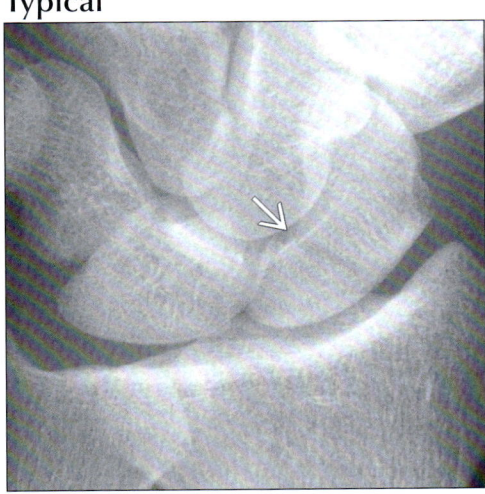 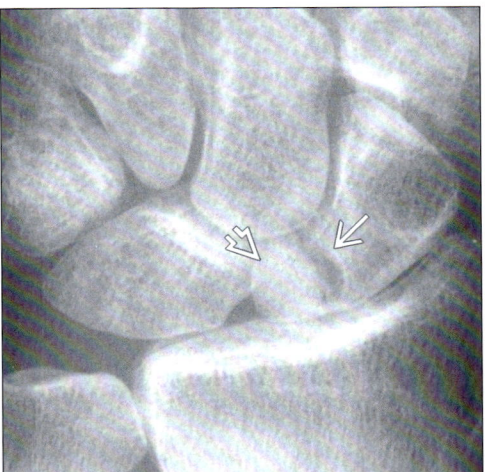

(Left) Posteroanterior radiograph shows fx of proximal pole of scaphoid ➡; it was recognized & appropriately immobilized. *(Right)* Posteroanterior radiograph obtained 4 months later, shows suggestion of sclerosis at fx site ➡, worrisome for impending nonunion. Proximal pole shows some resorption but is also relatively dense ➡. This density is not diagnostic of AVN, as was once thought, as it may recover.

CARPAL FRACTURES, OTHER THAN SCAPHOID

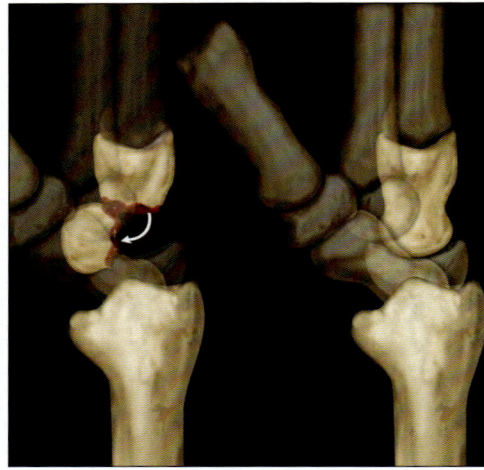

Graphic shows a fractured capitate (left) with typical proximal fragment rotation (may be 90° as this one, or 180°). Capitate fx is difficult to see due to overlapping bones. Normal comparison is shown on the right.

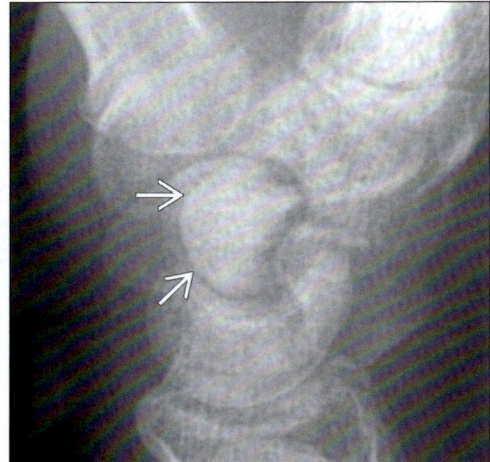

Lateral radiograph shows a fracture at the waist of the capitate. This is a typical location. The proximal fracture fragment has rotated 90 degrees; the proximal cortex is seen directed volarly ➡.

TERMINOLOGY

Abbreviations and Synonyms
- No synonyms; named by bone: Triquetrum, pisiform, hamate, capitate, lunate, trapezium, trapezoid

Definitions
- Cortical/trabecular fracture through osseous structure

IMAGING FINDINGS

General Features
- Best diagnostic clue: Fracture line; best positioning depends on carpal bone & type of fracture
- Location: Depends on structure & whether due to direct blow or avulsion
- Size: Variable; rarely significantly diastased
- Morphology
  ○ Triquetrum
    ▪ Dorsal chip or avulsion: Most common pattern
    ▪ Transverse (more common) or vertical
    ▪ Osteochondral fx at radial aspect of base of triquetrum
    ▪ Osteochondral fx at volar distal ulnar surface
  ○ Pisiform
    ▪ Vertical or transverse
  ○ Hamate
    ▪ Fx of hook is most common
    ▪ Fx of body (usually osteochondral)
    ▪ Fx of dorsum (usually IV and/or V carpometacarpal fx-dislocation)
  ○ Capitate
    ▪ Waist
  ○ Lunate
    ▪ Body
    ▪ Avulsion at volar pole
  ○ Trapezium
    ▪ Transverse or longitudinal (usually intraarticular)
    ▪ Volar-trapezial ridge avulsion injury
  ○ Trapezoid
    ▪ Rare, owing to its stable articulations, especially with 2nd metacarpal

Radiographic Findings
- Many carpal fx are occult by radiography
- **Triquetrum**
  ○ Triquetral dorsal chip best seen on lateral

Other Carpal Fractures

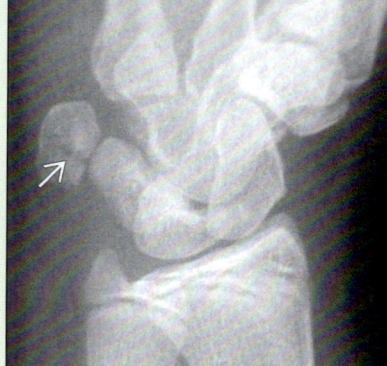

Pisiform, on Supinated Oblique

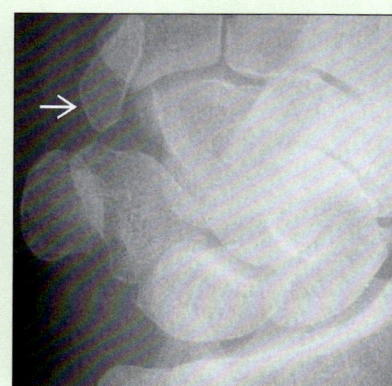

Os Hamuli Proprium

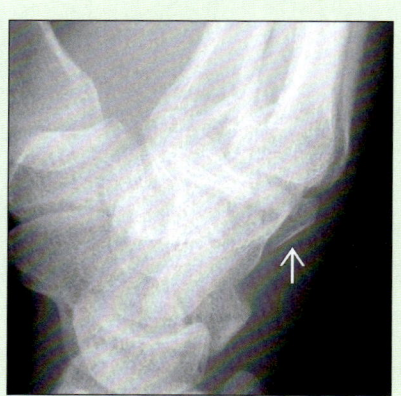

Dorsal Hamate Fx-Dislocation

CARPAL FRACTURES, OTHER THAN SCAPHOID

Key Facts

Imaging Findings
- Triquetral dorsal chip best seen on lateral
- Pisiform vertical or transverse fx seen on PA or semisupinated oblique
- Small osteochondral fragment in pisotriquetral joint recess is suggestive of pisiform fx
- Hook of hamate fx suspected on PA radiograph if the round hook is not visualized or appears smudgy
- Direct view of hook of hamate fx with semisupinated oblique or carpal tunnel view
- Subtle waist fx of capitate seen on PA or lateral
- Proximal pole capitate fx may be rotated 90° to 180°; watch for the rounded proximal cortex in an abnormal position (directed volarly or distally)

Diagnostic Checklist
- Radiographs alone likely significantly underestimate the number & extent of carpal fractures
- CT would increase sensitivity for subtle & small fractures; however, conservative treatment may not be significantly different
- Even specialized images (carpal tunnel, supinated oblique) may not show fx at base of hook of hamate; do not be overconfident in your ability to rule out fx based on radiograph alone
- Axial CT may have abnormalities related to partial volume; sagittal & coronal reformats needed to confirm small fx fragments
- MR may show edema, but fracture may be too small to visualize

---

- o Transverse or vertical best seen on posteroanterior (PA) view
- o Radial or ulnar chip very difficult to visualize
- **Pisiform**
  - o Pisiform vertical or transverse fx seen on PA or semisupinated oblique
  - o Small osteochondral fragment in pisotriquetral joint recess is suggestive of pisiform fx
- **Hamate**
  - o Hook of hamate fx suspected on PA radiograph if the round hook is not visualized or appears smudgy
  - o Direct view of hook of hamate fx with semisupinated oblique or carpal tunnel view
- **Capitate**
  - o Subtle waist fx of capitate seen on PA or lateral
  - o Proximal pole capitate fx may be rotated 90° to 180°; watch for the rounded proximal cortex in an abnormal position (directed volarly or distally)
- **Lunate**
  - o Extremely subtle; dorsal cortical lines of all adjacent bones overlap the lunate, making interruption of lunate cortex difficult to see
  - o Watch for any break in cortex or offset/double density in any surface
  - o Tiny avulsion fx at the proximal radial aspect indicates scapholunate ligament injury/avulsion
- **Trapezium**
  - o PA or oblique most useful for the routine fx pattern
  - o Volar avulsion injury: Carpal tunnel view or CT
- **Trapezoid**: Rare fx usually associated with 2nd metacarpal dislocation, which is more easily seen

CT Findings
- Thin-section CT with reformats useful to demonstrate occult fx, especially chip or avulsions
- With suspected high degree of insensitivity of radiography for carpal fx, CT should be readily used if suspicion is high

MR Findings
- T1 MR: Low signal fracture line; may be subtle
- Fluid sensitive sequences: Edema, may or may not visualize a fracture line

- Small avulsions: Fracture fragment likely to be missed; surrounding edema suggestive of the injury

Nuclear Medicine Findings
- Bone scan shows regional uptake

Imaging Recommendations
- Best imaging tool
  - o Radiographic series of wrist
  - o If negative & pain is on ulnar and volar side, add semisupinated oblique images and/or carpal tunnel
  - o If still negative & strong clinical suspicion, CT
- Protocol advice
  - o Special views to evaluate hook of hamate & pisiform
    - Carpal tunnel (hyperextended wrist, axial view): Difficult to perform effectively to see base of hook of hamate
    - Semisupinated oblique: May need to angle at slightly different degrees of supination to view base of hook of hamate
    - Radial deviated lateral with thumb abducted

DIFFERENTIAL DIAGNOSIS

Carpal Fracture Dislocation
- Evaluate carpal arcs on PA and coaxial alignment of radius/lunate/capitate on lateral views

Os Hamulus Proprius (Unfused Ossification Center)
- May mimic hook of hamate fx
- Differentiated by rounding of base and circumferential cortication

PATHOLOGY

General Features
- Etiology
  - o Triquetrum dorsal chip or avulsion
    - FOOSH with impingement from ulnar styloid
    - Shear forces

CARPAL FRACTURES, OTHER THAN SCAPHOID

- Avulsion by strong ligamentous attachments
  - Triquetral body fracture (transverse): FOOSH, often with carpal dislocation
  - Triquetral chip fx off radial proximal corner: Likely part of a perilunate fx-dislocation
  - Triquetral chip fx off distal volar & ulnar surface: Shear force from a dislocated/subluxed pisiform
  - Pisiform
    - Direct impact from FOOSH
    - Fatigue fracture in volleyball players
  - Hook of hamate
    - Direct blow: FOOSH, direct impact such as catching a ball or hitting club on ground
    - Avulsive force through transverse carpal ligament: Usually associated with racquet sports & golf (repetitive stress): Dominant hand in racquet sports, nondominant hand in baseball, hockey, or golf
  - Body of hamate: Carpal fracture-dislocation (shearing or impaction against lunate or triquetrum)
  - Dorsal hamate: 4th and/or 5th carpometacarpal fracture-dislocation (punching injury, force propagated along metacarpal shaft)
  - Capitate: Direct trauma or FOOSH with fracture-dislocation (fractured waists of scaphoid and capitate termed scaphocapitate syndrome)
  - Lunate: FOOSH or else scapholunate injury with avulsion from lunate
    - FOOSH, often with dislocation
    - Scapholunate injury causes avulsion from lunate
  - Trapezium: High energy impact, often transverse loading injury through an adducted thumb
    - High energy impact, often transverse loading injury through an adducted thumb
    - Avulsion injury by transverse carpal ligament
  - Trapezoid: Fx usually a fx-dislocation pattern at base of 2nd metacarpal
- Epidemiology
  - Fx of carpals & metacarpals account for 6% of all fxs
    - Occult fractures would increase this percentage if their prevalence could be determined
  - Scaphoid fx account for 60-70% of all carpal fx
    - This followed by triquetrum & pisiform (rare, but frequency is likely underestimated)
    - Followed (in approximate order) by: Hamate, capitate, lunate, trapezium, trapezoid

Gross Pathologic & Surgical Features
- Fx body usually has involvement of articular surfaces
- Hook of hamate fx at base: Good blood supply
- Hook of hamate fx located more palmarly: More likely displaced & greater risk of nonunion

CLINICAL ISSUES

Presentation
- Most common signs/symptoms
  - Fall on outstretched hand (FOOSH) injury
  - Grip weakness and pain
  - Hook of hamate or pisiform
    - Pain with resistance to flexion of the fifth finger
    - Paresthesia of 4th & 5th fingers
  - Injury of flexor digitorum profundus muscle occasionally is present

Demographics
- Age: Young, active patients, especially athletes
- Gender: M > F, related to rates of participation in baseball, hockey, golf, & tennis

Natural History & Prognosis
- Generally heal satisfactorily with immobilization
- Hook of hamate fx at risk for nonunion if fracture is located more palmarly than at base
- Undetected (and unreduced) hamate carpometacarpal fx-dislocation: Loss of power grip
- Proximal pole of capitate fracture is covered with hyaline cartilage & rarely may progress from fx to AVN
- Kienbock disease (AVN of lunate) may be a chronic manifestation of lunate fracture; follow-up of any fracture is warranted
- Trapezium fx often associated with wrist injuries or 1st metacarpal intraarticular injuries; at risk for developing early OA

Treatment
- Immobilization (casting/splinting) usually sufficient
- Displaced hook of hamate fx: Internal fixation or surgical resection
- If associated with carpal fracture-dislocation, open reduction internal fixation is usually required
- With persistent pain and non-union, surgical excision of fracture fragment occasionally required

DIAGNOSTIC CHECKLIST

Consider
- Radiographs alone likely significantly underestimate the number & extent of carpal fractures
- CT would increase sensitivity for subtle & small fractures; however, conservative treatment may not be significantly different

Image Interpretation Pearls
- Even specialized images (carpal tunnel, supinated oblique) may not show fx at base of hook of hamate; do not be overconfident in your ability to rule out fx based on radiograph alone
- Axial CT may have abnormalities related to partial volume; sagittal & coronal reformats needed to confirm small fx fragments
- MR may show edema, but fracture may be too small to visualize

SELECTED REFERENCES

1. Blum AG et al: Pathologic conditions of the hypothenar eminence: evaluation with multidetector CT and MR imaging. Radiographics. 26(4):1021-44, 2006
2. Hirano K et al: Classification and treatment of hamate fractures. Hand Surg. 10(2-3):151-7, 2005
3. Rosner JL et al: Imaging of athletic wrist and hand injuries. Semin Musculoskelet Radiol. 8(1):57-79, 2004
4. Goldfarb CA et al: Wrist fractures: what the clinician wants to know. Radiology. 219(1):11-28, 2001

CARPAL FRACTURES, OTHER THAN SCAPHOID

IMAGE GALLERY

Typical

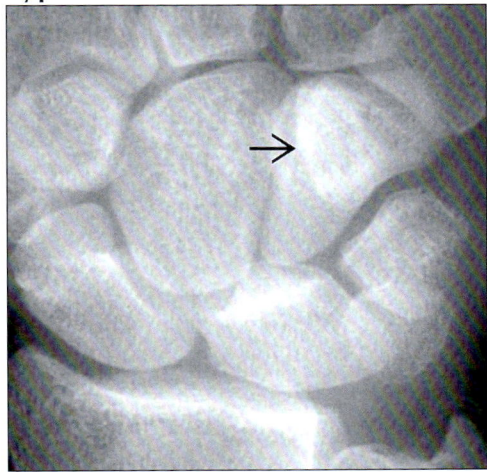
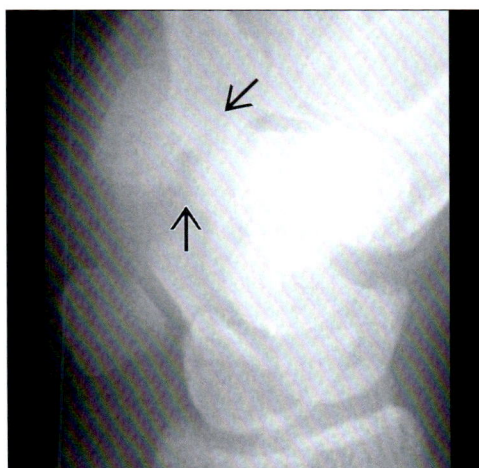

(Left) Posteroanterior radiograph allows inference of a hook of hamate fracture. The hook appears sclerotic and "fuzzy" in its outline ➡. Many, though not all, hook of hamate fractures give this indistinct appearance of the hook due to slight displacement. *(Right)* Semi-supinated oblique radiograph confirms the fracture at the base of the hook ➡. This obliquity can profile the hamate nicely and may obviate the need for a CT.

Typical

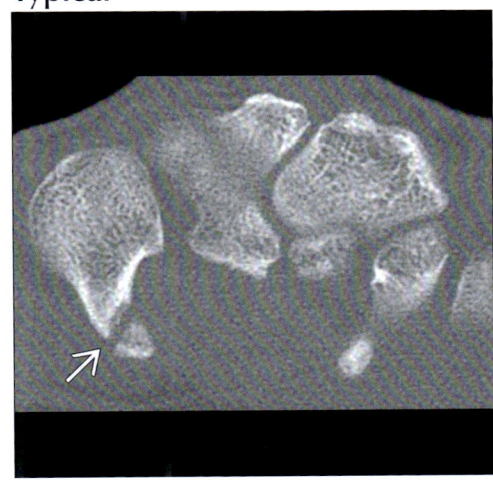
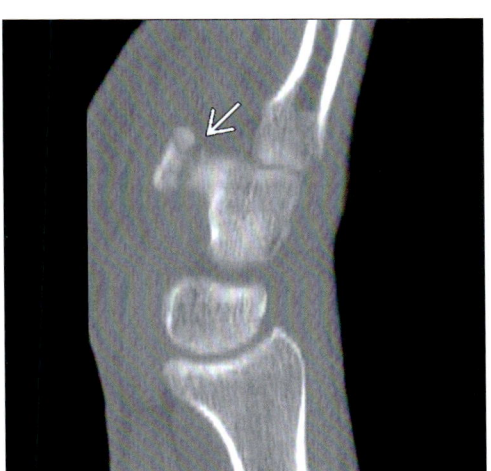

(Left) Axial bone CT shows a fracture at the distal end of the hook of hamate ➡. This is an acute injury. *(Right)* Sagittal bone CT reformat confirms the distal location of the fracture ➡. This site is less well-vascularized than a base of hook fracture, and is at greater risk for displacement and nonunion.

Typical

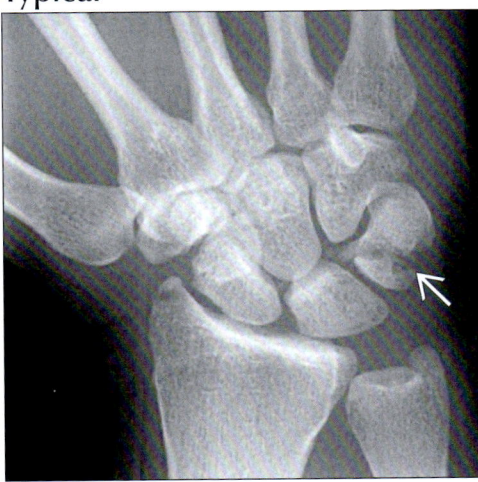
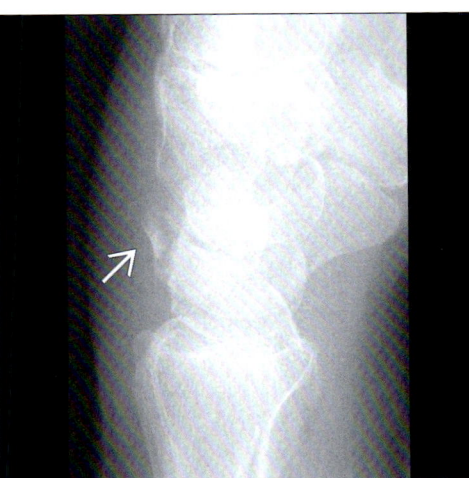

(Left) Posterioranterior radiograph shows transverse fracture of the triquetrum ➡. There is no associated carpal dislocation pattern, so this likely resulted from a direct blow FOOSH type of injury. *(Right)* Lateral radiograph shows a large dorsal chip fracture of the triquetrum ➡. A fracture in this location is virtually always triquetral, resulting from FOOSH injury, often from impingement with the ulnar styloid.

CARPAL DISLOCATIONS

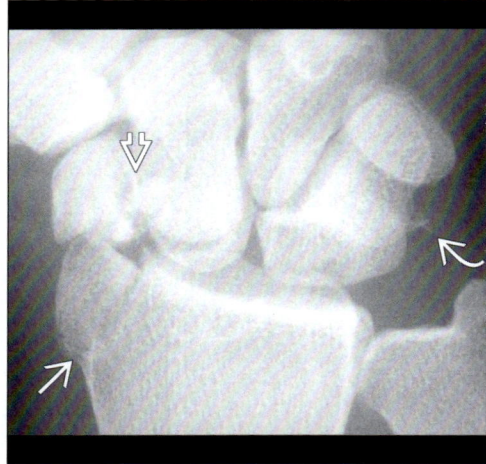

Posteroanterior radiograph shows a fx pattern following the zone of vulnerability: Fx of the radial styloid ➡, scaphoid ➡, & triquetrum ➡. There is disruption of the 1st & 2nd carpal arcs, indicating dislocation.

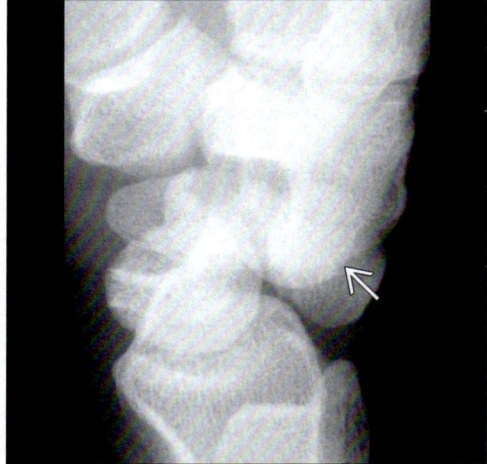

Lateral radiograph shows perilunate dislocation ➡, with dorsal dislocation of the capitate but intact radial-lunate articulation. The diagnosis is transradial, transscaphoid, transtriquetral, perilunate fracture-dislocation.

TERMINOLOGY

Abbreviations and Synonyms
- Types: Perilunate, midcarpal, & lunate dislocations

Definitions
- Dislocation requires complete dissociation of the articular surfaces
- Subluxation or angulation are not the same as dislocation
- Fractures are often associated; the terminology is very specific when this occurs
  - Fractures are named in the order of occurrence, from the radial side towards the ulnar side
  - The term "trans-" is placed in front of each bone that is fractured
  - This is followed by the type of dislocation
  - This is followed by the term "fracture-dislocation"
    - e.g., Transradial, transscaphoid, perilunate fracture-dislocation
    - e.g., Transscaphoid, transcapitate, transhamate, lunate fracture-dislocation

IMAGING FINDINGS

General Features
- Best diagnostic clue
  - Carpal dislocations are frequently & easily missed
  - Dislocation should be suspected based on disruption of the proximal row as seen on posteroanterior views
  - Critical evaluation of a technically good lateral radiograph is required
    - Must be able to pick out a lack of normal articulation between lunate & capitate and radius & lunate
    - Watch for dorsal placement of capitate
    - Watch for volar placement & rotation of lunate
  - Associated fractures must be sought; usually best seen on posteroanterior view
- Location
  - Perilunate dislocation: Dislocation is at midcarpal row
  - Midcarpal dislocation: Dislocation at midcarpal row, subluxation at radius-lunate articulation
  - Lunate dislocation: Dislocation at both radius-lunate articulation & midcarpal row

Other Carpal Dislocations

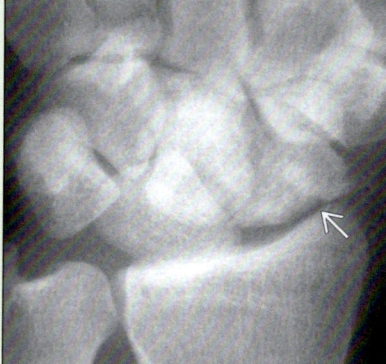

Transscaphoid Lunate Fx/Dis

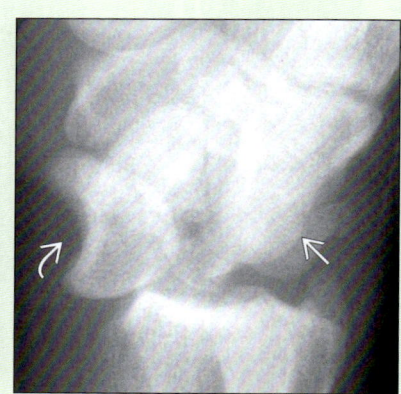

Lateral of Previous Case

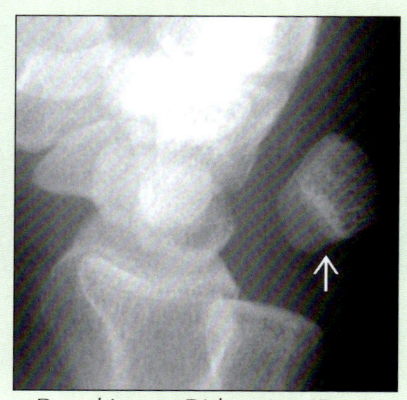

Dorsal Lunate Dislocation (Rare)

CARPAL DISLOCATIONS

Key Facts

Terminology
- Types: Perilunate, midcarpal, & lunate dislocations
- Dislocation requires complete dissociation of the articular surfaces
- Fractures are often associated; the terminology is very specific when this occurs

Imaging Findings
- Posteroanterior view: Disruption of carpal arcs 1 & 2
- Lateral view: Dislocation of carpal bones

Pathology
- Injury patterns follow either greater arc or lesser arc patterns; the patterns may be combined in a fracture-dislocation
- Carpal dislocations much less frequent than carpal fractures
- Perilunate dislocations are most frequent & have the least severe ligamentous damage
- Lunate dislocations are least frequent & have the most severe ligamentous damage

Diagnostic Checklist
- Carpal dislocations often go unrecognized in the ER; a high degree of suspicion may prevent this
- **Posteroanterior view: Evaluate the carpal arcs for disruption**
- Watch for associated fractures: Radial styloid, scaphoid, and on to others around the greater arc
- **Lateral view: Pick out the relevant bones and make certain there is appropriate articulation**
- Radius must articulate with proximal lunate
- Lunate distal articular surface must articulate with capitate

---

- Size: Ranges from perilunate dislocation (least damage) through lunate dislocation (most damage)
- Morphology: Crucial axis is the coaxial articulation of the distal radius-lunate-capitate

Radiographic Findings
- Posteroanterior view: Disruption of carpal arcs 1 & 2
  - Carpal arc 1 describes smooth contour of proximal aspect of proximal carpal row
  - Carpal arc 2 describes smooth contour of distal aspect of proximal carpal row
  - With disruption of these two carpal arcs, the lunate usually assumes a triangular appearance
- Lateral view: Dislocation of carpal bones
  - Simplify search by looking for relationship of distal radius, lunate, & capitate
  - There is a normal coaxial relationship, with radius articulating with lunate & lunate articulating with capitate
  - Perilunate dislocation
    - Capitate dislocates from lunate in a dorsal direction
    - Remainder of carpus follows capitate
    - Lunate remains articulating with radius
  - Midcarpal dislocation
    - Capitate dislocates from lunate in dorsal direction
    - Capitate drifts proximally towards radius, nudging lunate volarly
    - Lunate is subluxed but not dislocated from the radius
  - Lunate dislocation
    - Capitate dislocated from lunate
    - Capitate drifts proximally towards articulation of radius
    - Lunate dislocated from radius in a volar direction, rotated 90° volarly
- Fractures are frequently associated with carpal dislocations & may be seen on either view

Imaging Recommendations
- Best imaging tool: Radiographs; a true lateral is required to make a correct diagnosis

DIFFERENTIAL DIAGNOSIS

Carpal Instability
- Anteroposterior radiograph may appear similar, with disrupted arcs 1 & 2 as well as lunate tilt (triangular appearance)
- Diagnosis is secured on lateral, where an instability pattern shows abnormal angulation of the carpals, but no true dislocation

PATHOLOGY

General Features
- General path comments
  - Injury patterns follow either greater arc or lesser arc patterns; the patterns may be combined in a fracture-dislocation
  - Greater arc
    - Runs through radial styloid, waist of scaphoid, waist of capitate, base of hamate, base of triquetrum, & ulnar styloid
    - Greater arc injuries extend as fractures through these sites, or through the ligaments adjacent to these bones
    - Common greater arc injury: Transscaphoid perilunate fracture-dislocation, in which arc of injury passes through scaphoid waist, across ligaments fixing distal carpal row & triquetrum to lunate, & ulnar styloid
    - More fractures may be encountered, generally starting from radial side and extending towards ulnar
    - Another example: Transradial, transscaphoid, transcapitate perilunate fracture-dislocation
  - Lesser arc (also termed perilunate injuries)
    - Confined to ligaments surrounding lunate, starting on radial side and extending towards ulnar side
    - Ligamentous injury becomes more severe as injuries extend from radial to ulnar side

CARPAL DISLOCATIONS

- Dislocation pattern advances through a staging, associated with sequence of ligamentous injuries
- Etiology
  - Significant fall on hyperextended hand
  - On impact, hand & wrist undergo hyperextension, ulnar deviation, & intercarpal supination (rotary motion between the proximal & distal carpal rows)
  - Ligamentous sling of carpus is loaded in tension from radial side, & sequence of injuries ensues
    - Stage 1: Scapholunate dissociation or rotary subluxation: Rupture of proximal ligamentous attachments of scaphoid, opening space of Poirier on radial side; may also fracture scaphoid
    - Stage 2: Pericapitate dislocation: Capitate dislocates from lunate dorsally, taking with it remainder of carpus; triquetral ligaments remain intact
    - Stage 3: Midcarpal dislocation: Under continued loading triquetral ligaments fail by tear or avulsion, separating triquetrum from lunate
    - Stage 4: Lunate dislocation: If there is sufficient force to tear dorsal radiocarpal ligament, dorsally dislocated carpus ejects lunate from radius volarly; capitate collapses proximally towards radial surface; dislocated lunate is rotated 90° volarly, still held to the radius by its volar ligaments
  - Most frequently associated with high energy trauma
    - Motor vehicle accident
    - Fall from height
    - Industrial-related accident
- Epidemiology
  - Carpal dislocations much less frequent than carpal fractures
  - Both carpal dislocations and carpal fractures less frequent than forearm fractures
  - Of the carpal dislocations, the frequency of occurrence is inversely related to the severity of ligamentous injury
    - Perilunate dislocations are most frequent & have the least severe ligamentous damage
    - Lunate dislocations are least frequent & have the most severe ligamentous damage

Gross Pathologic & Surgical Features

- Intrinsic ligamentous disruption, frequently associated with fracture

CLINICAL ISSUES

Presentation
- Most common signs/symptoms: Pain and deformity following significant trauma

Demographics
- Age: Young adults involved in high energy trauma
- Gender: Male > female, related to likelihood of high energy trauma

Natural History & Prognosis
- Even with adequate reduction and healing of fractures, long term results usually show wrist compromise
  - Grip strength reduced
  - Instability
  - Associated osteoarthritis

Treatment
- Prompt recognition is required
- Immediate reduction, usually requiring distraction of the wrist
- Stable temporary internal fixation
  - Open reduction, arthroscopic reduction, & fluoroscopically-aided percutaneous techniques can all be successful

DIAGNOSTIC CHECKLIST

Consider
- Carpal dislocations often go unrecognized in the ER; a high degree of suspicion may prevent this

Image Interpretation Pearls
- **Anteroposterior view: Evaluate the carpal arcs for disruption**
- Watch for associated fractures: Radial styloid, scaphoid, and on to others around the greater arc
- **Lateral view: Pick out the relevant bones and make certain there is appropriate articulation**
  - Radius must articulate with proximal lunate
  - Lunate distal articular surface must articulate with capitate

SELECTED REFERENCES

1. Givissis P et al: Neglected trans-scaphoid trans-styloid volar dislocation of the lunate. Late result following open reduction and K-wire fixation. J Bone Joint Surg Br. 88(5):676-80, 2006
2. Grabow RJ et al: Carpal dislocations. Hand Clin. 22(4):485-500; abstract vi-vii, 2006
3. Leung YF et al: Transscaphoid transcapitate transtriquetral perilunate fracture-dislocation: a case report. J Hand Surg [Am]. 31(4):608-10, 2006
4. Osti M et al: Scaphoid and capitate fracture with concurrent scapholunate dissociation. J Hand Surg [Br]. 31(1):76-8, 2006
5. Weil WM et al: Open and arthroscopic treatment of perilunate injuries. Clin Orthop Relat Res. 445:120-32, 2006
6. Amaravati RS et al: Greater arc injury of the wrist with fractured lunate bone: a case report. J Orthop Surg (Hong Kong). 13(3):310-3, 2005
7. Park MJ et al: Arthroscopically assisted reduction and percutaneous fixation of dorsal perilunate dislocations and fracture-dislocations. Arthroscopy. 21(9):1153, 2005
8. Tomaino MM: Preliminary lunate reduction and pinning facilitates restoration of carpal height when treating perilunate dislocation, scaphoid fracture and nonunion, and scapholunate dissociation. Am J Orthop. 33(3):153-4, 2004
9. Herzberg G et al: Acute dorsal trans-scaphoid perilunate fracture-dislocations: medium-term results. J Hand Surg [Br]. 27(6):498-502, 2002
10. Gilula LA: Carpal injuries: analytic approach and case exercises. AJR Am J Roentgenol. 133(3):503-17, 1979

CARPAL DISLOCATIONS

IMAGE GALLERY

Typical

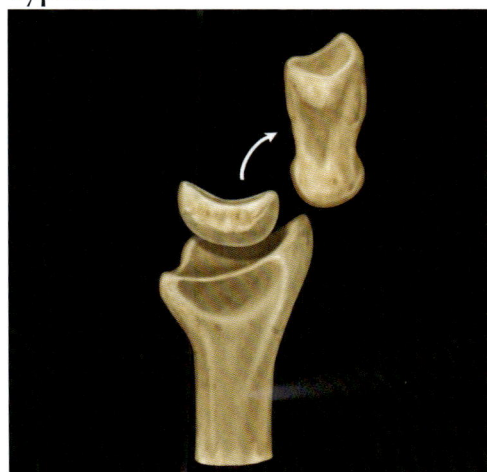 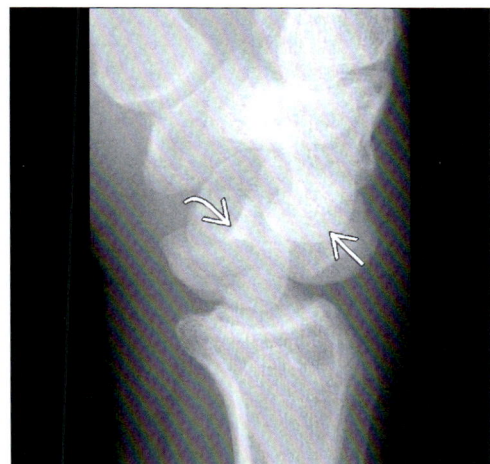

(Left) Lateral graphic shows a perilunate dislocation. The capitate dislocates from the lunate in a dorsal direction (taking the remainder of the carpus with it); the lunate maintains its normal articulation with the radius. *(Right)* Lateral radiograph of a perilunate dislocation. The lunate articulates normally with the radius. However, the capitate ➡ is dislocated relative to the lunate ➡. Note that the remainder of the carpus moves dorsally with the capitate.

Typical

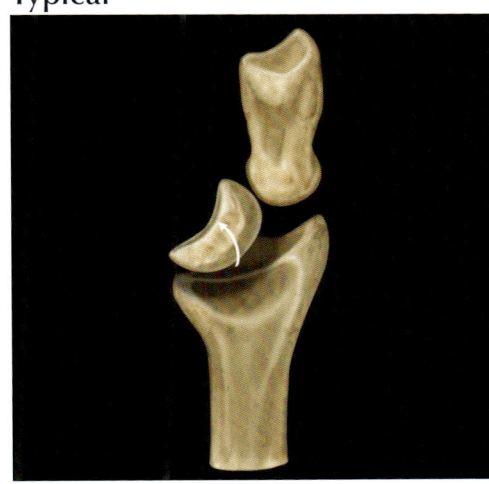 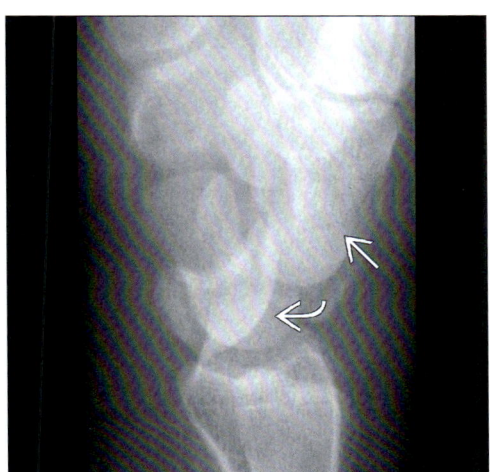

(Left) Lateral graphic shows a midcarpal dislocation. This is the next step following perilunate dislocation. The dislocated capitate nudges the lunate volarly, but the lunate is not yet dislocated from the radius. *(Right)* Lateral radiograph of a midcarpal dislocation, where the posteriorly dislocated capitate ➡ sinks proximally and pushes the lunate slightly volarly ➡. The lunate is not completely dislocated from the radius, but is subluxated.

Typical

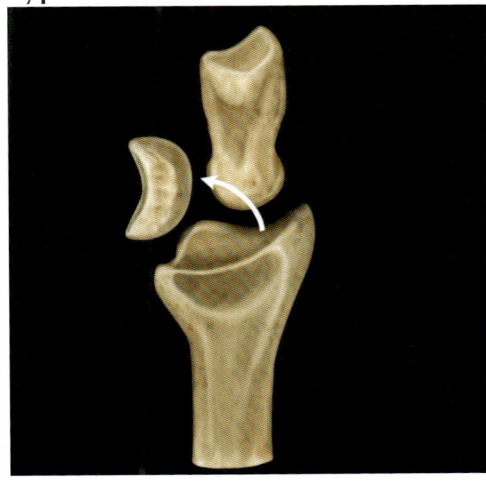 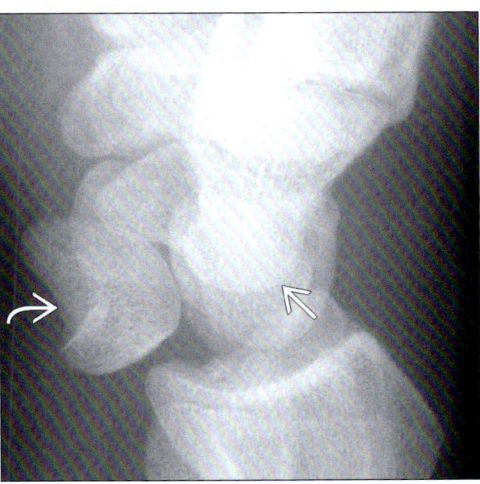

(Left) Lateral graphic of a lunate dislocation, the next stage of carpal dislocation. As the dislocated capitate sinks proximally towards the radius, it pushes the lunate volarly. As the lunate dislocates, it typically tilts 90° in the volar direction. *(Right)* Lateral radiograph shows a typical lunate dislocation, with dorsal dislocation of the capitate ➡ relative to the lunate, as well as the lunate dislocated from the radius. As the lunate dislocates volarly, it rotates 90 degrees ➡.

CARPAL INSTABILITIES

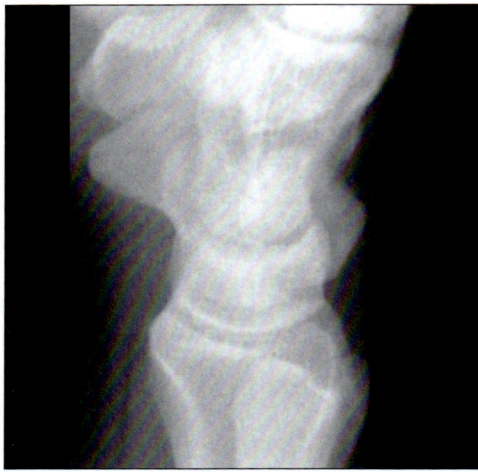

Lateral radiograph shows the normal expected coaxial alignment of the radius, lunate, and capitate. The capitate-lunate angle should be less than 20° and the scapholunate angle should range from 30-60°.

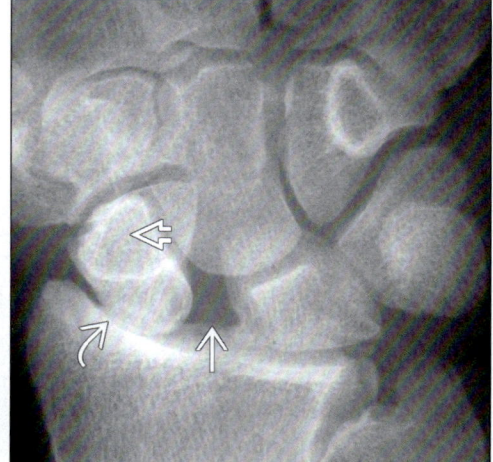

Posteroanterior radiograph shows S-L dissociation ➡. Abnormal volar subluxation of the scaphoid is inferred from the "target" or "ring" seen at the distal pole ➡. There is associated OA of the radiocarpal joint ➡.

TERMINOLOGY

Abbreviations and Synonyms
- Dorsiflexion instability, dorsal intercalated segmental instability (DISI)
- Volarflexion instability, volar intercalated segmental instability (VISI)
- Capitolunate instability pattern (CLIP)
- Scapholunate advanced collapse (SLAC)
- Palmar midcarpal instability (PMCI)

Definitions
- Instability: Inability to withstand normal loading
- Static instability: Seen on routine images, without motion needed for detection
- Dynamic instability: Requires motion (fluoroscopy) or force (clenched fist, deviation) to be detected
- Translocation: Shift of the entire carpus from its normal position relative to the radius
- Dissociation: Abnormal motion between bones within the same carpal row, often in association with interruption of the corresponding interosseous ligament
- Intercalated segment instability: Instability between carpal rows (particular focus on alignment between lunate & capitate)
- Carpal columns: Run perpendicular to carpal rows
  - Central column: Radius-lunate-capitate
  - Radial column: Radius-scaphoid-trapezium
  - Ulnar column: Ulna-triquetrum-hamate

IMAGING FINDINGS

General Features
- Best diagnostic clue: Abnormal alignment of carpal bones, either static or dynamic, with associated ligamentous injuries
- Morphology
  - **Scapholunate dissociation with rotary subluxation of scaphoid**
    - Scapholunate widening > 3 mm
    - Scapholunate angle on lateral > 60°
    - Disruption of scapholunate ligament + extrinsic radioscaphocapitate ligament
  - DISI: Axes of radius, lunate, & capitate (central column) assume a zigzag configuration

SLAC Wrist with Hamato-Lunate Impingement & Radiocarpal OA

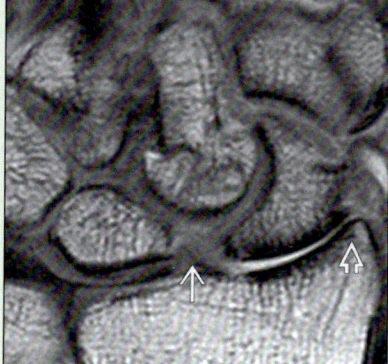

S-L Tear & Radiocarpal OA

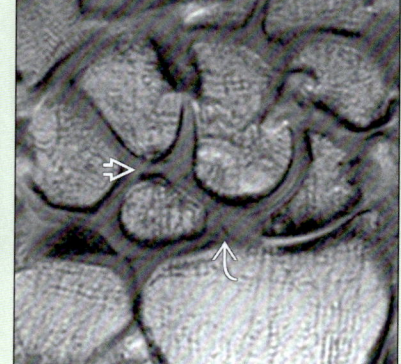

SLAC & Hamato-Lunate OA

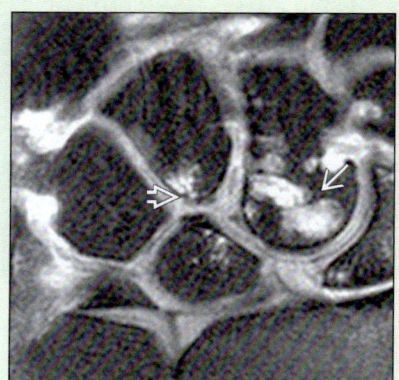

Associated Cyst Formation

CARPAL INSTABILITIES

Key Facts

Imaging Findings
- Best diagnostic clue: Abnormal alignment of carpal bones, either static or dynamic, with associated ligamentous injuries
- **Scapholunate dissociation with rotary subluxation of scaphoid**
- Scapholunate widening > 3 mm
- Scapholunate angle on lateral > 60°
- **DISI: Axes of radius, lunate, & capitate (central column) assume a zigzag configuration**
- Dorsal angulation (dorsiflexion) of lunate relative to radius
- Results in abnormal angulations: Capitolunate angle > 20°, scapholunate angle > 60°
- **VISI: Axes of radius, lunate, & capitate (central column) assume a reverse zigzag configuration**
- Volar angulation (volarflexion) of lunate relative to radius
- Results in abnormal angulations: Capitolunate angle > 20°, scapholunate angle < 30°
- **CLIP: Dynamic instability of the central column**
- **Triquetrohamate instability**: Dynamic instability of the ulnar column; ulnar-sided pain & reproducible click
- **Carpal translocation**: May occur in any direction, but ulnar most frequent; extrinsic ligament tears

Pathology
- Often overlooked initially as "wrist sprain" if no fracture seen at initial imaging & time of injury
- Inflammatory arthritis (particularly RA) can cause enough ligamentous damage to result in instability

---

- Dorsal angulation (dorsiflexion) of lunate relative to radius
- Volar angulation of capitate relative to lunate
- Radial side abnormalities, rotary subluxation of scaphoid is a frequent component
- Results in abnormal angulations: Capitolunate angle > 20°, scapholunate angle > 60°
○ **VISI: Axes of radius, lunate, & capitate (central column) assume a reverse zigzag configuration**
  - Volar angulation (volarflexion) of lunate relative to radius
  - Dorsal angulation of capitate relative to lunate
  - Ulnar side ligamentous abnormalities, including lunotriquetral (intrinsic) & ulnar arm arcuate, dorsal radiolunotriquetral, or volar radioscaphocapitate ligaments
  - Initially is a dynamic instability (palmar midcarpal instability = PMCI)
  - Results in abnormal angulations: Capitolunate angle > 20°, scapholunate angle < 30°
○ **CLIP: Dynamic instability of the central column**
○ **Triquetrohamate instability**: Dynamic instability of the ulnar column; ulnar-sided pain & reproducible click
○ **Carpal translocation**: May occur in any direction, but ulnar most frequent; extrinsic ligament tears

Radiographic Findings
- Posteroanterior view: Signs of instability
  ○ Loss of scapholunate articular parallelism; lunate may assume a triangular appearance
  ○ Scapholunate diastasis > 3 mm for scapholunate dissociation
  ○ Target or ring sign with scaphoid foreshortening if scaphoid is abnormally volarly flexed
- Lateral view: Signs of instability
  ○ Dorsal or volarflexion of lunate with abnormal capitolunate angle (> 20°) and scapholunate angle (< 30° or > 60°): VISI or DISI, respectively
  ○ Radioscaphoid angle > 80°: Abnormal volarflexion of scaphoid (often seen with scapholunate dissociation & DISI)
- Clenched fist views (in AP, ulnar, and radial deviation) may show a dynamic instability pattern

Fluoroscopic Findings
- Manipulation under fluoroscopy may be needed to demonstrate extent of injury or presence of dynamic instability

MR Findings
- T1 MR: Loss of osseous alignment; reactive change in bone
- Fluid sensitive sequences
  ○ Intrinsic ligament tear or thinning
  ○ Synovitis or disruption extrinsic ligament (especially volar radiocarpal)
- MR arthrogram (direct or indirect): Improves visualization of intrinsic ligament tear, perforation in extrinsic ligaments, cartilage thinning

Imaging Recommendations
- Best imaging tool
  ○ Radiographs for static instability
  ○ Fluoroscopy for dynamic instability
  ○ MR for evaluation of intrinsic & extrinsic ligaments
- Protocol advice
  ○ Manipulation under fluoroscopy can evaluate for specific instabiities by the following maneuvers
    - Scapholunate dissociation: Widening of scapholunate interval, generally provoked with clenched fist or ulnar deviation
    - Midcarpal instability (dynamic process prior to fixed VISI): Loss of normal physiologic VISI to DISI when move from radial to ulnar deviation; reproducible clunk
    - CLIP: In lateral position, stabilize patient's forearm with the wrist in slight ulnar deviation; grasp patient's hand at the metacarpals & apply alternating dorsal and volar oriented force; observe for subluxation at the capitolunate articulation

CARPAL INSTABILITIES

- Triquetrum-hamate instability: During radial to ulnar deviation, proximal carpal row abruptly shifts from palmar flexion to dorsi flexion just before extreme ulnar flexion is achieved; hamate may slide against the triquetrum

DIFFERENTIAL DIAGNOSIS

Carpal Dislocation
- Triangular appearance of lunate on PA radiograph & loss of articular parallelism may suggest dislocation
- Lateral view differentiates abnormal angulation from dislocation at the middle carpal column

Inflammatory Arthritis
- Pyrophosphate arthropathy may result in SLAC wrist
- Rheumatoid arthritis may result in any deformity, but particularly ulnar translocation & VISI

PATHOLOGY

General Features
- General path comments
  - Relevant anatomy
    - In neutral position, the axes of radius, lunate, & capitate are collinear on lateral images
    - With flexion or extension, half the normal motion occurs between lunate & radius; half between capitate & lunate
    - Normal scapholunate angle on lateral: 30-60°
    - Normal capitolunate angle on lateral: ≤ 20°
    - Extrinsic carpal ligaments provide gross stability
    - Intrinsic carpal ligaments: "Fine tuning" of carpal stability
    - Scapholunate ligament: Dorsal portion most important to carpal stability
    - Lunatetriquetral ligament: Volar portion most important to carpal stability
    - Extrinsic ligaments: Organized thickenings of dorsal & volar capsules
    - Volar extrinsic ligaments important to carpal stability: Radioscaphocapitate (interdigitates with ulnocapitate & triquetrocapitate to form arcuate), radiolunotriquetral, ulnotriquetral, ulnar collateral
    - Dorsal extrinsic ligaments important to carpal stability, particularly dorsal radiocarpal
- Etiology
  - Axial compression/hyperextension & intercarpal supination
  - FOOSH or backward fall on pronated hand
  - Often overlooked initially as "wrist sprain" if no fracture seen at initial imaging & time of injury
  - Inflammatory arthritis (particularly RA) can cause enough ligamentous damage to result in instability
    - Most common etiology of ulnar translocation
    - VISI more common than DISI
- Epidemiology
  - Scapholunate tear leads to most common types of carpal instabilities
  - Ligament injuries resulting in instability may be either isolated or residua of old perilunate injury

CLINICAL ISSUES

Presentation
- Most common signs/symptoms
  - Acute instability
    - Pain & swelling, related to site of injury
    - Painful clicking/clunk, reproducible
  - Chronic instability
    - History of "wrist sprain"
    - Pain & instability
    - Decreased grip strength
    - Post-traumatic arthritis
    - Painful clicks

Demographics
- Age: Adult population
- Gender
  - M = F in younger population
  - Older women with rheumatoid arthritis

Natural History & Prognosis
- Scapholunate dissociation can progress to SLAC wrist deformity
  - Due to chronic abnormal motion
  - Medial scaphoid & lateral lunate collapse, with capitate interposed
- Midcarpal instability (dynamic) can progress to fixed VISI

Treatment
- Conservative: Activity modification, NSAIDs, steroid injection, wrist immobilization
- Surgical if continued pain & instability
  - Acute: Closed reduction + internal fixation
  - Ligament reconstruction: Acute or chronic
  - Chronic: Capsular tightening
  - Chronic: Limited arthrodesis

DIAGNOSTIC CHECKLIST

Consider
- Clinical exam of characteristic sites of pain, clunk on exam, assessed in combination with imaging findings
- Clicking of carpus is common in asymptomatic wrists

SELECTED REFERENCES

1. Bencardino JT et al: Sports-related injuries of the wrist: an approach to MRI interpretation. Clin Sports Med. 25(3):409-32, vi, 2006
2. Kaufmann RA et al: Kinematics of the midcarpal and radiocarpal joint in flexion and extension: an in vitro study. J Hand Surg [Am]. 31(7):1142-8, 2006
3. Schmitt R et al: Carpal instability. Eur Radiol. 16(10):2161-78, 2006
4. Theumann NH et al: Association between extrinsic and intrinsic carpal ligament injuries at MR arthrography and carpal instability at radiography: initial observations. Radiology. 238(3):950-7, 2006
5. Cerezal L et al: Wrist MR arthrography: how, why, when. Radiol Clin North Am. 43(4):709-31, viii, 2005
6. Theumann NH et al: Extrinsic carpal ligaments: normal MR arthrographic appearance in cadavers. Radiology. 226(1):171-9, 2003

CARPAL INSTABILITIES

IMAGE GALLERY

Typical

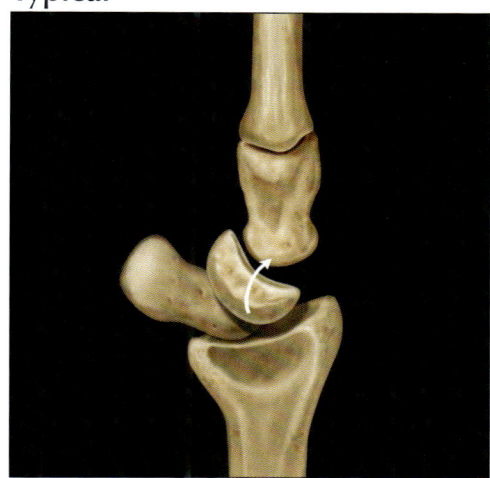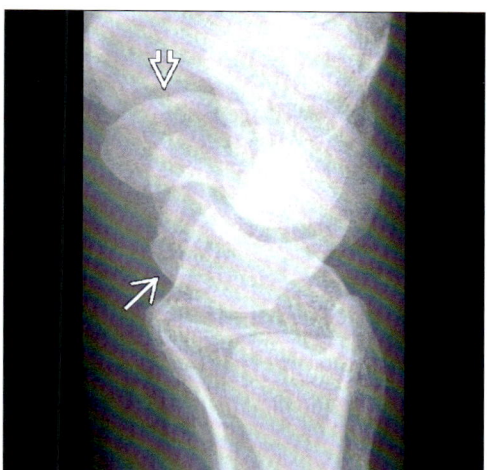

(Left) Lateral graphic shows a DISI pattern. The lunate is tilted dorsally & the scaphoid usually rotates volarly (as in this case). This results in an increased lunate-capitate angle (> 20°) & an increased scapholunate angle (> 60°). *(Right)* Lateral radiograph of a DISI pattern, with dorsal tilt of the lunate ⇨ & volar tilt of the scaphoid ⇨. The lunate-capitate angle measures > 20° & the scapholunate angle measures 90°. Note that the bones are tilted but not subluxed or dislocated.

Typical

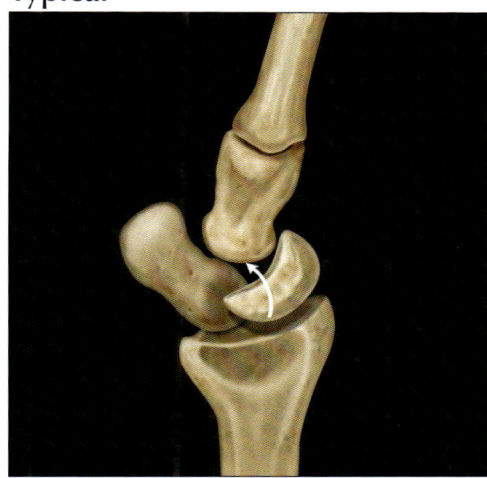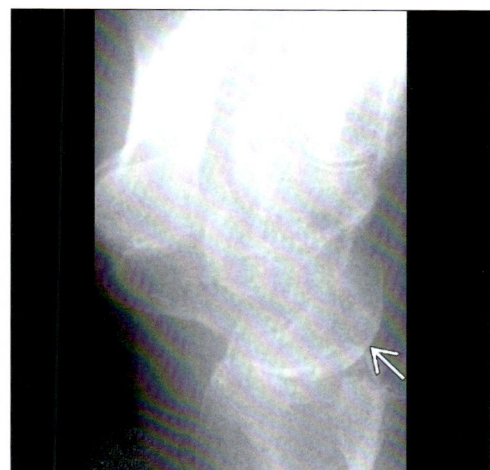

(Left) Lateral graphic shows a VISI pattern. The lunate is volarly tilted (but remains articulating with both the radius & capitate). This results in a lunate-capitate angle > 20° and scapholunate angle < 30°. *(Right)* Lateral radiograph shows a VISI pattern. The lunate is tilted volarly ⇨, resulting in a lunate-capitate angle which far exceeds 20°. The scapholunate angle is far reduced, approaching 0°. Note that this is an abnormality in angulation, not a dislocation.

Typical

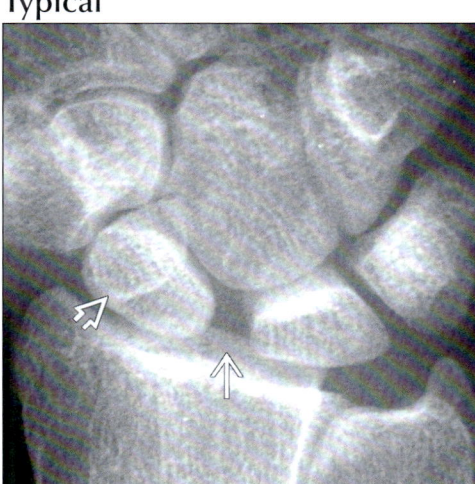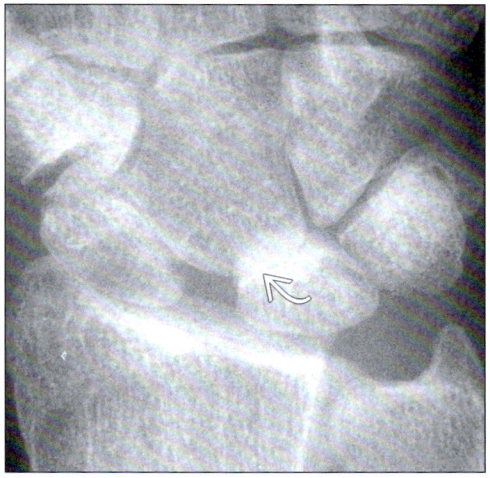

(Left) Posteroanterior radiograph shows scapholunate dissociation ⇨, with volar rotation of the scaphoid seen as a "target sign" of the distal pole ⇨. No arthritic changes are seen. *(Right)* Posteroanterior radiograph obtained one year later shows that the scapholunate dissociation has progressed to a SLAC (scapholunate advanced collapse) deformity, with the capitate displaced proximally ⇨ and OA at both the midcarpal and radiocarpal joints.

METACARPAL FRACTURES AND DISLOCATIONS

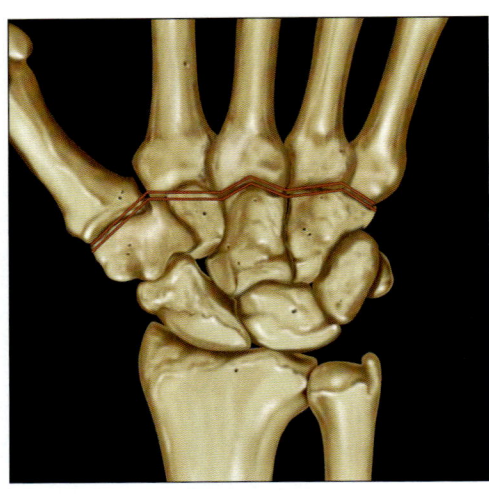

Posteroanterior graphic shows the "zig-zag" or "M" pattern outlining the carpometacarpal joints. Disruption of these articulations is usually subtle; checking this articulation carefully at each joint is crucial.

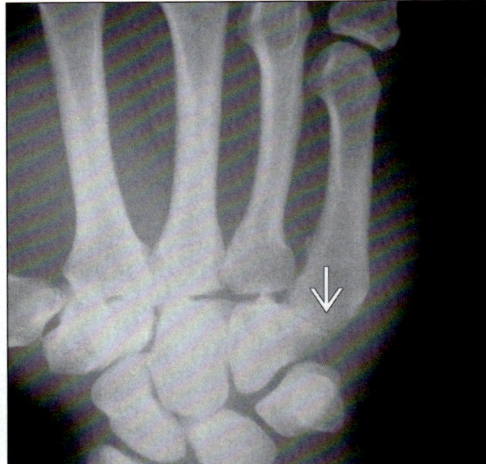

Posteroanterior radiograph shows disruption of the "zig-zag" pattern of the CMC joint at the 5th, with overlap of the base of the 5th MC and its hamate articulation ➡. This is a dislocation.

TERMINOLOGY

Abbreviations and Synonyms
- Carpometacarpal joint (CMC)
- Metacarpal (MC)
- Metacarpal-phalangeal joint (MCP)
- Bennett fracture: Single intraarticular fracture at base of 1st MC
- Rolando fracture: Intraarticular fracture at base of 1st MC, comminuted
- Boxer's fracture: Transverse fx neck MC, generally 5th and/or 4th

Definitions
- Fracture of metacarpal shaft
- Intraarticular fracture at metacarpal base
- Fracture/dislocation at CMC joint (fracture can be at either carpal bone or MC base)

IMAGING FINDINGS

General Features
- Best diagnostic clue
  - MC neck fx: Apex dorsal angulation best seen on lateral view
  - MC shaft fx: Shortening best seen on posteroanterior (PA) view
  - CMC dislocation: Loss of parallelism and symmetry at CMC joints
    - "Parallel M" or "zig-zag" pattern of CMC joints
    - Overlap at 2nd to 5th CMC joint margins
    - Loss of distinct cortical rim at apposing articular margins
  - CMC dislocation: Associated fractures of dorsal capitate and/or hamate
  - CMC dislocation: Disruption of the longitudinal axis seen on the lateral view (usually dorsal dislocation)
- Location
  - Neck of MC: Transverse
  - Shaft of MC: Oblique or spiral
  - Base of MC: Usually intraarticular
  - CMC joint: Generally dorsal dislocation MC, often with associated fracture of carpal bone
- Size: Fractures at base of MC generally small and subtle
- Morphology
  - Direction of CMC dislocations

Other Carpometacarpal Injuries

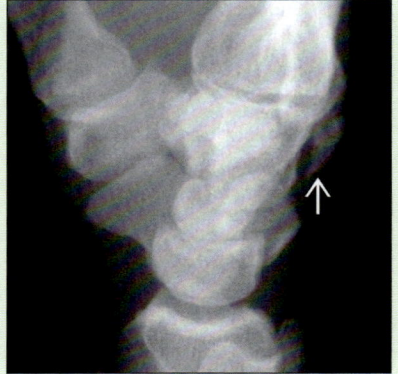

5th CMC Fx/Dislocation

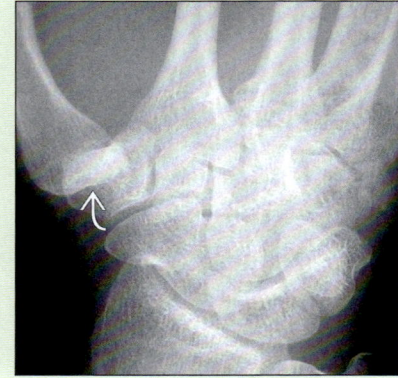

1st CMC Dislocation

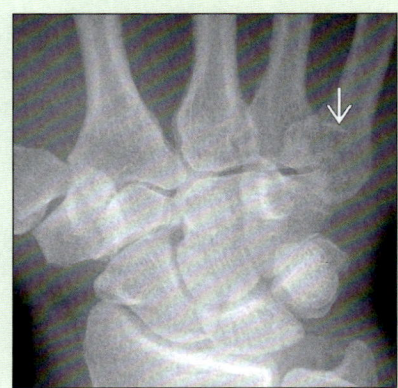

Intraarticular Fx Base 5th MC

METACARPAL FRACTURES AND DISLOCATIONS

Key Facts

Terminology
- Bennett fracture: Single intraarticular fracture at base of 1st MC
- Rolando fracture: Intraarticular fracture at base of 1st MC, comminuted

Imaging Findings
- CMC dislocation: Loss of parallelism and symmetry at CMC joints
- CMC dislocation: Associated fractures of dorsal capitate and/or hamate
- CMC dislocation: Disruption of the longitudinal axis seen on the lateral view (usually dorsal dislocation)

Pathology
- Majority CMC dislocations are multiple (60%)

- If CMC dislocations multiple, 30% involve 4th & 5th CMC

Clinical Issues
- Greater fx deformity of MC neck is tolerated in the ring & 5th finger than in the 2nd & 3rd MCs

Diagnostic Checklist
- Infection should be considered in patient with punching type of injury to MC head/neck
- If MCP contacts opponent's teeth, the skin can be broken and bacteria introduced into joint
- Fx of the dorsal surface of the distal carpal bones or of the MC bases suggests a CMC dislocation
- Angulated fx of the MC shaft suggests a dislocation at the corresponding CMC or adjacent CMC joint

---

- Dorsal: 60%
- Volar: 20%
- Ulnar: 15%
  - 5th CMC dislocation
    - Typically dorsal; occasionally volarly dislocated (two types)
    - Volar radial type: All ligamentous & tendon attachments are torn (more frequent of the volar types)
    - Volar ulnar type: Pisometacarpal ligament & flexor carpi ulnaris tendon attachments remain intact
    - In addition to dorsal displacement of MC, the extensor carpi ulnaris frequently displaces the MC proximally
  - Bennett fracture
    - Volar and ulnarly located fracture fragment remains located relative to trapezium (volar beak ligament holds it in alignment with trapezium)
    - Remainder of 1st MC subluxes radially relative to trapezium (displaced by abductor pollicis tendons)
  - MC neck fractures: Generally transverse, with apex dorsal angulation & associated shortening
  - MC spiral fractures
    - Often associated shortening
    - Rotation can be difficult to assess radiographically; clinical evaluation by flexing MCP and IP joints is more reliable

Radiographic Findings
- Routine 3 views of hand usually adequate for diagnosis of injuries to digits 2-5
- Thumb injuries require 3 views specifically of thumb
- Check alignment at CMC joint particularly carefully on PA view
- Check for dorsal dislocation or fx around CMC joints on lateral view
- Use lateral view to assess apex dorsal angulation of shaft or neck fx

CT Findings
- Generally not needed for initial diagnosis, though small fractures at CMC may be occult by radiograph

- Used in search for occult fx or in follow-up of reduction
  - Fracture-dislocation
  - Intraarticular fractures

Imaging Recommendations
- Best imaging tool: Radiograph
- Protocol advice
  - PA view must be obtained with wrist & hand flat
    - If fingers flexed or wrist hyperextended, CMC joint line will be obscured
  - Lateral view must be positioned well so that dorsal subluxation of base of MC will be seen in CMC fx-dislocation
  - If clinical concern is thumb
    - 3 views of thumb rather than of hand are required for evaluation
    - Routine 3 views of hand show the thumb all in a similar obliquity & injury may be missed
  - CT requires sub-mm slice acquisition with reformats
  - When CT done on small bones such as the CMC or MCP joints, routine axial acquisition is suboptimal
    - Very few cuts through the region of interest may be obtained with axial position
    - Use the Principle of Obliquity: Place the region of interest obliquely in the scan plane; will result in more cuts through the region of interest and therefore improved reformatting

DIFFERENTIAL DIAGNOSIS

Dislocation vs. Fx-Dislocation at CMC
- Dislocations often have small fx fragments which may be occult but should be sought

Dislocation vs. Subluxation at 1st CMC Joint
- 1st CMC is a saddle joint, allowing for significant multidirectional motion
- Results in normal & acceptable "subluxation", or mismatch of articular surface; must differentiate from complete dislocation

METACARPAL FRACTURES AND DISLOCATIONS

PATHOLOGY

General Features
- Etiology
  - Generally sports injuries
  - 5th MC
    - Direct force (punching injury in Boxer's fx)
    - Indirect force from torsion or bending of the finger distally
  - Bennett and Rolando: Axial loading across a partially flexed thumb (often in fist fight)
- Epidemiology
  - Carpometacarpal dislocations: Relative frequency
    - Majority CMC dislocations are multiple (60%)
    - If multiple, 30% involve 2nd through 5th CMC, inclusive
    - If CMC dislocations multiple, 30% involve 4th & 5th CMC
    - If solitary, 50% are 5th CMC
    - If solitary, 25% are 2nd CMC
  - Most frequently fractured bone in hand: 5th MC (20% of total)
- Associated abnormalities
  - MC dislocation: Associated carpal fracture is most frequent abnormality
    - Hamate > capitate > all others
  - MC dislocation: Associated MC fracture less frequent than carpal fx
    - Of these, 4th MC fractures most often

CLINICAL ISSUES

Presentation
- Most common signs/symptoms: Pain and deformity following trauma

Demographics
- Age: Adolescent & young adults, relating to sports participation
- Gender: M > F, relating to sports participation

Natural History & Prognosis
- Most simple nonarticular MC fractures heal without complication when treated conservatively
- Open or multiple fx require more aggressive treatment
- Fracture-dislocation usually requires internal fixation
- Bennett or Rolando fx: Inadequate reduction leads to malunion & secondary osteoarthritis

Treatment
- Most metacarpal fractures result from low energy trauma & can be treated non-operatively
- Open fractures have worse prognosis (infection & nonunion); may require more aggressive treatment
- Athlete's demands to return to activity may result in surgical fixation
- Metacarpal fx of the ring & middle finger are more inherently stable than index & 5th
  - Dual support from the radial & ulnar deep transverse intermetacarpal ligaments
- MC neck fractures
  - Typically unstable due to
    - Dorsal angulation of the fracture apex
    - Comminution
  - The more distal the fx, the greater the degree of dorsal angulation tolerated
  - Greater fx deformity of MC neck is tolerated in the ring & 5th finger than in the 2nd & 3rd MCs
    - < 50° of apex dorsal angulation can be tolerated in 4th & 5th MC
    - 30° angulation is acceptable in 2nd & 3rd MC
  - Open reduction for irreducible fx, soft tissue entrapment, or high energy trauma
- Midshaft, transverse, minimally displaced MC fx often treated with closed reduction & immobilization
- Open reduction internal fixation performed for most open fractures & in presence of multiple closed fx
- Oblique & spiral fx may result in MC shortening
  - If > 5 mm shortening, open reduction performed
- Extraarticular fx of 1st MC tends to maintain anatomic alignment
  - Owing to muscle attachments resisting fragment displacement
  - Treated in cast or splint
- Base of 1st MC fractures
  - Bennett (2 part intraarticular fx base of thumb)
    - If injury involves less than 20% of articular surface, closed reduction with pinning is often adequate
    - Greater involvement of articular surface in Bennett, or malalignment may necessitate open reduction and internal fixation
  - Rolando (comminuted) fx
    - The greater the degree of comminution, the less amenable the fx is to adequate result with open reduction and internal fixation
    - Highly comminuted fx may be treated closed

DIAGNOSTIC CHECKLIST

Consider
- Infection should be considered in patient with punching type of injury to MC head/neck
  - If MCP contacts opponent's teeth, the skin can be broken and bacteria introduced into joint
  - Signs
    - Cartilage destruction
    - Indistinctness of cortex of MC head
    - 4th & 5th MCP most frequently involved

Image Interpretation Pearls
- Fx of the dorsal surface of the distal carpal bones or of the MC bases suggests a CMC dislocation
- Angulated fx of the MC shaft suggests a dislocation at the corresponding CMC or adjacent CMC joint

SELECTED REFERENCES

1. Leggit JC et al: Acute finger injuries: part II. Fractures, dislocations, and thumb injuries. Am Fam Physician. 73(5):827-34, 2006
2. Rosner JL et al: Imaging of athletic wrist and hand injuries. Semin Musculoskelet Radiol. 8(1):57-79, 2004
3. Fisher M et al: A systematic approach to the diagnosis of carpometacarpal dislocations. Radiographics. 2(4):612-27, 1982

METACARPAL FRACTURES AND DISLOCATIONS

IMAGE GALLERY

Typical

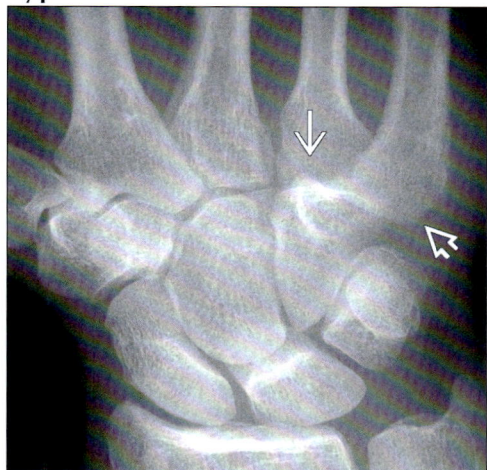
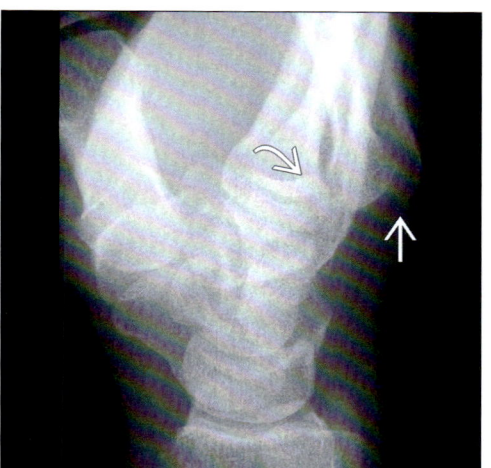

(Left) Anteroposterior radiograph shows loss of the normal joint space at the 4th metacarpal articulation ➡ with the hamate, as well as significant ulnar subluxation of the 5th metacarpal ➡. *(Right)* Lateral radiograph confirms the dislocation of both the 4th & 5th metacarpals ➡ in a dorsal direction. The articular surface of the hamate is seen ➡, without any metacarpal aligning with it.

Typical

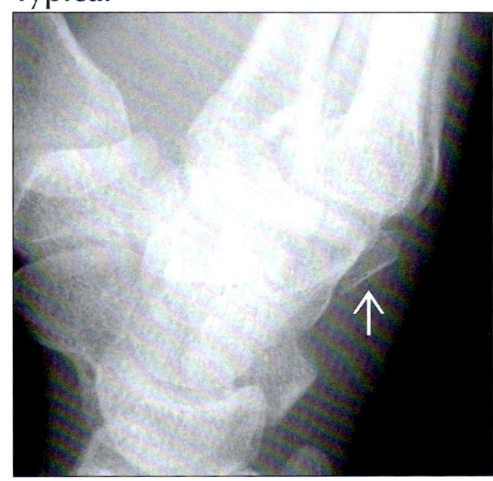
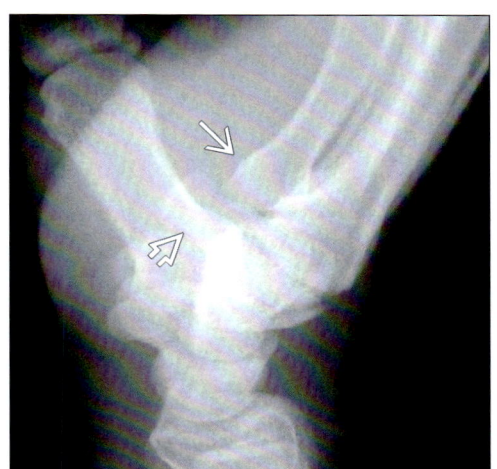

(Left) Lateral radiograph shows a dorsal intraarticular fracture of the hamate, with both the 4th & 5th metacarpals subluxing in a dorsal direction, along with the fragment ➡. *(Right)* Lateral radiograph shows the less common volar dislocation of the 5th metacarpal. Note the base of the MC ➡ which is volar in location relative to the other metacarpals, and which appears to articulate with the hook of hamate ➡.

Typical

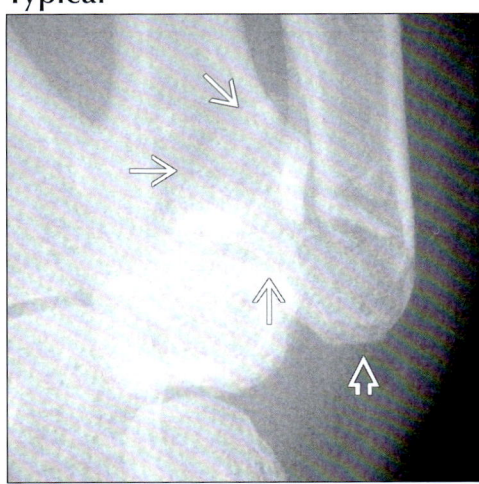
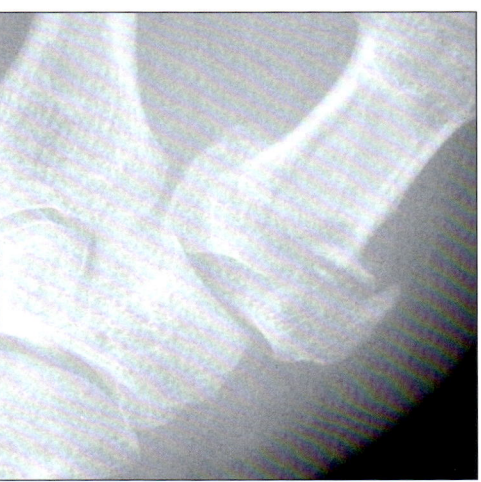

(Left) Anteroposterior radiograph shows a Bennett fx, which consists of an intraarticular fx at the base of the first metacarpal, with the large fragment ➡ remaining in position relative to the trapezium, and the remainder of the thumb subluxing proximally ➡. *(Right)* Anteroposterior radiograph shows a Rolando fracture, with significant intraarticular involvement and comminution. Surgical reduction of these fractures is often not successful, and results in early onset OA.

ULNAR COLLATERAL LIGAMENT TEAR, THUMB

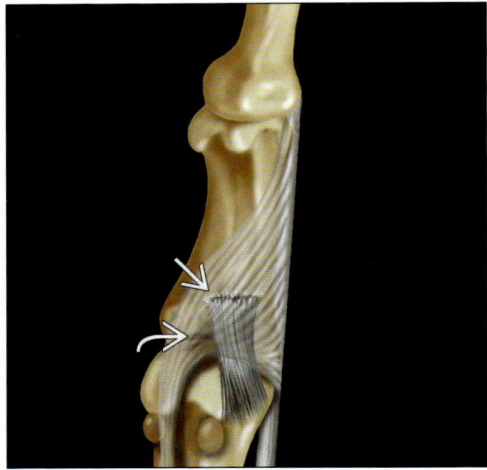

Lateral graphic shows UCL tear ➡ without displacement or retraction. The adductor aponeurosis is intact ➡ over the UCL. This represents a gamekeeper's thumb.

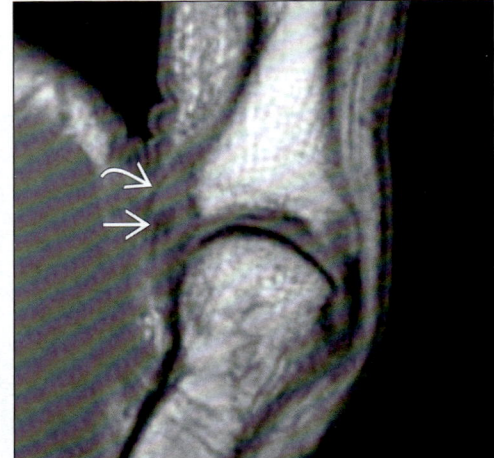

Coronal oblique T1WI MR shows a slightly displaced UCL tear ➡. Although the UCL is proximally retracted by 2 mm, the overlying adductor aponeurosis remains intact ➡, & the lesion may be treated by splinting.

TERMINOLOGY

Abbreviations and Synonyms
- UCL rupture, gamekeeper's thumb, ulnar collateral ligament rupture, skier's thumb

Definitions
- Disruption of the ulnar collateral ligament of the thumb, with or without associated avulsion fx

IMAGING FINDINGS

General Features
- Best diagnostic clue: Discontinuity of ulnar collateral ligament attachment to proximal phalanx, ± avulsion fx
- Location: 1st metacarpophalangeal (MCP) joint
- Size
  - Varies from partial thickness tear to full thickness tear
  - UCL may be retracted deep or superficial to adductor aponeurosis: Stener lesion
- Morphology
  - Thickened, foreshortened UCL with proximal retraction
  - Mass-like tissue vs. horizontally directed UCL in Stener lesion

Radiographic Findings
- Radiography
  - Obtain prior to stressing the MCP joint
  - Avulsion fragments uncommonly seen on radiograph (12% of UCL injuries)
  - Nondisplaced to minimal displacement (< 2 mm) avulsion fracture of proximal phalanx base = UCL avulsion without Stener lesion
  - Roberts view = hyperpronated anteroposterior view (true AP view of thumb)
  - Some concern that stress radiographs may transform nonsurgical (nondisplaced) injuries into surgical ones
  - Could underestimate degree of injury in a two-level UCL injury (rare)
    - Consists of both an undisplaced avulsion fragment & a displaced ligament tear
    - Osseous fragment may mislead one to a diagnosis of nondisplaced tear

DDx: Ulnar Collateral Ligament Tear, Thumb

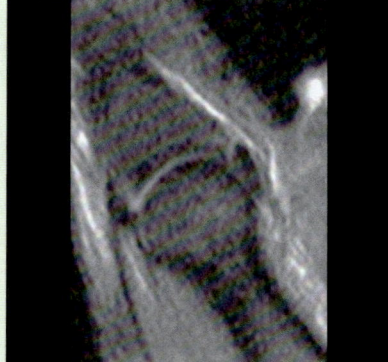

UCL Sprain

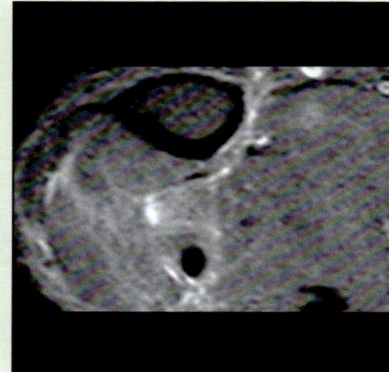

Thenar Sprain

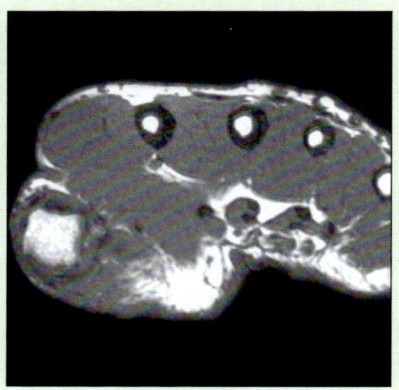

FPL Tear

ULNAR COLLATERAL LIGAMENT TEAR, THUMB

Key Facts

Imaging Findings
- Best diagnostic clue: Discontinuity of ulnar collateral ligament attachment to proximal phalanx, ± avulsion fx
- Varies from partial thickness tear to full thickness tear
- UCL may be retracted deep or superficial to adductor aponeurosis: Stener lesion
- Thickened, foreshortened UCL with proximal retraction
- Mass-like tissue vs. horizontally directed UCL in Stener lesion
- Avulsion fragments uncommonly seen on radiograph (12% of UCL injuries)
- "Yo-yo on a string" appearance of Stener lesion = retracted & balled-up UCL (yo-yo) with the more proximal linear adductor aponeurosis (the string)
- US accurate for evaluation of tear, displacement, Stener lesion
- Best imaging tool: MR or US identifies UCL morphology, location, retraction, & position relative to adductor aponeurosis

Pathology
- Gamekeeper's thumb = chronic injury to UCL (vs. acute trauma of skier's thumb)

Clinical Issues
- Most common signs/symptoms: MCP joint pain
- Mass = displaced UCL stump on ulnar side of MCP joint or proximal to MCP joint

Diagnostic Checklist
- Identify retracted UCL with folded or horizontally directed fibers

---

- Clue: A poorly visualized smaller bone fragment situated more proximally

MR Findings
- T1WI
  - Incomplete rupture or complete rupture without a Stener lesion
    - Hypo to intermediate signal intensity UCL remains deep to overlying hypointense adductor aponeurosis
    - Discontinuity at UCL attachment to proximal aspect proximal phalanx (thumb)
    - Intermediate signal intensity edema & fluid superficial & deep to UCL
    - UCL orientation remains along long axis of 1st ray (thumb)
  - Complete rupture with a Stener lesion
    - Intermediate signal intensity in retracted mass of UCL
    - UCL trapped beneath adductor aponeurosis
    - UCL directed superficial to linear adductor aponeurosis
- T2WI
  - Incomplete or complete rupture without Stener lesion
    - Thickened hypointense UCL with central signal inhomogeneity (focal hyperintense areas of edema)
    - Hyperintense fluid interposed between various planes of bone, ligament, & adductor aponeurosis
    - Hyperintense subchondral edema ± osseous avulsion at UCL distal attachment to proximal phalanx
  - Complete rupture with Stener lesion
    - Gross displacement of hypo or intermediate signal UCL medial to adductor aponeurosis
    - Trapped UCL either completely superficial to or intersecting the overlying adductor aponeurosis
    - UCL directional vector with increased horizontal orientation (no longer parallel to long axis of 1st digit)
  - "Yo-yo on a string" appearance of Stener lesion = retracted & balled-up UCL (yo-yo) with the more proximal linear adductor aponeurosis (the string)

Ultrasonographic Findings
- Normal UCL is hyperechoic structure spanning the ulnar side of the first MCP joint
- Superficially, it is covered by a thin hyperechoic band: Adductor pollicis aponeurosis (variably visualized)
- US accurate for evaluation of tear, displacement, Stener lesion

Imaging Recommendations
- Best imaging tool: MR or US identifies UCL morphology, location, retraction, & position relative to adductor aponeurosis
- Protocol advice
  - MR: T1, PD & FS PD FSE (vs. STIR or T2* gradient echo) in true coronal orthogonal plane through MCP joint
    - Axial images next most important plane
    - Sagittal - may document retracted UCL & mass-like effect on ulnar-sided images
  - US technique: Hand placed flat on table
    - MHz linear probe used with gel
    - US probe is slid from the 2nd finger onto the 1st MCP joint
    - Obtain transverse or longitudinal image of UCL at this site

DIFFERENTIAL DIAGNOSIS

MCP Joint Capsular Trauma
- Capsule: Proper radial & UCLs (UCL sprain)
- Volar (palmar) plate = anterior or glenoid ligament
  - Two asymmetric checkrein ligaments; sesamoid bones associated
  - Origin = volar distal thumb metacarpal
  - Insertion = palmar edge proximal phalanx

MCP Joint Dislocations
- Hyperextension with dorsal subluxation/dislocation

ULNAR COLLATERAL LIGAMENT TEAR, THUMB

- Associated volar plate injury & thenar sprain

Dorsal Hood Injury
- Ulnar displacement of the extensor pollicis longus

Thenar Muscle Injury
- Abductor pollicis brevis, flexor pollicis brevis, opponens pollicis, adductor pollicis

PATHOLOGY

General Features
- General path comments
  - Relevant anatomy = MCP joint of the thumb
    - Capsule - reinforced by volar plate, collateral ligaments, adductor aponeurosis, & extensor pollicis brevis tendon
- Etiology
  - Hyperabduction of thumb
  - Hyperextension stress to UCL of thumb
  - Fall (skier's thumb) with hyperextension + abduction = UCL tear
  - Gamekeeper's thumb = chronic injury to UCL (vs. acute trauma of skier's thumb)
- Epidemiology
  - UCL injury of thumb MCP joint is common
  - UCL rupture - majority occur distally
  - Stener lesion - 50 to 70% of complete tears
  - Increased incidence of Stener lesions in skiers (80%)

Gross Pathologic & Surgical Features
- Partial vs. complete tears UCL, ± Stener, ± avulsed fragment
- Nondisplaced UCL tear = discontinuity without retraction + intact adductor aponeurosis covering distal UCL
- Displaced UCL = Stener lesion with proximal retraction (ligament folding) proximal to MCP joint
- Proximal margin of adductor aponeurosis intersects or abuts folded UCL in Stener lesion
- Distal UCL end turned 180° & directed proximally in Stener lesion

Staging, Grading or Classification Criteria
- Partial tears
  - Grade I: Stretching
  - Grade II: Incomplete but discrete tear
- Complete rupture
  - Grade III (with or without Stener lesion)

CLINICAL ISSUES

Presentation
- Most common signs/symptoms: MCP joint pain
- Clinical Profile
  - Swelling, pain at 1st MCP, worst on ulnar side
  - Weakness in pinch & grasp strength
  - Mass = displaced UCL stump on ulnar side of MCP joint or proximal to MCP joint
  - Abnormal thumb rotation (rotation of proximal phalanx on intact axis of radial collateral ligament)
  - Absent endpoint on stress test = complete tear UCL
  - Instability in MCP flexion = proper collateral lig tear with intact accessory collateral + volar plate
  - Instability in flexion & extension = complete ulnar complex disruption
  - Stability ≤ 10° of opening
  - Instability ≥ 30° abduction arc on stress relative to contralateral side

Demographics
- Age
  - Young to middle aged adults
  - Activity related age groups
    - Football, hockey, wrestling, basketball & skiing
- Gender
  - M > F
  - Activity related

Natural History & Prognosis
- Partial tears & complete without Stener lesion may heal without surgery
- Fibrosis & granulation tissue in complete tears may delay or preclude ligament reattachment

Treatment
- Conservative
  - Partial tears (grade I & II)
  - Thumb spica cast vs. custom splint
  - Complete rupture without Stener lesion or significant displacement
- Surgical
  - Complete rupture with displacement or Stener lesion
  - Volar subluxation proximal phalanx
  - Primary repair of torn UCL - acute/subacute injuries
  - Reconstruction of chronic complete UCL ruptures
- Complications
  - Superficial branch of radial nerve injury
  - Failure of UCL repair
  - Loss of joint motion & osteoarthritis

DIAGNOSTIC CHECKLIST

Consider
- Evaluation of UCL tears & Stener lesions require coronal images through MCP parallel to the collateral ligament plane
- Identify retracted UCL with folded or horizontally directed fibers

SELECTED REFERENCES

1. Ebrahim FS et al: US diagnosis of UCL tears of the thumb and Stener lesions: technique, pattern-based approach, and differential diagnosis. Radiographics. 26(4):1007-20, 2006
2. Miller MD et al: Surgical atlas of sports medicine. Treatment of skier's/gamekeeper's thumb. Philadelphia Pennsylvania, WB Saunders, (67): 491-6, 2003
3. Plancher KD et al: Role of MR imaging in the management of "skier's thumb" injuries. Magn Reson Imaging Clin N Am. 7(1):73-84, viii, 1999
4. Heyman P et al: Injuries of the ulnar collateral ligament of the thumb metacarpophalangeal joint. Biomechanical and prospective clinical studies on the usefulness of valgus stress testing. Clin Orthop Relat Res. (292):165-71, 1993

ULNAR COLLATERAL LIGAMENT TEAR, THUMB

IMAGE GALLERY

Typical

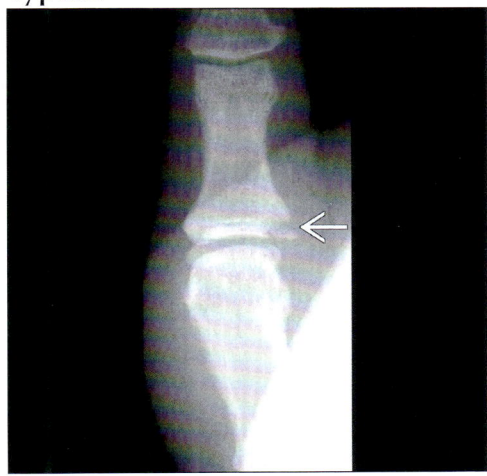 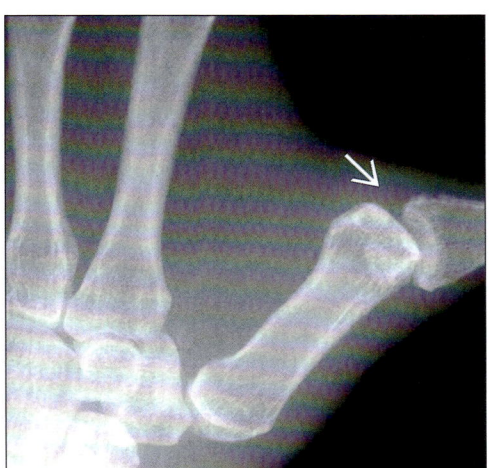

(Left) Anteroposterior radiograph shows intra-articular fracture from the ulnar aspect of the base of proximal phalanx of the thumb ➔. This avulsion resulted from a ski pole injury resulting in hyperabduction of the thumb. *(Right)* Anteroposterior radiograph shows no evidence of avulsion fracture, but significant subluxation ➔. This degree of subluxation indicates a significant injury; further evaluation by MR or US should be obtained.

Typical

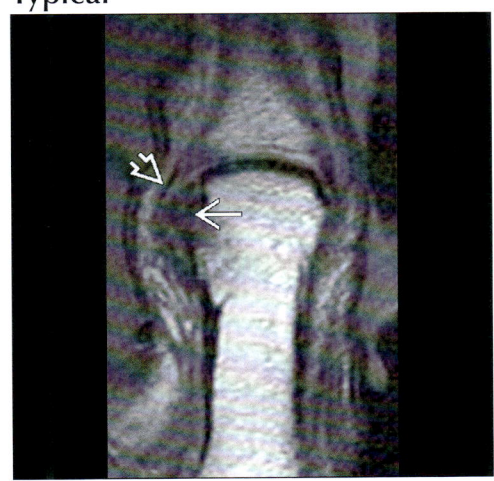 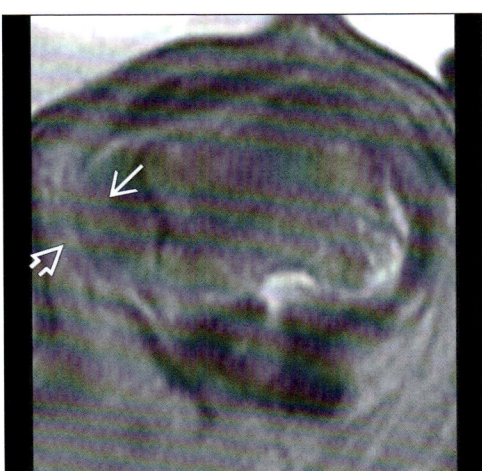

(Left) Coronal T1WI MR shows a UCL tear with significant retraction ➔. This is a chronic injury, and presents with a mass suspicious for Stener lesion. However, the adductor aponeurosis ➔ remains intact overlying the disrupted UCL. *(Right)* Axial PD/Intermediate FS MR of the same patient confirms that the adductor aponeurosis is partially torn ➔, but remains in place overlying the retracted and horizontally directed UCL ➔.

Typical

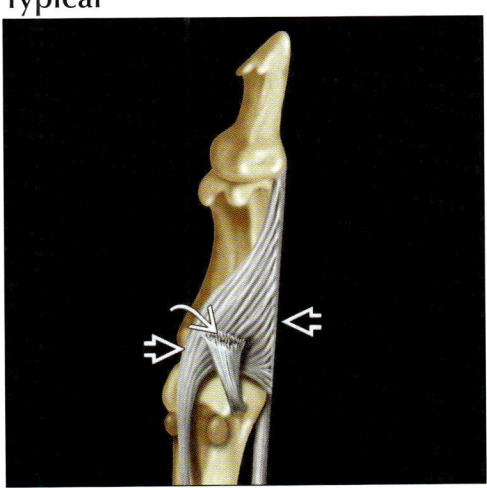 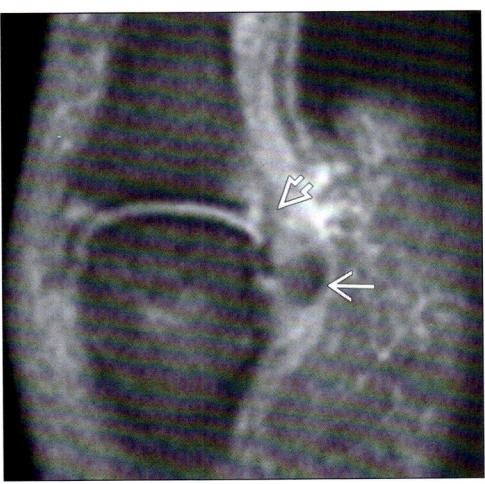

(Left) Oblique lateral graphic shows displacement of the retracted UCL ➔ superficial to the overlying adductor aponeurosis ➔ in a Stener lesion. *(Right)* Coronal T2* GRE MR shows a retracted torn UCL ➔ lying superficial to the adductor aponeurosis ➔. This case beautifully demonstrates the "yo-yo" sign of the balled-up UCL seemingly attached to the "string" of the aponeurosis. This is a Stener lesion.

FLEXOR ANNULAR PULLEY TEARS

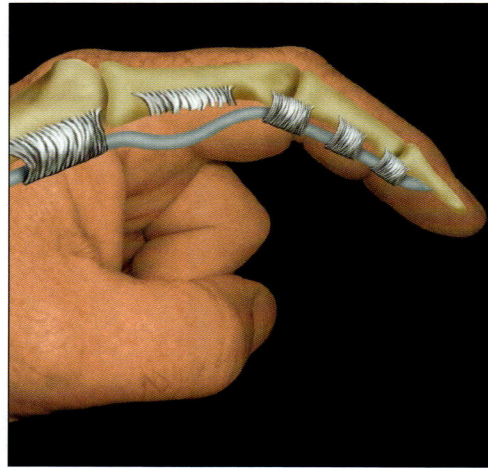

Lateral graphic shows disruption of the A2 pulley with volar bowstringing of the flexor tendon. This pulley must be intact to effectively flex the finger.

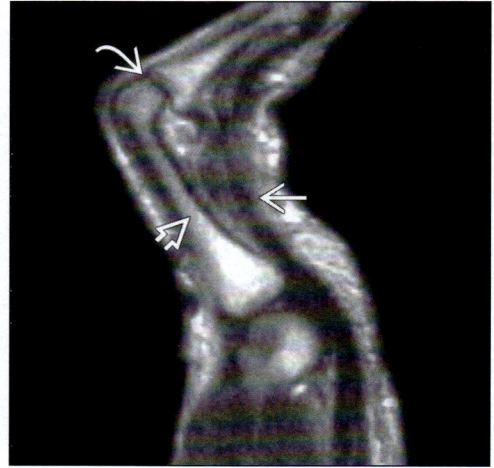

Sagittal T2WI MR shows separation of the flexor profunda and superficialis tendons ➡ from the proximal phalanx ▶ and proximal interphalangeal joint ➤ indicating rupture of the A2 and A3 pulleys.

TERMINOLOGY

Abbreviations and Synonyms
- Digital annular pulley (DAP) tears, flexor pulley tears

Definitions
- Lesion of fibro-osseous theca or flexor tendon sheath

IMAGING FINDINGS

General Features
- Best diagnostic clue: Attenuation or rupture of flexor tendon sheath pulley on axial images
- Location
  ○ Long finger (baseball) & ring finger
  ○ A4 pulley (annular)
  ○ Interval between A2 & A4 pulley
  ○ A5 pulley
  ○ First two cruciate pulleys
- Size: Attenuation to frank disruption
- Morphology: Severe injury = overt bowstringing

Radiographic Findings
- Radiography
  ○ Not diagnostic
  ○ Nonspecific soft tissue swelling
  ○ No evidence of fracture or cortical avulsion

MR Findings
- T1WI
  ○ Bowstringing from proximal interphalangeal (PIP) joint to base of proximal phalanx on sagittal images = complete rupture of A2 pulley
  ○ Bowstringing from PIP - not reaching base of proximal phalanx = incomplete rupture of A2 pulley
  ○ Bowstringing at level of proximal phalanx to region distal to PIP joint = A2 + A3 rupture
  ○ Bowstringing at level of middle phalanx = A4 rupture
  ○ Hypointense to intermediate signal fluid associated with affected pulley
  ○ Hypointense cysts
  ○ Hypo to intermediate signal intensity fibrous tissue
- T2WI
  ○ Hyperintense fluid associated with affected tendon pulley

DDx: Flexor Annular Pulley Tears

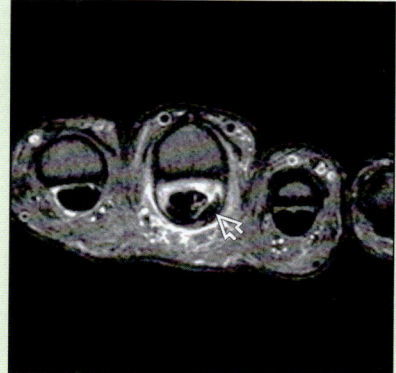

Flexor Digitorum Profundus Tear

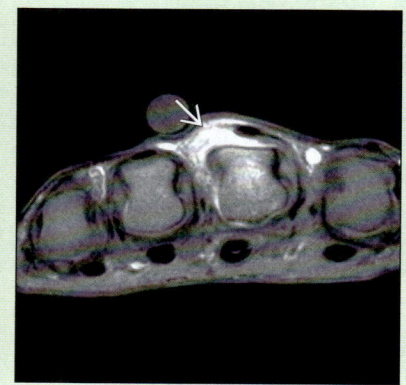

Extensor Tenosynovitis

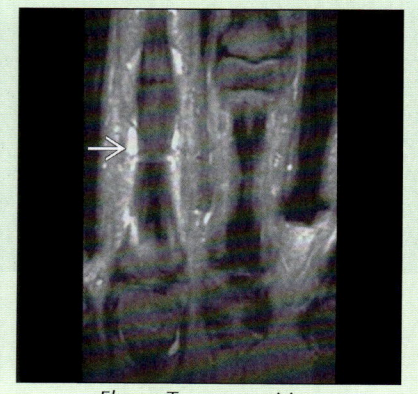

Flexor Tenosynovitis

FLEXOR ANNULAR PULLEY TEARS

Key Facts

Imaging Findings
- Best diagnostic clue: Attenuation or rupture of flexor tendon sheath pulley on axial images
- Long finger (baseball) & ring finger
- Morphology: Severe injury = overt bowstringing

Top Differential Diagnoses
- Tenosynovitis
- Flexor Tendon Tear
- Degenerative Arthritis
- Inflammatory Arthritis
- Joint Trauma

Pathology
- Forcible contraction flexor digitorum profundus (FDP) against extreme force
- Professional baseball injury (pitching)
- Rock climbing injury
- Pulley tears = 50% of lesions in elite climbers
- Ring & middle finger affected in climbing vs. middle finger in baseball pitchers
- Bowstringing of flexor tendon
- Failure A4 pulley
- Disruption of interval between A2 & A4
- A5 pulley & first 2 cruciate pulleys involved

Clinical Issues
- Most common signs/symptoms: Pain & tenderness over palmar (volar) & lateral aspects of flexor tendon
- ± DIP flexion with discomfort
- Restricted range of motion

Diagnostic Checklist
- Evaluate flexor tendon bowing on sagittal images

- ○ Discontinuity of pulley on axial images
- ○ Tendon displacement
  - Anterior displacement relative to proximal aspect proximal phalanx in A2 pulley area
  - Anterior displacement relative to middle phalanx in A4 pulley area
  - ± Medial or lateral subluxation
  - Hypointense fibrous scar tissue
- ○ Hyperintense
  - PIP or distal interphalangeal (DIP) joint fluid
  - Tenosynovitis
  - Tendon sheath cyst

Ultrasonographic Findings
- Dynamic studies
- Scan with resisted flexion
- Measurement of flexor tendon bowstringing
  - ○ Flexor tendon - phalanx (TP) distance > 1.0 mm = pulley injury
  - ○ TP measurement (with forced flexion) > 3.0 mm = complete rupture of A2 pulley
  - ○ TP distance (with forced flexion) > 5 mm = rupture A2 & A3 pulley
  - ○ TP distance ≥ 2.5 mm at middle phalanx = complete rupture A4 pulley
- Assessment of tendon gliding (superficialis, profundus & sheaths)

Imaging Recommendations
- Best imaging tool
  - ○ MR and dynamic ultrasound
  - ○ MR resolution allows direct pulley visualization
- Protocol advice
  - ○ T1, FS PD FSE, T2* gradient echo axial images
  - ○ T1 & FS PD FSE sagittal and coronal images

DIFFERENTIAL DIAGNOSIS

Tenosynovitis
- Inflammation of tendon sheath
- Fluid within tendon sheath (hyperintense on T2WI)
- ± Thickened sheath
- ± Associated tendon degeneration
- ± Tendon fraying
- Fluid intermediate on T2WI with chronic changes

Flexor Tendon Tear
- Avulsion of flexor digitorum profundus
  - ○ Type I: Retracts to palm
  - ○ Type II: Retracts to PIP joint
  - ○ Type III: Osseous avulsion + retraction to A4 pulley

Degenerative Arthritis
- Sclerosis
- Osteophytosis
- Joint space narrowing
- Subluxation
- Reactive subchondral marrow edema
- DIP or PIP joints most common

Inflammatory Arthritis
- Rheumatoid
- Rheumatoid variants
- Tenosynovitis + intermediate signal intensity synovial hypertrophy on T2WI (FS PD FSE)

Joint Trauma
- Dislocations of metacarpophalangeal (MCP) joint (± avulsion fracture)
  - ○ Lateral (coronal plane) injury
  - ○ Dorsal MCP dislocations
  - ○ Volar MCP dislocations
- Proximal interphalangeal joint dislocation
  - ○ Coach's finger = jammed finger
  - ○ Collateral ligaments - accessory & proper
  - ○ Dorsal & volar dislocation
- Pilon fractures
  - ○ Middle phalanx
  - ○ Axial loading
  - ○ Intraarticular comminution & displacement
- Distal interphalangeal dislocations
  - ○ Ball-handling & contact sports
  - ○ Dorsal dislocation

FLEXOR ANNULAR PULLEY TEARS

PATHOLOGY

General Features
- General path comments
  - Relevant anatomy = fibrous portion of fibro-osseous flexion tunnel
    - Five digital annular pulleys (DAP) (condensations of transversely oriented fibrous bands)
    - Annular pulleys A1 to A5
    - Cruciate pulleys C1 to C3
    - A2 (proximal aspect proximal phalanx) & A4 (mid aspect middle phalanx) = most important function of DAP
    - DAP: Stabilizes flexor tendons during flexion & resist ulnar/radial displacement as well as palmar bowing
- Etiology
  - Forcible contraction flexor digitorum profundus (FDP) against extreme force
  - Professional baseball injury (pitching)
    - Distal tip of long finger for control
    - Increased angular velocity in throwing mechanism
  - Rock climbing injury
    - Support of body weight with DIP joint in flexion
    - High stress
    - Repetitive microtrauma
    - Local trauma varies with grip techniques (loads up to 700N)
    - Crimped technique: MCP joint extension, PIP flexion & DIP extension = excessive forces on A2 & A3 DAP
- Epidemiology
  - Pulley tears = 50% of lesions in elite climbers
  - Ring & middle finger affected in climbing vs. middle finger in baseball pitchers
  - 30% of finger injuries

Gross Pathologic & Surgical Features
- Bowstringing of flexor tendon
  - Failure A4 pulley
  - Disruption of interval between A2 & A4
  - A5 pulley & first 2 cruciate pulleys involved
- Combined injury of A2 & A4 pulleys less common
- Partial tears - no tendon bowstringing
- Volar subluxation of tendon = DAP tear
- Associated tenosynovitis
- Fibrous tissue
- A2 & A3 pulley injuries (proximal phalanx) vs. A2 pulley rupture; requires forced flexion to differentiate

Microscopic Features
- Inflammatory infiltrate
- Fibrous tissue
- Tendons - low resistance to shear forces
- Tendon failure at end of linear portion of load-deformation relationship
- Collagen breakdown

CLINICAL ISSUES

Presentation
- Most common signs/symptoms: Pain & tenderness over palmar (volar) & lateral aspects of flexor tendon
- Clinical Profile
  - Increased tenderness associated with inflammation
  - Tendon fullness - fluid or hemorrhage
  - ± DIP flexion with discomfort
  - Weakness
  - Pitcher - decreased velocity of pitches
  - Tendon bowstringing
  - Soft tissue swelling
  - Restricted range of motion

Demographics
- Age
  - Young adult
  - At risk age groups includes professional baseball pitchers (20-30 years) & rock climbers (20-40 years)
- Gender: M > F (related to activities with forcible contraction of FDP)

Natural History & Prognosis
- Delayed diagnosis = fixed contractures of PIP joint
- Fibrosis/scar tissue
- Weakness
- Tenosynovitis or partial tear of DAP - treated conservatively

Treatment
- Conservative
  - Immobilization
  - Anti-inflammatory medication
  - ± Steroid injection if strong inflammatory component (may alter healing process)
  - Indicated in absence of bowstringing
- Surgical
  - Complete rupture of flexor pulley system = reconstruction

DIAGNOSTIC CHECKLIST

Consider
- Evaluate flexor tendon bowing on sagittal images
- Evaluate pulley integrity directly on axial images

SELECTED REFERENCES

1. Klauser A et al: Finger pulley injuries in extreme rock climbers: depiction with dynamic US. Radiology. 222(3):755-61, 2002
2. McCue FC III et al: The wrist in the adult. Orthopaedic sports medicine. vol 1. 2nd ed. Philadelphia PA, Saunders, (24):1337-63, 2002
3. Hauger O et al: Pulley system in the fingers: normal anatomy and simulated lesions in cadavers at MR imaging, CT, and US with and without contrast material distention of the tendon sheath. Radiology. 217(1):201-12, 2000
4. Martinoli C et al: Sonographic evaluation of digital annular pulley tears. Skeletal Radiol. 29(7):387-91, 2000
5. Klauser A et al: Finger injuries in extreme rock climbers. Assessment of high-resolution ultrasonography. Am J Sports Med. 27(6):733-7, 1999

FLEXOR ANNULAR PULLEY TEARS

IMAGE GALLERY

Typical

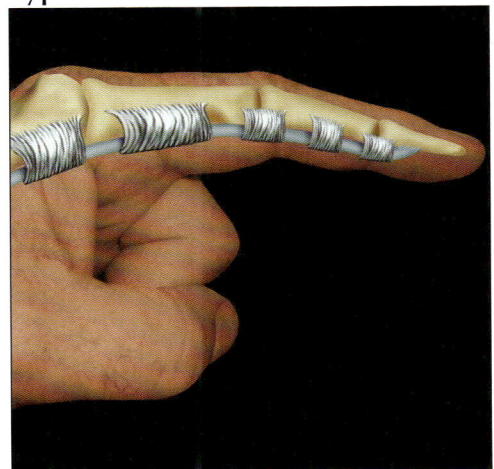
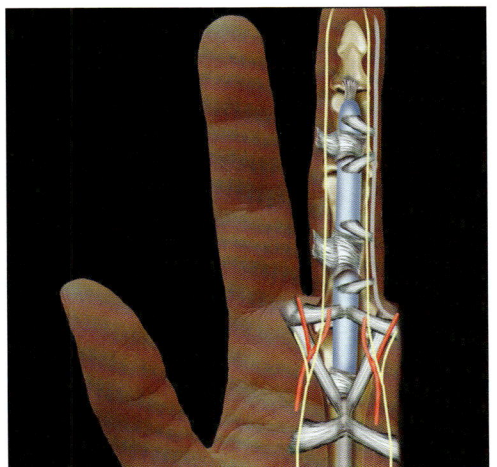

(Left) Lateral graphic shows a normal intact annular pulley system of the finger. A2 & A4 pulleys are at the midshaft of the proximal and middle digits, respectively. A1, A3, & A5 are superficial to the MCP, PIP, and DIP joints, respectively. *(Right)* Anterior graphic shows normal volar digital fascial anatomy with intact cruciate & annular pulleys.

Typical

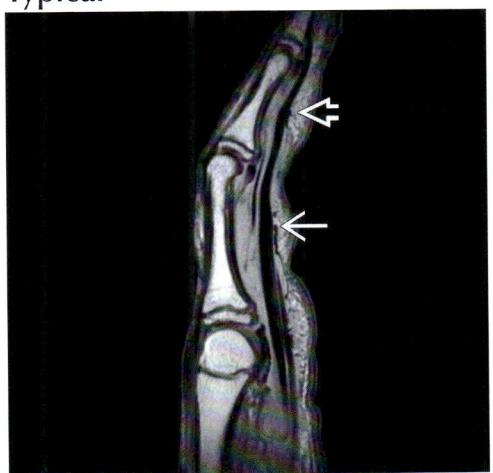
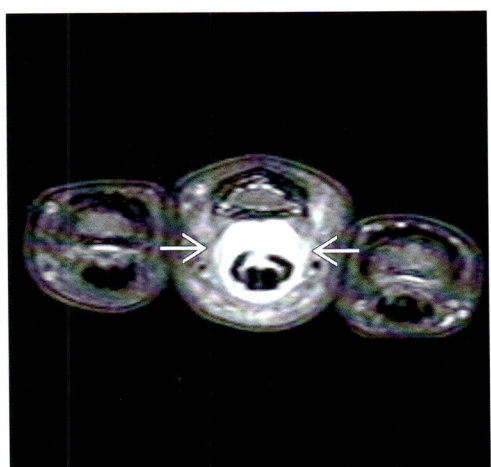

(Left) Sagittal PD/Intermediate MR shows typical "bowstring" appearance of flexor tendon, which is displaced away from bone in the region of the A2 ➡ and A4 ➡ pulleys. The A3 pulley over the PIP must be disrupted as well. *(Right)* Axial T2WI FS MR at level of the middle phalanx shows displacement of tendons and nonvisualization of the A4 pulley ➡. A large amount of fluid is present around the intact flexor tendons.

Typical

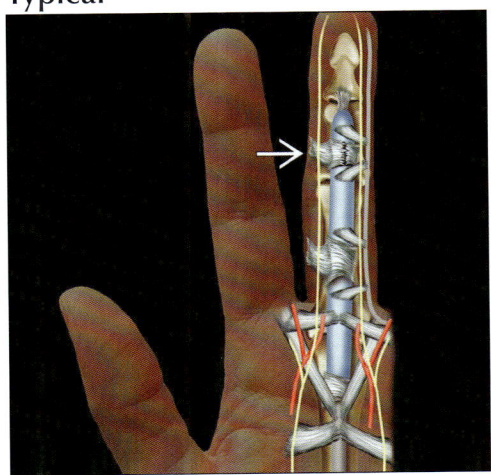
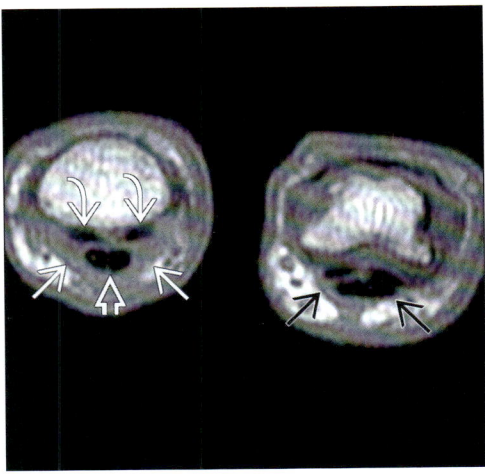

(Left) Anterior graphic depicts disruption of the A4 pulley ➡ at the level of the middle phalanx. The A2 & A4 pulleys are considered critical for finger flexion. *(Right)* Axial T1WI MR shows sprain of the A2 pulley of the ring finger without complete rupture. There is edema in the A2 pulley ➡, with intact flexor digitorum profundus ➡ & flexor digitorum superficialis ➡; they are not displaced away from the phalanx. The normal fifth finger A2 pulley ➡ is shown for comparison.

AVULSION FRACTURES, FINGER

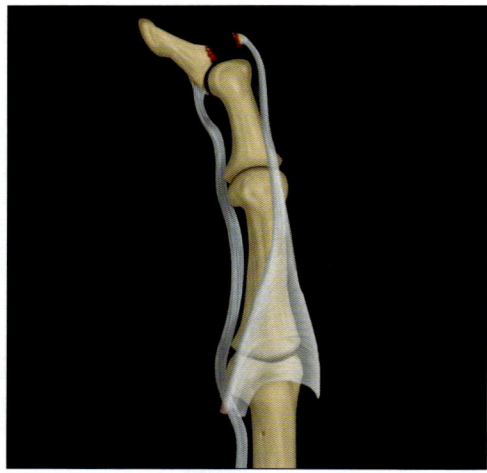

Lateral graphic shows a Mallet finger avulsion. The terminal extensor tendon has avulsed an intra-articular osseous fragment from the dorsal base of the distal phalanx. The finger will have a DIP flexion deformity.

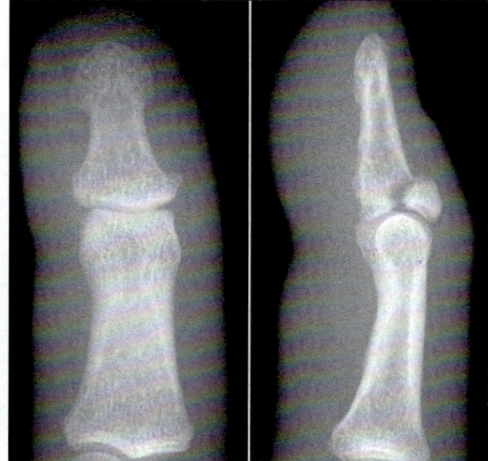

AP & lateral radiographs show a Mallet finger injury. The abnormality is barely visible on the AP view, but the intraarticular nature of the avulsion fracture is easily seen on the lateral. Note mild flexion of the DIP.

TERMINOLOGY

Abbreviations and Synonyms
- Mallet finger, Baseball finger, Jersey finger, flexor digitorum profundus (FDP) avulsion, Volar plate, Boutonniere, collateral ligament avulsion

Definitions
- Intraarticular fracture fragments avulsed from the base of proximal or middle phalanges, either on the dorsal, volar, or side (radial or ulnar)

IMAGING FINDINGS

General Features
- Best diagnostic clue
  - Fracture fragment, often triangular in shape, with donor site being the articular aspect of the base of distal or middle phalanx
  - Fracture fragment may be variably displaced from the donor site; FDP avulsions typically are displaced the farthest from the donor site
  - Associated deformities of joint related to the stabilizing structure which is disrupted
  - If tendon disruption without bony avulsion, deformity will be the indirect clue on radiograph; MR or US needed to directly image the abnormality
- Location: Articular portion of base of either proximal phalanx or middle phalanx
- Size: Disruption varies from large fracture fragment (50% of articular surface), through tiny fracture fragment, through isolated soft tissue disruption
- Morphology
  - Mallet or Baseball finger (terminal extensor tendon)
    - Avulsion fx of dorsal base of distal phalanx, or
    - Tear of distal terminal extensor tendon without fx
    - Results in flexion deformity DIP, even when PIP held in extension
  - Jersey finger (flexor digitorum profundus)
    - Avulsion of FDP from volar base of distal phalanx
    - May be a soft tissue tear of FDP, or bony avulsion
    - Either will generally retract; extent of retraction depends on whether the tendon or fragment is impeded by one of the annular pulleys
    - Results in extension deformity of DIP
  - Volar plate avulsion

Volar Plate Fracture

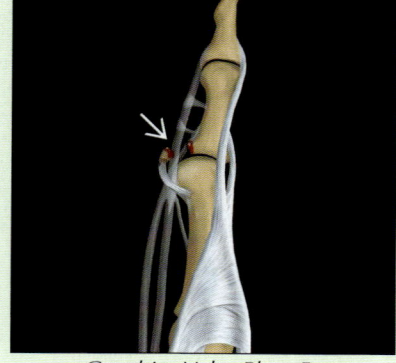

Graphic: Volar Plate Fx

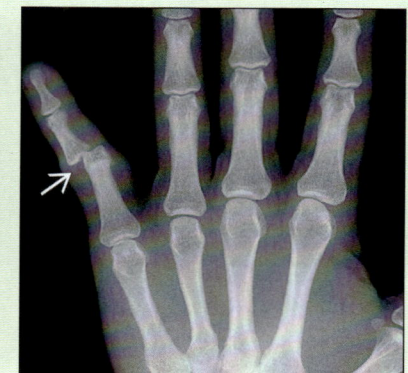

Injury: Dislocation

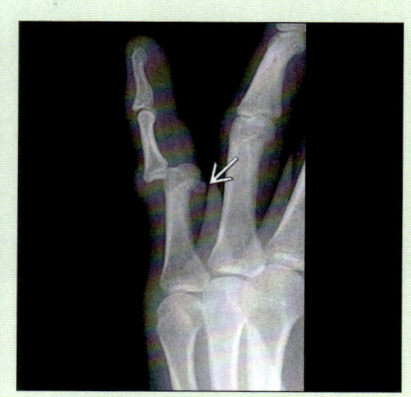

Dislocation/Volar Plate Fx

AVULSION FRACTURES, FINGER

Key Facts

Imaging Findings
- Fracture fragment, often triangular in shape, with donor site being the articular aspect of the base of distal or middle phalanx
- Fracture fragment may be variably displaced from the donor site; FDP avulsions typically are displaced the farthest from the donor site
- Associated deformities of joint related to the stabilizing structure which is disrupted
- If tendon disruption without bony avulsion, deformity will be the indirect clue on radiograph; MR or US needed to directly image the abnormality
- Radiograph best demonstrates avulsion and/or joint deformity
- MR or US to demonstrate tendon, ligament, or volar plate disruption if no bony fragment is present

Pathology
- PIP is most commonly injured joint in hand
- Extensor > flexor apparatus injuries
- Most common sports closed tendon injury: Mallet
- Volar plate injuries: Classified according to degree of articular instability
- Jersey (FDP) finger: 4 main types characterized by degree of retraction

Diagnostic Checklist
- Watch for fracture fragments about the IP joints
- Watch for unnatural angulation of the IP joints to suggest soft tissue disruption
- Hyperextended PIP: Volar plate
- Hyperflexed PIP + hyperextended DIP: Boutonniere
- Hyperflexed DIP when PIP is extended: Mallet finger
- Hyperextended DIP: Jersey finger

- Avulsion fx at volar base of middle phalanx
- May present as soft tissue disruption at distal aspect of volar plate, without bony fragment
- PIP may be hyperextended
- Rare type: Disruption of volar plate from proximal phalanx; causes a flexion deformity of PIP with intact extensor mechanism (pseudo-boutonniere)
  - Central slip extensor tendon injury (Boutonniere)
    - Avulsion of the dorsal base of the middle phalanx
    - May be a soft tissue disruption of the central slip
    - Initially the lateral bands that are dorsal to the axis of the PIP can maintain active extension
    - Untreated cases result in flexion deformity PIP (buttonhole) & eventual hyperextension of DIP
  - Collateral ligament injuries
    - Seen as > 10° medial or lateral angulation at the extended joint; avulsion fragment rarely seen

Radiographic Findings
- AP & lateral to show osseous avulsions
- Flexion or extension deformities at PIP or DIP
  - If presents in unnatural position without fracture fragment, suggests soft tissue disruption of associated flexor or extensor structure
- Ulnar or radial deformity: Collateral ligament injury

MR Findings
- T1 MR: Low signal tendinous/ligamentous structures; watch for disruption or retraction
- Fluid sensitive sequences: Low signal structures with disruption, fluid surrounding
- MR excellent to depict anatomy & soft tissue tears

Ultrasonographic Findings
- Tendons hypoechoic structures; follow anatomy to evaluate for disruption; dynamic study may be useful

Imaging Recommendations
- Best imaging tool
  - Radiograph best demonstrates avulsion and/or joint deformity
  - MR or US to demonstrate tendon, ligament, or volar plate disruption if no bony fragment is present

DIFFERENTIAL DIAGNOSIS

Dislocations without Avulsion or Tendon Disruptions
- Check for injuries following reduction, particularly volar plate injury

PATHOLOGY

General Features
- General path comments
  - Anatomy: Main stabilizers of PIP and DIP are surrounding soft tissues
    - Collateral ligaments proper & accessory collateral
    - Volar plate: Thick fibrocartilaginous structure that constitutes the volar aspect of the joint capsule; firmly attached distally but more elastic proximally
    - Volar flexor apparatus (stabilized by annular pulley system, with insertion at volar base distal phalanx)
    - Dorsal extensor apparatus (at MCP, extensor tendons are stabilized by extensor hood, at PIP, central slip with lateral slips that are connected by retinacular ligaments; at DIP, lateral bands have converged to form the terminal tendon)
- Etiology
  - Mallet finger (dorsal DIP)
    - Frequent: Acute forceful flexion of extended DIP
    - Less frequent: Direct trauma to dorsal DIP
    - Less frequent: Volar subluxation of distal phalanx with respect to middle phalanx
  - Jersey finger (volar DIP)
    - Forced extension of the flexed DIP
    - Classic: Player grabs a moving player's jersey
  - Volar plate disruption
    - Most common: Hyperextension of PIP, often from dislocation of either DIP or PIP
    - Less frequent: Rotational longitudinal compression of semi-flexed PIP
  - Boutonniere deformity

AVULSION FRACTURES, FINGER

- Forced flexion of the extended PIP: Basketball players or martial artists who use open hand blocking techniques
  - Volar dislocation of middle phalanx at PIP
- Collateral ligament injury
  - Abducting or adducting force applied to IP while finger is extended
- Epidemiology
  - PIP is most commonly injured joint in hand
  - Extensor > flexor apparatus injuries
  - Most common sports closed tendon injury: Mallet

Staging, Grading or Classification Criteria
- Volar plate injuries: Classified according to degree of articular instability
  - Type I: Isolated volar plate avulsion
  - Type II: Involvement of periarticular soft tissues, with volar plate avulsion + a major split between the components of the collateral ligament complex; more unstable, with dorsal subluxation
  - Type III: Fx-dislocation of volar base of middle phalanx; unstable if > 40% of articular surface involved
- Jersey (FDP) finger: 4 main types characterized by degree of retraction
  - Type I: Retraction of tendon into palm
  - Type II: Tendon ± avulsed fx retracts to PIP joint
  - Type III: Avulsion of large bone fragment, held in place by A4 pulley
  - Type IV: Type III + avulsion FDP from the fragment

CLINICAL ISSUES

Presentation
- Most common signs/symptoms
  - Mallet finger: Flexion deformity of DIP (full range of passive extension of distal phalanx may be maintained in the acute setting)
  - Jersey finger: Inability to actively flex the DIP
  - Volar plate: Sports injury, often with IP dislocation
  - Boutonniere: Initially will be able to maintain active extension of PIP, so injury may be clinically inapparent; deformity not seen for first 7-10 days

Demographics
- Age: Adolescents, young adults, related to sports activity
- Gender: Male > female, related to sports participation

Natural History & Prognosis
- Untreated Mallet finger progresses to "swan neck" deformity: Hyperextension of PIP results from the unopposed extensor pull of the central slip attachment to base middle phalanx
- Untreated Jersey finger results in fixed hyperextension of DIP
- Most volar plate injuries heal well with treatment; a few will develop contractures or joint laxity, which results in difficulty flexing the finger from a hyperextended position
- Untreated Boutonniere injuries progress to typical deformity: Hyperflexed PIP, hyperextended DIP
  - Initially the lateral bands that are dorsal to the axis of the PIP can maintain active extension
  - Eventually, the central slip will retract, causing lateral bands to move into a volar position, resulting in the deformity
  - Patient will still be able to passively extend the PIP

Treatment
- Mallet finger
  - Continuous splinting of DIP in extension, 6 weeks
  - Surgery reserved for fx involving > 50% of articular surface, or failure of conservative therapy
- Jersey finger
  - Most treated surgically
  - Degree of tendon retraction, presence and size of bony fragment, & integrity of blood supply determine the prognosis
- Volar plate
  - Most treated with short-term immobilization & early range of motion
  - May be unstable if fx > 40% of articular surface & the collateral ligaments remain attached to fx fragment; these require open reduction, internal fixation
- Boutonniere
  - Treated by continuous splinting of the PIP in extension for at least 4 weeks
  - DIP should be excluded from splint to avoid contractures
  - Surgical therapy reserved for cases that fail conservative management
- Collateral ligament injuries: Conservative, with short term immobilization followed by protected range of motion

DIAGNOSTIC CHECKLIST

Consider
- Watch for fracture fragments about the IP joints
- Watch for unnatural angulation of the IP joints to suggest soft tissue disruption
  - Hyperextended PIP: Volar plate
  - Hyperflexed PIP + hyperextended DIP: Boutonniere
  - Hyperflexed DIP when PIP is extended: Mallet finger
  - Hyperextended DIP: Jersey finger
  - Ulnar or radial angulation on AP view: Collateral ligament injury

SELECTED REFERENCES
1. Rosner JL et al: Imaging of athletic wrist and hand injuries. Seminars in Musculoskeletal. Radiology. 8(1):57-79, 2004
2. Clavero JA et al: MR imaging of ligament and tendon injuries of the fingers. Radiographics. 22:237-56, 2002
3. Graham TJ et al: Athletic injuries of the adult hand. Orthopaedic sports medicine. vol 1. 2nd ed. Philadelphia PA, WB Saunders. (24):1381-1430, 2002
4. Perron AD et al: Orthopedic pitfalls in the emergency department. J of Emerg Med. 19(1):76-80, 2001
5. VanHolsbeeck MT et al: Musculoskeletal ultrasound. 2nd ed. St. Louis MO, Mosby. 541-7, 2001

AVULSION FRACTURES, FINGER

IMAGE GALLERY

Typical

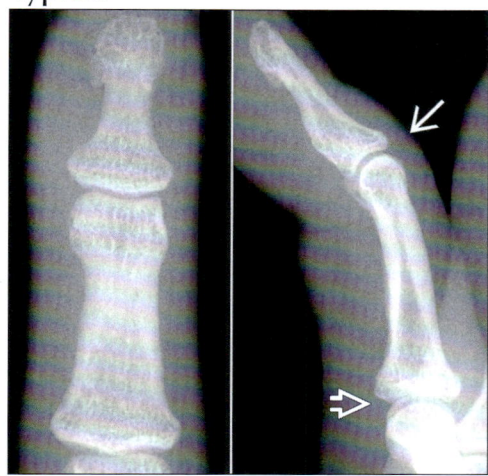
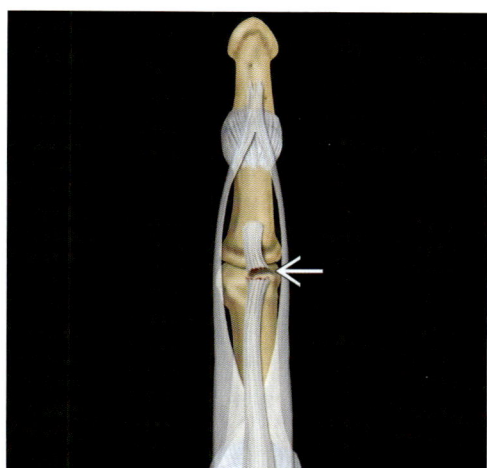

(Left) AP & lateral radiographs show flexion at the DIP ➡ with the PIP held in extension ➡. This is not a normal position, & suggests a soft tissue mallet finger injury (extensor digitorum tendon avulsion). (Right) Posterior graphic shows a tear at the distal middle slip of the extensor mechanism ➡. This is a soft tissue Boutonniere injury. Note the lateral slips converging to form the terminal extensor tendon which inserts at the base of the distal phalanx.

Typical

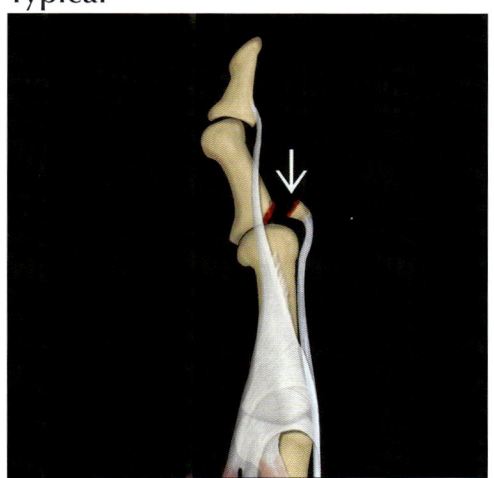
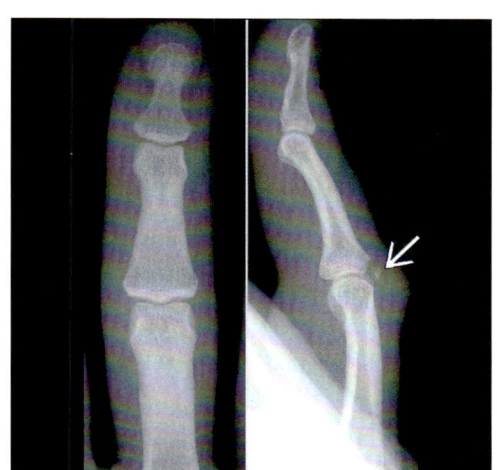

(Left) Lateral graphic shows an avulsion of the dorsal aspect of the base of the middle phalanx ➡, a Boutonniere fx. This fracture results in the typical deformity of PIP flexion & DIP hyperextension. (Right) AP & lateral radiographs show a Boutonniere injury, matching the graphic. There is soft tissue swelling & avulsion fx at the PIP joint ➡. The fragment is avulsed by the middle slip of the extensor tendon, resulting in the typical deformity.

Typical

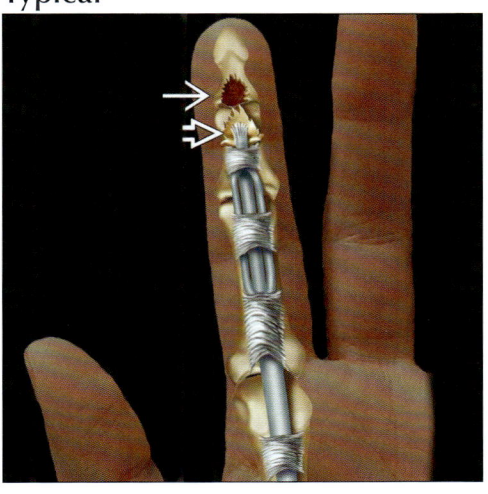
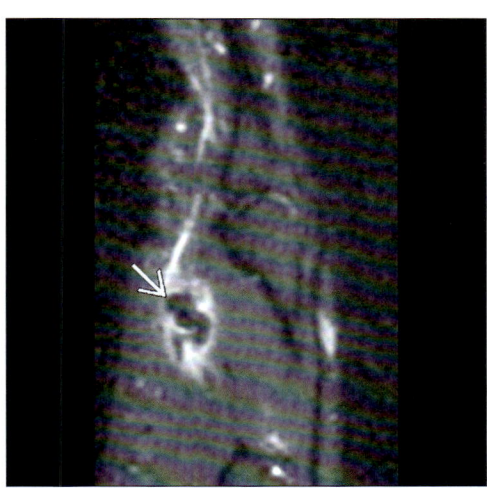

(Left) Anterior graphic depicts a type III flexor digitorum profundus avulsion. The donor site of the large bony fragment is the volar aspect of the base of the distal phalanx ➡; there is retraction of the tendon, with the fragment ➡ lodged at the level of the A4 pulley. (Right) Sagittal STIR MR shows a ruptured flexor digitorum profundus tendon ➡, which has retracted to the level of the A4 pulley. An avulsed bony fragment would be difficult to see without radiograph.

AVULSION FRACTURES, PELVIC

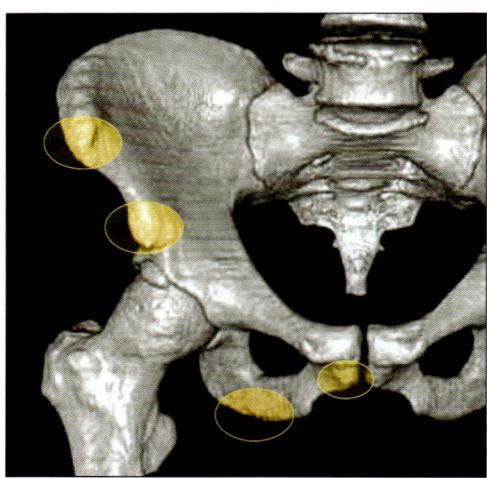

Frontal bone CT reformat shows common sites for pelvic avulsion fx. Counterclockwise from upper left: ASIS, AIIS, ischial tuberosity, pubic symphysis/inferior pubic ramus. Watch for adjacent subtle fx fragments.

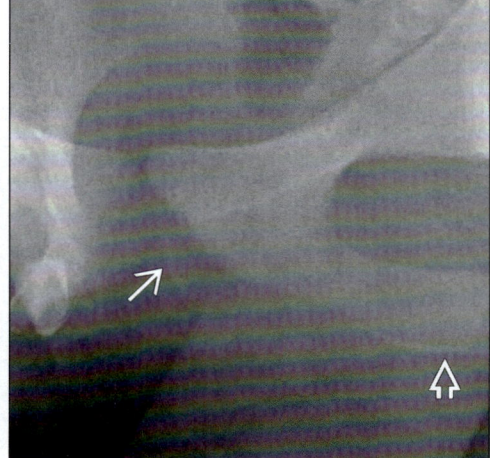

Oblique radiograph shows avulsion from the pubis by the adductors ➡. Crescentic shape & very faintly seen fragment is typical. Note the normal apophysis at the ischial tuberosity ➡.

TERMINOLOGY

Abbreviations and Synonyms
- Avulsion injury, tug injury, tug lesion, pelvic avulsion

Definitions
- Apophysis: Growth center at site of tendinous attachment; extraarticular
- Fracture at an apophysis resulting from a force applied by a musculotendinous unit

IMAGING FINDINGS

General Features
- Best diagnostic clue: Thin crescentic fragment or subtle discoid fragment adjacent to site of apophysis
- Location
  o Anterior superior iliac spine (ASIS): Avulsion by sartorius
  o Anterior inferior iliac spine (AIIS): Avulsion by rectus femoris
  o Inferior pubic symphysis: Avulsion by adductors
  o Ischial tuberosity: Avulsion by hamstrings
  o Less common avulsion sites
    ▪ Greater trochanter: Avulsion by glutei
    ▪ Lesser trochanter: Avulsion by iliopsoas
    ▪ Iliac crest: Abdominal muscles
- Size: Variable, relates to age & osseous development of the apophysis
- Morphology: Displaced fragment appears either crescentic or discoid, depending on whether it is viewed in profile or en face

Radiographic Findings
- Osseous fragment identified adjacent to donor site
  o If viewed in profile, will be a thin crescent shape
  o If viewed en face, will be thinner discoid shape & much less distinctly seen
  o Most fragments (ASIS, ischial tuberosity, pubic ramus) generally are not displaced > 1 cm from donor site
  o AIIS may be displaced > 1 cm from donor site (distally)
  o ASIS, AIIS, ischial tuberosity, greater & lesser tuberosity avulsions best seen on anteroposterior radiographs

Other Pelvic Avulsions

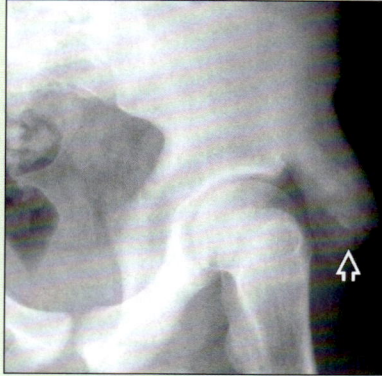

Mature AIIS Avulsion

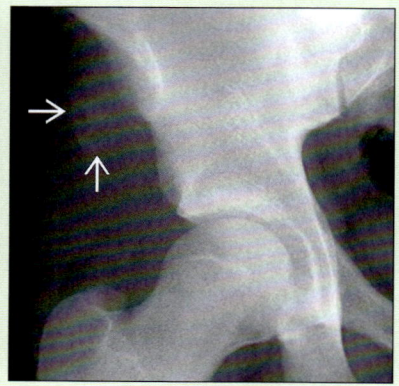

Subtle ASIS Avulsion

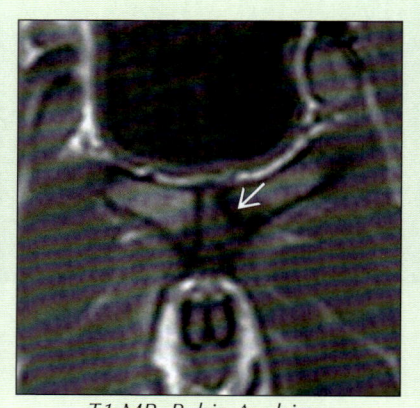

T1 MR, Pubic Avulsion

AVULSION FRACTURES, PELVIC

Key Facts

Terminology
- Fracture at an apophysis resulting from a force applied by a musculotendinous unit

Imaging Findings
- Osseous fragment identified adjacent to donor site
- If viewed in profile, will be a thin crescent shape
- If viewed en face, will be thinner discoid shape & much less distinctly seen
- Most fragments (ASIS, ischial tuberosity, pubic ramus) generally are not displaced > 1 cm from donor site
- AIIS may be displaced > 1 cm from donor site (distally)
- No radiographic abnormality seen if apophysis not yet ossified (~ < age 15)
- MR confirms a diagnosis if apophysis not yet ossified
- T1 may identify avulsion fragment by high (marrow) signal intensity
- Hyperintense marrow edema at donor site
- Laxity of avulsing musculotendinous unit

Top Differential Diagnoses
- Amorphous osteoid formation with early healing has the same morphology of osteoid formation in osteosarcoma
- Tendon Tear
- Stress Fracture

Diagnostic Checklist
- Watch for these avulsions particularly in the 15-25 year age range
- Location is the key; scan soft tissues in region of ASIS, AIIS, pubis, & ischial tuberosity

---

  - Pubic ramus avulsion may require oblique (Judet) view to be visualized
- If necessary, contralateral views distinguish open apophysis from avulsion fracture
- No radiographic abnormality seen if apophysis not yet ossified (~ < age 15)
- Healing response is exuberant callus
  - 4-6 weeks: Callus is immature osteoid & may give the appearance of aggressive osteoid formation
  - > 6 weeks, osteoid begins to mature, eventually resulting in a bony excrescence at the site
  - Bony excrescence may slowly resorb with time, or remain unchanged

CT Findings
- Osseous detail of fracture fragment & donor site
- May view contralateral side if need to distinguish between normal open apophysis & avulsion fracture
- Callus visualized; may simulate aggressive lesion when it is immature, as does radiograph

MR Findings
- MR confirms a diagnosis if apophysis not yet ossified
- May distinguish avulsed fragment from normal open apophysis
- T1 weighted MR
  - T1 may identify avulsion fragment by high (marrow) signal intensity
  - Adjacent soft tissue & hematoma signal may obscure small apophyseal fragment
  - May see hypointense edema in adjacent marrow (donor site)
  - May see low fluid signal in adjacent tissues
  - Avulsing musculotendinous unit may show laxity
- Fluid sensitive sequences
  - Hyperintense marrow edema at donor site
  - Hyperintense fluid, soft tissue edema, & hemorrhage at site of avulsion
  - Laxity of avulsing musculotendinous unit
  - Associated muscle strain: Hyperintense signal
  - Avulsed osseous fragment may be obscured, hypointense

Imaging Recommendations
- Best imaging tool
  - Diagnosis should be made by radiography
  - MR
    - If radiograph is negative, shows donor site edema & may show avulsed fragment
    - Documents status of musculotendinous unit
  - CT if searching for subtle small & barely ossified avulsion fragment
- Protocol advice
  - T1 optimizes marrow signal
  - Fluid sensitive sequence
  - Coronal & axial planes used most frequently
  - Sagittal plane helpful for rectus femoris injuries of straight head (AIIS) & reflected head (upper rim acetabulum)

DIFFERENTIAL DIAGNOSIS

Osteosarcoma
- Amorphous osteoid formation with early healing has the same morphology of osteoid formation in osteosarcoma
- Amorphous appearance closely related to time of injury; most aggressive appearing approximately 4-6 weeks following injury
- Beyond 6 weeks, will begin to mature both radiographically & histologically

Tendinosis
- Thickening of tendon origin & insertions
- Intermediate signal on T1 & T2 MR

Tendon Tear
- Common in hamstring & adductors
- Watch for retraction of tendon

Stress Fracture
- Repetitive stress
- Pubic ramus - long distance runners & joggers
- Sacral stress fractures - insufficiency vs. stress (runners)

AVULSION FRACTURES, PELVIC

Lesser Trochanter Avulsion in Older Adult
- Must exclude metastatic disease/tumor

PATHOLOGY

General Features
- General path comments
  ○ Relevant anatomy: Pelvic apophyses
    ▪ Do not ossify until middle teen years (~ age 14)
    ▪ Do not fuse until young adult years (~ age 25)
    ▪ Pelvic apophyses therefore at greatest risk for avulsion during this age range (14-25 years)
  ○ Relevant anatomy: Muscle origins
    ▪ Sartorius origin: ASIS & upper half iliac notch
    ▪ Rectus femoris: AIIS (straight head) & upper acetabular rim (reflected head)
    ▪ Biceps femoris, semitendinosus, & semimembranosus: Ischial tuberosity
    ▪ Gracilis, adductor longus, adductor brevis: Pubic symphysis & inferior pubic ramus
- Etiology
  ○ Adolescents: Traction on unfused apophysis
  ○ Fracture secondary to forceful concentric or eccentric muscle contraction
  ○ Fracture secondary to extreme passive stretch (dancers & gymnasts)
  ○ Less common: Avulsions secondary to chronic repetitive microtrauma
- Epidemiology: Avulsion fractures = 13.4% of children's pelvic fractures

Gross Pathologic & Surgical Features
- Displacement of ASIS limited by fascia lata & lateral inguinal ligament
- Displacement of AIIS limited by dual origin of straight head of rectus & reflected head
- Ischial apophysis displacement limited by sacrotuberous ligament

Microscopic Features
- Hematoma
- Revascularization & resorption of devascularized bone fragment
- Callus & fibrous scar tissue
- Biopsy should be avoided
  ○ May show mitoses & osteoid in healing bone
  ○ If pathologist does not know circumstance & location of biopsy, could mistake for high grade malignancy

CLINICAL ISSUES

Presentation
- Most common signs/symptoms: Local pain, often related to trauma
- Clinical Profile
  ○ Late teen or early adult
  ○ Swelling and pain after activity
  ○ Limitation of activity
  ○ Iliac crest avulsion rarely causes RLQ pain mimicking appendicitis
  ○ Point tenderness
  ○ Discoloration secondary to hematoma
  ○ Altered gait
  ○ Pain & weakness of involved muscle when placed under stress
  ○ Most commonly related to athletic injury
  ○ If in adult & atraumatic, exclude metastatic or insufficiency fracture (especially at lesser trochanter)

Demographics
- Age: Age 14-25 years most common
- Gender: M > F
- Related activity
  ○ ASIS: Forceful contraction of sartorius in kicking sports, jumping, or running
  ○ AIIS: Rectus femoris in kicking sports
  ○ Ischial tuberosity: Hamstring in dancers, gymnasts, sprinting, hurdling, & football

Natural History & Prognosis
- Most injuries heal with conservative treatment
- Poor healing results in chronic pain secondary to repetitive micromotion
- Surgery for recalcitrant pain or severely displaced fragments

Treatment
- Conservative
  ○ Recovery slow: Average 4-8 weeks up to 4 months
  ○ Initial bedrest to non-weight bearing + crutches
  ○ Ice, anti-inflammatories
  ○ Physical therapy: Gradual strengthening + progressive weight bearing
  ○ Reinjury if return to high level activity prematurely
- Surgical
  ○ Reattachment of severely displaced avulsed fragment
  ○ Chronic pain: Resection of weak bony union & surgical reattachment

DIAGNOSTIC CHECKLIST

Image Interpretation Pearls
- Watch for these avulsions particularly in the 15-25 year age range
- Location is the key; scan soft tissues in region of ASIS, AIIS, pubis, & ischial tuberosity
- Acute avulsion is subtle
  ○ Extremely thin disc if viewed en face
  ○ Crescentic if viewed in profile

SELECTED REFERENCES
1. Moeller JL: Pelvic and hip apophyseal avulsion injuries in young athletes. Curr Sports Med Rep. 2(2):110-5, 2003
2. Bui-Mansfield LT et al: Nontraumatic avulsions of the pelvis. AJR Am J Roentgenol. 178(2):423-7, 2002
3. Rossi F et al: Acute avulsion fractures of the pelvis in adolescent competitive athletes: prevalence, location and sports distribution of 203 cases collected. Skeletal Radiol. 30(3):127-31, 2001
4. Stevens MA et al: Imaging features of avulsion injuries. Radiographics. 19(3):655-72, 1999

AVULSION FRACTURES, PELVIC

IMAGE GALLERY

Typical

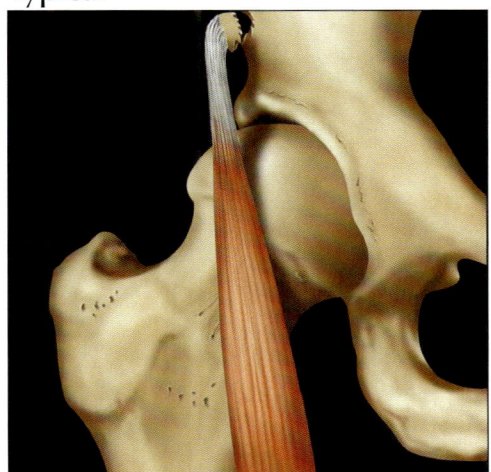
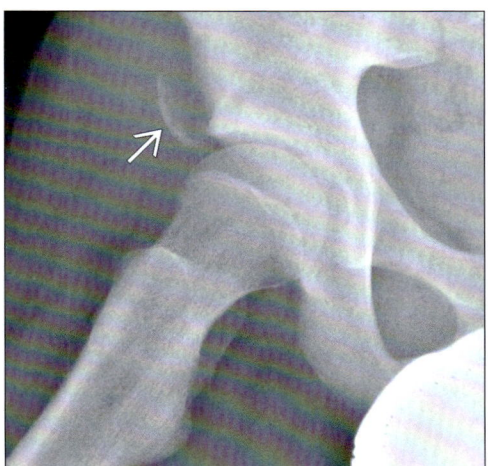

(Left) Anterior graphic shows avulsion of the anterior inferior iliac spine with origin of the straight head of the rectus femoris. *(Right)* Frog lateral radiograph shows avulsion fx of the anterior inferior iliac spine (AIIS) ➡. The location of the fragment in this nearly skeletally mature patient makes the diagnosis. The crescentic shape is typical when viewed in profile. Note that the fragment has displaced some distance inferiorly.

Typical

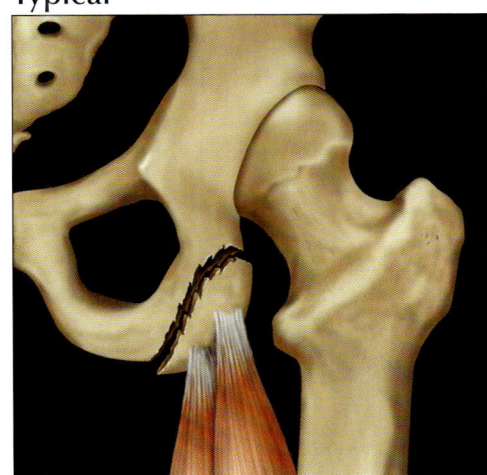
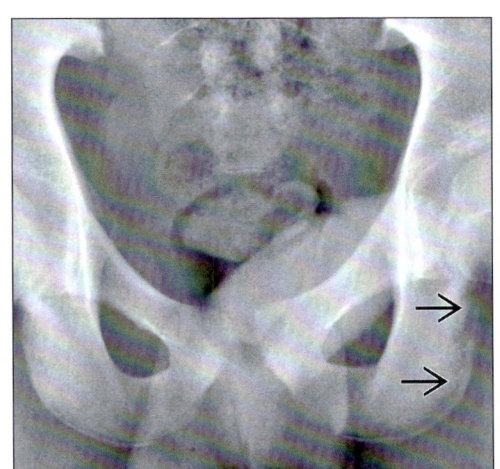

(Left) Anterior graphic shows osseous avulsion of the hamstring tendon attachment to the ischial tuberosity. *(Right)* Anteroposterior radiograph shows widening & irregularity of the left ischial apophysis ➡, compared to the normal right side. This indicates a subacute or chronic avulsion, with healing.

Typical

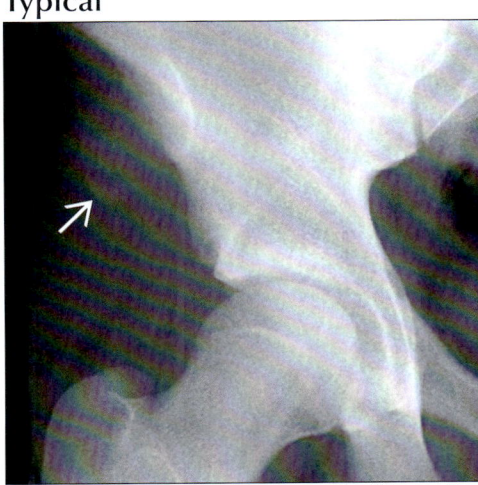
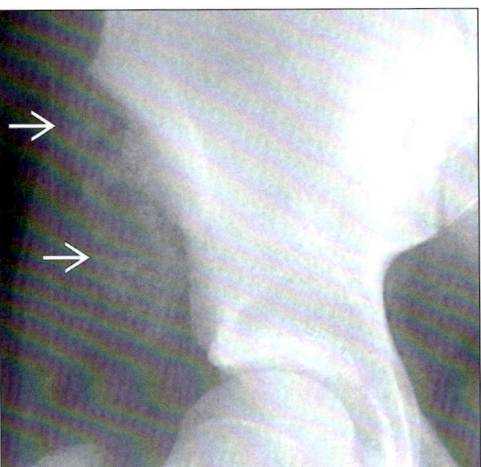

(Left) Anteroposterior radiograph shows a faint disc-shaped ossific density ➡ which is an acute avulsion of the anterior superior iliac spine (ASIS). Note that visualization is difficult when the fragment is viewed en face. *(Right)* Anteroposterior radiograph of the same patient 4 weeks later shows interval progression in maturation of the healing osteoid ➡. Care must be taken to avoid a mistaken diagnosis of osteosarcoma.

PELVIC FRACTURES, STABLE

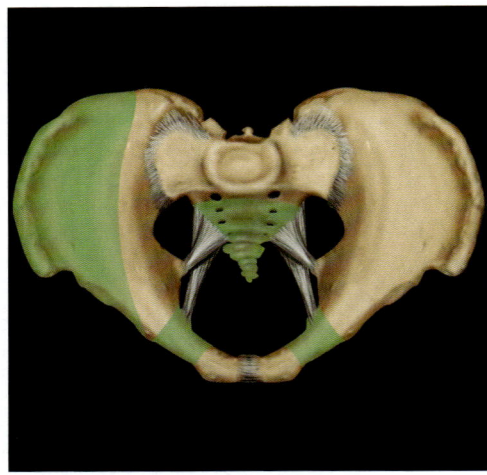

Stable pelvic fxs (green) include iliac wing, transverse sacral and pubic rami fxs which spare the posterior arch (SI ligaments, portions of ilium and sacrum).

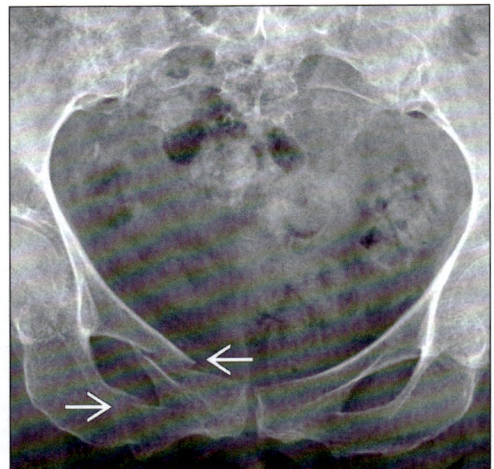

Anteroposterior radiograph shows transverse rami fxs ➡ in an elderly osteoporotic woman after a mechanical fall onto the right hip. The posterior arch is intact (type A2.2).

TERMINOLOGY

Abbreviations and Synonyms
- Duverney fx (iliac wing), pubic ramus fx, butterfly or straddle fx, avulsion fx, transverse sacral fx, Tile type A

Definitions
- Stable: Fracture sparing posterior arch; pelvic ring able to withstand normal physiological stress without displacement

IMAGING FINDINGS

General Features
- Best diagnostic clue: Posterior pelvic arch intact
- Location
  - Avulsion fx of innominate bone (includes ilium, ischium and pubic bones)
  - Iliac wing fx not extending through pelvic ring
  - Pubic rami fxs
  - Transverse fx of sacrum or coccyx
  - Nondisplaced posterior arch fx may be stable if sacroiliac (SI) ligaments intact
- Morphology
  - Iliac wing fx: Vertically/obliquely oriented fx line not extending through ring; seen with lateral compression (LC) force
  - Rami fxs
    - Typically horizontal/coronal fx line with lateral compression (LC) force
    - Typically vertical/sagittal fx line with anterior posterior compression (APC) or vertical shear (VS) force
  - Sacral/coccygeal fx: Transversely oriented; seen with direct trauma (in seated position)

Radiographic Findings
- Inlet/outlet pelvis views
  - Obtained with X-ray beam angled 45° caudal (inlet) and 45° cranial (outlet) relative to pelvis
  - Evaluates anteroposterior (inlet) and superoinferior (outlet) fx displacement
- "Judet" views
  - Iliac oblique obtained at 45° to pelvis with side of interest down; used to demonstrate fx of ilioischial (posterior) column, anterior acetabular rim and iliac wing

Partially Stable Pelvic Fx (Posterior Arch Partially Disrupted)

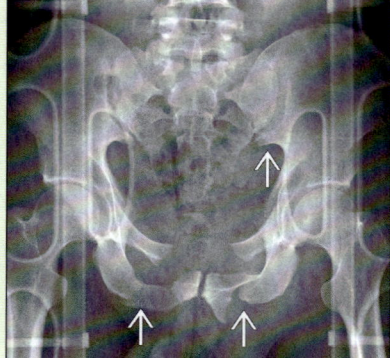

APC II Injury

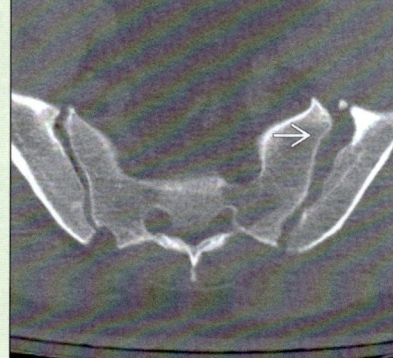

Wide SI Joint

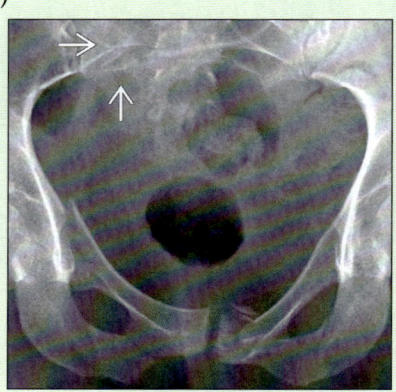

Arcuate Disruption

PELVIC FRACTURES, STABLE

Key Facts

Terminology
- Stable: Fracture sparing posterior arch; pelvic ring able to withstand normal physiological stress without displacement

Imaging Findings
- Most fxs (90%) detected on AP view; outlet and lateral view best for transverse sacral fxs
- CT ± CT cystogram in stable polytrauma patients

Pathology
- General path comments: Pelvic bones (sacrum and innominate) have no inherent stability; sacroiliac ligaments provide majority of ring stability

Clinical Issues
- Young athletes: Avulsion and pubic rami stress fxs
- Older osteoporotic women: Unilateral (typically superior) pubic rami fxs s/p fall
- Sacroiliac pain not explainable on radiograph may represent occult impaction fx; consider CT or MR
- Uncomplicated stable pelvic fxs with minimal displacement (< 5 mm) typically demonstrate full recovery in 6-8 weeks with conservative treatment
- Sacral fxs require neurosurgical or orthopedic consult for possible ORIF, particularly in cases of neurologic injury

Diagnostic Checklist
- Must exclude associated hemorrhagic, neurologic, genitourinary, orthopedic and infectious complications

---

  o Obturator oblique obtained at 45° to pelvis with side of interest up; demonstrates fx of iliopubic (anterior) column and posterior acetabular rim
- Slight offset at the pubic symphysis can be normal, particularly at the superior aspect of the pubic body
- Sacral arcuate lines and sacroiliac distance will be preserved in stable fxs

CT Findings
- CECT
  o Evaluate associated organ injuries
    - Arterial hemorrhage as a blush of contrast
    - Bladder tear as extravasation on CT cystogram
    - Bowel or vaginal tear as extraluminal air
- Bone CT
  o Accurately identifies complex injury patterns
    - Occult posterior ring injuries (sacral fx, SI joint diastasis)
    - Extension of iliac wing or pubic rami fx into acetabulum

MR Findings
- Generally not used in acute setting as edema and fluid can obscure ligamentous detail

Imaging Recommendations
- Best imaging tool
  o Most fxs (90%) detected on AP view; outlet and lateral view best for transverse sacral fxs
  o CT ± CT cystogram in stable polytrauma patients
    - Study of choice in cases of bilateral pubic rami fxs due to associated injuries of posterior arch and genitourinary (GU) tract
  o In stable polytrauma patients destined for CT, pelvic radiographs are not necessary for dx
- Protocol advice
  o CT
    - 1-3 mm axial pelvic reformats, ± IV contrast if concern for vascular/solid organ injury
  o CT cystogram (bladder catheterization required)
    - Follow CT with retrograde gravitational filling of bladder using dilute water soluble contrast until patient cannot tolerate or 500 cc filled
    - Contrast extravasation from bladder injury will limit visualization in fluoroscopic pelvic angiography

DIFFERENTIAL DIAGNOSIS

Partially Stable Pelvic Fracture
- Posterior arch partially disrupted

Muscle Strain, Hip
- Muscle pain without fx, high T2 signal on MR in affected muscle group

Sacral Insufficiency Fractures
- Normal forces on abnormal (insufficient) bone

Pubic Rami Stress Fractures
- Abnormal repetitive forces (stress) on normal bone

PATHOLOGY

General Features
- General path comments: Pelvic bones (sacrum and innominate) have no inherent stability; sacroiliac ligaments provide majority of ring stability
- Etiology
  o Avulsion fxs
    - Muscular traction secondary to contraction or stretching
    - More common in adolescents before closure of the corresponding physis occurs
  o Iliac wing fx
    - Direct trauma from lateral compressive force such as T-bone MVA or auto-pedestrian impact
  o Unilateral pubic rami fxs
    - Single horizontal/coronal superior ramus fx is the most common pelvic fx
    - Usually seen from lateral compression after a fall in elderly osteoporotic patients
  o Bilateral pubic rami fxs (butterfly or straddle fx)

PELVIC FRACTURES, STABLE

- Indicative of high energy injury (lateral or anterior-posterior compressive force)
    - Coccygeal and transverse sacral fx
        - Direct trauma often from fall in seated position
- Epidemiology: Pelvic fxs account for 3% of all skeletal fxs and 2% of orthopedic hospital admissions
- Associated abnormalities
    - Unilateral rami/iliac wing fxs from lateral compression associated w/occult sacral impaction fx
    - Bilateral rami fxs associated with posterior arch, GU and arterial injury; (especially if fx displaced > 5 mm)
    - Transverse sacral fx S3 and above
        - Associated with neurologic (21-34%) and rectal injury

Staging, Grading or Classification Criteria
- Goal of classification is to provide understanding of pelvic stability and direction of corrective forces needed to realign pelvic ring
- Orthopedic Trauma Association Classification (OTA); combines features of Tile (continuum of stability) and Young-Burgess (vector force) classification
    - Type A (stable): Lesion sparing (or with no displacement of) posterior arch
        - A1: Avulsion fx of innominate bone
        - A2: Fx of innominate bone involving rami or iliac wing (Duverney)
        - A3: Transverse fx/dislocation of sacrum/coccyx
    - Type B (partially stable): Incomplete disruption of posterior arch (typically posterior SI ligaments intact)
        - B1: Unilateral, partial disruption of posterior arch, external rotation (anterior posterior compression II)
        - B2: Unilateral, partial disruption of posterior arch, internal rotation (lateral compression I, II)
        - B3: Bilateral, partial disruption of posterior arch (APC II, LC III)
    - Type C (unstable): Complete disruption of posterior arch (sacrum, SI ligaments or posterior ilium)
        - C1: Unilateral, complete disruption of posterior arch (APC III, LC II, vertical shear)
        - C2: Bilateral; ipsilateral complete, contralateral incomplete (LC III, Combined Mechanism Injury)
        - C3: Bilateral, complete disruption (APC III, LC III, VS, CMI)

CLINICAL ISSUES

Presentation
- Most common signs/symptoms: Local pain, swelling, bruising, weakness of associated muscle origins
- Other signs/symptoms: Must exclude potential associated complications (hemorrhagic, GU, orthopedic, neurologic) and open fx (via communication with bowel, vagina, skin) in all cases of stable pelvic ring injuries
- Clinical Profile
    - Young athletes: Avulsion and pubic rami stress fxs
    - Older osteoporotic women: Unilateral (typically superior) pubic rami fxs s/p fall
- Sacroiliac pain not explainable on radiograph may represent occult impaction fx; consider CT or MR

Natural History & Prognosis
- Uncomplicated stable pelvic fxs with minimal displacement (< 5 mm) typically demonstrate full recovery in 6-8 weeks with conservative treatment
    - Associated myotendinous injury may cause prolonged pain and recovery time
- Displaced pubic rami fxs have poorer prognosis due to associated posterior arch, vascular and GU injuries
    - GU injuries (bladder rupture and/or urethral tear) occur with about 1/3 of bilateral rami fxs
    - Increased incidence of significant hemorrhage with fx displacement ≥ 5 mm, older patients (> 55 yo), osteoporotic patients
- Transverse sacral fxs S3 and above have higher associated morbidity due to neurologic damage (21-34%)
- Open fractures involving perineum, vagina or bowel have up to 50% mortality

Treatment
- Depends largely on associated injuries
- Uncomplicated stable fxs treated conservatively
- Instability of pelvic ring, intraarticular or displaced fx (> 5 mm) requires orthopedic consult for potential ORIF
- Sacral fxs require neurosurgical or orthopedic consult for possible ORIF, particularly in cases of neurologic injury
- Open fxs involving bowel require diverting ostomy

DIAGNOSTIC CHECKLIST

Consider
- Must exclude associated hemorrhagic, neurologic, genitourinary, orthopedic and infectious complications

Image Interpretation Pearls
- AP, inlet and outlet views can be obtained without moving the patient and allow for timely identification and classification of > 90% of pelvic fractures
- Transverse sacral fxs often missed on AP view, consider lateral and AP sacral (similar to outlet pelvis) views

SELECTED REFERENCES

1. Avey G et al: Radiographic and clinical predictors of bladder rupture in blunt trauma patients with pelvic fracture. Acad Radiol. 13(5):573-9, 2006
2. Durkin A et al: Contemporary management of pelvic fractures. Am J Surg. 192(2):211-23, 2006
3. Bucholz et al: Rockwood and Green's: Fractures In Adults. Vol 2. 6th ed. Philadelphia, Lippincott Williams & Wilkins, 1584-1664, 2005
4. Park J et al: Imaging of pelvic trauma. Contemporary Diagnostic Radiology. 28(24):1-6, 2005
5. Yoon W et al: Pelvic arterial hemorrhage in patients with pelvic fractures: detection with contrast-enhanced CT. Radiographics. 24(6):1591-605; discussion 1605-6, 2004
6. Stevens MA et al: Imaging features of avulsion injuries. Radiographics. 19(3):655-72, 1999

PELVIC FRACTURES, STABLE

IMAGE GALLERY

Typical

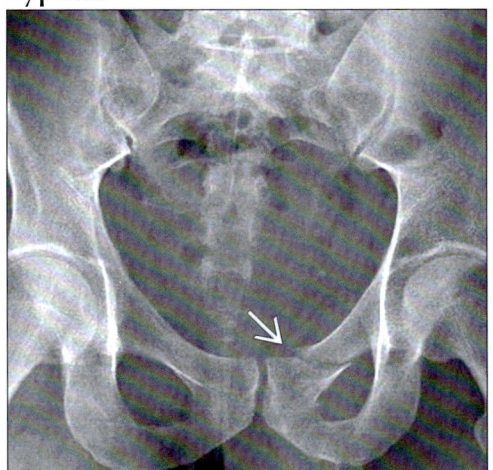
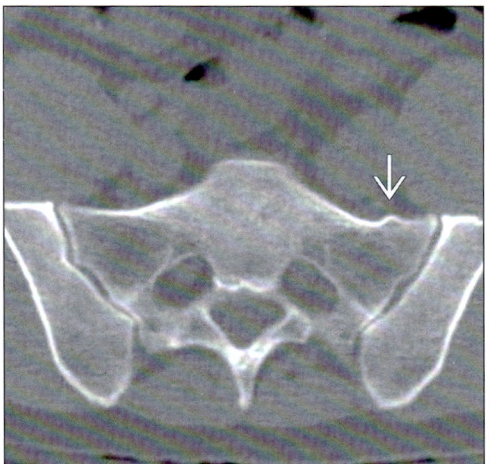

(Left) Anteroposterior radiograph shows a transverse superior ramus fx ➔ following a T-bone MVA. Patient also described posterior left SI pain but a fx was not seen on radiograph. *(Right)* Axial bone CT shows the associated sacral buckle fx ➔ = lateral compression I, type B2.1 = potentially unstable. However, pelvis was stable clinically and managed conservatively.

Typical

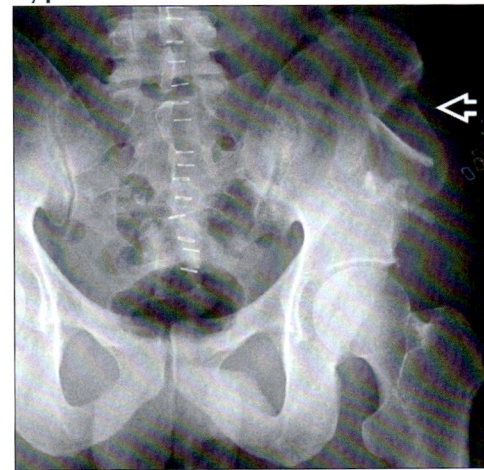
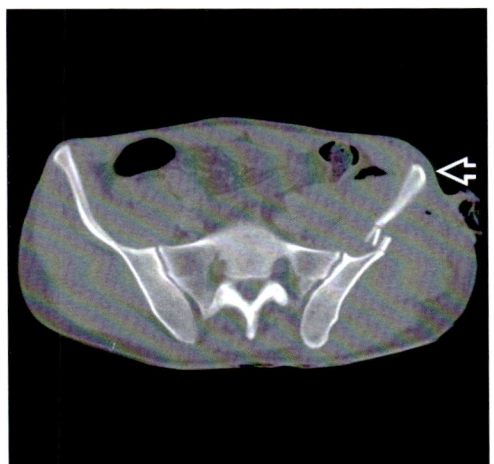

(Left) Anteroposterior radiograph shows a stable, open iliac wing fx ➔ (type A2.1, Duverney) post debridement. This type of open pelvic fx has a relatively low mortality rate (0-5%). *(Right)* Axial CECT correlation shows direction ➔ of lateral compression and air within the soft tissues surrounding the stable open iliac wing fracture. The SI joints and sacrum are normal.

Typical

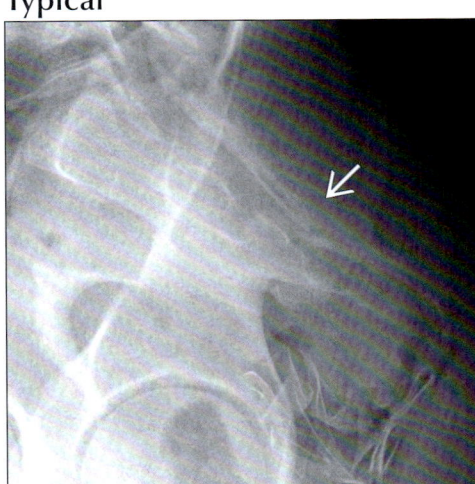
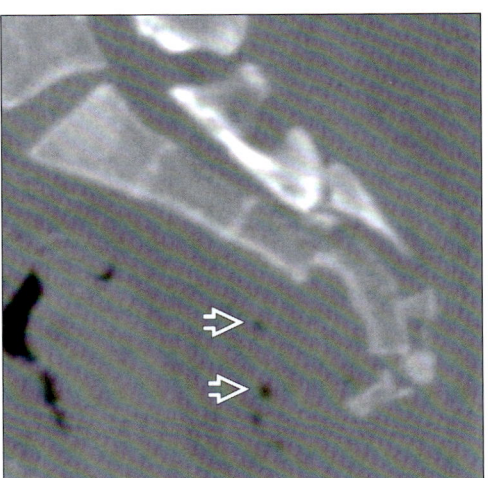

(Left) Lateral radiograph shows angulation ➔ of an open transverse sacral fx after a fall in seated position. Retroperitoneal packing was performed due to associated venous bleeding. *(Right)* Sagittal bone CT shows posterior displacement of the sacrum (type A3.3) inferior to S3 that was not appreciated on radiograph. Air in the presacral space ➔ indicates an open fx.

PELVIC FRACTURES, UNSTABLE

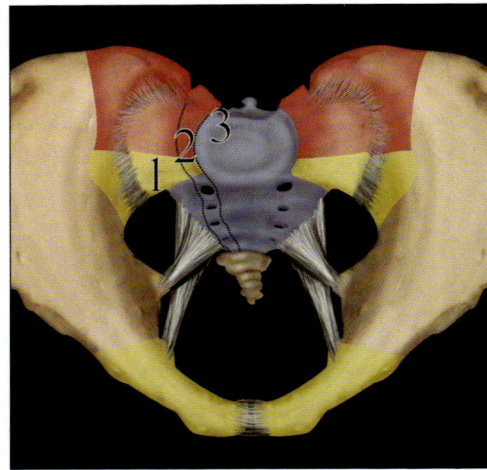

Distribution of partially stable (yellow) and unstable (yellow + red) pelvic ring disruption. Stability of sacral fx (blue) depends on fx line and ligamentous integrity. Denis classification (1, 2, 3) of sacral fxs.

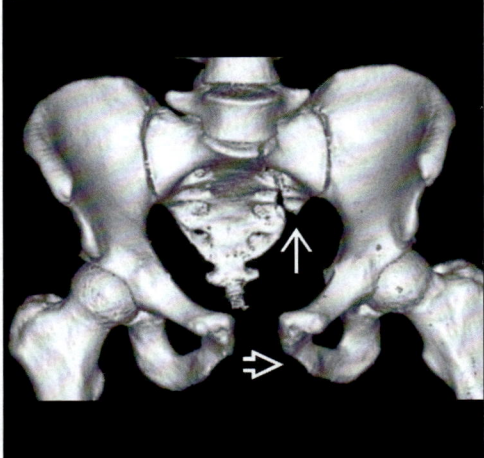

Bone CT with 3D surface rendering shows pubic diastasis ➡ and a Denis II sacral fx ➡. Posterior SI ligaments were intact (vertically stable, rotationally unstable) = APC II injury.

TERMINOLOGY

Abbreviations and Synonyms
- Tile type B and C; lateral compression (LC) II, III; anterior posterior compression (APC) II, III; vertical shear (VS); combined mechanism injury (CMI); open-book, malgaigne, bucket handle, crescent fx, windswept pelvis

Definitions
- Partially stable: Posterior osteoligamentous integrity partially maintained (rotationally unstable, vertically stable)
- Unstable: Complete loss of posterior osteoligamentous integrity (rotationally and vertically unstable)

IMAGING FINDINGS

General Features
- Best diagnostic clue
  - Posterior arch disruption (involves sacrum, posterior ilium and/or sacroiliac (SI) ligaments)
  - Displaced pubic rami fxs (> 5 mm) infer posterior arch injury
- Location: Anterior and posterior arch injury
- Morphology: Rotational and vertical instability inferred by rotational and vertical hemipelvis displacement

Radiographic Findings
- Pubic symphysis normally 5 mm wide; diastasis > 1 cm abnormal (exceptions for postpartum and skeletally immature)
- LC forces typically create horizontal/coronal rami fxs with medial rotational hemipelvis displacement
- APC forces typically create vertical/sagittal rami fxs with lateral rotational hemipelvis displacement (open-book)
- VS forces typically create vertical/sagittal rami fxs with vertical hemipelvis displacement

CT Findings
- CECT
  - Evaluate posterior arch and associated injuries
  - May demonstrate open fx or ongoing arterial hemorrhage as a blush

Injuries Associated with Pelvic Fractures

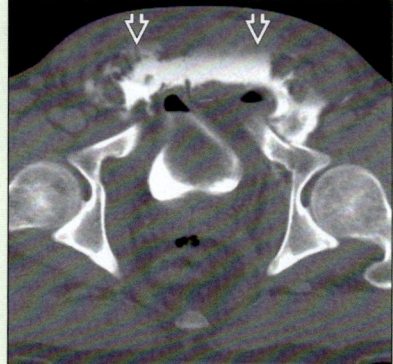

Bladder Rupture

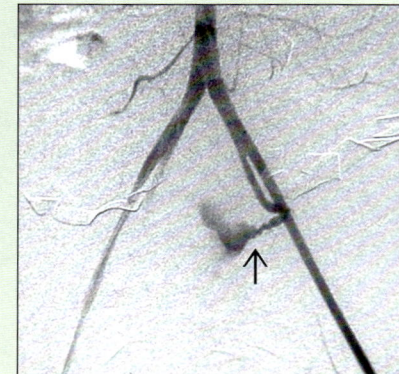

Arterial Bleed

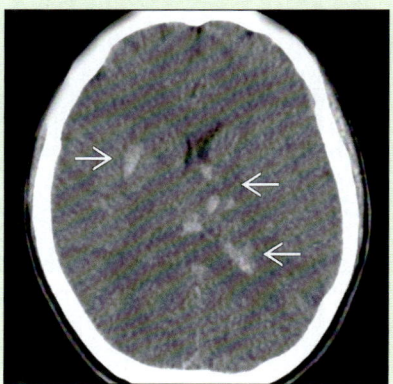

Closed Head Injury

PELVIC FRACTURES, UNSTABLE

Key Facts

Terminology
- Partially stable: Posterior osteoligamentous integrity partially maintained (rotationally unstable, vertically stable)
- Unstable: Complete loss of posterior osteoligamentous integrity (rotationally and vertically unstable)

Imaging Findings
- Posterior arch disruption (involves sacrum, posterior ilium and/or sacroiliac (SI) ligaments)
- If patient stable: CT to evaluate fx pattern, posterior arch integrity and associated injuries
- If patient unstable: Fx identification and classification accurately obtained with portable AP, inlet and outlet views

Pathology
- Sacroiliac ligaments provide majority of pelvic stability
- Significant pelvic bleeding can occur with stable and unstable fx patterns
- Young-Burgess classification of pelvic fxs: Focuses on direction of force

Diagnostic Checklist
- Assess associated injuries and determine most immediate threat to life
- Open wounds must be identified because mortality significantly increases with involvement of bowel, vagina or perineum

Ultrasonographic Findings
- Focused Abdominal Sonography for Trauma (FAST)
  - 4 views: Hepatorenal fossa, splenorenal fossa, retrovesical space, pericardial space
  - Most sensitive in retrovesical space (200 cc intraperitoneal fluid detectable)
  - Insensitive for retroperitoneal hemorrhage

Angiographic Findings
- Traumatic dissection, pseudoaneurysm, thrombosis, vasospasm or extravasation of injured artery

Other Modality Findings
- Retrograde urethrogram: Posterior urethral injury (membranous, prostatic) in pelvic fxs; anterior (bulbous) urethral injury in straddle trauma

Imaging Recommendations
- Best imaging tool
  - If patient stable: CT to evaluate fx pattern, posterior arch integrity and associated injuries
  - If patient unstable: Fx identification and classification accurately obtained with portable AP, inlet and outlet views
    - Inlet pelvis view obtained at 40-45° caudal tilt demonstrates anteriorposterior and rotational displacement
    - Outlet pelvis view obtained at 40-45° cephalad tilt demonstrates vertical displacement and fxs of the sacrum
- Protocol advice
  - Trauma protocol CT
    - Multiphase CT ± CT cystogram, pelvic and spine reformats at 1-3 mm

PATHOLOGY

General Features
- General path comments
  - Bony pelvis (sacrum and 2 innominate bones) has no inherent stability without ligamentous support
  - Sacroiliac ligaments provide majority of pelvic stability
  - Pelvic arteries at risk by location
    - Internal iliac artery and branches span the SI joint
    - Obturator and internal pudendal branches are adjacent to the pubic rami
- Etiology: High energy impact (motorcycle, fall > 15 ft)
- Epidemiology
  - Fx patterns in order of most to least common
    - Lateral compression > anterior posterior compression > acetabulum > combined mechanism injury > vertical shear
- Associated abnormalities
  - Injury to brain, long bones, thorax, abdominal organs, vessels and spine
  - Hemorrhagic complications (only 15% of mortality related to pelvic fx hemorrhage is arterial)
    - Significant pelvic bleeding can occur with stable and unstable fx patterns
  - GU complications
    - High association with displaced rami fxs, straddle fx and pubic symphysis diastasis
  - Orthopedic complications
    - Open, intraarticular, displaced fx (> 5 mm) or unstable posterior arch
  - Neurologic complications
    - Found in about 22% of sacral and 13% of acetabular fxs
  - Infectious complications
    - Open pelvic fx involving perineum, vagina or bowel have up to 50% mortality
    - Open pelvic fx not involving perineum, vagina or bowel (i.e., skin laceration with iliac wing fx) have 0-5% mortality

Staging, Grading or Classification Criteria
- Young-Burgess classification of pelvic fxs: Focuses on direction of force
  - Lateral compression: Transverse rami fx +
    - I: Sacral impaction fx on side of impact (typically stable)
    - II: Iliac wing fx extending through ring (crescent fx) on side of impact, (partial to unstable)

PELVIC FRACTURES, UNSTABLE

- III: Type I or II injury on side of impact with contralateral open-book injury = windswept pelvis, (partial to unstable)
  - Anterior posterior compression: Symphyseal diastasis or vertical rami fx +
    - I: Slight widening of symphysis (< 2.5 cm) and/or SI joint anteriorly; felt to represent stretched but intact SI ligaments, (stable)
    - II: Symphyseal diastasis > 2.5 cm, anterior SI diastasis; felt to represent torn anterior SI ligaments but intact posterior SI ligaments (partially stable)
    - III: Complete disruption of posterior arch including posterior SI ligaments (unstable)
  - Vertical shear: Symphyseal diastasis or vertical rami fx +
    - Complete disruption of posterior arch/SI ligaments and vertical displacement of hemipelvis (unstable)
  - Combined mechanism injury: Any combination of above injuries
- Denis classification of sacral fxs
  - Associates sacral fx with risk of neurologic injury
    - Zone I: Alar fx lateral to sacral foramina, 6% risk
    - Zone II: Transforaminal fx, 28% risk
    - Zone III: Central fx medial to sacral foramina, 56% risk

CLINICAL ISSUES

Presentation
- Most common signs/symptoms
  - Pelvic stability may be assessed clinically with anteroposterior and lateral compression; leg length discrepancy
  - Indicators of ongoing pelvic fx bleeding assuming other sources excluded
    - Pre-hospital hypotension (SBP < 90)
    - Admission base deficit ≥ 5
    - Persistent tachycardia in face of normal oxygenation and adequate pain control
    - Recurrent hypotension during resuscitation
    - Requirement for > 6 units blood during first 24 hours
  - Signs of bladder/urethral injury
    - Inability to void despite a full bladder; blood at the urethral meatus
  - Neurologic complication
    - Loss of rectal tone or bulbocavernosus reflex
    - Loss of lower extremity motor and sensory function
  - Internal open pelvic fx
    - Blood in vaginal vault and/or rectum
  - Morel-Lavalle lesion (fluctuance under the skin of the involved area)
    - Represents a large area of hematoma and fat necrosis under degloved skin
    - Associated with high rates of bacterial contamination
    - Can be considered a contraindication to ORIF (treated with debridement and drainage before operative intervention)

Natural History & Prognosis
- Mortality rates 5-50% depending largely on severity of pelvic fx bleeding and associated injuries
- Diverse assortment of morbidities (chronic pain, impotence, urethral stricture, infection) depending on associated injuries

Treatment
- Use of classification system based on force vectors allows surgeon to apply external fixation and corrective forces in an appropriate manner
  - External fixation shown to decrease mortality associated with pelvic fx hemorrhage
- Algorithm dependent on associated injuries
  - Stable pelvic ring
    - LC I, APC I: Typically conservative treatment (rx)
  - Partially stable ring
    - ± External fixation initially
    - APC II may be rx with anterior arch ORIF only
    - LC II, III definitive rx is variable, often with anterior and posterior arch ORIF
  - Unstable ring (completely disrupted posterior arch)
    - ± External fixation initially
    - APC III, LC III, VS, CMI: Rx with anterior and posterior arch ORIF
- Hemorrhage
  - Once other sources are excluded (chest and abdomen), pelvic bleeding may be approached with a combination of transfusion ±
    - External fixation to decrease pelvic volume
    - Retroperitoneal packing vs. catheter angiography/embolization

DIAGNOSTIC CHECKLIST

Consider
- Assess associated injuries and determine most immediate threat to life
- Open wounds must be identified because mortality significantly increases with involvement of bowel, vagina or perineum
- Retroperitoneal hemorrhage in hemodynamically unstable patients if thoracic or abdominal source not found

SELECTED REFERENCES

1. Durkin A et al: Contemporary management of pelvic fractures. Am J Surg. 192(2):211-23, 2006
2. Marx J et al: Rosen's Emergency Medicine: Concepts and Clinical Practice. Vol 1. 6th ed. St Louis, Mosby. 717-35, 2006
3. Bucholz et al: Rockwood and Green's: Fractures In Adults. Vol 2. 6th ed. Philadelphia, Lippincott Williams & Wilkins. 1584-1664, 2005
4. Park J et al: Imaging of pelvic trauma. Contemporary Diagnostic Radiology. 28(24):1-6, 2005
5. Demetrios D et al: Pelvic fractures: Epidemiology and predictors of associated abdominal injuries and outcomes. Am Coll of Surg. 195(1):1-10, 2002
6. Coppola PT et al: Emergency department evaluation and treatment of pelvic fractures. Emerg Med Clin North Am. 18(1):1-27, 2000

PELVIC FRACTURES, UNSTABLE

IMAGE GALLERY

Typical

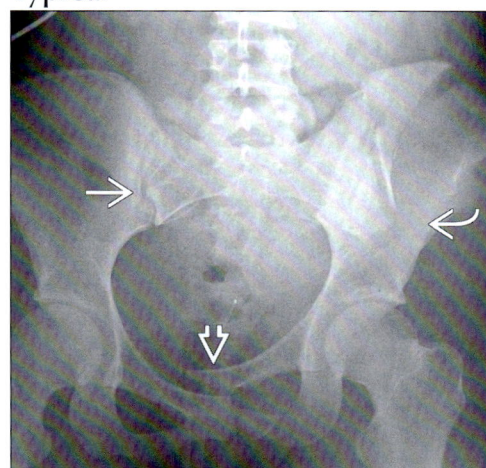 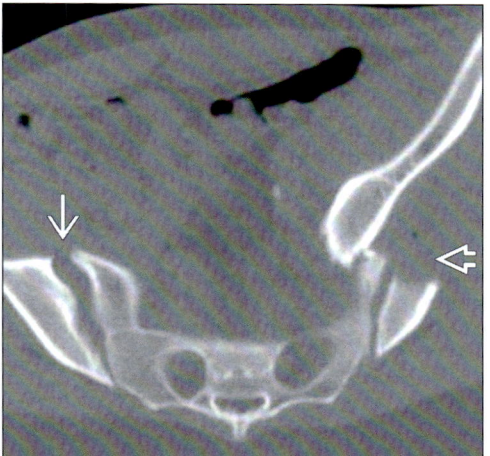

(Left) Anteroposterior radiograph shows overriding pubic rami ➔, rotated left innominate ➔, and widened right SI ➔ (LC III = windswept pelvis) in a patient driven over by a car. *(Right)* Axial bone CT better defines posterior arch injuries with a medially displaced left innominate crescent fx ➔ and anterior right SI widening ➔ = LC III, windswept pelvis.

Typical

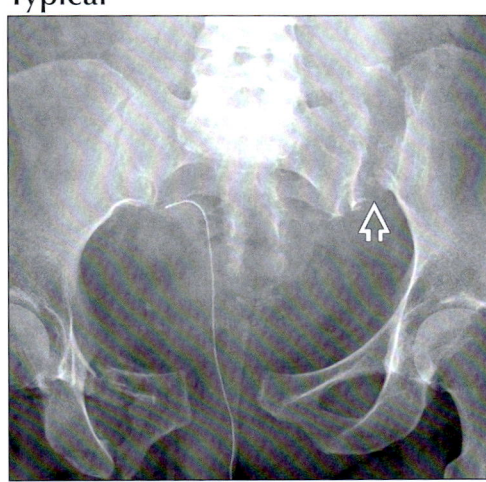 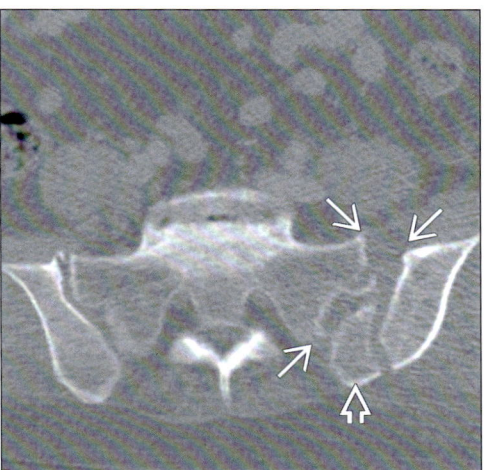

(Left) Anteroposterior radiograph shows complete left SI disruption ➔ and superior hemipelvis displacement with pubic symphysis diastasis and right rami fxs in this APC III injury. *(Right)* Axial bone CT correlation shows the SI joint diastasis ➔ with displaced and rotated intraarticular fx fragment from the posterior superior iliac spine ➔ = APC III injury.

Typical

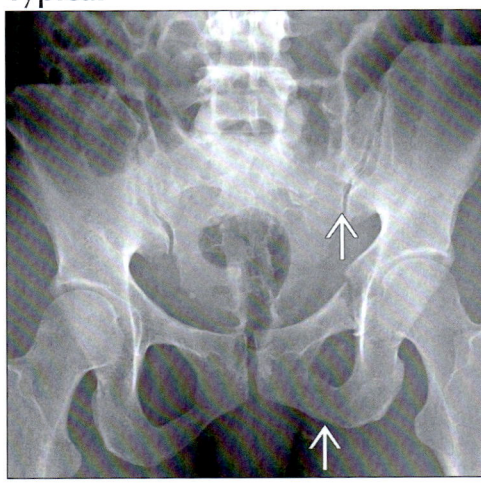 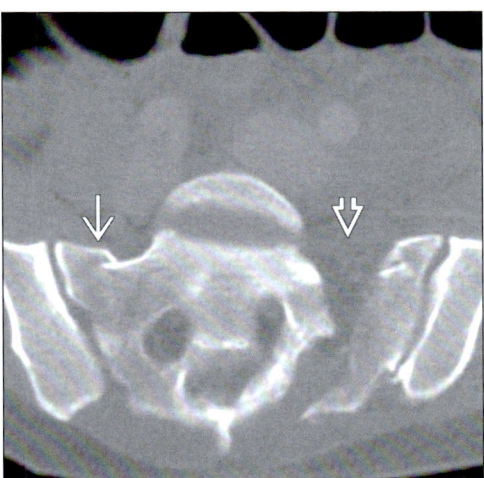

(Left) Outlet view radiograph shows vertical left rami and left sacral fx with superior hemipelvis displacement ➔ due to vertical shear force in this patient who fell 30 feet. *(Right)* Axial bone CT shows the unstable displaced left sacral fx ➔ (VS). The right sacral impaction fx ➔ (LC I) is better seen on CT. Left VS + right LC I = combined mechanism injury.

ACETABULAR FRACTURES

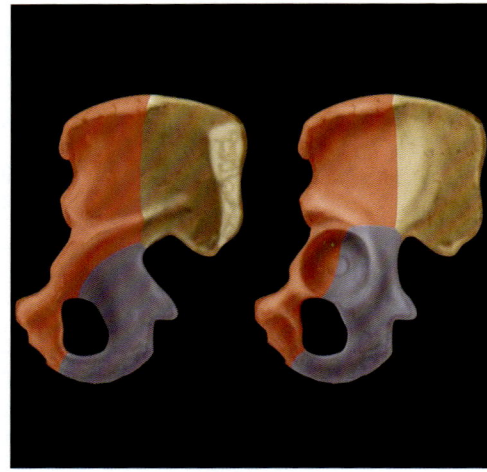

Sagittal graphic representation of acetabular column anatomy. On the left is a medial view and on the right is a lateral view with the femur removed. Blue: Posterior column. Red: Anterior column.

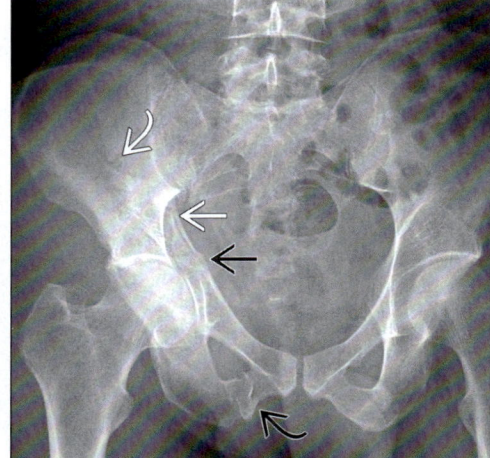

Frontal radiograph shows fractures through anterior ➡ and posterior ➡ columns as well as the obturator ring ➡ and iliac wing ➡; a both-column fracture involving the right acetabulum.

TERMINOLOGY

Abbreviations and Synonyms
- Both-column fracture, aka floating acetabulum

Definitions
- Acetabular fx = fx of anterior/posterior columns or walls/rims involving acetabular fossa of pelvis
- Sciatic buttress = thickened strut of bone extending toward sacrum that links acetabulum to axial skeleton

IMAGING FINDINGS

General Features
- Best diagnostic clue
  - Fx iliopubic (iliopectineal) line = anterior column
  - Fx ilioischial line = posterior column
- Location
  - Anterior column includes
    - Superior pubic ramus
    - Anterior half of acetabulum
    - Anterior superior/inferior iliac spines
    - Anterior iliac crest
  - Posterior column
    - Ischium: From ischiopubic junction of obturator foramen → greater sciatic notch
    - Posterior half of acetabulum
- Size
  - Anterior column fx may exit from below anterior inferior iliac spine to above iliac crest
  - > 40% fx of posterior wall (rim) → surgery
  - < 2 mm fx offset in weight-bearing dome → consider non-operative treatment
- Morphology
  - Judet-Letournel description
    - Anterior column fx
    - Posterior column fx
    - Anterior wall (rim) fx
    - Posterior wall (rim) fx (isolated); most common
    - Transverse fx
    - Both-column fx
    - Posterior column + posterior wall (rim) fx
    - Transverse + posterior wall (rim) fx
    - T-shaped fx
    - Anterior column + posterior hemi-transverse fx

Both-Column Fracture: Sequential Images

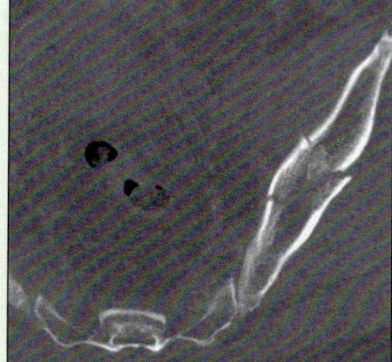

Fx Ilium Anterior to Sciatic Buttress

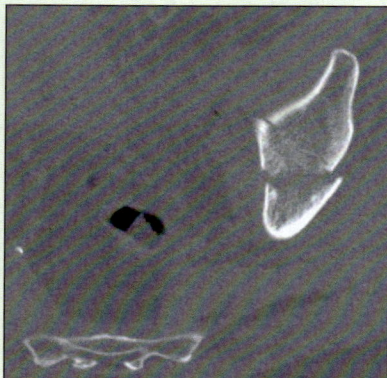

Coronal Fx Above Acetabulum

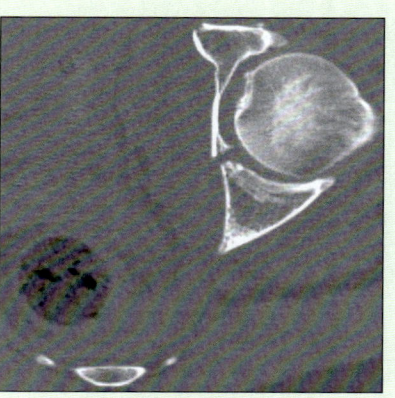

Coronal Fx Through Acetabulum

ACETABULAR FRACTURES

Key Facts

Imaging Findings
- Anterior column fx
- Posterior column fx
- Anterior wall (rim) fx
- Posterior wall (rim) fx (isolated); most common
- Transverse fx
- Both-column fx
- Transverse + posterior wall (rim) fx
- T-shaped fx
- Both-column fx: Coronal line through iliac wing
- Transverse or T-shaped fx: Sagittal oblique line through/just above acetabulum
- Best imaging tool: AP radiograph + CT; Judet optional

Top Differential Diagnoses
- Pelvic Ring Fracture
- Avulsion Fracture
- Hip Dislocation

Clinical Issues
- ATLS primary survey and resuscitation
- Emergent closed reduction of dislocation with anesthesia and fluoroscopy

Diagnostic Checklist
- Hip dislocation (emergent reduction)
- Nerve (e.g., sciatic) or arterial (superior gluteal) injury
- Pelvic rim fx: Vascular/visceral (e.g., urethra) injury
- Evaluate iliopubic/ilioischial lines, anterior/posterior walls/rims, & acetabular roof/teardrop
- Obturator ring fx: Column (single/both) or T-shaped
- Iliac wing fx: Separate both-column from T-shaped fx
- Spur sign is unique to both-column fx

Radiographic Findings
- Six lines on AP radiograph
  - Iliopubic = anterior column fx
  - Ilioischial = posterior column fx
  - Anterior rim/wall; posterior rim/wall
  - Acetabular roof/dome
  - Acetabular teardrop defines medial wall
- Judet views
  - Obturator oblique (internal oblique)
    - Evaluate anterior column & posterior rim
    - See obturator foramen en face
  - Iliac oblique (external oblique)
    - Evaluate posterior column & anterior rim
    - See iliac wing en face
- Fx iliopubic AND ilioischial line
  - Both-column, transverse, or T-shaped fx
- Obturator ring fracture
  - Does not imply acetabular fx
  - Anterior/posterior column fx
  - Both-column or T-shaped fx
- Iliac wing fracture
  - Does not imply acetabular fx
  - Anterior or both column fx
  - Not found in transverse/T-shaped fx
- Spur sign: Unique to both-column fx
  - Inferior-lateral point of the ilium still attached to sacrum that projects lateral to medially displaced acetabulum and head

CT Findings
- Anterior/both column fx: Coronal fx through ilium
- Both-column fx: Coronal line through iliac wing
  - Divides acetabulum into anterior & posterior halves
  - Acetabulum not connected to sacrum/axial skeleton
  - Fx lines separate columns from each other & sacrum
- Transverse or T-shaped fx: Sagittal oblique line through/just above acetabulum
  - Divides acetabulum into superior & inferior halves
  - Fx does not extend into iliac wing
- Note sacroiliac joint, pubic symphysis, sacrum: Ring fx

Imaging Recommendations
- Best imaging tool: AP radiograph + CT; Judet optional
- Protocol advice: CT: Thin (< 1 mm) axial imaging; coronal, sagittal, & 3D reconstructions (bone algorithm) for surgical planning

DIFFERENTIAL DIAGNOSIS

Pelvic Ring Fracture
- Anterior-posterior (AP) compression injury
  - Vertical fx through pubic rami
- Lateral compression (LC) injury
  - Horizontal oblique fx through pubic rami
- Vertical shear (VS) injury
  - AP pattern & distinctive cephalad displacement at fx
- Evaluate pubic rami fx, pubic symphysis/sacroiliac joint diastasis/compression, & sacral/iliac wing fx
- Attention to sacral arcuate lines & sacroiliac joints

Avulsion Fracture
- Anterior superior iliac spine: Sartorius muscle
- Anterior inferior iliac spine: Rectus femoris
- Ischial tuberosity: Hamstring muscles

Proximal Femoral Fracture
- Head: Sheared/impacted fragment 2° to dislocation
- Neck: Subcapital, midcervical, or basicervical
- Intertrochanteric fx

Hip Dislocation
- 90% posterior
- Associated with posterior rim fx

Insufficiency Fracture
- Commonly sacrum, pubic ramus, or femoral neck
- Mixed density on radiographs
- Radiographically occult: CT, MR, or bone scan
- Found in superior acetabulum following radiation

ACETABULAR FRACTURES

PATHOLOGY

General Features
- Etiology
  - Dashboard-type injury (flexed hip & knee) → posterior wall and column fx
  - Direct blow to greater trochanter
    - Femoral head externally rotated → anterior fx
    - Femoral head internally rotated → posterior fx
- Epidemiology
  - ~ 3-6/100,000 population/year
  - Associated with ~ 15-20% of pelvic ring fx
  - Isolated posterior wall/rim fx ~ 30-35%
  - Both column fx ~ 20-25%
  - Transverse + posterior wall/rim fx ~ 20-25%
  - 5 most common patterns (include T-shaped & transverse fx) account for 90%

Staging, Grading or Classification Criteria
- Judet-Letournel classification
  - 5 simple fracture types
    - Anterior/posterior column or wall, & transverse
  - 5 associated (combination) fx types
    - Includes T-shaped & both column fx
- AO (fracture workgroup) classification
  - Type A: Wall (rim)/column fx
  - Type B: T-shaped, transverse, hemi-transverse fx
  - Type C: Both-column fx
  - + Dislocation/impaction/articular surface modifiers
- Prognosis & treatment based on classification AND
  - Direction and amount of displacement
  - Degree of comminution
  - Femoral head dislocation
  - Intraarticular fragments
  - Injury weight-bearing dome or femoral head cartilage

CLINICAL ISSUES

Presentation
- Most common signs/symptoms
  - Hematoma at knee or greater trochanter
  - Posterior dislocation: Hip flexed & internally rotated
  - Anterior dislocation: Hip externally rotated & abducted
  - Dashboard knee injury: Patella fx & posterior cruciate ligament injury
- Other signs/symptoms
  - Evidence of multisystem trauma
  - Sciatic nerve injury
    - 10-30% of acetabular fractures
    - More common with posterior dislocation
  - Superior gluteal artery injury (in sciatic notch) is rare

Demographics
- Age
  - Young (majority): Trauma with associated injuries
  - Elderly patients: Fall & poor bone mineralization

Natural History & Prognosis
- Good clinical outcome (surgery & non-operative) in up to 90% of perfectly anatomic (< 1 mm offset) fx
- Arthritis: 10-20% if < 1 mm; 30-50% if 1-3 mm offset

Treatment
- Emergency treatment
  - ATLS primary survey and resuscitation
  - Emergent closed reduction of dislocation with anesthesia and fluoroscopy
  - Indications for urgent surgery
    - Irreducible dislocation
    - Increasing neurologic deficit
    - Associated vascular injury
    - Open fx (washout with later ORIF)
- Surgical treatment (< 7 days)
  - Anatomic reduction, stable fixation, & early motion
  - Instability or incongruity of head/acetabulum
    - > 40% posterior wall/rim fracture
    - Wall fracture + instability (sedated exam)
    - > 2 mm offset of weight-bearing dome
    - Both-column fx involving dome & incongruity
    - Transverse fx through weight-bearing dome
    - Bone/soft tissue fragments preventing congruity
- Nonoperative treatment
  - Minimally or non-displaced congruous fx (may include secondarily congruous both column fx)
  - Very poor medical/post-traumatic status
  - Severe osteoporosis/comminution
  - Lack of surgical expertise
- Complications
  - Mortality ~ 1-2% with surgery
  - PE/symptomatic DVT ~ 2-6%
  - Wound infection ~ 2-5%
  - Avascular necrosis femoral head ~ 2-10%
  - Nonunion < 1%
  - Heterotopic ossification: 2-70% (surgical technique)
  - Osteoarthritis: 5-50% (depends on fx offset)

DIAGNOSTIC CHECKLIST

Consider
- Hip dislocation (emergent reduction)
- Nerve (e.g., sciatic) or arterial (superior gluteal) injury
- Pelvic rim fx: Vascular/visceral (e.g., urethra) injury

Image Interpretation Pearls
- Evaluate iliopubic/ilioischial lines, anterior/posterior walls/rims, & acetabular roof/teardrop
- Obturator ring fx: Column (single/both) or T-shaped
- Iliac wing fx: Separate both-column from T-shaped fx
- Spur sign is unique to both-column fx

SELECTED REFERENCES
1. Bucholz RW et al: Rockwood and Green's Fractures in Adults. 6th ed. Philadelphia, Lippincott Williams & Wilkins. 1665-1714, 2007
2. Durkee NJ et al: Classification of common acetabular fractures: radiographic and CT appearances. AJR Am J Roentgenol. 187(4):915-25, 2006
3. Laird A et al: Acetabular fractures: a 16-year prospective epidemiological study. J Bone Joint Surg Br. 87(7):969-73, 2005
4. Tile M et al: Fractures of the Pelvis and Acetabulum. 3rd ed. Philadelphia, Lippincott Williams & Wilkins. 419-816, 2003

ACETABULAR FRACTURES

IMAGE GALLERY

Typical

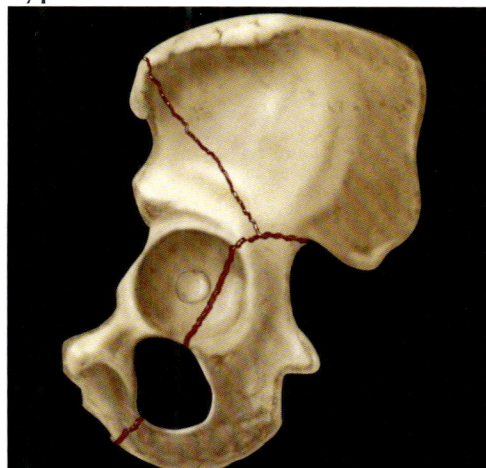
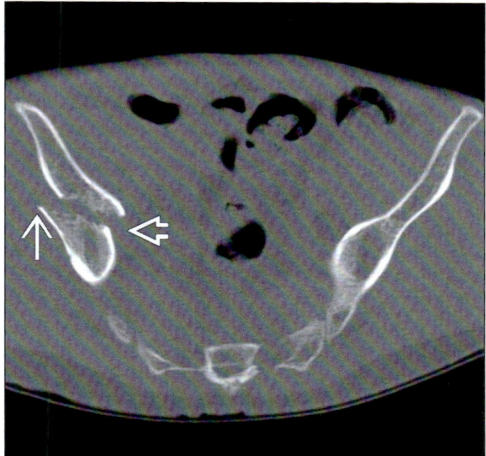

(Left) Lateral Sagittal representation of a both-column fracture, with fracture lines separating the columns & isolating the acetabulum from sacrum. *(Right)* Axial bone CT shows both-column fx with coronal iliac wing fx ➡ dividing the more inferior acetabulum (not shown) & extending through obturator ring (not shown). A lateral spur ➡ of bone connects to the sciatic buttress at a more superior position.

Typical

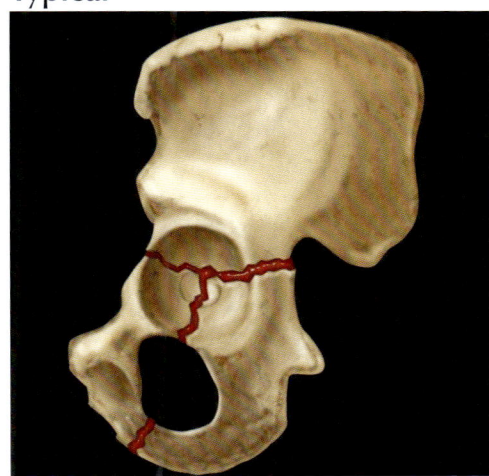
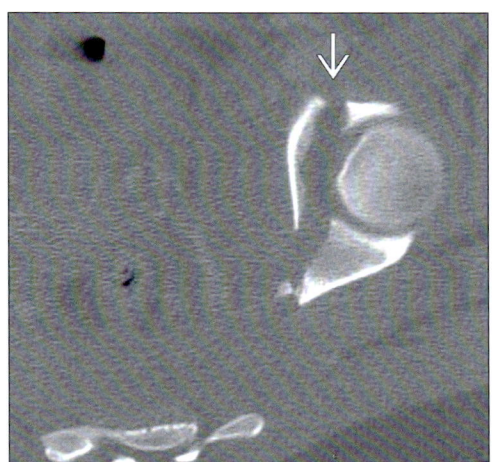

(Left) Lateral representation of a T-shaped fx with transverse portion through acetabulum, breaking anterior & posterior columns & a vertical portion through obturator ring. The iliac wing is spared. *(Right)* Transverse fx through acetabulum ➡ is in the sagittal plane of the pelvis. A perpendicular continuous fx line (not shown) breaks the more inferior obturator ring, making this a T-shaped fracture.

Typical

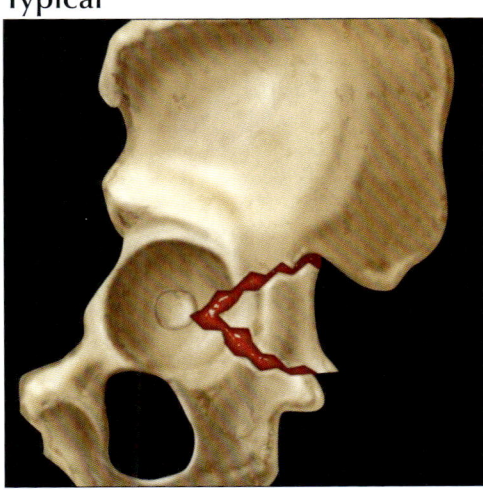
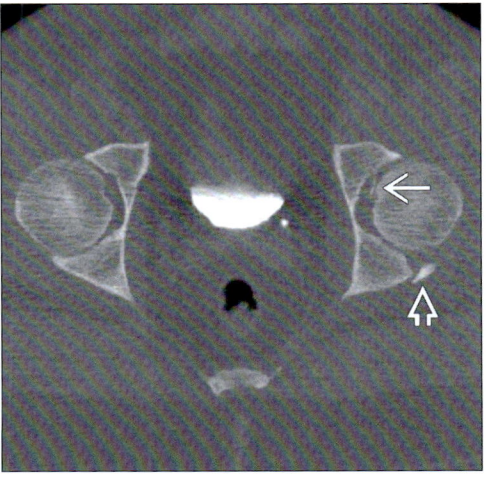

(Left) Lateral representation of a posterior wall (rim) fracture. Following reduction, rim fragments may be carried into the acetabulum to become intraarticular loose bodies. *(Right)* Axial bone CT shows a posterior wall (rim) fx ➡ and intra-articular fracture fragment ➡. There is contrast in the bladder.

HIP DISLOCATION

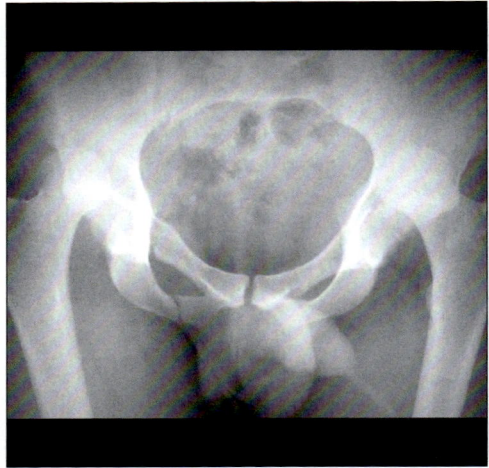

AP radiograph shows bilateral posterior hip dislocations. Both hips characteristically show posterior, superior locations, with internal rotation. Pubic ramus, right SI joint, & left acetabular disruption also present.

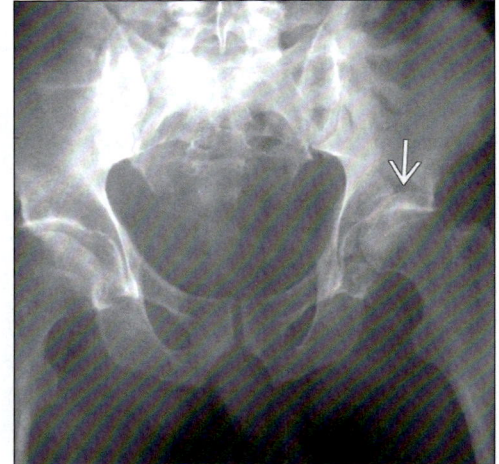

AP radiograph shows anterior (iliac) dislocation of left hip. Femoral head overlies superior part of acetabulum ➡. Position of hip in abduction & external rotation is typical of anterior dislocations.

TERMINOLOGY

Abbreviations and Synonyms
- Anterior hip dislocation, posterior hip dislocation

Definitions
- Dislocation (complete lack of articulation) of femoral head relative to acetabulum

IMAGING FINDINGS

General Features
- Best diagnostic clue: Lack of congruence of femoral head within acetabulum
- Location
  - Posterior: Most common
  - Anterior: Uncommon
    - Obturator
    - Iliac
  - Medial: Misnomer; this is actually impaction of femoral head into medial acetabular wall fx rather than dislocation
- Morphology
  - Posterior dislocation: 90% of hip dislocations
    - Femoral head posterior & slightly superiorly positioned
    - Femur in internal rotation
  - Anterior dislocation: Obturator or iliac position

Radiographic Findings
- Posterior dislocation
  - Femoral head posterior, usually slightly superior
  - Internal rotation: Greater trochanter is profiled, lesser trochanter obscured
  - Dislocated femoral head appears smaller than contralateral head since posterior position places it closer to the cassette
- **Anterior dislocation: Obturator**
  - Femoral head positioned medially & inferiorly, overlying obturator foramen
  - Femur in flexed & abducted position
- **Anterior dislocation: Iliac**
  - Femoral head superior to acetabulum (similar to posterior dislocation)
  - Femur extended & externally rotated (lesser trochanter profiled, greater trochanter obscured)

Missed Dislocation, with Sequelae of AVN

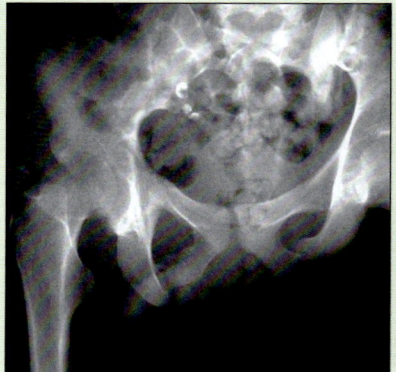
Anterior Dislocation

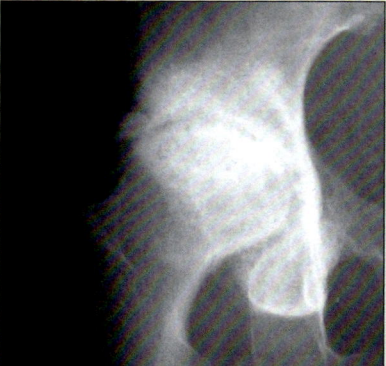
1 Year Later, AVN

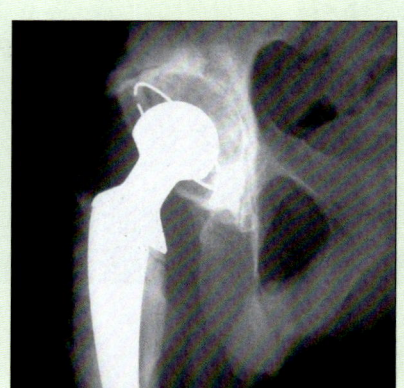
Arthroplasty Required

HIP DISLOCATION

Key Facts

Imaging Findings
- Posterior dislocation: 90% of hip dislocations
- Femoral head posterior, usually slightly superior
- Internal rotation: Greater trochanter is profiled, lesser trochanter obscured
- Dislocated femoral head appears smaller than contralateral head since posterior position places it closer to the cassette
- **Anterior dislocation: Obturator**
- Femoral head positioned medially & inferiorly, overlying obturator foramen
- **Anterior dislocation: Iliac**
- Femoral head superior to acetabulum (similar to posterior dislocation)
- Femur extended & externally rotated (lesser trochanter profiled, greater trochanter obscured)
- CT refines diagnosis of associated fracture extent, fragmentation, & intraosseous fragments

Clinical Issues
- Orthopedic emergency
- Reduce as soon as patient is otherwise stabilized
- High incidence of avascular necrosis with prolonged dislocation (50% if hip not reduced within 24 hours)

Diagnostic Checklist
- **After relocation, watch for:**
- Fracture of head and/or acetabular rim
- Increased distance between acetabular teardrop & medial femoral head, indicating retained intraarticular fracture fragments or soft tissue
- In follow-up of a dislocation, watch for early signs of AVN of the femoral head (MR may be required)

- AP view is diagnostic, Judet (oblique) or lateral views confirmatory
- Associated femoral head or acetabular rim fractures

CT Findings
- Associated acetabular rim fragmentation
- Associated femoral head shear or impaction fx
- Intraarticular osseous fragments

MR Findings
- MR is generally not indicated for initial diagnosis
- Useful for later evaluation for complication of avascular necrosis, labral, or chondral injury

Imaging Recommendations
- Best imaging tool
  - Radiograph (AP) makes initial diagnosis
  - CT refines diagnosis of associated fracture extent, fragmentation, & intraosseous fragments
- Protocol advice: CT: < 1 mm slice thickness, bone algorithm, coronal & sagittal reformats

DIFFERENTIAL DIAGNOSIS

None

PATHOLOGY

General Features
- General path comments
  - Relevant anatomy
    - Iliofemoral, pubofemoral, ischiofemoral, transverse + femoral head ligaments maintain femoral head in acetabulum
    - Blood supply to femoral head via femoral neck from branches of circumflex arteries; these at risk with prolonged dislocation
- Etiology
  - High velocity force required to dislocate hip
    - Posterior dislocation most frequently related to motor vehicle accidents: Flexed knee strikes dashboard, driving the flexed hip posteriorly
  - Posterior dislocation with contralateral anterior hip dislocation occurs with stepping from a dock onto a moving boat
- Associated abnormalities
  - Acetabular rim fracture
  - Femoral head fracture
    - Impaction (generally anterior cortex)
    - Shear fx
    - Avulsion fx at ligamentum teres insertion on head
  - Intraarticular osseous fragments from rim or head fx

Gross Pathologic & Surgical Features
- Osseous fragments
- Joint space widening

Microscopic Features
- Fracture; vascular disruption

Staging, Grading or Classification Criteria
- Pipkin classification used for hip dislocation with fracture of femoral head
  - Pipkin I: Fracture of femoral head below central fossa
  - Pipkin II: Fracture femoral head involving central fossa
  - Pipkin III: Fracture femoral head + neck
  - Pipkin IV: Fracture femoral head + superoposterior acetabular rim

CLINICAL ISSUES

Presentation
- Most common signs/symptoms: Pain, deformity following significant trauma
- Clinical Profile
  - Posterior dislocation
    - Hip & gluteal pain
    - Hip adducted, internally rotated
    - Lower extremity appears shortened

HIP DISLOCATION

- Lack of range of motion, inability to bear weight
- Sciatic nerve injury: Loss of sensation posterior leg/foot, + inability to dorsiflex/plantarflex foot
- Hematoma, soft tissue swelling
○ Anterior dislocation: Obturator
  - Hip, gluteal, groin pain
  - Hip externally rotated, abducted, flexed
  - Lower extremity may appear long compared with contralateral
  - Inability to walk/bear weight
  - Femoral nerve injury: Loss of motor function, absent reflexes
  - Femoral artery injury: Pain, pallor, pulseless
○ Anterior dislocation: Iliac
  - Hip, gluteal, groin pain
  - Hip extended & externally rotated
  - Lower extremity appears shortened
  - Inability to bear weight
  - Neurovascular injuries less likely

Demographics
- Age
  ○ Traumatic injuries due to motor vehicle accidents: < 35 years most common
  ○ Trauma secondary to falls > 65 years
- Gender: M > F

Natural History & Prognosis
- Orthopedic emergency
  ○ Reduce as soon as patient is otherwise stabilized
  ○ High incidence of avascular necrosis with prolonged dislocation (50% if hip not reduced within 24 hours)
- High morbidity/mortality
  ○ MVA associated intraabdominal, intrapelvic, & head injuries
  ○ Often associated pelvic ring fractures & severe hemorrhage
- Uncomplicated cases: Closed reduction successful (76-93%)
- Poorer prognosis when fractures present
- Recurrent dislocations if ligamentous support disrupted
- Complications
  ○ Avascular necrosis
  ○ Osteoarthritis
  ○ Sciatic nerve injuries (posterior dislocation)
  ○ Femoral nerve/artery injuries (anterior dislocation)
  ○ Deep venous thrombosis

Treatment
- Conservative
  ○ Closed reduction
  ○ Maneuvers to recreate deforming force + apply longitudinal traction
    - Posterior dislocation: Flexion, adduction, internal rotation/Stimson maneuver (prone)/Allis maneuver (supine)
    - Anterior dislocation: Abduction, external rotation, extension
- Surgical required for
  ○ Failed closed reduction
  ○ Intraarticular loose bodies
  ○ Interposed soft tissue (such as labrum)
  ○ Concomitant femoral head/neck fractures

DIAGNOSTIC CHECKLIST

Consider
- In patient post motor vehicle accident, there may be many obvious fractures, but look carefully for a hip dislocation; immediate relocation is required
- Direct posterior hip dislocation occasionally is not superiorly displaced
  ○ Watch for congruence of head and acetabulum so these are not missed
- Anterior hip dislocation in the iliac position may have a similar superior displacement to a posterior hip dislocation
  ○ Differentiate the two by direction of hip rotation: It will be internally rotated in a posterior dislocation and externally rotated in an anterior dislocation
  ○ Dislocated head will appear smaller than the contralateral head in a posterior dislocation, larger in an anterior dislocation

Image Interpretation Pearls
- After relocation, watch for:
  ○ Fracture of head and/or acetabular rim
  ○ Increased distance between acetabular teardrop & medial femoral head, indicating retained intraarticular fracture fragments or soft tissue
- In follow-up of a dislocation, watch for early signs of AVN of the femoral head (MR may be required)

SELECTED REFERENCES

1. Geusens E et al: Imaging in trauma of the pelvis and hip region. JBR-BTR. 87(4):190-202, 2004
2. Giza E et al: Hip fracture-dislocation in football: a report of two cases and review of the literature. Br J Sports Med. 38(4):E17, 2004
3. Hillyard RF et al: Sciatic nerve injuries associated with traumatic posterior hip dislocations. Am J Emerg Med. 21(7):545-8, 2003
4. Kim YT et al: Acetabular labrum entrapment following traumatic posterior dislocation of the hip. J Orthop Sci. 8(2):232-5, 2003
5. Sahin V et al: Traumatic dislocation and fracture-dislocation of the hip: a long-term follow-up study. J Trauma. 54(3):520-9, 2003
6. Pallia CS et al: Traumatic hip dislocation in athletes. Curr Sports Med Rep. 1(6):338-45, 2002
7. Rubel IF et al: MRI assessment of the posterior acetabular wall fracture in traumatic dislocation of the hip in children. Pediatr Radiol. 32(6):435-9, 2002
8. Alonso JE et al: A review of the treatment of hip dislocations associated with acetabular fractures. Clin Orthop Relat Res. (377):32-43, 2000
9. Brooks RA et al: Diagnosis and imaging studies of traumatic hip dislocations in the adult. Clin Orthop Relat Res. (377):15-23, 2000
10. Pape HC et al: Hip dislocation in patients with multiple injuries. A followup investigation. Clin Orthop Relat Res. (377):99-105, 2000
11. Rodriguez-Merchan EC: Osteonecrosis of the femoral head after traumatic hip dislocation in the adult. Clin Orthop Relat Res. (377):68-77, 2000
12. Poggi JJ et al: Changes on magnetic resonance images after traumatic hip dislocation. Clin Orthop Relat Res. (319):249-59, 1995

HIP DISLOCATION

IMAGE GALLERY

Typical

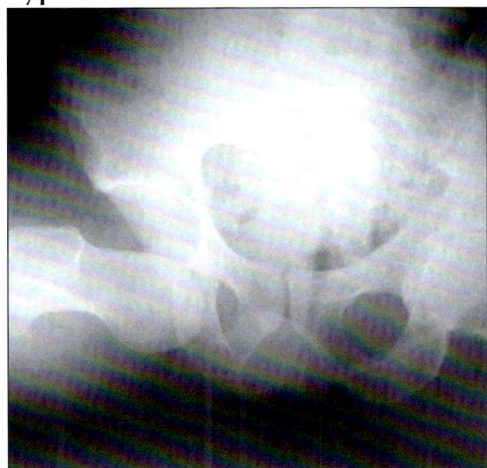 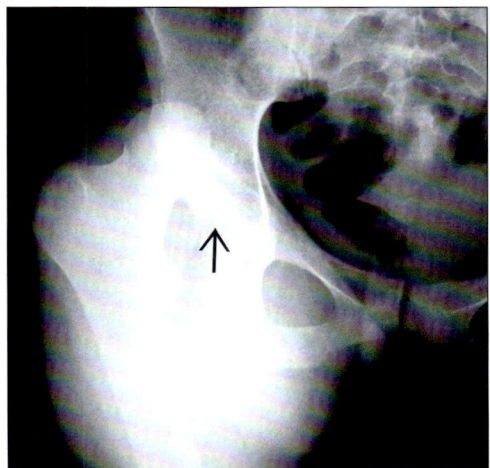

(Left) Anteroposterior radiograph shows anterior (obturator) hip dislocation. Hip is abducted and externally rotated, with femoral head superimposed over obturator foramen. (Right) Anteroposterior radiograph shows posterior hip dislocation. Head appears small & is proximally displaced. Hip is in neutral rotation; more typically it would be in a more severely internally rotated position. There is a large fragment of the femoral head remaining in acetabulum ➡.

Typical

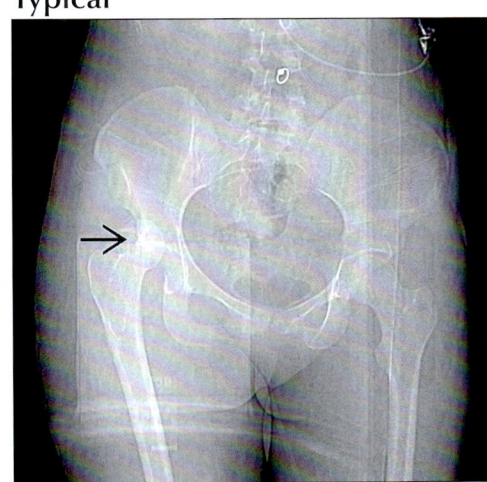 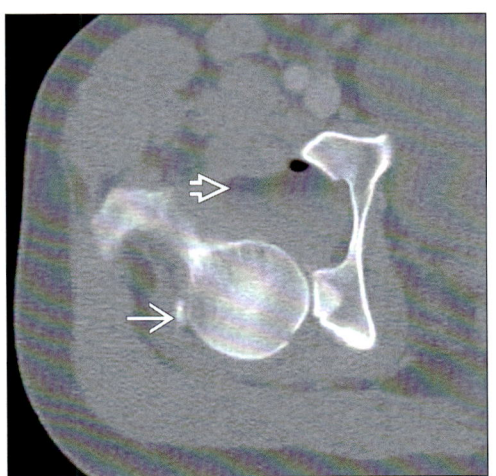

(Left) Anteroposterior radiograph shows the typical internal rotation and proximal placement of a posterior hip dislocation ➡. (Right) Axial bone CT of the same case confirms the posterior position of the head. A bone fragment arising from the posterior acetabular rim is seen ➡; upon relocation, these fragments often are pulled intra-articularly. A lipohemarthrosis is seen within the joint ➡.

Typical

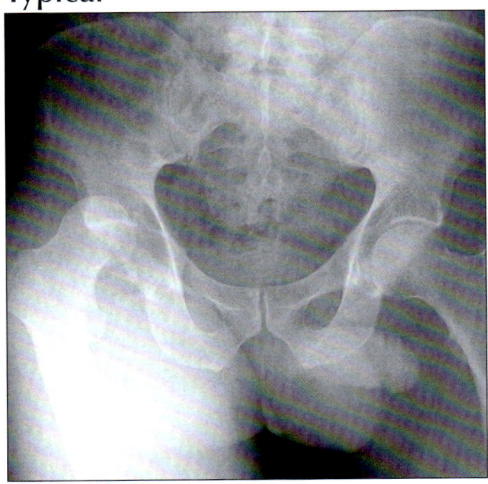 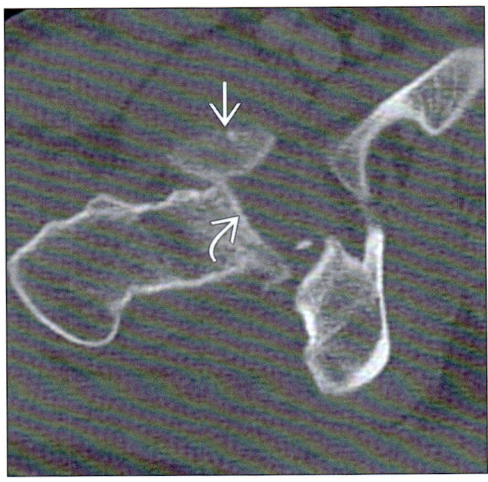

(Left) Anteroposterior radiograph shows a right hip dislocation (posterior), with the head appearing relatively small and the hip adducted and flexed. Only small bone fragments are seen. (Right) Axial bone CT obtained following reduction, shows that in fact there was a very large fracture of the anteroinferior femoral head ➡, with associated defect at the donor site ➡. Although the fracture fragment is large, this is classed as a Pipkin I since it is entirely below the fovea.

FEMORAL HEAD FRACTURES

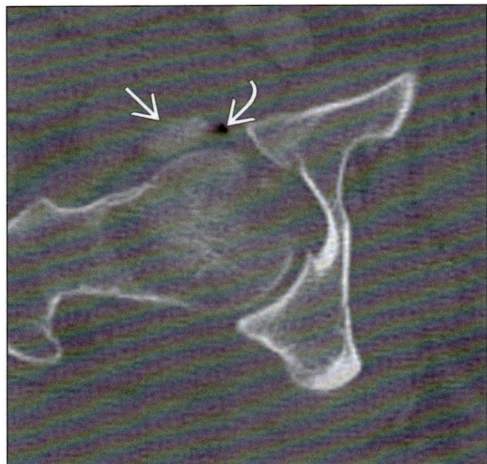

Axial bone CT shows large defect in femoral head following hip dislocation. Osseous fragment is displaced anteriorly ➡. Air bubble located anteriorly in joint ➡ is indicative of prior hip dislocation.

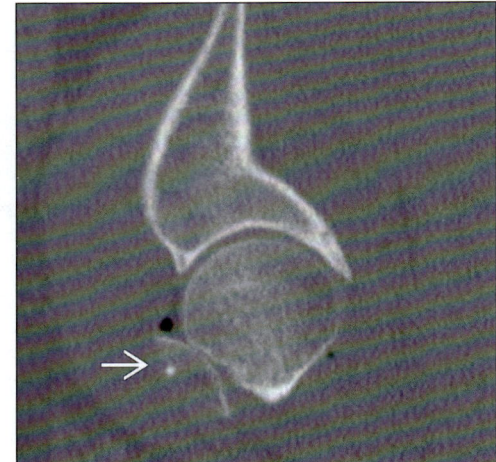

Sagittal bone CT shows large anterior osseous fragment ➡ with adjacent air bubble. Fx is entirely located below level of ligamentum teres; there is no acetabular fx. This represents a Pipkin I fx.

TERMINOLOGY

Abbreviations and Synonyms
- Capital fracture; subchondral fracture femoral head

Definitions
- Fracture of femoral head, involving the chondral surface but not primarily the femoral neck
  - Related to:
    - Posterior dislocation femoral head
    - Fatigue fracture
    - Insufficiency fracture

IMAGING FINDINGS

General Features
- Best diagnostic clue
  - In patient with posterior hip dislocation, look carefully for femoral head fracture on radiographs or CT
  - In osteoporotic patient with hip pain, perform MR to look for insufficiency fracture of femoral head
- Location: Femoral head
- Size: Variable
- Morphology: Oblique to vertical fracture line as viewed in coronal plane

Radiographic Findings
- Traumatic fracture related to dislocation ranges from obvious displaced fracture to subtle impaction of the anterior femoral cortex
- Insufficiency fracture unlikely to be diagnosed by radiograph

CT Findings
- Traumatic fracture related to dislocation ranges from obvious displaced fracture to subtle impaction of the anterior femoral cortex
- CT also used to assess degree of posterior acetabular rim fragmentation and presence of intraarticular fragments
- Insufficiency fracture may be missed on CT due to indistinctness of osteoporotic trabeculae

MR Findings
- T1WI: Hypointense fracture line
- STIR: Hyperintense femoral head edema; same for other fluid sensitive sequences

Insufficiency Fracture Femoral Head

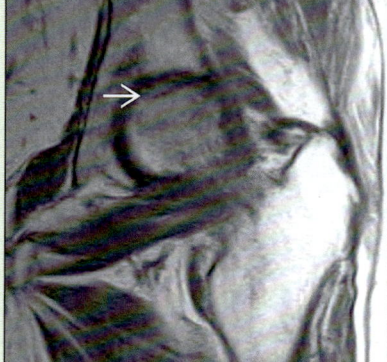

Cortical Fracture

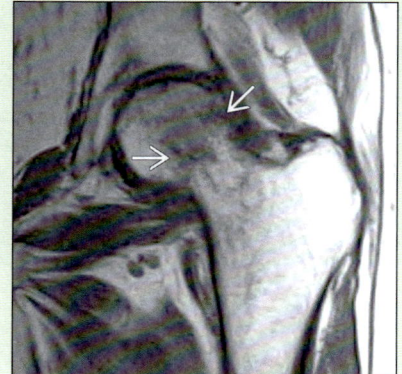

Fx Extension to Head

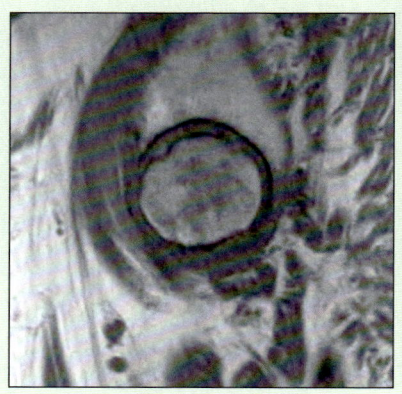

Irregular Cortex; Sagittal

FEMORAL HEAD FRACTURES

Key Facts

Terminology
- Fracture of femoral head, involving the chondral surface but not primarily the femoral neck
- Related to:
- Posterior dislocation femoral head
- Fatigue fracture
- Insufficiency fracture

Imaging Findings
- In patient with posterior hip dislocation, look carefully for femoral head fracture on radiographs or CT
- In osteoporotic patient with hip pain, perform MR to look for insufficiency fracture of femoral head
- Traumatic fracture related to dislocation ranges from obvious displaced fracture to subtle impaction of the anterior femoral cortex
- Insufficiency fracture unlikely to be diagnosed by radiograph
- CT also used to assess degree of posterior acetabular rim fragmentation and presence of intraarticular fragments
- Insufficiency fracture may be missed on CT due to indistinctness of osteoporotic trabeculae

Pathology
- Traumatic: Associated with posterior dislocation
- **Insufficiency:**
- Senile osteoporosis
- Corticosteroids
- Metabolic disease
- Rheumatoid arthritis
- Fatigue (stress): Overexertion, most often described in military recruits

Imaging Recommendations
- Best imaging tool
  - Radiograph is first imaging procedure
  - In case of dislocation, CT used to evaluate posterior rim acetabulum and femoral head fracture
  - If occult by radiograph, MR is more sensitive than CT, especially in osteopenic patient
- Protocol advice
  - CT: < 1 mm sections, bone algorithm, with reformats
  - MR: Coronal, axial, & sagittal T1 and STIR (or similar fluid sensitive sequence)

DIFFERENTIAL DIAGNOSIS

Avascular Necrosis
- Usually fractures in the immediate subchondral portion of femoral head (crescent sign)
- Occasionally will collapse with a more transverse/oblique femoral head fracture
  - Look for other signs of AVN, including central femoral head sclerosis on radiograph

Rapidly Destructive Osteoarthritis of Hip
- Rapid (months) onset of severe hip pain
- Rapid chondrolysis (50% joint space or > 2 mm cartilage loss in 1 year)
- No evidence of other etiologies (septic hip, AVN, inflammatory or deposition-related arthritis, neuropathic hip)
- MR shows effusion, cartilage thinning, femoral head flattening, cystic defects in subchondral region, & occasional thin low SI lines coursing parallel to the articular surface
  - Epiphyseal low SI lines similar to those seen with subchondral femoral head insufficiency fx related to osteopenia
  - Osteopenic insufficiency fracture, as a possible etiology for rapidly destructive osteoarthritis of the hip, does not explain the rapid chondrolysis which precedes the development of fracture

PATHOLOGY

General Features
- Etiology
  - Traumatic: Oblique fracture from shearing force from dislocation
  - Traumatic: Anterior femoral head impaction from posterior dislocation
  - Traumatic: Generally high velocity injuries, most commonly motor vehicle accident
  - Insufficiency fractures: Normal weight-bearing on osteopenic bone
  - Fatigue (stress) fracture with overuse
- Epidemiology
  - Traumatic: Associated with posterior dislocation
  - **Insufficiency:**
    - Senile osteoporosis
    - Corticosteroids
    - Metabolic disease
    - Rheumatoid arthritis
  - Fatigue (stress): Overexertion, most often described in military recruits

Gross Pathologic & Surgical Features
- Fragmentation of surrounding osseous & cartilaginous structures
- With dislocation, may have fragments entrapped in joint

Microscopic Features
- Fracture, callus formation
- No evidence of avascular necrosis or sepsis

Staging, Grading or Classification Criteria
- Pipkin classification for femoral head fracture
  - I: Below ligamentum teres; no associated injuries
  - II: Above ligamentum teres; no associated injuries
  - III: Either below or above ligamentum teres; associated femoral neck fracture
  - IV: Either below or above ligamentum teres; associated acetabular fracture

FEMORAL HEAD FRACTURES

CLINICAL ISSUES

Presentation
- Most common signs/symptoms
  - Hip pain
  - Clinical profile: Fracture related to dislocated hip
    - High energy trauma
    - Must be reduced ASAP; incidence of avascular necrosis increases significantly if reduction delayed > 12 hours
    - Maximum 2-3 attempts at closed reduction due to risk of AVN and iatrogenic injury
    - Associated morbidity/mortality secondary to associated head, abdominal, & pelvic trauma
  - Clinical profile: Fatigue fracture
    - Overexertion, most frequently in military recruits
  - Clinical profile: Insufficiency fracture
    - Senile osteoporosis
    - Other risk factors: Rheumatoid arthritis, corticosteroids, metabolic disease (renal osteodystrophy), anorexia, transient osteoporosis
    - Low-energy fall

Demographics
- Age
  - Traumatic: Young adults; high-energy trauma victims
  - Fatigue: Young adults
  - Insufficiency: Elderly
- Gender
  - Traumatic: Males
  - Fatigue: Males
  - Insufficiency: Females

Natural History & Prognosis
- Traumatic & fatigue femoral head fractures
  - Anatomic or near anatomic fracture reduction essential
    - Preserve function
    - Avoid avascular necrosis
    - Avoid early development of osteoarthritis
  - Outcome dependent on
    - Femoral head fracture type
    - Associated fractures (acetabular, femoral neck, pelvic ring)
    - Length of time until reduction
  - Pipkin I & II have better prognosis than III & IV
  - Open reduction indications
    - Failed closed reduction
    - Femoral neck fracture
    - Incongruent reduction
    - Intraarticular fragments
- Insufficiency femoral head fracture: Continued collapse

Treatment
- Traumatic & fatigue femoral head fractures
  - Pipkin I: Conservative
    - Closed reduction preferred
    - Displaced inferior fragment acceptable if it does not involve weight-bearing portion of head
  - Pipkin II: Conservative or surgical
    - Closed reduction only if fracture fragments are congruent
    - Open reduction with internal fixation (ORIF) for displaced/unstable fracture fragments
  - Pipkin III: Surgical
    - ORIF for younger patients (rigid pinning)
    - Hemiprosthesis for older patients
  - Pipkin IV: Surgical
    - ORIF for displaced/unstable acetabular & femoral head fractures in young patient
    - Total hip arthroplasty in older patient
  - Complications for fracture related to hip dislocation
    - Avascular necrosis
    - Post-traumatic arthritis
    - Recurrent dislocation
    - Sciatic nerve injury
- Insufficiency femoral head fractures: Hemiarthroplasty

DIAGNOSTIC CHECKLIST

Consider
- Association of femoral head fractures with posterior dislocation
- Fatigue fracture of femoral head should be considered in young patient with overexertion in absence of other pelvic/femoral neck stress fractures
- Insufficiency fracture of femoral head in elderly patient with pain suggesting femoral neck fracture; head fractures much less common than neck fx

Image Interpretation Pearls
- Watch for subtle anterior femoral head impaction fracture in CT for hip dislocation
- Include femoral head in search pattern on MR for femoral neck fractures
- With rapid cartilage loss, once septic hip is ruled out, consider diagnosis of rapidly destructive hip osteoarthritis & watch for collapse/resorption of femoral head

SELECTED REFERENCES

1. Miyanishi K et al: A subchondral fracture in transient osteoporosis of the hip. Skeletal Radiol. 2007
2. Chan CC et al: Subchondral insufficiency fracture of the femoral head. Hong Kong Med J. 12(6):460-2, 2006
3. Yamamoto T et al: Subchondral insufficiency fracture of the femoral head in younger adults. Skeletal Radiol. 2006
4. Asghar FA et al: Femoral head fractures: diagnosis, management, and complications. Orthop Clin North Am. 35(4):463-72, 2004
5. Khanna AJ et al: Rapidly destructive osteoarthropathy of the hip. Am J Orthop. 33(5):243-7, 2004
6. Legroux Gerot I et al: Subchondral fractures of the femoral head: a review of seven cases. Joint Bone Spine. 71(2):131-5, 2004
7. Song WS et al: Subchondral fatigue fracture of the femoral head in military recruits. J Bone Joint Surg Am. 86-A(9):1917-24, 2004
8. Boutry N et al: Rapidly destructive osteoarthritis of the hip: MR imaging findings. AJR Am J Roentgenol. 179(3):657-63, 2002
9. Watanabe W et al: Early MRI findings of rapidly destructive coxarthrosis. Skeletal Radiol. 31(1):35-8, 2002

FEMORAL HEAD FRACTURES

IMAGE GALLERY

Typical

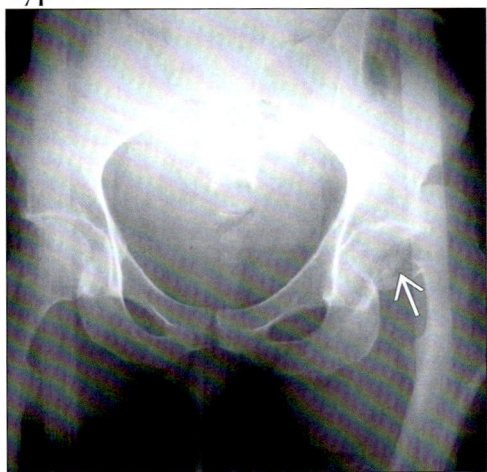
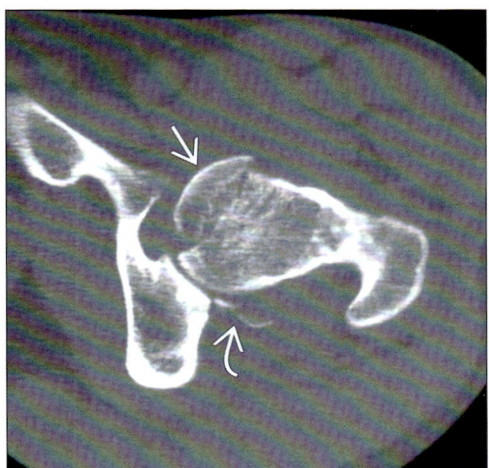

(Left) Anteroposterior radiograph shows a posterior hip dislocation; the adducted position of the femur is typical of a posterior dislocation. The donor site of the fracture fragment ➔ is the anterior femoral head. *(Right)* Axial bone CT shows the relocated femoral head, with the shear fracture fragment ➔ located below the ligamentum teres. This is classified as a Pipkin I fracture. Small intraarticular fracture fragments are noted as well ➔.

Typical

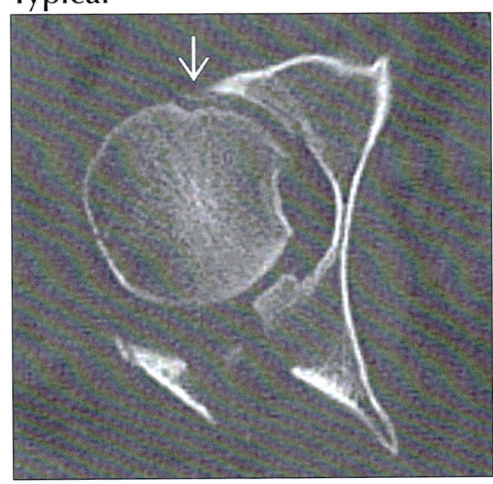
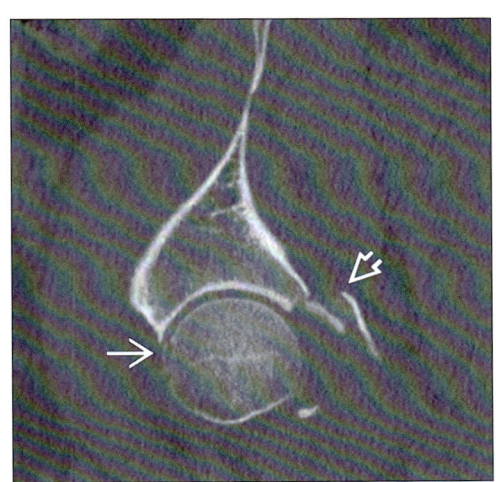

(Left) Axial bone CT shows extensive posterior acetabular rim fragmentation following dislocation. There is an associated impaction fracture of the anterior femoral head ➔, with minor fragmentation. *(Right)* Sagittal bone CT confirms the anterior femoral head impaction ➔, as well as the severe fragmentation and displacement of the posterior rim ➔. This case demonstrates a subtle impaction associated with dislocation.

Typical

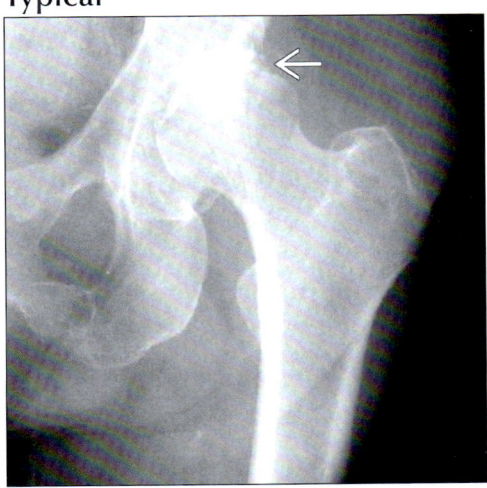
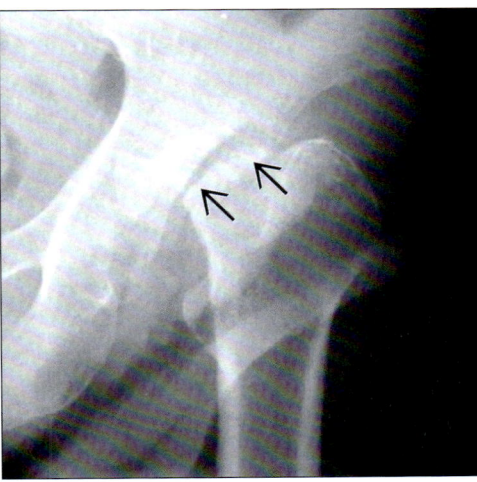

(Left) Anteroposterior radiograph shows severe cartilage loss ➔. Because of the patient's severe pain, aspiration was performed. Cultures & gram stain were negative. Work-up for inflammatory arthritides was negative. *(Right)* Anteroposterior radiograph obtained 5 months later shows severe destruction of the femoral head, neck ➔, & acetabulum. Rapid progression & otherwise negative work-up allows a diagnosis of rapidly destructive osteoarthritis.

FEMORAL NECK FRACTURES

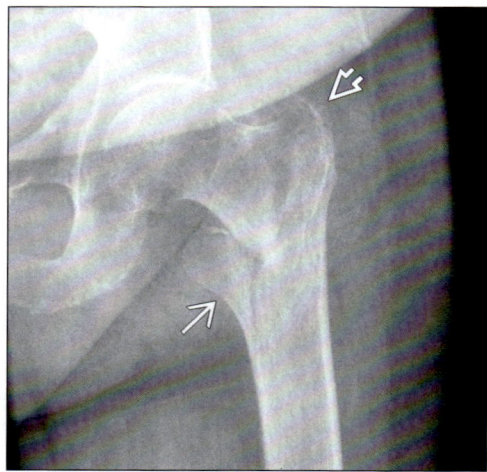

Anteroposterior radiograph shows a typical, displaced, 4 part intertrochanteric fx. The major fx line is oblique, resulting in varus angulation; greater ➡ & lesser ➡ trochanteric fragments often accompany the oblique fx.

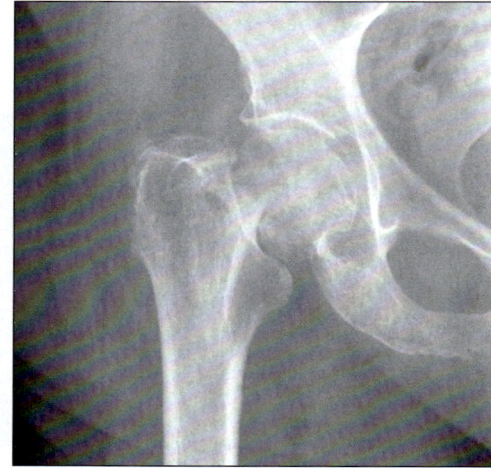

Anteroposterior radiograph shows a Garden IV subcapital fracture. The fracture is displaced, in varus angulation, and the shaft is proximally displaced. Note the external rotation of the shaft, which is typical.

TERMINOLOGY

Abbreviations and Synonyms
- Fracture (fx) of the proximal femur, subcapital, stress fracture, insufficiency fracture, midcervical, transcervical, basicervical, intertrochanteric

Definitions
- Intracapsular femoral neck fractures
  - Subcapital: Femoral head/neck junction
  - Midcervical (transcervical)
  - Basicervical: Base of femoral neck
- Extracapsular femoral neck fracture
  - Intertrochanteric

IMAGING FINDINGS

General Features
- Best diagnostic clue
  - If incomplete or non-displaced, may be extremely subtle on radiograph
    - Change of alignment of trabeculae
    - Subtle buckle of cortex
    - Smudgy sclerosis from impaction
  - MR makes the definitive diagnosis
- Location: Ranges from junction of femoral head & neck to intertrochanteric site; named accordingly
- Size: Ranges from incomplete, nondisplaced to displaced & comminuted
- Morphology
  - Subcapital
    - Slightly oblique, following line of femoral head/neck junction
    - Lucent fracture line is rarely seen
    - May be impacted, manifest as a sclerotic line
    - May see only a buckle of cortex, either medially or laterally
    - May see only subtle alteration of trabecular direction at fracture line
  - Midcervical: Mildly oblique, perpendicular to femoral neck
  - Basicervical
    - Fairly transverse at medial cortex
    - Extends obliquely to the lateral basicervical region
  - Intertrochanteric
    - Oblique, extending from greater trochanter superolaterally to lesser trochanter inferomedially

Subtle Subcapital Fracture

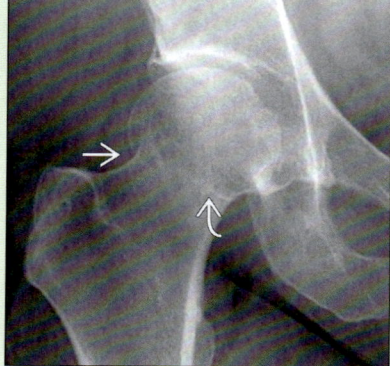

Acute Angulation at Cortex

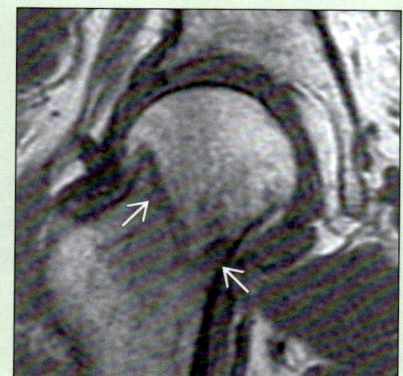

T1 MR Confirms Fracture

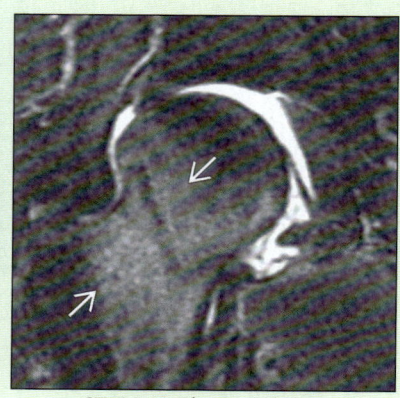

STIR MR Shows Edema

FEMORAL NECK FRACTURES

Key Facts

Imaging Findings
- Nondisplaced or incomplete fractures may be extremely subtle on radiograph
- Most of these patients are osteopenic; CT (even optimally imaged & with reformats) is significantly less sensitive than MR for nondisplaced fractures
- Bone scan is insensitive in osteoporotic patients for the first 72 hours
- If radiograph is negative and clinical suspicion high, MR should be performed

Clinical Issues
- Low grade subcapital fx may be stable, but bed rest puts patient at risk for other morbidities (pneumonia, pulmonary embolus)
- Higher grade subcapital fx: At risk for displacement, avascular necrosis
- Basicervical stress fractures at risk for completion
- Basicervical fx (complete) at risk for delayed or non-union
- Incomplete intertrochanteric fx at risk for completion

Diagnostic Checklist
- Femoral neck fractures are common, particularly in runners and osteoporotic individuals
- Subcapital & incomplete intertrochanteric insufficiency fractures may be missed on radiograph
- Basicervical stress fracture may be occult on radiograph
- If hip fx is a strong consideration clinically, but radiograph is negative, MR should be performed
- Patient often holds fractured hip in flexion & internal rotation; this can mask a subcapital fracture
- Subcapital fx lines mimicked by ring osteophytes

- Ranges from 2-part to 4-part, including each of the trochanters
- Severe comminution posteromedially, in calcar region, resulting in varus angulation
- Incomplete intertrochanteric fx is being recognized now as relatively common

Radiographic Findings
- Nondisplaced or incomplete fractures may be extremely subtle on radiograph
- Watch for
  - Subtle sclerosis
  - Abrupt cortical angulation
  - Change in trabecular alignment

CT Findings
- Most of these patients are osteopenic; CT (even optimally imaged & with reformats) is significantly less sensitive than MR for nondisplaced fractures

MR Findings
- T1WI
  - Hypointense linear signal at fracture line
  - May or may not extend entirely across femoral neck
- STIR: Hyperintense marrow edema; may obscure the fracture line; other fluid sensitive sequences are similar

Nuclear Medicine Findings
- Bone scan is insensitive in osteoporotic patients for the first 72 hours
- For a timely and specific diagnosis, MR is preferred to bone scan

Imaging Recommendations
- Best imaging tool
  - Radiograph is first line of imaging
  - If radiograph is negative and clinical suspicion high, MR should be performed
    - 27-40% of cases of clinically suspected hip fx but normal radiograph show hip or pelvic fx on MR
    - 50-65% of cases of clinically suspected hip fx but normal radiograph show soft tissue injury or fracture by MR
- Protocol advice: MR: T1 coronal & fluid sequence such as STIR

DIFFERENTIAL DIAGNOSIS

Radiographic
- Sclerosis in subcapital fracture may be mimicked by sclerotic ring osteophyte in osteoarthritis

Clinical
- Other reasons for groin/hip pain, including muscle strain, avascular necrosis, arthritis, intraarticular etiologies

PATHOLOGY

General Features
- Etiology
  - Subcapital
    - Fall; rarely direct trauma
    - Usually insufficiency: Senile osteoporosis is most common
    - Rarely, insufficiency from other etiologies such as anorexia or corticosteroids
  - Midcervical: Rare fracture, related to trauma
  - Basicervical
    - Rarely, direct and significant trauma
    - More frequently, stress fracture in runners (cyclic loading + torsional force)
    - Coxa vara predisposes athlete to risk of fracture
  - Intertrochanteric
    - Fall; rarely direct trauma
    - Usually insufficiency, with significant comminution
- Epidemiology
  - Insufficiency fractures (subcapital & intertrochanteric)
    - Extremely common in the elderly, paralleling the high prevalence of osteoporosis
  - Stress fractures (usually basicervical)
    - 15% of runners develop a stress fracture

FEMORAL NECK FRACTURES

- 5-10% of stress fractures involve the femoral neck
- Associated abnormalities: Falls resulting in femoral neck fractures in the elderly are highly associated with fractures of distal radius & proximal humerus

Microscopic Features
- Often vascular disruption of bone in subcapital fx
- Resorption, healing with callus

Staging, Grading or Classification Criteria
- Subcapital fx: Garden classification
  - Garden I: Incomplete with lateral impaction (slight valgus orientation of femoral neck)
  - Garden II: Complete but non-displaced
  - Garden III: Complete with partial displacement (slight varus orientation of fracture line)
  - Garden IV: Complete and displaced (femoral shaft externally rotated & telescoped)
- Stress fx: Blickenstaff/Morris classification
  - Type I: Endosteal or periosteal callus without fracture line
  - Type II: Fracture line
  - Type III: Displaced fracture

CLINICAL ISSUES

Presentation
- Most common signs/symptoms
  - Pain in groin, anterior thigh, or knee
  - Hip held in flexion, external rotation
  - Pain increased with axial compression or greater trochanter percussion

Demographics
- Age
  - Insufficiency femoral neck fractures (subcapital, intertrochanteric): Elderly, osteoporotic
    - By age 80, 10% of Caucasian women & 5% of Caucasian men sustain a hip fracture
    - By age 90, these rates double
- Gender
  - Elderly osteoporotic fractures: M < F
  - Stress fractures in military population: M > F
  - Stress fractures in athletes: M < F (anorexia, amenorrhea, premature osteoporosis)

Natural History & Prognosis
- Low grade subcapital fx may be stable, but bed rest puts patient at risk for other morbidities (pneumonia, pulmonary embolus)
- Higher grade subcapital fx: At risk for displacement, avascular necrosis
- Basicervical stress fractures at risk for completion
- Basicervical fx (complete) at risk for delayed or non-union
- Incomplete intertrochanteric fx at risk for completion

Treatment
- Subcapital
  - Garden I or II: Percutaneous pinning
  - Garden III or IV: Endoprosthesis (hemiarthroplasty)
    - For Garden IV fracture, there is > 40% nonunion rate & 30% rate of AVN
- Basicervical
  - Stress reaction or medial compression (incomplete): Conservative; non weight-bearing; healing 6-12 months
  - Traumatic or complete: Internal fixation
- Intertrochanteric
  - Complete: Dynamic plate & screw fixation
  - Incomplete: Non weight-bearing if < 50% width; otherwise, dynamic plate & screw fixation

DIAGNOSTIC CHECKLIST

Consider
- Femoral neck fractures are common, particularly in runners and osteoporotic individuals
- Subcapital & incomplete intertrochanteric insufficiency fractures may be missed on radiograph
- Basicervical stress fracture may be occult on radiograph
- If hip fx is a strong consideration clinically, but radiograph is negative, MR should be performed

Image Interpretation Pearls
- Patient often holds fractured hip in flexion & internal rotation; this can mask a subcapital fracture
- Subcapital fx lines mimicked by ring osteophytes
- Isolated lesser trochanteric fracture should be considered pathologic until proven otherwise

SELECTED REFERENCES
1. Parker MJ et al: Incidence of Fracture-healing Complications after Femoral Neck Fractures. Clin Orthop Relat Res. 2007
2. Bjorgul K et al: Incidence of hip fracture in southeastern Norway : A study of 1,730 cervical and trochanteric fractures. Int Orthop. 2006
3. Dharmarajan TS et al: Hip fracture. Risk factors, preoperative assessment, and postoperative management. Postgrad Med. 119(1):31-8, 2006
4. Hagino T et al: Prognosis of proximal femoral fracture in patients aged 90 years and older. J Orthop Surg (Hong Kong). 14(2):122-6, 2006
5. Holmberg AH et al: Risk factors for fragility fracture in middle age. A prospective population-based study of 33,000 men and women. Osteoporos Int. 17(7):1065-77, 2006
6. Johnell O et al: An estimate of the worldwide prevalence and disability associated with osteoporotic fractures. Osteoporos Int. 17(12):1726-33, 2006
7. Lesic A et al: Epidemiology of hip fractures in Belgrade, Serbia Montenegro, 1990-2000. Arch Orthop Trauma Surg. 2006
8. Lofthus CM et al: Young patients with hip fracture: a population-based study of bone mass and risk factors for osteoporosis. Osteoporos Int. 17(11):1666-72, 2006
9. Newman JS et al: MRI of the painful hip in athletes. Clin Sports Med. 25(4):613-33, 2006
10. Orwig DL et al: Hip fracture and its consequences: differences between men and women. Orthop Clin North Am. 37(4):611-22, 2006
11. Pihlajamaki HK et al: Displaced femoral neck fatigue fractures in military recruits. J Bone Joint Surg Am. 88(9):1989-97, 2006
12. Sorbie C: Sub-capital hip fracture: best treatment options. J Orthop Surg (Hong Kong). 14(3):237-9, 2006

FEMORAL NECK FRACTURES

IMAGE GALLERY

Typical

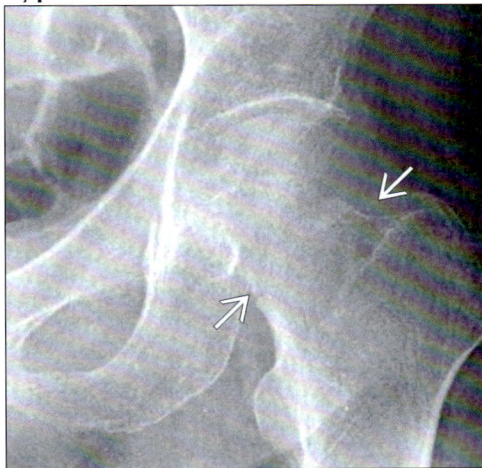
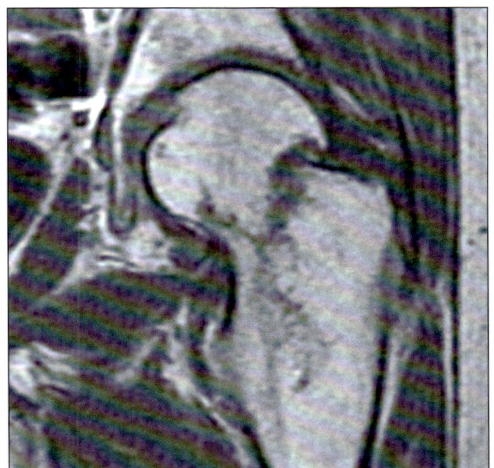

(**Left**) Anteroposterior radiograph shows a subtle nondisplaced subcapital fx. The head/neck angle is in slight valgus, and there is a buckle at the cortex ➔. This confirms the diagnosis. (**Right**) Coronal T1WI MR gives further confirmation of the subcapital fx. MR should not have been necessary in this case. T1 shows the fracture line, which can be obscured by intense edema in STIR imaging.

Typical

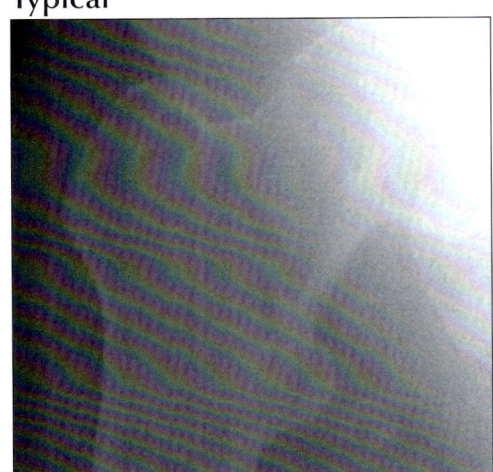
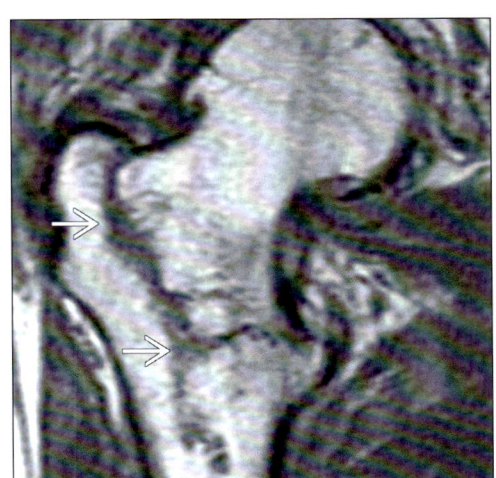

(**Left**) Anteroposterior radiograph shows no hint of either subcapital or intertrochanteric fracture in this elderly woman who fell. Clinical suspicion was high, and MR was performed. (**Right**) Coronal T1WI MR performed at the same setting shows a nondisplaced and nearly complete intertrochanteric fracture ➔. These fractures are becoming recognized more frequently since MR is obtained in the setting of high clinical suspicion but normal radiograph.

Typical

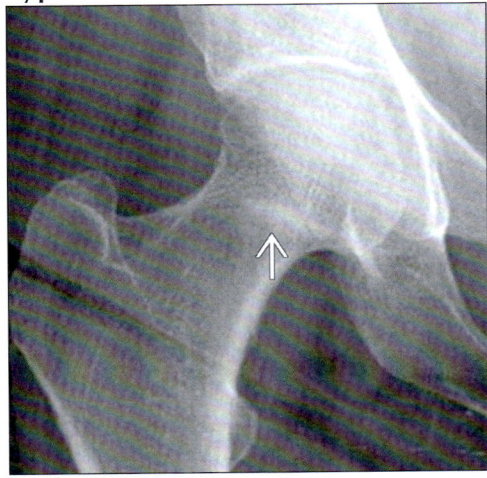
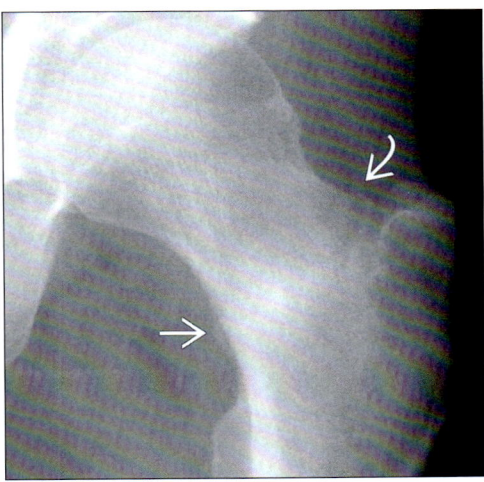

(**Left**) AP radiograph shows linear sclerosis at the medial subcapital site ➔. This is an insufficiency fracture in a 28 yo anorexic woman runner. Subcapital fractures in young adults are unusual & reasons for osteopenia should be sought. (**Right**) AP radiograph shows a basicervical fracture in a marathon runner. The fracture began as a typical stress fracture at the medial basicervical cortex ➔. The patient decided to "run through" his pain & completed the fracture ➔.

KNEE AVULSION FX: INTERNAL DERANGEMENT

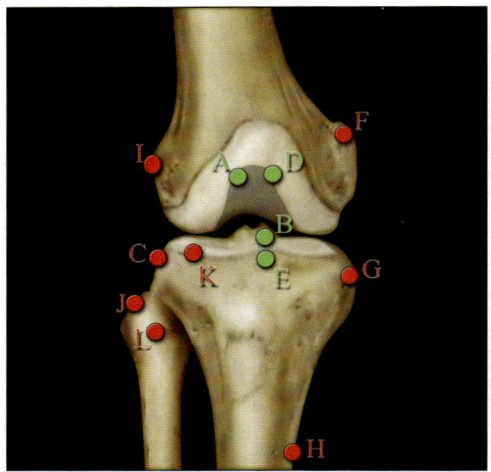

Graphic shows sites of avulsion fracture. Each suggests an internal derangement; confirmation is by MR. Red: Those seen on the surface on an AP view. Green: Those in intercondylar notch or posterior (E). Key: See text.

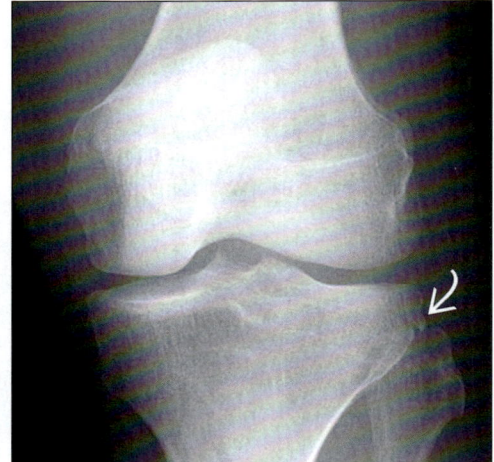

Anteroposterior radiograph shows subtle Segond fx ➔ arising from the lateral tibial plateau. This fx itself is not significant, but the injury which produces it often also results in ACL rupture. The ACL should be examined.

TERMINOLOGY

Abbreviations and Synonyms
- Anterior/posterior cruciate ligament (ACL/PCL)
- Medial/lateral collateral ligament (MCL/LCL)
- Iliotibial band (ITB)

Definitions
- Avulsion fracture: Bony fragment pulled from donor site by attached ligament or tendon
  - Avulsion sites around knee are predictable based on knowledge of origins & insertions
  - Understanding associated soft tissue injury patterns allows inference of extent of injury
- Impaction fracture: Impaction of bone on bone
  - Sites around knee are predictable based on patterns related to knee injury
  - Specific impaction sites are suggestive of associated ligamentous or tendon injuries
- Instability of the knee may also be predicted based on alignment of joint
  - Anterior-posterior shift suggests at least cruciate ligament injury, + likely secondary restraint injury
  - Medial-lateral shift or gap suggests medial or lateral support system disruption

IMAGING FINDINGS

General Features
- Best diagnostic clue
  - Fragment of bone at expected anatomic locations
  - Impaction at expected anatomic locations
  - Gap or displacement along joint line
- Location
  - Avulsions specific to origins & insertions of ligaments/tendons (see radiographic findings)
  - Impactions specific to pattern of injury
- Size: Avulsion fracture fragments about knee are generally small (< 1 cm) & impaction fx subtle (2 mm)

Radiographic Findings
- Avulsion fractures
  - ACL origin: Intercondylar notch at posterior aspect lateral femoral condyle ("A" on graphic)
  - ACL insertion: Medial aspect tibial spine ("B")
    - May involve entire spine, or only a portion

Other Avulsion Fractures Indicating Internal Derangement

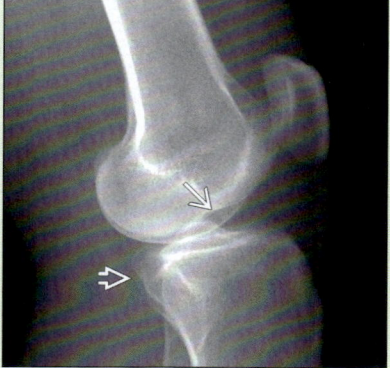

Lat. Recess Impaction, Ant. Drawer

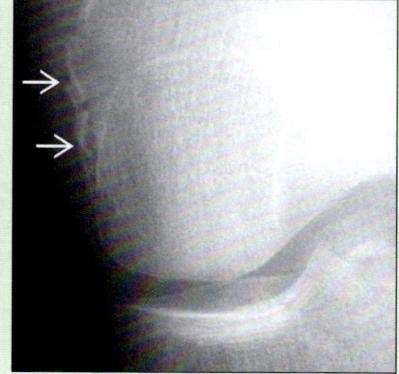

Medial Collateral Ligament

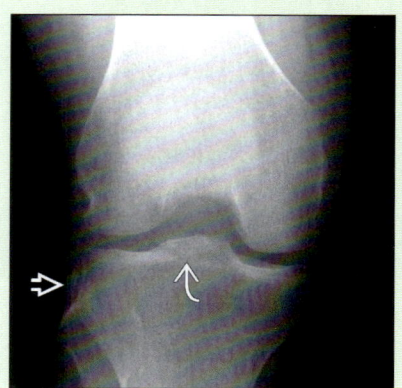

Tibial Spine & Segond

KNEE AVULSION FX: INTERNAL DERANGEMENT

Key Facts

Imaging Findings
- **Avulsion fractures**
- ACL origin: Intercondylar notch at posterior aspect lateral femoral condyle ("A" on graphic)
- ACL insertion: Medial aspect tibial spine ("B")
- Segond fx: Lateral capsular avulsion from lateral proximal tibia, adjacent to joint line ("C")
- PCL origin: Intercondylar notch at anterior-mid aspect medial femoral condyle ("D" on graphic)
- PCL insertion: Posterior mid tibial plateau, extraarticular ("E" on graphic)
- MCL origin: Medial femoral condyle, immediately distal to adductor tubercle ("F" on graphic)
- MCL insertion, deep meniscofemoral ligament (coronary ligament): Medial proximal tibia, adjacent to joint line ("G" on graphic)
- MCL insertion, superficial fibers: Anteromedial proximal tibia, approximately 5 cm distal to joint line ("H" on graphic)
- LCL origin: Lateral femoral condyle ("I" on graphic)
- Arcuate ligament (and popliteofibular, fabellofibular) insertion: Fibular styloid ("J" on graphic)
- ITB insertion (Gerdy tubercle): Anterolateral tibial plateau, adjacent to joint line ("K" on graphic)
- Conjoint tendon (LCL & biceps femoris) insertion: Fibular head & anterolateral tibia ("L" on graphic)

Diagnostic Checklist
- Location of bone fragments around knee are usually avulsions rather than "chip" fx
- Stimulates search for further internal derangement

  - Segond fx: Lateral capsular avulsion from lateral proximal tibia, adjacent to joint line ("C")
    - High association with ACL trauma because of injury mechanism
  - PCL origin: Intercondylar notch at anterior-mid aspect medial femoral condyle ("D" on graphic)
  - PCL insertion: Posterior mid tibial plateau, extraarticular ("E" on graphic)
    - Do not mistake for fabella; avulsion fragment is not as oval or regular in appearance as fabella & avulsion is located behind the notch on AP while fabella is located behind lateral femoral condyle (more proximal and lateral than the PCL avulsion)
  - MCL origin: Medial femoral condyle, immediately distal to adductor tubercle ("F" on graphic)
  - MCL insertion, deep meniscofemoral ligament (coronary ligament): Medial proximal tibia, adjacent to joint line ("G" on graphic)
  - MCL insertion, superficial fibers: Anteromedial proximal tibia, approximately 5 cm distal to joint line ("H" on graphic)
  - LCL origin: Lateral femoral condyle ("I" on graphic)
  - Arcuate ligament (and popliteofibular, fabellofibular) insertion: Fibular styloid ("J" on graphic)
    - Small crescentic fx arising from tip of styloid
  - ITB insertion (Gerdy tubercle): Anterolateral tibial plateau, adjacent to joint line ("K" on graphic)
  - Conjoint tendon (LCL & biceps femoris) insertion: Fibular head & anterolateral tibia ("L" on graphic)
    - Transverse fx through fibular head
  - Inferior patellar tendon origin: Sleeve avulsion from inferior patella
  - Inferior patellar tendon insertion: Tibial apophysis
- **Impaction fractures**
  - Lateral femoral condylar recess
    - Normal shallow concavity at anterior-mid lateral femoral condyle with thin cartilage
    - Impaction if indentation > 2 mm, ± fragmentation
    - High association with ACL injury
  - Anteromedial tibial rim fracture: High association with posterolateral corner injury
  - Medial patella: Associated with lateral patellar dislocation
- **Knee joint malalignment**
  - Anterior drawer sign: Anterior displacement of tibia relative to femur
    - Indicates ACL laxity + secondary restraint disruption
  - Posterior drawer sign: Posterior displacement of tibia relative to femur
    - Indicates PCL laxity + secondary restraint disrupted
  - Lateral gap: Lateral stabilizing structures disrupted
  - Medial gap: Medial stabilizing structures disrupted

MR Findings
- Avulsion fractures
  - T1WI: May show marrow signal in avulsed fragment if fragment is large enough
  - Fluid sensitive sequences: Shows associated bone bruise and extent of internal derangement
  - ACL femoral origin avulsion
    - Small triangular osseous fragment displaced a few mm posterior & inferior to donor site
    - ACL slightly retracted & concave relative to Blumensaat line, with attached fragment
    - Avulsion from ACL origin generally easier to see on MR than radiograph
  - ACL tibial insertion avulsion
    - Tibial spine fragment may be small, or very large, extending posteriorly to PCL insertion
    - Tibial spine fragment may be flipped 90 or 180°, particularly in skeletally immature patients
  - Segond fracture
    - Small oval or triangular osseous fragment arising from lateral tibial plateau, with minimal retraction
    - Associated ACL injury is usually intrasubstance
  - PCL femoral origin avulsion
    - Osseous fragment seen within the notch, slightly proximally displaced
    - PCL slightly retracted posteroinferiorly, with attached fragment
    - Avulsion from PCL origin generally easier to see on MR than radiograph

KNEE AVULSION FX: INTERNAL DERANGEMENT

- PCL tibial insertion avulsion
  - Fragment small, so difficult to see as bone marrow signal; edema at posterior tibial donor site
  - Pattern of PCL retraction from tibial insertion proximally & superiorly should suggest avulsion
- MCL avulsion
  - Bony fragment may be too small to see on MR
  - Deep or superficial MCL avulsion fx may be isolated, without involving the other portion
- Lateral complex avulsions
  - Differentiate ITB avulsion at Gerdy tubercle (anterolateral tibial plateau) from Segond fx (lateral tibial plateau) by location along tibia
  - Arcuate avulsion fragment may be too small to see on MR; watch for edema at fibular styloid
- Inferior patellar sleeve avulsion
  - Fragment has osseous & cartilaginous portions
  - Associated abnormal signal ± tear in proximal inferior patellar tendon
- Impaction fractures: Fragments may be too small to see, but bone bruise pattern is evident with either T1 or fluid-sensitive sequences
  - Lateral femoral condylar recess
    - Edema at recess, & likely associated bone bruise at posterior tibial plateau
    - ACL rupture, usually intrasubstance
  - Anteromedial tibial rim
    - Edema at rim impaction site, often "kissing" edema at anterior femoral condyle from hyperextension injury
    - Posterolateral structure injuries: PCL, LCL, popliteus tendon, arcuate ligament
  - Medial patella
    - Edema at medial patella & lateral femoral condyle
    - Disruption of medial retinaculum

Imaging Recommendations
- Best imaging tool
  - Radiograph to show most avulsions
  - MR to document the associated internal derangement (generally not emergent)
    - If posterolateral corner injury is suspected, MR and orthopedics consult should be performed relatively urgently (not necessarily same day)

DIFFERENTIAL DIAGNOSIS

Dystrophic Calcification
- Differentiation between bony and non-osseous calcification is usually possible
- Avulsions are location specific

PATHOLOGY

General Features
- Epidemiology
  - ACL avulsions
    - Avulsion rare compared with intrasubstance tear
    - Avulsion at tibial spine insertion more common than at femoral condylar origin
    - Avulsion relatively more frequent in skeletally immature patient than adult patient
  - Segond avulsions
    - Relatively common as a secondary sign of ACL disruption, but vast majority of ACL injuries do not have associated Segond fx
  - PCL avulsions
    - Avulsions rare relative to intrasubstance tear
    - Avulsions are relatively more common for PCL than ACL injury (however, ACL injury is so much more frequent that ACL avulsions are absolutely more frequent than PCL avulsions)
    - PCL avulsion at tibial insertion more frequent than at femoral origin
  - MCL avulsions: Rare; origin at femoral condyle more frequent than either insertion site on tibia
  - Lateral complex avulsions
    - Intrasubstance tear more common than avulsion
    - Origin of LCL: Rare
    - Insertion of conjoint tendon: Relatively rare
    - Insertion of arcuate: Relatively rare
    - Insertion of ITB: Rare
  - Patellar tendon avulsion: Rare compared with tear
  - Impaction fractures: Actual fractures are rare relative to bone marrow edema pattern at these sites
  - Knee joint malalignment
    - Rare relative to the number of internal derangement injuries
    - Joint line gap/displacement usually requires disruption of both primary & secondary restraints

CLINICAL ISSUES

Presentation
- Most common signs/symptoms: Pain, ± instability

Demographics
- Age
  - Young adults, relating to frequency of sports injuries
  - Avulsion fx generally are relatively more frequent than ligament/tendon injuries in adolescents
- Gender: M > F, relating to frequency of sports injuries

Treatment
- Most can be effectively treated; conservative vs. surgical treatment relates to type and extent of injury as well as patient activity demands
- Most can be stabilized at time of injury & sent for orthopedic evaluation in an outpatient setting
- Concern for posterolateral corner injury should lead to a more urgent consultation with orthopedics & MR

DIAGNOSTIC CHECKLIST

Consider
- Location of bone fragments around knee are usually avulsions rather than "chip" fx
- Stimulates search for further internal derangement

SELECTED REFERENCES

1. Bahk MS et al: Physical examination and imaging of the lateral collateral ligament and posterolateral corner of the knee. Sports Med Arthrosc. 14(1):12-9, 2006

KNEE AVULSION FX: INTERNAL DERANGEMENT

IMAGE GALLERY

Typical

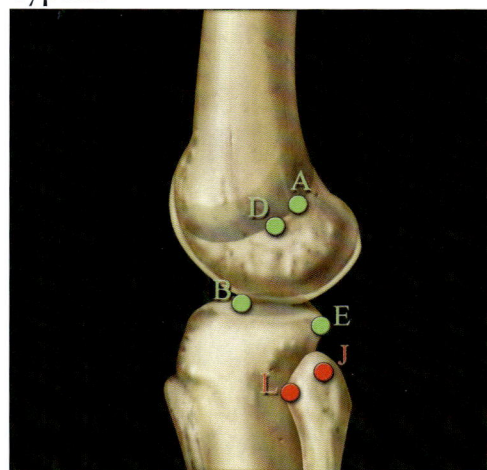
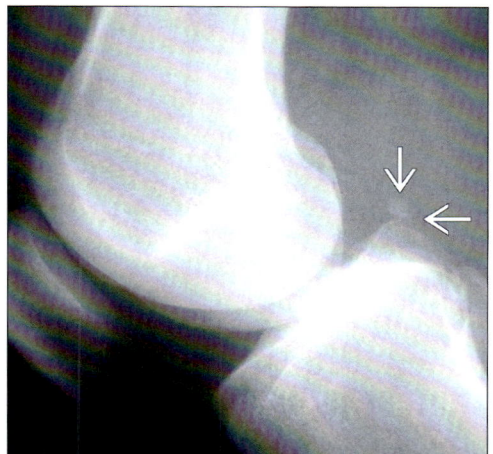

(Left) Graphic shows avulsion fx sites seen on lateral view. Red: Surface of fibula. Green: Intercondylar notch or posterior tibia (E). Type of internal derangement is inferred from the avulsion. Key: See text. *(Right)* Lateral radiograph shows an avulsion of the PCL ➔ from its insertion at the posterior mid tibial plateau. It has retracted proximally by about 1 cm.

Typical

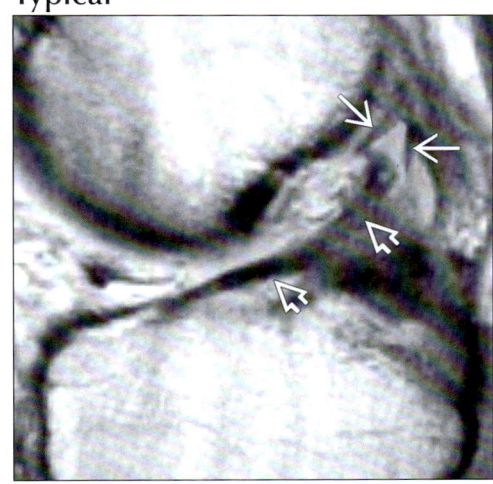
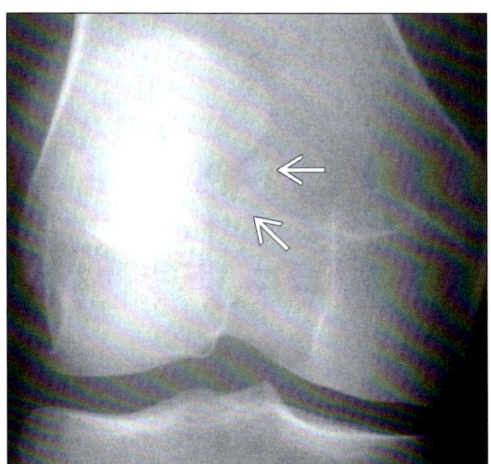

(Left) Sagittal PD/Intermediate MR shows avulsion of ACL from the femoral insertion site. The avulsion fragment ➔ is retracted from the donor site and the ACL is bowed inferiorly ➔ but itself is not disrupted. This avulsion fragment could not be seen on radiograph. *(Right)* Anteroposterior radiograph shows fragmentation at the medial patella ➔. This represents prior lateral patellar dislocation & must not be mistaken for a multipartite patella.

Typical

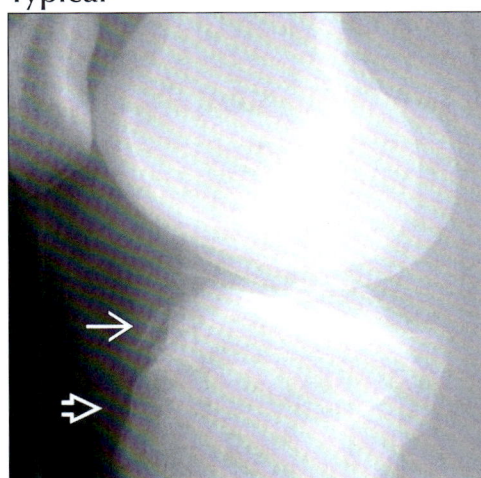
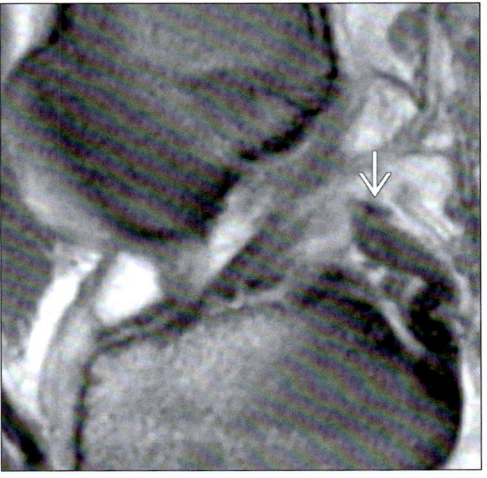

(Left) Lateral radiograph shows fragmentation of the anteromedial tibial rim ➔ & posterior displacement of the tibia relative to the femur ➔. The fragmentation suggests direct blow or hyperextension injury & should suggest associated posterior cruciate ligament (PCL) and/or posterolateral corner soft tissue injury. *(Right)* Sagittal PD/Intermediate FS MR confirms the PCL disruption ➔. Other images showed posterolateral soft tissue injury as well.

PATELLAR FRACTURE

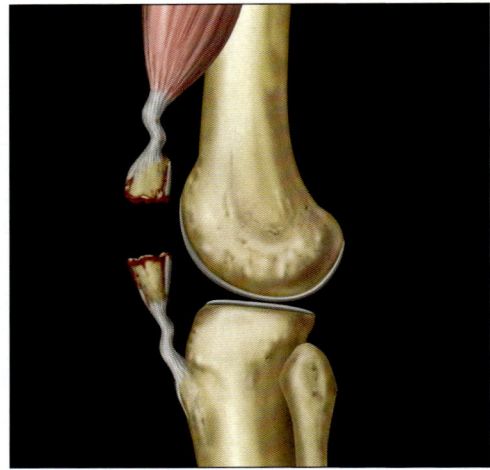

Lateral graphic shows a transverse fracture with separation caused by the opposing forces of the patellar and quadriceps tendons.

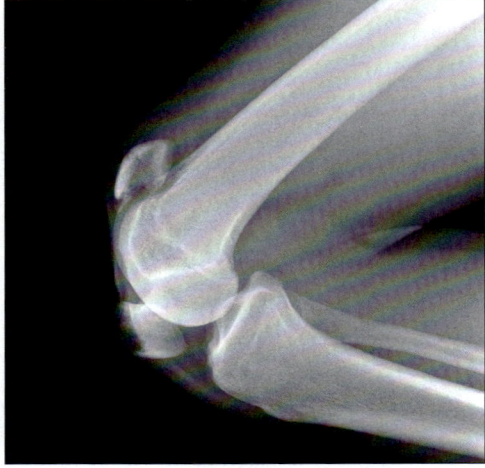

Lateral radiograph shows a distracted transverse fracture with mild comminution caused by an indirect injury. The extent of distraction indicates retinacular disruption.

TERMINOLOGY

Abbreviations and Synonyms
- Patellar sleeve fracture in children and adolescents
- Other types: Burst, transverse, vertical, chip

Definitions
- Patella fracture ± extensor mechanism disruption
- Extensor mechanism = quadriceps, patella, and patellar tendon
- Osteochondral fx = fx of articular cartilage + bone

IMAGING FINDINGS

General Features
- Best diagnostic clue
  - Fracture line/displacement on radiograph
  - Patella alta (look for small inferior pole avulsion)
- Location
  - Transverse fx usually mid-lower patella
  - Chip fx usually medial facet cortex
- Morphology
  - Transverse fx (50-80%)
  - Stellate (comminuted) fx (30-35%)
  - Vertical fx (12-17%)
  - Polar fx (quadriceps/patellar tendon insertion)
  - Osteochondral fx (secondary to lateral dislocation)
  - Sleeve fx
    - Variety of osteochondral fx
    - Most common patellar fx < 16 years
    - Avulsed cartilage ± bone at superior/inferior pole

Radiographic Findings
- Lateral radiograph
  - Transverse fracture line ± diastasis
    - Diastasis relates to disruption of retinacula
  - Fracture displacement and comminution
    - Separation > 3 mm → surgery
  - Articular surface incongruity
    - > 2 mm articular offset → surgery
  - Small avulsed fragment
    - Polar - superior or inferior
    - ± Visible calcified avulsion in sleeve fx
  - Patella alta
    - Patella height:patellar tendon height < 0.8
    - Suggests patellar tendon rupture
    - Look for small inferior polar fracture

DDx: Patella Fracture

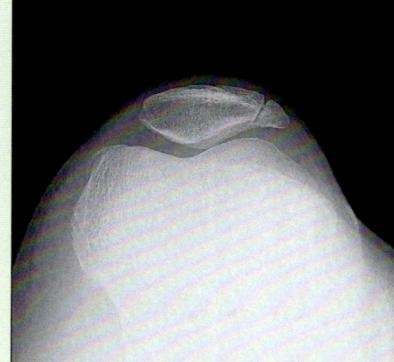

Bipartite Patella

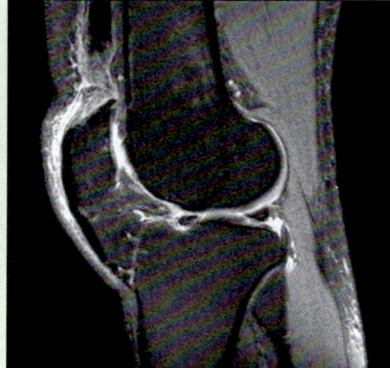

Quadriceps Tear

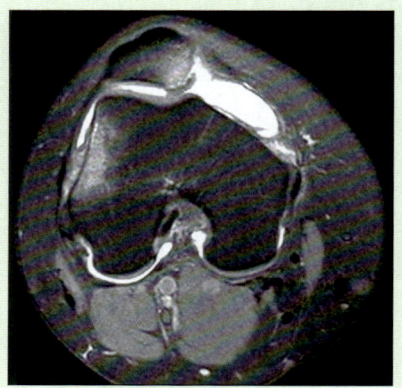

Patellar Dislocation

PATELLAR FRACTURE

Key Facts

Terminology
- Osteochondral fx = fx of articular cartilage + bone

Imaging Findings
- Transverse fx (50-80%)
- Stellate (comminuted) fx (30-35%)
- Vertical fx (12-17%)
- Polar fx (quadriceps/patellar tendon insertion)
- Osteochondral fx (secondary to lateral dislocation)
- Sleeve fx
- Separation > 3 mm → surgery
- > 2 mm articular offset → surgery
- Bone scan/MR may be useful for stress fx or bipartite patella synchrosis fx

Top Differential Diagnoses
- Bipartite Patella
- Quadriceps/Patellar Tear/Tendinopathy
- Transient Patellar Dislocation

Pathology
- Direct fx: Forceful blow to patella & flexed knee
- Indirect fx: Forceful jump, twist, fall, or near fall

Clinical Issues
- Pain, swelling, & ↓ extension strength
- Obtain radiographs before attempting extension
- Examine extensor mechanism & check for open fx
- < 16 years: Sleeve fracture most common
- Bipartite patella ≈ 9:1 M:F
- Open fracture is surgical emergency
- Non-operative: Splint/cast in extension for 4-6 weeks

Diagnostic Checklist
- Possibility of open fracture

- Seen with sleeve fx also
- Patella baja
  - Low patella
  - Suggests quadriceps tendon rupture
  - Look for small superior polar fracture
  - May be seen in sleeve fx
- Soft tissue mass of retracted tendons
- Joint effusion
- AP and merchant (sunrise) radiographs
  - Fracture displacement and comminution
  - Vertical fracture line
  - ± Calcified osteochondral fx of medial patellar facet or lateral femoral condyle after lateral dislocation

CT Findings
- Radiographically occult fracture
- Intraarticular bone fragment
- Associated femur/tibia fx
- Articular facet malalignment (tracking)

MR Findings
- Fx line ↓ T1 surrounded by ↑ T2 signal
- Joint effusion (↑ T2 signal)
- Articular cartilage involvement (↑ T2 signal)
- ± Tear of medial/lateral retinaculum
- ± ↑ T2 signal/laxity/discontinuity patella tendon & quadriceps
- ± Bone bruise & fx (↑ T2) adjacent tibia and femur
- Osteochondral fracture
  - Evidence of transient lateral patellar dislocation
    - Bone bruise (↑ T2 FS signal) of medial patella & lateral femoral condyle
    - ± Tear/injury (↑ T2 signal/discontinuity) of medial retinaculum, medial patellofemoral ligament (MPFL) & vastus medialis obliquus (VMO) muscle
  - ↓ Signal fragment in joint space or adjacent to patella on all sequences
  - Concave deformity of inferomedial patella
- Sleeve fracture
  - Separation through ossifying cartilage joining patella and tendon
  - Posterior articular cartilage (sleeve) of patella follows polar fragment & separates from patella
  - ↓ Signal cartilage ± bone fragment in joint space or adjacent to patella on all sequences

Nuclear Medicine Findings
- Bone Scan
  - Bone scan/MR may be useful for stress fx or bipartite patella synchrosis fx
  - Acute diffuse ↑ patella uptake (hyperemia)
  - Localized/linear ↑ uptake for several months
  - Often shows ↑ uptake at 1 year
  - Nonspecific, but 100% sensitive (study at 1 week)

Imaging Recommendations
- Best imaging tool
  - Lateral radiographs most sensitive but do not detect vertical or osteochondral fx
  - MR to evaluate extensor mechanism
  - Pre-operative CT for highly comminuted fx
- Protocol advice
  - CT: Bone algorithm with axial < 1 mm; sagittal and coronal reformats
  - MR: Axial T1/T2, axial T2 FS, coronal STIR

DIFFERENTIAL DIAGNOSIS

Bipartite Patella
- Smooth osseous margins on radiographs
- May be multipartite
- Osseous fragments may not appear contiguous, but overlying cartilage is smooth
- Usually superior-lateral patella
- 2-8% of population
- 40-45% bilateral: Consider contralateral knee radiograph
- Synchondrosis of 2° ossification centers can be injured
- Bone scan for synchondrosis fracture

Quadriceps/Patellar Tear/Tendinopathy
- ↑ T2 signal and thickening of tendon = tendinitis
- Discontinuity of laminated muscle layers = tear
- Abnormal T1 signal/mass at tear = hematoma & edema
- Occurs at tendinous-osseous junction

PATELLAR FRACTURE

- Complete tear usually diagnosed by physical exam

Transient Patellar Dislocation
- MR: Bone bruise (↑ T2 FS signal) of medial patella & lateral femoral condyle
- ± Medial retinaculum tear/injury (↑ T2 signal)
- ± Injury/tear of MPFL and/or VMO muscle
- Joint effusion
- Search for associated osteochondral fx & intraarticular fragments
- Presents as swelling & pain after twisting valgus injury

PATHOLOGY

General Features
- Etiology
  - Direct fx: Forceful blow to patella & flexed knee
    - Common cause of stellate and vertical fractures
    - More comminuted
    - Less displaced
    - More articular cartilage damage
  - Indirect fx: Forceful jump, twist, fall, or near fall
    - Transverse fracture
    - Patellar retinaculum tear → fx diastasis
  - Secondary to ACL reconstruction
    - Autologous tibia-patellar tendon-patella bone graft harvesting weakens patella
    - Usually indirect transverse fx < 2 months post-op
    - Occurs in 1% of patients
  - Pathologic fracture
    - Tumor (giant cell, chondroblastoma, lymphoma)
    - Metabolic (Brown tumor, gout)
- Epidemiology
  - 1% of all skeletal fractures
  - Majority are direct fractures
  - Osteochondral fx with 5% of dislocations
- Associated abnormalities: Hip dislocation, femoral neck/shaft/condyle fx, tibia fx with direct injury

CLINICAL ISSUES

Presentation
- Most common signs/symptoms
  - Pain, swelling, & ↓ extension strength
  - Large joint effusion or hemarthrosis
  - Inability to straight-leg raise
  - Point tenderness
  - Defect in smooth patellar cortex on palpation
- Evaluation
  - Obtain radiographs before attempting extension
  - Examine extensor mechanism & check for open fx
    - Intraarticular lidocaine may help patient extend
    - May inject joint and look for skin leak
  - Medial & lateral retinacula may be intact & allow extension with minimally distracted cortical fragments

Demographics
- Age
  - < 16 years: Sleeve fracture most common
  - Osteochondral fx at inferior or superior pole usually child or adolescent
  - Patella begins ossifying at 3-5 years
- Gender
  - M:F ≈ 2:1
  - Bipartite patella ≈ 9:1 M:F

Natural History & Prognosis
- Persistent pain and arthritis in approximately 50%
- 50-80% good/excellent surgical results reported
- Patellectomy → knee instability & ↓ extension strength

Treatment
- Acute
  - Open fracture is surgical emergency
  - Extension splinting and ice
  - Drainage of hemarthrosis for pain relief
  - Intraarticular local anesthetic for pain
- Surgery
  - Indications
    - > 3 mm separation of fx fragments
    - > 2 mm incongruity at articular surface
    - Disruption of extensor mechanism
    - Open fracture
  - Goals: Restore extensor mechanism & reduce complications (arthritis)
  - Techniques: Tension band, cerclage wire, screw fixation, partial/total patellectomy
    - Modified tension band = most stable fixation of transverse fx
    - Make every attempt to salvage patella
- Non-operative: Splint/cast in extension for 4-6 weeks

DIAGNOSTIC CHECKLIST

Consider
- Possibility of open fracture
- Integrity of extensor mechanism

Image Interpretation Pearls
- AP radiograph often falsely negative
- Osteochondral & sleeve fxs in child/adolescent may not have calcified fragment on radiograph
- Measure articular surface & fx fragment displacement

SELECTED REFERENCES
1. Bucholz RW et al: Rockwood and Green's Fractures in Adults. 6th ed. Philadelphia, Pennsylvania, Lippincott Williams & Wilkins. 1969-1997, 2007
2. Sanders TG et al: MRI of osteochondral defects of the lateral femoral condyle: incidence and pattern of injury after transient lateral dislocation of the patella. AJR Am J Roentgenol. 187(5):1332-7, 2006
3. Hunt DM et al: A review of sleeve fractures of the patella in children. Knee. 12(1):3-7, 2005
4. DeLee J et al: DeLee and Drez's Orthopaedic Sports Medicine. 2nd ed. Philadelphia, Pennsylvania, Saunders. 1760-7, 2003
5. Elias DA et al: Acute lateral patellar dislocation at MR imaging: injury patterns of medial patellar soft-tissue restraints and osteochondral injuries of the inferomedial patella. Radiology. 225(3):736-43, 2002
6. Yu JS et al: MR imaging of injuries of the extensor mechanism of the knee. Radiographics. 14(3):541-51, 1994

PATELLAR FRACTURE

IMAGE GALLERY

Typical

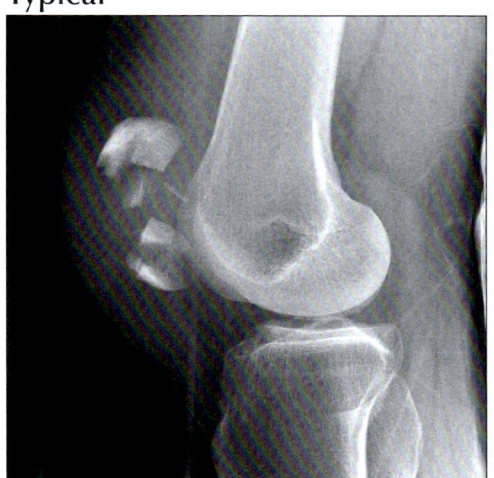
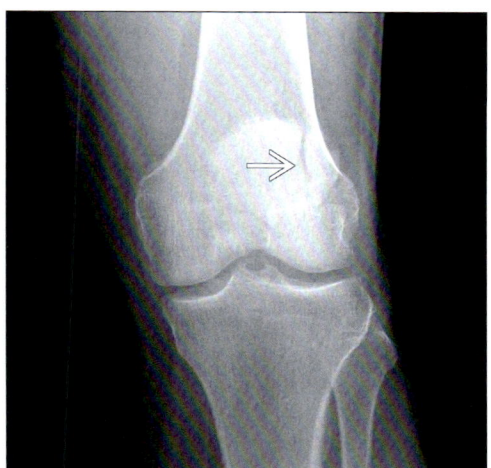

(Left) Lateral radiograph shows a comminuted, slightly distracted fracture with massive soft tissue swelling following a direct injury. *(Right)* Anteroposterior radiograph shows a vertical, nondisplaced fracture through the lateral articular facet ➔. A bipartite patella would be more oblique, with sclerosis along the lucency.

Typical

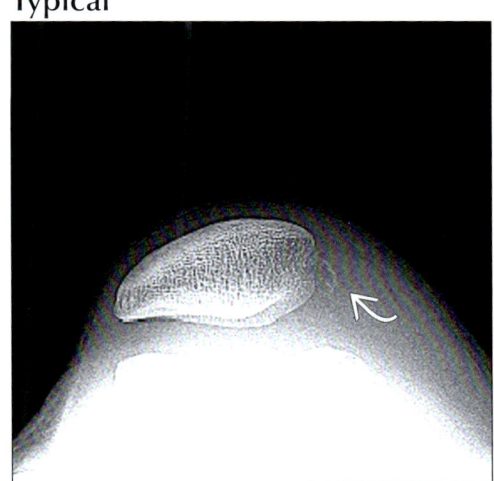
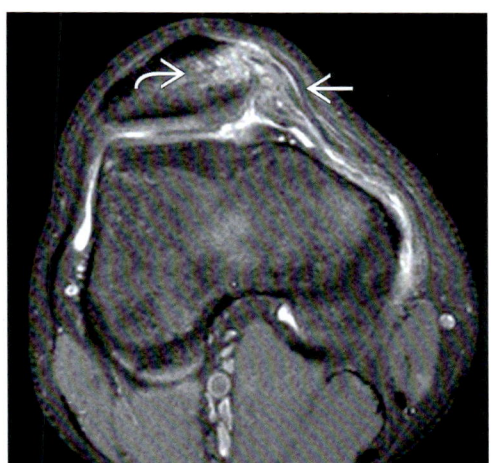

(Left) Sunrise radiograph shows an osteochondral fragment ➔ arising from the medial patella. The donor site is not always seen. *(Right)* Axial T2WI FS MR in the same patient as previous image, shows a medial patellar contusion ➔ with medial retinacular edema and tear ➔. The fracture fragment was too small to visualize on MR. The accompanying femoral condyle bruise is in a more cephalad position.

Typical

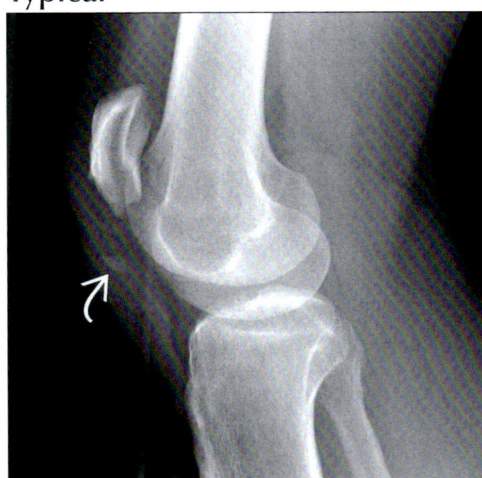
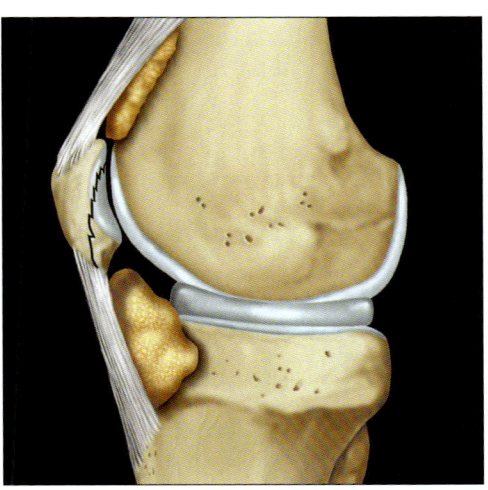

(Left) Lateral radiograph shows patella alta & an inferior pole fragment ➔ in an adult. The same radiographic appearance is consistent with a sleeve fracture in a child or adolescent. *(Right)* Lateral graphic shows a sleeve fx with separation in the ossifying cartilage between tendon and bone. The posterior articular cartilage (sleeve) follows the polar fragment away from the patella.

PATELLAR TENDON TEARS & TENDINOSIS

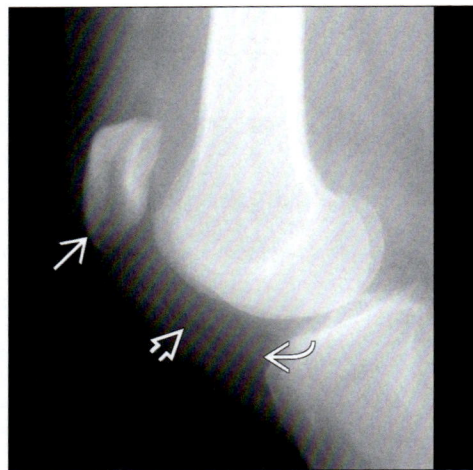

Lateral radiograph of an inferior patellar tendon tear shows patellar alta ➡, associated with absence of a sharp, distinct inferior patellar tendon ➡. Note also the absence of a well-defined Hoffa fat pad ➡.

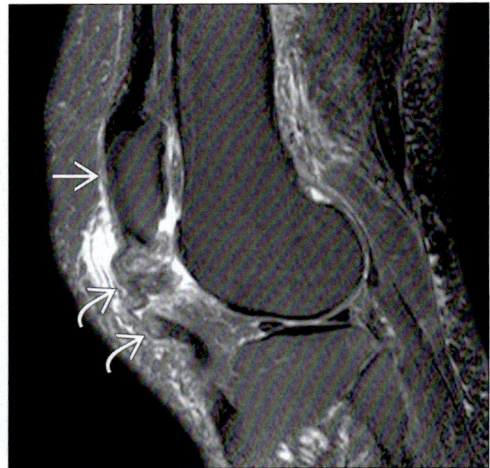

Sagittal PD/Intermediate FS MR confirms the patella alta ➡, retracted by the quadriceps tendon. The inferior patellar tendon is completely ruptured at its proximal aspect ➡ and retracted inferiorly.

TERMINOLOGY

Abbreviations and Synonyms
- Patellar tendon tear: Patellar tendon rupture
- Patellar tendinosis: Jumper's knee, chronic patellar tendinitis, patellar tendinopathy

Definitions
- Tear: Disruption of the patellar tendon
- Tendinosis: Focal degeneration, microtears of patellar tendon

IMAGING FINDINGS

General Features
- Best diagnostic clue
  - Tear: Gap in patellar tendon
    - ± Hemorrhage & granulation tissue
    - ± Patella alta
    - If patella alta present, radiograph may also show concavity in soft tissues at expected site of patellar tendon
  - Tendinosis: MR shows high signal within tendon without full thickness tear
    - ± Patellar tendon thickening
    - Signal abnormality more prominent on PD than T2 sequences indicative of tendinosis rather than partial tear
    - Unlikely to show abnormality on radiograph
- Location
  - Proximal third of the patellar tendon (most common)
    - Posterior fibers of proximal tendon
  - Inferior pole of patella: Uncommon
- Size
  - Tendon is thickened
  - Range from few mm signal abnormality to several cms involvement with retraction of torn fibers
- Morphology
  - Tear: Irregular thickened tendon edges, retracted to a variable degree, resulting in patellar alta
    - Patellar sleeve avulsion may be associated (cartilaginous avulsion from lower pole patella)
  - Tendinosis: Increased signal intensity of thickened tendon on short TE sequence

DDx: Patellar Tendon Tears

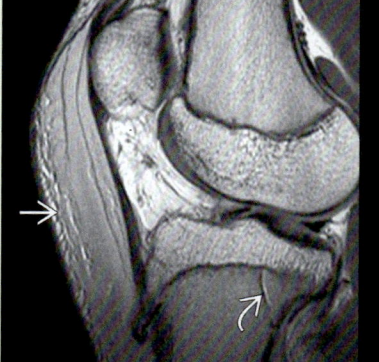
Prepatellar Hematoma + Salter II

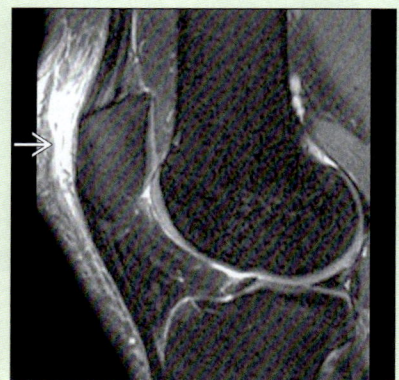
Prepatellar Bursitis

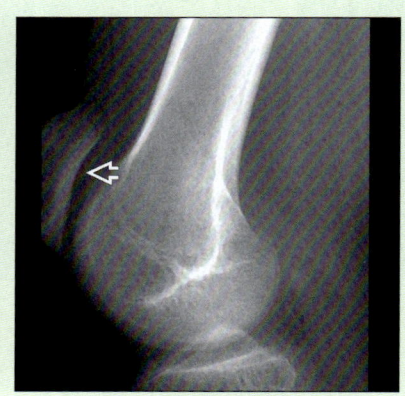
C-Shaped: Cerebral Palsy

PATELLAR TENDON TEARS & TENDINOSIS

Key Facts

Terminology
- Tear: Disruption of the patellar tendon
- Tendinosis: Focal degeneration, microtears of patellar tendon

Imaging Findings
- Proximal third of the patellar tendon (most common)
- Tear: Gap in tendon
- Early tendinosis: Hyperintense edema in peritenon without visible change in tendon itself
- Chronic tendinosis: Thickening & areas of intermediate (collagen degeneration) to hyperintense signal (partial tears) on fluid sensitive sequence
- Radiograph may show abnormal position of patella & morphologic abnormality of patellar tendon
- MR to document tendinosis vs partial vs complete tear, and document amount of retraction

Pathology
- Chronic overuse tendinosis often due to sports with jumping activities (basketball)
- Collagen vascular diseases may be related, as well as other diseases that weaken tendons

Clinical Issues
- Complete tear results in inability to extend knee
- Partial tear: Incomplete knee extension
- Complete tear requires surgical repair and is often considered an orthopedic emergency

Diagnostic Checklist
- Partial tear in the setting of peripatellar pain
- Tendinosis with increased signal in proximal tendon especially on short TE sequences

Radiographic Findings
- Radiography
  - Tear of inferior patellar tendon
    - Patellar alta
    - Thickened & irregular tendon may have anterior concavity
    - ± Avulsion
  - Tendinosis: Generally normal; ± tendon thickening

MR Findings
- T1WI
  - Tear: Gap in tendon
    - ± Fracture fragment
    - Low signal within adjacent Hoffa fat pad
  - Tendinosis: Thickening of tendon
    - Areas of intermediate signal intensity (collagen degeneration); high signal also seen on PD sequence with tendinosis
    - Decreased (normal) signal may indicate fibrosis if chronic
    - Low signal within adjacent Hoffa fat pad & inferior pole patella
- Fluid sensitive sequences
  - Tear: Gap in tendon
    - Fluid fills defect
    - High signal in adjacent Hoffa fat pad & bone
  - Early tendinosis: Hyperintense edema in peritenon without visible change in tendon itself
  - Chronic tendinosis: Thickening & areas of intermediate (collagen degeneration) to hyperintense signal (partial tears) on fluid sensitive sequence
    - T2 sequence may show no greater signal intensity than PD in tendinosis
    - T2 shows higher signal intensity than PD in partial tear; differentiates from tendinosis
    - FS T2 or STIR generally show higher signal than either PD or T2 in both tendinosis and partial tear
  - Increased signal in adjacent Hoffa fat pad & inferior pole of patella

Ultrasonographic Findings
- Thickened hypoechoic tendon
- Extent of tendon retraction can be evaluated

Imaging Recommendations
- Best imaging tool
  - Radiograph may show abnormal position of patella & morphologic abnormality of patellar tendon
  - MR to document tendinosis vs partial vs complete tear, and document amount of retraction
- Protocol advice: PD & FS T2 helps to differentiate tendinosis and partial tendon tears

DIFFERENTIAL DIAGNOSIS

Hematoma, Bursitis
- Increased signal mass on T2WI, in pre-patellar tissues
- ± Hyperintensity on T1WI related to hemorrhage
- Hemosiderin in hypointense rim or blooming on gradient echo sequences

Prepatellar Bursitis (Housemaid's or Preacher's Knee)
- Occupational history
- Fluid and inflammatory debris in prepatellar bursa
- Tendon and Hoffa fat pad normal and undisturbed

Sinding-Larsen-Johansson Disease
- Traction apophysitis at inferior pole of patella; tendon is normal
- Osseous fragments may be multiple and irregular
- May be painful during adolescence

Osgood Schlatter Disease
- Osteochondrosis
- Variable fragmentation of tibial apophysis
- May be painful in childhood, with associated swelling
- If symptomatic, ± associated infrapatellar bursitis

Cerebral Palsy
- If patient does not ambulate, may develop patella alta
- Shape of patella is distinctive: "C" shaped, concave

PATELLAR TENDON TEARS & TENDINOSIS

Salter Fracture in Adolescent
- An injury which may cause tendon tear in an adult is more likely to cause a physeal injury in a skeletally immature patient; Salter II most frequent

Magic Angle Artifact
- In tendons at 55° to external magnetic field
- Any portion of patellar tendon may demonstrate this
- High signal on short TE sequences (T1, PD, GRE)
- No associated tendon thickening or pain

PATHOLOGY

General Features
- General path comments
  - Chronic overload on patellar tendon because of strain from the quadriceps muscle group
    - Results in microtears & focal degeneration
  - Degeneration & deterioration are predisposing factor to tendon rupture
    - Tensile & viscoelastic properties of the patellar tendon, however, remain relatively stable between younger and older age groups
- Etiology
  - Chronic overuse tendinosis often due to sports with jumping activities (basketball)
  - Collagen vascular diseases may be related, as well as other diseases that weaken tendons
    - Rheumatoid arthritis
    - End stage renal disease
  - Steroid injections increase risk for tendon rupture
  - Some association with malalignment syndromes
  - ACL bone-patellar tendon-bone graft harvesting leaves the inferior patellar tendon at risk since 1/3 of tendon is harvested

Gross Pathologic & Surgical Features
- Thickened, indurated tendon edges with discontinuity if complete tear

Microscopic Features
- Collagen degeneration without significant influx of inflammatory cells
  - "Tendinosis" is more appropriate term than "tendinitis"

Staging, Grading or Classification Criteria
- Grade I: Pain after activity
- Grade II: Pain/discomfort during activity, without interfering with sports participation
- Grade III: Pain during & after participation, which interferes with activity
- Grade IV: Complete tendon disruption

CLINICAL ISSUES

Presentation
- Most common signs/symptoms
  - Complete tear: Pain, physical examination reveals palpable defect in patellar ligament
  - Tendinosis: Pain & tenderness over patellar tendon, especially with resisted extension
- Clinical Profile
  - Complete tear results in inability to extend knee
  - Partial tear: Incomplete knee extension

Demographics
- Age
  - Physically active patients < 40 years
  - Older patients with underlying disease predisposing to tendon weakness
- Gender: M > F for complete tears

Natural History & Prognosis
- Complete tear requires surgical repair and is often considered an orthopedic emergency
- Tendinosis will heal/improve with cessation of jumping sports
  - Without conservative treatment, may progress to complete tear

Treatment
- Conservative: Partial tear can be treated with immobilization for 3-6 weeks
  - Rest, ice, nonsteroidal anti-inflammatory agents (steroids may increase risk for completion of tear)
- Surgical: Repair using end-to-end sutures, ± delayed or late repair
  - Complete tear: Repair using end-to-end sutures
  - Persistent pain with tendinosis: May do Maquet procedure
    - Vertical osteotomy tibial apophysis, interposed bone graft to elevate anterior tibial tubercle
    - Procedure has moderate risk of nonunion

DIAGNOSTIC CHECKLIST

Consider
- Partial tear in the setting of peripatellar pain
- Tendinosis with increased signal in proximal tendon especially on short TE sequences
- Magic angle artifact may mimic tendon degeneration

Image Interpretation Pearls
- FS PD combined with T2 sagittal images demonstrate tendon tear morphology & helps to differentiate tendinosis from partial & complete tears

SELECTED REFERENCES

1. McGrory JE: Disruption of the extensor mechanism of the knee. J Emerg Med. 24(2):163-8, 2003
2. Panni AS et al: Overuse injuries of the extensor mechanism in athletes. Clin Sports Med. 21(3):483-98, ix, 2002
3. Casey MT Jr et al: Neglected ruptures of the patellar tendon. A case series of four patients. Am J Sports Med. 29(4):457-60, 2001
4. Enad JG et al: Primary patellar tendon repair and early mobilization: results in an active-duty population. J South Orthop Assoc. 10(1):17-23, 2001
5. Kasten P et al: Rupture of the patellar tendon: a review of 68 cases and a retrospective study of 29 ruptures comparing two methods of augmentation. Arch Orthop Trauma Surg. 121(10):578-82, 2001
6. Sonin AH: Magnetic resonance imaging of the extensor mechanism. Magn Reson Imaging Clin N Am. 2(3):401-11, 1994

PATELLAR TENDON TEARS & TENDINOSIS

IMAGE GALLERY

Typical

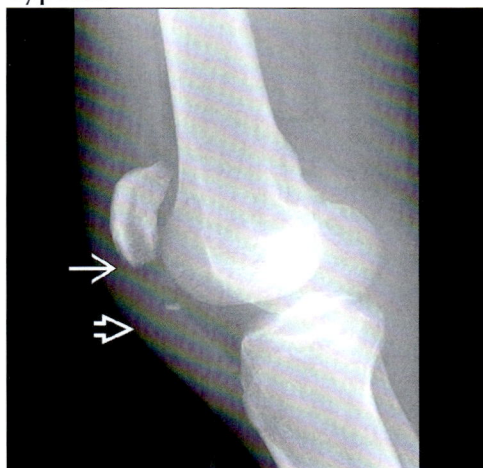 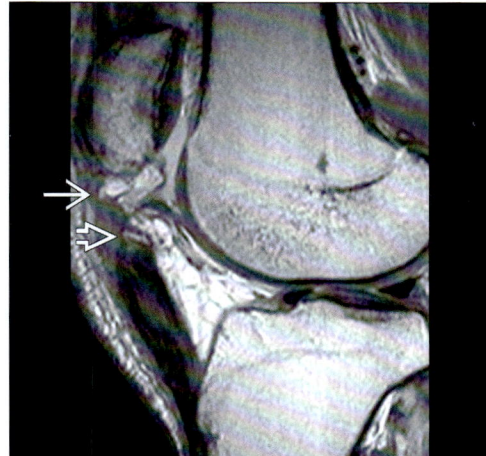

(Left) Lateral radiograph shows patellar alta ➡, with a small fx fragment & severe thickening of the inferior patellar tendon ➡. This is diagnostic of a patellar tendon tear associated with a patellar sleeve avulsion. *(Right)* Sagittal PD/Intermediate MR confirms the proximal tear ➡, and a 1.5 cm gap between the patella and the small fracture fragment ➡; this fragment corresponds to that seen on the radiograph. This patient sustained a direct blow to the knee.

Typical

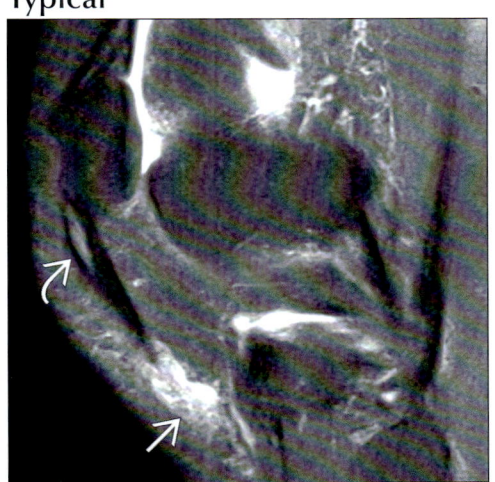 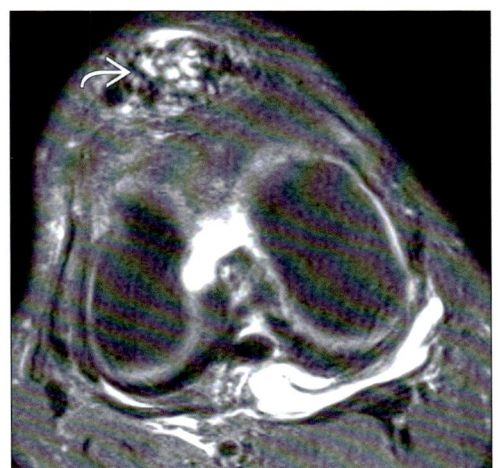

(Left) Sagittal T2WI FS MR shows acute inferior patellar tendon tear ➡ in a patient who has chronic longitudinal partial tears in the proximal portion of the tendon ➡. The inferior site of the complete tear is unusual. *(Right)* Axial T2WI FS MR confirms the extensive longitudinal tears within the proximal portion of the tendon ➡. This patient has chronic renal disease, representing one of the typical etiologies of extensor mechanism tear.

Typical

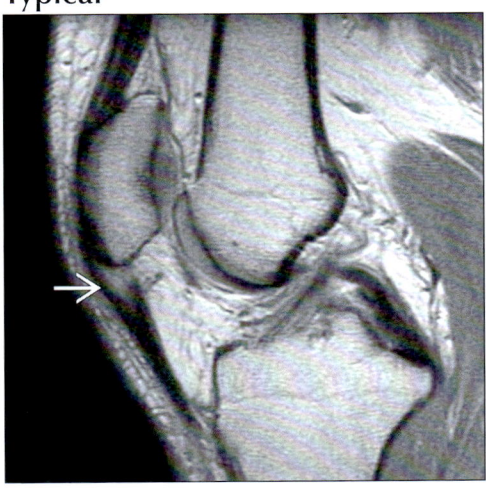 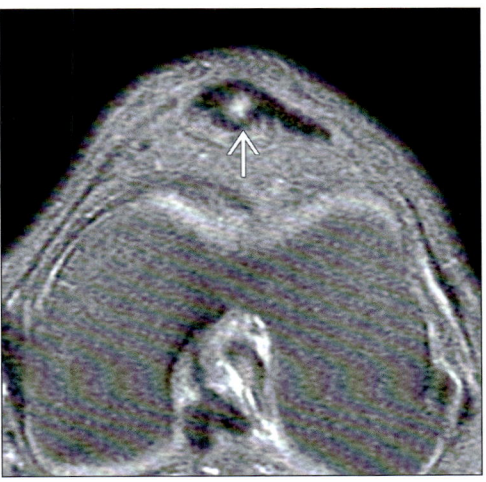

(Left) Sagittal PD/Intermediate MR shows a typical case of "jumper's knee", also called patellar tendinosis. There is fusiform swelling of the proximal inferior patellar tendon, due to chronic degeneration, with intermediate signal intensity on the proton density image ➡. *(Right)* Axial T2WI FS MR shows the region to have high signal ➡, representing a combination of degeneration & superimposed micro & macro tearing.

TIBIAL PLATEAU FRACTURE

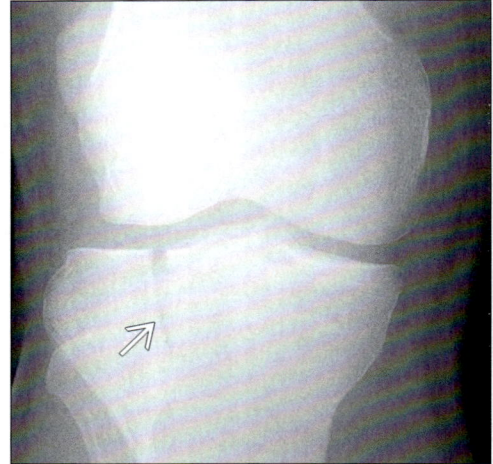 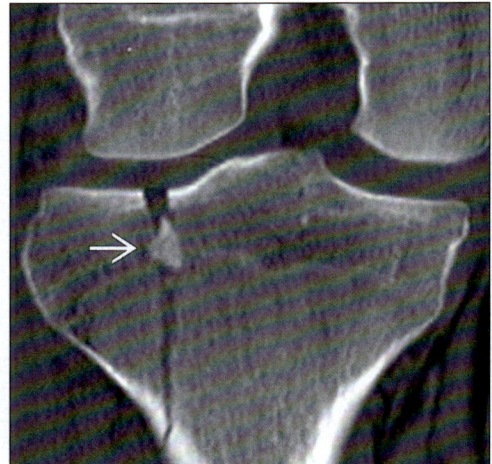

Anteroposterior radiograph shows a vertical split lateral plateau fracture ➡. Schatzker type I. Note the bone density is normal; this is a young patient who sustained a high-energy impact.

Coronal bone CT reformat gives additional information; there is an impacted cortical bone fragment ➡ wedged within the split fracture. This must be removed in order to obtain an anatomic reduction at the articular surface.

TERMINOLOGY

Abbreviations and Synonyms
- Lateral tibial plateau fx also known as "bumper" or "fender" fx

Definitions
- Fx of the plateau due to axial loading, ± rotational injury, ± valgus angulation

IMAGING FINDINGS

General Features
- Best diagnostic clue
  - Fat-fluid level in suprapatellar bursa
  - Oblique or vertical linear fx line on radiograph
  - Sclerotic horizontal line below the level of the cortex of either lateral or medial tibial plateau
- Location
  - Tibial plateau with variable extension medially or laterally
  - May involve tibial eminence
  - More severe plateau fx also has a transverse metaphyseal fx
- Size: Varies from trabecular injury to small nondisplaced fx to comminuted depressed fx
- Morphology
  - Younger patients: Vertical split fracture
  - Older osteoporotic patients: Depressed fractures with variable extension

Radiographic Findings
- Most plateau fractures can be diagnosed by conventional radiography, especially if there is a depressed fragment
- Lipohemarthrosis seen on cross table lateral or axial view of patella
  - Fat-fluid line
  - Lipohemarthrosis will not be seen on conventional lateral radiograph
- Oblique radiograph may enhance detection
- Depressed fragment may be seen as a sclerotic line below the level of the cortex, without lucent fx line
  - Sclerotic line is the cortex of depressed fragment

CT Findings
- Bone CT

Other Tibial Plateau Fractures

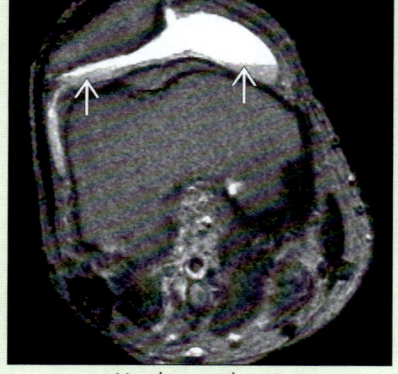 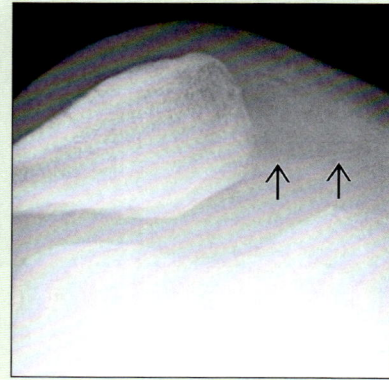 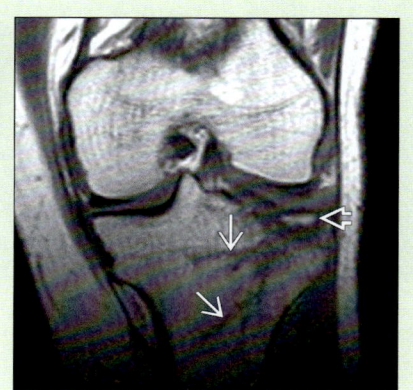

Lipohemarthrosis *Lipohemarthrosis* *Extends Medially*

TIBIAL PLATEAU FRACTURE

Key Facts

Terminology
- Lateral tibial plateau fx also known as "bumper" or "fender" fx

Imaging Findings
- Younger patients: Vertical split fracture
- Older osteoporotic patients: Depressed fractures with variable extension
- Most plateau fractures can be diagnosed by conventional radiography, especially if there is a depressed fragment
- CT with reformats detects radiographically occult plateau fractures
- Soft tissue injuries often underestimated without MR

Pathology
- 75-80% tibial plateau fractures are lateral
- Schatzker classification; generally I-III are low energy, IV-VI high energy

Diagnostic Checklist
- Compartment syndrome of leg must be ruled out
- Open wounds must be identified
- Varus/valgus stress test to knee in full extension to determine laxity which indicates articular depression or ligament injury
- Watch for lipohemarthrosis as a hint of an occult intraarticular fracture
- Watch for sclerotic line within cancellous subchondral bone which indicates an occult depressed fragment
- Evaluate and measure degree of depression with CT; injuries are underestimated with radiographs

---

- Assists in diagnosis of radiographically occult plateau fx
- Confirms anatomic relationship of fx fragments in complex cases
  - Complete description of fracture line extensions: Inferior, vertical, horizontal, medial, & lateral propagation
  - Accurate measurement of size and extent of plateau fragment depression
- Surgical planning for either elevation of depressed fragments or for Schatzker type IV-VI fx

MR Findings
- T1WI
  - Decreased signal intensity fracture line
  - Decreased signal intensity surrounding edema
  - Low signal intensity cortical bone depressed into central cancellous bone
  - High signal fat in lipohemarthrosis
  - May have associated meniscal tear
- T2WI
  - Decreased signal intensity fracture line with surrounding high signal edema
  - Contralateral collateral ligament tear: Thickening, increased signal, or discontinuity
  - Effusion with fluid-fluid level
- T2WI FS: Same as T2WI; fracture line may be obliterated by edema
- PD/Intermediate FS: Evaluate for associated internal derangement (menisci, ligaments, cartilage damage)
- STIR: Same as T2WI; fracture line may be obliterated by edema
- If markedly comminuted fracture, MR is limited for evaluation of relative orientation of osseous fragments
- MR excellent for associated internal derangement

Imaging Recommendations
- Best imaging tool
  - Radiographs performed initially
    - Internal oblique may be added to routine series if plateau fracture is suspected
    - Cross table lateral should be requested to look for lipohemarthrosis
  - CT with reformats detects radiographically occult plateau fractures
  - CT with reformats should be performed in all plateau fractures; radiographs underestimate both degree of depression & grade of fracture
  - Soft tissue injuries often underestimated without MR
- Protocol advice
  - Multidetector CT
    - High mAs (milliamperage-second)
    - Small axial slice thickness (≤ 1 mm) with coronal and sagittal reformats

DIFFERENTIAL DIAGNOSIS

Radiographic
- Floating knee: Ipsilateral distal femoral and proximal tibial fractures
  - Fraser I: Extraarticular fractures both femur and tibia
  - Fraser II: At least one intraarticular component
    - IIA: Femoral shaft fracture, intraarticular tibial fracture
    - IIB: Intraarticular femoral fracture, tibial shaft fracture
    - IIC: Intraarticular femoral and tibial fractures
- Clinical
  - Internal derangement of knee
  - Femoral condylar fracture

PATHOLOGY

General Features
- General path comments
  - Lateral plateau is convex, slightly higher, & smaller than medial
    - Results in asymmetric load distribution at knee, with more stress at medial side
    - Leads to increased strength & inherent protection for medial plateau
  - 75-80% tibial plateau fractures are lateral
    - Medial plateau is stronger than lateral

TIBIAL PLATEAU FRACTURE

- Varus stresses (leading to medial plateau fx) less common than valgus stresses (leading to lateral plateau fx) due to carrying angle of knee and protection by other extremity
  - Lateral plateau fractures have different morphology in young and elderly patients
    - Elderly: Usually low energy, resulting in depressed fragments
    - Young: High energy, resulting in split or wedge fracture pattern
- Etiology
  - Trauma with axial load ± bending force
    - Fall, with twisting or valgus force
    - Motor vehicle accident
    - Auto vs. pedestrian, "bumper" or "fender" fracture (etiology in 25%)
- Epidemiology: Approximately 1% of fractures
- Associated abnormalities
  - Lateral plateau fracture: Valgus force may also result in disruption of
    - Anterior cruciate ligament
    - Medial cruciate ligament
  - Medial plateau fracture: High energy, so also may result in disruption of
    - Lateral plateau
    - Posterior cruciate ligament
    - Posterolateral corner
    - Lateral collateral ligament
    - Popliteal artery (rare)

Staging, Grading or Classification Criteria
- Schatzker classification; generally I-III are low energy, IV-VI high energy
  - Schatzker I: Split fracture with no depression (usually younger patients)
  - Schatzker II: Lateral split/wedge fracture with depression of weight-bearing portion (usually older patients with osteoporosis)
  - Schatzker III: Focal depression of articular surface, no associated split (elderly, osteoporotic patients)
  - Schatzker IV: Medial plateau split, with or without depression; may involve tibial spines; associated soft tissue injuries & poor prognosis
  - Schatzker V: Split fracture of both medial and lateral plateau (bicondylar)
  - Schatzker VI: Bicondylar split fracture with dissociation of metaphysis from diaphysis

CLINICAL ISSUES

Presentation
- Most common signs/symptoms: Knee effusion, pain, inability to bear weight following trauma

Demographics
- Age: Older patients, related to osteoporosis
- Gender
  - Older patients: M < F, related to osteoporosis
  - Younger patients: M > F, related to high-energy sports injuries

Natural History & Prognosis
- Non-depressed fractures may heal with conservative treatment
- If uncorrected, depressed or non-reduced fragments and ligamentous instability result in osteoarthritis

Treatment
- Goal of treatment is anatomic reduction & early mobilization
- Depends on comorbidities; may opt for non-surgical treatment if
  - Diastasis < 3-4 mm
  - Depression < 4-5 mm
- Immediate surgery for
  - Open fracture
  - Neurovascular injury
  - Compartment syndrome
- If severely comminuted, may initially use external fixator & do definitive internal fixation after swelling is reduced

DIAGNOSTIC CHECKLIST

Consider
- Compartment syndrome of leg must be ruled out
- Open wounds must be identified
- Varus/valgus stress test to knee in full extension to determine laxity which indicates articular depression or ligament injury

Image Interpretation Pearls
- Watch for lipohemarthrosis as a hint of an occult intraarticular fracture
- Watch for sclerotic line within cancellous subchondral bone which indicates an occult depressed fragment
- Evaluate and measure degree of depression with CT; injuries are underestimated with radiographs

SELECTED REFERENCES

1. W Mui L et al: Comparison of CT and MRI in patients with tibial plateau fracture: can CT findings predict ligament tear or meniscal injury? Skeletal Radiol. 2006
2. Mustonen AO et al: Acute knee trauma: analysis of multidetector computed tomography findings and comparison with conventional radiography. Acta Radiol. 46(8):866-74, 2005
3. Cameron HU: Tibial plateau fractures. Can J Surg. 47(2):149, 2004
4. Dirschl DR et al: Injury severity assessment in tibial plateau fractures. Clin Orthop Relat Res. (423):85-92, 2004
5. Lawler LP et al: Multi- and single detector CT with 3D volume rendering in tibial plateau fracture imaging and management. Crit Rev Comput Tomogr. 43(4):251-82, 2002
6. Shepherd L et al: The prevalence of soft tissue injuries in nonoperative tibial plateau fractures as determined by magnetic resonance imaging. J Orthop Trauma. 16(9):628-31, 2002
7. Yacoubian SV et al: Impact of MRI on treatment plan and fracture classification of tibial plateau fractures. J Orthop Trauma. 16(9):632-7, 2002

TIBIAL PLATEAU FRACTURE

IMAGE GALLERY

Typical

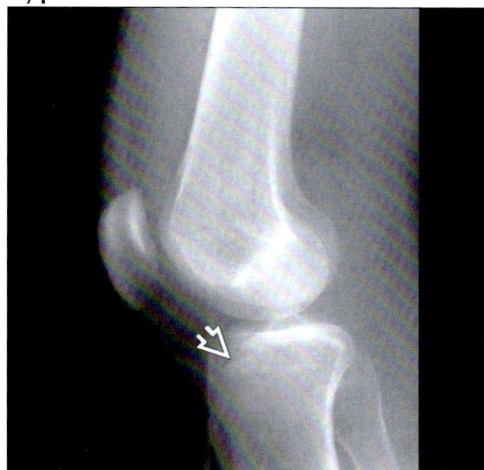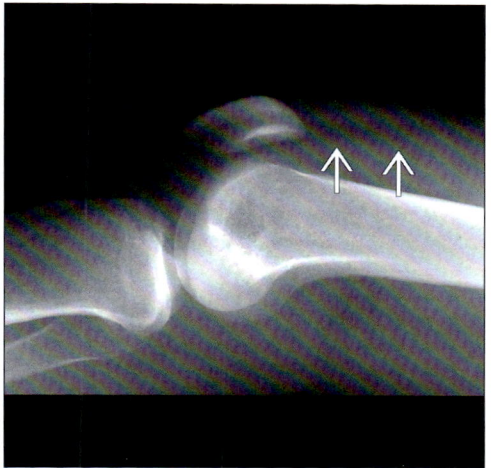

(Left) Lateral radiograph shows how subtle these lateral tibial plateau fractures may be. The impacted plateau fracture ➔ is seen as a linear sclerosis, impacted into the plateau. This is the only osseous finding; no fracture line is seen. *(Right)* Lateral radiograph is exactly the same image as previous, but displayed as a cross-table lateral, the way it was filmed. In this position, it is easier to see the fat-blood level ➔ which indicates there must be an intraarticular fracture.

Typical

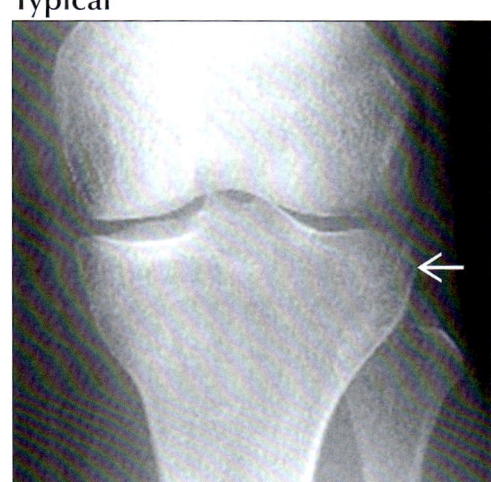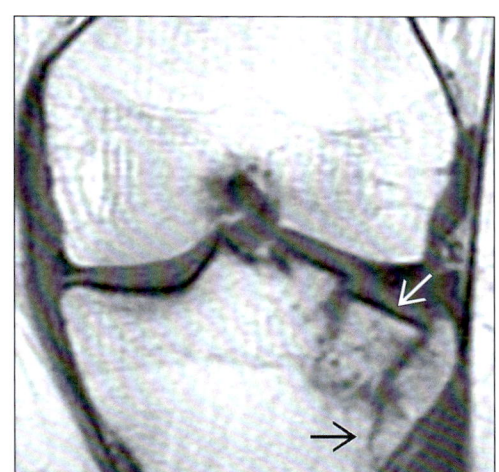

(Left) Anteroposterior radiograph shows no definite fracture line. There is some cortical indistinctness laterally ➔ and a hint of adjacent trabecular disruption. *(Right)* Coronal T1WI MR shows a split lateral plateau fracture ➔ with a depressed fragment ➔ (Schatzker type II) in this older osteoporotic patient. The diagnostic advantage of MR is clear.

Typical

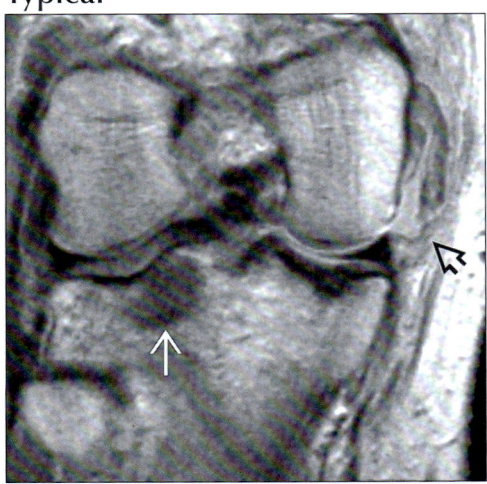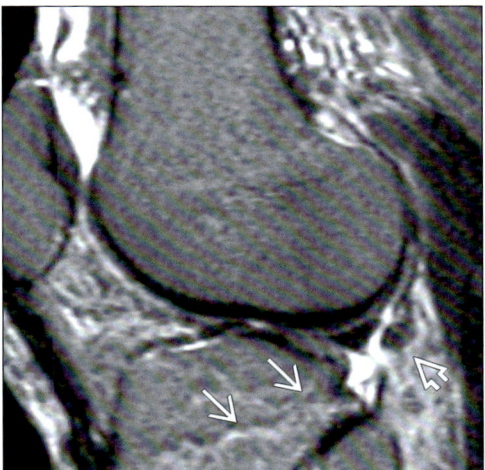

(Left) Coronal PD/Intermediate MR shows a depressed fracture fragment in the posterior portion of the lateral plateau ➔. There is an associated medial collateral ligament rupture ➔ with retraction. *(Right)* Sagittal T2WI MR shows the lateral plateau fracture propagating anteriorly ➔, as well as rupture and retraction of the popliteus tendon ➔ and adjacent arcuate and popliteofibular ligaments.

ANKLE FRACTURES

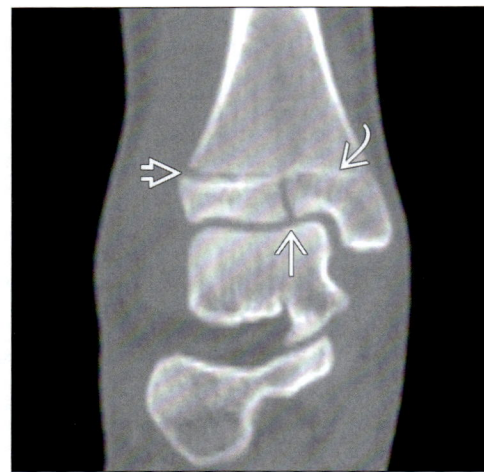

Coronal bone CT shows a classic juvenile Tillaux fx (Salter-Harris III). Note the epiphyseal fx line ➡ which extends into a widened physeal fx ➡. The medial physis is fused ➡, providing it protection from fx.

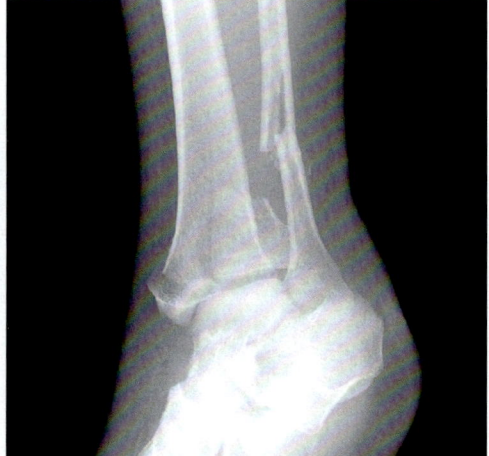

Oblique radiograph shows a comminuted, intraarticular distal tibial fracture; a Reudi III pilon fracture. There is a comminuted fibular fracture as well.

TERMINOLOGY

Abbreviations and Synonyms
- Open reduction internal fixation (ORIF)

IMAGING FINDINGS

General Features
- Best diagnostic clue: Visible fracture line
- Associated findings
  o Ankle joint effusion
    - Best seen anterior to the tibiotalar joint on the lateral view
    - Appears as a tongue-shaped soft tissue density that is convex superiorly
    - Presence of an ankle joint effusion requires a careful search for a fracture
  o Medial clear space
    - Measurement of medial mortise from medial aspect of talus to lateral aspect of medial malleolus
    - Should be uniform in width and < 4 mm
  o Lateral clear space (tibiofibular clear space)
    - Measured 1 cm proximal to the tibial plafond
    - Measured from the medial edge of the fibula to the lateral edge of the **posterior** tibia
    - Measurements of the lateral clear space in excess of 5 mm on either the AP or mortise view suggests some disruption of the syndesmosis
  o Lateral ankle soft tissue swelling should prompt an evaluation of the base of the 5th metatarsal for possible fracture

Imaging Recommendations
- Best imaging tool
  o Lateral and mortise view radiographs at a minimum
    - Mortise view is an AP oblique taken in 15-20° internal rotation
  o Most institutions also add an AP view
  o At least one view of the ankle radiograph series should include the base of the 5th metatarsal
- Stress views
  o May be useful to evaluate for stability
  o Medial talar tilt > 15° with applied varus stress suggests lateral collateral ligament disruption (normal medial tilt is 10-12°)

Additional Ankle Fracture Images

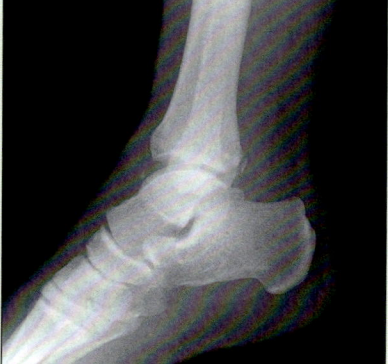

Posterior Malleolar Fracture

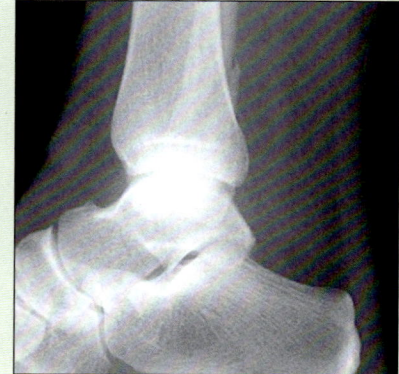

"Posterior Spike"

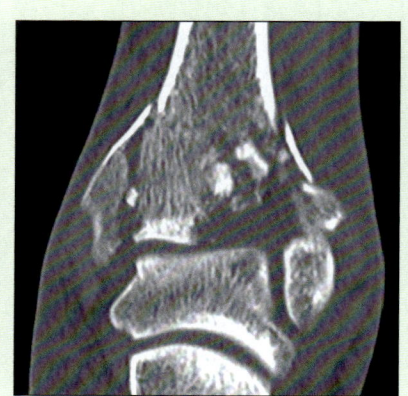

CT: Pilon Fx, Reudi Stage III

ANKLE FRACTURES

Key Facts

Imaging Findings
- Presence of an ankle joint effusion requires a careful search for a fracture
- Lateral ankle soft tissue swelling should prompt an evaluation of the base of the 5th metatarsal for possible fracture
- At least one view of the ankle radiograph series should include the base of the 5th metatarsal

Pathology
- With the Lauge-Hansen classification system, the characteristics of the fibular fracture (if present) are the easiest way to categorize the overall fracture pattern, as the fibular fractures are relatively unique for each category

- If radiographs demonstrate a medial injury (medial malleolar fracture or medial mortise widening), a posterior malleolar fracture, or lateral clear space widening, either alone or in combination, and no fibular fx is identified on the ankle films, the entire fibula must be examined for a fracture

Clinical Issues
- Ottawa rules are used to determine the need for radiographic evaluation
- Ankle fracture is considered unstable if any two of the three limbs of the ankle triangle are disrupted
- In the medial and lateral limbs of the ankle triangle, if either the bony OR ligamentous component is disrupted, the limb is considered disrupted

---

  - Anteriorly directed force applied to the posterior calcaneus may cause the talus to sublux anteriorly (anterior drawer)
    - An anterior drawer > 1 cm suggests anterior tibiofibular ligament disruption
- CT can be used for better characterization of some complex, comminuted fractures (e.g., pilon and triplane fractures)
- MR has little role in acute management of ankle fractures, but can be a useful adjunct for evaluation in the setting of continued pain despite normal radiographs

PATHOLOGY

General Features
- Epidemiology
  - Incidence of ankle fractures is increasing
  - Of all ankle injuries evaluated in the ER, only approximately 15% will have fractures

Staging, Grading or Classification Criteria
- **Lauge-Hansen classification of ankle fractures**
  - Classifies ankle fractures based on mechanism of injury
  - Useful to direct reduction as reduction forces should be opposite mechanism forces
  - Useful to direct radiographic evaluation as injuries occur in a predictable sequence
    - Although the injury sequence may arrest at any stage within a category, stages cannot be skipped
  - With the Lauge-Hansen classification system, the characteristics of the fibular fracture (if present) are the easiest way to categorize the overall fracture pattern, as the fibular fractures are relatively unique for each category
    - Stage can then be looked up if not memorized
    - On the AP radiograph, the two fibular fractures most difficult to distinguish from one another are those of the SER and PA injury patterns
    - On the lateral, SER fractures usually demonstrate a "**posterior spike**" whereas PA fractures are usually very difficult or impossible to see
  - **Supination Adduction (SA)**
    - **Stage I (stable):** Transverse fracture of lateral malleolus below tibial plafond (Weber A) OR lateral collateral ligament disruption (may be radiographically occult but can see lateral mortise widening)
    - **Stage II (unstable):** Oblique fracture of medial malleolus
  - **Supination external rotation (SER)**
    - **Stage I (stable):** Disruption of the anterior tibiofibular ligament (usually radiographically occult)
    - **Stage II (stable):** Fracture of the fibula at the level of the tibial plafond (Weber B), usually oblique running from anterior to posterior & best seen on the lateral, but may be spiral
    - **Stage III (variably stable):** Disruption of the posterior tibiofibular ligament (usually radiographically occult) OR posterior malleolar fx
    - **Stage IV (unstable):** Transverse fx of medial malleolus OR deltoid ligament disruption (may be radiographically occult but can see medial mortise widening)
  - **Pronation external rotation (PER)**
    - **Stage I (stable):** Transverse fx of medial malleolus OR deltoid ligament disruption (may be radiographically occult but can see medial mortise widening)
    - **Stage II (stable):** Disruption of the anterior tibiofibular ligament (usually radiographically occult) with extension into the interosseus ligament
    - **Stage III (unstable):** Spiral fx of the fibula above (typically six or more cm) the tibial plafond (Weber C)
    - **Stage IV (unstable):** Disruption of the posterior tibiofibular ligament (usually radiographically occult) OR posterior malleolar fracture
  - **Pronation abduction (PA)**

ANKLE FRACTURES

- **Stage I (stable):** Transverse fx of medial malleolus OR deltoid ligament disruption (may be radiographically occult but can see medial mortise widening)
- **Stage II (stable):** Combination of any of the following: Disruption of anterior and/or posterior tibiofibular ligaments (usually radiographically occult) OR posterior malleolar fx
- **Stage III (unstable):** Oblique fracture (from medial to lateral) of the distal fibula just above the tibial plafond (Weber C); best seen on AP radiograph
- **Danis-Weber classification of ankle fractures**
  - Classification is based on the relationship of the medial aspect of the fibular fx to the tibial plafond (roof)
  - Some consider this classification an oversimplification as it fails to take into account medial and syndesmotic involvement
    - Modification of this classification, known as the AO-Weber classification, subdivides the classes based on these additional injuries
    - Deficiencies of the Weber classification system can be overcome by either using the Lauge-Hansen classification system, or by simply describing additional injuries
  - **Class A:** Fibular fx line distal to the tibial plafond
    - Equivalent to Lauge-Hansen SA injury
    - Medial malleolar fracture is equivalent to an SA stage III injury, and is unstable
  - **Class B:** Fibular fx line at the level of the tibial plafond
    - Equivalent to Lauge-Hansen SER injury
    - Medial involvement (medial mortise widening or medial malleolar fx) suggests an SER stage IV injury, and therefore, instability
    - Medial involvement may be present without radiographic abnormality; if there is moderate-to-severe point tenderness over the deltoid ligament, medial involvement should be suspected
  - **Class C:** Fibular fx line above the level of the plafond
    - Equivalent to Lauge-Hansen PER stage III or IV injury or PA stage III injury
- **Maisonneuve fracture**
  - Although an oversimplification, can be considered any fibular fracture proximal enough to not be included on ankle films & which can be predicted based on radiographic ankle injury pattern
  - If radiographs demonstrate a medial injury (medial malleolar fracture or medial mortise widening), a posterior malleolar fracture, or lateral clear space widening, either alone or in combination, and no fibular fx is identified on the ankle films, the entire fibula must be examined for a fracture
  - Is an unstable fracture
- **Pilon fracture**
  - Comminuted fracture of the distal tibia with intraarticular extension into the plafond
  - **Reudi-Allgower classification**
  - **Type I:** Nondisplaced, T-shaped fracture in which inferior aspect of the "T" extends to the plafond
  - **Type II:** Same as type I, but with displacement of the intraarticular component
  - **Type III:** Multifragmented intraarticular extension
- **Tillaux fracture**
  - Salter-Harris III fracture of the **lateral** distal tibia
  - Unique to early adolescents, generally 12-14 years
  - Distal tibial physis fuses medial to lateral, leaving the lateral physis relatively weak and more prone to fracture in this age group

CLINICAL ISSUES

Presentation
- Most common signs/symptoms: Pain, swelling, inability to bear weight, and ± ecchymosis
- Ottawa ankle rules
  - Ottawa rules are used to determine the need for radiographic evaluation
  - Radiographs are warranted if there is pain in the malleolar zone **AND** at least one of the following
    - Bone pain to palpation along the posterior distal 6 cm of the fibula
    - Bone pain to palpation along the posterior distal 6 cm of the tibia
    - Inability to bear weight for 4 steps at the time of injury as well as in the ER
  - Malleolar zone extends from approximately 6 cm above the malleoli to approximately the margins of the talus

Treatment
- Although not absolute, if any of the following is present, the fracture will generally require ORIF
  - Open (compound) fracture
  - Comminuted intraarticular fracture
  - Intraarticular fracture with stepoff or diastasis > 2 mm
  - Stable fracture in which adequate closed reduction is not achieved
  - Unstable fracture
- Ankle "triangle" principle of stability
  - Ankle fracture is considered unstable if any two of the three limbs of the ankle triangle are disrupted
  - Ankle "triangle" is comprised of medial and lateral limbs and the syndesmosis
    - Medial limb is comprised of the medial malleolus & medial collateral ligament
    - Lateral limb is comprised of the lateral malleolus & lateral collateral ligament
  - In the medial and lateral limbs of the ankle triangle, if either the bony **OR** ligamentous component is disrupted, the limb is considered disrupted

SELECTED REFERENCES

1. Chen SH et al: Long-term results of pilon fractures. Arch Orthop Trauma Surg. 127(1):55-60, 2007
2. Thomsen NO et al: Observer variation in the radiographic classification of ankle fractures. J Bone Joint Surg Br. 73(4):676-8, 1991
3. Arimoto HK et al: Classification of ankle fractures: an algorithm. AJR Am J Roentgenol. 135(5):1057-63, 1980

ANKLE FRACTURES

IMAGE GALLERY

Typical

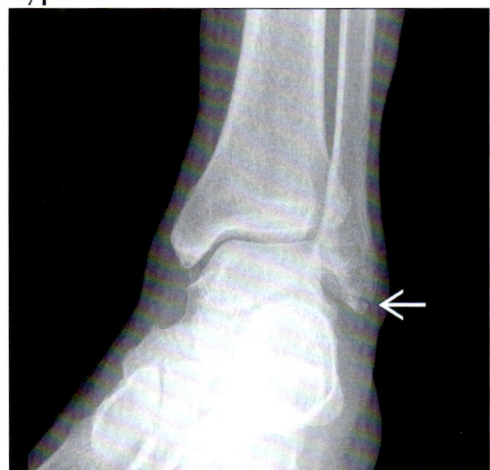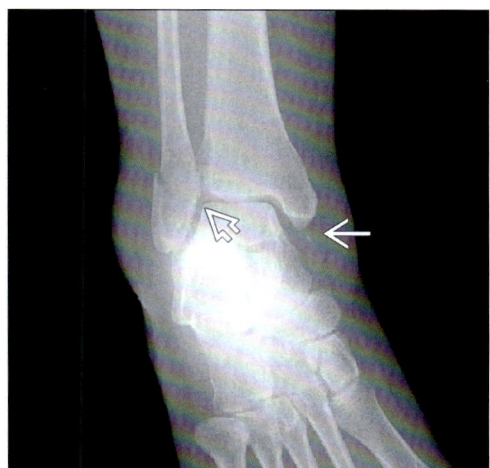

(Left) Oblique radiograph shows a Weber A/Lauge-Hansen SA stage I fracture of the distal fibula (below the plafond) ➡. *(Right)* Anteroposterior radiograph shows an oblique fibular fracture ➡ at the level of the plafond, a Weber B/Lauge-Hansen SER injury. Medial involvement ➡ makes this stage IV.

Typical

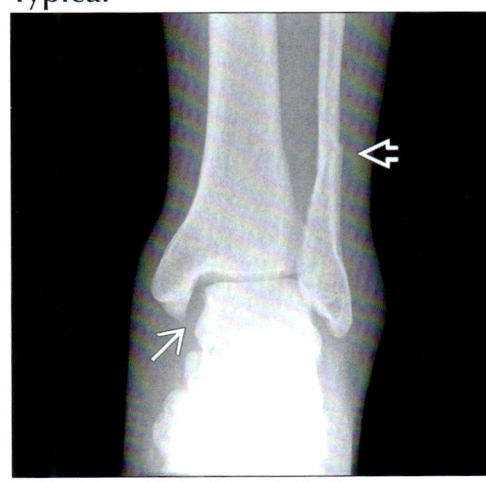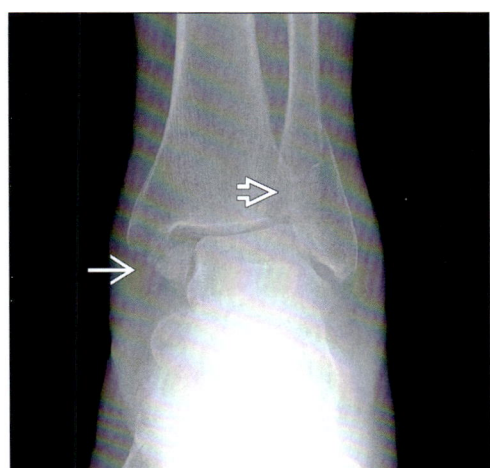

(Left) Anteroposterior radiograph shows a proximal fibular spiral fx ➡; Weber C/Lauge-Hansen PER injury. Medial involvement (mortise widening) ➡ is stage I. Fibular fx is stage III. *(Right)* Anteroposterior radiograph shows an oblique fibular fracture just above the plafond ➡; Weber C/Lauge-Hansen PA injury. Medial involvement ➡ is stage I. Fibular fracture is stage III.

Typical

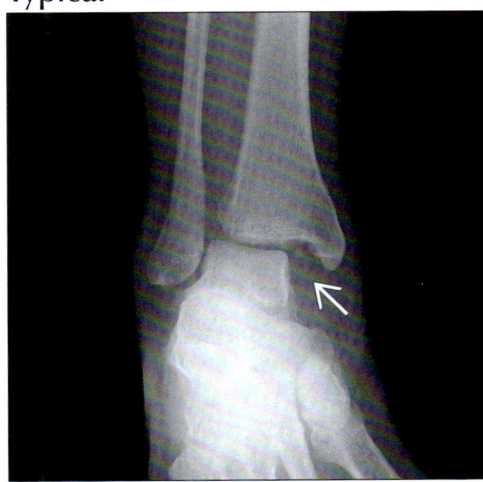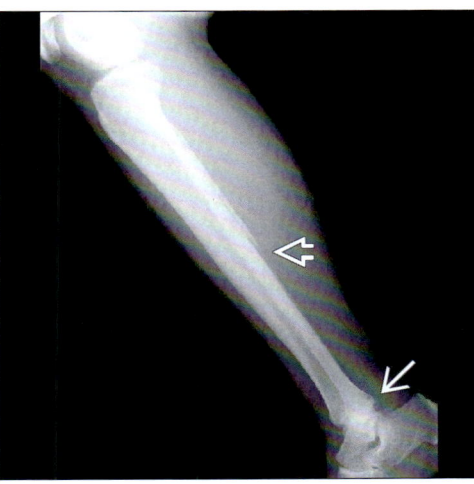

(Left) Anteroposterior radiograph shows medial mortise widening ➡ consistent with deltoid ligament disruption. No fibular fracture is seen, so the entire fibula must be examined for fracture. *(Right)* Lateral radiograph in same patient as previous image shows a more proximal fibular fracture ➡ making this a Maisonneuve fracture. Posterior malleolar fracture ➡ is also present.

ACHILLES TENDON TEAR & TENDINOPATHY

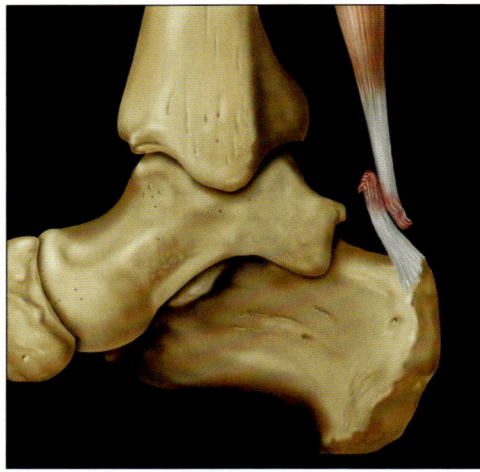

Lateral graphic shows complete Achilles tendon rupture with overlapping of proximal & distal tendon segments. Following rupture, segments may overlap but are more frequently distracted, which may dictate type of surgery.

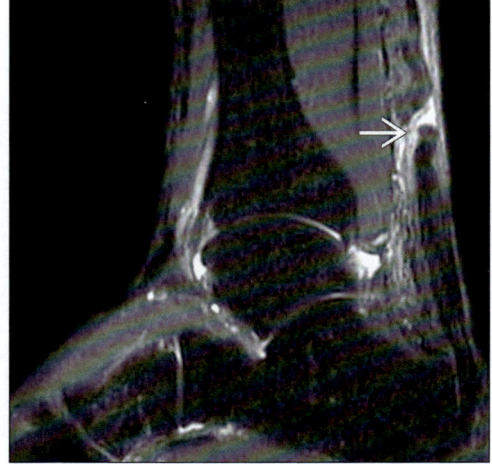

Sagittal STIR MR shows complete disruption of the Achilles tendon ➔ at the musculotendinous junction. The hyperintense edema in the gap between proximal & distal fibers allows estimation of the extent of diastasis.

TERMINOLOGY

Abbreviations and Synonyms
- Achilles tendon rupture
- Achilles tendinosis (preferable term to tendinitis), paratendinitis, peritendinitis

Definitions
- A spectrum of abnormalities, ranging from early degeneration to complete rupture
- Achilles tendinosis (tendinitis) subdivided into non-insertional & insertional

IMAGING FINDINGS

General Features
- Best diagnostic clue: Abnormal signal within Achilles tendon, or complete/incomplete disruption
- Location
  - Generally the vascular "watershed" area, 2-6 cm proximal to insertion (non-insertional type)
  - Insertional type: Site of insertion on posterior calcaneus

Radiographic Findings
- Achilles not visualized directly by radiograph, but is outlined anteriorly by Kager fat pad
- Complete tear of Achilles with retraction may result in posterior concavity which may be diagnosed on lateral view
- Thickening of Achilles may be noted in tendinopathy

MR Findings
- T1WI: General
  - Normal: Low signal; may contain higher signal punctate areas outlining fascicles
  - May show slightly higher signal as magic angle effect
  - Axial sequence used to evaluate cross-sectional shape of Achilles: Should be concave anteriorly
  - Evaluate abnormal signal in peritendinous fat pad
- Fluid sensitive sequences
  - Normal: Low signal, may contain higher signal punctate areas (interfascicular membranes)
  - No magic angle effect
- Across spectrum of Achilles disorders, ↑ in cross-sectional diameter of tendon is seen

DDx: Achilles Tendon Tear/Tendinopathy

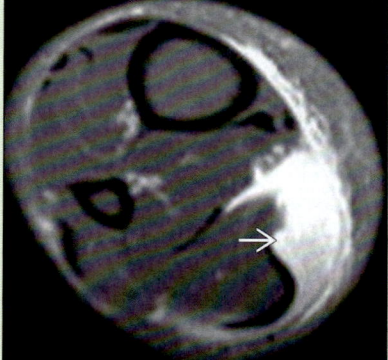

Rupture Medial Head Gastroc.

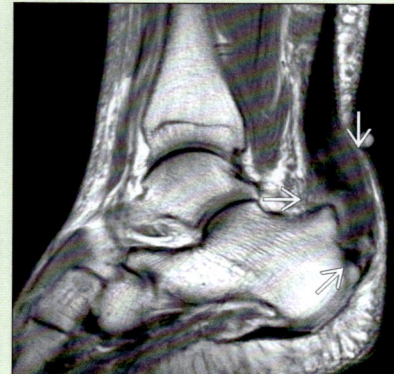

Haglund Syndrome

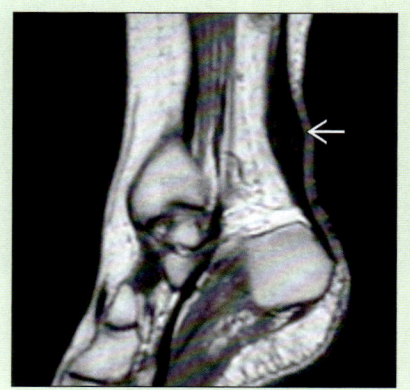

Xanthofibroma

ACHILLES TENDON TEAR & TENDINOPATHY

Key Facts

Imaging Findings
- Across spectrum of Achilles disorders, ↑ in cross-sectional diameter of tendon is seen
- Paratenonitis: First symptomatic stage of degenerative Achilles disorders
- Fibromatous (hypoxic) degeneration: Tendon thickening, usually without internal signal on MR
- Achilles tendon tears range in spectrum from interstitial tears, to partial tear, to complete tear
- Interstitial tears: High signal parallel to long axis of tendon, with intact surrounding fibers
- Partial tears: Heterogeneous high signal & tendon thickening without complete interruption
- Complete tear: Fibers may overlap or may be distracted; hyperintense fluid between torn fibers
- US can distinguish complete from partial tears with 92% accuracy

Pathology
- Blood supply is diminished 2-6 cm proximal to calcaneal insertion (watershed area): Proximal & distal tears uncommon
- Anterior margin concave below soleus insertion
- Tears: Indirect trauma; significant association with leisure activities
- Most commonly injured ankle tendon; 3rd most frequent tendon rupture overall

Clinical Issues
- 20-25% complete tears are missed clinically due to swelling obscuring the tendon gap and retention of weak plantarflexion

---

- Paratenonitis: First symptomatic stage of degenerative Achilles disorders
  - Partially circumferential high signal around Achilles on fluid sensitive sequence
  - Fat-suppression fluid sensitive sequences generally needed to visualize this
  - Kager fat pad may be irregular
  - Tendon itself is normal
- Fibromatous (hypoxic) degeneration: Tendon thickening, usually without internal signal on MR
- Mucoid (myxoid) degeneration: Beginning of interstitial tear
  - Tendon thickening
  - Linear area of increased signal on T1 or PD: More prominent than on T2
  - Fluid sensitive sequences: Areas of increased signal are interrupted & irregular; may not be as prominently seen as on PD unless fat-suppressed T2 or STIR
- Achilles tendon tears range in spectrum from interstitial tears, to partial tear, to complete tear
  - Tears more prominent on fluid-sensitive sequences than T1 or PD
  - Interstitial tears: High signal parallel to long axis of tendon, with intact surrounding fibers
  - Partial tears: Heterogeneous high signal & tendon thickening without complete interruption
  - Complete tear: Fibers may overlap or may be distracted; hyperintense fluid between torn fibers
- Insertional tendonitis: Likely the only "true" tendinitis
  - Edema at Achilles insertion, development of enthesophyte
  - Achilles thickened distally, ill-defined longitudinal high signal at insertion site (may mimic partial tear)

Ultrasonographic Findings
- US can distinguish complete from partial tears with 92% accuracy
  - Signs of complete tear
    - Undetectable tendon
    - Tendon retraction
    - Posterior acoustic shadowing

Imaging Recommendations
- Best imaging tool: MR for superior soft tissue contrast
- Protocol advice
  - Requires both T1 (or PD) and fluid sensitive (preferably fat suppressed) sequences
  - Requires both sagittal & axial planes

DIFFERENTIAL DIAGNOSIS

Xanthofibromatosis
- Lipidosis seen in inherited metabolic diseases
  - Type 2 & 3 hyperproteinemia and cerebrotendinous xanthomatosis
- Focal thickening of Achilles (may also occur in other tendons, usually dorsal)
- Low signal on all sequences

Tear Medial Head Gastrocnemius or Plantaris
- In differential for "tennis leg"

Haglund Disease
- Retro-Achilles bursa compressed against posterior lateral calcaneal prominence
- Calcaneal tuberosity focally enlarged
- Fluid in retrocalcaneal bursa & retro-Achilles bursa

PATHOLOGY

General Features
- General path comments
  - Relevant anatomy
    - Achilles is enclosed within a paratenon; does not require the lubrication of a tendon sheath since it does not change its axis of motion
    - Paratenon is analogous to synovium: Provides nutrition for tendon
    - Blood supply is diminished 2-6 cm proximal to calcaneal insertion (watershed area): Proximal & distal tears uncommon

ACHILLES TENDON TEAR & TENDINOPATHY

- Retrocalcaneal bursa: True synovial bursa; horseshoe-shaped, surrounded anteriorly by Kager fat pad; protects distal Achilles from frictional wear against posterior calcaneus
- Retro-Achilles bursa: Acquired posterior to calcaneal enthesis
- Average thickness is 6 mm
- Anterior margin straight or convex just above soleus insertion into Achilles
- Anterior margin concave below soleus insertion
- Etiology
  - Tears: Indirect trauma; significant association with leisure activities
    - Running sports, especially with pivot motion (basketball, tennis)
    - Jogging, soccer
    - Intermittent stress on ischemic region
  - Overtraining: Eccentric loading of a fatigued muscle-tendon unit
  - Hyperpronation/forefoot varus/cavus foot/equinus deformities
  - Direct trauma
  - Systemic arthropathy: Rheumatoid, spondyloarthropathies
  - Fibromatous (hypoxic) degeneration occurs after multiple symptomatic episodes
  - Mucoid degeneration: Mucoid patches & vacuoles between thinned degenerated tendon fibers
    - Coalescence of these areas is beginning of interstitial tear
  - Insertional tendinitis: Common in runners (may be only true form of acute Achilles tendinitis)
- Epidemiology
  - 7 cases per 100,000
  - Most commonly injured ankle tendon; 3rd most frequent tendon rupture overall
  - Non-insertional tendinopathy in 6-18% of runners

Gross Pathologic & Surgical Features

- Intratendinous degeneration without a significant inflammatory response
  - No true synovial sheath, so no true inflammatory process within tendon
  - Term "tendinosis" preferred to "tendinitis"
- Tendon is nodular & yellow, with edema & fibrillation
- Because of intimate association of distal Achilles & retrocalcaneal bursa, Achilles may be secondarily affected by inflammatory process originating in bursa
- Achilles paratenon may be affected by systemic inflammatory diseases such as rheumatoid arthritis

Staging, Grading or Classification Criteria

- Weinstabi classification
  - Type I: Inflammatory reaction
  - Type II: Degenerative changes
  - Type III: Partial tear
  - Type IV: Complete tear

CLINICAL ISSUES

Presentation

- Most common signs/symptoms
  - Pain, soft tissue swelling, hyperdorsiflexion
  - Occasional palpable tendon defect
  - Clinical signs are not straightforward to allow differentiation along spectrum of disease
    - Mucoid degeneration can mimic a tear
    - Silent Achilles disorders often have microscopic tears
    - 20-25% complete tears are missed clinically due to swelling obscuring the tendon gap and retention of weak plantarflexion

Demographics

- Age
  - Mean age of 36; rare in adolescents
  - Insertional tendinitis tends to occur in older, less active individuals
- Gender: M > F, 5-6:1 for complete rupture secondary to indirect trauma

Natural History & Prognosis

- Chronic tendinopathy
  - 90% symptomatic
  - May be precursor to partial or complete tendon tear
- Tear
  - Non-surgical rate of rerupture: 21%
  - Surgical rate of rerupture: 1.7%

Treatment

- Tendinosis
  - May be treated conservatively: Rest, stretching exercises, orthoses, antiinflammatory medications
  - Some are treated as interstitial tear: Debridement of degenerative center & oversewing of preserved peripheral fibers
- Partial tears: Often surgically repaired
  - Cast immobilization: Above knee with equinus
- Complete tears: Usually surgically repaired
  - May immobilize with cast acutely or if related to use of steroids
  - Partial tear or complete tear with < 3cm diastasis: end-to-end anastomosis
  - > 3 cm diastasis often requires tendon graft
  - Intratendinous fluid seen up to 6 months post-op

DIAGNOSTIC CHECKLIST

Consider

- Evaluate paratenon for inflammatory change
- Identify proximal & distal ends on sagittal images
- Use axial images to identify contour abnormalities
- Use axial images to confirm complete rupture & to differentiate intact plantaris from intact Achilles fiber

SELECTED REFERENCES

1. Dobson MH et al: Treatment of acute Achilles tendon ruptures. A meta-analysis of randomized, controlled trials. J Bone Joint Surg Am. 88(5):1160; author reply 1160, 2006
2. Hartgerink P et al: Full- versus partial-thickness Achilles tendon tears: sonographic accuracy and characterization in 26 cases with surgical correlation. Radiology 220:406-12, 2001
3. Schweitzer ME et al: MR imaging of disorders of the Achilles tendon. AJR. 175:613-25, 2000

ACHILLES TENDON TEAR & TENDINOPATHY

IMAGE GALLERY

Typical

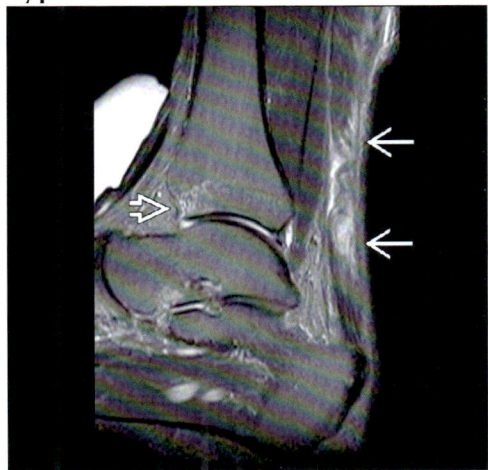
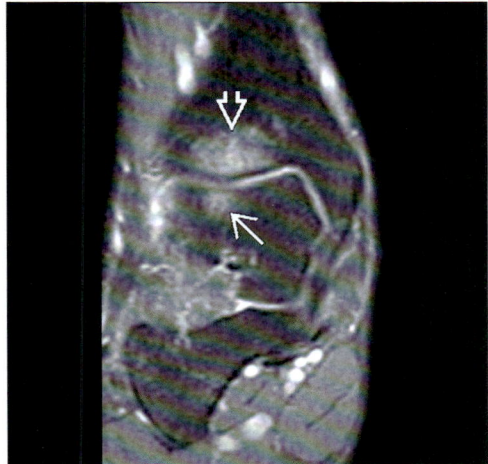

(Left) Sagittal T2WI FS MR shows complete Achilles rupture with significant diastasis of fibers ➡. There is an anterior tibial bone bruise ➡. (Right) Coronal T2WI FS MR located far anteriorly confirms "kissing" bone bruises in the anterior tibia ➡ & talus ➡. This indicates hyper-dorsiflexion as the mechanism of injury in this Rugby player.

Typical

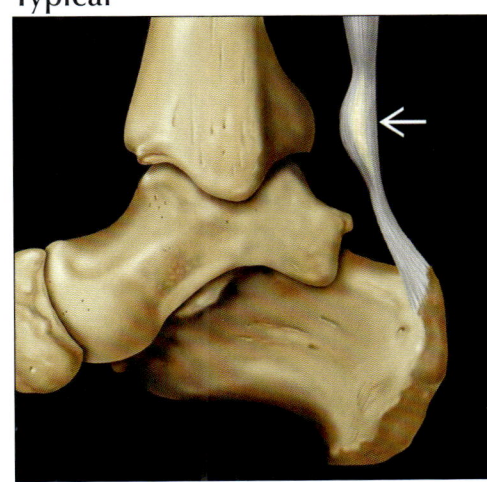
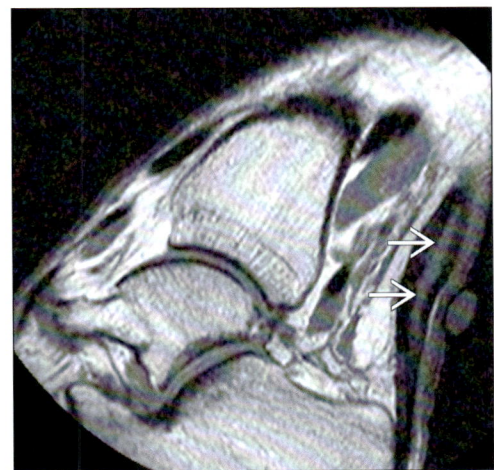

(Left) Lateral graphic shows non-insertional Achilles tendinosis with anterior tendon rounding at the musculotendinous junction. Mucoid degeneration is depicted in yellow ➡. (Right) Sagittal PD/Intermediate MR shows high signal longitudinally within the tendon ➡. The fibers are intact around it. The signal was not as prominent on T2 and indicates tendinopathy.

Typical

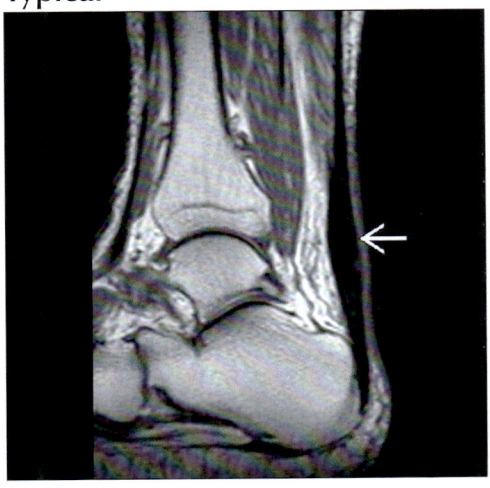
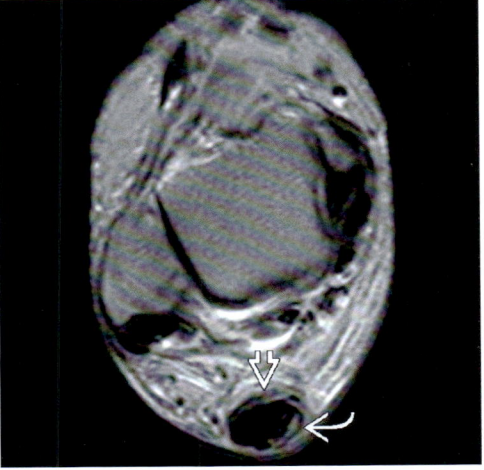

(Left) Sagittal PD MR shows enlargement & very subtle signal within the Achilles tendon ➡ approximately 4 cm proximal to the calcaneal insertion site, in the hypovascular (watershed) region of the tendon. (Right) Axial T2WI MR shows rounding of the normally concave anterior Achilles ➡. Additionally, there is high signal within the enlarged tendon ➡. With the signal appearing more prominent on T2 than the PD sequence, this represents a small partial tear.

CALCANEAL FRACTURES

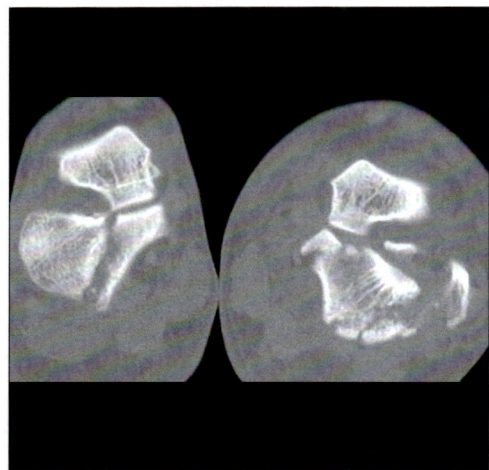

Axial bone CT shows bilateral intraarticular calcaneal fractures in a patient who sustained a fall from a height of 15 feet. The right side is classified as a Sanders IIC and the left a Sanders IV (both are Rowe type V).

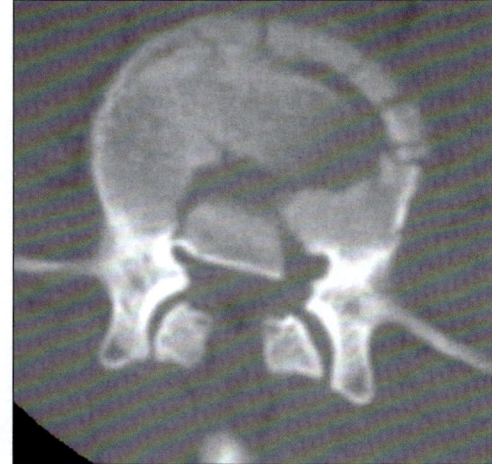

Axial NECT shows a burst fracture at L1, with severe cord compression. Severe fractures of the calcaneus should stimulate imaging of the lumbar spine, since this is a highly associated injury.

TERMINOLOGY

Abbreviations and Synonyms
- Don Juan fracture, lover's fracture

Definitions
- Fracture of the calcaneus; may be intraarticular, extraarticular, stress, insufficiency, or avulsion

IMAGING FINDINGS

General Features
- Best diagnostic clue: Fracture line, ± Boehler's angle flattening
- Location
  - Traumatic: Posterior tuberosity, ± involvement posterior facet
  - Avulsion: Anterosuperior, anterolateral, posteromedial, posterior tuberosity
  - Stress: Posterior tuberosity
- Size: Ranges from small avulsion to severe comminution
- Morphology
  - Traumatic extraarticular: Anterior process, posterior process, sustentaculum tali
  - Anterior process avulsion
    - Anterior superior aspect of anterior calcaneus
    - Origin of bifurcate ligament
  - Anterolateral avulsion
    - Located slightly lateral to anterior process, anterolaterally on anterior calcaneus
    - Origin of extensor digitorum brevis
  - Medial process avulsion
    - Medial plantar aspect of posterior calcaneus
    - Origin of abductor hallucis, flexor digitorum, & plantar fascia
  - Stress fracture calcaneus
    - Posterior 1/3 calcaneus
    - Incomplete linear sclerosis orthogonal to major trabeculae
  - Calcaneal insufficiency avulsion (CIA fracture): Posterior tuberosity avulsion
  - **Intraarticular calcaneal fx:**
    - Two fracture lines contribute, which can result in 2 different fx patterns
    - Primary fx line is a shear fx in the sagittal plane

Other Calcaneal Fractures

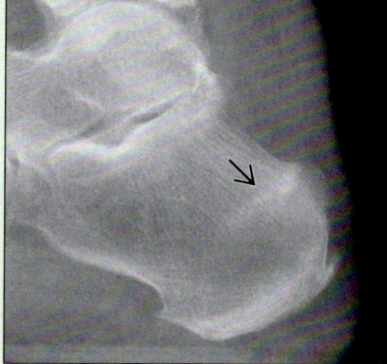

Stress Fracture

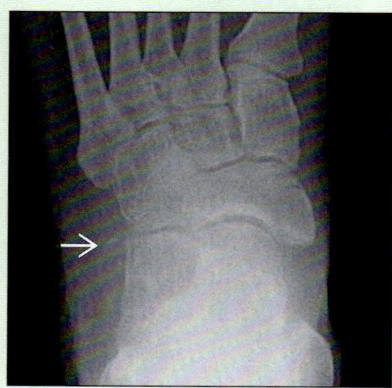

Extensor Digitorum Brevis Avulsion

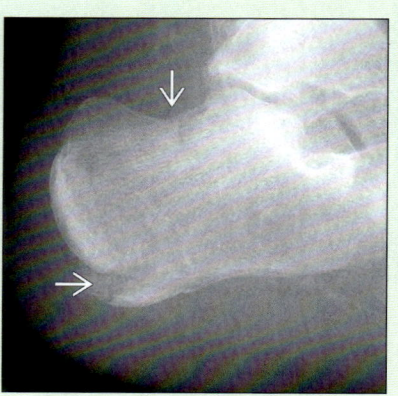

Calcaneal Insufficiency Avulsion

CALCANEAL FRACTURES

Key Facts

Imaging Findings
- Avulsion: Anterosuperior, anterolateral, posteromedial, posterior tuberosity
- Stress: Posterior tuberosity
- Calcaneal insufficiency avulsion (CIA fracture): Posterior tuberosity avulsion
- **Intraarticular calcaneal fx:**
- Two fracture lines contribute, which can result in 2 different fx patterns
- Primary fx line divides calcaneus into anteromedial (generally nondisplaced) & posterolateral (generally displaced) fragments
- Secondary fx line begins at angle of Gissane (deep angle seen on lateral between posterior & anterior facets) & extends posteriorly
- Tongue type: Occurs when the secondary fx line extends directly posteriorly producing a large superior, posterior, and lateral fragment with the rest of the body forming the inferior fragment
- Depressed type (more frequent): Secondary fx line begins at crucial angle & extends posteriorly but deviates dorsally to exit just posterior to posterior articular facet (fragment contains most of posterior facet)

Diagnostic Checklist
- Associated injuries may exist (i.e., in thoracolumbar spine, pelvis, opposite calcaneus)
- Radiography often underestimates degree of displacement & depression of posterolateral fx fragment
- CT required for full evaluation of intraarticular fx

- Primary fx line runs from plantar aspect obliquely upwards into the posterior facet
- Primary fx line divides calcaneus into anteromedial (generally nondisplaced) & posterolateral (generally displaced) fragments
- Secondary fx line is a compression fx in the coronal plane
- Secondary fx line begins at angle of Gissane (deep angle seen on lateral between posterior & anterior facets) & extends posteriorly
- Tongue type: Occurs when the secondary fx line extends directly posteriorly producing a large superior, posterior, and lateral fragment with the rest of the body forming the inferior fragment
- Depressed type (more frequent): Secondary fx line begins at crucial angle & extends posteriorly but deviates dorsally to exit just posterior to posterior articular facet (fragment contains most of posterior facet)

Radiographic Findings
- Lateral and axial (Harris Beath) views
- 87% sensitivity for calcaneal fx
- Anterior process avulsion (bifurcate ligament)
  - Seen on oblique or lateral
  - Sensitivity by radiography is poor
- Anterolateral avulsion (extensor digitorum brevis)
  - Tiny fragment seen 2 cm distal to lateral malleolus on AP ankle radiograph
  - May be seen lateral to the anterior calcaneus on AP foot radiograph
- Medial process avulsion: Seen on axial view; fx is posteromedial
- Stress fx: Sclerotic line in posterior calcaneus
  - Perpendicular to major trabeculae, best seen on lateral radiograph
- Calcaneal insufficiency avulsion: Posterior 1/3 of calcaneus, usually displaced 10-30 mm & partially rotated
- Intraarticular fx
  - Axial shows widening of calcaneus, with fx extension into posterior facet
  - Lateral shows fx line posterior tuberosity, with decreased Boehler's angle (normal 28-48°)
    - Boehler's angle: Intersection of two lines (one connects the superior margin of the anterior process & posterior margin of the posterior articular facet; other extends from that point to posterosuperior calcaneal tuberosity)
  - Severity of intraarticular fx usually underestimated by radiograph

CT Findings
- Multidetector CT with reformats reveals extent of fx & position of dislocated posterior calcaneal facet far better than radiography
- Axial plane may demonstrate entrapped tendons (particularly peroneals)
- Evaluate
  - Degree of involvement of posterior facet
    - Number of fragments/fracture lines entering facet
    - Diastasis & angulation of posterolateral fragment
    - Degree of depression of posterolateral fragment
    - Extension of fracture lines & degree of comminution

MR Findings
- Particularly useful to evaluate subtle avulsions, such as anterior process
- T1WI: Low signal fx lines and edema
- Fluid sensitive sequences: High signal edema
- Evaluates adjacent soft tissues (tendons, ligaments)

Imaging Recommendations
- Best imaging tool
  - First imaging is usually radiographs
  - Any intraarticular fx requires CT with reformats for complete evaluation
  - In high-energy trauma with high suspicion of calcaneal fx, may immediately CT
- Protocol advice: For Sanders classification: CT with < 1 mm slices; reformat parallel and perpendicular to the anatomic posterior facet off the sagittally reconstructed images

CALCANEAL FRACTURES

DIFFERENTIAL DIAGNOSIS

Clinical Differential Anterolateral Calcaneal Region
- Extensor digitorum brevis & anterior process avulsion fx may be indistinguishable by clinical exam

PATHOLOGY

General Features
- Etiology
  - Anterior process fracture: 2 etiologies
    - Avulsion of origin of bifurcate ligament by forceful inversion & plantarflexion of foot
    - Compression of anterior process by the cuboid secondary to eversion & dorsiflexion of foot
  - Anterolateral avulsion fracture: Avulsion by extensor digitorum brevis due to inversion of foot
  - Medial process fracture: Fall from a height with vertical sheer when foot is in valgus position
  - Stress fracture: Jogging; may be insufficiency as well
  - Calcaneal insufficiency avulsion fracture: Achilles avulsive injury in long time insulin-dependent diabetics
  - Intraarticular fracture: Axial loading that produces shear & compression fx lines
    - Jump from height (75%) or high-impact accident
- Epidemiology
  - 2% of all fractures
  - 25-30% extraarticular; 70-75% intraarticular
  - Prevalence of complex injuries increasing, perhaps as a result of increased use of automobile safety devices & ↓ mortality
  - When due to fall, bilateral in 5-9%
  - Low sensitivity on radiographs for avulsion fx (anterior & anterolateral calcaneus)
- Associated abnormalities
  - Fx from falls associated with thoracolumbar fx in 10%
  - Fx from falls associated with compartment syndrome in 10%

Staging, Grading or Classification Criteria
- Rowe classification: Types I-III are extraarticular, types IV-V intraarticular
  - Type I: Fx of calcaneal tuberosity, sustentaculum tali, or anterior process (20%)
  - Type II: Horizontal fx of calcaneal tuberosity (4%)
  - Type III: Oblique fx without extension to subtalar joint (20%)
  - Type IV: Fx extending to subtalar joint (25%)
  - Type V: Intraarticular with depression of subtalar joint or significant comminution (31%)
- Sanders classification of intraarticular fx: Based on CT scan with reformats
  - Type I: Nondisplaced
  - Type II: Split into 2 parts at posterior facet
    - A, B, C based on where the fracture enters facet (A: Lateral, B: Mid-facet, C: Medial)
  - Type III: Depressed and/or split into 3 parts
  - Type IV: Highly comminuted

CLINICAL ISSUES

Presentation
- Most common signs/symptoms
  - Traumatic fx: Severe pain & swelling, inability to bear weight
  - Stress & insufficiency fx: Pain & decreased ability to bear weight
  - Anterior process fx & extensor digitorum brevis avulsion fx: Point of maximum tenderness 1 cm inferior & 2-3 cm anterior to talofibular ligament

Demographics
- Age: Working age population (30-50 years)
- Gender: M:F = 5:1

Natural History & Prognosis
- Delay of diagnosis & conservative treatment of anterior process fx: Painful non-union
- Good to excellent results in 65-75%
  - Prognostic factors: Anatomic reduction at subtalar joint; overall shape of calcaneus
- Sanders type IV does poorly regardless of treatment
  - Poor results include limited ankle motion, pain, osteoarthritis, peroneal tendinitis, causalgia (nerve entrapment)

Treatment
- Most extraarticular fx: Conservative
- Anterior process fx: Displaced fx involving > 25% of calcaneocuboid articular surface usually treated with open reduction internal fixation; otherwise conservative
- Medial process fx: Usually open reduction internal fixation
- Displaced intraarticular (Sanders type II, III): Open reduction, internal fixation

DIAGNOSTIC CHECKLIST

Consider
- Associated injuries may exist (i.e., in thoracolumbar spine, pelvis, opposite calcaneus)
- Entrapped tendons

Image Interpretation Pearls
- Radiography often underestimates degree of displacement & depression of posterolateral fx fragment
- CT required for full evaluation of intraarticular fx

SELECTED REFERENCES
1. Silhanek AD et al: The effect of primary fracture line location on the pattern and severity of intraarticular calcaneal fractures: a retrospective radiographic study. J Foot Ankle Surg. 45(4):211-9, 2006
2. Sormaala MJ et al: Stress injuries of the calcaneus detected with magnetic resonance imaging in military recruits. J Bone Joint Surg Am. 88(10):2237-42, 2006
3. Bajammal S et al: Displaced intra-articular calcaneal fractures. J Orthop Trauma. 19(5):360-4, 2005
4. Daftary A et al: Fractures of the calcaneus: a review with emphasis on CT. Radiographics. 25(5):1215-26, 2005

CALCANEAL FRACTURES

IMAGE GALLERY

Typical

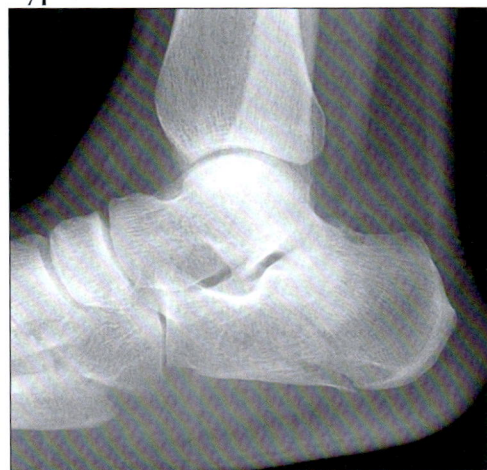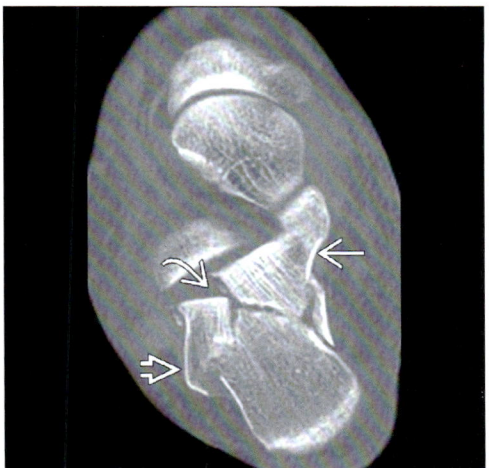

(Left) Lateral radiograph shows a calcaneal fracture. Though the fracture line is not visualized to be intraarticular, it is recognized as such because Boehler's angle is flattened. Posterior facet interruption can be assumed. (Right) Axial bone CT shows the fx entering at the posterior facet ➔. Note that the anteromedial fragment ➔ maintains normal alignment with the talus; the posterolateral fragment ➔ is depressed & angulated. This is a Sanders type IIB (Rowe type V).

Typical

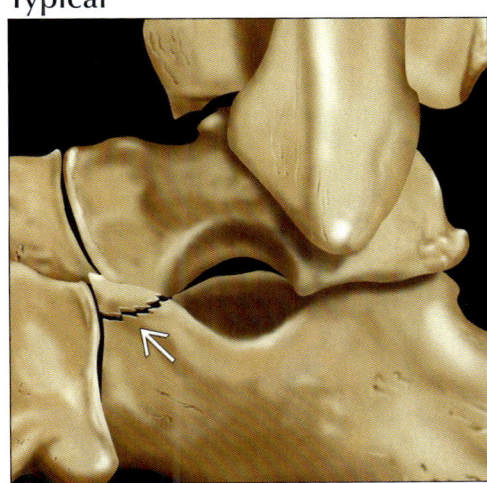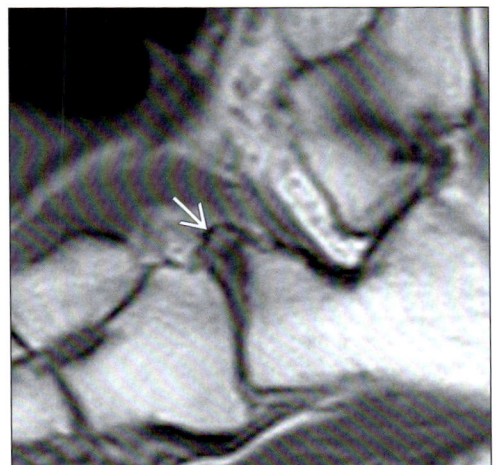

(Left) Lateral graphic shows the site of an anterior process fracture ➔. This is at the anterior and superior portion of the calcaneus. It is the site of origin of the bifurcate ligament. (Right) Sagittal T1WI MR shows an anterior process fracture ➔, corresponding with the graphic. This is an adjacent but distinct site of avulsion by the bifurcate ligament, compared with an avulsion of extensor digitorum brevis, which is slightly more lateral.

Typical

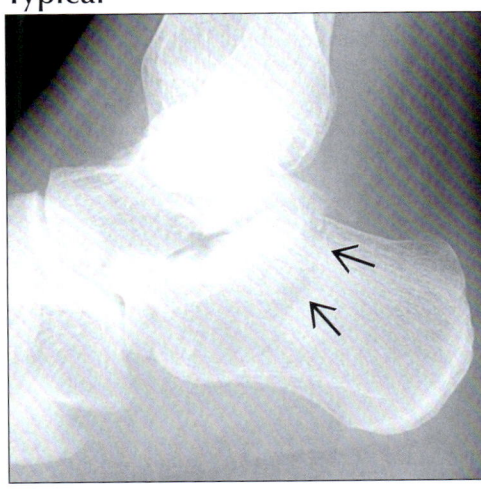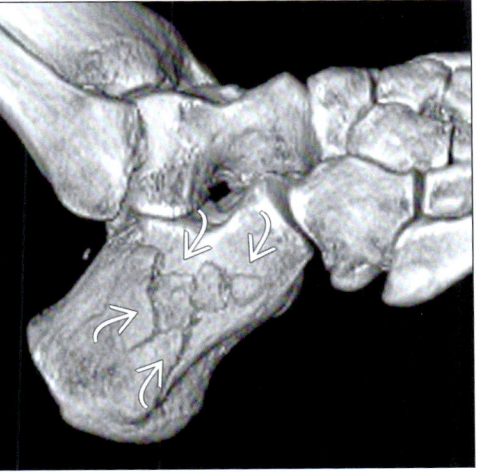

(Left) Lateral radiograph shows an extraarticular fracture of the calcaneus ➔. Note that Boehler's angle is intact, indicating that there is no substantial intraarticular extension of the fracture. (Right) 3D volume rendered NECT of the same case shows the fracture line to be complex ➔, but nonetheless it does not involve the articular surface. Although comminuted, it is nondisplaced and may be treated non-surgically.

TALUS FRACTURES

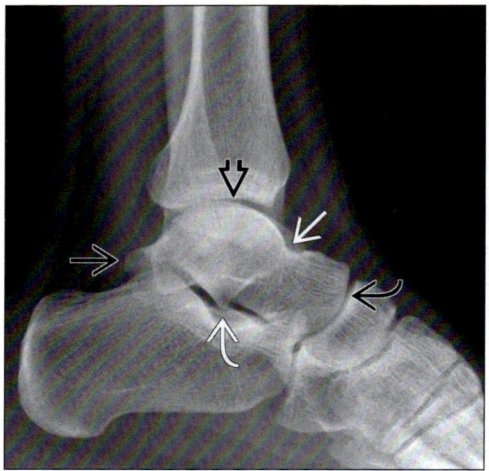

Lateral radiograph shows normal talar anatomy. Talar head ➡. Talar body ➡. Lateral process of the talus ➡. Posterior process of the talus ➡. Talar neck ➡.

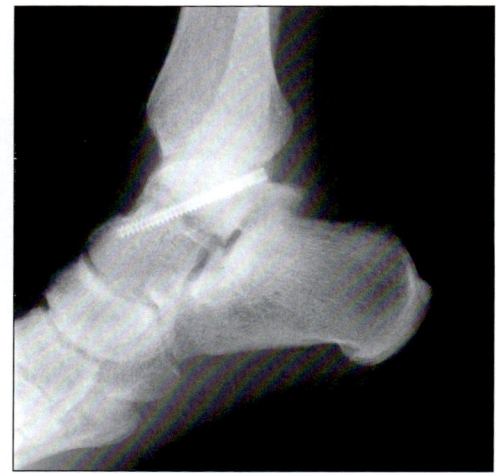

Lateral radiograph shows a fixed, yet diastased talar neck fracture with sclerosis of the talar body indicating AVN.

TERMINOLOGY

Abbreviations and Synonyms
- Avascular necrosis (AVN)
- Open reduction internal fixation (ORIF)

IMAGING FINDINGS

General Features
- Best diagnostic clue: Visualized fracture line
- Location
  o Major talar fx: Neck most frequent site
    - Isolated neck fx most common (over 50%)
    - Neck & body fx next most common (over 30%)
    - Isolated body fx next most common (over 11%)
    - Talar head fx uncommon; when present, usually associated with other talar fractures (most commonly neck)
  o Minor talar fx: Osteochondral injuries most common, usually talar dome
    - Lateral talar dome osteochondral injuries tend to be anterior
    - Medial talar dome osteochondral injuries tend to be posterior

Radiographic Findings
- Standard 3 view foot (AP, mortise, lateral): Sensitivity 24-33% compared with MDCT
- Broden view (45° internal oblique): Useful for evaluation of talar body or lateral process fx
  o Also useful to evaluate posterior facet subtalar joint subluxation
- Detection of osteochondral lesions of talar dome ↑ if mortise views performed in plantar & dorsiflexion

CT Findings
- Bone CT
  o Allows detection of fx not diagnosed by radiograph
  o CT often upgrades severity of fx (greater # fragments or associated subluxations)

MR Findings
- MR: Edema shown in early osteochondral injuries & posterior or lateral process injuries
- Fx line shown with surrounding edema
- Additional soft tissue injuries visualized well

DDx: Fracture Mimics

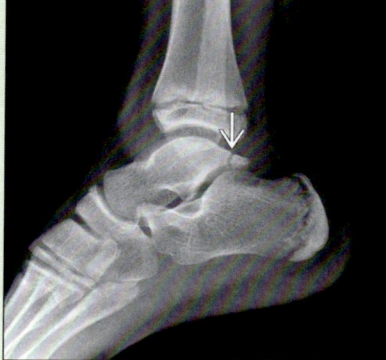

Unfused Posterior Process

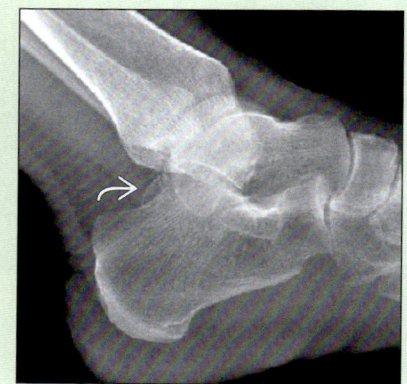

Os Trigonum

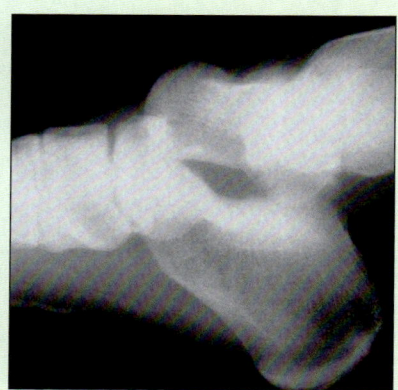

Swivel Type Subtalar Dislocation

TALUS FRACTURES

Key Facts

Imaging Findings
- Standard 3 view foot (AP, mortise, lateral): Sensitivity 24-33% compared with MDCT
- Broden view (45° internal oblique): Useful for evaluation of talar body or lateral process fx
- CT often upgrades severity of fx (greater # fragments or associated subluxations)
- MR: Edema shown in early osteochondral injuries & posterior or lateral process injuries

Pathology
- Fractures of the talar neck and body are associated with an increased risk of AVN of the talar body
- Hawkins' sign indicates an intact talar body blood supply & therefore, that AVN will not develop

- Os trigonum or unfused posterior process ossification center can be confused for a fracture of the posterior process
- Talar dome osteochondral injury classification best determined on marrow edema sensitive MR sequences (T2 fat-sat, STIR, or PD fat-sat)

Diagnostic Checklist
- **Always** evaluate the posterior process of the talus on the lateral radiograph
- **Always** evaluate the lateral process of the talus on **both** the lateral and AP radiographs
- **Always** evaluate the talar dome for osteochondral injuries
- **Always** evaluate the talar neck for subtle fractures

Imaging Recommendations
- Best imaging tool
  - Initial assessment should be with radiographs, but beware poor sensitivity
  - CT is useful for evaluation of complex fractures, evaluation of intraarticular extension, & detection of radiographically occult fractures
  - MR useful for evaluation of radiographically occult osteochondral lesions or other fractures as well as soft tissue clinical mimics
- Protocol advice
  - For CT evaluation of talar fractures thin reconstructions in all three planes is recommended
  - Talar dome osteochondral injury classification best determined on marrow edema sensitive MR sequences (T2 fat-sat, STIR, or PD fat-sat)
    - Osteochondral injuries are usually best seen on sagittal and coronal imaging

DIFFERENTIAL DIAGNOSIS

Radiographic
- Os trigonum or unfused posterior process ossification center can be confused for a fx of the posterior process

Clinical
- Focal tenderness inferior to the lateral malleolus can be seen with lateral collateral ligament injury, fx base of 5th metatarsal, or fx lateral process of the talus

PATHOLOGY

General Features
- General path comments
  - Fractures of the talar neck and body are associated with an increased risk of AVN of the talar body
    - Talar body blood supply is predominately retrograde from arteries in the sinus tarsi that enter at the talar neck
    - Fractures of the talar neck (the most common site of major talar fractures) may, therefore, disrupt blood supply to the body
  - **Hawkins' sign:** Thin zone of subcortical lucency of the talar dome
    - Hawkins' sign indicates an intact talar body blood supply & therefore, that AVN will not develop
- Etiology
  - Talar neck fractures are usually the result of a dorsally directed force on the foot while it is planted
    - Currently, this is usually seen in head on collision motor vehicle accidents when the patient is "standing" on the brake
    - Additional mechanism: Axial load + inversion
  - Talar dome osteochondral injuries (both medial and lateral) are the result of inversion
  - Fractures of the lateral process of the talus are usually due to eversion but may be caused by inversion/dorsiflexion; snowboarding injuries often implicated
  - Fractures of the posterior process of the talus are due to either extreme plantarflexion or avulsion by the posterior talofibular ligament (as may be seen in inversion)
- Epidemiology: 3-14% of all foot fx
- **Fractures of the posterior process of the talus**
  - Posterior process is composed of lateral & medial tubercles, between which runs the tendon of the flexor hallucis longus
    - Problems with, or injuries to the flexor hallucis longus may occur in the setting of fx of posterior process of the talus
  - Lateral tubercle is more frequently fractured
    - Also known as shepherd's fracture
  - Os trigonum or unfused posterior process ossification center can be confused for a fracture of the posterior process
    - Ossification center of the posterior process forms between ages 8 & 13 and usually fuses to the posterior talus within 1 year

TALUS FRACTURES

- If no bony fusion it becomes an accessory ossicle known as the os trigonum, articulating with the lateral tubercle via a synchondrosis
- Os trigonum usually has smooth, corticated (sclerotic) margins whereas a fracture has irregular margins without sclerosis
- Occasionally the margins of the synchondrosis between the os trigonum & talus are irregular (but usually well corticated & sclerotic)
- Repetitive microtrauma to the os trigonum or its synchondrosis (by extreme plantar flexion) can result in point tenderness which can cloud the clinical picture
- If clinical correlation does not distinguish between fracture & variant, MR can be useful
- **Fractures of the lateral process of the talus**
  - Also known as snowboarder's fracture
  - Increasing in incidence
  - Presentation of lateral process of the talus fx (tenderness and swelling inferior and slightly anterior to distal fibular tip) may be dismissed clinically as lateral collateral ligament injury
  - Often undetected radiographically due to lack of awareness of its location & incomplete evaluation

Staging, Grading or Classification Criteria
- **Hawkins' classification of talar neck fractures**
  (Incidence of talar body AVN included in parentheses)
  - **Type I:** Nondisplaced talar neck fx (0-13%)
  - **Type II:** Displaced talar neck fx **AND** subluxed or dislocated subtalar joint (20-50%)
  - **Type III:** Displaced talar neck fx **AND** subluxation or dislocation of **BOTH** the subtalar **AND** tibiotalar joints (69-100%)
  - **Type IV:** Displaced talar neck fx **AND** subluxation or dislocation talonavicular joint (approaches 100%)
    - When a talar body fx is present in combination with a neck fx, the incidence of AVN increases above that of an isolated neck fx
- **Classification of talar dome osteochondral fx**
  - Based on a modification of Berndt and Harty's original radiographic classification system
    - Radiographic findings included in parentheses
  - Talar dome osteochondral injury classification best determined on marrow edema sensitive MR sequences (T2 fat-sat, STIR, or PD fat-sat)
    - **Type I:** Subchondral marrow edema without definite fracture line (radiographs normal)
    - **Type II:** Incomplete or complete semicircular fracture line without complete rim of fluid signal (radiographs may show lucency or fx line)
    - **Type III:** Complete rim of fluid signal surrounding nondisplaced fragment (radiographs may show lucency or fx line)
    - **Type IV:** Fragment displaced from donor site (radiographs may show empty concave donor site, loose body, or both)

CLINICAL ISSUES

Presentation
- Most common signs/symptoms: Pain & instability

Demographics
- Age
  - Talar dome osteochondral injuries, posterior process fxs, and lateral process fxs are seen more often in younger, athletic patients
  - Other talar fractures are without age predilection

Natural History & Prognosis
- Because of the high risk of AVN in the setting of talar neck and/or body fractures, a dedicated assessment for AVN should always be performed in follow-up
  - Although radiographic follow-up may be used to assess for development of AVN, MR detects AVN earlier (sometimes as early as 3 weeks post injury)
    - MR evaluation of AVN in talar fractures may be limited following ORIF

Treatment
- Talar neck fractures
  - Hawkins' I: Usually treated conservatively
  - Hawkins' II: If post reduction alignment acceptable, conservative management may be attempted
    - Up to 50% treated conservatively will eventually require ORIF
  - Hawkins' III and IV fractures: ORIF is the rule
- Talar body fractures
  - If articular incongruence, especially diastasis or step-off of > 2 mm, ORIF is usually performed
  - If there is no articular incongruence, the classification of an associated talar neck fracture (present more often than not) may dictate the need for surgical reduction
- Lateral process fractures
  - Comminuted fx, displaced fx, & fx with a fragment > 1 cm are usually treated surgically
  - Nondisplaced fx (without the characteristics above) may undergo a trial of conservative management
- Posterior process fractures
  - Usually treated conservatively
  - Fragment excision may be performed if continued pain or nonunion

DIAGNOSTIC CHECKLIST

Image Interpretation Pearls
- **Always** evaluate the posterior process of the talus on the lateral radiograph
- **Always** evaluate the lateral process of the talus on **both** the lateral and AP radiographs
- **Always** evaluate the talar dome for osteochondral injuries
- **Always** evaluate the talar neck for subtle fractures

SELECTED REFERENCES
1. Pearce DH et al: Avascular necrosis of the talus: a pictorial essay. Radiographics. 25(2):399-410, 2005
2. Sanders TG et al: Fracture of the lateral process of the talus: appearance at MR imaging and clinical significance. Skeletal Radiol. 28(4):236-9, 1999
3. Wechsler RJ et al: Helical CT of talar fractures. Skeletal Radiol. 26(3):137-42, 1997

TALUS FRACTURES

IMAGE GALLERY

Typical

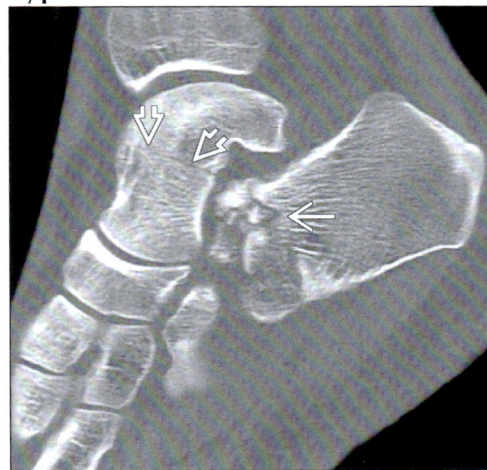
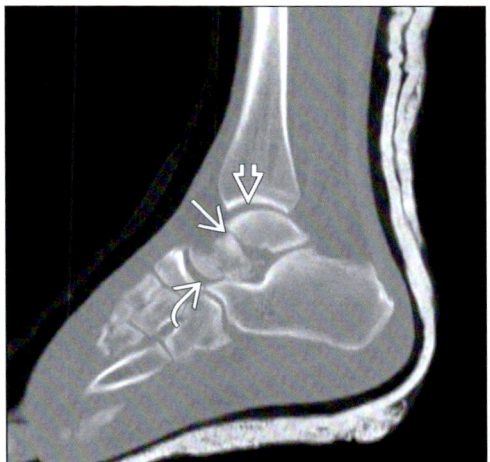

(Left) Sagittal bone CT shows a Hawkins' class I talar neck fracture ➡ (which was not visible on radiograph). CT was performed to evaluate the calcaneal fracture ➡. (Right) Sagittal bone CT shows a displaced talar neck fracture ➡ with diastased talonavicular ➡ & tibiotalar joints ➡ (both of which were also subluxed). This is a Hawkins' class IV injury.

Typical

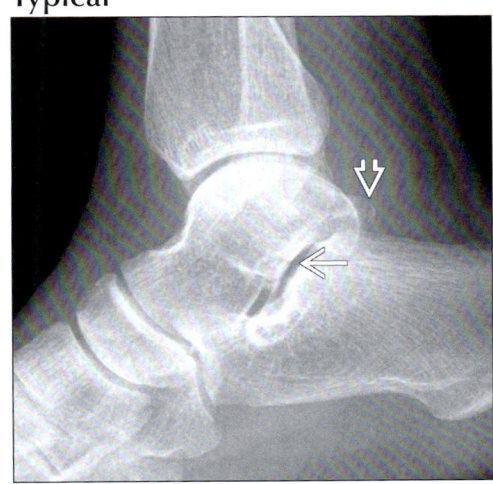
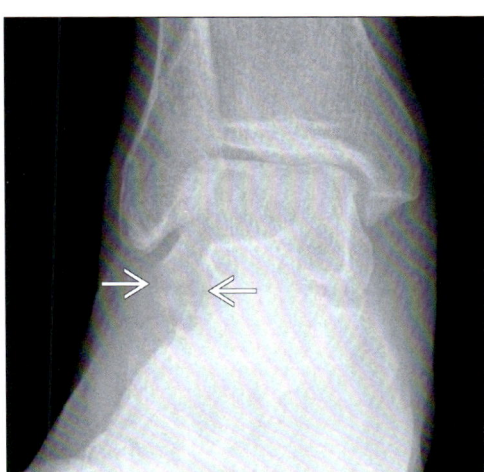

(Left) Lateral radiograph shows a vertical fracture line through the posterior process ➡ & a horizontal fracture line through the lateral process ➡. (Right) Anteroposterior radiograph of the same patient as previous image, shows a fracture line through the lateral process ➡. Both the posterior and lateral process fractures were confirmed on CT.

Typical

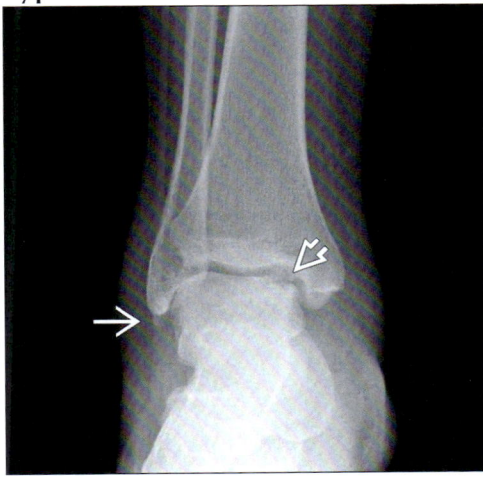
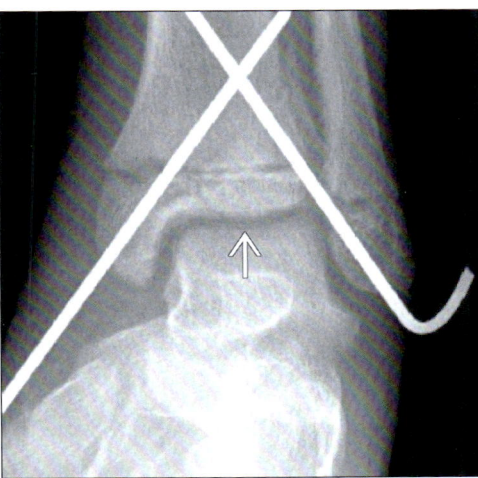

(Left) Anteroposterior radiograph shows a medial talar dome osteochondral injury ➡. There is also a Weber A (Lauge-Hansen supination-adduction) fracture ➡. Both result from inversion injuries. (Right) Anteroposterior radiograph shows a thin rim of talar dome subcortical lucency (Hawkins' sign) ➡. In the setting of talar fx, this indicates an intact blood supply to the talus and that AVN will not occur.

NAVICULAR FRACTURES

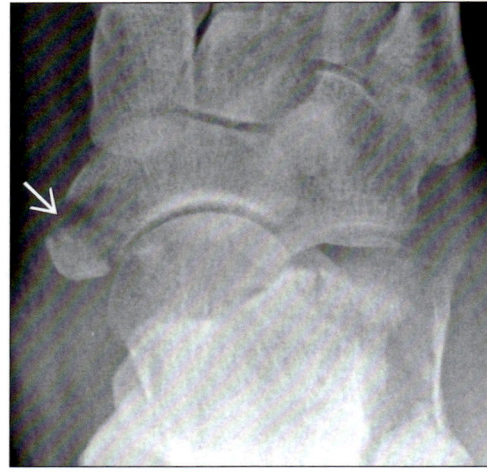

Anteroposterior radiograph shows an avulsion fx ➡ through the medial navicular. This is the site of insertion of the posterior tibial tendon. The degree of diastasis is approaching 1 cm, which would require surgery.

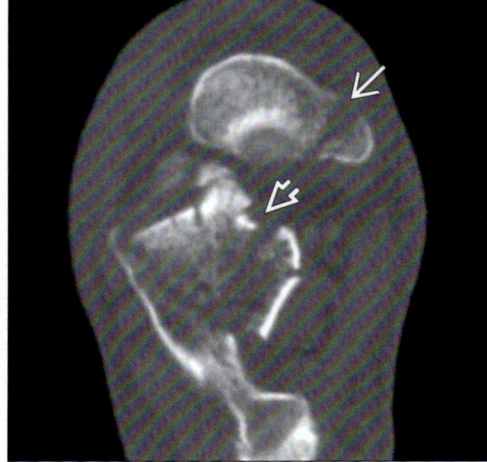

Axial bone CT shows navicular avulsion fracture ➡ and comminuted intraarticular calcaneus fracture ➡. Note that the pertinent tendons can be visualized on CT to evaluate for entrapment.

TERMINOLOGY

Abbreviations and Synonyms
- Navicular fracture

Definitions
- Four types of fractures
  - Navicular tuberosity avulsion: Posterior tibial tendon avulsion
  - Dorsal cortical avulsion: Talonavicular capsular avulsion
  - Body: Undisplaced or displaced (3 types)
  - Stress: Partial or complete fracture in sagittal plane

IMAGING FINDINGS

General Features
- Best diagnostic clue
  - Navicular tuberosity: Avulsed bone fragment
  - Dorsal cortical avulsion: Avulsed bone fragment
  - Body: Fracture line
  - Stress: Often negative radiograph ± fracture line ± small ossicles
- Location
  - Navicular tuberosity: Medial
  - Dorsal cortical avulsion: Dorsal
  - Body: Fracture within body varies by type
  - Stress: Junction of medial two thirds + lateral third of navicular
- Size: Varies by type from mild avulsion to significant comminuted fracture-dislocation
- Morphology
  - Avulsion: Associated with significant ligamentous injuries
  - Body: Associated with other midfoot fractures
  - Stress: Many are non-displaced, incomplete, vertical

Radiographic Findings
- Fracture line, avulsed bone fragment, or normal
  - Avulsion: Best seen on AP + medial oblique views
  - Body: Often seen on only lateral view
  - Stress: Often normal, radiographs 33% sensitive
- Often seen on only one view
- Often missed due to relative rarity, physician unfamiliarity, and multiple concurrent injuries

CT Findings
- Bone CT

DDx: Navicular Fracture

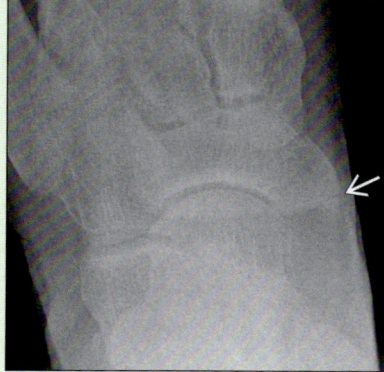

Accessory Navicular

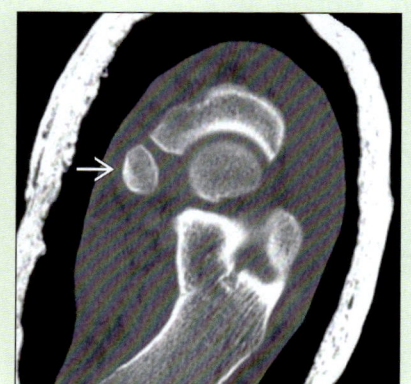

Accessory Navicular

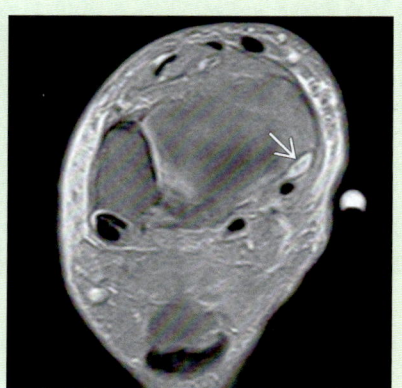

Posterior Tibial Tendon Tear

NAVICULAR FRACTURES

Key Facts

Terminology
- Four types of fractures
- Navicular tuberosity avulsion: Posterior tibial tendon avulsion
- Dorsal cortical avulsion: Talonavicular capsular avulsion
- Body: Undisplaced or displaced (3 types)
- Stress: Partial or complete fracture in sagittal plane

Imaging Findings
- Size: Varies by type from mild avulsion to significant comminuted fracture-dislocation

Top Differential Diagnoses
- Normal Variants
- Ligament or Tendon Tears
- Other Midfoot Fractures

Pathology
- Avulsion fractures most common: 47-67% of navicular fractures
- Body fractures commonly associated with other midfoot injuries

Clinical Issues
- Most common signs/symptoms: Midfoot pain
- Other signs/symptoms: Pain with passive eversion + active inversion

Diagnostic Checklist
- Perform CT with persistent midfoot pain
- Normal radiograph does not rule out navicular fracture
- Often seen on only one radiographic view

- ○ Identify radiographically occult fracture line
- ○ Delineate extent/pattern of fracture prior to surgery

MR Findings
- T1WI: Low signal intensity fracture line and edema
- T2WI: High signal intensity fracture line and edema
- Diagnostic for stress fractures
- Useful in identifying related soft tissue injury
- High sensitivity and specificity

Nuclear Medicine Findings
- Bone Scan
  - Increased uptake at navicular
  - Sensitive, but not specific

Imaging Recommendations
- Best imaging tool
  - Avulsion and body fractures
    - Radiographs: Best initial study
    - CT or MR: Identify fracture if negative radiograph + persistent clinical suspicion, determine extent
  - Stress fracture
    - Radiographs: Best initial study, but often negative
    - CT or MR: Standard for definitive diagnosis
- Protocol advice
  - Radiographs: AP, lateral, and oblique views
  - CT: Thin slices (≤ 1 mm) angled through the plane of the talonavicular joint; reformats in other planes

DIFFERENTIAL DIAGNOSIS

Normal Variants
- Accessory navicular or bipartite tarsal navicular
- Smooth, rounded edges allow differentiation from avulsion or body fracture

Ligament or Tendon Tears
- Posterior tibial tendon tear
  - Mimics navicular tuberosity avulsion fracture
- Plantar calcaneonavicular (spring) ligament tear
  - Associated with medial navicular avulsion
- Deltoid ligament sprain
  - Mimics dorsal avulsion fracture

- MR to evaluate integrity of tendon or ligament

Other Midfoot Fractures
- Cuboid fracture
  - Associated with navicular tuberosity avulsion; known as "nutcracker fracture"
- Cuneiform fracture

Köhler Disease
- Self limiting avascular necrosis of navicular in child < 6 years
- Collapsed navicular or normal navicular with increased density + fragmentation

PATHOLOGY

General Features
- General path comments
  - Navicular tuberosity
    - Non-displaced most common
    - Associated with compression fracture of cuboid
  - Dorsal cortical avulsion: May contain articular cartilage
  - Body
    - Non-displaced most common
    - Force required often results in subluxation or dislocation of navicular + other midfoot injuries
  - Stress
    - 96% are incomplete
    - ± Small ossicles at proximal dorsal border of navicular
- Etiology
  - Navicular tuberosity: Posterior tibial tendon pull from acute trauma consisting of pronation, external rotation, or dorsiflexion
  - Dorsal cortical avulsion: Caused by twisting force (usually eversion), capsular avulsion of talonavicular joint
  - Body: Caused by indirect axial load
    - Fall from a height
    - Motor vehicle accidents
  - Stress: Caused by repetitive impact load

NAVICULAR FRACTURES

- Push-off activities predispose: Jumping + sprinting
- Central one-third of navicular is avascular (↑ risk stress fracture + nonunion)
- Junction of medial two-thirds + lateral third of navicular experiences most shear stress
- Epidemiology
  - Avulsion fractures most common: 47-67% of navicular fractures
  - Body fractures commonly associated with other midfoot injuries
  - Navicular stress fractures
    - 14-35% of all stress fractures in one series
    - 59% are track and field athletes
    - Uncommon in general population
- Associated abnormalities
  - Tendon and ligament injuries
  - Midfoot fractures

Staging, Grading or Classification Criteria
- Body fractures (displaced)
  - Type I: Transverse fracture in coronal plane
  - Type II: Dorsal-lateral to plantar-medial fracture with medial forefoot displacement (most common)
  - Type III: Comminuted fracture with lateral forefoot displacement
- Stress fractures: CT based classification
  - Type I: Dorsal cortical break
  - Type II: Propagation into navicular body
  - Type III: Propagation into another cortex

CLINICAL ISSUES

Presentation
- Most common signs/symptoms: Midfoot pain
- Other signs/symptoms: Pain with passive eversion + active inversion
- Clinical Profile
  - Navicular tuberosity
    - Acute pain + swelling along medial arch of foot
    - Difficult or unable to walk
    - Pain out of proportion to radiographic findings
  - Dorsal cortical avulsion: Pain + swelling at fracture
  - Body: Mid-medial arch pain, tenderness, swelling
  - Stress
    - "N" spot tenderness: Proximal dorsal navicular
    - Insidious onset of pain
    - Resolves with rest, returns when activity resumed
    - Minimal swelling

Demographics
- Age: Stress fracture: Younger patient, sports-related
- Gender: Stress fractures: Female gender ↑ risk

Natural History & Prognosis
- Navicular tuberosity
  - Persistent pain
    - Significant ligamentous injury that was not fully appreciated at presentation
    - Unidentified occult articular injury
- Dorsal cortical avulsion: Full recovery at 4-6 months after injury with conservative treatment
- Body
  - Type III has worst prognosis
  - Late arthritis common in those treated with surgery
- Stress
  - Delayed diagnosis is common
  - 86% of non-displaced stress fractures heal
  - Up to 14% treated correctly do not return to previous activities
  - Time to return to sport
    - Non-operative management: 3-4 months
    - Operative management: 5-6 months
- Complications stress fx: Delayed union, nonunion, talonavicular degenerative joint disease, progression to fracture-dislocation
  - Early intervention can prevent
  - Can lead to prolonged pain, disability, arthritis
  - May need surgical correction

Treatment
- Navicular tuberosity: Surgery if > 1 cm proximal displacement, immobilization if non-displaced
- Dorsal cortical avulsion: Immobilization + restricted weight bearing for 6-12 weeks
- Body
  - Undisplaced: Immobilization + restricted weight bearing for 8-12 weeks
  - Displaced: Surgery for ≥ 1 mm displacement
- Stress
  - Immobilization + restricted weight bearing for 6 weeks, then functional rehabilitation
  - Type III may require surgery
  - Surgery: Complete/comminuted fractures, non-healing incomplete fractures, high level athlete

DIAGNOSTIC CHECKLIST

Consider
- Navicular fracture with other midfoot injuries
- Stress fracture with persistent pain
- Perform CT with persistent midfoot pain
- Early treatment can prevent complications
- Complications of untreated or under-treated navicular fractures can be career-ending for elite athletes

Image Interpretation Pearls
- Normal radiograph does not rule out navicular fracture
- Often seen on only one radiographic view
- CT is often needed

SELECTED REFERENCES
1. Coris EE et al: Tarsal navicular stress fractures. Am Fam Physician. 67(1):85-90, 2003
2. Jameson BH et al: Bilateral navicular body fractures. J Trauma. 54(6):1231-4, 2003
3. Pinney SJ et al: Fractures of the tarsal bones. Orthop Clin North Am. 32(1):21-33, 2001
4. Prokuski LJ et al: Challenging fractures of the foot and ankle. Radiol Clin North Am. 35(3):655-70, 1997
5. Davis CA et al: Midtarsal fracture-subluxation. Case report and review of the literature. Clin Orthop Relat Res. (292):264-8, 1993
6. Nyska M et al: Fractures of the body of the tarsal navicular bone: case reports and literature review. J Trauma. 29(10):1448-51, 1989

NAVICULAR FRACTURES

IMAGE GALLERY

Typical

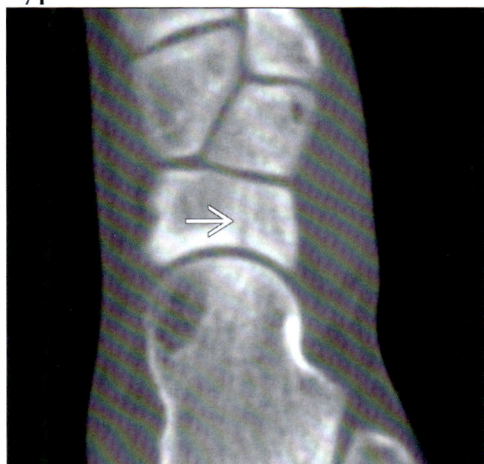
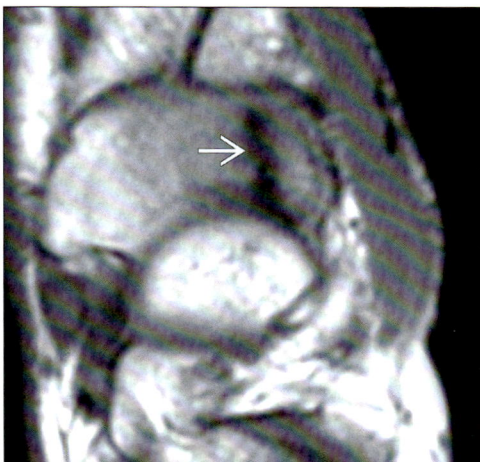

(Left) Axial NECT shows a typical example of incomplete fatigue stress fracture of the dorsum of the navicular ➔. *(Right)* Axial T1WI MR shows another typical example of fatigue stress fracture of the navicular, with a low signal intensity fracture line ➔ and surrounding marrow edema. Note that in both of these cases, the fracture line is in the most frequent location: Sagittal and at the junction of the middle & lateral thirds of the navicular.

Typical

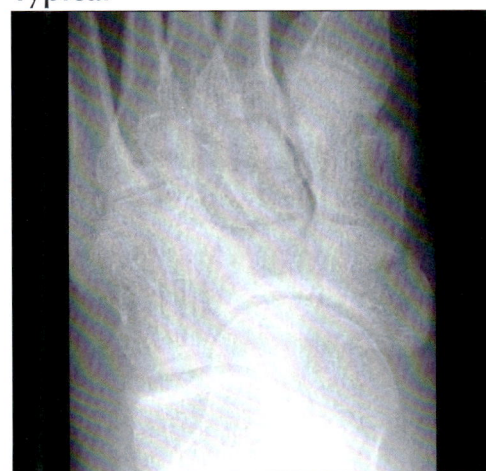
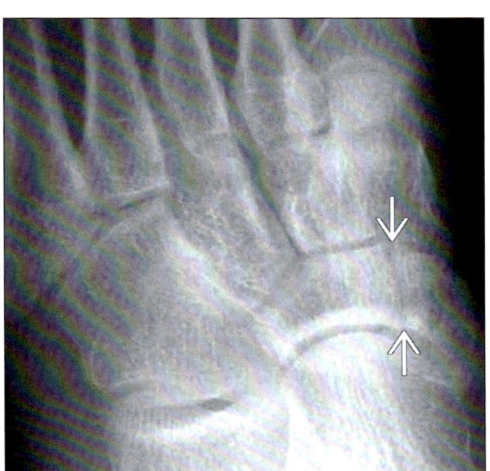

(Left) Anteroposterior radiograph shows how difficult it can be to see a vertical navicular fracture. The AP radiograph appears completely normal. *(Right)* Oblique radiograph shows the non-displaced vertical navicular fracture ➔ which was not apparent on the AP radiograph. Non-displaced fractures are under-diagnosed by radiography. CT or MR are often required to make the diagnosis.

Typical

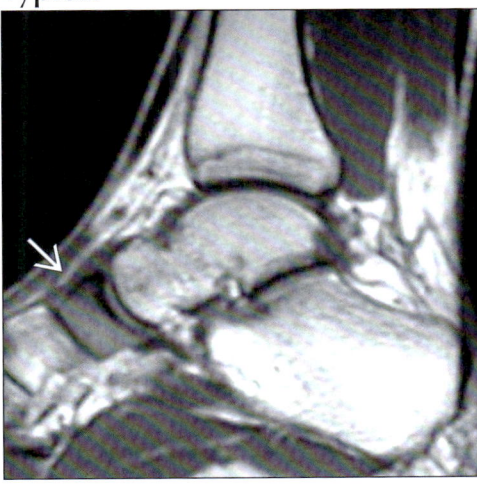
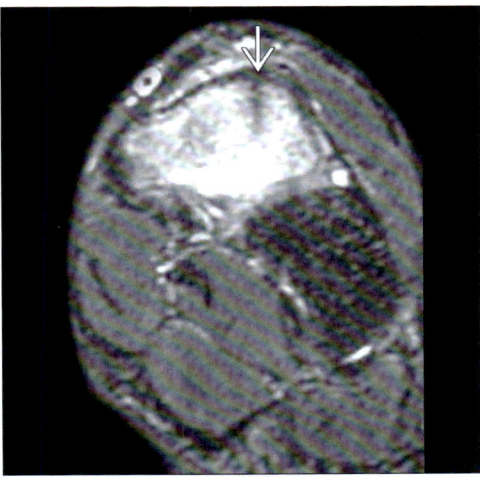

(Left) Sagittal T1WI MR shows low signal edema ➔ from a stress fracture of the navicular. The actual fracture line is in the sagittal plane, so is not expected to be seen on a sagittal image. *(Right)* Axial STIR MR shows a low signal intensity vertical fx line ➔, and surrounding edema typical of a navicular stress fx. Since this fx is nondisplaced and vertical, it can be impossible to visualize on radiographs. Because it is dorsal & propagating into the body, it is classified as type II.

LISFRANC FRACTURE-DISLOCATION

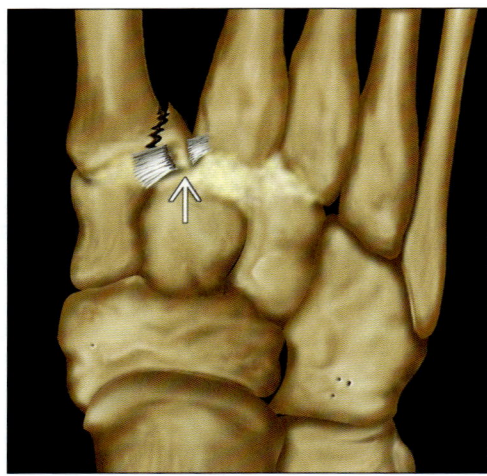

Anterior graphic shows disruption of the Lisfranc ligament between the medial cuneiform and recessed 2nd MT ➜, resulting in lateral displacement of MT 2-5 along with a fragment from MT 1.

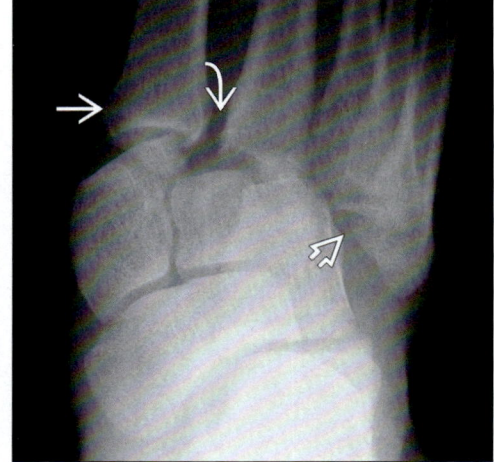

Anteroposterior radiograph shows a similar homolateral Lisfranc injury, with lateral displacement of all 5 MT ➜, as well as a gap between the bases of MT 1 & 2 ➜. Note the complete dislocation of MT 4 & 5 ➜.

TERMINOLOGY

Abbreviations and Synonyms
- Tarsometatarsal fx-dislocation
- Metatarsal: MT
- Tarsometatarsal: TMT

Definitions
- Dorsal dislocation metatarsals relative to tarsals
- Convergent (homolateral): All MT's sublux together in a lateral direction
- Divergent: 1st MT subluxes medially while MT 2-4 sublux laterally

IMAGING FINDINGS

General Features
- Best diagnostic clue: Radiograph: Offset at the TMT joints
- Location: TMT joints
- Size
  ○ Severity can be quite variable
    ■ Least severe: Subtle submillimeter fragmentation at TMT joint
    ■ Subtle (< 2 mm) gap at bases of 1st & 2nd MT or between medial & middle cuneiforms
    ■ Most severe: Complete subluxation/dislocation of all TMT joints, generally laterally and dorsally
- Morphology
  ○ Alignment of the TMT joints must be assessed carefully so as to not miss a subtle Lisfranc injury
    ■ Evaluation requires AP, oblique, & lateral views
    ■ There should be no gap between 1st & 2nd MT bases
    ■ There should be no gap between medial & middle cuneiform
    ■ On AP view, lateral cortex of 1st MT must align perfectly with lateral cortex of medial cuneiform
    ■ On AP view, medial cortex of 2nd MT must align perfectly with medial cortex of middle cuneiform
    ■ Lateral 3 TMT joints not evaluated on AP view because of transverse arch of foot
    ■ On oblique view, medial cortex of 3rd MT must align perfectly with medial cortex of lateral cuneiform

Extremely Subtle Lisfranc, Seen Only by CT

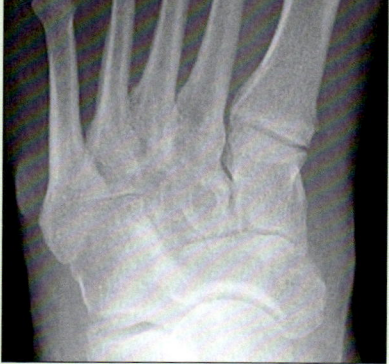

Normal AP

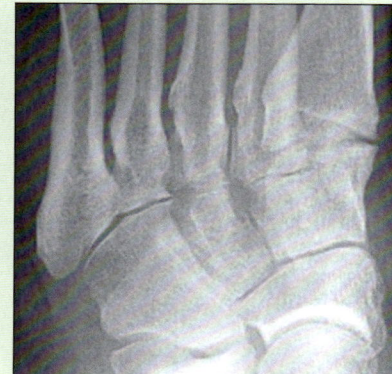

Normal Oblique

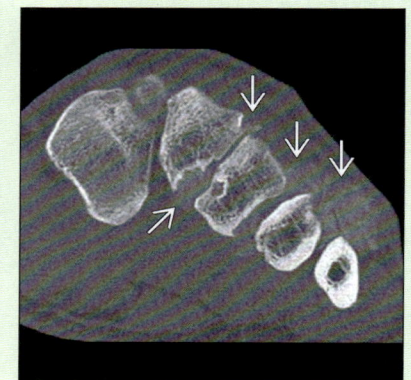

Fragmentation All T-MT Joints

LISFRANC FRACTURE-DISLOCATION

Key Facts

Terminology
- Convergent (homolateral): All MT's sublux together in a lateral direction
- Divergent: 1st MT subluxes medially while MT 2-4 sublux laterally

Imaging Findings
- Alignment of the TMT joints must be assessed carefully so as to not miss a subtle Lisfranc injury
- Evaluation requires AP, oblique, & lateral views
- There should be no gap between 1st & 2nd MT bases
- On AP view, lateral cortex of 1st MT must align perfectly with lateral cortex of medial cuneiform
- On AP view, medial cortex of 2nd MT must align perfectly with medial cortex of middle cuneiform
- On oblique view, medial cortex of 3rd MT must align perfectly with medial cortex of lateral cuneiform
- On oblique view, medial cortex of 4th MT must align perfectly with medial cortex of cuboid
- On oblique view, articular surface of 5th MT aligns with articular surface of cuboid; the nonarticular portion of the base of 5th MT projects laterally
- Lateral view is usually normal, despite severe disruption; if abnormal, the MT's sublux dorsally
- 20-25% missed by radiographic evaluation
- Even if radiograph shows injury, CT detects significantly more fractures in both tarsals and MT

Pathology
- 2nd MT base is recessed between 1st & 3rd MT bases
- Transverse ligaments unite the bases of MT 2-5
- Oblique (Lisfranc) ligament has 3 portions, all extending from anterolateral aspect of medial cuneiform to medial base of 2nd MT

  - On oblique view, medial cortex of 4th MT must align perfectly with medial cortex of cuboid
  - On oblique view, articular surface of 5th MT aligns with articular surface of cuboid; the nonarticular portion of the base of 5th MT projects laterally
  - Lateral view is usually normal, despite severe disruption; if abnormal, the MT's sublux dorsally

Radiographic Findings
- Routine 3 views necessary to fully evaluate alignment of TMT joints (see morphology, above)
- Even subtle offset must be considered abnormal
  - 20-25% missed by radiographic evaluation
  - Many of these may be detected retrospectively
- Weight-bearing radiographs do not appear to improve sensitivity

CT Findings
- Axial CT may show subtle osseous fragmentation at TMT joints that is not detectable by radiograph
- Axial CT with coronal & sagittal reformats demonstrates subtle subluxation at TMT joints or between medial & middle cuneiform
  - Should diagnose subluxation as small as 2 mm
- Significantly more sensitive than radiographs
  - May detect injury not seen by radiograph
  - Even if radiograph shows injury, CT detects significantly more fractures in both tarsals and MT
    - Radiographs showed only 62% of MT and 49% of tarsal fractures shown by CT in one study

MR Findings
- T1WI:
  - Axial: Lateral displacement MT's relative to respective tarsals
  - Fracture fragments hypointense
  - Hypointense edema at sites of osseous injury
- Fluid sensitive sequences
  - Hyperintense marrow edema at sites of fracture or injury
  - Oblique (Lisfranc) ligament disrupted, with surrounding high signal
  - Displacement in the various planes

Imaging Recommendations
- Best imaging tool
  - Radiographs generally abnormal, though it may be subtle
  - CT if high suspicion and radiographs are normal
  - CT should be obtained as primary imaging tool prior to surgery since it has much higher degree of sensitivity for additional fracture fragments
    - Detection of greater number of fractures & disruption may change the plan from conservative treatment to surgical procedure
  - MR generally not required for diagnosis or therapeutic planning, but is the only method capable of showing ligament disruption & osseous edema
    - Disrupted Lisfranc ligament virtually always accompanied by malalignment, detectable on radiograph or CT
    - MR may miss subtle fracture fragments, identifying injury as edema rather than fracture

DIFFERENTIAL DIAGNOSIS

Lateral Ligamentous Sprain
- Partial or complete tear localized to anterior talofibular ligament (ATFL) or calcaneofibular ligament (CFL)
- Thickened or attenuated scarred ligaments
- Inversion of plantarflexed ankle

Jones Fracture
- Fifth metatarsal base fracture
- Avulsion force + supination of foot

Navicular Fracture
- May involve naviculocuneiform & calcaneocuboid joints
- Repetitive stress (running, jumping)
- Body fractures due to axial compression
- Avulsion fracture of tuberosity: Pull of tibialis posterior
- Dorsal avulsion: Talonavicular or deltoid

LISFRANC FRACTURE-DISLOCATION

Subtalar Sprain
- Mild to complete subtalar & talonavicular dislocation
- Associated with lateral ankle sprain

Bifurcate Sprain
- Ligament extends from anterior process of calcaneus to navicular & cuboid
- May have anterior process fracture

PATHOLOGY

General Features
- Etiology
  - Majority are motor vehicle or industrial accidents
  - Forced plantar flexion of forefoot on hindfoot (as in stepping off curb)
  - Plantarflexed foot + longitudinal force (as in equestrian injury with foot caught in stirrup)
  - Direct blow or crush
  - Lisfranc fracture-dislocation is most frequent site of neuropathic joint in diabetic patients
    - Osteoporotic
    - Vascular calcification
    - Atrophic (osseous fragments resorbed)
- Epidemiology
  - 0.2% of all fractures
  - < 1% of all dislocations
- Relevant anatomy
  - 2nd MT base is recessed between 1st & 3rd MT bases
    - Position likely the reason the 2nd MT base is the most frequent site of MT fx in Lisfranc injury
  - Transverse ligaments unite the bases of MT 2-5
    - This arrangement favors displacement of 2nd-5th MT bases as a unit
  - There is no transverse ligament extending between the bases of MT 1 & 2
    - Oblique (Lisfranc) ligament has 3 portions, all extending from anterolateral aspect of medial cuneiform to medial base of 2nd MT
    - Lisfranc ligament serves to stabilize the 2nd MT & middle cuneiform relative to 1st MT & medial cuneiform
  - Metatarsal bases are wedge-shaped, forming the transverse arch
    - This configuration predisposes the MT bases to dorsal subluxation with injury

Gross Pathologic & Surgical Features
- Lisfranc ligament disruption
- ± Avulsion fracture
- Various displacement patterns
  - Homolateral displacement of all rays laterally, or of rays 2-5
  - Gap between bases of MT 1 & 2 or medial & middle cuneiforms
  - Divergent displacement: 1st MT displaced medially & 2-5 MT displaced laterally
  - Dorsal subluxation MT bases
- Associated fractures
  - Base of MT, particularly 2nd
  - Tarsal bones (particularly lateral aspect of cuboid) fractured in 50-90% of cases

CLINICAL ISSUES

Presentation
- Most common signs/symptoms: Pain TMT joint, midfoot
- Clinical Profile
  - Pop or snap
  - Edema or ecchymosis midfoot
  - Pain with weightbearing
  - Shortening or abduction/adduction forefoot
  - Excessive range of motion TMT

Demographics
- Age
  - High energy trauma not age specific
  - Athletic injury: Younger patient population
  - Charcot Lisfranc: Older diabetic population
- Gender: Male > female, relating to athletic activity

Natural History & Prognosis
- 20-25% missed diagnosis originally
- Delayed treatment → chronic instability
- Chronic instability → osteoarthritis
- Long term morbidity high

Treatment
- Conservative
  - Reserved for partial tear ligament /stretched capsule
  - Non-weightbearing, ice, compression, elevation
- Surgical
  - Unstable but nondisplaced: Percutaneous K-wire fixation
  - Unstable displaced: Open reduction, internal fixation
  - Anatomic reduction improves clinical outcome

DIAGNOSTIC CHECKLIST

Consider
- Always check alignment of MT's with associated tarsals

Image Interpretation Pearls
- There should be no gap between 1st & 2nd TMT joint
- Cannot evaluate lateral 3 TMT joints adequately on AP
- Radiographs seriously underestimate number of associated fractures

SELECTED REFERENCES

1. Desmond EA et al: Current concepts review: Lisfranc injuries. Foot Ankle Int. 27(8):653-60, 2006
2. Haapamaki V et al: Ankle and foot injuries: analysis of MDCT findings. AJR 183: 615-622, 2004
3. Haapamaki V et al: Lisfranc fracture-dislocation in patients with multiple trauma: diagnosis with multidetector computed tomography. Foot Ankle Int. 25(9):614-9, 2004
4. Peicha G et al: The anatomy of the joint as a risk factor for Lisfranc dislocation and fracture-dislocation. An anatomical and radiological case control study. J Bone Joint Surg Br 84(7):981-5, 2002
5. Preidler KW et al: Conventional radiography, CT, and MR imaging in patients with hyperflexion injuries of the foot: Diagnostic accuracy in the detection of bony and ligamentous changes. AJR 173(5):1673-7, 1999

LISFRANC FRACTURE-DISLOCATION

IMAGE GALLERY

Typical

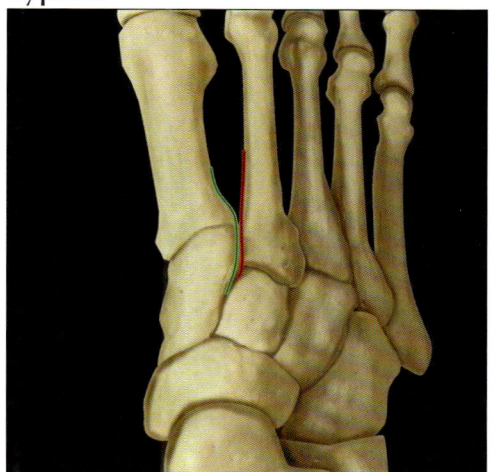 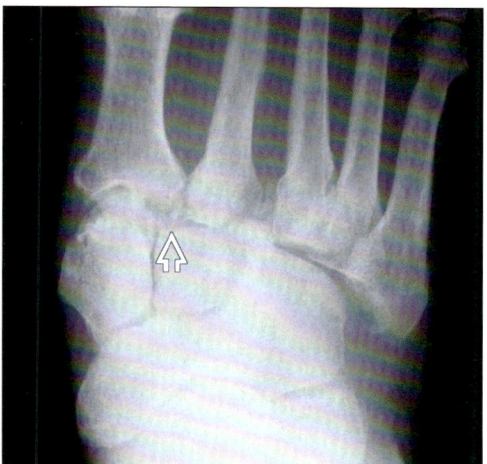

(Left) Anteroposterior graphic of the TMT joints shows normal alignment of the base of 1st MT with its medial cuneiform (green line) & base of 2nd MT with the middle cuneiform (red line). *(Right)* Anteroposterior radiograph shows that neither the 1st nor 2nd MT align properly with their respective medial and middle cuneiforms ➡. Although this case is easy to diagnose, others are more subtle & must rely on the integrity of these relationships.

Typical

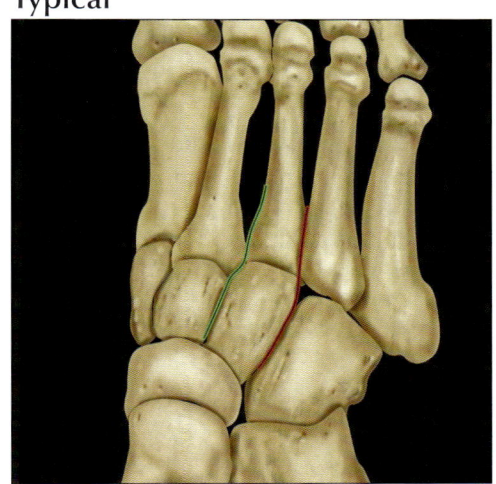 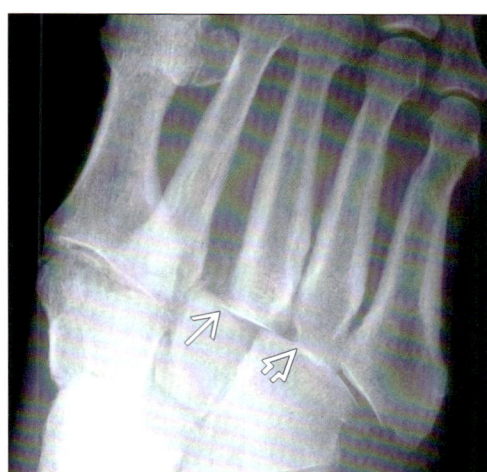

(Left) Oblique graphic of the TMT joints shows how the 3-5 TMT alignment is evaluated. The 3rd MT base must align perfectly with the medial aspect of the lateral cuneiform (green line) and the 4th MT base with the medial aspect of the cuboid (red line). The 5th MT has a nonarticular portion which is lateral to the cuboid. *(Right)* Oblique radiograph of the prior patient confirms the dislocation of both the 3rd MT ➡ and 4th MT ➡ relative to the lateral cuneiform & cuboid.

Typical

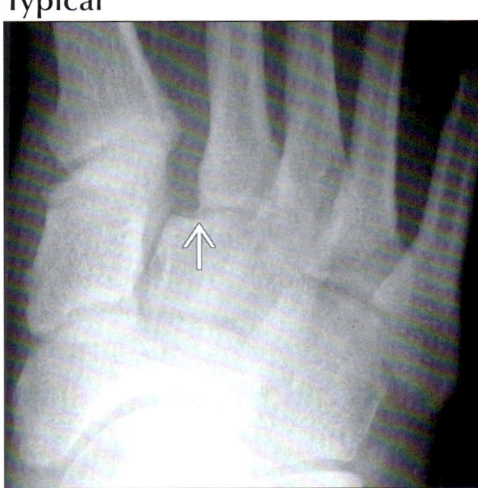 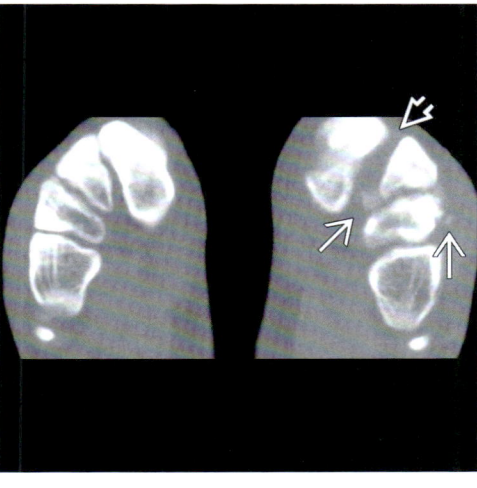

(Left) This athlete's Lisfranc fx/dislocation went undiagnosed for a number of weeks. The diagnosis is clear on the AP radiograph, which shows several mm of displacement of the 2nd MT base relative to the middle cuneiform ➡. The other MT joints retained their normal relationships. Though the abnormality is subtle, it must be noted. *(Right)* Axial NECT confirms the injury, with gap seen between the 1st & 2nd MT bases ➡ and small osseous fragments at other sites ➡.

METATARSAL FRACTURES

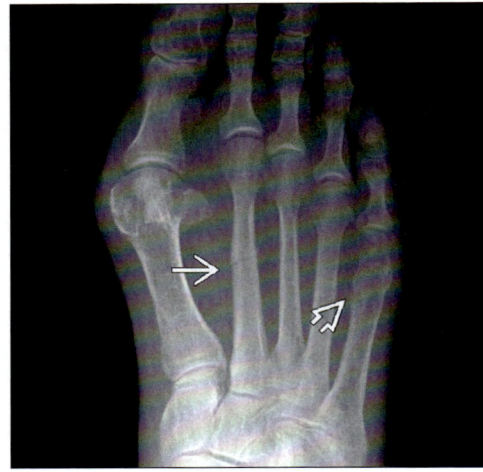

Anteroposterior radiograph shows a subacute (7 days out) stress fx in the 2nd metatarsal ➡. The fx line is faintly seen, with minimal callus. There is an old healed stress fx in the 5th MT ➡ in this osteoporotic patient.

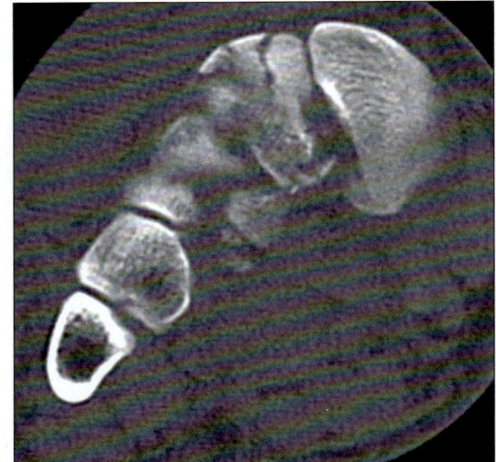

Coronal bone CT shows highly comminuted fractures involving the 2nd cuneiform & base of 3rd metatarsal which were occult on radiograph in this patient who had a crush injury. CT is valuable in such cases.

TERMINOLOGY

Abbreviations and Synonyms
- Jones, dancer: Fx of proximal 5th MT diaphysis
- Lisfranc: Fracture-dislocation of tarsometatarsal joints

Definitions
- Metatarsal fracture: Stress, traumatic, or avulsion

IMAGING FINDINGS

General Features
- Best diagnostic clue: Bone marrow edema + fx line
- Location
  - Stress: Proximal third, common in dancers
  - Stress: Middle & distal third, common in walker/runners
  - Location of proximal 5th MC traumatic fx is related to fracture type & prognosis
- Size
  - Variable
    - Stress: Transverse
    - Head: ± Shortening in impaction injuries
    - Neck: ± Displacement & ± multisegment involvement
    - Mid shaft: Size related to oblique, transverse, spiral & comminuted patterns
    - Base: Usually minimal displacement & anatomic alignment
- Morphology
  - Stress: Transverse ± angulation ± periosteal reaction/exuberant callus, related to age of fx
  - Head: ± Angulation or rotation
  - Neck: ± Plantar + lateral displacement
  - Mid shaft: Oblique, transverse, spiral or comminuted
  - Base
    - May be associated with Lisfranc fx-dislocation
    - May be highly comminuted, yet extremely subtle
  - First: Direct trauma has comminution vs. indirect with avulsion
  - **Fifth MT: 3 types of fracture at the proximal portion; all transverse**
    - Tuberosity avulsion fx: The most proximal & generally extraarticular (1/10 intraarticular)
    - Jones fracture: At junction of diaphysis and metaphysis; always extraarticular

Jones Fracture Progressing to Nonunion

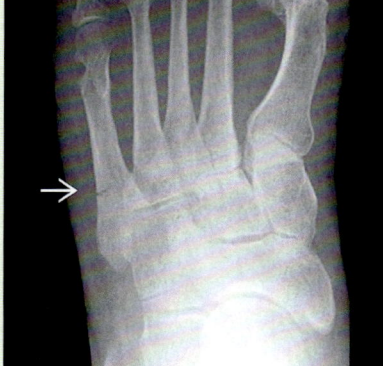

Fracture at Time of Injury

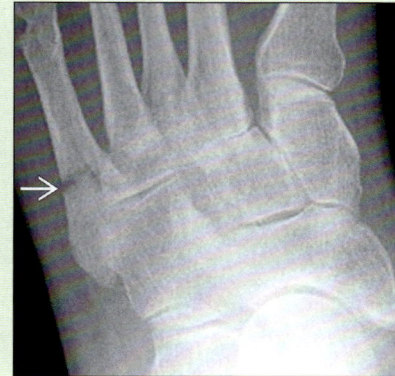

4 Months: Ununited

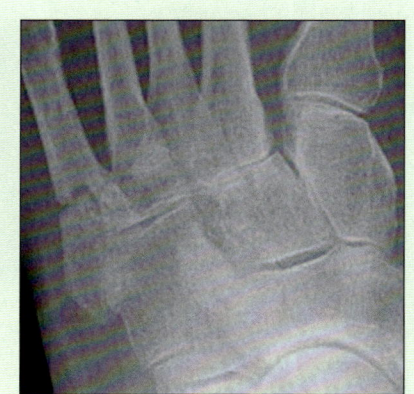

6 Months: Nonunion

METATARSAL FRACTURES

Key Facts

Imaging Findings
- Best diagnostic clue: Bone marrow edema + fx line
- **Fifth MT: 3 types of fracture at the proximal portion; all transverse**
- Tuberosity avulsion fx: The most proximal & generally extraarticular (1/10 intraarticular)
- Jones fracture: At junction of diaphysis and metaphysis; always extraarticular
- Stress fx: Proximal diaphysis, distal to Jones
- **Stress fx usually nondisplaced**
- May not be visible at time of initial pain/injury
- May be seen only as periosteal reaction/callus formation 7-10 days post injury
- Radiograph is initial study, but nondisplaced fx may be occult
- MR to identify marrow edema in nondisplaced fx

Clinical Issues
- Age: Stress fractures: Young runners, dancers, marchers
- Jones fracture (proximal diaphysis 5th MT, not intraarticular) is at particular risk for nonunion

Diagnostic Checklist
- MT marrow edema often indicative of a stress fracture
- Do not misinterpret soft tissue & marrow edema of stress fx seen on MR as tumor
- Do not misinterpret longitudinal ununited apophysis of base of 5th MT as fx
- Be sure to distinguish Jones fx from base of 5th MT tuberosity fx
- Twisting injuries of the ankle may result in fx of base of 5th MT; be certain to look at this site on lateral ankle radiograph

---

- Stress fx: Proximal diaphysis, distal to Jones

Radiographic Findings
- Radiography
  - Confirms fracture location
  - Three views recommended
  - **Stress fx usually nondisplaced**
    - May not be visible at time of initial pain/injury
    - May be seen only as periosteal reaction/callus formation 7-10 days post injury

CT Findings
- Bone CT
  - Documents subtle fx at base MT which may not be seen by radiograph
  - May be used to evaluate fx displacement or associated tarsometatarsal dislocation

MR Findings
- T1WI
  - Stress fracture
    - Subchondral hypointensity
    - Asymmetric thickening of hypointense cortex (subacute)
    - Hypointense fracture line (single or multiple)
    - Usually perpendicular to metatarsal long axis
  - Head: Hypointense edema ± dislocation
  - Neck: Hypointense oblique/transverse fx & edema, ± plantar displacement
  - Mid shaft: Oblique/transverse fx & edema, ± shortening, angulation, displacement
  - Base: Hypointense marrow edema; identify multiple MT involvement
  - First
    - ± Extensive soft tissue effacement with hypointense edema/hemorrhage
    - Comminution in direct injuries
    - Avulsion fragment
  - Fifth: Hypointensity of base ± extension into proximal diaphysis
- Fluid sensitive sequences: All sites
  - Watch for displacement, shortening, involvement adjacent bones, as in T1WI
  - Marrow edema may obscure fracture line
  - May have extensive soft tissue edema surrounding fx
- Pitfall: Stress fx seen on MR misinterpreted as tumor
  - Fx line subtle or not seen
  - Edema prominent both within marrow and in surrounding soft tissues
  - Use location to strongly consider stress fracture rather than tumor

Imaging Recommendations
- Best imaging tool
  - Radiograph is initial study, but nondisplaced fx may be occult
  - MR to identify marrow edema in nondisplaced fx
- Protocol advice
  - T1 + fluid sequence
    - Direct axial for Lisfranc joint
    - Coronal for displacement & dislocation
    - Sagittal for shortening and angulation

DIFFERENTIAL DIAGNOSIS

Lisfranc Fracture-Dislocation
- Tarsometatarsal involvement rather than MT only
- Homolateral vs. divergent displacement

Navicular Fracture
- Dorsal avulsion
- Tuberosity
- Body

Cuboid & Cuneiform Fracture
- Cuneiform associated with tarsometatarsal dislocations
- Cuboid associated with fractures of calcaneus, fifth metatarsal or navicular

Metatarsal Tumor
- Mistaken diagnosis may be made since fx line is subtle in stress fx
- Marrow edema & surrounding soft tissue edema is prominent

METATARSAL FRACTURES

PATHOLOGY

General Features
- General path comments
  - Relevant anatomy
    - MT structure = base, diaphysis, neck & head
    - Base: Broad & cancellous with strong plantar ligaments
    - Diaphysis: Origin of intrinsic foot muscles
    - Neck: Strong intermetatarsal ligaments
    - Metatarsal heads: Weightbearing
    - Poor blood supply of proximal metadiaphyseal region of 5th MT; relates to healing complications
    - Proximal apophysis 5th MT: Oriented longitudinally
- Etiology
  - Direct vs. indirect force
    - Direct: Crushing, blunt trauma or penetrating injuries
    - Indirect: Axial loading
  - Stress
    - Overuse: Running or dancing
    - Decreased bone density: Amenorrhea, senile osteoporosis
  - Head: Direct trauma
  - Neck: Shearing force vs. direct trauma
  - Mid shaft: Direct, blunt vs. torsional
  - Base: Direct trauma = motor vehicle accident or fall from a height
  - First metatarsal: Crush vs. twisting
  - Central metatarsals: Direct impact or crushing
  - Fifth metatarsal
    - Avulsion tuberosity fx: Inversion of plantarflexed foot; avulsion by conjoined fibers of lateral component plantar aponeurosis + peroneus brevis
    - Jones fx: Large adduction force to the forefoot with the ankle in plantarflexion; fx occurs between insertion of peroneus brevis & peroneus tertius
    - Proximal diaphyseal stress fx: Running or dancing, repetitive injury
- Epidemiology
  - 35% of foot fractures involve metatarsal
  - Base 5th: Tuberosity avulsion > Jones > stress fx
  - 5th MT > 3rd > 2nd > 1st > 4th

Gross Pathologic & Surgical Features
- Stress mechanism to complex trauma
- Malalignment post fracture = displacement, shortening, or angulation

CLINICAL ISSUES

Presentation
- Most common signs/symptoms
  - Pain at fracture site
  - Patient often complains of "twisting ankle" but fx is in fact at base of 5th MT rather than at ankle
- Clinical Profile
  - Stress: Focal tenderness + pain with activity (diaphysis or neck most common)
  - First metatarsal: Altered gait

Demographics
- Age: Stress fractures: Young runners, dancers, marchers
- Gender
  - Females more susceptible in military context (thinner cortices)
  - Level of fitness & degree of osteoporosis most important determinants (stress fractures)

Natural History & Prognosis
- Bridging callus: Good prognosis
- Complications: Nonunion, malunion, continued pain
- Jones fracture (proximal diaphysis 5th MT, not intraarticular) is at particular risk for nonunion

Treatment
- Conservative
  - Stress fracture: Decreased/altered activity to immobilization
  - Head: Closed treatment if intact nondisplaced articular surface
  - Neck, base, central, fifth = immobilization/cast for nondisplaced fractures
- Surgical
  - Open reduction with internal fixation (ORIF) for significant displacement
  - Internal fixation for ununited Jones fracture

DIAGNOSTIC CHECKLIST

Consider
- MT marrow edema often indicative of a stress fracture

Image Interpretation Pearls
- Do not misinterpret soft tissue & marrow edema of stress fx seen on MR as tumor
- Do not misinterpret longitudinal ununited apophysis of base of 5th MT as fx
- Be sure to distinguish Jones fx from base of 5th MT tuberosity fx
- Twisting injuries of the ankle may result in fx of base of 5th MT; be certain to look at this site on lateral ankle radiograph

SELECTED REFERENCES

1. Theodorou DJ et al: Fractures of proximal portion of fifth metatarsal bone: anatomic and imaging evidence of a pathogenesis of avulsion of the plantar aponeurosis and the short peroneal muscle tendon. Radiology. 226(3):857-65, 2003
2. Ashman CJ et al: Forefoot pain involving the metatarsal region: differential diagnosis with MR imaging. Radiographics. 21(6):1425-40, 2001
3. Banks A et al: McGlamry's comprehensive textbook of foot and ankle surgery. Metatarsal fractures. vol 1. 3rd ed. Philadelphia PA, Lippincott Williams & Wilkins, (55):1775-90, 2001
4. Harmath C et al: Stress fracture of the fifth metatarsal. Orthopedics. 24(2):111, 204-8, 2001
5. Chowchuen P et al: Stress fractures of the metatarsal heads. Skeletal Radiol. 27(1):22-5, 1998
6. Harrington T et al: Overuse ballet injury of the base of the second metatarsal. A diagnostic problem. Am J Sports Med. 21(4):591-8, 1993

METATARSAL FRACTURES

IMAGE GALLERY

Typical

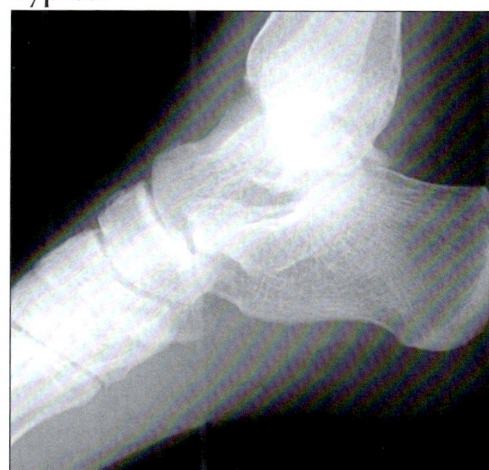 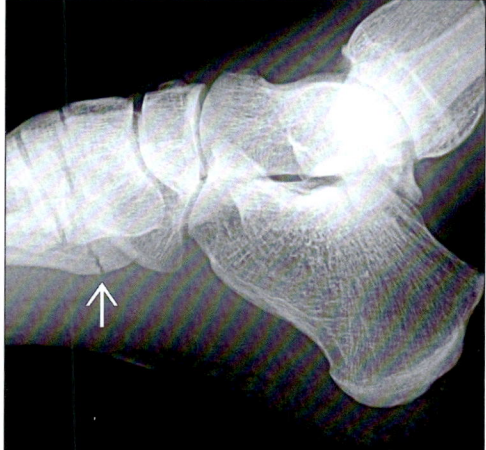

(Left) Lateral radiograph of the ankle appears normal. However, it is poorly positioned (note anterior placement of fibula and overlap of metatarsal bases), which can mask pathology. *(Right)* Lateral radiograph of the same patient which is properly positioned shows a typical avulsion fx at the base tuberosity of the 5th metatarsal ➡. This fracture can present clinically as ankle pain.

Typical

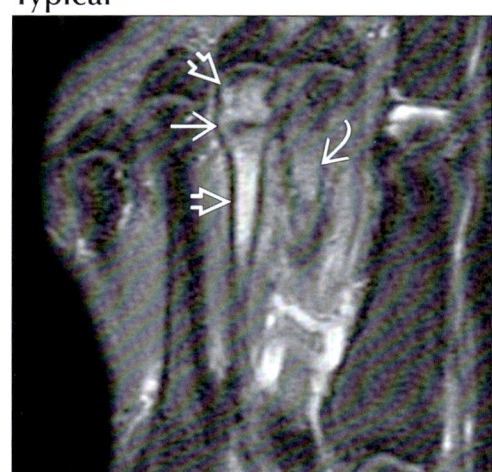 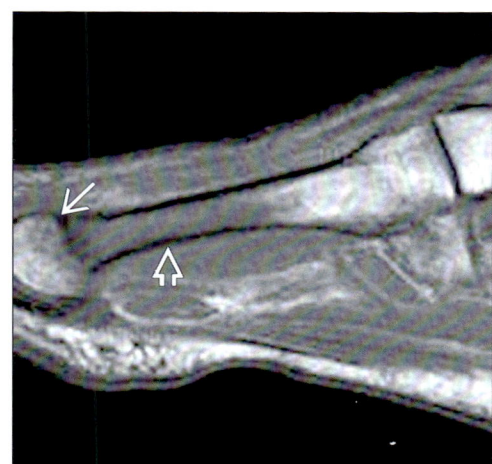

(Left) Axial STIR MR shows low signal fx line ➡ in this 3rd MT stress fx, surrounded by marrow edema ➡. Note the first and 4th MT low signal, which is the normal STIR appearance of marrow. There is slight increased signal in the 2nd MT, suggesting stress injury at that site ➡ as well. *(Right)* Sagittal T1WI MR confirms the stress fx ➡ and edema pattern ➡. The radiographs were normal.

Typical

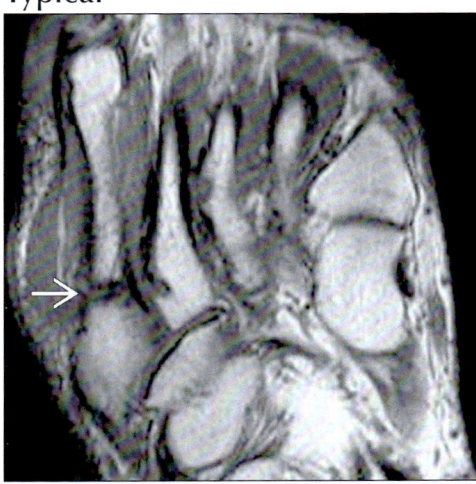 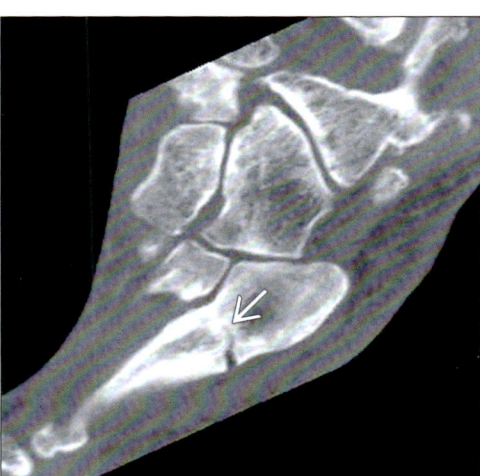

(Left) Axial T1WI MR shows sclerosis at the edges of an ununited subacute proximal shaft fracture of the 5th MT ➡. *(Right)* Sagittal bone CT reformat confirms both the chronic nature of this injury and its features of nonunion ➡. A fracture in this location of the 5th MT (junction of the diaphysis & metaphysis) is known as a Jones or dancer's fracture, and is at risk for nonunion.

PHYSEAL FRACTURES, PEDIATRIC

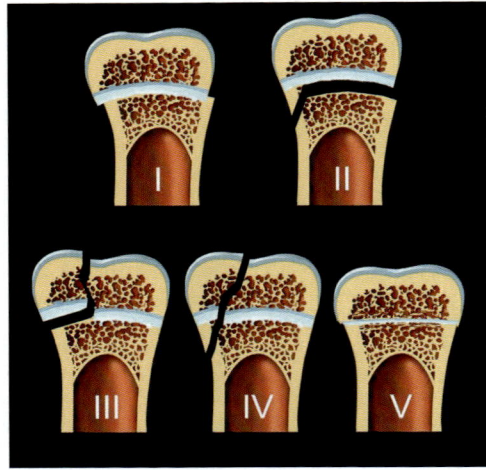

Graphic shows the relationship of the epiphyseal, physeal, and metaphyseal components of the 5 types of Salter-Harris fractures.

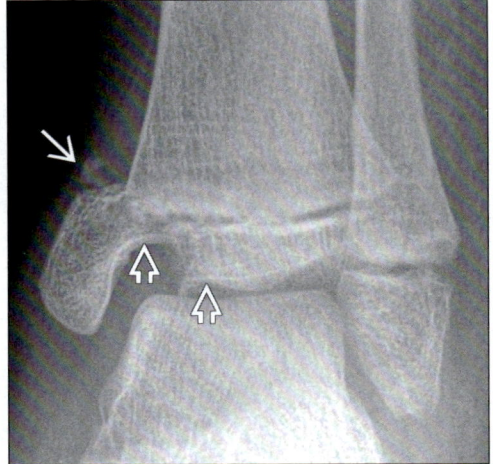

Anteroposterior radiograph shows Salter-Harris type IV fracture. Fracture traverses epiphysis ➡, physis, and metaphysis. A small metaphyseal fragment ➡ is also present.

TERMINOLOGY

Abbreviations and Synonyms
- Salter-Harris fractures
- Salter fractures

Definitions
- Immature-skeleton fractures affecting physis

IMAGING FINDINGS

General Features
- Location
  - Incidence of various physeal fractures in children's hospital population (percent of all physeal fractures)
  - Upper extremity
    - Distal radius: 28%
    - Fingers: 26%
    - Distal humerus: 7%
    - Proximal radius: 5%
    - Distal ulna: 5%
    - Metacarpals: 4%
    - Proximal humerus: 2%
    - Clavicle: 1%
    - Proximal ulna: 1%
  - Lower extremity
    - Distal tibia: 9%
    - Toes: 7%
    - Distal fibula: 3%
    - Metatarsals: 1%
    - Proximal tibia: 1%
    - Distal femur: 1%

Radiographic Findings
- Radiography
  - Physeal widening, associated fracture lines within epiphysis and metaphysis
  - If persistent physeal widening (physeal gap) > 3 mm post-reduction, periosteal entrapment in fracture likely
    - Lower tibial fractures: Premature physeal closure rate increases to 17-60% if physeal gap present
    - Requires open reduction to remove trapped periosteum

CT Findings
- Evaluate anatomic extent and degree of displacement

DDx: Complicated Physeal Fractures

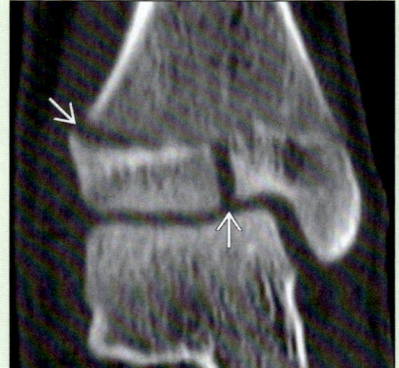

Tillaux

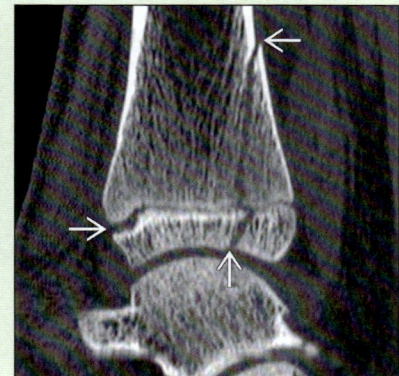

Triplane Sagittal

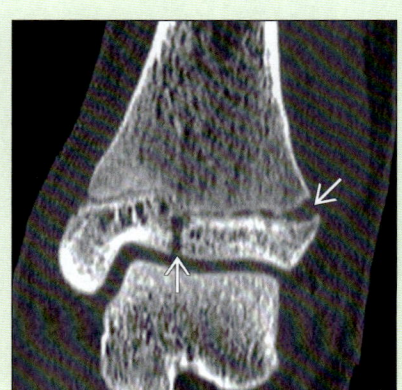

Triplane Coronal

PHYSEAL FRACTURES, PEDIATRIC

Key Facts

Imaging Findings
- Detection of subtle or occult fractures may change Salter-Harris staging and orthopedic management
- Protocol advice: Opposite-side comparison radiographs may help determine whether Salter-Harris type I fracture is present

Top Differential Diagnoses
- Distal radial physis stress injury: Occurs in 17% of gymnasts' wrists

Pathology
- 18% of childhood fractures involve physeal injury
- Causes of distal tibial physeal fractures: Nonspecific fall (25%), skateboard accident (16%), motor vehicle accident (12%), football (12%), soccer (8%)

Clinical Issues
- Percentage of physeal fractures in both boys and girls: 18%
- Overall complication rate: ~14%
- Complications: Premature early or complete epiphyseal closure, limb shortening or angulation, persistently trapped periosteum, joint incongruity
- Most substantial complications occur at knee and ankle
- Prolonged immobilization (3-18 months) may be needed in children with myelodysplasia

Diagnostic Checklist
- Follow knee and ankle fractures for at least a year or until skeletal maturity for early detection of premature closure of epiphyses

---

  - Most commonly used with triplane fractures of distal tibia

MR Findings
- T2WI: Increased edema in surrounding marrow and soft tissues
- May identify physeal fractures in patients evaluated for sports-related injuries or pain
- Detection of subtle or occult fractures may change Salter-Harris staging and orthopedic management
- Cartilage visualization permits immediate recognition of joint-surface incongruity
- Fracture may be seen as low signal line on T1 weighted images extending into region of physis
- Facilitates detection of premature post-traumatic physeal closure
  - Quantification of closure as percentage of physis that is closed

Ultrasonographic Findings
- Evaluation of physeal birth injuries presenting as "pseudodislocation" in long bones with unformed ossification centers
  - Proximal and distal humerus, proximal femur most common

Imaging Recommendations
- Protocol advice: Opposite-side comparison radiographs may help determine whether Salter-Harris type I fracture is present

DIFFERENTIAL DIAGNOSIS

Triplane Fracture of Distal Tibia
- Vertical: Epiphyseal fracture
- Horizontal: Physis cleavage/fracture
- Oblique: Metaphysis fracture
- Frequently requires internal fixation

Tillaux Fracture of Distal Tibia
- Salter-Harris type III fracture of distal tibia
  - Stress through anterior inferior tibio-fibular ligament → avulsion of anterolateral tibial epiphysis (distal anterior tibial tubercle)
  - Forced external rotation of foot in 12-14 year old
  - Open reduction if bone/cartilage gap of > 2 mm on tibial articular surface remains

Stress Injury
- Distal radial physis stress injury: Occurs in 17% of gymnasts' wrists
- Widened physis mimicking Salter-Harris type I fractures
- Metaphyseal irregularity and sclerosis
- May be premature physeal closure or bridge formation
- Physeal cartilage may extend into metaphysis
- Metaphyseal bone bruising

PATHOLOGY

General Features
- General path comments
  - Physis involved in up to 18% of extremity fractures in children
  - Joint capsule and ligamentous structures are stronger than physis in children
    - Ligamentous strain injuries in adults are physeal fractures in children
- Etiology
  - Structure of normal epiphysis
    - Germinal zone closest to epiphyseal ossification center: Small active chondrocytes emerge from resting chondrocytes
    - Proliferative zone: Flattened chondrocytes arranged in columns
    - Hypertrophic zone: Swollen chondrocytes arranged in columns
    - Provisional calcification zone: Chondrocytes die, cartilage matrix calcifies, osteoclasts form osteoid
    - Perichondral ring: Layer of cartilaginous tissue contiguous with adjacent periosteum of metaphysis and epiphysis

PHYSEAL FRACTURES, PEDIATRIC

- Surface of metaphyses' and epiphyses' physeal face is irregular or corrugated: Consists of small bony projections, undulations, knobs and ridges (mammillary processes)
- Metaphysis and epiphysis receive most arterial supply from separate sources: Fracture through physis does not interfere with blood supply of either epiphysis or metaphysis (exception: Femoral capital and radial head epiphyses, which are intra-articular)
○ Structure of physeal fracture
- Damage due to shear, grinding, compression force
- Fracture plane undulates within proliferative, hypertrophic and provisional calcification zones
- Fibrin appears within cleavage, cartilaginous cells continue to grow, epiphyseal plate thickens as cellular columns lengthen
- Fibrin gone and normal growth pattern restored in about 21 days
- Epidemiology
○ 18% of childhood fractures involve physeal injury
○ Relative incidence of Salter-Harris fractures
- Type I: 8.5%
- Type II: 73% (most common)
- Type III: 6.5%
- Type IV: 12%
- Type V: 0% (rarest)
○ Exceptions to general relative incidence
- Distal humerus: Almost all fractures are type IV
- Distal tibia: Types II, III, and IV equally common
○ Causes of distal tibial physeal fractures: Nonspecific fall (25%), skateboard accident (16%), motor vehicle accident (12%), football (12%), soccer (8%)

Staging, Grading or Classification Criteria
- Type I: Involves only physis
- Type II: Involves physis and metaphysis
- Type III: Involves physis and epiphysis
- Type IV: Involves physis, metaphysis, and epiphysis
- Type V: Crush fracture involving all or part of physis (rare)
○ Usually first recognized when cone epiphyses or partial epiphyseal arrest becomes apparent later
- Type VI-IX, as described by Ogden 1981 (rare)
○ Perichondral ring injury (type VI), intra-epiphyseal fracture not involving physis (type VII), metaphysis fracture not involving physis directly but → ischemic growth disturbance (type VIII), periosteal injury → disturbed diaphyseal growth (type IX)

CLINICAL ISSUES

Presentation
- Most common signs/symptoms: Pain, swelling, point tenderness, limited range of motion, inability to bear weight

Demographics
- Age
○ Peak age: 11-12 years
○ Ages 16 and 17: Physeal fractures more common in males; physes have closed in females
- Gender
○ Average age: Girls = 11 years; boys = 12 years
○ Percentage of physeal fractures in both boys and girls: 18%

Natural History & Prognosis
- Overall complication rate: ~14%
- Complications: Premature early or complete epiphyseal closure, limb shortening or angulation, persistently trapped periosteum, joint incongruity
- Most substantial complications occur at knee and ankle
- Prognosis worse in lower extremities regardless of Salter-Harris classification
- Premature epiphyseal closure in lower tibial fractures
○ 27% overall rate
○ 21% in triplane fractures, rare in Tillaux fractures

Treatment
- Casting for low Salter-Harris categories
- Open reduction and internal fixation often required with higher categories
- Prolonged immobilization (3-18 months) may be needed in children with myelodysplasia

DIAGNOSTIC CHECKLIST

Consider
- Follow knee and ankle fractures for at least a year or until skeletal maturity for early detection of premature closure of epiphyses

SELECTED REFERENCES

1. Craig JG et al: The distal femoral and proximal tibial growth plates: MR imaging, three-dimensional modeling and estimation of area and volume. Skeletal Radiol. 33(6):337-44, 2004
2. Swischuk LE et al: Frequently missed fractures in children (value of comparative views). Emerg Radiol. 11(1):22-8, 2004
3. Barmada A et al: Premature physeal closure following distal tibia physeal fractures: a new radiographic predictor. J Pediatr Orthop. 23(6):733-9, 2003
4. Ecklund K et al: Patterns of premature physeal arrest: MR imaging of 111 children. AJR Am J Roentgenol. 178(4):967-72, 2002
5. Koury SI et al: Recognition and management of Tillaux fractures in adolescents. Pediatr Emerg Care. 15(1):37-9, 1999
6. Carey J et al: MRI of pediatric growth plate injury: correlation with plain film radiographs and clinical outcome. Skeletal Radiol. 27(5):250-5, 1998
7. Rodgers WB et al: Chronic physeal fractures in myelodysplasia: magnetic resonance analysis, histologic description, treatment, and outcome. J Pediatr Orthop. 17(5):615-21, 1997
8. Shih C et al: Chronically stressed wrists in adolescent gymnasts: MR imaging appearance. Radiology. 195(3):855-9, 1995
9. Rogers LF et al: Imaging of epiphyseal injuries. Radiology. 191(2):297-308, 1994
10. Ogden JA: Injury to the growth mechanisms of the immature skeleton. Skeletal Radiol. 6(4):237-53, 1981
11. Salter RB et al: Injuries involving the epiphyseal plate. J Bone Joint Surg Am. 45:587-622, 1963

PHYSEAL FRACTURES, PEDIATRIC

IMAGE GALLERY

Typical

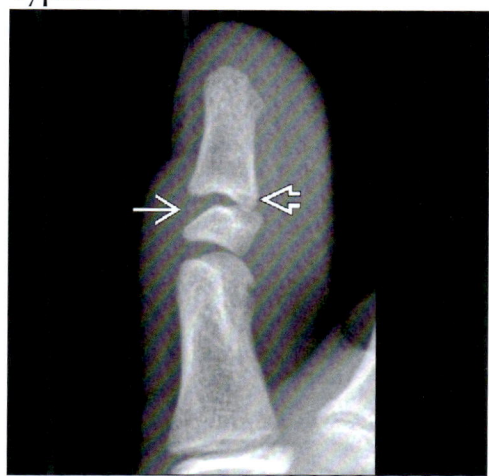
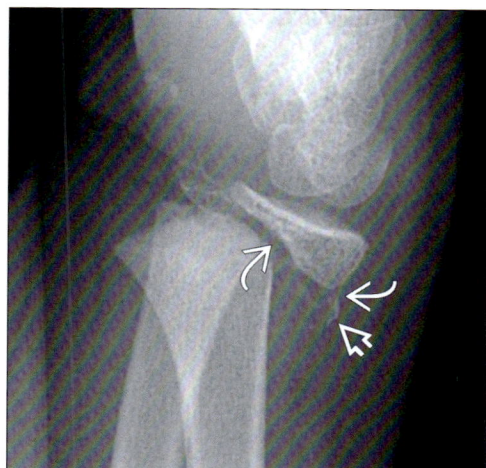

(Left) Oblique radiograph shows Salter-Harris type I fracture of distal phalanx of hallux. The space between epiphysis and diaphysis is widened ➡, with slight bony offset ➡. *(Right)* Lateral radiograph shows a Salter-Harris type II distal radius fracture. The fracture traverses physis ➡ and metaphysis, leaving a small metaphyseal fragment ➡.

Typical

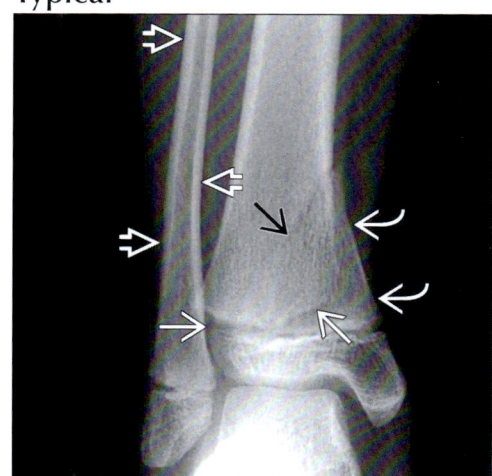
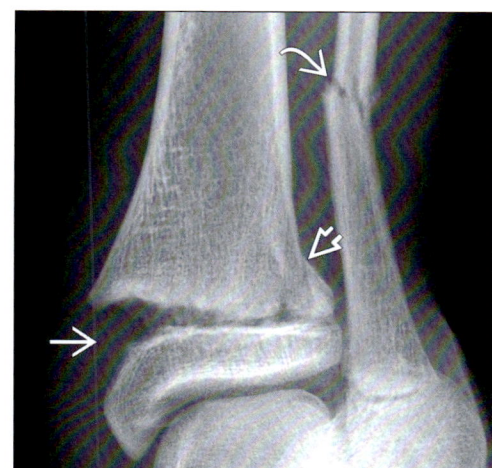

(Left) Anteroposterior radiograph shows Salter-Harris type II fracture traversing physis ➡ and metaphysis ➡, and breaking off large metaphyseal fragment ➡. Plastic bowing fibular fracture ➡ also present. *(Right)* Oblique radiograph shows Salter-Harris type II fracture involving physis ➡ and metaphysis ➡. Fibular diaphyseal fracture ➡ is also seen.

Typical

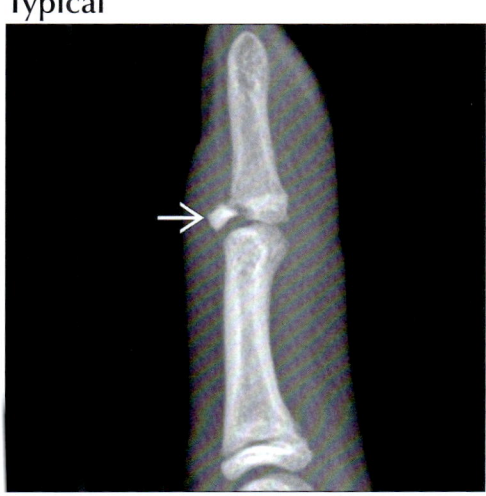
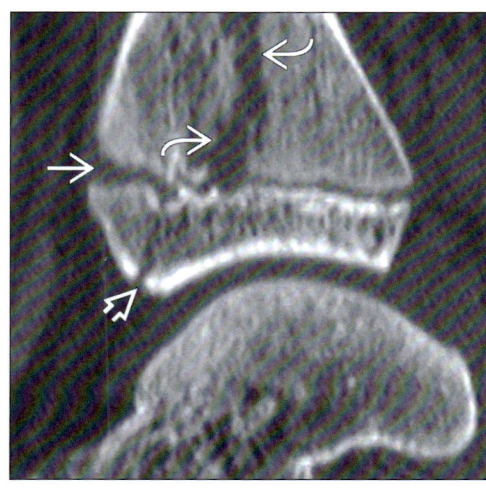

(Left) Lateral radiograph shows a Salter-Harris type III fracture ➡ of epiphysis and physis of terminal phalanx. *(Right)* Sagittal NECT shows Salter-Harris type IV tibial fracture. The fracture runs through metaphysis ➡, physis ➡, and epiphysis ➡.

CHILD ABUSE, METAPHYSEAL FRACTURE

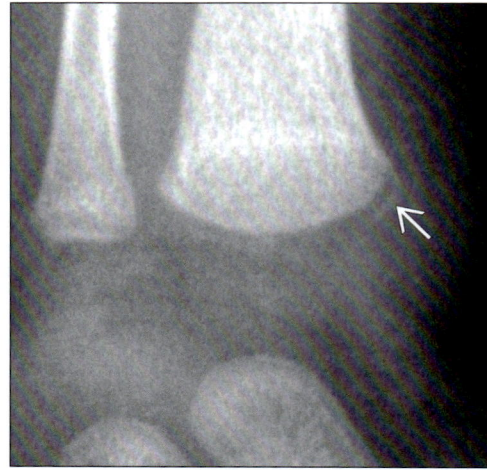

Oblique radiograph shows distal tibial metaphyseal fracture ➔ with features of both corner & bucket handle fractures: At a corner, has circumferential length.

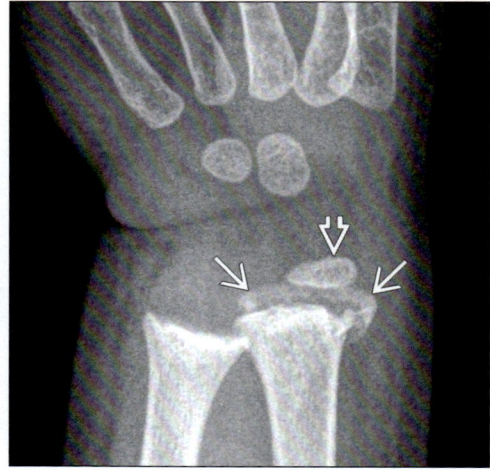

Anteroposterior radiograph of wrist shows bucket handle fracture ➔ with accompanying lateral offset of distal radial ossification center ➔.

TERMINOLOGY

Abbreviations and Synonyms
- Child abuse: Nonaccidental trauma, battered child syndrome
- Metaphyseal corner fracture; metaphyseal lesion; bucket-handle fracture; metaphyseal infraction; avulsion fracture; metaphyseal flag

Definitions
- Injury of a child by violent act of another human being
  - Shaken, squeezed, jerked, twisted, punched, burned, bitten, punctured, and/or thrown
  - Abuse may be psychologically devastating, but this is not an indication for imaging
  - Perpetrators usually have parental or parent-like relationship to child
  - Confession by perpetrator is rare, so mechanism of injury usually is not known

IMAGING FINDINGS

General Features
- Best diagnostic clue: Bucket-handle fracture on radiographs
- Location
  - Metaphyses of long bones
  - Most common in lower femur, upper and lower tibia, upper humerus
- Size: Often subtle

Radiographic Findings
- Radiography
  - Metaphyseal corner fractures highly specific for child abuse
    - Triangular bit of bone seen at corner of metaphysis close to physis
    - May be subtle prior to callus formation
  - Radiographic appearance depends upon angle at which fractured metaphyseal rim visualized
    - If viewed tangential to plane of physis, fracture will appear as corner fracture
    - If viewed obliquely, corner fracture may turn into bucket-handle fracture

DDx: Diseases with Multiple Fractures or Fracture-Like Appearance

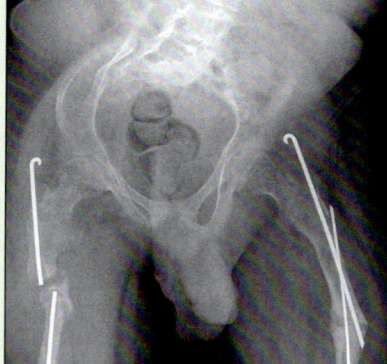
Osteogenesis Imperfecta

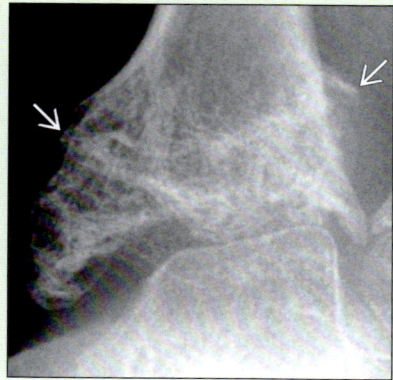
Spondylometaphyseal Dysplasia

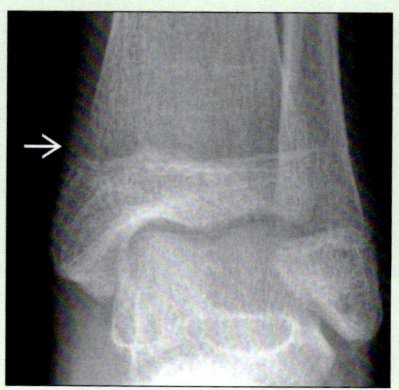
Leukemia

CHILD ABUSE, METAPHYSEAL FRACTURE

Key Facts

Imaging Findings
- Best diagnostic clue: Bucket-handle fracture on radiographs
- Metaphyseal corner fractures highly specific for child abuse
- If viewed obliquely, corner fracture may turn into bucket-handle fracture
- Bucket-handle fractures similar to corner fractures, but involve more of metaphyseal circumference
- Other fractures highly specific for child abuse in infants: Rib, scapula, spinous process, sternum, metaphysis
- Bone scintigraphy extremely helpful in first week post-injury: Shows areas of subperiosteal hemorrhage before subperiosteal new bone may become visible
- Scintigraphy excellent for detecting rib fractures
- Radiographs superior to scintigraphy for finding metaphyseal and skull fractures
- When abuse suspected, obtain skeletal survey to document abuse findings for legal means to remove child from abuser
- Repeat skeletal survey in two weeks to identify healing, previously occult fractures and subperiosteal new bone formation

Top Differential Diagnoses
- Osteogenesis Imperfecta
- Rickets
- Myelomeningocele
- Leukemia

Clinical Issues
- Most children < 1 year old at presentation

- Bucket-handle fractures similar to corner fractures, but involve more of metaphyseal circumference
  - Bucket-handle fracture may be seen when metaphysis viewed obliquely to plane of epiphysis
  - Will appear as one or two corner fractures if X-ray beam is parallel to physis
  - Crescentic or annular rim of bone from metaphysis just underneath "periosteal collar" where cortical bone is resorbed as part of bone remodeling during growth
  - May be seen only as corner fracture when X-ray beam is in plane of epiphysis
- Other bone fractures
  - Other fractures highly specific for child abuse in infants: Rib, scapula, spinous process, sternum, metaphysis
  - Moderately specific for child abuse in infants/children: Multiple fractures (especially bilateral); fractures of different ages; epiphyseal separations; vertebral-body fractures; finger fractures; complex skull fractures
  - Common but low specificity: Subperiosteal new bone formation; clavicular, long-bone diaphysis, and linear skull fractures
  - Spiral femoral fractures before walking

CT Findings
- Rib and lung injuries
- Liver, spleen, pancreas injury
- Duodenal hematoma
- Bowel rupture
- Subdural hematoma

MR Findings
- Brain injury
  - Shaken baby syndrome

Ultrasonographic Findings
- Grayscale Ultrasound
  - Subdural hematoma
  - Intracerebral hemorrhage
  - Liver, spleen, kidney, and pancreas injury
  - Duodenal hematoma

Nuclear Medicine Findings
- Bone scintigraphy extremely helpful in first week post-injury: Shows areas of subperiosteal hemorrhage before subperiosteal new bone may become visible
  - Scintigraphy excellent for detecting rib fractures
  - Difficult in regions of physes as these are normally high in activity
  - Radiographs better for skull fractures and metaphyseal fractures

Imaging Recommendations
- Best imaging tool
  - Skeletal survey using radiographs
  - Radiographs superior to scintigraphy for finding metaphyseal and skull fractures
- Protocol advice
  - When abuse suspected, obtain skeletal survey to document abuse findings for legal means to remove child from abuser
  - Identification and reporting of radiographic findings of abuse is important task
  - False-positive findings may result in removal of nonabused child from family
  - False-negative findings may result in returning child to dangerous environment
- Other tests that may be used to document findings of abuse
  - Repeat skeletal survey in two weeks to identify healing, previously occult fractures and subperiosteal new bone formation
  - Skeletal scintigraphy
  - Abdominal and chest CT
  - Brain MR

DIFFERENTIAL DIAGNOSIS

Osteogenesis Imperfecta
- Multiple fractures, wormian bones

CHILD ABUSE, METAPHYSEAL FRACTURE

Rickets
- Metaphyseal irregularity and fractures, subperiosteal new bone formation

Congenital Indifference to Pain
- Metaphyseal injuries common

Myelomeningocele
- Metaphyseal injuries in leg bones due to decreased pain sensation

Leukemia
- Metaphyseal fractures due to osteopenia, subperiosteal new bone formation

Menkes Syndrome
- Osteopenia, metaphyseal fractures, Wormian bones

Spondylometaphyseal (SM) Dysplasia
- Metaphyseal irregularities resembling corner fractures due to abnormal endochondral ossification

Metaphyseal Chondrodysplasia
- Metaphyseal irregularities resembling corner fractures due to abnormal endochondral ossification

PATHOLOGY

General Features
- General path comments
  - Metaphyseal corner fractures
    - Occur in plane of physis
    - Extend though primary spongiosa of metaphysis
    - Weakest area of bone; most prone to fracture
    - Thought to be 2° forceful twisting or shaking of extremity
    - Ring-like configuration along metaphyseal edge; radiographic appearance depends upon angle at which fracture is visualized
  - Bucket-handle fractures: Crescentic or annular rim of bone from metaphysis just underneath "periosteal collar" where cortical bone is resorbed as part of bone remodeling during growth
  - Subperiosteal new bone: Response to subperiosteal hemorrhage
    - May be seen in 5-14 days after trauma
    - May be seen in femur, tibia, humerus, forearm of normal infants
    - Usually thin and bilateral
- Epidemiology
  - Estimated more than 1 million children seriously injured and 5,000 murdered annually 2° abuse in USA alone
  - 30% of fractures in infants are 2° abuse
  - Rib fractures most common from birth to 18 months
  - Skull fractures most common in children over 1 year, compared to those less than one year

Microscopic Features
- Child's bones weakest at metaphyseal-physeal chondro-osseous junction
  - Vascular invasion of zone of hypertrophic chondrocytes occurring

CLINICAL ISSUES

Presentation
- Most common signs/symptoms
  - Clinically occult without symptoms
  - Apnea, seizures, fussiness
    - Retinal hemorrhages in shaken babies
  - Bruises
    - Bruises on buttocks, back, genitals, back of hands
  - Cigarette burns; scald burns from immersion in hot water
- Other signs/symptoms
  - Cause of death
    - Brain injury most common cause of death
    - Intra-abdominal injury second most common

Demographics
- Age
  - Most children < 1 year old at presentation
  - Almost all children < 6 years of age
  - Rib fractures, metaphyseal injuries common in first year
    - Average age 4 months
  - Long-bone diaphyseal fractures most common after first year

Treatment
- Recognition that child has been abused is keystone
- Documentation of abuse
- Removal of child from hostile environment
- Postmortem imaging may be vital to future protection of siblings

SELECTED REFERENCES

1. Mandelstam SA et al: Complementary use of radiological skeletal survey and bone scintigraphy in detection of bony injuries in suspected child abuse. Arch Dis Child. 88(5):387-90; discussion 387-90, 2003
2. Boal DK: Metaphyseal fractures. Pediatr Radiol. 32(7):538-9, 2002
3. Kleinman PK et al: A regional approach to the classic metaphyseal lesion in abused infants: the distal femur. AJR Am J Roentgenol. 170(1):43-7, 1998
4. Kleinman PK et al: A regional approach to classic metaphyseal lesions in abused infants: the distal tibia. AJR Am J Roentgenol. 166(5):1207-12, 1996
5. Kleinman PK et al: A regional approach to the classic metaphyseal lesion in abused infants: the proximal humerus. AJR Am J Roentgenol. 167(6):1399-403, 1996
6. Kleinman PK et al: A regional approach to the classic metaphyseal lesion in abused infants: the proximal tibia. AJR Am J Roentgenol. 166(2):421-6, 1996
7. Kleinman PK et al: Follow-up skeletal surveys in suspected child abuse. AJR Am J Roentgenol. 167(4):893-6, 1996
8. Kleinman PK et al: Inflicted skeletal injury: a postmortem radiologic-histopathologic study in 31 infants. AJR Am J Roentgenol. 165(3):647-50, 1995
9. Kleinman PK et al: Relationship of the subperiosteal bone collar to metaphyseal lesions in abused infants. J Bone Joint Surg Am. 77(10):1471-6, 1995

CHILD ABUSE, METAPHYSEAL FRACTURE

IMAGE GALLERY

Typical

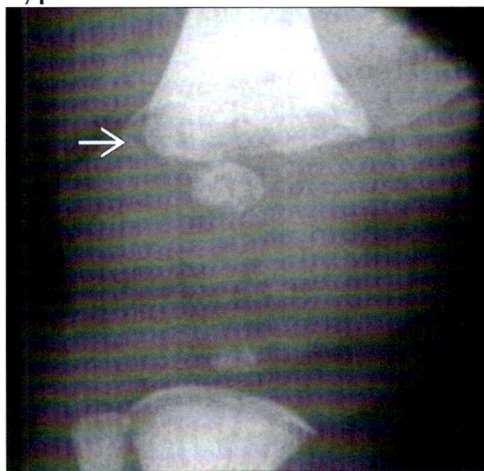
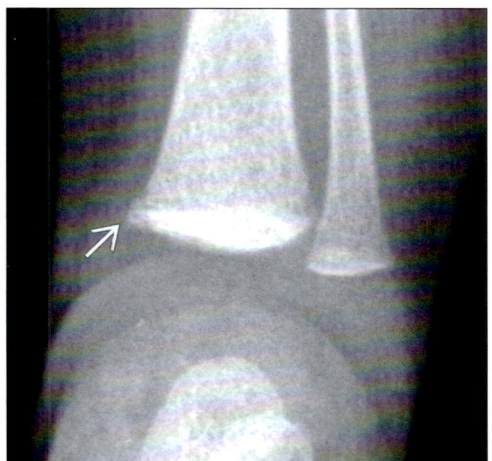

(Left) Anteroposterior radiograph of knee shows bucket handle fracture ➡ of femur. This will become more conspicuous in 10 days after callus is formed. *(Right)* Anteroposterior radiograph of ankle shows subtle metaphyseal corner fracture ➡ of tibia. Subsequently, periosteal reaction will be visible in this area.

Typical

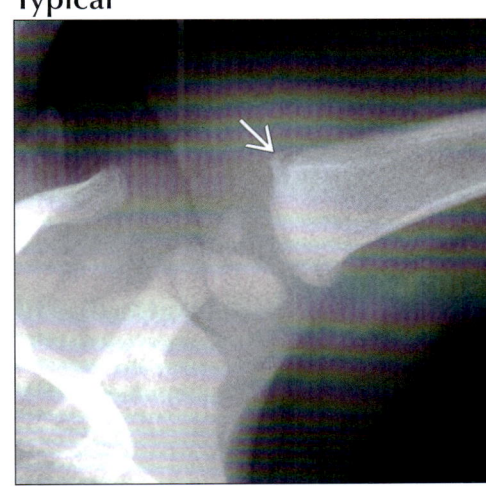
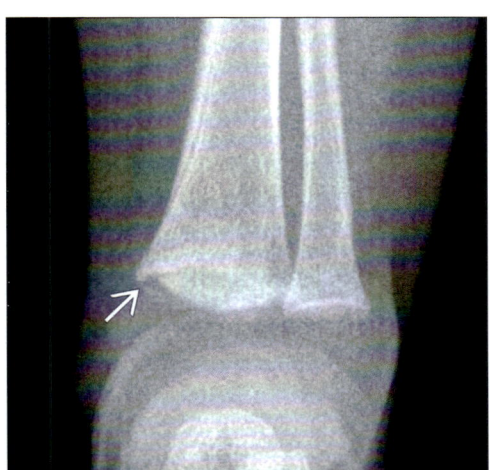

(Left) Anteroposterior radiograph shows metaphyseal corner fracture ➡ of humerus. Proximal humerus and distal radius are common sites for metaphyseal fractures in the upper extremity. *(Right)* Anteroposterior radiograph of the ankle shows a metaphyseal fracture of the tibia ➡.

Typical

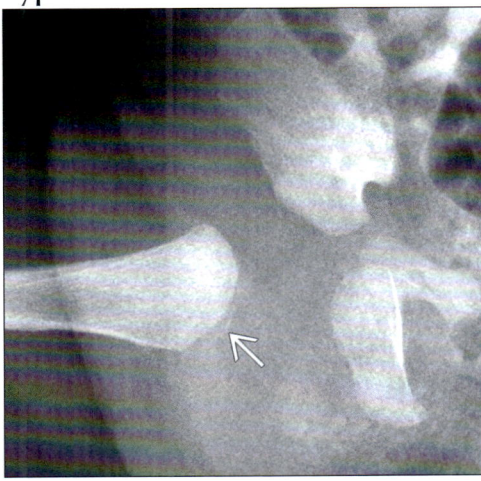
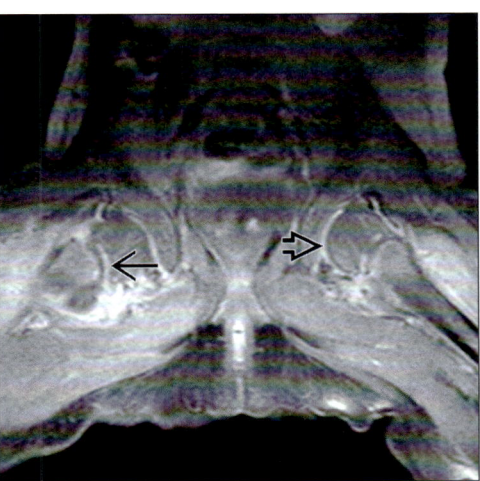

(Left) Frog lateral radiograph of hip shows femoral metaphyseal fracture ➡. This subtle finding gives only a hint of the injuries revealed by the MR study. *(Right)* Coronal T1 C+ FS MR in same infant as previous image, shows capital physeal fracture ➡ of right femur, as well as traumatic synovitis ➡ with bone and soft tissue injury on left.

INCOMPLETE FRACTURES, PEDIATRIC

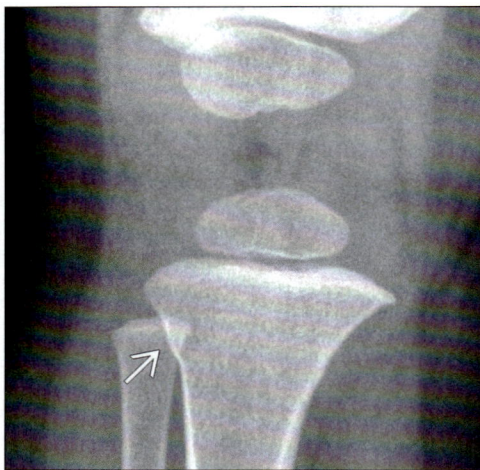
Anteroposterior radiograph shows a buckle fracture ➡ of tibial metaphysis.

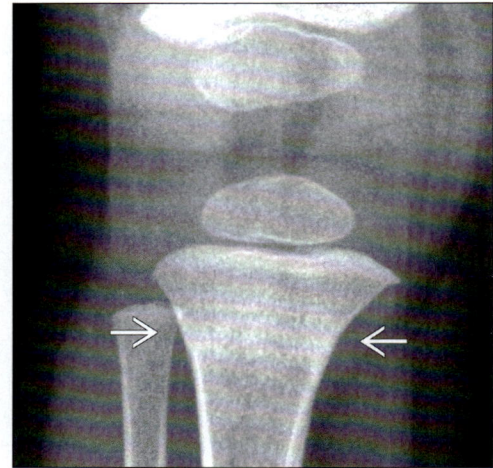
Anteroposterior radiograph 25 days later in the same child as previous image, shows sclerotic band ➡ due to microtrabecular callus.

TERMINOLOGY

Abbreviations and Synonyms
- Buckle, torus, greenstick, plastic bowing, plastic bending, toddler, impaction, stress, and hairline fractures

Definitions
- Pediatric bones are more elastic than adult bone, greater propensity to bow or bend before breaking
- Incomplete fracture: Does not involve entire circumference
  - Buckle fractures
    - Buckle fracture: Bone cortex bulges out or in on compression side; cortex usually intact on tension side
    - Bone cortex folds either in or out when buckles
    - Buckled in (concave): "Buckle fracture" or "angle buckle fracture"
    - Buckled out (convex): "Buckle fracture", also may be termed "torus fracture"
  - Plastic bending fractures: Bone bent without cortical deformity or visible fracture line
  - Greenstick fractures
    - Plastic bowing fracture variant: One or several incomplete fractures occur on tension side
    - Appearance of bending a "green stick"
  - Impaction fractures: Due to longitudinal compression
  - Hairline fractures: Tiny fractures close to limit of system's resolution
  - Stress fractures
    - Incomplete fracture initially due to repetitive stress; either invisible or hairline at onset of symptoms
    - May progress to complete fracture
  - Toddler fractures
    - Incomplete lower extremity fracture without known trauma in young child who recently began to walk
  - Salter-Harris physeal fractures types II-IV not considered incomplete fractures because joint and physeal involvement demands different orthopedic management

DDx: Bent Bones

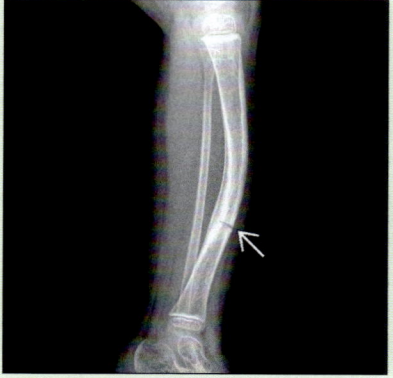
Osteogenesis Imperfecta

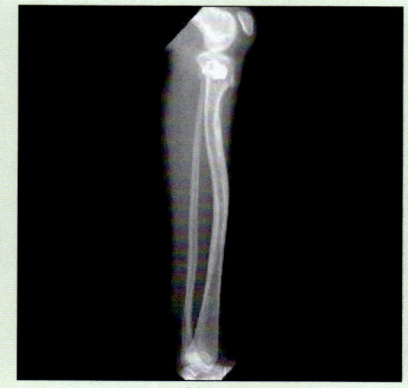
Neurofibromatosis

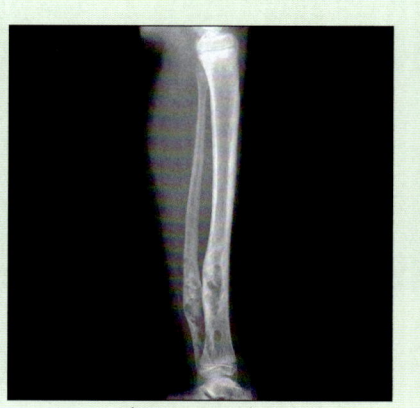
Fibrous Dysplasia

INCOMPLETE FRACTURES, PEDIATRIC

Key Facts

Terminology
- Incomplete fracture: Does not involve entire circumference
- Buckle fracture: Bone cortex bulges out or in on compression side; cortex usually intact on tension side
- Plastic bending fractures: Bone bent without cortical deformity or visible fracture line
- Plastic bowing fracture variant: One or several incomplete fractures occur on tension side

Imaging Findings
- Monteggia-equivalent fracture: Bending fracture of ulna with anterior dislocation of radial head
- Plastic bending fractures may be subtle: Comparison views of contralateral bones may assist diagnosis
- Often accompanied by complete or plastic bending fracture of companion bone in forearm and lower leg
- Bone scan shows increased uptake in all incomplete fractures including plastic bending
- Best imaging tool: Radiographs
- Comparison radiographs of opposite normal side may assist in evaluation of subtle fractures

Pathology
- Absorption of fracture energy may occur along length of immature bone → plastic bowing and greenstick fractures

Clinical Issues
- Decreased range of pronation-supination in plastic bending forearm fractures

IMAGING FINDINGS

General Features
- Best diagnostic clue: Cortical bump or angulation at site of pain or injury
- Location
  - Buckle fractures
    - Most often in humerus, radius, ulna, carpal scaphoid, metacarpals, fingers, tibia, fibula, metatarsals, toes
  - Plastic bending fractures
    - Most common in radius, ulna, clavicle, fibula
    - Also reported in neonatal femur
    - Monteggia-equivalent fracture: Bending fracture of ulna with anterior dislocation of radial head
    - Slow to remodel if untreated, especially in older children
  - Greenstick fractures
    - Most common in forearm
  - Impaction fractures
    - Type-II toddler fracture in tibia, cuboid, carpal scaphoid
  - Hairline fractures
    - Small bones of hands and feet, tibial diaphysis, tibial proximal metaphysis, proximal ulna
  - Stress fractures
    - Most common in legs and feet
  - Toddler fractures
    - Found in legs and feet

Radiographic Findings
- Radiography
  - Buckle fracture
    - Angular deformity or buckle of cortex
    - Found on cortical side subjected to compression
    - Subtle angulation may be seen at buckle site
  - Plastic bending fracture
    - Typically in midshaft of bones
    - Most common in radius and ulna
    - Plastic bending fractures may be subtle: Comparison views of contralateral bones may assist diagnosis
    - Often accompanied by complete or plastic bending fracture of companion bone in forearm and lower leg
    - Periosteal reaction absent during recovery (neonates may be exception)
    - Rarely occurs in adults
  - Greenstick fracture
    - Visible hairline (or larger) fractures in convex cortical side subjected to tension; bone and periosteum intact on concave (compression) side

CT Findings
- NECT: Useful if physeal fracture suspected or evaluating area of sclerosis in setting of unclear subacute fracture

MR Findings
- Useful if physeal fracture suspected

Nuclear Medicine Findings
- Bone Scan
  - Bone scan shows increased uptake in all incomplete fractures including plastic bending
    - Increased osteoblastic activity

Imaging Recommendations
- Best imaging tool: Radiographs
- Protocol advice
  - Comparison radiographs of opposite normal side may assist in evaluation of subtle fractures
    - Can be helpful in plastic bending fractures
    - Contralateral views not recommended as part of routine imaging

DIFFERENTIAL DIAGNOSIS

Bone Bending Due to Skeletal Disease
- Bone dysplasia
  - Osteogenesis imperfecta (OI)
  - Fibrous dysplasia
  - Neurofibromatosis, type I
  - Many other dysplasias
- Metabolic bone disease

INCOMPLETE FRACTURES, PEDIATRIC

- Hyperparathyroidism
- Hyperphosphatemia
- Hypophosphatasia
- Rickets

Normal Variation
- Comparison views may be helpful

PATHOLOGY

General Features
- General path comments
  - Developing skeleton is more elastic, less brittle than adult bone
    - Absorption of fracture energy may occur along length of immature bone → plastic bowing and greenstick fractures
- Etiology
  - Plastic bending fractures: Axial load on long bone
  - Scaphoid impaction fracture: Fall on hyperextended wrist
  - Buckle fractures: Angular loading, often with rotational component

Microscopic Features
- Torus fracture
  - Periosteum intact but variably elevated 2° subperiosteal hemorrhage
  - Cortical fracture propagates through vascular foramina
  - Longitudinal splits along osteoid seams
- Greenstick and plastic bending fractures
  - Splitting and widening of developing Haversian system
  - Compressive distortion along osteoid seams

CLINICAL ISSUES

Presentation
- Most common signs/symptoms
  - Pain, swelling, tenderness
  - Refusal to walk
- Decreased range of pronation-supination in plastic bending forearm fractures

Natural History & Prognosis
- Usually complete healing
- Development of small subperiosteal post-traumatic cortical defects in radius is rare phenomenon
  - 1-10 months post-injury
  - Usually in cortex which was compressed during injury
  - MR signal consistent with blood or fat in defect
- Remodeling corrects angular bone deformities, may not correct rotational deformities
- Greenstick fracture: Median nerve entrapment and transection may occur

Treatment
- Immobilization (casting)
- Most heal without internal fixation
- Manipulation of plastic bending forearm fractures to restore full range of pronation-supination
  - Normal range: Supination is 80-120° from neutral; pronation is 50-80° from neutral

DIAGNOSTIC CHECKLIST

Image Interpretation Pearls
- Ball-bearing rule: Imagine a ball bearing rolling down bone's surface on radiograph; if bearing bounces, positive for buckle fracture

SELECTED REFERENCES

1. Sai S et al: Radial head dislocation with acute plastic bowing of the ulna. J Orthop Sci. 10(1):103-7, 2005
2. Swischuk LE et al: Frequently missed fractures in children (value of comparative views). Emerg Radiol. 11(1):22-8, 2004
3. Hernandez JA et al: The angled buckle fracture in pediatrics: a frequently missed fracture. Emerg Radiol. 10(2):71-5, 2003
4. Hernandez JA et al: Scaphoid (navicular) fractures of the wrist in children: attention to the impacted buckle fracture. Emerg Radiol. 9(6):305-8, 2002
5. Roach RT et al: Paediatric post-traumatic cortical defects of the distal radius. Pediatr Radiol. 32(5):333-9, 2002
6. Proubasta IR et al: Entrapment of the median nerve in a greenstick forearm fracture. A case report and review of the literature. Bull Hosp Jt Dis. 58(4):220-3, 1999
7. Noonan KJ et al: Forearm and distal radius fractures in children. J Am Acad Orthop Surg. 6(3):146-56, 1998
8. Sclamberg J et al: Acute plastic bowing deformation of the forearm in an adult. AJR Am J Roentgenol. 170(5):1259-60, 1998
9. Wass AR et al: Cortical bone cyst following a greenstick radial fracture. J Accid Emerg Med. 13(1):63-4, 1996
10. Ogden JA et al: The pathology of acute chondro-osseous injury in the child. Yale J Biol Med. 66(3):219-33, 1993
11. Gordon L et al: Acute plastic deformation of the ulna in a skeletally mature individual. J Hand Surg [Am]. 16(3):451-3, 1991
12. Aponte JE Jr et al: Acute plastic bowing deformity: a review of the literature. J Emerg Med. 7(2):181-4, 1989
13. Zionts LE et al: Plastic bowing of the femur in a neonate. J Pediatr Orthop. 4(6):749-51, 1984
14. Miller JH et al: Scintigraphy in acute plastic bowing of the forearm. Radiology. 142(3):742, 1982
15. Martin W 3rd et al: Acute plastic bowing fractures of the fibula. Radiology. 131(3):639-40, 1979
16. Borden S 4th: Roentgen recognition of acute plastic bowing of the forearm in children. Am J Roentgenol Radium Ther Nucl Med. 125(3):524-30, 1975

INCOMPLETE FRACTURES, PEDIATRIC

IMAGE GALLERY

Typical

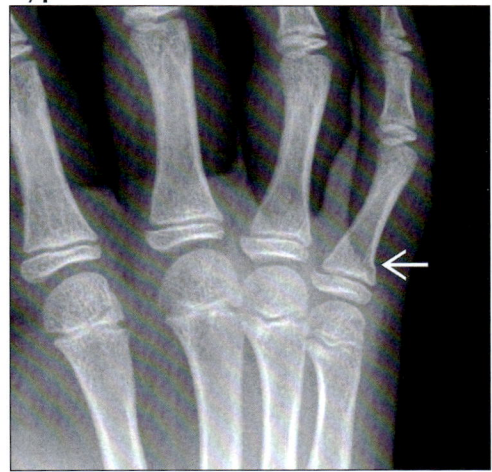
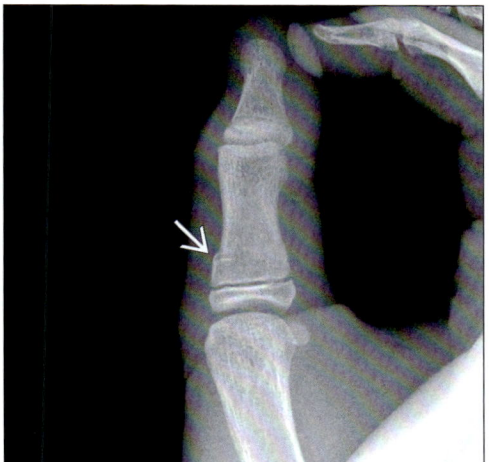

(Left) Anteroposterior radiograph shows buckle fracture ➡ of proximal phalanx of little finger. Such subtle fractures often are only seen on one radiograph. Also, they may be multiple. *(Right)* Oblique radiograph shows a buckle fracture ➡ of proximal phalanx of thumb. Watch for occurrence of osteomyelitis if there is a skin laceration.

Typical

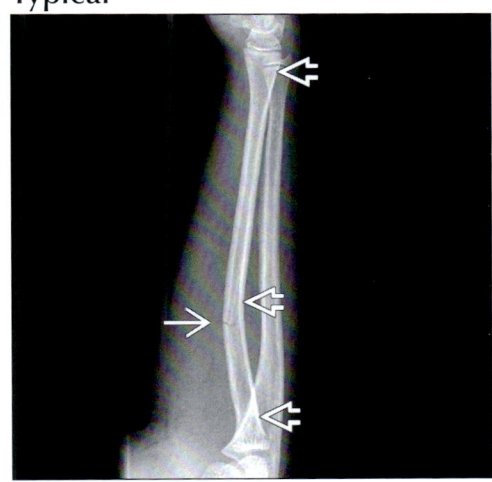
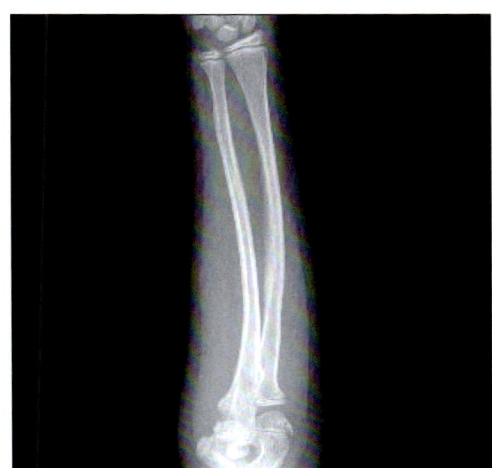

(Left) Lateral radiograph shows greenstick fracture of radius with both a plastic bowing fracture ➡ and incomplete hairline fracture ➡ on tension side of bowing. In the lower leg, a fibular plastic bowing fracture often accompanies a transverse tibial fracture. *(Right)* Anteroposterior radiograph shows plastic bowing fracture of both radius and ulna. Pronation and supination are limited in such cases.

Typical

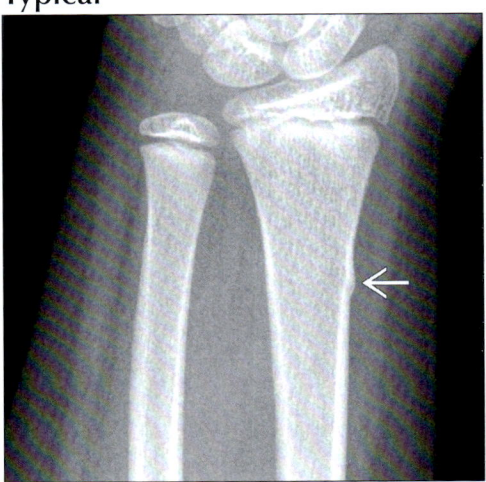
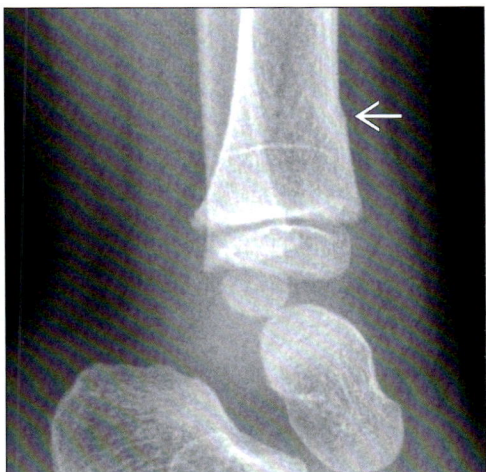

(Left) Anteroposterior radiograph shows a buckle fracture ➡ of radius. A ball bearing rolling down radius would "bounce" here. The osseous base of a small osteochondroma can resemble a buckle fracture. *(Right)* Lateral radiograph shows buckle fracture ➡ of tibia. A ball bearing rolling down the anterior surface of the tibia would bounce at the cortical buckle.

SUPRACONDYLAR FRACTURE, PEDIATRIC

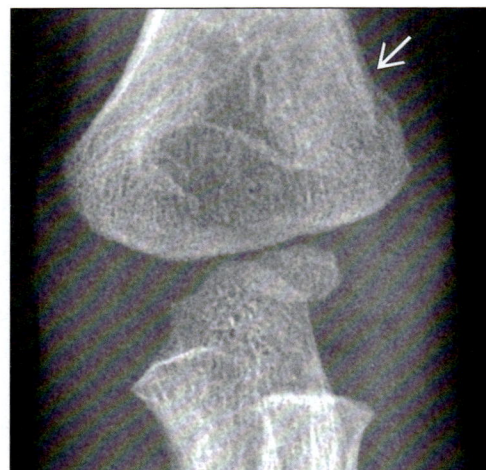

Anteroposterior radiograph shows a lateral cortical buckle fracture ➡. Child's lateral radiograph is on your right.

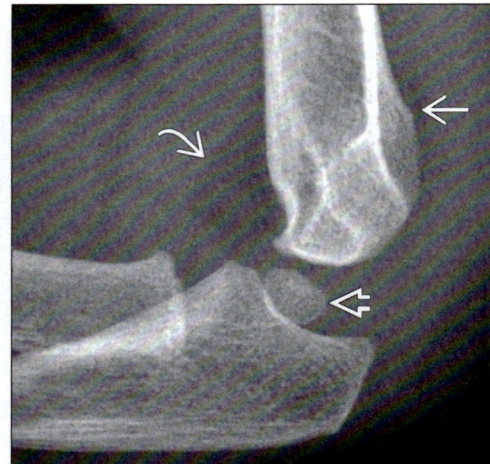

Lateral radiograph shows type I extension fracture with cortical buckle ➡, anterior fat pad sign ➡, and posterior displacement of capitellum ➡ relative to anterior humeral line.

TERMINOLOGY

Abbreviations and Synonyms
- Gartland fracture

Definitions
- Transverse fracture of distal humerus from a bending force usually in hyperextension
- Often due to fall on outstretched arm

IMAGING FINDINGS

General Features
- Best diagnostic clue
  - Radiographs
    - Positive fat pad sign
    - Transverse metaphyseal lucency (fracture line)
    - Mid-capitellum not crossed by anterior humeral line
  - Linear decreased signal intensity surrounded by edema on PD FSE/T2WI of supracondylar humerus
- Location
  - Thin distal humerus at risk between olecranon and coronoid fossae
  - Extraarticular in children
- Size: Involves entire distal humerus above condylar epiphyses
- Morphology
  - Plastic deformity of distal humerus
  - Posterior angulation/displacement usually
  - Fracture line angles from anterior distal to posterior proximal

Radiographic Findings
- Radiography
  - Fracture line in metaphysis on anteroposterior (AP) or angled AP view
  - Fracture line may not be visible in up to 25%
  - Positive fat pad sign on lateral view
  - Anterior humeral line projects anterior to middle third of capitellum in 94%
    - Anterior humeral line: Line that is drawn along anterior cortex of humerus normally bisects the capitellum

DDx: Supracondylar Fracture

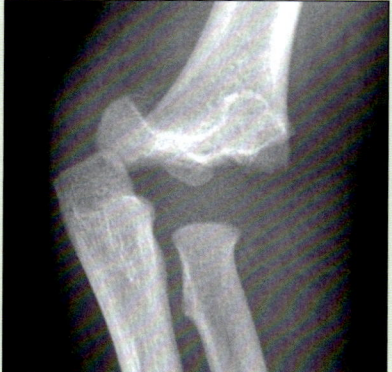
Fracture-Dislocation

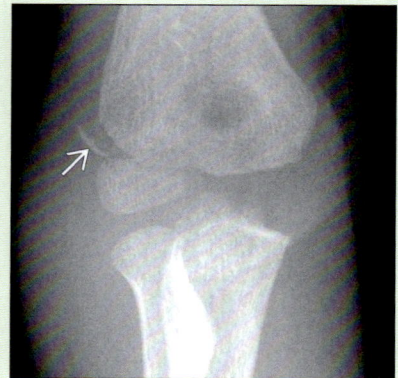
Lateral Condyle

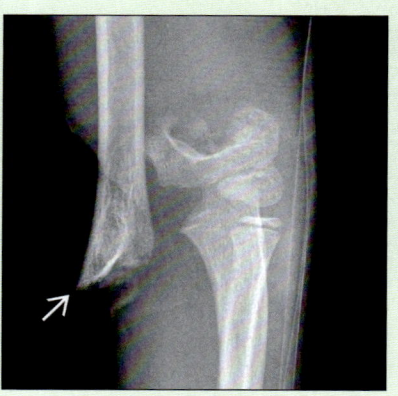
Open Fracture

SUPRACONDYLAR FRACTURE, PEDIATRIC

Key Facts

Terminology
- Gartland fracture
- Transverse fracture of distal humerus from a bending force usually in hyperextension

Imaging Findings
- Mid-capitellum not crossed by anterior humeral line
- Fracture line in metaphysis on anteroposterior (AP) or angled AP view
- Fracture line may not be visible in up to 25%
- Positive fat pad sign on lateral view
- Anterior humeral line projects anterior to middle third of capitellum in 94%

Top Differential Diagnoses
- Lateral Condylar Fracture

- T-condylar = supracondylar with intraarticular extension

Pathology
- Extension injury more common (95% of cases) than flexion type
- Type I: Nondisplaced fracture (30%)
- Type II: Displaced but intact posterior cortex (24%)
- Type III: Displaced plus complete cortical disruption (45%)

Diagnostic Checklist
- Presence of other fractures, especially olecranon and medial epicondyle
- Associated vascular and neural injuries

CT Findings
- NECT: Linear lucencies in distal humeral metaphysis indicating fracture
- CTA: Use to assess vascular injury

MR Findings
- T1WI
  - Decreased marrow signal indicating bone edema
  - Low signal line indicating fracture line
    - Sagittal: ± Fragment rotation/displacement
  - Low-signal joint effusion
- T2WI
  - Increased marrow signal indicating edema
  - FS PD FSE: Visualization improved by using FS
  - High-signal joint effusion
    - ± Periarticular extension of fluid with capsular rupture and vascular injury
  - Low-signal fracture lines surrounded by edema
- STIR
  - Very sensitive for bony injury shown as high signal areas in marrow space
  - Especially useful at mid- and low-field
- T2* GRE
  - Thin slice capability useful for detailed analysis of fragment and adjacent soft tissues
  - Susceptibility decreases utility for detection of edema in bone

Imaging Recommendations
- Best imaging tool: Radiographs

DIFFERENTIAL DIAGNOSIS

Lateral Condylar Fracture
- Fall on an outstretched hand, with impaction of radial head
- Varus stress with elbow flexed/supinated, avulsion by common extensor action
- 17% of distal humerus fractures
- Common in age 5-10 years (peak = 6 years)

Other Distal Humerus Fractures
- Medial epicondyle
  - Varus force on extended arm
- Medial condyle
  - Uncommon; avulsion with forced varus and direct impact on flexed elbow
- T-condylar and lateral epicondyle fractures
  - Less common distal humerus fractures
  - T-condylar = supracondylar with intraarticular extension

Olecranon Fracture
- Fall on a flexed, supinated forearm
- Olecranon epiphysis fuses at 16-18 years
- Direct trauma; throwing injury (pitchers)

Valgus Injury
- Throwing activities
- Includes trabecular injury
- ± Bone trabecular injury of the capitellum
- ± Medial collateral ligament (MCL) tear

Capitellum Osteochondritis Dissecans
- Necrosis of the bone followed by healing response and reossification
- 12-16 year age group (after ossification of capitellum)
- 20% bilateral
- Chronic valgus stress with lateral impaction seen in gymnasts and adolescent pitchers
- Panner disease (age 7-10 years) as an osteochondrosis

Posterior Dislocation
- Ulna and radius displaced proximally
- ± Extensor tendon tear
- ± Fractures: Coronoid, radial head; capitellum
- Lateral ulnar collateral ligament (LUCL) tear common
- LUCL tear, posterolateral rotating instability (PLRI) predisposing
- Supracondylar fracture associated

SUPRACONDYLAR FRACTURE, PEDIATRIC

PATHOLOGY

General Features
- General path comments
  - Extension injury more common (95% of cases) than flexion type
  - Extraarticular in children but may be intraarticular in adults
  - Brachial artery and median nerve are vulnerable to traction over angulated fracture fragment
- Etiology
  - Hyperextension form: Fall onto extended forearm
  - Flexion type: Fall onto point of elbow
- Epidemiology
  - Accounts for about 60% of pediatric elbow fractures
  - Rare in adults (< 3%)
  - Common in nondominant side (1.5:1)
- Associated abnormalities
  - Other elbow fractures, especially olecranon and medial condylar
  - Distal radial fracture (5-6%)
  - Olecranon avulsion fracture; medial condyle impaction
  - Traction injuries to brachial artery (0.5%) and anterior interosseous branch of median nerve (4%)

Gross Pathologic & Surgical Features
- Oblique transverse fracture through thin aspect of distal humerus between medial and lateral pillars
- Failure of anterior cortex (tensile side)
- Plastic deformity of posterior cortex (compression side)
- Posterior rotation; ± varus malalignment

Microscopic Features
- Disruption of cortex and trabeculae
- Hemorrhage with cellular infiltrate ranging from osteoblasts and osteoclasts to inflammatory cells
  - Infiltrate contains osteoblasts, osteoclasts, and inflammatory cells
  - Depends on fracture age

Staging, Grading or Classification Criteria
- Flexion or extension fracture (extension in 96% of fractures)
- Based on classification of Gartland (for extension injuries)
  - Type I: Nondisplaced fracture (30%)
  - Type II: Displaced but intact posterior cortex (24%)
  - Type III: Displaced plus complete cortical disruption (45%)

CLINICAL ISSUES

Presentation
- Most common signs/symptoms
  - Pain and loss of function
  - Swelling and discoloration
  - Decreased distal pulse

Demographics
- Age
  - Common in children < 10 years old
  - Median age of incidence = 6 years
  - Only when seen in non-ambulatory infants are such fractures suggestive of abuse
- Gender: M > F

Natural History & Prognosis
- Return of function in over 90%
- Temporary nerve impairment in 10-16%
- Return of range of motion may take a year
- Neurovascular injuries in displaced supracondylar fractures
  - Anterior interosseous branch of median nerve
  - Radial nerve
  - Brachial artery
- Use of crossed pins may ↑ incidence of nerve injury
- Olecranon osteotomy reduces functional outcome compared to triceps splitting approach to open reduction with internal fixation (ORIF)

Treatment
- Conservative
  - Type I, splinting in 90° flexion
- Surgical
  - Type II and III = percutaneous lateral pin fixation or ORIF with cross pinning
    - ORIF may be needed in up to 20%
- Complications
  - Failure of reduction
  - Vascular injury (rare)
  - Median nerve injury (traumatic and iatrogenic – up to 5%)
  - Volkmann contracture secondary to unrecognized untreated acute vascular injury
  - Cubitus varus most common complication (Baumann angle 2-5° greater than unaffected side)

DIAGNOSTIC CHECKLIST

Consider
- Presence of other fractures, especially olecranon and medial epicondyle
- Associated vascular and neural injuries

SELECTED REFERENCES
1. Pudas T et al: Magnetic resonance imaging in pediatric elbow fractures. Acta Radiol. 46(6):636-44, 2005
2. Gosens T et al: Neurovascular complications and functional outcome in displaced supracondylar fractures of the humerus in children. Injury. 34(4):267-73, 2003
3. Cheng JC et al: Epidemiological features of supracondylar fractures of the humerus in Chinese children. J Pediatr Orthop B. 10(1):63-7, 2001
4. Skaggs DL et al: Operative treatment of supracondylar fractures of the humerus in children. The consequences of pin placement. J Bone Joint Surg Am. 83-A(5):735-40, 2001
5. McKee MD et al: Functional outcome after open supracondylar fractures of the humerus. The effect of the surgical approach. J Bone Joint Surg Br. 82(5):646-51, 2000
6. O'Hara LJ et al: Displaced supracondylar fractures of the humerus in children. Audit changes practice. J Bone Joint Surg Br. 82(2):204-10, 2000
7. Sonin A: Fractures of the elbow and forearm. Semin Musculoskelet Radiol. 4(2):171-91, 2000

SUPRACONDYLAR FRACTURE, PEDIATRIC

IMAGE GALLERY

Typical

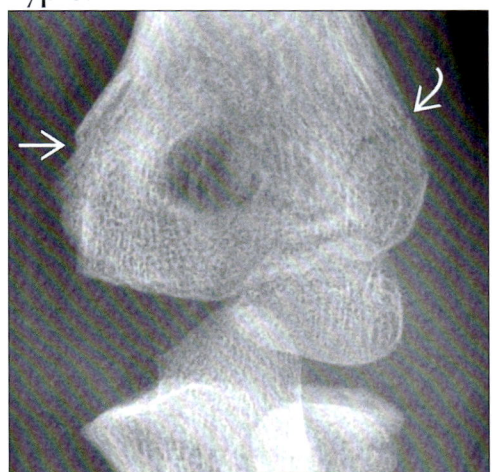
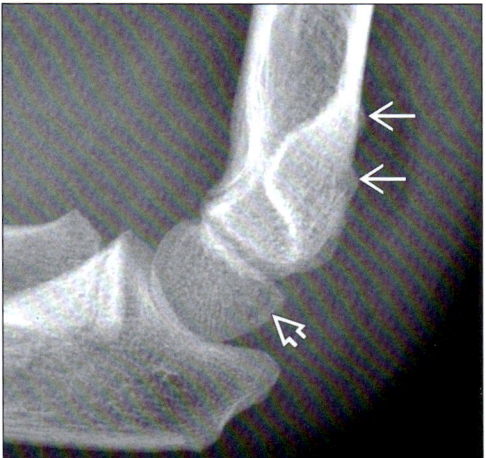

(Left) Anteroposterior radiograph shows medial buckle ➡ and lateral cortical hairline ➡ fracture components. *(Right)* Lateral radiograph shows type I extension fracture with 2 cortical buckle fractures ➡ but no displacement of capitellum ➡ relative to anterior humoral line in same child.

Typical

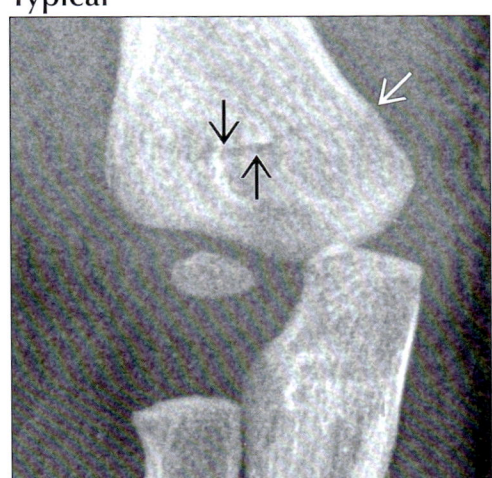
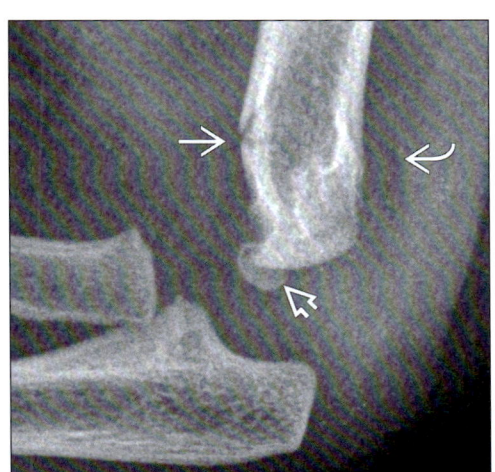

(Left) Anteroposterior radiograph shows a transverse fracture line ➡ and a medial cortical buckle fracture ➡. *(Right)* Lateral radiograph shows type II extension fracture with anterior cortical fracture ➡, posterior displacement of the capitellum ➡, and posterior fat pad sign ➡ in the same child as previous image.

Typical

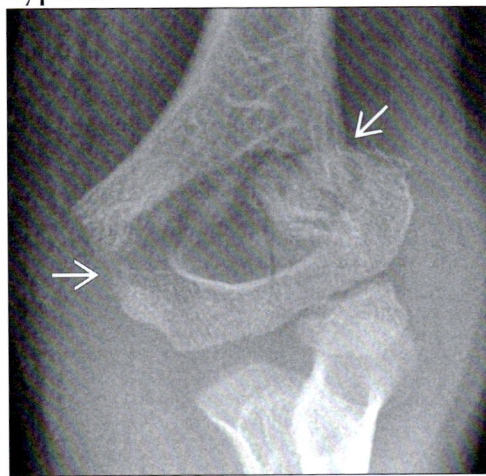
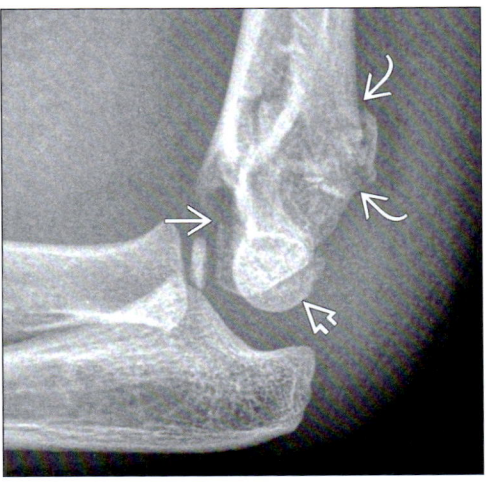

(Left) Anteroposterior radiograph shows transverse comminuted supracondylar fracture ➡. *(Right)* Lateral radiograph shows type III extension fracture with disruption of anterior ➡ and posterior ➡ cortex. Capitellum ➡ is posteriorly displaced relative to anterior humoral line in the same child as previous image.

TODDLER'S FRACTURES

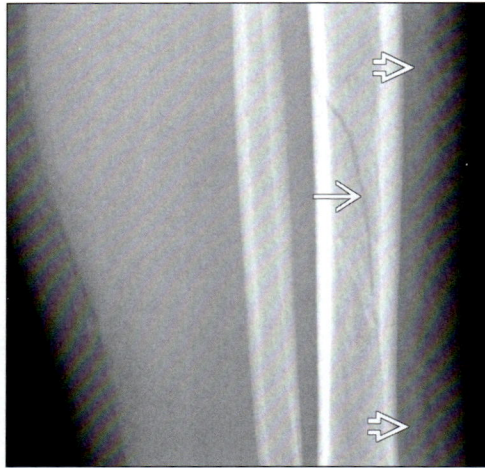

Lateral radiograph shows spiral fracture ➡ of the tibia with adjacent subcutaneous edema ➡.

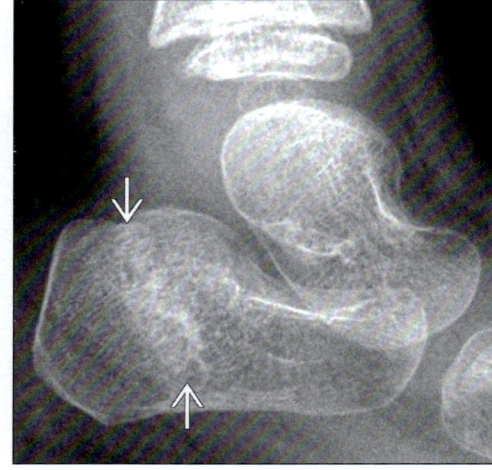

Lateral radiograph shows a band ➡ of increased density due to microtrabecular callus that was not present 25 days before in the calcaneus.

TERMINOLOGY

Definitions
- Clinically subtle lower extremity fracture in a toddler or young child that results in refusal to bear weight, gait disturbance, or inability to walk
- Most common sites for a toddler's fracture are midshaft of tibia, proximal tibia, cuboid, and calcaneus

IMAGING FINDINGS

General Features
- Best diagnostic clue: Hairline spiral fracture of tibia or sclerotic band in a tarsal bone
- Location
  ○ Tibia
    ■ Toddler's fracture, type 1: Twisting of foot on leg → spiral fracture, usually in distal third
    ■ Toddler's fracture, type 2: Knee hyperextension → upper tibial metadiaphysis distraction fracture of posterior cortex and compression of anterior cortex
    ■ Type 2 may be due to child abuse: Consider possibility if seen in non-ambulatory child
    ■ Buckle fracture: Distal metaphysis
  ○ Fibula
    ■ Distal metadiaphysis
  ○ Calcaneus
    ■ Near apophysis (vertical) or along base (horizontal)
  ○ Talus
    ■ Neck and body
  ○ Cuboid
    ■ Near calcaneus head
  ○ Metatarsals
    ■ Shafts and bases
- Size: Usually subtle

Radiographic Findings
- Radiography
  ○ Overview
    ■ Normality or only subtle soft tissue swelling may be present in first 7-10 days after injury
    ■ Periosteal reaction and callus appear eventually (except in fibular plastic-bowing fractures) in tibia, fibula, and metatarsals after 10-14 days

DDx: Lesions Causing Leg Pain

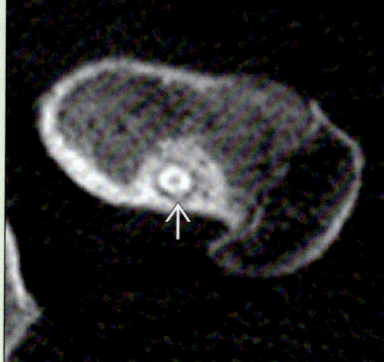
Osteoid Osteoma

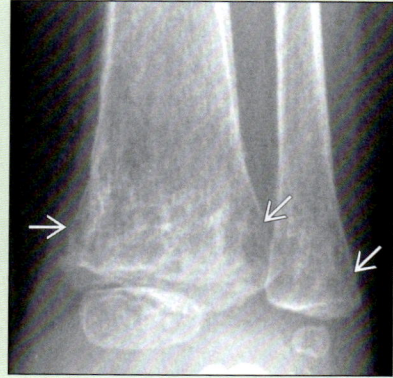
Leukemia

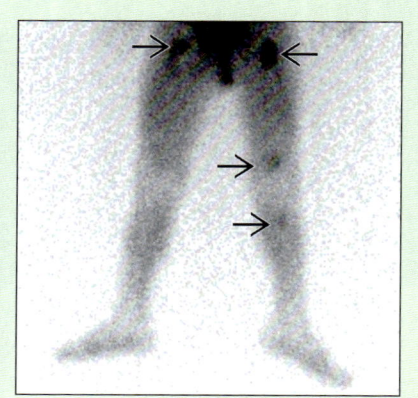
Neuroblastoma

TODDLER'S FRACTURES

Key Facts

Terminology
- Clinically subtle lower extremity fracture in a toddler or young child that results in refusal to bear weight, gait disturbance, or inability to walk

Imaging Findings
- Best diagnostic clue: Hairline spiral fracture of tibia or sclerotic band in a tarsal bone
- Periosteal reaction and callus appear eventually (except in fibular plastic-bowing fractures) in tibia, fibula, and metatarsals after 10-14 days
- Type 1 tibial fracture: Spiral hairline fracture often better seen on oblique views
- Type 2 tibial fracture: Buckling of anterior cortex, deepening of tibial tubercle notch, anterior tilt of epiphyseal plate, transverse fracture of posterior cortex

- Bone scan highly sensitive
- > 50% of bone-scan leg abnormalities in children ≤ 5 years are in tarsal bones

Clinical Issues
- Tibia spiral fracture: Gently twisting foot with knee stable (→ tibial torsion) causes pain
- Tarsal fracture: Direct pressure painful
- Metatarsal fracture: Pain when squeezing metatarsals, or when applying axial pressure from each toe towards heel
- Age: 9 months to 5 years

Diagnostic Checklist
- Normal-side comparison views when subtle plastic bowing or buckle fractures suspected

---

- Sclerotic bands due to trabecular microcallus appear during healing in metatarsals, tarsals, and tibia
- Plastic bowing fractures may heal without callus or periosteal reaction
- Often initial radiographs may be normal and sclerosis or callus formation seen on follow-up radiographs
  - Tibia
    - Type 1 tibial fracture: Spiral hairline fracture often better seen on oblique views
    - Soft tissue swelling frequent
    - Cortical sclerosis and periosteal reaction eventually
    - Type 2 tibial fracture: Buckling of anterior cortex, deepening of tibial tubercle notch, anterior tilt of epiphyseal plate, transverse fracture of posterior cortex
    - May appear as lucent line or sclerotic band
  - Fibula
    - Plastic-bowing and buckle fractures
  - Tarsals
    - Cortical: Cortical interruption or buckle fractures
    - Cancellous: Trabecular interruption or compression fractures
  - Calcaneus
    - Vertical sclerotic band parallel to apophysis of calcaneus in subcortical marrow space
    - Horizontal sclerotic band parallel to base of calcaneus
    - Similar lesion may occur after cast removed for other fracture and activity resumed
  - Cuboid
    - Sclerotic band in subcortical marrow parallel to most proximal cortex
    - Similar lesion may occur after cast removed for other fracture and activity resumed
  - Metatarsals
    - Buckle or corner fracture of first metatarsal due to jumping
    - Metatarsal buckle fractures may be multiple

CT Findings
- NECT
  - Thin collimation (1.25 or 2.5 mm)
  - Reconstructed sagittal and coronal images may be helpful in identifying fracture line
  - Often best to include both extremities in field of view for contralateral comparison
    - Abnormal areas of sclerosis or lucency may be more obvious with comparison side present
  - May be used to demonstrate fracture when tumor or osteomyelitis are other possibilities
  - If subacute, may show surrounding sclerotic band, cortical thickening or periosteal reaction

Nuclear Medicine Findings
- Bone Scan
  - Bone scan highly sensitive
    - Become positive in 1-2 days
    - Useful for demonstrating all the various toddler's fractures
  - Wide field of view
  - > 50% of bone-scan leg abnormalities in children ≤ 5 years are in tarsal bones

Other Modality Findings
- MR
  - T1WI: Marrow edema and hemorrhage are hypointense
  - T2WI: Marrow edema and hemorrhage are hyperintense
  - Fracture seen as hypointense linear structure with marked surrounding soft tissue and marrow edema

Imaging Recommendations
- Best imaging tool
  - Radiographs initially, bone scan if radiographs normal
  - Consider repeat radiographs in 10-14 days if persistent unexplained symptoms
  - CT for evaluation/further characterization of sclerotic lesions
- Protocol advice

TODDLER'S FRACTURES

- CT
  - Thin collimation
  - Sagittal and coronal reformats of axial data

DIFFERENTIAL DIAGNOSIS

Osteomyelitis
- Most common in children < 5 years of age
  - Femur, tibia, fibula frequently involved
- If chronic, may present with sclerosis but will not typically be linear
- May have sequestrum or sinus tract

Osteoid Osteoma
- Area of sclerosis and cortical thickening
- Central lucent nidus (round) rather than linear lucency

Leukemia and Neuroblastoma
- May stop walking due to bone pain
- Horizontal lucent line/band in metaphysis
- Typically wider and more poorly-defined compared with stress fracture

Septic Arthritis
- Most commonly in the hip joint
- Age peak during infancy

Toxic Synovitis of the Hip
- Occurs most commonly < 10 years of age

Juvenile Rheumatoid Arthritis
- Peak age of onset 1-3 years of age
- Commonly affects knee and hip

Child Abuse
- Very uncommon for abuse to mimic a toddler's fracture

PATHOLOGY

General Features
- Etiology
  - Compression
    - Tarsal and metatarsal fractures
    - Plastic-bowing fractures of long bones
    - Jumping from a height may → first metatarsal corner or buckle fracture (bunk-bed fracture)
  - Torsion
    - Tibial type 1 spiral fracture
  - Bending
    - Tibial buckle fracture
    - Fibular buckle and plastic bowing fractures
  - Forceful hyperextension of knee
    - Tibial type 2 distraction-compression fracture
  - Forceful foot dorsiflexion
    - Talus neck fracture caused by tibial impingement
  - Forceful foot plantarflexion
    - Cuboid compression fracture
- Epidemiology
  - Toddler's type 1 fractures are youngest part of a spectrum of childhood accidental spiral tibial fractures occurring in children age 1-8 years
  - Mean age 4 years to 3 months
  - M:F = 69:31

CLINICAL ISSUES

Presentation
- Most common signs/symptoms
  - Refusal to walk or bear weight
  - Physical examination
    - Tibia spiral fracture: Gently twisting foot with knee stable (→ tibial torsion) causes pain
    - Tarsal fracture: Direct pressure painful
    - Metatarsal fracture: Pain when squeezing metatarsals, or when applying axial pressure from each toe towards heel

Demographics
- Age: 9 months to 5 years

Natural History & Prognosis
- Rapid healing without deformity
  - Theoretical exception could be persistent anterior angulation of tibial epiphysis in tibial type 2 fractures

Treatment
- Options range from no treatment to long-leg cast

DIAGNOSTIC CHECKLIST

Consider
- Normal-side comparison views when subtle plastic bowing or buckle fractures suspected

Image Interpretation Pearls
- Toddler who refrains from bearing weight will commonly have toddler's fracture involving tibia or tarsal bones

SELECTED REFERENCES

1. Senaran H et al: Cuboid fractures in preschool children. J Pediatr Orthop. 26(6):741-4, 2006
2. Swischuk LE et al: Frequently missed fractures in children (value of comparative views). Emerg Radiol. 11(1):22-8, 2004
3. Connolly LP et al: Skeletal scintigraphy in the multimodality assessment of young children with acute skeletal symptoms. Clin Nucl Med. 28(9):746-54, 2003
4. Donnelly LF: Toddler's fracture of the fibula. AJR Am J Roentgenol. 175(3):922, 2000
5. Kleinman PK: Occult hyperextension "toddler's" fracture by Swischuk, et al. Pediatr Radiol. 29(9):720, 1999
6. Swischuk LE et al: Upper tibial hyperextension fractures in infants: another occult toddler's fracture. Pediatr Radiol. 29(1):6-9, 1999
7. John SD et al: Expanding the concept of the toddler's fracture. Radiographics. 17(2):367-76, 1997
8. Schindler A et al: Occult fracture of the calcaneus in toddlers. J Pediatr Orthop. 16(2):201-5, 1996
9. Neumann L: Acute plastic bowing fractures of both the tibia and the fibula in a child. Injury. 21(2):122-3, 1990

TODDLER'S FRACTURES

IMAGE GALLERY

Typical

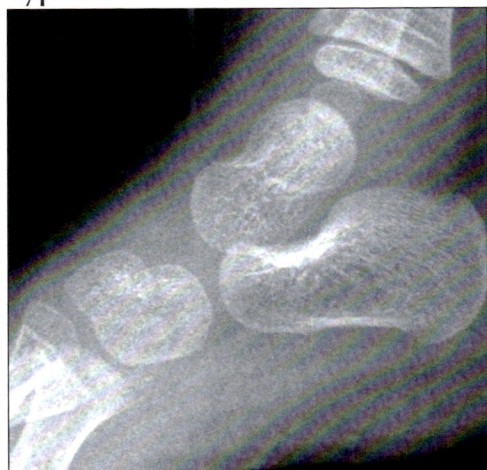
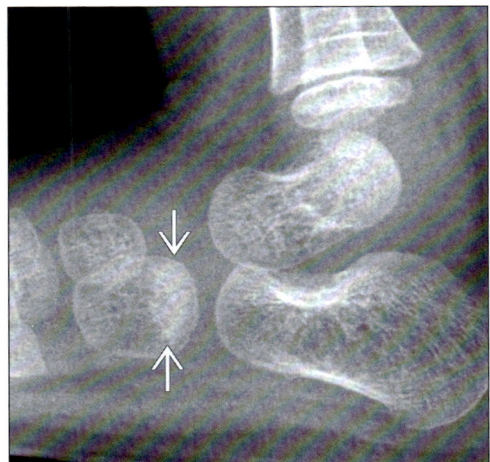

(Left) Lateral radiograph shows a normal tarsal bone at the time of injury. *(Right)* Lateral radiograph shows cuboid sclerosis ➡ in the same child as previous image, 15 days later.

Typical

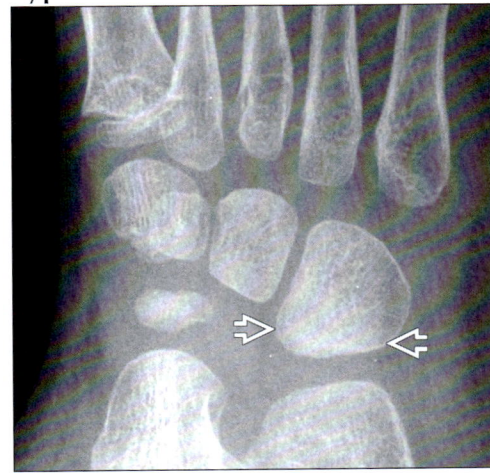
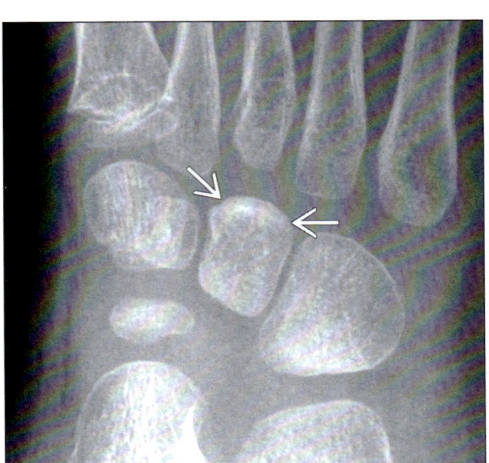

(Left) Anteroposterior radiograph shows midfoot bones at the time of injury. The sclerotic band in the cuboid ➡ is probably a remote healed stress fracture. *(Right)* Anteroposterior radiograph shows new sclerosis ➡ in the lateral cuneiform bone 12 days later in the same child as previous image.

Typical

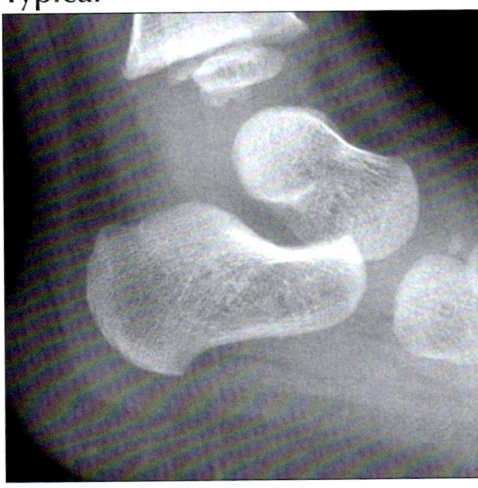
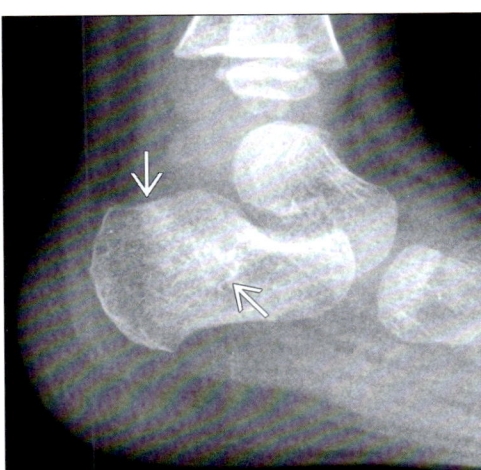

(Left) Lateral radiograph shows normal hindfoot bones at the time of injury. *(Right)* Lateral radiograph shows a sclerotic band ➡ 25 days later in the calcaneus.

STRESS FRACTURE, PEDIATRIC

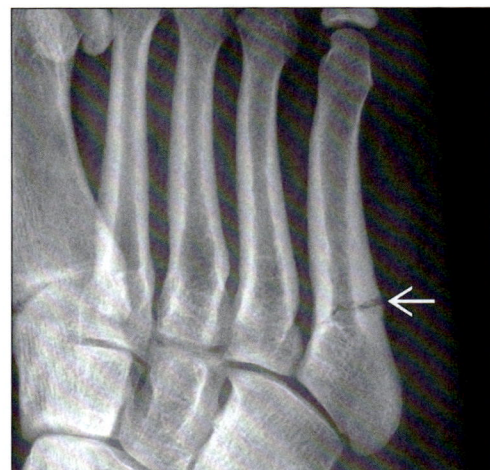

Oblique radiograph shows stress fracture ➡ of fifth metatarsal.

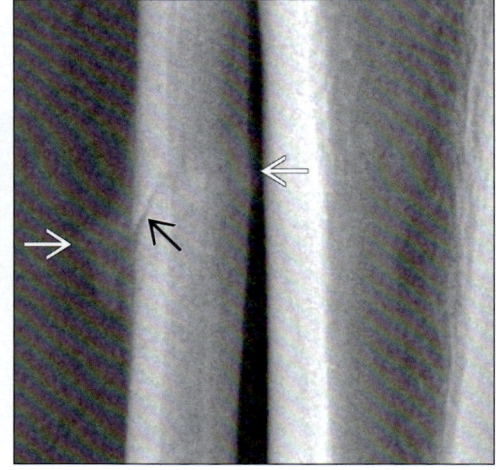

Lateral radiograph shows stress fracture ➡ of fibular diaphysis with circumferential periosteal reaction ➡.

TERMINOLOGY

Abbreviations and Synonyms
- March fracture, exhaustion fracture, spontaneous fracture, crack fracture, insufficiency fracture, pseudofracture

Definitions
- Fatigue fracture
  - Normal bone subject to repetitive stresses, incapable of producing a fracture on its own, leading to mechanical failure over time
- Insufficiency fracture: Normal stress applied to abnormal bone
  - Osteopenia/osteoporosis, osteogenesis imperfecta, rickets/osteomalacia, hyperparathyroidism

IMAGING FINDINGS

General Features
- Best diagnostic clue: Persistent pain in athlete, refusal to walk in toddler
- Location
  - Upper extremity
    - Coracoid process of scapula: Trapshooting
    - Scapula: Running with handheld weights
    - Humerus: Throwing, racquet sports
    - Olecranon: Pitching, javelin, gymnastics, weight lifting
    - Ulna: Tennis, gymnastics, volleyball, swimming, softball, wheelchair sports
  - Axial skeleton
    - First rib: Pitching
    - Ribs 2-10: Rowing, kayaking
    - Pars interarticularis: Gymnastics, ballet, soccer, cricket, volleyball, springboard diving
    - Pubic ramus: Distance running, ballet
  - Lower extremity
    - Femoral neck: Distance running, jumping, ballet
    - Femoral shaft: Distance running
    - Patella: Running, hurdles
    - Tibial plateau: Running
    - Tibial shaft: Running, ballet
    - Fibula: Running, aerobics, race walking, ballet
    - Medial malleolus: Basketball, running
  - Foot: Calcaneus

DDx: Lesions with Bone Sclerosis

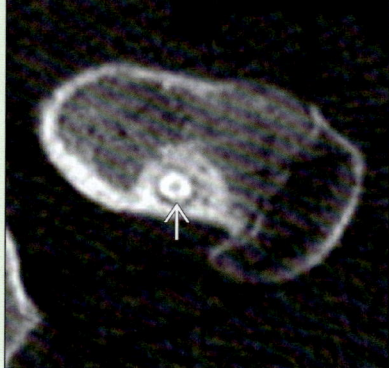

Osteoid Osteoma

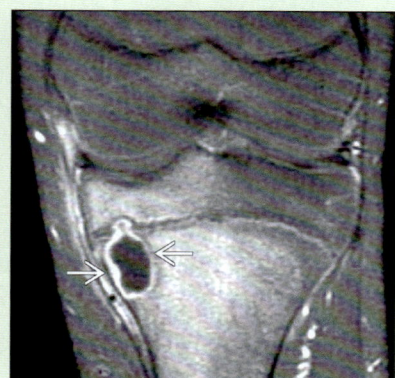

Brodie Abscess

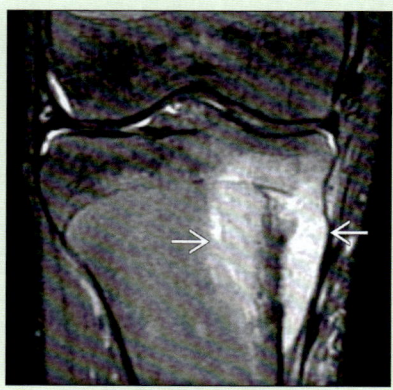

Osteosarcoma

STRESS FRACTURE, PEDIATRIC

Key Facts

Terminology
- Normal bone subject to repetitive stresses, incapable of producing a fracture on its own, leading to mechanical failure over time

Imaging Findings
- Subperiosteal new bone at any stage except earliest may be only radiographic sign
- Sclerotic bands: Cancellous bone trabecular microcallus
- Pars interarticularis fracture → spondylolysis → spondylolisthesis
- IR, FSE, FS: Areas of marrow hyperintensity against dark background of suppressed fat
- Radiography → bone scan → MR
- CT for high-risk locations such as femoral neck, or when MR negative

Pathology
- Stress fractures: Microdamage rate exceeds repair rate
- Track & field: 64% of stress fractures in females, 50% in males
- Microfracture → osteoclasts form resorption cavities adjacent to osteons → cavities coalescence → stress fracture
- Microfractures, stress fractures → periosteal stimulation → subperiosteal new bone formation
- Trabecular microfractures → microcallus → sclerotic cancellous bone

Clinical Issues
- Prognosis poorer in anterior tibial and tarsal navicular fractures

---

- Calcaneus: Baseball, soccer, basketball, gymnastics, military marching
- Talus: Pole vaulting
- Navicular: Sprinting, middle-distance running, hurdles, long- or triple-jumping, football
- Metatarsals: Running, ballet, marching
- Second metatarsal base: Ballet
- Fifth metatarsal: Tennis, ballet
- Foot sesamoids: Running, ballet, basketball, skating

Radiographic Findings
- Initially subtle, poor cortical definition, intracortical lucent striations
  - Due to osteoclastic activity
  - Hairline fracture progresses to complete fracture
- Subperiosteal new bone at any stage except earliest may be only radiographic sign
- Sclerotic bands: Cancellous bone trabecular microcallus
- Spine
  - Pars interarticularis fracture → spondylolysis → spondylolisthesis
- Pelvis and sacrum
  - Cancellous bone sclerosis common
- Femoral neck
  - Compression stress fracture
    - Lower medial femoral neck: Cortex and cancellous bone sclerotic, rarely progress to complete break
  - Distraction stress fracture
    - Upper femoral neck: Starts as hairline fractures, may progress to complete break
- Tibia
  - Anterior midshaft
    - Distraction fracture; hairline fracture may progress to complete fracture
  - Posterior superior metadiaphysis
    - Compression fracture causing cortical thickening and cancellous sclerosis; heals with rest
  - Inferior metadiaphysis
    - Cancellous bone sclerosis
- Tarsals
  - Sclerotic bands of cancellous bone sclerosis

CT Findings
- Best modality for showing pars interarticularis stress fractures
- Hairline fractures, areas of intracortical radiolucency, subperiosteal new bone

Nuclear Medicine Findings
- Bone scan: Sensitivity ~ 100%
  - Intense cortical uptake
  - Abnormal in 6-72 hours
  - Multiple areas may be seen
- Pars interarticularis stress fracture
  - Increased uptake at fracture: Scan becomes normal when lesion progresses to chronic phase of spondylolysis

Other Modality Findings
- MR: Sensitivity ~ 100%
  - T1WI and T2WI: Areas of marrow hypointensity due to edema, hemorrhage
  - IR, FSE, FS: Areas of marrow hyperintensity against dark background of suppressed fat

Imaging Recommendations
- Best imaging tool: Bone scan or MR when radiographs normal
- Protocol advice
  - Radiography → bone scan → MR
  - CT for high-risk locations such as femoral neck, or when MR negative

DIFFERENTIAL DIAGNOSIS

Bone Tumor
- Cortical destruction
- Soft tissue mass outside bone

Osteoid Osteoma
- Sclerosis with lucent nidus
- Night pain relieved by aspirin

STRESS FRACTURE, PEDIATRIC

Brodie Abscess
- Sclerosis with lucent nidus

Shinsplints (Medial Tibial Stress Syndrome)
- MR with fat-suppression
  - High signal along medial posterior surface of tibia (traction periostitis)
  - High signal in longitudinally oriented region of bone marrow within medial part of tibial diaphysis (microdamage and repair)

PATHOLOGY

General Features
- Etiology
  - Normal response of stressed bone: Microdamage with subsequent repair: Normal response of stressed bone
    - Runner's shin pain → fewer kilometers run per week → restoration of microdamage-microrepair equilibrium
  - Stress fractures: Microdamage rate exceeds repair rate
- Epidemiology
  - Stress fractures in athletes
    - Tibia: 19-63%
    - Cuboid-calcaneus-talus: 8-63%
    - Fibula: 0-30%
    - Tarsal navicular: 0-29%
    - Femur: 0-23%
    - Pelvis: 0-11%
    - Track & field: 64% of stress fractures in females, 50% in males
  - Females: Stress fracture incidence rate (case rate)
    - Track & field: 31%, crew: 8%, basketball: 4%, lacrosse: 3%, soccer: 3%
  - Males: Stress fracture incidence rate
    - Track & field: 10%, lacrosse: 4%, crew: 2%, football: 1%
  - Sports medicine practice
    - Up to 10% of cases are stress fractures
  - Most frequent cause of stress fractures: Running
  - Risk factors
    - New, different, or rigorous activity
    - Race: Relative risk ratio Caucasian: African-American = 2-25:1

Microscopic Features
- Cortical or compact bone
  - Microfracture → osteoclasts form resorption cavities adjacent to osteons → cavities coalescence → stress fracture
    - Bone loss (resorption cavity formation) maximal at 3 weeks
    - Bone reconstruction (filling resorption cavities with lamellar bone) maximal at 90 days
    - Microfractures, stress fractures → periosteal stimulation → subperiosteal new bone formation
- Cancellous or spongy bone
  - Trabecular microfractures → microcallus → sclerotic cancellous bone

CLINICAL ISSUES

Presentation
- Most common signs/symptoms
  - Pain, swelling, warmth, discoloration
  - Palpable periosteal thickening
- Other signs/symptoms
  - Bone percussion → pain
  - Pars interarticularis fracture: Back pain for several weeks, pain with spinal extension
  - Pelvic stress fracture: Hopping → groin pain
  - Sacral stress fracture: Buttock pain
- After lower extremity cast removal, second insufficiency fx may occur 2° to disuse osteopenia
  - Most common locations: Calcaneus, cuboid, tibia
- Young child with refusal to bear weight may have stress/insufficiency fracture
  - Most common locations: Calcaneus, cuboid, tibia

Demographics
- Gender: M < F

Natural History & Prognosis
- Recurrence rate: 10-60%
- Prognosis poorer in anterior tibial and tarsal navicular fractures

Treatment
- Prevention paramount
  - Gradual, deliberate increase in new activity
  - Prompt activity reduction when pain occurs
- Combination of reduced activity, rest, immobilization, casting, internal fixation
  - Compression fractures: Reduced activity and rest
  - Tension fractures: Internal fixation likely
- Pars interarticularis stress fracture
  - Boston brace or warm-n-form orthosis
  - No bracing with activity modification
  - Majority result in non-union, but can return to full athletic activity except weight lifting

SELECTED REFERENCES

1. Jones GL: Upper extremity stress fractures. Clin Sports Med. 25(1):159-74, xi, 2006
2. Lee SH et al: Stress fractures of the femoral diaphysis in children: a report of 5 cases and review of literature. J Pediatr Orthop. 25(6):734-8, 2005
3. Ahovuo JA et al: Fatigue stress fractures of the sacrum: diagnosis with MR imaging. Eur Radiol. 14(3):500-5, 2004
4. Lehman RA Jr et al: Tension-sided femoral neck stress fracture in a skeletally immature patient. A case report. J Bone Joint Surg Am. 86-A(6):1292-5, 2004
5. Ogden JA et al: Sever's injury: a stress fracture of the immature calcaneal metaphysis. J Pediatr Orthop. 24(5):488-92, 2004
6. Biedert R et al: Stress fractures of the medial great toe sesamoids in athletes. Foot Ankle Int. 24(2):137-41, 2003
7. Iwamoto J et al: Stress fractures in athletes: review of 196 cases. J Orthop Sci. 8(3):273-8, 2003
8. Parr TJ et al: Overuse injuries of the olecranon in adolescents. Orthopedics. 26(11):1143-6, 2003
9. Ishibashi Y et al: Comparison of scintigraphy and magnetic resonance imaging for stress injuries of bone. Clin J Sport Med. 12(2):79-84, 2002

STRESS FRACTURE, PEDIATRIC

IMAGE GALLERY

Typical

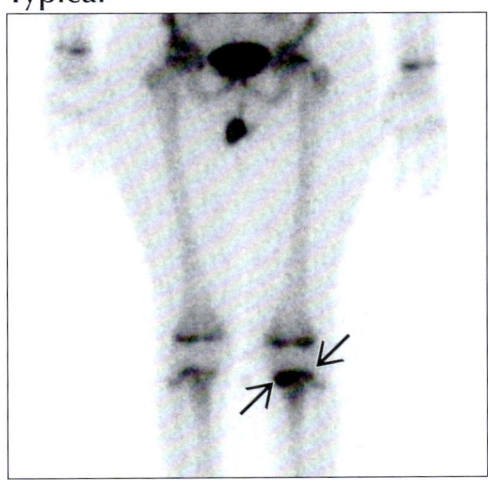
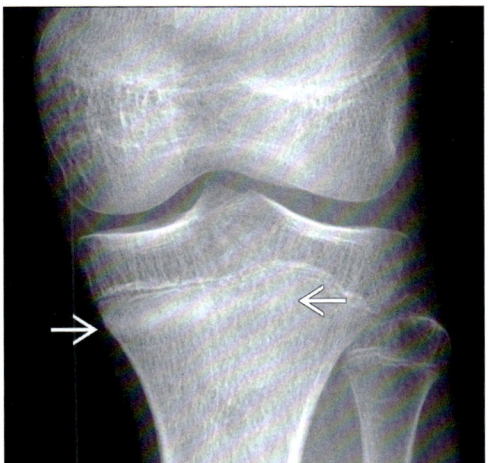

(Left) Anteroposterior bone scan shows increased radiotracer activity ➡ in vicinity of tibial physis. *(Right)* Anteroposterior radiograph in same child as previous image, shows band of sclerosis ➡ due to healing microtrabecular stress fracture. Radiograph taken 14 days before was normal.

Typical

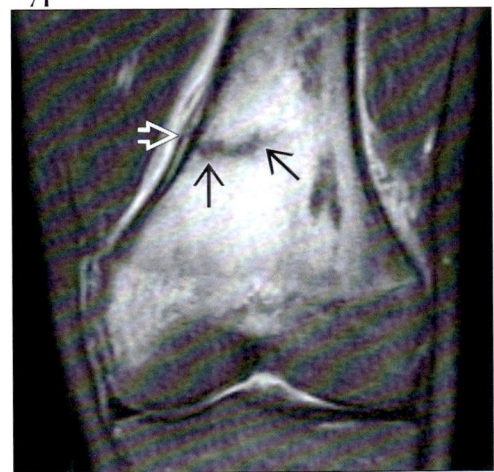
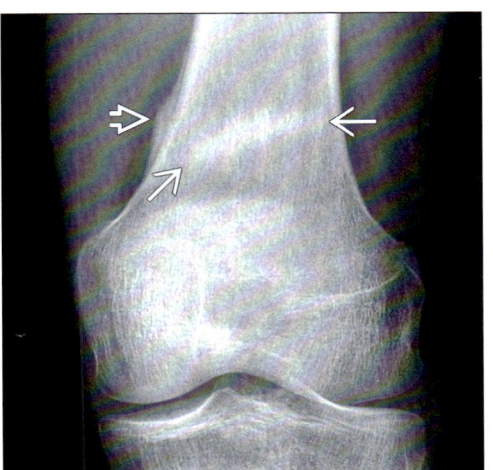

(Left) Coronal T2WI TSE FS MR shows hypointense line ➡ of stress fracture within hyperintense marrow; slight periosteal elevation ➡ is also seen. Radiographs were normal at this time. *(Right)* Anteroposterior radiograph 31 days later in same patient as previous image, shows periosteal reaction ➡ and new band ➡ of trabecular sclerosis.

Typical

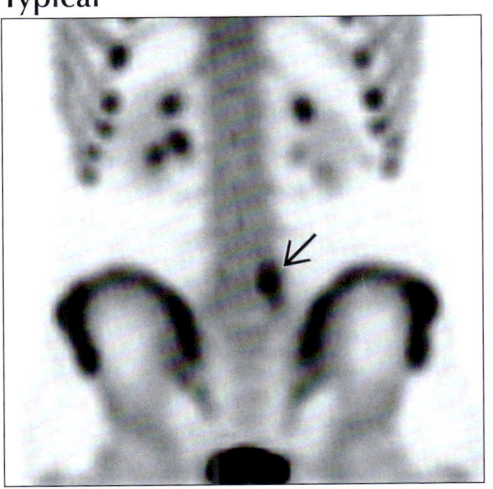
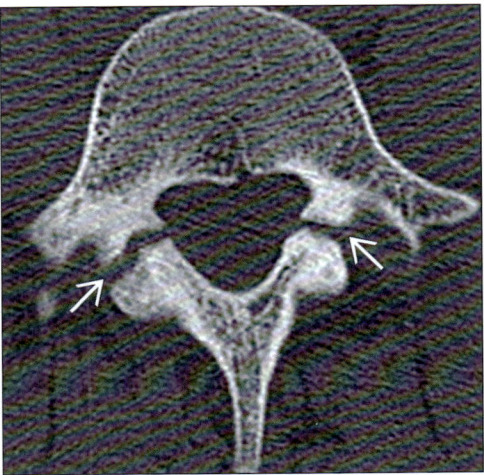

(Left) Anteroposterior SPECT shows focal radiotracer uptake ➡ on left side of L5. *(Right)* Axial NECT in same patient as previous image, shows spondylolysis with bilateral pars interarticularis stress fractures ➡.

MEDIAL EPICONDYLE AVULSION, PEDIATRIC

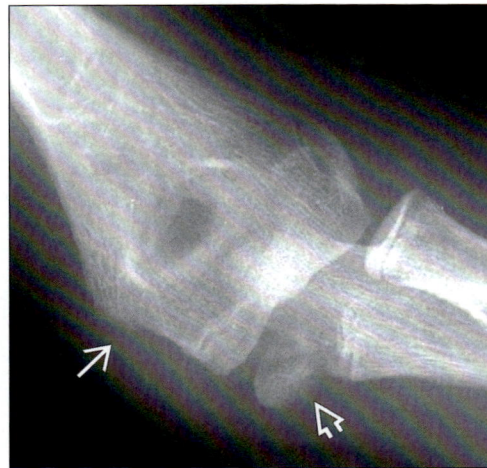

Anteroposterior radiograph shows no ME ossification center ➡ in its normal location despite trochlear ossification. The entrapped ME fragment ➡ is seen within the medial elbow joint.

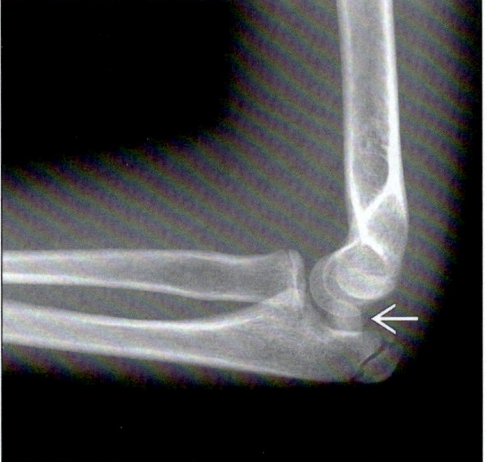

Lateral radiograph in the same child shows a rounded bone fragment, the entrapped ME ossification center ➡ between the olecranon and trochlea.

TERMINOLOGY

Abbreviations and Synonyms
- Medial epicondyle (ME) avulsion, medial epicondylitis (apophysitis), little leaguer's elbow, pitcher's elbow, golfer's elbow, medial tennis elbow

Definitions
- Acute injury
  - Medial epicondylar avulsion
- Chronic stress injury: Golfer's elbow, pitcher's elbow, little leaguer's elbow, medial tennis elbow
  - Degeneration of the common flexor tendon secondary to overload caused by chronic valgus stress

IMAGING FINDINGS

General Features
- Best diagnostic clue: Displaced medial epicondyle ossification center in the acute injury
- Location
  - Medial elbow
  - ± Entrapped between olecranon & trochlea after elbow dislocation
- Size: Displacement > 5 mm, surgical open reduction
- Morphology
  - Ossification pattern on radiographs
    - Capitellum 1st: 1-2 years old
    - Medial epicondyle: 4-7 years old
    - Trochlea: 8 years
    - Lateral epicondyle: 10-11 years
    - Radial head: 3-6 years
    - Olecranon: 6-12 years
  - Should see medial epicondyle on AP radiograph if trochlea is identified
    - Helps to exclude an entrapped medial epicondyle, can simulate the trochlear ossification center
  - Medial epicondyle apophysis fuses with medial condyle by 18-20 years old
    - Does not contribute to longitudinal growth

Radiographic Findings
- Radiography
  - Displacement of the medial epicondyle in acute injuries

DDx: Spectrum of Radiographic Findings in Adolescent Pitchers

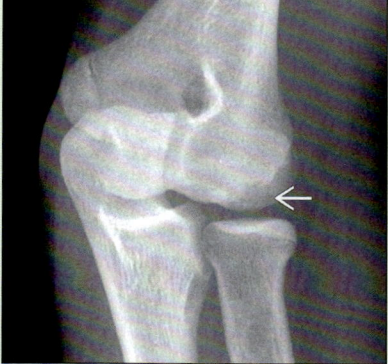
Capitellar OCD

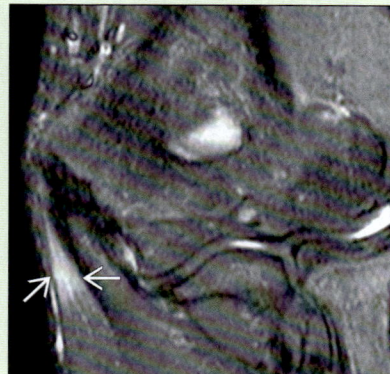
Palmaris Longus Strain

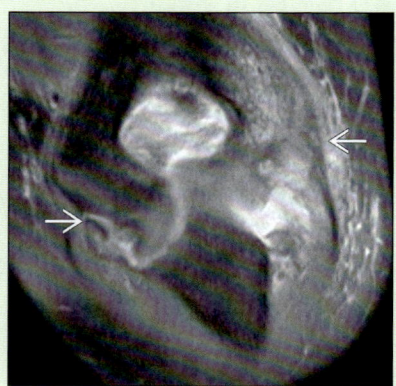
MCL Tear

MEDIAL EPICONDYLE AVULSION, PEDIATRIC

Key Facts

Terminology
- Medial epicondyle (ME) avulsion, medial epicondylitis (apophysitis), little leaguer's elbow, pitcher's elbow, golfer's elbow, medial tennis elbow
- Acute injury
- Medial epicondylar avulsion
- Chronic stress injury: Golfer's elbow, pitcher's elbow, little leaguer's elbow, medial tennis elbow
- Degeneration of the common flexor tendon secondary to overload caused by chronic valgus stress

Imaging Findings
- Should see medial epicondyle on AP radiograph if trochlea is identified
- Helps to exclude an entrapped medial epicondyle, can simulate the trochlear ossification center
- AP & lateral radiographs to exclude an acute avulsion
- T1, FS PD FSE (best), FS T2 FSE &/or STIR for ligament/tendon evaluation

Pathology
- Medial epicondyle avulsion; incidence of up to 50% in elbow dislocations
- Ulnar nerve injury in dislocation (25-50%)
- Trapped medial epicondyle in the elbow joint following dislocation (up to 20%)

Diagnostic Checklist
- Should see medial epicondyle when trochlear ossification center is identified
- Displaced medial epicondyle can simulate the trochlear ossification center

---

   - Enlargement, sclerosis, fragmentation, widened physis in chronic repetitive injuries
   - Unreliable fat pad sign
     - Children > 2 year old, medial epicondyle may become extracapsular
     - May be positive if there are other fractures
     - ± In elbow dislocation, depends on if the capsule is disrupted
- **MR Findings**
- T2WI
  - Medial tension overload
    - Increased signal intensity within the common flexor tendon origin at the medial epicondyle
    - Thickened tendon
  - Hyperintense water signal intensity within the tendon in the case of a partial tear or complete tears
    - FS T2WI FSE or STIR images demonstrate the increased signal to best advantage
    - Hyperintense signal within the common flexor muscle belly in the case of muscle strain
    - Avulsion of medial epicondyle in skeletally immature individuals
    - Strains & tears of the ulnar collateral ligament
  - Ulnar neuritis
    - Hyperintense T2WI signal & thickening of the ulnar nerve usually within the cubital tunnel
  - Lateral compression
    - Osteochondral injuries of the humeral capitellum
    - Hyperintense signal in capitellum on T2 weighted images
    - May see chondromalacia & underlying bone marrow edema or cysts
    - Loose bodies may be present
  - Hyperintense signal in the medial epicondyle in little leaguer's elbow
    - Often associated tendon strain
- T2* GRE: Widened & irregular physis in chronic injuries

Ultrasonographic Findings
- Grayscale Ultrasound: To assess displacement prior to ossification center appearing radiographically

Imaging Recommendations
- Best imaging tool
  - AP & lateral radiographs 1st
    - If still questionable 10-15° oblique view for acute avulsion
    - Avulsed fragment usually displaces inferiorly
- Protocol advice
  - AP & lateral radiographs to exclude an acute avulsion
  - T1, FS PD FSE (best), FS T2 FSE &/or STIR for ligament/tendon evaluation

DIFFERENTIAL DIAGNOSIS

Medial Collateral Ligament Injury
- Valgus extension, overload injury
- Tear: Disruption of continuous linear hypointense signal
  - Best imaging sequence: FS PD FSE
  - Partial tears: "T" sign
- Strain: Continuous linear hypointense signal

Flexor or Pronator Muscle Injury/Strain
- Common in throwing athlete

Olecranon Stress Injury
- Common in throwing athlete, valgus stress
- Marrow edema with olecranon T2WI or STIR

Capitellar Osteochondritis Dissecans
- 12-17 year old, valgus stress
- Lateral elbow pain, diffuse elbow pain worsens with activity

Ulnar Neuritis
- Hyperintense T2WI signal & thickening of the ulnar nerve usually within the cubital tunnel

Flexor or Pronator Muscle Strain/Tear
- Medial elbow pain
- Throwing athlete

MEDIAL EPICONDYLE AVULSION, PEDIATRIC

Loose Bodies
- Acute or repetitive injury

PATHOLOGY

General Features
- Etiology
  - Chronic injury
    - Overuse syndrome found in athletes participating in throwing sports
    - Due to repeated valgus stress causing tendon degeneration
    - Strain → tendinosis → tear
  - Children
    - In children the injury is often to the medial epicondyle itself manifesting as a stress fracture or avulsion of the epicondyle
  - Mechanism for avulsion
    - Forceful contraction of the pronator & flexor muscle groups of the forearm
    - Fall on an outstretched arm with the elbow flexed & hand extended
    - Posterior/lateral elbow dislocation (50-55%)
- Epidemiology: Avulsion: 10% of all elbow fractures
- Associated abnormalities
  - Medial epicondyle avulsion; incidence of up to 50% in elbow dislocations
    - Ulnar nerve injury in dislocation (25-50%)
  - Trapped medial epicondyle in the elbow joint following dislocation (up to 20%)

Gross Pathologic & Surgical Features
- Thickening of the tendon, ± macroscopic partial tearing or through-and-through tearing
- Avulsed epicondyle in the case of some children
- May include tear of the ulnar collateral ligament

Microscopic Features
- Microscopic tendon degeneration with macroscopic partial or complete tear surrounded by hemorrhage and inflammation

CLINICAL ISSUES

Presentation
- Most common signs/symptoms: Elbow pain
- Other signs/symptoms
  - Palpable freely mobile medial epicondyle
  - Crepitus
  - Athlete participating in throwing sports with onset of medial elbow pain
  - Medial epicondylar pain, increased by valgus stress to elbow (little leaguer's elbow)

Demographics
- Age
  - Avulsion injury: 9-14 year old
  - Older children, near skeletal maturity tend to injure tendons/ligaments similar to adults
- Gender: M > F = 4:1

Natural History & Prognosis
- Good prognosis
- If nonunion occurs may lead to instability

Treatment
- Medial epicondyle avulsion, acute injury
  - Minimally displaced: Immobilization
  - > 5 mm open reduction & pin fixation
  - Surgery for valgus instability
- Chronic tension stress injury
  - Physical therapy and steroid injection with decrease in physical activity
  - Tendon release
  - Tendon repair

DIAGNOSTIC CHECKLIST

Image Interpretation Pearls
- Should see medial epicondyle when trochlear ossification center is identified
  - Displaced medial epicondyle can simulate the trochlear ossification center

SELECTED REFERENCES

1. Ahmad CS et al: Valgus extension overload syndrome and stress injury of the olecranon. Clin Sports Med. 23(4):665-76, x, 2004
2. Kijowski R et al: Magnetic resonance imaging of the elbow. Part I: normal anatomy, imaging technique, and osseous abnormalities. Skeletal Radiol. 33(12):685-97, 2004
3. Williams RJ 3rd et al: Medial collateral ligament tears in the throwing athlete. Instr Course Lect. 53:579-86, 2004
4. Cain EL Jr et al: Elbow injuries in throwing athletes: a current concepts review. Am J Sports Med. 31(4):621-35, 2003
5. Parr TJ et al: Overuse injuries of the olecranon in adolescents. Orthopedics. 26(11):1143-6, 2003
6. Gilchrist AD et al: Valgus instability of the elbow due to medial epicondyle nonunion: treatment by fragment excision and ligament repair--a report of 5 cases. J Shoulder Elbow Surg. 11(5):493-7, 2002
7. Klingele KE et al: Little league elbow: valgus overload injury in the paediatric athlete. Sports Med. 32(15):1005-15, 2002
8. Chen FS et al: Medial elbow problems in the overhead-throwing athlete. J Am Acad Orthop Surg. 9(2):99-113, 2001
9. Kocher MS et al: Upper extremity injuries in the paediatric athlete. Sports Med. 30(2):117-35, 2000
10. Ciccotti MG: Epicondylitis in the athlete. Instr Course Lect. 48:375-81, 1999
11. Fritz RC: MR imaging of sports injuries of the elbow. Magn Reson Imaging Clin N Am. 7(1):51-72, viii, 1999
12. Fowles JV et al: Elbow dislocation with avulsion of the medial humeral epicondyle. J Bone Joint Surg Br. 72(1):102-4, 1990
13. Harrison RB et al: Radiographic clues to fractures of the unossified medial humeral condyle in young children. Skeletal Radiol. 11(3):209-12, 1984
14. Loomer RL: Elbow injuries in athletes. Can J Appl Sport Sci. 7(3):164-6, 1982

MEDIAL EPICONDYLE AVULSION, PEDIATRIC

IMAGE GALLERY

Typical

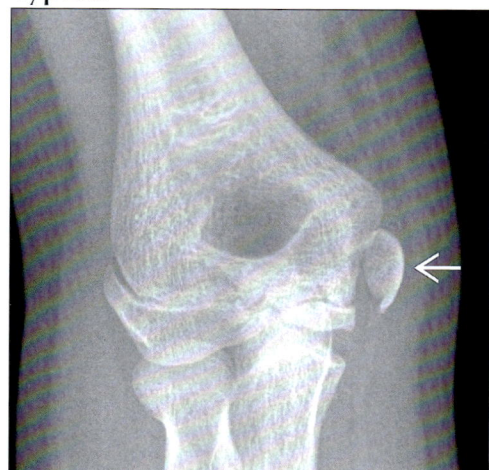
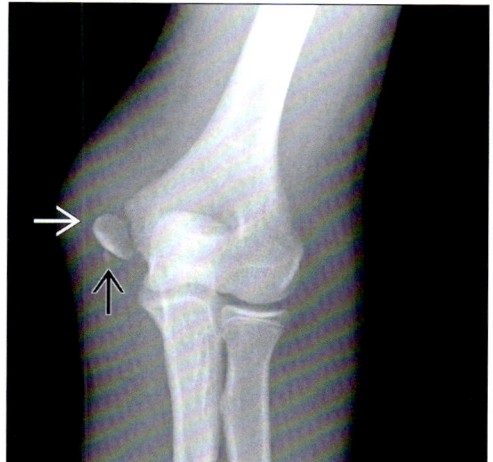

(Left) Anteroposterior radiograph shows an acute avulsion injury of ME ➔ with mild rotation of the ME fragment. *(Right)* Anteroposterior radiograph shows acute avulsion injury of ME ➔ with overlying soft tissue swelling and small bone fragments ➔ inferior to ME from prior or repetitive injury.

Typical

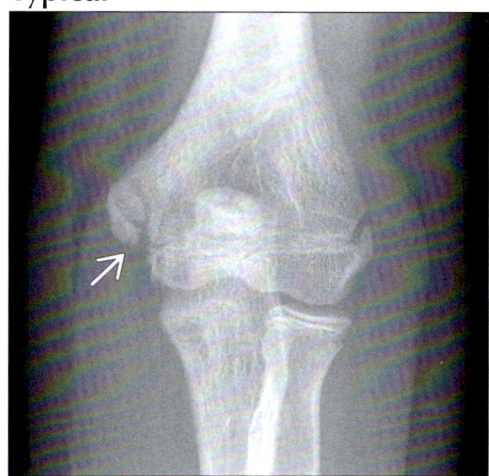
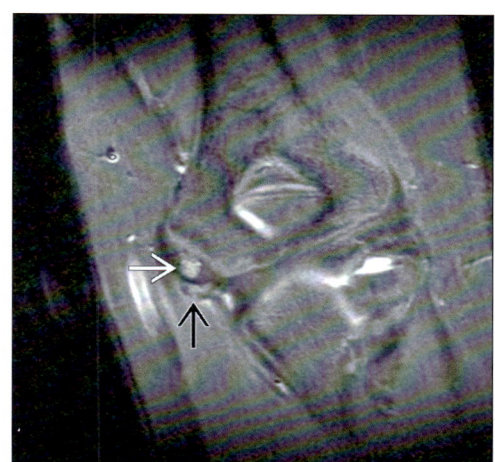

(Left) Anteroposterior radiograph shows subtle small fragments ➔ inferior to the ME from chronic repetitive injury in this young baseball pitcher with medial elbow pain. *(Right)* Coronal STIR MR in the same child shows hyperintense signal ➔ within the ME, and partial tear or strain of ulnar collateral ligament ➔ in a child with little leaguer's elbow.

Typical

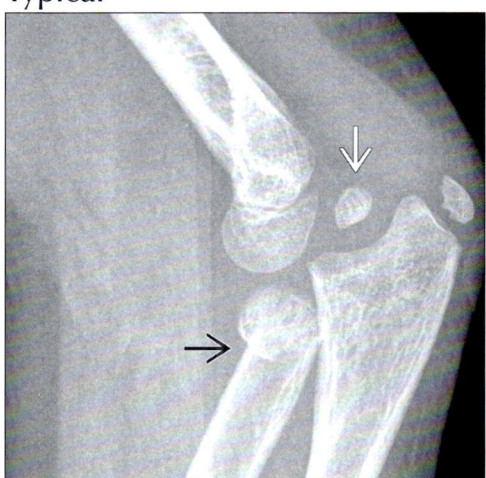
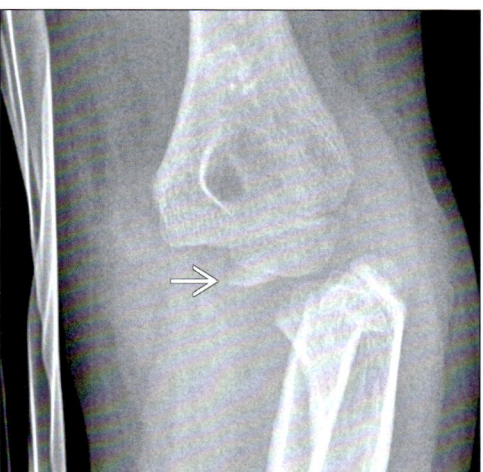

(Left) Lateral radiograph shows acute avulsion injury, displaced ME ➔. There is also radial neck fracture ➔ and elbow dislocation. After reduction, it is important to assure ME fragment does not get entrapped. *(Right)* Anteroposterior radiograph in the same child shows ME fragment ➔ displaced into the elbow joint.

PART II
Non-Trauma

CNS 1

Chest/Cardiovascular 2

Abdomen/Pelvis 3

Musculoskeletal 4

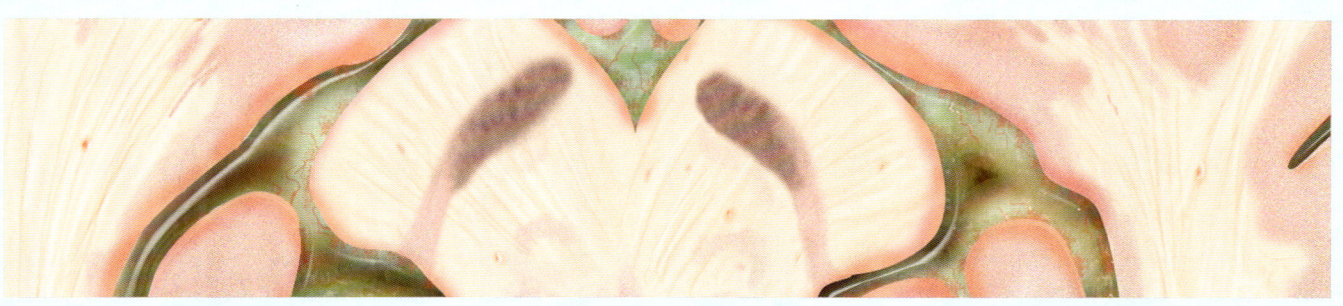

SECTION 1: CNS

Introduction and Overview
CNS Imaging Issues, Non-Trauma	II-1-2

Brain
Aneurysmal Subarachnoid Hemorrhage	II-1-4
Nonaneurysmal Perimesencephalic SAH	II-1-6
Saccular Aneurysm	II-1-8
Fusiform Aneurysm	II-1-12
Blood Blister-like Aneurysm	II-1-14
Intracerebral Hematoma	II-1-16
Spontaneous Intracranial Hemorrhage	II-1-20
Hypertensive Intracranial Hemorrhage	II-1-24
Acute Hypertensive Encephalopathy, PRES	II-1-28
Acute Cerebral Ischemia-Infarction	II-1-32
Dural Sinus Thrombosis	II-1-36
Neonatal Meningitis	II-1-40
Meningitis	II-1-44
Abscess	II-1-48
Extra-Axial Empyema	II-1-52
Herpes Encephalitis	II-1-56
Opportunistic Infection, AIDS	II-1-60
Drug Abuse	II-1-64
Hydrocephalus	II-1-68
Inborn Errors of Metabolism	II-1-72
Near-Drowning	II-1-76
Carbon Monoxide Poisoning	II-1-78

Head & Neck
Necrotizing External Otitis	II-1-80
Complicated Otitis Media	II-1-84
Idiopathic Orbital Inflammatory Disease	II-1-88
Subperiosteal Abscess, Orbit	II-1-92
Acute Rhinosinusitis	II-1-96
Fungal Sinusitis, Invasive	II-1-100
Parotitis, Acute	II-1-104
Retropharyngeal Space Abscess	II-1-108

Spine
Pyogenic Osteomyelitis, Spine	II-1-112
Granulomatous Osteomyelitis, Spine	II-1-116
Epidural Paravertebral Abscess	II-1-120
Spinal Cord Infarction	II-1-124

CNS IMAGING ISSUES, NON-TRAUMA

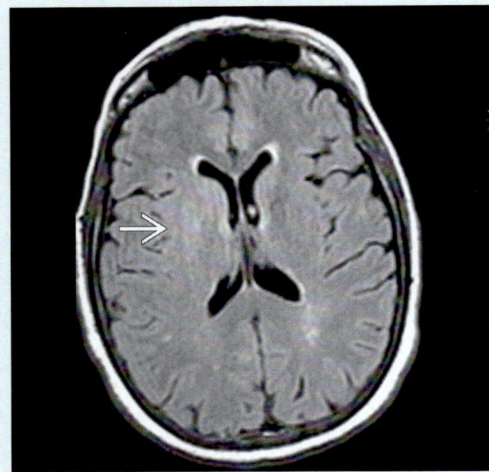

Axial FLAIR MR of acute infarction, relatively normal 4 hours after onset of left hemiplegia. In retrospect there is subtle hyperintensity in right basal ganglia ➡ compared to left.

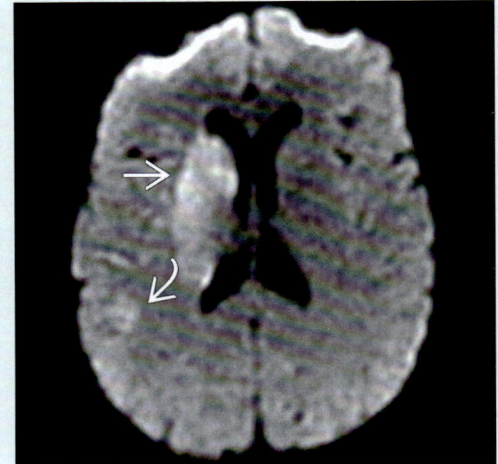

Axial DWI MR in same case previous image shows obvious DWI hyperintensity due to restricted diffusion in right basal ganglia ➡ and minimal hyperintensity in right parietal lobe ➡.

PATHOLOGY-BASED IMAGING ISSUES

Key Concepts or Questions
- Cerebral infarction
  - Hyperacute (< 6 hours)
    - CT: Loss of gray matter density (cortical ribbon) without mass effect; dense vessel (MCA or basilar) due to acute embolus; sensitivity 45%
    - Multimodal CT: CT angiography & CT perfusion increases sensitivity, allows detection of ischemic penumbra (salvageable brain)
    - MR: Hyperintense on diffusion-weighted images (DWI), iso- to hyperintense on FLAIR; lack of flow-related hyperintensity in artery on gradient echo (GRE); sensitivity > 90%
    - MR angiography (MRA) and MR perfusion (MRP): Delineation of vascular abnormality, detection of ischemic penumbra
  - Acute (6-24 hours)
    - CT: Progressive CT hypodensity with mild sulcal effacement; dense artery; early hemorrhagic transformation if occluded artery recanalized
    - MR: Progressive T2 hyperintensity (FLAIR & T2WI); marked hyperintensity on DWI with restricted diffusion; hemorrhagic conversion hypointense on GRE (most sensitive test)
- Spontaneous intracerebral hemorrhage
  - Etiology
    - Hypertension: Deep gray matter, brain stem, cerebellum
    - Cerebral amyloid angiopathy (CAA): Lobar hemorrhage; multiple hemorrhages of different ages
    - Underlying mass (glioma, metastases) or vascular malformation (arteriovenous malformation, cavernous malformation)
    - Dural sinus thrombosis
  - Imaging features
    - CT: Hyperdense mass; progressive edema
    - MR: Hyperacute (< 8 hours): Mildly hyperintense on T1WI & T2WI; peripheral hypointensity on GRE
    - MR: Acute (8 hours-3 days): Mildly hypointense on T1WI; hypointense on T2WI & GRE
    - Underlying mass or vascular lesion may be visible on enhanced images and/or CTA/MRA
- Aneurysmal subarachnoid hemorrhage
  - Most common locations: Anterior communicating artery, posterior communicating artery, middle cerebral artery trifurcation, basilar tip
  - Imaging features
    - Hyperdensity in basal cisterns (95% sensitivity in first 48 hours)
    - Intraventricular hemorrhage common
    - Mild hydrocephalus common
    - FLAIR more sensitive than CT for detection of SAH; may confirm or exclude diagnosis
- Venous sinus thrombosis
  - Etiology
    - Children: Dehydration, meningitis, polycythemia
    - Adults: Pregnancy, birth-control pills, Inflammatory bowel, collagen vascular disease
  - Clinical features
    - Non-specific: Headache, obtundation, seizures, focal neurologic deficit
  - Imaging features
    - CT: Hyperdense dural sinus, focal or diffuse edema, subcortical hematoma near occluded sinus
    - CT venogram: Filling defect in sinus and/or cortical veins
    - MR: Superior to CT; intensity of clot dependent on age; acute is T1 isointense, T2 hypointense, GRE markedly hypointense; edema hyperintense on T2WI, isointense on DWI
    - MRV & enhanced MR confirm diagnosis
- Posterior reversible encephalopathy syndrome (PRES)
  - Etiology
    - Acute hypertension, pre-eclampsia, cyclosporin toxicity, toxic uremic syndrome
    - Loss of autonomic control of cerebral vascular autoregulation

CNS IMAGING ISSUES, NON-TRAUMA

Key Facts

- MR superior to CT for evaluation of most acute neurologic conditions, with exception of aneurysmal SAH (CT/CTA allow for accurate diagnosis, therapeutic decisions)
- DWI critical for correct diagnosis of acute infarction (DWI +) posterior reversible encephalopathy syndrome (PRES) (DWI -) & abscess (DWI +)
- GRE critical for identification of hyperacute hemorrhage, microbleeds and acute embolic occlusion of major vessels
- Addition of perfusion information extends therapeutic window for thrombolytic therapy in acute infarction to 6 hours
- Advanced imaging tools (CT, MR perfusion, angiography) increasingly important in work-up of emergent neurologic conditions

---

  - Imaging features
    - CT: Hypodensity predominantly in posterior subcortical white matter
    - MR: T2 hyperintensity in posterior subcortical white matter and cortex; isointense on DWI (vasogenic edema without restricted diffusion)
- Infection
  - Abscess: Focal necrotic mass with T2 hyperintense rim, smooth peripheral enhancement, central hyperintensity on DWI (restricted diffusion)
  - Herpes encephalitis: T2 and DWI hyperintensity in inferior temporal lobe insula and hippocampus

Imaging Approaches
- Hyperacute infarction (6 hours)
  - Multi-modal CT or MR (MR more sensitive)
- Acute infarction (8-24 hours)
  - MR or CT (MR more sensitive)
- Aneurysmal SAH
  - CT & CT angiography (CTA) at presentation
  - Catheter angiography for endovascular treatment
  - MR/MRA in angiographically occult SAH: Thrombosed aneurysm, perimesencephalic SAH
- Venous thrombosis
  - MR and MR venography (MRV) best test
  - CT and CT venogram if MR cannot be done
- Other
  - MR superior to CT for detection of PRES and infection

Imaging Pitfalls
- Infarction
  - Loss of cortical density often subtle; narrow CT windows accentuate gray-white differences
- Aneurysmal SAH
  - Isodense SAH → loss of normal cisternal CSF density in suprasellar cistern, mild prominence of anterior 3rd ventricle & temporal horns of lateral ventricles
  - Pseudo-SAH: Diffuse hypodensity 2° to severe anoxia/brain death; preserved vessel density at skull base dura and leptomeninges mimics SAH

CLINICAL IMPLICATIONS

Clinical Importance
- Failure to detect aneurysmal SAH results in devastating outcome: Untreated ruptured aneurysms have high rate of recurrent hemorrhage, high morbidity/mortality
- Early detection can lead to effective treatment, improved outcome in venous thrombosis, PRES, metabolic abnormalities, infection

RELATED REFERENCES
1. Albers GW et al: Magnetic resonance imaging profiles predict clinical response to early reperfusion: the diffusion and perfusion imaging evaluation for understanding stroke evolution (DEFUSE) study. Ann Neurol. 60(5):508-17, 2006
2. Mullins ME et al: CT and conventional and diffusion-weighted MR imaging in acute stroke: study in 691 patients at presentation to the emergency department. Radiology. 224(2):353-60, 2002

IMAGE GALLERY

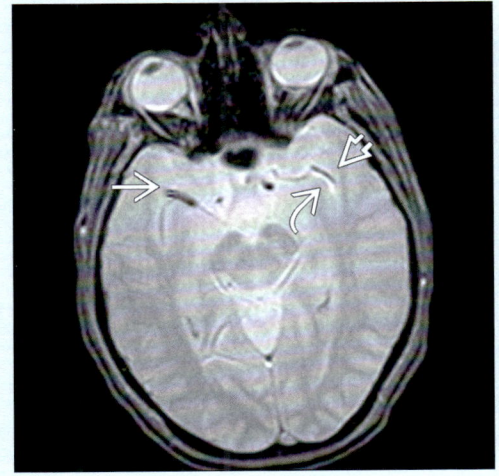 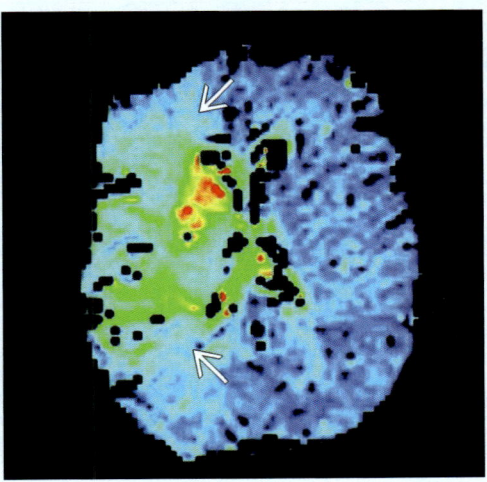

(Left) Axial T2* GRE MR in same case as previous images shows hypointense clot ➡ in right MCA. Patent left MCA has normal hyperintense flow-related enhancement ➡ adjacent to flow void ➡. *(Right)* Axial MR perfusion study in same case previous image shows diffusion perfusion mismatch. Area of decreased perfusion ➡ is larger than area of DWI abnormality and represents salvageable brain.

ANEURYSMAL SUBARACHNOID HEMORRHAGE

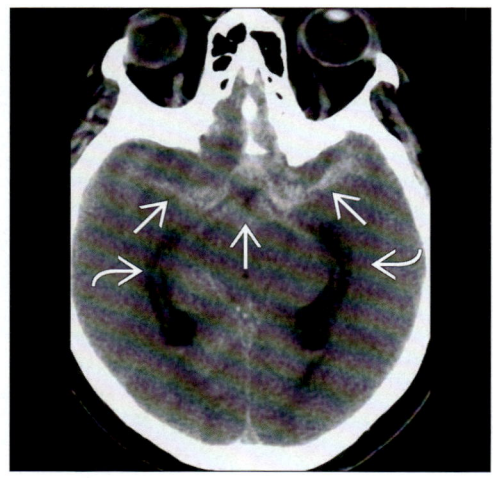

Axial NECT shows symmetric hyperdensity in basal cisterns ➡ 2° to rupture of anterior communicating artery aneurysm; hydrocephalus also present ➡.

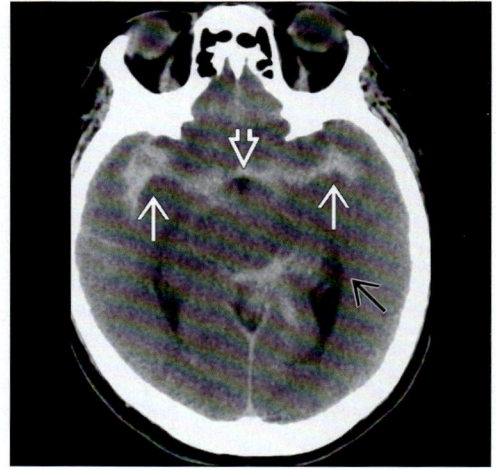

Axial NECT shows asymmetric SAH in basal cisterns ➡ 2° to posterior communicating or middle cerebral artery aneurysm. Note 3rd ➡ & lateral ventricles ➡ dilation.

TERMINOLOGY

Abbreviations and Synonyms
- Aneurysmal subarachnoid hemorrhage (aSAH)

Definitions
- SAH caused by ruptured aneurysm

IMAGING FINDINGS

General Features
- Best diagnostic clue: Hyperdense CSF on NECT
- Location
  ○ Suprasellar, basal, sylvian & interhemispheric cisterns most common location
    ▪ Hemorrhage most extensive at site of aneurysm

CT Findings
- NECT: 95% positive in first 24 hr, < 50% by 1 week
- CTA: CTA 90-95% positive if aneurysm ≥ 2 mm

MR Findings
- FLAIR: Hyperintense; FLAIR more sensitive than CT but less specific
- MRA: 85-95% sensitive: Insufficient detail for surgery
- Difficult to see on T1WI, T2WI & GRE
  ○ T1WI: CSF mildly hyperintense ("dirty")

Angiographic Findings
- Conventional
  ○ Negative in 15% of aSAH; repeat positive < 5%
  ○ For endovascular therapy or if CTA equivocal

Imaging Recommendations
- Best imaging tool
  ○ Best tool: NECT & CTA
    ▪ Surgery or coiling based on CTA
- Protocol advice: MR when CT negative & strong clinical suspicion

DIFFERENTIAL DIAGNOSIS

Nonaneurysmal SAH
- Occult trauma, dissection
- Perimesencephalic SAH

"Pseudo-SAH"
- Hypodense brain: Severe cerebral edema

DDx: Aneurysmal SAH Mimics

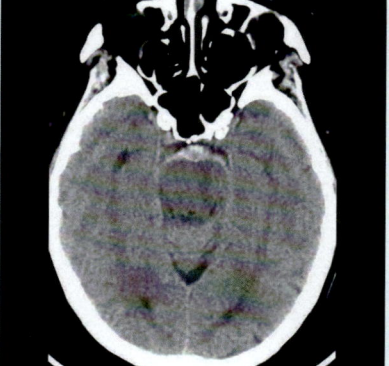

Perimesencephalic SAH

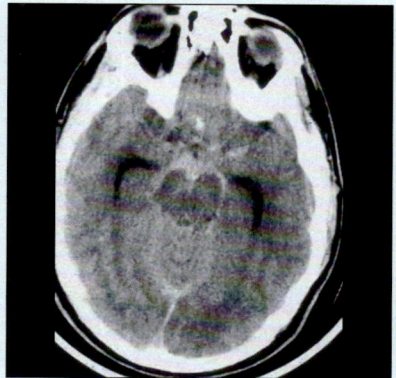

Traumatic SAH

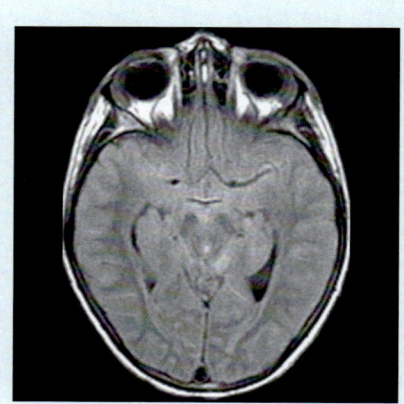

O₂ Therapy

ANEURYSMAL SUBARACHNOID HEMORRHAGE

Key Facts

Imaging Findings
- Best diagnostic clue: Hyperdense CSF on NECT
- Suprasellar, basal, sylvian & interhemispheric cisterns most common location
- Best tool: NECT & CTA

Top Differential Diagnoses
- Nonaneurysmal SAH
- "Pseudo-SAH"

Pathology
- Epidemiology: 85% spontaneous SAH

Clinical Issues
- Most common signs/symptoms: Sudden onset severe headache: "Thunderclap"

Diagnostic Checklist
- Isodense SAH: Anterior 3rd ventricle & temporal horns only CSF density structures at base of brain

---

- Hyperdense CSF: Intrathecal contrast; meningitis

Non-SAH Causes of High CSF Signal on FLAIR
- Meningeal infection or neoplasm
- O₂ therapy, pulsation artifact

PATHOLOGY

General Features
- Etiology
  ○ Saccular & dissecting intracranial aneurysms
  ○ ↑ Risk: Smoking, family history aSAH, polycystic kidney disease
- Epidemiology: 85% spontaneous SAH

Gross Pathologic & Surgical Features
- Blood in basal cisterns, sulci & ventricles

Staging, Grading or Classification Criteria
- Clinical: Hunt and Hess grade 0-5
  ○ Asymptomatic unruptured aneurysm → comatose

CLINICAL ISSUES

Presentation
- Most common signs/symptoms: Sudden onset severe headache: "Thunderclap"
- Clinical Profile: Middle-aged: "Worst headache of life"

Demographics
- Age: Peak = 40-60 y
- Gender: F > M

Natural History & Prognosis
- 50% mortality, 15% rebleed within first 24 hr
- Vasospasm + ischemia = delayed morbidity, mortality
  ○ Severity correlates with extent of SAH
  ○ Onset: 3-5 days; maximal 5-8 days
- 90% hydrocephalus at presentation
  ○ ~ 10% require permanent shunt

Treatment
- Locate, clip/coil ruptured aneurysm
- Prevent/treat vasospasm
- Temporary or permanent CSF diversion

DIAGNOSTIC CHECKLIST

Image Interpretation Pearls
- Isodense SAH: Anterior 3rd ventricle & temporal horns only CSF density structures at base of brain

SELECTED REFERENCES
1. Hansen-Schwartz J: Receptor changes in cerebral arteries after subarachnoid haemorrhage. Acta Neurol Scand. 109(1):33-44, 2004

IMAGE GALLERY

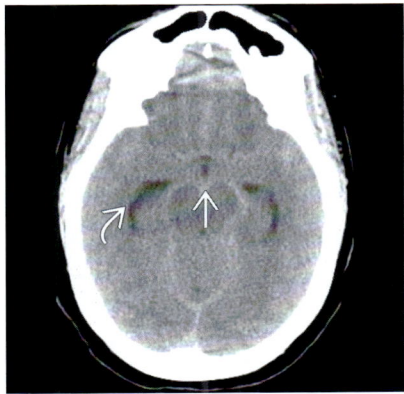 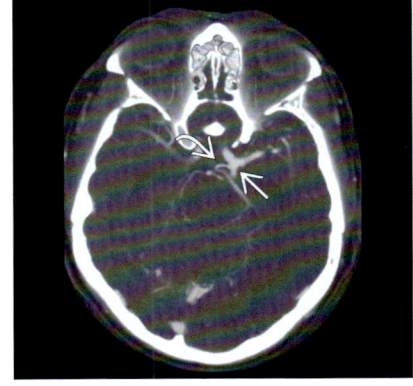 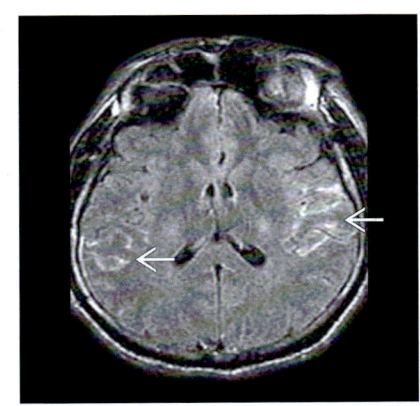

(Left) Axial NECT shows loss of normal CSF density (subtle hyperintensity) in basal cisterns. Temporal horns ➡ & anterior 3rd ventricle ➡ dilated & "jump out" as only CSF density structures. *(Center)* Axial CTA shows posterior communicating artery aneurysm ➡ arising from communicating artery ➡. CTA provides sufficient detail for surgical planning. *(Right)* Axial FLAIR MR reveals marked sulcal hyperintensity ➡ 2° to SAH 3 days after onset of severe headache; CT was normal.

NONANEURYSMAL PERIMESENCEPHALIC SAH

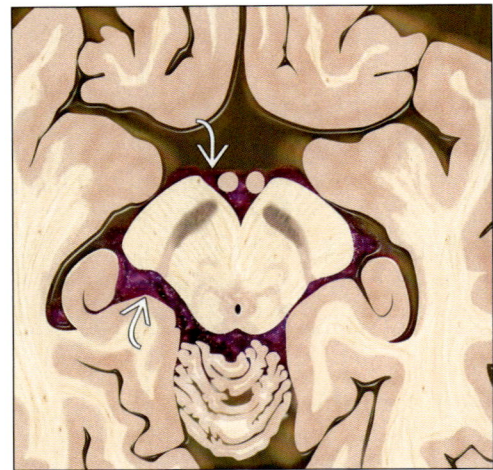

Axial graphic shows classic pnSAH. Hemorrhage is confined to interpeduncular fossa and ambient (perimesencephalic) cisterns ➔. Source is usually venous. Contrast with aSAH.

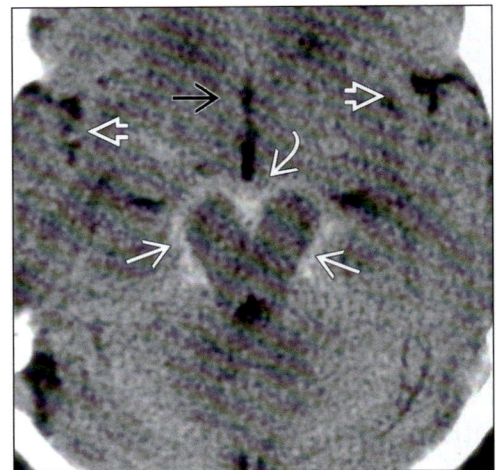

Axial NECT shows diffuse SAH in interpeduncular ➔ and perimesencephalic ➔ cisterns. There is no SAH in sylvian ➔ or interhemispheric fissures ➔.

TERMINOLOGY

Abbreviations and Synonyms
- Perimesencephalic nonaneurysmal SAH (pnSAH)
- Benign perimesencephalic SAH

Definitions
- Clinically benign SAH confined to perimesencephalic, prepontine cisterns
- No source demonstrated at angiography

IMAGING FINDINGS

General Features
- Best diagnostic clue: Hyperdense prepontine, perimesencephalic CSF
- Location: Anterior to pons & around midbrain

CT Findings
- NECT
  - High attenuation anterior to pons & around midbrain
  - No supratentorial extension
- CTA
  - CTA/MRA/DSA
    - No source of hemorrhage identified

MR Findings
- T1WI: Focal hyperintense clot around basilar artery
- T2WI: Hypointense clot around basilar artery
- FLAIR
  - Hyperintense CSF posterior fossa
    - Mimicked by CSF pulsation artifact
- T2* GRE: Hypointense clot around basilar artery

Angiographic Findings
- Conventional: Normal DSA required to confirm dx

Imaging Recommendations
- Best imaging tool
  - Best screening for pnSAH: NECT
  - MR/MRA may confirm diagnosis & negate need for repeat DSA
- Protocol advice
  - NECT with CTA
  - MR/MRA may help confirm diagnosis

DDx: Nonaneurysmal Perimesencephalic SAH

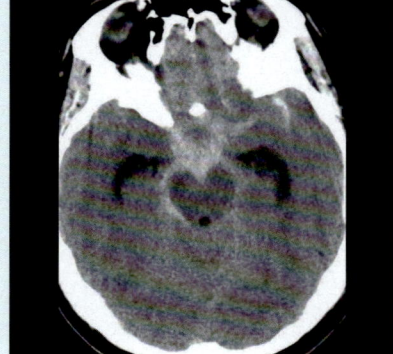
Ruptured Aneurysm

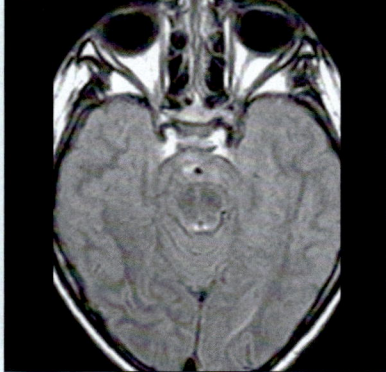
FLAIR Artifact/O₂ Therapy

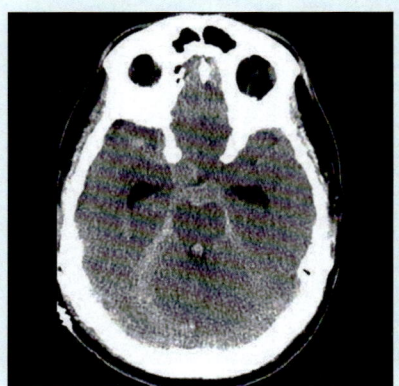
Traumatic SAH 2° Dissection

NONANEURYSMAL PERIMESENCEPHALIC SAH

Key Facts

Terminology
- Clinically benign SAH confined to perimesencephalic, prepontine cisterns

Imaging Findings
- Best diagnostic clue: Hyperdense prepontine, perimesencephalic CSF
- No source of hemorrhage identified
- T1WI: Focal hyperintense clot around basilar artery
- Conventional: Normal DSA required to confirm dx

Top Differential Diagnoses
- Aneurysmal SAH (aSAH)
- Traumatic SAH (tSAH)
- Artifact: FLAIR

Pathology
- Etiology: Most likely cause: Ruptured perimesencephalic/prepontine vein

DIFFERENTIAL DIAGNOSIS

Aneurysmal SAH (aSAH)
- More extensive hemorrhage
- Posterior circular aneurysms may have pnSAH pattern

Traumatic SAH (tSAH)
- Perisylvian, convexity > pretruncal pattern

Artifact: FLAIR
- Incomplete CSF suppression
- > 50% O_2 concentration

PATHOLOGY

General Features
- General path comments: Similar to aSAH
- Etiology: Most likely cause: Ruptured perimesencephalic/prepontine vein
- Epidemiology: Majority of angiogram-negative SAH

Gross Pathologic & Surgical Features
- Clotted blood in perimesencephalic cisterns

CLINICAL ISSUES

Presentation
- Most common signs/symptoms
  - Headache (usually Hunt/Hess grade 1 or 2)
    - Often post-coital

Demographics
- Age: 50-60 years
- Gender: M = F

Natural History & Prognosis
- Benign course: Rebleed rare (< 1%); no vasospasm

Treatment
- No further treatment

DIAGNOSTIC CHECKLIST

Consider
- Occult trauma, vertebral dissection

Image Interpretation Pearls
- Angiography necessary to exclude aneurysm
- Focal clot around basilar artery on MR

SELECTED REFERENCES

1. Matsumaru Y et al: Significance of a small bulge on the basilar artery in patients with perimesencephalic nonaneurysmal subarachnoid hemorrhage. Report of two cases. J Neurosurg. 98(2):426-9, 2003

IMAGE GALLERY

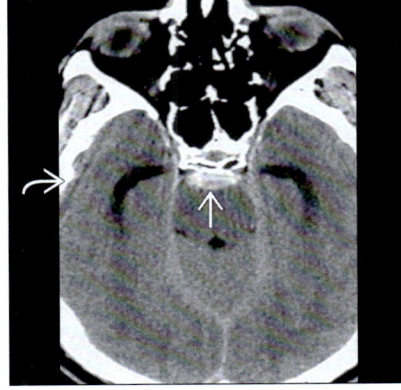
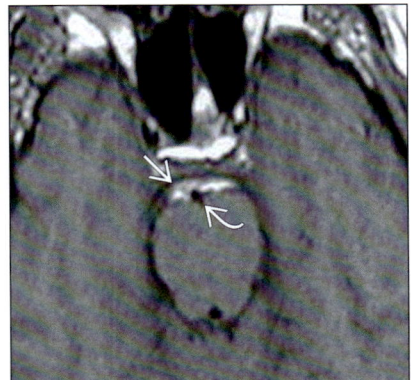
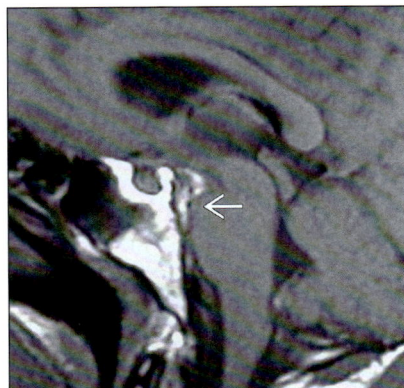

(Left) Axial NECT shows focal SAH anterior to pons ➡ with hydrocephalus present ➡. *(Center)* Axial T1WI MR same case as previous image, shows focal clot ➡ surrounding distal basilar artery ➡. *(Right)* Sagittal T1WI MR shows focal hyperintense clot ➡ in prepontine and interpeduncular cisterns around basilar artery.

SACCULAR ANEURYSM

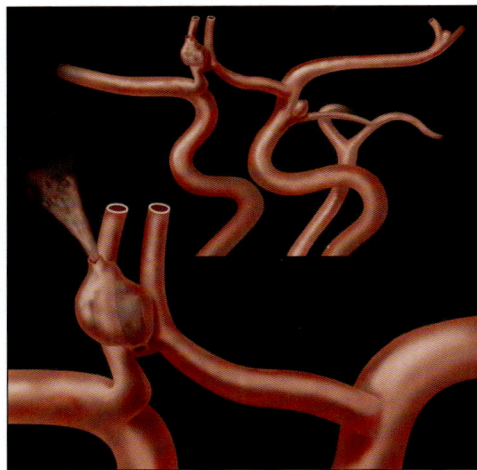

Graphic of the COW shows a large ACoA aneurysm with long aspect ratio. The "tit" at its apex has ruptured, causing SAH. A second small IC-PCoA aneurysm is present.

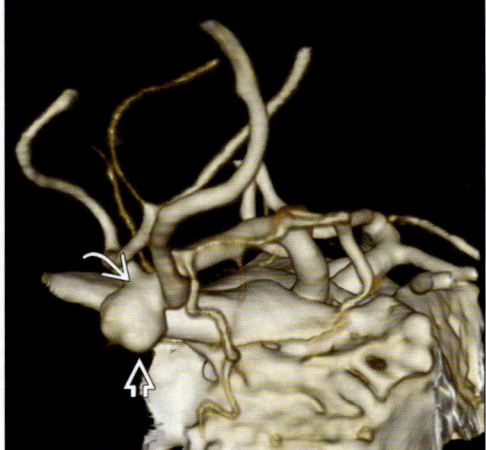

Left posterior oblique CTA shows a lobulated left MCA bifurcation saccular aneurysm with demarcation of neck ➔ and dome ➔; aneurysm was surgically clipped.

TERMINOLOGY

Abbreviations and Synonyms
- Intracranial saccular aneurysm (SA), true aneurysm

Definitions
- Dilatation or outpouching of arterial vascular lumen caused by weakness of all vessel wall layers

IMAGING FINDINGS

General Features
- Best diagnostic clue: Round/lobulated vascular outpouching from arterial bifurcation of circle of Willis (COW) or MCA bifurcation
- Location
  - 90% arise from COW
    - 90% anterior circulation (IC-PCoA, ACoA most common sites)
    - 10% posterior (BA bifurcation, PICA most common sites)
    - 1-3% miscellaneous sites distal to COW (often traumatic, mycotic, oncotic)
  - Vessel bifurcation > lateral wall
- Size: Small (2-3 mm) to giant (> 2.5 cm)
- Morphology
  - Round, lobulated or bleb-like outpouching
  - Narrow or broad-based origin from parent vessel

CT Findings
- NECT
  - Ruptured SAs have high-density blood in basal cisterns, sulci
    - Pattern of SAH helps localize SA location
  - Patent aneurysm
    - Well-delineated round/lobulated extra-axial mass
    - Slightly hyperdense to brain (may have mural Ca++)
  - Partially/completely thrombosed aneurysm
    - Moderately hyperdense (Ca++ common)
- CECT
  - Lumen of patent SA enhances uniformly
  - Completely thrombosed SA may have reactive rim enhancement
- CTA
  - Multislice CTA positive in 95% of aSAH patients

DDx: Saccular Intracranial Aneurysm Mimics

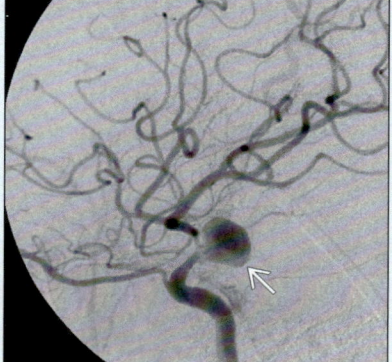
Pseudoaneurysm

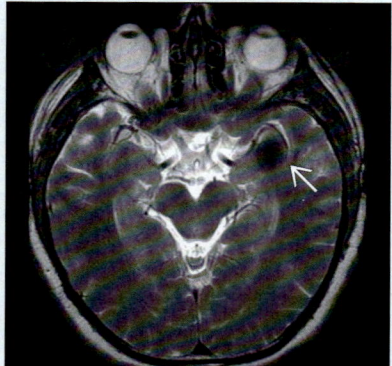
Cavernoma

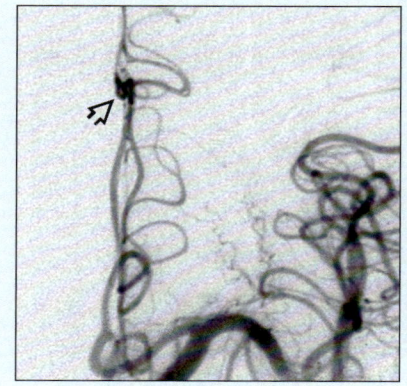
Vascular Loop

SACCULAR ANEURYSM

Key Facts

Imaging Findings
- Best diagnostic clue: Round/lobulated vascular outpouching from arterial bifurcation of circle of Willis (COW) or MCA bifurcation
- 90% arise from COW
- Ruptured SAs have high-density blood in basal cisterns, sulci
- Multislice CTA positive in 95% of aSAH patients
- Typically hypointense on T2WI
- FLAIR: Acute aSAH: High signal in sulci, cisterns
- Increases phase artifact in patent SAs
- 3D DSA with shaded-surface display optimal
- Best imaging tool: NECT for aSAH + CTA

Top Differential Diagnoses
- Vessel Loop
- Infundibulum
- Pseudoaneurysm
- "Flow Void" Mimic on MR
- Short T1 on MRA

Pathology
- 1-2% incidental finding of unruptured SA at autopsy, angiography
- 15-20% multiple

Clinical Issues
- Critical size for aneurysm rupture: 4-7 mm
- Estimated risk of rupture: 1-2% year cumulative for unruptured aneurysms
- Giant aneurysms have lower rate of rupture, symptoms related to mass effect
- ISUIA: 22.6% relative, 6% absolute risk reduction (coiling vs surgery); others show little/no difference

---

  - If screening for unruptured SA: Negative CTA = very low probability of "clinically important" aneurysm

MR Findings
- T1WI
  - Patent aneurysm (signal varies)
    - 50% have "flow void" on T1WI
    - 50% iso-/heterogeneous signal (slow/turbulent flow; saturation effects; phase dispersion)
  - Partially/completely thrombosed aneurysm
    - Signal depends on age(s) of thrombus
    - Common: Mixed signal, laminated thrombus
- T2WI
  - Typically hypointense on T2WI
  - May be laminated with very hypointense rim
- FLAIR: Acute aSAH: High signal in sulci, cisterns
- DWI: ± Restricted parenchymal diffusion 2° vasospasm, ischemia
- T1 C+
  - Slow flow in patent lumen may enhance
  - Increases phase artifact in patent SAs
- MRA
  - 3D TOF: DSA for aneurysms 3 mm or greater
  - 3T TOF better than 1.5T
  - Short T1 substances such as subacute hemorrhage may simulate flow

Angiographic Findings
- Conventional
  - Role of DSA
    - Identify SA, define neck
    - Identify perforating arteries arising from dome
    - Assess potential for collateral circulation
    - Detect multiple aneurysms
    - Assess for vasospasm
  - Multiple projections with cross-compression needed for complete COW delineation
    - Round/lobulated, focal outpouching, may have apical "tit"
    - Narrow or broad-based
    - Rare: Contrast extravasation with active SAH
  - 3D DSA with shaded-surface display optimal

Imaging Recommendations
- Best imaging tool: NECT for aSAH + CTA
- Protocol advice
  - Thin slices, low pitch CTA; 3D TOF MRA
  - If CTA/MRA negative, DSA

DIFFERENTIAL DIAGNOSIS

Vessel Loop
- Use multiple projections

Infundibulum
- < 3 mm, conical, small PCoA arises directly from apex

Pseudoaneurysm
- Often arises distal to COW
- May be indistinguishable from true SA

"Flow Void" Mimic on MR
- Aerated anterior clinoid or supraorbital cell
- Cavernous malformation (cavernoma)

Short T1 on MRA
- Lipoma
- Pituitary gland (contrast-enhanced MRA)
- Subacute hemorrhage

PATHOLOGY

General Features
- General path comments: SA development and rupture risk reflect complex combination of inherited susceptibility + acquired mechanically-mediated vessel wall stresses
- Genetics
  - General inheritance pattern
    - Autosomal recessive 57%, dominant 36%
  - Abnormal expression/polymorphism of some genes
    - Endoglin, MMP-9, apolipoprotein(a), eNOS genes

SACCULAR ANEURYSM

- Overexpression of other genes encoding extracellular matrix components (collagen, α2(I) elastin)
  - Familial intracranial aneurysms (FIAs)
    - No known heritable connective tissue disorder
    - Occur in "clusters" (two first-order relatives)
    - 10% prevalence in FIAs
    - Younger patients, no female predominance compared to sporadic SAs
- Etiology
  - Flow-related "bioengineering fatigue" in vessel wall
  - Abnormal vascular hemodynamics
    - Arises at areas of high biomechanical stress
    - Higher/disturbed flow, increased pulsatility
- Epidemiology
  - 1-2% incidental finding of unruptured SA at autopsy, angiography
  - 15-20% multiple
  - Annual risk of de novo aneurysm following previous clipping: 0.8%
- Associated abnormalities
  - Hereditary/connective tissue disorders
    - Fibromuscular dysplasia
    - Autosomal dominant polycystic kidney disease (10%)
    - Ehlers-Danlos type IV, NF1 (usually fusiform, not SA)
  - Anomalous/aberrant vessel
    - Intraoptic A1 ACA
    - Persistent trigeminal artery
    - ± Fenestrated vessel
  - Flow-related (30-35% on feeding pedicle of AVM)
  - Trauma, infection, tumor, etc. (usually pseudoaneurysms)

Gross Pathologic & Surgical Features
- Round/lobulated sac, thin or thick wall, ± SAH

Microscopic Features
- Disrupted/absent internal elastic lamina
- Muscle layer absent
- May have "tit" of fragile adventitia

CLINICAL ISSUES

Presentation
- Most common signs/symptoms
  - 80-90% of nontraumatic SAH caused by ruptured SA
  - Headache (often "thunderclap")
  - Cranial neuropathy 15-30%
    - Pupil-involving CN3 palsy (PCoA aneurysm)
- Other signs/symptoms: "Migraine", TIA, seizure
- Clinical Profile: Middle-aged patient with "worst headache of my life"

Demographics
- Age
  - From 1.22/100,000 persons/yr (age 0-34) to 44.47/100,000 persons/yr (age 65-74)
  - Rare in children
    - 1-2% of all aneurysms
    - Different location (ICA bifurcation, M2 MCA)
    - Often associated with trauma, infection
- Gender: M < F (especially with multiple aneurysms)

Natural History & Prognosis
- Rupture risk
  - Size most important (but not only) factor
    - Critical size for aneurysm rupture: 4-7 mm
    - Estimated risk of rupture: 1-2% year cumulative for unruptured aneurysms
    - 20-50% of ruptured untreated aneurysms rebleed within 2 weeks
  - Configuration vs rupture risk increased if
    - Multilobed > round/ovoid shape
    - Apical "tit" or "bleb" present
    - Aspect ratio (length vs neck) > 1.6
  - Other (hypertension, female gender, smoking)
- Untreated "giant" aneurysm (> 2.5 cm)
  - Slow growth by recurrent internal hemorrhage, laminated thrombus of varying ages
  - Giant aneurysms have lower rate of rupture, symptoms related to mass effect

Treatment
- Endovascular (coiling, liquid, embolics)
  - ISUIA: 22.6% relative, 6% absolute risk reduction (coiling vs surgery); others show little/no difference
- Clipping (high-volume institutions and surgeons have significantly lower morbidity)

DIAGNOSTIC CHECKLIST

Consider
- aSAH vs nonaneurysmal SAH or pseudoSAH

Image Interpretation Pearls
- "Angiogram-negative" SAH may be caused by "blister-like" aneurysm
  - Look for asymmetric hemispheric bulge
- ACoA most frequent site of "initially occult aneurysm"

SELECTED REFERENCES

1. Barker FG 2nd et al: Age-dependent differences in short-term outcome after surgical or endovascular treatment of unruptured intracranial aneurysms in the United States, 1996-2000. Neurosurgery. 54(1):18-28; discussion 28-30, 2004
2. Gibbs GF et al: Improved image quality of intracranial aneurysms: 3.0-T versus 1.5-T time-of-flight MR angiography. AJNR Am J Neuroradiol. 25(1):84-7, 2004
3. Henkes H et al: Endovascular coil occlusion of 1811 intracranial aneurysms: early angiographic and clinical results. Neurosurgery. 54(2):268-80; discussion 280-5, 2004
4. Juvela S: Treatment options of unruptured intracranial aneurysms. Stroke. 35(2):372-4, 2004
5. Rasmussen PA et al: Defining the natural history of unruptured aneurysms. Stroke. 35(1):232-3, 2004
6. Nanda A et al: Management of intracranial aneurysms: factors that influence clinical grade and surgical outcome. South Med J. 96(3):259-63, 2003
7. Wiebers DO et al: Unruptured intracranial aneurysms: natural history, clinical outcome, and risks of surgical and endovascular treatment. Lancet. 362(9378):103-10, 2003
8. Gonsoulin M et al: Death resulting from ruptured cerebral artery aneurysm: 219 cases. Am J Forensic Med Pathol. 23(1):5-14, 2002

SACCULAR ANEURYSM

IMAGE GALLERY

Typical

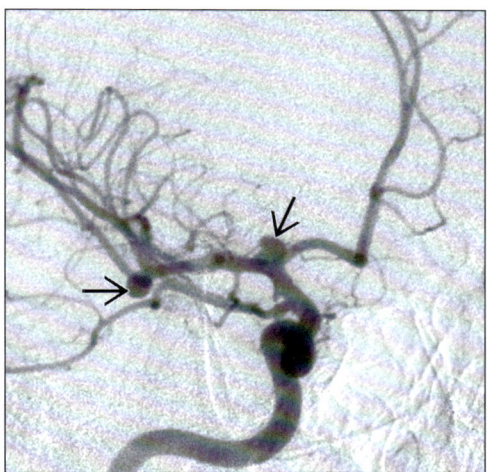

(Left) Axial NECT shows a ruptured, peripherally calcified ICA terminus aneurysm ➡ with extensive SAH ➡ and IVH ➡, as well as development of hydrocephalus. *(Right)* Coronal oblique angiography demonstrates right ICA terminus and right MCA bifurcation aneurysms ➡. Aneurysms are multiple in 15-20% of cases, with strong female predominance.

Variant

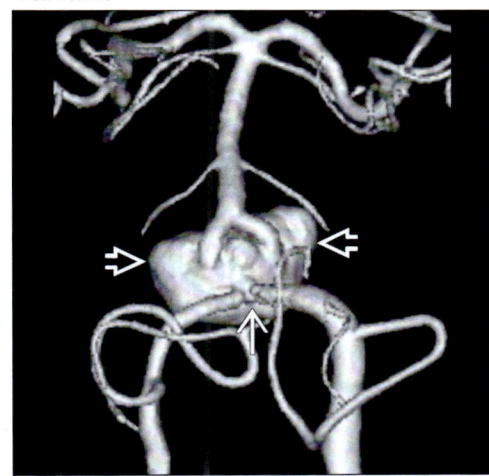
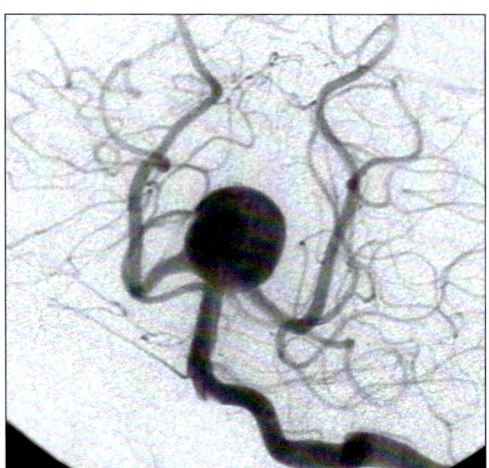

(Left) Anterior 3D DSA shows large saccular aneurysm ➡ originating from fenestrated basilar artery ➡, an uncommon variant predisposing to aneurysm formation. *(Right)* Anteroposterior angiography shows large basilar tip aneurysm during early arterial phase of left vertebral artery injection. Approximately 5% of aneurysms occur at basilar tip.

Variant

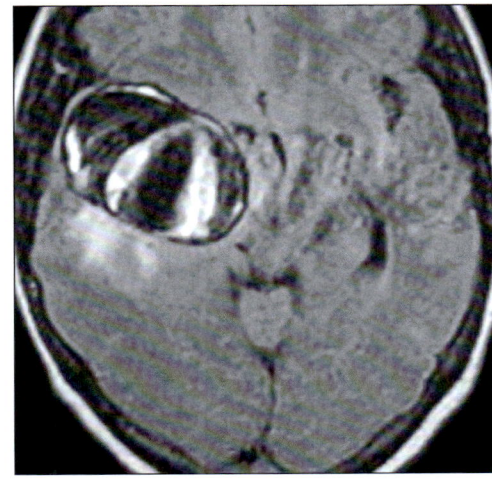
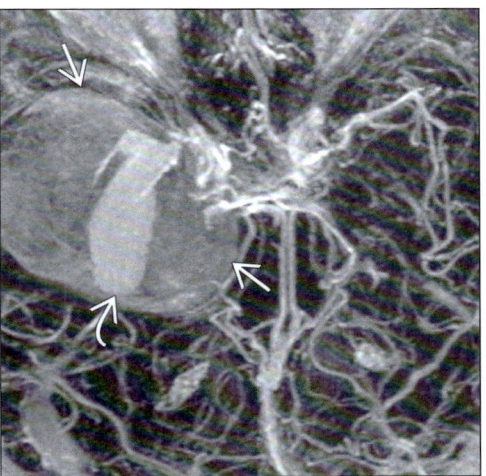

(Left) Axial FLAIR MR shows giant, mostly thrombosed aneurysm. Mass contains multiple laminated layers of variable signal intensity. Central flow void is causing phase artifact across image. *(Right)* Axial contrast-enhanced MRA shows patent residual lumen ➡ within much larger thrombosed aneurysm ➡.

FUSIFORM ANEURYSM

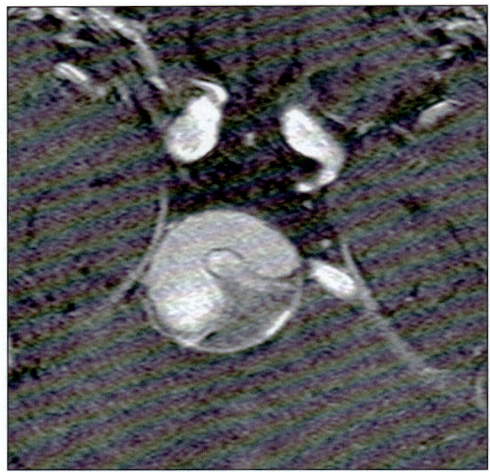

Axial CE-MRA of partially thrombosed basilar ASVD fusiform aneurysm. Distal aspect of aneurysm appears more saccular with contrast layering caused by slow intraluminal flow.

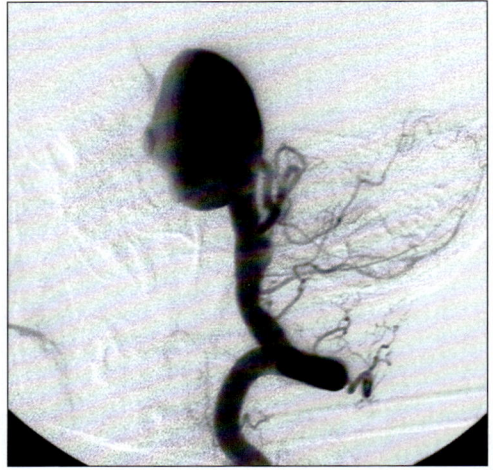

Lateral angiography of partially thrombosed distal basilar ASVD fusiform aneurysm. Proximal vertebral artery is enlarged, ectatic and somewhat irregular.

TERMINOLOGY

Abbreviations and Synonyms
- Atherosclerotic fusiform aneurysm (ASVD FA); aneurysmal dolichoectasia

Definitions
- Ectasia with focal aneurysmal outpouching

IMAGING FINDINGS

General Features
- Best diagnostic clue: Long segment irregular fusiform or ovoid arterial dilatation
- Location: Vertebrobasilar > carotid circulation
- Size: Usually large; may be giant (> 2.5 cm)
- Morphology: Solitary/multifocal dolichoectatic vessel with focal aneurysmal dilatation

CT Findings
- NECT: Hyperdense; rim Ca++ common
- CECT: Lumen enhances; intramural clot does not
- CTA: Exaggerated arterial ectasia with focal fusiform/saccular enlargement

MR Findings
- T1WI: Signal varies with flow, hematoma presence/age
- T2WI: Lumen, clot often hypointense
- T1 C+: Residual lumen enhances strongly
- MRA: Pre-contrast 3D-TOF may be inadequate because of flow saturation, phase dispersion

Imaging Recommendations
- Best imaging tool: Dynamic CE-MRA or CTA
- Protocol advice: Giant ASVD FAs require dynamic T1 C+ sequences for accurate delineation

DIFFERENTIAL DIAGNOSIS

Atherosclerotic Dolichoectasia
- No focal fusiform/saccular dilatation
- Posterior circulation most commonly affected

Giant Serpentine Aneurysm (GSA)
- Large, partially thrombosed mass, no definable neck
- May be indistinguishable from ASVD FA

DDx: Fusiform Aneurysm Mimics

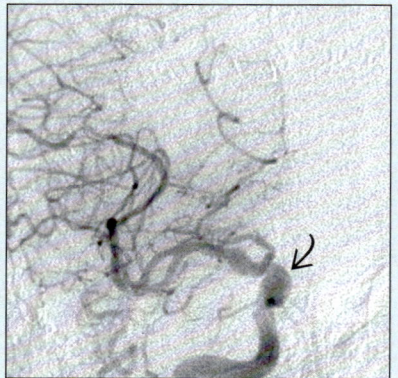

Atherosclerosis

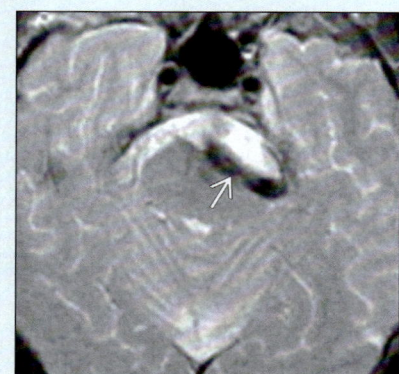

Dolichoectasia

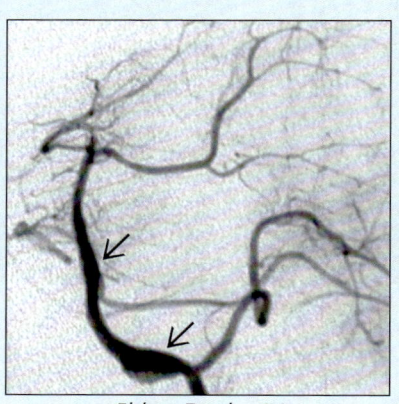

Ehlers-Danlos IV

FUSIFORM ANEURYSM

Key Facts

Imaging Findings
- Best diagnostic clue: Long segment irregular fusiform or ovoid arterial dilatation
- Location: Vertebrobasilar > carotid circulation
- NECT: Hyperdense; rim Ca++ common
- CECT: Lumen enhances; intramural clot does not
- Best imaging tool: Dynamic CE-MRA or CTA

Top Differential Diagnoses
- Atherosclerotic Dolichoectasia
- Giant Serpentine Aneurysm (GSA)
- Nonatherosclerotic Fusiform Vasculopathy
- Dissecting Aneurysm

Diagnostic Checklist
- Complex flow in lumen may give heterogeneous signal
- DSA or CE-MRA/CTA to delineate patent lumen

Nonatherosclerotic Fusiform Vasculopathy
- Younger patient with vasculopathy, immune disorder

Dissecting Aneurysm
- Vertebral > basilar artery; no ASVD changes in other vessels

PATHOLOGY

General Features
- Etiology: Atherosclerosis usual cause of basilar FA in older adults
- Epidemiology: ASVD FA less common than vertebrobasilar dolichoectasia (VBD) or SA

Gross Pathologic & Surgical Features
- Generalized ASVD with focally dilated fusiform ectasia

Microscopic Features
- Plaques of foam cells, thickened intima, organized thrombus

CLINICAL ISSUES

Presentation
- Most common signs/symptoms: Vertebrobasilar TIAs > cranial neuropathy
- Clinical Profile: Elderly patient with hypertension and ASVD

Demographics
- Age: Peak age: 7th, 8th decades

Natural History & Prognosis
- Slow but progressively increasing ectasia, enlargement

Treatment
- Sometimes none; endovascular occlusion or stenting of vessel

DIAGNOSTIC CHECKLIST

Image Interpretation Pearls
- Complex flow in lumen may give heterogeneous signal
- DSA or CE-MRA/CTA to delineate patent lumen

SELECTED REFERENCES

1. Findlay JM et al: Non-atherosclerotic fusiform cerebral aneurysms. Can J Neurol Sci. 29(1):41-8, 2002
2. Sakata N et al: Different roles of arteriosclerosis in the rupture of intracranial dissecting aneurysms. Histopathology. 38(4):325-37, 2001
3. Jager HR et al: Contrast-enhanced MR angiography of intracranial giant aneurysms. AJNR Am J Neuroradiol. 21(10):1900-7, 2000
4. Nakatomi H et al: Clinicopathological study of intracranial fusiform and dolichoectatic aneurysms : insight on the mechanism of growth. Stroke. 31(4):896-900, 2000

IMAGE GALLERY

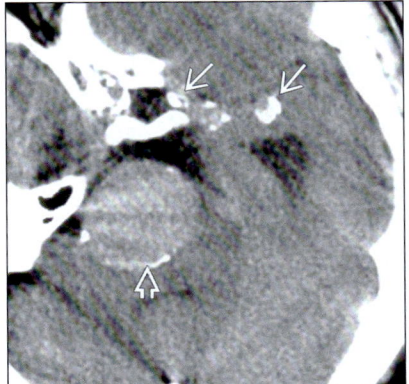
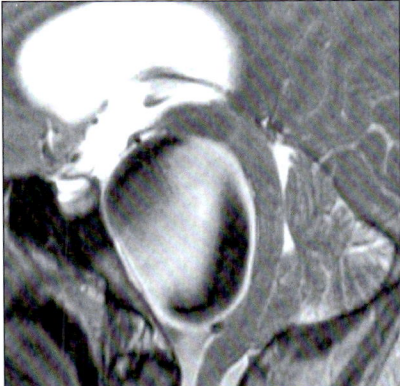
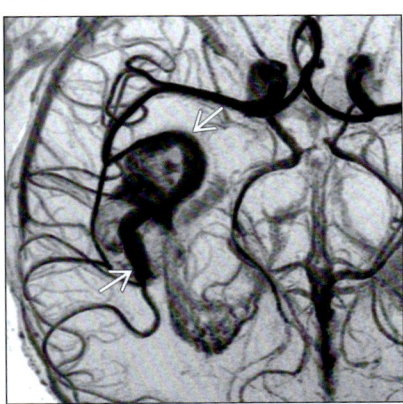

(Left) Axial NECT shows extensive mural calcifications of left ICA & MCA ➡, as well as large hyperdense posterior fossa mass with peripheral calcifications ➡, consistent with ASVD FA. *(Center)* Sagittal T2WI MR shows large basilar artery ASVD FA compressing brainstem. *(Right)* Axial CE-MRA shows unusual NASVD partially thrombosed middle cerebral artery FA ➡. Young age, atypical location suggest underlying vasculopathy.

BLOOD BLISTER-LIKE ANEURYSM

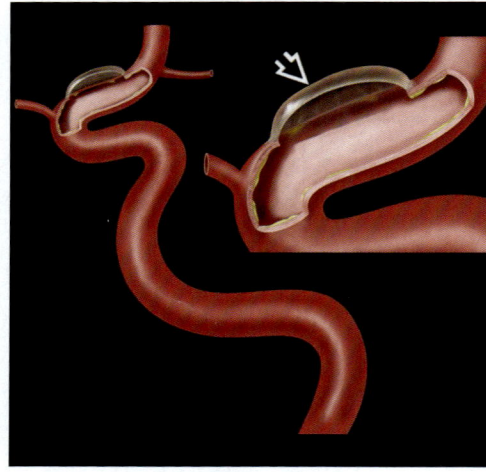

Sagittal graphic shows blood blister-like aneurysm arising from dorsal (superolateral) wall of supraclinoid ICA ➡. BBA is covered only by thin fibrous wall.

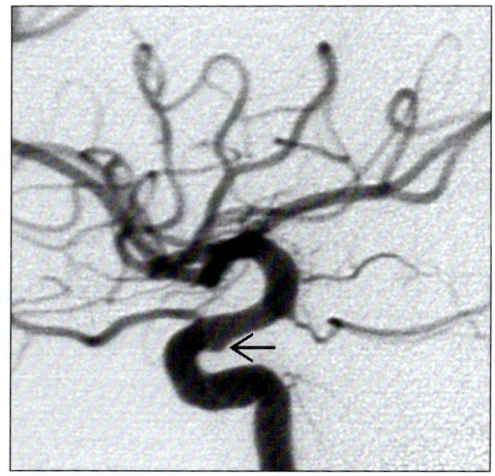

Lateral angiography shows subtle outpouching along inferior aspect of supraclinoid ICA ➡; initially dismissed as atherosclerosis.

TERMINOLOGY

Abbreviations and Synonyms
- Blood blister-like aneurysm (BBA); blister-like pseudoaneurysm; trunk aneurysm

Definitions
- Broad-based, "side-wall" aneurysm composed primarily/exclusively of fibrous tissue

IMAGING FINDINGS

General Features
- Best diagnostic clue: Small broad-based hemispherical bulge of lateral arterial wall
- Location: Supraclinoid ICA is most common site
- Size: Usually small (< 10 mm)
- Morphology: Asymmetrical bulge in vessel wall

CT Findings
- NECT: Aneurysmal subarachnoid hemorrhage (aSAH)
- CTA: ± Asymmetric bulging of supraclinoid ICA below terminal bifurcation

MR Findings
- T1WI: CSF may appear isointense to brain if subarachnoid hemorrhage (SAH) present
- FLAIR: Hyperintense CSF if SAH present
- MRA: ± Visualized on high-resolution MRA

Angiographic Findings
- Conventional
  - DSA
    - Initial angiogram often read as normal
    - Slight irregularity/small focal bulge of arterial wall

Imaging Recommendations
- Best imaging tool: High-resolution DSA, 3D DSA, CTA
- Protocol advice: Obtain multiple obliques, angled lateral views of circle of Willis on DSA

DIFFERENTIAL DIAGNOSIS

Saccular Aneurysm (SA)
- Usually arises at arterial bifurcation/branching point
- Round, lobulated, narrow base

DDx: Blood Blister-Like Mimics

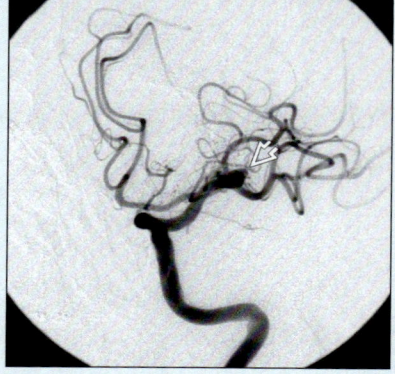

Saccular Aneurysm

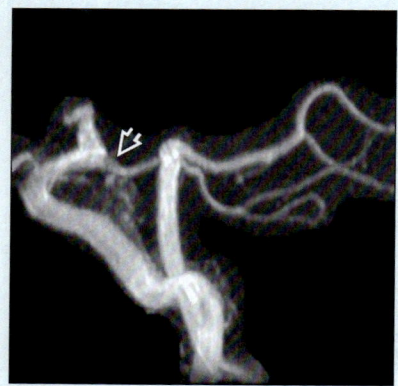

PCoA Infundibulum

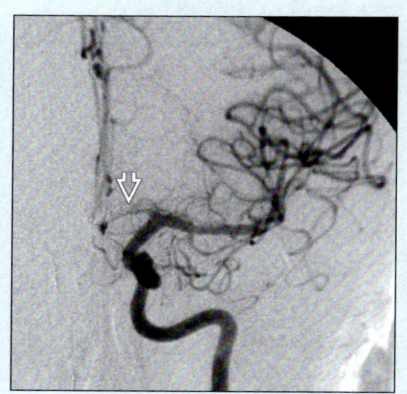

Vasospasm

BLOOD BLISTER-LIKE ANEURYSM

Key Facts

Imaging Findings
- Best diagnostic clue: Small broad-based hemispherical bulge of lateral arterial wall
- Location: Supraclinoid ICA is most common site
- Size: Usually small (< 10 mm)
- CTA: ± Asymmetric bulging of supraclinoid ICA below terminal bifurcation
- Initial angiogram often read as normal

Top Differential Diagnoses
- Saccular Aneurysm (SA)
- Vasospasm
- Atherosclerotic Vascular Disease (ASVD)
- PCoA Infundibulum

Clinical Issues
- Tend to rupture earlier, at smaller size than SA
- High surgical mortality/morbidity

Vasospasm
- Usually symmetrical, concentric narrowing of vessel

Atherosclerotic Vascular Disease (ASVD)
- Common in patients with BBA, difficult to distinguish

PCoA Infundibulum
- Funnel-shaped, PCoA arises from apex, < 3 mm

PATHOLOGY

General Features
- General path comments: Blister-like pseudoaneurysm
- Etiology: ASVD with ulceration, hematoma formation
- Epidemiology: < 1% of all intracranial aneurysms

Gross Pathologic & Surgical Features
- Focal arterial wall defect covered with fibrous tissue

Microscopic Features
- Dome of fibrous tissue/adventitia
- Significant ASVD in parent vessel common

CLINICAL ISSUES

Presentation
- Most common signs/symptoms: aSAH
- Clinical Profile: Middle-aged patient with "angiogram-negative" aSAH

Demographics
- Age: Peak incidence in mid 50s
- Gender: M:F = 1:2

Natural History & Prognosis
- Tend to rupture earlier, at smaller size than SA
- High surgical mortality/morbidity
  - Small size, very thin wall, wide base
  - Avulse readily, intraoperative rupture common

Treatment
- "Trapping", stenting or surgical wrapping

DIAGNOSTIC CHECKLIST

Consider
- "Angiogram-negative" aSAH may be caused by BBA

Image Interpretation Pearls
- Look for subtle asymmetry/bulging of supraclinoid ICA wall when SA not seen in patient with aSAH

SELECTED REFERENCES
1. Nutik SL: Subclinoid aneurysms. J Neurosurg. 98(4):731-6, 2003
2. McNeely PD et al: Endovascular treatment of a "blister-like" aneurysm of the internal carotid artery. Can J Neurol Sci. 27(3):247-50, 2000
3. Kobayashi S et al: Blisterlike aneurysms. J Neurosurg. 91(1):164-6, 1999

IMAGE GALLERY

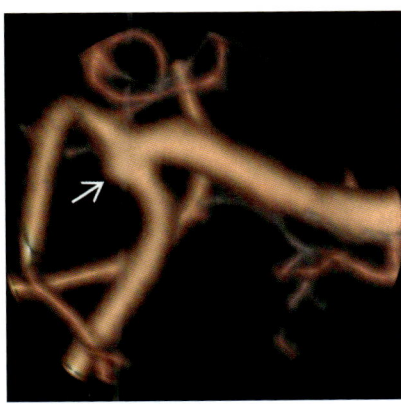 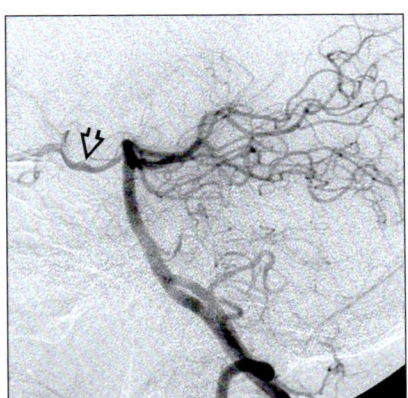 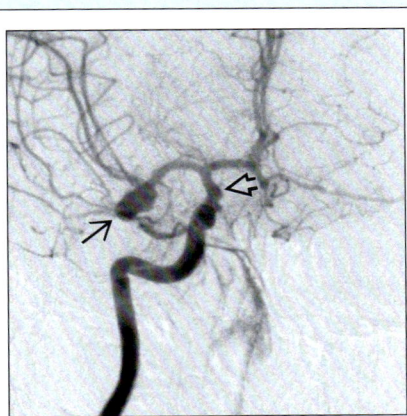

(Left) Axial oblique CTA shows small but definite hemispherical bulge at right MCA bifurcation ➡. Images can be viewed from many different perspectives, significant advantage of CTA over DSA. *(Center)* Lateral angiography shows typical BBA in unusual location. Transient reflux of contrast opacifies posterior communicating artery demonstrating small hemispheric bulge ➡. *(Right)* Anteroposterior angiography shows subtle BBA ➡ seen in context of much larger, more obvious SA ➡. Multiple aneurysms seen in 15-20% of all cases.

INTRACEREBRAL HEMATOMA

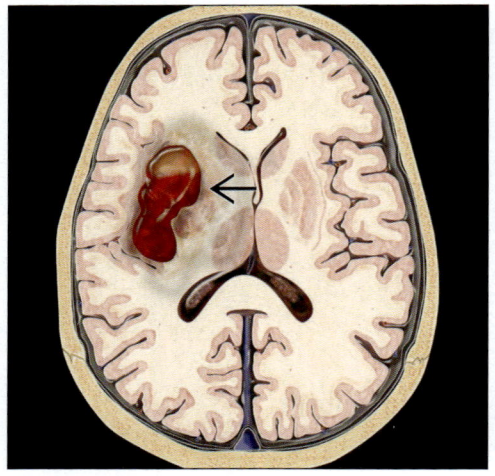

Axial graphic shows right basal ganglia acute hematoma with early peripheral edema (gray). Mild mass effect partially effaces right lateral ventricle; heme-fluid level is forming ➡.

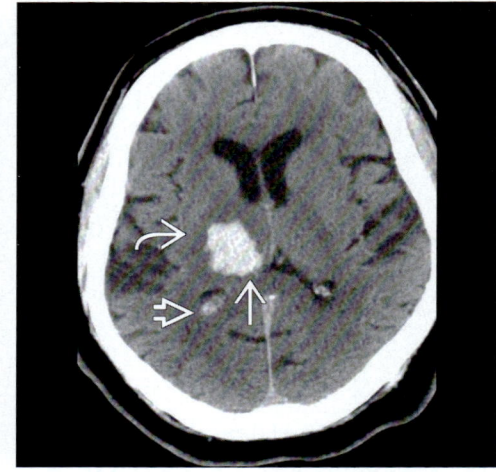

Axial NECT shows acute right thalamic hematoma ➡ with intraventricular extension ➡ and peripheral edema ➡, features typical for hypertensive hemorrhage of 1-2 days duration.

TERMINOLOGY

Abbreviations and Synonyms
- Intracerebral hematoma (ICH)

Definitions
- Parenchymal blood collection

IMAGING FINDINGS

General Features
- Best diagnostic clue
  - Hyperdense (50-70 HU) mass on CT; peripheral edema develops over first days
  - MR: ICH staging based on signal characteristics
  - Factors influencing ICH appearance on MR
    - Intrinsic: Clot macroscopic structure, Hgb oxidative state, RBC integrity, clot hydration, size/location, edema
    - Extrinsic: Pulse sequence, field strength
- Location: Supratentorial > infratentorial brain
- Size: Near-microscopic to very large; solitary > multiple
- Morphology: Ovoid; larger hematomas more irregular

CT Findings
- NECT
  - Acute: Hyperdense mass 0-3 days
    - Rapidly growing hematoma → unretracted semiliquid clot with central hypodensity
    - More hyperdense over first few hours 2° to clot retraction
    - Isodense if Hgb < 8-10 (hemophilia, renal failure)
    - Fluid-fluid levels with coagulopathies or thrombolytic therapy
    - Edema & mass effect initially mild (< 3 hours)
  - Subacute: 3-10 days
    - Progressive decreased attenuation beginning at margin (↓ 1.5 HU/day)
    - Edema peaks at ~ 5 days
    - Isodense in 1-2 weeks, dependent on original size
  - Chronic: > 10 days
    - Hypodense lesion without mass effect; subtle hyperdense rim may be present
    - Residua: ↓ Attenuation foci (37%), no residua (27%), slit-like lesions (25%), calcifications (10%)
- CECT
  - Active bleeding: Contrast pooling

DDx: Acute Hematoma Mimics

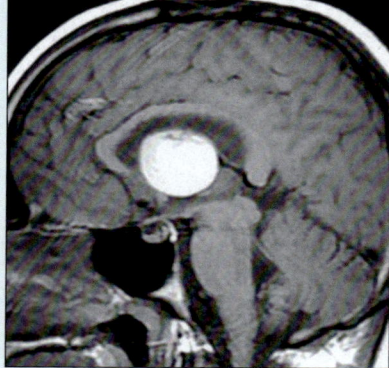

Colloid Cyst

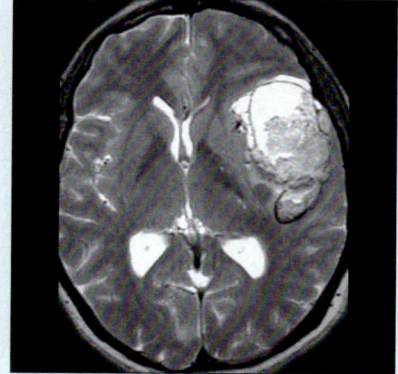

Dermoid

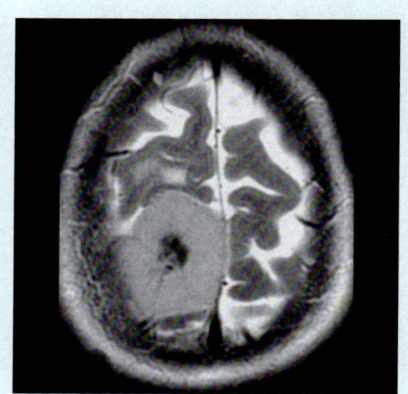

Calcified Meningioma

INTRACEREBRAL HEMATOMA

Key Facts

Terminology
- Parenchymal blood collection

Imaging Findings
- Hyperdense (50-70 HU) mass on CT; peripheral edema develops over first days
- MR: ICH staging based on signal characteristics
- MR: Signal change proceeds peripherally to centrally on all sequences
- Hyperacute: Initially hypointense margin; critical feature to differentiate hemorrhage from other masses at this stage
- Most sensitive technique for detecting acute intracranial hemorrhage
- Initial diagnosis: NECT or MR
- Staging/work-up: MR, MRA, MRV
- GRE necessity to evaluate for hemorrhage

Top Differential Diagnoses
- Fat-Containing Lesions (Dermoid, Lipoma)
- Calcified Lesions (Dural Plaque, Meningioma, Mineralized Basal Ganglia, Partially Thrombosed Aneurysm)
- Proteinaceous Fluid Collections (Colloid Cyst, Craniopharyngioma, Rathke Cleft Cyst)

Clinical Issues
- Clinical Profile: HTN, ↑ age most important risk factors
- Rebleed: Enlargement, ↑ morbidity/mortality

Diagnostic Checklist
- MR more sensitive, more accurate aging of ICH than CT

  - Subacute-chronic: Rim-enhancement (breakdown in blood brain barrier) 3 days to 1 month
  - Chronic: Enhancement disappears 2-6 months

MR Findings
- T1WI
  - MR: Signal change proceeds peripherally to centrally on all sequences
    - ICH rim "ages" faster than center
  - Hyperacute (< 8 hours): Isointense
  - Acute (8 hours to 3 days): Mildly hypointense
  - Early subacute (3-6 days): Initially hyperintense at hematoma margin
  - Late subacute/early chronic (6-21 days): More diffuse hyperintensity
  - Chronic-late (> 21 days): Iso- to hypointense
- T2WI
  - Hyperacute: Hyperintense, may have subtle hypointense rim, hyperintense peripheral edema
  - Acute: Markedly hypointense, increased hyperintense edema
  - Early subacute: Hypointensity slightly decreased, edema increased
  - Late subacute/early chronic: Progressive increase in central intensity, progressive peripheral hypointensity
  - Late chronic: Hypointense rim or cleft, no edema
- FLAIR
  - Same as on T2WI
  - Hyperintense CSF in subarachnoid hemorrhage (SAH)
    - More sensitive than CT for SAH
- T2* GRE
  - Hyperacute: Initially hypointense margin; critical feature to differentiate hemorrhage from other masses at this stage
    - Most sensitive technique for detecting acute intracranial hemorrhage
    - More sensitive than CT for hemorrhagic infarction
  - Acute: Marked diffuse hypointensity
    - Insensitive to acute SAH unless blood clots
  - Early subacute: Persistent hypointensity (> T2WI & FLAIR)
  - Late subacute/early chronic: Increasing hypointense rim (hemosiderin)
  - Late chronic: Persistent marked hypointense nodule or cleft
    - Microbleeds: Punctate foci of chronic hemorrhage
- DWI
  - Hypointense: Susceptibility effects "trump" diffusion effects during acute-subacute phase
  - Significant correlation between ICH volume & degree of ADC elevation in perihematoma edema
  - B° images (T2, susceptibility weighted) show marked hypointensity in acute hematoma
    - Not adequate to detect subtle hemorrhage within infarction or identify microbleeds
- T1 C+: Subacute: Peripheral enhancement within few days

Imaging Recommendations
- Best imaging tool
  - Initial diagnosis: NECT or MR
  - Staging/work-up: MR, MRA, MRV
  - Angiography if no clear cause, or in young, normotensive, stable surgical candidates
- Protocol advice
  - GRE necessity to evaluate for hemorrhage
    - Susceptibility weighted imaging (SWI) more sensitive than GRE

DIFFERENTIAL DIAGNOSIS

Fat-Containing Lesions (Dermoid, Lipoma)
- Mimics subacute ICH (hyperintense on T1WI, hypointense on T2WI)
- Chemical shift artifact, lack of edema, loss of intensity on fat-suppressed images confirm diagnosis

Calcified Lesions (Dural Plaque, Meningioma, Mineralized Basal Ganglia, Partially Thrombosed Aneurysm)
- Hypointense on T2WI & GRE, variable on T1WI

INTRACEREBRAL HEMATOMA

Proteinaceous Fluid Collections (Colloid Cyst, Craniopharyngioma, Rathke Cleft Cyst)
- Mildly hyperintense on T1WI, hypointense on T2WI

PATHOLOGY

General Features
- General path comments
  - Vasogenic edema forms rapidly, progresses up to 3 days
  - May decompress into ventricles/subarachnoid space
- Etiology
  - Very common: HTN, cerebral amyloid angiopathy (CAA), trauma, hemorrhagic vascular malformations
  - Common: Infarct with reperfusion, coagulopathy, blood dyscrasia, drug abuse, tumor (high grade glioma, metastases)
  - Less common: Dural sinus thrombosis, eclampsia, endocarditis with septic emboli, fungal infection (aspergillosis, mucormycosis), encephalitis

Gross Pathologic & Surgical Features
- Acute to early subacute: Blood-filled cavity surrounded by vasogenic edema, inflammation
- Early subacute to early chronic: Organizing clot, vascularized wall
- Late chronic: Hemosiderin scar surrounding region of gliosis

Microscopic Features
- Immediate
  - Liquid hematoma; 95-98% Oxy-Hgb
  - Unretracted fibrin mass forms gel matrix
  - RBCs, WBCs, platelet clumps, serum
- Hyperacute
  - Peripheral edema
  - Hemoconcentration (hematocrit ↑ 70-90%), clot retraction
  - RBCs form spherocytes, contain Oxy-Hgb (no magnetic susceptibility effects)
- Acute
  - RBCs shrink, lose spherical shape
    - Intracellular Deoxy-Hgb in intact RBCs
    - Susceptibility effects of unpaired electrons in deoxy-HgB sequestered in cells → T2WI & GRE hypointensity
  - Severe edema
- Early subacute
  - Intact cells containing met-Hgb
  - Unpaired electrons in met-HgB cause
    - Susceptibility effects (T2WI & GRE hypointensity)
    - T1 shortening 2° dipole interactions between unpaired electrons on molecule surface adjacent water protons (T1WI hyperintensity)
  - Met-HgB formation begins at hematoma surface → T1 hyperintensity initially seen at margin
- Late subacute-early chronic
  - RBC lysis → release met-Hgb into extracellular space
  - Cell lysis → homogeneous distribution of met-Hgb, loss of susceptibility effect; persistent T1WI hyperintensity, ↑ intensity on T2WI & FLAIR
  - Edema & mass effect decrease
  - Perivascular inflammation; macrophages in clot wall
- Chronic
  - Edema, inflammation resolve
  - Met-Hgb resorbed: Decreased central hyperintensity
  - Activated macrophages in vascularized wall contain ferritin & hemosiderin → hypointense rim on T2WI, most marked on GRE
  - Residual cysts and clefts with hemosiderin scar persist indefinitely

CLINICAL ISSUES

Presentation
- Most common signs/symptoms
  - HTN (90%), vomiting, (50%), ↓ consciousness (50%), headache (40%), seizures (10%)
  - Acute focal neurologic deterioration; clot size & location determine deficit
    - 51-63% patients have symptom progression
- Clinical Profile: HTN, ↑ age most important risk factors

Natural History & Prognosis
- No rebleed: Evolution with retraction to scar
- Rebleed: Enlargement, ↑ morbidity/mortality
  - 14-38% expand within first 24 hours
- 50% rupture into ventricles; poor prognosis when entire ventricular system filled
- 50% of deaths occur in first 2 days
- 35-52% were dead at 1 month
- 10% independent at 1 month; 20% at 6 months

Treatment
- Surgical evacuation as needed

DIAGNOSTIC CHECKLIST

Image Interpretation Pearls
- MR more sensitive, more accurate aging of ICH than CT

SELECTED REFERENCES
1. Kamal AK et al: Temporal evolution of diffusion after spontaneous supratentorial intracranial hemorrhage. AJNR Am J Neuroradiol. 24(5):895-901, 2003
2. Atlas S et al: MR Detection of of Hyperacute Parenchymal Hemorrhage of the Brain. AJNR. 19:1471-77, 1998
3. Clark RA et al: Acute Hematomas: Effects of Deoxygenation, Hematocrit, and Fibrin-Clot Formation and Retraction on T2 Shortening. Radiology. 175:201-6, 1990
4. Zimmerman RD et al: Acute intracranial hemorrhage: intensity changes on sequential MR scans at 0.5 T. AJR Am J Roentgenol. 150(3):651-61, 1988
5. Scott WR et al: Computerized Axial Tomography of Intracerebral and Intraventricular Hemorrhage. Radiology. 112:73-80, 1974

INTRACEREBRAL HEMATOMA

IMAGE GALLERY

Typical

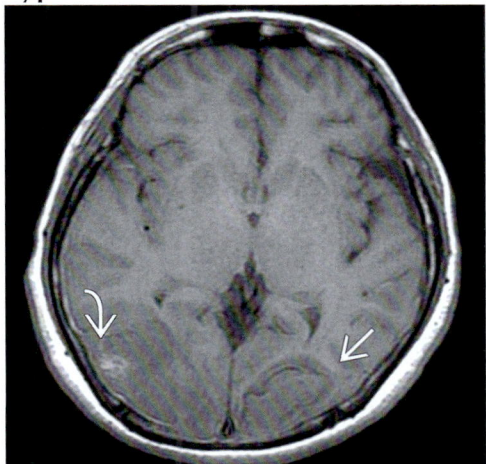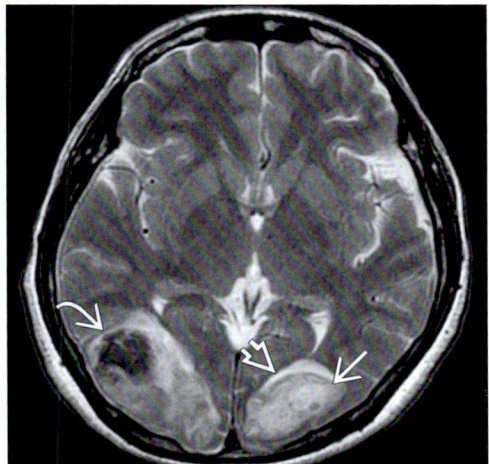

(Left) Axial T1WI MR shows hyperacute left & acute right ICH. Left ICH is isointense ➡, right ICH is mildly hypointense with hyperintense focus ➡ (oldest component). *(Right)* Axial T2WI MR in same case as left shows hyperintense left ICH ➡ with subtle hypointense rim ➡. Acute right ICH is heterogeneous with lateral focus of marked hypointensity ➡.

Typical

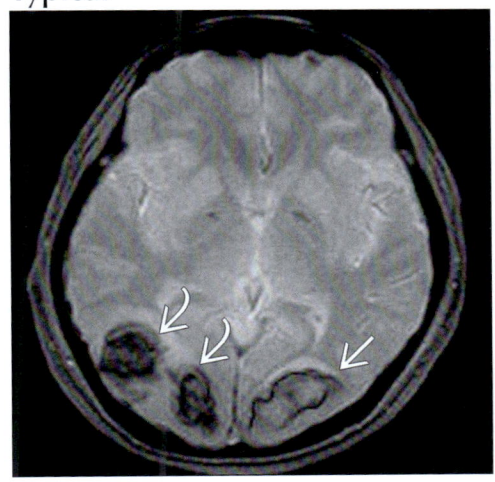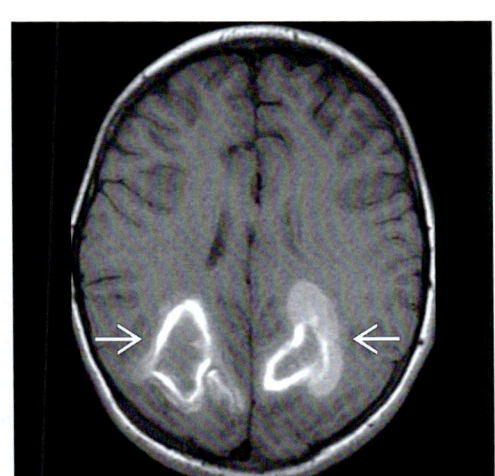

(Left) Axial T2* GRE MR in same case as prior shows left hyperacute hematoma ➡ with hypointense rim, mildly hyperintense center. Acute right hematoma is diffusely hypointense ➡. *(Right)* Axial T1WI MR shows bilateral subacute hematomas. T1WI hyperintensity is present at margins of both hematomas ➡, which are centrally isointense.

Typical

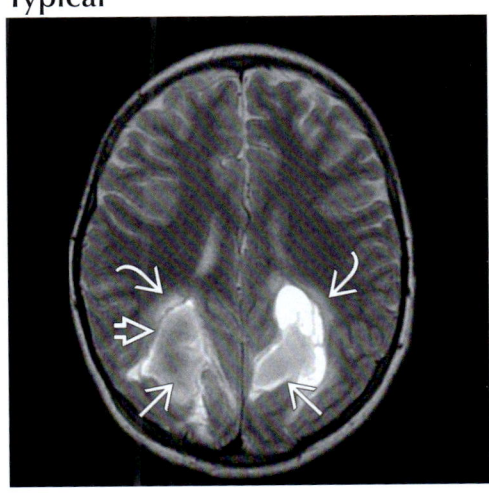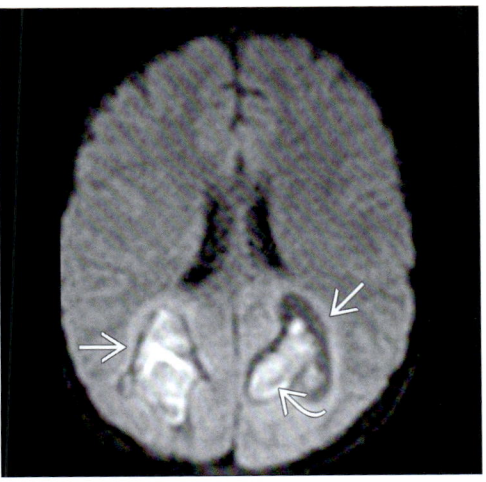

(Left) Axial T2WI FS MR in same case as previous image shows central mild hypointensity ➡, mildly hypointense rim ➡, and mild hyperintense vasogenic edema ➡. *(Right)* Axial DWI MR in same case as left shows hypointense rim ➡ due to susceptibility effect. Hyperintense core of ICH ➡ reflects combination of diffusion, T1 & T2 effects.

SPONTANEOUS INTRACRANIAL HEMORRHAGE

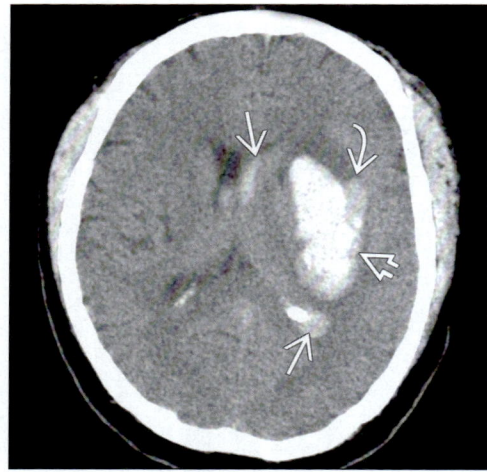

Axial NECT shows classic hypertensive ICH with striatocapsular hematoma ⇒, rupture into lateral ventricle ⇒, fluid-fluid level ⇒. Elderly hypertensive anticoagulated patient.

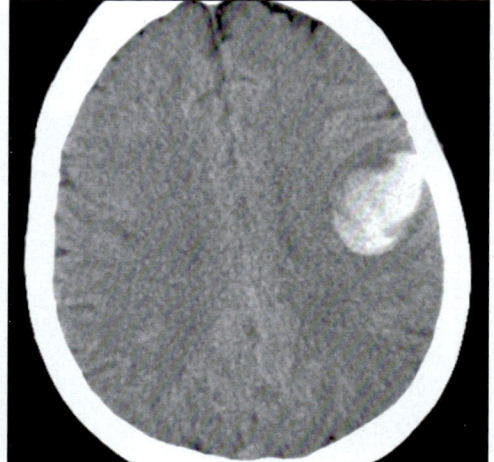

Axial NECT shows lobar hematoma in a 68 y normotensive, demented patient. Differential diagnosis includes CAA, underlying neoplasm, cortical vein occlusion, and coagulopathy.

TERMINOLOGY

Abbreviations and Synonyms
- Primary intracranial hemorrhage (pICH); stroke

Definitions
- Acute nontraumatic ICH
  - Etiology often initially unknown

IMAGING FINDINGS

General Features
- Best diagnostic clue: Acute intracerebral hematoma without history of trauma
- Location
  - Varies with etiology
    - Hypertension (HTN): Deep gray matter (basal ganglia, thalamus) pons, cerebellar hemisphere
    - Cerebral amyloid angiopathy (CAA): Lobar (cortical and subcortical)
    - Arteriovenous malformation (AVM): Any location
    - Cavernous malformation: Any location - common in brainstem
    - Venous sinus thrombosis: Subcortical white matter adjacent to occluded sinus
    - Neoplasm (location varies)
- Size: Sub-centimeter "microbleeds" to multiple centimeters
- Morphology
  - Usually typically round or oval; when large often irregular
  - Two types seen with HTN & CAA
    - Acute focal hematoma
    - Multiple subacute/chronic "microbleeds" in deep gray matter (HTN > CAA) or subcortical white matter (CAA > HTN)
    - Microbleeds typically seen only on GRE MR scans

CT Findings
- NECT
  - Acute usually round/elliptical, hyperdense
  - May be mixed iso-/hyperdense
  - May have fluid-fluid level (rapid bleeding, coagulopathy)
  - Peripheral low density (edema)
  - Deep (ganglionic) ICH may extend into lateral ventricle

DDx: Less Common ICHs

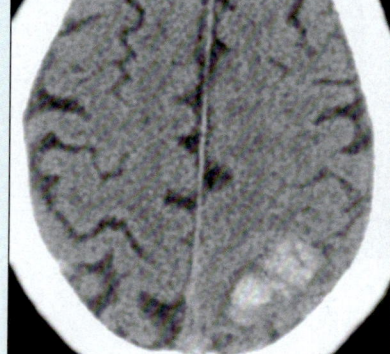
Venous Thrombosis

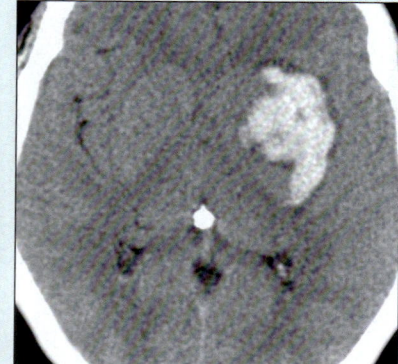
Drug Abuse

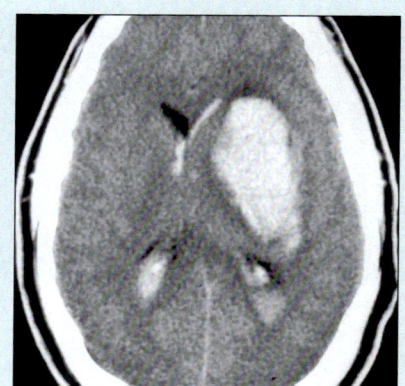
Vasculitis

SPONTANEOUS INTRACRANIAL HEMORRHAGE

Key Facts

Terminology
- Primary intracranial hemorrhage (pICH); stroke

Imaging Findings
- Best diagnostic clue: Acute intracerebral hematoma without history of trauma
- Screening: NECT
- Optional: Standard MR (include T2*, DWI)

Top Differential Diagnoses
- Cerebral Amyloid Disease
- Underlying Neoplasm
- Vascular Malformation
- Cortical Venous Thrombosis
- Anticoagulation
- Drug Abuse
- Vasculitis

Pathology
- Numerous causes; vary with age
- Patients < 45 y: Vascular malformation, drug abuse, venous thrombosis, vasculitis
- Patients > 45 y: HTN, CAA, venous thrombosis, neoplasm (primary--often glioblastoma--or metastatic), coagulopathy

Diagnostic Checklist
- Consider underlying etiology for hemorrhage (CVM, CAA, neoplasm, drug use, etc.)
- Any unexplained ICH should prompt search for microbleeds on T2* MR
- Fluid-fluid level, iso/mildly hyperdense clot may indicate coagulopathy

---

- CECT: No pathologic enhancement
- CTA
  - Usually normal
  - +/- Underlying vascular malformation

MR Findings
- T1WI
  - Hyperacute (< 6 hrs)
    - Isointense center (oxygenated hematoma)
    - Isointense periphery (deoxygenated Hgb, clot tissue interface)
    - Hypointense rim (vasogenic edema)
- T2WI
  - Hyperacute (< 6 hrs)
    - Iso-/hyperintense, heterogeneous center
    - Hypointense periphery
    - Hyperintense rim of edema
- T2* GRE
  - Profoundly hypointense
  - Look for multifocal hypointense lesions ("black dots")
    - Basal ganglionic suggests HTN
    - Peripheral, subcortical WM suggests CAA
- DWI: T2 "shine-through" common
- T1 C+
  - Usually none in acute ICH
  - May enhance if underlying neoplasm, vascular malformation
- MRA: Usually normal
- MRV: Look for dural sinus thrombosis

Angiographic Findings
- DSA
  - Usually negative
  - Look for dural sinus occlusion, "stagnating vessels" (thrombosed AVM)

Imaging Recommendations
- Best imaging tool
  - Screening: NECT
    - If older patient with HTN, striatocapsular hematoma, stop
    - CTA if MR shows atypical hematoma
  - Optional: Standard MR (include T2*, DWI)
    - If no clear cause of hemorrhage, or atypical appearance on CT
    - If T2* shows multifocal "black dots," stop
    - T1 C+ if hematoma appears atypical, bizarre
    - MRA if standard study suggests vascular etiology
  - Follow-up: Repeat MR if etiology unclear +/- DSA if initial MRA/CTA negative
- Protocol advice
  - Atypical hematoma or unclear history: MR (with T2*, DWI, T1 C+ contrast)
  - Add MRV if venous infarction suspected
  - DSA if thrombosed CVM suspected

DIFFERENTIAL DIAGNOSIS

Hypertensive Intracranial Hemorrhage
- Patients usually older
- Basal ganglionic hematoma most common finding

Cerebral Amyloid Disease
- Older patients (70 y, normotensive, often demented)
- Lobar >> basal ganglionic hemorrhage
- Look for microbleeds ("black dots") on T2*
- Confluent white matter hyperintensity usually present

Underlying Neoplasm
- Causes 2-15% of nontraumatic ICHs
- Can be primary (glioblastoma multiforme) or metastatic tumor
- Disordered hemorrhage evolution
- May show enhancing foci

Vascular Malformation
- AVM, cavernous malformation most common causes
- ICH rate in patients with AVM of basal ganglia or thalamus (9.8% per year) much higher than in patients with AVM in other locations
- High risk of incurring neurological deficit with each hemorrhagic event

Cortical Venous Thrombosis
- Adjacent dural sinus often thrombosed

SPONTANEOUS INTRACRANIAL HEMORRHAGE

Anticoagulation
- "Growing" hematoma, fluid-fluid levels common
- Check history

Drug Abuse
- May have hypertensive striatocapsular hemorrhage
- Less common = ruptured cortical pseudoaneurysm

Vasculitis
- Rare cause of spontaneous ICH
- Patients usually younger

PATHOLOGY

General Features
- General path comments: Can be arterial or venous, cortical or deep, gross or microscopic
- Genetics: MMP-9, cytokine gene expression ↑ after acute spontaneous ICH
- Etiology
  - Numerous causes; vary with age
    - Patients < 45 y: Vascular malformation, drug abuse, venous thrombosis, vasculitis
    - Patients > 45 y: HTN, CAA, venous thrombosis, neoplasm (primary--often glioblastoma--or metastatic), coagulopathy
- Epidemiology: Causes 15-20% of acute strokes

Gross Pathologic & Surgical Features
- Findings range from petechial "microbleeds" to gross parenchymal hematoma

Microscopic Features
- Co-existing microangiopathy common in amyloid, HTN

Staging, Grading or Classification Criteria
- Clinical "ICH score" correlates with 30 day mortality
  - Admission GCS
  - Age > 80 y, ICH volume
  - Infratentorial
  - Presence of IVH

CLINICAL ISSUES

Presentation
- Most common signs/symptoms
  - 90% of patients with recurrent pICH are hypertensive
  - Large ICHs present with sensorimotor deficits, impaired consciousness

Demographics
- Age: Perinatal through elderly
- Gender: No gender predisposition

Natural History & Prognosis
- Prognosis related to location, size of ICH
- Hematoma enlargement common in first 24-48 hrs
  - Risk factors: EtOH, low fibrinogen, coagulopathy, irregularly shaped hematoma, disturbed consciousness
- Edema associated with poor outcome
- Mortality 30-55% in first month
- 30% rebleed within 1 year
- Recovery poor; most survivors have significant deficits

Treatment
- Control of ICP, hydrocephalus
- Surgical evacuation controversial

DIAGNOSTIC CHECKLIST

Consider
- Consider underlying etiology for hemorrhage (CVM, CAA, neoplasm, drug use, etc.)

Image Interpretation Pearls
- Any unexplained ICH should prompt search for microbleeds on T2* MR
- Microbleeds may signal diffuse hemorrhage-prone vasculopathy
- Fluid-fluid level, iso/mildly hyperdense clot may indicate coagulopathy

SELECTED REFERENCES

1. Harden SP et al: Cranial CT of the unconscious adult patient. Clin Radiol. 62(5):404-15, 2007
2. Chao CP et al: Cerebral amyloid angiopathy: CT and MR imaging findings. Radiographics. 26(5):1517-31, 2006
3. Finelli PF: A diagnostic approach to multiple simultaneous intracerebral hemorrhages. Neurocrit Care. 4(3):267-71, 2006
4. Leach JL et al: Imaging of cerebral venous thrombosis: current techniques, spectrum of findings, and diagnostic pitfalls. Radiographics. 26 Suppl 1:S19-41; discussion S42-3, 2006
5. Thanvi B et al: Sporadic cerebral amyloid angiopathy--an important cause of cerebral haemorrhage in older people. Age Ageing. 35(6):565-71, 2006
6. Chalela JA et al: Multiple cerebral microbleeds: MRI marker of a diffuse hemorrhage-prone state. J Neuroimaging. 14(1):54-7, 2004
7. Abilleira S et al: Matrix metalloproteinase-9 concentration after spontaneous intracerebral hemorrhage. J Neurosurg. 99(1):65-70, 2003
8. Fewel ME et al: Spontaneous intracerebral hemorrhage: a review. Neurosurg Focus. 15(4):E1, 2003
9. Kalaria RN et al: Introduction: Non-atherosclerotic cerebrovascular disorders. Brain Pathol. 12(3):337-42, 2002
10. Skidmore CT et al: Spontaneous intracerebral hemorrhage: epidemiology, pathophysiology, and medical management. Neurosurg Clin N Am. 13(3):281-8, v, 2002
11. Woo D et al: Spontaneous intracerebral hemorrhage: epidemiology and clinical presentation. Neurosurg Clin N Am. 13(3):265-79, v, 2002
12. Bernardini GL et al: Critical care of intracerebral and subarachnoid hemorrhage. Curr Neurol Neurosci Rep. 1(6):568-76, 2001
13. Qureshi AI et al: Spontaneous intracerebral hemorrhage. N Engl J Med. 344(19):1450-60, 2001
14. Roob G et al: Magnetic resonance imaging of cerebral microbleeds. Curr Opin Neurol. 13(1):69-73, 2000

SPONTANEOUS INTRACRANIAL HEMORRHAGE

IMAGE GALLERY

Typical

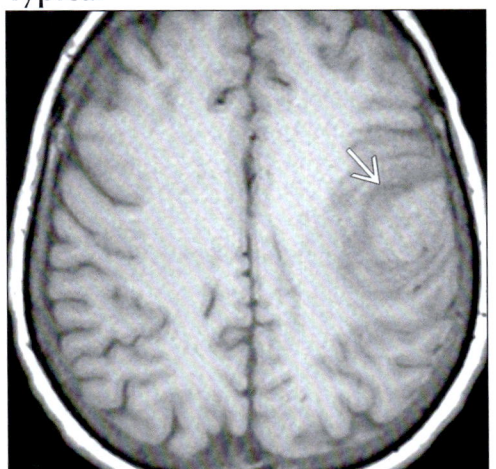
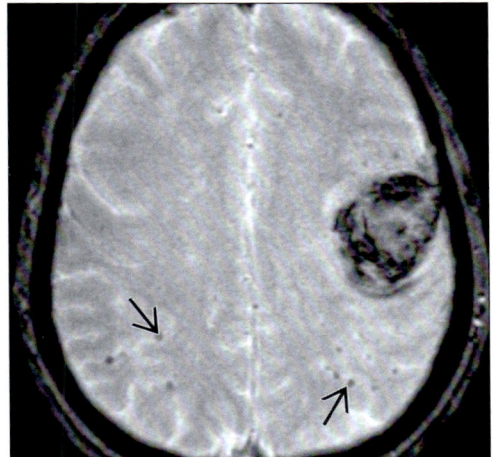

(Left) Axial T1WI MR shows a mostly isointense left anterior parietal mass ➡. No other abnormalities were seen on this sequence. *(Right)* Axial T2* GRE MR in the same case shows hematoma blooms strongly but inhomogeneously. Note multifocal cortical/subcortical hypointensities ("black dots") ➡. Probable CAA.

Typical

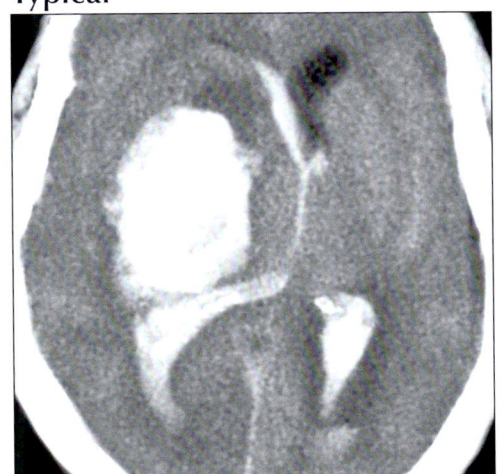
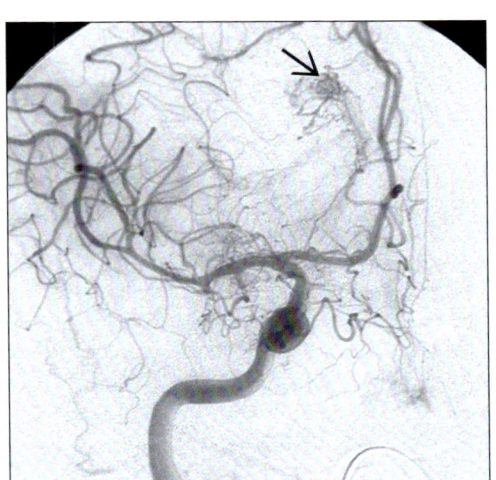

(Left) Axial NECT in a 46 y mildly hypertensive male shows basal ganglionic hemorrhage with intraventricular blood. No history of drug abuse could be elicited. *(Right)* DSA was performed to look for an underlying vascular lesion. Note tangle of abnormal arteries ➡. Mostly thrombosed arteriovenous malformation was confirmed at surgery.

Typical

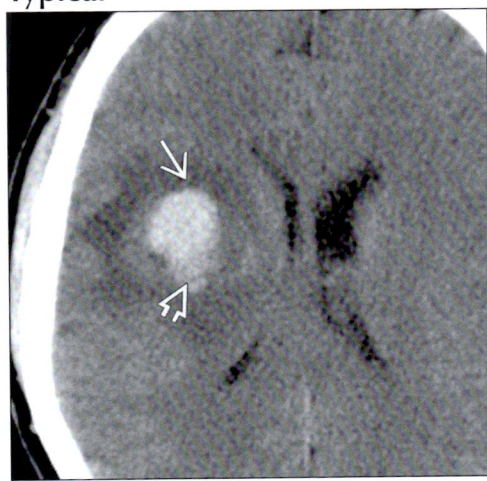
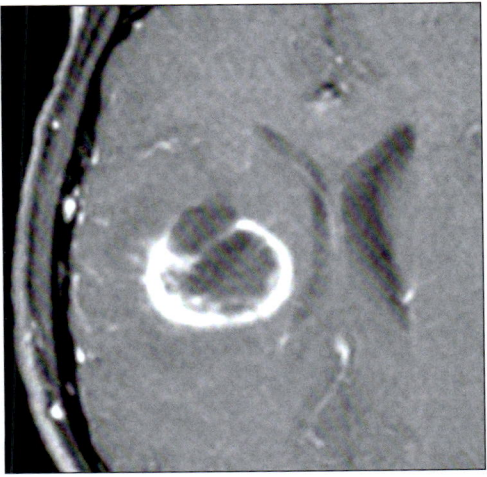

(Left) Axial NECT in an elderly patient shows a hyperdense mass in the right centrum semiovale ➡. Significant cerebral edema ➡ is present surrounding the lesion. *(Right)* Axial T1 C+ MR in the same case shows a thick, irregular rind of enhancement around the hematoma. GBM was found at surgery.

HYPERTENSIVE INTRACRANIAL HEMORRHAGE

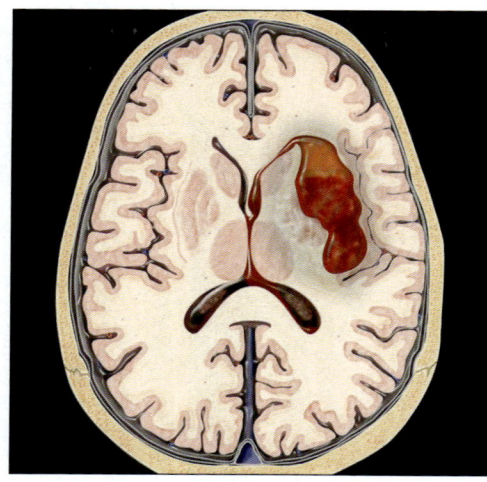

Axial graphic shows acute hypertensive basal ganglionic/external capsule hemorrhage with dissection into the lateral ventricle. Hemorrhage extends through foramen of Monro to 3rd ventricle.

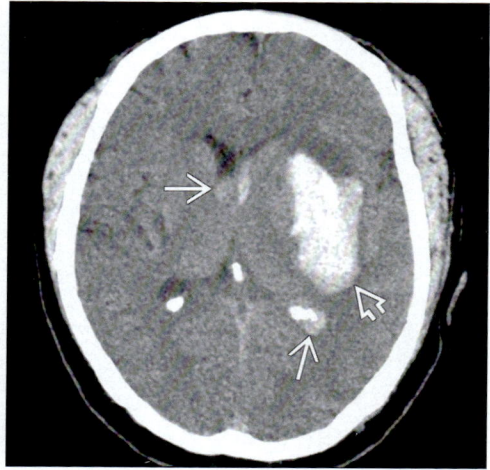

Axial NECT shows a classic acute putaminal/external capsule hemorrhage ➡ in this patient with untreated hypertension. Note blood in the lateral ventricles ➡.

TERMINOLOGY

Abbreviations and Synonyms
- Hypertensive intracranial hemorrhage (hICH)
- "Stroke"

Definitions
- Acute nontraumatic ICH secondary to systemic hypertension (HTN)

IMAGING FINDINGS

General Features
- Best diagnostic clue
  - Round/elliptical high density mass with epicenter in basal ganglia/external capsule
  - Most characteristic sign = putamen/external capsule hematoma in patient with HTN
- Location
  - Striatocapsular (putamen/external capsule) 60-65%
  - Thalamus 15-25%
  - Pons, cerebellum 10%
  - Lobar 5-15%
  - Multifocal "microbleeds" 1-5%
- Size: Varies from sub-centimeter ("microbleeds") to multiple centimeters
- Morphology
  - Typically rounded or oval-shaped
  - Two distinct patterns seen with hICH
    - Acute focal hematoma
    - Multiple subacute/chronic "microbleeds"

CT Findings
- NECT
  - Elliptical high density parenchymal mass
  - Acute ICH usually hyperdense
  - Mixed density if coagulopathy, active bleeding
  - Other: Hydrocephalus, IVH, herniation
- CECT: No enhancement in acute hICH
- CTA: Avascular mass effect unless underlying vascular lesion (AVM, aneurysm)

MR Findings
- T1WI
  - Varies with age of clot
    - Hyperacute hematoma (< 6 hrs): Oxyhemoglobin (Hgb) (iso-/hypointense)

DDx: Hypertensive Intracranial Hemorrhage

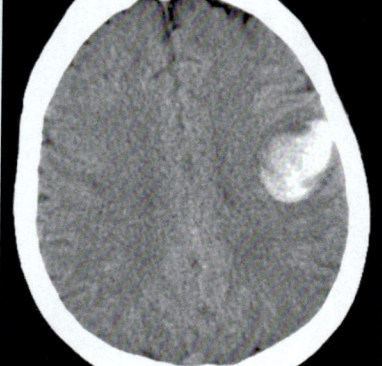

Amyloid

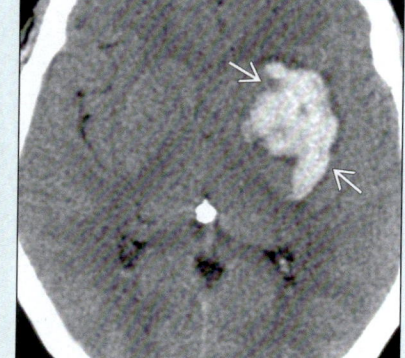

Cocaine Overdose

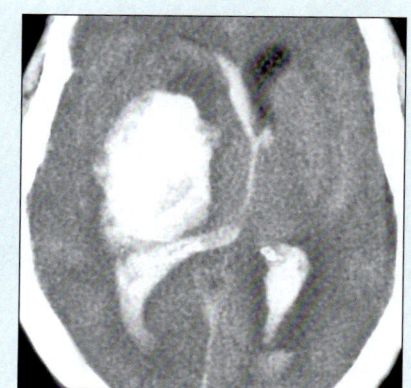

Arteriovenous Malformation

HYPERTENSIVE INTRACRANIAL HEMORRHAGE

Key Facts

Terminology
- Acute nontraumatic ICH secondary to systemic hypertension (HTN)

Imaging Findings
- Round/elliptical high density mass with epicenter in basal ganglia/external capsule
- Striatocapsular (putamen/external capsule) 60-65%
- Thalamus 15-25%
- Pons, cerebellum 10%
- Lobar 5-15%
- Multifocal "microbleeds" 1-5%
- Appearance of hematoma varies with stage
- "White matter hyperintensities" are ICH risk markers

Top Differential Diagnoses
- Cerebral Amyloid Angiopathy
- Vascular Malformation
- Drug Abuse
- Coagulopathy
- Cortical Venous Thrombosis
- Deep Cerebral Venous Thrombosis
- Hemorrhagic Neoplasm

Pathology
- 50% of primary nontraumatic ICHs caused by hypertensive hemorrhage
- HTN most common cause of spontaneous ICH between 45-70 years
- 10-15% of all cases of "stroke"; associated with highest mortality rate

Clinical Issues
- 80% mortality in massive ICH with IVH

- Acute hematoma (48-72 hrs): DeoxyHgb (iso-/hyperintense)
- Subacute hematoma (several days): Intracellular metHgb (hyperintense)
- Chronic hematoma (week-months): Extracellular metHgb (hyperintense)
- T2WI
    - Appearance of hematoma varies with stage
        - Hyperacute hematoma (< 6 hrs): OxyHgb (hyperintense)
        - Acute hematoma (hrs-several days): DeoxyHgb (hypointense)
        - Subacute hematoma (first several days): Intracellular metHgb (hypointense)
        - Chronic hematoma (several days-months): Extracellular metHgb (hyperintense)
        - Remote hematoma (months-yrs): Hypointense hemosiderin scar ± small central hyperintense cavity
    - "White matter hyperintensities" are ICH risk markers
- T2* GRE
    - Multifocal hypointense lesions ("black dots") on T2*
    - Common with longstanding HTN
    - Also commonly seen with amyloid angiopathy
- DWI: Hypo- or mixed hypo/hyperintense (early hematoma)
- T1 C+
    - Typically no enhancement
    - Contrast extravasation = active hemorrhage, growing hematoma
- MRA: Negative

Angiographic Findings
- Conventional
    - DSA usually normal if history of HTN + deep ganglionic hemorrhage
        - May show avascular mass effect
        - Rare: "Bleeding globe" microaneurysm on lenticulostriate artery (LSA)
    - Co-existing vascular abnormalities
        - Increased prevalence of unruptured intracranial aneurysms
        - More common in females

Imaging Recommendations
- Best imaging tool
    - If older patient with HTN and high suspicion for hICH, NECT
    - If hyperacute ischemic "stroke" suspected, MR with T2* and DWI
    - If MR shows classic hematoma + co-existing multifocal "black dots," stop
    - If MR shows atypical hematoma, CTA
    - If CTA inconclusive, consider DSA
- Protocol advice
    - Initial screen = NECT in patients with HTN
    - Otherwise MR (include T2* sequences, DWI, + MRA; T1 C+ optional)

DIFFERENTIAL DIAGNOSIS

Cerebral Amyloid Angiopathy
- Lobar > basal ganglionic
- Usually elderly, demented, normotensive
- Only 5-15% of hICHs are lobar but HTN so common that it is always a diagnostic consideration

Vascular Malformation
- Patients usually normotensive, younger
- Most common = cavernous malformation
    - Look for "black dots" (multiple lesions) on T2* (GRE, SWI) scans
- Less common = thrombosed hemorrhagic AVM or dAVF
    - Look for stagnating vessels, early draining veins on DSA

Drug Abuse
- Cocaine may cause sudden ↑↑ HTN
- Be suspicious if unexplained basal ganglionic bleed in young patient

Coagulopathy
- Elderly patients on anticoagulant therapy

HYPERTENSIVE INTRACRANIAL HEMORRHAGE

Cortical Venous Thrombosis
- May have history of dehydration, "flu," pregnancy/BCPs
- Causes lobar hematoma
- Look for hyperdense dural sinus (not always present)

Deep Cerebral Venous Thrombosis
- Less common than dural sinus or cortical vein thrombosis
- Look for
  o Low density thalami, basal ganglia on NECT
  o Hyperdense (clotted) ICVs, intraventricular hemorrhage

Hemorrhagic Neoplasm
- Secondary (metastasis) and primary (GBM)

PATHOLOGY

General Features
- General path comments
  o Striatocapsular hematoma most common autopsy finding
  o Diffuse "microbleeds" also common
- Etiology
  o Chronic HTN with atherosclerosis, fibrinoid necrosis, abrupt wall rupture ± pseudoaneurysm formation
  o "Bleeding globe" (penetrating LSA aneurysm)
- Epidemiology
  o 50% of primary nontraumatic ICHs caused by hypertensive hemorrhage
  o HTN most common cause of spontaneous ICH between 45-70 years
  o 10-15% of all cases of "stroke"; associated with highest mortality rate
  o 10-15% of hypertensive patients with spontaneous ICH have underlying aneurysm or AVM

Gross Pathologic & Surgical Features
- Large ganglionic hematoma ± IVH
- Subfalcine herniation, hydrocephalus common
- Co-existing small chronic hemorrhages, ischemic lesions common

Microscopic Features
- Fibrous balls (fibrosed miliary aneurysm)
- Severe arteriosclerosis with hyalinization, pseudoaneurysm (lacks media/IEL)

CLINICAL ISSUES

Presentation
- Most common signs/symptoms
  o 10-20% of patients with "stroke" have hICH
  o Large ICHs present with sensorimotor deficits, impaired consciousness
- Clinical Profile: Major risk factor = HTN (increases risk of ICH 4x)

Demographics
- Age: Elderly
- Gender: Males
- Ethnicity: African-American most common

Natural History & Prognosis
- Bleeding can persist for up to 6 hr following ictus
- Neurologic deterioration common within 48 hr
  o Increasing hematoma
  o Edema
  o Development of hydrocephalus
  o Herniation syndromes
- Recurrent hICH in 5-10% of cases, usually different location
- Prognosis related to location, size of ICH
- 80% mortality in massive ICH with IVH
- Only one-third of patients with hICH survive first year
- One-third of survivors are severely disabled

Treatment
- Control of ICP and hydrocephalus
- Large met-analysis failed to show benefit of surgery over conservative treatment

DIAGNOSTIC CHECKLIST

Consider
- Does the patient have a history of poorly-controlled systemic HTN?
- Could there be an underlying coagulopathy, hemorrhagic neoplasm or vascular malformation?
- Check for history of substance abuse in young patients with unexplained hICH

Image Interpretation Pearls
- The underlying cause of lobar intracerebral hemorrhage (ICH) is often difficult to determine
- Subarachnoid extension of hematoma on CT strongly indicates a non-hypertensive cause more specifically, it suggests lobar ICH caused by vascular abnormalities
- The definite diagnosis of CAA vs HTN-related hemorrhage requires histopathological confirmation and should not be based solely on hemorrhage pattern interpretation

SELECTED REFERENCES
1. Ferro JM: Update on intracerebral haemorrhage. J Neurol. 253(8):985-99, 2006
2. Sakuma I et al: Dural arteriovenous fistulas of the cavernous sinus with onset of intracerebral haemorrhage mimicking hypertensive putaminal hemorrhage. Acta Neurochir (Wien). 148(8):915-8, 2006
3. Hanley DF et al: Critical care and emergency medicine neurology. Stroke. 35(2):365-6, 2004
4. Hiroki M et al: Link between linear hyperintensity objects in cerebral white matter and hypertensive intracerebral hemorrhage. Cerebrovasc Dis. 18(2):166-73, 2004
5. Matsumoto K et al: Co-existence of unruptured cerebral aneurysms in patients with hypertensive intracerebral hemorrhage. Acta Neurochir (Wien). 146(10):1085-9; discussion 1089, 2004
6. Ohtani R et al: Clinical and radiographic features of lobar cerebral hemorrhage: hypertensive versus non-hypertensive cases. Intern Med. 42(7):576-80, 2003

HYPERTENSIVE INTRACRANIAL HEMORRHAGE

IMAGE GALLERY

Typical

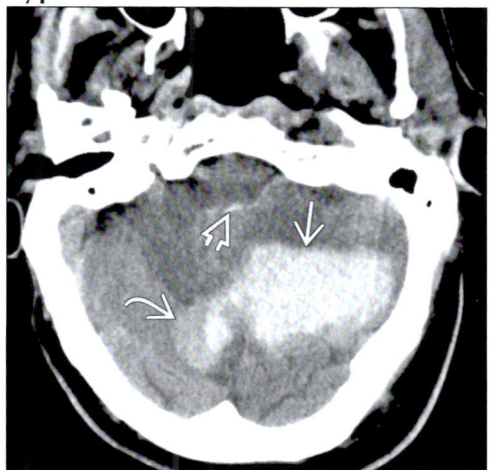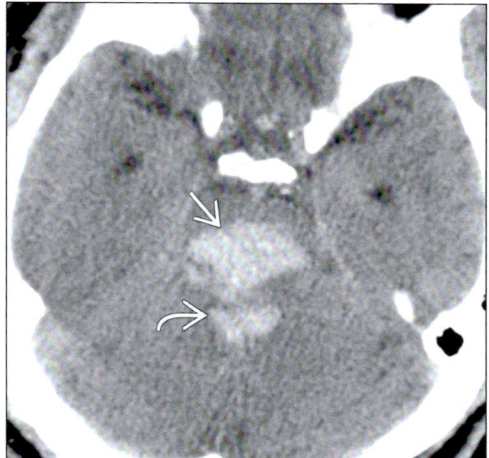

(Left) Axial NECT shows large hypertensive bleed in left cerebellum ➔ with adjacent area of lesser hyperdensity ➔ indicating active bleeding. Blood is also in the lower 4th ventricle ➔. *(Right)* Axial NECT illustrates classic intrapontine high density characteristic of hypertensive brainstem hemorrhage ➔. Note blood has dissected into the fourth ventricle ➔.

Typical

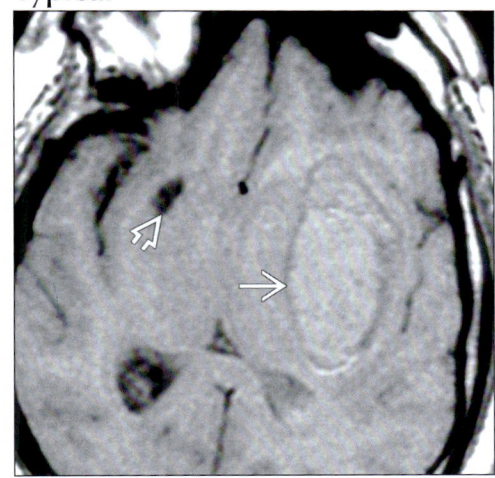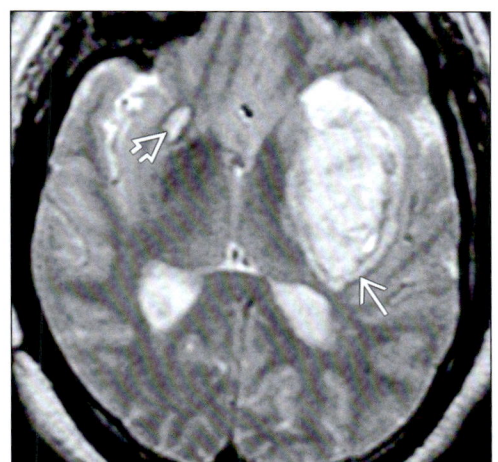

(Left) Axial T1WI MR in a 38 year old male with uncontrolled hypertension shows a mostly isointense mass in the left basal ganglia ➔. Note possible old right basal ganglionic infarct ➔. *(Right)* Axial T2WI MR in the same case shows acute, inhomogeneously hyperintense hemorrhage in the left basal ganglia ➔ and a chronic right basal ganglia infarct surrounded by hemosiderin ➔.

Typical

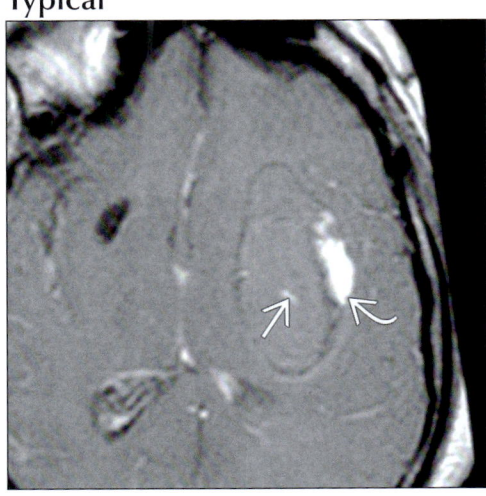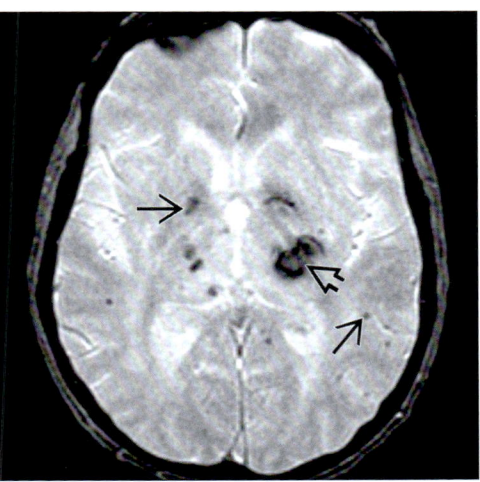

(Left) Axial T1 C+ MR in the same case shows a linear enhancing focus ➔ with contrast accumulating in the outside margin of the clot ➔. The lesion is actively bleeding. *(Right)* Axial T2* GRE MR in another case shows old left thalamic/internal capsule hemorrhage ➔. Innumerable "black dots" ➔ represent residua from hypertensive microbleeds.

ACUTE HYPERTENSIVE ENCEPHALOPATHY, PRES

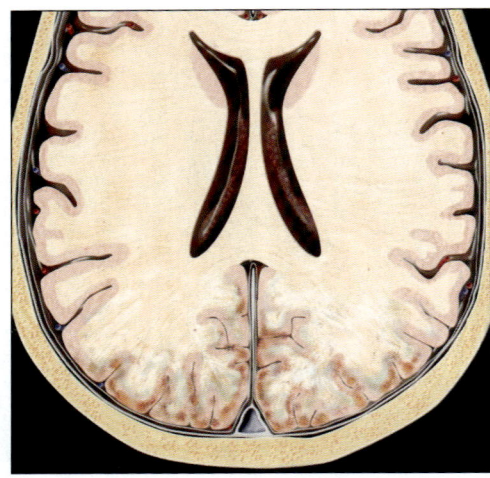

Axial graphic shows the classic posterior circulation cortical/subcortical vasogenic edema characteristic of PRES. Petechial hemorrhage occurs in some cases but is unusual.

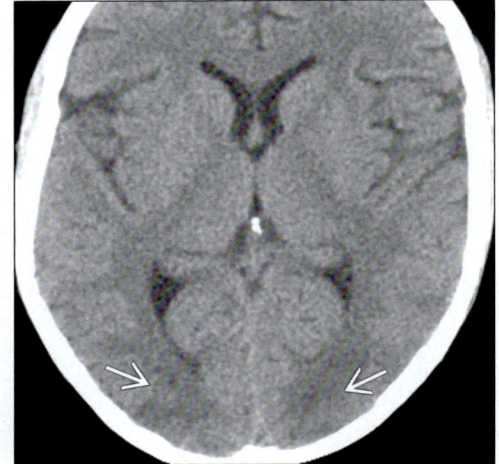

Axial NECT in an eclamptic female shows bilateral hypodensities in the occipital lobes ➔ characteristic of PRES.

TERMINOLOGY

Abbreviations and Synonyms
- Hypertensive encephalopathy; posterior reversible encephalopathy syndrome (PRES); reversible posterior leukoencephalopathy syndrome (RPLS)

Definitions
- Variant of hypertensive encephalopathy characterized by headache, visual disturbances, altered mental function
- Cerebrovascular autoregulatory disorder
  - Multiple etiologies
  - Most caused by acute hypertension (HTN)

IMAGING FINDINGS

General Features
- Best diagnostic clue: Patchy cortical/subcortical PCA territory lesions in a patient with severe acute/subacute HTN
- Location
  - Most common: Cortex, subcortical white matter
    - Predilection for posterior circulation (parietal, occipital lobes, cerebellum)
    - At junctions of vascular watershed zones
    - Usually bilateral, often somewhat asymmetric
  - Less common: Basal ganglia
  - Rare: Predominate/exclusive brainstem involvement
- Size: Extent of abnormalities highly variable
- Morphology: Patchy > confluent

CT Findings
- NECT
  - Patchy bilateral nonconfluent hypodense foci
    - Posterior parietal, occipital lobes > basal ganglia, brainstem
  - Less common: Petechial cortical/subcortical or basal ganglionic hemorrhage
- CECT: With or without mild patchy/punctate enhancement
- CTA
  - Usually normal
  - Rare: Vasospasm with multifocal areas of arterial narrowing

MR Findings
- T1WI: Hypointense cortical/subcortical lesions

DDx: Gyral Hyperintensity

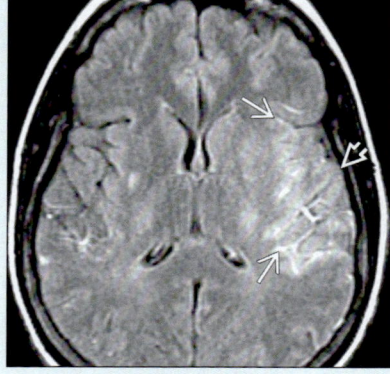
Acute Ischemia

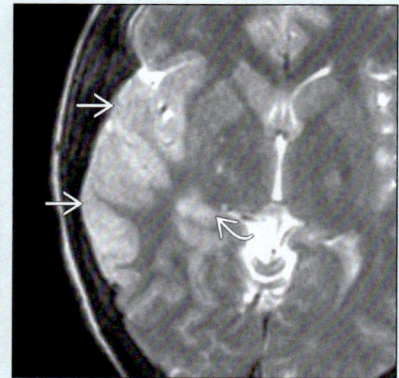
Status Epilepticus

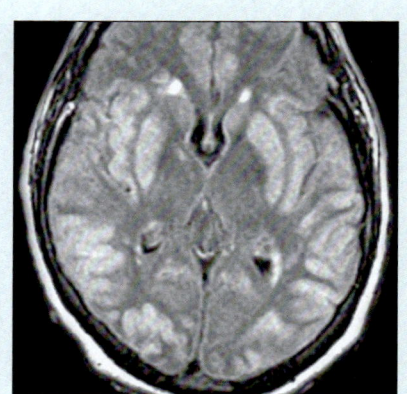
Severe Hypoglycemia

ACUTE HYPERTENSIVE ENCEPHALOPATHY, PRES

Key Facts

Imaging Findings
- Best diagnostic clue: Patchy cortical/subcortical PCA territory lesions in a patient with severe acute/subacute HTN
- Parieto-occipital hyperintense cortical lesions in 95%
- DWI: Usually normal
- ADC map: Markedly elevated (bright areas)
- T1 C+: Variable patchy enhancement

Top Differential Diagnoses
- Cerebral Ischemia-Infarction, Acute
- Status Epilepticus
- Gliomatosis Cerebri

Pathology
- Diverse causes, clinical entities with HTN as common component
- Breakthrough of autoregulation causes BBB disruption
- Result = vasogenic (not cytotoxic) edema
- Acute/subacute systemic HTN
- Preeclampsia, eclampsia
- Uremic encephalopathies
- Drug toxicity (many reported)

Clinical Issues
- Headache, seizure, altered mental status
- Caution: Some patients, especially children, may be normotensive/minimally elevated BP!
- Favorable outcome with prompt recognition, treatment of HTN
- Delayed diagnosis/therapy can result in chronic neurologic sequelae

---

- T2WI
  - Hyperintense cortical/subcortical lesions
  - Less common
    - Extensive brain stem hyperintensity
    - Generalized white matter edema
- PD/Intermediate: Multifocal hyperintensities
- FLAIR
  - Parieto-occipital hyperintense cortical lesions in 95%
  - +/- Symmetric lesions in basal ganglia
  - Does not discriminate between vasogenic, cytotoxic edema (both have increased signal intensity)
- T2* GRE: Blooms if hemorrhage present
- DWI
  - DWI: Usually normal
    - Most common: Normal (no restriction)
    - Less common: High signal on DWI with "pseudonormalized" ADC (may indicate irreversible infarction)
  - ADC map: Markedly elevated (bright areas)
  - DTI (diffusion tensor imaging)
    - Shows foci of increased diffusion representing anisotropy loss
    - Vasogenic edema due to cerebrovascular autoregulatory dysfunction
  - Perfusion scans may show increased microvascular CBF
- T1 C+: Variable patchy enhancement
- MRS
  - May show widespread metabolic abnormalities
    - Increased Cho, Cr
    - Mildly decreased NAA
    - Usually return to normal within 2 months

Nuclear Medicine Findings
- SPECT
  - Variable findings reported; some show hyper-, others hypoperfusion in affected areas

Imaging Recommendations
- Best imaging tool: Contrast-enhanced MR + DWI
- Protocol advice: Repeat scan after BP normalized

DIFFERENTIAL DIAGNOSIS

Cerebral Ischemia-Infarction, Acute
- MCA distribution >> PCA
- DWI usually shows restriction (high signal)

Status Epilepticus
- May cause transient gyral edema, enhancement
- Can mimic PRES, stroke, infiltrating neoplasm

Acute Cerebral Hyperemia Syndromes, Miscellaneous
- Rapid decompression of chronic SDH
  - Generally localized to cortex under the SDH
- Postcarotid endarterectomy, angioplasty or stenting
  - Hyperperfusion syndrome occurs in 5-9% of cases
  - Perfusion MR or CT scans show elevated rCBF
  - Aggressive control of BP associated with clinical, radiological improvement

Hypoglycemia
- Also other metabolic derangements (e.g., dialysis disequilibrium syndrome)
- Locations somewhat different
  - Pons, basal ganglia, white matter in osmotic demyelination
  - Posterior circulation in PRES, porphyria

Gliomatosis Cerebri
- Entire lobe(s) involved rather than patchy cortical/subcortical
- Can mimic brainstem PRES

PATHOLOGY

General Features
- Etiology
  - Diverse causes, clinical entities with HTN as common component
  - Acute HTN damages vascular endothelium
  - Breakthrough of autoregulation causes BBB disruption

ACUTE HYPERTENSIVE ENCEPHALOPATHY, PRES

- Primarily at arteriolar level with HTN, diabetic vasculopathy, etc.
  - Result = vasogenic (not cytotoxic) edema
    - Arteriolar dilatation with cerebral hyperperfusion
    - Hydrostatic leakage (extravasation, transudation of fluid and macromolecules through arteriolar walls)
    - Interstitial fluid accumulates in cortex, subcortical white matter
    - Posterior circulation sparsely innervated by sympathetic nerves (predilection for parietal, occipital lobes)
  - Frank infarction with cytotoxic edema rare in PRES
- Epidemiology
  - Pre-eclampsia in 5% of pregnancies
  - Eclampsia lower (< 1%)
- Associated abnormalities
  - Acute/subacute systemic HTN
  - Preeclampsia, eclampsia
    - Typically occurs after 20 weeks gestation
    - Rare: Headache, seizures up to several weeks postpartum
  - Uremic encephalopathies
    - Acute glomerulonephritis
    - HUS/TTP
    - Lupus nephropathy, etc.
  - Drug toxicity (many reported)
    - Cyclosporin or FK-506
    - Tacrolimus
    - Cisplatin
    - Interferon-alpha
    - Erythropoietin
  - Severe infection
    - 20-25% of patients with sepsis, shock develop PRES
    - Blood pressure can be normal or elevated
  - Tumor lysis syndrome

Gross Pathologic & Surgical Features
- Common
  - Cortical/subcortical edema
  - +/- Petechial hemorrhage in parietal, occipital lobes
- Less common: Lesions in basal ganglia, cerebellum, brain stem, anterior frontal lobes

Microscopic Features
- Usually no residual abnormalities after HTN corrected
- Autopsy in severe cases shows microvascular fibrinoid necrosis, ischemic microinfarcts, variable hemorrhage
- Chronic HTN associated with mural thickening, deposition of collagen, laminin, fibronectin in cerebral arterioles

CLINICAL ISSUES

Presentation
- Most common signs/symptoms
  - Headache, seizure, altered mental status
  - Caution: Some patients, especially children, may be normotensive/minimally elevated BP!
- Clinical Profile
  - Young female with acute/subacute systemic HTN, headache +/- seizure
  - Child with kidney disease or transplant

Demographics
- Age: Any age but young > old
- Gender: M < F

Natural History & Prognosis
- Most cases resolve with adequate treatment
  - Reversibility not spontaneous but related to blood pressure normalization
  - Brainstem, deep white matter lesions less reversible than cortical/subcortical
  - Eclampsia more reversible > drug-related PRES
- May be life-threatening
- Permanent infarction rare
- 4% of patients develop recurrent PRES

Treatment
- Favorable outcome with prompt recognition, treatment of HTN
- Delayed diagnosis/therapy can result in chronic neurologic sequelae

DIAGNOSTIC CHECKLIST

Consider
- Patchy bilateral low density foci in occipital lobes may be earliest manifestation of PRES

Image Interpretation Pearls
- Major ddx of PRES is cerebral ischemia; DWI is positive in the latter, usually negative in the former

SELECTED REFERENCES

1. Sweany JM et al: "Recurrent" posterior reversible encephalopathy syndrome: report of 3 cases--PRES can strike twice! J Comput Assist Tomogr. 31(1):148-56, 2007
2. Bartynski WS et al: Posterior reversible encephalopathy syndrome in infection, sepsis, and shock. AJNR Am J Neuroradiol. 27(10):2179-90, 2006
3. Ishikura K et al: Posterior reversible encephalopathy syndrome in children: its high prevalence and more extensive imaging findings. Am J Kidney Dis. 48(2):231-8, 2006
4. Mirza A: Posterior reversible encephalopathy syndrome: a variant of hypertensive encephalopathy. J Clin Neurosci. 13(5):590-5, 2006
5. Narbone MC et al: PRES: posterior or potentially reversible encephalopathy syndrome? Neurol Sci. 27(3):187-9, 2006
6. Pande AR et al: Clinicoradiological factors influencing the reversibility of posterior reversible encephalopathy syndrome: a multicenter study. Radiat Med. 24(10):659-68, 2006
7. Kaito E et al: The role of tumor lysis in reversible posterior leukoencephalopathy syndrome. Pediatr Radiol. 35(7):722-7, 2005
8. Striano P et al: Clinical spectrum and critical care management of Posterior Reversible Encephalopathy Syndrome (PRES). Med Sci Monit. 11(11):CR549-53, 2005
9. Kinoshita T et al: Diffusion-weighted MR imaging of posterior reversible leukoencephalopathy syndrome: a pictorial essay. Clin Imaging. 27(5): 307-15, 2003
10. Thambisetty M et al: Hypertensive brainstem encephalopathy: clinical and radiographic features. J Neurol Sci. 208(1-2):93-9, 2003

ACUTE HYPERTENSIVE ENCEPHALOPATHY, PRES

IMAGE GALLERY

Typical

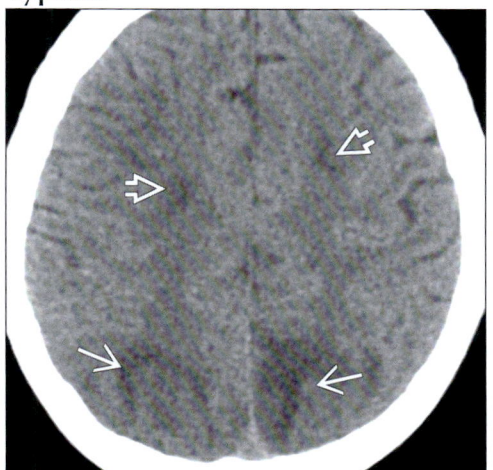
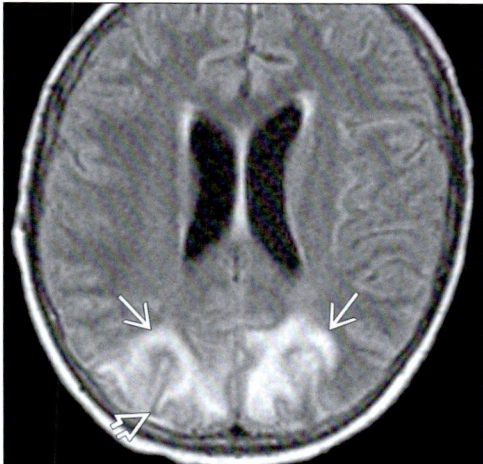

(Left) Axial NECT shows bioccipital ➡ as well as watershed ⇨ hypodensities in this patient with severe hypertension. *(Right)* Axial FLAIR MR in the same case shows hyperintensity in the white matter of both occipital lobes ➡. Subtle cortical hypointensity ➡ may represent petechial hemorrhage.

Typical

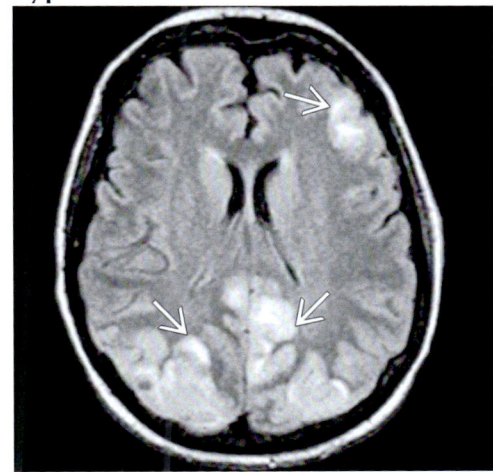
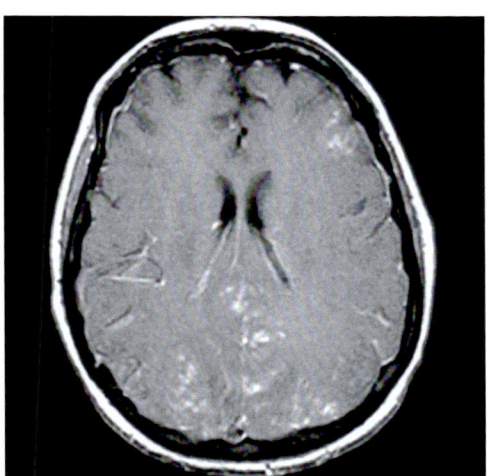

(Left) Axial FLAIR MR shows cortical and subcortical edema in both occipital lobes as well as the posterior left frontal lobe ➡. *(Right)* Axial T1 C+ MR in the same case shows multifocal punctate areas of enhancement indicating active blood-brain barrier disruption in this case of PRES.

Variant

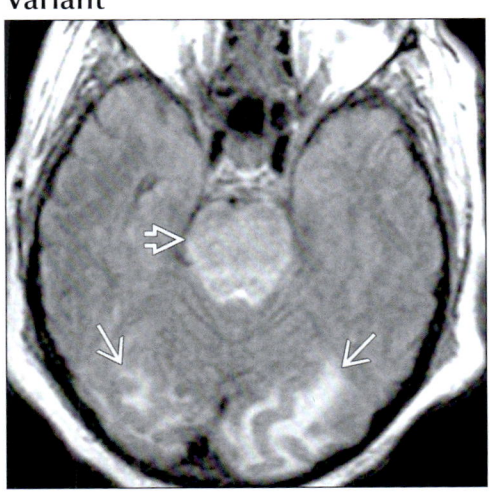
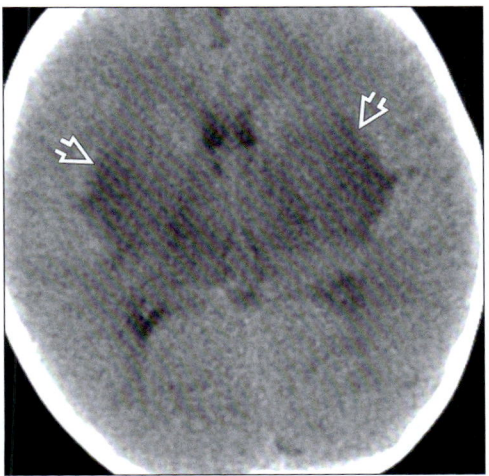

(Left) Axial FLAIR MR shows bilateral occipital hyperintensity in the cortex and subcortical white matter ➡. There is striking hyperintensity in the pons ➡. *(Right)* Axial NECT in a 4 year old hypertensive child with hemolytic-uremic syndrome and renal failure shows hypodensity in basal ganglia, thalami ➡. Occipital lobes are normal.

ACUTE CEREBRAL ISCHEMIA-INFARCTION

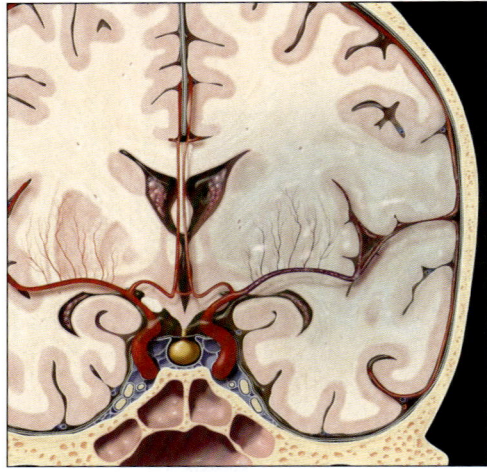

Coronal graphic illustrates left M1 occlusion. Proximal occlusion affects entire MCA territory, including deep nuclei, which are perfused by lenticulostriate arteries.

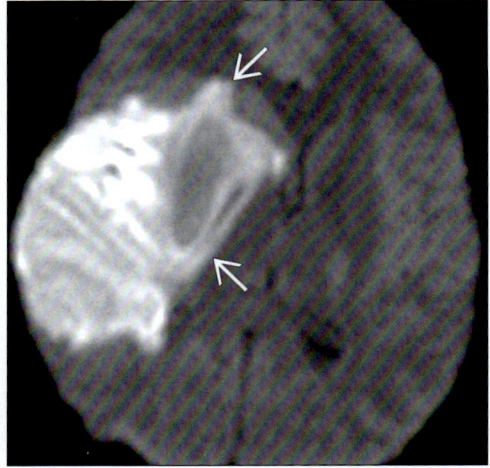

Axial DWI MR demonstrates acute right middle cerebral artery (MCA) infarction. MCA occlusion is proximal (M1 segment) because basal ganglia ➡ are included in infarction.

TERMINOLOGY

Abbreviations and Synonyms
- Stroke, cerebrovascular accident (CVA), brain attack

Definitions
- Interrupted blood flow to brain resulting in cerebral ischemia/infarction with variable neurologic deficit

IMAGING FINDINGS

General Features
- Best diagnostic clue: Diffusion restriction with correlating ADC map
- Location: One or more vascular territories, or at border-zones ("watershed")
- Size: Dependent on degree of compromise and collateral circulation
- Morphology: Wedge-shaped if gray matter (GM) involved, variable if white matter (WM) involved

CT Findings
- NECT
  - Hyperdense vessel (high specificity, low sensitivity)
    - Acute thrombus in cerebral vessel(s)
    - Hyperdense M1 MCA in 35-50%
    - "Dot sign": Occluded MCA branches in Sylvian fissure (16-17%)
  - Loss of GM-WM distinction in first 3 hrs (50-70%)
    - Obscuration of deep nuclei
    - Loss of cortical "ribbon"
  - Parenchymal hypodensity
    - If > 1/3 MCA territory initially, large lesion later
    - Temporary transition to isodensity (up to 54%) at 2-3 weeks post-ictus (CT "fogging")
  - Gyral swelling, sulcal effacement 12-24 hrs
  - "Hemorrhagic transformation" in 15-45%
    - Delayed onset (24-48 hrs) most typical
    - Can be gross (parenchymal) or petechial
- CECT
  - Enhancing cortical vessels: Slow flow or collateralization acutely
  - Absent vessels: Occlusion
  - Triphasic perfusion CT: Assess ischemic core vs. penumbra, identify patients who benefit most from revascularization

DDx: Mimics of Acute Cerebral Ischemia

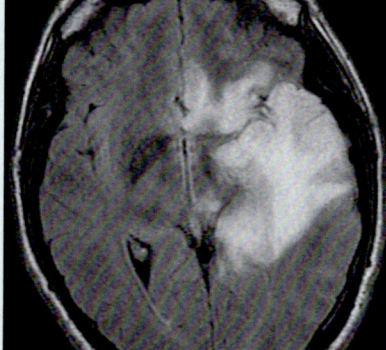

Herpes Simplex Virus Encephalitis

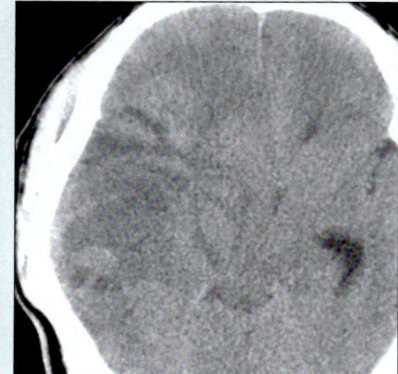

Astrocytoma

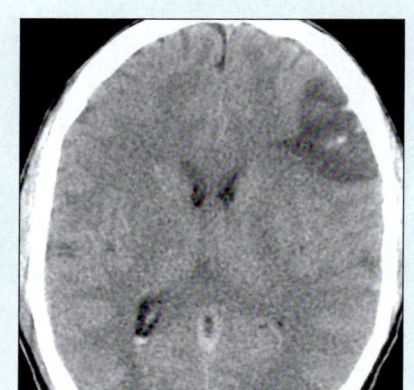

Cerebral Contusion

ACUTE CEREBRAL ISCHEMIA-INFARCTION

Key Facts

Terminology
- Interrupted blood flow to brain resulting in cerebral ischemia/infarction with variable neurologic deficit

Imaging Findings
- Best diagnostic clue: Diffusion restriction with correlating ADC map
- Location: One or more vascular territories, or at border-zones ("watershed")
- Morphology: Wedge-shaped if gray matter (GM) involved, variable if white matter (WM) involved
- Hyperdense vessel (high specificity, low sensitivity)
- Loss of GM-WM distinction in first 3 hrs (50-70%)
- "Hemorrhagic transformation" in 15-45%
- DWI/PWI "mismatch": "Penumbra" or "at-risk" tissue
- Conventional MR sequences positive in 70-80%
- Restricted diffusion improves accuracy to 95%

Top Differential Diagnoses
- Hyperdense Vessel Mimics
- Parenchymal Hypodensity (Nonvascular Causes)

Pathology
- Second most common worldwide cause of death
- Number-one cause of US morbidity

Clinical Issues
- Focal acute neurologic deficit
- Clinical diagnosis inaccurate in 15-20% of strokes
- "Time is brain": IV rTPA window < 3 hrs; IA rTPA window < 6 hrs

Diagnostic Checklist
- DWI positive for acute stroke only if ADC correlates

- Perfusion CT determines perfused CBV and/or CBF, mean transit time (MTT)
  - Cortical/gyral enhancement after 48-72 hrs
- CTA: Identify occlusions, dissections, stenoses, status of collaterals

MR Findings
- T1WI: Early cortical swelling & hypointensity, loss of GM-WM borders
- T2WI
  - Early cortical swelling, hyperintensity in affected distribution
  - May normalize 2-3 weeks post-ictus (MR "fogging")
- FLAIR
  - Parenchymal hyperintensity in affected distribution when other sequences normal (up to 6 hrs post-ictus)
  - Intra-arterial FLAIR hyperintensity is early sign of major vessel occlusion or slow flow
- T2* GRE
  - Detection of acute blood products
  - Arterial "blooming" (thrombosed vessel) from clot susceptibility
  - Loss of normal misregistration flow artifact
- DWI
  - Hyperintense restriction from cytotoxic edema
    - Improves hyperacute stroke detection to 95%
    - Usually correlates to "ischemic core" (final infarct size); some diffusion abnormalities reversible (TIA, migraine)
    - May have reduced sensitivity in brainstem and medulla in first 24 hours
    - High signal can persist up to 57 days post-ictus, (after 10 days, T2 effect may predominate over low ADC: T2 "shine-through")
  - Corresponding low signal on ADC maps
    - May normalize after tissue reperfusion
    - Hyperintensity on ADC map (T2 "shine-through") may mimic diffusion restriction
  - Distinguish cytotoxic from vasogenic edema in complicated cases; helpful to evaluate new deficits after tumor resection
- T1 C+
  - Variable enhancement patterns evolve over time
    - Hyperacute: Intravascular enhancement (stasis from slow antegrade or retrograde collateral flow)
    - Acute: Meningeal enhancement (pial collateral flow appears in 24-48 hrs, resolves over 3-4 days)
    - Subacute: Parenchymal enhancement (appears after 24-48 hrs, can persist for weeks/months)
- MRA: Major vessel occlusions, stenoses, status of collaterals
- MRS
  - Elevated lactate, decreased NAA
    - At mid-TE (e.g., 135) lactate doublet inverts
- Perfusion MR
  - Bolus-tracking T2* gadolinium perfusion imaging (PWI) with rCBV map
    - ↓ Perfusion; 75% larger than DWI abnormality
    - Calculate rCBF, rMTT with arterial input
  - DWI/PWI "mismatch": "Penumbra" or "at-risk" tissue
- Conventional MR sequences positive in 70-80%
  - Restricted diffusion improves accuracy to 95%

Angiographic Findings
- Conventional
  - Vessel occlusion (cutoff, tapered, tram track)
  - Slow antegrade flow, retrograde collateral flow
- Neurointerventional
  - IA rTPA fibrinolytic therapy for treatment of selected acute nonhemorrhagic stroke within 6 hr window
  - IA mechanical clot removal with retriever device

Imaging Recommendations
- Best imaging tool: MR + DWI, T2* GRE
- Protocol advice
  - MR with FLAIR, GRE, DWI, MRA, PWI
  - NECT, CTP, CTA
  - DSA with thrombolysis in selected patients

DIFFERENTIAL DIAGNOSIS

Hyperdense Vessel Mimics
- High hematocrit (polycythemia)
- Microcalcification in vessel wall

ACUTE CEREBRAL ISCHEMIA-INFARCTION

- Diffuse cerebral edema makes vessels appear relatively hyperdense
- Normal circulating blood always slightly hyperdense to normal brain

Parenchymal Hypodensity (Nonvascular Causes)
- Infiltrating neoplasm (e.g., astrocytoma)
- Cerebral contusion
- Inflammation (cerebritis, encephalitis)
- Evolving encephalomalacia
- Dural venous thrombosis with parenchymal venous congestion and edema

PATHOLOGY

General Features
- Etiology
  - Many causes (thrombotic vs. embolic, dissection, vasculitis, hypoperfusion)
  - Early: Critical disturbance in CBF
    - Severely ischemic core has CBF < (6-8 cm^3)/(100 g/min) [normal ~ (60 cm^3)/(100 g/min)]
    - Oxygen depletion, energy failure, terminal depolarization, ion homeostasis failure
    - Bulk of final infarct → cytotoxic edema, cell death
  - Later: Evolution from ischemia to infarction depends on many factors (e.g., hyperglycemia influences "destiny" of ischemic brain tissue)
  - Ischemic "penumbra" CBF between (10-20 cm^3)/(100 g/min)
    - Theoretically salvageable tissue
    - Target of thrombolysis, neuroprotective agents
- Epidemiology
  - Second most common worldwide cause of death
  - Number-one cause of US morbidity
  - Newly identified stroke risk factors: C-reactive protein, homocysteine
- Associated abnormalities: Cardiac disease, prothrombotic states

Gross Pathologic & Surgical Features
- Acute thrombosis of major vessel
- Pale, swollen brain; GM-WM boundaries "smudged"

Microscopic Features
- After 4 hrs: Eosinophilic neurons with pyknotic nuclei
- 15-24 hrs: Neutrophils invade, necrotic nuclei look like "eosinophilic ghosts"
- 2-3 days: Blood-derived phagocytes
- 1 week: Reactive astrocytosis, ↑ capillary density
- End result: Fluid-filled cavity lined by astrocytes

CLINICAL ISSUES

Presentation
- Most common signs/symptoms
  - Focal acute neurologic deficit
  - Paresis, aphasia, decreased mental status

Demographics
- Age
  - Usually older adults
  - Consider underlying disease (sickle cell, moyamoya, NF1, cardiac, drugs) in children, young adults
- Gender: No gender predilection

Natural History & Prognosis
- Clinical diagnosis inaccurate in 15-20% of strokes
- Malignant MCA infarct (coma, death)
  - Up to 10% of all stroke patients
  - Fatal brain swelling with increased ICP

Treatment
- "Time is brain": IV rTPA window < 3 hrs; IA rTPA window < 6 hrs
- Patient selection most important factor in outcome
  - Symptom onset < 6 hrs
  - No parenchymal hematoma on CT
  - < 1/3 MCA territory hypodensity

DIAGNOSTIC CHECKLIST

Consider
- Add DWI to all brain MRs: Time cost < 1 minute

Image Interpretation Pearls
- DWI positive for acute stroke only if ADC correlates

SELECTED REFERENCES

1. Bourekas EC et al: Intraarterial thrombolytic therapy within 3 hours of the onset of stroke. Neurosurgery. 54(1):39-44; discussion 44-6, 2004
2. Diaz J et al: Cerebral ischemia: new risk factors. Cerebrovasc Dis. 17 Suppl 1:43-50, 2004
3. Fiebach JB et al: Stroke magnetic resonance imaging is accurate in hyperacute intracerebral hemorrhage: a multicenter study on the validity of stroke imaging. Stroke. 35(2):502-6, 2004
4. Fiehler J et al: Predictors of apparent diffusion coefficient normalization in stroke patients. Stroke. 35(2):514-9, 2004
5. Gass A et al: Diffusion-weighted MRI for the "small stuff": the details of acute cerebral ischaemia. Lancet Neurol. 3(1):39-45, 2004
6. Kelly PJ et al: Inflammation, homocysteine, and vitamin B6 status after ischemic stroke. Stroke. 35(1):12-5, 2004
7. Mahagne MH et al: Voxel-based mapping of cortical ischemic damage using Tc 99m L,L-ethyl cysteinate dimer SPECT in acute stroke. J Neuroimaging. 14(1):23-32, 2004
8. Nakajima M et al: Relationships between angiographic findings and National Institutes of Health stroke scale score in cases of hyperacute carotid ischemic stroke. AJNR Am J Neuroradiol. 25(2):238-41, 2004
9. Borisch I et al: Preoperative evaluation of carotid artery stenosis: comparison of contrast-enhanced MR angiography and duplex sonography with digital subtraction angiography. AJNR Am J Neuroradiol. 24(6):1117-22, 2003
10. Eastwood JD et al: Quantitative assessment of the time course of infarct signal intensity on diffusion-weighted images. AJNR Am J Neuroradiol. 24(4):680-7, 2003
11. Leary MC et al: Validation of computed tomographic middle cerebral artery "dot"sign: an angiographic correlation study. Stroke. 34(11):2636-40, 2003
12. Toyoda K et al: Fluid-attenuated inversion recovery intraarterial signal: an early sign of hyperacute cerebral ischemia. AJNR Am J Neuroradiol. 22(6):1021-9, 2001

ACUTE CEREBRAL ISCHEMIA-INFARCTION

IMAGE GALLERY

Typical

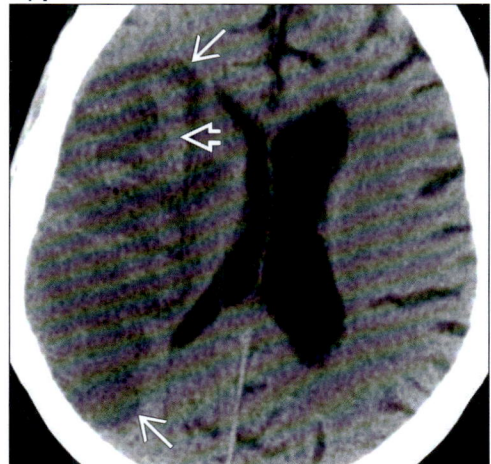
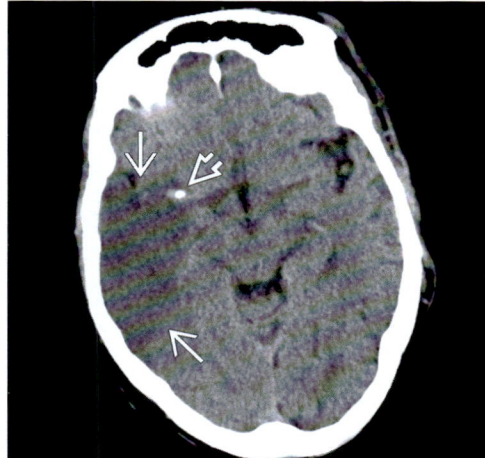

(Left) Axial CECT demonstrates abnormal lucency, loss of GM-WM differentiation and mass effect consistent with subacute infarction ➔. Note petechial hemorrhagic transformation ➔. *(Right)* Axial NECT shows wedge-shaped region of acute infarction ➔ with mild mass effect (sulcal effacement) secondary to mid-right M1 calcified embolus ➔.

Typical

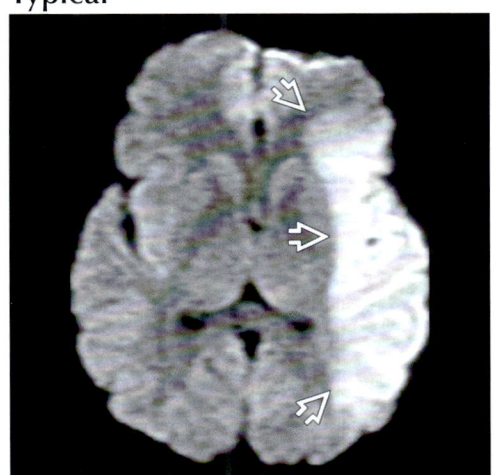
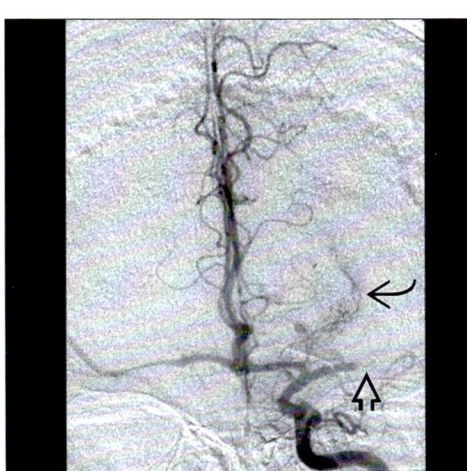

(Left) Axial DWI MR shows wedge-shaped hyperintensity consistent with acute restricted water diffusion ➔ in left MCA distribution & sparing of basal ganglia, consistent with distal M1 occlusion. *(Right)* Anteroposterior angiography in same patient as previous image confirms suspected distal M1 occlusion ➔ and demonstrates associated prominent lenticulostriate vessels ➔.

Typical

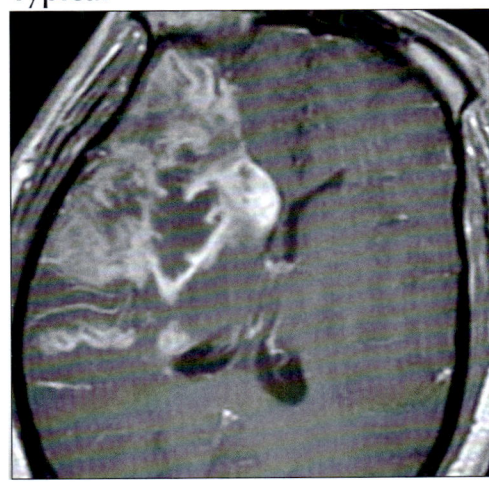
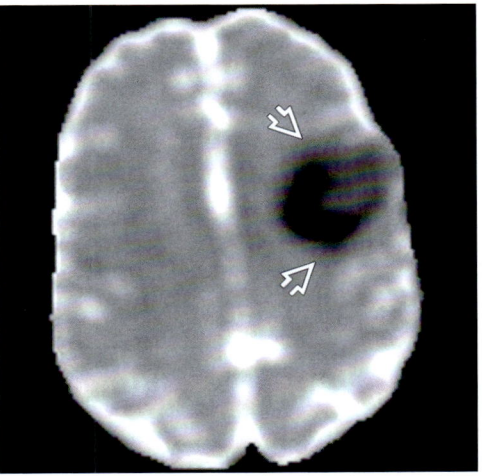

(Left) Axial T1 C+ MR shows heterogeneous gyriform enhancement in right MCA territory due to breakdown of BBB in subacute infarction. This appearance can mimic glioblastoma. *(Right)* Axial ADC map shows focal region of restricted water diffusion in left MCA territory ➔ consistent with acute infarction. Same region was "light-bulb" bright on DWI.

DURAL SINUS THROMBOSIS

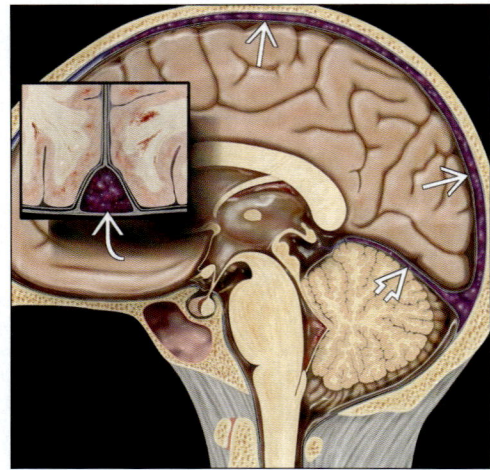

Sagittal graphic shows thrombosis of the superior sagittal sinus (SSS) ➡ and straight sinus ➡. Inset in upper left reveals thrombus in SSS in cross section ("empty delta" sign) ➡.

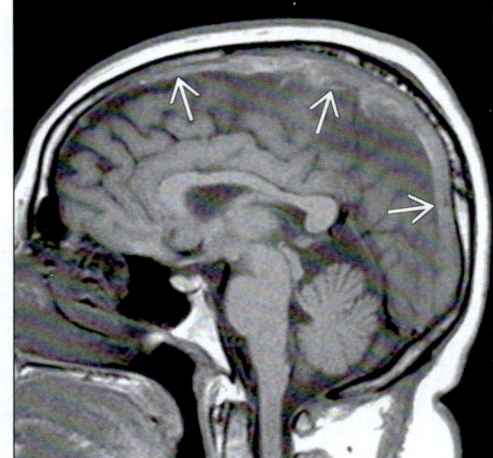

Sagittal T1WI MR reveals intermediate to high intensity clot ➡ filling the swollen superior sagittal sinus. This signal would indicate the thrombosis is subacute in age.

TERMINOLOGY

Abbreviations and Synonyms
- Dural sinus thrombosis (DST), cerebral vein thrombosis (CVT)

Definitions
- Thrombotic occlusion of intracranial dural sinuses

IMAGING FINDINGS

General Features
- Best diagnostic clue
  - "Empty delta sign" on CECT, CE MR
  - Early imaging findings often subtle
- Location: Thrombus in dural sinus ± adjacent cortical vein(s)

CT Findings
- NECT
  - Hyperdense dural sinus > cortical vein: **Cord sign**
  - Venous infarct present in 50% of cases
    - Cortical/subcortical petechial hemorrhages, edema
  - If straight sinus (SS)/internal cerebral veins (ICV) occlude, thalami/basal ganglia hypodense
- CECT
  - "**Empty delta sign**" in 25-30%
    - Enhancing dura surrounds non-enhancing thrombus
  - Shaggy, irregular veins (collateral channels)
- CTA: CT venogram (CTV): Filling defect (thrombus) in dural sinus

MR Findings
- T1WI
  - Acute thrombus: Isointense
  - Subacute thrombus: Hyperintense
  - Chronic thrombus: Isointense
- T2WI
  - Acute thrombus: Hypointense
    - Warning: Hypointense thrombus can mimic normal sinus flow void!
  - Subacute thrombus: Hyperintense
  - Chronic thrombus: Hyperintense
  - Chronically thrombus: Fibrotic dural sinus eventually appears isointense

DDx: Dural Sinus Thrombosis Mimics

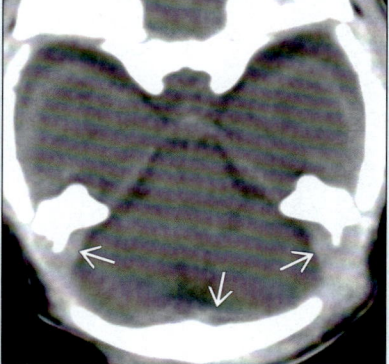

Normal Infant Sinuses

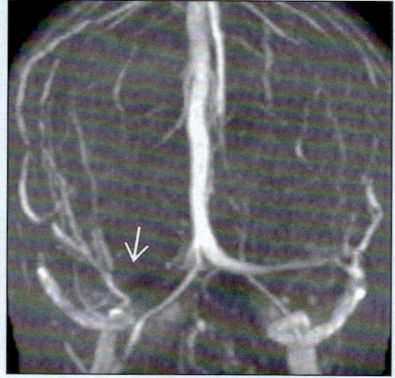

Transverse Sinus Hypoplasia

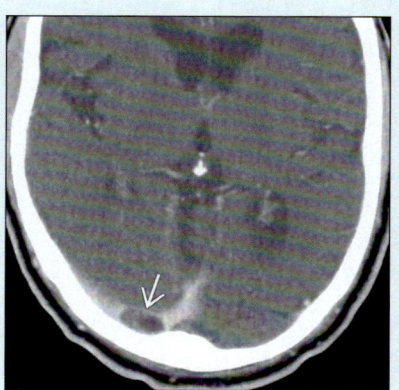

Arachnoid Granulation

DURAL SINUS THROMBOSIS

Key Facts

Terminology
- Thrombotic occlusion of intracranial dural sinuses

Imaging Findings
- "**Empty delta sign**" on CECT, CE MR
- Early imaging findings often subtle
- Hyperdense dural sinus > cortical vein: **Cord sign**
- Cortical/subcortical petechial hemorrhages, edema
- Acute thrombus: Isointense
- Hypointense thrombus "**blooms**"
- 40% have hyperintense clot in occluded vessel
- Absence of flow in occluded sinus on 2D TOF MRV
- If CT negative, MR with MRV
- If MRV equivocal, cerebral angiography

Top Differential Diagnoses
- Normal Dural Sinuses
- Dural Sinus Hypoplasia-Aplasia
- Arachnoid Granulations, "Giant"
- Venous infarct can enhance, mimic neoplasm

Pathology
- Resistance to activated protein C (typically due to factor V Leiden mutation): Most common cause of sporadic CVT
- Epidemiology: 1% of acute strokes
- **Venous ischemia grading**
- Type 1: No abnormality
- Type 2: Hyperintense on T2/FLAIR; no enhancement
- Type 3: Hyperintense on T2/FLAIR; enhancement
- Type 4: Hemorrhage or venous infarction

Clinical Issues
- Up to 50% of cases progress to venous infarction

- Venous infarct: Mass effect with mixed hypointense and hyperintense signal in adjacent parenchyma
- PD/Intermediate
  - Loss of normal flow voids
  - More sensitive than T2WI, less sensitive than FLAIR
- FLAIR
  - Hyperintense thrombus
  - Hyperintense venous infarcts
- T2* GRE
  - Hypointense thrombus "**blooms**"
  - Hypointense petechial ± parenchymal hemorrhages
- DWI
  - 40% have hyperintense clot in occluded vessel
  - DWI/ADC findings in parenchyma variable, heterogeneous
    - Mixture of vasogenic and cytotoxic edema; cytotoxic edema may precede vasogenic edema
    - Parenchymal abnormalities more frequently reversible than arterial occlusions
- T1 C+
  - Peripheral enhancement around acute clot
  - Chronic sinus thrombosis can enhance due to organizing fibrous tissue
- MRV
  - Absence of flow in occluded sinus on 2D TOF MRV
    - Frayed or shaggy appearance of venous sinus
    - Abnormal collateral channels (e.g., enlarged medullary veins)
  - T1 hyperintense (subacute) clot can masquerade as flow on MRV; evaluate standard sequences, source images to exclude artifacts
  - Contrast-enhanced MRV (CE-MRV) better demonstrates thrombus, small vein detail, collaterals much faster than 2D TOF
  - Phase contrast MRV not limited by T1 hyperintense thrombus

Angiographic Findings
- Occlusion of involved sinus
- Slow flow in adjacent patent cortical veins
- Collateral venous drainage develops

Imaging Recommendations
- Best imaging tool
  - NECT, CECT scans ± CTV as initial screening
  - MR, MRV (include T2*, DWI, T1 C+)
- Protocol advice
  - If CT negative, MR with MRV
  - If MRV equivocal, cerebral angiography

DIFFERENTIAL DIAGNOSIS

Normal Dural Sinuses
- Blood in vessels normally slightly hyperdense on NECT
- Common in newborns (unmyelinated low density brain, physiologic polycythemia)

Dural Sinus Hypoplasia-Aplasia
- Congenital hypoplastic/aplastic transverse sinus
  - Transverse sinus flow gaps 31%; nondominant sinus
  - Right transverse sinus dominant in 59%, left dominant in 25%, codominant in 16%
- "High-splitting" tentorium

Arachnoid Granulations, "Giant"
- Round/ovoid filling defect (clot typically long, linear)
- Cerebrospinal fluid (CSF) density/signal intensity
- Normal in 24% of CECT, 13% of MR
  - Transverse sinus most common location by imaging, L > R
  - SSS most common location for arachnoid granulations on histopathology (lateral lacunae, not well seen by imaging)

Acute Subdural Hematoma
- Layered blood on tentorium cerebelli may mimic transverse sinus thrombosis

Neoplasm
- Venous infarct can enhance, mimic neoplasm
- Intravascular lymphomatosis (rare)

DURAL SINUS THROMBOSIS

PATHOLOGY

General Features
- Genetics
  - Resistance to activated protein C (typically due to factor V Leiden mutation): Most common cause of sporadic CVT
  - Protein S deficiency
  - Prothrombin (factor II) gene mutation (G20210A)
- Etiology
  - Wide spectrum of predisposing causes
    - Trauma, infection, inflammation
    - Pregnancy, oral contraceptives
    - Metabolic (dehydration, thyrotoxicosis, cirrhosis)
    - Hematological (coagulopathy)
    - Collagen-vascular disorders (APLA syndrome)
    - Vasculitis (Behçet)
  - Most common pattern
    - Thrombus forms in dural sinus
    - Clot propagates into cortical veins
    - Venous drainage obstructed, venous pressure elevated
    - Blood brain barrier breakdown with vasogenic edema, hemorrhage
    - Venous infarct with cytotoxic edema
- Epidemiology: 1% of acute strokes
- Associated abnormalities: Dural AVF; venous occlusive disease may be underlying etiologic factor

Gross Pathologic & Surgical Features
- Sinus occluded, distended by acute clot
- Thrombus in adjacent cortical veins
- Edematous adjacent cortex; petechial hemorrhage

Microscopic Features
- Thrombosis of veins, proliferative fibrous tissue in chronic thromboses

Staging, Grading or Classification Criteria
- **Venous ischemia grading**
  - Type 1: No abnormality
  - Type 2: Hyperintense on T2/FLAIR; no enhancement
  - Type 3: Hyperintense on T2/FLAIR; enhancement
  - Type 4: Hemorrhage or venous infarction

CLINICAL ISSUES

Presentation
- Most common signs/symptoms
  - Headache, nausea, vomiting ± neurologic deficit
  - Clinical diagnosis often elusive

Demographics
- Age: Any age can be affected
- Gender: M < F

Natural History & Prognosis
- Extremely variable: Asymptomatic to coma, death
  - Up to 50% of cases progress to venous infarction
  - Can be fatal if severe brain swelling, herniation

Treatment
- Inpatient heparin followed by outpatient Coumadin
- In more severe cases, endovascular mechanical thrombectomy ± local heparin infusion

DIAGNOSTIC CHECKLIST

Consider
- Angiography for patients with suspected chronic DST
- Venous filling defect from arachnoid granulation

Image Interpretation Pearls
- Review MRV source images
- Transverse sinus common site for hypoplastic segment variations mimicking occlusion

SELECTED REFERENCES

1. Klingebiel R et al: Comparative evaluation of 2D time-of-flight and 3D elliptic centric contrast-enhanced MR venography in patients with presumptive cerebral venous and sinus thrombosis. Eur J Neurol. 14(2):139-43, 2007
2. Leach JL et al: Partially recanalized chronic dural sinus thrombosis: findings on MR imaging, time-of-flight MR venography, and contrast-enhanced MR venography. AJNR Am J Neuroradiol. 28(4):782-9, 2007
3. Rodallec MH et al: Cerebral venous thrombosis and multidetector CT angiography: tips and tricks. Radiographics. 26 Suppl 1:S5-18; discussion S42-3, 2006
4. Oppenheim C et al: Subarachnoid hemorrhage as the initial presentation of dural sinus thrombosis. AJNR Am J Neuroradiol. 26(3):614-7, 2005
5. Alper F et al: Importance of anatomical asymmetries of transverse sinuses: an MR venographic study. Cerebrovasc Dis. 18(3):236-9, 2004
6. Favrole P et al: Diffusion-weighted imaging of intravascular clots in cerebral venous thrombosis. Stroke. 35(1):99-103, 2004
7. Ferro JM et al: Prognosis of cerebral vein and dural sinus thrombosis: results of the International Study on Cerebral Vein and Dural Sinus Thrombosis (ISCVT). Stroke. 35(3):664-70, 2004
8. Soleau SW et al: Extensive experience with dural sinus thrombosis. Neurosurgery. 52(3):534-44; discussion 542-4, 2003
9. Hinman JM et al: Hypointense thrombus on T2-weighted MR imaging: a potential pitfall in the diagnosis of dural sinus thrombosis. Eur J Radiol. 41(2):147-52, 2002
10. Kawaguchi T et al: Classification of venous ischaemia with MRI. J Clin Neurosci. 8 Suppl 1:82-8, 2001
11. Liang L et al: Evaluation of the intracranial dural sinuses with a 3D contrast-enhanced MP-RAGE sequence: prospective comparison with 2D-TOF MR venography and digital subtraction angiography. AJNR Am J Neuroradiol. 22(3):481-92, 2001
12. Ayanzen RH et al: Cerebral MR venography: normal anatomy and potential diagnostic pitfalls. AJNR Am J Neuroradiol. 21(1):74-8, 2000
13. Provenzale JM et al: Dural sinus thrombosis: findings on CT and MR imaging and diagnostic pitfalls. AJR Am J Roentgenol. 170(3):777-83, 1998
14. Kim SY et al: Direct endovascular thrombolytic therapy for dural sinus thrombosis: infusion of alteplase. AJNR Am J Neuroradiol. 18(4):639-45, 1997
15. Leach JL et al: Normal appearance of arachnoid granulations on contrast-enhanced CT and MR of the brain: differentiation from dural sinus disease. AJNR Am J Neuroradiol. 17(8):1523-32, 1996

DURAL SINUS THROMBOSIS

IMAGE GALLERY

Typical

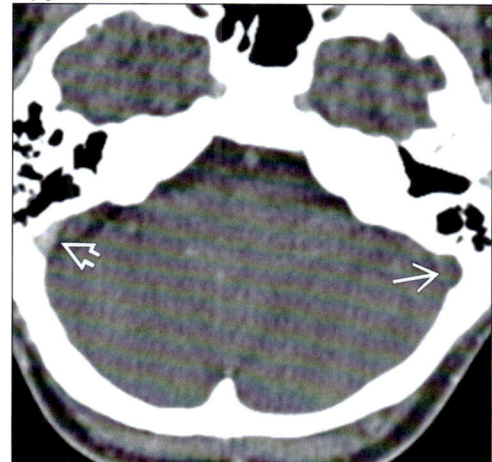
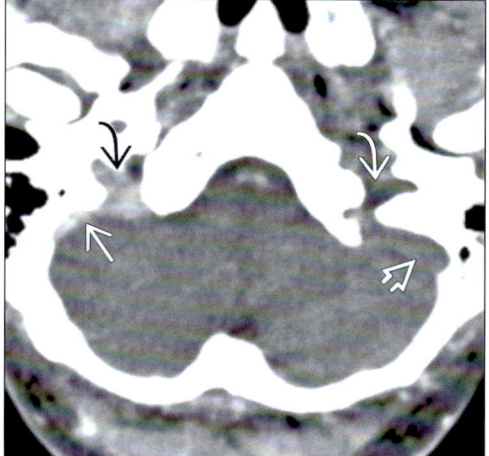

(Left) Axial CTA demonstrates low density clot in the left transverse sinus ➡. The normal right transverse sinus is filled with contrasted blood ➡. (Right) Axial CTA shows sigmoid sinus ➡ and jugular foramen thrombosis ➡ on the left. Notice the normal right enhancing sigmoid sinus ➡ and jugular bulb ➡.

Typical

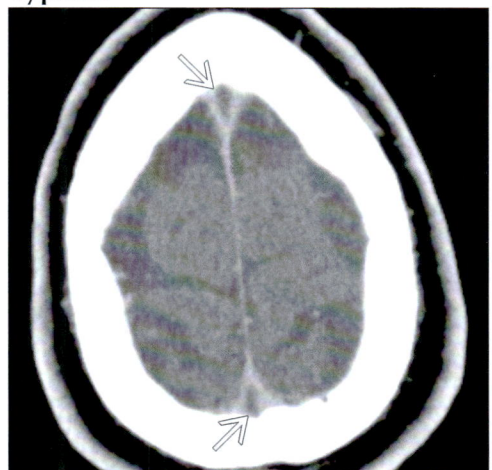
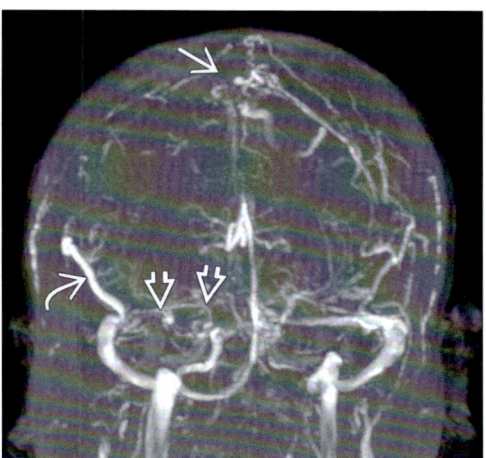

(Left) Axial CECT demonstrates a double "empty delta signs" ➡ at the anterior and posterior margins of the superior sagittal sinus. Complete superior sagittal sinus thrombosis was present. (Right) Coronal MRV reveals superior sagittal sinus thrombosis ➡ with right transverse sinus thrombosis ➡. Note right vein of Labbe ➡ is large as it provides collateral flow.

Typical

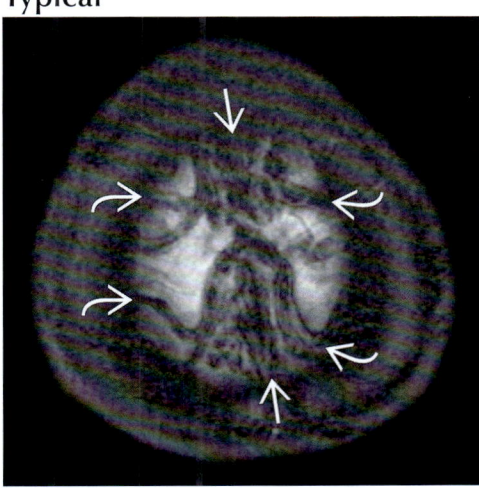
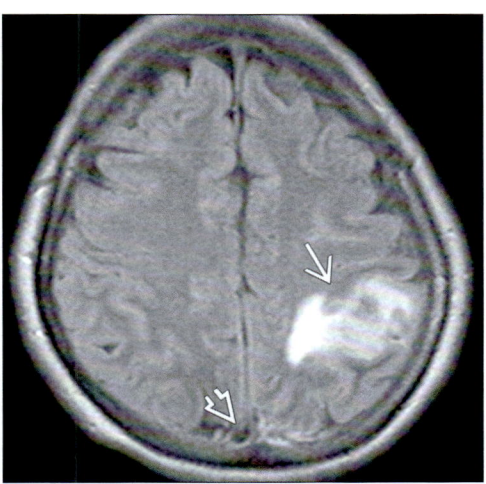

(Left) Axial T2* GRE MR shows blooming (overly large low signal) in the thrombosed superior sagittal sinus ➡ and in the associated cortical veins ➡. Cerebral infarction may result. (Right) Axial FLAIR MR reveals high signal in the high left hemisphere ➡ secondary to cerebral vein thrombosis associated with the superior sagittal sinus thrombosis ➡.

NEONATAL MENINGITIS

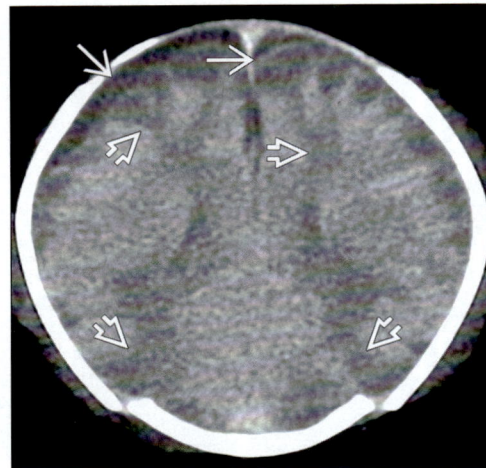

Axial NECT in a 3 week old with seizure and fever caused by group B strep meningitis shows fluid collections over the frontal lobes ➡ and multiple foci of decreased attenuation ➡.

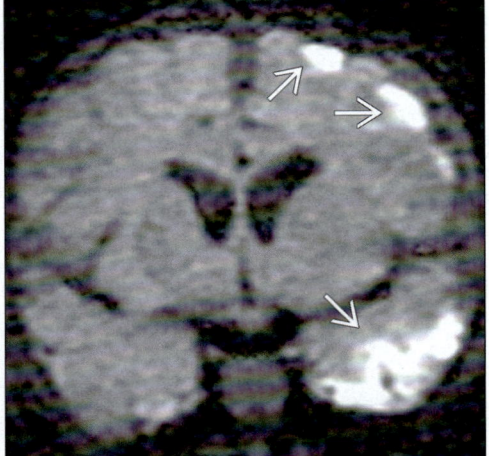

Coronal DWI MR shows multiple regions of restricted diffusion in the periphery of the left temporal and frontal lobes ➡ in this 3 month old with group B streptococcal meningitis.

TERMINOLOGY

Definitions
- Bacterial meningitis in neonates and infants caused by a number of organisms that infrequently cause CNS infection in older children and adults
  - Group B strep (GBS)
  - Escherichia coli (E. coli)
  - Listeria monocytogenes
  - Citrobacter species, Serratia species, Enterobacter species, Klebsiella species

IMAGING FINDINGS

General Features
- Best diagnostic clue: Multifocal regions of decreased attenuation on CT in a neonate
- Location: Cerebral hemispheres and deep gray matter
- Size: Extensive, panlobar involvement typical
- Morphology: Multifocal involvement

CT Findings
- NECT
  - Acutely causes scattered hypodensities in gray matter (GM), white matter (WM), basal ganglia
  - Occasional hyperdense foci reflect hemorrhagic venous infarcts or laminar necrosis
  - Subacutely subdural collections can develop
    - Subdural empyema (purulent) vs. sympathetic subdural effusion (non-inflamed, hypocellular)
  - Intra-axial fluid collections can develop
    - Frank abscesses (purulent) vs. non-inflamed cavitation (hypocellular)
  - Hydrocephalus ± dependent debris in ventricles
  - Bacterial induced pneumocephalus has been reported with Citrobacter infection
- CECT
  - Dural, leptomeningeal, parenchymal enhancement variably present
    - Rim-enhancement around subdural empyemas and abscesses
    - Little or no enhancement around effusions or cavities
  - Ependymal enhancement indicates ventriculitis

MR Findings
- T1WI

DDx: Destructive Brain Lesions in Neonates

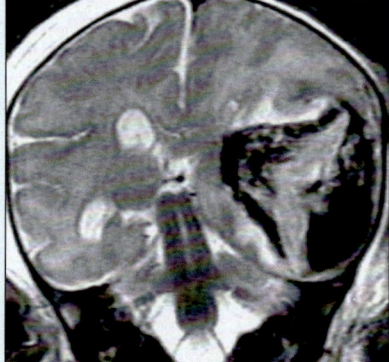

Venous Infarct

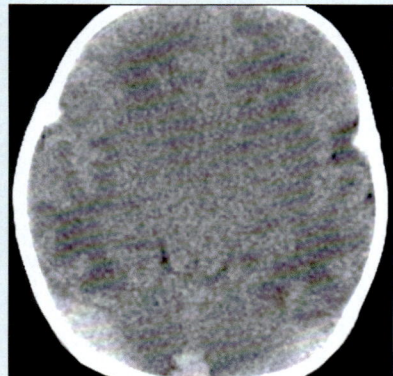

Hypoxic Ischemic Encephalopathy

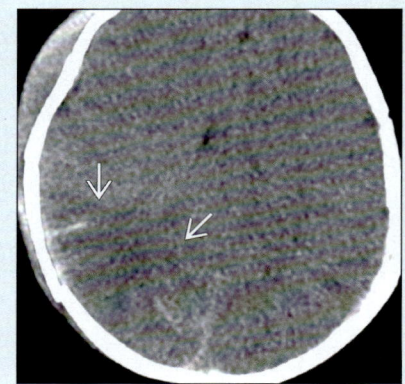

Child Abuse

NEONATAL MENINGITIS

Key Facts

Terminology
- Group B strep (GBS)
- Escherichia coli (E. coli)
- Listeria monocytogenes
- Citrobacter species, Serratia species, Enterobacter species, Klebsiella species

Imaging Findings
- Best diagnostic clue: Multifocal regions of decreased attenuation on CT in a neonate
- Size: Extensive, panlobar involvement typical
- Dural, leptomeningeal, parenchymal enhancement variably present
- Ependymal enhancement indicates ventriculitis
- MRV: Up to 30% will have sinus or cortical vein thrombosis

Pathology
- Neonatal meningitis occurs in approximately 3 per 10,000 live births
- GBS accounts for nearly 50%
- **All neonatal meningitides have a propensity to cause abscesses/cavitation**
- Citrobacter species are especially noted for this complication

Clinical Issues
- Fever, apnea, hypotension, lethargy, irritability
- Seizures are typically late findings
- Typical signs/symptoms of meningitis subtle or absent in neonate
- Mortality of neonatal meningitis approaches 25%
- Up to 30% of survivors have neurological sequelae

- ○ Hypo- and hyperintense parenchymal foci
  - ■ Hypointensities = edema, ischemia, infarction
  - ■ Hyperintensities = laminar necrosis, hemorrhagic venous infarction
- T2WI
  - ○ Hyperintensities in WM
  - ○ Multifocal loss of gray-white differentiation
- FLAIR
  - ○ WM edema may be dark on FLAIR, unlike in older children or adults
    - ■ Complete suppression due to lack of normal myelination
  - ○ Purulent collections in parenchyma (abscess) and subdural space (empyema) characteristically hyperintense on FLAIR
    - ■ Cavities and effusions typically not hyperintense
- T2* GRE: Blooming of hemorrhagic foci
- DWI
  - ○ Restriction in infarcted parenchyma
  - ○ Restricted diffusion in focal cerebritis
  - ○ Restricted diffusion in abscesses and empyemas
    - ■ Little or no diffusion restriction in effusions or sterile cavities
- T1 C+: More sensitive than CECT for dural, leptomeningeal, parenchymal, ependymal enhancement
- MRA: Irregular arterial stenoses, vasculitis
- MRV: Up to 30% will have sinus or cortical vein thrombosis
- MRS
  - ○ ↑ Choline, ↓ NAA in injured parenchyma
  - ○ (+) Lactate in areas of ischemia/infarction/abscess

Ultrasonographic Findings
- Grayscale Ultrasound
  - ○ Patchy regions of increased echogenicity
  - ○ Debris/septations may be visible in ventricles
  - ○ Cavities often anechoic

Imaging Recommendations
- Best imaging tool: Contrast-enhanced MR with DWI and MRV
- Protocol advice: CT useful for rapid initial assessment

DIFFERENTIAL DIAGNOSIS

Hypoxic Ischemic Encephalopathy (HIE)
- Preterm
  - ○ Injury to periventricular WM (mild)
  - ○ Injury to thalami, basal ganglia, brainstem (severe)
- Term
  - ○ Injury to mature vascular watershed zones (mild)
  - ○ Diffuse lobar injury (severe)

Inborn Errors of Metabolism
- Some metabolic diseases will present in neonatal period with lethargy and encephalopathy
  - ○ Maple syrup urine disease (MSUD)
    - ■ Involvement of brainstem, cerebellar WM, thalamus greater than cerebrum
  - ○ Nonketotic hyperglycinemia
    - ■ May show evidence of prenatal injury
  - ○ Neonatal hypoglycemia (multiple etiologies)
    - ■ Urea cycle disorders
- Most will cause multiple regions of altered attenuation on CT
  - ○ Frequently symmetric
  - ○ Frequently involve deep nuclear structures
    - ■ Brainstem, thalami, basal ganglia

Neonatal Stroke
- Arterial infarct
  - ○ Low apgar scores, focal neurologic findings
  - ○ May be associated with birth trauma, nuchal cord
  - ○ Often inapparent clinically
- Venous infarct associated with hypercoagulable state
  - ○ Lateral temporal location classic for thrombosis of vein of Labbé
  - ○ May present with decreased hematocrit, seizure

Traumatic Brain Injury
- Child abuse ⇒ multifocal regions of decreased GM/WM hypodensity, subdural hematomas
- Subdural hematomas
- Skull, rib fractures

NEONATAL MENINGITIS

Congenital Infections (TORCH)
- Cytomegalovirus, toxoplasmosis, rubella: Infection occurs in-utero with chronic sequelae present in neonate/infant
- Herpes simplex virus type 2 (HSV 2): Infection acquired during passage through birth canal; presents in first 2-4 wks of life

PATHOLOGY

General Features
- Etiology
  - Most infections occur during labor and delivery
    - Onset of bacteremia is facilitated by immature neonatal immune system
- Epidemiology
  - Neonatal meningitis occurs in approximately 3 per 10,000 live births
  - E. coli accounts for 20%
  - GBS accounts for nearly 50%
    - 10-30% pregnant women have asymptomatic GBS colonization of genital/GI tract
    - Incidence remains high in mothers with negative screening
    - GBS agalactiae serotype III responsible for majority of GBS meningitis

Gross Pathologic & Surgical Features
- Debris, exudates at subarachnoid space/ventricles; ventricular septations
  - Meningeal/arachnoid inflammatory response is increased in older infant compared to neonate
- Parenchymal infarction/encephalomalacia
- **All neonatal meningitides have a propensity to cause abscesses/cavitation**
  - Citrobacter species are especially noted for this complication

Microscopic Features
- GBS: Gram (+) diplococci
- E. coli: Gram (-) enteric bacteria
- Citrobacter: Gram (-) enteric bacteria
- Klebsiella: Encapsulated rod-shaped, gram (-) bacteria
- Listeria: Gram (+) rods

CLINICAL ISSUES

Presentation
- Most common signs/symptoms
  - Fever, apnea, hypotension, lethargy, irritability
  - Seizures are typically late findings
- Other signs/symptoms
  - Late onset disease typically presents with more obvious neurologic findings
    - Impaired consciousness, seizure
- Clinical Profile
  - Newborn with sepsis
  - Typical signs/symptoms of meningitis subtle or absent in neonate

Demographics
- Age
  - Can have early-onset (EOD) or late-onset (LOD) disease
    - Early onset disease ⇒ 0-48 hr
    - Late onset disease ⇒ > 7 days

Natural History & Prognosis
- Mortality of neonatal meningitis approaches 25%
- Up to 30% of survivors have neurological sequelae

DIAGNOSTIC CHECKLIST

Image Interpretation Pearls
- Normal low density WM on neonate CT is symmetric
- Asymmetric low density is worrisome for edema/encephalitis
  - Especially with asymmetric extra-axial fluid collections

SELECTED REFERENCES
1. Agrawal D et al: Vertically acquired neonatal citrobacter brain abscess - case report and review of the literature. J Clin Neurosci. 12(2):188-90, 2005
2. Puopolo KM et al: Early-onset group B streptococcal disease in the era of maternal screening. Pediatrics. 115(5):1240-6, 2005
3. Shah DK et al: Cerebral white matter injury in the newborn following Escherichia coli meningitis. Eur J Paediatr Neurol. 9(1):13-7, 2005
4. Heath PT et al: Neonatal meningitis. Arch Dis Child Fetal Neonatal Ed. 88(3):F173-8, 2003
5. Stevens JP et al: Long term outcome of neonatal meningitis. Arch Dis Child Fetal Neonatal Ed. 88(3):F179-84, 2003
6. Gotoff SP: Group B streptococcal infections. Pediatr Rev. 23(11):381-6, 2002
7. Volpe JJ: Bacterial and Fungal Intracranial Infections. Neurology of the Newborn, 4th Ed. W.B. Saunders, Philadelphia. 774-810, 2001

NEONATAL MENINGITIS

IMAGE GALLERY

Typical

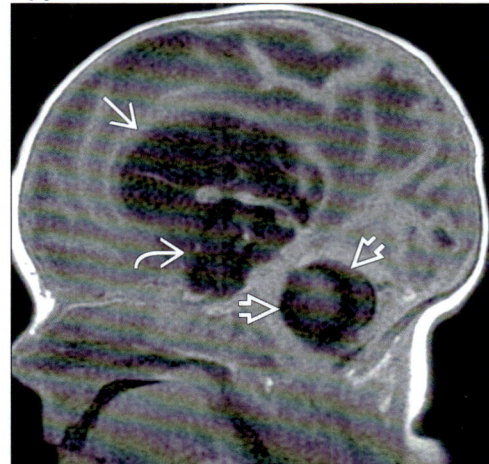
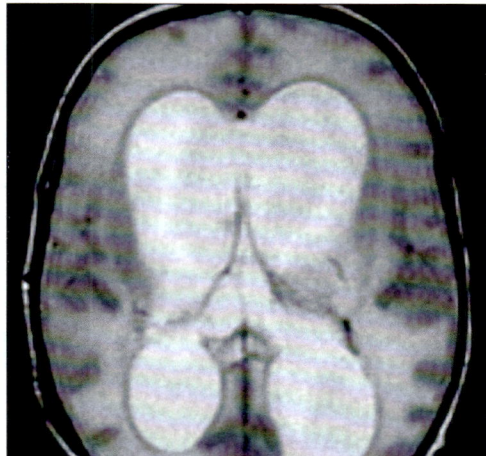

(Left) Sagittal T1WI MR in a 4 week old with E. coli meningitis shows marked dilation of the 3rd ➡, 4th ➡, and lateral ➡ ventricles due to ependymal inflammation caused by the infection. *(Right)* Axial T2WI MR in the same child again shows ventricular enlargement, along with marked edema throughout the white matter.

Typical

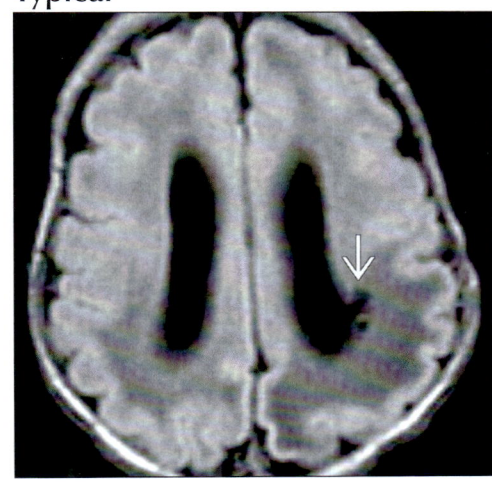
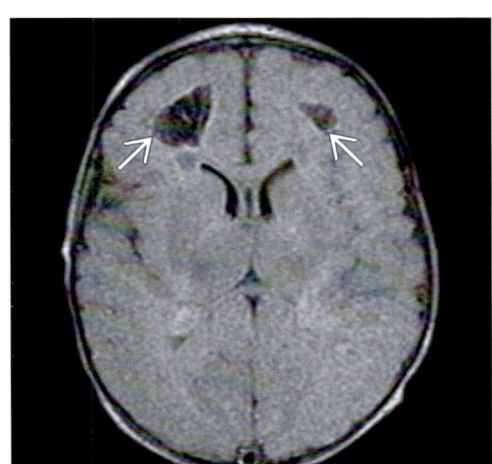

(Left) Axial FLAIR MR in a neonate with Citrobacter meningitis shows hypointense white matter edema in the parietal lobes, with early cavity formation on the left ➡. *(Right)* Axial FLAIR MR in a 3 week old with Citrobacter meningitis shows bilateral cavity formation in the frontal lobes ➡. Rapid necrosis and cavitation is characteristic of this infection.

Typical

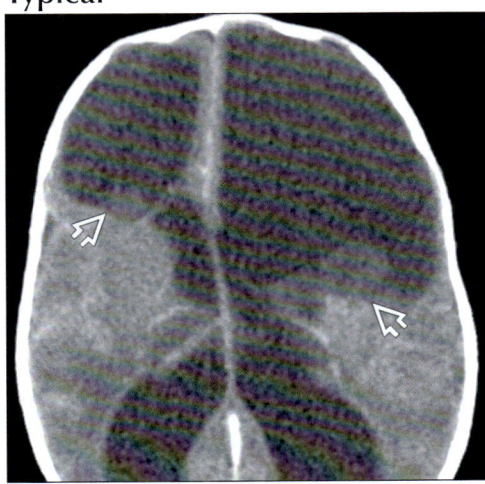
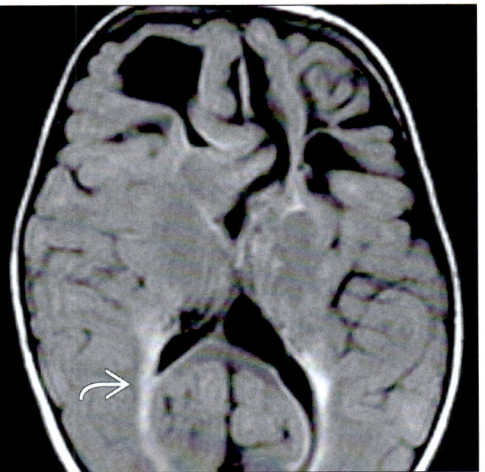

(Left) Axial CECT in a former premature infant with a history of meningitis caused by Serratia marcescens shows large frontal cavities with debris ➡, contiguous with the frontal horns. *(Right)* Axial FLAIR MR in the same child several months later shows collapse of the cavities and loss of frontal white matter volume. Note gliosis in periventricular white matter posteriorly ➡.

MENINGITIS

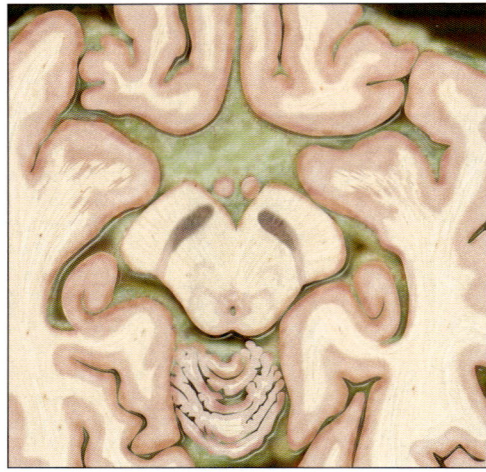

Axial graphic shows diffuse inflammatory exudate involving the leptomeninges, filling the basal cisterns and sulci. This results in increased density/signal intensity on imaging studies.

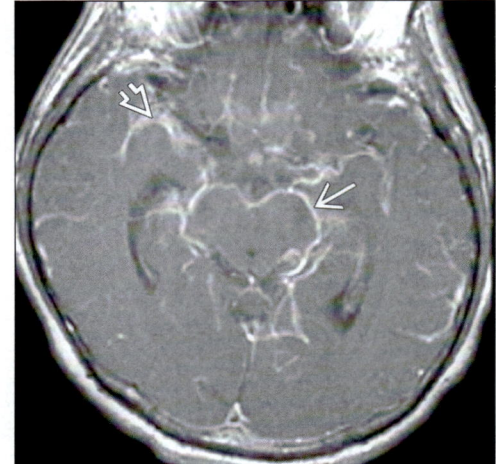

Axial T1 C+ MR shows diffusely thickened, enhancing pia ⇒ as well as sulcal-cisternal enhancement seen best in the right sylvian fissure ⇒. Tuberculous meningitis.

TERMINOLOGY

Abbreviations and Synonyms
- Leptomeningitis

Definitions
- Inflammatory infiltration of pia, arachnoid, CSF
- Acute pyogenic (bacterial); lymphocytic (viral); chronic (tuberculosis)

IMAGING FINDINGS

General Features
- Best diagnostic clue: Positive CSF by lumbar puncture
- Location: Subarachnoid cisterns, pia
- Morphology
  ○ Typically smooth ± thick, intense sulcal-cisternal enhancement
  ○ Tuberculosis (TB), fungal meningitis often basilar/confluent; may be nodular
- Imaging may be normal early
- Imaging findings nonspecific
- Imaging best delineates complications
  ○ Hydrocephalus (often early complication)
  ○ Cerebritis/abscess
  ○ Empyema

CT Findings
- NECT
  ○ Most common = normal
  ○ Mild ventricular enlargement common
  ○ Sulci, basal cisterns may appear effaced
- CECT
  ○ Enhancing exudate in sulci, cisterns
  ○ Low-density areas related to ischemic complications
- CTA: Arterial narrowing, occlusion

MR Findings
- T1WI: Isointense exudate
- T2WI: Hyperintense exudate
- FLAIR: Hyperintense signal in sulci, cisterns (nonspecific!)
- DWI
  ○ Variable, may show restriction
  ○ Most useful for vascular complications
- T1 C+: Exudate, brain surface (pia) enhance
- MRA: Arterial narrowing, occlusion

DDx: FLAIR Hyperintense CSF

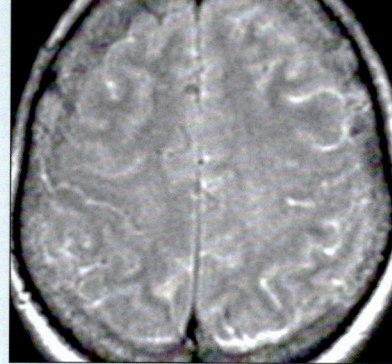

Aneurysmal SAH

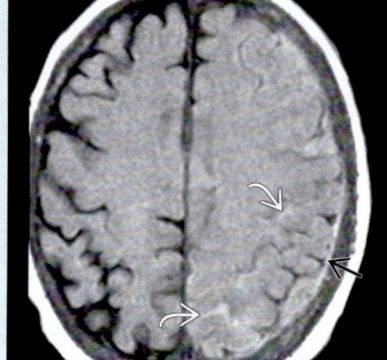

Metastases

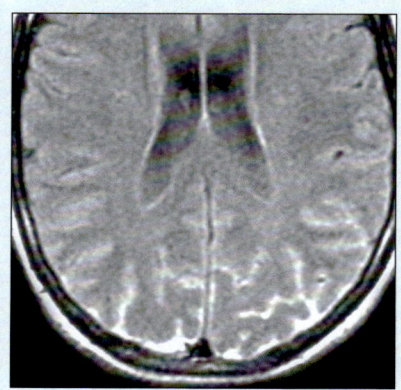

Artifact

MENINGITIS

Key Facts

Terminology
- Inflammatory infiltration of pia, arachnoid, CSF

Imaging Findings
- Best diagnostic clue: Positive CSF by lumbar puncture
- Imaging may be normal early
- Imaging best delineates complications
- FLAIR: Hyperintense signal in sulci, cisterns (nonspecific!)
- T1 C+: Exudate, brain surface (pia) enhance
- Delayed enhanced FLAIR most sensitive sequence for leptomeningeal disease

Top Differential Diagnoses
- Neoplastic Meningitis
- Neurosarcoidosis
- Increased FLAIR Signal in CSF

Pathology
- Gross pathology generally same regardless of agent

Clinical Issues
- Adults: Headache, fever, nuchal rigidity, ± altered mental status
- Children: Fever, irritability, nuchal rigidity
- Effective antimicrobial agents have reduced but not eliminated mortality, morbidity
- Complications occur in 50% of adult patients
- Infectious: Cerebritis/abscess, ventriculitis, empyema, effusion
- Vascular: Ischemia related to arterial spasm or infectious arteritis, dural venous thrombosis
- Mortality 20-25%

Ultrasonographic Findings
- Sulcal enlargement, echogenic deposits in subarachnoid space in infants
- Abnormally thickened meninges

Angiographic Findings
- Conventional
  - Arterial narrowing, occlusion related to infectious arteritis
  - Venous thrombosis may be seen

Imaging Recommendations
- Best imaging tool
  - Contrast-enhanced MR
    - Best for evaluating complications
- Protocol advice
  - Include FLAIR, DWI, T1 C+
  - Delayed enhanced FLAIR most sensitive sequence for leptomeningeal disease

DIFFERENTIAL DIAGNOSIS

Neoplastic Meningitis
- Primary tumor often known (exception = lymphoma)
- Breast, lung most common extracranial sources
- Primary CNS tumors: GBM, medulloblastoma, pineal tumors, choroid plexus tumors

Neurosarcoidosis
- Lacy leptomeningeal enhancement
- May have ventricular, dural-base enhancing masses

Increased FLAIR Signal in CSF
- Nonspecific; many causes
  - Subarachnoid hemorrhage (SAH)
  - High inspired oxygen
  - Acute stroke (parenchymal edema, vascular congestion)
  - Artifact
  - Retained gadolinium in CSF
    - Dialysis-dependent patient with end-stage renal disease

PATHOLOGY

General Features
- General path comments
  - Gross pathology generally same regardless of agent
  - Pia penetrated by inflammatory cells, BBB altered
  - Meningitis-associated brain injury
    - Cytokines, reactive nitrogen species, hippocampal apoptosis (cell death)
  - Basilar meningitis typical of pyogenic infections, TB, cryptococcus, neurosyphilis, sarcoid, lymphoma
- Etiology
  - Hematogenous
    - Most common
    - Spread from remote infection (heart, teeth, etc.)
    - Some may enter CNS via choroid plexus (lacks blood-brain barrier)
  - Direct extension
    - Less common
    - Sinusitis, otitis media, orbital infection
    - Skull base fracture
  - Penetrating injury (least common)
- Epidemiology
  - Bacterial meningitis increase in last 30 years related to nosocomial infection
    - Approximately 3/100,000 in US
  - Meningitis most common form of CNS infection in children
  - Incidence of bacteria based on age
    - Elderly: Listeria monocytogenes, Streptococcus pneumoniae, Neisseria meningitidis, gram-negative bacilli
    - Adults: S. pneumoniae, N. meningitidis, group B streptococcus
    - Children: N. meningitidis
    - Infants: S. pneumoniae, N. meningitidis
    - Neonates: Group B streptococcus, Escherichia coli
  - Vaccine has markedly decreased incidence of Haemophilus influenzae meningitis
  - Viral meningitis: Enteroviruses most common
  - Chronic meningitis
    - TB most common

MENINGITIS

- High morbidity, mortality common in spite of treatment
  - Fungal meningitis: Cryptococcus neoformans (AIDS) and Coccidioides immitis most common
- Associated abnormalities
  - Complications
    - Extraventricular obstructive hydrocephalus (EVOH)
    - Ventriculitis, choroid plexitis
    - Cerebritis, abscess
    - Post-meningitis subdural fluid collections (empyema, effusion)
  - Cerebrovascular complications
    - Arteritis, ischemia
    - Frank infarction
    - Venous thrombosis (cortical, dural sinus)

Gross Pathologic & Surgical Features

- Cisterns, sulci filled with cloudy CSF, then purulent exudate
- Pia-arachnoid congested, may mimic SAH
- Cortex may be edematous

Microscopic Features

- Meningeal exudate
  - Polymorphonuclear neutrophils (PMNs), fibrin, intra/extracellular bacteria
- Vessels within exudate may show fibrinoid necrosis, thrombosis
- Foci of cortical necrosis
- Infection may extend into perivascular spaces, ventricles
- Subpial microglial, astrocytic proliferation

CLINICAL ISSUES

Presentation

- Most common signs/symptoms
  - Adults: Headache, fever, nuchal rigidity, ± altered mental status
    - Brudzinski sign: Hips and knees flex involuntarily when neck is flexed
    - Kernig sign: Flex hips and knees, try to extend knees; pain in hamstrings, patient resistance
  - Children: Fever, irritability, nuchal rigidity
  - Infants: Fever, lethargy, irritability
  - Seizures in 30%
- Clinical Profile
  - CSF shows increased white blood cells (leukocytosis)
    - Elevated CSF protein, decreased glucose typical of infectious meningitis
  - Purpuric rash may develop in N. meningitidis (meningococcal) meningitis, highly morbid

Demographics

- Age: Occurs at all ages

Natural History & Prognosis

- Effective antimicrobial agents have reduced but not eliminated mortality, morbidity
- Impaired CSF resorption may cause EVOH
- Elevated ICP, cerebral perfusion alterations can be early complications
- Complications occur in 50% of adult patients
  - Infectious: Cerebritis/abscess, ventriculitis, empyema, effusion
    - Effusion may be difficult to differentiate from empyema
  - Vascular: Ischemia related to arterial spasm or infectious arteritis, dural venous thrombosis
  - Labyrinthine ossificans is uncommon complication
    - Infection of labyrinth via cochlear aqueduct from subarachnoid space
    - Typically results in bilateral hearing loss
- Mortality 20-25%

Treatment

- Intravenous antibiotics
  - Empiric therapy based on age
    - < 1 month: Ampicillin and Cefotaxime
    - > 1 month: Ceftriaxone or Cefotaxime + Vancomycin + Dexamethasone
  - Specific therapy based on culture and sensitivity
  - Ceftriaxone or Cefotaxime ± Vancomycin: Treatment of choice for most bacterial meningitides
  - Penicillin or Ampicillin: N. meningitidis, L. monocytogenes, group B streptococcus
  - Amphotericin B ± Fluconazole or Flucytosine: Fungal meningitis
  - TB meningitis requires combination therapy: Isoniazid, Pyrazinamide, Rifampin
  - Viral meningitis: Supportive care; except for herpes meningitis (Acyclovir)
- Surgery for complications (hydrocephalus, empyema, etc.)

DIAGNOSTIC CHECKLIST

Consider

- Imaging may be normal, most useful for complications

Image Interpretation Pearls

- Meningitis is a clinical/laboratory diagnosis, not imaging diagnosis!
  - Meningitis can occur in presence of normal imaging studies
- T1 C+, FLAIR often complementary in diagnosis
- Delayed contrast-enhanced FLAIR best for subtle disease

SELECTED REFERENCES

1. Smirniotopoulos JG et al: Patterns of contrast enhancement in the brain and meninges. Radiographics. 27(2):525-51, 2007
2. Gleissner B et al: Neoplastic meningitis. Lancet Neurol. 5(5):443-52, 2006
3. Kremer S et al: Accuracy of delayed post-contrast FLAIR MR imaging for the diagnosis of leptomeningeal infectious or tumoral diseases. J Neuroradiol. 33(5):285-91, 2006
4. Meyer S et al: Tuberculous meningitis. Lancet. 367(9523):1682, 2006
5. Migirov L et al: Otogenic intracranial complications: a review of 28 cases. Acta Otolaryngol. 125(8):819-22, 2005
6. Overturf GD: Defining bacterial meningitis and other infections of the central nervous system. Pediatr Crit Care Med. 6(3 Suppl):S14-8, 2005

MENINGITIS

IMAGE GALLERY

Typical

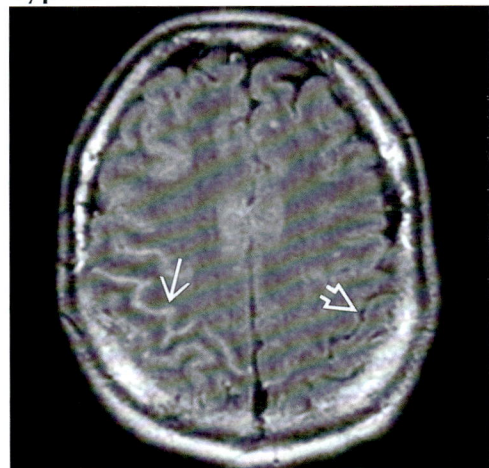
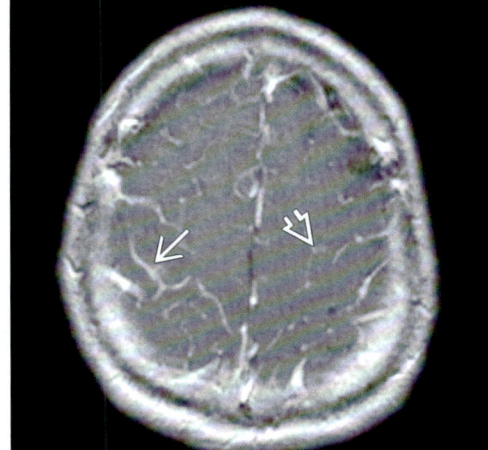

(Left) Axial FLAIR MR shows hyperintensity in the right parietal sulci ➔ compared to the nearly normal hypointense CSF on the left ➔. CSF normally suppresses on FLAIR. *(Right)* Axial T1 C+ MR in the same case shows striking enhancement in the right sulci ➔ but even the left sulci ➔ enhance although more subtly. Pyogenic meningitis.

Typical

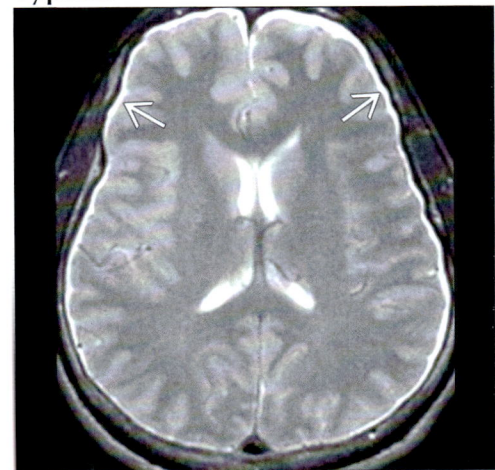
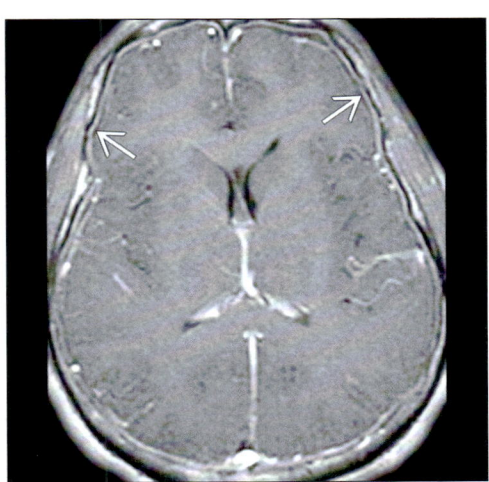

(Left) Axial T2WI MR in a child with proven pyogenic meningitis shows smooth, very hyperintense thickened dura ➔. *(Right)* Axial T1 C+ MR in the same case shows thickened dura enhances diffusely ➔. Dura-arachnoid enhancement is significantly less common than pia-subarachnoid space enhancement in meningitis.

Typical

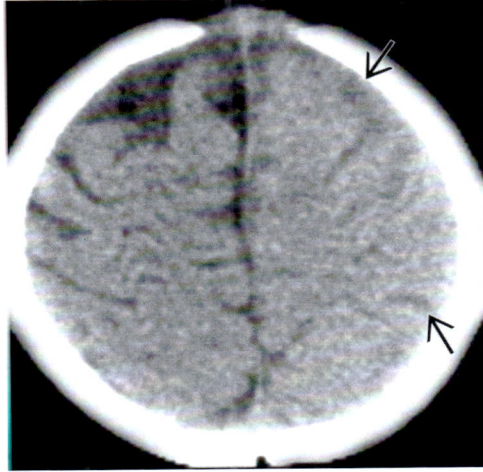
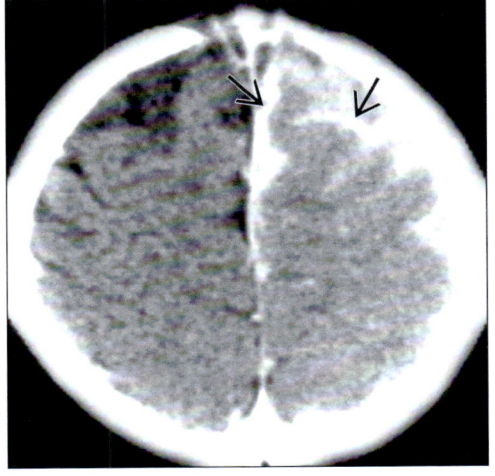

(Left) Axial NECT shows CSF over right hemisphere is normal. Sulci over left hemisphere ➔ are poorly seen as they are filled with nearly isodense proteinaceous CSF. *(Right)* Axial CECT in the same case shows diffuse enhancement of the sulci over the left hemisphere ➔ while the right hemispheric sulci show no enhancement.

ABSCESS

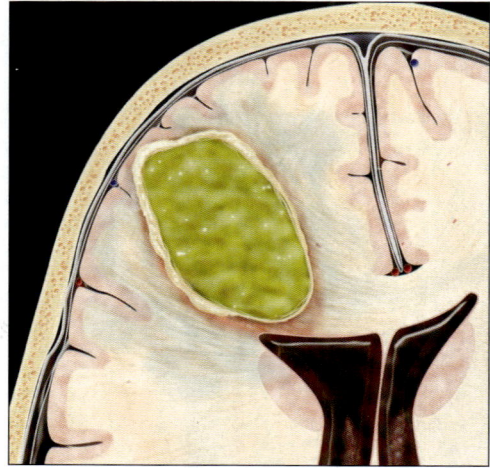

Axial graphic shows early capsule formation with central liquified necrosis and inflammatory debris. Collagen and reticulin form the well-defined abscess wall. Note the surrounding edema.

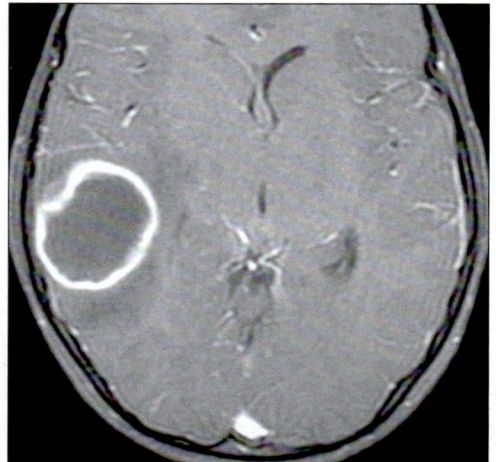

Axial T1 C+ FS MR in a 12 y/o with "flu-like" illness, headache, nausea and vomiting shows a complete rim of thin-walled enhancing tissue surrounding a nonenhancing central core.

TERMINOLOGY

Definitions
- Focal pyogenic infection of brain parenchyma, typically bacterial; fungal or parasitic less common
- Four pathologic stages: Early cerebritis, late cerebritis, early capsule, late capsule

IMAGING FINDINGS

General Features
- Best diagnostic clue
  - Imaging varies with stage of abscess development
  - Early capsule: Well-defined, thin-walled enhancing rim
  - Ring-enhancing lesion: High signal on DWI, low ADC
  - T2 hypointense rim with surrounding edema
- Location
  - Typically supratentorial; up to 14% infratentorial
  - Frontal, parietal lobes most common
  - Usually at gray-white junction (hematogenous)
  - Multiple lesions may represent septic emboli
- Size: 5 mm up to several cm
- Morphology: Thin-walled, well-delineated, ring-enhancing cystic-appearing mass

CT Findings
- NECT
  - Early cerebritis: Ill-defined hypodense subcortical lesion with mass effect; may be normal early
  - Late cerebritis: Central low-density area; peripheral edema, mass effect increase
  - Early capsule: Hypodense mass with moderate vasogenic edema and mass effect
  - Late capsule: Edema, mass effect diminish
  - Gas-containing abscess rare
- CECT
  - Early cerebritis: ± Mild patchy enhancement
  - Late cerebritis: Irregular rim-enhancement
  - Early capsule
    - Low-density center with thin, distinct enhancing rim
    - Deep part of capsule thinnest; thickest near cortex
  - Late capsule
    - Cavity shrinks
    - Capsule thickens

DDx: Ring-Enhancing Mass

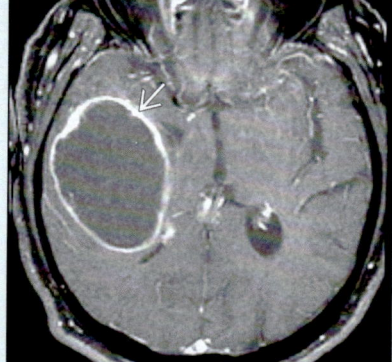

Glioblastoma

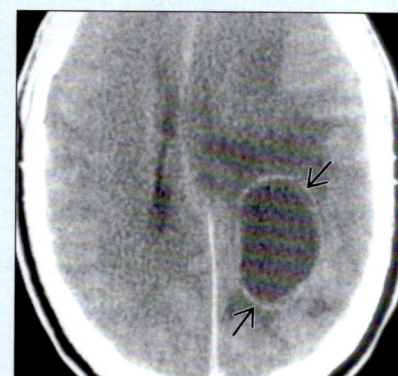

Metastasis

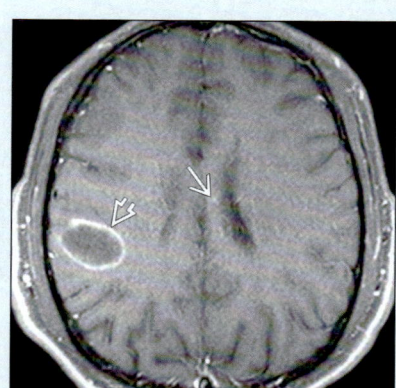

Multiple Sclerosis

ABSCESS

Key Facts

Terminology
- Four pathologic stages: Early cerebritis, late cerebritis, early capsule, late capsule

Imaging Findings
- Imaging varies with stage of abscess development
- Ring-enhancing lesion: High signal on DWI, low ADC
- T2 hypointense rim with surrounding edema
- Late capsule
- Multiplanar MR without and with contrast, DWI
- MRS to distinguish abscess from neoplasm

Top Differential Diagnoses
- Glioblastoma Multiforme
- Parenchymal Metastases
- Demyelinating Disease
- Resolving Intracerebral Hematoma
- Subacute Cerebral Infarction

Clinical Issues
- Headache (up to 90%)
- Fever in only 50%
- Age: Most common during third and fourth decades, but 25% occur in patients < 15 years
- Potentially fatal but treatable lesion
- Intraventricular rupture, ventriculitis
- Mass effect, herniation
- Primary therapy: Surgical drainage and/or excision
- If < 2.5 cm or early phase cerebritis: Antibiotics only

Diagnostic Checklist
- DWI, MRS helpful to distinguish abscess from mimics
- Search for local cause (sinusitis, otitis media, mastoiditis)

- May have "daughter" abscesses

MR Findings
- T1WI
  - Early cerebritis: Poorly marginated, mixed hypo-/isointense mass
  - Late cerebritis: Hypointense center, iso-/mildly hyperintense rim
  - Early capsule: Rim iso-/hyperintense to WM; center hyperintense to CSF
  - Late capsule: Cavity shrinks, capsule thickens
- T2WI
  - Early cerebritis: Ill-defined hyperintense mass
  - Late cerebritis: Hyperintense center, hypointense rim; hyperintense edema
  - Early capsule: Hypointense rim
    - Related to collagen, hemorrhage, or paramagnetic free radicals
  - Late capsule: Edema and mass effect diminish
  - Resolving abscess
    - Hyperintense on T2WI, FLAIR; hypointense rim resolves
    - Small ring/punctate enhancing focus may persist for months
- DWI
  - Increased signal intensity in cerebritis and abscess
  - ADC map: Markedly decreased signal centrally within abscess
- T1 C+
  - Early cerebritis: Patchy enhancement
  - Late cerebritis: Intense, irregular rim enhancement
  - Early capsule: Well-defined, thin-walled enhancing rim
  - Late capsule
    - Cavity collapses, capsule thickens
    - Capsule thinnest on ventricular side
- MRS: Central necrotic area may show presence of acetate, lactate, alanine, succinate, pyruvate, amino acids

Nuclear Medicine Findings
- PET: FDG and Carbon-11-Methionine have shown increased uptake in brain abscess

Imaging Recommendations
- Best imaging tool: Contrast-enhanced MR
- Protocol advice
  - Multiplanar MR without and with contrast, DWI
  - MRS to distinguish abscess from neoplasm

Other Modality Findings
- Perfusion MR shows low rCBV in capsule (vs. high for neoplasms)

DIFFERENTIAL DIAGNOSIS

Glioblastoma Multiforme
- Thick, nodular > thin wall
- Low signal on DWI (sometimes high, mimics abscess)
- Hemorrhage common
- Other cystic primary neoplasms can also mimic abscess

Parenchymal Metastases
- Thick-walled
- Often multiple

Demyelinating Disease
- Multiple sclerosis, ADEM
- Ring enhancement often incomplete ("horseshoe")
- Characteristic lesions elsewhere in brain
- Mass effect small for size of lesion

Resolving Intracerebral Hematoma
- History of trauma or vascular lesion
- Blood products present on MR

Subacute Cerebral Infarction
- History of stroke
- Vascular distribution
- Gyriform >> ring enhancement (rare)

ABSCESS

PATHOLOGY

General Features
- General path comments
  - Cerebritis: Unencapsulated zone of vessels, inflammatory cells, edema; necrotic foci gradually coalesce
  - Capsule: Well-defined capsule develops around necrotic core; edema/mass effect decreases as abscess matures
- Etiology
  - Hematogenous from extracranial location (pulmonary infection, endocarditis, urinary tract infections)
  - Direct extension from calvarial or meningeal infection
    - Paranasal sinus, middle ear, teeth infections (via valveless emissary veins)
  - Penetrating trauma (bone fragments > metal)
  - Post-operative
  - Right-to-left shunts (congenital cardiac malformations, pulmonary arteriovenous fistulas)
  - 20-30% have no identifiable source (cryptogenic)
    - Often polymicrobial (streptococci, staphylococci, anaerobes)
- Epidemiology
  - Uncommon; approximately 2,500 cases/year in U.S.
  - Bacterial: Staphylococcus, Streptococcus, Pneumococcus
  - Diabetic: Klebsiella pneumoniae
  - Post-transplant: Nocardia, Aspergillus, Candida
  - AIDS: Toxoplasmosis, Mycobacterium Tuberculosis
  - Neonates: Citrobacter, Proteus, Pseudomonas, Serratia, Staphylococcus aureus

Gross Pathologic & Surgical Features
- Early cerebritis (3-5 days)
  - Infection focal but not localized
  - Unencapsulated mass of PMNs, edema, scattered foci of necrosis, petechial hemorrhage
- Late cerebritis (4-5 days-2 weeks)
  - Necrotic foci coalesce
  - Rim of inflammatory cells, macrophages, granulation tissue, fibroblasts surrounds central necrotic core
  - Vascular proliferation, surrounding vasogenic edema
- Early capsule (begins about 2 weeks)
  - Well-delineated collagenous capsule
  - Liquified necrotic core, peripheral gliosis
- Late capsule (weeks-months)
  - Central cavity shrinks
  - Thick wall (collagen, granulation tissue, macrophages, gliosis)

Microscopic Features
- Early cerebritis: Hyperemic tissue with PMNs, necrotic blood vessels, microorganisms
- Late cerebritis: Progressive necrosis of neuropil, PMN destruction, and inflammatory cells
- Early capsule: Granulation tissue proliferation around necrotic core
- Late capsule: Multiple layers of collagen & fibroblasts

CLINICAL ISSUES

Presentation
- Most common signs/symptoms
  - Headache (up to 90%)
  - Fever in only 50%
- Other signs/symptoms
  - Seizures, altered mental status, focal neurologic deficits
  - Increased erythrocyte sedimentation rate (ESR) (75%), elevated WBC count (50%)

Demographics
- Age: Most common during third and fourth decades, but 25% occur in patients < 15 years
- Gender: M:F = 2:1

Natural History & Prognosis
- Potentially fatal but treatable lesion
  - Stereotactic surgery + medical therapy have greatly reduced mortality
- Complications of inadequately or untreated abscesses
  - Intraventricular rupture, ventriculitis
    - May be fatal
    - Ventricular debris with irregular fluid level
    - Hydrocephalus
    - Ependymal enhancement typical
  - Meningitis, "daughter" lesions
  - Mass effect, herniation
- Factors affecting prognosis
  - Size, location, virulence of infecting organism(s)
  - Systemic conditions
- Mortality variable: 0-30%

Treatment
- Primary therapy: Surgical drainage and/or excision
- If < 2.5 cm or early phase cerebritis: Antibiotics only
- Steroids to treat edema and mass effect
- Lumbar puncture hazardous; pathogen often can't be determined from CSF

DIAGNOSTIC CHECKLIST

Consider
- DWI, MRS helpful to distinguish abscess from mimics

Image Interpretation Pearls
- Search for local cause (sinusitis, otitis media, mastoiditis)
- T2 hypointense abscess rim resolves before enhancement in successfully treated patients

SELECTED REFERENCES
1. Fertikh D et al: Discrimination of capsular stage brain abscesses from necrotic or cystic neoplasms using diffusion-weighted magnetic resonance imaging. J Neurosurg. 106(1):76-81, 2007
2. Plotnik AN et al: Multiple cystic ring-enhancing cerebral lesions. J Clin Neurosci. 13(9):933, 976, 2006
3. Reddy JS et al: The role of diffusion-weighted imaging in the differential diagnosis of intracranial cystic mass lesions: a report of 147 lesions. Surg Neurol. 66(3):246-50; discussion 250-1, 2006

ABSCESS

IMAGE GALLERY

Typical

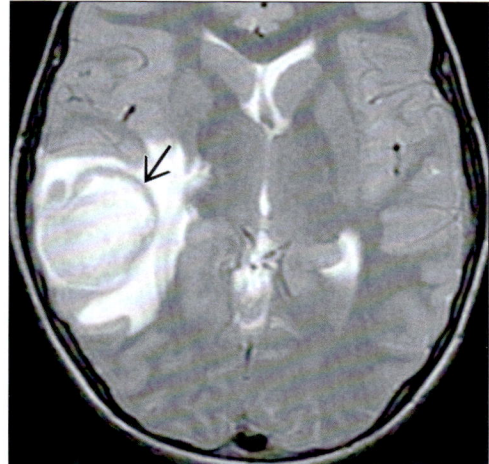
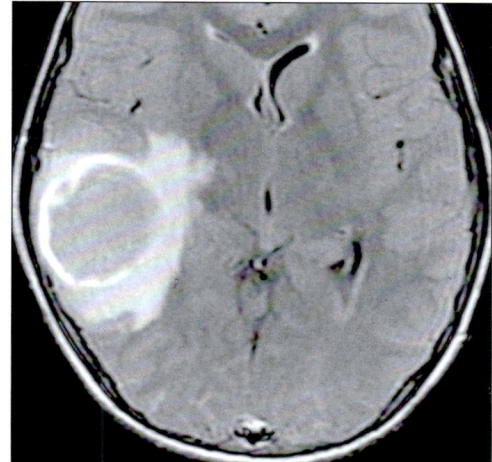

(Left) Axial T2WI MR in the same patient as previous image shows a hypointense rim ➔ surrounding an inhomogeneously hyperintense central core. Moderate edema, mass effect are present. *(Right)* Axial FLAIR MR in the same patient as previous image shows that rim appears hyperintense and the central core does not suppress, indicating probable proteinaceous, necrotic contents.

Typical

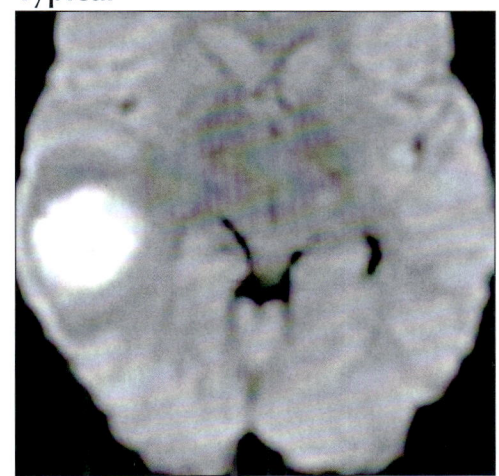
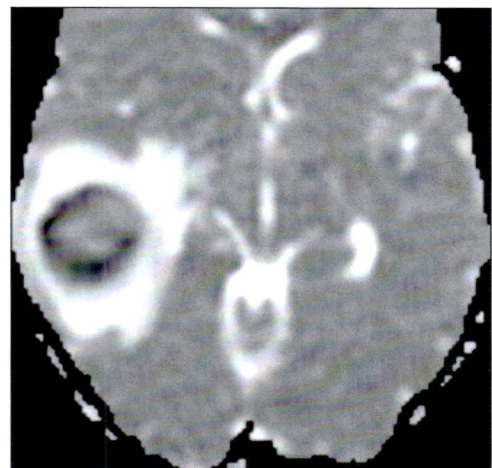

(Left) Axial DWI MR shows that the central cystic component appears hyperintense on trace diffusion MR. *(Right)* Axial ADC shows the lesion appears markedly hypointense, representing restricted diffusion.

Typical

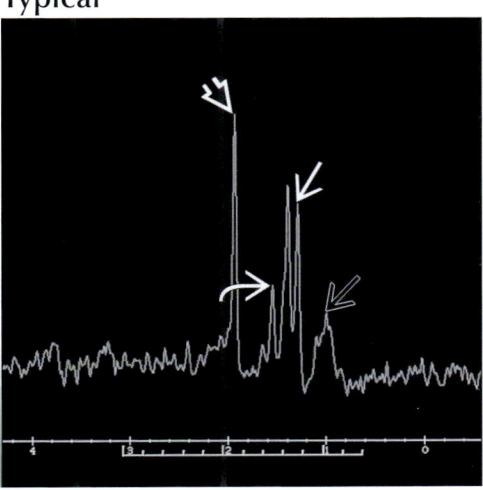
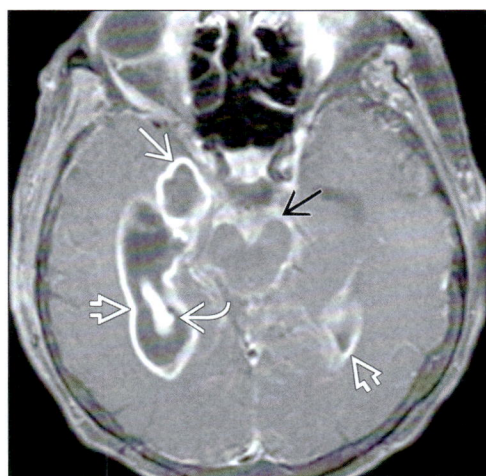

(Left) MRS (TR2000/TE288) shows large lactate peak at 1.3 ppm ➔. Acetate is present at 2 ppm ➔. Alanine is seen at 1.5 ppm ➔. Peak at .9 ppm ➔ represents cytosolic amino acids. *(Right)* Axial T1 C+ MR in another case shows a right temporal lobe abscess ➔ that has ruptured into the temporal horn, causing ventriculitis ➔, choroid plexitis ➔ and meningitis ➔.

EXTRA-AXIAL EMPYEMA

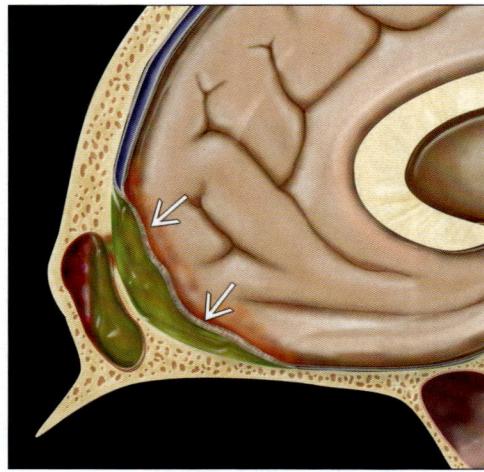

Sagittal graphic shows frontal sinus purulence and direct extension to epidural space ➡, resulting in epidural empyema (EDE). Note inflammation in the adjacent frontal lobe.

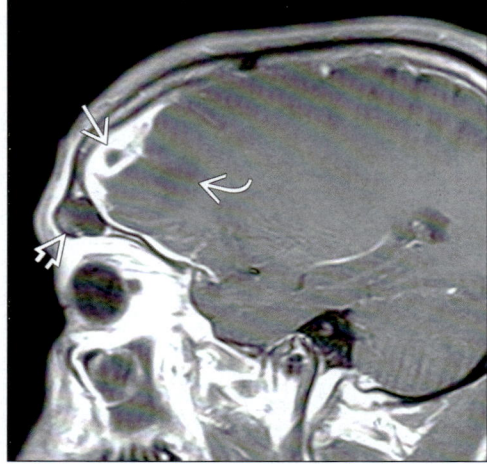

Sagittal T1 C+ FS MR reveals subdural empyema ➡ secondary to acute rhinosinusitis ➡. Note lack of low signal rim to indicate pus is epidural. Underlying frontal lobe cerebritis ➡.

TERMINOLOGY

Abbreviations and Synonyms
- Subdural empyema (SDE), epidural empyema (EDE), epidural abscess
- Epidural empyema = epidural abscess

Definitions
- Loculated collection of pus in subdural or epidural space, or both

IMAGING FINDINGS

General Features
- Best diagnostic clue: Extra-axial collection with C+ rim
- Location
  - Supratentorial typical
    - SDE: Convexity in > 50%, parafalcine in 20%
    - EDE: Often adjacent to frontal sinus
  - Infratentorial (up to 10%)
    - Often associated with mastoiditis
    - > 90% associated with hydrocephalus
- Morphology
  - SDE: Crescentic typical; may be lens-shaped (lentiform) on coronal images
  - EDE: Biconvex, lentiform

CT Findings
- NECT
  - Extra-axial collection, iso- to hyperdense to CSF
  - SDE: Crescentic iso- to hyperdense collection, confined by falx
    - Frequently bilateral
    - Warning: Can be small, easily overlooked!
  - EDE: Biconvex low-density collection between dura, calvarium; contained by cranial sutures
    - Often continuous across midline
- CECT
  - Strong peripheral rim enhancement
  - Posterior fossa EDE
    - Typically at sinodural angle
    - Tegmen tympani ± sigmoid plate eroded
    - Pus may extend into cerebellopontine angle
- Bone CT
  - **Sinusitis** common in **supratentorial** SDE-EDE
  - **Otomastoiditis** common in **infratentorial** SDE-EDE

DDx: Extra-Axial Collections

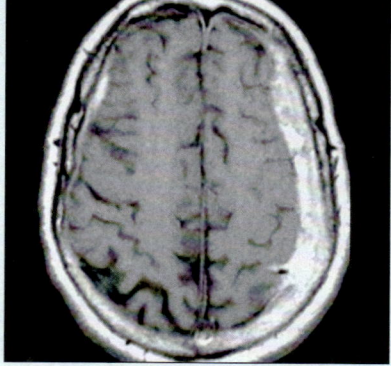

Chronic Subdural Hematoma

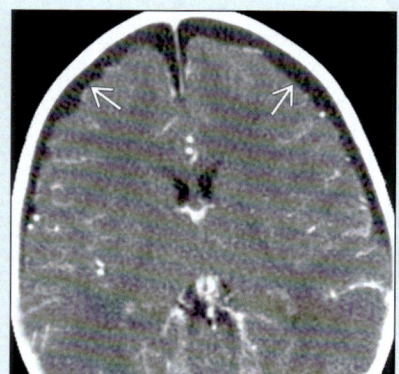

Subdural Effusions

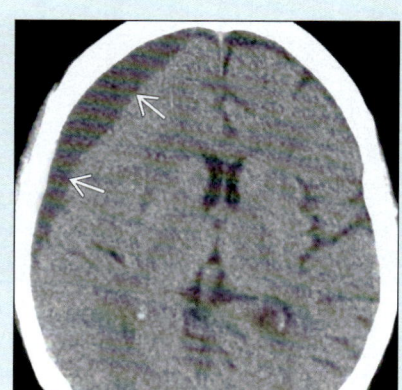

Subdural Hygroma

EXTRA-AXIAL EMPYEMA

Key Facts

Terminology
- Loculated collection of pus in subdural or epidural space, or both

Imaging Findings
- Best diagnostic clue: Extra-axial collection with C+ rim
- Supratentorial typical
- Infratentorial (up to 10%)
- Extra-axial collection, iso- to hyperdense to CSF
- Underlying brain may be hyperintense
- Best imaging tool: **MR with DWI** best to demonstrate presence, nature, extent, complications

Top Differential Diagnoses
- Chronic Subdural Hematoma
- Subdural Effusion
- Subdural Hygroma
- Dural Metastasis

Pathology
- SDE much more common than EDE
- 15% of cases have both EDE & SDE
- Infants, young children: Complication of **bacterial meningitis**
- Older children, adults: Related to **paranasal sinus disease** (> 2/3)

Clinical Issues
- EDE, SDE rare, yet highly lethal
- Progresses rapidly, **neurosurgical emergency**
- **Mortality 10-15%**
- Surgical drainage via wide craniotomy is gold standard

MR Findings
- T1WI
  - Extra-axial collection, hyperintense to CSF
  - SDE: Crescentic extra-axial collection
  - EDE: Lentiform bifrontal or convexity collection
    - Inwardly displaced dura seen as **hypointense line** between fluid and brain
    - May cross midline in frontal region
- T2WI
  - Iso- to hyperintense to CSF
  - SDE: Crescentic collection, underlying brain may be hyperintense
  - EDE: Lentiform bifrontal or convexity collection
    - Inwardly displaced dura seen as hypointense line between fluid and brain
    - Underlying brain usually spared
- FLAIR
  - Hyperintense to CSF
  - SDE: Crescentic collection, underlying brain may be hyperintense
  - EDE: Lentiform bifrontal or convexity collection
    - Underlying brain may be hyperintense
- DWI
  - SDE: **Restricted diffusion** (↑ signal intensity) typical
  - EDE: Variable signal with hyperintense components
- T1 C+
  - Prominent enhancement at margin related to granulomatous tissue and inflammation
  - SDE: Encapsulating membranes enhance strongly, may be loculated with internal fibrous strands
  - EDE: Strong enhancement of collection margins
  - May see enhancement of adjacent brain parenchyma (cerebritis/abscess)
  - Subgaleal phlegmon or abscess ("Pott puffy tumor")
- MRV: Venous thrombosis may be seen as lack of flow

Ultrasonographic Findings
- Useful in infants
- Heterogeneous echogenic convexity collection with mass effect
  - Hyperechoic fibrous strands
  - Thick hyperechoic inner membrane
  - Increased echogenicity of pia-arachnoid and exudates in subarachnoid space

Imaging Recommendations
- Best imaging tool: **MR with DWI** best to demonstrate presence, nature, extent, complications
- Protocol advice
  - Contrast-enhanced multiplanar MR with DWI
  - **DWI** helpful to evaluate extent and complications

DIFFERENTIAL DIAGNOSIS

Chronic Subdural Hematoma
- MR shows blood products; may be loculated
- Often enhances along edge; usually thinner than SDE
- May be indistinguishable; history may help

Subdural Effusion
- Sterile, CSF-like collection associated with meningitis
- Follows CSF on all MR sequences
- Usually nonenhancing; may enhance mildly
- Frontal and temporal regions common, often bilateral

Subdural Hygroma
- Nonenhancing CSF collection, often trauma history

Dural Metastasis
- Primary tumor often known, typically breast, prostate
- Often diffuse, nodular enhancement
- May have associated bone metastases

PATHOLOGY

General Features
- General path comments
  - SDE much more common than EDE
  - SDE more commonly complicated by abscess and venous thrombosis (> 10%)
  - 15% of cases have both EDE & SDE
- Etiology
  - Infants, young children: Complication of **bacterial meningitis**

EXTRA-AXIAL EMPYEMA

- Older children, adults: Related to **paranasal sinus disease** (> 2/3)
  - Direct spread via posterior wall of frontal sinus
  - Retrograde spread through **valveless bridging emissary veins** of extra-, intracranial spaces
- **Mastoiditis** (± cholesteatoma) in 20%
- Complication of head trauma or neurosurgical procedure (rare)
- Complication of meningitis in adults (very rare)
- Causative organism: Streptococci, H. influenzae, S. aureus, S. epidermidis most common
- Anaerobic or microaerophilic organisms (strep, bacteroides) common
- Epidemiology
  - Uncommon; occur 1/4 to 1/2 as often as abscess
  - SDE and EDE account for approximately 30% of intracranial infections
  - SDE: Sinusitis in 67%, mastoiditis in 10%

Gross Pathologic & Surgical Features
- Encapsulated, yellowish, purulent collection
- Spreads widely but may be loculated
- Osteitis in 35%

Microscopic Features
- Inflammatory infiltrate-granulomatous tissue

CLINICAL ISSUES

Presentation
- Most common signs/symptoms
  - Majority have fever, headaches
  - Meningismus common, may mimic meningitis
  - Sinusitis often present
  - Cerebritis-brain abscess cause neurologic signs
- Clinical Profile
  - Sinus or ear infection in > 75% of cases
  - Frontal subgaleal abscess ("Pott puffy tumor") in up to 1/3; typically adolescent males
  - Periorbital swelling may be seen
  - Confused with meningitis; delayed diagnosis
  - EDE, SDE rare, yet highly lethal

Demographics
- Age: Can occur at any age

Natural History & Prognosis
- Progresses rapidly, **neurosurgical emergency**
- Rapidly evolving, fulminant course
- EDE may occasionally have indolent course, as dura mater functions as barrier between infection and brain
  - Much better prognosis than SDE
- Can be fatal unless recognized, treated
  - **Lumbar puncture** can be fatal!
  - CSF can be normal
- Complications common
  - Cerebritis and brain abscess: Approximately 5%
  - Cortical vein, dural sinus thrombosis (ischemia)
  - Cerebral edema
  - Hydrocephalus (> 90% of infratentorial SDE)
- **Mortality 10-15%**

Treatment
- Surgical drainage via wide craniotomy is gold standard
- Intravenous antibiotics
- Sinus drainage + antibiotics possible in small sinus-related EDE

DIAGNOSTIC CHECKLIST

Consider
- Chronic subdural hematoma may be difficult to differentiate from SDE; history may help
- Look for empyema in patient with sinusitis and neurologic symptoms
- If SDE or EDE discovered, look also for sinusitis, otomastoiditis, dural sinus thrombosis, brain abscess

Image Interpretation Pearls
- MR with contrast and **DWI** is most sensitive; CT may miss small collections
- DWI differentiates SDE from subdural effusions
- MR with DWI may be use to monitor treatment response

SELECTED REFERENCES

1. Osborn MK et al: Subdural empyema and other suppurative complications of paranasal sinusitis. Lancet Infect Dis. 7(1):62-7, 2007
2. Fanning NF et al: Serial diffusion-weighted MRI correlates with clinical course and treatment response in children with intracranial pus collections. Pediatr Radiol. 36(1):26-37, 2006
3. Venkatesh MS et al: Pediatric infratentorial subdural empyema: analysis of 14 cases. J Neurosurg. 105(5 Suppl):370-7, 2006
4. Wong AM et al: Diffusion-weighted MR imaging of subdural empyemas in children. AJNR Am J Neuroradiol. 25(6):1016-21, 2004
5. Heran NS et al: Conservative neurosurgical management of intracranial epidural abscesses in children. Neurosurgery. 53(4):893-7; discussion 897-8, 2003
6. Lim CC et al: Diffusion-weighted MR imaging in intracranial infections. Ann Acad Med Singapore. 32(4):446-9, 2003
7. Tsai YD et al: Intracranial suppuration: a clinical comparison of subdural empyemas and epidural abscesses. Surg Neurol. 59(3):191-6; discussion 196, 2003
8. Tsuchiya K et al: Diffusion-weighted MRI of subdural and epidural empyemas. Neuroradiology. 45(4):220-3, 2003
9. Guzman R et al: Use of diffusion-weighted magnetic resonance imaging in differentiating purulent brain processes from cystic brain tumors. J Neurosurg. 97(5):1101-7, 2002
10. Rohde V et al: Complications of burr-hole craniostomy and closed-system drainage for chronic subdural hematomas: a retrospective analysis of 376 patients. Neurosurg Rev. 25(1-2):89-94, 2002
11. Bambakidis NC et al: Intracranial complications of frontal sinusitis in children: Pott's puffy tumor revisited. Pediatr Neurosurg. 35(2):82-9, 2001
12. Nathoo N et al: Cranial extradural empyema in the era of computed tomography: a review of 82 cases. Neurosurgery. 44(4):748-53; discussion 753-4, 1999
13. Chen CY et al: Subdural empyema in 10 infants: US characteristics and clinical correlates. Radiology. 207(3):609-17, 1998

EXTRA-AXIAL EMPYEMA

IMAGE GALLERY

Variant

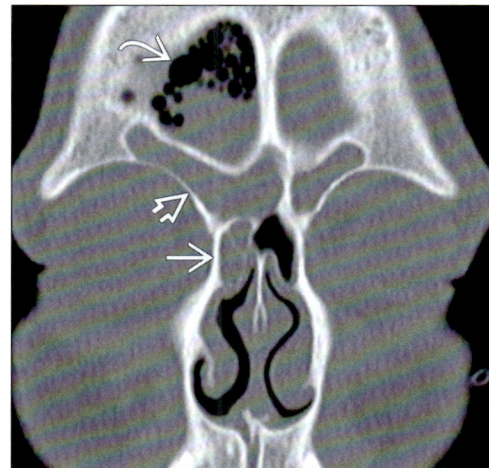
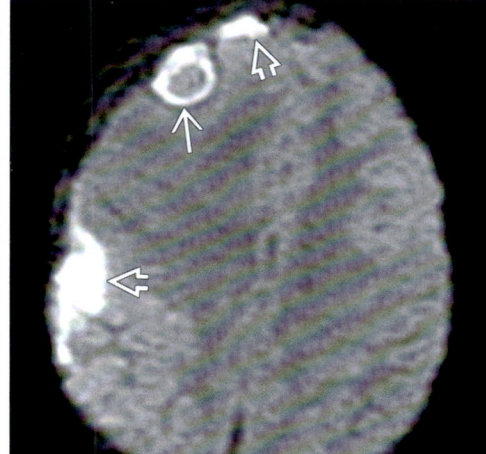

(Left) Coronal bone CT demonstrates agger nasi ➡ and frontal sinus ➡ opacification. Intracranial air ➡ should signal the possibility of serious complication from the patient's sinusitis. *(Right)* Axial DWI MR shows restricted diffusion of both epidural empyema (EDE) ➡ and subdural empyema (SDE) ➡. EDE circumscribed by its dural margin while SDE flows in subarachnoid space.

Variant

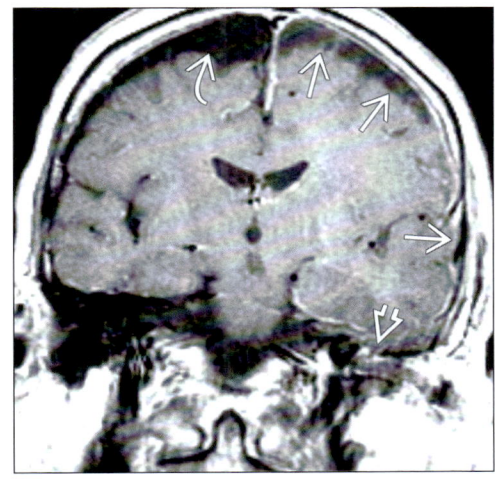
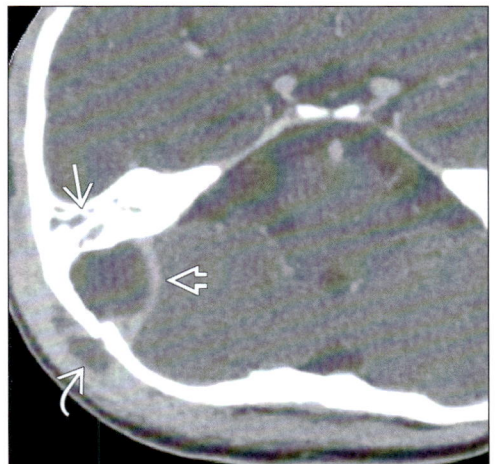

(Left) Coronal T1 C+ MR shows subdural empyema around left hemisphere ➡ with tegmen tympani dehiscence ➡ from otomastoiditis. Note higher signal empyema compared to opposite hygroma ➡. *(Right)* Axial CECT shows mastoid opacification ➡ with associated epidural empyema-abscess in the posterior fossa ➡ as well as subgaleal abscess ➡. Cholesteatoma is often associated.

Variant

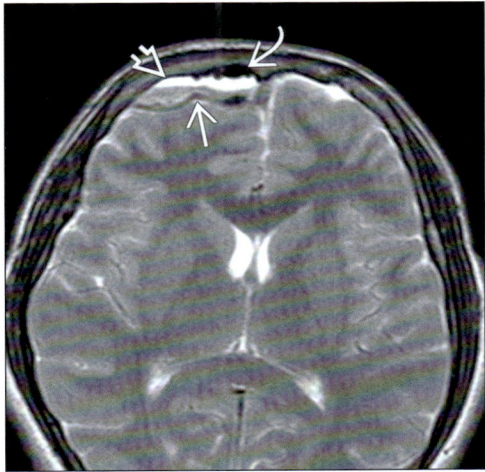
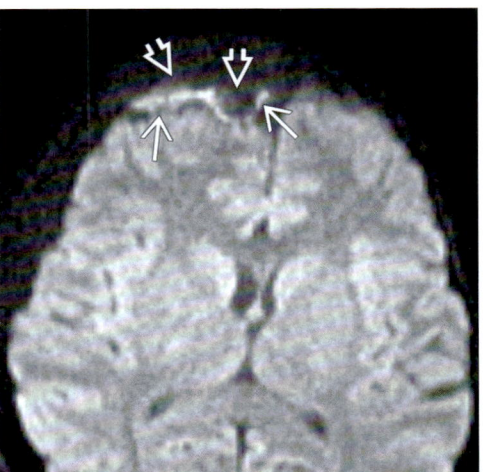

(Left) Axial T2WI FS MR shows hemorrhagic epidural empyema confined by dura ➡ containing a fluid-fluid level ➡ and air ➡. The dural provides a protective barrier for the brain. *(Right)* Axial DWI MR demonstrates mixed signal of frontal epidural empyema. Restricted diffusion high signal ➡ mix with low signal areas ➡ due to air and blood product susceptibility blooming.

HERPES ENCEPHALITIS

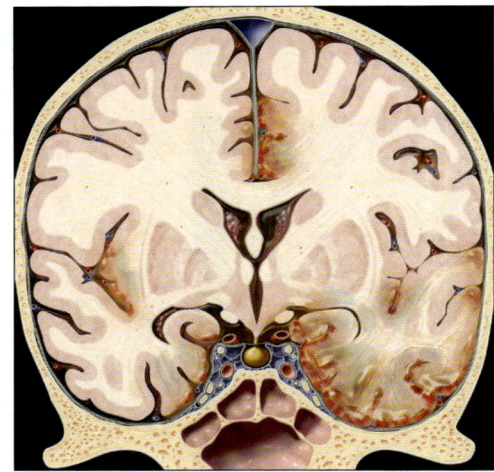

Coronal graphic shows inflammation in the temporal lobes, left cingulate gyrus, and right insula. Bilateral, asymmetric involvement of gray & white matter, typical of herpes encephalitis.

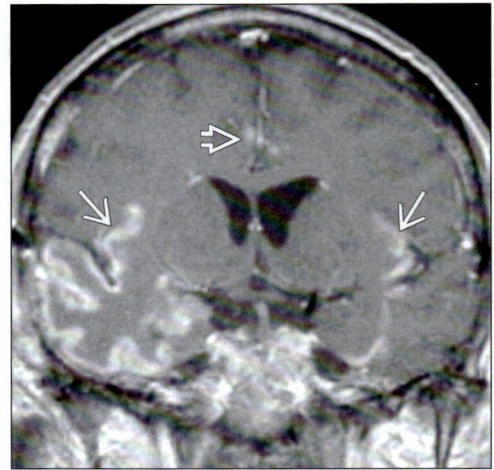

Coronal T1 C+ MR shows striking bilateral but asymmetric enhancement in the temporal lobe and insular cortex ➡. Subtle lesions are seen in the cingulate gyri ➡. Classic HE.

TERMINOLOGY

Abbreviations and Synonyms
- Herpes simplex encephalitis (HSE)

Definitions
- Brain parenchyma infection caused by herpes simplex virus type 1 (HSV-1)
- Typically reactivation in immunocompetent patients

IMAGING FINDINGS

General Features
- Best diagnostic clue
  - Hyperintense medial temporal, inferior frontal cortex
  - Involvement of cingulate gyrus, contralateral temporal lobe highly suggestive
- Location
  - Limbic system: Temporal lobes, insula, subfrontal area, cingulate gyri typical
  - Cerebral convexity, posterior occipital cortex may become involved
  - Typically bilateral disease, but asymmetric
  - Basal ganglia usually spared
  - Atypical patterns seen in infants, children
    - May primarily affect cerebral hemispheres
  - Rarely affects midbrain and pons (mesenrhombencephalitis)

CT Findings
- NECT
  - CT often normal early!
    - Low attenuation, mild mass effect in medial temporal lobes, insula
    - Hemorrhage typically late feature
  - Predilection for limbic system; basal ganglia spared
  - Earliest CT findings at 3 days after symptom onset
- CECT: Patchy or gyriform enhancement of temporal lobes (late acute/subacute feature)

MR Findings
- T1WI
  - Cortical swelling with loss of gray-white junction, mass effect
  - May see subacute hemorrhage as increased signal within edematous brain

DDx: Gyriform Hyperintensity

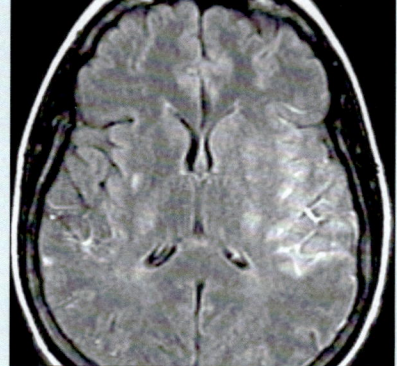

Ischemia/Infarct

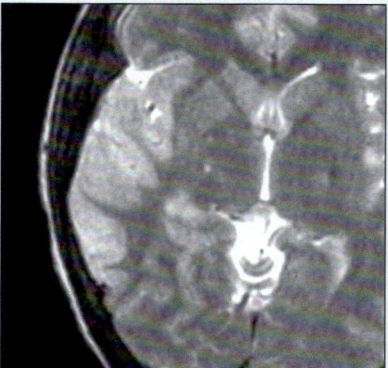

Status Epilepticus

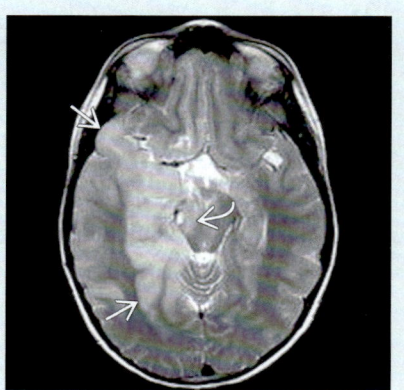

Gliomatosis Cerebri

HERPES ENCEPHALITIS

Key Facts

Imaging Findings
- Hyperintense medial temporal, inferior frontal cortex
- Involvement of cingulate gyrus, contralateral temporal lobe highly suggestive
- CT often normal early!
- Restricted diffusion with hyperintensity in limbic system
- Best imaging tool: MR (positive 24-48 h earlier than CT)

Top Differential Diagnoses
- Cerebral Ischemia-Infarction, Acute
- Status Epilepticus
- Infiltrating Neoplasm
- Limbic Encephalitis
- Other Encephalitides

Pathology
- HSV-1 in adults, children
- Most common cause of fatal sporadic encephalitis
- Hemorrhagic, necrotizing encephalitis

Clinical Issues
- Fever, headache, seizures, ± viral prodrome
- Children often present with nonspecific symptoms
- Altered mental status
- Focal or diffuse neurologic deficit (< 30%)
- Polymerase chain reaction (PCR) of CSF most accurate diagnosis
- 50-70% mortality rate

Diagnostic Checklist
- Start IV Acyclovir immediately if HSE suspected
- MR most sensitive for early diagnosis

  - Atrophy, encephalomalacia in late subacute/chronic cases
- T2WI
  - Cortical, subcortical hyperintensity with relative white matter sparing
  - May see subacute hemorrhage as increased signal within edematous brain
- PD/Intermediate: Increased signal in affected areas
- FLAIR
  - Cortical hyperintensity
  - May see changes earlier than on T2WI
- T2* GRE: If hemorrhagic, hypointensity "blooms" within edematous brain
- DWI
  - Restricted diffusion with hyperintensity in limbic system
  - Look for bilateral disease
- T1 C+
  - May see mild, patchy enhancement early
  - Gyriform enhancement usually seen 1 week after initial symptoms
  - Meningeal enhancement occasionally seen
  - Enhancement seen in temporal lobes, insular cortex, subfrontal area, cingulate gyrus

Imaging Recommendations
- Best imaging tool: MR (positive 24-48 h earlier than CT)
- Protocol advice: Multiplanar MR with coronal T2 and/or FLAIR, DWI, T2* GRE, contrast

DIFFERENTIAL DIAGNOSIS

Cerebral Ischemia-Infarction, Acute
- Typical vascular distribution (MCA, ACA, PCA)
- Hyperacute symptoms vs 2-3 d history of "flu-like" illness

Status Epilepticus
- Active seizures may disrupt BBB, cause signal abnormalities and enhancement
- Temporal lobe epilepsy hyperperfusion may mimic HSE

Infiltrating Neoplasm
- Low grade gliomas often involve medial temporal lobe and cause epilepsy
- Gliomatosis cerebri may involve frontal and temporal lobes, may be bilateral
- Onset usually indolent

Limbic Encephalitis
- Rare paraneoplastic syndrome associated with primary tumor, often lung
- Predilection for limbic system, often bilateral
- Hemorrhage not present
- Imaging may be indistinguishable
- Symptom onset weeks to months, vs acute in HSE

Other Encephalitides
- Limbic system not typically involved
- Neurosyphilis can affect medial temporal lobes, mimic HSE
  - May involve meninges, blood vessels (obliterative endarteritis)
- West Nile can mimic clinically but typically involves basal ganglia

PATHOLOGY

General Features
- General path comments
  - HSV-1 in adults, children
  - HSV-2 more common in neonates
  - HSV-1 is DNA virus
  - Viruses are obligate intracellular pathogens
  - Herpes viruses include: HSV-1, HSV-2, Epstein-Barr virus (EBV), cytomegalovirus (CMV), varicella-zoster virus (VZV), B virus, HSV-6, HSV-7
- Etiology
  - Initial HSV-1 infection usually occurs in oronasopharynx via contact with infected secretions

HERPES ENCEPHALITIS

- HSV-1 invades along cranial nerves (via lingual nerve, division of trigeminal nerve) to ganglia
- HSV-1 remains dormant in trigeminal ganglion
- New infection with genetically distinct HSV > reactivation of dormant virus (entry portal probably CN1)
- HSV-1 reactivation may occur spontaneously or be precipitated by various factors
  - Local trauma, immunosuppression, hormonal fluctuations, emotional stress
- HSV-1 causes acute hemorrhagic, necrotizing encephalitis (primarily involving limbic system)
- Epidemiology
  - HSV-1 causes 95% of all HSE
  - Most common cause of fatal sporadic encephalitis
  - Most common nonepidemic cause of viral meningoencephalitis
  - In adults, typically related to viral reactivation
  - Incidence: 1-3 cases/million

Gross Pathologic & Surgical Features
- Hemorrhagic, necrotizing encephalitis
  - Severe edema, massive tissue necrosis with hemorrhage typical
  - Involvement of temporal lobes, insular cortex, orbital surface of frontal lobes
  - Less frequent involvement of cingulate gyrus and occipital cortex

Microscopic Features
- Intense perivascular cuffing, interstitial lymphocytic inflammation
- Intranuclear inclusion bodies in infected cells (neurons, glia, endothelial cells)
  - Typically eosinophilic Cowdry A nuclear inclusions
- Immunohistochemistry shows viral antigens, antibodies to HSV-1
- Chronic cases, microglial nodules form

CLINICAL ISSUES

Presentation
- Most common signs/symptoms
  - Fever, headache, seizures, ± viral prodrome
  - Children often present with nonspecific symptoms
    - Behavioral changes, fever, headaches, seizures
  - Patients typically immunocompetent
    - HSV-1 uncommon in AIDS
- Other signs/symptoms
  - Altered mental status
  - Focal or diffuse neurologic deficit (< 30%)
- Clinical Profile
  - CSF studies show lymphocytic pleocytosis, ↑ protein
  - Polymerase chain reaction (PCR) of CSF most accurate diagnosis
    - Sensitivity/specificity nearly 95-100%
    - False negatives can occur very early after disease onset
  - EEG shows temporal lobe activity
  - Brain biopsy may be required for diagnosis

Demographics
- Age
  - Any age
  - Highest incidence in adolescents and young adults
  - Approximately one-third of all patients < 20 years old
- Gender: No gender predominance

Natural History & Prognosis
- May progress to coma and death
  - 50-70% mortality rate
  - Rapid diagnosis, early treatment with antiviral agents can decrease mortality, may improve outcome
- Despite Acyclovir therapy, nearly two-thirds of survivors have significant neurological deficits
- Survival complicated by memory difficulties, hearing loss, medically intractable epilepsy, personality changes

Treatment
- Antiviral therapy with intravenous Acyclovir

DIAGNOSTIC CHECKLIST

Consider
- Start IV Acyclovir immediately if HSE suspected
- Unilateral disease may mimic stroke or tumor, history often helpful
- Limbic encephalitis if all clinical HSE tests negative and subacute onset of symptoms
- Acute onset of HSE helps differentiate from other etiologies

Image Interpretation Pearls
- MR most sensitive for early diagnosis
- FLAIR, DWI are most sensitive sequences
- Imaging often key in diagnosis

SELECTED REFERENCES

1. Rimon A et al: West Nile encephalitis mimicking herpes encephalitis. Pediatr Neurol. 35(1):62-4, 2006
2. Whitley RJ: Herpes simplex encephalitis: adolescents and adults. Antiviral Res. 71(2-3):141-8, 2006
3. Kuker W et al: Diffusion-weighted MRI in herpes simplex encephalitis: a report of three cases. Neuroradiology. 46(2):122-5, 2004
4. Kaga K et al: Auditory agnosia in children after herpes encephalitis. Acta Otolaryngol. 123(2):232-5, 2003
5. Cakirer S et al: MR imaging in epilepsy that is refractory to medical therapy. Eur Radiol. 12(3):549-58, 2002
6. Bash S et al: Mesiotemporal T2-weighted hyperintensity: neurosyphilis mimicking herpes encephalitis. AJNR Am J Neuroradiol. 22(2):314-6, 2001
7. Kleinschmidt-DeMasters BK et al: The expanding spectrum of herpesvirus infections of the nervous system. Brain Pathol. 11(4):440-51, 2001
8. Teixeira J et al: Diffusion imaging in pediatric central nervous system infections. Neuroradiology. 43(12):1031-9, 2001
9. Leonard JR et al: MR imaging of herpes simplex type 1 encephalitis in infants and young children: a separate pattern of findings. AJR Am J Roentgenol. 174(6):1651-5, 2000

HERPES ENCEPHALITIS

IMAGE GALLERY

Typical

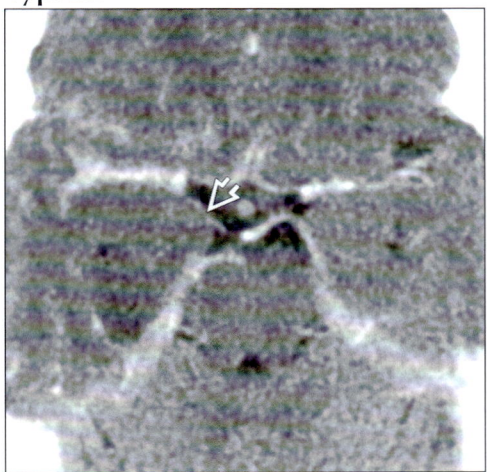
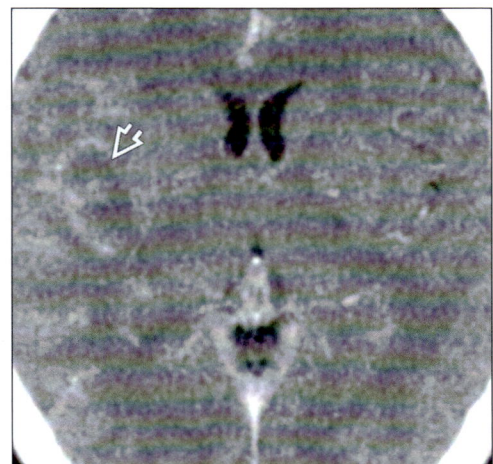

(Left) Axial CECT shows low density right medial temporal lobe, insular cortex ➡ in this elderly female with fever, confusion, decreased consciousness and seizure. *(Right)* Axial CECT in same case shows involvement of insular cortex ➡. Herpes encephalitis was suggested on the basis of CT scan and acyclovir therapy was begun immediately.

Typical

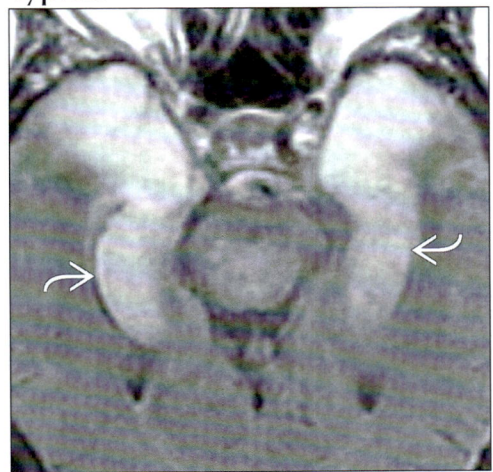
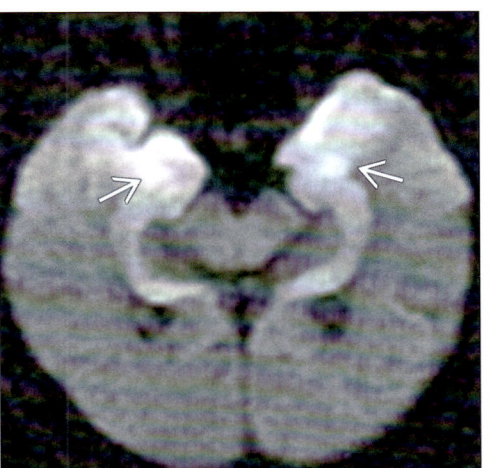

(Left) Axial FLAIR MR shows typical findings of bilateral temporal lobe hyperintensity ➡ in herpes encephalitis. Note gyral edema with relative sparing of underlying white matter. *(Right)* Axial DWI MR in the same case shows restricted diffusion in both temporal lobes ➡ and hippocampal cortex.

Typical

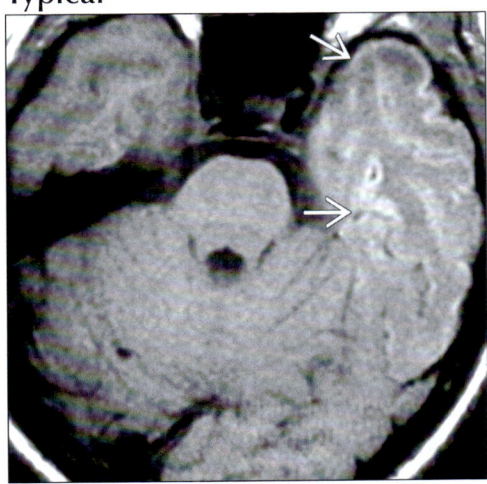
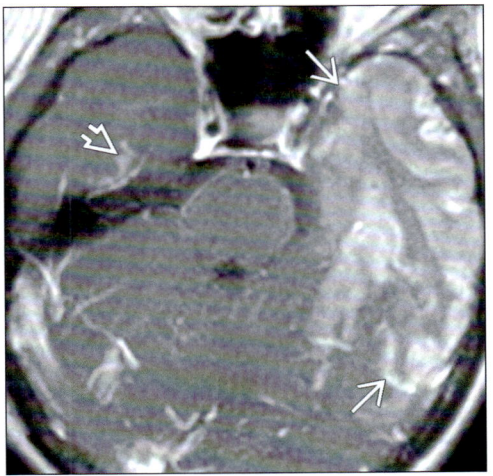

(Left) Axial T1WI MR in a case of herpes encephalitis imaged several days after symptom onset shows gyral hyperintensity ➡ characteristic of petechial hemorrhage at this stage of the disease. *(Right)* Axial T1 C+ MR in the same case shows striking gyriform enhancement in the left temporal lobe ➡ and subtle enhancement in the right temporal lobe cortex ➡.

OPPORTUNISTIC INFECTION, AIDS

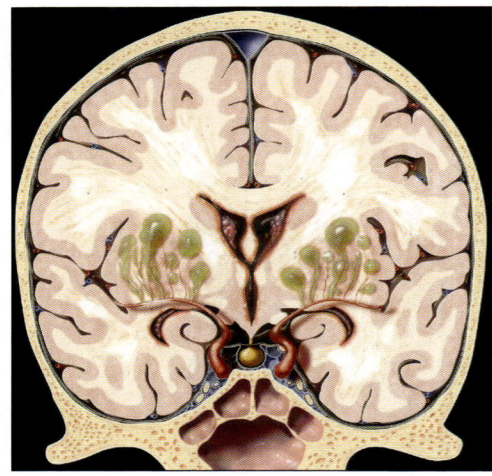
Coronal graphic shows gelatinous pseudocysts due to cryptococcus extending within perivascular spaces adjacent to small perforating arteries.

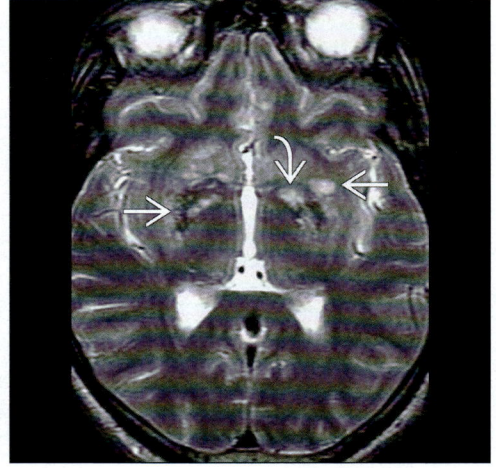
Axial T2WI FS MR shows cryptococcal gelatinous pseudocysts. Multiple foci of T2 hyperintensity ➡ surround anterior commissure ➡ without mass effect.

TERMINOLOGY

Abbreviations and Synonyms
- Opportunistic infections (OIs)

Definitions
- CNS infections in patients with impaired cell-mediated immunity
  - HIV (AIDS) debilitation, hematopoietic neoplasms, chronic immunosuppressive therapy
- Viral disease
  - HIV encephalitis
  - Progressive multifocal leukoencephalopathy (PML)
  - Cytomegalovirus (CMV) infection: Ventriculitis, encephalitis
- Parasitic disease
  - Toxoplasmosis (Toxo)
- Granulomatous disease: Fungal & bacterial
  - Aspergillosis
  - Cryptococcosis (crypto): Leptomeningeal, parenchymal
  - Tuberculosis (TB): Meningitis, tuberculoma

IMAGING FINDINGS

General Features
- Best diagnostic clue
  - Toxo: Multiple ring-enhancing lesions of varying size with surrounding edema in deep and superficial brain
    - Most common cause of focal lesion in HIV+
  - HIV: Rapidly progressive atrophy, diffuse symmetric periventricular white-matter (WM) change
  - PML: Large multifocal subcortical WM lesions without mass effect, enhancement
  - Aspergillosis: Hemorrhagic, multifocal, poorly defined, rim-enhancing lesions
  - Crypto: Multiple small fluid-intensity foci in basal ganglia (BG)
  - TB: Basal meningeal enhancement, hydrocephalus, deep infarcts
- Location
  - Toxo: Cerebral hemispheres, deep gray matter (GM)
  - Crypto: Virchow-Robin spaces (VRSs), mostly BG, superior brain stem
  - PML: Supratentorial subcortical WM most common
    - Posterior fossa & thalamus less common

DDx: Opportunistic Infection Mimics

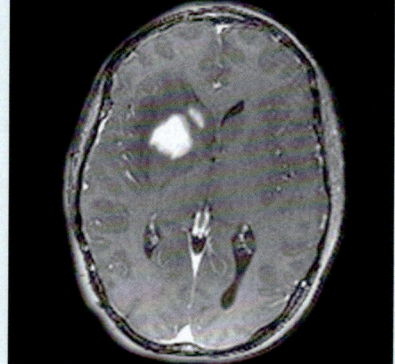
Lymphoma

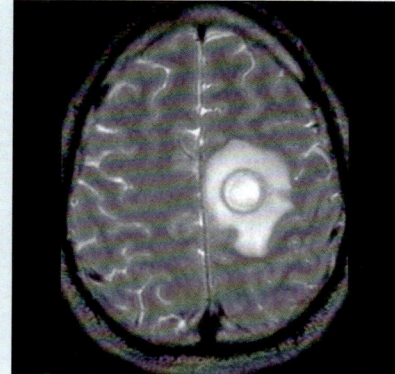
Pyogenic Abscess

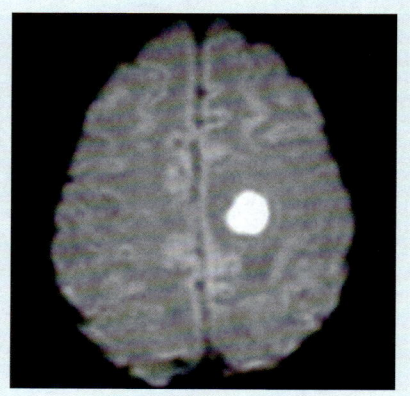
Pyogenic Abscess

OPPORTUNISTIC INFECTION, AIDS

Key Facts

Terminology
- CNS infections in patients with impaired cell-mediated immunity

Imaging Findings
- Toxo: Multiple ring-enhancing lesions of varying size with surrounding edema in deep and superficial brain
- HIV: Rapidly progressive atrophy, diffuse symmetric periventricular white-matter (WM) change
- PML: Large multifocal subcortical WM lesions without mass effect, enhancement
- Crypto: Multiple small fluid-intensity foci in basal ganglia (BG)
- Toxo: Rim-enhancement; smooth, nodular or target (central nodule & peripheral rim)
- Aspergillosis & TB granuloma: Solid or rim-enhancing
- Best imaging tool: MR better than CT
- Protocol advice: T1 C+, FLAIR, T2WI, GRE & DWI

Top Differential Diagnoses
- Diffuse/Patchy WM Abnormalities in AIDS: HIV Encephalitis, PML, CMV
- Focal/Multifocal Brain Lesions in AIDS: Toxo, Lymphoma, Tuberculoma Fungal & Abscess

Clinical Issues
- Highly active antiretroviral therapy improves prognosis

Diagnostic Checklist
- Use contrast in any CT/MR imaging of AIDS patients
- Diffusion more restricted within lymphoma lesions than toxo lesions

---

- Size: Variable

CT Findings
- NECT
  - HIV: Atrophy ± subtle periventricular hypodensity
  - PML: Multifocal, scalloped WM hypodensities without mass effect, edema
    - Rapid increase in size, number of lesions
  - Toxo: Usually multiple hypo-/isodense lesions with edema, mass effect
    - Follow-up CT: Complete resolution or residual lucency or calcification
  - TB meningitis: Extraventricular obstructive hydrocephalus (> 50%)
    - Vasculitis → deep gray infarct
  - Cryptococcal pseudocysts: Multifocal, small, fluid-density cysts around anterior commissure, BG
  - TB & fungal: Focal, solid, mildly hyperdense or hypodense cystic mass with variable edema
    - Aspergillosis: Multifocal, small, hemorrhagic masses
- CECT
  - Toxo: Rim or "target" enhancement
  - CMV: Smooth ventricular lining enhancement
  - TB meningitis: Basal meningeal and/or superficial sulcal enhancement
  - TB & fungal masses: Poorly marginated solid or rim-enhancement
  - PML & Crypto: Usually nonenhancing

MR Findings
- T1WI
  - HIV: Isointense
  - PML: Hypointense with cortical sparing
  - Toxo & Tuberculoma: Focal hypointense mass
    - Healed toxo lesions often hyperintense
  - Cryptococcal pseudocysts: CSF intensity
  - Aspergillus: Hypo- to hyperintense (hemorrhage)
  - TB meningitis: Mild hyperintensity ("dirty CSF")
- T2WI
  - HIV: Bilateral confluent hyperintense periventricular lesions
  - PML: Hyperintense subcortical lesions
  - Toxo & Tuberculoma: Focal hyperintense lesions ± hypointense rim
  - Aspergillus: Hypointense rim or center (hemorrhage)
    - Hypointensity more marked on GRE
  - CMV: Subependymal hyperintensity
  - TB meningitis: CSF isointense on T2WI, hyperintense on FLAIR
- DWI
  - HIV: Isointense
  - PML: May have lead edge DWI hyperintensity
  - Toxo, Tuberculoma, Aspergillus: Variable signal (rim hyperintensity may be seen)
  - TB meningitis: CSF hyperintense
- T1 C+
  - Toxo: Rim-enhancement; smooth, nodular or target (central nodule & peripheral rim)
  - HIV: No enhancement
  - PML: Typically does not enhance, occasional cases of mild peripheral enhancement
  - Aspergillosis & TB granuloma: Solid or rim-enhancing
    - Enhancement may be minimal in Aspergillosis
  - TB meninigitis: Avid enhancement of basal meninges or superficial sulci
  - Crypto: Typically does not enhance

Nuclear Medicine Findings
- SPECT thallium differentiates between toxo & lymphoma

Imaging Recommendations
- Best imaging tool: MR better than CT
- Protocol advice: T1 C+, FLAIR, T2WI, GRE & DWI

DIFFERENTIAL DIAGNOSIS

Diffuse/Patchy WM Abnormalities in AIDS: HIV Encephalitis, PML, CMV
- HIV encephalitis: Atrophy and confluent symmetric, periventricular/diffuse WM disease
- PML: Patchy multifocal lesions
- Ischemic WM change

OPPORTUNISTIC INFECTION, AIDS

- Healed toxoplasmosis lesions

Focal/Multifocal Brain Lesions in AIDS: Toxo, Lymphoma, Tuberculoma Fungal & Abscess
- Primary CNS lymphoma: Second most common cause of focal mass in AIDS
  - Intraparenchymal mass(es) ± leptomeningeal/intraventricular extension
  - Solitary/multifocal mass, predilection for deep GM, corpus callosum
    - Mildly hypointense on T1WI, isointense on T2WI
    - Occasionally hyperintense on T1WI due to hemorrhage or necrosis
    - Solid or ring-enhancing
  - Positive 201Tl-SPECT (most solitary mass lesions in HIV+ are lymphoma, especially if subependymal)
- Granulomas
  - Tuberculoma, Aspergillosis
- Pyogenic abscess
  - T2 hypointense rim, smooth enhancement, marked central restricted diffusion (hyperintense on DWI, hypointense on ADC)
- Tumefactive demyelination: Multiple sclerosis, acute disseminated encephalomyelitis ADEM)
  - WM mass lesions, irregular rim-enhancement

Meningeal Involvement in AIDS
- Acute aseptic HIV meningitis
- Fungal & TB meningitis
- Lymphoma: Multifocal involvement of cranial nerves

PATHOLOGY

General Features
- Etiology
  - HIV virus
  - PML: JC virus (polyoma) with tropism for oligodendrocytes (reactivation)
  - CMV: Cytomegalic inclusion virus
  - Toxo: Reactivated obligate intracellular protozoan toxo gondii
  - Fungal infection: Cryptococcus, Aspergillosis
  - TB: Mycobacterium tuberculosis
- Epidemiology
  - 40 million AIDS patients worldwide
  - CNS toxo in 3-40% of AIDS patients
    - Decreased incidence with improved anti-HIV treatment
  - Crypto in 5-10%
  - PML in 2-5%

Gross Pathologic & Surgical Features
- HIV: Late demyelination
- PML: Multifocal gray/brownish discoloration of WM (myelin loss)
- Toxo: Three morphological lesion types
  - Necrotizing, organizing, chronic abscess
- Aspergillosis: Ill-defined hemorrhagic mass
- Cryptococcus: Gelatinous material in basal cisterns and VR spaces at base of brain
- TB meningitis: Viscous CSF

Microscopic Features
- Toxo: Initial focus of encephalitis ⇒ parenchymal abscesses with necrosis, surrounding inflammation
  - Tachyzoites at lesion periphery
- HIV: Microglial nodule and myelin pallor; late demyelination
- PML: Enlarged astrocytes with lobulated hyperchromatic nuclei
  - Intranuclear JC inclusions within oligodendrocytes
- Crypto: Dilated VRSs filled with fungi, no invasion of surrounding brain
  - Waxy cell membrane produces gelatinous appearance

CLINICAL ISSUES

Presentation
- Most common signs/symptoms
  - HIV: Dementia, seizures
  - PML: Headache, visual disturbance, dementia, hemiparesis, cognitive impairment, seizure
  - Mass lesions (Toxo, Aspergillosis, Tuberculoma): Headache, seizures, focal deficits
  - Meningeal disease (Crypto, TB): Headache, obtundation, signs of increased intracranial pressure

Demographics
- Age: Young adults most common; OI uncommon in pediatric & neonatal populations

Natural History & Prognosis
- Highly active antiretroviral therapy improves prognosis
- Toxo: 70-95% response to specific therapy (evidence of improvement within 2 weeks)
- PML may respond to anti-viral treatment (improved immune system)

DIAGNOSTIC CHECKLIST

Image Interpretation Pearls
- Use contrast in any CT/MR imaging of AIDS patients
- MR > CT; obtain contrast-enhanced scans
- Diffusion more restricted within lymphoma lesions than toxo lesions

SELECTED REFERENCES
1. Collazos J: Opportunistic infections of the CNS in patients with AIDS: diagnosis and management. CNS Drugs. 17(12):869-87, 2003
2. Haimes AB et al: MR Imaging of Brain Abscesses. AJNR. 10:279-91, 1989
3. Post MJD et al: CT, MR and Pathology of HIV Encephalitis and Meningitis. AJNR. 9:469-476, 1988
4. Jinkins JR et al: Cranial Manifestations of Aspergillosis. Neuroradiology. 29:181-5, 1987
5. Gaston A et al: Cerebral Toxoplasmosis in acquired Immunodeficiency Syndrome. Neuroradiology. 27:83-86, 1985

OPPORTUNISTIC INFECTION, AIDS

IMAGE GALLERY

Typical

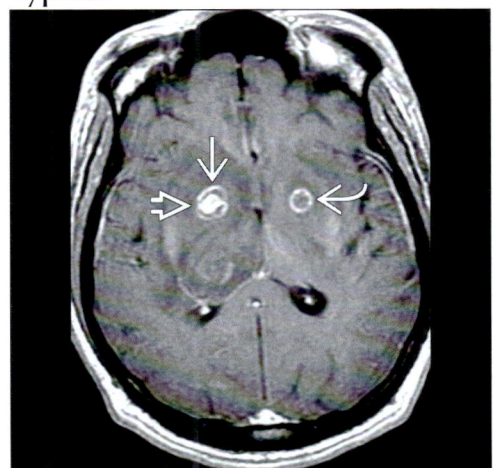 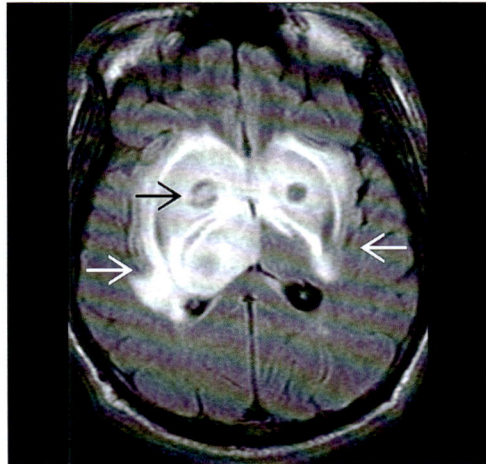

(Left) Axial T1 C+ MR in toxoplasmosis shows multiple deep gray lesions. Note smooth rim-enhancement ⇒ in left lesion, central (target) ⇒ & rim-enhancement ⇒ in right ganglionic lesion. (Right) Axial FLAIR MR same case as previous image shows focal lesions with hypointense rims ⇒, extensive peripheral edema ⇒.

Typical

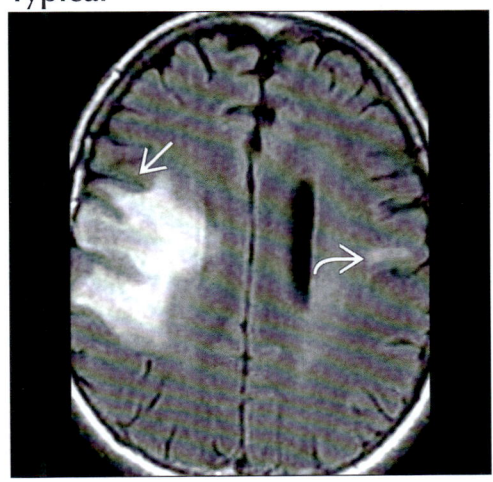 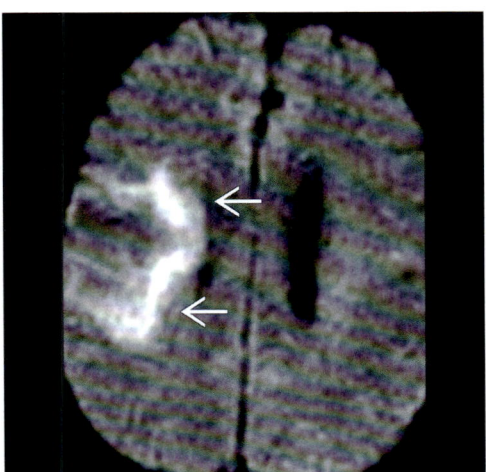

(Left) Axial FLAIR MR in patient with PML shows right subcortical hyperintensity sparing adjacent GM ⇒ without mass effect, and second small left frontal lesion ⇒. (Right) Axial DWI MR same case as previous image shows peripheral hyperintensity ⇒ due to restricted diffusion at "active" margin of lesion.

Typical

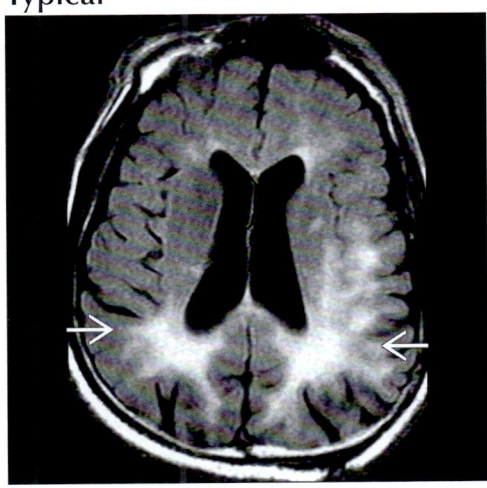 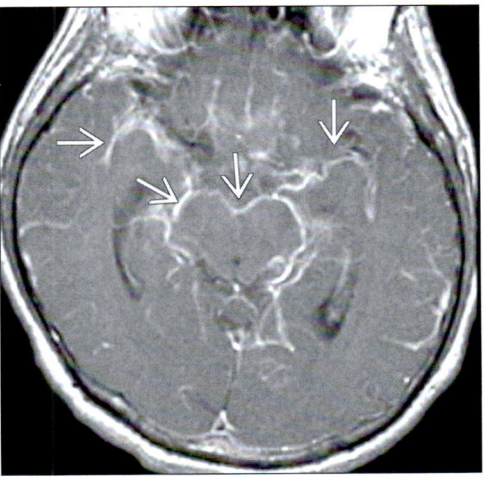

(Left) Axial FLAIR MR shows HIV encephalitis with atrophy and bilateral diffuse periventricular hyperintensity ⇒ without mass effect. (Right) Axial T1 C+ MR in a patient with TB meningitis shows leptomeningeal enhancement of basal cisterns ⇒.

DRUG ABUSE

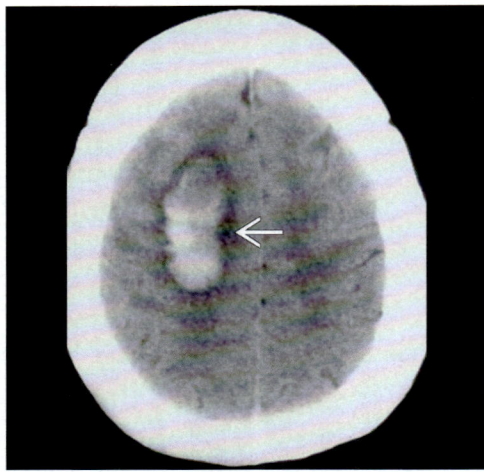

Axial NECT shows left frontal subcortical hematoma ➡ in patient shortly after using cocaine.

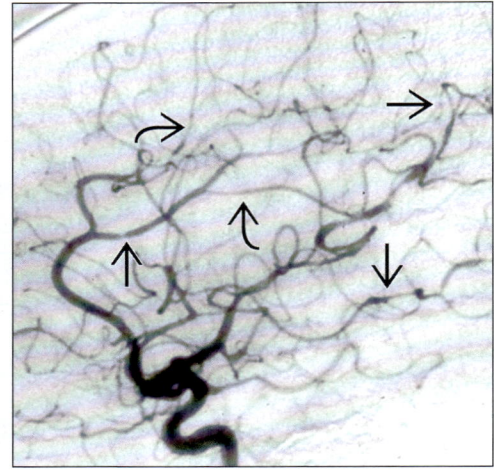

Lateral catheter angiography in same case as previous shows multiple regions of focal ➡ and diffuse ➡ arterial narrowing due to vasculitis.

TERMINOLOGY

Definitions
- Many drugs (prescription, illicit or "street") have adverse CNS effects
  - Major pathology generally vascular or metabolic
  - Polydrug abuse (including ETOH) common
- Cerebrovascular disease caused by illicit drug use
  - Cocaine: Intranasal, intravenous (IV), intramuscular, smoked, transplacental transfer
    - Cocaine hydrochloride (HCl) not smokable
    - Alkaloid form ("freebase", "crack") smokable
  - Amphetamines: Oral, intranasal, parenteral use
    - 3-, 4-Methylenedioxymethamphetamine (MDMA, "ecstasy")
  - Heroin: IV use, inhaled ("chasing the dragon")
  - ETOH abuse: Interference with normal clotting increases risk of spontaneous hemorrhage and extent of hemorrhage due to primary pathology
    - Traumatic brain injury
    - Hypertensive cerebral vascular disease
- May interfere with critical metabolic pathways
  - Nitrous oxide (NO_2) abuse → inactivates vitamin B12 → subacute combined degeneration
- May lead to nutritional deficiencies
  - Chronic ETOH abuse → thiamine deficiency → Wernicke encephalopathy
- Organ damage from chronic drug abuse
  - ETOH → liver failure → manganese deposition in basal ganglia (BG)

IMAGING FINDINGS

General Features
- Best diagnostic clue: Young/middle-aged adult with ischemic or hemorrhagic stroke in close temporal proximity to drug administration
- Location
  - Hemorrhage: Intracranial (ICH), subarachnoid (SAH), intraventricular (IVH)
  - Nonhemorrhagic ischemic stroke: MCA territory most common
  - Cocaine: Infarctions in cerebrum, thalamus, brainstem, cerebellum, retina
  - Heroin, MDMA: Globus pallidus (GP) ischemia
  - Amphetamines: Hemorrhage, vasculitis, pseudoaneurysm, infarcts

DDx: Drug Abuse Mimics

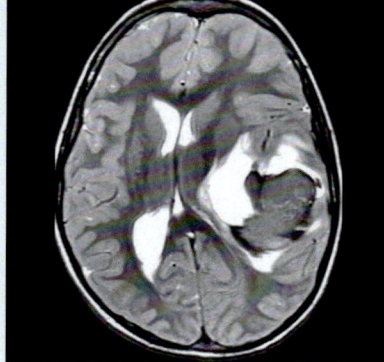

ICH due to AVM

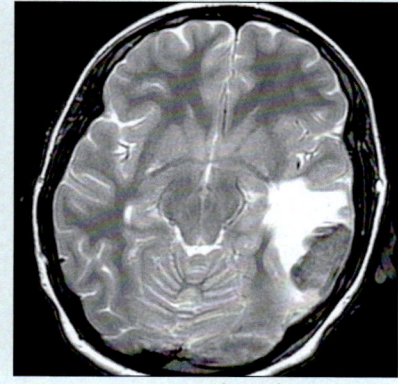

Transverse Sinus Thrombosis ICH

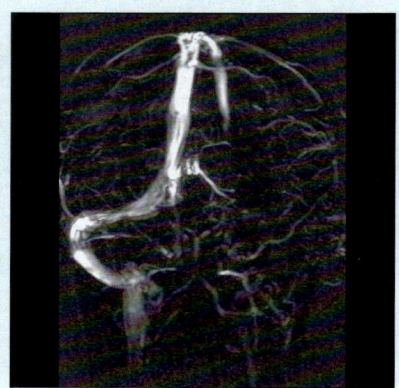

Transverse Sinus Thrombosis ICH

DRUG ABUSE

Key Facts

Terminology
- Cerebrovascular disease caused by illicit drug use

Imaging Findings
- Heroin inhalation: Symmetric hypodensity in cerebellar white matter (WM), posterior cerebral hemisphere WM, posterior limb of internal capsule
- Cocaine: May have severe T2 hyperintense lesions
- Cerebral, insular subcortex WM lesions
- DWI: DWI may show restricted diffusion in acute ischemic and metabolic lesions

Top Differential Diagnoses
- Hypertension (HTN): BG hemorrhages
- Vascular malformations
- Intratumoral hemorrhage
- Dural sinus thrombosis with hemorrhagic infarct

Pathology
- Cocaine HCl: Hemorrhagic (80%) > ischemic stroke
- Alkaloidal cocaine: Hemorrhagic = ischemic stroke
- Amphetamines: Hemorrhagic > ischemic stroke
- Heroin: Cerebral infarctions (MCA area, not watershed distribution), toxic leukoencephalopathy
- Up to 30% of strokes in young patients (15-44 years) are drug-related
- Drug-related ICH frequently related to underlying vascular malformation (cerebral aneurysm, AVM)

Diagnostic Checklist
- Drug abuse in young/middle-aged patient with stroke
- Drug-related hemorrhages may indicate underlying vascular abnormality

---

- o Wernicke: Bilateral posterior thalamus, mammillary bodies, posterior mesencephalon
- o Liver failure: BG
- o NO2: Posterior spinal cord

CT Findings
- NECT
  - o Cocaine: ICH, SAH, IVH
  - o Heroin inhalation: Symmetric hypodensity in cerebellar white matter (WM), posterior cerebral hemisphere WM, posterior limb of internal capsule
    - ▪ GP ischemic change (hypodensity)
- CTA: May show segmental narrowing in vasculitis

MR Findings
- T1WI
  - o Heroin vapor inhalation: Leukoencephalopathy
  - o Hepatic encephalopathy: Hyperintense BG
- T2WI
  - o Cocaine: May have severe T2 hyperintense lesions
    - ▪ Cerebral, insular subcortex WM lesions
    - ▪ Transient arterial occlusion in MCA territory: Small infarctions
  - o Heroin vapor inhalation
    - ▪ Hyperintense cerebral, cerebellar tracts
    - ▪ WM cerebellum, posterior cerebral, posterior limb of internal capsule
    - ▪ Sparing of subcortical WM & dentate nuclei
  - o Wernicke encephalopathy
    - ▪ Hyperintensity in medial thalami tectum, periaqueductal gray matter (GM) mammillary bodies, rarely cortex
  - o Subacute combined degeneration
    - ▪ Hyperintensity in posterior spinal cord (cervical & thoracic)
- T2* GRE: Hemorrhagic lesions have decreased signal
- DWI: DWI may show restricted diffusion in acute ischemic and metabolic lesions
- MRA
  - o Arterial spasm and/or vasculitis
    - ▪ Vasculitis difficult to diagnose on MRA unless high quality; 3T MRA > 1.5T MRA

Imaging Recommendations
- Best imaging tool: CT, MR
- Protocol advice
  - o NECT for suspected hemorrhage
  - o If CT reveals hemorrhage, CTA/MRA/DSA
  - o MR: Include T1 C+, GRE

DIFFERENTIAL DIAGNOSIS

Spontaneous ICH in Young Adults
- Hypertension (HTN): BG hemorrhages
- Vascular malformations
  - o Cavernous hemangiomas
  - o Arteriovenous malformations (AVMs)
- Intratumoral hemorrhage
  - o Seen in ~ 1% of brain tumors, usually malignant
    - ▪ Incomplete hemosiderin rings, enhancing nodule
    - ▪ Persistent mass effect disproportionate to amount of hemorrhage
- Dural sinus thrombosis with hemorrhagic infarct
  - o Underlying coagulable state often present (e.g., activated protein C deficiency)
  - o Infarcts typically hemorrhagic, subcortical
- Severe posterior reversible encephalopathy syndrome (PRES) with secondary hemorrhage
- Mycotic aneurysm with parenchymal hemorrhage

PATHOLOGY

General Features
- General path comments
  - o Cocaine HCl: Hemorrhagic (80%) > ischemic stroke
  - o Alkaloidal cocaine: Hemorrhagic = ischemic stroke
  - o Amphetamines: Hemorrhagic > ischemic stroke
  - o Heroin: Cerebral infarctions (MCA area, not watershed distribution), toxic leukoencephalopathy
- Etiology
  - o Cocaine, amphetamines

DRUG ABUSE

- Systemic vasoconstriction ⇒ acute arterial HTN ⇒ hemorrhagic stroke (rupture of preexisting aneurysms, bleeding from AVM)
- Cerebral vasoconstriction, vasculitis ⇒ infarction
  o Parenteral drugs
    - Infective endocarditis (IE) ⇒ emboli ⇒ cerebral infarction, hemorrhage, abscess, mycotic aneurysm
    - Bacteremia in absence of IE: Brain abscess
    - Hepatitis: Bleeding diathesis
  o Cocaine
    - ↑ Platelet aggregation with thrombosis
    - Heart disease: Source of emboli
  o MDMA abuse: Loss of serotoninergic neurons
  o Heroin: Toxic leukoencephalopathy, hypoxic brain injury, ischemic stroke, brain abscess
    - Generalized hypoxia and hypotension
    - Possible immunologic-mediated vasculitis
    - Nephropathy ⇒ severe HTN
  o Wernicke encephalopathy: ↓ Thiamine affects membrane function → failure to maintain osmotic gradients
  o Subacute combined degeneration
    - NO_2 inactivates B12 so serum B12 levels normal; may obscure diagnosis
  o Concomitant alcohol use may potentiate illicit drug effects (↓ hepatic metabolism)
- Epidemiology
  o 4% of all strokes occur in patients < 45 years
  o Up to 30% of strokes in young patients (15-44 years) are drug-related
  o Estimated relative risk for stroke among drug abusers (after controlling for other stroke risk factors): 6.5
  o Subacute combined degeneration
    - Individuals with access to medical NO_2
    - Abuse of NO_2 canisters (poppers)
- Associated abnormalities
  o Drug-related ICH frequently related to underlying vascular malformation (cerebral aneurysm, AVM)
  o Drug-induced IE, vasculitis

Gross Pathologic & Surgical Features
- Amphetamine, cocaine: Arterial spasm/vasculitis
- Cocaine in pregnancy: Fetal infarctions in BG, ↑ rate of neural tube closure defects
- Amphetamine, cocaine, MDMA: ICH, SAH
- MDMA: Vasoconstriction in recent users, vasodilatation in ex-users
  o Bilateral GP necrosis (2° prolonged vasospasm)

Microscopic Features
- Amphetamines: Inflammatory vasculitis + vessel wall necrosis ("speed arteritis") similar to PAN
- Cocaine: Vasculitis affecting CNS
- Heroin: Vasculitis (rare), probably related to drug contaminants
  o Inhaled heroin vapors: Symmetric spongiform degeneration in cerebral/cerebellar WM, corticospinal and solitary tracts

CLINICAL ISSUES

Presentation
- Most common signs/symptoms
  o Cocaine, MDMA, amphetamines: Stroke, headache, seizures
  o Heroin: BG damage (Parkinsonism, hemiballism)
    - Toxic leukoencephalopathy: Cerebellar, pyramidal & pseudobulbar signs, spasms, death
  o Wernicke: Obtundation & ataxia
  o Subacute combined degeneration: Loss of proprioception
- Clinical Profile
  o Cerebral infarcts, TIAs, ICH, SAH
    - Temporal proximity of stroke to drug use

Demographics
- Age: 85-90% of drug-related strokes occur in 4th-5th decade

Natural History & Prognosis
- Time interval between drug use & stroke onset: Up to one week
  o Stroke risk highest within first 6 hours after drug use
- IE-related strokes may be delayed
  o 20% mortality for IE-associated strokes
  o 67% mortality for hemorrhagic strokes
- Cocaine worsens presentation & outcome of aneurysmal SAH patients

Treatment
- Management of drug-related stroke largely supportive
- Antibiotics for embolic stroke due to IV-drug-induced IE ↓ risk of recurrent infarction
- Aggressive addiction rehabilitation
- Experimentally, magnesium reverses cocaine-induced vasospasm
- Wernicke: Supplementary thiamine
- Subacute combined degeneration: B12 injection

DIAGNOSTIC CHECKLIST

Consider
- Drug abuse in young/middle-aged patient with stroke

Image Interpretation Pearls
- Drug-related hemorrhages may indicate underlying vascular abnormality
- Vasculitis can be very difficult to distinguish from drug-related vasospasm

SELECTED REFERENCES
1. Keogh CF et al: Neuroimaging features of heroin inhalation toxicity: "chasing the dragon". AJR Am J Roentgenol. 180(3):847-50, 2003
2. Bartzokis G et al: The incidence of T2-weighted MR imaging signal abnormalities in the brain of cocaine-dependent patients is age-related and region-specific. AJNR Am J Neuroradiol. 20(9):1628-35, 1999
3. Kokkinos J et al: Stroke. Neurol Clin. 11(3):577-90, 1993
4. Wojak JC et al: Intracranial hemorrhage and cocaine use. Stroke. 18(4):712-5, 1987

DRUG ABUSE

IMAGE GALLERY

Typical

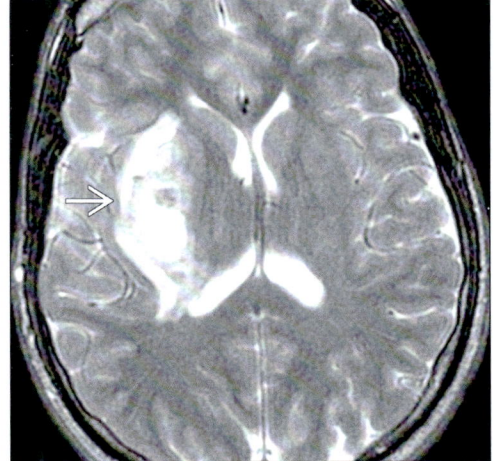 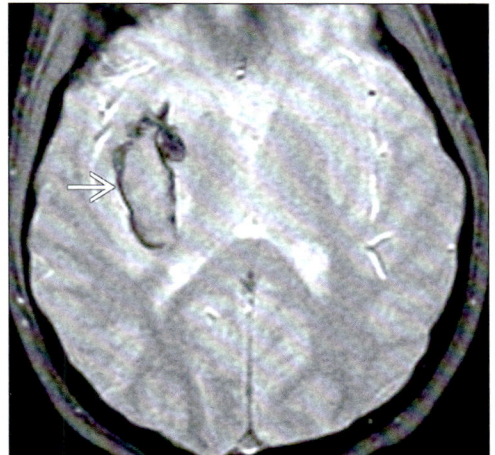

(Left) Axial T2WI MR shows hyperacute (3 hours) basal ganglia hemorrhage ➜ in 26 y/o with history of ecstasy abuse. *(Right)* Axial T2* GRE MR in same case as previous shows typical features of hyperacute hematoma with markedly hypointense rim ➜.

Variant

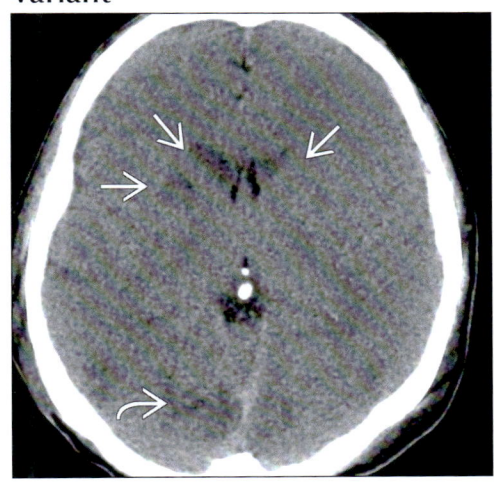 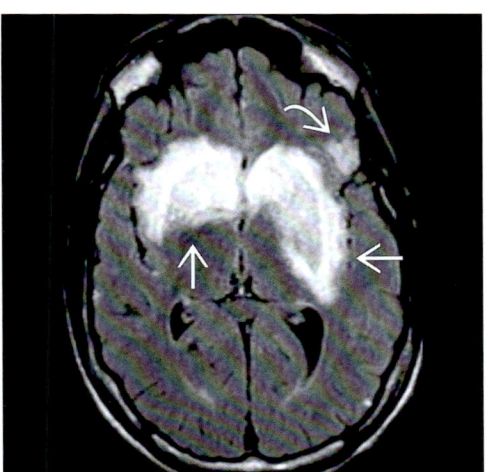

(Left) Axial NECT in comatose patient after cocaine abuse shows focal hypodensity in basal ganglia ➜ & occipital lobe ➜. Note diffuse loss of GM-WM differentiation due to severe anoxia. *(Right)* Axial FLAIR MR in a patient with history of amphetamine abuse shows bilateral basal ganglia ➜ & frontal lobe ➜ edema due to vasculitis.

Typical

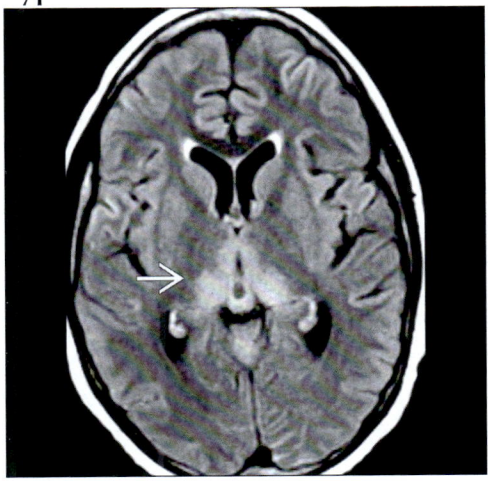 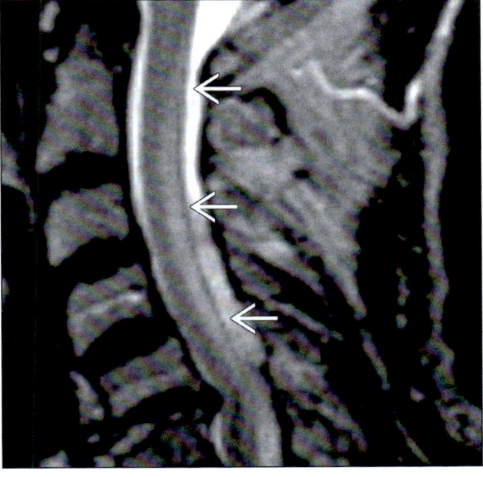

(Left) Axial FLAIR MR in obtunded ETOH abuser shows bilateral medial thalamic edema ➜, indicative of Wernicke encephalopathy. *(Right)* Sagittal T2WI MR in a patient with history of NO₂ abuse shows hyperintensity ➜ in posterior portion of spinal cord, indicative subacute combined degeneration.

HYDROCEPHALUS

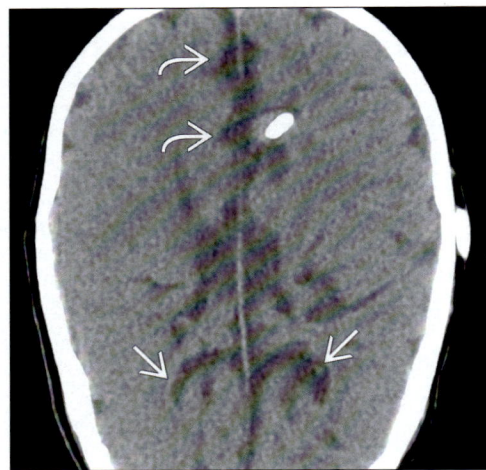
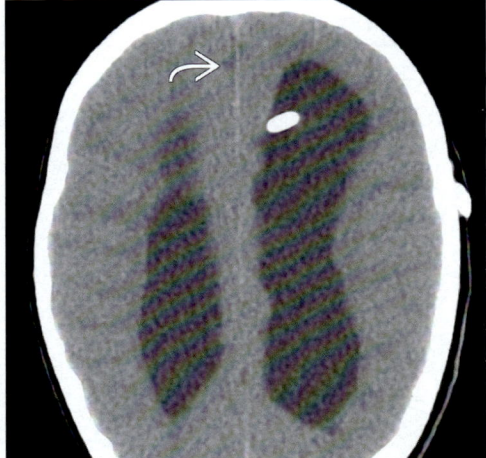

Axial NECT in a child with shunted hydrocephalus caused by the Chiari 2 malformation, shows collapse of the lateral ventricles ➡. Note prominent interhemispheric sulci ➡.

Axial NECT in the same child, shows malfunction of the shunt, with enlarged ventricles and effaced sulci ➡. It is important to assess extra-axial spaces when considering shunt malfunction.

TERMINOLOGY

Abbreviations and Synonyms
- Obstructive hydrocephalus, intraventricular obstructive hydrocephalus (IVOH)
- Communicating hydrocephalus, external hydrocephalus, extraventricular obstructive hydrocephalus (EVOH)

Definitions
- Excess volume of intracranial cerebrospinal fluid (CSF)
  - Due to obstruction of CSF flow within ventricular system ⇒ IVOH
  - Due to decreased resorption into dural sinuses ⇒ EVOH
  - Due to overproduction
- Ventriculomegaly does not equal hydrocephalus!

IMAGING FINDINGS

General Features
- Best diagnostic clue
  - IVOH ⇒ enlarged ventricles with decreased extra-axial spaces
  - EVOH ⇒ enlarged ventricles with enlarged extra-axial spaces
  - In children with open sutures, hydrocephalus always causes macrocrania
  - In children with closed sutures, hydrocephalus always causes increased intracranial pressure (ICP)
- Location
  - IVOH ⇒ obstructing lesions at key points in ventricular system
    - Foramen of Monro: Subependymal giant cell astrocytoma, colloid cyst
    - Posterior 3rd ventricle: Pineal germinoma
    - Cerebral aqueduct: Tectal glioma, aqueductal stenosis
    - Fourth ventricle: Medulloblastoma, cerebellar pilocytic astrocytoma
    - "Trapped" temporal horn by mass effect on trigone
  - EVOH ⇒ obstruction at level of arachnoid granulations
    - Prior intracranial hemorrhage (ICH) or meningitis
    - Elevated pressure in venous sinuses
- Size: Ventriculomegaly does not equal hydrocephalus!

DDx: Tumors that Obstruct the Ventricular System

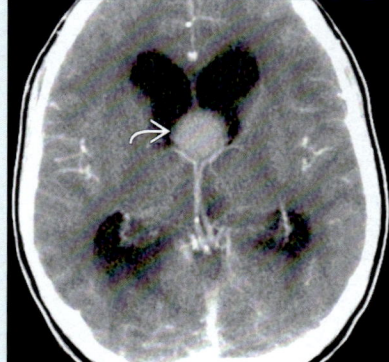
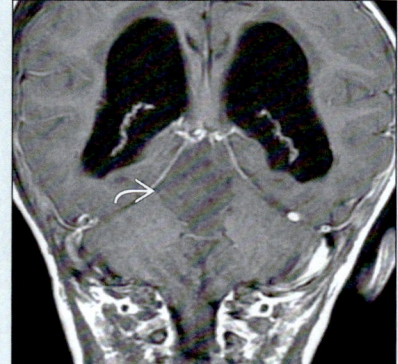
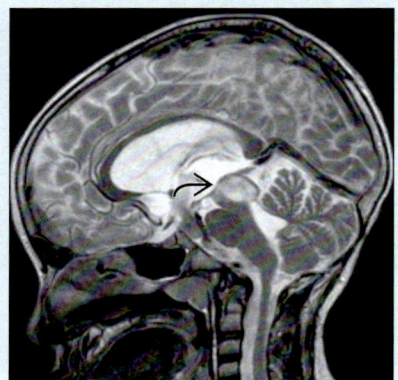

Colloid Cyst

Medulloblastoma

Tectal Glioma

HYDROCEPHALUS

Key Facts

Terminology
- Excess volume of intracranial cerebrospinal fluid (CSF)
- Ventriculomegaly does not equal hydrocephalus!

Imaging Findings
- In children with open sutures, hydrocephalus always causes macrocrania
- In children with closed sutures, hydrocephalus always causes increased intracranial pressure (ICP)
- IVOH ⇒ obstructing lesions at key points in ventricular system
- EVOH ⇒ obstruction at level of arachnoid granulations
- NECT is most repeatable, efficient, and consistent means of evaluating ventricle size

Top Differential Diagnoses
- Obstructing Tumor
- Shunt Malfunction
- Benign Macrocrania

Pathology
- Epidemiology: Most common neurosurgical procedure in children = CSF shunting for hydrocephalus

Clinical Issues
- Decompensation due to failure of ventricular drainage system ⇒ shunt malfunction
- Acute presentation of new obstructive hydrocephalus caused by a focal mass lesion ⇒ tumor

---

- Morphology
  - As ventricles enlarge, they lose angular margins
    - Frontal horns and third ventricle become rounder
  - LaPlace law applies ⇒ as pressure increases, regions with larger radius are under more tension and preferentially dilate
    - Trigones enlarge first when lateral ventricles obstructed

Radiographic Findings
- Shunt series is mainstay of evaluating integrity of ventricular drainage systems
  - Anteroposterior (AP) and lateral skull, AP chest, and AP abdomen radiographs

CT Findings
- NECT
  - Enlarged and rounded ventricles
  - Periventricular halo of low-attenuation ⇒ transependymal edema
  - Basal cisterns and sulci compressed in IVOH
  - Basal cisterns and sulci enlarged in EVOH
- CECT: May help show subarachnoid vessels in enlarged extra-axial spaces in EVOH

MR Findings
- T1WI
  - Enlarged and rounded ventricles
  - Corpus callosum thinned, stretched upward
  - Optic recess of 3rd ventricle herniated into expanded sella
  - Bright signal in frontal horns or posterior third ventricle may reflect pulsatile CSF flow
- T2WI
  - Morphologic findings like T1WI
  - Transependymal edema
    - Hyperintense "stain" spreading from acute ventricular margins
    - Accentuated at corners, minimized at lateral walls
    - May reduce or resolve in chronic obstruction (compensated)
- FLAIR: Best modality for showing transependymal edema

- MRV
  - Dural sinus thrombosis can cause EVOH
    - More likely to cause pseudotumor cerebri
- MR Cine
  - Ideal for demonstrating patency of 3rd ventriculostomy defects
    - Third ventriculostomy ⇒ hole created in floor of third ventricle via ventriculoscope
    - Allows passage of CSF from 3rd ventricle into subarachnoid space

Imaging Recommendations
- Best imaging tool
  - NECT is most repeatable, efficient, and consistent means of evaluating ventricle size
  - Fast and motion-reducing MR sequences may replace CT
    - No radiation
    - Less well tolerated by non-sedated children
- Protocol advice: All CT studies must be acquired at consistent levels and angles

DIFFERENTIAL DIAGNOSIS

Obstructing Tumor
- Colloid cyst
- Tectal glioma
- Medulloblastoma
- Ependymoma

Shunt Malfunction
- Kinked or disrupted catheter tubing
  - Intracranial cracks can cause pseudocysts in brain
- Faulty or misapplied valve
  - Pressure too high, facing wrong direction
- Pseudocyst around distal tubing
  - < 5% incidence
  - Questionable association with infection
- Erosion of distal tube into viscus
  - May precipitate meningitis
- Occluded proximal catheter
  - More common in former premature infants

HYDROCEPHALUS

Choroid Plexus Papilloma (CPP)
- Usually located in the trigones of the lateral ventricles
- Can over-produce CSF or obstruct ventricle

Benign Macrocrania
- Self-limited form of EVOH common in children 6-24 months of age
- Large-headed child with large-headed parents
- Head circumference measurements abnormal, but parallel normal growth curve
- No associated symptoms

Ventriculomegaly from Parenchymal Volume Loss
- Diffuse enlargement of sulci, cisterns
- Normal to small head circumference
- Thickened cranium with closed sutures (chronic)

Hemimegalencephaly
- Causes increase in volume of parenchyma and ventricle on same side
- Gray matter is dysplastic and thickened

PATHOLOGY

General Features
- General path comments: Large ventricles without loss/dysgenesis of brain tissue
- Etiology
  - CSF is produced by choroid and seeps into ventricles from interstitium
  - Migrates from ventricles into subarachnoid spaces
  - Transported into dural sinuses via arachnoid granulations
    - Energy-dependent active transport
  - Obstruction or failure at any point causes hydrocephalus
  - Inflammatory processes can render arachnoid granulations impaired
    - ICH, meningitis
- Epidemiology: Most common neurosurgical procedure in children = CSF shunting for hydrocephalus
- Associated abnormalities
  - Common sequela of congenital brain malformations
    - Chiari 2, agenesis of corpus callosum

Gross Pathologic & Surgical Features
- Ependyma and adjacent white matter secondarily injured

Microscopic Features
- Ependymal lining damaged or lost

CLINICAL ISSUES

Presentation
- Most common signs/symptoms: Macrocrania, headache, papilledema
- Other signs/symptoms: Nausea, irritability, seizures

Demographics
- Age
  - Tectal gliomas typically present in school-age or older children
    - CSF diversion may be only treatment necessary
- Gender: Some congenital causes or tumors are gender biased (x-linked aqueductal stenosis, germinoma)

Natural History & Prognosis
- Emergency presentation of hydrocephalus in children falls into two scenarios
  - Decompensation due to failure of ventricular drainage system ⇒ shunt malfunction
  - Acute presentation of new obstructive hydrocephalus caused by a focal mass lesion ⇒ tumor
- Typically fatal if untreated and sutures closed
  - Untreated hydrocephalus may become compensated
- Complications of ventricular shunting are a frequent cause of emergency imaging

Treatment
- CSF diversion (shunt), third ventriculostomy, septation fenestration

DIAGNOSTIC CHECKLIST

Consider
- Consider MR for routine assessment to reduce life-long radiation dose to patients with shunts
- Tectal glioma can be very subtle on CT
  - Use MR to evaluate unexplained lateral and third ventriculomegaly

Image Interpretation Pearls
- Always correlate ventriculomegaly with head circumference measurements
- Size of ventricles generally correlates poorly with intracranial pressure
- Pulsatile CSF may create confusing signal intensity, even mimic intraventricular mass
- Ventricular asymmetry is normal

SELECTED REFERENCES

1. Duhaime AC: Evaluation and management of shunt infections in children with hydrocephalus. Clin Pediatr (Phila). 45(8):705-13, 2006
2. Sacar S et al: A retrospective study of central nervous system shunt infections diagnosed in a university hospital during a 4-year period. BMC Infect Dis. 6:43, 2006
3. Winston KR et al: CSF shunt failure with stable normal ventricular size. Pediatr Neurosurg. 42(3):151-5, 2006
4. Mangano FT et al: Early programmable valve malfunctions in pediatric hydrocephalus. J Neurosurg. 103(6 Suppl):501-7, 2005
5. Mobley LW 3rd et al: Abdominal pseudocyst: predisposing factors and treatment algorithm. Pediatr Neurosurg. 41(2):77-83, 2005
6. Grunert P et al: The role of third ventriculostomy in the management of obstructive hydrocephalus. Minim Invasive Neurosurg. 46(1):16-21, 2003

HYDROCEPHALUS

IMAGE GALLERY

Typical

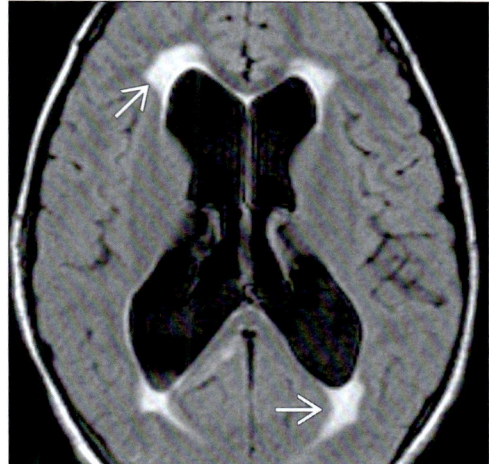 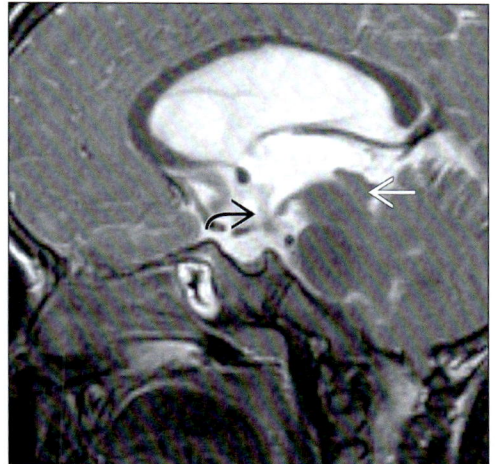

(Left) Axial FLAIR MR shows transependymal edema ➡ capping the occipital and frontal horns, caused by increased ventricular pressure that prevents drainage of fluid from the interstitium. *(Right)* Sagittal T2WI MR shows a jet of CSF flow ➡ through a patent ventriculostomy defect in the floor of the 3rd ventricle in a child with aqueductal stenosis ➡.

Typical

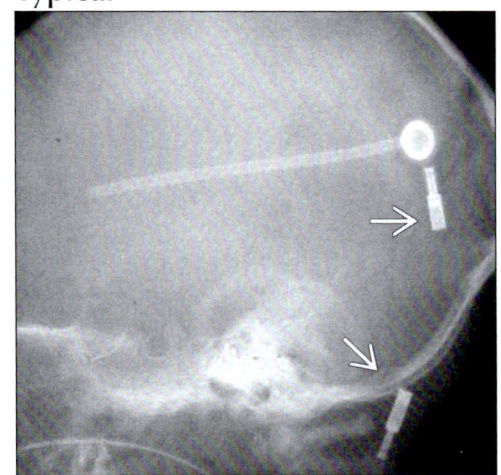 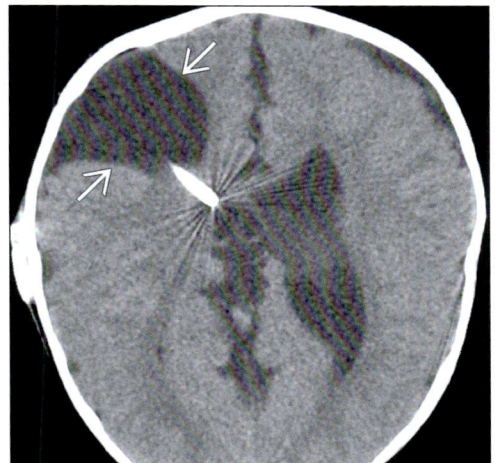

(Left) Lateral radiograph of the skull in a child with a shunt disconnection ➡, shows abnormal widening and angulation between metallic connectors in the scalp. *(Right)* Axial NECT shows an extra-axial cyst ➡ formed around a leaking shunt catheter. The right lateral ventricle is preferentially decompressed because the leak is proximal to the shunt valve.

Other

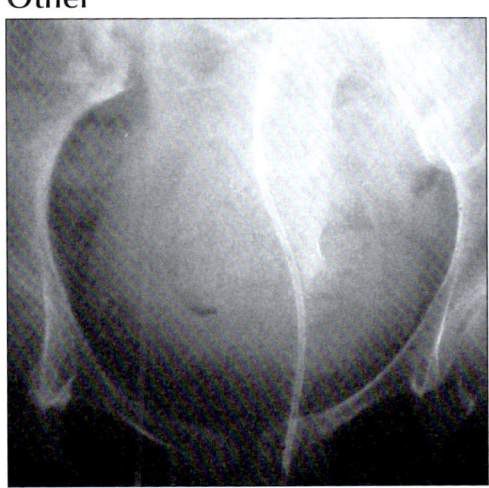 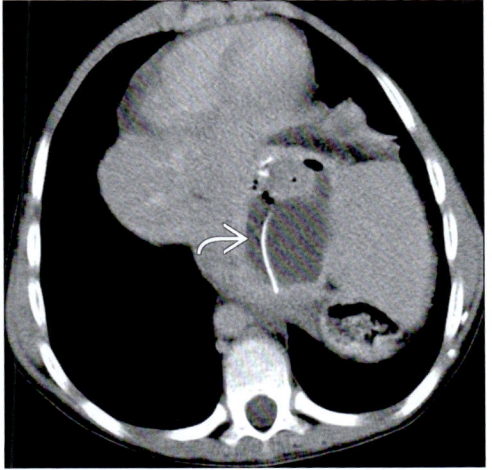

(Left) Anteroposterior radiograph of the pelvis in a child with shunt malfunction shows the end of the distal shunt catheter that has eroded into the rectum and was observed on physical exam. *(Right)* Axial NECT shows a pseudocyst ➡ in the upper abdomen of a child with shunt malfunction. In children these usually result in neurological symptoms; in adults they cause abdominal symptoms.

INBORN ERRORS OF METABOLISM

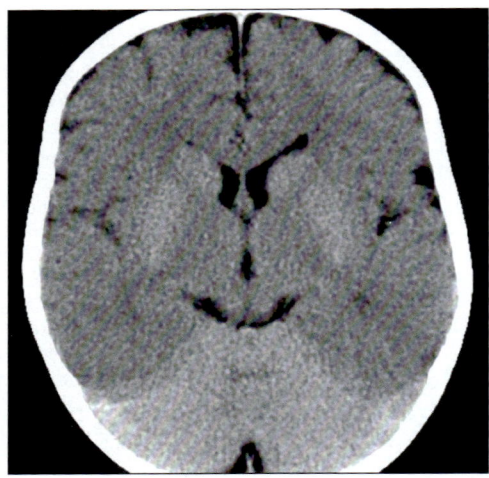

Axial NECT in a 2 year old who presented to the emergency department unresponsive with a glucose of 27 mg/dL shows diffuse decreased attenuation of the supratentorial brain. MCAD deficiency.

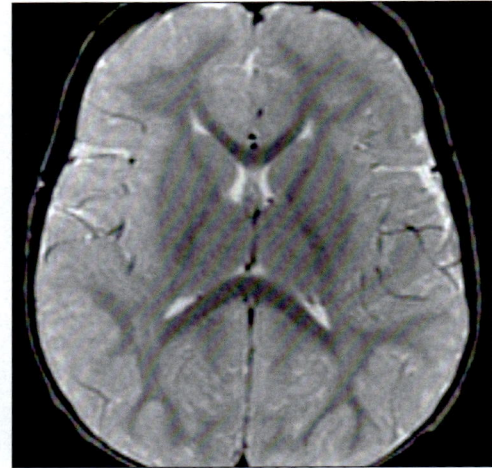

Axial T2WI MR in the same child shows swelling and increased signal of cerebral cortex. Diffuse cortical injury with marked hypoglycemia should prompt investigation for MCAD deficiency.

TERMINOLOGY

Definitions
- Genetically based disorders that acutely present with neurological dysfunction
  - Mitochondrial encephalopathies (MEMs)
    - Leigh syndrome (LS), glutaric aciduria type 1 (GA-1), mitochondrial myopathy, encephalopathy, lactic acidosis, and stroke-like episodes (MELAS), Kearns-Sayre syndrome (KSS)
  - Disorders of fatty acid oxidation
    - Medium chain acyl CoA dehydrogenase (MCAD) deficiency
  - Disorders of amino acid metabolism
    - Maple syrup urine disease (MSUD)
  - Urea cycle disorders
    - Ornithine transcarbamylase (OTC) deficiency, arginase deficiency, N-acetylglutamate synthetase deficiency, several others

IMAGING FINDINGS

General Features
- Best diagnostic clue
  - MEM ⇒ well-defined regions of hypodensity (on CT) and metabolic acidosis
  - MCAD deficiency ⇒ diffuse cortical swelling and marked hypoglycemia
  - Amino acid disorders ⇒ white matter (WM) edema in a neonate, especially dorsal brainstem
  - Urea cycle disorders ⇒ cerebral edema in a neonate with elevated urine ammonia and respiratory alkalosis

CT Findings
- NECT
  - Focal hypodensities
    - Bilateral and symmetric basal ganglia lesions in MEMs
    - Peripheral stroke-like lesions in MELAS
  - Diffusely decreased density of WM
    - Accentuate gray-white differentiation in hemispheres
    - Notable in dorsal brainstem in MSUD

DDx: Multifocal Lesions in Infants

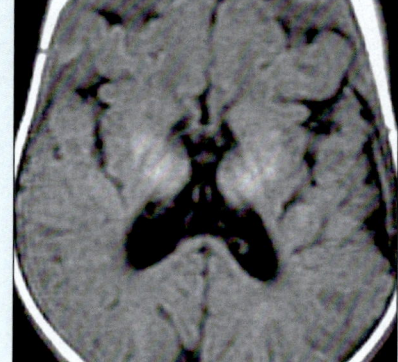

Perinatal Hypoxic-Ischemic Injury

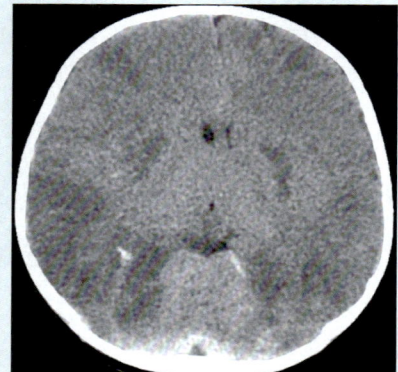

Child Abuse

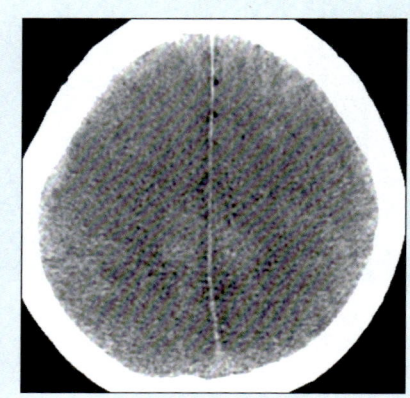

CO Poisoning

INBORN ERRORS OF METABOLISM

Key Facts

Terminology
- Mitochondrial encephalopathies (MEMs)
- Medium chain acyl CoA dehydrogenase (MCAD) deficiency
- Maple syrup urine disease (MSUD)
- Urea cycle disorders

Imaging Findings
- MEM ⇒ well-defined regions of hypodensity (on CT) and metabolic acidosis
- MCAD deficiency ⇒ diffuse cortical swelling and marked hypoglycemia
- Amino acid disorders ⇒ white matter (WM) edema in a neonate, especially dorsal brainstem
- Urea cycle disorders ⇒ cerebral edema in a neonate with elevated urine ammonia and respiratory alkalosis

Top Differential Diagnoses
- Child Abuse
- Encephalitis
- Perinatal Hypoxic-Ischemic Injury (HIE)

Clinical Issues
- MEMs may be unmasked by metabolic stressors (infection, exercise)
- MCAD deficiency classically presents after period of fasting or viral infection
- Urea cycle disorders: Encephalopathy at 24-48 hours

Diagnostic Checklist
- Think of MEMs when encountering an atypical presentation of stroke, severe encephalitis, or seizure
- Infant/child with cerebral edema and hypoglycemia ⇒ MCAD deficiency

---

- Diffuse brain swelling with effacement of sulci
  - Typical of MCAD deficiency and urea cycle disorders
- GA-1 ⇒ volume loss with subdural collections
  - Subdural collections in GA-1 mimic subdural hematomas from child abuse

MR Findings
- T1WI
  - Hypointense lesions
    - Foci of hyperintensity may reflect Ca++, blood products, myelin breakdown
    - Urea cycle disorders can cause ↑ signal in globi pallidi, insular cortex
  - Enlarged sylvian fissures in GA-1, with frontal and temporal lobe atrophy
- T2WI
  - MEMs typically cause hyperintense lesions on T2WI and FLAIR
    - LS typically causes a speckled pattern in deep nuclei
  - MSUD causes characteristic hyperintensity (edema) in cerebellar WM, brainstem, and globi pallidi
  - Urea cycle disorders can cause ↑ signal in globi pallidi, insular cortex, base of frontal sulci
- DWI
  - MEMs may or may not cause foci of restricted diffusion
  - MSUD causes restricted diffusion in WM in hyperacute phase
- MRS
  - Detection of lactate characteristic of MEMs
    - Absence of lactate does not exclude diagnosis, however
  - MSUD causes broad peak at 0.9 ppm
  - Elevated glutamine/glutamate peak in urea cycle disorders

Imaging Recommendations
- Best imaging tool
  - NECT is valuable in acute assessment for focal lesions or diffuse swelling
  - MR is modality of choice in investigation of suspected metabolic disease of any sort
- Protocol advice
  - Abnormalities best shown by T2WI and FLAIR
  - MRS can be helpful, although often nonspecific

DIFFERENTIAL DIAGNOSIS

Child Abuse
- Diffuse cerebral edema seen in > 70% of abused infants with head injuries
  - Multifactorial ⇒ shear, post-traumatic hyperemia, hypoxia-ischemia

Near Drowning
- High lactate implies poorer prognosis

Encephalitis
- Viral encephalidites can cause symmetric basal ganglia T2 prolongation
- Acute disseminated encephalomyelitis (ADEM) is typically less symmetric

Carbon Monoxide (CO) Poisoning
- Symmetric basal ganglia hypodensities

Perinatal Hypoxic-Ischemic Injury (HIE)
- Central pattern of injury affects ventrolateral thalamus and basal ganglia
  - T2 signal abnormalities can be difficult to identify in the unmyelinated brain
  - T1 hyperintensity seen acutely ⇒ myelin breakdown/clumping?

Neurofibromatosis Type 1
- Signal abnormalities in basal ganglia most common brain manifestation
- Evolve/resolve over time

Stroke
- True arterial or venous infarcts difficult to distinguish from MELAS

INBORN ERRORS OF METABOLISM

○ Must maintain a clinical presumption of a vascular etiology unless proven otherwise

PATHOLOGY

General Features
- General path comments
  ○ Many inborn errors of metabolism can present with acute neurologic symptoms
    ▪ Most are superimposed upon a history of developmental delay and/or decline
  ○ The entities discussed here have a tendency to present acutely, often without recognized pre-existing symptoms
- Genetics
  ○ MEMs ⇒ can be caused by defects in mitochondrial DNA or nuclear DNA
  ○ MCAD deficiency ⇒ mutations in the ACADM gene on the short arm of chromosome 1
  ○ Urea cycle disorders ⇒ multiple autosomal recessive gene mutations
    ▪ Exception: OTC deficiency is X-linked
  ○ MSUD ⇒ mutations in genes for enzymes of branched-chain α-ketoacid dehydrogenase (BCKD) complex
- Etiology
  ○ MEMs reduce the ability of the mitochondrion to synthesize ATP via the Krebs cycle and respiratory chain
    ▪ Diversion to anaerobic metabolism with build-up of lactate
  ○ MCAD deficiency prevents the entry of medium-chain fatty acids into the beta oxidation cycle
    ▪ Inability to utilize these fatty acids results in severe hypoglycemia in the face of metabolic stress or fasting
  ○ Urea cycle disorders result from enzyme deficiencies that disrupt incorporation of nitrogen into urea for excretion
    ▪ Cause a build up of toxic nitrogen products
  ○ MSUD reduces activity of BCKD complex, causing build-up of branched chain amino acids and metabolites
    ▪ Build-up of leucine is especially neurotoxic
- Epidemiology
  ○ MEMs are relatively common ~ 1:8,500
  ○ MCADD has a prevalence of ~ 1:12,500
  ○ OTC deficiency is the most common of the urea cycle disorders ~ 1:14,000
- Associated abnormalities
  ○ KSS ⇒ ophthalmoplegia, heart block, retinitis pigmentosa
  ○ Urea cycle disorders may have hypertension, electrolyte abnormalities, coarse hair
  ○ MSUD has "comb-like" rhythms on EEG

CLINICAL ISSUES

Presentation
- Most common signs/symptoms
  ○ Seizures, ataxia, ophthalmoplegia, vomiting, dystonia
    ▪ MEMs may be unmasked by metabolic stressors (infection, exercise)
    ▪ MCAD deficiency classically presents after period of fasting or viral infection
    ▪ Urea cycle disorders: Encephalopathy at 24-48 hours

Demographics
- Age
  ○ MSUD and urea cycle disorders typically present in the neonatal period with acute encephalopathy
    ▪ MSUD presentation may be delayed in breast-fed babies
    ▪ Partial urea cycle defects may present later in childhood or as adults
  ○ Most MEMs present in infancy
    ▪ Age at onset and severity correlates with degree of enzyme deficit
  ○ MCAD deficiency typically presents in infancy
    ▪ May be induced by stopping of nighttime feeds, viral infection

Treatment
- Urea cycle disorders ⇒ liver transplant
- MSUD ⇒ dietary modification
- MCAD deficiency ⇒ carbohydrate supplementation, avoid fasting
- MEMs ⇒ supportive care

DIAGNOSTIC CHECKLIST

Image Interpretation Pearls
- Think of MEMs when encountering an atypical presentation of stroke, severe encephalitis, or seizure
  ○ Don't forget to consider GA-1 when an infant presents with subdurals
- Infant/child with cerebral edema and hypoglycemia ⇒ MCAD deficiency

SELECTED REFERENCES

1. Kolker S et al: Guideline for the diagnosis and management of glutaryl-CoA dehydrogenase deficiency (glutaric aciduria type I). J Inherit Metab Dis. 30(1):5-22, 2007
2. Abe K et al: Comparison of conventional and diffusion-weighted MRI and proton MR spectroscopy in patients with mitochondrial encephalomyopathy, lactic acidosis, and stroke-like events. Neuroradiology. 46(2):113-7, 2004
3. Christodoulou J: Clinical evaluation and emergency management of inborn errors of metabolism presenting in the newborn. Southeast Asian J Trop Med Public Health. 34 Suppl 3:189-97, 2003
4. Nyhan WL et al: Treatment of the acute crisis in maple syrup urine disease. Arch Pediatr Adolesc Med. 152(6):593-8, 1998
5. Smith ET Jr et al: Medium-chain acylcoenzyme-A dehydrogenase deficiency. Not just another Reye syndrome. Am J Forensic Med Pathol. 14(4):313-8, 1993

INBORN ERRORS OF METABOLISM

IMAGE GALLERY

Typical

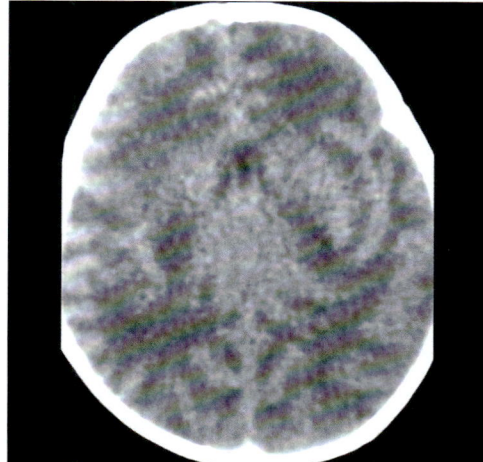 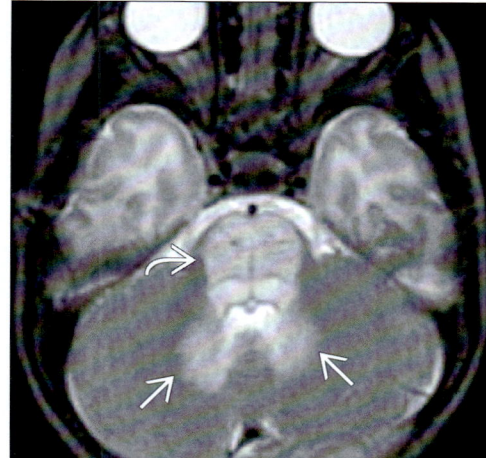

(Left) Axial NECT in a neonate with MSUD shows diffuse acute brain swelling and hypodense WM. These findings should suggest the disorder even before the classic subacute MSUD pattern appears. *(Right)* Axial T2WI MR shows characteristic pattern of edema seen in MSUD, with abnormal bright signal in cerebellar WM ➡ and brainstem ➡.

Typical

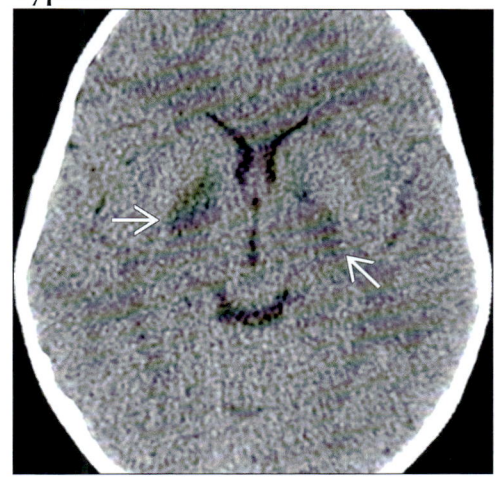 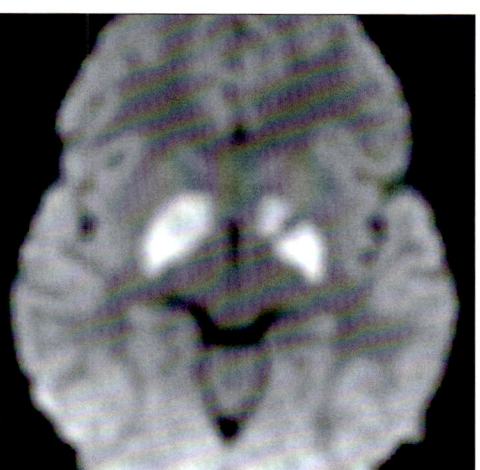

(Left) Axial NECT in a 4 year old with respiratory failure and metabolic acidosis shows bilateral low density globus pallidus lesions ➡ strongly suggestive of mitochondrial encephalopathy. *(Right)* Axial DWI MR shows restricted diffusion in the lesions, indicating an acute injury, likely ischemic. The symmetric distribution and presentation in a child is virtually diagnostic for MEM.

Typical

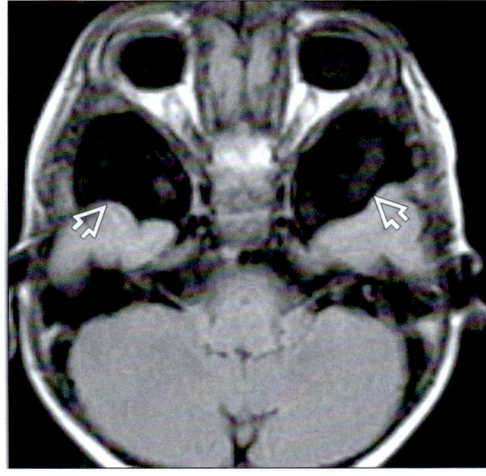 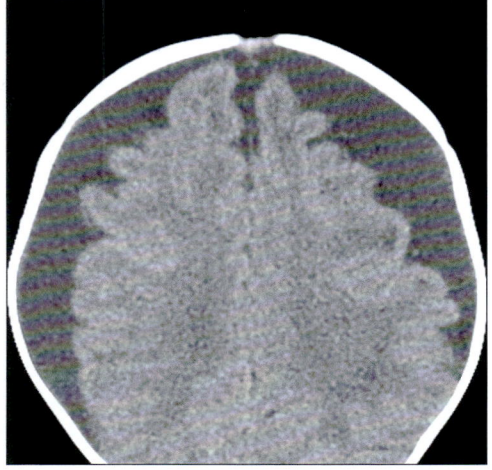

(Left) Axial FLAIR MR in a child with GA-1 shows enlarged subdural spaces in the middle cranial fossae ➡. These collections can raise concern for traumatic brain injury, delaying diagnosis. *(Right)* Axial NECT shows bifrontal hyperdense subdural collections in a child with GA-1. This entity causes cerebral atrophy which leads to the formation of subdurals.

NEAR-DROWNING

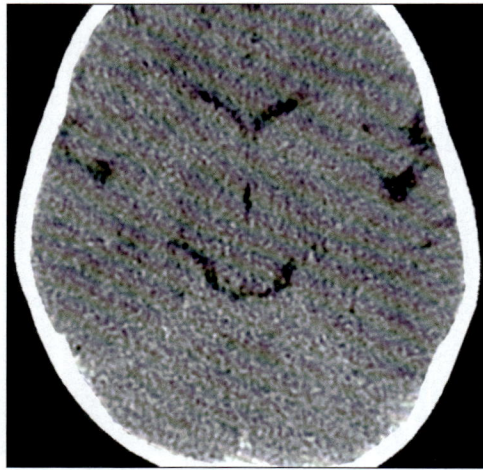

Axial NECT in a 2 year old found in a wading pool shows poor gray-white differentiation throughout the cerebrum. Abnormalities on initial CT are a very poor prognostic indicator.

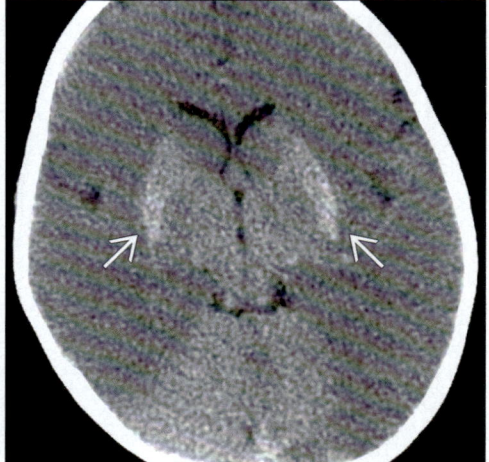

Axial NECT in the same child 8 days later, shows diffuse decreased attenuation with hyperdensity in the basal ganglia and thalamus ➡ indicating petechial hemorrhage or calcification.

TERMINOLOGY

Abbreviations and Synonyms
- Submersion injury

Definitions
- Brain injury caused by asphyxiation in water
  - Pattern and severity of injury may be mitigated by "diving reflex"
- Wet drowning ⇒ some water/fluid is aspirated into lungs
- Dry drowning ⇒ laryngospasm prevents any water from entering lungs (20%)

IMAGING FINDINGS

General Features
- Best diagnostic clue: Hyperintensity on T2WI in basal ganglia (BG)

CT Findings
- NECT
  - Can show decreased attenuation in BG, peripheral cortex
  - Presence of diffuse edema ⇒ very poor outcome
  - Valuable to detect unsuspected hemorrhage or other traumatic lesions

MR Findings
- T2WI
  - Patchy bright signal in BG
  - Bright signal and swelling in peripheral cortex
    - Most commonly occipital
- DWI
  - Restricted diffusion in regions of affected cortex
  - May be falsely normal-appearing in BG
- MRS
  - Decreased absolute levels of NAA (< 75% of normal) indicates poor prognosis
  - ↑ Lactate indicates poor prognosis

Imaging Recommendations
- Best imaging tool: MR with MR spectroscopy
- Protocol advice
  - Initial CT still of value to assess for hemorrhage
  - MR with MRS and DWI at 24-48 hours
    - Imaging too early may be falsely reassuring

DDx: Bilateral Basal Ganglia Lesions in Children

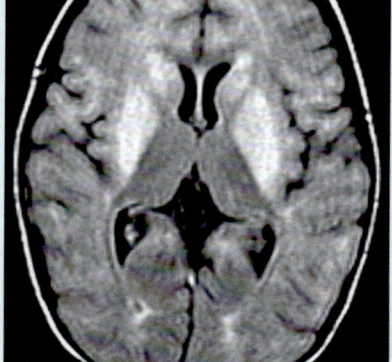

Encephalitis

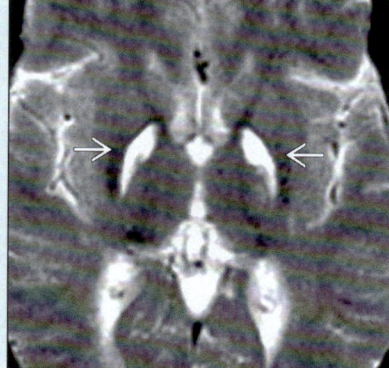

Carbon Monoxide Poisoning

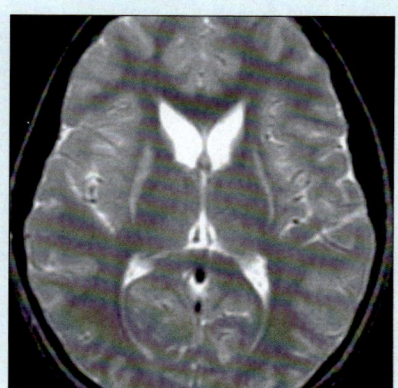

Huntington Disease

NEAR-DROWNING

Key Facts

Imaging Findings
- Presence of diffuse edema ⇒ very poor outcome
- Patchy bright signal in BG
- Decreased absolute levels of NAA (< 75% of normal) indicates poor prognosis
- Initial CT still of value to assess for hemorrhage

Top Differential Diagnoses
- Carbon Monoxide Poisoning
- Metabolic Brain Disease

Pathology
- 2nd only to motor vehicle collisions as a cause of injury and death in children 1 month-14 years

Clinical Issues
- 35% of submersion episodes in children are fatal
- Another 45% have neurological sequelae
- Long term follow-up of children with "good" outcomes indicate problems with memory and cognition

DIFFERENTIAL DIAGNOSIS

Carbon Monoxide Poisoning
- Can cause same pattern of injury

Encephalitis
- Viral pathogens can cause patchy signal abnormalities in BG and cortex

Metabolic Brain Disease
- Mitochondrial encephalopathies
- Huntington disease
- Pantothenate kinase associated neurodegeneration (PKAN, Hallervorden-Spatz)

Hypoxic Ischemic Encephalopathy
- Essentially the same diagnosis with a different etiology

PATHOLOGY

General Features
- General path comments: Prolonged hypoxemia leads to acidosis
- Etiology
  - < 1 year ⇒ bathtub
  - 1-6 years ⇒ pools
  - Teenagers ⇒ natural bodies of water
- Epidemiology
  - 8000+ cases per year in US
    - 1500+ in children
    - 3.22 per 100,00 under 4 years of age
  - 2nd only to motor vehicle collisions as a cause of injury and death in children 1 month-14 years
- Associated abnormalities
  - Intracranial hemorrhage (subdural, epidural hematoma)
  - Fungal infection with brain abscesses (Pseudallescheria boydii)

CLINICAL ISSUES

Natural History & Prognosis
- 35% of submersion episodes in children are fatal
- Another 45% have neurological sequelae
- Long term follow-up of children with "good" outcomes indicate problems with memory and cognition

SELECTED REFERENCES

1. Panichpisal K et al: Central nervous system pseudallescheriasis after near-drowning. Clin Neurol Neurosurg. 108(4):348-52, 2006
2. Pierro MM et al: Anoxic brain injury following near-drowning in children. Rehabilitation outcome: three case reports. Brain Inj. 19(13):1147-55, 2005
3. Dubowitz DJ et al: MR of hypoxic encephalopathy in children after near drowning: correlation with quantitative proton MR spectroscopy and clinical outcome. AJNR Am J Neuroradiol. 19(9):1617-27, 1998
4. Romano C et al: Assessment of pediatric near-drowning victims: is there a role for cranial CT? Pediatr Radiol. 23(4):261-3, 1993

IMAGE GALLERY

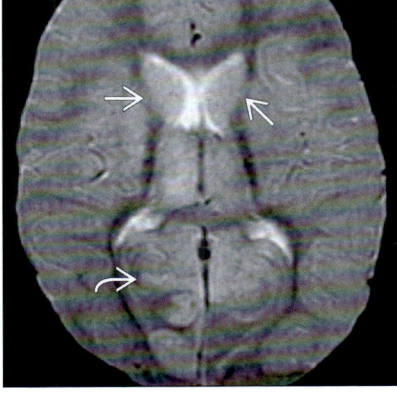
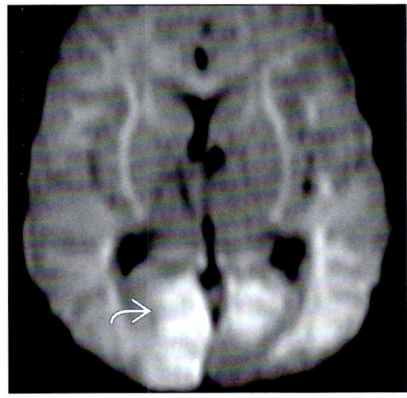
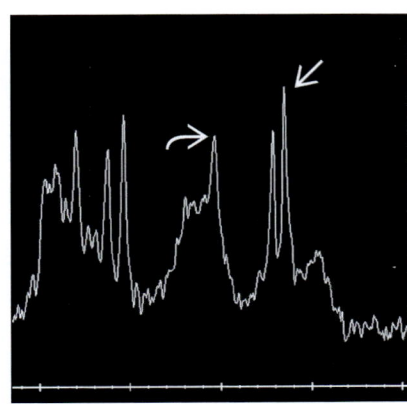

(**Left**) Axial FLAIR MR shows patchy abnormally hyperintense signal throughout the basal ganglia ➡ and in the peripheral cortex ➡. (**Center**) Axial DWI MR in the same child shows restricted diffusion in peripheral cortex ➡. Basal ganglia injury can be subtle or inapparent on DWI. (**Right**) Short-echo MR spectroscopy acquired in the basal ganglia of the same child shows reduction in NAA ➡, and an abnormal prominent lipid/lactate doublet ➡.

CARBON MONOXIDE POISONING

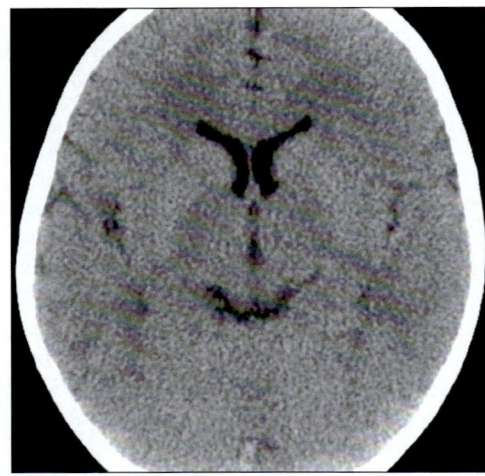

Axial NECT in a 2 year old with carbon monoxide poisoning shows an essentially normal appearance of the brain parenchyma. Initial imaging in CO poisoning is often unremarkable.

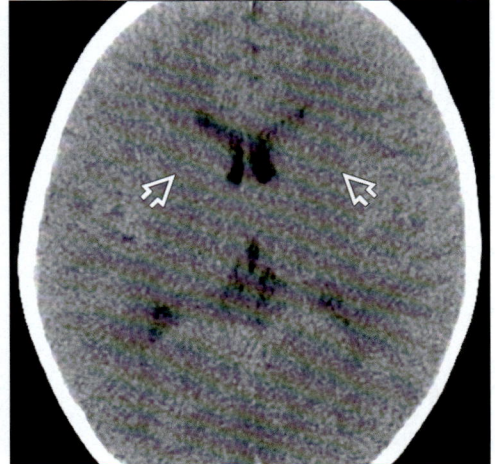

Axial NECT in the same child 2 days later, shows complete loss of differentiation of the basal ganglia ➡, with no definition of the internal or external capsules.

TERMINOLOGY

Definitions
- Cerebral injury due to acute or chronic exposure to carbon monoxide (CO)

IMAGING FINDINGS

General Features
- Best diagnostic clue: Bilateral and symmetric globus pallidus lesions
- Location
  - Globus pallidus, putamen, thalamus
  - More widespread white matter (WM) involvement, (delayed)

CT Findings
- NECT: Bilateral and symmetric low-attenuation in basal ganglia

MR Findings
- T1WI
  - Hypointense lesions in basal ganglia
  - Hyperintensity indicates hemorrhagic necrosis
- T2WI
  - Acute
    - Hyperintense symmetric basal ganglia lesions
  - Chronic
    - Symmetric hyperintensity in centrum semiovale, internal and external capsules, and corpus callosum
    - Hippocampal lesions may be apparent
- DWI
  - Restricted diffusion evident in injured white matter
  - May reverse in milder cases
- MRS
  - Elevated lactate and reduced NAA indicate irreversible injury
  - Increased choline has been reported, thought to reflect ongoing demyelination

Imaging Recommendations
- Best imaging tool: MR imaging with DWI and MRS
- Protocol advice: Include gradient echo imaging to identify hemorrhagic lesions

DDx: Striatal Lesions in Children

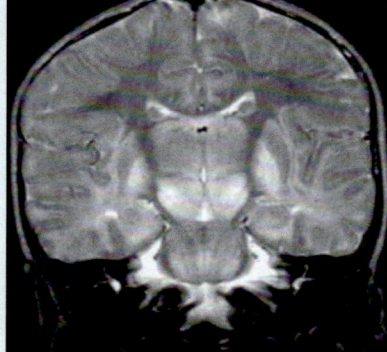

Maple Syrup Urine Disease

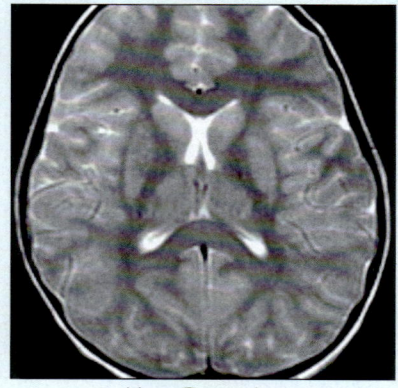

Near Drowning

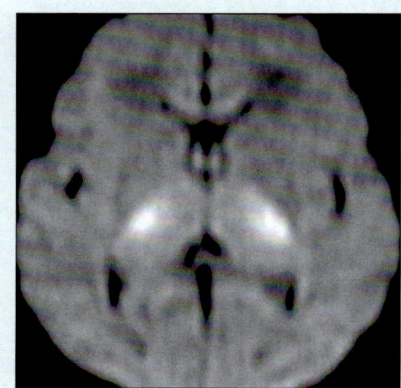

Hypoxic Ischemic Encephalopathy

CARBON MONOXIDE POISONING

Key Facts

Terminology
- Cerebral injury due to acute or chronic exposure to carbon monoxide (CO)

Imaging Findings
- Best diagnostic clue: Bilateral and symmetric globus pallidus lesions
- Restricted diffusion evident in injured white matter
- Elevated lactate and reduced NAA indicate irreversible injury

Top Differential Diagnoses
- Near Drowning
- Hypoxic Ischemic Encephalopathy (HIE)
- Mitochondrial encephalopathies

Diagnostic Checklist
- Consider CO poisoning, metabolic disease, and near drowning in children with bilateral basal ganglia lesions

DIFFERENTIAL DIAGNOSIS

Near Drowning
- Causes very similar bilateral basal ganglia lesions

Hypoxic Ischemic Encephalopathy (HIE)
- Ventrolateral thalamus more classically involved

Inborn Errors of Metabolism
- Mitochondrial encephalopathies
  - Leigh syndrome, MELAS, pantothenate kinase associated neurodegeneration (PKAN)
- Maple syrup urine disease (MSUD)

PATHOLOGY

General Features
- Etiology
  - Accidental: Leaks from heaters, poorly ventilated charcoal grills
  - Purposeful: Suicide attempts with car exhaust
  - Secondary to house fires
- Epidemiology: Leading cause of accidental poisoning in North America and Europe

Gross Pathologic & Surgical Features
- CO binds with hemoglobin (carboxyhemoglobin), reducing oxygen carrying capacity
- CO binds with myoglobin, causing myocardial depression
- CO binds with cytochrome c and P450

CLINICAL ISSUES

Presentation
- Most common signs/symptoms
  - Acute: Headache, nausea, lethargy, coma
  - Postanoxic delayed encephalopathy in 1-12% of cases

DIAGNOSTIC CHECKLIST

Consider
- Consider CO poisoning, metabolic disease, and near drowning in children with bilateral basal ganglia lesions

SELECTED REFERENCES
1. Hopkins RO et al: Basal ganglia lesions following carbon monoxide poisoning. Brain Inj. 20(3):273-81, 2006
2. Weaver LK et al: Hemorrhagic infarction in white matter following acute carbon monoxide poisoning. Neurology. 64(6):1101; author reply 1101, 2005
3. Kim JH et al: Delayed encephalopathy of acute carbon monoxide intoxication: diffusivity of cerebral white matter lesions. AJNR Am J Neuroradiol. 24(8):1592-7, 2003
4. Sener RN: Acute carbon monoxide poisoning: diffusion MR imaging findings. AJNR Am J Neuroradiol. 24(7):1475-7, 2003

IMAGE GALLERY

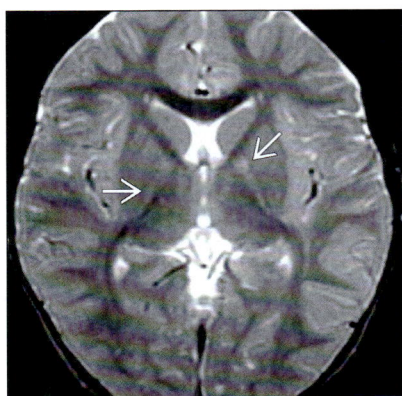 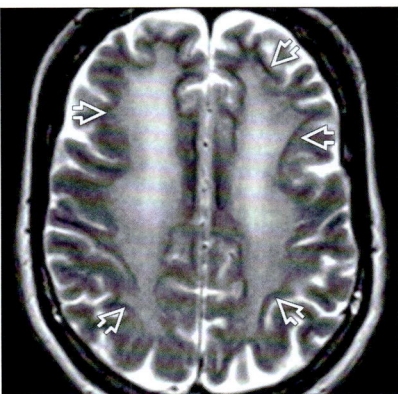 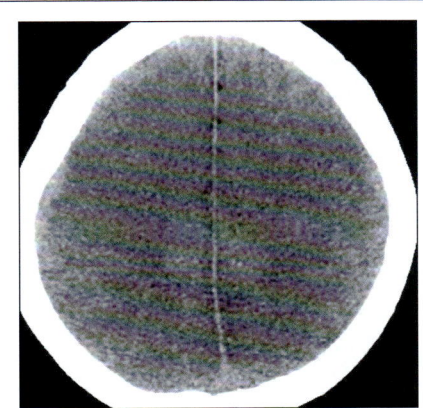

(Left) Axial T2WI MR shows subtle regions of abnormal hyperintensity in the globus pallidus on each side ➡. *(Center)* Axial T2WI MR shows bilateral diffuse hyperintensity throughout the white matter with sparing of the subcortical U-fibers ➡. *(Right)* Axial NECT shows decreased attenuation of both gray and white matter with loss of gray-white differentiation in a 4 year old, 48 hours after presenting with CO poisoning from a house fire.

NECROTIZING EXTERNAL OTITIS

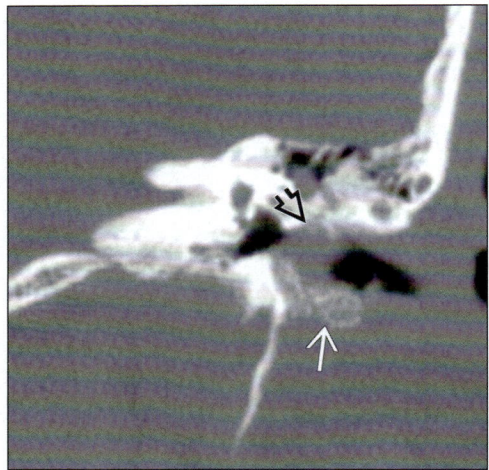

Coronal bone CT shows destruction of floor ➡ and roof ⇗ of bony EAC.

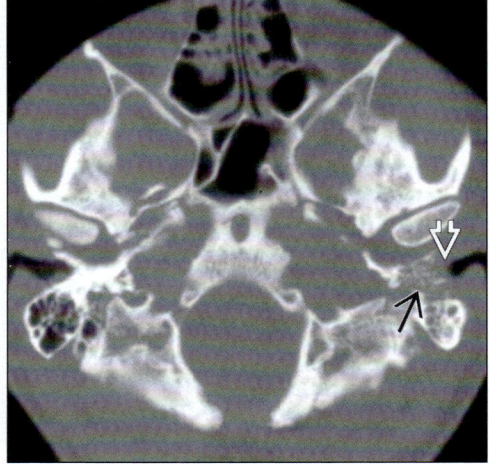

Axial bone CT shows destruction of floor of left EAC ⇗ just lateral to osseous/cartilaginous junction ➡.

TERMINOLOGY

Abbreviations and Synonyms
- Necrotizing external otitis (NEO)
- Malignant external otitis, malignant otitis externa

Definitions
- NEO: Severe invasive infection of external auditory canal (EAC), adjacent soft tissues and skull base

IMAGING FINDINGS

General Features
- Best diagnostic clue: Swollen EAC soft tissues with bony erosion & adjacent cellulitis or abscess
- Location: EAC and surrounding soft tissues
- Size: Variable depending on spread of infectious process into adjacent soft tissues
- Morphology: Variable based on route of spread

CT Findings
- NECT
  - T-bone CT
    - Early: Thickened mucosa of EAC & auricle
    - Late: Bone destruction in EAC (especially floor) and skull base
- CECT: Enhancement of thickened soft tissue, ring enhancement of abscesses

MR Findings
- T1WI
  - Thickened EAC, auricle & adjacent soft tissues
  - Replacement of normal fatty marrow signal in infected bone (skull base)
- T2WI
  - Diffuse trans-spatial, high signal suggests cellulitis
  - Focal high signal areas suggest abscess
- STIR: Increased signal intensity within inflamed EAC, auricle, adjacent soft tissues, and infected bone
- T1 C+ FS
  - Tissues of EAC & auricle diffusely enhance
  - Heterogeneous enhancement with cellulitis in adjacent soft tissues
  - Abscesses present as rim-enhancing fluid collections
- MRV: NEO may be complicated by cerebral venous sinus thrombosis

DDx: Mimics of Necrotizing External Otitis

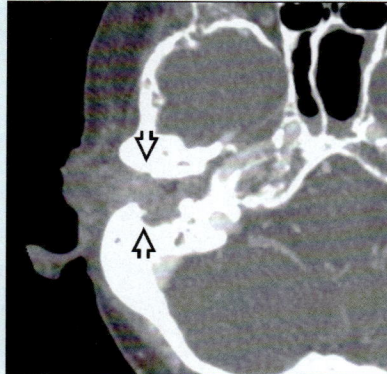

Squamous Cell Carcinoma

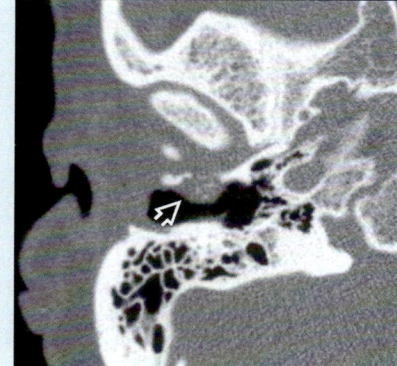

EAC Cholesteatoma

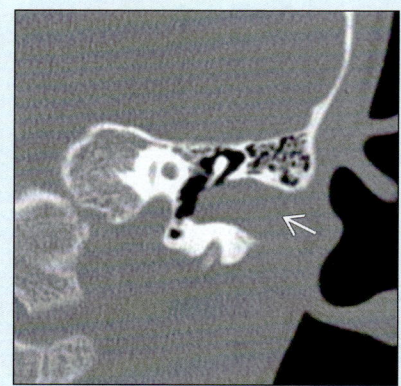

Keratosis Obturans

NECROTIZING EXTERNAL OTITIS

Key Facts

Terminology
- NEO: Severe invasive infection of external auditory canal (EAC), adjacent soft tissues and skull base

Imaging Findings
- Best diagnostic clue: Swollen EAC soft tissues with bony erosion & adjacent cellulitis or abscess

Top Differential Diagnoses
- EAC Squamous Cell Carcinoma (EAC SCC)
- EAC Cholesteatoma
- Post-Inflammatory Medial Canal Fibrosis
- Keratosis Obturans

Pathology
- Severe infectious changes involving EAC & adjacent soft tissues
- Iatrogenic procedures (e.g., aural irrigation)
- Immunosuppression, neoplasm, dermatitis

Clinical Issues
- Clinical Profile: Afebrile elderly diabetic patient with severe otalgia disproportionate to physical findings
- Begins as soft tissue EAC infection, progresses into surrounding osseous structures, including TMJ

Diagnostic Checklist
- SCC can have similar appearance to NEO and both may coexist; biopsy may be required for definitive differentiation
- Small, early cortical erosions best seen with CT at initial diagnosis
- Look for sigmoid sinus thrombosis if CN9-11 affected, cavernous sinus thrombosis if CN5 or 6 affected

Nuclear Medicine Findings
- Bone Scan
  - Technetium Tc-99m MDP: Binds to osteoblasts, increased uptake in bony EAC & adjacent skull base with osteomyelitis, but nonspecific
    - Spatial resolution improved with SPECT
    - Scintigraphic abnormalities may persist for many months despite effective therapy
  - Gallium-67 citrate binds to granulocytes and bacteria
    - Low specificity, false-negative case reports in recurrent disease
    - Gallium scan correlates better with therapeutic response than Tc-99m

Imaging Recommendations
- Best imaging tool
  - Bone CT may identify subtle cortical erosions signaling early osteomyelitis
  - MR more sensitive for intracranial complications, bone marrow edema, extent of extracranial soft tissue involvement
  - Follow-up treatment
    - NM studies: Gallium scan correlates most specifically with treatment response
    - Bone changes persist on CT for up to a year
    - Resolution of soft tissue and marrow changes on MR may be better marker of treatment response
- Protocol advice
  - Axial bone HRCT with coronal reconstruction
  - Contrast HRCT (soft tissue algorithm) useful for evaluation of soft tissues, venous sinuses

DIFFERENTIAL DIAGNOSIS

EAC Squamous Cell Carcinoma (EAC SCC)
- May have history of cutaneous SCC; ESR not ↑; no Pseudomonas on culture
- May be impossible to differentiate from NEO radiographically, and two can coexist

EAC Cholesteatoma
- Mass composed of exfoliated keratin with stratified squamous epithelium
- Unilateral soft tissue mass with underlying bony destruction, intramural bony "flakes"

Post-Inflammatory Medial Canal Fibrosis
- Characterized by formation of fibrous tissue in medial aspect of bony EAC without bony erosion
- Chronic otitis externa or surgical procedure causal

Keratosis Obturans
- Rare condition with abnormal accumulation & obstruction of bony EAC from desquamated keratin
- Homogeneous soft tissue filling EAC with mild enlargement, no aggressive bony changes
- Classically seen in patients with chronic sinusitis & bronchiectasis

PATHOLOGY

General Features
- General path comments
  - Severe infectious changes involving EAC & adjacent soft tissues
  - Embryology/anatomy
    - Typically extends inferiorly from EAC via fissures of Santorini
    - Vertically oriented fissures in cartilaginous EAC allow flexibility, also present inferior route of infectious spread
  - Cellulitis & abscesses may spread in any direction
    - Inferiorly: Parotid, masticator & parapharyngeal spaces
    - Posteriorly: Mastoid air cells
    - Medially: Middle ear cavity/petrous apex
    - Anteriorly: Temporomandibular joint
- Etiology
  - Diabetic vasculopathy and immune dysfunction
  - Pseudomonas aeruginosa is infecting organism in > 98% of cases

NECROTIZING EXTERNAL OTITIS

- Aggressive EAC cellulitis + osteomyelitis
- Extra-/subtemporal spread via fissures of Santorini
- Aspergillus fumigatus, other organisms may be a cause in immunosuppressed/AIDS patients
- Other predisposing factors
  - Iatrogenic procedures (e.g., aural irrigation)
  - Immunosuppression, neoplasm, dermatitis
- Epidemiology
  - 95% of adults with NEO have diabetes (predisposition equal for types I and II)
  - Most patients elderly
  - Children with NEO more frequently immunocompromised due to malignancy, malnutrition
  - More common in warm, humid climates

Gross Pathologic & Surgical Features
- EAC edema with granulation tissue along floor of bony-cartilaginous EAC junction
- Granulation tissue may not be seen in immunosuppressed/AIDS patients

Microscopic Features
- Severe inflammation with necrosis in subcutaneous tissues in EAC

CLINICAL ISSUES

Presentation
- Most common signs/symptoms
  - Exquisite otalgia and otorrhea
  - Pain extends to TMJ, exacerbated by chewing
- Other signs/symptoms
  - Intractable temporal headaches
  - Cranial neuropathies due to inflammation or neurotoxin elaborated by Pseudomonas species
  - CN7 paresis, though rare, is most common cranial neuropathy (inferior spread of infection)
  - CN9-12 cranial neuropathy: Extension to jugular foramen, hypoglossal canal, or carotid space
  - CN5, 6 can be affected by petrous apex extension of disease
  - WBC normal or mildly ↑, ESR invariably ↑ (but is **not** ↑ in EAC SCC or uncomplicated acute external otitis)
- Clinical Profile: Afebrile elderly diabetic patient with severe otalgia disproportionate to physical findings

Demographics
- Age
  - Middle-aged or elderly (> 60 y)
  - Immunocompromised patients (e.g., HIV) with NEO tend to be younger, non-diabetic
- Gender: M:F = 2:1

Natural History & Prognosis
- Begins as soft tissue EAC infection, progresses into surrounding osseous structures, including TMJ
- May progress to frank skull base osteomyelitis
- Potentially lethal if untreated
- Intracranial extension can lead to venous sinus thrombosis, meningitis, brain abscess, empyema, high mortality rate
- 20% recurrence rate (usually due to inadequate length of therapy)
- Lower cranial nerve involvement associated with high mortality in older reports, but may not be with optimized antibiotic regimens

Treatment
- Glucose control, aggressive & meticulous granulation debridement, topical and systemic antibiotic therapy
  - 6-8 weeks of oral quinolone (Ciproflaxin); resistant cases require antipseudomonal β-lactam agent ± aminoglycoside
  - Adjuvant therapy with hyperbaric oxygenation may be considered
- Surgical drainage of any deep facial abscess

DIAGNOSTIC CHECKLIST

Consider
- SCC can have similar appearance to NEO and both may coexist; biopsy may be required for definitive differentiation

Image Interpretation Pearls
- Small, early cortical erosions best seen with CT at initial diagnosis
- Look for sigmoid sinus thrombosis if CN9-11 affected, cavernous sinus thrombosis if CN5 or 6 affected

SELECTED REFERENCES
1. Mani N et al: Cranial nerve involvement in malignant external otitis: implications for clinical outcome. Laryngoscope. 117(5):907-10, 2007
2. Rubin Grandis J et al: The changing face of malignant (necrotising) external otitis: clinical, radiological, and anatomic correlations. Lancet Infect Dis. 4(1):34-9, 2004
3. Soldati D et al: Necrotizing otitis externa caused by Staphylococcus epidermidis. Eur Arch Otorhinolaryngol. 256(9):439-41, 1999
4. Grandis JR et al: Necrotizing (malignant) external otitis: prospective comparison of CT and MR imaging in diagnosis and follow-up. Radiology. 196(2):499-504, 1995
5. Weinroth SE et al: Malignant otitis externa in AIDS patients: case report and review of the literature. Ear Nose Throat J. 73(10):772-4, 777-8, 1994
6. Grandis JR et al: Simultaneous presentation of malignant external otitis and temporal bone cancer. Arch Otolaryngol Head Neck Surg. 119(6):687-9, 1993
7. Guy RL et al: Computed tomography in malignant external otitis. Clin Radiol. 43(3):166-70, 1991
8. McElroy EA Jr et al: Fatal necrotizing otitis externa in a patient with AIDS. Rev Infect Dis. 13(6):1246-7, 1991
9. Shupak A et al: Hyperbaric oxygenation for necrotizing (malignant) otitis externa. Arch Otolaryngol Head Neck Surg. 115(12):1470-5, 1989
10. Cunningham M et al: Necrotizing otitis externa due to Aspergillus in an immunocompetent patient. Arch Otolaryngol Head Neck Surg. 114(5):554-6, 1988

NECROTIZING EXTERNAL OTITIS

IMAGE GALLERY

Typical

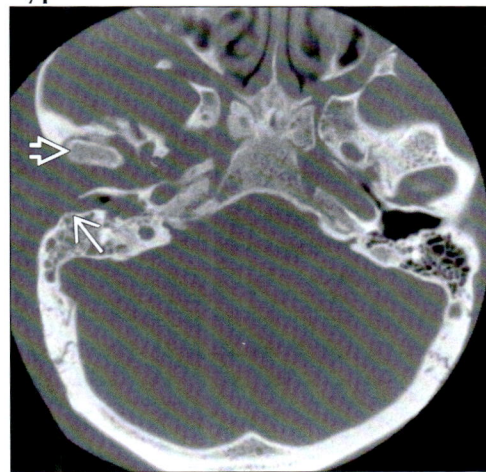
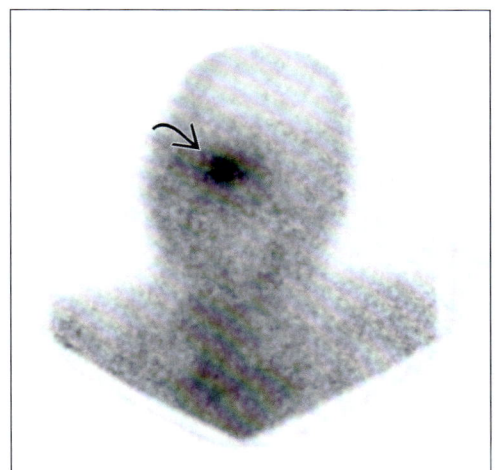

(Left) Axial bone CT shows inflammatory soft tissue changes in/about right EAC ➡ with extension into right TM with anterior displacement of condyle ➡. *(Right)* Anteroposterior cranial gallium scan shows increased uptake in region of right mastoid ➡, consistent with NEO.

Typical

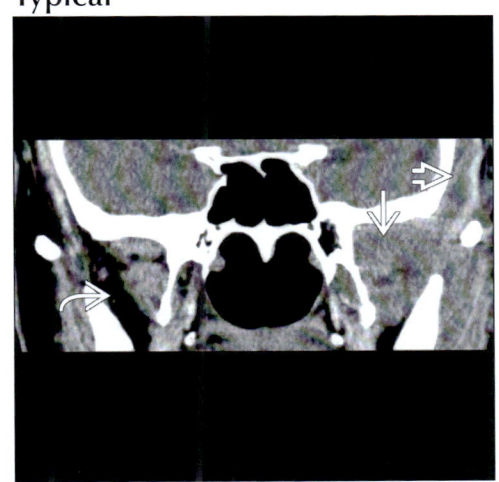
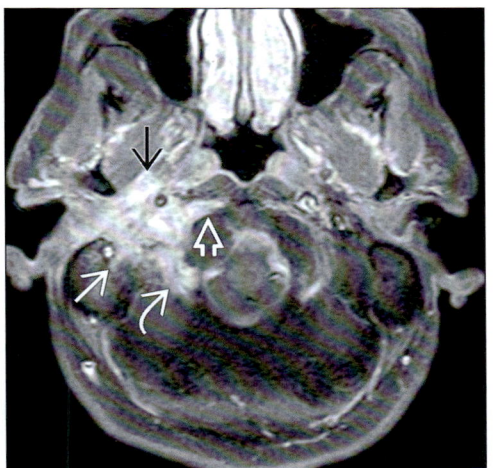

(Left) Coronal NECT shows NEO extension into left infrazygomatic ➡ and suprazygomatic masticator spaces ➡ (temporalis muscle). Note normal-appearing fat planes on right side ➡. *(Right)* Axial T1 C+ FS MR shows enhancing tissue extending from right EAC into parapharyngeal space ➡, prevertebral space ➡, occipital bone ➡, and stylomastoid foramen ➡ in patient with NEO.

Typical

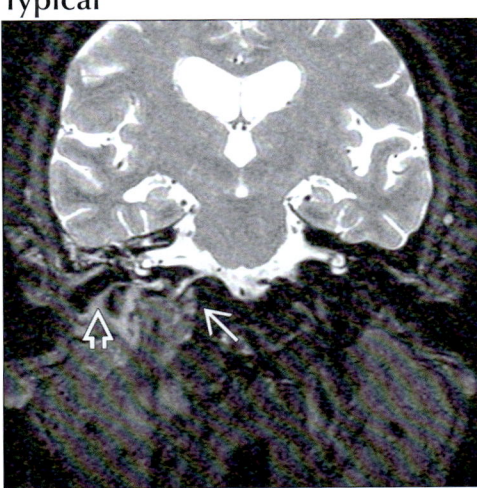
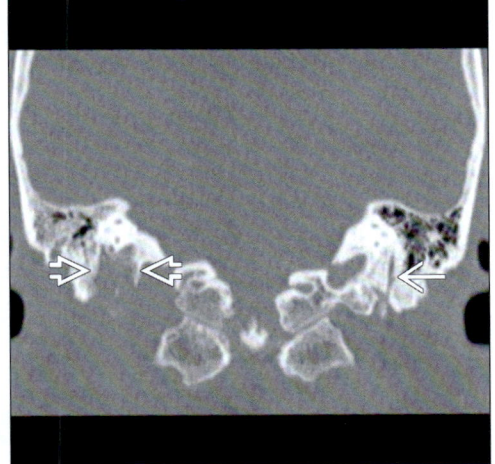

(Left) Coronal T2WI FS MR shows increased signal in soft tissue surrounding R EAC ➡, extending to right occipital bone ➡ and affecting all intervening tissues in a patient with NEO. *(Right)* Coronal bone CT shows bone destruction ➡ surrounding right mastoid facial nerve canal in a patient with NEO and right CN7 paralysis. Note normal facial nerve canal on left ➡.

COMPLICATED OTITIS MEDIA

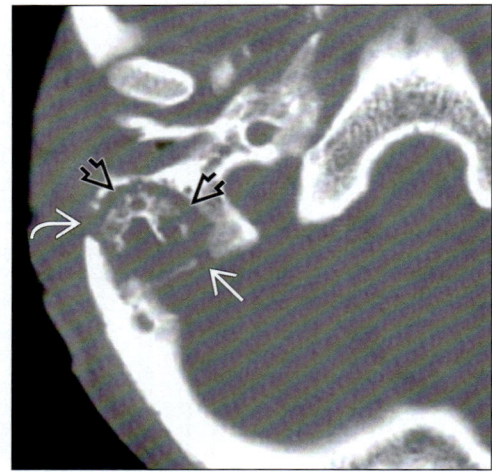

Axial bone CT shows erosion of lateral mastoid cortex ➔, floating osseous sequestrum ➔, and erosion of sigmoid plate ➔ in a patient with coalescent otomastoiditis.

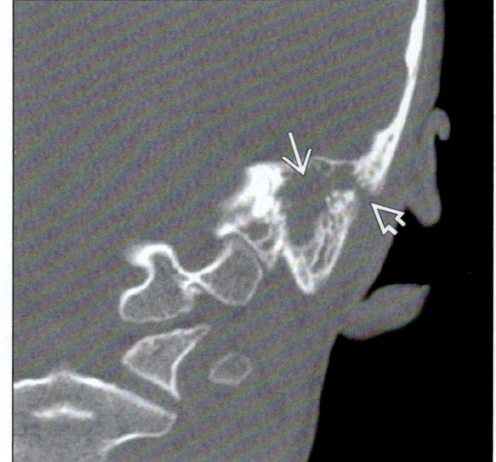

Coronal bone CT shows mastoid trabecular destruction ➔ and lateral cortical dehiscence ➔ due to CM. Dehiscence is potential route for subperiosteal abscess formation.

TERMINOLOGY

Abbreviations and Synonyms
- Acute otomastoiditis or acute otitis media (AOM); chronic otitis media or otomastoiditis (COM)
- Coalescent otomastoiditis (CM)
- Coalescent otomastoiditis with abscess (CM-A)

Definitions
- Definitions
  - AOM, COM: Acute or chronic infection in middle ear & mastoid air cells without bone destruction
  - CM: Destruction of mastoid trabeculae/cortex due to intramastoid empyema
  - CM-A: Extratemporal (subperiosteal, epidural, subdural) abscess/empyema complicating CM

IMAGING FINDINGS

General Features
- Best diagnostic clue
  - CM: Middle ear/mastoid air cell opacification with erosion of mastoid septations, coalescent cells
  - CM-A: Otomastoid opacification + adjacent extratympanic rim-enhancing fluid collection
- Location
  - CM: Middle ear, mastoid, petrous apex
  - CM-A: Subperiosteal, epidural, subdural, or temporal lobe

CT Findings
- NECT
  - AOM: Opacified middle ear/mastoid, air-fluid levels
  - CM: Destruction of mastoid trabeculae ± cortex
  - Scalloped erosion of bone with cholesteatoma
- CECT
  - AOM: Enhancement of inflammatory debris in middle ear & mastoid
  - CM-A: Rim-enhancing fluid collection adjacent to opacified mastoid air cells
- CTA: May show dural sinus thrombosis

MR Findings
- T2WI
  - Hyperintense debris in middle ear, mastoid
    - Cholesteatoma relatively hypointense
  - CM-A: Hyperintense loculated fluid collection
- T1 C+

DDx: Mimics of Complicated Otitis Media

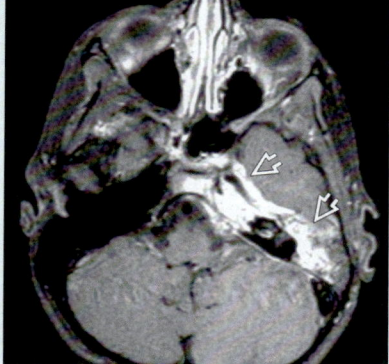

Apical Petrositis

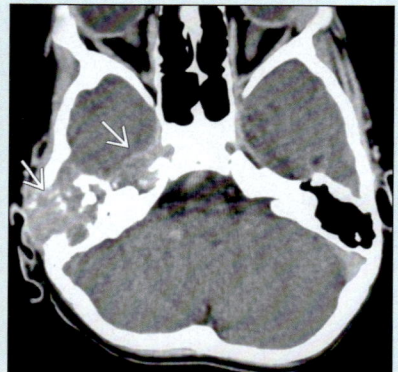

Langerhans Cell Histiocytosis

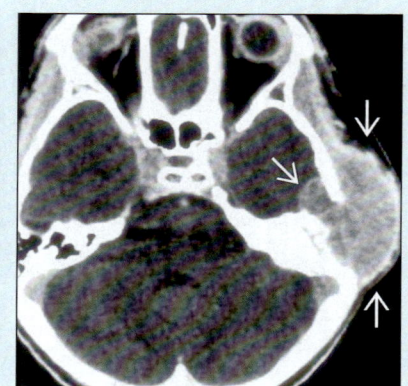

Rhabdomyosarcoma

COMPLICATED OTITIS MEDIA

Key Facts

Terminology
- Coalescent otomastoiditis (CM)
- AOM, COM: Acute or chronic infection in middle ear & mastoid air cells without bone destruction
- CM: Destruction of mastoid trabeculae/cortex due to intramastoid empyema

Imaging Findings
- CM: Middle ear/mastoid air cell opacification with erosion of mastoid septations, coalescent cells
- CM-A: Otomastoid opacification + adjacent extratympanic rim-enhancing fluid collection
- Best imaging tool: Computed tomography

Top Differential Diagnoses
- Acute Uncomplicated Otomastoiditis
- Apical Petrositis
- Congenital Cholesteatoma
- Acquired Cholesteatoma
- Langerhans Cell Histiocytosis (LCH)
- Rhabdomyosarcoma

Pathology
- Luminal pus under pressure → ischemia, acidosis, increased osteoclastic activity → CM
- Most CM 2° incompletely treated AOM; 25% of cases occur with COM + cholesteatoma
- Dehiscent bone facilitates spread of infection

Diagnostic Checklist
- Use side-to-side symmetry to guide interpretation of trabecular changes
- Detection of abscesses, cholesteatoma has critical surgical implications

---

- Enhancement of inflammatory debris
- Enhancement of adjacent inflamed meninges
- Rim-enhancement of abscesses
- CN7 enhancement with facial paralysis
- Labyrinthine enhancement with labyrinthitis
- MRA: Petrous carotid pseudoaneurysm rare
- MRV: May show dural sinus thrombosis

Imaging Recommendations
- Best imaging tool: Computed tomography
- Protocol advice
  - Axial bone HRCT (≤ 1.0 mm), coronal reformats
    - HR CECT in soft-tissue algorithm for CM-A, sinovenous thrombosis
  - MR optimal for intracranial complications
    - Include multiplanar T1 C+ FS MR, MRA, MRV

DIFFERENTIAL DIAGNOSIS

Acute Uncomplicated Otomastoiditis
- Painful ear, infectious symptoms
- No osseous destruction

Apical Petrositis
- CN6 palsy, retroauricular pain, otomastoiditis
- Coalescent changes in petrous apex on CT, mucosal and meningeal enhancement on MR

Congenital Cholesteatoma
- No infectious symptoms; white retrotympanic mass, intact TM
- Large lesions → significant bone erosion

Acquired Cholesteatoma
- Tympanic membrane perforation with middle ear/lateral epitympanic mass
- May cause ossicular erosion, scutum, mastoid trabecular & cortical destruction
- Does not enhance on T1 C+

Langerhans Cell Histiocytosis (LCH)
- Usually systemic; child with draining ear and periauricular mass, usually no cranial neuropathy
- Significant bone destruction, often bilateral, on bone CT
- Enhancing mass on T1 C+ MR

Rhabdomyosarcoma
- Presentation similar to CM, may have cranial nerve deficits (CN7)
- Bone destruction, intracranial extension
- Enhancing middle ear mass

PATHOLOGY

General Features
- Etiology
  - Luminal pus under pressure → ischemia, acidosis, increased osteoclastic activity → CM
  - Most CM 2° incompletely treated AOM; 25% of cases occur with COM + cholesteatoma
  - Dehiscent bone facilitates spread of infection
  - Abscesses may form without bone dehiscence due to septic thrombophlebitis of emissary veins
  - Extracranial abscess sites
    - Subperiosteal mastoid abscess: Via lateral mastoid wall, postauricular > preauricular
    - Bezold abscess: Deep to or within sternocleidomastoid muscle via mastoid tip
    - Subperiosteal zygomatic abscess: Adjacent to zygomatic process of temporal bone
    - Luc abscess: Via/through periosteum of EAC to collect beneath temporalis muscle
    - Citelli abscess: Subperiosteal in occipital bone
  - Intracranial abscesses occur in temporal lobe, epidural or subdural compartments
  - Bacteria involved
    - Streptococcus pneumoniae, Haemophilus influenzae, Streptococcus pyogenes
  - Fungal disease: Consider invasive Aspergillosis in immunocompromised patients
- Epidemiology
  - 46% children have > 2 episodes AOM by age 3
  - 0.24% patients with AOM develop CM

COMPLICATED OTITIS MEDIA

Gross Pathologic & Surgical Features
- CM: Soft osteomyelitic bone with pus filling confluent mastoid air cells

Microscopic Features
- Offending organism often not cultured (prior antibiotic treatment)
- CM-A: Polymicrobial aerobes & anaerobes, Streptococcus species common

CLINICAL ISSUES

Presentation
- Most common signs/symptoms: Otalgia, otorrhea
- Other signs/symptoms
  - Fever, malaise
  - Postauricular edema (Griesinger sign); lateralized auricle (displaced by abscess)
  - Conductive > sensorineural hearing loss
  - Meningeal signs, seizures if intracranial complications
  - ↑ WBC, ↑ ESR
- Clinical Profile: CM, CM-A (extracranial): Young child with otalgia, post-auricular swelling, fever, otorrhea

Demographics
- Age
  - AOM and complications more common in young children
  - Complications due to COM ± cholesteatoma more common in older children and adults
- Gender: M > F

Natural History & Prognosis
- Uncomplicated CM typically has excellent prognosis
- Extracranial complications (subperiosteal abscess)
  - Excellent prognosis with prompt therapy, worse with incomplete antibiotic therapy, virulent organism or immunocompromised host
- Intracranial complications worsen prognosis
  - More common with COM + cholesteatoma than isolated AOM or COM
  - Bone erosion by cholesteatoma may facilitate intracranial spread of infection
  - Meningitis & brain abscess (temporal lobe > cerebellum), epidural abscess, subdural empyema
  - Sigmoid sinus thrombosis/thrombophlebitis (SST)
    - Can occur due to bone erosion into, or emissary venous seeding of, perisinus space
  - Otitic hydrocephalus
    - Communicating hydrocephalus due to obstruction of arachnoid granulations or venous sinus thrombosis
- Temporal bone complications
  - Serous or suppurative labyrinthitis
    - Pathogens enter round window → vertigo, sensorineural hearing loss
  - Apical petrositis: May occur in up to 30% of individuals who have pneumatized petrous apex
  - Facial nerve paralysis: Usually related to inflammation of tympanic segment

Treatment
- AOM
  - Antibiotics, myringotomy tube placement
  - AOM + abscess (but no CM): Needle aspiration or incision and drainage without mastoidectomy
- CM
  - Recently myringotomy and IV antibiotics advocated as alternative to mastoidectomy
  - Presence of cholesteatoma requires surgery
- CM-A
  - IV antibiotics, myringotomy, incision and drainage (vs. needle aspiration) of abscess
  - Mastoidectomy if underlying cholesteatoma
- Brain abscesses
  - Address causative temporal bone pathology
  - Surgical drainage of abscess

DIAGNOSTIC CHECKLIST

Consider
- Carefully seek complications of CM

Image Interpretation Pearls
- Use side-to-side symmetry to guide interpretation of trabecular changes
- Detection of abscesses, cholesteatoma has critical surgical implications
- Rhabdomyosarcoma or LCH usually cause more destruction & have a more solidly enhancing soft tissue component than CM or CM-A

SELECTED REFERENCES

1. Smith JA et al: Complications of chronic otitis media and cholesteatoma. Otolaryngol Clin North Am. 39(6):1237-55, 2006
2. Penido Nde O et al: Intracranial complications of otitis media: 15 years of experience in 33 patients. Otolaryngol Head Neck Surg. 132(1):37-42, 2005
3. Migirov L: Computed tomographic versus surgical findings in complicated acute otomastoiditis. Ann Otol Rhinol Laryngol. 112(8):675-7, 2003
4. Vazquez E et al: Imaging of complications of acute mastoiditis in children. Radiographics. 23(2):359-72, 2003
5. Tarantino V et al: Acute mastoiditis: a 10 year retrospective study. Int J Pediatr Otorhinolaryngol. 66(2):143-8, 2002
6. Zapalac JS et al: Suppurative complications of acute otitis media in the era of antibiotic resistance. Arch Otolaryngol Head Neck Surg. 128(6):660-3, 2002
7. Dobben GD et al: Otogenic intracranial inflammations: role of magnetic resonance imaging. Top Magn Reson Imaging. 11(2):76-86, 2000
8. Go C et al: Intracranial complications of acute mastoiditis. Int J Pediatr Otorhinolaryngol. 52(2):143-8, 2000
9. Antonelli PJ et al: Computed tomography and the diagnosis of coalescent mastoiditis. Otolaryngol Head Neck Surg. 120(3):350-4, 1999
10. Spiegel JH et al: Contemporary presentation and management of a spectrum of mastoid abscesses. Laryngoscope. 108(6):822-8, 1998

COMPLICATED OTITIS MEDIA

IMAGE GALLERY

Typical

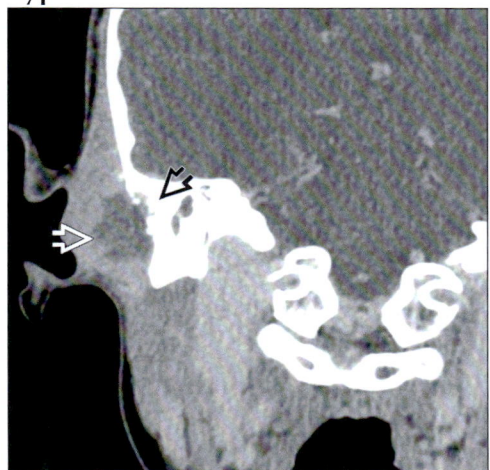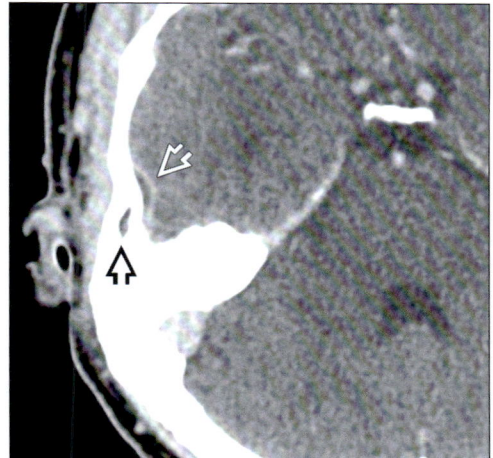

(Left) Axial CECT shows erosion of lateral wall of right mastoid ➔ with overlying abscess ➔ (CM-A). *(Right)* Axial HRCT shows tiny epidural abscess ➔ adjacent to opacified air cell ➔. High-resolution CECT is helpful in detecting abscesses and evaluating venous sinuses.

Typical

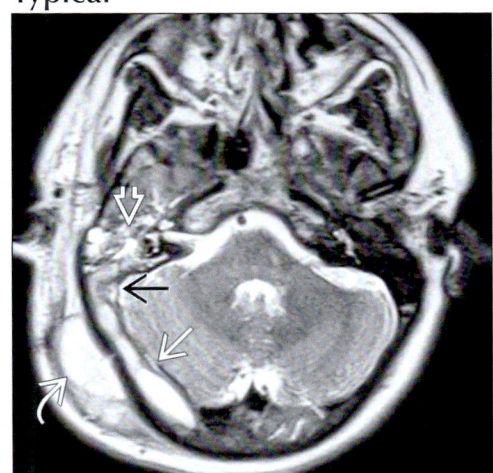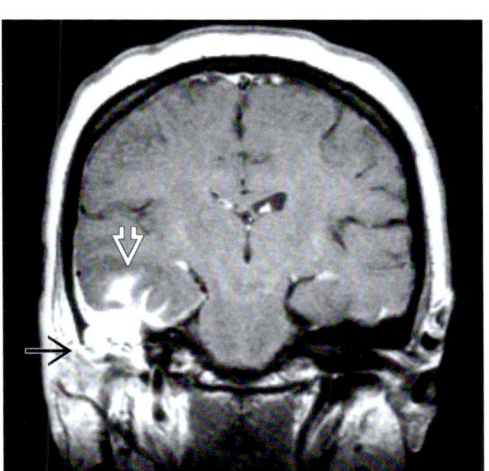

(Left) Axial T2WI MR shows subperiosteal ➔, epidural ➔ abscesses complicating right sided otomastoiditis ➔. Absent signal void in right sigmoid sinus ➔ suggests thrombosis. *(Right)* Coronal T1 C+ MR shows evolving overlying right temporal lobe abscess/encephalitis ➔ in this patient with severe right CM ➔.

Typical

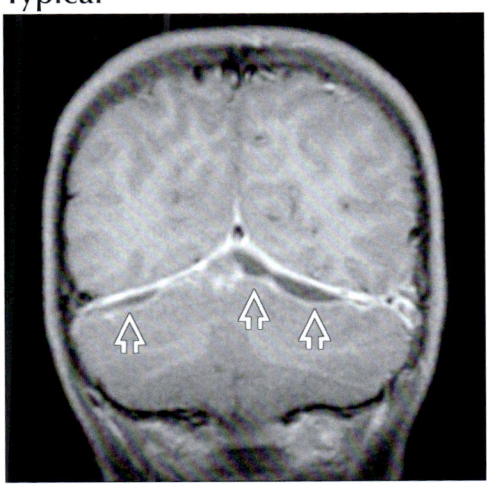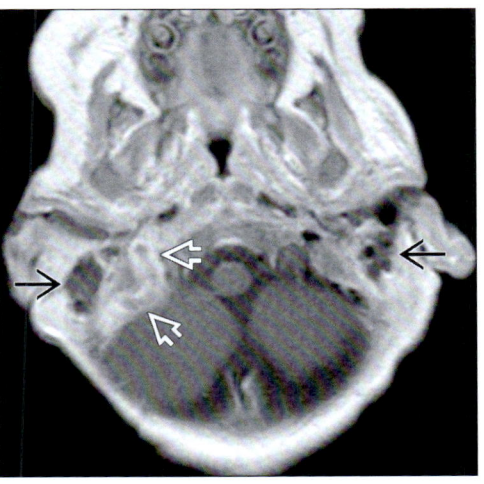

(Left) Coronal T1 C+ FS MR shows subdural empyema along tentorium ➔ complicating left otomastoiditis/cholesteatoma with tegmen dehiscence. *(Right)* Axial T1 C+ MR shows tubular thrombus ➔ in right sigmoid sinus complicating bilateral otomastoiditis ➔.

IDIOPATHIC ORBITAL INFLAMMATORY DISEASE

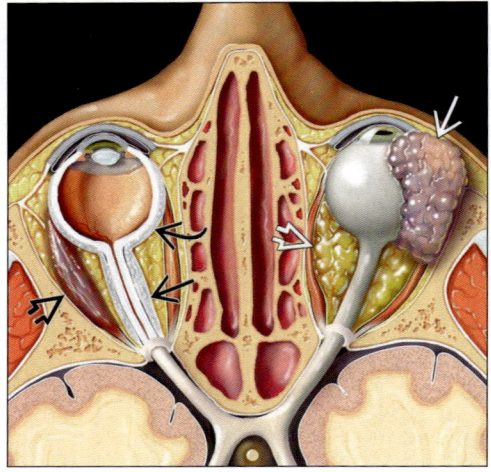

Axial graphic depicts inflammation of extraocular muscles, orbital fat, lacrimal gland, sclera, and optic sheath.

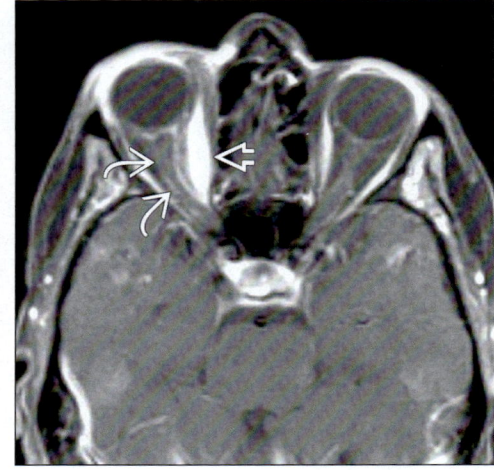

Axial T1 C+ FS MR shows enlarged enhancing right medial rectus muscle (myositis). There is also enhancement of adjacent optic nerve sheath, suggesting perineuritis.

TERMINOLOGY

Abbreviations and Synonyms
- Idiopathic orbital inflammatory disease (IOID)
- Synonyms: Idiopathic orbital inflammatory syndrome, orbital pseudotumor

Definitions
- Orbital inflammation not due to infection, lymphoproliferative lesions (LPLs), granulomatous diseases, thyroid orbitopathy, vasculitides, or other systemic illnesses

IMAGING FINDINGS

General Features
- Best diagnostic clue: Poorly marginated mass-like enhancing soft tissue involving any area of orbit
- Location: Most commonly involves extraocular muscle (EOM) or lacrimal gland; bilateral in 25% of cases
- Morphology
  ○ May be focally mass-like or diffuse
  ○ Irregular margins, infiltrative features may mimic neoplasm or aggressive infection
- Categorized by area(s) of involvement
  ○ Myositic (EOMs)
    ▪ Most common pattern
    ▪ Any muscle affected, superior complex and medial rectus most frequent
    ▪ Involves tendinous insertions, tubular configuration, shaggy margins
  ○ Lacrimal gland
    ▪ Second most common pattern
    ▪ Diffuse enlargement of gland in AP dimension
    ▪ May be impossible to differentiate from LPLs or sarcoidosis by imaging alone
  ○ Anterior (globe, retrobulbar orbit)
    ▪ Third most common pattern
    ▪ Uveal-scleral (episcleritis or sclerotenonitis): Thickened sclera with shaggy enhancement
    ▪ Variable involvement of retrobulbar fat and nerve
    ▪ Perineuritis (least common type): Irregular nerve sheath thickening and enhancement; differentiate from optic neuritis
  ○ Diffuse (intra-, extraconal, or both)
    ▪ Overlaps with other patterns

DDx: Idiopathic Orbital Inflammatory Disease Mimics

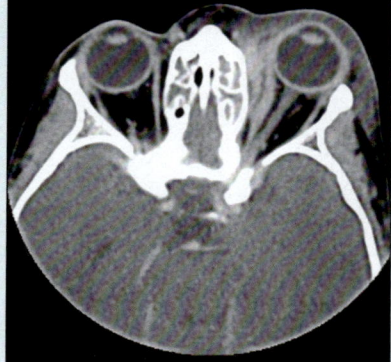

Orbital Cellulitis

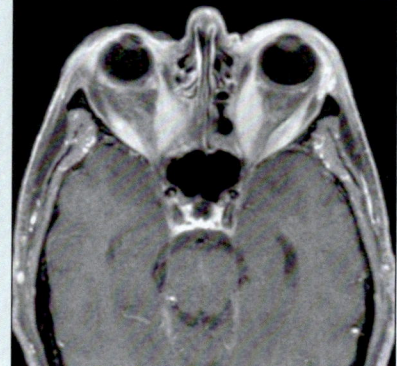

Thyroid Orbitopathy

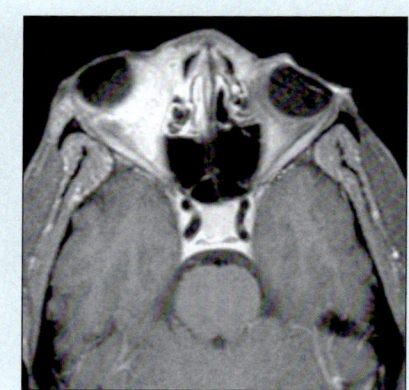

Sarcoidosis

IDIOPATHIC ORBITAL INFLAMMATORY DISEASE

Key Facts

Imaging Findings
- Best diagnostic clue: Poorly marginated mass-like enhancing soft tissue involving any area of orbit
- Myositic (EOMs)
- Lacrimal gland
- Anterior (globe, retrobulbar orbit)
- Diffuse (intra-, extraconal, or both)
- Apical (orbital apex, intracranial extension)

Top Differential Diagnoses
- Thyroid-Associated Orbitopathy
- Sarcoidosis
- Wegener Granulomatosis
- Lymphoproliferative Lesions

Pathology
- Most common painful orbital mass in adults

Clinical Issues
- Proptosis and globe displacement
- Uveitis, sclerotenonitis, retinal detachments
- Cranial nerve palsies (III, IV, V, VI) with Tolosa-Hunt syndrome
- Steroids effective in most patients
- Radiotherapy for nonresponsive or refractory cases or when steroids contraindicated

Diagnostic Checklist
- IOID is diagnosis of exclusion; exclude infectious orbital cellulitis, CCF in acute cases
- Atypical onset or recurrences should prompt biopsy for confirmation

---

  - Frequently mass-like, but tends not to distort globe or erode bone
  - Apical (orbital apex, intracranial extension)
    - Less common; involves orbital apex with posterior extension through fissures
    - Tolosa-Hunt considered intracranial variant of IOID involving cavernous sinus

CT Findings
- NECT
  - Lacrimal, EOM or orbital mass
  - Focal or infiltrative; poorly circumscribed
  - May rarely erode bone
- CECT
  - Moderate diffuse enhancement
  - Dynamic CT: Attenuation increases into late phase (lymphoma's attenuation decreases)

MR Findings
- T1WI: Hypointense to normal muscle
- T2WI: Findings with fat suppression similar to STIR
- STIR
  - Isointense or slightly hyperintense to muscle
  - Hypointense compared to many orbital lesions due to cellular infiltrate ± fibrosis
  - Lower signal portends worse treatment response
- T1 C+: Marked, diffuse, irregular enhancement
- MRA: Tolosa-Hunt may be associated with cavernous ICA narrowing that reverses with effective therapy

Ultrasonographic Findings
- Reduced reflectivity, regular internal echoes, weak attenuation, similar to lymphoproliferative lesions

Imaging Recommendations
- Best imaging tool: Enhanced axial helical CT with coronal reformats
- Protocol advice: T1 C+ FS MR for apical and cavernous sinus disease

DIFFERENTIAL DIAGNOSIS

Orbital Infection
- Adjacent sinusitis or prior orbital trauma, surgery
- Subperiosteal or intraconal phlegmon or abscess

Thyroid-Associated Orbitopathy
- Most patients hyperthyroid
- 80-90% bilateral and more than one muscle, uncommonly painful
- Affects muscle belly, spares tendons

Sarcoidosis
- Multiple organ granulomatous inflammation
- Orbit involvement in 25%, especially lacrimal

Wegener Granulomatosis
- Necrotizing vasculitis (respiratory tract, kidneys)
- Paranasal sinus disease with orbital extension, bone destruction
- Commonly bilateral

Idiopathic Orbital Sclerotic Inflammation
- Similar but distinct entity from IOID
- Often bilateral, may extend into adjacent sinuses
- Fibrosis; very hypointense on T1 and T2 MR

Lymphoproliferative Lesions
- Lymphoid hyperplasia: Benign (reactive) or atypical (borderline)
- Non-Hodgkin lymphoma: Most common malignant orbital tumors in adults
- May involve muscles, lacrimal gland; may be diffuse; 25% bilateral

Carotid Cavernous Fistula (CCF)
- Pulsatile exophthalmos, chemosis, orbital bruit, usually not acutely painful
- Direct (traumatic ICA tear, ruptured cavernous ICA aneurysm) or indirect (dural AVM) fistula
- Enlarged orbital veins and cavernous sinus(es) with signal voids on MR, no discrete orbital mass

IDIOPATHIC ORBITAL INFLAMMATORY DISEASE

PATHOLOGY

General Features
- General path comments: Polymorphous infiltration of inflammatory cells with variable fibrosis
- Etiology: Pathogenesis unknown; probably related to underlying immune-mediated processes
- Epidemiology
  - Most common painful orbital mass in adults
  - 5% of all orbital lesions, third most common orbital disorder after thyroid orbitopathy and LPLs
- Associated abnormalities
  - Secondary angle-closure glaucoma
  - Autoimmune disorders: Crohn disease, SLE, RA, IDDM, myasthenia gravis, ankylosing spondylitis
  - Churg-Strauss syndrome

Gross Pathologic & Surgical Features
- Typically soft, compressible mass
- Occasionally hard, fibrotic; particularly chronic

Microscopic Features
- Acute: Mixed population of lymphocytes, plasma cells, macrophages, eosinophils
- Chronic: Lymphoid follicles with germinal centers in background of fibrosis

CLINICAL ISSUES

Presentation
- Most common signs/symptoms: Acute to subacute onset of orbital pain, inflammation, edema, restricted eye motion, diplopia, proptosis
- Other signs/symptoms: Impaired vision (perineuritis)
- Clinical Profile
  - Myositic
    - Proptosis, lid swelling, chemosis
    - Diplopia; painful limitation of ocular movement
    - Conjunctival injection at muscle insertions
  - Lacrimal
    - Enlarged, tender gland
    - Proptosis and globe displacement
    - More likely to have systemic disorder (50%)
  - Anterior
    - Proptosis, ptosis, lid swelling, injection
    - Uveitis, sclerotenonitis, retinal detachments
    - Decreased vision and limited movement
    - More likely in younger patients
  - Apical
    - Milder signs of inflammation
    - Decreased vision; optic neuropathy
    - Cranial nerve palsies (III, IV, V, VI) with Tolosa-Hunt syndrome

Demographics
- Age
  - Any age may be affected; mean in 5th decade
  - More commonly bilateral in children
- Gender: M = F overall, except myositic form (2:1 F:M)

Natural History & Prognosis
- Intermittent disease more likely in younger patients
- 5-10% resolve spontaneously
- Steroids effective in most patients
  - Dramatic and rapid improvement typical in majority
  - No response in 15%, recurrence after initial response in 25%
- Pattern of involvement affects prognosis
  - Recurrence, associated systemic disorder more likely with multiple muscles, bilateral disease
  - Systemic association in up to half with lacrimal disease, particularly if chronic or tumefactive
  - Negative visual outcome more likely in apical and diffuse disease
- Chronic sclerosing disease not as responsive, but therapy may slow progression

Treatment
- Systemic steroids are first-line therapy
- Radiotherapy for nonresponsive or refractory cases or when steroids contraindicated
- Immunosuppressive chemotherapy (e.g., Methotrexate) for recalcitrant cases

DIAGNOSTIC CHECKLIST

Consider
- IOID is diagnosis of exclusion; exclude infectious orbital cellulitis, CCF in acute cases
- Consider other systemic causes with bilateral, multifocal, lacrimal, and apical involvement
- Atypical onset or recurrences should prompt biopsy for confirmation

Image Interpretation Pearls
- Isolated lateral rectus enlargement is most likely IOID, essentially never thyroid orbitopathy

SELECTED REFERENCES

1. Gordon LK: Diagnostic dilemmas in orbital inflammatory disease. Ocul Immunol Inflamm. 11(1):3-15, 2003
2. Yuen SJ et al: Idiopathic orbital inflammation: distribution, clinical features, and treatment outcome. Arch Ophthalmol. 121(4):491-9, 2003
3. Jacobs D et al: Diagnosis and management of orbital pseudotumor. Curr Opin Ophthalmol. 13(6):347-51, 2002
4. Wasmeier C et al: Idiopathic inflammatory pseudotumor of the orbit and Tolosa-Hunt syndrome--are they the same disease? J Neurol. 249(9):1237-41, 2002
5. Yuen SJ et al: Idiopathic orbital inflammation: ocular mechanisms and clinicopathology. Ophthalmol Clin North Am. 15(1):121-6, 2002
6. Bernardino CR et al: Angle-closure glaucoma in association with orbital pseudotumor. Ophthalmology. 108(9):1603-6, 2001
7. Smith JR et al: A role for methotrexate in the management of non-infectious orbital inflammatory disease. Br J Ophthalmol. 85(10):1220-4, 2001
8. Maalouf T et al: What has become of our idiopathic inflammatory pseudo-tumors of the orbit? Orbit. 18(3):157-166, 1999
9. Weber AL et al: Pseudotumor of the orbit. Clinical, pathologic, and radiologic evaluation. Radiol Clin North Am. 37(1):151-68, xi, 1999
10. Rootman J et al: Idiopathic sclerosing inflammation of the orbit. A distinct clinicopathologic entity. Ophthalmology. 101(3):570-84, 1994

IDIOPATHIC ORBITAL INFLAMMATORY DISEASE

IMAGE GALLERY

Typical

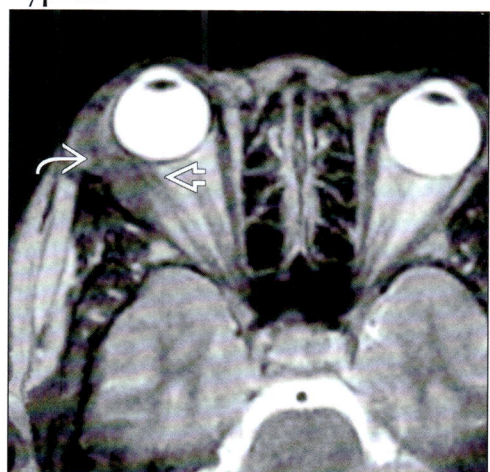
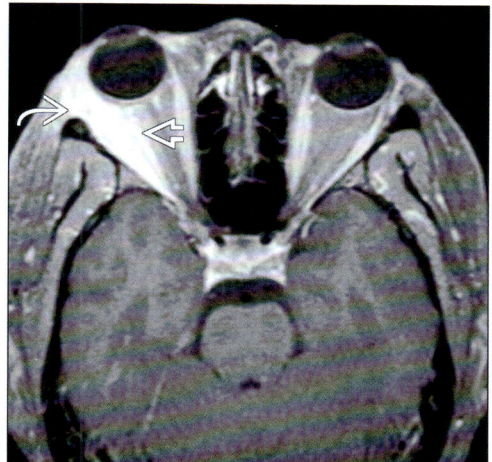

(Left) Axial T2WI MR shows enlarged, poorly marginated hypointense right lacrimal gland ➡ (dacryoadenitis). Inflammatory process extends to adjacent lateral rectus muscle ➡. *(Right)* Axial T1 C+ FS MR in the same patient as previous image, shows intense poorly marginated enhancing lacrimal gland ➡ and contiguous right lateral rectus muscle ➡. Combined myositis and dacryoadenitis.

Variant

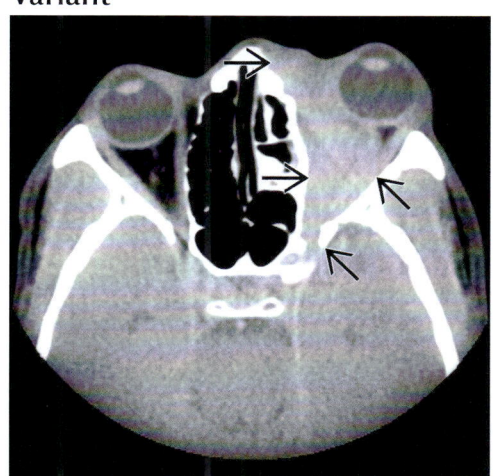
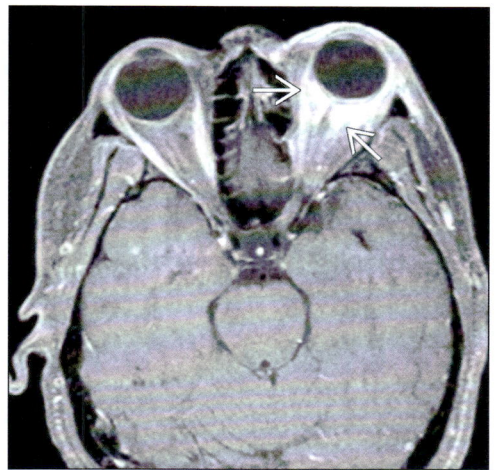

(Left) Axial CECT shows mass nearly filling left orbit from preseptal region to orbital apex ➡ (diffuse orbital pseudotumor). Despite proptosis, left ocular shape is preserved. *(Right)* Axial T1 C+ FS MR shows marked "shaggy" enhancement of Tenon capsule and anterior optic nerve sheath ➡ on left, as well as left-sided proptosis. Episcleritis and perineuritis.

Variant

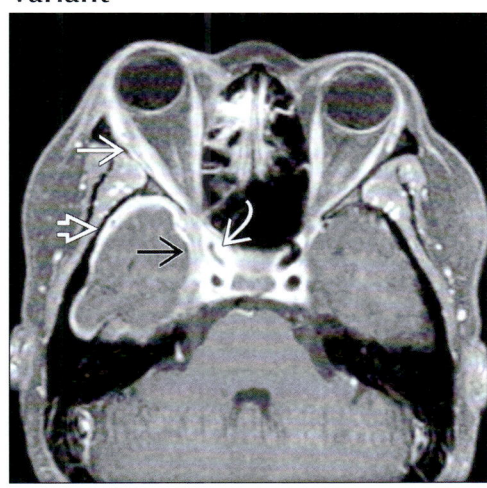
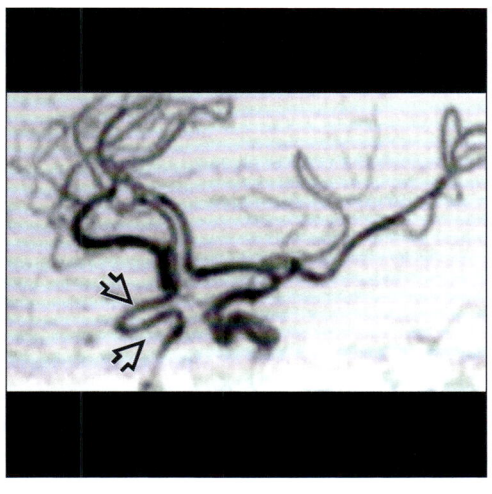

(Left) Axial T1 C+ FS MR shows enlarged right lateral rectus ➡, widened right cavernous sinus ➡. Note thickened middle fossa dura ➡ and narrow RICA ➡. Tolosa-Hunt syndrome. *(Right)* Left anterior oblique MRA in the same patient as previous image, shows cavernous, supraclinoid RICA narrowing ➡, associated with right-sided Tolosa-Hunt syndrome.

SUBPERIOSTEAL ABSCESS, ORBIT

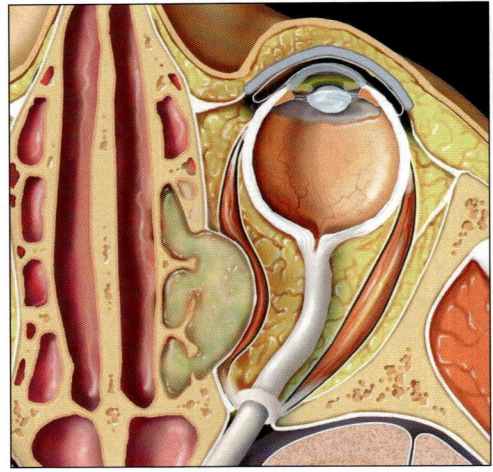

Coronal graphic depicts infection spread from ethmoid sinuses through lamina papyracea into medial orbit. Subperiosteal abscess results, putting optic nerve at risk.

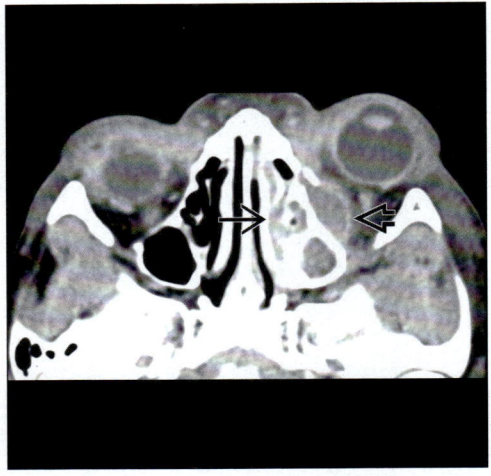

Axial CECT shows left medial orbital subperiosteal abscess ➡. Note adjacent ethmoid and maxillary sinusitis ➡.

TERMINOLOGY

Abbreviations and Synonyms
- Orbital subperiosteal abscess (SPA)

Definitions
- Pus accumulation between bony orbital wall, periorbita

IMAGING FINDINGS

General Features
- Best diagnostic clue: Lentiform, rim-enhancing collection in medial orbit with adjacent sinusitis
- Location
  - Medial extraconal orbit, along lamina papyracea
  - Lateral or posterior extension with progression

CT Findings
- NECT
  - Confluent density in medial orbit
  - Ethmoid ± maxillary sinus opacification
  - Inflammatory stranding of orbital fat ("dirty fat")
  - Gas in collection suggests anaerobes
  - Bone CT: Demineralization of lamina papyracea
- CECT
  - Rim-enhancing hypodense fluid collection
  - Prominently enhancing paranasal sinus mucosa
  - Enhancing swollen extraocular muscles
  - Lateral margin of abscess bordered by enhancing periosteum and displaced lateral rectus

MR Findings
- T1WI
  - Hypodense fluid signal in abscess
  - Moderately hypointense inflammatory changes
- T2WI
  - Similar to STIR if T2WI FS MR
  - Fat obscures findings unless suppressed
- STIR
  - Hyperintense fluid signal in abscess
  - Hyperintense edema in adjacent fat
- T1 C+
  - Rim-enhancing fluid collection in medial orbit
  - Intraorbital and periorbital enhancement

DDx: Mimics of Subperiosteal Abscess

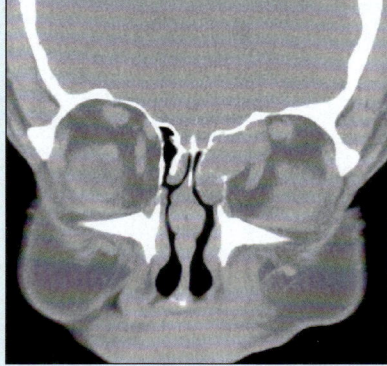

Mucocele

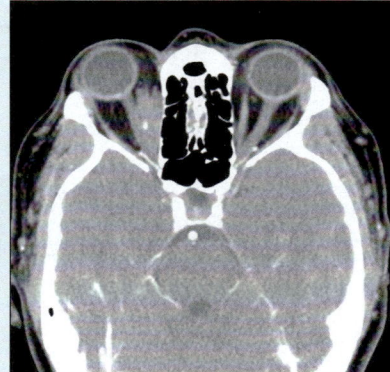

Lymphangioma

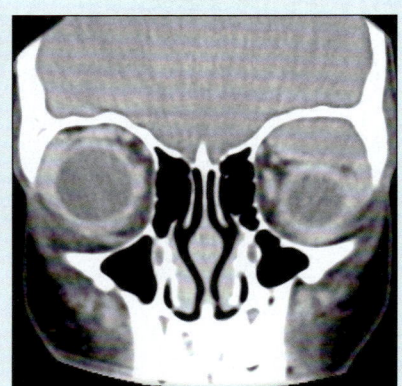

Subperiosteal Hematoma

SUBPERIOSTEAL ABSCESS, ORBIT

Key Facts

Imaging Findings
- Best diagnostic clue: Lentiform, rim-enhancing collection in medial orbit with adjacent sinusitis
- Bone CT: Demineralization of lamina papyracea
- Best imaging tool: CECT
- Enhanced MR for potential intracranial complications

Top Differential Diagnoses
- Lymphangioma
- Dermoid Cyst
- Dacryocystocele
- Mucocele (Ethmoid)
- Subperiosteal Hematoma

Pathology
- Secondary to acute sinusitis, particularly ethmoid
- Hematogenous transmission of bacteria through valveless orbital veins
- Orbital complications in 3% of sinusitis

Clinical Issues
- Most common signs/symptoms: Orbital edema, painful proptosis with fever
- IV antibiotics with drainage when indicated results in excellent prognosis in most cases

Diagnostic Checklist
- Requires immediate attention (may cause blindness)
- Improvement on CT may lag behind clinical picture
- Orbit disease may be first sign of sinusitis in children
- Gas in collection suggests anaerobic infection (exclusion criterion for non-surgical management in some centers)

Ultrasonographic Findings
- Fusiform collection between bone and highly reflective periosteum, adjacent to muscle

Imaging Recommendations
- Best imaging tool: CECT
- Protocol advice
  - Thin slice (≤ 1 mm) axial helical CECT, coronal planar reconstructions, bone & soft tissue algorithm
  - Enhanced MR for potential intracranial complications

DIFFERENTIAL DIAGNOSIS

Lymphangioma
- Congenital malformation of lymphatic vessels
- Poorly marginated cystic mass, irregular enhancement, fluid-fluid levels

Dermoid Cyst
- Developmental epithelial inclusion cyst
- Typically lateral; may be medial (25%)
- Pathognomic if fat-density (50%)
- Inflammatory changes if ruptured

Dacryocystocele
- Nasolacrimal imperforation or obstruction
- Fluid-signal mass in enlarged lacrimal fossa and canal

Mucocele (Ethmoid)
- Long-standing obstruction; inspissated secretions
- Expanded sinus; contents vary from fluid to concretion

Subperiosteal Hematoma
- Post-traumatic, post-surgical, or post-partum
- Similar CT appearance to abscess, less-associated inflammation

Other Pediatric Orbital Diseases
- Orbital pseudotumor: Any area of orbit; painful proptosis without fever or leukocytosis
- Orbital rhabdomyosarcoma: Inflammatory changes at presentation (25%)

PATHOLOGY

General Features
- General path comments
  - Secondary to acute sinusitis, particularly ethmoid
  - Uncommonly due to trauma, bacteremia, skin infection
- Etiology
  - Microbiology
    - Under 10 years old: Commonly single aerobes
    - 10-15 years old: Mixed, mostly aerobes
    - Over 15 years old: Mixed aerobes and anaerobes
  - Pathogenesis of abscess
    - Ethmoid sinusitis induces periostitis
    - Relatively avascular subperiosteal space limits antibiotic penetration
    - Pus may rapidly accumulate in subperiosteal space
    - Development of orbital phlegmon; orbital cellulitis may precede abscess
  - Mechanisms of spread from sinus into orbit
    - Hematogenous transmission of bacteria through valveless orbital veins
    - Direct extension through congenital or acquired dehiscence in lamina papyracea
- Epidemiology
  - Orbital complications in 3% of sinusitis
  - Abscess represents 20% of orbital complications
- Associated abnormalities
  - Cystic fibrosis, ciliary dyskinesia
  - Mechanical sinonasal obstruction

Gross Pathologic & Surgical Features
- Pocket of yellow-green fluid in expanded space between bone and periosteum

Microscopic Features
- Necrotic debris with inflammatory cells, microorganisms

SUBPERIOSTEAL ABSCESS, ORBIT

Staging, Grading or Classification Criteria
- Chandler classification of sinus-related orbital disease (does not imply order of disease progression)
  - 85%: I (preseptal cellulitis) and II (orbital cellulitis)
  - 15%: III (subperiosteal) and IV (orbital abscess)
  - Rare: V (cavernous sinus thrombosis)

CLINICAL ISSUES

Presentation
- Most common signs/symptoms: Orbital edema, painful proptosis with fever
- Clinical Profile
  - Sinusitis, upper respiratory infection, fever
  - Eye swelling, erythema, gaze restriction
  - Visual disturbance in 15-30%
    - Optic neuritis due to intraconal extension; may occur with minimal orbital signs
    - Ischemia related to increased intraorbital pressure
    - Retinal ischemia from central artery occlusion or thrombophlebitis

Demographics
- Age: Orbital complications of sinusitis more common in children than adults

Natural History & Prognosis
- Rapidly progressive, potentially blinding disease
- IV antibiotics with drainage when indicated results in excellent prognosis in most cases
- Progression leads to intraorbital abscess
  - Increased proptosis, increased pressure
  - Worsening vision, ophthalmoplegia
- May lead to blindness if untreated (up to 10%)
- Other complications
  - Superior ophthalmic vein thrombosis
  - Cavernous sinus thrombosis; rare but devastating
    - High morbidity
    - Bilateral cranial neuropathies, CNS signs
  - Intracranial extension
    - Spread through diploic vessels
    - Meningitis, subdural empyema, cerebritis, brain abscess

Treatment
- Under 10 years: Antibiotics alone often adequate
- 10-15 years: May respond to antibiotics alone
- Over 15 years: Generally require surgical draining
- Medical therapy (IV antibiotics)
  - Antibiotics without surgery appropriate in about 25% of patients
    - Children under 10-15 years
    - Without visual signs, other surgical indications
    - Phlegmon without abscess
  - Antibiotic regimen
    - Broad polymicrobial coverage
    - 2nd or 3rd generation cephalosporins, β-lactamase-resistant penicillin combinations, carbapenems
    - Add clindamycin for anaerobe coverage, particularly over 10-15 years old
- Surgical indications
  - Emergent (immediate drainage): Optic nerve or retinal compromise; intracranial involvement
  - Urgent (antibiotics alone contraindicated)
    - Age over 10-15 years; immunocompromised
    - Visual compromise
    - Superior or inferior extension of abscess
    - Frontal sinus origin
    - Disproportionate pain
  - Expectant (after failed medical therapy)
    - Visual changes at any time
    - Persistent fever after 36 hours
    - Clinical deterioration after 48 hours
    - No improvement after 72 hours
- Surgical options
  - Endoscopic drainage: Small abscesses in medial orbit
  - Direct external drainage: Larger abscesses; abscesses extending along roof or floor of orbit
  - Transcaruncular approach: Alternative to direct orbital, alone or with endoscopy

DIAGNOSTIC CHECKLIST

Consider
- Requires immediate attention (may cause blindness)
- Serial CTs helpful for monitoring response, but with increased lens dose
- Improvement on CT may lag behind clinical picture
- Orbit disease may be first sign of sinusitis in children

Image Interpretation Pearls
- Gas in collection suggests anaerobic infection (exclusion criterion for non-surgical management in some centers)

SELECTED REFERENCES
1. Pelton RW et al: Cosmetic considerations in surgery for orbital subperiosteal abscess in children. Arch Otolaryngol Head Neck Surg. 129(6):652-5, 2003
2. Rahbar R et al: Management of orbital subperiosteal abscess in children. Arch Otolaryngol Head Neck Surg. 127(3):281-6, 2001
3. Garcia GH et al: Criteria for nonsurgical management of subperiosteal abscess of the orbit: analysis of outcomes 1988-1998. Ophthalmology. 107(8):1454-6; discussion 1457-8, 2000
4. Curtin HD et al: Extension to the orbit from paraorbital disease. The sinuses. Radiol Clin North Am. 36(6):1201-13, xi, 1998
5. Pereira KD et al: Management of medial subperiosteal abscess of the orbit in children--a 5 year experience. Int J Pediatr Otorhinolaryngol. 38(3):247-54, 1997
6. Harris GJ: Subperiosteal abscess of the orbit. Age as a factor in the bacteriology and response to treatment. Ophthalmology. 101(3):585-95, 1994
7. Arjmand EM et al: Pediatric sinusitis and subperiosteal orbital abscess formation: diagnosis and treatment. Otolaryngol Head Neck Surg. 109(5):886-94, 1993
8. Patt BS et al: Blindness resulting from orbital complications of sinusitis. Otolaryngol Head Neck Surg. 104(6):789-95, 1991
9. Chandler JR et al: The pathogenesis of orbital complications in acute sinusitis. Laryngoscope. 80(9):1414-28, 1970

SUBPERIOSTEAL ABSCESS, ORBIT

IMAGE GALLERY

Typical

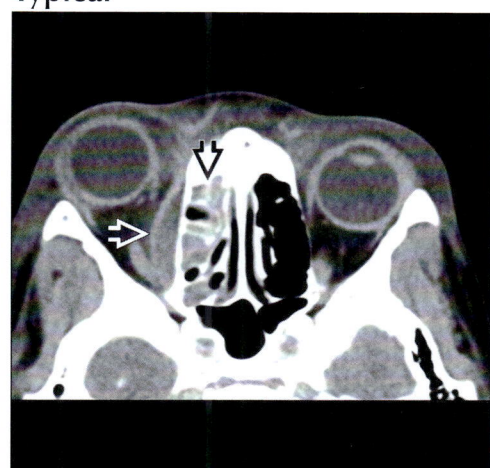
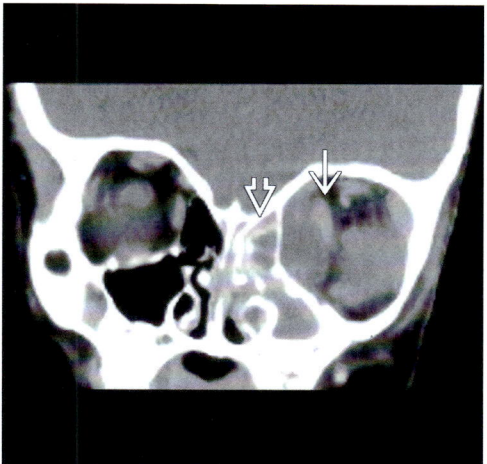

(Left) Axial CECT shows right medial subperiosteal orbital abscess ➡ associated with ethmoid sinusitis ➡. *(Right)* Coronal CECT shows ethmoid and maxillary sinusitis ➡ complicated by large left medial subperiosteal abscess. Medial rectus ➡ is displaced laterally by abscess.

Variant

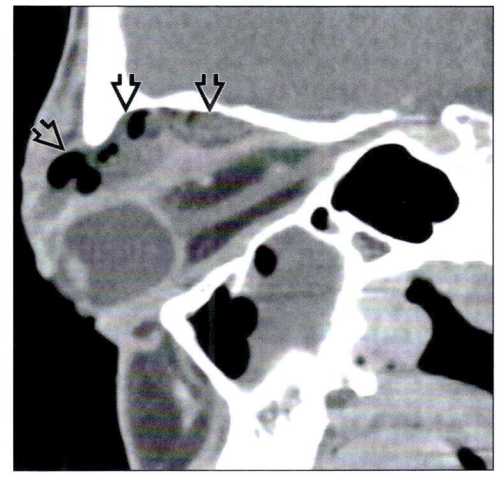
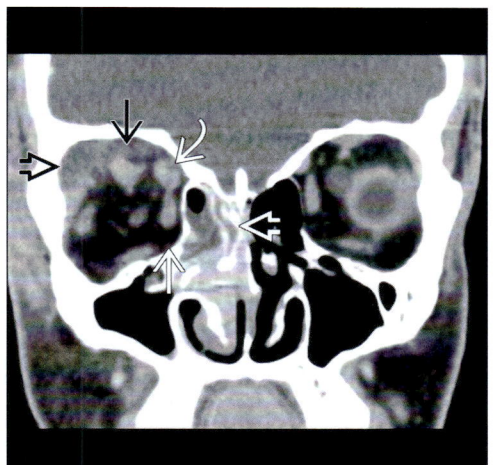

(Left) Sagittal oblique CECT shows depression of globe and muscle cone by superiorly located gas-containing abscess ➡. Patient had ipsilateral frontal, ethmoid, and maxillary sinusitis. *(Right)* Coronal CECT shows superior subperiosteal abscess ➡, ethmoid sinusitis ➡. Note depression of superior muscle complex ➡, superior oblique muscle ➡, normal medial orbital fat ➡.

Variant

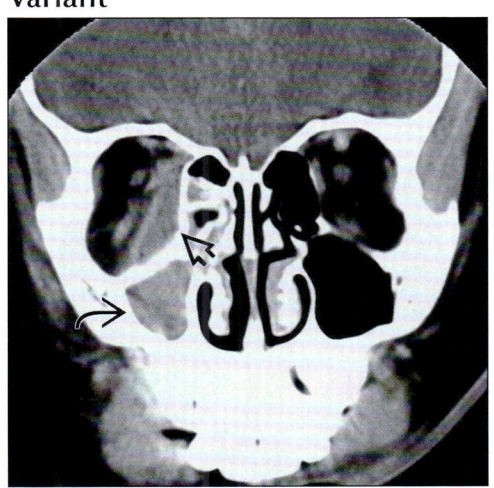
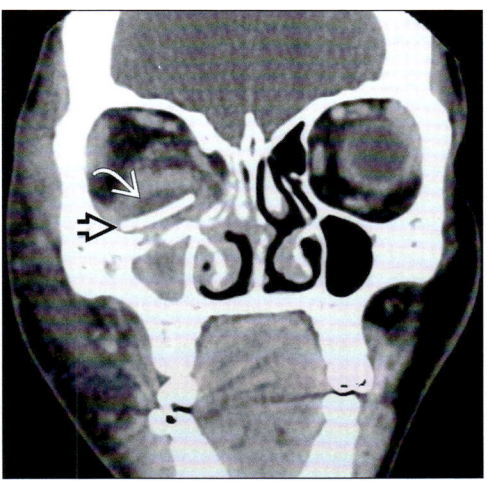

(Left) Coronal CECT of subperiosteal orbital abscess ➡ complicating maxillary sinusitis ➡, with only mild ethmoid disease. Most cases result from ethmoid sinusitis. *(Right)* Coronal CECT shows abscess ➡ surrounding infected prosthesis ➡ surgically implanted to repair orbital floor fracture.

ACUTE RHINOSINUSITIS

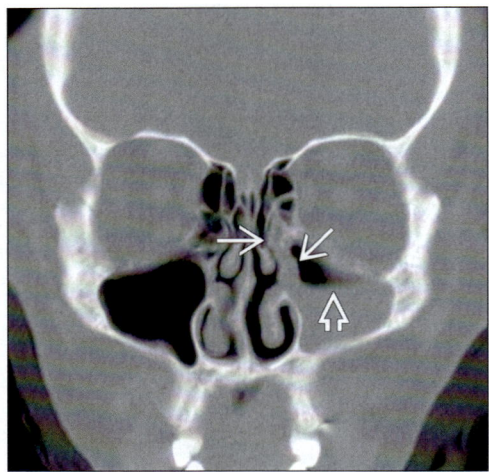

Coronal NECT shows left maxillary sinus air-fluid level ⮕ and mucosal thickening occluding left ethmoid infundibulum and hiatus semilunaris ⮕.

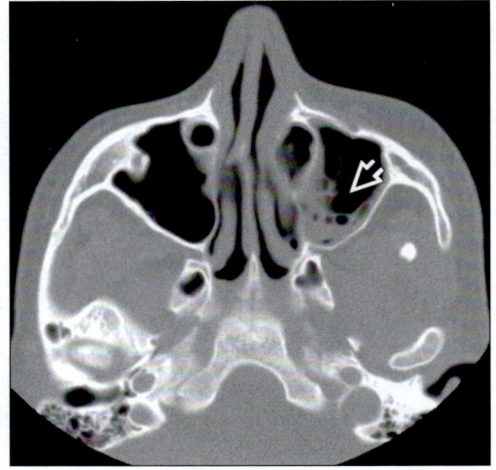

Axial NECT shows "bubbly" left maxillary sinus luminal contents ⮕ in a patient with left maxillary sinusitis.

TERMINOLOGY

Abbreviations and Synonyms
- Acute rhinosinusitis (ARS)
- Acute bacterial rhinosinusitis (ABRS)

Definitions
- ARS: Acute inflammatory process of sinonasal mucosa lasting ≤ 4 weeks

IMAGING FINDINGS

General Features
- Best diagnostic clue: Air-fluid level, bubbly or strandy-appearing secretions within sinus with mucosal thickening
- Location: Most common in ethmoid, maxillary sinuses
- Size
  - Normal sinus lumen size
    - No expansion (mucocele) or reduced volume (chronic rhinosinusitis)

Radiographic Findings
- Radiography
  - Mucosal thickening, opacification of sinus
  - Air-fluid level in maxillary sinus; difficult to identify in other sinuses
  - Inaccurate in assessing extent of inflammation, particularly in ethmoid, frontal & sphenoid sinuses

CT Findings
- NECT
  - Air-fluid level, bubbly or strandy-appearing secretions
  - Mucosal thickening
  - Inflammatory tissue obstructing drainage pathways of ostiomeatal complex (OMC)
- CECT
  - Enhancement of inflamed mucosa
  - Central secretions do not enhance

MR Findings
- T1WI
  - Mucosal thickening isointense to other soft tissues
  - Fluid signal layering within sinus

DDx: Opacified Sinus, Facial Discomfort

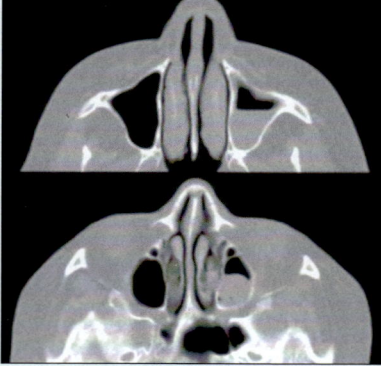

Mucus Retention Cyst

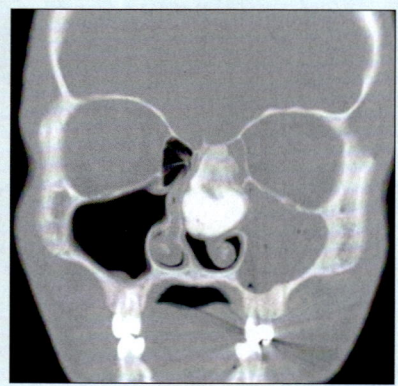

Obstructed Secretions (Osteoma)

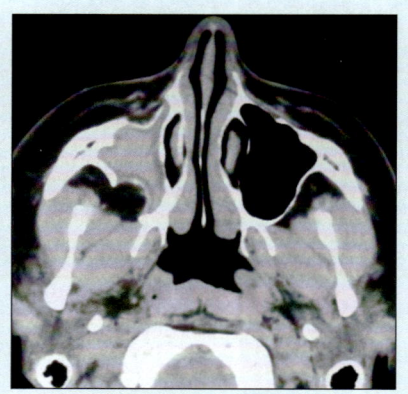

Silent Sinus Syndrome

ACUTE RHINOSINUSITIS

Key Facts

Terminology
- Acute rhinosinusitis (ARS)
- ARS: Acute inflammatory process of sinonasal mucosa lasting ≤ 4 weeks

Imaging Findings
- Best diagnostic clue: Air-fluid level, bubbly or strandy-appearing secretions within sinus with mucosal thickening
- Location: Most common in ethmoid, maxillary sinuses
- Diagnosis often made clinically without imaging
- CT: Confirm diagnosis, evaluate for complications, anatomic variants, masses
- Axial helical CT ≤ 1 mm slice thickness with coronal, sagittal reconstructions to evaluate OMC and frontal recess, respectively

Top Differential Diagnoses
- "Pseudo" Fluid Level
- Post-Traumatic Blood Level
- Post-Obstructive Secretions

Pathology
- Most cases of ARS follow viral upper respiratory infections (URI)

Clinical Issues
- Symptoms: Nasal congestion & purulent discharge, facial pain/pressure, headache, olfactory dysfunction, fever, cough

Diagnostic Checklist
- Look for signs of invasive fungal sinusitis if immunocompromised patient

---

- Serous secretions increase in signal with elevated protein content
- Air, cortical bone appear as signal voids
- T2WI
  - Fluid & mucosal thickening hyperintense
  - Serous secretions decrease in signal with elevated protein content/inspissation
- T1 C+
  - Enhancement of inflamed peripheral mucosa
  - Central secretions do not enhance

Imaging Recommendations
- Best imaging tool
  - Diagnosis often made clinically without imaging
  - CT: Confirm diagnosis, evaluate for complications, anatomic variants, masses
  - MR: Useful to evaluate for orbital or intracranial complications, fungal disease, neoplasm
- Protocol advice
  - Axial helical CT ≤ 1 mm slice thickness with coronal, sagittal reconstructions to evaluate OMC and frontal recess, respectively
  - Axial plane useful for evaluating sphenoid & posterior ethmoid regions, posterior wall of frontal sinus

DIFFERENTIAL DIAGNOSIS

"Pseudo" Fluid Level
- Flaccid mucus retention cyst (MRC) mimics air-fluid level
- Fluid level not persistent through entire sinus; rounded edge usually found

Post-Traumatic Blood Level
- Increased attenuation of blood
- Associated sinus wall fractures

Post-Obstructive Secretions
- Lesion obstructs sinus drainage pathway, trapping fluid

- Mass may be increased density compared to trapped fluid on NECT
- Tumor enhances on CECT
- MR easily differentiates tumor from obstructed secretions

Silent Sinus Syndrome
- Chronic maxillary sinus atelectasis with painless enophthalmos, diplopia, facial asymmetry
- Due to infundibular occlusion, uncinate process displaced laterally against inferomedial orbital wall
- Middle meatus enlarged, sinus appears "imploded"

PATHOLOGY

General Features
- Genetics: Cystic fibrosis (autosomal recessive disorder) predisposes to rhinosinusitis
- Etiology
  - Most cases of ARS follow viral upper respiratory infections (URI)
    - Viral symptoms usually improve in 7-10 days; symptoms > 10 days or worsening after 5-7 days suggest bacterial disease
    - May be caused by vasomotor dysfunction or associated with physical or barotrauma
    - Common organisms: Streptococcus pneumonia, Haemophilus influenzae, Moraxella catarrhalis
  - URI ⇒ mucosal swelling ⇒ sinus outflow obstruction ⇒ infection
  - Other important cause: Odontogenic sinusitis (erosion of dental periapical granuloma or abscess into sinus)
- Epidemiology
  - Common cold causes viral RS; 90% of patients with colds have viral or bacterial RS
  - > 1 billion cases of viral & bacterial RS annually in US
- Associated abnormalities
  - Allergies, immunoglobulin deficiency, immotile cilia syndrome, cystic fibrosis
  - Anatomic abnormalities

ACUTE RHINOSINUSITIS

- Septal deviation & spurs, uncinate process, middle turbinate, frontal recess, anterior ethmoid anatomic variants

Gross Pathologic & Surgical Features
- Edematous, erythematous mucosa with ostial obstruction, purulent secretions

Microscopic Features
- Tissue-invasive bacteria
- Luminal exudate of neutrophils, eosinophils
- Microabscess formation, epithelial degeneration
- Mucosal infiltration with lymphocytes, neutrophils, plasma cells
- Interleukins 1, 6, & 8 present in exudate

Staging, Grading or Classification Criteria
- Can be classified according to etiology: Viral, bacterial, vasomotor

CLINICAL ISSUES

Presentation
- Most common signs/symptoms
  - Symptoms: Nasal congestion & purulent discharge, facial pain/pressure, headache, olfactory dysfunction, fever, cough
  - Signs: Facial swelling & erythema, nasal turbinate edema, nasal crusting, purulent nasal cavity/pharynx
    - Worst in morning, improves as patient is upright, symptoms worsen when bending over
- Other signs/symptoms
  - Maxillary: Infraorbital, cheek, upper teeth or gum pain
  - Ethmoid: Lacrimal, periorbital or temporal region tenderness
  - Frontal: Headache localized to forehead, supraorbital region
  - Sphenoid: Pain radiates to occiput ± skull vertex; infection near cavernous sinus may cause CN2-4, V1, V2 or 6 dysfunction
- Clinical Profile: Pediatric or adult patient with nasal discharge & obstruction frequently following viral URI; lasting ≤ 4 weeks
- Laboratory results
  - Nasal cultures nonspecific, often contaminated with S. aureus
  - Endoscopic paranasal sinus aspiration more specific

Demographics
- Age
  - Typically follows viral URI in children
    - Lack of previous exposure to viruses that attack upper respiratory tract, proximity of mucosal surfaces, small size of ostia

Natural History & Prognosis
- Usually self-limited if viral
- Bacterial ARS course may be shortened by medical therapy, surgical drainage
- Untreated bacterial ARS may become complicated

  - Orbital cellulitis, subperiosteal abscess, meningitis, subdural empyema, brain abscess, venous sinus thrombosis

Treatment
- Medical therapy
  - Saline nasal sprays & irrigants, mucolytics
  - Topical steroids
  - Decongestants, antihistamines, antibiotics
- Surgical therapy
  - More often performed for chronic RS
  - Drainage procedures performed in acute disease (frontal and sphenoid) to prevent development of complications

DIAGNOSTIC CHECKLIST

Consider
- Use ≤ 1 mm axial CT scans; coronal and sagittal reformations
- CT cannot differentiate viral from bacterial disease
- High incidence of sinus CT abnormalities in asymptomatic patients

Image Interpretation Pearls
- Fluid levels are most specific indicator in absence of recent nasal lavage or presence of NG tube
- Normal nasal mucosal cycle may be impossible to distinguish from ARS mucosal thickening on MR
- Look for signs of invasive fungal sinusitis if immunocompromised patient

SELECTED REFERENCES

1. Anand VK: Epidemiology and economic impact of rhinosinusitis. Ann Otol Rhinol Laryngol Suppl. 193:3-5, 2004
2. Kaplan BA et al: Diagnosis and pathology of unilateral maxillary sinus opacification with or without evidence of contralateral disease. Laryngoscope. 114(6):981-5, 2004
3. Piccirillo JF: Clinical practice. Acute bacterial sinusitis. N Engl J Med. 351(9):902-10, 2004
4. Zinreich SJ: Imaging for staging of rhinosinusitis. Ann Otol Rhinol Laryngol Suppl. 193:19-23, 2004
5. Aalokken TM et al: Conventional sinus radiography compared with CT in the diagnosis of acute sinusitis. Dentomaxillofac Radiol. 32(1):60-2, 2003
6. Reider JM et al: Do imaging studies aid diagnosis of acute sinusitis? J Fam Pract. 52(7):565-7; discussion 567, 2003
7. Illner A et al: The silent sinus syndrome: clinical and radiographic findings. AJR Am J Roentgenol. 178(2):503-6, 2002
8. Kenny TJ et al: Prospective analysis of sinus symptoms and correlation with paranasal computed tomography scan. Otolaryngol Head Neck Surg. 125(1):40-3, 2001
9. Varonen H et al: Comparison of ultrasound, radiography, and clinical examination in the diagnosis of acute maxillary sinusitis: a systematic review. J Clin Epidemiol. 53(9):940-8, 2000
10. Larson TL: Sinonasal inflammatory disease: pathophysiology, imaging, and surgery. Semin Ultrasound CT MR. 20(6):379-90, 1999
11. Thorp MA et al: Complicated acute sinusitis and the computed tomography anatomy of the ostiomeatal unit in childhood. Int J Pediatr Otorhinolaryngol. 49(3):189-95, 1999

ACUTE RHINOSINUSITIS

IMAGE GALLERY

Typical

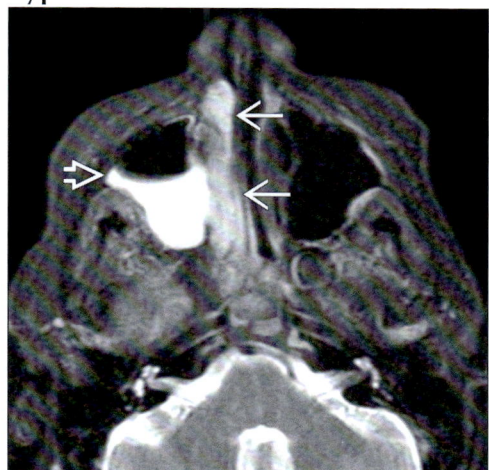
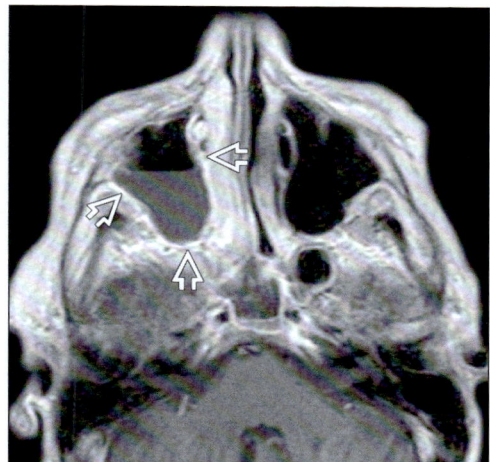

(Left) Axial T2WI FS MR shows air-fluid level in right maxillary sinus ➡, with swelling of right nasal turbinate mucosa ➡. *(Right)* Axial T1 C+ MR shows prominent enhancement of inflamed right maxillary sinus mucosa ➡.

Variant

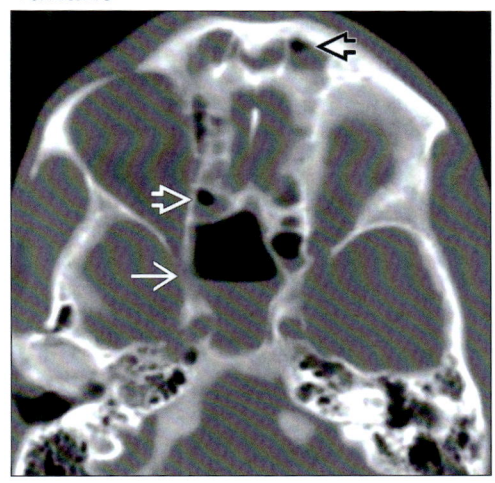
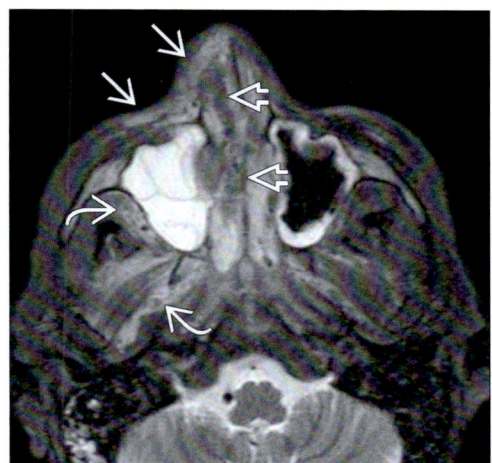

(Left) Axial NECT shows "pansinusitis" in HIV-positive patient. Note air-fluid levels in frontal ➡, ethmoid ➡, and sphenoid ➡ sinuses. *(Right)* Axial T2WI FS MR shows mucosal thickening in right antrum, edema in skin ➡ and infratemporal fossa ➡. Nasal fungal disease appears hypointense ➡. Invasive fungal sinusitis.

Variant

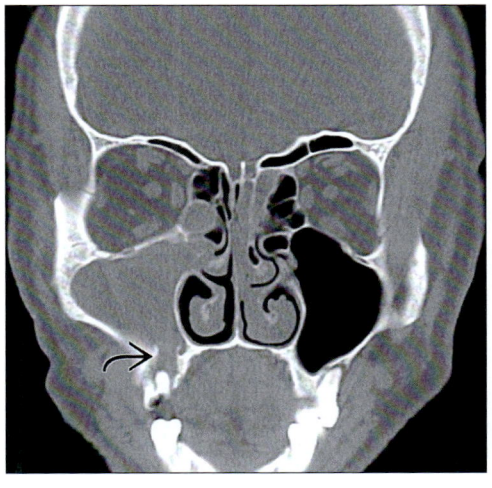
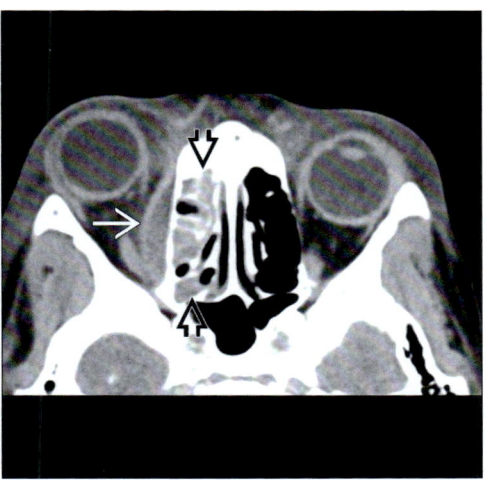

(Left) Coronal NECT shows right maxillary sinusitis associated with carious right maxillary tooth. Periapical dental abscess has eroded into alveolar recess ➡ producing "apical sinusitis". *(Right)* Axial CECT shows right ethmoid sinusitis ➡ in a child, complicated by medial subperiosteal abscess ➡. Orbital disease may be first symptom of sinusitis in children.

FUNGAL SINUSITIS, INVASIVE

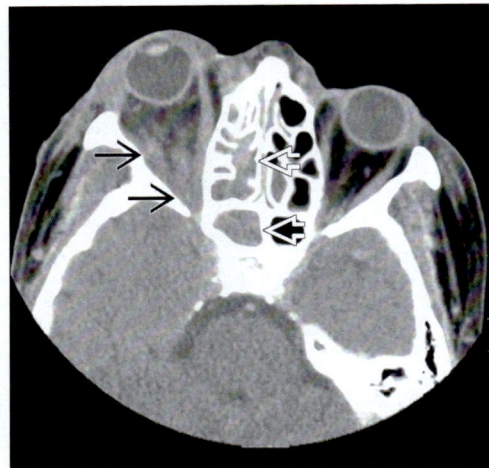

Axial CECT shows right orbital apical soft-tissue density ➡, right ethmoid & sphenoid opacification ⇨ in a patient with acute leukemia and acute invasive Mucor sinusitis.

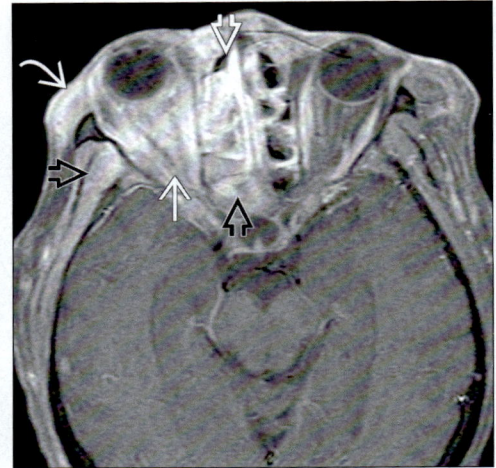

Axial T1 C+ FS MR in same patient as previous image shows diffusely enhancing right orbital contents ➡, periorbital soft tissues ➡, temporalis muscle ➡, ethmoid & sphenoid sinus mucosa ➡.

TERMINOLOGY

Abbreviations and Synonyms
- Invasive fungal sinusitis (IFS)

Definitions
- Acute/fulminant (focus of this chapter): Rapidly progressive fungal infection of sinuses; infection crosses mucosa to involve blood vessels, bone, adjacent soft tissues, orbit, intracranial cavities
- Chronic: Dense hyphal accumulation resembling mycetoma (from which it may arise), associated with orbital apex syndrome, diabetes mellitus, corticosteroid therapy
- Granulomatous: Rarely seen in US; indolent but profuse fungal growth with noncaseating granulomas

IMAGING FINDINGS

General Features
- Best diagnostic clue: Sinus opacification with focal bone erosion, adjacent soft tissue infiltration
- Location
  - Most common in maxillary & ethmoid sinuses followed by sphenoid sinus
  - Spread from sinuses can extend in any direction
    - Laterally into masticator space-infratemporal fossa
    - Posteriorly into pterygopalatine fossa
    - Laterally (ethmoid) or superiorly (maxillary) into orbit
    - Via venous or arterial connections into intracranial cavity
- Morphology: Ill-defined soft-tissue involvement

CT Findings
- NECT
  - Complete or partial soft-tissue opacification of affected sinus; mucosal thickening
  - Hyperattenuation of secretions suggests fungal infection; more typical of chronic than acute
  - Focal areas of sinus wall erosion
  - Soft-tissue infiltration of adjacent fat, soft tissue
    - Maxillary sinus: Perimaxillary fat infiltration (anterior, pre-maxillary, or retroantral fat)
    - Can be present without bone destruction via perivascular channels

DDx: Acute Onset Orbital Pain and Swelling

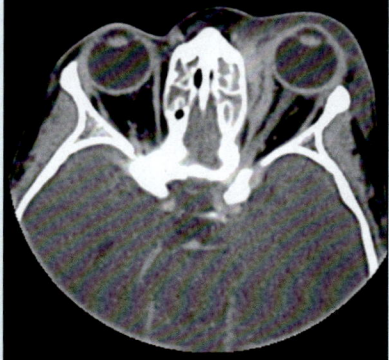

Orbital Cellulitis

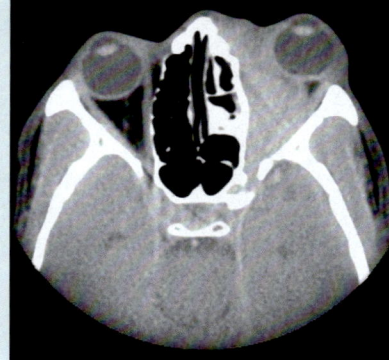

Pseudotumor

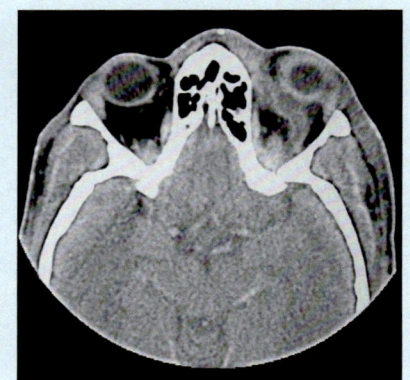

Orbital Vein Thrombosis

FUNGAL SINUSITIS, INVASIVE

Key Facts

Terminology
- Acute/fulminant (focus of this chapter): Rapidly progressive fungal infection of sinuses; infection crosses mucosa to involve blood vessels, bone, adjacent soft tissues, orbit, intracranial cavities
- Chronic: Dense hyphal accumulation resembling mycetoma (from which it may arise), associated with orbital apex syndrome, diabetes mellitus, corticosteroid therapy

Imaging Findings
- Best diagnostic clue: Sinus opacification with focal bone erosion, adjacent soft tissue infiltration
- Best imaging tool: CECT with soft tissue & bone windows to evaluate bone erosion, soft-tissue infiltration
- T1 C+ FS MR images recommended to map disease spread beyond sinuses

Top Differential Diagnoses
- Acute Rhinosinusitis Complication
- Idiopathic Orbital Inflammatory Disease
- Orbital Vein, Cavernous Sinus Thrombosis

Pathology
- Spread from sinuses via vascular invasion

Clinical Issues
- Most common signs/symptoms: Acute onset fever, epistaxis, sinus pain, headache, cough, nasal mucosal ulcerations, crusting
- Can be rapidly progressive & fatal without appropriate surgical-medical therapy

---

- May be due to edema from vascular congestion, tissue infiltration by fungal elements
- CECT: Periantral soft tissues, adjacent musculature may enhance
- CTA: May show arterial or venous narrowing, occlusion

MR Findings
- T1WI
  - Variable signal of material within involved sinus
    - Depends on protein/water content, presence of fungal elements
  - Diminished signal, similar to soft tissue, within periantral fat
- T2WI
  - Variable signal of sinus secretions; fungal elements may cause hypointense T2 signal
  - High signal edema in involved soft tissues may be seen with fat suppression
- T1 C+: Enhancement of involved soft tissues
- MRA: Vascular involvement (narrowing, dissection, thrombosis)

Angiographic Findings
- Vascular involvement (narrowing, dissection, thrombosis)

Imaging Recommendations
- Best imaging tool: CECT with soft tissue & bone windows to evaluate bone erosion, soft-tissue infiltration
- Protocol advice
  - Axial helical CECT ≤ 1 mm slice thickness reconstructed in bone & soft tissue algorithm, coronal reconstructions
  - T1 C+ FS MR images recommended to map disease spread beyond sinuses

DIFFERENTIAL DIAGNOSIS

Acute Rhinosinusitis Complication
- Patient may not be immunocompromised
- Bone erosion unlikely
- Homogeneous air-fluid level, peripheral mucosal thickening

Idiopathic Orbital Inflammatory Disease
- Non-immunocompromised patient
- No paranasal sinus disease
- Bone erosion unusual

Orbital Vein, Cavernous Sinus Thrombosis
- Enlarged superior orbital vein ± cavernous sinus with luminal thrombus
- May have coincident paranasal sinusitis
- No bone destruction

Carotid Cavernous Fistula
- Orbital proptosis, chemosis, not usually acutely painful, no sign of infection
- No paranasal sinus disease
- Enlarged orbital veins, cavernous sinus with signal voids on MR

PATHOLOGY

General Features
- General path comments: Rapidly progressive invasive fungal infection in immunocompromised patient, spread from sinuses via vascular invasion
- Etiology
  - Rarely seen in healthy individuals
  - Saprophytic fungi become invasive in patients with variety of predisposing conditions
    - Diabetes mellitus, diabetic ketoacidosis
    - Leukemia, bone-marrow transplant
    - Severe malnutrition
    - Malignancy-related neutropenia
    - End-stage renal disease
    - Prolonged corticosteroid or antibiotic use, chronic immunosuppressive therapy
    - Hemochromatosis
  - Most common organisms: Mucorales, aspergillus fumigatus

FUNGAL SINUSITIS, INVASIVE

  ○ Spread from sinuses via vascular invasion
- Epidemiology: Diabetic or immunocompromised patients with predisposing conditions

Gross Pathologic & Surgical Features
- Necrotic involved tissue, discoloration 2° presence of fungus

Microscopic Features
- Invasion of mucosa, submucosa & blood vessels by fungal hyphae
- Prominent tissue necrosis
- Mucormycosis & aspergillosis have affinity for arterial invasion
- Growth along internal elastic lamina → dissection from media; growth into vessel lumen → endothelial damage/thrombosis
- Variable associated inflammatory infiltrate
- Most cases have superimposed bacterial infection

CLINICAL ISSUES

Presentation
- Most common signs/symptoms: Acute onset fever, epistaxis, sinus pain, headache, cough, nasal mucosal ulcerations, crusting
- Other signs/symptoms: Periorbital swelling, proptosis, mental status changes
- Clinical Profile
  ○ Diabetic, immunocompromised patient with onset of facial pain ± headache
  ○ Nasal mucosa appears pale at endoscopy
  ○ Mucormycosis may show dark pigmentation on mucosa at endoscopy
  ○ Diagnosis requires identification of invasive fungi from biopsy samples of mucosa, submucosa, bone

Demographics
- Age: Typically in adults

Natural History & Prognosis
- Can be rapidly progressive & fatal without appropriate surgical-medical therapy
- Fair prognosis if limited to sinus & immediately adjacent tissues
- Orbital & intracranial involvement are most dreaded complications
- IFS of sphenoid sinus can lead to cavernous sinus thrombosis, carotid occlusion, mycotic aneurysm formation, cranial nerve dysfunction, cerebral infarction
- Poor prognosis if intracranial involvement

Treatment
- Radical debridement until histopathologically normal tissue reached
- Antifungal therapy with amphotericin B (Mucor species not sensitive to "azole" antifungals)
- Treat underlying condition responsible for immunocompromised state

DIAGNOSTIC CHECKLIST

Consider
- IFS in immunocompromised patient with maxillary disease, "dirty" periantral fat even if no bone erosion present

Image Interpretation Pearls
- Do not confuse normal variability in volume of periantral fat from side-to-side with fat infiltration
- Do not confuse normal musculature (orbicularis oculi, temporalis, pterygoid) with fat infiltration around antrum
- Evaluate orbit, intracranial cavities for involvement
- Closely examine cavernous sinus, internal carotid artery in sphenoid IFS

SELECTED REFERENCES

1. Granville L et al: Fungal sinusitis: histologic spectrum and correlation with culture. Hum Pathol. 35(4):474-81, 2004
2. Kargi S et al: Invasive fungal sinusitis. Plast Reconstr Surg. 113(3):1067-9, 2004
3. Parikh SL et al: Invasive fungal sinusitis: a 15-year review from a single institution. Am J Rhinol. 18(2):75-81, 2004
4. DelGaudio JM et al: Computed tomographic findings in patients with invasive fungal sinusitis. Arch Otolaryngol Head Neck Surg. 129(2): 236-40, 2003
5. Malani PN et al: Invasive and Allergic Fungal Sinusitis. Curr Infect Dis Rep. 4(3): 225-232, 2002
6. Howells RC et al: Usefulness of computed tomography and magnetic resonance in fulminant invasive fungal rhinosinusitis. Am J Rhinol. 15(4): 255-61, 2001
7. Hurst RW et al: Mycotic aneurysm and cerebral infarction resulting from fungal sinusitis: imaging and pathologic correlation. AJNR Am J Neuroradiol. 22(5): 858-63, 2001
8. Ruoppi P et al: Paranasal sinus mucormycosis: a report of two cases. Acta Otolaryngol. 121(8): 948-52, 2001
9. Ferguson BJ: Definitions of fungal rhinosinusitis. Otolaryngol Clin North Am. 33(2): 227-35, 2000
10. Gillespie MB et al: An algorithmic approach to the diagnosis and management of invasive fungal rhinosinusitis in the immunocompromised patient. Otolaryngol Clin North Am. 33(2): 323-34, 2000
11. Hunt SM et al: Invasive fungal sinusitis in the acquired immunodeficiency syndrome. Otolaryngol Clin North Am. 33(2): 335-47, 2000
12. Lund VJ et al: Fungal rhinosinusitis. J Laryngol Otol. 114(1): 76-80, 2000
13. Rizk SS et al: Aggressive combination treatment for invasive fungal sinusitis in immunocompromised patients. Ear Nose Throat J. 79(4): 278-80, 282, 284-5, 2000
14. Fatterpekar G et al: Fungal diseases of the paranasal sinuses. Semin Ultrasound CT MR. 20(6): 391-401, 1999
15. Silverman CS et al: Periantral soft-tissue infiltration and its relevance to the early detection of invasive fungal sinusitis: CT and MR findings. AJNR Am J Neuroradiol. 19(2): 321-5, 1998
16. deShazo RD et al: A new classification and diagnostic criteria for invasive fungal sinusitis. Arch Otolaryngol Head Neck Surg. 123(11): 1181-8, 1997

FUNGAL SINUSITIS, INVASIVE

IMAGE GALLERY

Typical

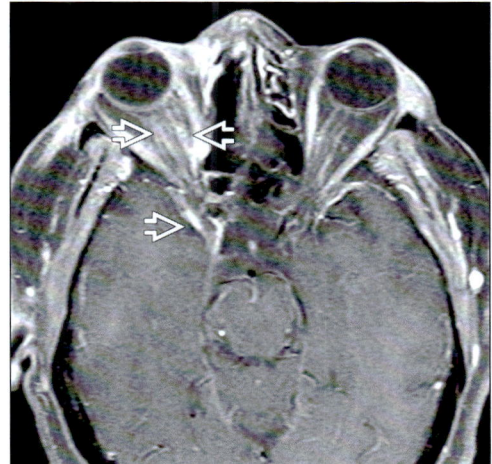 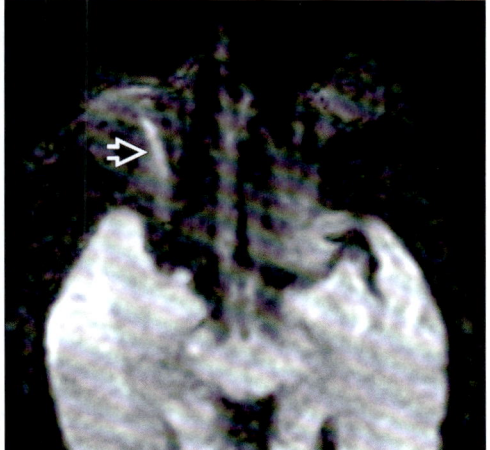

(Left) Axial T1 C+ FS MR shows enhancement along right optic nerve & anterior clinoid process ➡ in a patient with diabetes and acute invasive Mucor sinusitis status post extensive debridement. (Right) Axial DWI MR in same patient as previous image shows restricted diffusion in infarcted right optic nerve ➡.

Typical

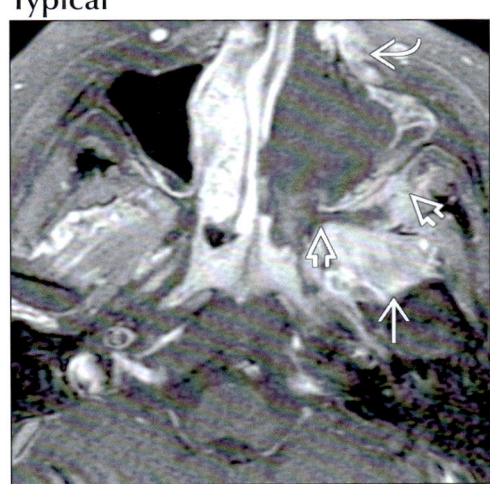 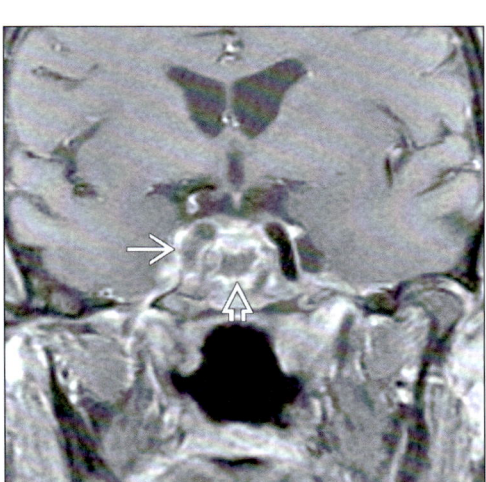

(Left) Axial T1 C+ FS MR of acute invasive left antral fungal sinusitis invading pterygopalatine fossa & pterygomaxillary fissure ➡, left premaxillary soft tissues ➡ & masticator space ➡. (Right) Coronal T1 C+ MR of invasive sphenoid fungal sinusitis ➡ extending into cavernous sinus with right internal carotid artery thrombosis (note loss of carotid signal void) ➡.

Variant

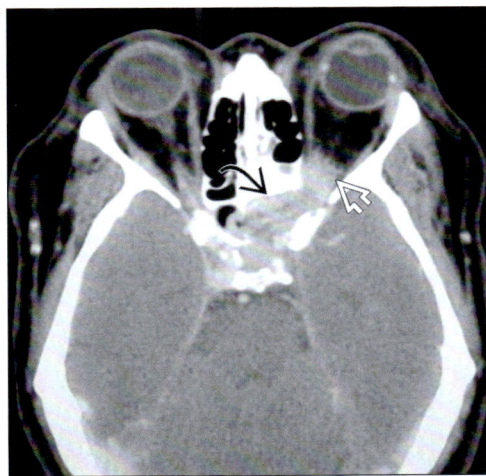 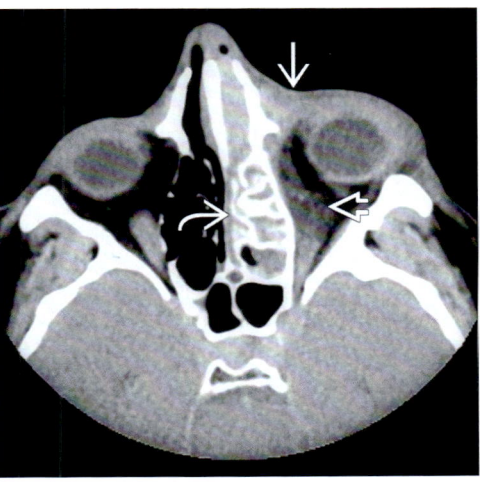

(Left) Axial CECT shows left orbital apex invasion ➡ by chronic left ethmoid and sphenoid Aspergillus sinusitis ➡ in a diabetic patient with chronic IFS. (Right) Axial CECT shows left periorbital ➡ & orbital ➡ invasion of chronic left ethmoid ➡ Aspergillus sinusitis without identifiable bone destruction in a diabetic patient with chronic IFS.

PAROTITIS, ACUTE

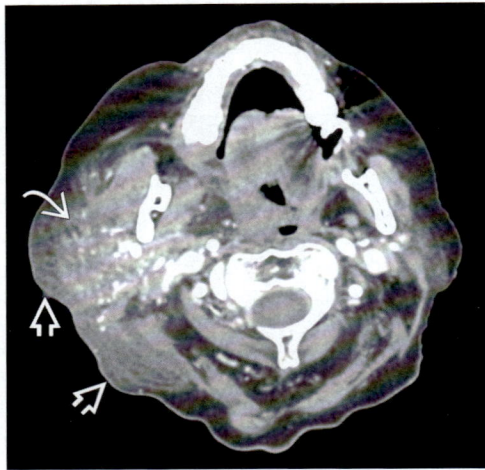

Axial CECT shows enlarged, "shaggy" right parotid gland ➔. Note marked parenchymal vascular enhancement, inflammation in adjacent fat ➔. Methicillin-resistant Staph aureus parotitis.

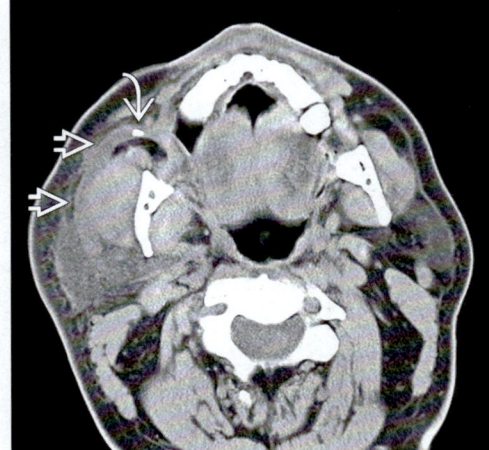

Axial NECT shows stone in right Stensen duct ➔. Dilated duct ➔ demonstrates graded attenuation due to settling of pus. Note enlarged dense parotid, stranding of subcutaneous fat.

TERMINOLOGY

Abbreviations and Synonyms
- Acute sialadenitis

Definitions
- Acute inflammation of parotid gland
  - Bacterial: Acute suppurative parotitis, localized infection
  - Viral: Acute viral parotitis, systemic viral infection
  - Calculus-induced parotitis: Due to ductal obstruction by stone

IMAGING FINDINGS

General Features
- Best diagnostic clue: Unilateral painful swelling of parotid & overlying soft tissues, purulent ostial discharge
- Location
  - Bacterial: Most commonly unilateral
  - Viral: 75% bilateral; submandibular & sublingual glands may also be involved
  - Calculus-induced: Radiopaque stone in parotid duct with unilateral intraparotid infection

CT Findings
- NECT
  - Bacterial: Hyperdense enlarged parotid, ill-defined margins
  - Viral: Hyperdense enlarged parotid glands
  - Calculus-induced: Parotid duct calculus usually obvious
- CECT
  - Bacterial: Enlarged diffusely enhancing parotid, inflammatory stranding of overlying soft tissues, ring enhancement of abscesses
  - Viral: Enlarged parotids with mild enhancement
  - Calculus-induced: Parotid duct dilated with enhancing walls

MR Findings
- T2WI: Diffuse high signal ± focal areas of high signal (abscesses or sialectasis)
- T1 C+
  - Enlarged parotid enhances moderately diffusely
  - Abscesses: Rim-enhancing fluid collections

DDx: Parotid Enlargement

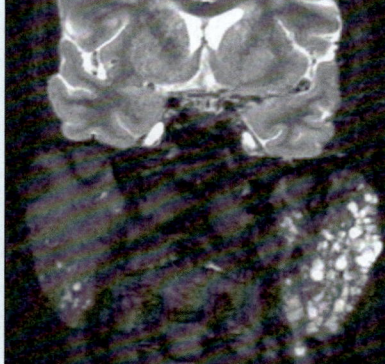

Sjögren Syndrome

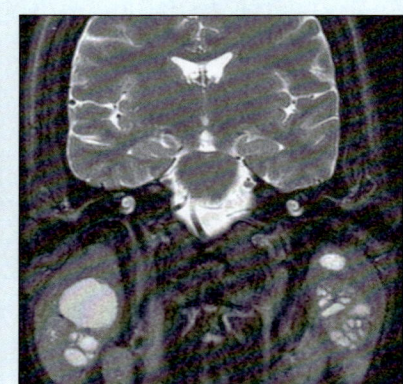

HIV Lesions

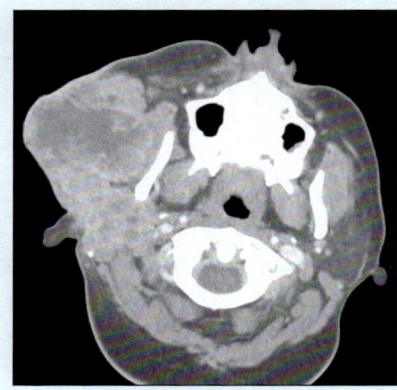

Carcinoma

PAROTITIS, ACUTE

Key Facts

Terminology
- Acute inflammation of parotid gland
- Bacterial: Acute suppurative parotitis, localized infection
- Viral: Acute viral parotitis, systemic viral infection
- Calculus-induced parotitis: Due to ductal obstruction by stone

Imaging Findings
- Best diagnostic clue: Unilateral painful swelling of parotid & overlying soft tissues, purulent ostial discharge

Top Differential Diagnoses
- Sjögren Syndrome
- Benign Lymphoepithelial Disease in HIV
- Parotid Benign Mixed Tumor
- Parotid Malignancy

Pathology
- Bacterial (suppurative) parotitis unilateral in 75-85%
- Viral parotitis more frequently bilateral
- Bacterial: Usually due to ascending infection

Clinical Issues
- Bacterial: > 50 years & neonates
- Viral: Most < 15 years; peak age 5-9 years
- Suppurative parotitis mortality may reach 20%
- Responds well to early treatment, though number of complications recognized

Diagnostic Checklist
- Carefully inspect entire parotid duct for calculus

Ultrasonographic Findings
- Enlarged hypoechoic heterogeneous gland
- Sensitive for detection of calculi
- Focal hypoechoic collection suggests abscess formation
  - US can be used to guide aspiration

Other Modality Findings
- Sialography contraindicated in acute suppurative parotitis, but useful in evaluating recurrent disease

Imaging Recommendations
- Best imaging tool
  - Bacterial & calculus-induced infection: CECT best for detection of calculi or abscess
  - Viral parotitis is clinical diagnosis; imaging rarely required
- Protocol advice
  - NECT unnecessary; calculus considerably more dense than contrast in vessels
  - Optimize CT scan plane (parallel to upper fillings) so dental amalgam artifact does not obscure calculus in parotid duct

DIFFERENTIAL DIAGNOSIS

Sialosis (Sialadenosis)
- Bilateral, prolonged, painless, soft parotid (and occasionally submandibular gland) enlargement
- Associated with alcoholism, endocrinopathies (especially diabetes mellitus), malnutrition (including anorexia nervosa, bulimia)

Sjögren Syndrome
- Dry eyes & mouth; rheumatoid arthritis or other associated collagen vascular disease
- Bilateral mixed cystic & solid intraparotid lesions ± calcifications
- Sialographically normal ducts early in disease

Benign Lymphoepithelial Disease in HIV
- May be found prior to detection of HIV
- Bilateral heterogeneous parotids, often with cystic & solid lesions
  - Prominent Waldeyer ring & cervical nodes

Parotid Benign Mixed Tumor
- Slow-growing "cheek" mass
- Well-defined, homogeneous intraparotid mass (typically T2-hyperintense, intensely enhancing)
  - Lobulated & inhomogeneous when large

Parotid Malignancy
- CN7 dysfunction should raise suspicion of malignant neoplasm
- Unilateral focal (low-grade) or ill-defined (high-grade) parotid mass
  - High-grade tumors associated with nodal metastases

PATHOLOGY

General Features
- General path comments
  - Bacterial (suppurative) parotitis unilateral in 75-85%
  - Viral parotitis more frequently bilateral
- Etiology
  - Bacterial: Usually due to ascending infection
    - Staph Aureus (50-90%) > streptococcus, Haemophilus, E. Coli, anaerobes
    - Neonatal suppurative parotitis may be bilateral, due to bacteremia; more common in premature infants, males
  - Viral: Mumps paramyxovirus most common cause; so-called "epidemic parotitis"
    - Also influenza, parainfluenza, Coxsackie A & B virus, ECHO virus, lymphocytic choriomeningitis virus
    - CMV, adenovirus reported with HIV infection
  - Recurrent parotitis of childhood
    - Recurrent episodes mimic mumps, usually begin by age 5; virtually all cases resolve by age 10-15
    - Patient often has unilateral symptoms but bilateral sialographic abnormalities
    - Sialographically mimics Sjögren syndrome

PAROTITIS, ACUTE

- Etiology unknown
- Epidemiology: Parotid is most commonly inflamed salivary gland (absence of bacteriostatic mucin in its serous secretions)
- Associated abnormalities: Parotid abscess

Microscopic Features
- Bacterial: Acinar degeneration with mixed neutrophil & round cell infiltrates
  - Microabscesses with necrotic amorphous debris & neutrophils
- Viral: Rarely examined microscopically
  - Lobular architecture maintained with interstitial subacute infiltrate

CLINICAL ISSUES

Presentation
- Most common signs/symptoms
  - Bacterial: Sudden onset parotid pain & swelling
    - Indurated, erythematous, tender gland, purulent ostial discharge
    - Patient may be toxic, febrile, dehydrated, confused
    - Leukocytosis with neutrophilia
    - Normal/slightly elevated amylase
  - Viral: Prodromal symptoms of headaches, malaise, myalgia followed by parotid pain, earache, trismus, dysphagia
    - Swollen parotid but not erythematous or warm
    - Involvement usually bilateral, but swelling may be asynchronous
    - May also experience orchitis, meningoencephalitis, pancreatitis, oophoritis, thyroiditis, mastitis
    - Leukocytopenia with relative lymphocytosis
    - Elevated serum amylase, especially first week
- Clinical Profile
  - Bacterial: Acutely painful enlarged parotid in debilitated patient or neonate
  - Predisposing factors
    - Dehydration, surgery, diuretics or anticholinergics reducing salivary flow
    - Duct obstruction by calculus
    - Immunosuppression, poor oral hygiene, malnutrition
  - Viral: More frequently seen in children who have not received MMR vaccine

Demographics
- Age
  - Bacterial: > 50 years & neonates
  - Viral: Most < 15 years; peak age 5-9 years
    - Adults usually immune from childhood exposure or MMR vaccine
- Gender: No gender predilection

Natural History & Prognosis
- Suppurative parotitis mortality may reach 20%
  - Due largely to occurrence in debilitated elderly patients
- Responds well to early treatment, though number of complications recognized
  - Early complications
    - Abscess formation ⇒ rupture to deep neck spaces, EAC or TMJ
    - Thrombophlebitis of retromandibular or facial veins ⇒ IJV thrombosis
    - CN7 dysfunction rarely found, usually resolves
  - Long-term complications
    - Sialectasis with recurrent infections, reduced salivation, pain
- Viral parotitis self-limited; swelling lasts ≤ 2 weeks
  - Systemic mumps paramyxovirus infection has many complications
    - Orchitis, meningoencephalitis, thyroiditis, sensorineural hearing loss, pancreatitis

Treatment
- Bacterial
  - Broad spectrum antibiotics, rehydration, good oral hygiene, sialogogues
  - Surgical drainage of abscesses
- Viral
  - Supportive treatment with rest, hydration
- Calculus-induced
  - Extract smaller stones from duct (perorally)
  - Larger proximal stones may require surgical removal ± parotidectomy

DIAGNOSTIC CHECKLIST

Consider
- Sialography for recurrent disease
  - Exclude autoimmune disease, ductal strictures
- Re-image parotid if residual mass after resolution of acute infection
  - Exclude underlying malignancy or abscess

Image Interpretation Pearls
- Carefully inspect entire parotid duct for calculus

SELECTED REFERENCES

1. Spiegel R et al: Acute neonatal suppurative parotitis: case reports and review. Pediatr Infect Dis J. 23(1):76-8, 2004
2. Brook I: Acute bacterial suppurative parotitis: microbiology and management. J Craniofac Surg. 14(1):37-40, 2003
3. Fattahi TT et al: Management of acute suppurative parotitis. J Oral Maxillofac Surg. 60(4):446-8, 2002
4. Mandel L et al: Bilateral parotid swelling: a review. Oral Surg Oral Med Oral Pathol Oral Radiol Endod. 93(3):221-37, 2002
5. Yousem DM et al: Major salivary gland imaging. Radiology. 216(1):19-29, 2000
6. Cohen MA et al: Acute suppurative parotitis with spread to the deep neck spaces. Am J Emerg Med. 17(1):46-9, 1999
7. McQuone SJ: Acute viral and bacterial infections of the salivary glands. Otolaryngol Clin North Am. 32(5):793-811, 1999
8. Pang YT et al: Acute suppurative parotitis and facial paralysis. J Laryngol Otol. 110(1):91-2, 1996
9. Nusem-Horowitz S et al: Acute suppurative parotitis and parotid abscess in children. Int J Pediatr Otorhinolaryngol. 32(2):123-7, 1995
10. Brook I: Diagnosis and management of parotitis. Arch Otolaryngol Head Neck Surg. 118(5):469-71, 1992

PAROTITIS, ACUTE

IMAGE GALLERY

Typical

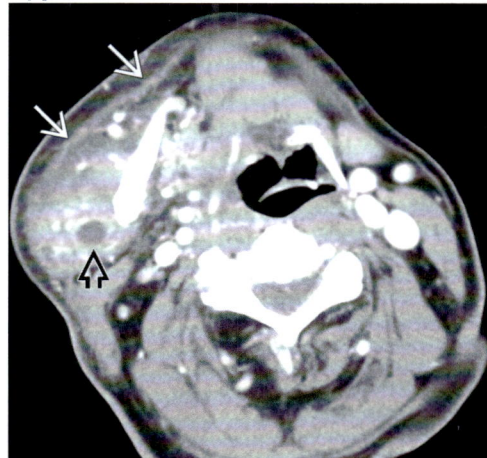
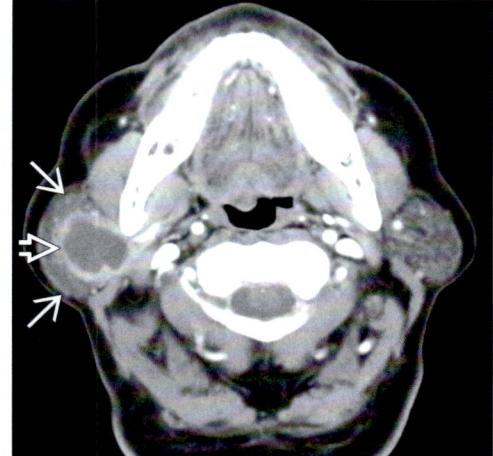

(Left) Axial CECT shows acute right parotitis with evolving abscess ➔ in tail of gland. Note thickened, shaggy overlying platysma ➔. *(Right)* Axial CECT shows subacute right parotid abscess in patient with incomplete response to antibiotic therapy. Note enlarged, enhancing parotid ➔, shaggy abscess capsule ➔.

Typical

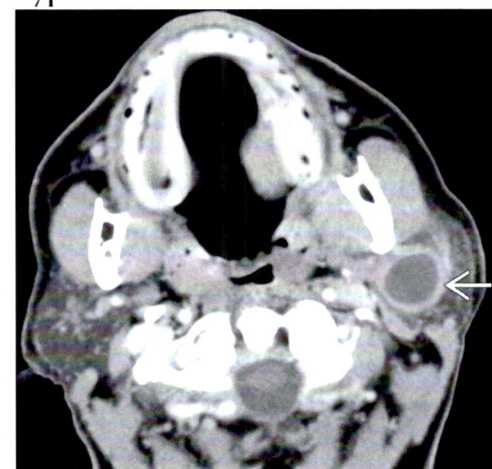
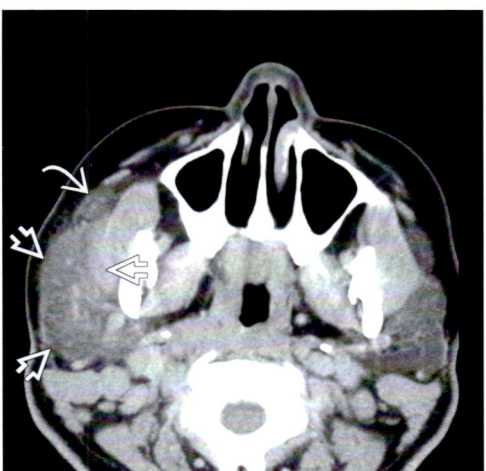

(Left) Axial CECT shows more evolved left parotid abscess. Left parotid gland is slightly higher in attenuation than right parotid. Note thick, well-formed abscess capsule ➔. *(Right)* Axial CECT shows enlarged enhancing right parotid gland. Margins of gland ➔ are slightly ill-defined. Note that accessory right parotid tissue ➔ is affected.

Typical

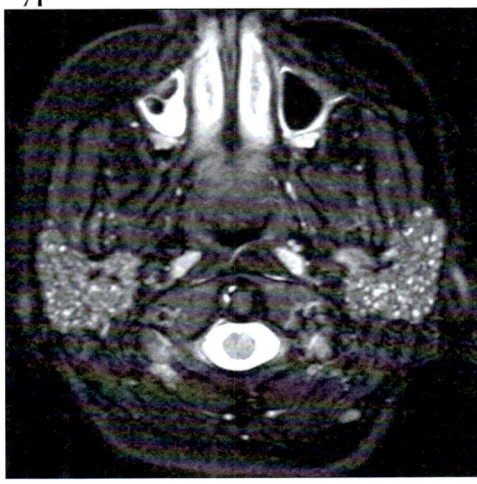
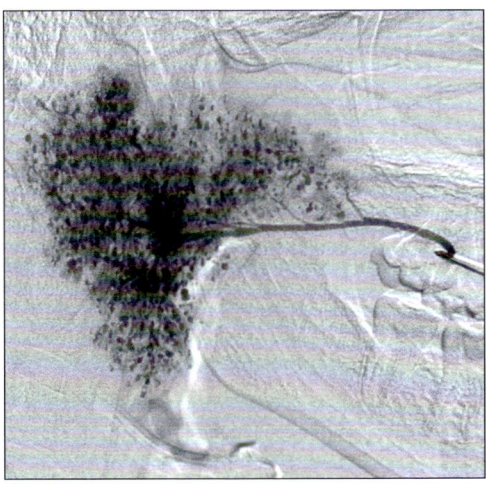

(Left) Axial T2WI FS MR shows tiny bilateral parotid "cysts" and minimal parotid enlargement in child with recurrent parotid enlargement. Presumed benign recurrent parotitis. *(Right)* Lateral sialogram shows diffuse globular contrast collections in right parotid. Patient is 23 yo female with parotid swelling & discomfort, Sjögren syndrome. Note relatively normal ducts.

RETROPHARYNGEAL SPACE ABSCESS

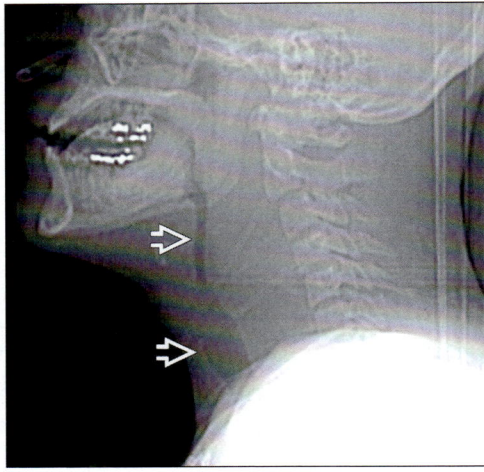

Lateral scout shows markedly anteriorly displaced airway ➡ in an adult patient with retropharyngeal abscess.

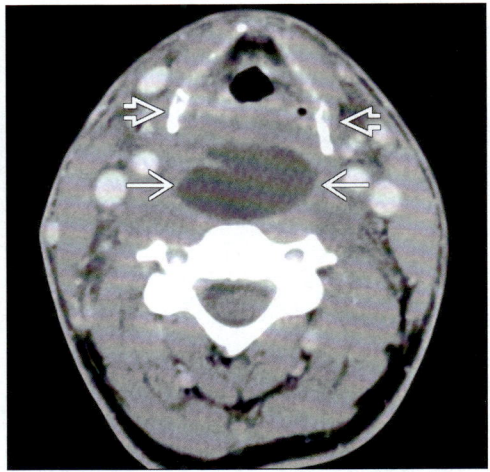

Axial CECT shows faintly enhancing rim ➡ of retropharyngeal abscess displacing larynx ➡ anteriorly.

TERMINOLOGY

Abbreviations and Synonyms
- Retropharyngeal space abscess (RPSA)

Definitions
- Extranodal purulent fluid collection in RPS

IMAGING FINDINGS

General Features
- Best diagnostic clue: Midline-spanning fluid collection distending RPS with variable rim-enhancement
- Location
  ○ Posterior to pharyngeal mucosal space, anterior to prevertebral space
  ○ Can extend inferiorly into mediastinum; must assess full craniocaudal extent
- Size: Variable
- Morphology: Variable shape on CT, depends on volume/distribution of collection

Radiographic Findings
- Radiography
  ○ Lateral plain X-ray frequent screening exam
  ○ Widened prevertebral distance; infrequently RPS air
  ○ Perform during inspiration with neck extension in children
  ○ Normal prevertebral soft tissue
    - C2: ≤ 7 mm at any age
    - C6: ≤ 14 mm in patients under 15 years, ≤ 22 mm in adults

CT Findings
- CECT
  ○ Fluid distends RPS with flattening of posterior prevertebral muscles
    - Variable peripheral enhancement of RPS collection
    - Thick enhancing wall suggests mature RPSA
    - CECT may not differentiate between early RPSA and effusion
    - Assess for complications (airway or vascular compromise, mediastinal extension)

DDx: Retropharyngeal Fluid

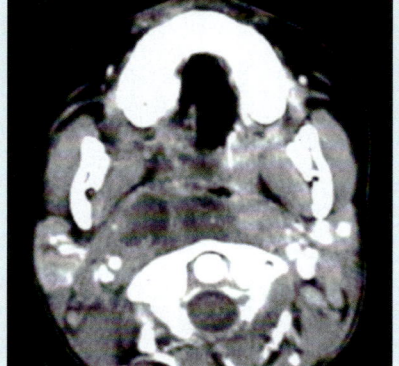

Retropharyngeal Adenitis

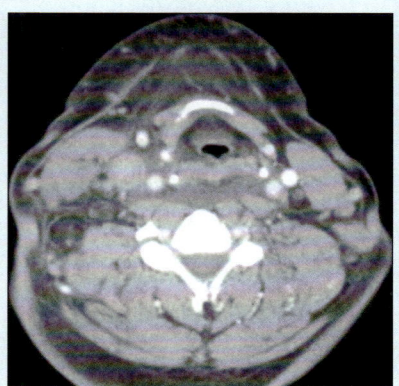

RIJV Occlusion, RP Effusion

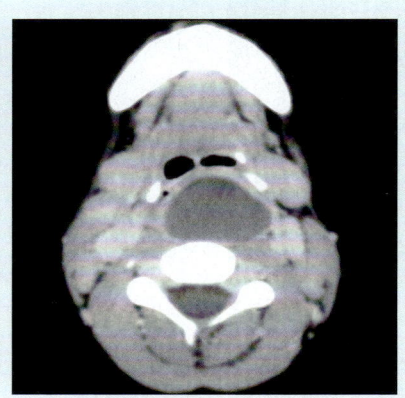

Subacute RP Hematoma

RETROPHARYNGEAL SPACE ABSCESS

Key Facts

Imaging Findings
- Best diagnostic clue: Midline-spanning fluid collection distending RPS with variable rim-enhancement

Top Differential Diagnoses
- RPS Effusion/Edema
- RPS Suppurative Node
- RPS Invasion from Neoplastic Process

Pathology
- Early RPS infection produces cellulitis without drainable pus collection
- Can be clinically & radiologically difficult to distinguish cellulitis from RPSA
- Head & neck (H&N) infection (pharyngitis, tonsillitis) seeds RPS lymph node
- Ventral spread of diskitis/osteomyelitis & prevertebral infection
- Pharyngeal penetrating foreign body

Clinical Issues
- Septic patient: Fever, chills, elevated WBC & ESR
- Increasing frequency in adult population
- Immunocompromised states: Diabetes, HIV, alcoholism, malignancy
- Prognosis generally excellent if early diagnosis, aggressive management

Diagnostic Checklist
- Rim-enhancement suggests abscess formation; not always present in early abscess
- ENT consultation imperative

MR Findings
- Rarely utilized in septic patient with tenuous airway, patient monitoring problematic
- Potentially advantageous to differentiate from cellulitis (more sensitive to contrast-enhancement)

Ultrasonographic Findings
- More accurate than CT & MR in differentiating RPSA from cellulitis
- Limited by operator experience, patient tolerance
- Not able to assess full extent of disease

Imaging Recommendations
- Best imaging tool: CECT: Readily available, allows rapid image acquisition
- Protocol advice
  - Helical axial CT from skull base to carina
  - Contrast prebolus before IV infusion improves soft tissue contrast with rapid helical scanning

DIFFERENTIAL DIAGNOSIS

RPS Effusion/Edema
- Venous or lymphatic obstruction (IJV thrombosis, prior node dissection, XRT), regional inflammation (pharyngitis, tonsillitis, longus colli tendinitis)
- RPS fluid without definable wall or rim-enhancement; RP vessels may traverse "collection"
- Impaired lymphatic drainage or excess lymph production
- Drainage not required

RPS Suppurative Node
- Sick child suspicious for RPSA
- Central hypodense node in lateral RPS with adjacent cellulitis on CECT
- Pus formation in reactive lymph node; intranodal abscess
- May progress to RPSA if inadequate medical therapy

RPS Invasion from Neoplastic Process
- Older non-septic patient with known pharyngeal SCCa
- Solid enhancing soft tissue mass of posterior pharyngeal wall on CECT
- Tumors involving posterior pharyngeal wall may extend into RPS, prevertebral tissues
  - Nasopharyngeal and posterior wall oro- & hypopharyngeal SCCa

PATHOLOGY

General Features
- General path comments
  - Early RPS infection produces cellulitis without drainable pus collection
  - Can be clinically & radiologically difficult to distinguish cellulitis from RPSA
- Etiology
  - Head & neck (H&N) infection (pharyngitis, tonsillitis) seeds RPS lymph node
    - H&N infection ⇒ reactive node ⇒ suppurative node (intranodal abscess)
    - Nodal rupture ⇒ RPSA
    - Most common organisms: Staph aureus, Haemophilus, streptococcus
  - Ventral spread of diskitis/osteomyelitis & prevertebral infection
    - More frequent cause of RPSA in adults
    - Pyogenic or tuberculous
  - Pharyngeal penetrating foreign body
    - Most often: Child running with penetrating object in mouth
- Epidemiology: RPSA less frequently seen; infection detected and treated in earlier cellulitic stage

Gross Pathologic & Surgical Features
- Yellow-green fluid draining from distended RPS
- Thick abscess wall of fibrous connective tissue

Microscopic Features
- Pus: Necrotic debris, polymorphonuclear leukocytes, lymphocytes, macrophages
- Abscess wall: Granulation tissue, fibrous connective tissue

RETROPHARYNGEAL SPACE ABSCESS

CLINICAL ISSUES

Presentation
- Most common signs/symptoms
  - Septic patient: Fever, chills, elevated WBC & ESR
  - Dysphagia, sore throat, poor oral intake, dehydration
  - Posterior pharyngeal wall edema or bulge, reactive cervical adenopathy (both less common in adults)
- Clinical Profile
  - Neck pain with limitation of movement, especially extension
  - Uncommonly present with signs of airway compromise (stridor)

Demographics
- Age
  - Most patients < 6 years old
  - Increasing frequency in adult population
    - Immunocompromised states: Diabetes, HIV, alcoholism, malignancy
    - Spine infection
    - Trauma (iatrogenic or foreign body impaction)
- Gender: M:F = 2:1

Natural History & Prognosis
- Prognosis generally excellent if early diagnosis, aggressive management
- Complications may result from spread to adjacent spaces
  - Narrowing of pharyngeal lumen ⇒ airway compromise
  - Inferior spread via danger space to mediastinum ⇒ mediastinitis ⇒ 50% mortality
  - Carotid space involvement
    - Jugular vein thrombosis or thrombophlebitis
    - Narrowing of ICA caliber often found; neurological sequelae infrequent
    - Potential for ICA pseudoaneurysm and rupture
  - Aspiration pneumonia
  - Grisel syndrome (nontraumatic atlanto-axial subluxation) rare complication
    - Distension or loosening of atlanto-axial ligaments after H&N inflammation
  - Extension to spine ⇒ epidural abscess

Treatment
- Early ENT consultation
- IV antibiotics, airway management, fluid resuscitation
- Surgical intervention if failure to improve or significant/complex abscess present

DIAGNOSTIC CHECKLIST

Consider
- Lateral plain film: First-line screening tool
- CECT to distinguish RPSA from effusion

Image Interpretation Pearls
- Rim-enhancement suggests abscess formation; not always present in early abscess
- Important to evaluate for full extent of abscess, presence of complications
- ENT consultation imperative

SELECTED REFERENCES

1. Shefelbine SE et al: Pediatric retropharyngeal lymphadenitis: differentiation from retropharyngeal abscess and treatment implications. Otolaryngol Head Neck Surg. 136(2):182-8, 2007
2. Craig FW et al: Retropharyngeal abscess in children: clinical presentation, utility of imaging, and current management. Pediatrics. 111(6 Pt 1):1394-8, 2003
3. McClay JE et al: Intravenous antibiotic therapy for deep neck abscesses defined by computed tomography. Arch Otolaryngol Head Neck Surg. 129(11):1207-12, 2003
4. Vural C et al: Accuracy of computerized tomography in deep neck infections in the pediatric population. Am J Otolaryngol. 24(3):143-8, 2003
5. Wang LF et al: Characterizations of life-threatening deep cervical space infections: a review of one hundred ninety-six cases. Am J Otolaryngol. 24(2):111-7, 2003
6. Cmejrek RC et al: Presentation, diagnosis, and management of deep-neck abscesses in infants. Arch Otolaryngol Head Neck Surg. 128(12):1361-4, 2002
7. Dawes LC et al: Retropharyngeal abscess in children. ANZ J Surg. 72(6):417-20, 2002
8. Elden LM et al: Accuracy and usefulness of radiographic assessment of cervical neck infections in children. J Otolaryngol. 30(2):82-9, 2001
9. Kirse DJ et al: Surgical management of retropharyngeal space infections in children. Laryngoscope. 111(8):1413-22, 2001
10. Chong VF et al: Radiology of the retropharyngeal space. Clin Radiol. 55(10):740-8, 2000
11. Boucher C et al: Retropharyngeal abscesses: a clinical and radiologic correlation. J Otolaryngol. 28(3):134-7, 1999
12. Stone ME et al: Correlation between computed tomography and surgical findings in retropharyngeal inflammatory processes in children. Int J Pediatr Otorhinolaryngol. 49(2):121-5, 1999
13. Hudgins PA et al: Internal carotid artery narrowing in children with retropharyngeal lymphadenitis and abscess. AJNR Am J Neuroradiol. 19(10):1841-3, 1998
14. Ide C et al: An early MR observation of carotid involvement by retropharyngeal abscess. AJNR Am J Neuroradiol. 19(3):499-501, 1998
15. Wetmore RF et al: Computed tomography in the evaluation of pediatric neck infections. Otolaryngol Head Neck Surg. 119(6):624-7, 1998
16. Tannebaum RD: Adult retropharyngeal abscess: a case report and review of the literature. J Emerg Med. 14(2):147-58, 1996
17. Glasier CM et al: CT and ultrasound imaging of retropharyngeal abscesses in children. AJNR Am J Neuroradiol. 13(4):1191-5, 1992

RETROPHARYNGEAL SPACE ABSCESS

IMAGE GALLERY

Typical

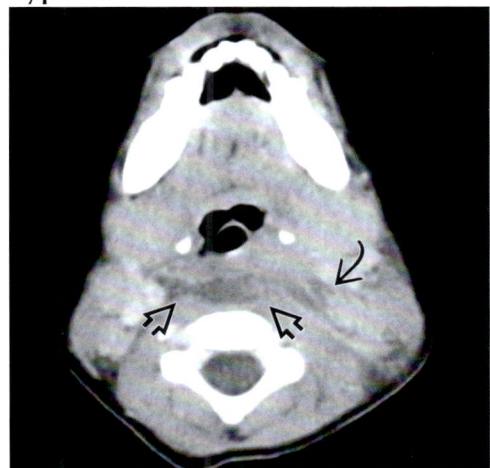
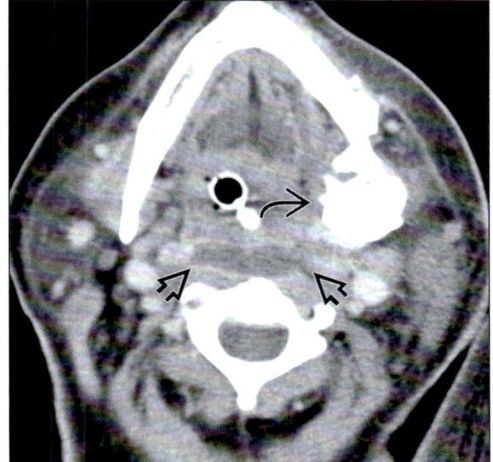

(Left) Axial CECT shows rim-enhancing retropharyngeal abscess ➔ in a child; patient also had suppurative retropharyngeal adenitis ➔ at higher levels. *(Right)* Axial CECT shows faintly enhancing rim of retropharyngeal abscess ➔ complicating left parapharyngeal abscess (surgical drain in place ➔).

Variant

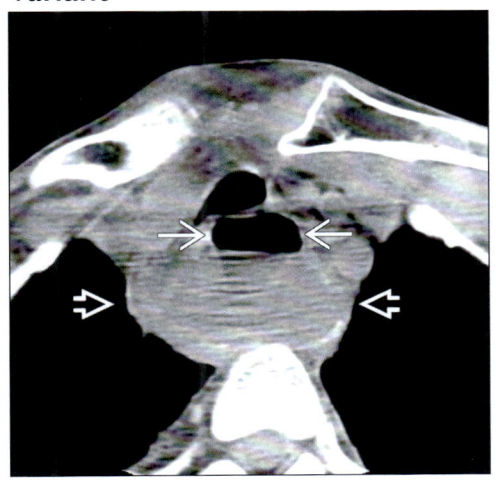
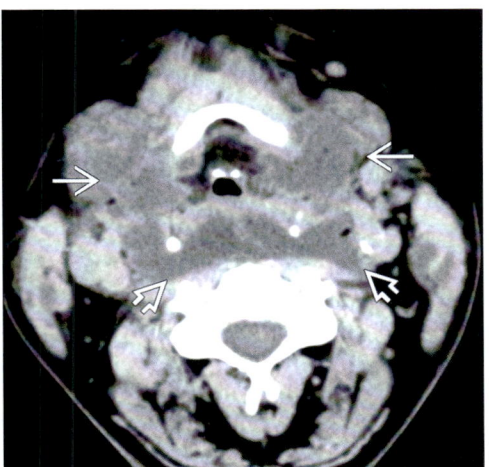

(Left) Axial NECT shows retropharyngeal abscess extending into mediastinum ➔. Note anteriorly displaced, air-filled esophagus ➔. *(Right)* Axial NECT shows multicompartmental abscesses with retropharyngeal abscess ➔ in a patient with Ludwig angina. Also note bilateral submandibular space abscesses ➔.

Variant

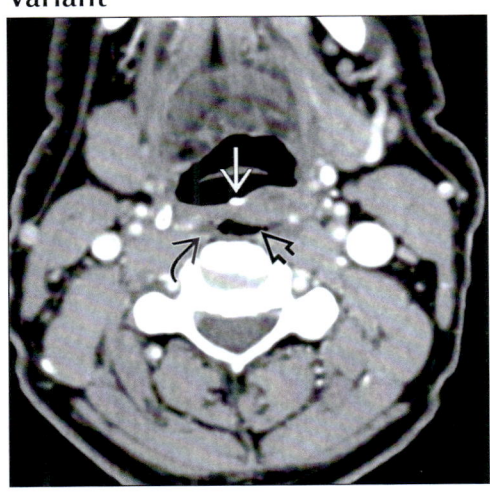
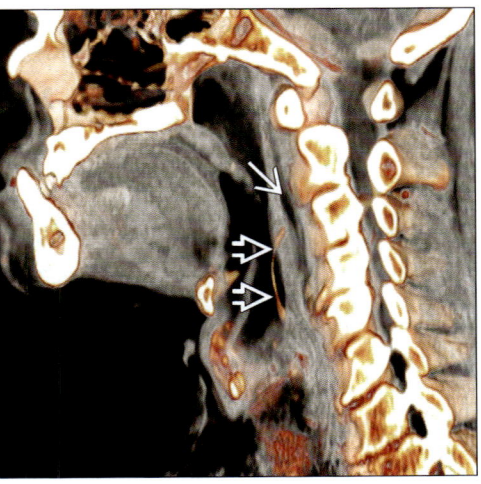

(Left) Axial CECT shows inadvertently ingested chicken bone ➔ embedded in posterior pharyngeal wall, retropharyngeal gas ➔ and fluid ➔. *(Right)* Sagittal 3D CT in the same patient as previous image, better demonstrates chicken bone ➔ embedded in the posterior pharyngeal wall, as well as retropharyngeal gas ➔.

PYOGENIC OSTEOMYELITIS, SPINE

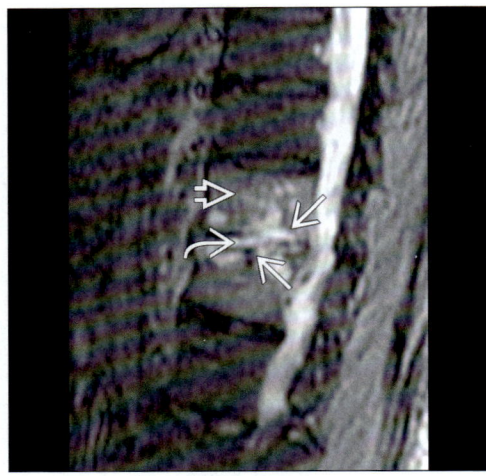

Sagittal T2WI FS MR shows irregularity ⇨ of contiguous endplates with marrow edema in vertebral bodies ➡. High signal in disc space indicates abscess ➡.

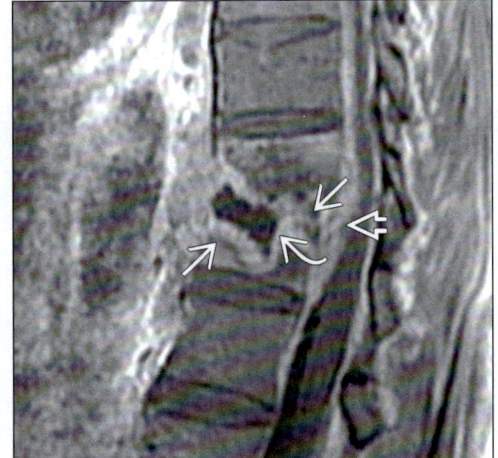

Sagittal T1 C+ FS MR shows endplate irregularity with enhancement of adjacent marrow ➡, as well as rim enhancement of disc space ➡. Note epidural extension of infection ⇨.

TERMINOLOGY

Abbreviations and Synonyms
- Pyogenic spondylodiscitis

Definitions
- Bacterial suppurative infection of vertebrae and intervertebral disc

IMAGING FINDINGS

General Features
- Best diagnostic clue: Ill-defined hypointense vertebral marrow on T1WI with loss of endplate definition on both sides of disc
- Location
  - All spinal segments involved
    - Lumbar (48%) > thoracic (35%) > cervical spine (6.5%)
- Size: Two adjacent vertebrae with intervening disc
- Morphology
  - Loss of disc height
  - Abnormal disc signal
  - Destruction of vertebral endplate cortex
  - Ill-defined marrow signal alteration
  - Vertebral collapse
  - Paraspinal ± epidural infiltrative soft tissue ± loculated fluid collection
    - Present in 75% of pyogenic vertebral osteomyelitis
  - Variable central canal narrowing

Radiographic Findings
- Radiography
  - Negative up to 2-8 weeks after onset of symptoms
  - Initial endplate & vertebral osteolysis followed by increased bone density
  - Paraspinal soft-tissue density
    - Loss of expected fat planes
  - Fusion across disc space late in disease course

CT Findings
- NECT
  - Endplate osteolytic/osteosclerotic changes
  - Spinal deformity best seen on coronal & sagittal reformation
  - Increase in iso- to hypodense paraspinal soft tissue
    - ± Soft-tissue gas

DDx: Pyogenic Osteomyelitis Mimics

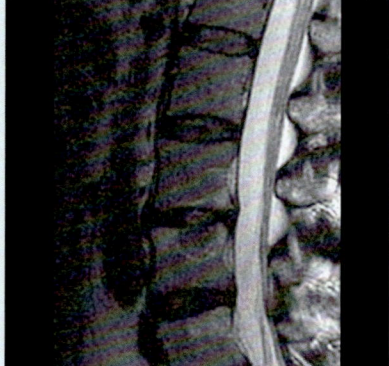
Degenerative Disease

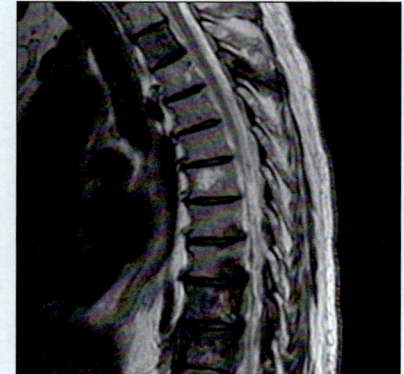
Metastases

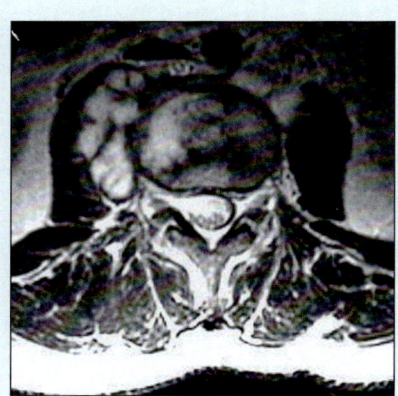
Tuberculous Spondylitis

PYOGENIC OSTEOMYELITIS, SPINE

Key Facts

Terminology
- Pyogenic spondylodiscitis
- Bacterial suppurative infection of vertebrae and intervertebral disc

Imaging Findings
- Best diagnostic clue: Ill-defined hypointense vertebral marrow on T1WI with loss of endplate definition on both sides of disc
- Lumbar (48%) > thoracic (35%) > cervical spine (6.5%)
- Loss of disc height
- Destruction of vertebral endplate cortex
- Ill-defined marrow signal alteration
- Paraspinal ± epidural infiltrative soft tissue ± loculated fluid collection
- CECT: Enhancing disc, marrow, & paravertebral soft tissue

Top Differential Diagnoses
- Degenerative Endplate Changes
- Tuberculous Vertebral Osteomyelitis
- Spinal Neuropathic Arthropathy
- Chronic Hemodialysis Spondyloarthropathy

Clinical Issues
- Acute or chronic back pain
- Focal spinal tenderness
- Fever

Diagnostic Checklist
- Diffusely enhancing disc, adjacent vertebral marrow, soft tissue with endplate erosion highly suggestive of vertebral osteomyelitis

---

- CECT: Enhancing disc, marrow, & paravertebral soft tissue

MR Findings
- Disc space
  - Hypointense on T1WI
  - Variable, typically hyperintense on T2WI
  - Diffuse or rim enhancement with gadolinium
  - Loss of height
- Vertebral marrow signal abnormality abutting disc
  - Hypointense on T1WI
  - Hyperintense on fat-saturated T2WI or STIR
  - Avid enhancement with gadolinium
- Paraspinal & epidural phlegmon or abscess
  - Isointense to muscle on T1WI
  - Hyperintense on T2WI
  - Diffuse or rim enhancement
- Cord compression

Nuclear Medicine Findings
- Bone Scan: Three-phase technetium Tc-99m diphosphonate scan shows increased activity in all phases
- Gallium Scan
  - Increased uptake of gallium citrate (Ga-67)
    - Increased sensitivity with SPECT
  - May be used in combination with bone scan
- WBC Scan
  - Often false-negative in patients with chronic vertebral osteomyelitis

Imaging Recommendations
- Best imaging tool
  - Sagittal and axial T2WI and T1WI MR
    - Sensitivity 96%, specificity 92%, accuracy 94%
  - SPECT Ga-67 scan good alternative
    - Sensitivity & specificity in low 90%
- Protocol advice
  - STIR or FSE T2 with fat suppression most sensitive for marrow edema, epidural involvement
  - Post-gadolinium T1WI with fat suppression also improves MR sensitivity
    - Improves evaluation of epidural & soft tissue spaces

DIFFERENTIAL DIAGNOSIS

Degenerative Endplate Changes
- Most common mimic
- Disc desiccation
  - Hypointense on T1WI & T2WI
  - Minimal or absent enhancement with gadolinium
- Vertebral endplates preserved
- Degenerative marrow pattern (Modic I-III)
- Disc aspiration in difficult cases

Tuberculous Vertebral Osteomyelitis
- Mid-thoracic or thoracolumbar > lumbar or cervical
- Vertebral collapse, gibbus deformity
- ± Endplate destructive changes
- Large dissecting paraspinal abscesses out of proportion to vertebral involvement

Spinal Neuropathic Arthropathy
- Sequela of spinal cord injury
- Disc space loss/T2 hyperintensity; endplate erosion/sclerosis; osteophytosis; soft tissue mass
  - Present in both spondylodiscitis and neuropathic spine
- Vacuum disc/rim enhancement; facet involvement; spondylolisthesis; debris; disorganization
  - More common in neuropathic spine

Chronic Hemodialysis Spondyloarthropathy
- Cervical spine most common
- Disc space loss, endplate erosion, vertebral destruction
- Vertebral marrow hypointense on both T1WI & T2WI
- Low to intermediate disc-signal intensity on T2WI
- ± Soft-tissue component
- Clinical history of renal disease, hemodialysis
- Presence of amyloid on biopsy

Spinal Metastases
- Discrete or ill-defined vertebral lesions
  - Hypointense on T1WI

PYOGENIC OSTEOMYELITIS, SPINE

- ○ Hyperintense on T2WI
- ○ Post-gadolinium enhancement
- Non-contiguous vertebral involvement
- Posterior elements commonly effected
- Disc space preserved

PATHOLOGY

General Features
- General path comments: Spectrum of suppurative infections involving disc, vertebrae, & adjacent soft tissue
- Etiology
  - ○ Predisposing factors
    - Intravenous drug use
    - Immunocompromised state
    - Chronic medical illnesses (renal failure, cirrhosis, cancer, diabetes)
  - ○ Staphylococcus aureus is most common pathogen
    - Escherichia coli most common within gram-negative bacilli
    - Salmonella more common in patients with sickle-cell disease
  - ○ Bacteremia from extraspinal primary source
    - Most common route of infection
    - GU or GI tract, lungs, cardiac, mucous/cutaneous sources
    - Vascularized subchondral bone adjacent to endplate seeded primarily
    - Secondary infection of intervertebral disc, adjacent vertebra
    - Intervertebral disc first site of infection in children due to presence of vascularity
  - ○ Direct inoculation from penetrating trauma, surgical intervention, or diagnostic procedures
    - Epidural injection/catheter
  - ○ Extension from adjacent infection in paraspinal soft tissues
    - Diverticulitis, appendicitis, inflammatory bowel disease
    - Pyelonephritis
- Epidemiology: 2-7% of osteomyelitis in US
- Associated abnormalities
  - ○ Spinal meningitis
  - ○ Myelitis

Gross Pathologic & Surgical Features
- Necrotic bone
- Suppurative soft tissue

Microscopic Features
- Bone/disc fragments
- Leukocytes, micro-organisms, cellular debris

CLINICAL ISSUES

Presentation
- Most common signs/symptoms
  - ○ Acute or chronic back pain
  - ○ Focal spinal tenderness
  - ○ Fever
- Other signs/symptoms
  - ○ Myelopathy if cord compromised
  - ○ Elevated erythrocyte sedimentation rate, C-reactive protein, white cell count
- Clinical Profile: Average duration of symptoms for 7 weeks before diagnosis

Demographics
- Age
  - ○ Bimodal distribution
    - Pediatric patients
    - 6th-7th decade
- Gender: Slight male predominance

Natural History & Prognosis
- Vertebral collapse
- Irreversible neurological deficits
- Mortality rate 2-12%
- Favorable outcome, resolution of symptoms if prompt diagnosis & treatment
  - ○ Residual functional deficits may be present in 15% of patients
- Recurrence due to incomplete treatment: 2-8%
- Improvement in imaging findings may lag behind clinical improvement

Treatment
- Early empiric antibiotics, broad spectrum coverage until causative pathogen isolated
  - ○ Should be effective against staphylococci, gram-negatives, anaerobes
- Organism-specific parenteral antibiotics for 6-8 weeks
- Spinal immobilization with bracing for 6-12 weeks
- Surgical treatment
  - ○ Laminectomy, debridement, ± stabilization
  - ○ Especially if epidural abscess, instability present

DIAGNOSTIC CHECKLIST

Image Interpretation Pearls
- Diffusely enhancing disc, adjacent vertebral marrow, soft tissue with endplate erosion highly suggestive of vertebral osteomyelitis

SELECTED REFERENCES

1. Ledermann HP et al: MR imaging findings in spinal infections: rules or myths? Radiology. 228(2):506-14, 2003
2. Love C et al: Diagnosing spinal osteomyelitis: a comparison of bone and Ga-67 scintigraphy and magnetic resonance imaging. Clin Nucl Med. 25(12):963-77, 2000
3. Wagner SC et al: Can imaging findings help differentiate spinal neuropathic arthropathy from disk space infection? Initial experience. Radiology. 214(3):693-9, 2000
4. Carragee EJ: The clinical use of magnetic resonance imaging in pyogenic vertebral osteomyelitis. Spine. 22(7):780-5, 1997
5. Dagirmanjian A et al: MR imaging of vertebral osteomyelitis revisited. AJR Am J Roentgenol. 167(6):1539-43, 1996
6. Thrush A et al: MR imaging of infectious spondylitis. AJNR Am J Neuroradiol. 11(6):1171-80, 1990
7. Modic MT et al: Vertebral osteomyelitis: assessment using MR. Radiology. 157(1):157-66, 1985

PYOGENIC OSTEOMYELITIS, SPINE

IMAGE GALLERY

Typical

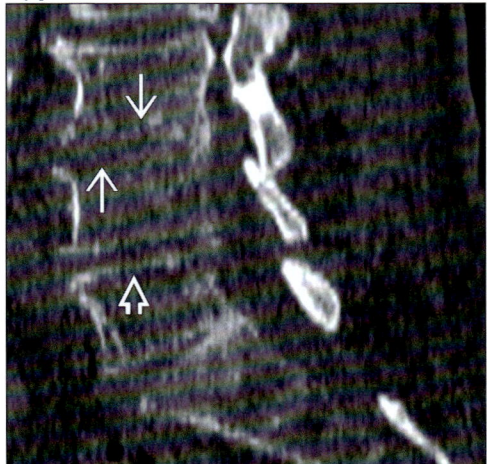
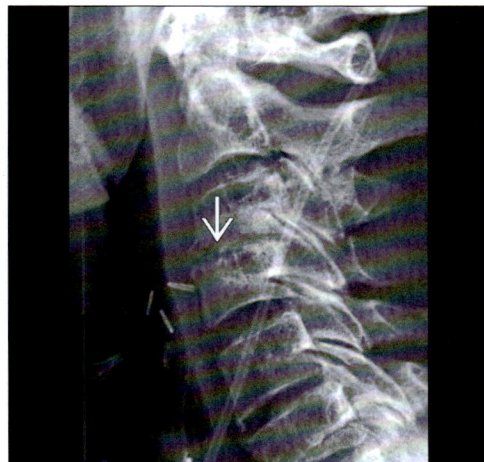

(Left) Sagittal NECT shows disc space narrowing at L3-4 with loss of cortical margins of endplates ➡. Note normal cortical margin at adjacent disc space ➡.
(Right) Lateral radiograph shows loss of C3-4 disc height with irregularity of endplates surrounding disc ➡.

Typical

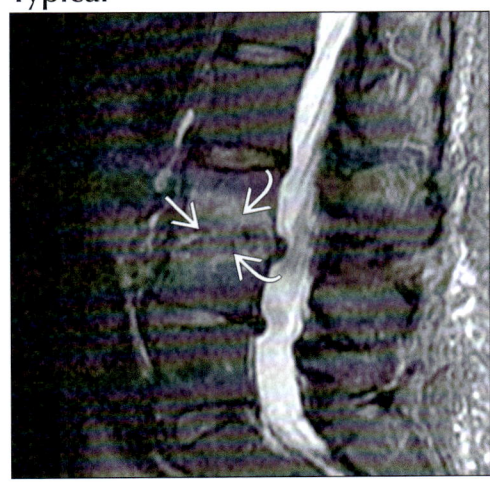
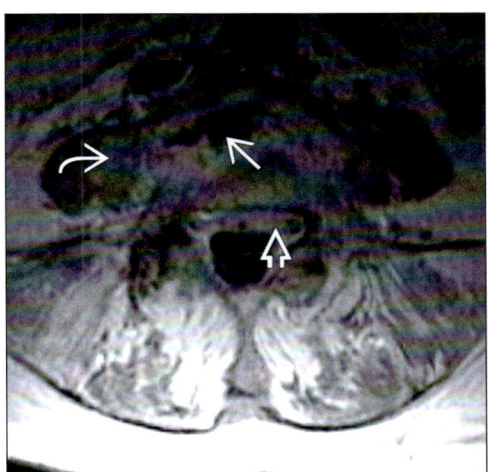

(Left) Sagittal T2WI FS MR shows loss of disc height with endplate destruction ➡ and increased marrow signal adjacent to endplates ➡.
(Right) Axial T1 C+ MR shows abnormal enhancement of disc with rim-enhancing abscess ➡. Note extension of phlegmon into paraspinal muscle ➡ & anterior epidural space ➡.

Typical

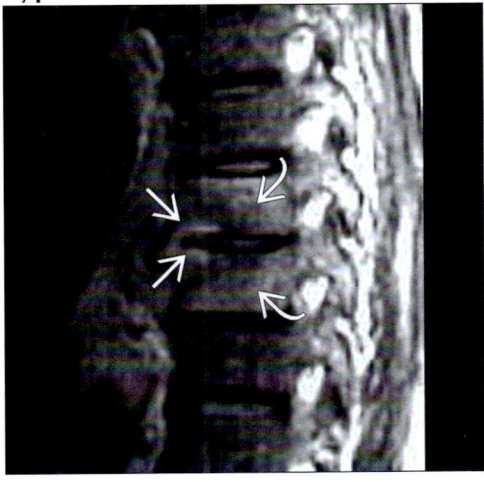
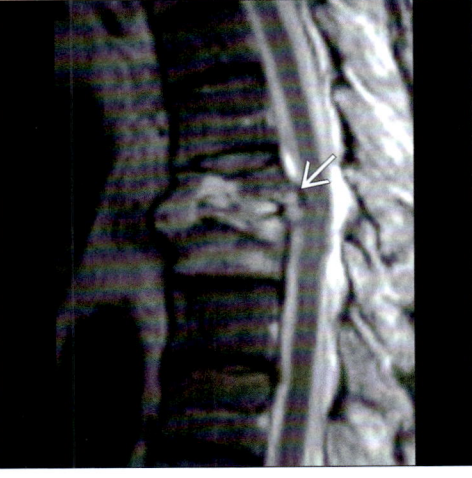

(Left) Sagittal T2WI FS MR shows bone marrow edema of two contiguous vertebral bodies ➡ with early endplate irregularity of anterior endplates ➡.
(Right) Sagittal T2WI FS MR in same patient as left shows progression to loss of disc height and vertebral body collapse. Note small focus of epidural extension ➡.

GRANULOMATOUS OSTEOMYELITIS, SPINE

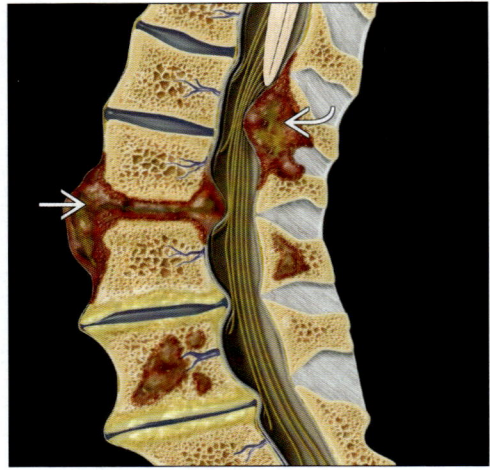

Sagittal graphic through lumbar spine depicts multifocal granulomatous osteomyelitis. Frank abscesses are present at L3-4 disc space ➡ and between spinous process of L2 and L3 ➡.

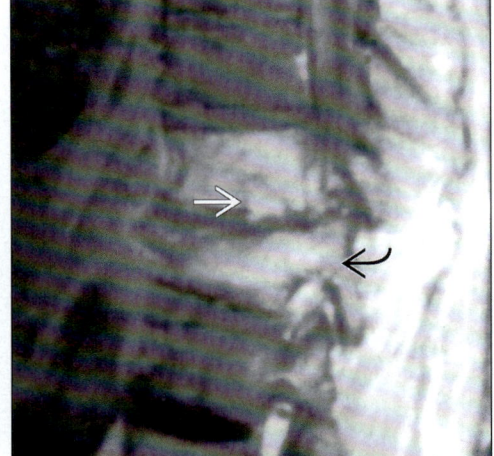

Sagittal T1 C+ FS MR shows endplate irregularity and vertebral body collapse of contiguous vertebrae ➡. There is diffuse marrow enhancement extending into posterior elements ➡.

TERMINOLOGY

Abbreviations and Synonyms
- Tuberculous spondylitis (TS): Pott disease
- Brucellar spondylitis (BS)

Definitions
- Granulomatous infection of spine and adjacent soft tissue typically 2° tuberculosis or brucellosis

IMAGING FINDINGS

General Features
- Best diagnostic clue
  - TS: Gibbus vertebrae with relatively intact intervertebral discs, large paraspinal abscesses
  - BS: Anterosuperior epiphysitis at L4 with associated sacroiliitis
- Location
  - TS
    - Mid-thoracic or thoracolumbar > lumbar, cervical
    - Anterior vertebral body
    - Isolated posterior element involvement possible
    - Laminae > pedicles > spinous process > transverse process
  - BS
    - Lower lumbar spine (L4) > cervical = thoracic
    - Sacroiliac joints
    - Posterior elements not affected
    - Anterior endplate at diskovertebral junction involved in focal BS
    - Entire vertebral body affected in diffuse BS
- Size: Multiple (non)contiguous vertebrae
- Morphology
  - TS
    - Vertebral collapse, gibbus deformity
    - ± Destruction of intervertebral discs
    - Epidural soft-tissue mass
    - Large dissecting paraspinal abscesses over considerable distance
  - BS
    - Vertebrae morphologically intact despite osteomyelitis
    - Spinal deformity rare
    - Destruction of intervertebral discs
    - Epidural soft-tissue mass
    - Paraspinal soft-tissues rarely affected

DDx: Granulomatous Osteomyelitis

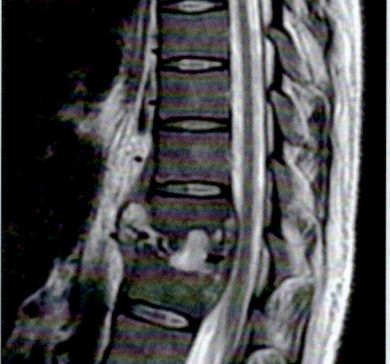
Pyogenic Osteomyelitis

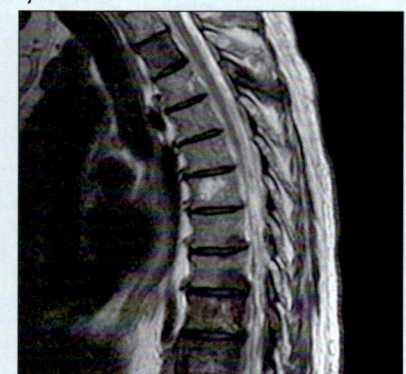
Metastases

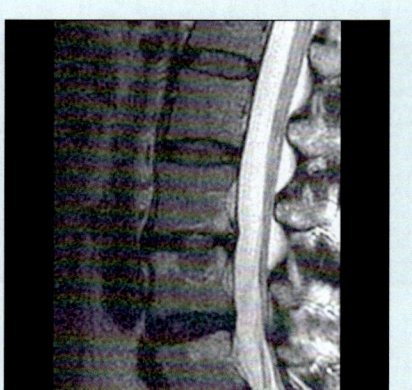
Degenerative Disc Disease

GRANULOMATOUS OSTEOMYELITIS, SPINE

Key Facts

Terminology
- Tuberculous spondylitis (TS): Pott disease
- Brucellar spondylitis (BS)
- Granulomatous infection of spine and adjacent soft tissue typically 2° tuberculosis or brucellosis

Imaging Findings
- TS: Gibbus vertebrae with relatively intact intervertebral discs, large paraspinal abscesses
- Endplate irregularity, osteolysis on radiographs
- Vertebral sclerosis on radiographs
- Fusion across disc space in late TS & BS on radiographs
- Endplate destruction on NECT
- T2WI: Hyperintense marrow, disc, phlegmon/abscess
- Marrow, subligamentous, discal, dural enhancement on T1 C+
- Diffusely enhancing soft-tissue (phlegmon) on T1 C+
- Gallium Scan: ↑ Radionuclide uptake in spine & paraspinal soft-tissue

Top Differential Diagnoses
- Pyogenic Spondylitis (PS)
- Fungal Spondylitis
- Degenerative Disc Disease
- Spinal Metastases

Clinical Issues
- Most common signs/symptoms: Chronic back pain, focal tenderness, fever

Diagnostic Checklist
- Thoracic spondylitis with posterior element involvement, large paraspinal abscesses suggest TS

Radiographic Findings
- Radiography
  - Endplate irregularity, osteolysis on radiographs
  - Vertebral sclerosis on radiographs
    - Focal in BS, diffuse in TS
  - Fusion across disc space in late TS & BS on radiographs
  - Findings may not be present until weeks after onset of infection

CT Findings
- NECT
  - Endplate destruction on NECT
  - Fragmentation of vertebral bodies
  - Calcifications of chronic paravertebral abscesses: TS > BS
- CECT: Diffuse or peripherally enhancing epidural and paraspinal soft-tissue

MR Findings
- T1WI
  - Hypointense marrow in contiguous vertebrae
  - Hypointense intraosseous, extradural, paraspinal abscesses
- T2WI: Hyperintense marrow, disc, phlegmon/abscess
- STIR: Hyperintense marrow, disc, phlegmon/abscess
- T1 C+
  - Marrow, subligamentous, discal, dural enhancement on T1 C+
  - Diffusely enhancing soft-tissue (phlegmon) on T1 C+
  - Peripherally enhancing soft-tissue (abscess)
- Cord displacement or compression from epidural abscess
- May have extradural infection without bone destruction
- Atypical findings in TS
  - Isolated vertebral body or posterior element involvement
  - Sacral involvement

Nuclear Medicine Findings
- Bone Scan
  - Increased spinal radionuclide uptake
  - Sensitive but not specific
- Gallium Scan: ↑ Radionuclide uptake in spine & paraspinal soft-tissue
  - Highly sensitive and specific for vertebral osteomyelitis

Imaging Recommendations
- Best imaging tool
  - Sagittal and axial T1WI, T2WI and T1 C+ MR
    - Evaluate extent of disease, assess response to treatment
- Protocol advice: Sagittal STIR or FSE T2 with fat-saturation most sensitive for bone marrow edema, epidural involvement

DIFFERENTIAL DIAGNOSIS

Pyogenic Spondylitis (PS)
- Peak incidence in older patients
- Predilection for lower lumbar spine
- Initial infection in subchondral bone adjacent to endplate
  - Intervertebral discs typically affected
- Posterior element involvement less common
- Soft-tissue calcifications and spinal deformity infrequent

Fungal Spondylitis
- May be indistinguishable from TS

Degenerative Disc Disease
- Modic type-I changes may mimic infection
  - Hypointense T1, hyperintense T2 signal
  - Inflammatory marrow change

Spinal Metastases
- Hypointense T1, hyperintense T2 signal
  - Post-gadolinium enhancement
  - Posterior elements typically involved

GRANULOMATOUS OSTEOMYELITIS, SPINE

- Extraosseous epidural or paraspinal extension
- Pathologic compression fractures
- Disc space preserved
- May be difficult to distinguish from isolated tuberculous, fungal, or brucellar spondylitis

PATHOLOGY

General Features
- General path comments: Granulomatous destruction of spinal column with adjacent soft-tissue infection
- Etiology
  - TS
    - Hematogenous spread or through lymphatics from pulmonary origin
    - Initial inoculum in anterior vertebral body
    - Spread to noncontiguous vertebral bodies beneath longitudinal ligaments
    - Sparing of intervertebral disc 2° lack of proteolytic enzymes
    - Paraspinal, subarachnoid dissemination of disease
  - BS
    - Access to spine via hematogenous dissemination
    - Direct extension to adjacent discs and vertebrae
  - Other pathogens causing granulomatous osteomyelitis (streptomyces, Madurella) uncommon
- Epidemiology
  - Rising incidence of tuberculosis in past two decades
  - TS in < 1% of patients with tuberculosis
  - Concomitant pulmonary tuberculosis in about 10% of patients
  - TS more aggressive in children
    - Kyphosis, cord compression more common
  - Brucellosis uncommon in US: 100-200 cases per year
    - Prevalent in Mediterranean, South and Central America, Middle East, with reported incidence 6-58%
- Associated abnormalities
  - Intramedullary abscess
  - Arachnoiditis

Microscopic Features
- Both TS and BS show caseating granulomas, nonspecific inflammatory reaction
- Acid-fast bacilli isolated < 50% of time
- Brucellar species very difficult to culture

CLINICAL ISSUES

Presentation
- Most common signs/symptoms: Chronic back pain, focal tenderness, fever
- Other signs/symptoms
  - Paraparesis, kyphosis, sensory disturbance
  - Bladder and bowel dysfunction
- Clinical Profile
  - Gradual, insidious onset of symptoms results in diagnostic delay
  - Fever relatively infrequent in TS
  - Neurologic deficits more common with TS compared to BS

Demographics
- Age
  - TS: Most prevalent in fifth decade
  - BS: More common in sixth decade
- Gender
  - M = F in TS
  - M:F = 2.4:1 in BS

Natural History & Prognosis
- Prognosis depends on early diagnosis and institution of appropriate therapy
- Proper treatment
  - Favorable outcome with resolution of symptoms
    - Particularly favorable if early presentation and lack of neurologic deficits or spinal deformity
- No treatment
  - Progressive vertebral collapse
  - Irreversible neurologic deficits
  - Death

Treatment
- Antibrucellar medications highly effective
  - Surgical debridement rarely indicated
- Long-term antituberculous medication for at least one year
- Surgical decompression in setting of neurologic deficits ± spinal deformity
  - Indicated in 10-25% of TS
  - Laminectomy and debridement in absence of vertebral destruction
  - Debridement and fusion if spinal deformity present

DIAGNOSTIC CHECKLIST

Image Interpretation Pearls
- Thoracic spondylitis with posterior element involvement, large paraspinal abscesses suggest TS
- BS should be differential diagnosis of L4 lumbar spondylitis with associated bilateral sacroiliitis

SELECTED REFERENCES

1. Akman S et al: Magnetic resonance imaging of tuberculous spondylitis. Orthopedics. 26(1):69-73, 2003
2. Narlawar RS et al: Isolated tuberculosis of posterior elements of spine: magnetic resonance imaging findings in 33 patients. Spine. 27(3):275-81, 2002
3. Gouliamos AD et al: MR imaging of tuberculous vertebral osteomyelitis: pictorial review. Eur Radiol. 11(4):575-9, 2001
4. Hadjipavlou AG et al: The effectiveness of gallium citrate Ga 67 radionuclide imaging in vertebral osteomyelitis revisited. Am J Orthop. 27(3):179-83, 1998
5. Sharif HS et al: Granulomatous spinal infections: MR imaging. Radiology. 177(1):101-7, 1990
6. Sharif HS et al: Brucellar and tuberculous spondylitis: comparative imaging features. Radiology. 171(2):419-25, 1989
7. Smith AS et al: MR imaging characteristics of tuberculous spondylitis vs vertebral osteomyelitis. AJR Am J Roentgenol. 153(2):399-405, 1989

GRANULOMATOUS OSTEOMYELITIS, SPINE

IMAGE GALLERY

Typical

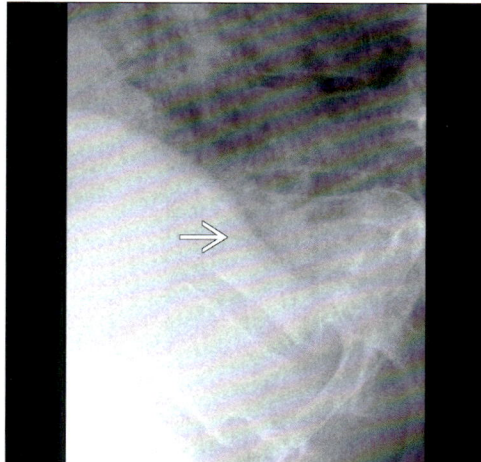
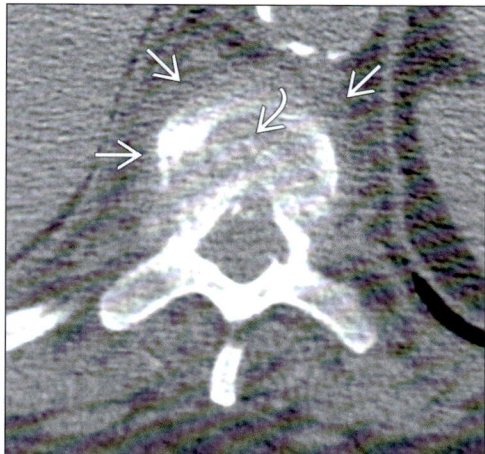

(Left) Lateral radiograph shows destruction of T11 and T12 vertebral bodies ➡ with resulting acute kyphosis (gibbus deformity). *(Right)* Axial NECT shows destruction and fragmentation of T12 vertebral body ➡ with increased paraspinal soft tissue ➡ indicating phlegmon.

Typical

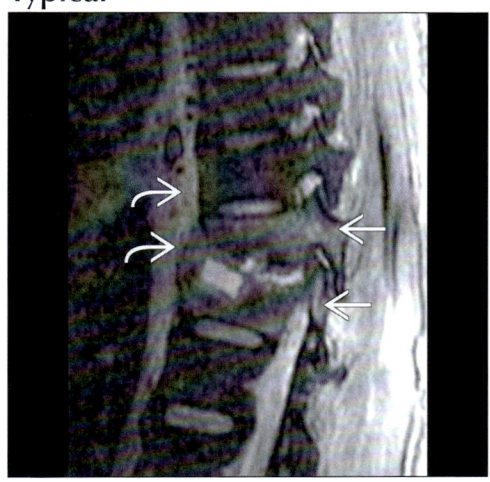
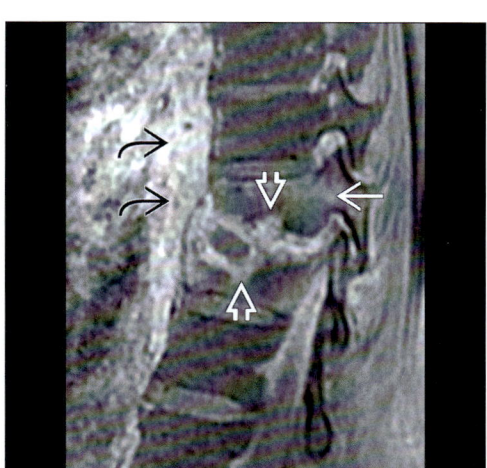

(Left) Sagittal STIR MR shows endplate destruction and marrow edema of two contiguous thoracic vertebrae affecting posterior elements ➡. Note prevertebral tissue edema ➡. *(Right)* Sagittal T1 C+ FS MR shows marked enhancement of paravertebral soft tissues ➡, consistent with infection. Note mild enhancement of vertebral endplates ➡ and bone marrow ➡.

Typical

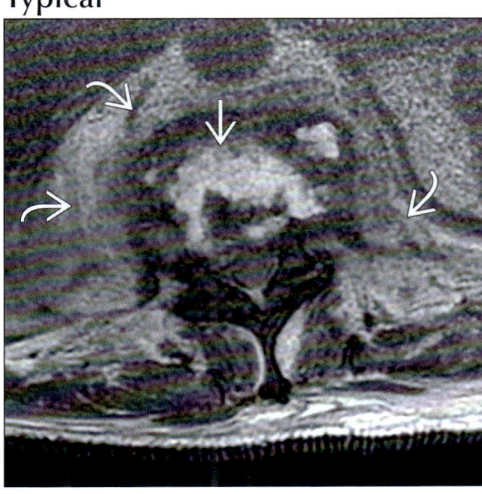
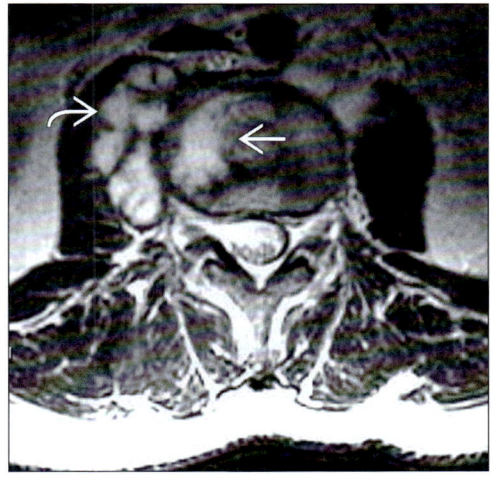

(Left) Axial T2WI FS MR shows fragmentation and increased signal within vertebral body ➡. Note extensive increased signal in paraspinal soft tissues ➡. *(Right)* Axial T2WI MR shows increased signal within vertebral body ➡ in patient with TB spondylitis. Notice loculated increased signal in right psoas ➡, indicating abscess.

EPIDURAL PARAVERTEBRAL ABSCESS

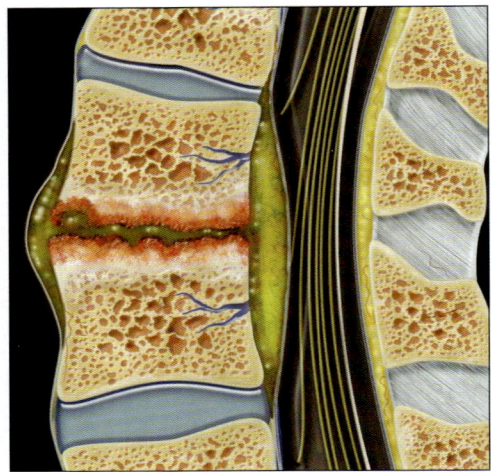

Sagittal graphic through lumbar spine demonstrates vertebral osteomyelitis with intervertebral abscess extending ventrally and dorsally, narrowing central canal.

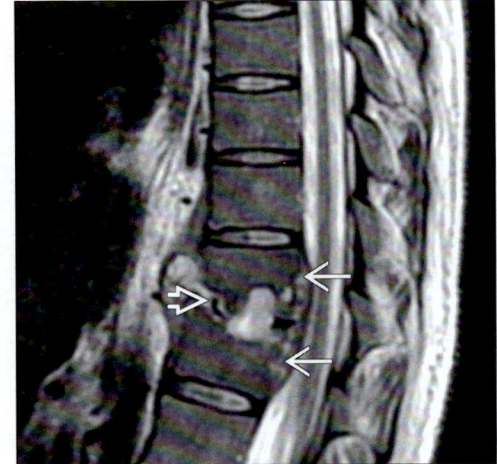

Sagittal T2WI MR shows spondylodiscitis of two lower thoracic vertebrae ➡. Note epidural extension of infection ➡ narrowing spinal canal.

TERMINOLOGY

Abbreviations and Synonyms
- Spinal epidural abscess (SEA)
- Spinal dural empyema

Definitions
- Extradural spinal infection with abscess formation

IMAGING FINDINGS

General Features
- Best diagnostic clue: Findings of spondylodiscitis with adjacent enhancing epidural phlegmon ± peripherally enhancing fluid collection
- Location
  - Posterior epidural space (80%), anterior (20%), circumferential (caudal to S2)
  - Lower thoracic and lumbar > cervical and upper thoracic
- Size: May extend over many segments
- Morphology: Focal or diffuse elongated epidural soft tissue

Radiographic Findings
- Radiography
  - Not directly visualized
  - Associated findings of spondylodiscitis: Endplate irregularity/destruction; disc height loss

CT Findings
- CECT: Enhancing epidural mass narrowing central canal
- Bone CT
  - Increased epidural soft tissue
  - May be difficult to distinguish from disc

MR Findings
- T1WI: Iso- to hypointense to cord
- T2WI: Hyperintense
- STIR: Hyperintense
- T2* GRE: Iso- to hyperintense
- DWI: Hyperintense
- T1 C+
  - Homogeneously or heterogeneously enhancing phlegmon on T1 C+
  - Peripherally enhancing necrotic abscess on T1 C+
  - Diffuse dural enhancement in extensive SEA

DDx: Epidural Abscess Mimics

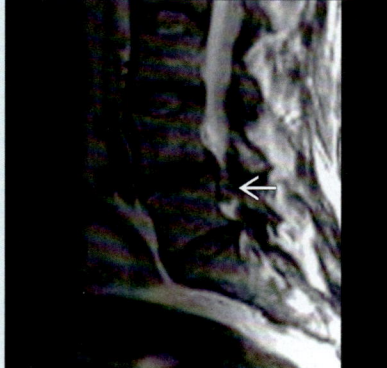

Disc Extrusion

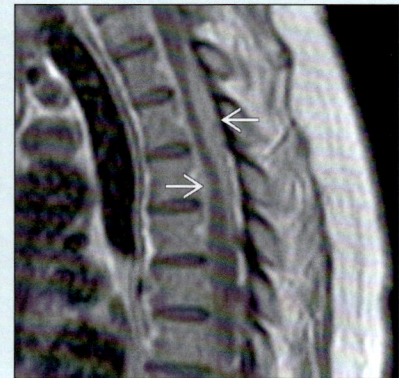

Epidural Tumor

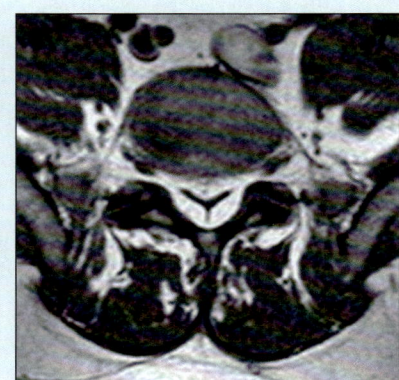

Epidural Lipomatosis

EPIDURAL PARAVERTEBRAL ABSCESS

Key Facts

Terminology
- Extradural spinal infection with abscess formation

Imaging Findings
- Best diagnostic clue: Findings of spondylodiscitis with adjacent enhancing epidural phlegmon ± peripherally enhancing fluid collection
- Posterior epidural space (80%), anterior (20%), circumferential (caudal to S2)
- Lower thoracic and lumbar > cervical and upper thoracic
- T1WI: Iso- to hypointense to cord
- T2WI: Hyperintense
- Homogeneously or heterogeneously enhancing phlegmon on T1 C+
- Peripherally enhancing necrotic abscess on T1 C+

Top Differential Diagnoses
- Extradural Metastasis
- Epidural Hematoma
- Extruded/Migrated Disc

Pathology
- Staphylococcus aureus is most common pathogen: 57-73% of reported cases
- Mycobacterium tuberculosis is next most frequent cause: 25% of reported cases
- Cord symptoms likely from combination of compressive & ischemic effects

Clinical Issues
- Most common signs/symptoms: Fever, acute or subacute spinal pain and tenderness

---

  - Enhancing prominent anterior epidural veins or basivertebral venous plexus above/below abscess
- Various degree of encroachment on central canal and intervertebral foramina
- Signal alteration in spinal cord 2° compression, ischemia or direct infection
- Persistent epidural enhancement without mass effect on follow-up MR imaging
  - Probable sterile granulation tissue or fibrosis
  - Correlation with erythrocyte sedimentation rate for disease activity

Non-Vascular Interventions
- Myelography: Epidural mass impeding cerebral spinal fluid flow

Nuclear Medicine Findings
- Gallium scan
  - Increased uptake in spinal or epidural area

Imaging Recommendations
- Best imaging tool: Sagittal and axial T1WI and T2WI MR with gadolinium
- Protocol advice: Sagittal STIR or T2WI with fat-saturation increases lesion conspicuity by suppressing signal from epidural fat and vertebral marrow

DIFFERENTIAL DIAGNOSIS

Extradural Metastasis
- Well-circumscribed extra-osseous soft-tissue mass
  - Hypointense on T1WI, hyperintense on T2WI
  - Diffuse enhancement
  - Often contiguous with vertebral lesion
    - Destruction of posterior vertebra/pedicle
  - Intervertebral discs unaffected
- Pathologic compression fractures
- Sparing of spinal column in some cases
  - Spinal epidural lymphoma

Epidural Hematoma
- Heterogeneously hyperintense on T2WI
- Acute hemorrhage isointense on T1WI
  - Subacute and chronic hemorrhage hyperintense
- No significant post-gadolinium enhancement
- Intact vertebrae in absence of trauma

Extruded/Migrated Disc
- Associated parent disc height loss, protrusion, degeneration
  - Iso- to hypointense on T2WI
- More focal appearance
- ± Mild peripheral post-gadolinium enhancement
- Vertebral endplates intact

Epidural Lipomatosis
- Excessive epidural fat in thoracic and lumbar canal
- Homogeneous and hyperintense on T1WI and T2WI
- Signal loss with fat suppression
- Mass effect on spinal cord

PATHOLOGY

General Features
- General path comments: Suppuration of epidural space from adjacent infection or bacteremia
- Genetics: No genetic predilection
- Etiology
  - Staphylococcus aureus is most common pathogen: 57-73% of reported cases
  - Mycobacterium tuberculosis is next most frequent cause: 25% of reported cases
  - Fungal infection less common
  - Predisposing factors
    - Intravenous drug abuse
    - Immunocompromised state
    - Diabetes mellitus, chronic renal failure, alcoholism, cancer, other chronic illnesses
  - Anterior SEA arises from adjacent discitis & vertebral osteomyelitis
  - Posterior SEA arises from GU or GI tract, lungs, cardiac, mucous/cutaneous sources through hematogenous dissemination

EPIDURAL PARAVERTEBRAL ABSCESS

- Direct inoculation from penetrating trauma, surgical intervention, or diagnostic procedures
  - Risk of SEA in epidural anesthesia: 5.5%
  - Extradural hematoma may become infected in blunt trauma
- Extension from adjacent infection in paraspinal soft tissues
  - Diverticulitis, appendicitis, pyelonephritis
- Anterior cranial-caudal epidural extension by tracking beneath posterior longitudinal ligament
- Tuberculous infection tends to spread beneath anterior longitudinal ligament
  - Intervertebral discs spared
- Cord symptoms likely from combination of compressive & ischemic effects
  - Cord ischemia from compromised epidural venous plexuses
- Epidemiology: 0.2 to 2.8 cases per 10,000
- Associated abnormalities: Discitis, osteomyelitis, paraspinal abscess, septic facet arthritis

Microscopic Features
- Granulation tissue, leukocytes, cellular debris

CLINICAL ISSUES

Presentation
- Most common signs/symptoms: Fever, acute or subacute spinal pain and tenderness
- Other signs/symptoms: Radiculopathy, paraparesis/paralysis, paresthesia, loss of bladder and bowel control
- Clinical Profile
  - In patients with septicemia or chronic illness, neurologic symptoms may be obscured by systemic complaints
  - Lumbar SEA mimics disc herniation
  - Abscess from hematogenous spread progresses rapidly
  - Abscess from discitis/osteomyelitis tends to smolder

Demographics
- Age
  - All ages reported
  - Peak incidence in sixth and seventh decades
- Gender: M:F = 1:0.56

Natural History & Prognosis
- Irreversible neurologic deficit and death if untreated or delayed treatment
- Factors influencing prognosis
  - Age
    - Better prognosis in children than adults
  - Severity of initial neurologic deficits
    - Thecal compression > 50% associated with poor prognosis
  - Duration between onset of neurologic deficits and surgical intervention
    - Early diagnosis & institution of treatment improve prognosis
  - Co-morbidities
- Mortality rate 12-30%

Treatment
- Emergent surgical decompression with abscess drainage
  - Even in absence of initial neurologic compromise
    - Rapid progression of neurologic deficits can occur despite appropriate medical therapy
- Early empiric antibiotics with broad-spectrum coverage until causative pathogen isolated
  - Should be effective against staphylococci, gram-negatives and anaerobes
- Organism-specific intravenous antibiotics followed by long-term parenteral antibiotics for 6-8 weeks
- Medical therapy alone if substantial operative risks, extensive cranial-caudal involvement of spinal canal, or paralysis > 3 days

DIAGNOSTIC CHECKLIST

Image Interpretation Pearls
- Epidural soft tissue with homogeneous or peripheral enhancement and adjacent spondylodiscitis characteristic of SEA

SELECTED REFERENCES

1. Eastwood JD et al: Diffusion-weighted imaging in a patient with vertebral and epidural abscesses. AJNR Am J Neuroradiol. 23(3):496-8, 2002
2. Varma R et al: Imaging of pyogenic infectious spondylodiskitis. Radiol Clin North Am. 39(2):203-13, 2001
3. Reihsaus E et al: Spinal epidural abscess: a meta-analysis of 915 patients. Neurosurg Rev. 23(4):175-204; discussion 205, 2000
4. Ruiz A et al: MR imaging of infections of the cervical spine. Magn Reson Imaging Clin N Am. 8(3):561-80, 2000
5. Sampath P et al: Spinal epidural abscess: a review of epidemiology, diagnosis, and treatment. J Spinal Disord. 12(2):89-93, 1999
6. Tung GA et al: Spinal epidural abscess: correlation between MRI findings and outcome. Neuroradiology. 41(12):904-9, 1999
7. Khanna RK et al: Spinal epidural abscess: evaluation of factors influencing outcome. Neurosurgery. 39(5):958-64, 1996
8. Numaguchi Y et al: Spinal epidural abscess: evaluation with gadolinium-enhanced MR imaging. Radiographics. 13(3):545-59; discussion 559-60, 1993
9. Nussbaum ES et al: Spinal epidural abscess: a report of 40 cases and review. Surg Neurol. 38(3):225-31, 1992
10. Sandhu FS et al: Spinal epidural abscess: evaluation with contrast-enhanced MR imaging. AJNR Am J Neuroradiol. 12(6):1087-93, 1991

EPIDURAL PARAVERTEBRAL ABSCESS

IMAGE GALLERY

Typical

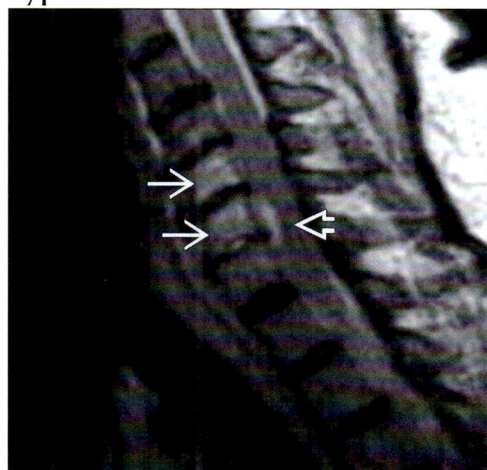
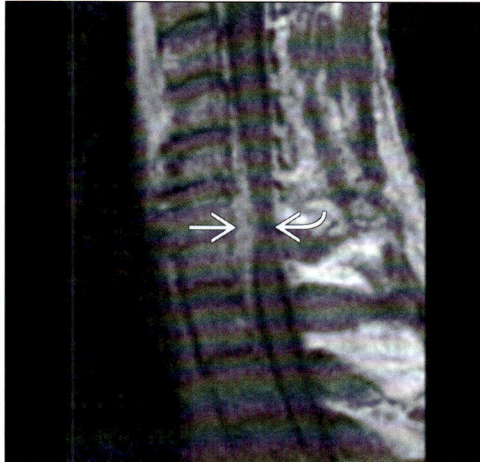

(Left) Sagittal T2WI MR shows increased signal in multiple vertebrae ➜ 2° osteomyelitis. Note epidural abscess posterior to C6-7 disc ➜ with mass effect on cord. *(Right)* Sagittal T1WI MR shows epidural abscess ➜ narrowing spinal canal and compressing cervical cord ➜. Abscess has high T1 signal due to proteinaceous pus.

Typical

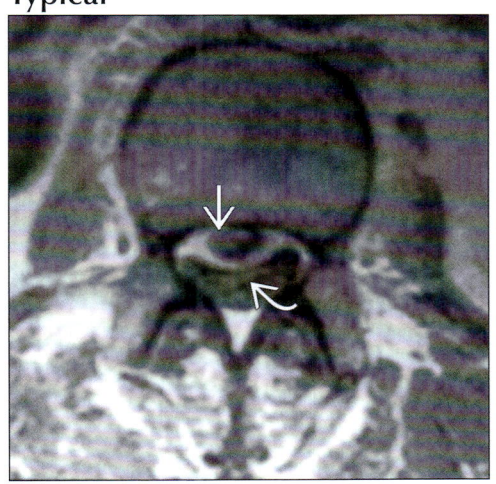
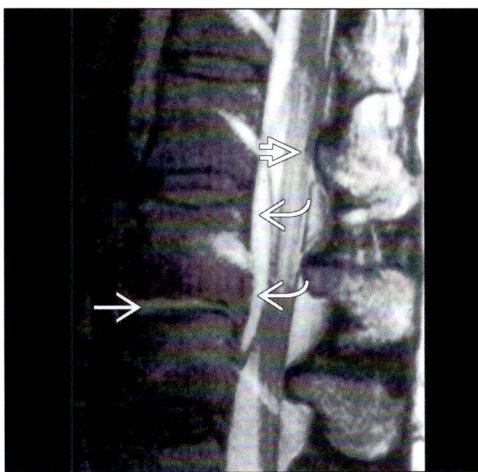

(Left) Axial T1 C+ FS MR shows rim-enhancing collection consistent with abscess ➜ compressing anterior thecal sac and cord ➜. *(Right)* Sagittal T2WI FS MR shows narrowing and increased signal of infected disc ➜ with extension to epidural space ➜. Note abnormal signal in nerve roots ➜.

Typical

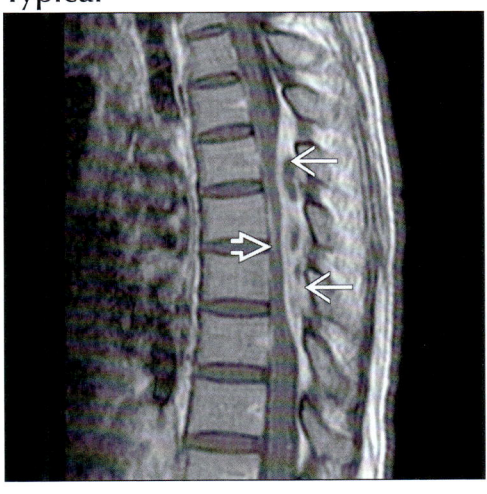
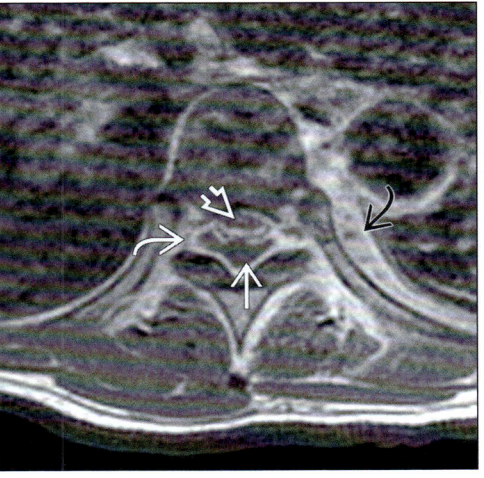

(Left) Sagittal T1 C+ MR shows rim-enhancing collection in posterior epidural space ➜ representing abscess. Note severe compression of thecal sac/spinal cord ➜. *(Right)* Axial T1 C+ MR in the same patient as previous image, again shows abscess ➜ and compressed cord ➜. Note extension into right foramen ➜ and left paraspinal collection ➜.

SPINAL CORD INFARCTION

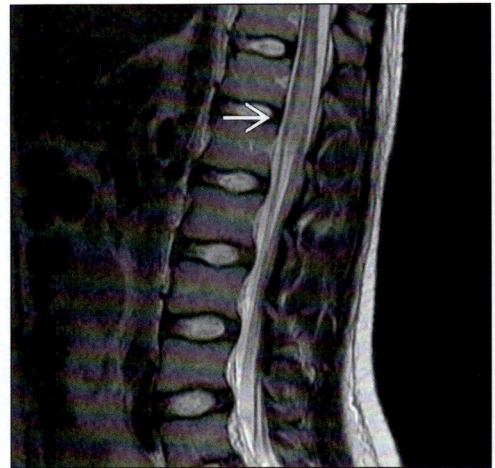

Sagittal T2WI MR shows central hyperintensity ➡ of conus.

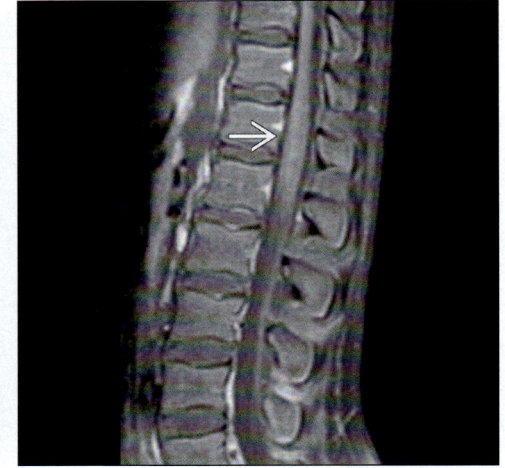

Sagittal T1 C+ MR shows expansion of conus ➡, no enhancement.

TERMINOLOGY

Abbreviations and Synonyms
- Spinal cord infarction (SCI); cord ischemia
- Cord infarction 2° vessel occlusion (radicular artery)

IMAGING FINDINGS

General Features
- Best diagnostic clue: Hyperintensity on T2WI
- Location: Thoracic cord → arterial border zone
- Size: Usually more than one vertebral body segment
- Morphology: Central hyperintensity on T2WI

CT Findings
- NECT: Noncontributory

MR Findings
- T1WI
  - Slight cord expansion
  - Hemorrhage conversion → hyperintense
- T2WI: Hyperintensity central GM or entire cross-sectional area
- DWI: Hyperintense
- MRA: Assess for dural arteriovenous fistula

Imaging Recommendations
- Protocol advice: T2WI sagittal & axial, DWI

DIFFERENTIAL DIAGNOSIS

Multiple Sclerosis (MS)
- Peripheral location, < two segments

Spinal Cord Neoplasm
- Expansion, enhancement, edema, cyst

Idiopathic Transverse Myelitis
- Central, usually > 2/3 cross-sectional area of cord
- 3-4 Segments, occupies > 2/3 of cord diameter

Type-I Dural Fistula
- Cord expansion & edema on T2WI
- Enlarged serpentine pial veins on cord surface

DDx: Spinal Cord Infarction Mimics

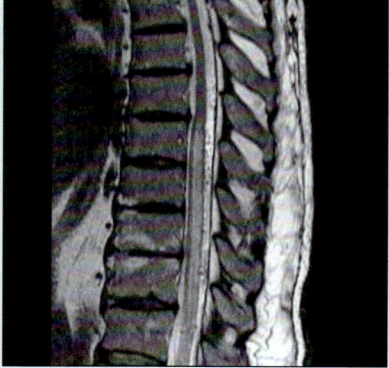

Dural AV Fistula

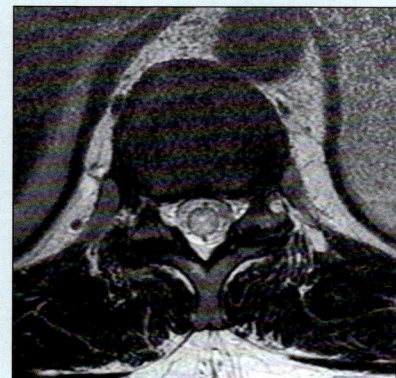

Dural AV Fistula

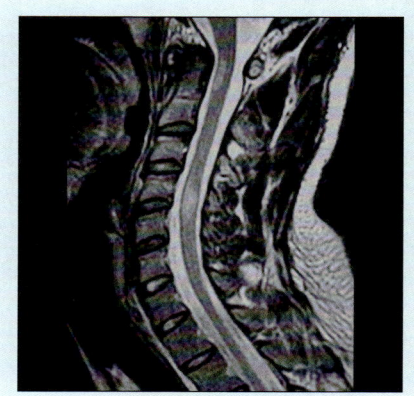

Multiple Sclerosis

SPINAL CORD INFARCTION

Terminology
- Spinal cord infarction (SCI); cord ischemia
- Cord infarction 2° vessel occlusion (radicular artery)

Imaging Findings
- Best diagnostic clue: Hyperintensity on T2WI
- Location: Thoracic cord → arterial border zone
- Size: Usually more than one vertebral body segment
- Slight cord expansion

Key Facts
- T2WI: Hyperintensity central GM or entire cross-sectional area
- DWI: Hyperintense
- Protocol advice: T2WI sagittal & axial, DWI

Top Differential Diagnoses
- Multiple Sclerosis (MS)
- Type-I Dural Fistula

PATHOLOGY

General Features
- General path comments
  - Embryology/anatomy
    - Radicular arteries → 1 anterior, 2 posterior spinal arteries
    - Anterior spinal artery branches supply GM, adjacent WM mantle
    - Posterior branches supply 1/3 cord periphery
- Etiology
  - Atherosclerosis → dissection or emboli
  - Thoracoabdominal aneurysm; aortic surgery
  - Systemic hypotension; spinal AVM
  - Vasculitis; decompression sickness

Gross Pathologic & Surgical Features
- Soft, pale, swollen tissue

Microscopic Features
- Acute: Ischemic neurons with cytotoxic + vasogenic edema, swelling of endothelial cells + astrocytes

CLINICAL ISSUES

Presentation
- Most common signs/symptoms
  - Anterior spinal syndrome: Paralysis, pain & temperature sensation loss, bladder & bowel dysfunction
  - Posterior spinal cord infarction: Loss of vibration sense, proprioception
  - Sudden onset
- Clinical Profile
  - Abrupt onset weakness, loss of sensation
  - Rapid progression; maximum deficit within hours

Demographics
- Age: > 50

Natural History & Prognosis
- Poor prognosis, with permanent disabling sequelae

Treatment
- Anticoagulation, steroids, systemic hypertension

DIAGNOSTIC CHECKLIST

Image Interpretation Pearls
- Classic imaging appearance: T2 hyperintensity involving anterior horn cells

SELECTED REFERENCES
1. Weidauer S et al: Spinal cord infarction: MR imaging and clinical features in 16 cases. Neuroradiology. 44(10): 851-7, 2002
2. Cheshire WP et al: Spinal cord infarction: etiology and outcome. Neurology. 47(2): 321-30, 1996

IMAGE GALLERY

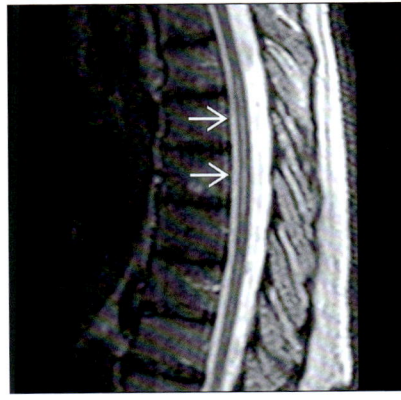 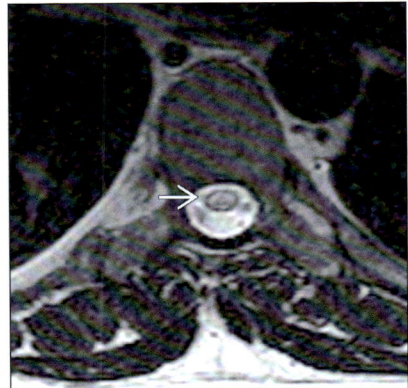 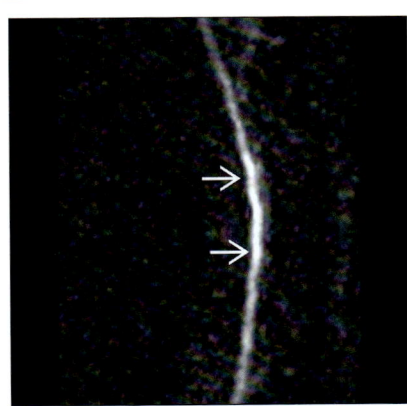

(Left) Sagittal T2WI MR shows hyperintensity in thoracic spinal cord ➡. (Center) Axial T2WI MR shows hyperintensity in anterior 2/3 of spinal cord ➡. (Right) Sagittal DWI MR shows hyperintensity in cord ➡ due to acute infarction.

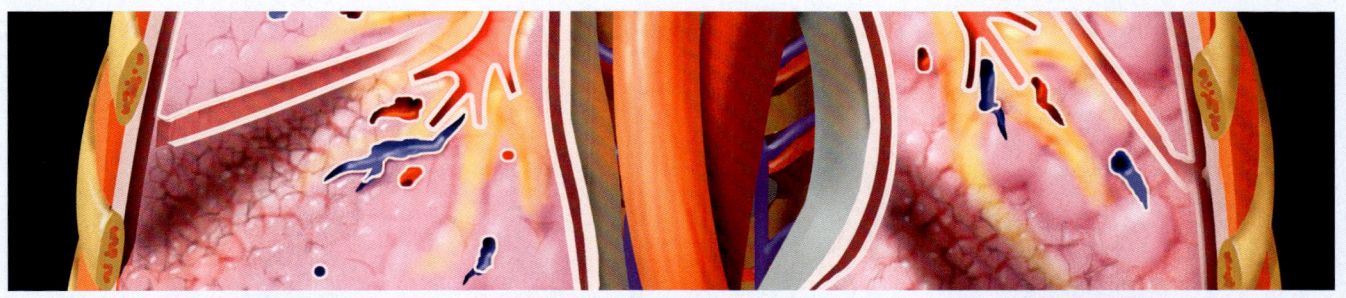

SECTION 2: Chest/Cardiovascular

Introduction and Overview

Chest Imaging Issues, Non-Trauma	II-2-2

Chest/Cardiovascular

Cardiogenic Pulmonary Edema	II-2-4
Mitral Regurgitation Pulmonary Edema	II-2-8
Noncardiac Pulmonary Edema	II-2-12
Smoke Inhalation	II-2-16
Silo-Filler's Disease	II-2-20
Community Acquired Pneumonia	II-2-24
Immunocompromised Pneumonia	II-2-28
Lung Abscess	II-2-32
Viral Lung Infection, Pediatric	II-2-36
Round Pneumonia, Pediatric	II-2-40
Neonatal Pneumonia	II-2-44
Exudative Tracheitis	II-2-48
Croup	II-2-52
Epiglottitis	II-2-56
Transient Tachypnea of the Newborn	II-2-60
Pulmonary Interstitial Emphysema, Pediatric	II-2-64
Diffuse Alveolar Hemorrhage	II-2-68
Vasculitis, Pulmonary	II-2-72
Sickle Cell, Acute Chest Syndrome	II-2-76
Eosinophilic Pneumonia	II-2-80
Acute Interstitial Pneumonia	II-2-84
Illicit Drug Abuse, Pulmonary	II-2-88
Talcosis, Pulmonary	II-2-92
Chronic Obstructive Pulmonary Disease	II-2-96
Asthma	II-2-100
Hypersensitivity Pneumonitis	II-2-104
Aspiration	II-2-108
Meconium Aspiration Syndrome	II-2-112
Bronchial Foreign Body, Pediatric	II-2-116
Pulmonary Emboli	II-2-120
Septic Emboli, Pulmonary	II-2-124
Aortic Dissection	II-2-128
SVC Syndrome	II-2-132
Pericardial Tamponade	II-2-136

CHEST IMAGING ISSUES, NON-TRAUMA

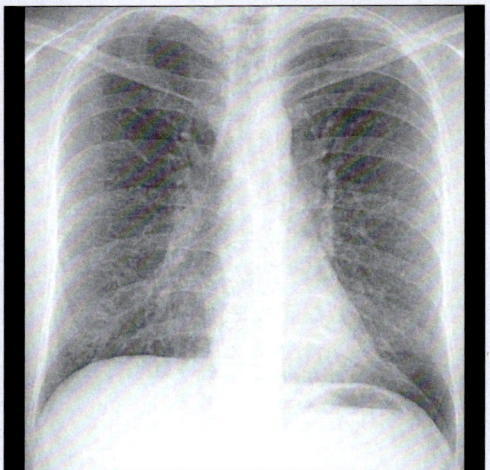

Frontal radiograph shows focal consolidation in left lower lobe ➡. Numerous air-bronchograms along medial edge of consolidation. Patient had cough and fever. Community acquired pneumonia.

Frontal radiograph is normal. Patient presented with wheezing and history of asthma. Patients often proceed onto to cross-sectional imaging to exclude other processes when chest radiographs are normal.

TERMINOLOGY

Abbreviations
- Deep venous thrombosis (DVT), pulmonary embolism (PE), tuberculosis (Tb)

CLINICAL IMPLICATIONS

Clinical Overview
- Pulmonary symptoms: Chest pain, shortness of breath, wheezing common cause of ER visits
- Nonspecificity of chest pain involves long and costly work-up to exclude life-threatening injuries
- Approximately 1/3rd of patients with cardiorespiratory symptoms will have abnormal chest radiograph
  - Highest incidence in patients with symptoms of congestive heart failure, dyspnea, hemoptysis, dysrhythmia, and hypertension
  - Lowest incidence in those with asthma
- Imaging used to decide between
  - Life threatening vs. non-life threatening
  - Portable radiographs often 1st test
    - Overview of heart, lungs, and pleural space
  - CECT often 2nd test
    - Effectively excludes pulmonary embolism, aortic dissection, and other life-threatening injuries
  - Diagnostic imaging has become modern physical examination
    - Risk of radiation dose often ignored
    - Chest radiograph dose: 0.10 mSv
    - CT dose: 18.0 mSv (180x that of chest radiograph)
  - Effective dose of 10 mSv (1 CT examination) increases risk of development of cancer 1 in 1,000
    - Most problematic in young patients
    - Repeat negative examinations from multiple separate visits to the emergency room needs to be addressed either through education or informed consent
- Nonthromboembolic findings on CTA to rule out pulmonary embolism (PE)
  - Current prevalence of PE < 10% (and trending lower)
  - Current prevalence of significant nonthromboembolic findings ~ 25%, most common findings:
    - Pneumonia
    - Aortic aneurysm or dissection
    - Mass suggesting malignancy

Top Ten Chest Pain Questions
- Past history of myocardial infraction or angina
- Quality of pain
- Principal location of pain
- Time elapsed since onset of pain
- Radiation of pain
- Presence of diaphoresis
- Presence of dyspnea
- Response to therapy
- Comparison of pain with past anginal pain
- Risk factors: Smoking, hypertension, family history

ER Decision Rule for Obtaining Chest Radiographs
- Short of breath (SO BREATH)
  - S: Saturation < 90%
  - O: Older than 59 years
  - B: Breath sounds decreased
  - R: Rales or respiratory rate > 24 breaths/min
  - E: Embolic disease (prior DVT or PE)
  - A: Alcohol abuse
  - T: Tuberculosis or temperature ≥ 38 °C
  - H: Hemoptysis
- Utility of decision rule
  - Reduce number of chest radiographs by 1/3rd
  - However, 5% false negative rate including missing congestive heart failure, pneumonia, and lung cancers
  - Interobserver agreement for history high (hemoptysis, history of Tb or DVT, alcohol abuse)
  - Interobserver agreement for physical exam findings poor (decreased breath sounds or rales)

CHEST IMAGING ISSUES, NON-TRAUMA

Key Facts

Acute Chest Pain Abnormal Radiographs
- Pneumothorax
- Pneumomediastinum
- Rib fractures (poor sensitivity)
- Vertebral compression fractures
- Pleural effusions
- Pneumonia
- Radio-opaque foreign bodies
- Aortic dissection

Acute Chest Pain Normal Radiographs
- Pulmonary embolism
- Myocardial infarction
- Aortic dissection
- Pericarditis
- Rib fractures
- Non-radio-opaque foreign bodies

○ For common presenting complaints: Chest pain, shortness of breath or cough; decision rule less useful either due to poor sensitivity (chest pain) or poor specificity (shortness of breath or cough)

Importance of Radiologist Interpretation
- Chest radiographs the most common examination to be misinterpreted
  ○ Typical discrepancy rates: 5-20%
  ○ Patients with radiologic signs of pneumonia discharged without treatment: 25%
  ○ Patients with radiologic signs of worsening congestive heart failure discharged without treatment: 20%
  ○ Most common missed findings
    - Pneumonia (10%)
    - Hilar mass (8%)
    - Lung nodule (7%)
    - Congestive heart failure (7%)

Imaging Trends
- Increase in number of radiologic examinations per patient
- Increase in number of cross-sectional imaging studies per patient
- Rationale includes
  ○ Diagnostic certainty: Fear of discharging patient with serious illness
  ○ Malpractice fears: High cost of litigation, insurance, jury awards
  ○ Speed & efficiency: Watchful waiting, a hospital strategy previously used to observe course of patients no longer a viable alternative

Future Trends
- "Triple-rule out" chest CTA for acute chest pain to evaluate for acute coronary syndrome, aortic dissection, and pulmonary embolism currently under investigation
  ○ Challenges include: Requirement for latest multidetector CT scanners
  ○ Heart rate monitoring: Requires slowing heart rate, regular rhythm, and EKG gating
  ○ Large data sets: Workstation processing and time-consuming to move across networks
  ○ Poor evaluation of esophageal or musculoskeletal causes of chest pain
- Sensitivity of technique for acute coronary syndrome unknown
- Outcomes of patients discharged with negative examinations unknown

RELATED REFERENCES
1. Gatt ME et al: Chest radiographs in the emergency department: is the radiologist really necessary? Postgrad Med J. 79(930):214-7, 2003
2. Rothrock SG et al: High yield criteria for obtaining non-trauma chest radiography in the adult emergency department population. J Emerg Med. 23(2):117-24, 2002

IMAGE GALLERY

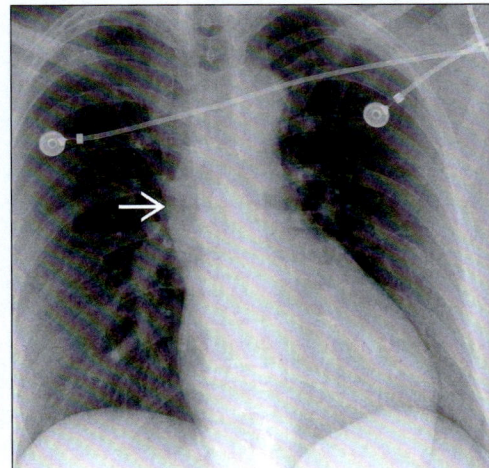
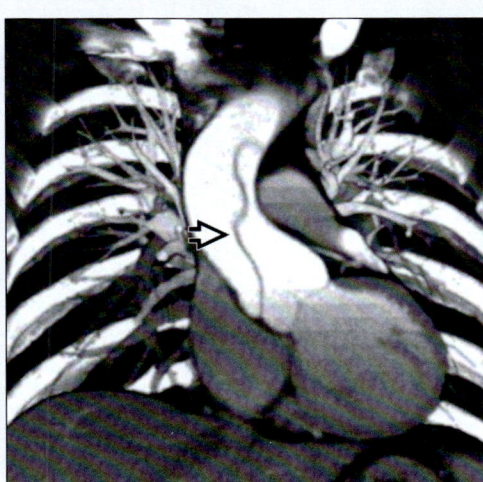

(Left) Anteroposterior radiograph shows prominent ascending aorta ➡. Acute chest pain. Differential includes life-threatening injuries requiring rapid work-up. Pertinent history of Marfan syndrome. (Right) Coronal CECT reconstruction shows intimal flap ➡ in ascending aorta from aortic dissection.

CARDIOGENIC PULMONARY EDEMA

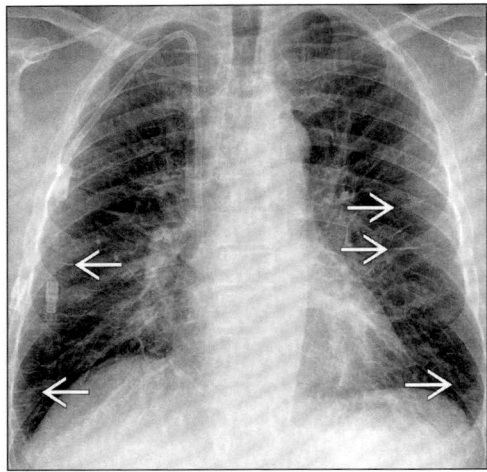

Frontal radiograph shows development of numerous Kerley B lines ➔ from acute pulmonary edema.

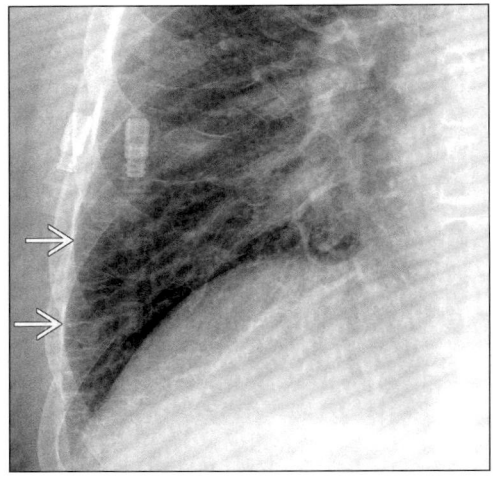

Frontal radiograph shows short horizontal Kerley B lines ➔ stair-stepping up the lateral chest wall.

TERMINOLOGY

Abbreviations and Synonyms
- Hydrostatic edema, hemodynamic edema, congestive heart failure (CHF)
- Pulmonary venous hypertension (PVHTN), pulmonary capillary wedge pressure (PCWP)

Definitions
- Increased fluid in extravascular compartment of lung from hemodynamic dysfunction

IMAGING FINDINGS

General Features
- Best diagnostic clue: Cardiomegaly, pulmonary venous hypertension (PVHTN), septal lines, & pleural effusions
- Location: Worse in gravity dependent or perihilar (batwing) locations

Radiographic Findings
- Radiographic precursor of edema: Vascular redistribution with PVHTN
  - Upper lobe vessels ≥ diameter of lower lobe vessels (erect position)
  - Increased pulmonary artery/bronchus ratio in upper lobes (erect position)
    - Vessel size varies with position (erect vs. supine)
  - Best indicator of increased preload left-ventricular filling pressure
    - Sensitivity 65%, specificity 65%; interreader agreement fair
- Interstitial edema
  - Edema not visible until lung water increases by 30%
  - Thickening of interlobular septa
    - **Kerley B**: Short (1-2 cm), peripheral, perpendicular lines in lower lobes (common)
    - Kerley A: Long lines (3-5 cm) in upper lobes radiating towards hilum (rare)
  - Peribronchial cuffing
  - Lower zonal & perihilar haze (ill-defined vessel margins)

DDx: Batwing Pattern

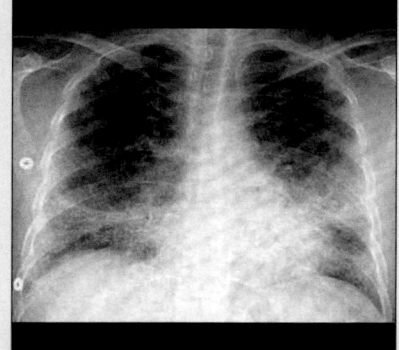
Pneumocystis

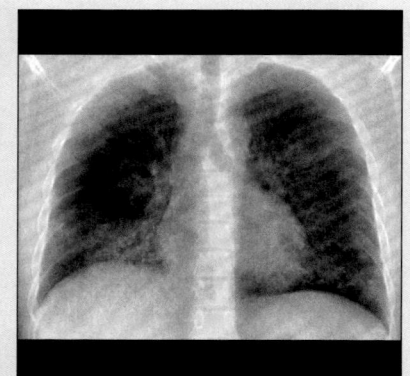
Alveolar Proteinosis

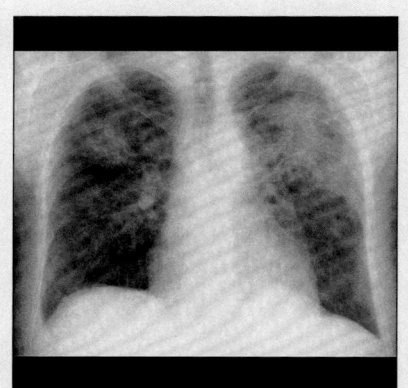
Uremia

CARDIOGENIC PULMONARY EDEMA

Key Facts

Terminology
- Increased fluid in extravascular compartment of lung from hemodynamic dysfunction

Imaging Findings
- Best diagnostic clue: Cardiomegaly, pulmonary venous hypertension (PVHTN), septal lines, & pleural effusions
- Location: Worse in gravity dependent or perihilar (batwing) locations
- Edema not visible until lung water increases by 30%
- Stepwise progression from PVHTN to interstitial edema to alveolar edema

Pathology
- Upper zone vascular distention with PCWP of 12-18 mm Hg
- Kerley lines develop when PCWP reach 20-25 mm Hg
- Alveolar edema develops with PCWP of > 25 mm Hg

Clinical Issues
- **Third heart sound** (S_3) (ventricular filling gallop) highly specific for elevated left ventricular end-diastolic pressure
- **PCWP**: Gold standard for determining cause of acute pulmonary edema
- **Brain natriuretic peptide** (BNP): Levels correlate with left ventricular end-diastolic pressure and PCWP

Diagnostic Checklist
- Appearance of cardiogenic pulmonary edema can be modified by noncardiogenic factors, especially emphysema

---

- ○ Fissural thickness either from subpleural edema (or pleural effusion)
- Alveolar edema
  - ○ Diffuse consolidation with fluffy margins
    - ▪ Usually more severe in the right lung
  - ○ Shifts gradually with position (gravitational shift test)
  - ○ Batwing (butterfly, perihilar) distribution
  - ○ Distribution altered by underlying disease that causes loss of capillary bed, particularly emphysema
- Pleural effusions
  - ○ Often bilateral, usually larger on right, rarely unilateral on left
  - ○ Blunting lateral costophrenic angle usually requires the accumulation of approximately 250 mL of fluid
- **Vascular pedicle width** (VPW)
  - ○ Left margin: Mediastinal edge where left subclavian artery exits from aortic arch
  - ○ Right margin: Mediastinal edge where SVC crosses right main stem bronchus
  - ○ Vascular pedicle = horizontal distance between left and right margin
  - ○ As blood volume increases, distensible right-sided veins increase in diameter, widening the vascular pedicle; correlates with circulating blood volume
  - ○ Absolute number varies widely primarily from body habitus (mean 48 ± 5 mm)
    - ▪ Supine position increases VPW 20%
    - ▪ Right oblique projection increases VPW 6%; conversely left oblique narrows VPW
    - ▪ Minimal change between inspiration and expiration
  - ○ Relative change in individual patient more meaningful as measure of circulating blood volume
  - ○ Measurable in 75%
- Cardiomegaly
  - ○ Heart size may be normal with acute edema
  - ○ Normal transverse diameter of the heart < ½ the thoracic diameter
  - ○ Best correlate for predicting reduced ejection fraction
    - ▪ Sensitivity 50%, specificity 80%; interreader agreement moderate
  - ○ Magnification error: AP position, short focal film distance (from supine positioning)
  - ○ Cardiac size often small in chronic obstructive pulmonary disease due to hyperinflation
    - ▪ Subsequent increases in heart size may not be beyond range which is considered normal
- Temporal relationship of pressure & volume
  - ○ Stepwise progression from PVHTN to interstitial edema to alveolar edema
  - ○ Acute PCWP elevation
    - ▪ Edema accumulates over 12 hour period
  - ○ Resolution elevated PCWP
    - ▪ Edema resolves hours to days; radiograph **lags** clinical course

CT Findings
- HRCT
  - ○ Ground-glass opacities
    - ▪ Gravitational distribution common but maybe subtle, parahilar batwing distribution uncommon)
    - ▪ Geographic distribution (spared lobules intermixed with abnormal lobules)
    - ▪ Ill-defined centrilobular nodules
  - ○ Interlobular septal thickening
    - ▪ Reticular linear opacities outlining secondary pulmonary lobules or thickened fissures (due to dilated subpleural lymphatics)
    - ▪ **Smooth** not nodular
    - ▪ Associated with peribronchovascular interstitial thickening
    - ▪ Does not have gravitational distribution
  - ○ Bronchovascular bundle thickening (peribronchovascular edema)
    - ▪ Bronchial wall thickening
    - ▪ Central pulmonary vessels larger than adjacent bronchus (from either dilatation artery or perivascular edema)
  - ○ Mediastinal lymph nodes mildly enlarged (< 2 cm) in 85%
    - ▪ Effacement mediastinal fat 60%

CARDIOGENIC PULMONARY EDEMA

- Combination of findings common, earliest solo finding ground-glass opacities

Echocardiographic Findings
- Normal echocardiography does not rule out cardiogenic pulmonary edema (especially edema from diastolic dysfunction)
- Procedure of choice to evaluate valvular function and left ventricular morphology

Imaging Recommendations
- Best imaging tool: Chest radiography usually suffices for diagnosis & treatment

DIFFERENTIAL DIAGNOSIS

Batwing Pattern
- Uremia
  - Renal disease with elevated creatinine
- Pneumocystis jiroveci pneumonia
  - Heart usually normal in size
  - Pneumonia will not shift with gravity
- Alveolar proteinosis
  - Patients often asymptomatic
  - Heart size normal with no pleural effusions

Septal Thickening
- Lymphangitic carcinomatosis
  - Normal heart size
  - Known history of malignancy
  - Usually not diffuse like pulmonary edema

Interstitial & Pleural Thickening & Cardiomegaly
- Erdheim-Chester disease (rare, non-Langerhans cell granulomatosis)
  - Will not respond to diuretics
  - Sclerotic symmetric bone lesions

PATHOLOGY

General Features
- Etiology
  - Rapid increase in hydrostatic pressure in pulmonary capillaries, usually from PVHTN
  - Pulmonary venous hypertension etiology
    - Myocardial infarction, ischemic cardiomyopathy
    - Mitral valve disease, left atrial myxoma
    - Fluid overload, renal failure
    - Veno-occlusive disease, fibrosing mediastinitis
  - Pulmonary venous hypertension usually due to left heart failure (elevated left ventricular end-diastolic pressure)
  - Rate of edema accumulation depends on hydrostatic & osmotic pressures in vessels, interstitium & lymphatics (Starling equation)
    - Lymphatic flow increases in chronic edema 10-fold, but not developed in acute edema
    - Normal lymphatics remove approximately 2 liters fluid/day
  - Pathophysiology
    - Upper zone vascular distention with PCWP of 12-18 mm Hg
    - Kerley lines develop when PCWP reach 20-25 mm Hg
    - Alveolar edema develops with PCWP of > 25 mm Hg

Microscopic Features
- Hemosiderin-containing macrophages called heart failure cells commonly seen in long-standing CHF

CLINICAL ISSUES

Presentation
- Most common signs/symptoms
  - Paroxysmal nocturnal dyspnea, dyspnea on exertion, orthopnea
  - Frothy, blood-tinged sputum
  - Physical examination
    - **Third heart sound** (S_3) (ventricular filling gallop) highly specific for elevated left ventricular end-diastolic pressure
    - S_3 gallop specificity 95%, sensitivity 10-50%
- Other signs/symptoms
  - PCWP: Gold standard for determining cause of acute pulmonary edema
    - > 18 mm Hg = cardiogenic pulmonary edema or volume overload
    - Rate of adverse complications 5-10%
  - **Brain natriuretic peptide** (BNP): Levels correlate with left ventricular end-diastolic pressure and PCWP
    - Secreted by ventricles in response to wall stretch
    - < 100 pg/mL CHF unlikely (negative predictive value > 90%)
    - > 500 pg/mL CHF likely (positive predictive value > 90%)

Natural History & Prognosis
- Onset can be acute or insidious
- Prognosis depends on severity & reversibility of underlying hemodynamic dysfunction

Treatment
- Diuretics and afterload reduction

DIAGNOSTIC CHECKLIST

Consider
- Appearance of cardiogenic pulmonary edema can be modified by noncardiogenic factors, especially emphysema

SELECTED REFERENCES

1. Wang CS et al: Does this dyspneic patient in the emergency department have congestive heart failure? JAMA. 294(15):1944-56, 2005
2. Ware LB et al: Clinical practice. Acute pulmonary edema. N Engl J Med. 353(26):2788-96, 2005
3. Gehlbach BK et al: The pulmonary manifestations of left heart failure. Chest. 125(2):669-82, 2004

CARDIOGENIC PULMONARY EDEMA

IMAGE GALLERY

Typical

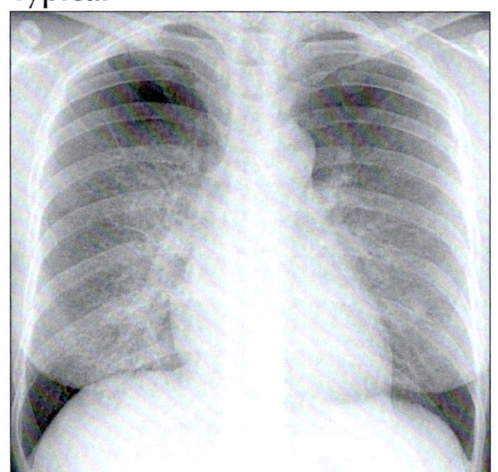
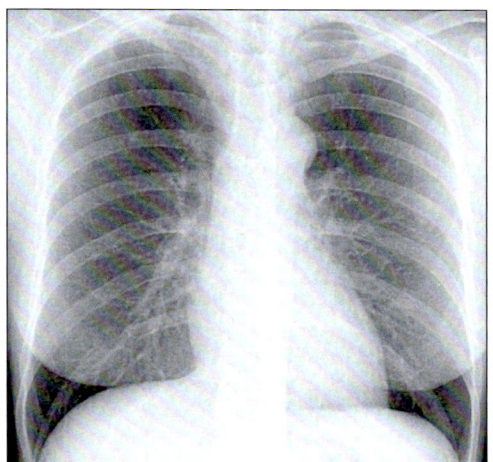

(Left) Frontal radiograph shows increased diffuse central linear opacities radiating peripherally in a batwing distribution. *(Right)* Frontal radiograph shows resolution after treatment.

Typical

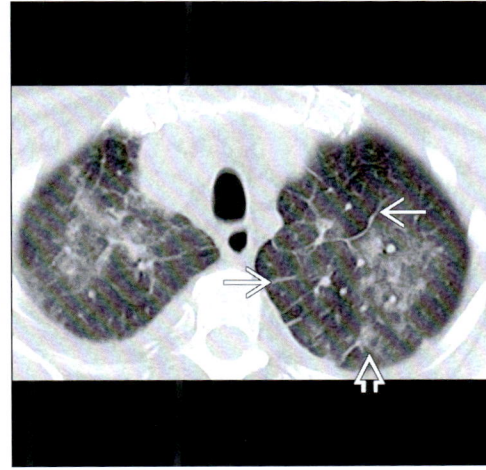
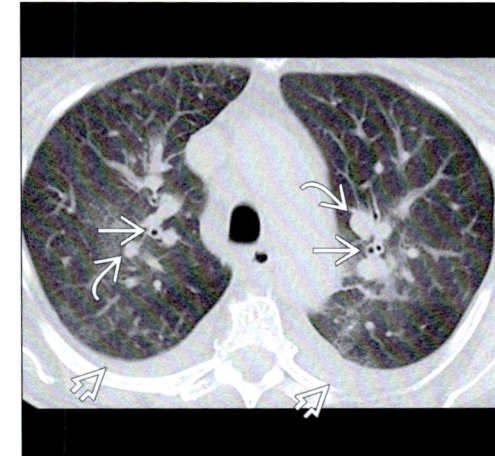

(Left) Axial CECT shows centrilobular ground-glass opacities ➡, smooth thickened interlobular septa ➡, consistent with interstitial edema. Small bilateral pleural effusions. Geographic pattern with abnormal lobules adjacent to uninvolved lobules. *(Right)* Axial CECT shows bronchial wall thickening ➡, enlarged vessels ➡, and small bilateral pleural effusions ➡.

Typical

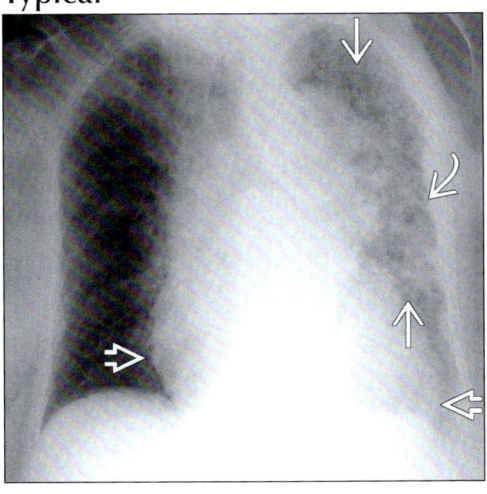
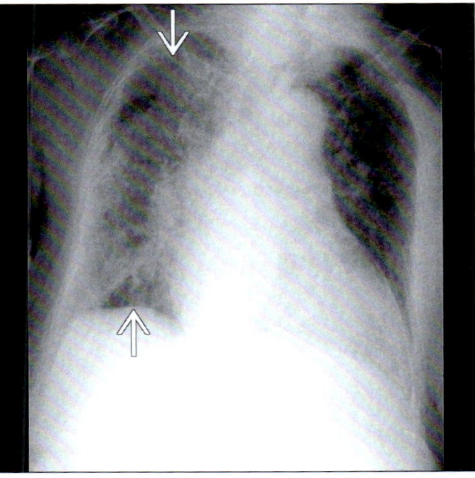

(Left) Anteroposterior radiograph in left lateral decubitus position for 2 hours shows diffuse interstitial thickening and consolidation in the left lung ➡. Small pleural effusion layers along the chest wall ➡. Heart moderately enlarged ➡. *(Right)* Anteroposterior radiograph in right lateral decubitus position for 2 hours shows shift of edema into the dependent right lung ➡. Positive gravitational shift test.

MITRAL REGURGITATION PULMONARY EDEMA

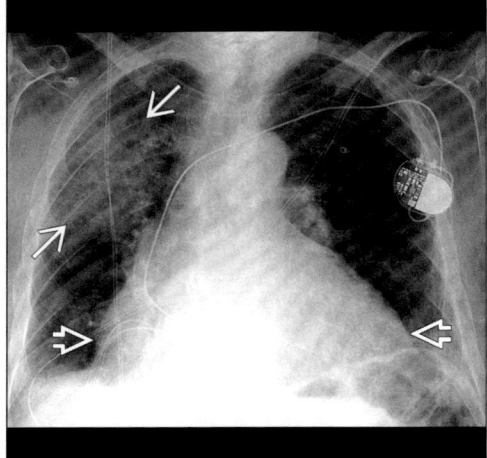

Frontal radiograph shows focal consolidation in the right upper lobe ➡. Mild cardiomegaly ➡. Edema resolved over 3 day period.

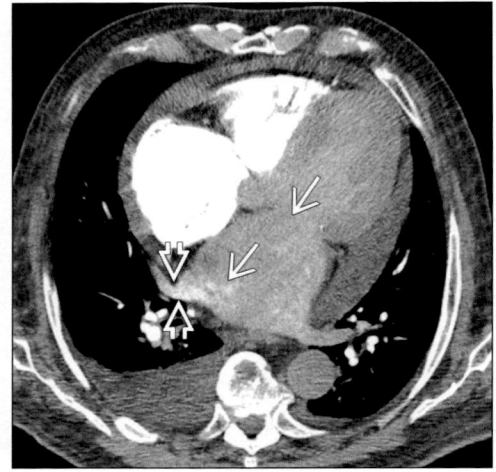

Axial oblique CECT reconstruction shows direction of flow ➡ across mitral valve to the right superior pulmonary vein ➡.

TERMINOLOGY

Abbreviations and Synonyms
- Left heart failure, congestive heart failure (CHF), asymmetric pulmonary edema

Definitions
- Asymmetric edema more severe in the right upper lobe due to left heart decompensation and mitral regurgitation

IMAGING FINDINGS

General Features
- Best diagnostic clue: Right upper lobe consolidation, mild diffuse edema elsewhere, and cardiomegaly
- Location
  o Right upper lobe with mitral regurgitation through native valve (10%)
  o Left upper lobe with perivalvular regurgitation around prosthetic valve (rare)

Radiographic Findings
- Radiography
  o Edema in a single lobe far out of proportion to edema elsewhere in the lung
    ▪ Right upper lobe, may also include right middle lobe
    ▪ Left upper lobe (rare): Usually associated with mitral valve prosthesis
  o Cardiomegaly, left atrium often selectively enlarged
    ▪ Enlarged left atrium only seen with chronic mitral regurgitation
    ▪ Heart size may be normal with acute mitral regurgitation
  o Pulmonary venous hypertension: Redistribution blood flow upper lobes, peribronchial cuffing, septal lines, pleural effusions
  o Mitral annulus calcification
    ▪ Age related degeneration common in elderly women
    ▪ May be a cause of mitral regurgitation
    ▪ C-shaped calcification overlying heart, easier to visualize on lateral projection
  o Cor pulmonale: Enlarged central pulmonary arteries

DDx: Right Upper Lobe Consolidation

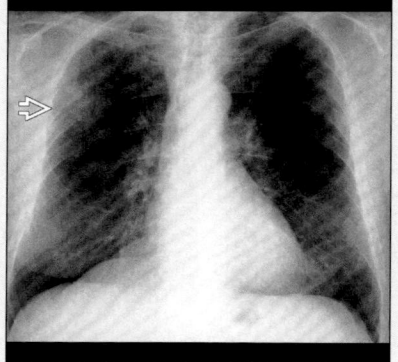

Aspiration

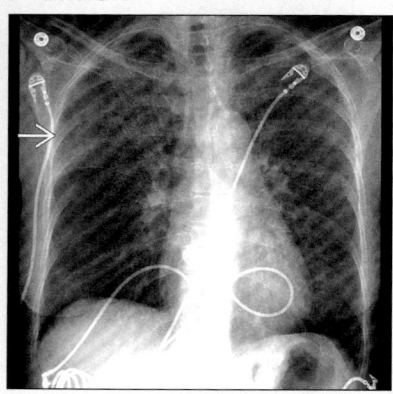

Neurogenic Pulmonary Edema

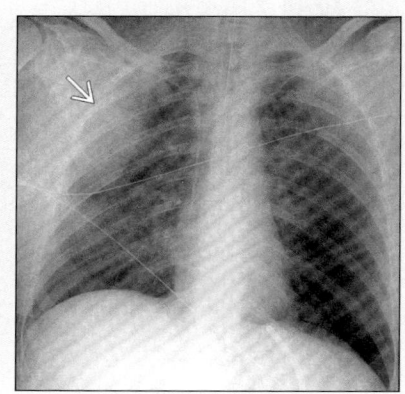

Smoke Inhalation

MITRAL REGURGITATION PULMONARY EDEMA

Key Facts

Terminology
- Asymmetric edema more severe in the right upper lobe due to left heart decompensation and mitral regurgitation

Imaging Findings
- Best diagnostic clue: Right upper lobe consolidation, mild diffuse edema elsewhere, and cardiomegaly
- Left upper lobe (rare): Usually associated with mitral valve prosthesis

Top Differential Diagnoses
- Pneumonia
- Aspiration
- Left Heart Failure
- Negative Pressure Pulmonary Edema
- Re-Expansion Pulmonary Edema

Pathology
- Mitral valve: Valve plane faces posterior, superior, and to the right
- Regurgitant stream is directed to the right superior pulmonary vein: Especially due to malfunction of posterior mitral valve leaflet
- Asymmetric right upper lobe edema in 10% in those with severe mitral regurgitation (20% in children)
- Gravitational: Patients with CHF prefer right lateral decubitus position

Diagnostic Checklist
- Pulmonary edema usually not thought of as a predominant cause of focal pulmonary consolidation
- Asymmetric edema in left upper lobe in patient with mitral valve prosthesis: Consider perivalvular leak

---

- Late finding in end-stage mitral regurgitation
- Resolution
  - With mitral valve replacement or medical therapy for CHF, resolution over 2-3 days

CT Findings
- More sensitive for calcification of mitral valve or annulus and size of atria and ventricles
- Pulmonary varices: Enlarged tortuous pulmonary veins entering left atrium; in mitral valve disease, right-sided pulmonary veins more commonly involved
- Lung edema: Spectrum from smooth septal thickening to ground-glass opacities to consolidation

MR Findings
- MR Cine
  - Through valve plane to evaluate valve morphology and qualitative evaluation of flow jets
  - Cine phase-contrast sequences for quantitative analysis of regurgitant flow and peak velocities
  - Long and short axis cine images through ventricles to measure ejection fraction, end-diastolic volume, and stroke volume
  - Grading mitral insufficiency (regurgitant volume in mL/heartbeat)
    - Mild: < 30
    - Moderate: 30-44
    - Moderately severe: 45-59
    - Severe: > 60

Echocardiographic Findings
- Color flow Doppler will demonstrate direction and flow of regurgitant stream
  - Severity of mitral regurgitation directly proportional to size of regurgitant jet
  - May underestimate regurgitant volume (Coanda effect results when jet impinges on atrial wall)
- Echocardiography will demonstrate status of mitral valve leaflets, dimensions of left atrial and ventricular enlargement, left ventricular wall thickness, and quantify degree of regurgitation

Imaging Recommendations
- Best imaging tool
  - Echocardiography or MR to evaluate mitral apparatus
    - MR advantage over echocardiography: Not limited by body habitus
    - MR disadvantage compared to echocardiography: Non-portable, not for those with pacemakers
- Protocol advice: Chest radiography usually suffices for monitoring response to therapy

DIFFERENTIAL DIAGNOSIS

Pneumonia
- Common in hospitalized patients
- Commonly arise from aspiration of oropharyngeal secretions
- Upper lobe location common

Aspiration
- Common in hospitalized or obtunded patients
- Upper lobe location common in supine or decubitus position (gravity dependent posterior segment of upper lobe)

Left Heart Failure
- Patients in congestive heart failure prefer the right lateral decubitus position
  - Edema will be predominantly right-sided

Neurogenic Pulmonary Edema
- CNS injury resulting in increased intracranial pressure
- Edema develops acutely often with upper lung zone predilection
- When unilateral, usually affects the right lung

Smoke Inhalation
- Toxic injury due to injurious effects of products of combustion
- Noncardiogenic edema often upper lung zone predilection, develops within hours of inhalation
- May have subglottic edema

MITRAL REGURGITATION PULMONARY EDEMA

Negative Pressure Pulmonary Edema
- Develops acutely following relief of upper airway obstruction, most commonly laryngospasm
- Edema often has upper lung zone predilection

Re-Expansion Pulmonary Edema
- Edema develops after within hours of evacuation large chronic pleural effusions or pneumothorax
- Ipsilateral to pleural process

High-Altitude Pulmonary Edema
- Noncardiogenic edema occurs at altitudes, generally above 3,000 meters (10,000 feet)
- Capillary stress failure due to hypoxic pulmonary artery vasoconstriction and permeability edema
- Variable distribution, often upper lung zones

Unilateral Pulmonary Edema
- Contralateral pulmonary edema
  - Opposite to major perfusion abnormality: Unilateral pulmonary thromboembolism, congenital absence pulmonary artery, Swyer-James syndrome
- Ipsilateral pulmonary edema
  - Ipsilateral: Dependent lung left ventricular dysfunction, acute mitral regurgitation, unilateral veno-occlusive disease, extrinsic pulmonary venous compression, left-to-right shunts
  - Noncardiogenic: Re-expansion following drainage pleural fluid or air, aspiration, contusion

PATHOLOGY

General Features
- General path comments
  - Mitral apparatus: Mitral annulus, anterior and posterior leaflets, chordae tendineae, anterior and posterior papillary muscles
  - Mitral valve: Valve plane faces posterior, superior, and to the right
    - Regurgitant stream is directed to the right superior pulmonary vein: Especially due to malfunction of posterior mitral valve leaflet
    - Right superior pulmonary vein may also drain right middle lobe
    - Regurgitant flow around malfunctioning mitral valve prosthesis directed to left upper lobe pulmonary veins
- Etiology
  - Mitral valve dysfunction
    - Acute: Ruptured chordae tendineae, ischemic papillary muscle dysfunction, infective endocarditis
    - Chronic: Myxomatous degeneration, rheumatic heart disease, mitral annular calcification, Marfan syndrome
  - Rheumatic heart most common cause of mitral regurgitation world wide
    - Myxomatous degeneration of valve most common in developed countries
- Epidemiology
  - Asymmetric right upper lobe edema in 10% in those with severe mitral regurgitation (20% in children)
  - Mitral regurgitation requiring surgery: 1 in 200 by age 50, increased to 3% by age 70
- Pathophysiology asymmetric edema
  - Gravitational: Patients with CHF prefer right lateral decubitus position
  - Alterations lung perfusion
    - Unilateral thromboembolism
    - Swyer-James syndrome
  - Alterations in ventilation
    - Bronchial obstruction

CLINICAL ISSUES

Presentation
- Most common signs/symptoms
  - Due to left heart failure: Dyspnea on exertion, orthopnea
  - Murmur of mitral regurgitation: Holosystolic murmur
  - Absence fever
- Other signs/symptoms: Swan-Ganz catheter: Large V wave common

Demographics
- Age: Average age mitral valve replacement 55
- Gender: M > F = 2:1

Treatment
- Medical therapy for left ventricular dysfunction: Diuretics, afterload reduction
  - Anticoagulant therapy for atrial fibrillation
  - Bacterial endocarditis prophylaxis
- Surgical replacement mitral valve for those failing medical therapy
  - Mortality 3-9%

DIAGNOSTIC CHECKLIST

Consider
- Pulmonary edema usually not thought of as a predominant cause of focal pulmonary consolidation

Image Interpretation Pearls
- Asymmetric edema in left upper lobe in patient with mitral valve prosthesis: Consider perivalvular leak

SELECTED REFERENCES

1. Chuang YS et al: Right upper lobe pulmonary edema after mitral valve replacement caused by paravalvular leakage recognized by bedside transesophageal echocardiography. Crit Care Med. 30(3):695-6, 2002
2. Young AL et al: Mitral valve regurgitation causing right upper lobe pulmonary edema. Tex Heart Inst J. 28(1):53-6, 2001
3. Lesieur O et al: Unilateral pulmonary oedema complicating mitral regurgitation: diagnosis and demonstration by transoesophageal echocardiography. Intensive Care Med. 26(4):466-70, 2000
4. Chen JC et al: Mitral regurgitation presenting as localised right middle lobe pulmonary oedema. J Accid Emerg Med. 16(1):72-3, 1999

MITRAL REGURGITATION PULMONARY EDEMA

IMAGE GALLERY

Typical

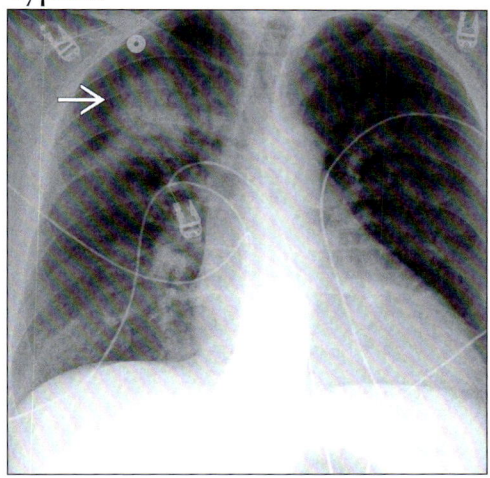 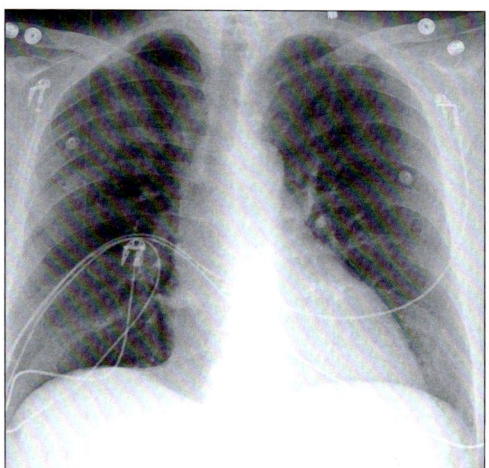

(Left) Anteroposterior radiograph shows diffuse pulmonary edema and focal consolidation right upper lobe ➡. Heart mildly enlarged. Acute MI. *(Right)* Anteroposterior radiograph 3 days later shows near complete resolution of pulmonary edema. Mitral regurgitation pulmonary edema.

Typical

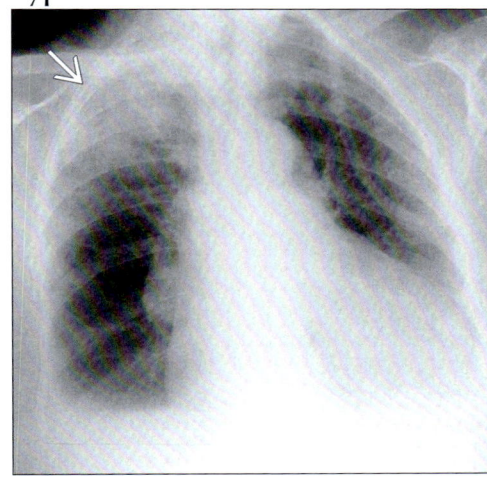 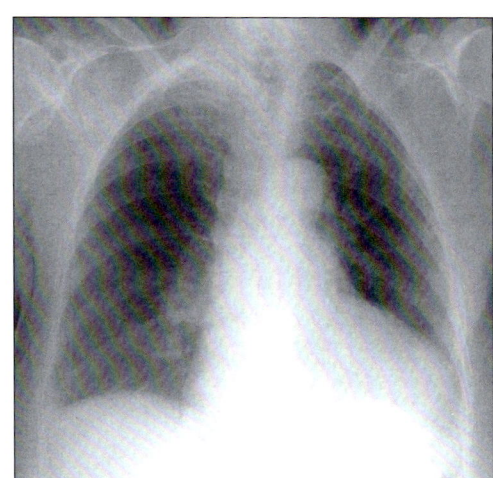

(Left) Anteroposterior radiograph shows focal consolidation in the right upper lobe ➡, marked cardiomegaly, and small bilateral pleural effusion. *(Right)* Anteroposterior radiograph several days later, right upper consolidation has nearly completely resolved and bilateral pleural effusions have decreased. Mitral regurgitation pulmonary edema.

Typical

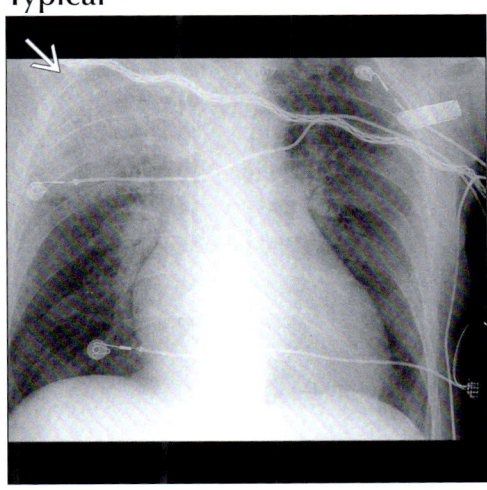 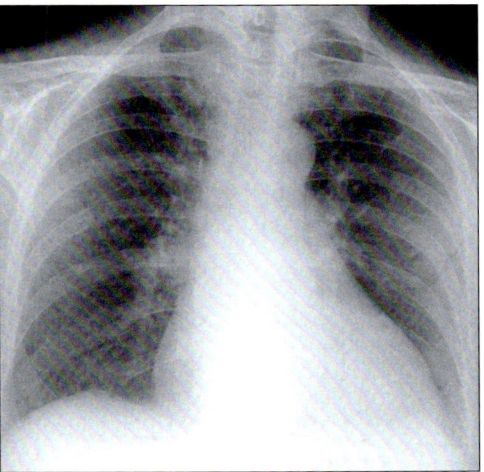

(Left) Anteroposterior radiograph shows diffuse consolidation in the right upper lobe ➡. Heart mildly enlarged. Mitral regurgitation pulmonary edema. *(Right)* Anteroposterior radiograph follow-up several days later, the lungs are now normal. Heart remained mildly enlarged.

NONCARDIAC PULMONARY EDEMA

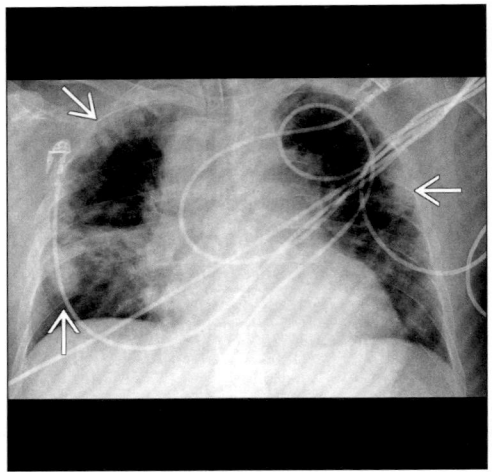

Anteroposterior radiograph shows peripheral consolidation ➡. Patient intubated for hypoxemia.

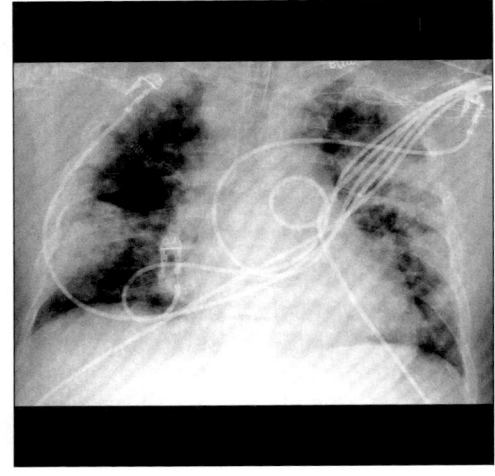

Anteroposterior radiograph 3 days later shows progression of noncardiac pulmonary edema.

TERMINOLOGY

Abbreviations and Synonyms
- Noncardiogenic pulmonary edema; increased permeability edema, adult respiratory distress syndrome (ARDS), acute lung injury, diffuse alveolar damage (DAD)

Definitions
- Extravascular lung water due to increased permeability of the alveolar-capillary barrier
- American-European Consensus Conference (AECC)
  - ARDS
    - Acute onset
    - $PaO_2/FIO_2 \leq 200$
    - Diffuse parenchymal abnormality chest radiograph
    - Pulmonary artery wedge pressure < 18 mm Hg
  - Acute lung injury same except $PaO_2/FIO_2 \leq 300$ mm Hg

IMAGING FINDINGS

General Features
- Best diagnostic clue: Diffuse symmetric bilateral air space opacification in intubated patient
- Location: Tends to be more peripheral than cardiogenic edema (which tends to be more central with a "bat's wing" distribution)

Radiographic Findings
- Radiography
  - Purpose of chest radiographs
    - Integral to the definition of ARDS
    - Evaluate extent and progress of parenchymal opacification
    - Ensure location of support and monitoring catheters
    - Detect complications of barotrauma
  - Because oxygenation severely impaired, patients nearly always intubated for respiratory support
    - Moderate or worse consolidation without intubation not likely to be due to ARDS
  - May be normal initially but rare
  - Diffuse bilateral airspace opacification

DDx: Noncardiogenic Pulmonary Edema

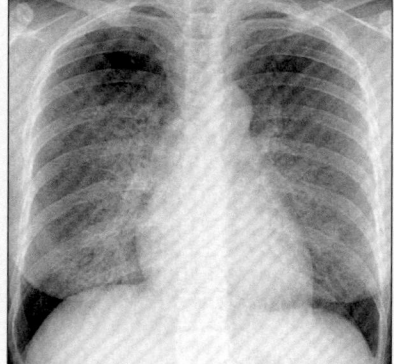

Cardiogenic Pulmonary Edema

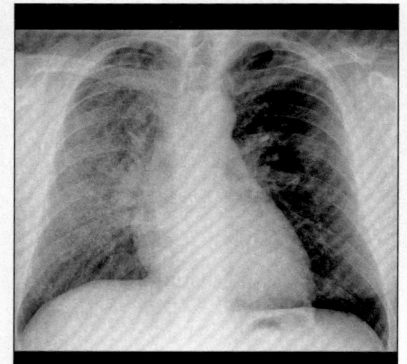

Hemorrhage

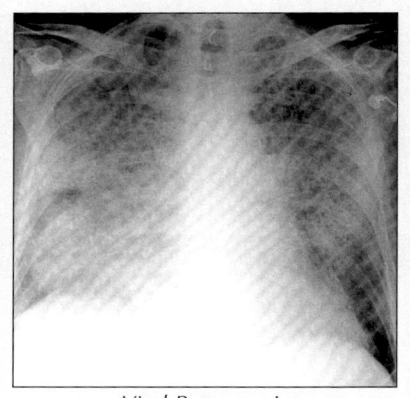

Viral Pneumonia

NONCARDIAC PULMONARY EDEMA

Key Facts

Terminology
- Extravascular lung water due to increased permeability of the alveolar-capillary barrier

Imaging Findings
- Best diagnostic clue: Diffuse symmetric bilateral air space opacification in intubated patient
- In contrast to radiography, strikingly inhomogeneous distribution on CT
- Nondependent lung sometimes hyperinflated (even showing cystic changes) from PEEP related overinflation

Top Differential Diagnoses
- Cardiogenic Edema
- Diffuse Pulmonary Hemorrhage
- Pulmonary Infection

Pathology
- Secondary (extrapulmonary) ARDS: Indirect injury to lungs secondary to systemic sepsis, massive transfusion, following (non-thoracic) surgery, eclampsia
- Primary (pulmonary) ARDS: Direct injury to lungs typically secondary to severe pulmonary infection, massive aspiration but also toxic fume inhalation and O_2 toxicity

Clinical Issues
- Survivors may have either restrictive or obstructive functional deficits

Diagnostic Checklist
- Usually patients rapidly intubated to support oxygenation even when severity of lung disease mild

---

- Often heterogeneous initially rapidly coalescing to severe homogeneous consolidation
- Usually symmetric with or without air bronchograms
- Nonsymmetric opacities may be secondary to pulmonary cause of ARDS or superimposed pneumonia
- Earliest stage, opacities can be considered to be either interstitial or alveolar
- Favors the lung periphery rather than perihilar lung as in cardiogenic edema
- Septal (Kerley B) lines less common than in cardiogenic edema
- Peribronchial cuffing less common than in cardiogenic edema
- Normal heart size
- No pulmonary vascular redistribution
- May have small pleural effusions but effusions less common than in cardiogenic edema
- Treatment related complications
  - Initial use of positive end-expiratory pressure (PEEP) may increase lung volume giving apparent radiographic "improvement"
  - Barotrauma common (50%) with PEEP: Pulmonary interstitial emphysema, pneumomediastinum, pneumothorax (often tension)
  - Superimposed (ventilator-related/nosocomial) pneumonia common, difficult to recognize and radiographic accuracy no different than coin toss
- Resolution
  - 80% return to normal over days to weeks
  - Mild chronic fibrosis and low lung volumes in 10%
  - Hyperinflation described but uncommon

CT Findings
- In contrast to radiography, strikingly inhomogeneous distribution on CT
- In secondary (extrapulmonary) ARDS, roughly symmetric changes seen more often than in primary (pulmonary) ARDS
- Typical pattern characterized by
  - Ground-glass opacification admixed with apparently normally aerated lung in the non-dependent lung
  - Dense parenchymal opacification in the dependent lung
  - Nondependent lung sometimes hyperinflated (even showing cystic changes) from PEEP related overinflation
- Lung compartments
  - Hyperinflated compartment (voxels CT number between -1000 HU and -901 HU)
  - Normal aerated compartment (voxels CT number between -900 HU and -501 HU)
  - Poorly aerated compartment (voxels CT number between -500 HU and -101 HU)
- Primary (pulmonary) ARDS, more often associated with an "atypical" pattern
  - Foci of dense parenchymal opacification in nondependent lung more common than in extrapulmonary ARDS
  - Foci of dense parenchymal opacification in dependent lung less common than in extrapulmonary ARDS
  - Diffuse ground-glass opacification and apparently normally lung (as with extrapulmonary ARDS)
  - Multiple thin-walled cysts more common than in extrapulmonary ARDS
- Survivors
  - Mild reticular fibrosis in non-dependent lung presumably due to damage from barotrauma

Imaging Recommendations
- Best imaging tool
  - Chest radiography adequate for monitoring course
  - CT used as problem solving tool
- Protocol advice
  - Portable chest radiograph: Notation of position and ventilator settings by technicians helpful in interpretation
  - Digital radiography superior to conventional film-screen combinations

NONCARDIAC PULMONARY EDEMA

DIFFERENTIAL DIAGNOSIS

Cardiogenic Edema
- Separation from cardiogenic pulmonary edema not always possible based on radiographic features
- Elements of cardiogenic and noncardiogenic pulmonary edema may coexist-exist in the same patient
- Signs more frequently associated with cardiac pulmonary edema include
  - Increased heart size
  - Central ("bat's wing") distribution
  - Septal (Kerley B) lines
  - Peribronchial cuffing
  - Pleural effusions

Diffuse Pulmonary Hemorrhage
- May have identical radiographic findings, patient often anemic with history of hemoptysis
- Normal heart size
- Diffuse distribution
- Not usually associated with pleural effusions
- Usually don't require intubation

Pulmonary Infection
- Fever and elevated white blood cell count
- No pulmonary vascular redistribution
- Normal heart size
- May result in ARDS

PATHOLOGY

General Features
- General path comments
  - DAD not a diagnosis but nonspecific reaction to a multitude of injurious agents that damage the alveolar-capillary membrane
  - ARDS represents the pathologic state of increased permeability edema associated with alveolar-capillary damage
- Etiology
  - Secondary (extrapulmonary) ARDS: Indirect injury to lungs secondary to systemic sepsis, massive transfusion, following (non-thoracic) surgery, eclampsia
  - Primary (pulmonary) ARDS: Direct injury to lungs typically secondary to severe pulmonary infection, massive aspiration but also toxic fume inhalation and O_2 toxicity
  - Sepsis syndrome most common predisposing risk factor
  - Causes of increased permeability edema not obviously associated with alveolar-capillary epithelial damage include
    - Rapid pulmonary re-expansion
    - Neurogenic pulmonary edema
    - Severe upper (extrathoracic) airway obstruction
    - High altitude pulmonary edema
- Epidemiology: 75 cases/100,000 persons/year

Microscopic Features
- Diffuse alveolar damage: 3 stages
  - Exudative phase (stage 1): Vascular congestion, exudation of proteinaceous fluid into interstitium and airspaces, microatelectasis, hyaline membrane formation over first 1-7 days
  - Proliferative phase (stage 2): Proliferation of myofibroblasts in airspace and interstitium, deposition of proteoglycans (and eventually collagen) in interstitium over 7-14 days
  - Fibrotic phase (stage 3): Hyperplasia type II pneumocyte, fibroblastic infiltration and fibrosis over 1-2 weeks
- Lung usually shows mixed stages in different areas of the lung

Staging, Grading or Classification Criteria
- Lung injury score (LIS)
  - 0-4 for chest radiograph, hypoxemia, respiratory system compliance, and PEEP
    - Chest radiograph: Alveolar consolidation score 1 for one quadrant, 2 for two quadrants, 3 for three quadrants, 4 for four quadrants
    - PaO_2/FIO_2: > 300 mm Hg score 0, 225-299 score 1, 175-224 score 2, 100-174 score 3, < 100 score 4
    - Compliance (mL/cmH_2O): > 80 score 0, 60-79 score 1, 40-59 score 2, 20-39 score 3, < 19 score 4
    - PEEP (cmH_2O): < 5 score 0, 6-8 score 1, 9-11 score 2, 12-14 score 3, > 15 score 4
  - ARDS defined as LIS > 2.5

CLINICAL ISSUES

Presentation
- Most common signs/symptoms
  - Onset of symptoms/signs may be insidious (over a few days) or relatively rapid (over a few hours) after an inciting pulmonary or extrapulmonary "event"
  - Typical symptoms/signs include: Breathlessness, tachypnea, dry cough, cyanosis, coarse crackles

Natural History & Prognosis
- In general, high mortality rate (30-40%)
- Survivors may have either restrictive or obstructive functional deficits

Treatment
- Supportive treatment in the intensive care unit with mechanical ventilation and PEEP
- Steroids or extracorporeal membrane oxygenation (ECMO) not shown to be beneficial

DIAGNOSTIC CHECKLIST

Consider
- Usually patients rapidly intubated to support oxygenation even when severity of lung disease mild

SELECTED REFERENCES
1. Rubenfeld GD et al: Epidemiology and outcomes of acute lung injury. Chest. 131(2):554-62, 2007
2. Dueck R: Alveolar recruitment versus hyperinflation: A balancing act. Curr Opin Anaesthesiol. 19(6):650-4, 2006

NONCARDIAC PULMONARY EDEMA

IMAGE GALLERY

Typical

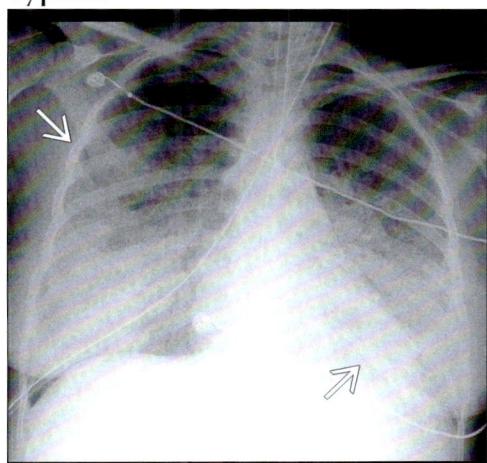
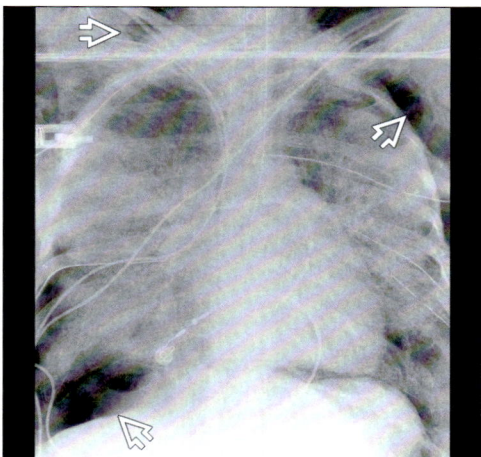

(Left) Anteroposterior radiograph shows diffuse symmetric pulmonary consolidation ➡. Intubated with PEEP. Viral pneumonia. *(Right)* Anteroposterior radiograph 3 days later shows subcutaneous emphysema and right pneumothorax ➡ from barotrauma. Edema unchanged.

Typical

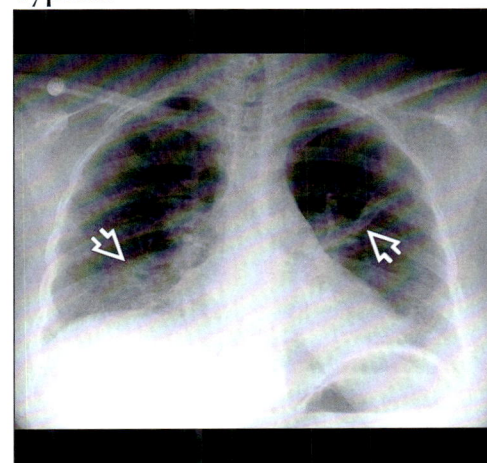
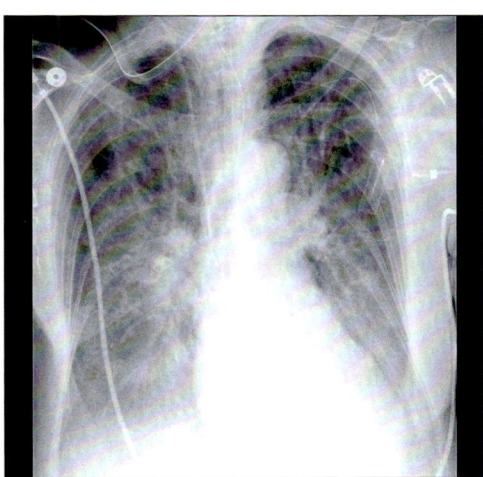

(Left) Frontal radiograph 6 months later shows residual scarring in the left mid-lung and right base ➡. Patient had mild mixed restrictive and obstructive pulmonary function tests. *(Right)* Anteroposterior radiograph shows diffuse consolidation and normal heart size. Intubated. Nonspecific pattern but consistent with ARDS.

Typical

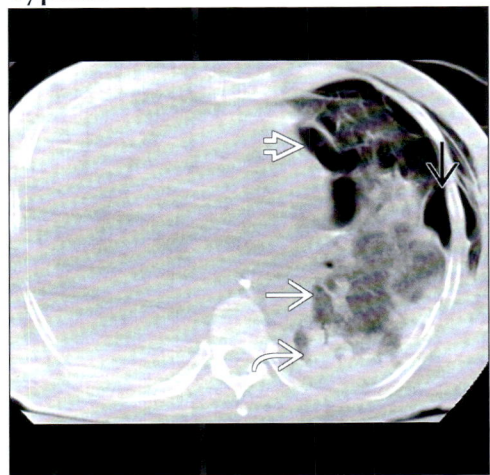
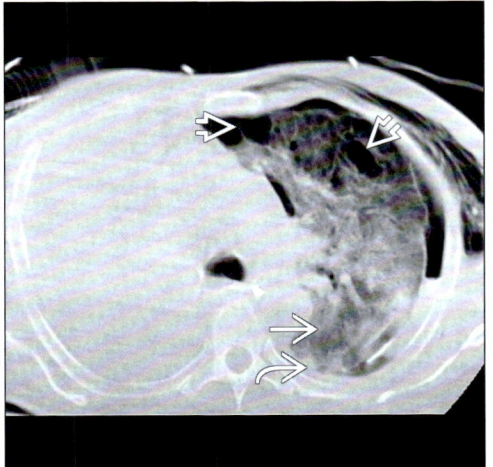

(Left) Axial NECT shows diffuse ground-glass ➡ and dependent consolidation ➡ from ARDS. Ventral lung contains cysts from barotrauma ➡. Pneumothorax ➡. Ventral lung not protected from high airway pressure (PEEP) and may become overdistended. *(Right)* Axial NECT shows diffuse ground-glass ➡ and dependent consolidation ➡ from ARDS. Ventral lung contains cysts from barotrauma ➡.

SMOKE INHALATION

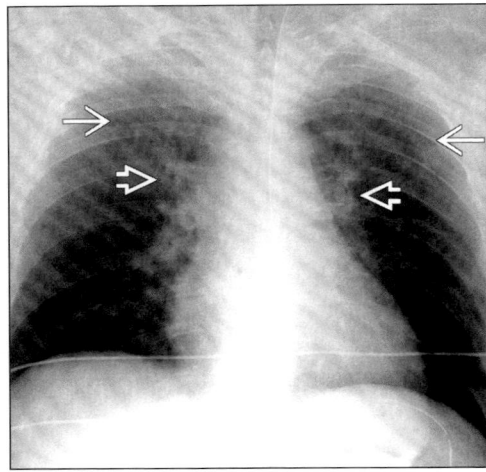

Anteroposterior radiograph shows faint consolidation in the upper lobes ➡ from smoke inhalation. Hila indistinct ⊟ probably from bronchial wall thickening.

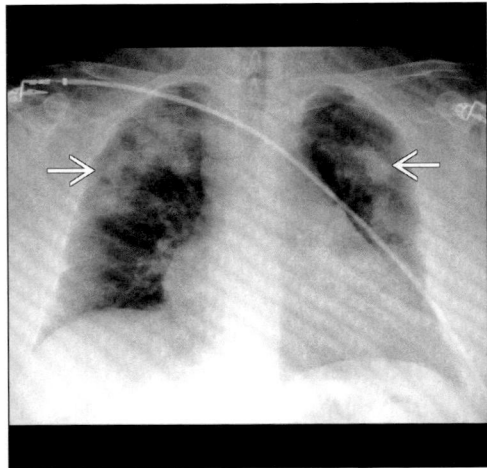

Anteroposterior radiograph focal consolidation in both upper lobes ➡ from smoke inhalation. 8 hours after rescue from house fire.

TERMINOLOGY

Definitions
- Inhalation injury to upper and lower respiratory tract due to thermal, chemical and particulate matter from products of combustion

IMAGING FINDINGS

Radiographic Findings
- Radiography
  - Severity of injury dependent on concentration and length of exposure, airways predominant manifestation 1st 24 hours followed by lung parenchyma over next 24-48 hours
  - Acute: Up to 48 hours
    - Initial radiograph often normal
    - Diffuse peribronchial wall thickening (85%)
    - Conical narrowing of the subglottic trachea from edema, never isolated: Will also have peribronchial wall thickening
    - Subsegmental atelectasis: Airways narrowed by mucosal edema
    - Consolidation predominantly in perihilar and upper lung zones
    - Uncomplicated course resolves over 3-5 days
    - Pleural effusions may develop without parenchymal abnormality, probably related to hypoproteinemia from skin burns
    - Soft tissue thickening from edema of skin burns
  - Subacute: 3 days to end of hospitalization
    - Barotrauma due to positive pressure ventilation common
    - Superimposed pneumonia common especially in those with cutaneous burns, suspect with worsening of parenchymal abnormalities after the first 48 hours, develops in up to 40%
    - Cardiogenic pulmonary edema commonly superimposed due to large volumes of administered fluid, especially in those with cutaneous burns
    - Adult respiratory distress syndrome (ARDS) a severe complication with high mortality rate
    - Pulmonary emboli after first 3 days
  - Delayed: Weeks to months after hospital discharge
    - Hyperinflation and small nodules in previously affected lung due to bronchiolitis obliterans (BO)

DDx: Smoke Inhalation

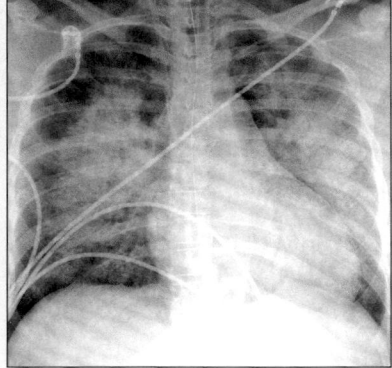

Cardiogenic Pulmonary Edema

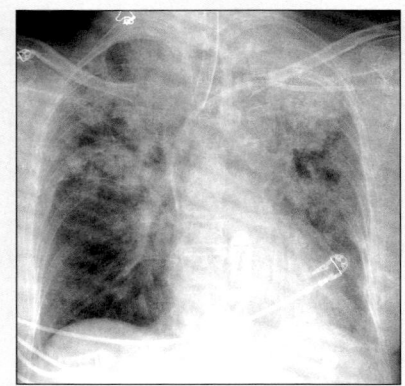

Negative Pressure Pulmonary Edema

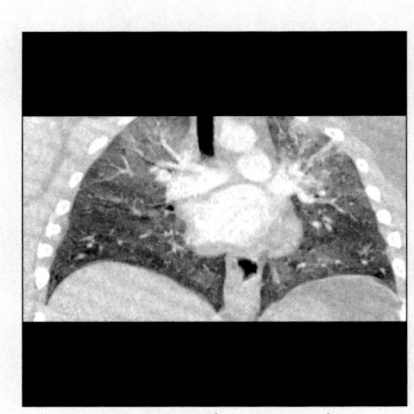

Neurogenic Pulmonary Edema

SMOKE INHALATION

Key Facts

Terminology
- Inhalation injury to upper and lower respiratory tract due to thermal, chemical and particulate matter from products of combustion

Imaging Findings
- Severity of injury dependent on concentration and length of exposure, airways predominant manifestation 1st 24 hours followed by lung parenchyma over next 24-48 hours
- Diffuse peribronchial wall thickening (85%)
- Conical narrowing of the subglottic trachea from edema, never isolated: Will also have peribronchial wall thickening
- Subsegmental atelectasis: Airways narrowed by mucosal edema
- Consolidation predominantly in perihilar and upper lung zones
- Superimposed pneumonia common especially in those with cutaneous burns, suspect with worsening of parenchymal abnormalities after the first 48 hours, develops in up to 40%

Top Differential Diagnoses
- Hydrostatic Pulmonary Edema
- Pneumonia
- Aspiration

Pathology
- Severity of chemical pneumonitis dependent on composition and concentration of smoke and length of exposure

CT Findings
- Acute
  - Rarely used initially but would be expected to be more sensitive
  - Bronchial wall thickening
  - Ground-glass opacities due to edema or mosaic perfusion from small airway occlusion
- Subacute
  - Problem solving tool for suspected complications such as pulmonary embolus
  - Helpful to investigate parenchymal abnormalities, especially in patients with a complicated clinical course
- Delayed
  - Bronchiectasis
  - Mosaic pattern of attenuation (air-trapping) from BO

Other Modality Findings
- Xenon-133 ventilation scanning
  - Delayed washout, incomplete washout within 120 seconds, or segmental hang-up
  - Maybe abnormal when chest radiograph normal, rarely used today

Imaging Recommendations
- Best imaging tool
  - Chest radiography surveillance to detect and monitor course of disease
  - CT as problem solving tool or to evaluate unexplained radiographic abnormalities

DIFFERENTIAL DIAGNOSIS

Hydrostatic Pulmonary Edema
- Smoke inhalation has proclivity for upper lung zones
- Fluid overload common in smoke inhalation due to massive fluid administration for burns

Pneumonia
- Clinical history different from entrapment in fire
- Superimposed pneumonia common in smoke inhalation, develops > 48 hours after admission

Aspiration
- Identical radiographic findings
- Hypoxic neurologically impaired victim of smoke inhalation at high risk for aspiration

Neurogenic Pulmonary Edema (NPE)
- Requires a central nervous system insult that will raise intracranial pressure
- Hypoxic neurologically impaired victim often requires head CT to exclude intracranial pathology

Mitral Regurgitant Pulmonary Edema (MRPE)
- Pulmonary edema due to heart failure in patient with incompetent mitral valve
- Edema diffuse but more severe in the right upper lobe due to directional back flow through the right superior pulmonary vein
- Enlarged heart, usually normal in smoke inhalation
- Responds quickly to diuretic and inotropic support

Negative Pressure Pulmonary Edema (NPPE)
- Develops acutely following relief of upper airway obstruction, most commonly laryngospasm
- Victims of smoke inhalation at risk for NPPE due to subglottic edema

PATHOLOGY

General Features
- General path comments
  - Smoke consists of gases and fine particulate material
    - Carbonaceous particles (soot) absorb noxious substances in the gas acting as a delivery vehicle to the respiratory mucosa
  - Water solubility of combustion products determines site of action
    - Highly water-soluble products are irritating and affect the upper airways: Ammonia, hydrogen chloride, sulfur dioxide

SMOKE INHALATION

- Less water-soluble products are non-irritating (do not evoke attempts to flee) and primarily affect the distal airway: Chlorine, nitrogen oxides, phosgene
  - Severity of chemical pneumonitis dependent on composition and concentration of smoke and length of exposure
    - Injury may occur from upper airways to pulmonary capillary bed
  - Airway wall
    - Spectrum beginning with edema and inflammatory cells, proceeding to hemorrhage, necrosis, ulceration and charring
  - Airway casts commonly cause widespread bronchial plugging
    - Casts composed of neutrophils, shed bronchial epithelium, mucin, and fibrin
    - Mean reduction in cross-sectional area: Bronchi (30%), bronchioles (10%) 48 hours after injury
  - Pathophysiology: General
    - Gas concentrations in the lung determined by ventilation perfusion ratio (V/Q)
    - Normal upright lung, V/Q ratio highest in upper lung zone, therefore concentration of inhaled gas concentrated in the nondependent lung
  - Pathophysiology: Thermal injury
    - Rare, inhaled gases rapidly cooled by the upper respiratory tract
    - If occurs, limited to the upper respiratory tract and larynx
    - Seen primarily with superheated steam and explosions
  - Pathophysiology: Asphyxiation due to carbon monoxide and carbon dioxide
    - Carbon monoxide displaces oxygen, produces profound hypoxemia, accounts for 50% of fire-related fatalities
    - Carbon dioxide reduces ambient oxygen concentration
  - Pathophysiology: Pyrolysis
    - Cyanide gas from natural and synthetic fabric and plastics (especially polyvinyl chloride-PVC)
    - Hydrogen chloride from combustion PVC combines with water to produce hydrochloric acid
- Etiology
  - Nitric oxide (NO)
    - Smoke-induced release from epithelial cells and alveolar macrophages
    - NO causes loss of hypoxic vasoconstriction and increased vascular permeability
  - Bronchial blood flow markedly increased (8x)
    - May contribute to pulmonary edema
    - In animal models, bronchial artery occlusion lessens severity of smoke injury

Gross Pathologic & Surgical Features
- Diffuse friable airway mucosa with ulceration and charring

Microscopic Features
- Acute: Diffuse alveolar damage with hyaline membrane formation
- Delayed: Bronchiolitis obliterans

CLINICAL ISSUES

Presentation
- Most common signs/symptoms: Dyspnea, wheezing, burns, singed nasal hairs, carbonaceous sputum
- Other signs/symptoms
  - Elevated carboxyhemoglobin (from carbon monoxide inhalation)
    - Increased mixed venous PO_2 and decreased arteriovenous oxygen difference suggests either carbon monoxide or hydrogen cyanide poisoning
  - Wheezing common due to airway narrowing
- Bronchoscopic findings in smoke inhalation, typically used acutely for diagnosis
  - Laryngeal edema, airway ulceration and charring
- Delayed symptoms months later: Dyspnea, nonproductive cough
- Pulmonary function tests
  - Decreased maximum expiratory flow volume and forced vital capacity

Demographics
- Age: Any age, favors those who are physically unable to escape a fire
- Firefighters
  - Long term risk of obstructive lung disease

Natural History & Prognosis
- Primary cause of death in 75% of burn injuries
- Mortality rate ranges from 50% to 80%
- Abnormal chest radiograph within 48 hours of exposure poor prognostic sign

Treatment
- Supportive, intubation and ventilation with supplemental oxygen to counter hypoxia
- Fluid management critical to support cardiac output and urine output
- Serial cultures for infectious surveillance
- Steroids may be detrimental, prophylactic antibiotics do not influence survival
- Promising: NO inhibitors and aerosolized acetylcysteine and heparin to reduce airway casts

DIAGNOSTIC CHECKLIST

Consider
- Hydrogen cyanide exposure in patients with unexplained respiratory failure or persistent anion gap metabolic acidosis

SELECTED REFERENCES

1. Koljonen V et al: Multi-detector computed tomography demonstrates smoke inhalation injury at early stage. Emerg Radiol. 2007
2. Reske A et al: Computed tomography--a possible aid in the diagnosis of smoke inhalation injury? Acta Anaesthesiol Scand. 49(2):257-60, 2005
3. Latenser BA et al: Smoke inhalation injury. Semin Respir Crit Care Med. 22(1):13-22, 2001
4. Teixidor HS et al: Smoke inhalation: radiologic manifestations. Radiology. 149(2):383-7, 1983

SMOKE INHALATION

IMAGE GALLERY

Typical

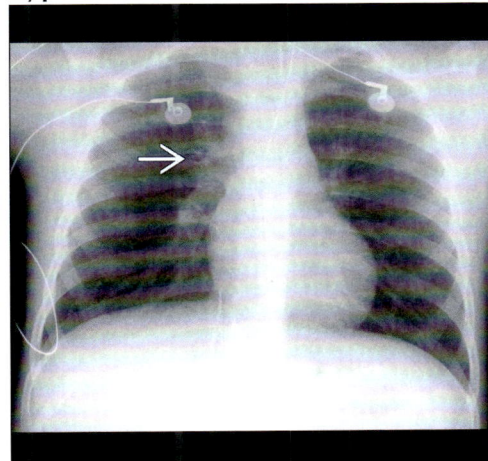
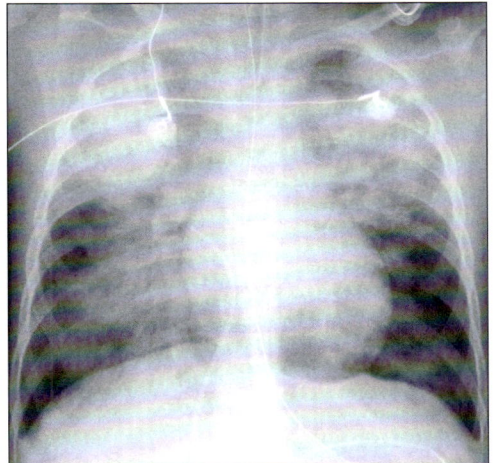

(Left) Anteroposterior radiograph shows subtle central bronchial wall thickening ➡. Intubated. Initial film from house fire. *(Right)* Anteroposterior radiograph 7 hours later shows diffuse pulmonary consolidation; more marked in the upper lung zones.

Typical

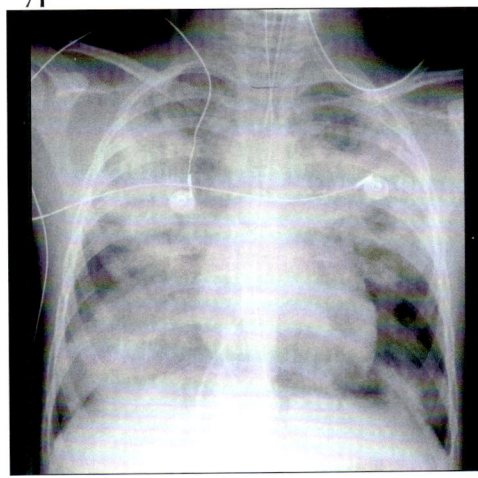
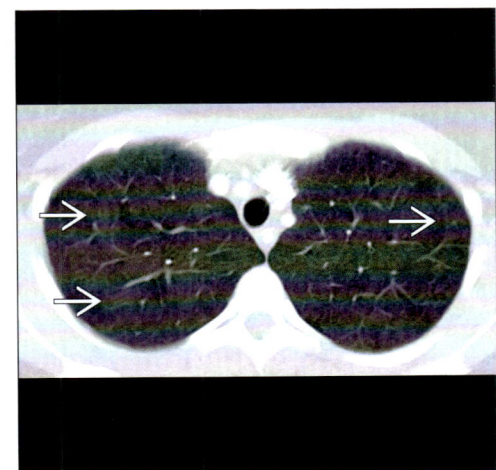

(Left) Anteroposterior radiograph 5 hours later shows progressive edema. Patient did not survive. *(Right)* Transverse CECT shows multiple, ill-defined and subtle air space nodules ➡ that show a tendency to coalesce after toxic fume inhalation.

Typical

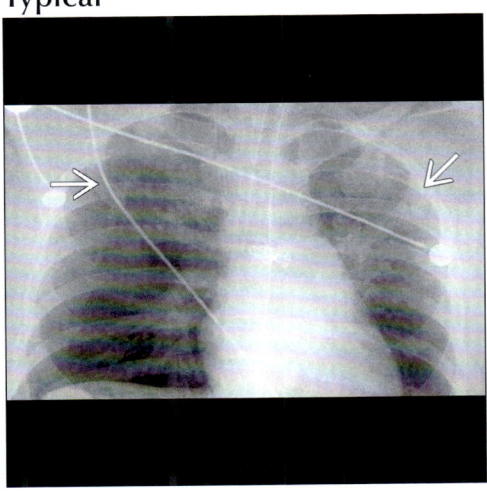
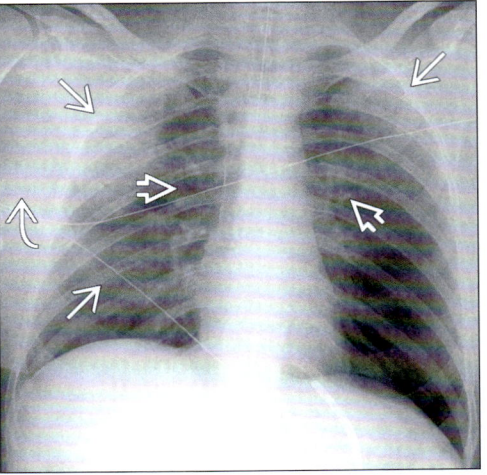

(Left) Anteroposterior radiograph on admission shows mild streaking in the upper lung zones ➡. Intubated with ET tube at carina. *(Right)* Anteroposterior radiograph 3 hours later shows progression to homogeneous peripheral consolidation ➡. Central airways are thickened ➡. Soft tissue thickening from burn ➡.

SILO-FILLER'S DISEASE

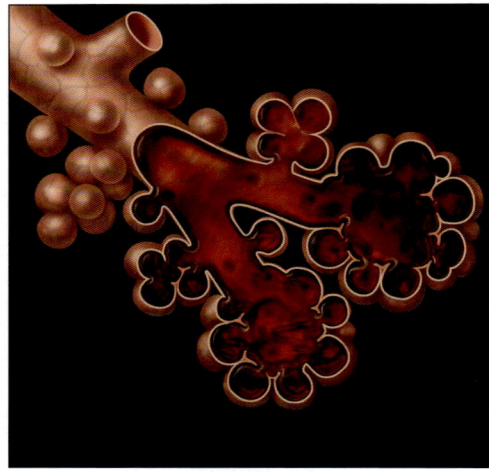

Graphic shows consequences of acute silo filler's disease. Diffuse alveolar damage with proteinaceous hemorrhagic fluid-filling alveoli. The small airways may be damaged leading to bronchiolitis obliterans.

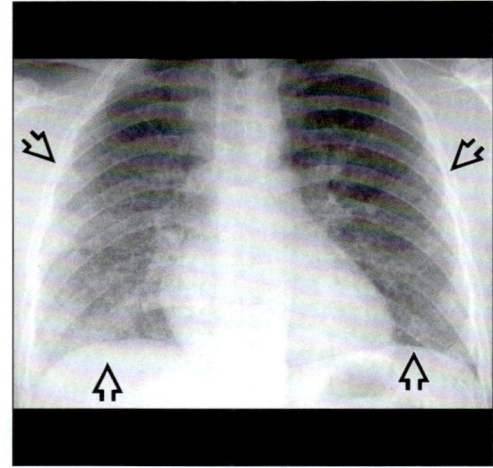

Frontal radiograph shows diffuse bibasilar ground-glass opacities from silo filler's disease ⊃. Normal heart size and no pleural effusions. Worked in freshly filled silo.

TERMINOLOGY

Abbreviations and Synonyms
- Silo filler's disease (SFD), nitrogen dioxide (NO_2), nitric oxide (NO), carbon dioxide (CO_2)

Definitions
- Occupational disease that results from pulmonary exposure to oxides of nitrogen
- Inhalation of toxic gases from freshly stored silage
  - Also formed during welding, glassblowing, Zamboni ice resurfacing, manufacture of lacquers, dyes, rocket propellants, and fertilizers, metal cleaning; rayon and food bleaching, nitrocellulose incineration

IMAGING FINDINGS

General Features
- Best diagnostic clue: Diffuse pulmonary edema within hours of toxic fume inhalation
- Morphology: Airspace disease; miliary to small nodules

Radiographic Findings
- Initial radiograph may be normal
- Acute findings
  - Parenchymal injury develops either immediate or up to first 48 hours (typically within 6 hours of exposure)
  - Noncardiogenic pulmonary edema (sometimes hemorrhagic)
    - 6-12 hours after exposure, usual
    - Ill-defined, alveolar opacities, nonspecific pulmonary edema pattern
  - Resolves over 3-5 days
    - Superimposed pneumonia common complication, develops 48 hours after admission
    - Any worsening of consolidation after 48 hours should be considered superinfection
  - Normal heart size
  - Pleural effusions uncommon
- Late findings
  - 2-4 weeks after exposure, usual (range, weeks to months)
  - Hyperinflation from bronchiolitis obliterans
  - Diffuse ill-defined small or miliary nodules

DDx: Toxic Fume Inhalation

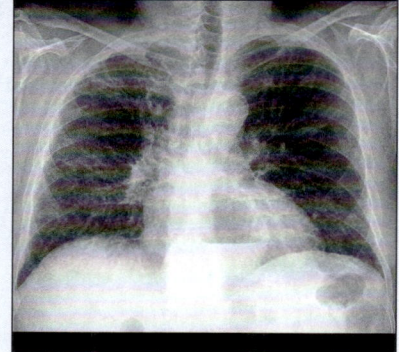

Farmer's Lung

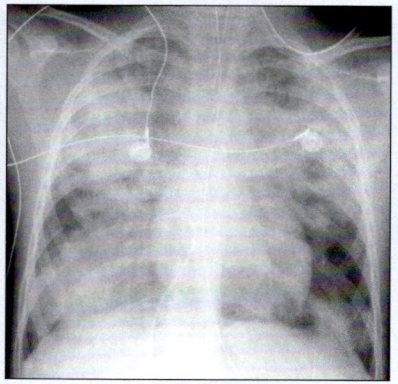

Smoke Inhalation

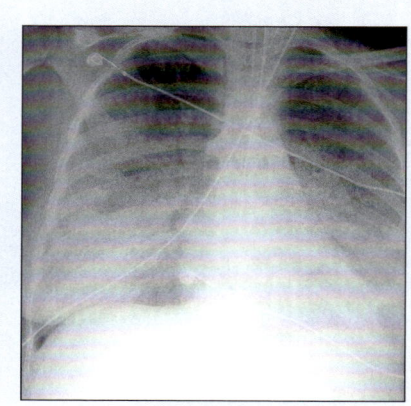

Viral Pneumonia

SILO-FILLER'S DISEASE

Key Facts

Terminology
- Occupational disease that results from pulmonary exposure to oxides of nitrogen

Imaging Findings
- Best diagnostic clue: Diffuse pulmonary edema within hours of toxic fume inhalation
- Initial radiograph may be normal
- Bronchiolitis obliterans, late

Top Differential Diagnoses
- Other Agricultural Lung Diseases
- Other toxic gases: Hydrogen sulfide (H_2S), ammonia, carbon dioxide, methane
- Organic dust toxicity syndrome
- Pesticide exposure
- Hypersensitivity Pneumonitis (Farmer's Lung)
- Smoke Inhalation

Pathology
- Dependent on composition and concentration of gas and length of exposure
- Nitrogen (corn has 5.5% free nitrates) in the plant undergoes 2 oxidation steps to form NO and then NO_2
- Hours after stored, toxic and lethal levels of NO_2 develop
- NO_2, heavier than air, settles on top of silage, yellowish-orange in appearance with bleach-like odor
- Harvest months, September to October

Clinical Issues
- Preventive: Avoid freshly-filled silo for 14 days (gases dissipate a few weeks after ensilage)

CT Findings
- HRCT
  - Nonspecific appearance
  - Bilateral airspace and ground-glass opacities, patchy or diffuse
  - Pleural effusions uncommon
  - Cryptogenic organizing pneumonia (COP) pattern
    - Peripheral wedge-shaped opacities (ground-glass or consolidation) with air bronchograms
  - Bronchiolitis obliterans, late
    - Mosaic attenuation: Geographic regions of ground-glass opacification and hyperlucency

Nuclear Medicine Findings
- V/Q Scan
  - Xenon-133 ventilation scanning
    - Air-trapping and delayed washout
    - Maybe abnormal when chest radiograph normal
    - Rarely used, replaced by CT

Imaging Recommendations
- Best imaging tool: Chest radiographs suffice for extent of injury and monitoring course
- Protocol advice: Serial radiographs, for initial 4 days and at 1 week, 1 month, and 3 months

DIFFERENTIAL DIAGNOSIS

Other Agricultural Lung Diseases
- Other toxic gases: Hydrogen sulfide (H_2S), ammonia, carbon dioxide, methane
  - Toxic swine and dairy manure exposure (dung lung)
    - Hydrogen sulfide acts as anesthetic leads to asphyxiation, aspiration, pneumonia
  - Anhydrous ammonia inhalation
    - From leaks in fertilizer tanks and hoses, and toxic levels in animal confinement buildings
    - Leads to chemical bronchitis, pneumonitis, asthma like symptoms, bronchiolitis obliterans
- Organic dust toxicity syndrome
  - Inflammation due to bacterial cell wall endotoxin inhalation, primarily gram-negative bacteria
  - Usually seen in the spring from moldy dust silage (silo-filler's disease in fall)
  - Radiographs usually normal, HRCT may show ill-defined centrilobular nodules
- Pesticide exposure
  - Paraquat lung: Usually absorbed through skin
  - Rapid pulmonary fibrosis, end stage lung within 30 days, often fatal

Hypersensitivity Pneumonitis (Farmer's Lung)
- Exposure to dust (not gas)
  - Allergic reaction to fungi (typically Actinomycetes) in silage or organic material
  - Not all workers exposed develop injury
- Similar symptoms but context different
  - Usually silo exposure in spring (residual moldy and dusty silage)
- Radiographs often normal
- CT: Lobular ground-glass opacities or centrilobular ground-glass nodules admixed with foci of hyperinflated lobules
- May result in chronic fibrosis

Smoke Inhalation
- Acutely, bronchial wall thickening and subglottic edema
- Perihilar and upper lung zone pulmonary edema
- Subsegmental atelectasis
- Skin burns

Cardiogenic Pulmonary Edema
- Similar radiographic findings
- Cardiac enlargement common
- Pleural effusions common

Pneumonia
- Similar radiographic findings
- Superimposed pneumonia common, develops 48 hours after admission

SILO-FILLER'S DISEASE

- Any worsening of consolidation after 48 hours should be considered superinfection

Aspiration
- Similar radiographic findings
- More common in dependent lung (depends on body habitus at time of aspiration)

PATHOLOGY

General Features
- General path comments
  - Severity of chemical pneumonitis
    - Dependent on composition and concentration of gas and length of exposure
    - Greatest injury to lower respiratory tract
  - Pathophysiology
    - Toxic gas concentrations dependent on V/Q ratio
    - Normal upright lung, V/Q ratio highest in upper lung zone
- Etiology
  - Production of nitrogen dioxide in top-unloading silo
    - Anaerobic bacteria ferment green forage crops in silo: Product of fermentation called silage
    - Nitrogen (corn has 5.5% free nitrates) in the plant undergoes 2 oxidation steps to form NO and then NO_2
    - Fumes form rapidly in farm silos filled with fresh organic material
    - Hours after stored, toxic and lethal levels of NO_2 develop
    - Gas continues to form during the first 10 days after filling the silo (concentration up to 100,000 ppm)
    - Grain grown under drought conditions with heavy fertilization, extremely high levels
    - NO_2, heavier than air, settles on top of silage, yellowish-orange in appearance with bleach-like odor
  - Silage used as feedstock for livestock during the winter
  - Inhalation of NO_2
    - NO_2 combines with water in lung to produce nitrous and nitric acid
    - Free radical generation, protein oxidation, lipid peroxidation, cell membrane damage
    - High levels of CO_2 in the silo stimulate deeper inspiration causing higher delivered dose
    - Concentration directly related to severity of lung injury
    - With high concentrations, farmer overcome within 2-3 minutes
- Epidemiology
  - 5 cases per 100,000 silo-associated farm workers per year
  - Under-reported (rural stoic population)
  - Harvest months, September to October

Microscopic Features
- Acute nonspecific findings: Diffuse alveolar damage with hyaline membrane formation
- Chronic findings: Small airways damage, bronchiolitis obliterans or cryptogenic organizing pneumonia

CLINICAL ISSUES

Presentation
- Most common signs/symptoms
  - Signs and symptoms depend on duration of exposure and concentration of gas
  - May be asymptomatic, 1/2 to 42 hours after exposure
  - Most symptomatic exposures are mild and self-limiting
    - Cough, light headedness, dyspnea, fatigue
  - Mucosal irritation less common because NO_2 less soluble than water
    - Runny nose, ocular irritation less common
    - Lack of mucosal irritation is one reason harmful effects of gas are ignored (lots of things on a farm stink)
  - Laryngeal spasm, wheezing, bronchiolar spasm, cyanosis, and loss of consciousness in severe exposures
  - Relapse of symptoms of dyspnea, nonproductive cough months later heralds onset of bronchiolitis obliterans
- Other signs/symptoms
  - Methemoglobinemia
    - NO_2 binds to hemoglobin to form nitrosyl hemoglobin which then oxidizes to methemoglobin

Natural History & Prognosis
- Variable, depends on extent of initial injury
- 1/3 with severe exposure die from pulmonary edema and bronchiolitis obliterans

Treatment
- Preventive: Avoid freshly-filled silo for 14 days (gases dissipate a few weeks after ensilage)
  - Education through state and county agricultural extension services
- Monitor those exposed for 48 hours
- Supportive, mechanical ventilation to maintain oxygenation
- Serial cultures for infectious surveillance
- Steroids, to prevent or treat cryptogenic organizing pneumonia and bronchiolitis obliterans (not proven effective)

DIAGNOSTIC CHECKLIST

Consider
- Any breathless farmer at harvest time

SELECTED REFERENCES
1. Leavey JF et al: Silo-Filler's disease, the acute respiratory distress syndrome, and oxides of nitrogen. Ann Intern Med. 141(5):410-1, 2004
2. Jackson L: Grain silo cleanup operation leads to two occupational deaths. Appl Occup Environ Hyg. 17(7):464-6, 2002
3. Stepanek J et al: Case in point. Silo fillers lung. Hosp Pract (Minneap). 33(1):70, 1998

SILO-FILLER'S DISEASE

IMAGE GALLERY

Typical

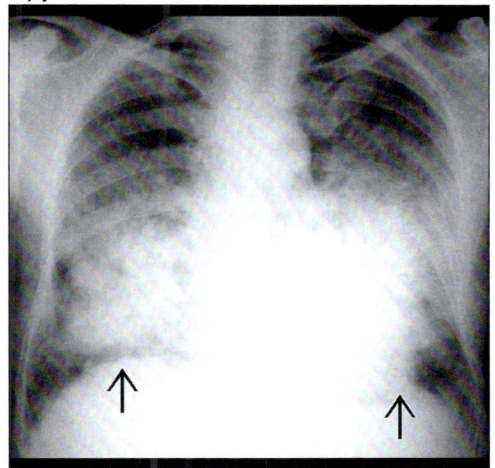
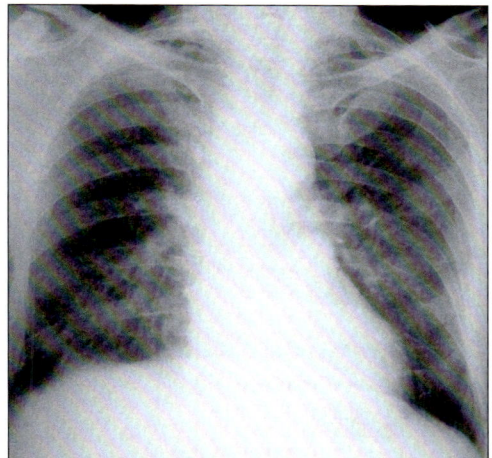

(Left) Anteroposterior radiograph shows dense bilateral consolidation ➔ developing within hours of working in a freshly filled silo. Hemorrhagic pulmonary edema. *(Right)* Frontal radiograph 1 week later shows near complete resolution of noncardiac pulmonary edema.

Typical

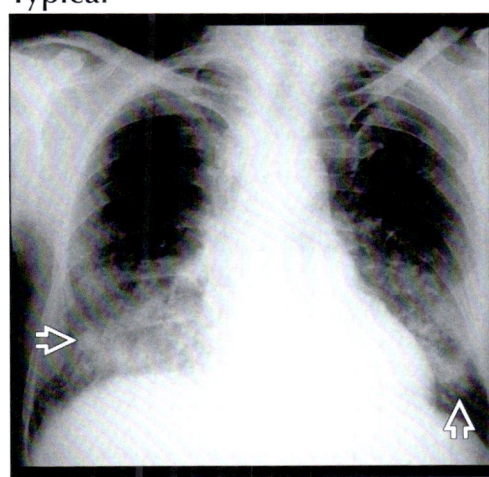
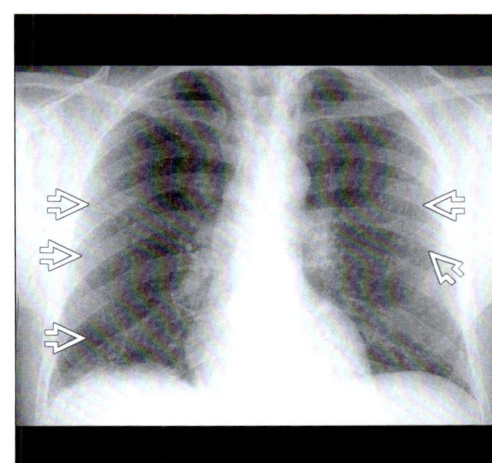

(Left) Frontal radiograph 1 month later shows new nodular areas of consolidation ➔ in areas which were most severely involved initially. Pathologic diagnosis: Cryptogenic organizing pneumonia. *(Right)* Frontal radiograph shows miliary nodules ➔. Patient had had a remote history of Silo-filler's disease.

Typical

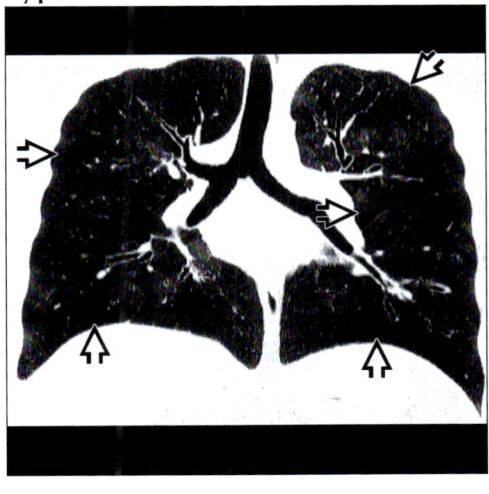
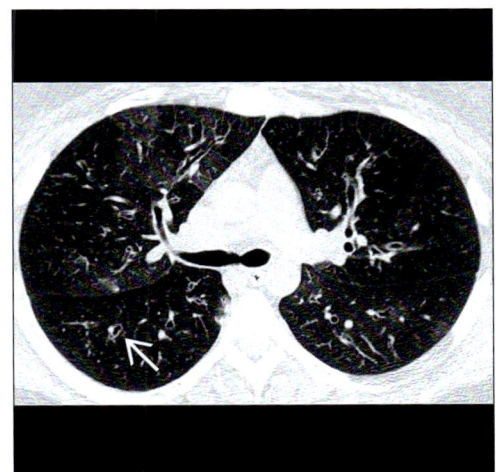

(Left) Coronal HRCT MinIP reconstruction shows widespread hypoattenuation ➔ from severe bronchiolitis obliterans. *(Right)* Axial HRCT shows mosaic attenuation. Vessels in the ground-glass attenuation larger than corresponding areas of hypoattenuation. Larger central airway walls are thickened and dilated ➔.

COMMUNITY ACQUIRED PNEUMONIA

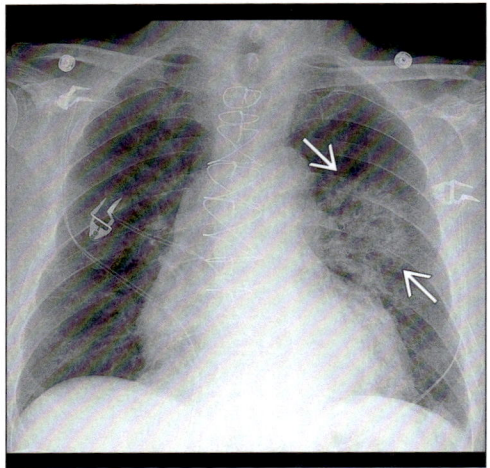

Anteroposterior radiograph shows focal consolidation in the left mid lung ➡. Differential includes pneumonia, aspiration, hemorrhage. Edema less likely because process is unilateral.

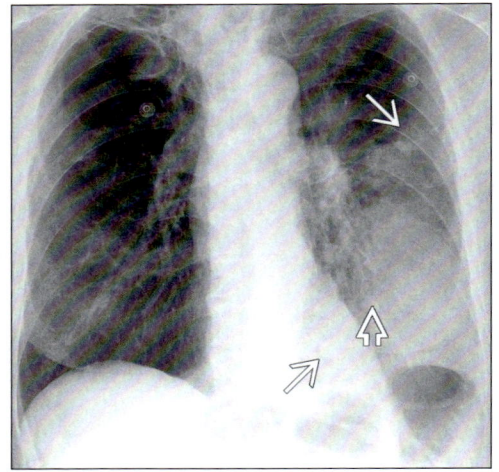

Frontal radiograph shows focal consolidation throughout left lower lobe ➡. Numerous air-bronchograms ⇨ along medial edge of consolidation. Classic lobar pneumonia pattern.

TERMINOLOGY

Definitions
- Clinical classification
  - Community-acquired pneumonia (CAP)
  - Aspiration pneumonia
  - Healthcare-associated pneumonia (HCAP)
    - Hospitalization > 2 days in preceding 90 days
    - Nursing home residence
    - Home infusion therapy
    - Long-term dialysis
    - Home wound care
    - Exposure to family members with multiple drug-resistant pathogens
  - Hospital acquired pneumonia (HAP)
    - 48 hours after hospital admission or within 48 hours discharge from hospital
  - Ventilator-associated pneumonia (VAP)

IMAGING FINDINGS

General Features
- Best diagnostic clue: Focal parenchymal abnormality in patient with fever

Imaging Recommendations
- Best imaging tool
  - Chest radiograph for detection, assessing extent of disease, detect complications, and evaluate treatment response
  - Limited value in predicting causative organism
- Protocol advice: CT problem solving tool for nondiagnostic chest radiographs, unresolved pneumonia, or suspected complications

Radiographic Findings
- Indications for chest radiograph
  - Fever, cough, sputum production, coarse crackles
- High sensitivity: May not have visible abnormality in
  - Immunocompromised, especially if neutropenic
  - Dehydration: Controversial; rare if it exists at all
- Typical distribution segmental consolidation: Unilateral or bilateral

DDx: Community Acquired Pneumonia

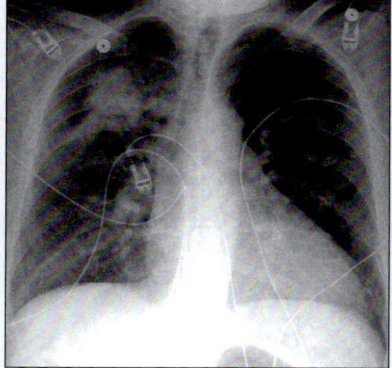

Mitral Regurgitant Edema

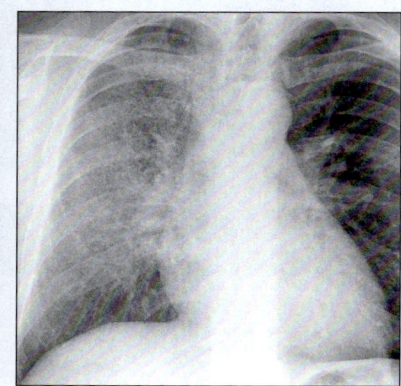

Diffuse Alveolar Hemorrhage

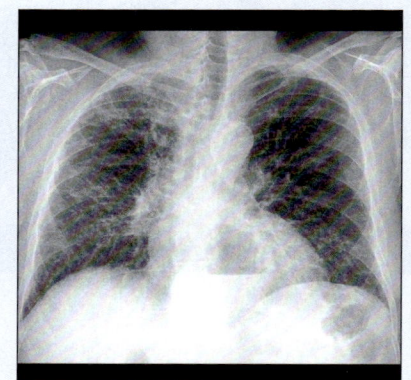

Hypersensitivity Pneumonitis

COMMUNITY ACQUIRED PNEUMONIA

Key Facts

Imaging Findings
- Best diagnostic clue: Focal parenchymal abnormality in patient with fever
- Significant interobserver variability in pattern recognition
- 50% resolution 2 weeks; 66% 4 weeks; 75% 6 weeks
- Mortality associated with 2 radiographic abnormalities: Bilateral pleural effusions and multilobar disease
- Centrilobular nodules in patchy distribution: Most helpful finding distinguishing infectious vs. noninfectious disease

Top Differential Diagnoses
- Cardiogenic Pulmonary Edema
- Hemorrhage
- Hypersensitivity Pneumonitis

Pathology
- Pneumonia Outcomes Research Team (PORT) severity Index useful in determining inpatient vs. outpatient treatment

Clinical Issues
- No individual or combinations of signs and symptoms from the history and physical examination can reliably confirm or refute the presence of pneumonia
- Pulmonary cavity in edentulous patient = lung Ca

Diagnostic Checklist
- Diagnosis based on culture (grayscale image does not substitute for Gram-stain)
- Absence of parenchymal abnormality excludes pneumonia (except in immunocompromised)

- Significant interobserver variability in pattern recognition
  - May have nearly any pattern from ground-glass, interstitial, to consolidation
  - Pattern not diagnostic of organism, single organism may cause multiple patterns
  - Poor agreement for pattern of disease, presence of air bronchogram, bronchial wall thickening
  - Good to excellent agreement for pleural effusion, extent of radiographic abnormalities
- Lobar vs. bronchopneumonia
  - Pathologic designation difficult to reliably identify radiographically
- Unusual patterns
  - Hyperinflation common with viral pneumonia (due to obstruction of distal airways)
  - Lobar enlargement with bulging fissures: Klebsiella pneumonia
  - Round pneumonia more common pattern of CAP in children
  - Pneumatoceles
    - Develop later in course of pneumonia (classically in S. aureus), may persist for months, resolve spontaneously
  - Hilar adenopathy
    - Rare, limits differential: Tuberculosis, mycoplasma, fungi, mononucleosis, measles, plague, tularemia, anthrax, pertussis
- Complications
  - Cavitation: Suggests bacterial disease (S. aureus, gram-negative bacteria, anaerobes)
  - Empyema
    - Pleural effusion in 20-60% reactive parapneumonic effusions
    - Up to 5% go on to empyema
    - Suspect if effusion enlarging or becomes loculated
- Resolution
  - Delayed with advancing age and involvement of multiple lobes
    - Faster resolution in nonsmokers and outpatients
  - Time table, expected
    - 50% resolution 2 weeks; 66% 4 weeks; 75% 6 weeks
- Mortality associated with 2 radiographic abnormalities: Bilateral pleural effusions and multilobar disease

CT Findings
- More sensitive and specific for complications
- Centrilobular nodules in patchy distribution: Most helpful finding distinguishing infectious vs. noninfectious disease
- Abscess vs. empyema
  - Abscess: Thick, irregular wall, round shape, small area of contact with chest wall
  - Empyema: Thin, uniform wall; lenticular shape, broad area of contact with chest, split pleura sign
- In those with recurrent pneumonia, consider: Bronchogenic carcinoma, bronchiectasis, COPD

DIFFERENTIAL DIAGNOSIS

Cardiogenic Pulmonary Edema
- Cardiomegaly and pulmonary venous hypertension
- Edema will shift with position (gravitational shift test)
- Focal edema in right upper lobe common with mitral regurgitation

Hemorrhage
- Patients usually anemic and often have hemoptysis

Aspiration
- May have predisposing condition such as esophageal motility disorder
- Gravitational dependent location

Cryptogenic Organizing Pneumonia
- Patients often treated for pneumonia for variable length of time
- Focal chronic bibasilar consolidation or interstitial thickening

Chronic Eosinophilic Pneumonia
- Typically chronic peripheral upper lobe consolidation

COMMUNITY ACQUIRED PNEUMONIA

- Will not respond to antibiotics

Hypersensitivity Pneumonitis
- Often mistaken as pneumonia
- History of antigen exposure
- Chest radiograph often normal
- CT: Diffuse ground-glass opacities, centrilobular nodules, and geographic hyperinflation of lobules

Pulmonary Infarction
- Resolution: Infarcts exhibit "melting snowball" sign, pneumonia in contrast "fades" away like a ghost

Atelectasis
- Fissural displacement or other signs of air loss

PATHOLOGY

General Features
- General path comments
  - Offending organism cultured in < 50%
  - Portal of entry inhalation or aspiration of oral secretions
- Etiology: Most common pathogens: Streptococcus pneumoniae (50%), Viral pneumonia (20%), Haemophilus influenzae (20%), Mycoplasma pneumoniae (5%), Chlamydia pneumoniae (15%), Legionella pneumophila
- Epidemiology: Pneumonia 6th most common cause of death

Gross Pathologic & Surgical Features
- Lobar vs. bronchopneumonia
  - Lobar
    - Alveolar flooding with inflammatory exudate, especially neutrophils
    - Rapidly spreads throughout lobe, only stopped by intact fissures
    - Usually peripheral in lung
  - Bronchopneumonia
    - Exudate centered on terminal bronchioles (centrilobular)
    - Respects septal boundaries
    - Patchy: Adjacent secondary pulmonary lobules may be normal, patchwork quilt patterns

Microscopic Features
- Nonspecific acute and or chronic inflammatory cells
- Organism identified with special stains (such as Gram or acid-fast)

Staging, Grading or Classification Criteria
- Pneumonia Outcomes Research Team (PORT) severity Index useful in determining inpatient vs. outpatient treatment
  - 5 severity classes (2-step process)
    - Step 1: Class I criteria: Age < 50 years with 0-5 comorbid conditions, normal or mildly deranged vital signs, normal mental status
    - Comorbid conditions: Neoplastic disease [30 points], liver disease [20 points], congestive heart failure [10 points], cerebrovascular disease [10 points], renal disease [10 points]
    - Step 2. If not class 1, stratify into class II-V on points assigned to: 5 comorbid conditions (see above)
    - 3 demographic variables: Age, sex, [men: Points = age in yrs; women: Points = age in yrs - 10], nursing home residency [10 points]
    - 5 physical examination findings: Pulse > 125 beats/min [10 points], respiratory rate ≥ 30 breaths/min [20 points], systolic blood pressure < 90 mm Hg [20 points], temperature < 35° C or ≥ 40° C [15 points], altered mental status [20 points]
    - 7 laboratory or radiographic findings: Arterial pH < 7.35 [30 points], BUN ≥ 30 mg/dL [20 points], sodium < 130 mmol/L [20 points], glucose ≥ 250 mg/dL [10 points], hematocrit < 30% [10 points], hypoxemia O_2 saturation < 90% (pulse oximetry) or < 60 mm HG (arterial blood gas) [10 points]; Pleural effusion initial radiograph [10 points]
  - Class I & II risk low (70 or fewer total points)
  - Class III risk low (71-90 points)
  - Class IV risk moderate (91-130 points)
  - Class V risk high (> 130 total points)

CLINICAL ISSUES

Presentation
- Most common signs/symptoms
  - No individual or combinations of signs and symptoms from the history and physical examination can reliably confirm or refute the presence of pneumonia
  - Classic findings: Fever, chills cough, sputum
  - Empyema: May be surprisingly free of toxic symptoms
  - Pulmonary cavity in edentulous patient = lung Ca
    - Lung abscess invariably associated with poor dentition

Natural History & Prognosis
- Depends or virulence of organism, antibiotic susceptibility and host

Treatment
- Appropriate antibiotics
- Drain empyemas, not abscesses

DIAGNOSTIC CHECKLIST

Consider
- Diagnosis based on culture (grayscale image does not substitute for Gram-stain)

Image Interpretation Pearls
- Absence of parenchymal abnormality excludes pneumonia (except in immunocompromised)

SELECTED REFERENCES
1. Mandell LA et al: Infectious Diseases Society of America/American Thoracic Society consensus guidelines on the management of community-acquired pneumonia in adults. Clin Infect Dis. 44 Suppl 2:S27-72, 2007

COMMUNITY ACQUIRED PNEUMONIA

IMAGE GALLERY

Typical

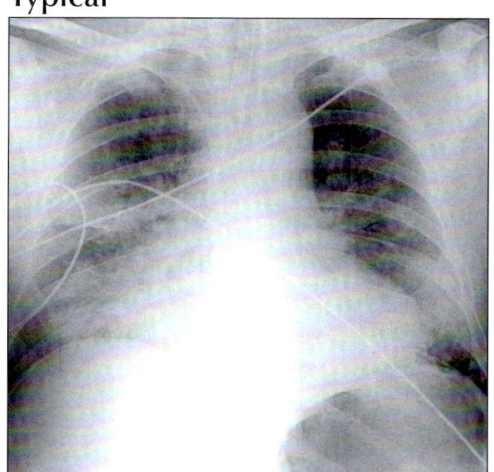
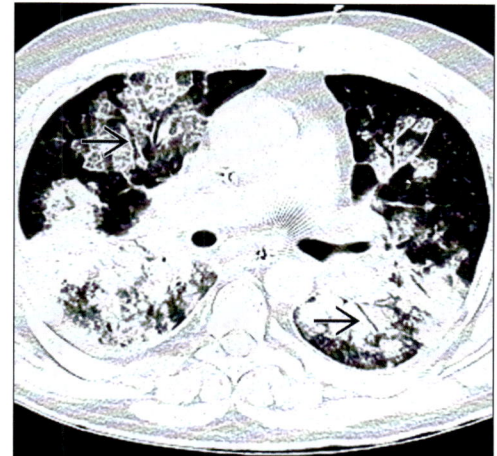

(Left) Anteroposterior radiograph shows dense bilateral heterogeneous lung consolidation from pneumonia. *(Right)* Axial NECT confirms the presence of dense bilateral pneumonia that obscures bronchial and vascular margins. Air bronchogram ➡ is produced by aerated bronchus outlined by dense adjacent pulmonary consolidation. Streptococcus pneumonia.

Typical

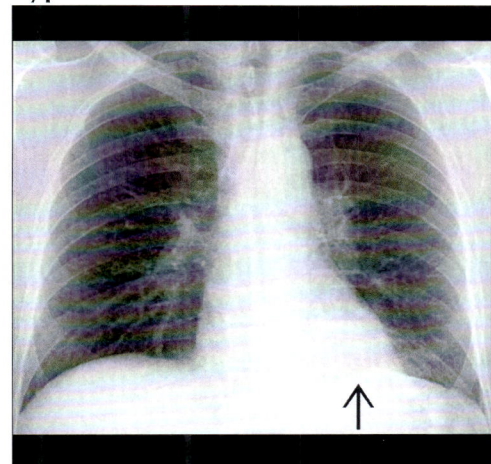
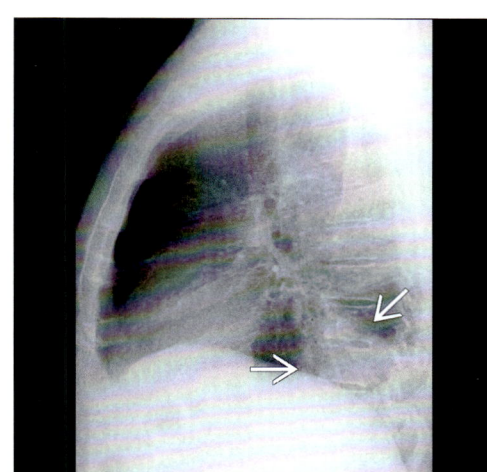

(Left) Frontal radiograph shows a faint opacity superimposed on the heart ➡. This would be easy to overlook. *(Right)* Lateral radiograph shows consolidation superimposed over the lower thoracic spine ➡.

Typical

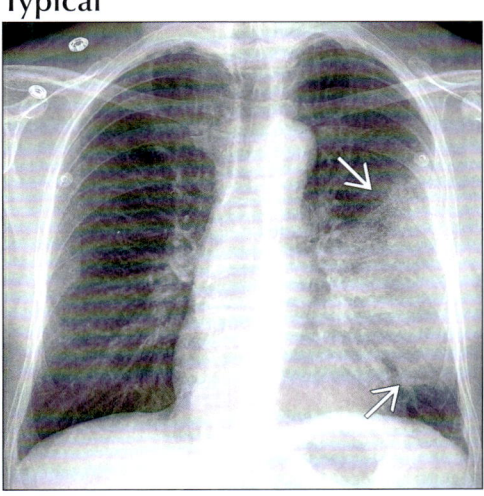
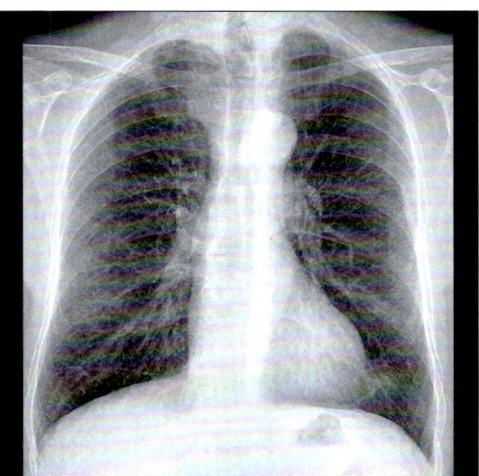

(Left) Frontal radiograph shows lingular lobar pneumonia ➡. No pleural effusion or other complicating findings. *(Right)* Frontal radiograph 6 weeks later shows complete resolution of pneumonia.

IMMUNOCOMPROMISED PNEUMONIA

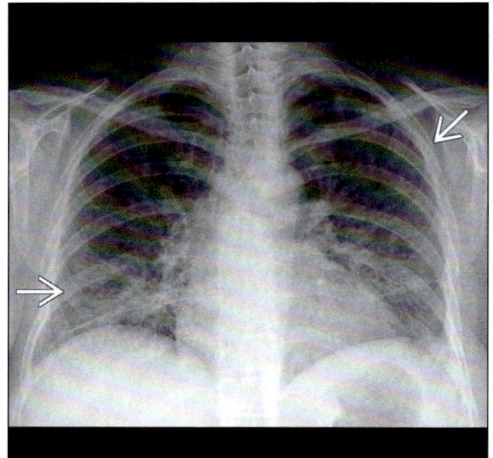

Frontal radiograph shows diffuse ground-glass opacities ➔ in AIDS patient with fever.

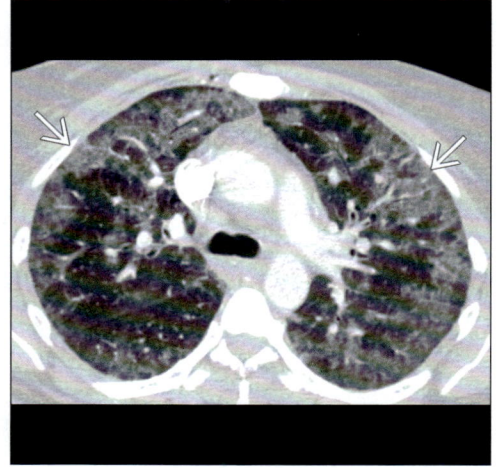

Axial CECT shows diffuse ground-glass opacities ➔. Lavage demonstrated Pneumocystis pneumonia.

TERMINOLOGY

Abbreviations and Synonyms
- Graft-vs-host disease (GVHD), cytomegalovirus (CMV), Pneumocystis jiroveci pneumonia (PCP), acquired immune deficiency syndrome (AIDS), human immunodeficiency virus (HIV), Ebstein-Barr virus (EBV)

Definitions
- Congenital or acquired abnormality of immune system putting patient at increased risk for life-threatening infection

IMAGING FINDINGS

Imaging Recommendations
- Best imaging tool
  ○ Chest radiograph useful surveillance tool prior to onset of symptoms
  ○ Sufficient in most cases to detect, find complications, and monitor response to therapy
- Protocol advice: CT more sensitive, will detect infection an average of 5 days before chest radiograph shows abnormalities

Radiographic Findings
- Sensitivity > 90%
- Nonspecific findings
  ○ Diagnostic interpretation correct in only 1/3rd
  ○ Accuracy of highly confident diagnosis 50% (toss up)
  ○ May be normal in PCP or mycobacterial infections in AIDS
- Consolidation
  ○ Focal or diffuse, subsegmental to diffuse, consider
    ▪ Bacterial, mycobacterial, or fungal pneumonia
    ▪ Hemorrhage
    ▪ Radiation pneumonitis
    ▪ Recurrent tumor: Lymphoma
  ○ Nodules, consider
    ▪ Fungal, nocardia, mycobacterial pneumonia
    ▪ Septic emboli
    ▪ Metastases
    ▪ Drug toxicity: Bleomycin, methotrexate

DDx: Fever in Immunocompromised

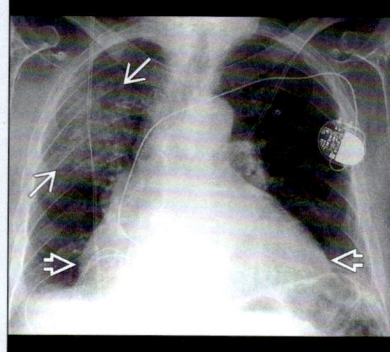

Mitral Regurgitant Pulmonary Edema

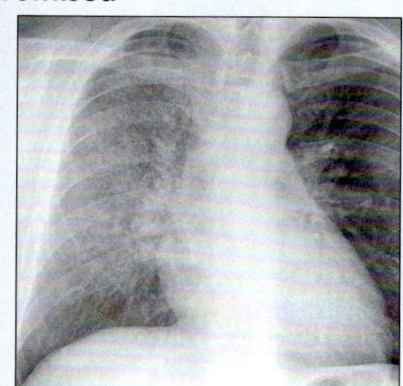

Diffuse Hemorrhage

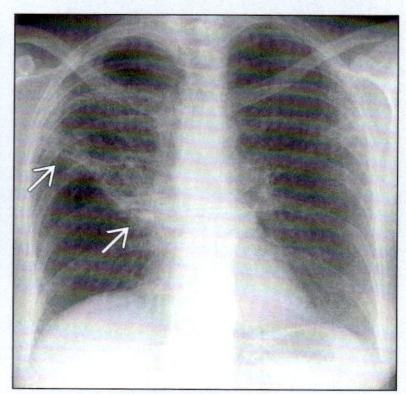

Radiation Pneumonitis

IMMUNOCOMPROMISED PNEUMONIA

Key Facts

Terminology
- Congenital or acquired abnormality of immune system putting patient at increased risk for life-threatening infection

Imaging Findings
- Protocol advice: CT more sensitive, will detect infection an average of 5 days before chest radiograph shows abnormalities
- Diagnostic interpretation correct in only 1/3rd
- Accuracy of highly confident diagnosis 50% (toss up)

Top Differential Diagnoses
- Edema (Cardiogenic and Noncardiogenic)
- Diffuse Hemorrhage
- Drug Toxicity
- Radiation Pneumonitis

Pathology
- 75% of all complications infections
- Up to 1/3rd have more than 1 complication
- Even with sampling, a precise cause not identified in 20%

Clinical Issues
- Most common signs/symptoms: Findings usually nonspecific, fever may not be due to infection
- Establishing a cause by an invasive procedure may not improve outcome by more than 20%

Diagnostic Checklist
- Statistics don't substitute for sampling
- Early diagnosis reduces mortality by more than 50%

- Post-transplant lymphoproliferative disorder (PTLD)
- Interstitial pattern, consider
  - PCP or viral pneumonia
  - Edema, cardiac and noncardiac: Kerley B lines more likely due to edema than infection
  - Drug toxicity
  - Lymphangitic metastases
- Pleural effusion, consider
  - Congestive heart failure
  - Bacterial pneumonia
  - Infarction
  - GVHD
  - Lymphoma especially in AIDS
- Cysts
  - Pneumatoceles seen in PCP or lymphocytic interstitial pneumonia in AIDS patients
- Adenopathy
  - Pneumonia: Mycobacterial or fungal, or bacillary angiomatosis
  - Kaposi
  - Lymphoma
- Rapid progression, focal nodules or consolidation
  - Bacterial, mycobacterial, fungal pneumonia
  - Infarction or hemorrhage
  - Septic emboli
- Rapid progression, diffuse
  - Pulmonary edema, hemorrhage
  - Fungal pneumonia, mycobacteria
- Subacute to chronic, focal
  - Mycobacterial or fungal pneumonia
  - Recurrent tumor
  - PTLD
- Subacute to chronic, diffuse
  - Viral, PCP pneumonia
  - Radiation pneumonitis
  - Lymphangitic tumor or Kaposi sarcoma

CT Findings
- Nodules
  - Centrilobular nodules < 1 cm usually infectious
  - Nodules > 1 cm usually neoplastic
  - Nodules with ground-glass halo: Invasive aspergillosis
  - Cavitation: Septic emboli, metastases, resolving angioinvasive aspergillosis
  - Pneumatoceles: PCP, lymphocytic interstitial pneumonia
  - Tree-in-bud: Infections
- Distribution
  - Peribronchovascular distribution: Kaposi sarcoma, lymphoma
  - Upper lobe ground-glass opacities: PCP
- Adenopathy
  - Enhancing adenopathy: Mycobacteria, bacillary angiomatosis
  - Amorphous nodal calcification: PCP

DIFFERENTIAL DIAGNOSIS

Edema (Cardiogenic and Noncardiogenic)
- Cardiomegaly and pleural effusions
- Kerley B lines: Edema more common than infection

Diffuse Hemorrhage
- Anemia and often expectoration of blood

Drug Toxicity
- Nearly any pattern, should always be considered in immunosuppressed

Radiation Pneumonitis
- Usually develops within 1 month of finishing treatment
- Radiation pneumonitis peaks 4 months after completion therapy, then evolves into scarring
- Radiographic abnormalities conforms to radiation port

PATHOLOGY

General Features
- Etiology
  - Macrophage or neutrophil disorder

IMMUNOCOMPROMISED PNEUMONIA

- Phagocytic defect often seen with bone marrow suppression, chemotherapy, leukemia, bone marrow transplant
  - B-cell disorder
    - Antibody defect either primary (x-linked agammaglobulinemia or immunoglobulin deficiency) or secondary from multiple myeloma, Waldenstrom, chronic lymphocytic leukemia
  - T-cell disorder
    - Cell-mediated defect either primary (DiGeorge or Nezelof syndrome) or secondary to AIDS, lymphoma, leukemia, aging
    - HIV infection depletes helper T cells (CD4) leading to immunosuppression
    - Typically CD4 count 800-1,000 cells/mm^3, HIV depletes 50 cells/year (prodromal period approximately 10 years)
  - Edema
    - Multifactorial: High volumes of fluid for chemotherapy, chemotherapy or radiation damage to heart, minor transfusion reactions, anemia
- Epidemiology
  - 75% of all complications infections
  - Up to 1/3rd have more than 1 complication
  - AIDS
    - 50% develop pulmonary complications: Infections and malignancy
    - Nearly 50% pneumonias bacterial
    - Non-Hodgkin lymphoma most common malignancy, Kaposi sarcoma on the decline (Kaposi also seen following solid organ transplantation)
- Type of immunosuppression
  - Mechanical
    - Mucosal disruption (chemotherapy), intubation (bypass nose and airway defenses), splenectomy
  - Cellular
    - Macrophages, neutrophil dysfunction: B-cell or T-cell dysfunction
- Bacteriology
  - Splenectomy
    - Encapsulated bacteria: Streptococcus, Haemophilus influenza, Staphylococcus
  - Mucosal disruption: Candida, gram-organisms
  - Phagocytic dysfunction at risk for
    - Staphylococcus, gram -'s, aspergillus and mucormycosis
  - Antibody dysfunction at risk for
    - Encapsulated bacteria: Staphylococcus, Haemophilus
  - Cell mediated dysfunction at risk for
    - Intracellular pathogens, Streptococcus, pseudomonas, mycobacteria, nocardia, Legionella, cryptococcus, Histoplasmosis, Coccidiomycosis, varicella-zoster, CMV, EBV, PCP, Toxoplasmosis

Microscopic Features
- Even with sampling, a precise cause not identified in 20%

CLINICAL ISSUES

Presentation
- Most common signs/symptoms: Findings usually nonspecific, fever may not be due to infection
- Other signs/symptoms
  - Graft vs. Host disease
    - Acute (donor T cell damage): Skin, liver, GI mucosa primary targets
    - Chronic (autoimmune): Aspects of Sjögren, systemic lupus erythematosus, scleroderma, esophageal motility, bronchiolitis obliterans, lichen planus, sicca syndrome

Natural History & Prognosis
- Solid organ transplantation
  - < 1 month: Aspiration, wound infection, line colonization
  - 1-4 months: CMV, PCP, aspergillus, nocardia, mycobacteria
  - > 4 months: Cryptococcus, PCP, legionella
- Bone marrow transplantation
  - < 30 days: Edema, pseudomonas, aspiration, hemorrhage
  - 30-100 days: CMV, PCP, drugs, radiation, edema, GVHD
  - > 100 days: Streptococcus, Staphylococcus, varicella-zoster, GVHD
- AIDS
  - Tuberculosis: Pattern of disease may vary with CD4 count
    - > 200 cells/mm^3: Post-primary pattern
    - 50-200 cells/mm^3: Primary pattern
    - < 50 cells/mm^3: Miliary interstitial pattern
    - Paradoxical response: Transient worsening of radiographic pattern with antiviral therapy (strengthened hypersensitivity response)
- Prognosis
  - Depends on underlying condition and response to therapy

Treatment
- Empiric therapy with antibiotics often used in immunosuppressed, if no response, more aggressive sampling used
- Empiric diuresis often tried to exclude edema
- Establishing a cause by an invasive procedure may not improve outcome by more than 20%

DIAGNOSTIC CHECKLIST

Image Interpretation Pearls
- Statistics don't substitute for sampling
- Early diagnosis reduces mortality by more than 50%

SELECTED REFERENCES
1. Grubb JR et al: The changing spectrum of pulmonary disease in patients with HIV infection on antiretroviral therapy. AIDS. 20(8):1095-107, 2006
2. Kotloff RM et al: Pulmonary complications of solid organ and hematopoietic stem cell transplantation. Am J Respir Crit Care Med. 170(1):22-48, 2004

IMMUNOCOMPROMISED PNEUMONIA

IMAGE GALLERY

Typical

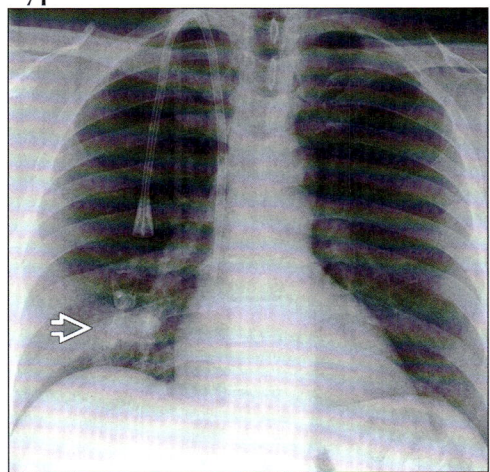
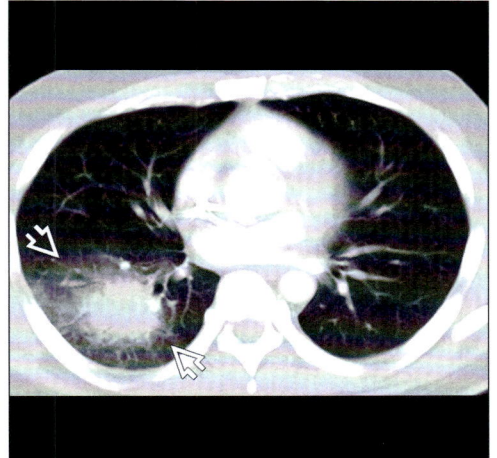

(Left) Frontal radiograph shows focal nonspecific vague opacity in the right lower lobe ⇨ in bone marrow transplant recipient. *(Right)* Axial NECT shows mass-like consolidation in the right lower lobe surrounded by ground-glass halo ⇨. Invasive aspergillosis.

Typical

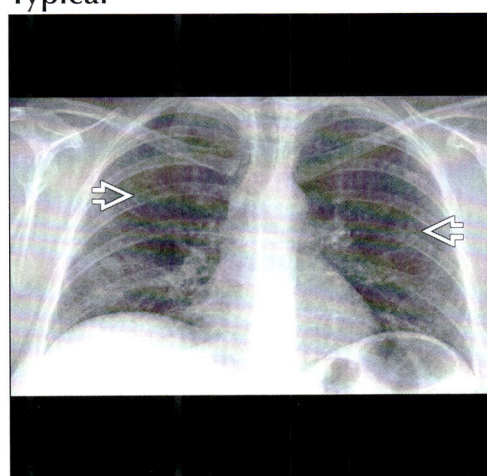
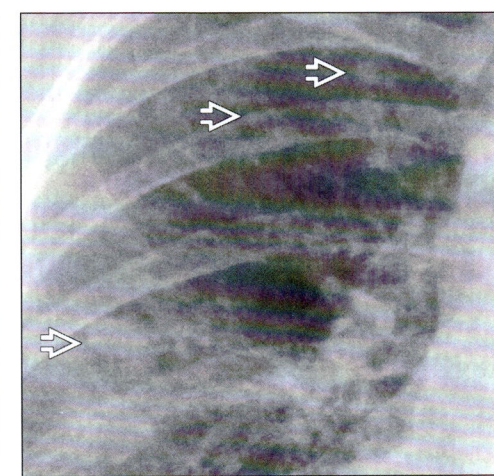

(Left) Frontal radiograph shows miliary nodules ⇨ uniformly distributed throughout the lungs. Heart size normal, no adenopathy or pleural effusions. *(Right)* Frontal radiograph magnified better shows miliary nodules ⇨ from varicella zoster pneumonia.

Typical

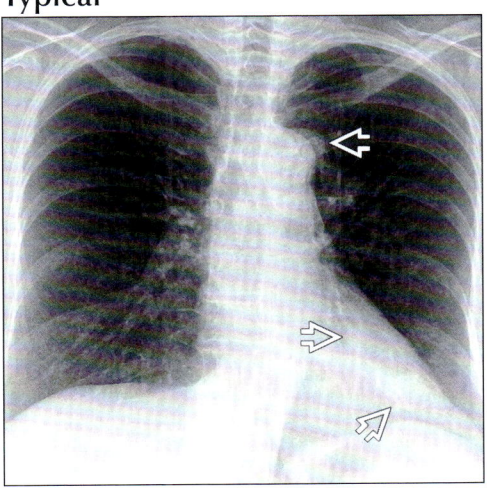
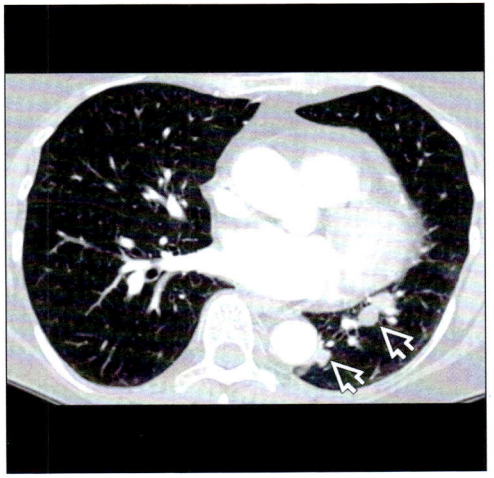

(Left) Frontal radiograph shows multiple pulmonary nodules ⇨ in immunosuppressed patient. *(Right)* Axial CECT shows multiple nodules ⇨ in left lung. Cryptococcal pneumonia.

LUNG ABSCESS

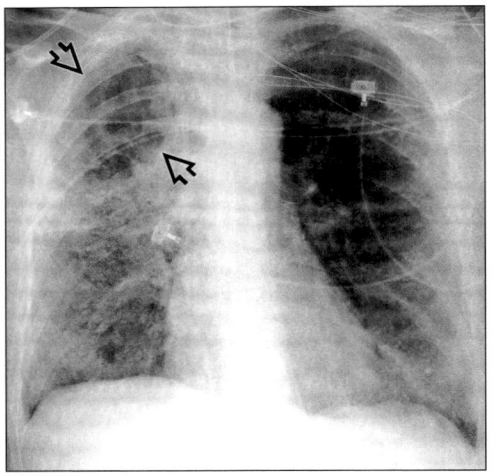

Anteroposterior radiograph shows large cavity ⇨ at the apex of the right lung.

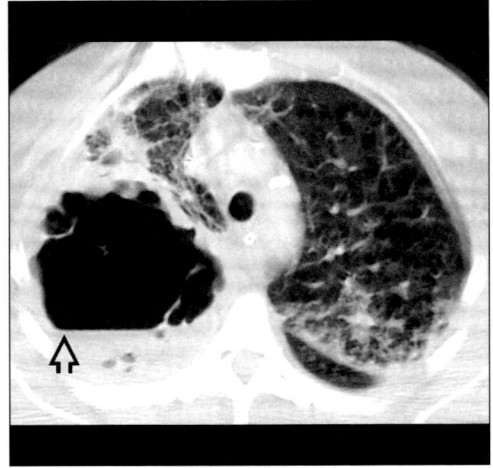

Axial CECT shows a large abscess cavity with an air-fluid level ⇨. Inner wall contour nodular.

TERMINOLOGY

Abbreviations and Synonyms
- Necrotizing pneumonia, pulmonary gangrene, lung cavity

Definitions
- Necrosis of lung by microbial infection
- Cavity refers to an air containing lesion with a relatively thick wall (> 4 mm) or within an area of a surrounding opacity or mass

IMAGING FINDINGS

General Features
- Best diagnostic clue: Irregular solitary thick-walled cavity, often containing air-fluid level
- Location: Gravitationally dependent segments after aspiration
- Morphology: Spherical thick-walled cavity with smooth inner margin surrounded by consolidated lung

Radiographic Findings
- Radiography
  - Consolidation from pneumonia typically evolves into abscess cavity over 7-14 days
  - Cavity
    - Often solitary
    - Wall thickness: < 4 mm (5%); 5-15 mm (80%); > 15 mm (15%)
    - Air-fluid level 75%
    - Often surrounded by consolidated lung (50%)
  - Location usually related to aspiration in gravitationally dependent locations
    - Supine position: Posterior segments upper lobes, superior segments lower lobes
    - Decubitus position: Posterior segments upper lobes, lateral basilar segments lower lobes
    - Upright position: Basilar segments lower lobes, right middle lobe
  - Lower lobe abscesses usually larger than upper lobe abscesses
  - Pleural effusions common (50%), may evolve into empyema
  - Multiple abscesses consider

DDx: Cavity

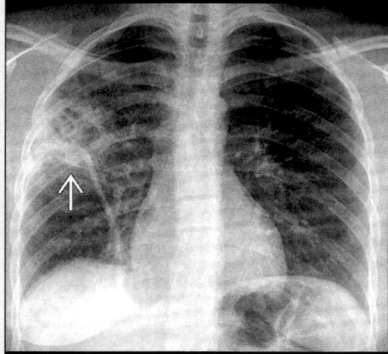

Pneumatoceles

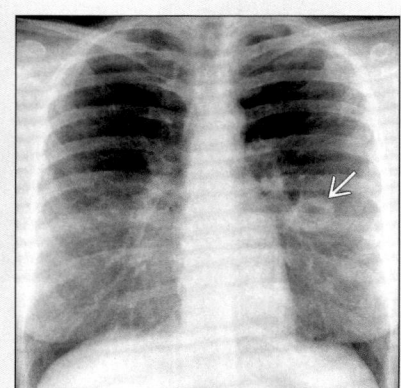

Wegener Granulomatosis

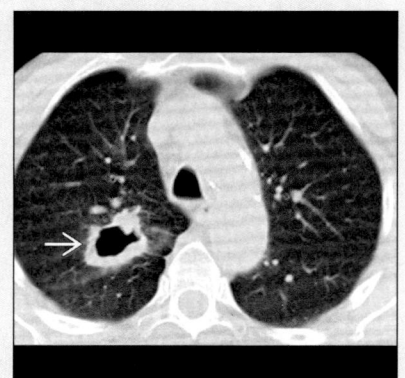

Lung Cancer

LUNG ABSCESS

Key Facts

Terminology
- Necrosis of lung by microbial infection
- Cavity refers to an air containing lesion with a relatively thick wall (> 4 mm) or within an area of a surrounding opacity or mass

Imaging Findings
- Morphology: Spherical thick-walled cavity with smooth inner margin surrounded by consolidated lung
- Consolidation from pneumonia typically evolves into abscess cavity over 7-14 days
- Location usually related to aspiration in gravitationally dependent locations
- Resolution with treatment prolonged often taking months
- Larger the abscess the longer to resolution
- Protocol advice: Antibiotics should be continued until chest radiograph shows resolution or stability

Top Differential Diagnoses
- Pneumatoceles
- Infected Bulla
- Bronchogenic Carcinoma
- Septic Embolism

Pathology
- High risk: Poor dentition, seizure disorder, alcoholism

Clinical Issues
- Cough, foul smelling sputum, periodontal disease

Diagnostic Checklist
- Lung cancer in edentulous patient (most abscesses arise from periodontal bacteria)

- Bronchogenic spread from initial abscess (daughter abscesses usually smaller than parent and located in areas gravitationally dependent from parent)
- **Lemierre syndrome**: Sore throat with thrombosis internal jugular vein, usually secondary to Fusobacterium
○ To distinguish abscess from empyema
  - Cavity: Spherical shape, air-fluid levels on frontal and lateral views equal length, acute angles with chest wall
  - Empyema: Lenticular shape, air-fluid levels on frontal and lateral views unequal length, obtuse angles with chest wall
  - 33% of lung abscesses accompanied by empyema
○ Resolution with treatment prolonged often taking months
  - Larger the abscess the longer to resolution

CT Findings
- Abscess may be fluid-filled
- Air-fluid level or central air collection indicates bronchial communication
- Cavity wall thickness: Variable, 4 mm to < 15 mm; thick wall more common
  ○ Luminal interior wall usually smooth (90%), shaggy (10%)
- Pericavitary opacification (airspace or ground-glass) may show air-bronchograms or tiny air bubbles
- Abscess vs. empyema
  ○ Abscess: Thick, irregular wall, spherical, narrow contact with chest wall, bronchovascular markings extend toward the abscess
  ○ Empyema: Thin uniform wall, lenticular shape, broad contact with chest wall, split pleura sign, adjacent compressed lung
- Reactive hilar and mediastinal lymphadenopathy common, nodes usually < 2.5 cm short axis diameter
- Bronchopleural fistula: Development of hydropneumothorax, empyema
- Air crescent: Suggests invasive aspergillosis or mycetoma in a pre-existing cavity

Imaging Recommendations
- Best imaging tool: CT to distinguish pulmonary abscess from empyema, and to evaluate for associated lung cancer
- Protocol advice: Antibiotics should be continued until chest radiograph shows resolution or stability

DIFFERENTIAL DIAGNOSIS

Pneumatoceles
- Difficult to distinguish from abscess, especially in Staphylococcal pneumonia

Mycobacterium Tuberculosis
- Bilateral upper lobe location

Infected Bulla
- Smoking and emphysema
- Thin-walled bulla with air-fluid level
- Considered a pneumonia variant, responds to antibiotics

Bronchogenic Carcinoma
- Cavity in edentulous patient more likely from carcinoma than lung abscess
- Thickest portion of cavity wall > 15 mm suggests tumor
- Wall more nodular
- Less likely to have pericavitary consolidation

Septic Embolism
- Endocarditis, extrathoracic site of infection, indwelling catheter or IV drug abuse
- Often multiple, consolidation rapidly evolves into cavities (24 hours)

Wegener Granulomatosis
- History of sinus disease, acute renal disease
- Nodules or masses, with or without cavitation, air-fluid levels rare
- Subglottic stenosis may be associated

LUNG ABSCESS

Necrobiotic Nodules
- History of rheumatoid arthritis, and/or dust inhalation
- Few, small and subpleural in location

Intralobar Sequestration
- Recurrent pneumonias at the same site especially medial basilar segments of lower lobes

PATHOLOGY

General Features
- Etiology
  - Aspiration: Often due to mixed aerobic and anaerobic polymicrobial bacterial infection originating from gingiva
  - Organisms leading to abscess
    - Anaerobes: Peptostreptococcus, Bacteroides, Fusobacterium, microaerophilic Streptococci
    - Aerobes: Staphylococcus aureus, Streptococcus pyogenes, Klebsiella pneumoniae, Haemophilus influenzae, Actinomyces, Nocardia and Mycobacterium species
    - Parasites: Paragonimus, entamoeba
    - Fungi: Aspergillus, Cryptococcus Histoplasma, Blastomyces, Coccidioides Immitis
- Epidemiology
  - High risk: Poor dentition, seizure disorder, alcoholism
  - Predisposition in patients with immune deficiency, bronchiectasis, malignancy, emphysema, steroid treatment
  - May develop in patients with inappropriate/inadequate antibiotic treatment of pneumonia
  - 70-80% are smokers; 12% have associated lung cancer, (infected lung cancer rare)
- Associated abnormalities: May progress to empyema and bronchopleural fistula

Gross Pathologic & Surgical Features
- Parenchymal destruction that heals with scarring, bronchiectasis, cyst formation
- Uncommon complication, pulmonary gangrene with necrotic lung fragments in abscess cavity (pulmonary sequestrum)

Microscopic Features
- Half the cases have anaerobic organisms alone that must be cultured with anaerobic techniques
  - Any antibiotic administration makes retrieval of anaerobes nearly impossible
- Gram stain of sputum classically polymicrobial with many neutrophils
- TB or Nocardia detected with acid fast stain; fungi detected with silver stain

CLINICAL ISSUES

Presentation
- Most common signs/symptoms
  - Often subacute illness of weeks to months
  - Fever, leukocytosis in 90% of patients
  - Cough, foul smelling sputum, periodontal disease
  - Hemoptysis can occur, may be fatal
- Other signs/symptoms
  - Diagnosis can be obtained with CT or ultrasound guided fine needle aspiration
    - No bronchoscopy in acute phase for abscess > 4 cm because of potential spillover of contents to normal lung

Demographics
- Age: Any age but more common in elderly
- Gender: M:F = 4:1

Natural History & Prognosis
- Good prognosis with early diagnosis and treatment
  - 33% mortality if untreated
- Aspiration leads to pneumonia, pneumonia progresses to lung abscess in 7-14 days
  - Resolution slower than non-cavitary pneumonia
  - Heals with scarring, bronchiectasis, cystic change
  - Mortality higher in elderly debilitated immunocompromised patients with large abscesses

Treatment
- Usually responds to antibiotics (Clindamycin 4-6 weeks of therapy), in contrast to abscesses elsewhere that usually require tube drainage
- Bronchoscopy to assess for an endobronchial lesion or foreign body if medical treatment has failed
- Less than 10% require surgery for non-resolving abscess
- Percutaneous drainage, controversial
  - Reserved for non-resolving abscess or empyema that abuts the chest wall (10-20%)

DIAGNOSTIC CHECKLIST

Consider
- Lung cancer in edentulous patient (most abscesses arise from periodontal bacteria)
- CT to evaluate for complications such as empyema and bronchopleural fistula

SELECTED REFERENCES

1. Bartlett JG: The role of anaerobic bacteria in lung abscess. Clin Infect Dis. 40(7):923-5, 2005
2. Lai C et al: Images in clinical medicine. Lemierre's Syndrome. N Engl J Med. 350(16):e14, 2004
3. Ryu JH et al: Cystic and cavitary lung diseases: focal and diffuse. Mayo Clin Proc. 78(6):744-52, 2003
4. Mueller PR et al: Complications of lung abscess aspiration and drainage. AJR Am J Roentgenol. 178(5):1083-6, 2002
5. Franquet T et al: Aspiration diseases: findings, pitfalls, and differential diagnosis. Radiographics. 20(3):673-85, 2000
6. Shaham D et al: Lemierre's syndrome presenting as multiple lung abscesses. Clin Imaging. 24(4):197-9, 2000
7. Marom EM et al: The many faces of pulmonary aspiration. AJR Am J Roentgenol. 172(1):121-8, 1999
8. Woodring JH et al: Solitary cavities of the lung: diagnostic implications of cavity wall thickness. AJR Am J Roentgenol. 135(6):1269-71, 1980

LUNG ABSCESS

IMAGE GALLERY

Typical

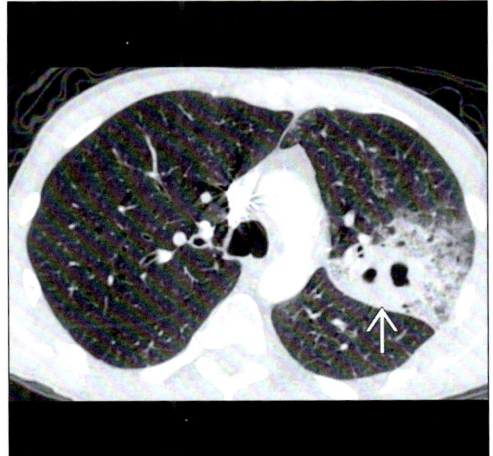
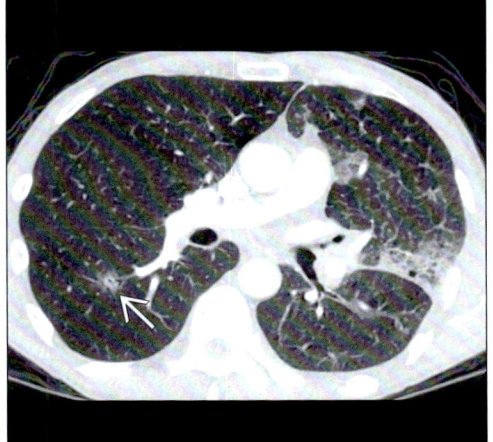

(Left) Axial CECT shows lung abscess ➡ surrounded by consolidated lung in the left upper lobe. Abscess wall is thick and the inner contour is smooth. *(Right)* Axial CECT shows bronchogenic spread into the opposite lung ➡. Abscess contents may spill into other dependent regions of the lung.

Typical

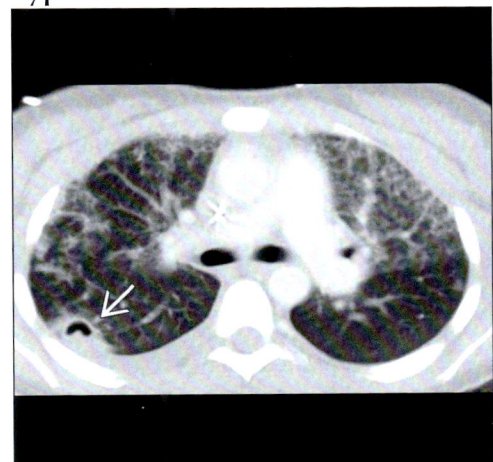
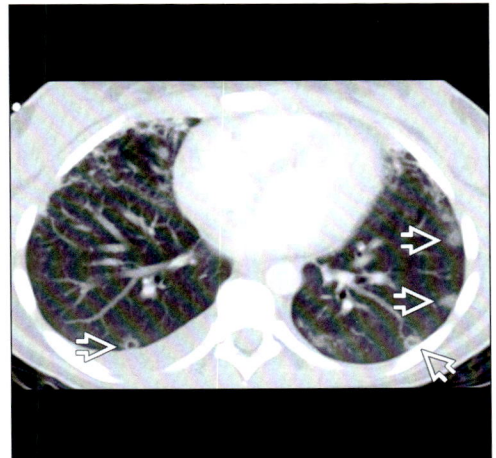

(Left) Axial CECT shows peripheral lung abscess ➡ and patchy reticular opacities in the nondependent lung. College student with sore throat for 3 weeks. *(Right)* Axial CECT shows smaller peripheral abscesses ➡. Culture positive Fusobacterium. Diagnosis: Lemierre syndrome.

Typical

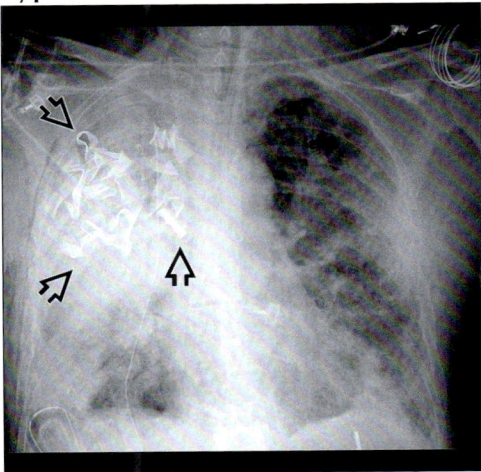
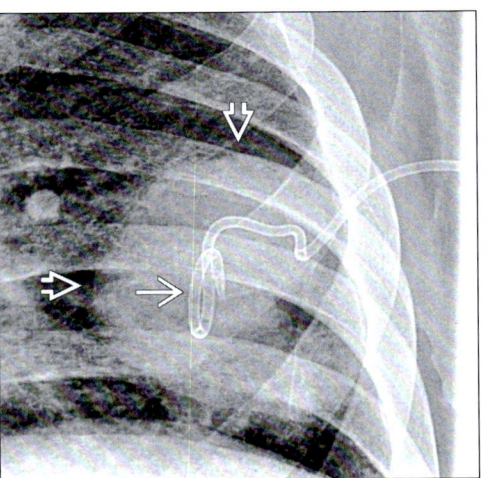

(Left) Anteroposterior radiograph shows surgical packing ➡ of large abscess cavity in right upper lobe. Diffuse consolidation from pneumonia. *(Right)* Frontal chest fluoroscopy shows well-defined mass ➡. Pigtail catheter ➡ placed in abscess for drainage.

VIRAL LUNG INFECTION, PEDIATRIC

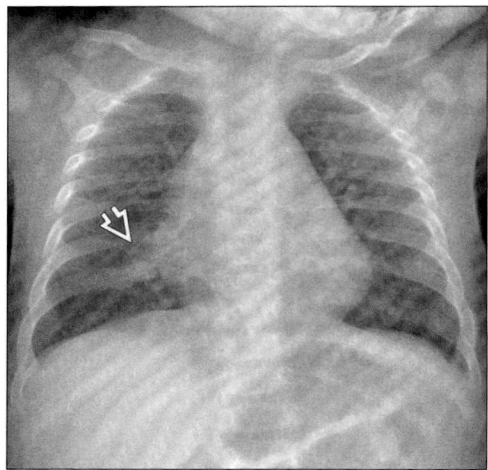

Frontal radiograph shows increased perihilar markings and subsegmental atelectasis ➔ in the right middle lobe.

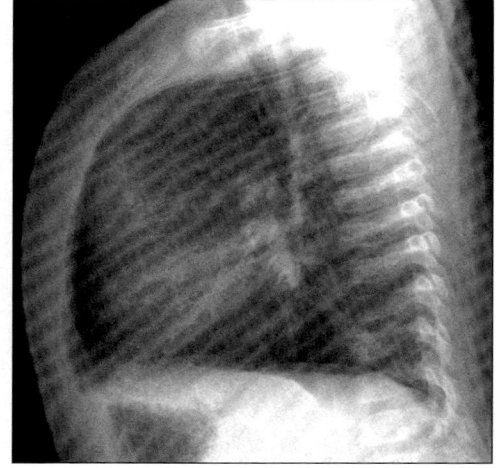

Lateral radiograph (same patient as previous) shows marked hyperinflation with increased AP diameter of the chest. There are also increased perihilar markings.

TERMINOLOGY

Abbreviations and Synonyms
- Bronchiolitis

Definitions
- Viral infection of the lower respiratory tract

IMAGING FINDINGS

General Features
- Best diagnostic clue: Increased peribronchial markings and hyperinflation
- Location: Bilateral and symmetric hyperinflation

Radiographic Findings
- Radiography
  - Major goal of imaging (chest radiography) is to differentiate viral from bacterial pneumonia
  - Best imaging clue for viral disease
    - Increased peribronchial markings
    - Hyperinflation
  - Lack of focal lung consolidation (hallmark for bacterial infection)
  - Increased peribronchial markings
    - Symmetric, coarse linear markings radiating from the hila into the lung
    - Central portions of the lungs may appear "dirty" or "busy"
    - Very subjective finding
    - Hila may appear prominent on lateral view
  - Hyperinflation
    - Hyperlucency
    - Depression of the diaphragm to more than 10 posterior ribs
    - Flattening of the hemi-diaphragms (best seen on lateral view)
    - Increased anteroposterior chest diameter (in infants chest wider than tall on lateral view)
    - Hyperinflation often much better appreciated on lateral view
  - Subsegmental atelectasis
    - Wedge-shaped or triangular areas of density most commonly seen in the mid or lower lung

DDx: Lower Respiratory Track Symptoms

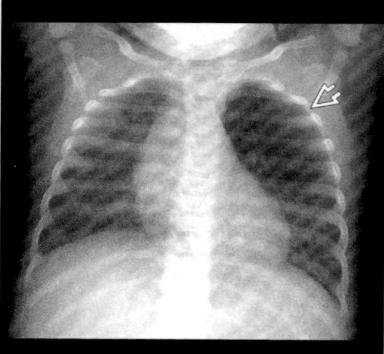

Foreign Body

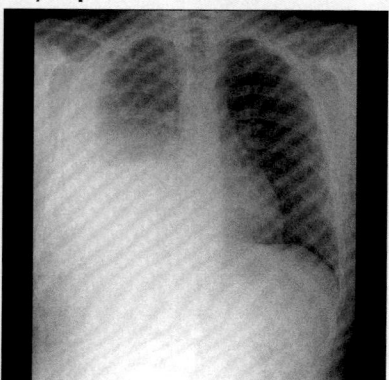

Bacterial Pneumonia

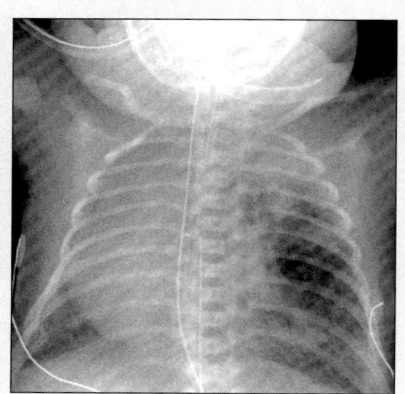

CCAM

VIRAL LUNG INFECTION, PEDIATRIC

Key Facts

Terminology
- Bronchiolitis

Imaging Findings
- Best diagnostic clue: Increased peribronchial markings and hyperinflation
- Lack of focal lung consolidation (hallmark for bacterial infection)
- Increased peribronchial markings
- Symmetric, coarse linear markings radiating from the hila into the lung
- Hyperinflation
- Hyperinflation often much better appreciated on lateral view
- Subsegmental atelectasis

Pathology
- Combination of narrowing of the lumen of small airways from edema and necrotic debris and mucus in the airway lumen leads to small airway occlusion
- Airway occlusion results in hyperinflation and areas of subsegmental atelectasis
- Anatomic consideration render small children more predisposed to air trapping and collapse
- < 2 years of age: 80% are viral
- > 2 years of age: 49% are viral

Clinical Issues
- Supportive
- Do not need antibiotics

- Misinterpretation of subsegmental atelectasis as opacities suspicious for bacterial pneumonia is one of the most common errors in pediatric radiology
  - Hilar lymphadenopathy
    - Can be seen in lower respiratory tract infection in children
    - Does not have as alarming significance in this setting, as when seen in adults

CT Findings
- Not used to make diagnosis of viral disease but CT may be obtained in patient with viral disease
- Prominent and ill-defined hila with peribronchial markings radiating into the lung
- Ground-glass opacities
- Increased interstitial markings
- Mild hilar lymphadenopathy may be present

Imaging Recommendations
- Best imaging tool
  - Chest radiography is the best diagnostic tool to try to differentiate bacterial from viral lower respiratory tract infection
  - Performance of chest radiography in identifying and excluding bacterial pneumonia
    - Positive predictive value 30%
    - Negative predictive value 92%
  - Since the goal is to treat all children with possible bacterial pneumonia with antibiotics while minimizing the number of children unnecessarily treated with antibiotics, the high negative predictive value of chest radiography is helpful

DIFFERENTIAL DIAGNOSIS

Bacterial Pneumonia
- Focal lung consolidation
- Lack of increased peribronchial markings
- Pleural effusions more common with bacterial infection

Asthma
- Increased peribronchial markings and hyperinflation
- Virtually identical appearance to viral lower respiratory tract infection
- Both asthma and viral disease are related to inflammation of the small airways

Left to Right Shunts
- In infants, left to right shunts may have similar appearance
- Increased pulmonary arterial flow may mimic increased peribronchial markings
- Shunts, like viral disease, typically have hyperinflation
- Shunts have associated cardiomegaly

Infected Congenital Lesions
- Congenital cystic adenomatoid malformations
- Sequestration
- May present with respiratory symptoms
- Focal solid or cystic mass present rather than diffuse bilateral process

Aspirated Bronchial Foreign Body
- May present with wheezing very similar to viral disease
- Asymmetric hyperinflation
- Static lung volume throughout respiratory cycle

PATHOLOGY

General Features
- General path comments
  - Viral infection involves the airways
  - Inflammation of the small airways results in peribronchial edema
  - Combination of narrowing of the lumen of small airways from edema and necrotic debris and mucus in the airway lumen leads to small airway occlusion
  - Airway occlusion results in hyperinflation and areas of subsegmental atelectasis
  - Anatomic consideration render small children more predisposed to air trapping and collapse

VIRAL LUNG INFECTION, PEDIATRIC

- Small airway lumen diameter
- Poorly developed collateral circulation of ventilation
- More abundant production of mucus
- Etiology
  - Most common viral infections in one series of community acquired pneumonia (2000)
    - Respiratory syncytial virus 29%
    - Rhinovirus 58%
    - Parainfluenza virus (1, 2, 3) 25%
    - Adenovirus 7%
    - Influenza A & B 4%
    - Coronavirus 3%
    - Human herpesvirus 3%
  - Most common bacterial
    - Streptococcus pneumoniae 37%
    - Haemophilus influenza 9%
    - Mycoplasma pneumoniae 7%
    - Chlamydia pneumoniae 3%
    - Staphylococcus pneumonia 0%
- Epidemiology
  - Respiratory tract infection is the most common cause of illness in children and continues to be a significant cause of morbidity and mortality
  - Evaluation of potential lower respiratory tract infection is one of the most common indications for imaging in children
  - Etiology of lower respiratory tract infection varies with age
  - Preschool children (4 months to 5 years)
    - Viruses majority of lower respiratory tract infections
  - School age children (> 5 years)
    - Viruses still most common
    - Mycoplasma pneumoniae 30%
    - Streptococcus pneumoniae becomes more frequent
  - Another study of lower respiratory tract infections showed
    - < 2 years of age: 80% are viral
    - > 2 years of age: 49% are viral
    - For all ages: 47% viral, 38% bacterial, 15% mixed viral/bacterial
- Associated abnormalities: May lead to bronchiolitis obliterans

CLINICAL ISSUES

Presentation
- Most common signs/symptoms
  - Cough
  - Wheezing
- Other signs/symptoms
  - Often upper respiratory tract (sinus) symptoms
  - May have fever
  - Hypoxia/respiratory failure in severe cases
  - Difficult to differentiate bacterial from viral lower respiratory tract infection on basis of physical exam or any other available laboratory tests

Demographics
- Age: Typical and striking radiographic findings of viral disease more often seen in young children (< 5 years of age)

Natural History & Prognosis
- Resolution of symptoms over time

Treatment
- Supportive
- Do not need antibiotics

DIAGNOSTIC CHECKLIST

Consider
- If any question of asymmetry, consider aspirated foreign body

SELECTED REFERENCES

1. Copley SJ: Application of computed tomography in childhood respiratory infections. Br Med Bull. 61:263-79, 2002
2. Virkki R et al: Differentiation of bacterial and viral pneumonia in children. Thorax. 57(5):438-41, 2002
3. Donnelly LF: Fundamentals of Pediatric Radiology. Philadelphia, W.B. Saunders, 2001
4. Donnelly LF: Practical issues concerning imaging of pulmonary infection in children. J Thorac Imaging. 16(4):238-50, 2001
5. Juven T et al: Etiology of community-acquired pneumonia in 254 hospitalized children. Pediatr Infect Dis J. 19(4):293-8, 2000
6. Markowitz RI et al: The spectrum of pulmonary infection in the immunocompromised child. Semin Roentgenol. 35(2):171-80, 2000
7. Donnelly LF: Maximizing the usefulness of imaging in children with community-acquired pneumonia. AJR Am J Roentgenol. 172(2):505-12, 1999
8. Katz DS et al: Radiology of pneumonia. Clin Chest Med. 20(3):549-62, 1999
9. Brunelle F: [Radiologic approach to community-acquired pneumonia] Arch Pediatr. 5 Suppl 1:26s-27s, 1998
10. Donnelly LF et al: Cavitary necrosis complicating pneumonia in children: sequential findings on chest radiography. AJR Am J Roentgenol. 171(1):253-6, 1998
11. Donnelly LF et al: The yield of CT of children who have complicated pneumonia and noncontributory chest radiography. AJR Am J Roentgenol. 170(6):1627-31, 1998
12. Donnelly LF et al: CT appearance of parapneumonic effusions in children: findings are not specific for empyema. AJR Am J Roentgenol. 169(1):179-82, 1997
13. Donnelly LF et al: Pneumonia in children: decreased parenchymal contrast enhancement--CT sign of intense illness and impending cavitary necrosis. Radiology. 205(3):817-20, 1997
14. Wahlgren H et al: Radiographic patterns and viral studies in childhood pneumonia at various ages. Pediatr Radiol. 25(8):627-30, 1995
15. Korppi M et al: Comparison of radiological findings and microbial aetiology of childhood pneumonia. Acta Paediatr. 82(4):360-3, 1993
16. Condon VR: Pneumonia in children. J Thorac Imaging. 6(3):31-44, 1991
17. Kirkpatrick JA: Pneumonia in children as it differs from adult pneumonia. Semin Roentgenol. 15(1):96-103, 1980

VIRAL LUNG INFECTION, PEDIATRIC

IMAGE GALLERY

Typical

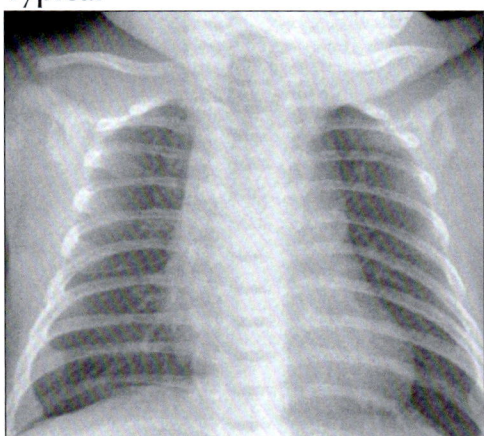
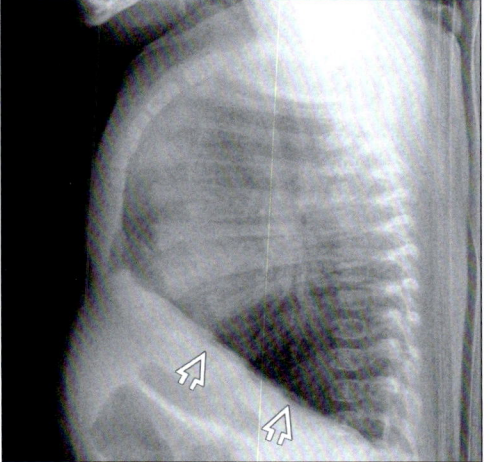

(Left) Frontal radiograph shows marked hyperinflation and increased peribronchial markings. *(Right)* Lateral radiograph in same patient as previous image, shows marked increased hyperinflation with flattening of the hemidiaphragms ➡, seen much better than on frontal view.

Typical

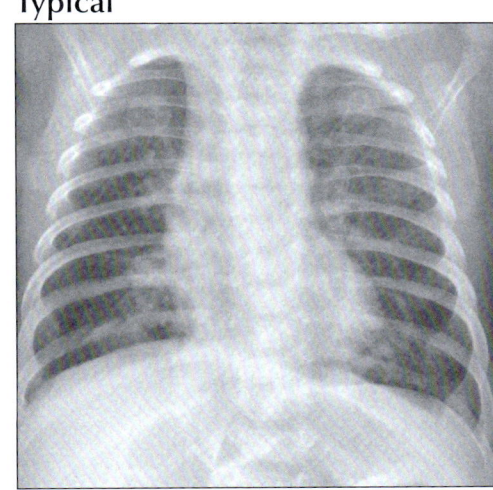
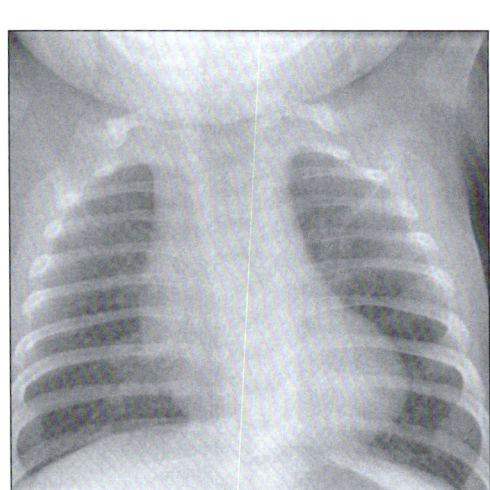

(Left) Frontal radiograph shows marked increased peribronchial markings as ropy densities radiating from the hila bilaterally. *(Right)* Frontal radiograph of same patient as previous image, from 5 days earlier, shows marked difference in appearance of the chest. Note lack of ropy markings, such as those seen on left when patient was acutely ill.

Typical

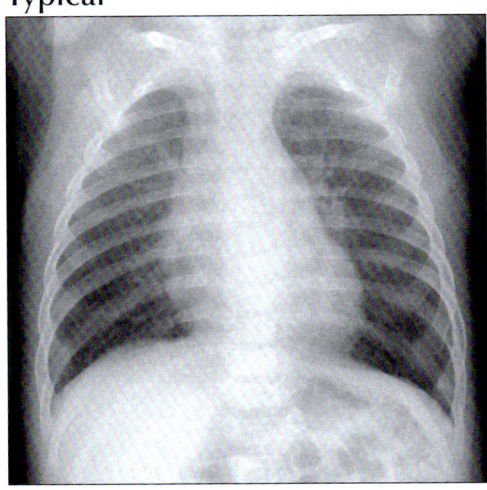
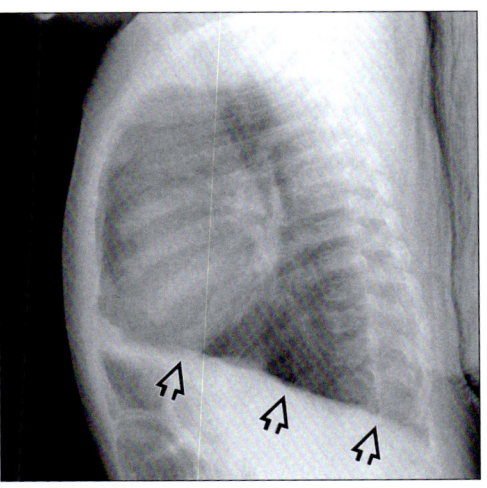

(Left) Frontal radiograph shows marked increased perihilar markings. It is difficult to appreciate the degree of hyperinflation on the frontal view. *(Right)* Lateral radiograph of same patient as previous image, shows marked hyperinflation with flattening of the hemidiaphragms ➡. Hyperinflation is much easier to appreciate here than on the frontal view.

ROUND PNEUMONIA, PEDIATRIC

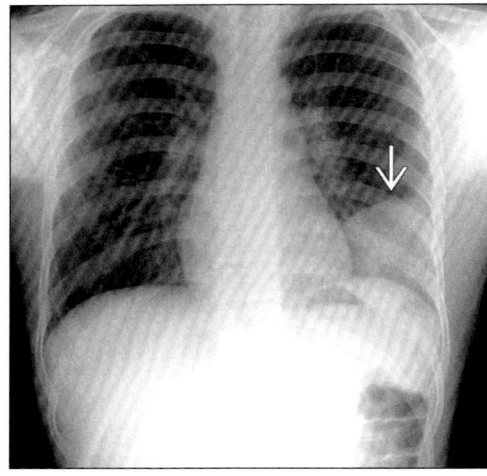

Anteroposterior radiograph shows left lower lobe round opacity ➡ with well-defined borders. Lesion has a very mass-like appearance.

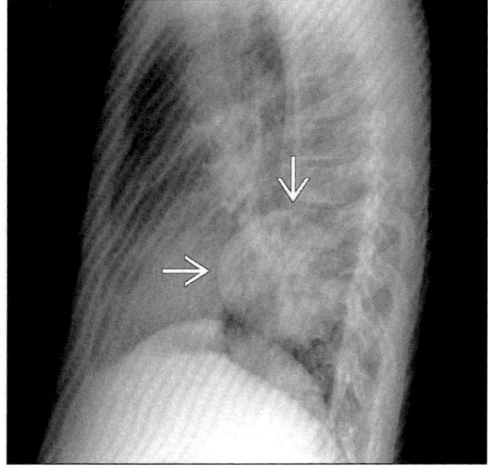

Lateral radiograph in same patient as on left shows round opacity ➡ to be located in posterior aspect of left lower lobe. Lesion resolved on follow-up radiography after antibiotics.

TERMINOLOGY

Definitions
- Bacterial pneumonia with a very round, well-defined appearance on chest radiography, simulating a mass
- Should typically only be seen up to approximately 8 years of age
- Typically occurs with streptococcal pneumoniae infection

IMAGING FINDINGS

General Features
- Best diagnostic clue: Round lung opacity with well-defined borders in a child less than 8 years of age
- Location
  - More common in lower lobes
  - Most common in superior segment of lower lobes
  - Most commonly posterior in location
  - No peripheral or central predisposition
- Size
  - May vary in size related to time of imaging diagnosis in relation to development of pneumonia
  - With growth, eventually may present as lobar pneumonia and no longer appear round
  - More commonly resolves with clearing rather than progression to lobar
  - Reported size varies between 1-7 cm
  - Most commonly single focus
  - Multiple (2 or 3) foci can occur but are uncommon

Radiographic Findings
- Radiography
  - Round lung opacity
  - Supportive findings of airspace disease
    - Air bronchograms
  - May progress to lobar pneumonia if child's illness progresses and serial films obtained
  - Respects lobar anatomy without crossing fissures

CT Findings
- NECT
  - CT not advocated in suspected cases of round pneumonia but may be obtained to evaluate for possibility of a mass
  - CT of abdomen obtained for pain may also show round pneumonia in lower lobes as cause of abdominal pain

DDx: Round Lung Mass

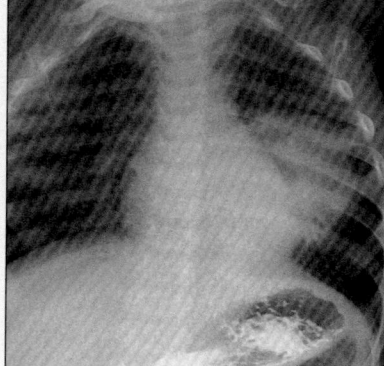
Bronchogenic Cyst

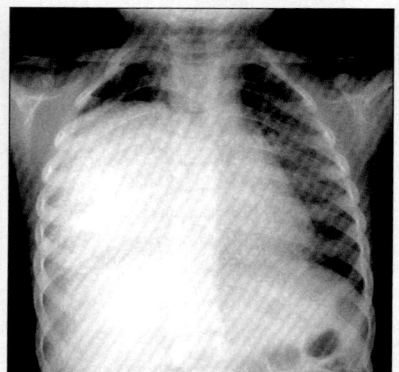
Neuroblastoma

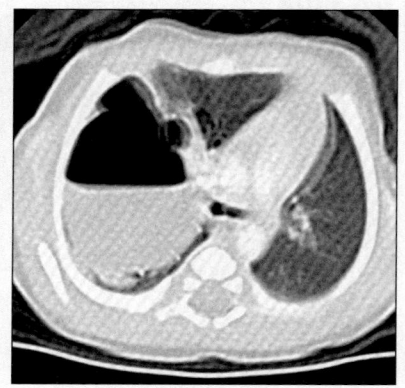
CCAM

ROUND PNEUMONIA, PEDIATRIC

Key Facts

Terminology
- Bacterial pneumonia with a very round, well-defined appearance on chest radiography, simulating a mass

Imaging Findings
- More common in lower lobes
- Reported size varies between 1-7 cm
- Air bronchograms
- Respects lobar anatomy without crossing fissures
- If child has symptoms of pneumonia and "round" density on chest radiograph, additional imaging with modalities such as CT not necessary
- Follow-up radiograph several weeks after antibiotic therapy may be helpful to document resolution of the process

- This is one of the few indications concerning pneumonia in children where a follow-up chest radiograph may be indicated even if the child becomes asymptomatic in order to exclude underlying mass

Pathology
- In children, collateral pathways of air circulation are not well-developed until approximately 8 years of age
- After 8 years of age, if round mass seen on chest radiograph, high suspicion for other pathology
- Etiology: Most commonly seen with streptococcal pneumoniae infection

Clinical Issues
- Cough and fever
- May present with abdominal pain

  - CT shows round opacity
  - Air-bronchograms may be present
  - Respects lobar anatomy and does not cross fissures
  - No other specific CT findings
- CECT
  - May show normal pulmonary vessels coursing through lesion
  - There will be no enhancing rim or wall
  - No systemic arterial supply from descending aorta (seen with sequestration)
  - Presence of central cavity favors alternative diagnosis

MR Findings
- Not utilized in work-up of round pneumonia
- If MR of chest performed because round mass suspected as neuroblastoma, findings may be encountered
- Round pneumonia will appear as high signal mass within pulmonary parenchyma

Imaging Recommendations
- If child has symptoms of pneumonia and "round" density on chest radiograph, additional imaging with modalities such as CT not necessary
- Follow-up radiograph several weeks after antibiotic therapy may be helpful to document resolution of the process
- This is one of the few indications concerning pneumonia in children where a follow-up chest radiograph may be indicated even if the child becomes asymptomatic in order to exclude underlying mass
- If greater than 8 years of age, increased suspicion for other causes of mass should be considered and CT obtained

DIFFERENTIAL DIAGNOSIS

Bronchogenic Cyst
- May appear as round, well-defined, soft tissue mass on chest radiography
- Very similar appearance to round pneumonia

- Only contains air or air fluid levels if infected
- Most common in perihilar areas
- CT: Well-defined mass that is water attenuated which may have an enhancing rim and no air bronchograms

Neuroblastoma
- If pneumonia is posterior, may simulate posterior mediastinal mass such as neuroblastoma
- Round pneumonia will have acute rather than obtuse borders with mediastinum
- Rib erosion/destruction seen with neuroblastoma
- Calcifications present in up to 85% of thoracic neuroblastoma
- Neuroblastoma may also appear as paraspinal mass with widening of paraspinal stripe on radiography

Congenital Cystic Adenomatoid Malformation (CCAM)
- May appear as solid appearing lesion typically soon after birth
- Most CCAM are cystic and communicate with the bronchial tree at birth and as a result quickly fill with air
- "Solid" type 3 CCAM are exceedingly rare

Pulmonary Sequestration
- Most common in the left lower lobe
- Present as recurrent pneumonia
- Round pneumonia almost never recurs in same location
- Systemic arterial supply to sequestration from descending aorta
- Sequestration typically do not appear as round

PATHOLOGY

General Features
- General path comments
  - In children, collateral pathways of air circulation are not well-developed until approximately 8 years of age
    - Channels of Lambert

ROUND PNEUMONIA, PEDIATRIC

- Pores of Kohn
  - Lack of well-developed collateral circulation thought to hinder spread of bacterial infection and predispose to "round" appearance on radiography
  - After 8 years of age, if round mass seen on chest radiograph, high suspicion for other pathology
  - There are rarely reported cases in adults
- Etiology: Most commonly seen with streptococcal pneumoniae infection

Gross Pathologic & Surgical Features
- Exudative opacification of pulmonary airspaces related to bacterial infection

CLINICAL ISSUES

Presentation
- Most common signs/symptoms
  - Cough and fever
  - If classic symptoms of pneumonia are present, other causes of mass do not need to be excluded with imaging
- Other signs/symptoms
  - May present with abdominal pain
  - General malaise

Demographics
- Age
  - Should only see round pneumonia in children less than 8 years of age
  - Mean age 5 years
  - Cases are rarely reported in older children and adults
    - Sometimes leads to biopsy
    - Course of antibiotics may be considered if round pneumonia is a possibility

Natural History & Prognosis
- If responds to antibiotics, opacity should progressively resolve within several weeks
- If resistant to antibiotics, may progress to lobar pneumonia infection

Treatment
- Antibiotics
- Follow-up radiograph several weeks following completion of antibiotic therapy to exclude other masses

DIAGNOSTIC CHECKLIST

Image Interpretation Pearls
- Round lung mass in a child less than 8 years, think round pneumonia

SELECTED REFERENCES
1. Copley SJ: Application of computed tomography in childhood respiratory infections. Br Med Bull. 61:263-79, 2002
2. Virkki R et al: Differentiation of bacterial and viral pneumonia in children. Thorax. 57(5):438-41, 2002
3. Donnelly LF: Fundamentals of Pediatric Radiology. Philadelphia, W.B. Saunders, 2001
4. Donnelly LF: Practical issues concerning imaging of pulmonary infection in children. J Thorac Imaging. 16(4):238-50, 2001
5. Juven T et al: Etiology of community-acquired pneumonia in 254 hospitalized children. Pediatr Infect Dis J. 19(4):293-8, 2000
6. Markowitz RI et al: The spectrum of pulmonary infection in the immunocompromised child. Semin Roentgenol. 35(2):171-80, 2000
7. Donnelly LF: Maximizing the usefulness of imaging in children with community-acquired pneumonia. AJR Am J Roentgenol. 172(2):505-12, 1999
8. Katz DS et al: Radiology of pneumonia. Clin Chest Med. 20(3):549-62, 1999
9. Price J: Round pneumonia and focal organizing pneumonia are different entities. AJR Am J Roentgenol. 172(2):549-50, 1999
10. Brunelle F: [Radiologic approach to community-acquired pneumonia] Arch Pediatr. 5 Suppl 1:26s-27s, 1998
11. Donnelly LF et al: Cavitary necrosis complicating pneumonia in children: sequential findings on chest radiography. AJR Am J Roentgenol. 171(1):253-6, 1998
12. Donnelly LF et al: The yield of CT of children who have complicated pneumonia and noncontributory chest radiography. AJR Am J Roentgenol. 170(6):1627-31, 1998
13. Wagner AL et al: Radiologic manifestations of round pneumonia in adults. AJR Am J Roentgenol. 170(3):723-6, 1998
14. Donnelly LF et al: CT appearance of parapneumonic effusions in children: findings are not specific for empyema. AJR Am J Roentgenol. 169(1):179-82, 1997
15. Donnelly LF et al: Pneumonia in children: decreased parenchymal contrast enhancement--CT sign of intense illness and impending cavitary necrosis. Radiology. 205(3):817-20, 1997
16. Katsumura Y et al: Pneumococcal spherical pneumonia multiply distributed in one lung. Eur Respir J. 10(10):2423-4, 1997
17. Wahlgren H et al: Radiographic patterns and viral studies in childhood pneumonia at various ages. Pediatr Radiol. 25(8):627-30, 1995
18. Korppi M et al: Comparison of radiological findings and microbial aetiology of childhood pneumonia. Acta Paediatr. 82(4):360-3, 1993
19. Kirkpatrick JA: Pneumonia in children as it differs from adult pneumonia. Semin Roentgenol. 15(1):96-103, 1980

ROUND PNEUMONIA, PEDIATRIC

IMAGE GALLERY

Variant

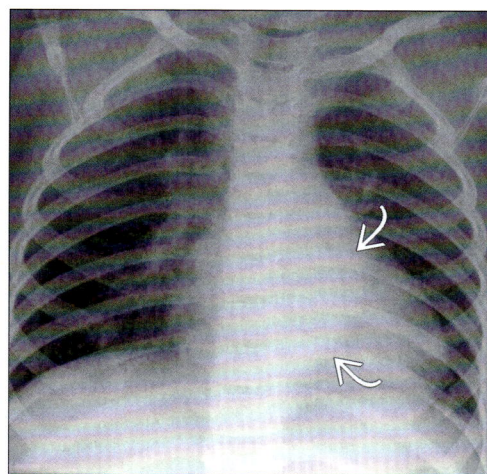
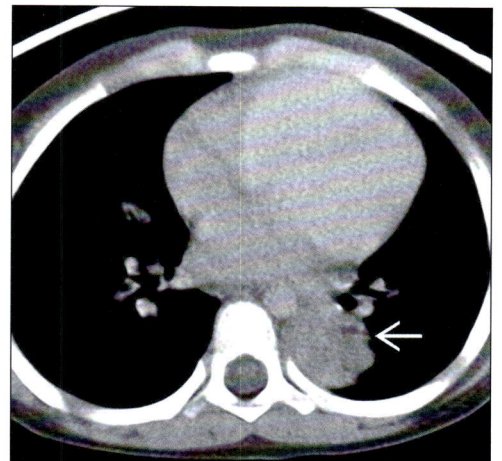

(Left) Anteroposterior radiograph shows rounded opacity ➡ in medial aspect of left retrocardiac area. *(Right)* Axial CECT in same patient shows rounded paraspinal mass ➡ with possible small air bronchogram. Important to note was the absence of spinal neural foraminal extension.

Typical

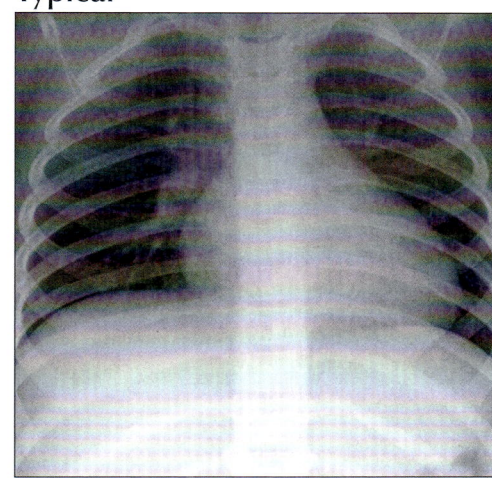
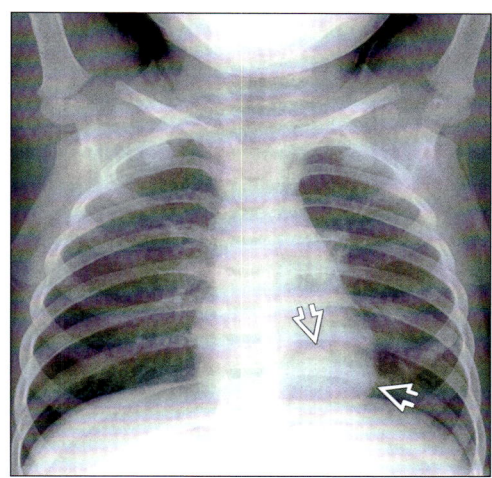

(Left) Anteroposterior radiograph after 2 weeks of antibiotic therapy shows resolution of the round pneumonia. *(Right)* Anteroposterior radiograph radiograph shows left lower lobe, rounded opacity ➡ consistent with round pneumonia, given the patient's symptoms.

Variant

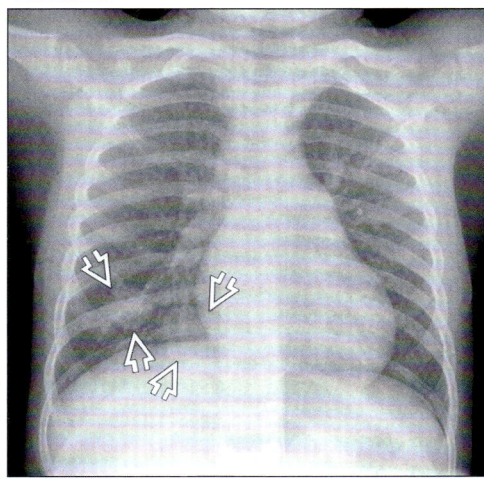
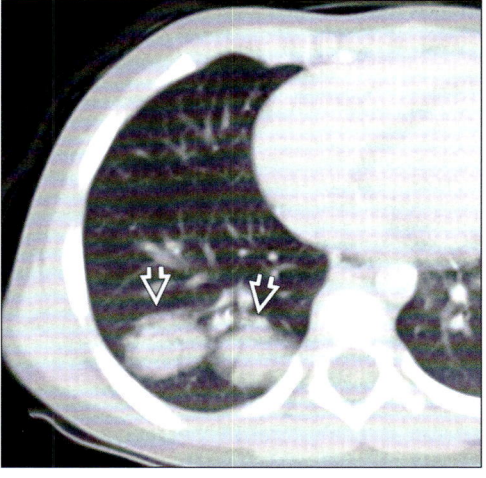

(Left) Frontal radiograph shows two very round foci of density ➡ in right lower lobe. *(Right)* Axial CECT in same patient as on left shows two round densities ➡ within right lower lobe which contain air-bronchograms. Multiple foci of round pneumonia can occur but is uncommon.

NEONATAL PNEUMONIA

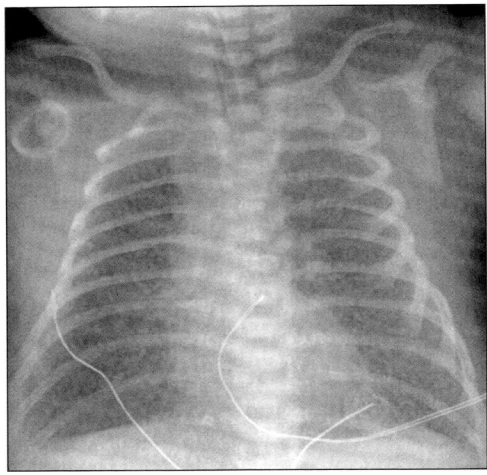

Anteroposterior radiograph in a newborn shows bilateral reticulonodular opacities which mimics surfactant deficiency disease in this patient with group B streptococcal infection.

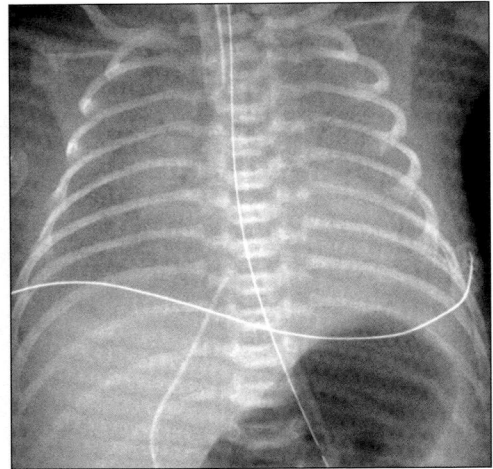

Anteroposterior radiograph in a newborn shows nonspecific bilateral perihilar hazy opacities. This patient was culture positive for group B streptococcal infection.

TERMINOLOGY

Definitions
- Pneumonia occurring in neonate within the first 28 days of life
- Lung infection occurs in utero, during delivery, or within the first month of life

IMAGING FINDINGS

General Features
- Best diagnostic clue
  - Patchy asymmetric perihilar densities and hyperinflation
  - May be unilateral or bilateral
  - May or may not have effusions
    - Approximately 25% of group B infections have effusions
  - May be reticulonodular in appearance
  - May have pulmonary hypoventilation
  - May be interstitial
  - Complications include pneumothorax, pneumomediastinum, pneumatoceles
- Location
  - Chest
  - May have other systemic signs of infection
    - Sepsis, hypovolemia and shock
    - Neonatal meningitis
    - Intracranial calcifications with toxoplasmosis, rubella, cytomegalovirus, herpes simplex virus (HSV) (TORCH)
    - Bone lesions can be seen in syphilis
    - Premature infants may have systemic candidiasis
- Size: Usually bilateral, can be unilateral

Radiographic Findings
- Radiography
  - Group B pneumonia
    - Most common neonatal pneumonia
    - Different appearance than other causes of neonatal pneumonia
    - Low lung volumes and granular opacities similar to surfactant deficiency
    - Pleural effusion in 25%: Only differentiating factor from surfactant deficiency
  - Other types of neonatal pneumonia
    - Bilateral hyperinflation

DDx: Mimics of Neonatal Pneumonia

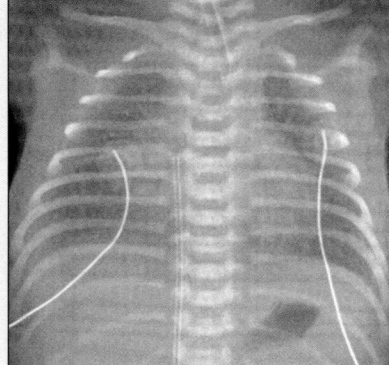
Transient Tachypnea

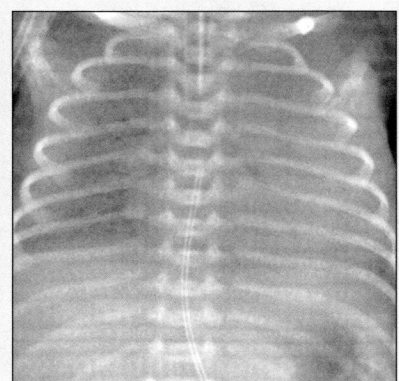
Surfactant Deficiency

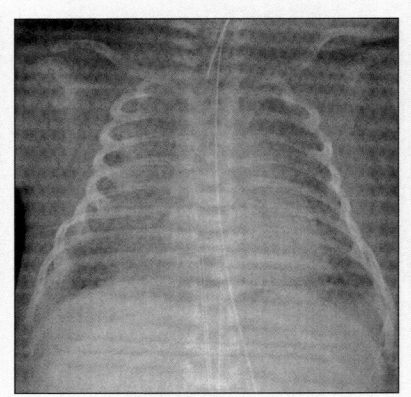
Meconium Aspiration

NEONATAL PNEUMONIA

Key Facts

Terminology
- Pneumonia occurring in neonate within the first 28 days of life
- Lung infection occurs in utero, during delivery, or within the first month of life

Imaging Findings
- Group B pneumonia
- Most common neonatal pneumonia
- Different appearance than other causes of neonatal pneumonia
- Low lung volumes and granular opacities similar to surfactant deficiency
- Pleural effusion in 25%: Only differentiating factor from surfactant deficiency
- Other types of neonatal pneumonia
- Bilateral hyperinflation
- Rope-like perihilar markings
- Best imaging tool: Chest radiography

Top Differential Diagnoses
- Surfactant Deficient Disease
- Congenital Cystic Adenomatoid Malformation (CCAM) of the Chest
- Meconium Aspiration Syndrome
- Transient Tachypnea of the Newborn
- Congenital Heart Disease

Pathology
- Occurs in approximately 1% of term neonates and 10% of preterm neonates

Diagnostic Checklist
- Usually bilateral diffuse disease
- Chest radiographs are nonspecific

- Rope-like perihilar markings
- Areas of atelectasis
- Pleural effusions not uncommon
- May have pneumothorax and other air-block complications

CT Findings
- HRCT: Occasionally done when infant is older to evaluate residual disease

Imaging Recommendations
- Best imaging tool: Chest radiography

DIFFERENTIAL DIAGNOSIS

Surfactant Deficient Disease
- Premature infants < 32 weeks gestation
- Reticulonodular densities in both lung
- Hypoinflation
- Mimics group B streptococcus infection
  - Should not have an associated effusion

Congenital Cystic Adenomatoid Malformation (CCAM) of the Chest
- Usually localized mass
- Cystic and/or solid component
- May have mass effect

Meconium Aspiration Syndrome
- History of meconium staining or aspiration
- Coarse lung markings bilaterally, frequently asymmetric
- Hyperinflation of the lungs
- Complications include pneumothorax, pneumomediastinum

Transient Tachypnea of the Newborn
- Occurs in term infants who have C-sections
- Prominent interstitial pattern with normal to hyperinflated lungs
  - Pleural effusions may be evident
- Benign course
  - Infants are usually well except for tachypnea
- Radiographs to exclude other causes of tachypnea

Congenital Heart Disease
- Echocardiography for diagnosis
- Infants present with tachypnea
  - Usually afebrile
- May have normal heart size
  - Example: Total anomalous pulmonary venous return with obstruction
    - Interstitial edema

PATHOLOGY

General Features
- Etiology
  - Before delivery: Congenital or transplacental infection
    - Hematogenous spread from mother to fetus in utero
    - Severe pneumonia occurs with congenital rubella
    - TORCH
    - Other rare causes: Varicella zoster, adenovirus, enteroviruses, mycobacterium tuberculosis (< 200 reported cases), and listeria
    - Syphilis presents with systemic signs
  - During delivery: Infection occurs during vaginal delivery
    - Occurs during birth or as a result of maternal infection
    - Etiologic agents are those colonizing maternal birth canal
    - Group B hemolytic streptococcus (GBS) is the most common organism
    - 25% of woman are colonized by the organism
    - Organisms include GBS, E. coli, Klebsiella, Proteus, Chlamydia, Candida, Bacteroides, HSV, enteroviruses
    - Chlamydia may have delayed appearance
  - Postnatal or after delivery
    - Viral: Respiratory syncytial virus influenza most common

NEONATAL PNEUMONIA

- Community acquired bacterial pneumonia (S. pneumoniae, H. influenza) may also occur
- Bacterial pneumonias are Pseudomonas, Klebsiella, Serratia, Enterobacter, Staphylococcus aureus (methicillin-sensitive and resistant)
- Fungal: Postnatal Candida pneumonia may occur in disseminated disease
  - Risk factors
    - Neonates have immature pulmonary anatomy and immature host defense mechanisms
    - Preterm infants more immature, therefore at increased risk
    - Anatomical anomalies predispose or may cause pneumonia such as tracheoesophageal fistula, cleft palate
    - Critically ill infants: Normal mucocutaneous barriers disrupted with invasive devices and procedures
    - Maternal fever
    - Maternal amniotitis, fever, sepsis
- Epidemiology
  - Occurs in approximately 1% of term neonates and 10% of preterm neonates
  - Mortality rate for perinatally acquired pneumonia: 20%
  - Mortality rate for postnatally acquired pneumonia: 50%
  - Bacteremia is present in as many as 46% of infants with perinatal pneumonia
  - Most common cause in the first week of life is GBS
    - 57% of infants with pneumonia have GBS isolated from blood or tracheal secretions
    - Vaginal colonization occurs in nearly 30% of pregnant women
    - Without chemoprophylaxis, 50% of newborns born to colonized women will acquire colonization
- Associated abnormalities: Most frequent cause of septicemia in neonate

CLINICAL ISSUES

Presentation
- Most common signs/symptoms
  - Respiratory distress
    - Nasal flaring, retractions, grunting, cyanosis
  - Symptoms usually begin within first 48 hours of life
    - Chlamydia pneumonia may have delayed onset
    - Most infants present with systemic signs not localized to chest
  - High risk
    - Premature infants
    - Infants with immunosuppression
    - Infants with congenital heart disease
- Other signs/symptoms
  - Tachycardia, hypothermia
  - Irritability, lethargy, poor feeding
  - Chlamydia pneumonia: Has long incubation (acquired at birth), but presents at 2-12 weeks
    - Presents with conjunctivitis and respiratory complaints
  - Candidal pneumonia: Infant often presents at birth with maculopapular rash
  - Herpes simplex pneumonia: Rapidly progressive and fatal
  - S. aureus may cause a severe necrotizing pneumonia with pneumatocele formation

Demographics
- Age: Neonates within first 28 days of life

Natural History & Prognosis
- Depends on organism and success of treatment: Early intervention and aggressive therapy are key
  - Usually associated with sepsis
  - May affect multiple organs
- Can be associated with intraventricular hemorrhage, neurological damage, and developmental delay

Treatment
- Perinatal screening and treatment prior to delivery
  - Maternal GBS vaccination to cause transplacental transfer of passive immunity
- GBS intrapartum chemoprophylaxis recommended
  - Positive perinatal screening culture
  - GBS during pregnancy
- Broad spectrum antibiotics (a penicillin + an aminoglycoside) until organism identified
- Viral pneumonia: Acyclovir; adjunctive hyperimmune immunoglobulin may improve outcome
- Surfactant replacement may be of benefit
- ECMO used as last resort

DIAGNOSTIC CHECKLIST

Image Interpretation Pearls
- Usually bilateral diffuse disease
- Chest radiographs are nonspecific

SELECTED REFERENCES
1. Kuhn JP et al: Caffey's Pediatric Diagnostic Imaging. 10th Ed. Volume I. Philadelphia, Mosby. 3:88-9, 2004
2. Apisarnthanarak A et al: Ventilator-associated pneumonia in extremely preterm neonates in a neonatal intensive care unit: characteristics, risk factors, and outcomes. Pediatrics. 112(6 Pt 1):1283-9, 2003
3. Campbell JR: Neonatal pneumonia. Semin Respir Infect. 11(3):155-62, 1996
4. Potter B et al: Neonatal radiology. Acquired diaphragmatic hernia with group B streptococcal pneumonia. J Perinatol. 15(2):160-2, 1995
5. Ablow RC et al: The radiographic features of early onset Group B streptococcal neonatal sepsis. Radiology. 124(3):771-7, 1977
6. Ablow RC et al: A comparison of early-onset group B steptococcal neonatal infection and the respiratory-distress syndrome of the newborn. N Engl J Med. 294(2):65-70, 1976

NEONATAL PNEUMONIA

IMAGE GALLERY

Typical

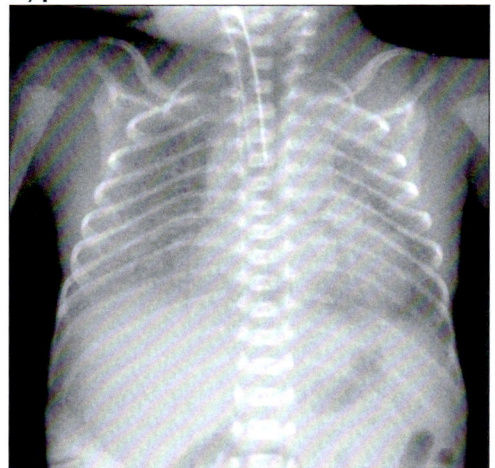
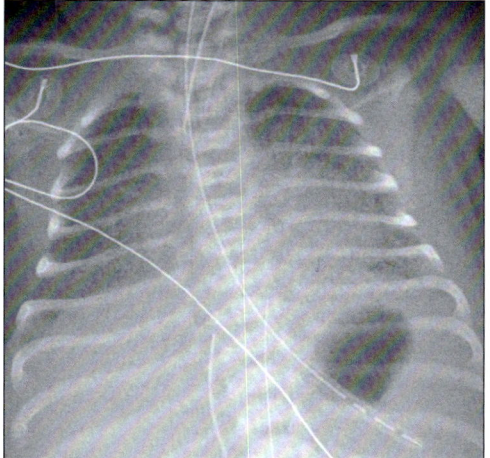

(Left) Anteroposterior radiograph shows hazy bilateral lung opacities, more severe within the lung bases in this patient with a neonatal pneumonia. *(Right)* Anteroposterior radiograph in a 2 day old shows bilateral perihilar opacities. This patient culture positive for group B streptococcal infection.

Typical

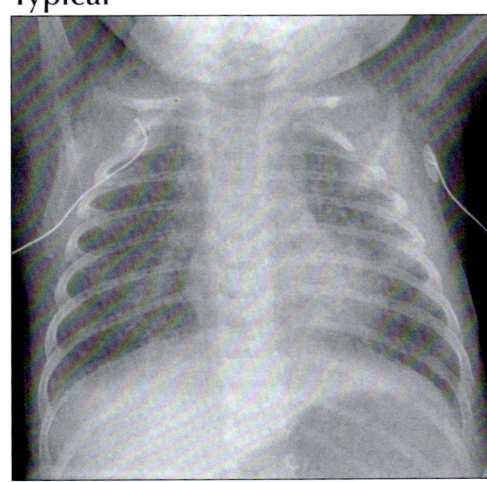
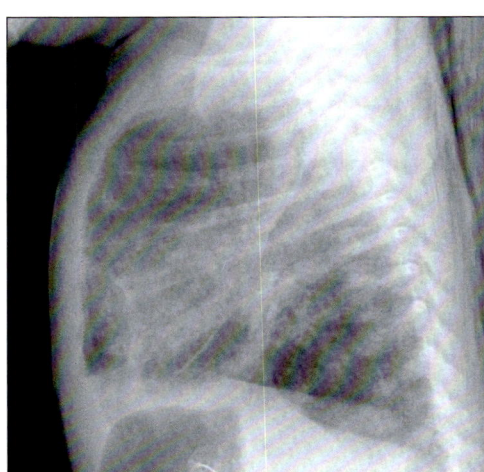

(Left) Anteroposterior radiograph shows perihilar coarse lung markings and more focal opacities within the lingula and left lower lobe in this patient who presented with conjunctivitis and tachypnea. *(Right)* Lateral radiograph in the same patient as previous image, shows the diffuse coarse lung opacities. The radiographic findings are nonspecific. Cultures were positive for Chlamydia.

Typical

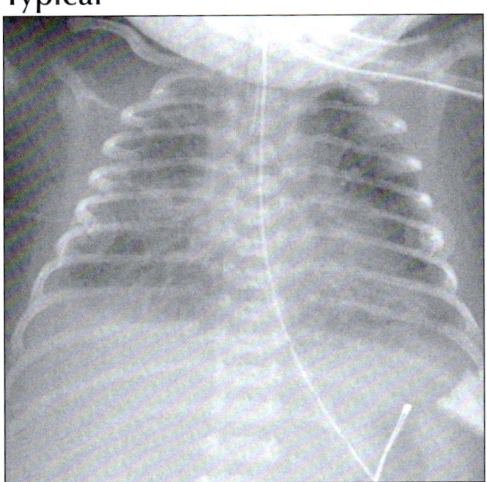
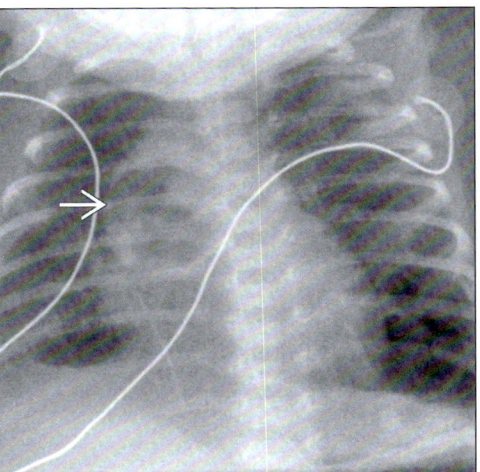

(Left) Anteroposterior radiograph shows diffuse perihilar and rope-like opacities in this patient with E. Coli sepsis. *(Right)* Anteroposterior radiograph (same patient as previous image) at 11 days of age, shows clearing of the bilateral rope-like opacities and a pneumatocele within the right hemithorax ➡. The pneumatocele was no longer seen on a follow-up radiograph at 8 months of age.

EXUDATIVE TRACHEITIS

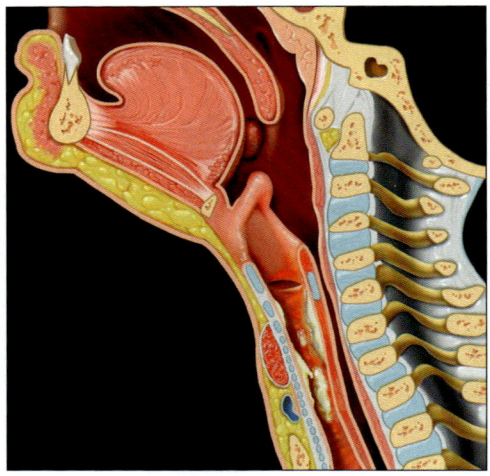

Graphic shows inflammation of trachea with formation of inflammatory plaques (membranes) along tracheal walls. These membranes may detach from tracheal wall and form intraluminal filling defect.

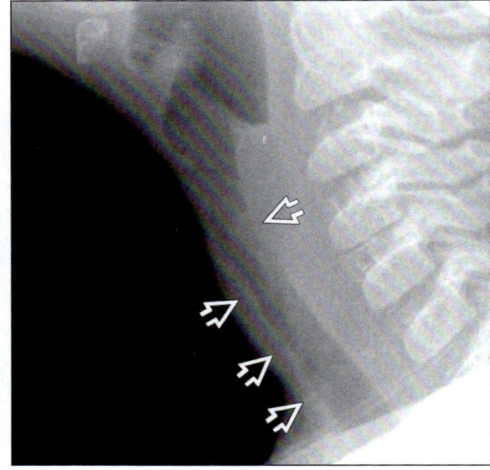

Lateral radiograph shows irregularity and poor definition ➡ of anterior and posterior walls of trachea.

TERMINOLOGY

Abbreviations and Synonyms
- Bacterial tracheitis, membranous croup, membranous laryngotracheobronchitis
- "Membranous croup" poor term as may become confused with more benign entity "croup"

Definitions
- Purulent infection of trachea that results in exudative plaques that form along tracheal walls and can slough and occlude airway
- Controversial disease
  - Seen much more frequently in certain medical centers and rarely ever seen in other centers of similar climate
  - No known cases of death in community without reaching medical center, as would be expected with life-threatening disease
  - While many documented "real" cases with associated morbidity/mortality have occurred, many questions over diagnosis and over treatment at certain centers

IMAGING FINDINGS

General Features
- Best diagnostic clue: Radiography demonstrates plaque-like irregularity of tracheal wall or linear filling defect (membrane) within the trachea
- Location: Purulent infection of the trachea which may extend to involve the larynx and bronchi
- Size: Variable
- Morphology: Soft tissue irregularities of the tracheal walls (plaques) and linear filling defects (membranes)

Radiographic Findings
- Radiography
  - Best diagnostic sign or clue: Presence of linear, soft tissue, filling defect within the airway (visualized membrane)
  - Plaque-like irregularity or loss of smooth contours of the tracheal walls seen on frontal or lateral is suggestive
  - Symmetric or asymmetric subglottic narrowing in a child older than typically seen with croup raises possibility of exudative tracheitis

DDx: Acute Stridor

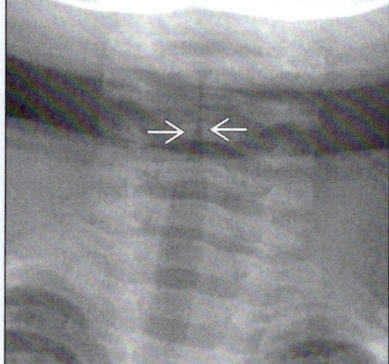

Croup

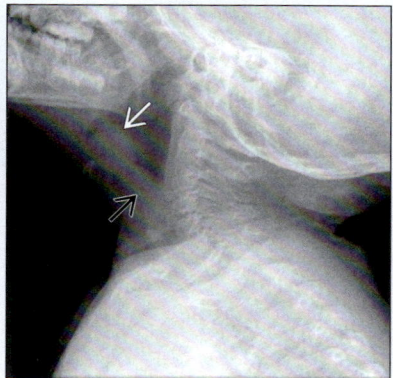

Epiglottitis

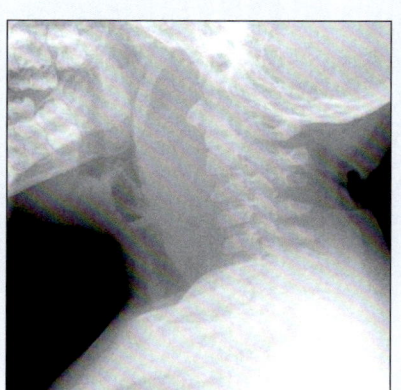

Retropharyngeal Abscess

EXUDATIVE TRACHEITIS

Key Facts

Terminology
- Bacterial tracheitis, membranous croup, membranous laryngotracheobronchitis
- Purulent infection of trachea that results in exudative plaques that form along tracheal walls and can slough and occlude airway
- While many documented "real" cases with associated morbidity/mortality have occurred, many questions over diagnosis and over treatment at certain centers

Imaging Findings
- Best diagnostic clue: Radiography demonstrates plaque-like irregularity of tracheal wall or linear filling defect (membrane) within the trachea
- Morphology: Soft tissue irregularities of the tracheal walls (plaques) and linear filling defects (membranes)

Pathology
- Uncommon but potentially life-threatening cause of acute upper airway obstruction
- Inflamed mucosa forms exudative plaques that can slough and lead to obstruction of the airway (much like airway obstruction seen in diphtheria)
- Has replaced epiglottitis as the most common life-threatening acute inflammatory airway disease since Haemophilus influenzae vaccine
- Affected children typically older and more ill than those with croup

Clinical Issues
- Because illness can lead to airway obstruction, respiratory failure and death, children are treated aggressively

---

  - Non-adherent mucus can mimic membranes but clears if patient coughs and film repeated

Imaging Recommendations
- Best imaging tool: Plaques and membranes can be detected on the lateral or frontal radiograph: Obtain both lateral and frontal when evaluating for suspected exudative tracheitis
- Protocol advice: If adherent mucus is suspected, radiograph should be repeated after the child has coughed to allow for clearing of the airway

DIFFERENTIAL DIAGNOSIS

Epiglottitis
- Severe, life-threatening condition
- Marked enlargement of epiglottis and aryepiglottic folds
- May cause symmetric subglottic narrowing on frontal view, similar in appearance to croup
- Similar age group to exudative tracheitis

Croup
- Benign, self-limited condition
- Most common such airway condition encountered
- Symmetric subglottic narrowing
- Younger age than exudative tracheitis
- Mean age of patients with croup = 1 year

Aspirated Bronchial Foreign Body
- Radiopaque foreign body seen in minority of cases
- Asymmetric lung aeration on chest radiographs

Retropharyngeal Abscess
- Thickening of the retropharyngeal soft tissues
- Often also have sore throat and drooling in addition to stridor

PATHOLOGY

General Features
- General path comments
  - Purulent infection of the larynx, trachea, and bronchi
  - Uncommon but potentially life-threatening cause of acute upper airway obstruction
  - Inflamed mucosa forms exudative plaques that can slough and lead to obstruction of the airway (much like airway obstruction seen in diphtheria)
- Etiology
  - Debate over whether infection is primary bacterial infection or super infection following compromise of the respiratory mucosa secondary to viral illness
  - Initial descriptions of disease suggested Staphylococcus aureus as most common etiology
  - More recent reports suggest that polymicrobial infection is often present, supporting the etiology of secondary infection
  - Hemophilus influenzae, Streptococcus pneumoniae, and Moraxella catarrhalis have been reported in cases of bacterial tracheitis
- Epidemiology
  - Has replaced epiglottitis as the most common life-threatening acute inflammatory airway disease since Haemophilus influenzae vaccine
  - Affected children typically older and more ill than those with croup

Gross Pathologic & Surgical Features
- Infectious inflammation of the trachea with purulent exudates producing plaques and membranes within the airway

Microscopic Features
- Infectious inflammation

CLINICAL ISSUES

Presentation
- Most common signs/symptoms: High grade fever, severe stridor and respiratory distress
- Other signs/symptoms: Usually preceded by several day history of viral upper respiratory tract infection, low grade fever, and cough

EXUDATIVE TRACHEITIS

- Patients present with stridor often accompanied by fever
- Initial descriptions described patients as severely toxic in appearance
- More recently encountered patients are not always severely ill
- If symptoms of croup are seen in child older than typical, exudative tracheitis should be suspected
- Child typically able to handle oral secretions and tolerates a supine position, unlike appearance in epiglottitis

Demographics
- Age: Typical age is 6-10 years, much older than patients who present with classic croup
- Gender: No predilection

Natural History & Prognosis
- Endoscopy showing subglottic edema, ulcerations, copious secretions and pseudomembrane formation is diagnostic
- Children suspected to have exudative tracheitis usually undergo further evaluation with endoscopy and possible intervention
- Severe systemic complications of bacterial tracheitis such as toxic shock syndrome, septic shock, pulmonary edema, and acute respiratory distress syndrome (ARDS) have been described

Treatment
- Because illness can lead to airway obstruction, respiratory failure and death, children are treated aggressively
- If exudative tracheitis is suspected clinically or radiographically, the child is evaluated with a flexible nasopharyngeal scope
- If membranes are visualized within the trachea, the patients undergo rigid bronchoscopy and "stripping" of the membranes
- Child is then observed under prophylactic tracheal intubation for several days while on antibiotics

DIAGNOSTIC CHECKLIST

Consider
- Repeat radiograph after the child has coughed, if adherent mucus is suspected

Image Interpretation Pearls
- Linear filling defects (membranes) and soft tissue irregularity of the tracheal walls (plaques) are very suggestive of the diagnosis

SELECTED REFERENCES
1. Hammer J: Acquired upper airway obstruction. Paediatr Respir Rev. 5(1):25-33, 2004
2. Rotta AT et al: Respiratory emergencies in children. Respir Care. 48(3):248-58; discussion 258-60, 2003
3. Steinman MA et al: Predictors of broad-spectrum antibiotic prescribing for acute respiratory tract infections in adult primary care. JAMA. 289(6):719-25, 2003
4. Ward MA: Emergency department management of acute respiratory infections. Semin Respir Infect. 17(1):65-71, 2002
5. Stroud RH et al: An update on inflammatory disorders of the pediatric airway: epiglottitis, croup, and tracheitis. Am J Otolaryngol. 22(4):268-75, 2001
6. Damm M et al: Management of acute inflammatory childhood stridor. Otolaryngol Head Neck Surg. 121(5):633-8, 1999
7. Bernstein T et al: Is bacterial tracheitis changing? A 14-month experience in a pediatric intensive care unit. Clin Infect Dis. 27(3):458-62, 1998
8. Brody AS et al: Membranous tracheitis: how accurate is the plain film diagnosis? Pediatr Radiol (Abstr). 27:705, 1997
9. Brook I: Aerobic and anaerobic microbiology of bacterial tracheitis in children. Pediatr Emerg Care. 13(1):16-8, 1997
10. Fayon MJ et al: Nosocomial pneumonia and tracheitis in a pediatric intensive care unit: a prospective study. Am J Respir Crit Care Med. 155(1):162-9, 1997
11. Britto J et al: Systemic complications associated with bacterial tracheitis. Arch Dis Child. 74(3):249-50, 1996
12. Gold SM et al: Radiological case of the month. Membranous laryngotracheobronchitis. Arch Pediatr Adolesc Med. 150(1):97-8, 1996
13. Horowitz IN: Staphylococcal tracheitis, pneumonia, and adult respiratory distress syndrome. Pediatr Emerg Care. 12(4):288-90, 1996
14. Bank DE et al: New approaches to upper airway disease. Emerg Med Clin North Am. 13(2):473-87, 1995
15. Eid NS et al: Bacterial tracheitis as a complication of tonsillectomy and adenoidectomy. J Pediatr. 125(3):401-2, 1994
16. Cox PN: Current management of laryngotracheobronchitis, bacterial tracheitis and epiglottitis. Intensive Care World. 10(1):8-12, 1993
17. Eckel HE et al: Airway endoscopy in the diagnosis and treatment of bacterial tracheitis in children. Int J Pediatr Otorhinolaryngol. 27(2):147-57, 1993
18. Seigler RS: Bacterial tracheitis: recognition and treatment. J S C Med Assoc. 89(2):83-7, 1993
19. John SD et al: Stridor and upper airway obstruction in infants and children. Radiographics. 12(4):625-43; discussion 644, 1992
20. Tan AK et al: Hospitalized croup (bacterial and viral): the role of rigid endoscopy. J Otolaryngol. 21(1):48-53, 1992
21. Walker P et al: Croup, epiglottitis, retropharyngeal abscess, and bacterial tracheitis: evolving patterns of occurrence and care. Int Anesthesiol Clin. 30(4):57-70, 1992
22. Han BK et al: Membranous laryngotracheobronchitis (membranous croup). AJR Am J Roentgenol. 133(1):53-8, 1979

EXUDATIVE TRACHEITIS

IMAGE GALLERY

Typical

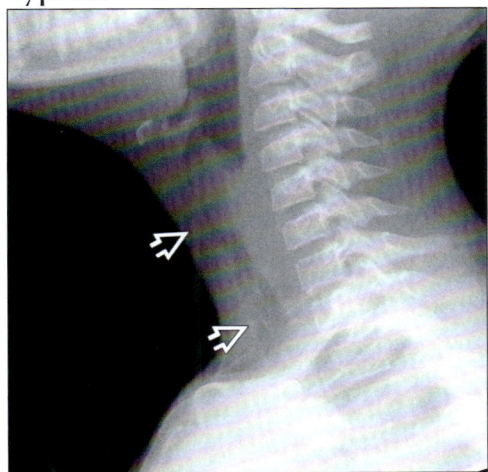
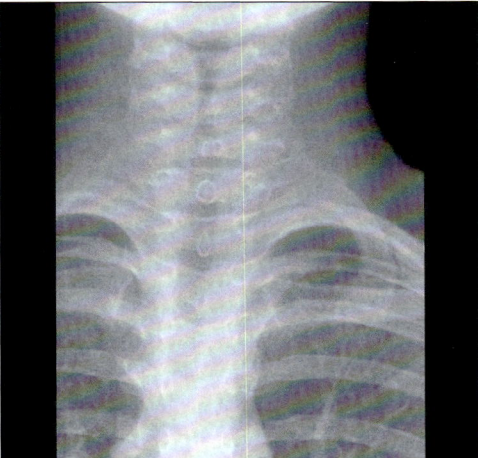

(Left) Lateral radiograph shows multiple filling defects ➡ within trachea as well as tracheal wall irregularity consistent with exudative tracheitis. *(Right)* Frontal radiograph of same patient as previous image, shows paucity of visualization of changes on frontal view. Sometimes even striking cases are seen only on one view.

Typical

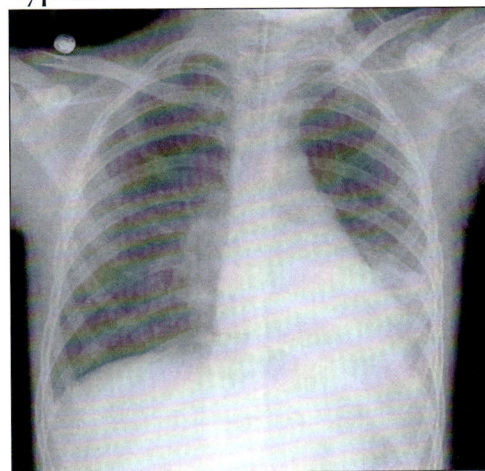
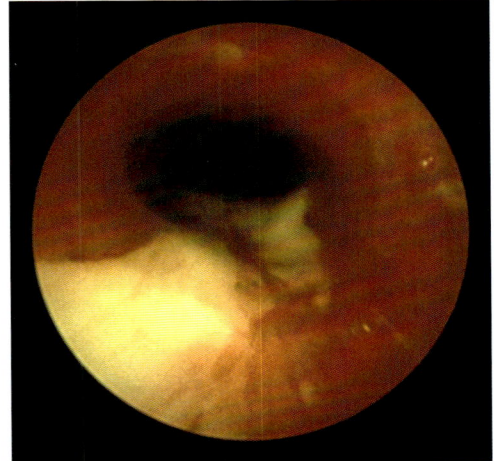

(Left) Frontal radiograph in same patient as previous image shows the patient is intubated and has developed left lower lobe opacity. *(Right)* Intra-operative photograph during endoscopy shows multiple exudative plaques, with purulent white appearance, along tracheal wall.

Typical

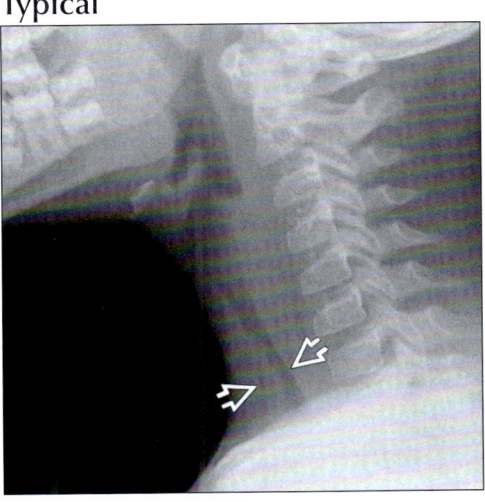
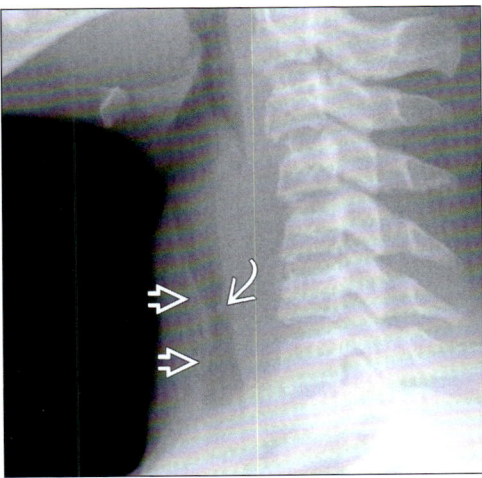

(Left) Lateral radiograph shows large intraluminal filling defect ➡ within lower trachea, consistent with exudative tracheitis. *(Right)* Lateral radiograph shows large anterior tracheal plaque ➡ and intraluminal filling defect ➡.

CROUP

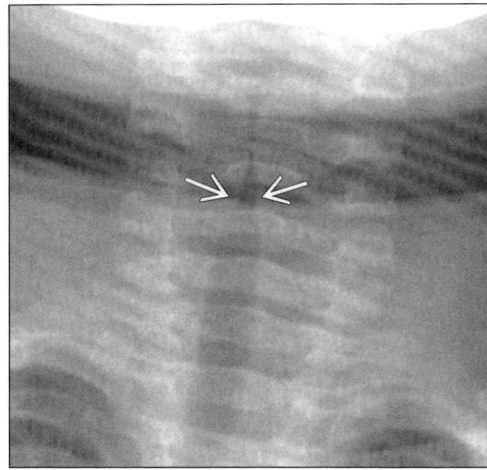

Anteroposterior radiograph shows symmetric narrowing ➡ of subglottic trachea resulting in a steeple appearance.

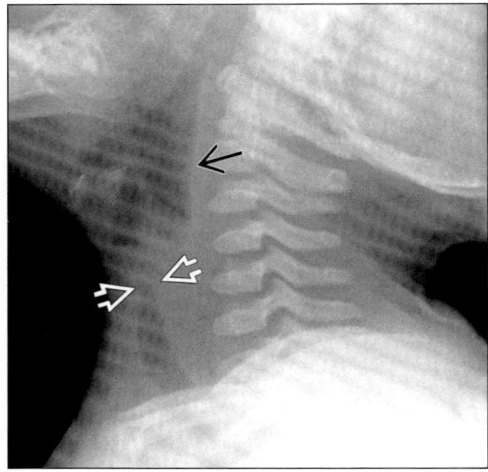

Lateral radiograph in same patient as on left, shows mild overdistension of the hypopharynx ➡. Note subglottic narrowing ➡, but not as well seen as on frontal view.

TERMINOLOGY

Abbreviations and Synonyms
- Acute laryngotracheobronchitis

Definitions
- Self-limited viral inflammation of the airways resulting in symmetric subglottic edema and croupy cough

IMAGING FINDINGS

General Features
- Best diagnostic clue: Symmetric subglottic narrowing on the anteroposterior (AP) projection with loss of normal shoulders of the subglottic trachea
- Location: Subglottic airway
- Size: Subglottic narrowing which extends beyond the inferior extent of the pyriform sinuses
- Morphology: "Steeple sign", "pencil tip", or inverted "V" on frontal radiograph

Radiographic Findings
- Radiography
  - Frontal radiograph
    - Purpose of radiographs is to exclude more serious causes of stridor
    - Loss of normal shoulders (lateral convexities) of the subglottic trachea secondary to subglottic edema: "Steeple sign" or inverted "V"
    - Symmetric, subglottic narrowing with narrow portion of airway extending more inferiorly than level of the pyriform sinuses on frontal view
    - Findings on frontal often more revealing than on lateral radiograph
  - Lateral radiograph
    - Narrowing of the subglottic trachea
    - Loss of definition of the subglottic trachea
    - Hypopharyngeal overdistention
    - Normal epiglottis and aryepiglottic folds
    - Hypopharynx may be collapsed with distention of the lower cervical trachea if expiratory image
  - Pertinent negatives
    - No radiopaque foreign body
    - No enlargement of epiglottis
    - No widening of retropharyngeal soft tissues
    - No tracheal wall irregularity of airway filling defects

DDx: Acute Stridor

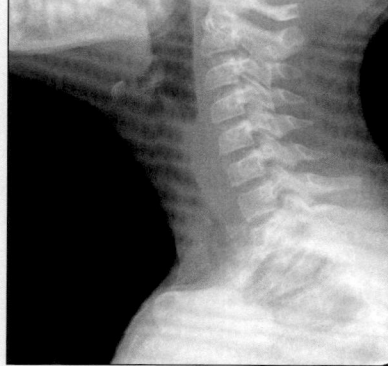

Exudative Tracheitis

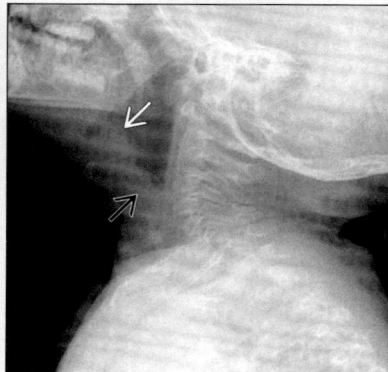

Epiglottitis

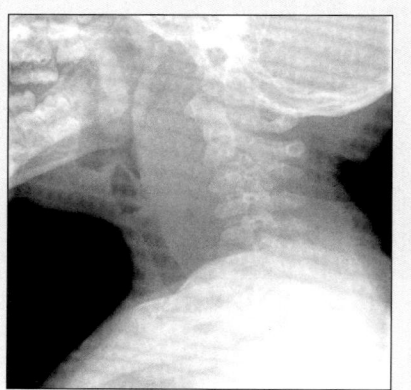

Retropharyngeal Abscess

CROUP

Key Facts

Terminology
- Acute laryngotracheobronchitis
- Self-limited viral inflammation of the airways resulting in symmetric subglottic edema and croupy cough

Imaging Findings
- Loss of normal shoulders (lateral convexities) of the subglottic trachea secondary to subglottic edema: "Steeple sign" or inverted "V"
- Symmetric, subglottic narrowing with narrow portion of airway extending more inferiorly than level of the pyriform sinuses on frontal view

Top Differential Diagnoses
- Aspirated Bronchial Foreign Body
- Epiglottitis
- Exudative Tracheitis

Pathology
- Benign, self-limited condition secondary to viral illness
- Most common cause of upper airway obstruction in young children

Clinical Issues
- Most common signs/symptoms: Acute clinical syndrome characterized by barky ("croupy") cough, inspiratory stridor, and hoarseness
- Peak age: 1 year
- Managed supportively as outpatients
- Oral or inhaled corticosteroids have become more routinely used as therapy for all children with croup

Imaging Recommendations
- Best imaging tool
  - Conventional frontal and lateral radiographs
  - Diagnosis can typically be made by frontal radiograph alone
  - Lateral radiograph may show overdistention of the hypopharynx and helps exclude other diagnoses
- Protocol advice: Ensure that the neck is extended and avoid imaging while the child is swallowing

DIFFERENTIAL DIAGNOSIS

Aspirated Bronchial Foreign Body
- Radiopaque foreign body seen in minority of cases
- Most common foreign body in main bronchi
- Tracheal foreign bodies rare
- Asymmetric lung aeration on chest radiographs

Epiglottitis
- Typically older than croup: Mean age of epiglottitis = 3 years
- Severe, life-threatening condition
- Marked enlargement of epiglottis and aryepiglottic folds
- May cause symmetric subglottic narrowing on frontal view: Similar in appearance to croup

Exudative Tracheitis
- Children typically older than those with croup
- Intraluminal filling defect (membrane)
- Tracheal wall plaque-like irregularity
- Asymmetric subglottic narrowing

PATHOLOGY

General Features
- General path comments
  - Inflammation and edema of subglottic airway
  - Secondary to viral infection
  - Redundant mucosa in this region predisposes to edema and narrowing
  - Swelling of the vocal cords results in hoarseness
  - Barky cough results from the inflammation of the larynx and trachea
  - Inspiratory stridor results because small children have proportionately small subglottic trachea which is predisposed to obstruction with edema
    - Same viral infections and edema does not compromise adult sized airway
- Etiology
  - Benign, self-limited condition secondary to viral illness
  - Parainfluenza virus types 1 and 2 account for the majority of cases
  - Influenza virus
  - Respiratory syncytial virus
  - Metapneumovirus
  - Adenovirus
  - Rhinovirus
  - Enterovirus and rarely herpes simplex virus types 1 and 2 and measles virus have been described
- Epidemiology
  - Most common cause of upper airway obstruction in young children
  - Seasonal occurrence with viral disease
  - Most prevalent in the fall and winter months

Gross Pathologic & Surgical Features
- Characterized by inflammatory edema of the subglottic airway walls

CLINICAL ISSUES

Presentation
- Most common signs/symptoms: Acute clinical syndrome characterized by barky ("croupy") cough, inspiratory stridor, and hoarseness
- Other signs/symptoms: May be preceded by a prodrome consisting of low-grade fever, mild cough, and rhinorrhea

CROUP

- Symptoms are characteristically worse at night and are aggravated by agitation and crying
- Barky ("croupy") or seal-like cough
- Occurs with other symptoms of lower respiratory tract infection
- May be febrile
- Typically child able to manage oral secretions

Demographics
- Age
  - Disease of young infants
  - Age range: 6 months to 3 years
  - Peak age: 1 year
  - Age > 3 years, other cause of stridor should be highly suspected
  - Much more common than other pathologic causes of stridor
- Gender: M:F = 3:2

Natural History & Prognosis
- Benign, self-limited disease
- Resolution within several days
- If persistence of symptoms → suspect other cause
- Radiographs obtained to exclude other disease such as
  - Aspirated foreign body
  - Epiglottitis
  - Exudative tracheitis
  - Subglottic hemangioma

Treatment
- Managed supportively as outpatients
- Parents "managed" with reassurance
- Oral or inhaled corticosteroids have become more routinely used as therapy for all children with croup
- Use of corticosteroids has significantly reduced the severity of symptoms, hospital admissions, and rates of return visit to the health care practitioner
- Only in severe cases is nebulized epinephrine or intubation required

DIAGNOSTIC CHECKLIST

Consider
- Best imaging modality is a frontal radiograph
- Bronchoscopy may be helpful in further evaluating children who present with atypical, prolonged or recurrent symptoms or who do not respond to medical therapy
- Younger age of presentation than seen with epiglottitis and exudative tracheitis
- Much more common than other causes of stridor

Image Interpretation Pearls
- Croup results in symmetric subglottic narrowing

SELECTED REFERENCES

1. Bjornson CL et al: A randomized trial of a single dose of oral dexamethasone for mild croup. N Engl J Med. 351(13):1306-13, 2004
2. Fisher JD: Out-of-hospital cardiopulmonary arrest in children with croup. Pediatr Emerg Care. 20(1):35-6, 2004
3. Hammer J: Acquired upper airway obstruction. Paediatr Respir Rev. 5(1):25-33, 2004
4. Henrickson KJ et al: National disease burden of respiratory viruses detected in children by polymerase chain reaction. Pediatr Infect Dis J. 23(1 Suppl):S11-8, 2004
5. Knutson D et al: Viral croup. Am Fam Physician. 69(3):535-40, 2004
6. Leung AK et al: Viral croup: a current perspective. J Pediatr Health Care. 18(6):297-301, 2004
7. Parker R et al: How long does stridor at rest persist in croup after the administration of oral prednisolone? Emerg Med Australas. 16(2):135-8, 2004
8. Principi N et al: Burden of influenza in healthy children and their households. Arch Dis Child. 89(11):1002-7, 2004
9. Rittichier KK: The role of corticosteroids in the treatment of croup. Treat Respir Med. 3(3):139-45, 2004
10. Russell K et al: Glucocorticoids for croup. Cochrane Database Syst Rev. (1):CD001955, 2004
11. Fitzgerald DA et al: Croup: assessment and evidence-based management. Med J Aust. 179(7):372-7, 2003
12. Yang TY et al: Clinical manifestations of parainfluenza infection in children. J Microbiol Immunol Infect. 36(4):270-4, 2003
13. Zoorob RJ et al: Acute dyspnea in the office. Am Fam Physician. 68(9):1803-10, 2003
14. Brown JC: The management of croup. Br Med Bull. 61:189-202, 2002
15. Chin R et al: Effectiveness of a croup clinical pathway in the management of children with croup presenting to an emergency department. J Paediatr Child Health. 38(4):382-7, 2002
16. Infosino A: Pediatric upper airway and congenital anomalies. Anesthesiol Clin North America. 20(4):747-66, 2002
17. Lichenstein R et al: Respiratory viral infections in hospitalized children: implications for infection control. South Med J. 95(9):1022-5, 2002
18. Neto GM et al: A randomized controlled trial of mist in the acute treatment of moderate croup. Acad Emerg Med. 9(9):873-9, 2002
19. Peltola V et al: Clinical courses of croup caused by influenza and parainfluenza viruses. Pediatr Infect Dis J. 21(1):76-8, 2002
20. Stannard W et al: Management of croup. Paediatr Drugs. 4(4):231-40, 2002
21. Wright RB et al: New approaches to respiratory infections in children. Bronchiolitis and croup. Emerg Med Clin North Am. 20(1):93-114, 2002
22. John SD et al: Stridor and upper airway obstruction in infants and children. Radiographics. 12(4):625-43; discussion 644, 1992
23. Dunbar JS: Upper respiratory tract obstruction in infants and children. Am J Roentgenol Radium Ther Nucl Med. 109(2):227-46, 1970
24. Capitanio MA et al: Upper respiratory tract obstruction in infants and children. Radiol Clin North Am. 6(2):265-77, 1968

CROUP

IMAGE GALLERY

Typical

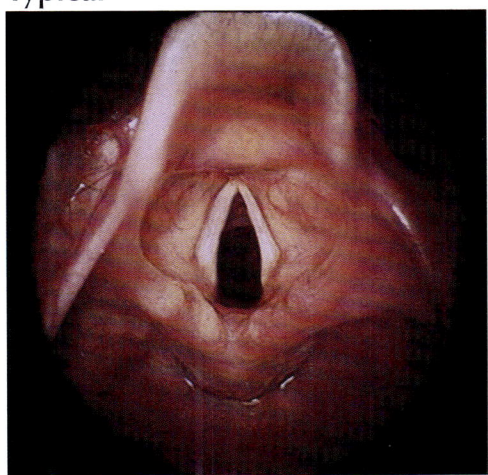
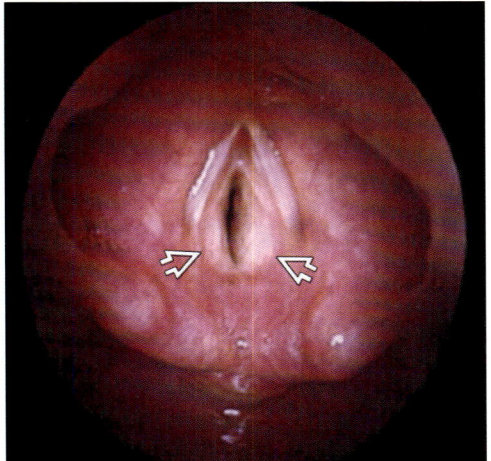

(Left) Endoscopic photograph shows normal subglottic airway. *(Right)* Endoscopic photograph in child with croup shows edematous subglottic mucosa ➡ and narrowing of the subglottic airway.

Typical

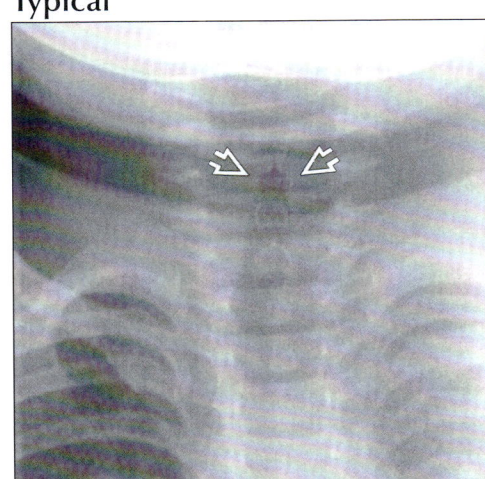
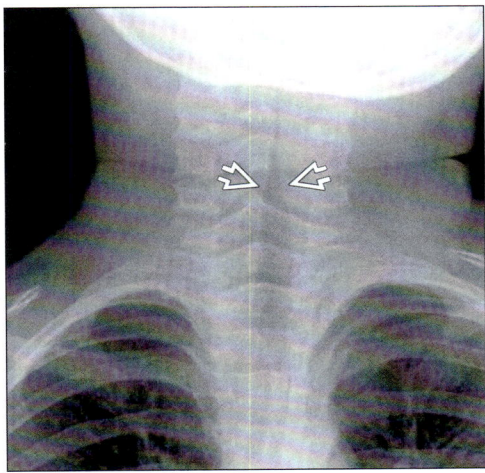

(Left) Frontal radiograph shows normal appearance of subglottic trachea. Note normal "shoulders" ➡ of subglottic trachea as outpouchings. In croup, edema obliterates these "shoulders". *(Right)* Anteroposterior radiograph shows croup with subglottic narrowing resulting in "steeple" like appearance of subglottic trachea. Note loss of normal "shoulders" of subglottic trachea ➡.

Typical

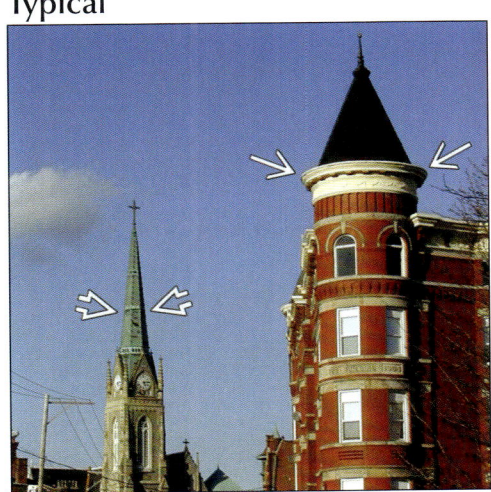
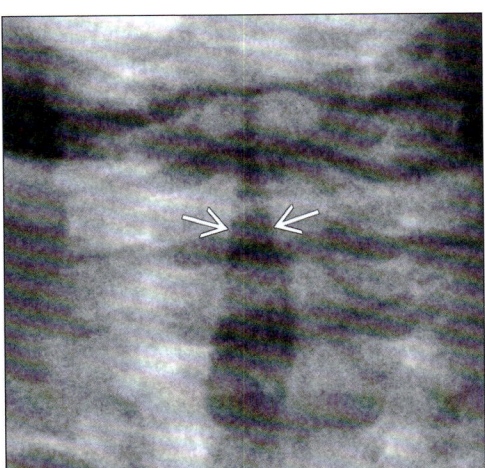

(Left) Photograph demonstrates potential confusion over "steeple" sign. Steeple on left ➡ has appearance of "croup". Steeple on right ➡ has appearance of normal airway. *(Right)* Frontal radiograph shows typical steeple sign of croup. Note symmetric subglottic narrowing ➡.

EPIGLOTTITIS

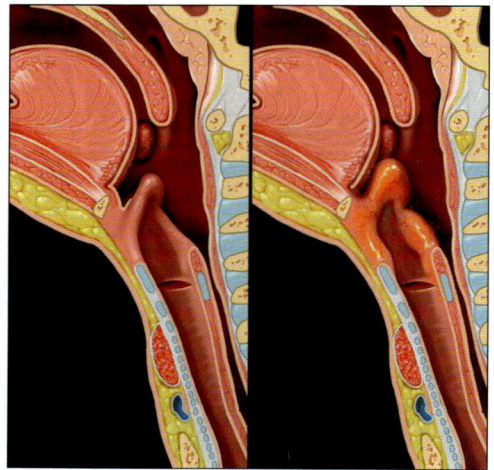

Sagittal graphic shows epiglottitis (right) as compared to normal epiglottis (left). Epiglottis and aryepiglottic folds are swollen and diffusely enlarged.

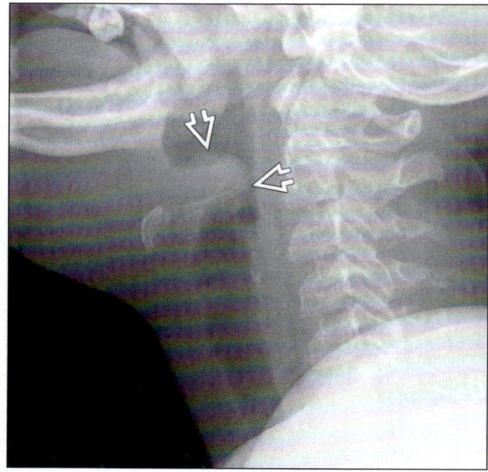

Lateral radiograph shows epiglottitis as markedly swollen epiglottis ➡ with "thumb-like" appearance, in patient with congenital insensitivity to pain.

TERMINOLOGY

Definitions
- Airway obstruction secondary to infectious inflammation of the epiglottis and surrounding tissues

IMAGING FINDINGS

General Features
- Best diagnostic clue
  - Classic imaging appearance: Lateral radiograph shows enlargement of epiglottis and thickening of the aryepiglottic folds
  - Not to be confused with "omega" epiglottis: Normal variant when epiglottis imaged obliquely
- Location: Serious, life threatening infection resulting in inflammation and swelling of the epiglottis and surrounding tissues (i.e. the aryepiglottic folds)
- Size: Diffuse enlargement and swelling of the epiglottis
- Morphology: Infectious inflammation of the epiglottitis results in "thumb sign" appreciated on lateral radiograph

Radiographic Findings
- Radiography
  - Lateral radiograph
    - Should be obtained with patient upright in comfortable position
    - Marked thickening of the epiglottis
    - Aryepiglottic folds: Become markedly thickened
    - Extend from epiglottis anterosuperiorly to arytenoid cartilage posteroinferiorly
    - Normally are thin and convex inferiorly
    - When thickened become convex superiorly
    - It is the swelling of these folds that actually leads to airway obstruction
    - Ballooning of the hypopharynx
  - Frontal radiograph
    - Only a lateral radiograph should be obtained when epiglottitis is highly suspected
    - Symmetric subglottic narrowing, similar to as seen in croup, may be seen on frontal radiograph when obtained
    - Swelling of epiglottis and aryepiglottic folds not seen on frontal view

DDx: Acute Stridor

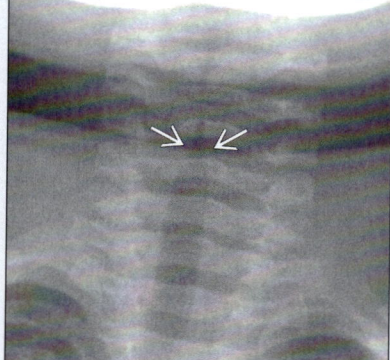
Croup

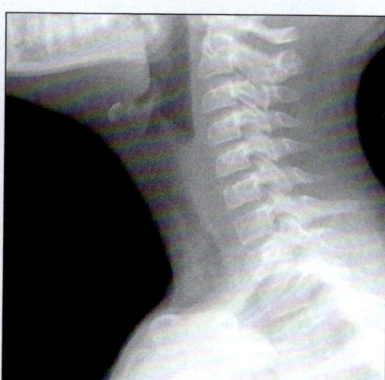
Exudative Tracheitis

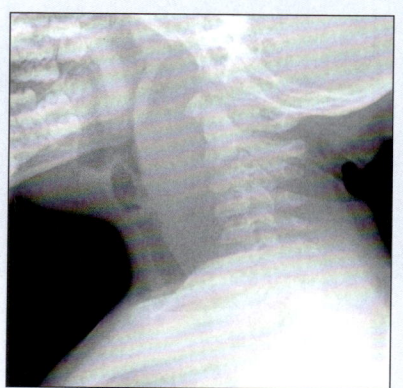
Retropharyngeal Abscess

EPIGLOTTITIS

Key Facts

Terminology
- Airway obstruction secondary to infectious inflammation of the epiglottis and surrounding tissues

Imaging Findings
- Classic imaging appearance: Lateral radiograph shows enlargement of epiglottis and thickening of the aryepiglottic folds
- Not to be confused with "omega" epiglottis: Normal variant when epiglottis imaged obliquely

Pathology
- Typically older than patients with croup
- Since vaccine for Haemophilus influenzae (Hib) is available, incidence of epiglottitis has markedly decreased
- More cases of epiglottitis resulting from other bacterial organisms, viral or combined viral-bacterial infections are now seen since introduction of Hib vaccination
- With introduction of Hib vaccine, epidemiology has shifted toward significantly older patients
- Epiglottitis may be seen in older patients and even those previously immunized against Hib

Clinical Issues
- Increased respiratory distress when recumbent (reason why radiographs obtained upright or whatever way patient comfortable)
- Life threatening disease often requiring emergent intubation

CT Findings
- NECT
  - Rarely indicated, but will show edematous, enlarged epiglottis with involvement of the aryepiglottic folds
  - May also note that due to the extensive inflammation and edema that the epiglottis is slightly lower in attenuation when compared to other soft tissue
- CECT
  - In rare cases may see a phlegmonous collection within the adjacent soft tissues associated with the epiglottis
  - May be helpful in evaluating for complications such as deep neck space infection

Imaging Recommendations
- Best imaging tool
  - Due to the serious, life-threatening infection and an airway emergency, most cases may go directly for direct laryngoscopy and bronchoscopy with intubation as indicated
  - If the patient is not unstable, only a lateral radiograph should be obtained in cases suspecting epiglottis
- Protocol advice
  - Child should be upright and comfortable
  - Patient may be drooling due to difficulty handling oral secretions and should not be agitated or placed supine
  - Patient with suspected epiglottis should be accompanied by physician with readily available supportive equipment to secure airway if necessary
  - Obtaining lateral radiograph should never interfere with securing airway given potential rapid and fatal outcome

DIFFERENTIAL DIAGNOSIS

Omega Epiglottis (Normal Variant)
- If epiglottis obliquely imaged, can appear artificially wide because left and right sides of epiglottis are being imaged adjacent to each other causing an "omega" shaped appearance
- Thickening of aryepiglottic folds is absent

Aspirated Bronchial Foreign Body
- Radiopaque foreign body seen in minority of cases
- Asymmetric lung aeration on chest radiographs

Croup
- Benign, self-limited condition
- Most common acute airway condition encountered
- Symmetric subglottic narrowing

Exudative Tracheitis
- Children typically older than those with croup
- Intraluminal filling defect (membrane), tracheal wall plaque-like irregularity, asymmetric subglottic narrowing

Retropharyngeal Abscess (RPA)
- Pyogenic infection of retropharyngeal space

PATHOLOGY

General Features
- General path comments
  - Typically older than patients with croup
  - Since vaccine for Haemophilus influenzae (Hib) is available, incidence of epiglottitis has markedly decreased
  - Can also rarely occur from noninfectious etiologies such as angioneurotic edema, trauma, Stevens-Johnson syndrome, caustic ingestion, bee stings
- Etiology
  - Most common etiologic agent remains Haemophilus influenzae

EPIGLOTTITIS

- More cases of epiglottitis resulting from other bacterial organisms, viral or combined viral-bacterial infections are now seen since introduction of Hib vaccination
- Other organism have been reported such as group A β-hemolytic Streptococcus pneumonia, Staphylococcus aureus, Klebsiella pneumonia, Moraxella catarrhalis, Pseudomonas species, Candida albicans, Pasturella multocida and Neisseria species
- Bacterial superinfections on top of virus infections such as herpes simplex, parainfluenzae, varicella-zoster, and Epstein-Barr have also been reported
- Epidemiology
  - With introduction of Hib vaccine, epidemiology has shifted toward significantly older patients
  - Incidence of epiglottitis has decreased
  - Epiglottitis may be seen in older patients and even those previously immunized against Hib

Gross Pathologic & Surgical Features
- Marked inflammation and edema of epiglottitis and aryepiglottic folds
- Complete airway obstruction may occur at any time

Microscopic Features
- Infectious inflammation of epiglottitis and surrounding tissues

CLINICAL ISSUES

Presentation
- Most common signs/symptoms: Abrupt onset of stridor often associated with dysphagia
- Other signs/symptoms
  - High fever, sore throat, dysphonia, hot potato voice, hoarseness, drooling, and stridor
  - Patients have toxic appearance with fever
  - Patients are described as anxious and uncomfortable
  - Older age group than those children with croup
  - Increased respiratory distress when recumbent (reason why radiographs obtained upright or whatever way patient comfortable)
  - May have characteristic "tripod position", sitting up with neck extended and leaning forward with jaw thrust out to maximize laryngeal opening

Demographics
- Age
  - Mean age has shifted from 3.5 years to 14.6 years since introduction of Hib vaccine
  - Significantly older than children with croup (mean age 1 year)
- Gender: M:F = 1:1

Natural History & Prognosis
- Life threatening disease often requiring emergent intubation
- Time period of intubation is usually short, 2-3 days
- Abrupt onset of stridor, dysphagia, fever, restlessness, toxic appearance
- Incidence markedly decreased because most cases secondary to Haemophilus influenzae, which is now preventable by immunization

Treatment
- Life-threatening if untreated
- Has evolved from tracheotomy in order to secure airway, to direct laryngoscopy and bronchoscopy with intubation being performed in controlled setting
- Emergent tracheal intubation to relieve/prevent airway obstruction and respiratory failure
- Steroids and broad-spectrum intravenous antibiotic therapy

DIAGNOSTIC CHECKLIST

Consider
- Lateral radiograph should only be obtained when patient quickly returns to emergency department
- Patient should remain in comfortable position

Image Interpretation Pearls
- Epiglottitis should not be confused with an "omega" epiglottis which is a normal variant seen when epiglottis imaged obliquely
- May present in older patients

SELECTED REFERENCES

1. Baines PB et al: Upper airway obstruction. Hosp Med. 65(2):108-11, 2004
2. Gilbert A et al: Epiglottic abscess. Ear Nose Throat J. 83(3):154-5, 2004
3. Hammer J: Acquired upper airway obstruction. Paediatr Respir Rev. 5(1):25-33, 2004
4. Krost WS: Pediatric pulmonary emergencies. Emerg Med Serv. 33(1):71-7; quiz 105, 2004
5. McVernon J et al: Trends in Haemophilus influenzae type b infections in adults in England and Wales: surveillance study. BMJ. 329(7467):655-8, 2004
6. Shah RK et al: Epiglottitis in the Hemophilus influenzae type B vaccine era: changing trends. Laryngoscope. 114(3):557-60, 2004
7. Berger G et al: The rising incidence of adult acute epiglottitis and epiglottic abscess. Am J Otolaryngol. 24(6):374-83, 2003
8. Garner D et al: Effectiveness of vaccination for Haemophilus influenzae type b. Lancet. 361(9355):395-6, 2003
9. McEwan J et al: Paediatric acute epiglottitis: not a disappearing entity. Int J Pediatr Otorhinolaryngol. 67(4):317-21, 2003
10. McVernon J et al: Immunologic memory in Haemophilus influenzae type b conjugate vaccine failure. Arch Dis Child. 88(5):379-83, 2003
11. Rotta AT et al: Respiratory emergencies in children. Respir Care. 48(3):248-58; discussion 258-60, 2003
12. Nakamura H et al: Acute epiglottitis: a review of 80 patients. J Laryngol Otol. 115(1):31-4, 2001
13. Stroud RH et al: An update on inflammatory disorders of the pediatric airway: epiglottitis, croup, and tracheitis. Am J Otolaryngol. 22(4):268-75, 2001
14. John SD et al: Stridor and upper airway obstruction in infants and children. RadioGraphics. 12:625-43, 1992
15. Dunbar JS: Upper respiratory tract obstruction in infants and children. AJR. 109:227-46, 1970

EPIGLOTTITIS

IMAGE GALLERY

Typical

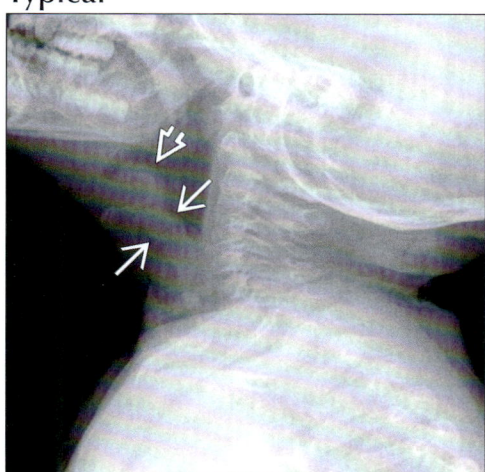
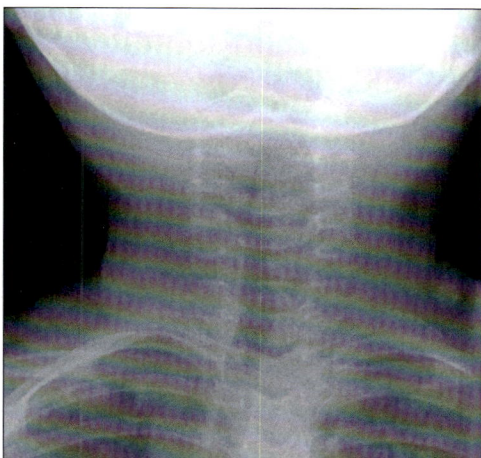

(Left) Lateral radiograph shows marked swelling of epiglottis ➡ and also thickening of aryepiglottic folds ➡. (Right) Anteroposterior radiograph in same patient as on left shows remarkably little, not atypical on frontal radiographs for epiglottitis. There is no significant subglottic narrowing appreciated.

Typical

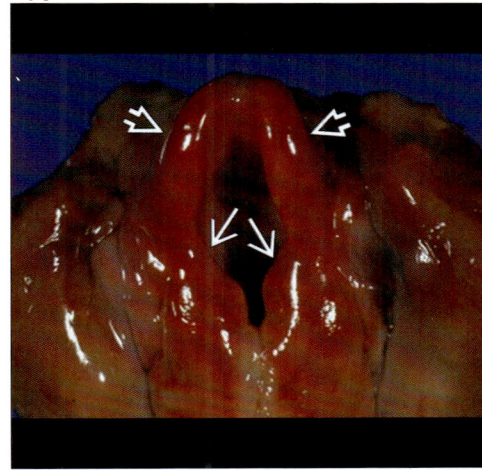
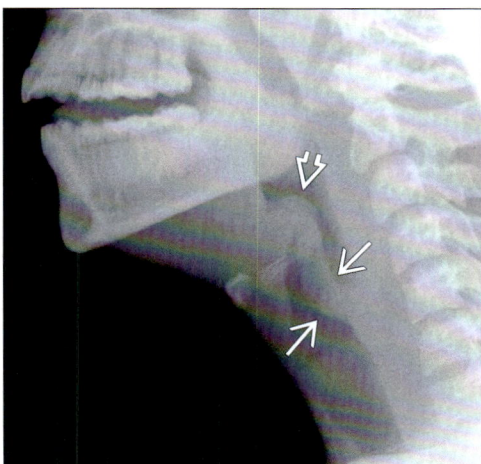

(Left) Gross pathology shows inflamed and edematous epiglottis ➡ and swollen aryepiglottic folds ➡. It is the swelling of the aryepiglottic folds that leads to airway obstruction. (Right) Lateral radiograph shows marked thickening of epiglottis ➡ and aryepiglottic folds ➡.

Typical

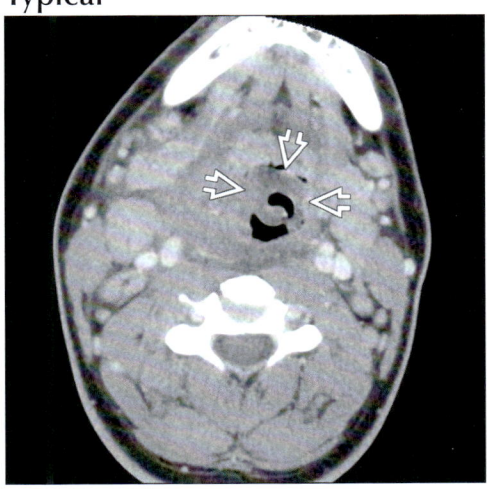
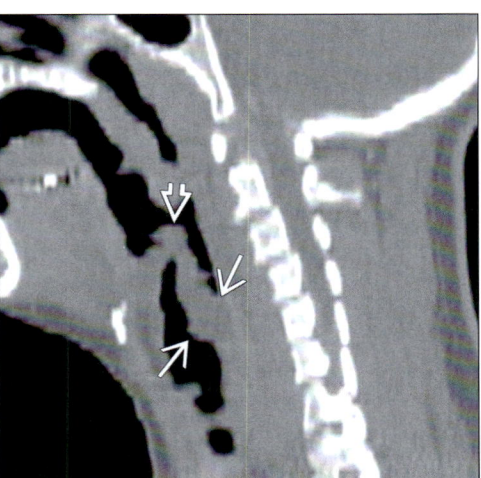

(Left) Axial CECT performed in same patient as previous image shows marked thickening of epiglottis ➡. CT is not indicated in these patients but shown for illustrative purposes. (Right) Sagittal reformat in same patient as on left shows thickening of epiglottis ➡ and aryepiglottic folds ➡.

TRANSIENT TACHYPNEA OF THE NEWBORN

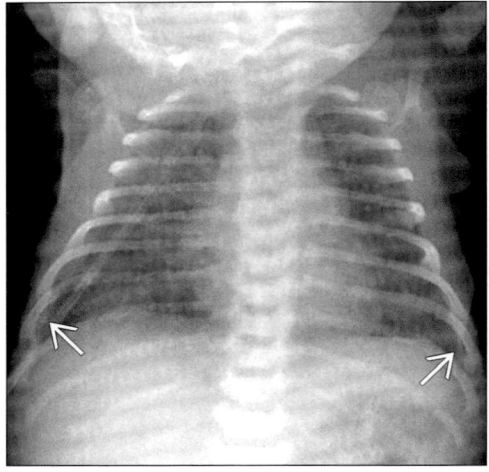

Anteroposterior radiograph shows prominent bilateral perihilar interstitial markings and minimal bilateral pleural effusions ➔ in this full term infant.

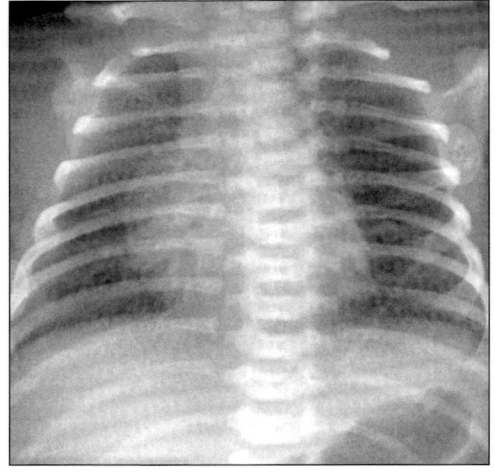

Anteroposterior radiograph shows asymmetric perihilar interstitial markings and hyperinflation, right greater than left in this infant with respiratory distress.

TERMINOLOGY

Abbreviations and Synonyms
- Transient tachypnea of the newborn (TTN), wet lung disease, retained fetal fluid

Definitions
- Transient tachypnea occurs when liquid in the fetal lung is removed slowly or incompletely from newborn lung and there is increased absorption by lymphatics and capillaries
  - Lack of normal thoracic compression that normally occurs during vaginal delivery and is bipassed by C-section
  - Lack of normal breathing may occur with sedated infants
- By definition there is no other cause for tachypnea
- Diagnosis of exclusion

IMAGING FINDINGS

General Features
- Best diagnostic clue: Prominent interstitial pattern in lung with history of C-section
- Location: Lungs
- Size: Usually term infants

Imaging Recommendations
- Best imaging tool
  - Chest radiographs
    - Findings similar to pulmonary edema
    - Normal heart size
    - Prominent intersitial markings
    - Diffuse, bilateral and commonly symmetric increased lung markings which becomes normal within 24-48 hours
    - ± Pleural effusion
    - ± Fluid in the fissures
    - Patients usually not intubated
    - Normal to ↑ lung volumes
    - Not associated with any chronic condition or lung disease

DDx: Interstitial Disease

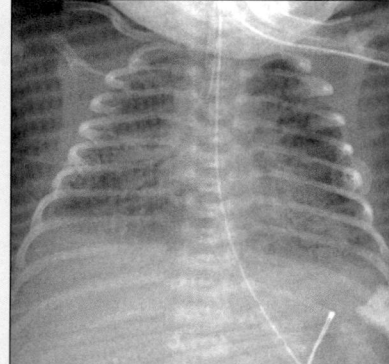

Neonatal Pneumonia

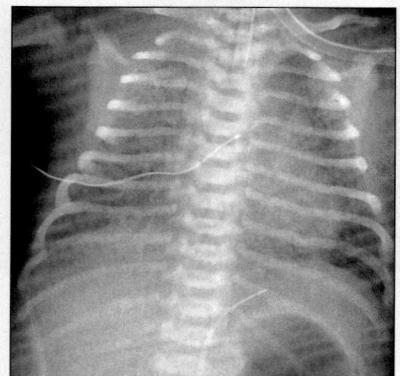

Meconium Aspiration

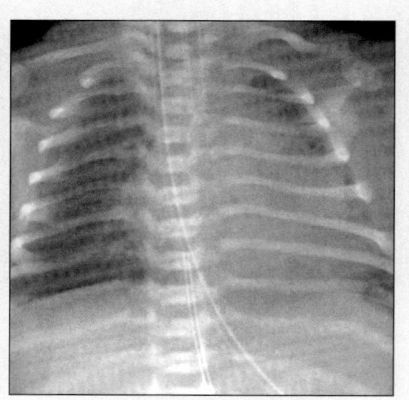

Hypoplastic Left Heart

TRANSIENT TACHYPNEA OF THE NEWBORN

Key Facts

Terminology
- Transient tachypnea of the newborn (TTN), wet lung disease, retained fetal fluid
- Transient tachypnea occurs when liquid in the fetal lung is removed slowly or incompletely from newborn lung and there is increased absorption by lymphatics and capillaries

Imaging Findings
- Findings similar to pulmonary edema
- Normal heart size
- Prominent intersitial markings
- Diffuse, bilateral and commonly symmetric increased lung markings which becomes normal within 24-48 hours
- ± Pleural effusion
- ± Fluid in the fissures

Top Differential Diagnoses
- Congenital Heart Disease (CHD)
- Meconium Aspiration Syndrome
- Congenital Lymphangiectasia
- Neonatal Pneumonia

Pathology
- Incidence is 11 per 1,000 live births
- Not associated with any mortality or morbidity

Clinical Issues
- Newborns
- Initial mild to moderate respiratory distress at birth or within six hours
- Relatively benign clinical course
- Exclude other causes of tachypnea in a term newborn

- Imaging occasionally necessary to exclude other causes
  - Echocardiography to exclude congenital heart disease
  - Intracranial ultrasound to exclude high flow shunt
  - Chest ultrasound or CT
  - Extremity imaging for anomalies
- Protocol advice
  - Anteroposterior chest radiograph
  - Clinical history is helpful

DIFFERENTIAL DIAGNOSIS

Congenital Heart Disease (CHD)
- Echocardiogram is the gold standard for making diagnosis
- Total anomalous pulmonary venous return (TAPVR)
  - With obstruction has normal heart size and interstitial edema
  - Cyanosis, acidosis
- Left-sided heart obstructions
  - Aortic interruption
  - Severe coarctation
  - Aortic stenosis
  - Endocardial fibroelastosis
  - Hypoplastic left heart
    - Most common
    - Radiograph may be normal initially
- Cardiac arrhythmias
  - Supraventricular tachycardia most common
  - Congenital heart block

Meconium Aspiration Syndrome
- Term infant
- Rope-like perihilar markings
- Hyperinflation

Congenital Anomalies in Thorax
- Lung hypoplasia or agenesis
- Tracheo-esophageal fistula with or without esophageal atresia

Congenital Lymphangiectasia
- Rare cause presenting with persistent tachypnea
- Persistent intersitial pattern

Neonatal Pneumonia
- Streptococcus is the most common
- Tuberculosis pneumonia in endemic areas
- Before delivery: Transplacental
  - Syphilis, herpes
- During delivery
  - Group B streptococcus, chlamydia, herpes
- After delivery
  - 30% premature infants colonized with Candida
  - Chlamydia pneumonia has delayed appearance
  - Staphylococcal, pseudomonas pneumonia

Neonatal Chest Masses
- Cystic adenomatoid malformation
  - Focal solid or cystic mass
  - Mediastinal shift, possible effusion
  - May have mass effect
- Diaphragmatic hernia
  - Cystic mass with mediastinal shift
  - Solid and cystic components
  - Abnormal position of stomach, spleen or liver, bowel
  - Usually diagnosed in-utero
- Lobar emphysema
  - Initially may appear solid
  - May shift mediastinum
- Duplication cysts

Many Extrathoracic Causes of Tachypnea
- Hematologic abnormalities
  - Polycythemia or severe anemia
- Arterial-venous malformations
  - Vein of Galen malformation
  - Hemangioendothelioma of liver
- Airway obstruction
  - Choanal atresia
  - Nasal aperture stenosis
  - Vocal cord paralysis

TRANSIENT TACHYPNEA OF THE NEWBORN

- ○ Diaphragmatic paralysis
- ○ Tracheal stenosis
- CNS abnormalities
  - ○ Cerebral anoxia or depression
  - ○ Birth trauma or cord injury
- Thoracic anomalies or congenital syndromes
  - ○ Asphyxiating thoracic dystrophy
  - ○ Thanatophoric dwarfism
  - ○ Osteogenesis imperfecta

Systemic Causes of Respiratory Distress
- Sepsis
- Hypovolemia
- Electrolyte abnormalities
- Severe acidosis, hypothermia

Neuromuscular Causes
- Werdnig Hoffman disease
- Muscular dystrophy

Intraabdominal Abnormalities
- Pneumoperitoneum
- Abdominal distension

PATHOLOGY

General Features
- Genetics: No predisposition
- Etiology
  - ○ During fetal life, lungs expanded with ultrafiltrate of fetal fluid
  - ○ During and after birth, the lung fluid is replaced with air
    - Chest is normally compressed and fluid expelled during vaginal delivery: "Vaginal squeeze" or thoracic squeeze
    - Pulmonary capillaries and lymphatics remove the remaining fluid
  - ○ Most infants with TTN are healthy and normal within 48 hours
- Epidemiology
  - ○ Incidence is 11 per 1,000 live births
  - ○ More common in C-section infants
    - Increased number of cases
- Associated abnormalities: Usually healthy infants with no other anomalies

Gross Pathologic & Surgical Features
- Not associated with any mortality or morbidity

CLINICAL ISSUES

Presentation
- Most common signs/symptoms
  - ○ Mild to moderate respiratory distress
  - ○ Frequent history of C-section
  - ○ Tachypnea occurs early after birth
    - Respiratory rates may exceed 60/min
  - ○ Expiratory grunting, chest retractions, nasal flaring
  - ○ Occasional cyanosis which is changed by minimal oxygen
  - ○ Typically do not require intubation
- Other signs/symptoms
  - ○ Usually healthy large infants
  - ○ Infants usually improve rapidly and are normal
    - Tachypnea is transient

Demographics
- Age
  - ○ Newborns
    - Tend to be term infants
    - Uncommon in premature infants
- Gender: More frequently in males

Natural History & Prognosis
- Initial mild to moderate respiratory distress at birth or within six hours
  - ○ Occasionally need oxygen for several hours
- Relatively benign clinical course
- Radiographic resolution usually by 24-48 hours
- Respiratory symptoms disappear usually by three days
- In healthy asymptomatic infant, follow-up films not necessary

Treatment
- Exclude other causes of tachypnea in a term newborn
- Normal support of infant
  - ○ Oxygen for mild cyanosis, normal feeding
- Some advocate IV furosemide but controversial

DIAGNOSTIC CHECKLIST

Image Interpretation Pearls
- Increased lung volumes, coarse streaky opacities, pleural fluid, fluid in fissure

SELECTED REFERENCES

1. Kuhn JP et al: Caffey's Pediatric Diagnostic Imaging. 10th Edition. Volume I. Philadelphia, Mosby. 3:72-3, 2004
2. Zanardo V et al: Neonatal respiratory morbidity risk and mode of delivery at term: influence of timing of elective caesarean delivery. Acta Paediatr. 93(5):643-7, 2004
3. Kugelman A et al: Familial neonatal pneumothorax associated with transient tachypnea of the newborn. Pediatr Pulmonol. 36(1):69-72, 2003
4. Lewis V et al: Furosemide for transient tachypnea of the newborn. Cochrane Database Syst Rev. (1):CD003064, 2002
5. Herting E et al: Surfactant treatment of neonates with respiratory failure and group B streptococcal infection. Members of the Collaborative European Multicenter Study Group. Pediatrics. 106(5):957-64; discussion 1135, 2000
6. Newman B. Related Articles et al: Imaging of medical disease of the newborn lung. Radiol Clin North Am. 37(6):1049-65, 1999
7. Cleveland RH. Related Articles et al: A radiologic update on medical diseases of the newborn chest. Pediatr Radiol. 25(8):631-7, 1995
8. Shaw D et al: Imaging Children. Edinburgh, Churchill Livingstone. 1-165, 1994

TRANSIENT TACHYPNEA OF THE NEWBORN

IMAGE GALLERY

Typical

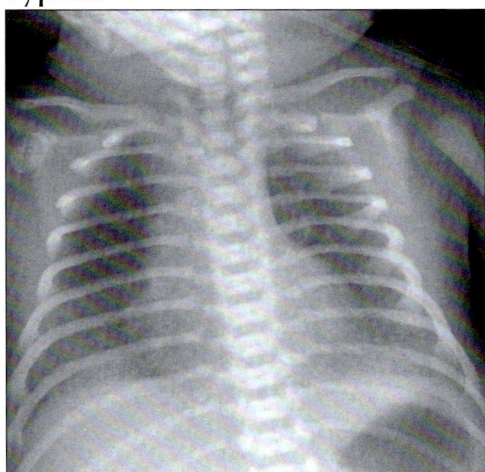
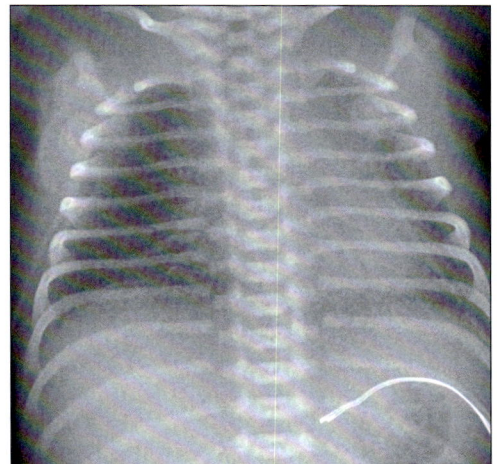

(Left) Anteroposterior radiograph shows asymmetric hazy opacities greatest at the lung bases and hyperinflation in a term infant with TTN and a history of mandibular hypoplasia and arthrogryposis. *(Right)* Anteroposterior radiograph shows upper normal inflation and prominent bilateral interstitial markings.

Typical

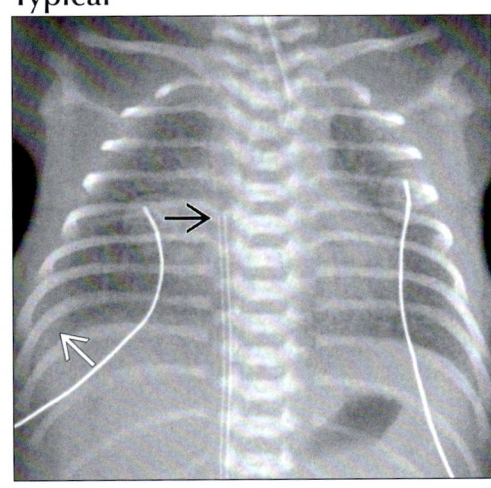
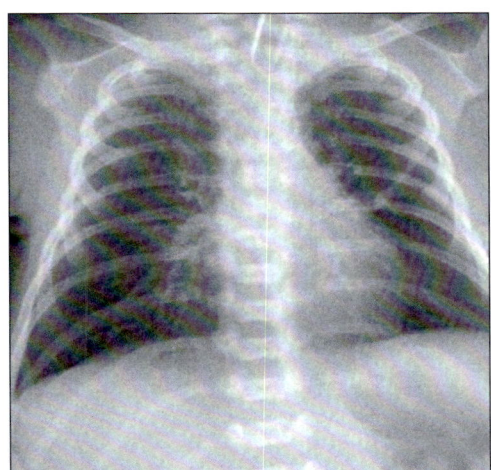

(Left) Anteroposterior radiograph infant delivered via C-section shows bilateral interstitial opacities with small right pleural effusion ➡. The umbilical venous catheter tip ➡ projects over the SVC/right atrial junction. *(Right)* Anteroposterior radiograph shows increased perihilar interstitial markings and mild hyperinflation in this patient with presumed transient tachypnea of the newborn.

Typical

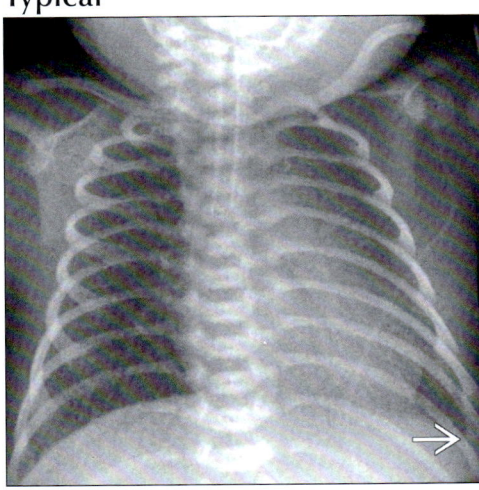
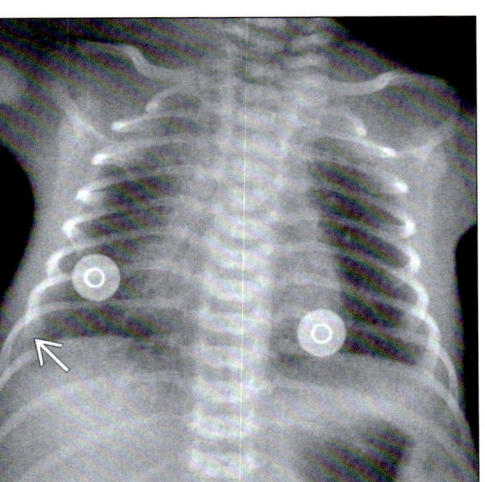

(Left) Anteroposterior radiograph in a term infant shows mild asymmetric interstitial prominence, left greater than right, and minimal left pleural effusion ➡. *(Right)* Anteroposterior radiograph shows hyperinflation and asymmetric perihilar interstitial markings, right greater than left. Notice the small right ➡ and possibly left pleural effusion.

PULMONARY INTERSTITIAL EMPHYSEMA, PEDIATRIC

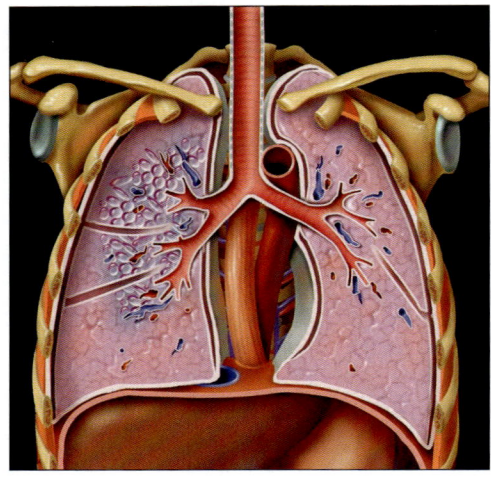

Graphic shows round and linear lucencies secondary to air escaping into the pulmonary interstitium.

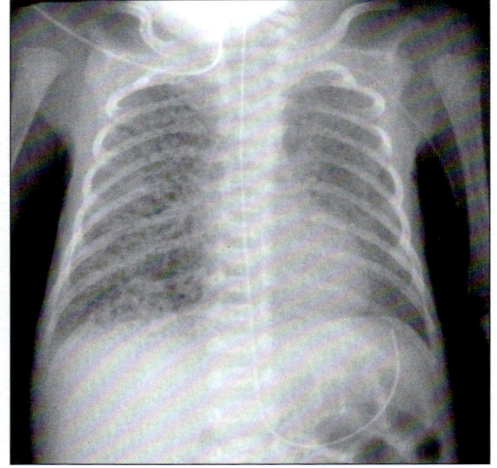

Frontal radiograph shows right-sided, bubble-like lucencies consistent with PIE.

TERMINOLOGY

Abbreviations and Synonyms
- Pulmonary interstitial emphysema (PIE)

Definitions
- Abnormal location of pulmonary air within the interstitium and lymphatics; usually secondary to barotrauma

IMAGING FINDINGS

General Features
- Best diagnostic clue: Bubble-like or linear lucencies within the lung

Radiographic Findings
- Radiography
  - Bubble-like or linear lucencies within the lung
  - Lucencies typically uniform in size
  - Often radiate from hilum
  - May be focal (one lobe) or diffuse and bilateral
  - Involved lung usually noncompliant: Static lung volume seen on multiple consecutive chest radiographs, even with change in volume of uninvolved lung from radiograph to radiograph
  - Serves as a warning sign for other pending air-block complications: Pneumothorax, pneumomediastinum
  - Finding is typically transient
  - Rarely, PIE may persist and form large air-filled cystic mass: Persistent pulmonary interstitial emphysema
    - May act as mass lesion and compress other thoracic structures and cause progressive respiratory distress
    - Initial management conservative: Decubitus positioning, selective intubation opposite lung
    - Usually affects single lobe
    - Most commonly left upper lobe
    - Sometimes requires surgical resection

CT Findings
- CT not obtained to evaluate routine typical PIE
  - PIE may be seen when CT obtained for other reasons

DDx: Lung Lucencies In Neonates

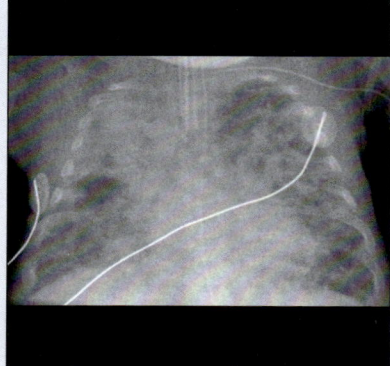

Bronchopulmonary Dysplasia

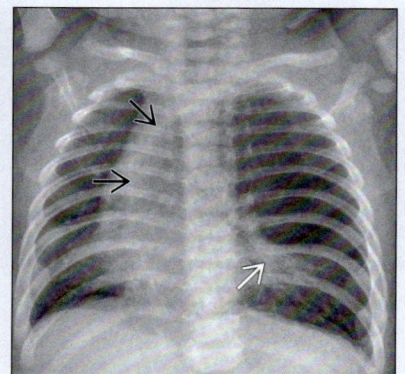

Lobar Emphysema

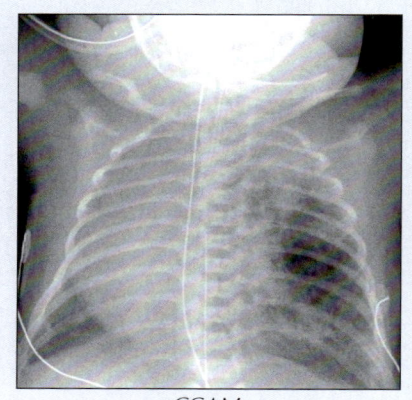

CCAM

PULMONARY INTERSTITIAL EMPHYSEMA, PEDIATRIC

Key Facts

Terminology
- Abnormal location of pulmonary air within the interstitium and lymphatics; usually secondary to barotrauma

Imaging Findings
- Best diagnostic clue: Bubble-like or linear lucencies within the lung
- Lucencies typically uniform in size
- Often radiate from hilum
- May be focal (one lobe) or diffuse and bilateral
- Involved lung usually noncompliant: Static lung volume seen on multiple consecutive chest radiographs, even with change in volume of uninvolved lung from radiograph to radiograph
- Serves as a warning sign for other pending air-block complications: Pneumothorax, pneumomediastinum
- Finding is typically transient
- CT findings: Air surrounds pulmonary arterial branches which are seen as soft tissue linear or dot-like densities surrounded by abnormal gas collections

Clinical Issues
- Presence influences care givers to alter support: Switching from conventional to high-frequency ventilation
- Usually occurs during first several days of life
- Almost always during first week of life
- Almost always occurs only in infants on ventilator support

- CT is often utilized to evaluate persistent PIE and differentiate from other neonatal causes of lucent lung masses
- CT findings: Air surrounds pulmonary arterial branches which are seen as soft tissue linear or dot-like densities surrounded by abnormal gas collections
  - This pattern of central linear and dot-like densities is characteristic for PIE
  - Characteristic pattern seen in 82% of patients with persistent PIE
  - Helps to differentiate persistent PIE from other hyperlucent lung masses in children such as congenital lobar emphysema, cystic adenomatoid malformation

DIFFERENTIAL DIAGNOSIS

Partially Treated Surfactant Deficiency Disease (SDD)
- With treatment of SDD with exogenous surfactant, there may be partial clearing of collapsed alveoli
- Pattern of alternating distended and collapsed acini may mimic pulmonary interstitial emphysema
- Important to know timing of surfactant therapy in relationship to time of radiograph

Developing Bronchopulmonary Dysplasia (Chronic Lung Disease)
- Bubble-like lucencies that are seen with developing bronchopulmonary dysplasia (BPD) can appear similar to PIE
- Age is helpful: PIE typically occurs during first week of life, BPD later
- Acuteness of onset: PIE is abrupt, BPD changes are gradual

Congenital Cystic Adenomatoid Malformation (CCAM)
- Typically present at birth
- Cysts often more variable in size and static
- PIE more transient and most typical bubble-like lucencies are small

Congenital Lobar Emphysema
- Typically seen at birth
- May present as fluid density on initial radiographs
- Generalized lucency of entire lobe rather than small focal lucencies seen with PIE

Congenital Diaphragmatic Hernia
- Not commonly confused with PIE
- Large lucencies with bowel-like appearance in chest
- Typically seen immediately after birth
- Position of support apparatus helpful
- Paucity of gas in abdomen

PATHOLOGY

General Features
- General path comments
  - Barotrauma results in increased alveolar pressure and alveolar rupture
  - Rupture of overdistended pulmonary alveoli leads to entry of air into pulmonary interstitium
  - Air escape into adjacent lung interstitium and lymphatics is referred to as pulmonary interstitial emphysema
  - Air is distributed along bronchovascular structures and appears on radiography as radiolucent bubble-like and linear densities
  - Air may further dissect and lead to pneumothorax or pneumomediastinum

CLINICAL ISSUES

Presentation
- Most common signs/symptoms: Usually asymptomatic
- Other signs/symptoms: Difficulty with ventilation secondary to development of pneumothorax
- Typically presents on routine neonatal unit radiographs prior to symptoms

PULMONARY INTERSTITIAL EMPHYSEMA, PEDIATRIC

- Serves as a warning sign for other pending air block complications: Pneumothorax, pneumomediastinum
- Presence influences care givers to alter support: Switching from conventional to high-frequency ventilation
- Usually occurs during first several days of life
- Almost always during first week of life
- Almost always occurs only in infants on ventilator support
- Usually is transient

Demographics
- Age
  - Premature infants
  - Usually during first days of life

Natural History & Prognosis
- Usually transient
- Can develop into persistent PIE

Treatment
- Often switching from conventional to high-frequency ventilation
- Increased frequency of clinical and radiographic monitoring for air-block complications such as pneumothorax
- For persistent pulmonary interstitial emphysema
  - Conservative management initial therapy
  - High frequency ventilation
  - Decubitus positioning with affected side down
  - Selective intubation of opposite lung
  - Surgery reserved for unmanageable respiratory distress
  - In one series, 53% of patients with persistent PIE required surgical resection

DIAGNOSTIC CHECKLIST

Consider
- Consider age of patient and rapidity of development to differentiate PIE from developing bronchopulmonary dysplasia

SELECTED REFERENCES
1. Corbett HJ et al: Pulmonary sequestration. Paediatr Respir Rev. 5(1):59-68, 2004
2. Johnson AM et al: Congenital anomalies of the fetal/neonatal chest. Semin Roentgenol. 39(2):197-214, 2004
3. Donnelly LF et al: CT findings and temporal course of persistent pulmonary interstitial emphysema in neonates: a multiinstitutional study. AJR Am J Roentgenol. 180(4):1129-33, 2003
4. Donnelly LF: Fundamentals of Pediatric Radiology. Philadelphia; W.B. Saunders, 2001
5. Frerking I et al: Pulmonary surfactant: functions, abnormalities and therapeutic options. Intensive Care Med. 27(11):1699-717, 2001
6. Suresh GK et al: Current surfactant use in premature infants. Clin Perinatol. 28(3):671-94, 2001
7. Khatua S et al: Advances in management of meconium aspiration syndrome. Indian J Pediatr. 67(11):837-41, 2000
8. Cohen MC et al: Solitary unilocular cyst of the lung with features of persistent interstitial pulmonary emphysema: report of four cases. Pediatr Dev Pathol. 2(6):531-6, 1999
9. Donnelly LF: Localized radiolucent chest lesions in neonates: causes and differentiation. AJR Am J Roentgenol. 172(6):1651-8, 1999
10. Newman B: Imaging of medical disease of the newborn lung. Radiol Clin North Am. 37(6):1049-65, 1999
11. Ogawa Y et al: Strategy for the prevention and treatment of chronic lung disease of the premature infant. Pediatr Pulmonol Suppl. 18:212-5, 1999
12. Agrons GA et al: Lung disease in premature neonates: impact of new treatments and technologies. Semin Roentgenol. 33(2):101-16, 1998
13. Breysem L et al: Bronchopulmonary dysplasia: correlation of radiographic and clinical findings. Pediatr Radiol. 27(8):642-6, 1997
14. Jabra AA et al: Localized persistent pulmonary interstitial emphysema: CT findings with radiographic-pathologic correlation. AJR Am J Roentgenol. 169(5):1381-4, 1997
15. Cleveland RH: A radiologic update on medical diseases of the newborn chest. Pediatr Radiol. 25(8):631-7, 1995
16. Wood BP: The newborn chest. Radiol Clin North Am. 31(3):667-76, 1993
17. Azizkhan RG et al: Acquired lobar emphysema (overinflation): clinical and pathological evaluation of infants requiring lobectomy. J Pediatr Surg. 27(8):1145-51; discussion 1151-2, 1992
18. Schneider JR et al: The changing spectrum of cystic pulmonary lesions requiring surgical resection in infants. J Thorac Cardiovasc Surg. 89(3):332-9, 1985

PULMONARY INTERSTITIAL EMPHYSEMA, PEDIATRIC

IMAGE GALLERY

Typical

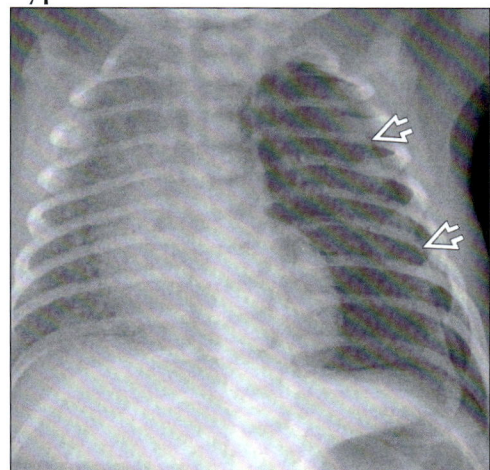
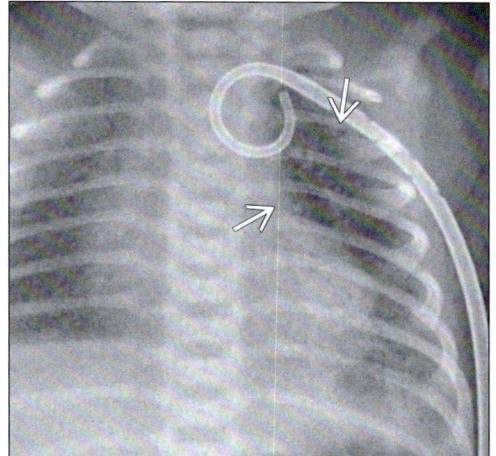

(Left) Frontal radiograph shows left pneumothorax ➡ and bubble-like lucencies in left lung consistent with PIE. *(Right)* Frontal radiograph in same patient as previous image after chest tube placement, shows persistent bubble-like lucencies ➡ in left upper lobe and resolution of pneumothorax.

Typical

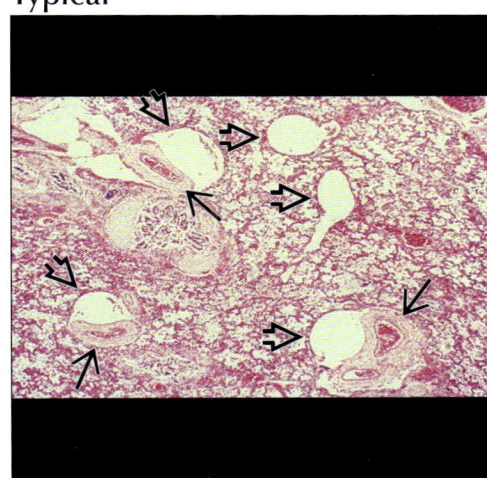
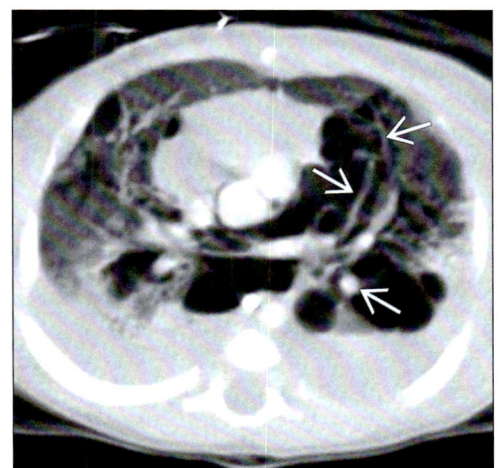

(Left) Microscopic image shows PIE as gas collections ➡ in pulmonary interstitium and lymphatics. Gas surrounds bronchial arteries ➡. *(Right)* Axial CECT shows lucencies in central portion of lung with gas surrounding vascular structures ➡: Consistent with PIE. Vascular structures appear as soft tissue density lines or dots depending upon orientation of CT plane to vessel.

Typical

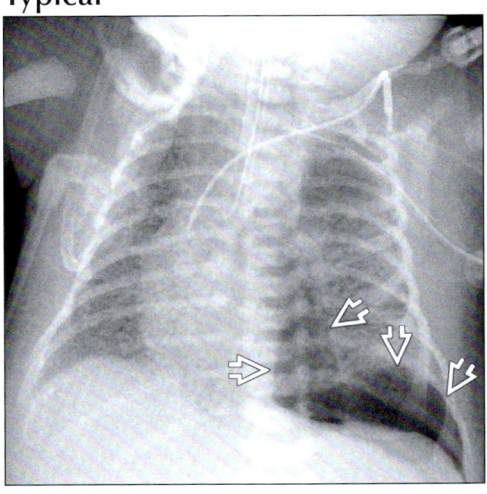
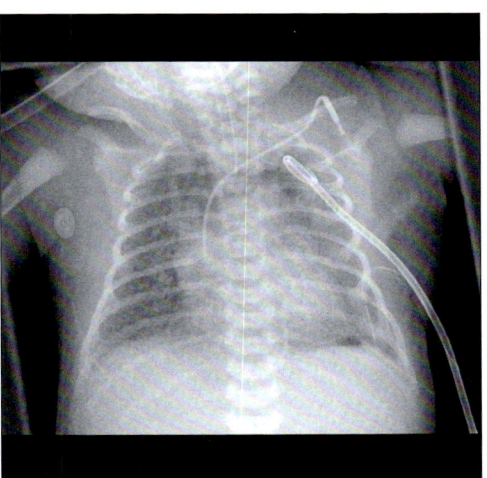

(Left) Frontal radiograph shows bubble-like lucencies throughout the bilateral hemithoraces consistent with PIE. There is also a pneumothorax on the left ➡. *(Right)* Frontal radiograph after chest tube placement in same patient as previous image, shows resolution of pneumothorax but persistent PIE, as bubble-like lucencies, now predominantly on right.

DIFFUSE ALVEOLAR HEMORRHAGE

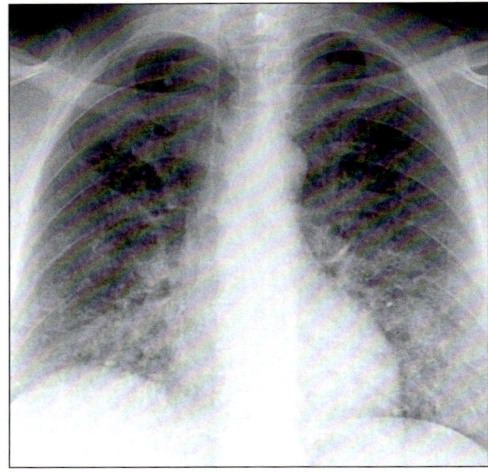

Frontal radiograph shows poorly-defined perihilar opacities. The heart size is normal.

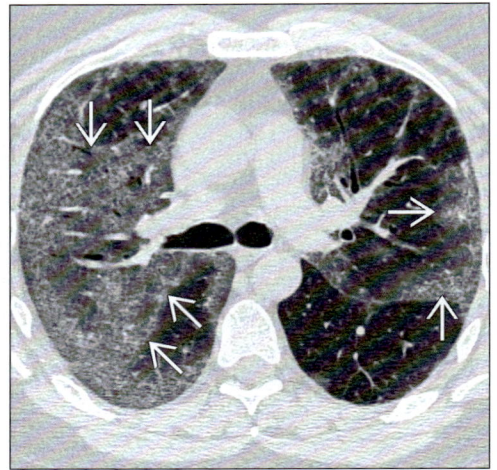

Axial HRCT shows asymmetric ground-glass opacities predominantly on the right ➡.

TERMINOLOGY

Abbreviations and Synonyms
- Diffuse alveolar hemorrhage (DAH), Wegener granulomatosis (WG), idiopathic pulmonary hemosiderosis (IPH), microscopic polyangiitis (MP), systemic lupus erythematosus (SLE)

Definitions
- Pulmonary hemorrhage that originates from alveolar capillaries
  - Classifications based on immune status, immune complexes, histology or presence of glomerulonephritis (pulmonary-renal syndrome)
- Must rule out aspiration of blood from localized source
  - Sources include bronchiectasis, angiosarcoma or Kaposi sarcoma, infections (angioinvasive aspergillosis), nasal, esophageal varices aspiration

IMAGING FINDINGS

General Features
- Best diagnostic clue: Acute onset of bilateral consolidation with apical sparing in an anemic patient

Radiographic Findings
- May be normal, abnormal radiographic findings not specific
- Acute bilateral consolidation with apical sparing
  - Typically perihilar distribution (bat-wing)
  - Consolidation may be focal or asymmetric
- Pleural effusions rare
- Prominent Kerley B lines: Consider mitral stenosis
- Resolution variable from 48 hours to several days
  - Consolidation evolves into interstitial pattern (Kerley lines)
  - Radiograph returns to normal
- Chronic bleeding or recurrent episodes may result in permanent reticular opacities (from fibrosis)
- 1st manifestation usually airspace (consolidation or ground-glass opacities)
  - May begin as reticulonodular interstitial thickening, especially in BMT

DDx: Perihilar Consolidation

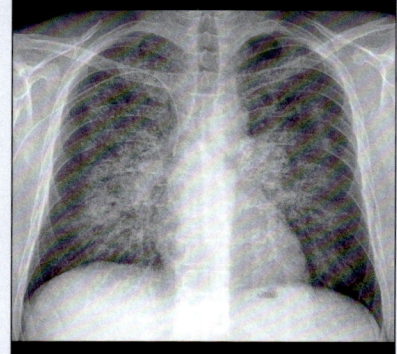

Acute Pulmonary Edema

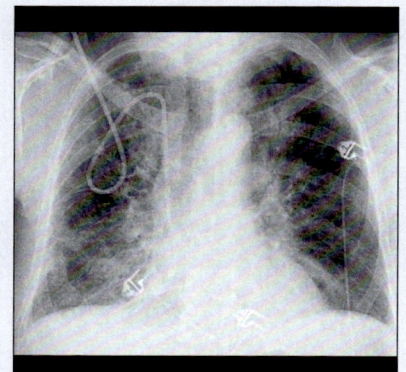

Noncardiac Pulmonary Edema

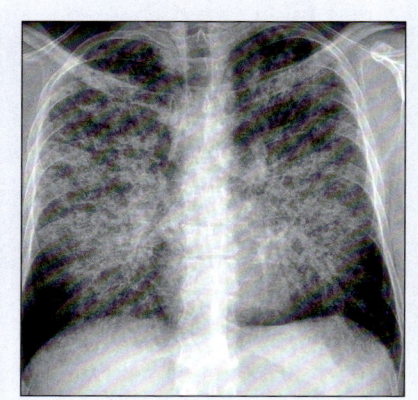

PCP Pneumonia

DIFFUSE ALVEOLAR HEMORRHAGE

Key Facts

Terminology
- Pulmonary hemorrhage that originates from alveolar capillaries

Imaging Findings
- Acute bilateral consolidation with apical sparing
- Resolution variable from 48 hours to several days
- Consolidation evolves into interstitial pattern (Kerley lines)
- Chronic bleeding or recurrent episodes may result in permanent reticular opacities (from fibrosis)

Top Differential Diagnoses
- Cardiogenic Pulmonary Edema
- Non-Cardiogenic Pulmonary Edema
- Pulmonary Infection: Viral or Pneumocystis

Pathology
- Hemorrhage in airspaces and hemosiderin-laden macrophages in airspaces and interstitium
- Hemosiderin appears within 48 hours after bleeding
- Anticoagulation rare cause of hemorrhage

Clinical Issues
- Cough, hemoptysis (66%), dyspnea, and decreased hemoglobin
- Iron deficiency anemia in chronic hemorrhage
- Bronchoalveolar lavage: Progressive bloody aliquots with hemosiderin macrophages

Diagnostic Checklist
- Evolution from airspace pattern (ground-glass, consolidation) to interstitial pattern (Kerley lines)

- Localized hemorrhage source
  - Focal abnormality (mass, cavity, atelectasis, consolidation) 60%

CT Findings
- HRCT
  - Radiographic findings not specific
  - Acute hemorrhage
    - Lobular ground-glass opacities to dense consolidation
    - Edge of opacity typically ground-glass
    - Ground-glass opacities and consolidation usually admixed
    - High density from acute hemorrhage rare
    - Opacities tend to be gravity dependent
    - Prominent segmental and subsegmental bronchi (dark bronchus sign)
    - Spares costophrenic angles and lung periphery
    - Prominent septal lines suggest underlying mitral stenosis or leukemic pulmonary involvement
    - Pleural effusions and mediastinal adenopathy rare
    - Heart size normal
  - Resolution
    - Over 24-48 hours develop interlobular & intralobular interstitial thickening superimposed on ground-glass opacities (crazy paving pattern)
    - Complete resolution from 48 hours to days
  - Interlude between hemorrhage
    - Ill-defined 1-3 mm centrilobular nodules from intraalveolar accumulation of macrophages
    - Nodules diffuse, no zonal predominance
  - Chronic hemorrhage
    - Interlobular thickening with traction bronchiectasis
    - Interstitial thickening may have nodular calcification (from hemosiderosis, especially in long-standing mitral stenosis)

MR Findings
- No important role in the evaluation of DAH
- Intermediate signal on T1 weighted sequences and low signal on T2 weighted (iron susceptibility effect)
  - Pulmonary edema and pneumonia often demonstrate high signal on T2

Imaging Recommendations
- Best imaging tool
  - Chest radiograph usually sufficient for detection
  - HRCT: More sensitive and possibly more specific

DIFFERENTIAL DIAGNOSIS

Cardiogenic Pulmonary Edema
- Cardiomegaly, bilateral gravity-dependent opacities, septal thickening and pleural effusions
  - Resolves rapidly with therapy
- Hemorrhage will not shift with gravity (gravitational shift test) as opposed to edema

Non-Cardiogenic Pulmonary Edema
- Septal lines less common
- Favors lung periphery

Pulmonary Infection: Viral or Pneumocystis
- Fever, chills, productive cough and elevated white blood cell count common
- Evolution from consolidation to a reticular pattern unusual

PATHOLOGY

General Features
- General path comments
  - Hemorrhage in airspaces and hemosiderin-laden macrophages in airspaces and interstitium
    - Hemosiderin appears within 48 hours after bleeding
- Etiology
  - Pathologic correlation
    - Hemorrhage into alveolar spaces (ground-glass opacities to consolidation)
    - Blood removed from alveoli by macrophages (2-3 days)

DIFFUSE ALVEOLAR HEMORRHAGE

- Macrophages migrate into interstitium (septal thickening)
- Macrophages removed by lymphatics (7-14 days) (lung returns to normal)
- Repeat or chronic hemorrhage: Mild to moderate fibrosis, hemosiderosis
- Epidemiology
  - Most common cause
    - Wegener (33%)
    - Goodpasture (15%)
    - SLE (15%)
    - Idiopathic pulmonary hemosiderosis (15%)
    - Microscopic polyangiitis (10%)
  - Anticoagulation rare cause of hemorrhage

Microscopic Features

- Bland pulmonary hemorrhage: Underlying lung preserved, no inflammatory cells
  - Coagulation disorders, especially disseminated intravascular coagulation or thrombocytopenic purpura
  - Mital stenosis
  - Idiopathic pulmonary hemosiderosis
- Pulmonary capillaritis: Neutrophils infiltrate interstitium, neutrophils die (leukocytoclasis) and fragment leaving nuclear fragments (dust) accumulating within lung
  - Goodpasture syndrome
  - Microscopic polyangiitis
  - Wegener
  - SLE
  - Henoch-Schönlein purpura
  - Cryoglobulinemia
  - Pauci-immune pulmonary capillaritis
  - Acute pulmonary allograft rejection
  - Drug-induced
    - Phenytoin, penicillamine, propylthiouracil
- Diffuse alveolar damage: Edema and hyaline membrane formation
  - Crack cocaine inhalation
  - BMT

Staging, Grading or Classification Criteria

- Immunocompetent host
  - Goodpasture, SLE, Wegener, IPH, coagulation disorders, drug reactions
- Immunocompromised host
  - Idiopathic diseases, leukemia, bone marrow transplantation

CLINICAL ISSUES

Presentation

- Most common signs/symptoms
  - Cough, hemoptysis (66%), dyspnea, and decreased hemoglobin
    - Hemoptysis may be mild even with massive hemorrhage
  - Iron deficiency anemia in chronic hemorrhage
  - Bronchoalveolar lavage: Progressive bloody aliquots with hemosiderin macrophages
- Other signs/symptoms: C-ANCA positive in 85-98% of patients with active Wegener granulomatosis
- Goodpasture syndrome
  - May follow influenza-illness
  - Usually seen in smokers
- Wegener granulomatosis
  - Hemorrhage presentation 8%
  - Occurs in absence of typical cavitary nodules
- Microscopic polyangiitis
  - Small vessel variant of polyarteritis nodosa
  - Hemorrhage in 10-30%
  - Glomerulonephritis 80-100%
  - P-ANCA 80%
- SLE
  - Renal involvement in 60-90% of patients
  - Hemorrhage 2%, usually occurs in those with already established disease
- BMT
  - Usually occurs during the marrow engraftment period (10-21 days following transplant)
- Idiopathic pulmonary hemosiderosis
  - May be associated with celiac disease
  - Diagnosis of exclusion, older reports probably misclassified

Demographics

- Age: IPH usually < 15 yo, Goodpasture syndrome often young adults, MP mean age 55 yo and Wegener most common 30-55 yo
- Gender
  - Goodpasture syndrome male predominance (9:1)
  - SLE female predominance (70%) also MP (1.5:1)

Natural History & Prognosis

- Survival 50%: IPH and SLE, 70% for microscopic polyangiitis
- Wegener granulomatosis has a 90% mortality if untreated, but up to 75% will experience complete remission following therapy

Treatment

- Options, risks, complications: Lung biopsy usually not necessary or helpful
- 50% of hemorrhagic episodes result in respiratory failure severe enough to require mechanical ventilation
- Immune complex diseases and inflammatory vasculitis
  - Immunosuppression: Especially cytotoxic drugs
  - Corticosteroid therapy
  - Plasmapheresis to remove circulating antibodies

DIAGNOSTIC CHECKLIST

Image Interpretation Pearls

- Evolution from airspace pattern (ground-glass, consolidation) to interstitial pattern (Kerley lines)

SELECTED REFERENCES

1. Marten et al: Pattern-based differential diagnosis in pulmonary vasculitis using volumetric CT. AJR. 184:720-33, 2005
2. Hansell D: Small-vessel diseases of the lung: CT-pathologic correlates. Radiology. 225:639-53, 2002

DIFFUSE ALVEOLAR HEMORRHAGE

IMAGE GALLERY

Typical

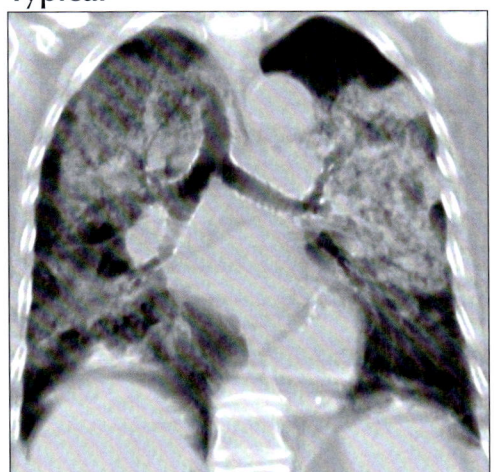 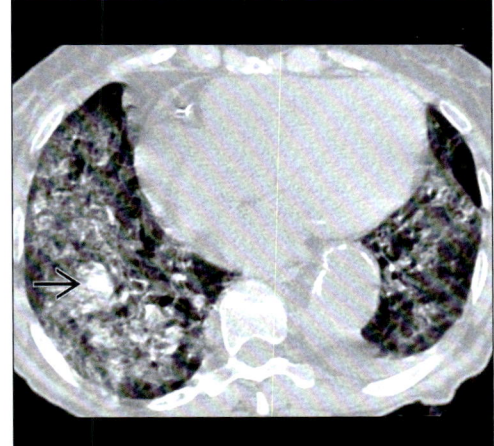

(Left) Coronal NECT shows distribution of perihilar (bat-wing) consolidation from diffuse hemorrhage. *(Right)* Axial NECT shows diffuse ground-glass opacities and focal consolidation ➡. Patient had hemoptysis and anemia.

Typical

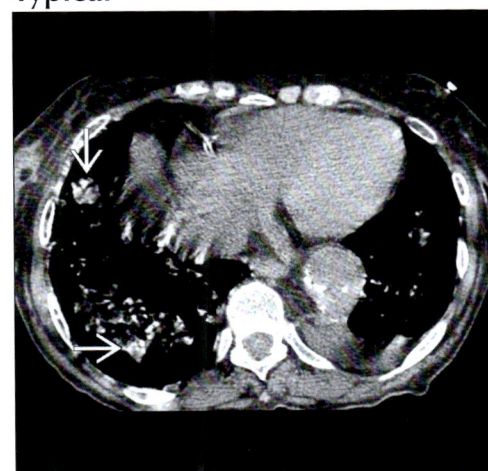 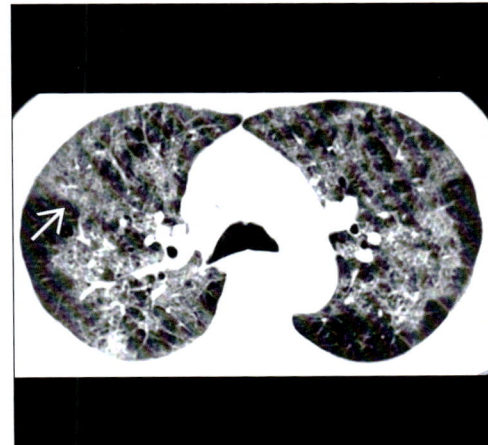

(Left) Axial NECT in same patient as previous image shows high density consolidation ➡ from acute hemorrhage. High density opacities from acute hemorrhage unusual radiographic finding. *(Right)* Axial NECT in a different patient with diffuse alveolar hemorrhage shows geographic distribution of ground-glass opacities ➡ and intralobular interstitial thickening from subacute diffuse hemorrhage.

Typical

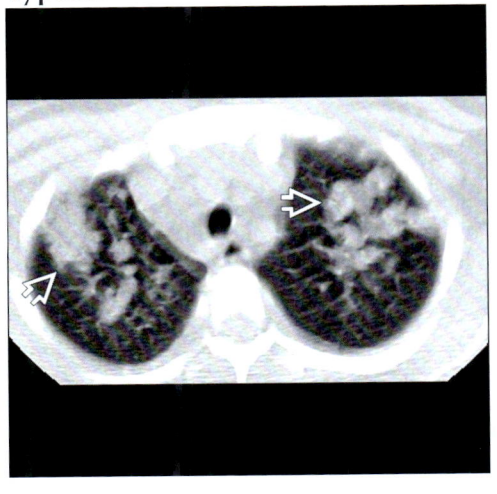 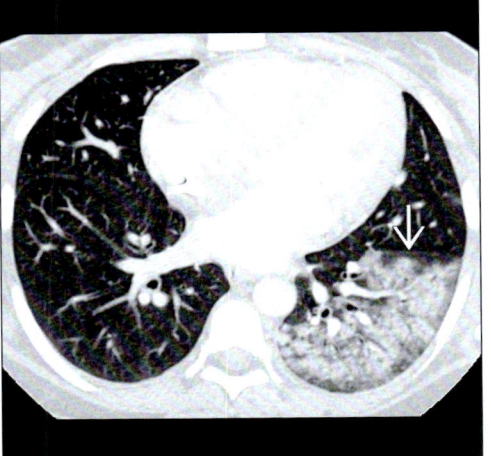

(Left) Axial NECT in patient with SLE shows lobular areas of consolidation ➡ from hemorrhage. *(Right)* Axial NECT 2 years later shows new area of hemorrhage in the left lower lobe ➡. Even with repeat hemorrhage, lung returned to normal.

VASCULITIS, PULMONARY

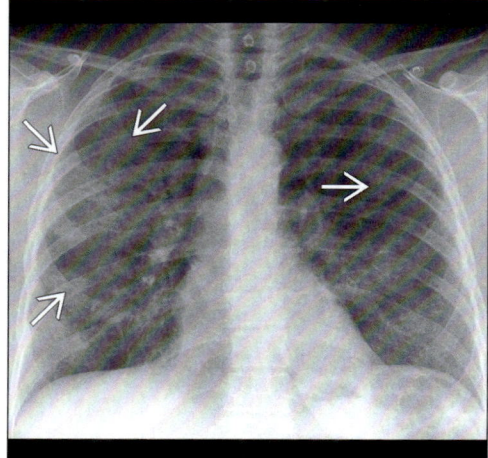

Frontal radiograph shows patchy areas of peripheral consolidation ➡. Normal lung volumes. History of asthma.

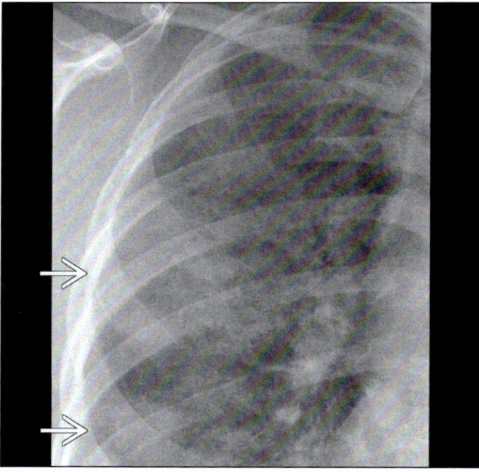

Frontal radiograph close-up shows homogeneous consolidation ➡ in the right upper lobe. Churg-Strauss vasculitis.

TERMINOLOGY

Abbreviations and Synonyms
- Diffuse alveolar hemorrhage (DAH), Wegener granulomatosis (WG), microscopic polyangiitis (MP), Churg-Strauss syndrome (CSS)

Definitions
- Vasculitis is inflammatory process involving blood vessels, lungs commonly affected because of large capillary bed
- Classified by smallest vessel involved: Large, medium, and small
  - Affects pulmonary arteries, capillaries, or veins
- Spectrum includes WG, Goodpasture disease and CSS, MP, Behçet disease, and Takayasu disease

IMAGING FINDINGS

General Features
- Best diagnostic clue: Pulmonary arterial hypertension in patient with diffuse alveolar hemorrhage

Radiographic Findings
- Radiography
  - Imaging features nonspecific
  - Large vessel vasculitis
    - Pulmonary artery aneurysms
  - Small and medium vessel vasculitis
    - Radiographic features of diffuse alveolar hemorrhage
    - Peripheral consolidation mirroring eosinophilic pneumonias
    - Multiple (often cavitary) nodules: Bilateral without zonal predominance, usually few in number (< 10), range up to 10 cm in diameter, thick irregular wall, air-fluid level uncommon
  - Pulmonary artery hypertension: Enlarged central pulmonary arteries with rapid tapering
    - Occurs with any size vessel vasculitis
  - Adenopathy rare
  - Kerley B lines uncommon
  - Pleural effusion variable, occur in 20% WG and 33% of CSS and Behçet syndrome

CT Findings
- Large vessel vasculitis

DDx: Peripheral Consolidation

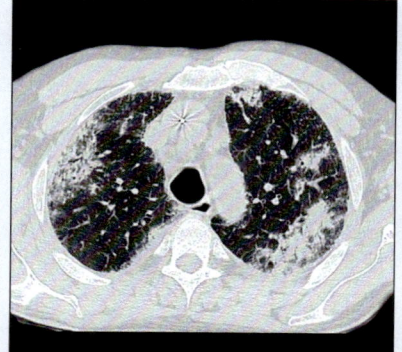

Eosinophilic Pneumonia

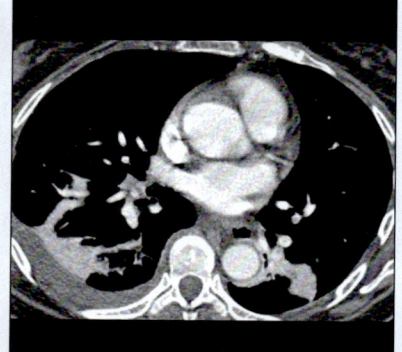

Pulmonary Infarction

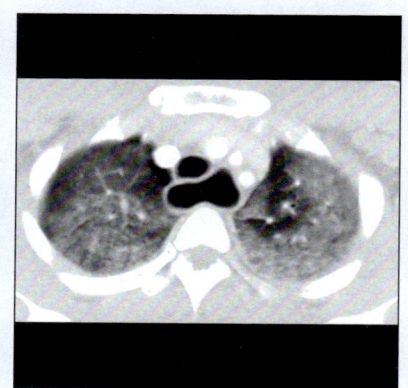

Neurogenic Pulmonary Edema

VASCULITIS, PULMONARY

Key Facts

Terminology
- Vasculitis is inflammatory process involving blood vessels, lungs commonly affected because of large capillary bed
- Spectrum includes WG, Goodpasture disease and CSS, MP, Behçet disease, and Takayasu disease

Imaging Findings
- Imaging features nonspecific

Top Differential Diagnoses
- Cardiogenic Pulmonary Edema
- Diffuse Pulmonary Infection
- Non-Cardiogenic Pulmonary Edema
- Chronic Pulmonary Emboli

Pathology
- Mixed and often nonspecific: Predominant cell types include granulomatous, eosinophilic, lymphoplasmacytic or neutrophilic

Clinical Issues
- ANCA useful to monitory disease activity
- Development pulmonary artery hypertension poor prognostic sign

Diagnostic Checklist
- Overlap features between vasculitis syndromes common
- Signs of pulmonary arterial hypertension superimposed on signs of diffuse alveolar hemorrhage highly suggestive of underlying vasculitis

---

  - Early: Pulmonary arterial wall thickening or irregularity and beading of arteries, wall may enhance with contrast administration
  - Late: Stenosis or aneurysms
  - Parenchymal: Mosaic oligemia or hemorrhage and infarction
- Small and medium vessel vasculitis
  - Alveolar hemorrhage
    - Diffuse lobular ground-glass opacities admixed with consolidation
    - Edge of opacity typically ground-glass
    - Gravity dependent distribution
    - Prominent segmental and subsegmental bronchi (dark bronchus sign)
    - Septal lines uncommon
    - Crazy-paving pattern (more common as hemorrhage resolves)
  - Eosinophilic pneumonia
    - Fleeting peripheral nonsegmental ground-glass opacities to consolidation
  - Tracheobronchial involvement
    - Wegener: Subglottic stenosis in 15%
  - Pulmonary arterial hypertension: Enlarged central arteries with distal pruning

Imaging Recommendations
- Best imaging tool: HRCT: More sensitive and specific
- Protocol advice: Chest radiographs usually suffice to monitor for complications and disease relapse

DIFFERENTIAL DIAGNOSIS

Cardiogenic Pulmonary Edema
- Cardiomegaly, bilateral gravity-dependent opacities, septal thickening and pleural effusions
  - Resolves rapidly with therapy

Diffuse Pulmonary Infection
- Fever, chills, productive cough and elevated white blood cell count common
- Requires culture to exclude

Non-Cardiogenic Pulmonary Edema
- Septal lines uncommon
- Favors lung periphery
- Usually severely hypoxemic, requiring mechanical ventilation

Chronic Pulmonary Emboli
- Pulmonary artery hypertension
- Central pulmonary artery walls thickened by chronic thrombus, usually much thicker than thickened walls from vasculitis
- No systemic symptoms

Cryptogenic Organizing Pneumonia
- Peripheral basilar rounded opacities
- Opacities may be migratory

PATHOLOGY

General Features
- General path comments
  - Pulmonary vasculitis usually part of systemic process
    - Idiopathic pauci-immune pulmonary capillaritis: Isolated to lung without systemic vasculitis
- Etiology
  - Unknown: May be autoimmune or response to infection or an environmental insult
  - Antineutrophil cytoplasmic antibodies (ANCA) circulating autoantibodies, titers directly reflect disease activity
    - C-ANCA: Proteinase-3 (Wegener)
    - p-ANCA: Perinuclear (Churg-Strauss, microscopic polyangiitis)
  - Wegener granulomatosis
    - Ear nose throat (ENT) symptoms 75% at presentation, eventually in 90%: Sinusitis, nasal stuffiness, otitis media, ear pain, oral ulcers
    - Pulmonary involvement (nodules often cavitary) 50% at presentation, during course 85%
    - Glomerulonephritis 20% at presentation, during course 80%

VASCULITIS, PULMONARY

- Churg-Strauss syndrome (allergic granulomatosis)
  - Medium and small vessel vasculitis
  - Asthmatics with eosinophilia
  - Cardiac: Pericarditis, myocarditis common
- Microscopic polyangiitis (MPA)
  - Affects kidneys, peripheral nerves, skin, and lungs
  - Small vessel variant of polyarteritis nodosa
  - Hemorrhage in 10-30%
  - Glomerulonephritis 80-100%
  - p-ANCA positive 80%
- Behçet disease
  - Widespread involvement of large and small vessels
  - Pulmonary aneurysms that may hemorrhage
  - Thromboemboli and superior vena cava thrombosis
  - Recurrent oral or genital ulcers
  - Hughes-Stovin syndrome: Variant of Behçet, does not have oral or genital ulcers
- Takayasu disease
  - Large vessel vasculitis of aorta and occasionally pulmonary arteries
  - Granulomatous inflammation
- Polyarteritis nodosa
  - "CLASH" associations: Cryoglobulinemia, hairy cell leukemia, rheumatoid arthritis, Sjögren syndrome, hepatitis B
- Infection
  - Hepatitis B and C and human immunodeficiency virus (HIV) sometimes associated with vasculitis
- Epidemiology
  - Incidence: 20-100 cases/million
  - Prevalence: 150-450 cases/million
  - Behçet disease common in Turkey and Asia
  - Takayasu disease common in Asia

Gross Pathologic & Surgical Features
- Mixed and often nonspecific: Predominant cell types include granulomatous, eosinophilic, lymphoplasmacytic or neutrophilic
- Classified by vessel size: Large, medium, and small
  - Large: Aorta and largest arterial branches
    - Takayasu arteritis, temporal (giant cell) arteritis
  - Medium: Main visceral arteries (renal, coronary, mesenteric)
    - Churg-Strauss, polyarteritis nodosa, Kawasaki
  - Small: Capillaries, venules, arterioles
    - Wegener granulomatosis, Churg-Strauss syndrome, microscopic polyangiitis
- Small-vessel vasculitides
  - Antineutrophil cytoplasmic antibody (ANCA) positive
    - Wegener granulomatosis
    - Churg-Strauss syndrome
    - Microscopic pulmonary angiitis

Microscopic Features
- Often nonspecific inflammatory cells in walls of arteries with variable thrombosis

CLINICAL ISSUES

Presentation
- Most common signs/symptoms
  - Clinical scenarios suggestive of vasculitis
    - Diffuse alveolar hemorrhage: Hemoptysis (80%), anemia
    - Acute glomerulonephritis
    - Pulmonary-renal syndrome
    - Destructive upper airway lesions
    - Palpable purpura
    - Mononeuritis multiplex
  - Organs commonly involved in vasculitis: Skin, joints, muscles, gastrointestinal tract, peripheral and central nervous system and the eye
- Other signs/symptoms
  - Sedimentation rate often elevated (normal does not rule out vasculitis)
  - ANCA useful to monitory disease activity
  - Anemia common with hemorrhage

Demographics
- Age: Any
- Gender: Takayasu disease much more common in women

Natural History & Prognosis
- Variable, depends on underlying illness
- Waxing and waning common, 50% with ANCA vasculitis suffer one or more flares despite therapy (most common with WG)
- Development pulmonary artery hypertension poor prognostic sign

Treatment
- Corticosteroids and immunosuppressant cytotoxic agents

DIAGNOSTIC CHECKLIST

Consider
- Overlap features between vasculitis syndromes common
- In presence of unexplained nodular or cavitary disease

Image Interpretation Pearls
- Signs of pulmonary arterial hypertension superimposed on signs of diffuse alveolar hemorrhage highly suggestive of underlying vasculitis

SELECTED REFERENCES

1. Brown KK: Pulmonary vasculitis. Proc Am Thorac Soc. 3(1):48-57, 2006
2. Manganelli P et al: Respiratory system involvement in systemic vasculitides. Clin Exp Rheumatol. 24(2 Suppl 41):S48-59, 2006
3. Deane KD et al: Antiphospholipid antibodies as a cause of pulmonary capillaritis and diffuse alveolar hemorrhage: a case series and literature review. Semin Arthritis Rheum. 35(3):154-65, 2005
4. Pesci A et al: Respiratory system involvement in ANCA-associated systemic vasculitides. Sarcoidosis Vasc Diffuse Lung Dis. 22 Suppl 1:S40-8, 2005
5. Ravenel JG et al: Pulmonary vasculitis: CT features. Semin Respir Crit Care Med. 24(4):427-36, 2003
6. Hansell DM: Small-vessel diseases of the lung: CT-pathologic correlates. Radiology. 225(3):639-53, 2002
7. Burns A: Pulmonary vasculitis. Thorax. 53(3):220-7, 1998

VASCULITIS, PULMONARY

IMAGE GALLERY

Typical

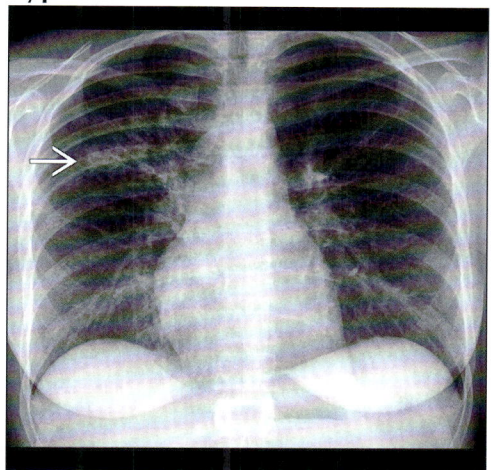
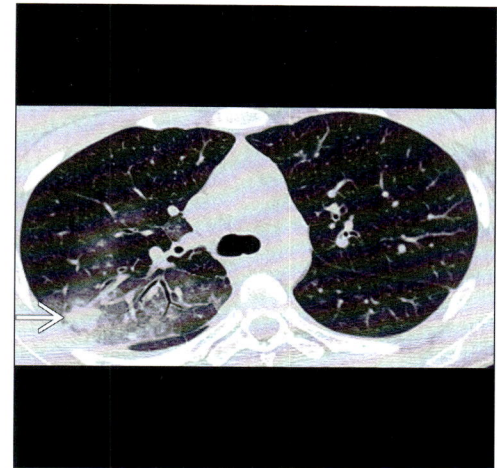

(Left) Frontal radiograph shows nonspecific focal consolidation ➡ in the right upper lobe. Patient has a genital ulcer. *(Right)* Axial CECT shows ground glass and nodular consolidation centered on pulmonary arteries ➡. Behçet vasculitis.

Typical

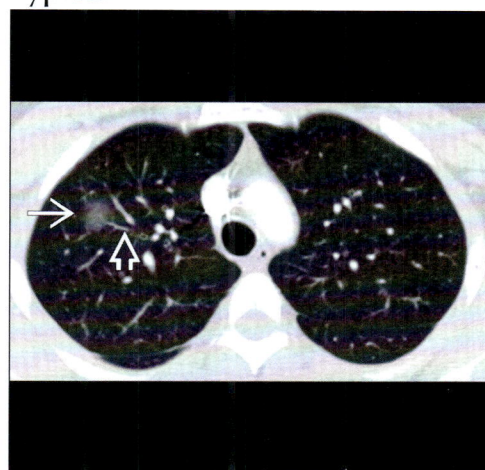
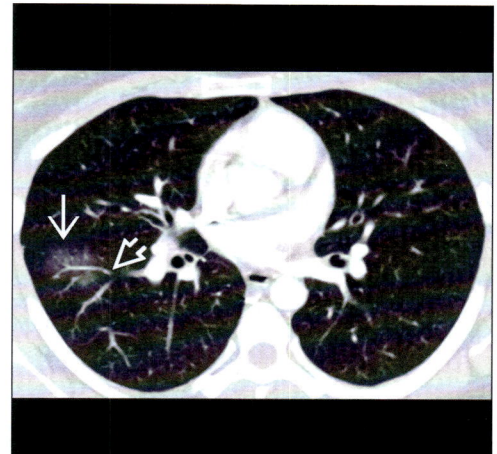

(Left) Axial CECT shows focal ground-glass opacities ➡ centered on pulmonary vessels ⇨. *(Right)* Axial CECT shows focal ground-glass opacities ➡ centered on pulmonary vessels ⇨. Associated glomerulonephritis. Diagnosis: Microscopic polyangiitis.

Typical

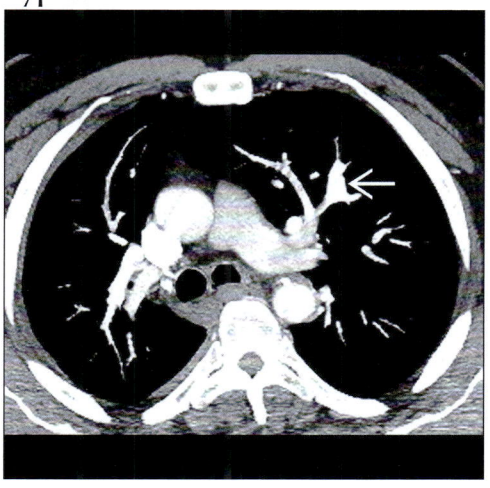
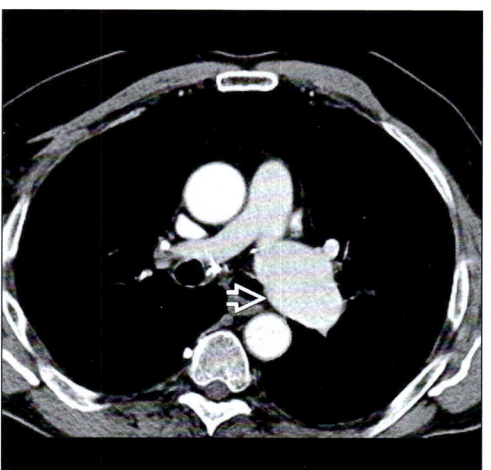

(Left) Axial CECT shows aneurysms in segmental sized pulmonary arteries ➡ probably mycotic etiology or large vessel vasculitis. Patient had multiple aneurysms. *(Right)* Axial CECT shows aneurysmal dilatation left pulmonary artery ➡. Hugh-Stovin syndrome.

SICKLE CELL, ACUTE CHEST SYNDROME

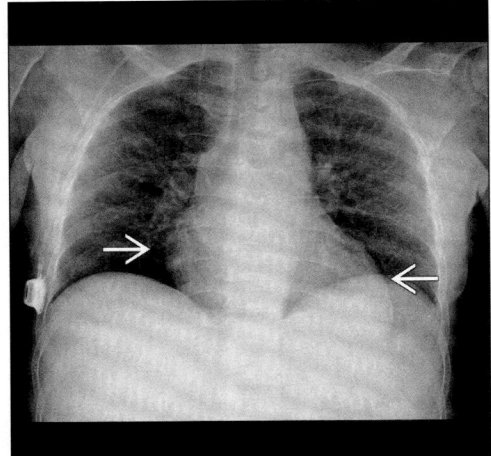

Frontal radiograph shows mild cardiomegaly ➡. Spleen absent. Long term indwelling catheter for transfusions and IV hydration.

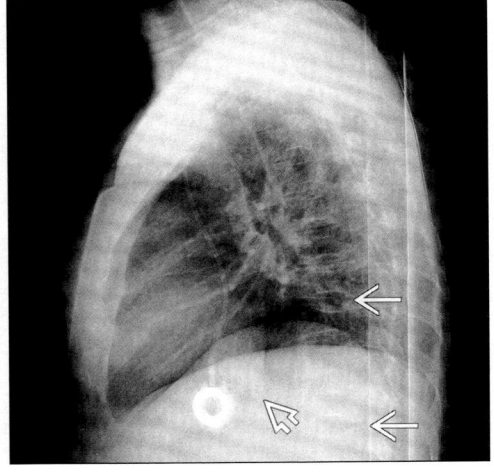

Lateral radiograph shows mild cardiomegaly ➡ and typical end-plate changes ➡ from sickle cell disease. Multiple episodes of ACS but lungs normal.

TERMINOLOGY

Abbreviations and Synonyms
- Acute chest syndrome (ACS), sickle cell disease (Hb SS)

Definitions
- Sickle cell disease due to abnormal hemoglobin which deforms when deoxygenated
- Appearance of new pulmonary opacity on chest radiograph accompanied by fever and respiratory symptoms (cough, tachypnea, and chest pain) in patient with Hb SS

IMAGING FINDINGS

General Features
- Best diagnostic clue: Pulmonary opacity in patient with Hb SS who has fever and respiratory symptoms
- Location: Lower lobes predominate
- Size: Variable extent of pulmonary opacification
- Morphology: Cardiomegaly and ill-defined air-space or interstitial opacities

Radiographic Findings
- Radiography
  - Lung parenchyma
    - Initial chest radiograph may be normal (50%)
    - Lobar, segmental, or subsegmental opacity due to pneumonia, atelectasis or infarct
    - Lower lobes predominate
    - Interstitial thickening due to acute edema or scarring from prior episodes of ACS
  - Pleura
    - Pleural effusions due to pneumonia, infarcts, or left heart failure
  - Heart
    - Cardiomegaly common due to chronic anemia and high output heart failure
  - Mediastinum
    - Posterior paraspinal mediastinal mass from extramedullary hematopoiesis
    - Unilateral or bilateral, smooth, sharply marginated
  - Skeletal
    - Avascular necrosis (AVN) humeral heads

DDx: Focal Pulmonary Airspace Opacities

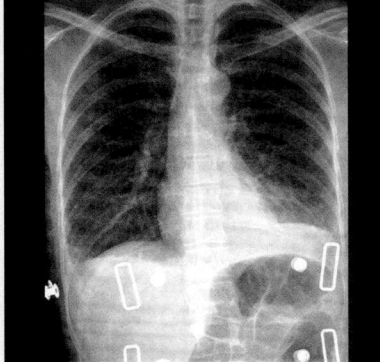

Pneumonia

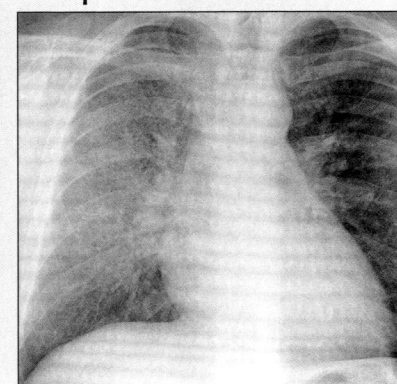

Hemorrhage

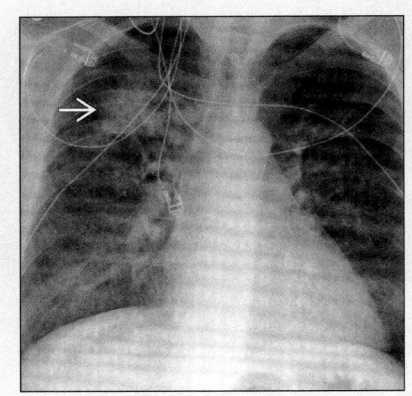

Mitral Regurgitant Pulmonary Edema

SICKLE CELL, ACUTE CHEST SYNDROME

Key Facts

Terminology
- Appearance of new pulmonary opacity on chest radiograph accompanied by fever and respiratory symptoms (cough, tachypnea, and chest pain) in patient with Hb SS

Imaging Findings
- Initial chest radiograph may be normal (50%)
- Lobar, segmental, or subsegmental opacity due to pneumonia, atelectasis or infarct
- Lower lobes predominate
- Cardiomegaly common due to chronic anemia and high output heart failure
- Avascular necrosis (AVN) humeral heads
- H-shaped vertebrae (10%): Step-off deformity superior and inferior endplates (Reynold sign)
- Small or absent spleen, may be calcified (autosplenectomy)
- Protocol advice: CT more sensitive for parenchymal changes but usually not necessary, excess radiation dose in the young

Pathology
- ACS: Pathogenesis multifactorial, exact cause rarely determined
- ACS occurs in up to 50% with Hb SS
- Recurrent episodes in 80%
- Children 100x more susceptible to pneumonia; recurrence rate 30%

Clinical Issues
- ACS: Difficult to distinguish infectious from noninfectious etiology

---

       - H-shaped vertebrae (10%): Step-off deformity superior and inferior endplates (Reynold sign)
       - Enlarged ribs due to marrow expansion
       - Bone sclerosis due to bone infarcts
     - Upper abdomen
       - Small or absent spleen, may be calcified (autosplenectomy)

CT Findings
- CT findings mirror those seen on chest radiography
- Mosaic perfusion due to microvascular occlusion
  - Geographic areas of hypoperfusion
    - Areas of decreased attenuation contain small vessels
  - Geographic areas of hyperperfusion
    - Areas of ground-glass opacities with normal-sized vessels (larger than those in areas of decreased attenuation)
    - Due to redistribution of flow to lung with less microvascular occlusion
  - Ground-glass opacities may also be due to hemorrhagic edema caused by reperfusion of ischemic lung
- CECT: High osmolarity contrast contraindicated which may induce sickling
- Acute chest syndrome sequelae
  - Parenchymal bands
  - Septal thickening
  - Peripheral wedge-shaped opacities
  - Architectural distortion
  - Traction bronchiectasis

Nuclear Medicine Findings
- Bone Scan
  - Often see foci of decreased or increased radiotracer uptake in ribs from bone infarction
  - Commonly see increased skull uptake
  - Increased spleen uptake due to calcification from autosplenectomy
  - Delayed renal uptake
- Tc-99m Sulfur Colloid: Will show uptake in extramedullary hematopoiesis
- V/Q Scan
  - Limited clinical use in ACS, findings resemble those of pulmonary emboli
    - Etiology may be sickling erythrocytes vs. pneumonia vs. fat emboli
    - Often resolve quickly with supportive therapy

Imaging Recommendations
- Best imaging tool: Chest radiographs usually suffice for evaluation and treatment
- Protocol advice: CT more sensitive for parenchymal changes but usually not necessary, excess radiation dose in the young

DIFFERENTIAL DIAGNOSIS

Chest Pain
- Pneumothorax
  - See visceral pleural line with lucency lateral to line
- Pulmonary edema related to high output heart failure
  - Opacities may be more diffuse and bilateral
  - May be radiographically indistinguishable
- Aspiration
  - Lower lobe opacities, similar to ACS
  - May resolve quickly, similar to ACS

H-Shaped Vertebra
- Gaucher disease
  - Spleen usually enlarged
- Paroxysmal nocturnal hemoglobinuria
  - Spleen normal, lung normal
- Alcoholism
  - Ribs may show bilateral rib fractures in various stages of healing
  - Portal hypertension may result in splenomegaly and paraspinal masses (from varices)

PATHOLOGY

General Features
- General path comments: Red blood cells sickle when deoxygenated

SICKLE CELL, ACUTE CHEST SYNDROME

- Genetics
  - Valine substitution for glutamic acid in hemoglobin beta subunit (Hb S)
    - Hb S has some protection from malaria
    - Normal hemoglobin (Hb A)
  - Sickle cell anemia (Hb SS)
    - Exposure to low oxygen tension → Hb S becomes less soluble and forms large polymers
    - Results in a distorted erythrocyte (sickle cell) → vaso-occlusion and hemolysis
  - May also occur in Hb SC, Hb SB°, Hb SB+
- Etiology
  - ACS: Pathogenesis multifactorial, exact cause rarely determined
    - Pneumonia and or infarctions from thrombosis or fat embolus
    - Rib infarction → pain → splinting → discoid atelectasis
    - Large vessel thrombosis possible but rare
  - Pneumonia
    - Documented in 30% of cases
    - More common cause of ACS in children
    - Most common pathogens: Chlamydia pneumoniae, Mycoplasma pneumoniae, respiratory syncytial virus
    - Pulmonary opacity persists longer than cases where infection not documented
    - Upper lobe consolidation more likely pneumonia because oxygen tension highest in upper lung zones due to high V/Q ratio
  - Pulmonary fat embolism
    - Emboli with fat and necrotic bone marrow in 10%
    - Frequently have bone pain, decreased hemoglobin and platelet count, increased plasma free fatty acids and phospholipase A2
    - Diagnosis supported by lipid-laden macrophages in bronchoalveolar lavage fluid
  - Rib infarction
    - High correlation between rib infarction and pulmonary opacity
    - Pain may result in splinting and atelectasis
    - Incentive spirometry may decrease atelectasis and prevent pulmonary complications of ACS
    - Analgesics may decrease splinting, but may cause hypoventilation
  - Left-ventricular dysfunction due to combination of
    - High output failure from anemia, especially when hemoglobin ≤ 7 gm/dL
    - Over-hydration with intravenous fluids may exacerbate
    - Fluid balance from renal insufficiency (from microinfarction of renal papilla)
  - Autosplenectomy: Impaired immunity due to functional asplenia
    - At risk for pneumonia from encapsulated organisms such as Streptococcus pneumoniae, Haemophilus influenzae
- Epidemiology
  - Hb SS most prevalent inherited disorder among African-Americans
    - Hb SS occurs in 0.15% African-American population
    - Hb SA in 8% African-American population
  - Average life expectancy 42 years for men and 48 years for women
  - Lung one of the major organs affected by Hb SS
  - ACS occurs in up to 50% with Hb SS
    - Recurrent episodes in 80%
    - Children 100x more susceptible to pneumonia; recurrence rate 30%

CLINICAL ISSUES

Presentation
- Most common signs/symptoms
  - ACS: Difficult to distinguish infectious from noninfectious etiology
    - Wheezing, cough, and fever most common in patients less than 10 years of age
    - Chest pain rare in pediatric age group
    - Fat embolism: Pulmonary findings preceded by bone pain
  - Adults: Dyspnea, arm and leg pain more common, frequently afebrile
- Other signs/symptoms: Hyper-reactive airway disease 40% children

Natural History & Prognosis
- ACS: Leading cause of death in Hb SS
  - Responsible for up to 25% of deaths
  - > 20% Have fatal pulmonary complications, thromboembolus seen in 25% of autopsies
  - Second most common cause of hospitalization in Hb SS patients
- Recurrent ACS long term sequelae
  - Sickle cell chronic lung disease 5%
  - High output cardiac failure
  - Pulmonary artery hypertension: 33%
    - Late in natural history of sickle cell disease

Treatment
- Supportive, because the cause remains largely unknown
  - Oxygen and adequate hydration
    - Overhydration may lead to pulmonary edema
  - Pain control
  - Incentive spirometry
  - Antibiotics for presumed pneumonia
  - Bronchodilators
  - Blood transfusions
  - Bronchodilators for hyper-reactive airway disease
- Prevention
  - Pneumococcal and Haemophilus influenza vaccination
    - At higher risk for pneumonia from encapsulated organisms because of poor or absent splenic function

SELECTED REFERENCES
1. Delclaux C et al: Factors associated with dyspnea in adult patients with sickle cell disease. Chest. 128(5):3336-44, 2005
2. Maitre B et al: Acute chest syndrome in adults with sickle cell disease. Chest. 117(5):1386-92, 2000

SICKLE CELL, ACUTE CHEST SYNDROME

IMAGE GALLERY

Typical

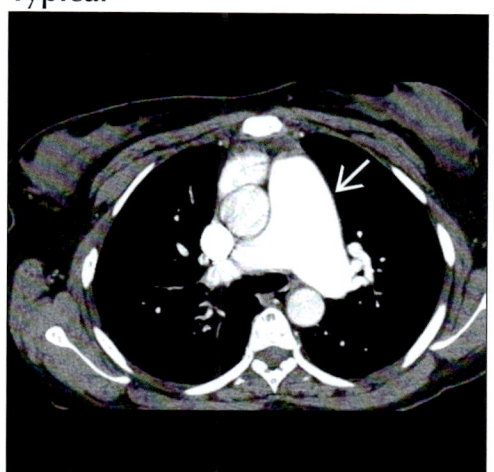
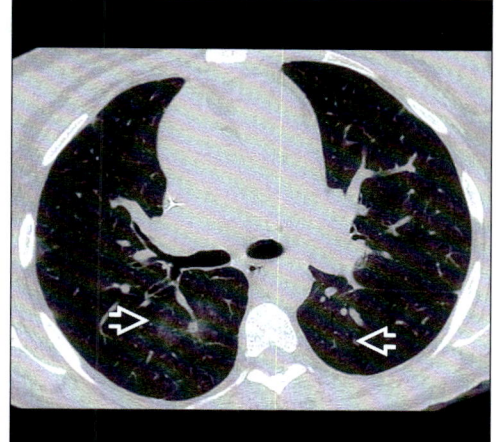

(Left) Axial CECT shows enlarged central pulmonary artery ➡. Patient with sickle cell disease. *(Right)* Axial HRCT mosaic attenuation ➡ from vascular disease. Ground-glass lung normal or hyperperfused lung. Chronic microvascular occlusion resulting in pulmonary arterial hypertension.

Typical

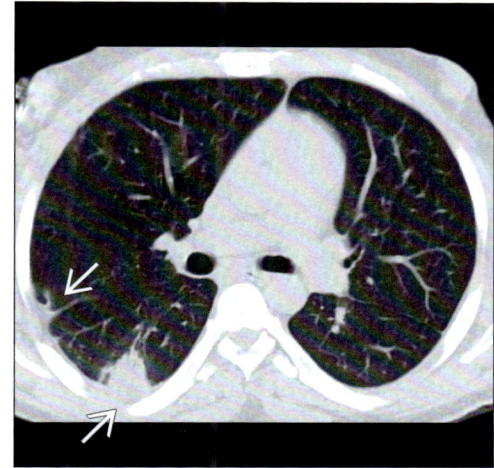
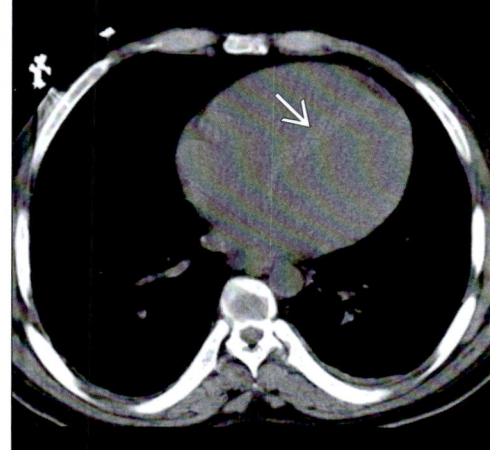

(Left) Axial NECT shows multiple peripheral linear and wedge-shaped opacities ➡ from previous infarcts or pneumonia. *(Right)* Axial NECT shows prominent interventricular septum ➡ from anemia from sickle cell disease.

Typical

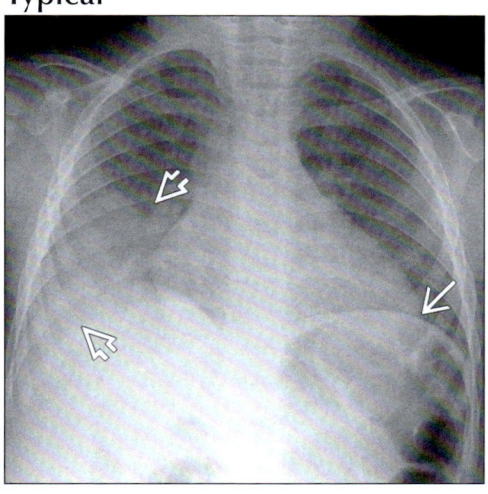
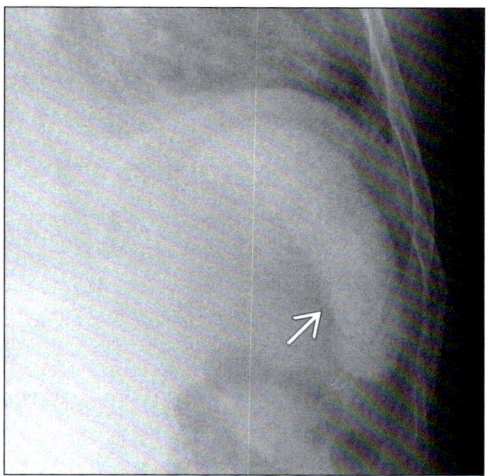

(Left) Frontal radiograph shows homogeneous consolidation ➡ in the right lower lobe from pneumonia. Lack of deviation of air-filled bowel loops in left upper quadrant suggests small or absent spleen ➡. *(Right)* Frontal radiograph shows small calcified spleen ➡ (autosplenectomy) from sickle cell disease.

EOSINOPHILIC PNEUMONIA

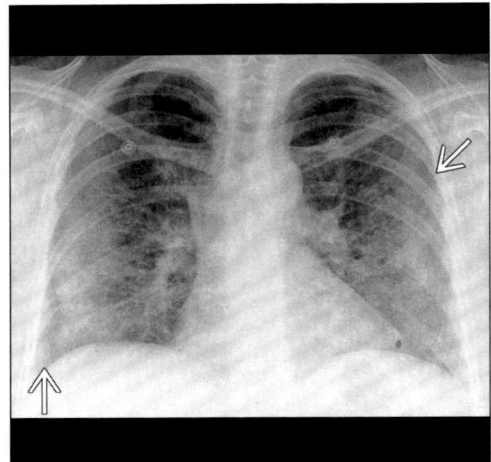

Frontal radiograph shows diffuse peripheral consolidation with subpleural sparing ➡. Peripheral eosinophilia.

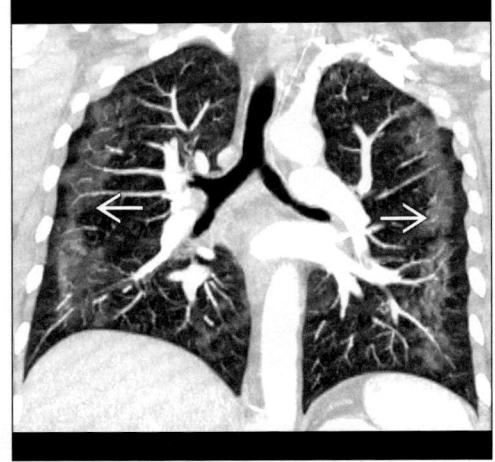

Coronal CECT shows peripheral ground-glass opacities ➡. Diffuse lung disease resolved 24 hours after administration steroids. Eosinophilic pneumonia.

TERMINOLOGY

Abbreviations and Synonyms
- Acute eosinophilic pneumonia (AEP), chronic eosinophilic pneumonia (CEP), idiopathic hypereosinophilic syndrome (IHS), allergic bronchopulmonary aspergillosis (APBA), bronchocentric granulomatosis (BG), pulmonary infiltration with eosinophilia (PIE), Löffler syndrome

Definitions
- Acute and chronic pneumonias due to eosinophilic infiltration with or without blood eosinophilia
  - Classified into those of unknown cause: Löffler syndrome, AEP, CEP, IHS, and eosinophilic lung disease of known cause (ABPA, BG, parasitic infections, Churg-Strauss vasculitis, drug reactions)
  - Individual patients often have overlap syndromes
- Eosinophils cause damage by recruitment, activation, and interaction with other inflammatory and immune cells

IMAGING FINDINGS

General Features
- Best diagnostic clue
  - AEP: Mimics pulmonary edema
  - CEP: Photographic negative of pulmonary edema (peripheral consolidation)
- Location
  - AEP: Lower lung zone predominant
  - CEP: Upper lung zone predominant

Radiographic Findings
- Radiography
  - Löffler syndrome
    - Consolidation: Single or multiple nonsegmental with peripheral distribution in mid and upper lung zones
    - Migratory and rapidly evolving over days, spontaneously clears within 1 month
  - AEP
    - Nonspecific combined alveolar and interstitial pattern with lower lung zone predominance
    - Rapid progression over hours to days
    - Small pleural effusions common (66%)

DDx: Peripheral Consolidation

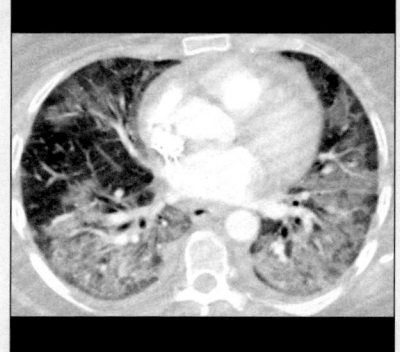

Methotrexate Toxicity

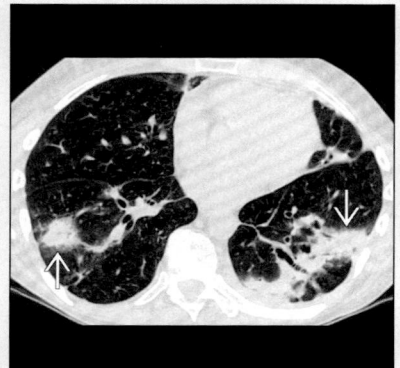

Cryptogenic Organizing Pneumonia

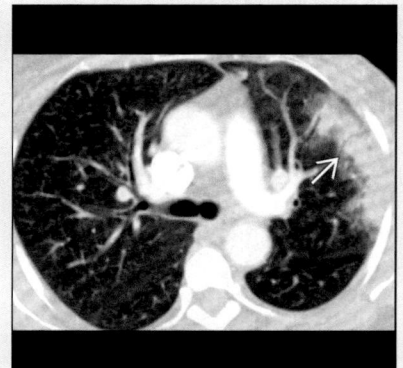

Radiation Pneumonitis

EOSINOPHILIC PNEUMONIA

Key Facts

Terminology
- Acute and chronic pneumonias due to eosinophilic infiltration with or without blood eosinophilia
- Classified into those of unknown cause: Löffler syndrome, AEP, CEP, IHS, and eosinophilic lung disease of known cause (ABPA, BG, parasitic infections, Churg-Strauss vasculitis, drug reactions)

Imaging Findings
- AEP: Mimics pulmonary edema
- CEP: Photographic negative of pulmonary edema (peripheral consolidation)

Top Differential Diagnoses
- Cryptogenic Organizing Pneumonia (COP)
- Diffuse Pulmonary Hemorrhage
- Migratory Pulmonary Opacities

Pathology
- Extrathoracic manifestations consider Churg-Strauss syndrome or IHE

Clinical Issues
- Often misdiagnosed as pneumonia with apparent "response" to antibiotics; this tends to delay the diagnosis for months or years
- Both AEP and CEP show rapid response to corticosteroid therapy
- Relapse unusual in AEP but common in CEP

Diagnostic Checklist
- Review of multiple old films often suggestive of the diagnosis
- Peripheral band-like opacities paralleling chest wall subtle clue to the diagnosis

---

- Rapid response to corticosteroid therapy
- CEP
  - Bilateral, nonsegmental, homogeneous consolidation with peripheral distribution and upper lung zone predominance (66%) **"photographic negative of pulmonary edema"**
  - May migrate from one area to another (25%)
  - May involve entirety of one lung
  - Usually persistent over time in absence of treatment, but sometimes transient/fleeting
  - When recurrent, often in same location
  - Pleural effusions rare (< 10%)
  - Rapid response to corticosteroid therapy
  - In response to therapy, the most peripheral areas of consolidation are typically the first to clear
  - As the peripheral areas of consolidation clear, residual band-like opacities may be visualized coursing parallel to pleural surface
- IHE
  - Pulmonary involvement 40%: Nonspecific focal or diffuse interstitial or alveolar opacities
  - Pleural effusions 50%
  - Edema common (due to endocardial fibrosis, restrictive cardiomyopathy, or valvular damage)

CT Findings
- AEP
  - Bilateral, lower-lobe predominant ground-glass opacities
  - Smooth interlobular septal thickening and thickening of bronchovascular bundles
  - Occasional localized areas of consolidation or small nodules
  - Small pleural effusions common
  - Band-like opacities paralleling chest wall that may even cross pleural fissures, nearly pathognomonic
- CEP
  - Peripheral distribution of consolidation more frequently detected with CT than with chest radiographs
  - Ground-glass opacities or nodules often seen in association with consolidation, may give rise to halo sign

Imaging Recommendations
- Best imaging tool
  - Chest radiograph usually suffices for diagnosis and follow-up
  - Characteristic peripheral distribution of CEP is more frequently detected with CT (95%) than with chest radiographs (65%)

DIFFERENTIAL DIAGNOSIS

Other Causes of Eosinophilic Lung Disease
- Eosinophilic lung disease due to specific causes may mimic AEP
  - Drugs
    - Antibiotics
    - Nonsteroidal anti-inflammatory agents
    - Agents used for treatment of inflammatory bowel disease
    - Inhaled non-therapeutic drugs including cocaine and heroin
  - Parasitic infestation
    - Most common cause of eosinophilic lung disease worldwide
    - Ascaris lumbricoides, Strongyloides stercoralis, Paragonimiasis westermani
  - Fungal infection
    - Allergic bronchopulmonary aspergillosis
- Churg-Strauss syndrome
  - Similar to CEP
    - CEP peripheral homogeneous consolidation, Churg-Strauss lobular consolidation
    - Churg-Strauss associated with centrilobular nodules in ground-glass opacities
  - Presence of systemic disease helps to distinguish from CEP

Cryptogenic Organizing Pneumonia (COP)
- Peripheral distribution of consolidation mimics CEP, but lower lung zones more commonly affected in COP
- COP may also demonstrate bronchovascular distribution in minority of cases

EOSINOPHILIC PNEUMONIA

Diffuse Pulmonary Hemorrhage
- Diffuse pulmonary consolidation, evolves into reticular interstitial pattern during resolution
- Anemia and hemoptysis (80%) common
- History renal disease common

Migratory Pulmonary Opacities
- Hemorrhage, vasculitis, cryptogenic organizing pneumonia, recurrent aspiration

Acute Eosinophilic Pneumonia
- Cardiogenic or noncardiogenic pulmonary edema, acute interstitial pneumonia, viral pneumonia

Chronic Eosinophilic Pneumonia
- Cryptogenic organizing pneumonia, Churg-Strauss syndrome

PATHOLOGY

General Features
- General path comments
  - Eosinophilic lung diseases either centered on airways or lung parenchyma
  - AEP: Diffuse alveolar damage (acute or organizing) associated with large number of interstitial and alveolar eosinophils
  - CEP: Filling of alveolar air spaces by inflammatory infiltrate with a high proportion of eosinophils
- Etiology
  - Pathogenesis unknown, but speculated to represent a hypersensitivity reaction to an unknown antigen
    - AEP clusters after exposure to dust (World Trade Center)
- Epidemiology
  - Prevalence: 1 case per 1,000,000 population per year
    - AEP may be increased in military deployments
- Associated abnormalities
  - Asthma in 50% of patients with CEP
  - Extrathoracic manifestations consider Churg-Strauss syndrome or IHE

Microscopic Features
- Alveoli flooded with eosinophils, macrophages, and mononuclear cells

Staging, Grading or Classification Criteria
- Diagnosis made by satisfying one of 3 criteria
  - Peripheral eosinophilia and chest radiographic abnormalities
  - Tissue eosinophilia confirmed by biopsy
  - Increased eosinophils (≥ 25%) in bronchoalveolar lavage (BAL)
    - Normal BAL fluid < 1% eosinophils
    - BAL differential 2-25% nonspecific

CLINICAL ISSUES

Presentation
- Most common signs/symptoms
  - Löffler syndrome: Minimal or no pulmonary symptoms
  - AEP: Acute febrile illness of < 5 days duration
    - Acute onset of fever, shortness of breath, myalgias and pleuritic chest pain
    - Hypoxemic respiratory failure
    - May be more common in smokers
  - CEP
    - Insidious onset fever (often at night), malaise, weight loss, dyspnea and cough (average of 7.7 months symptoms before diagnosis made)
    - Nearly 50% have asthmatic symptoms
    - 20% chronic rhinitis or sinusitis
    - 90% nonsmokers
- Other signs/symptoms
  - Laboratory data
    - AEP: Peripheral eosinophilia absent but marked increase in eosinophils on bronchoalveolar lavage (> 30-40% eosinophils)
    - CEP: Peripheral eosinophilia present > 90%; increase in eosinophils on bronchoalveolar lavage (> 25% eosinophils)
  - Pulmonary function tests
    - Restriction: AEP, CEP, parasitic
    - Obstructive: ABPA, Churg-Strauss syndrome

Demographics
- Age: CEP peak incidence during 4th decade; AEP all ages
- Gender: CEP women affected twice as frequently as men; AEP no gender predominance, IHS male-female ratio 7:1

Natural History & Prognosis
- AEP may be life-threatening
- Often misdiagnosed as pneumonia with apparent "response" to antibiotics; this tends to delay the diagnosis for months or years
- Rapid clearing with steroids over a period of days (complete resolution in a week)

Treatment
- Both AEP and CEP show rapid response to corticosteroid therapy
- Relapse unusual in AEP but common in CEP

DIAGNOSTIC CHECKLIST

Consider
- Always consider specific causes of eosinophilic lung disease such as drugs, parasitic infestation and fungal infection

Image Interpretation Pearls
- CEP: Photographic negative of pulmonary edema
- Review of multiple old films often suggestive of the diagnosis
- Peripheral band-like opacities paralleling chest wall subtle clue to the diagnosis

SELECTED REFERENCES
1. Jeong YJ et al: Eosinophilic lung diseases: a clinical, radiologic, and pathologic overview. Radiographics. 27(3):617-37; discussion 637-9, 2007

EOSINOPHILIC PNEUMONIA

IMAGE GALLERY

Typical

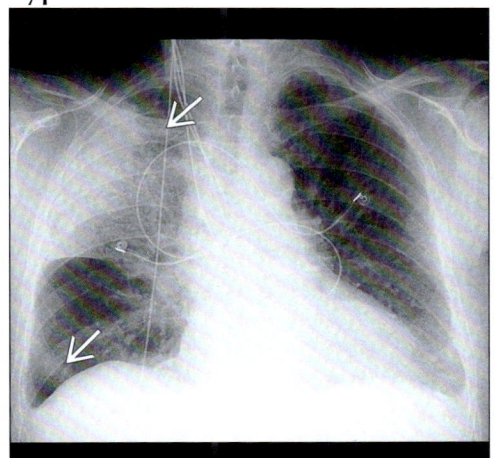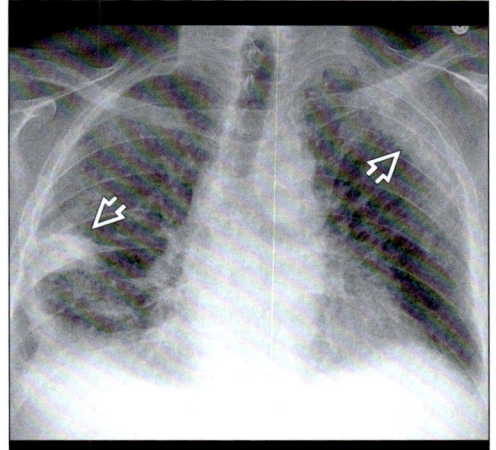

(Left) Frontal radiograph shows peripheral consolidation in the right upper lobe and faint band-like opacity in the right costophrenic angle ➡. *(Right)* Frontal radiograph 2 months later shows new peripheral consolidation in the left upper lobe and right base ➡. Right upper lobe consolidation has resolved. Migratory lung disease from eosinophilic pneumonia.

Typical

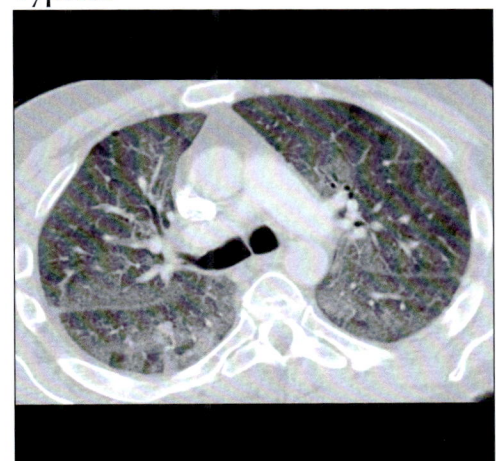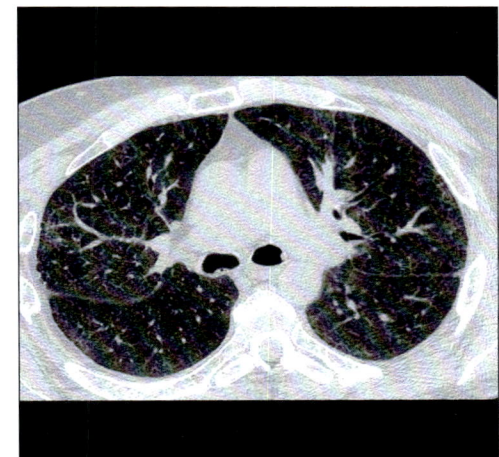

(Left) Axial CECT shows diffuse ground-glass opacities. No adenopathy or pleural effusion. *(Right)* Axial CECT shows marked resolution 4 days following steroid administration. Acute eosinophilic pneumonia.

Typical

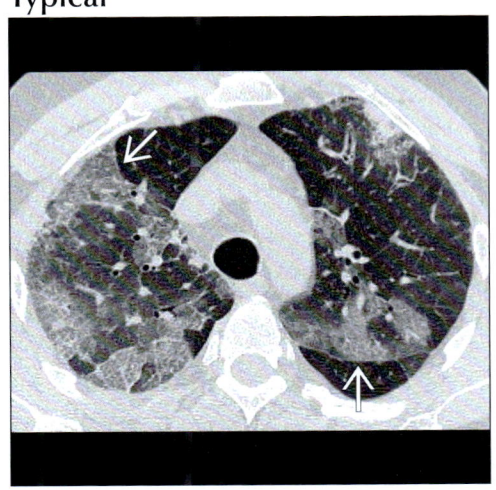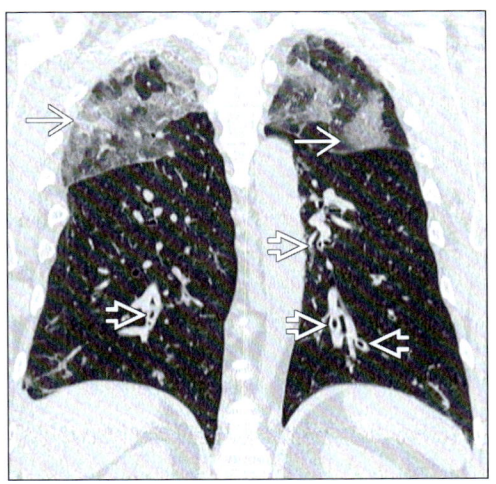

(Left) Axial HRCT shows lobular ground-glass opacities and crazy-paving pattern ➡ predominantly in the upper lobes. *(Right)* Coronal HRCT reconstruction shows ground-glass opacities in the upper lobes ➡ and bronchial wall thickening in the lower lobes ➡. Asthma and Churg-Strauss vasculitis.

ACUTE INTERSTITIAL PNEUMONIA

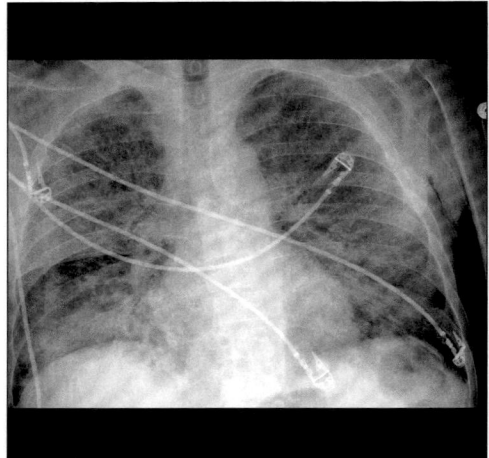

Anteroposterior radiograph shows severe, symmetric, homogeneous, diffuse, ground-glass opacities. Duration of illness short.

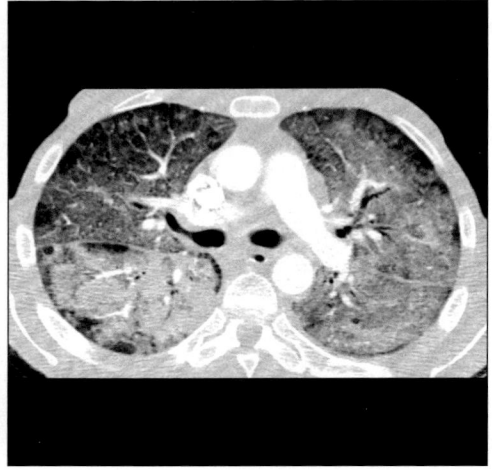

Axial CECT shows diffuse ground-glass opacities involving nearly the entire lung. No honeycombing, pleural effusions or loss of volume.

TERMINOLOGY

Abbreviations and Synonyms
- Acute interstitial pneumonia (AIP), Hamman-Rich syndrome, noncardiogenic pulmonary edema, diffuse alveolar damage (DAD), adult respiratory distress syndrome (ARDS)

Definitions
- Rapidly progressive respiratory failure of unknown etiology occurring in patients without pre-existing lung disease, resembles ARDS
- Formerly called Hamman-Rich syndrome
- Criteria for diagnosis
  - Acute illness of less than 2 months
  - Radiographs show diffuse opacification
  - DAD on lung biopsy
  - No known inciting condition, especially infections, toxic exposures, connective tissue disease, or pre-existing interstitial lung disease

IMAGING FINDINGS

General Features
- Best diagnostic clue
  - Radiograph: Diffuse symmetrical air space opacification
  - CT: Extensive ground-glass opacities combined with traction bronchiectasis
- Location: Lower lung zones
- Size: Usually more than 50% lung involved
- Morphology: Ground-glass more extensive than consolidation

Radiographic Findings
- Radiography
  - Nonspecific diffuse bilateral and symmetrical air space opacification
    - Usually intubated on mechanical ventilation
    - No particular zonal predilection
    - Pleural effusions and septal lines less common than in cardiogenic edema
    - Honeycombing rare

DDx: Acute Interstitial Pneumonia

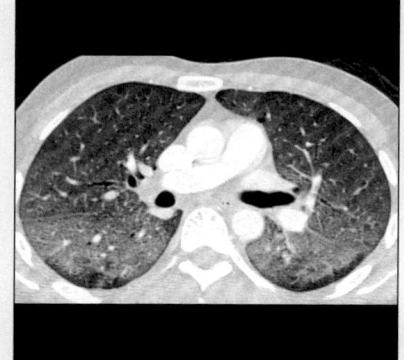

Pneumocystis Pneumonia

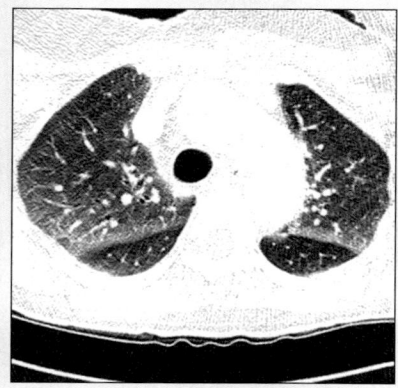

Cardiogenic Edema

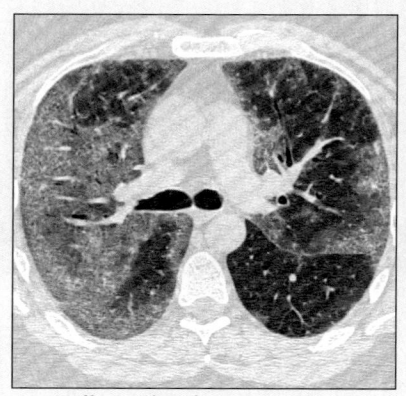

Diffuse Alveolar Hemorrhage

ACUTE INTERSTITIAL PNEUMONIA

Key Facts

Terminology
- Rapidly progressive respiratory failure of unknown etiology occurring in patients without pre-existing lung disease, resembles ARDS

Imaging Findings
- Ground-glass opacification exceeds consolidation
- Traction bronchiectasis involves central airways more commonly than peripheral
- Traction bronchiectasis out of proportion to degree of reticular opacities and honeycombing

Top Differential Diagnoses
- Acute Respiratory Distress Syndrome (ARDS)
- Known history of immunocompromise
- Accelerated Idiopathic Pulmonary Fibrosis (IPF)
- Diffuse Alveolar Hemorrhage

Pathology
- Diffuse alveolar damage not specific to AIP, seen with
- Temporal uniformity suggests single (overwhelming) injury

Clinical Issues
- Acute onset (over a period of 1-3 weeks)
- Majority flu-like prodrome: Headache, myalgia, sore throat, malaise, dry cough
- Poor prognosis (mortality rate usually ≥ 50%; most deaths within 2 months of onset)

Diagnostic Checklist
- Traction bronchiectasis combined with predominantly ground-glass opacification

CT Findings
- More sensitive than radiography
- Ground-glass opacification predominant abnormality
  - Extent: 50% of lung
  - Ground-glass opacification exceeds consolidation
  - Distribution
    - Lower lung zone (40%)
    - Upper lung zone (15%)
  - Symmetry the rule
  - May be seen in all phases of AIP
  - Likely reflects differing histopathologic processes
  - More extensive ground-glass opacification (without traction bronchiectasis/bronchiolectasis) associated with better outcome
- Consolidation
  - Involves 25% of lung
  - Also may be seen in all phases of AIP
  - More extensive air space opacification (without traction bronchiectasis/bronchiolectasis) associated with better outcome
- Honeycombing
  - Rare, (but more common than in ARDS)
- Traction bronchiectasis/bronchiolectasis
  - Typically combined with ground-glass opacities
  - Traction bronchiectasis involves central airways more commonly than peripheral
    - Primarily segmental and subsegmental airways
    - Traction bronchiectasis out of proportion to degree of reticular opacities and honeycombing
  - Develop in the proliferative/fibrotic phases
  - Correlates with disease duration
  - Associated with poorer outcome
  - May persist in survivors
- Architectural distortion
  - May be seen in the proliferative/fibrotic phases
- Less common CT findings include
  - Interlobular septal thickening
  - "Crazy paving" appearance
  - Nodular opacities
  - Thickening of bronchovascular bundles
  - Pleural effusions (30%)
  - Lymphadenopathy (5%)

Imaging Recommendations
- Best imaging tool: CT for characterization of diffuse pulmonary disease

DIFFERENTIAL DIAGNOSIS

Acute Respiratory Distress Syndrome (ARDS)
- Associated with a known cause
- Consolidation exceeds ground-glass opacities
- Honeycombing less common in ARDS
- Lower zone and symmetric distribution less common in ARDS

Disseminated Infection (e.g., Pneumocystis Jiroveci Pneumonia)
- Variable appearances but typically bilateral ground-glass opacification
- Known history of immunocompromise

Accelerated Idiopathic Pulmonary Fibrosis (IPF)
- Rare complication of IPF
  - Criteria: Exacerbation of dyspnea within 1 month, new diffuse pulmonary opacities, worsening hypoxemia (minimum 10 mmHg), absent of infectious agent or heart failure
- Diffuse but patchy ground-glass opacification on background of characteristic changes of IPF
- Honeycombing more profuse than the superimposed ground-glass opacity
- Poor prognosis

Diffuse Alveolar Hemorrhage
- Diffuse ground-glass opacification, often evolves into reticular pattern
- Features of pulmonary fibrosis may be seen but generally only with repeated episodes
- Anemia and hemoptysis (80%) common

Hydrostatic Pulmonary Edema
- Bilateral air space opacification

ACUTE INTERSTITIAL PNEUMONIA

- Enlarged heart
- Pleural effusion
- History of cardiac disease

Alveolar Proteinosis
- Geographical areas of ground-glass opacification and thickened smooth interlobular septa
- No particular zonal distribution
- Paucity of symptoms striking (compared to degree of radiographic abnormalities)

Desquamative Interstitial Pneumonia
- Smokers
- Symptoms indolent, does not require mechanical ventilation

Connective Tissue Disease
- Typically systemic lupus erythematosus
- Arthralgias common
- DAD rare complication of underlying disease

Bronchoalveolar Cell Carcinoma
- Diffuse bilateral ground-glass opacification
- No signs of fibrosis (parenchymal distortion, traction bronchiectasis/bronchiolectasis)
- Insidious onset and progressive course
- Does note require mechanical ventilation

PATHOLOGY

General Features
- General path comments
  - Diffuse alveolar damage not specific to AIP, seen with
    - Acute hypersensitivity pneumonitis
    - ARDS
    - Connective tissue disease: Systemic lupus erythematosus, rheumatoid arthritis
    - Microscopic polyarteritis
    - Drug-induced: Bleomycin, crack cocaine, methotrexate, nitrofurantoin
    - Infection: Mycoplasma pneumonia, viruses, legionella pneumophila
    - Toxins: Nitrogen dioxide, oxygen toxicity, paraquat, chlorine gas
- Etiology
  - Temporal uniformity suggests single (overwhelming) injury
  - Not associated with smoking

Microscopic Features
- Acute exudative phase (1st week)
  - Edema
  - Hemorrhagic fluid in air spaces
  - Type I pneumocyte necrosis
  - Hyaline membranes
- Proliferative phase (after 2nd week)
  - Type II pneumocyte proliferation
  - Collagen deposition
  - Myofibroblast proliferation
- Fibrotic phase
  - Fibrosis within alveoli and interstitium (may be severe)
  - Predominantly fibroblasts, relatively little collagen (just the opposite of usual interstitial pneumonia)

CLINICAL ISSUES

Presentation
- Most common signs/symptoms
  - Acute onset (over a period of 1-3 weeks)
    - 50% seek help within 1 week onset
    - 25% more indolent, seek help 30 days after onset of symptoms
    - Rapid progression to respiratory failure requiring mechanical ventilation
    - Similar presentation to ARDS except no etiologic factor identifiable
  - Majority flu-like prodrome: Headache, myalgia, sore throat, malaise, dry cough
  - Dyspnea (95%), dry cough (70%)
  - Tachypnea and hypoxemic (mean PaO_2 45 mm Hg)
- Other signs/symptoms: Bronchoalveolar lavage: Increased red blood cells, neutrophils, occasional lymphocytes

Demographics
- Age: Mean age 50, from pediatrics to adults
- Gender: M = F

Natural History & Prognosis
- Poor prognosis (mortality rate usually ≥ 50%; most deaths within 2 months of onset)
- Survivors may have complete recovery of lung function
  - Persistent stable restrictive physiology also common
  - Recurrence seen but extremely rare

Treatment
- No known treatment effective
- Steroids typically administered, never shown to be useful
- Supportive care mainstay
  - Mean duration of mechanical ventilation 30 days

DIAGNOSTIC CHECKLIST

Image Interpretation Pearls
- Traction bronchiectasis combined with predominantly ground-glass opacification

SELECTED REFERENCES

1. Kim DS et al: Classification and natural history of the idiopathic interstitial pneumonias. Proc Am Thorac Soc. 3(4):285-92, 2006
2. Visscher DW et al: Histologic spectrum of idiopathic interstitial pneumonias. Proc Am Thorac Soc. 3(4):322-9, 2006
3. Pipavath S et al: Imaging of the chest: idiopathic interstitial pneumonia. Clin Chest Med. 25(4):651-6, v-vi, 2004
4. Vourlekis JS: Acute interstitial pneumonia. Clin Chest Med. 25(4):739-47, vii, 2004
5. Wittram C et al: CT-histologic correlation of the ATS/ERS 2002 classification of idiopathic interstitial pneumonias. Radiographics. 23(5):1057-71, 2003

ACUTE INTERSTITIAL PNEUMONIA

IMAGE GALLERY

Typical

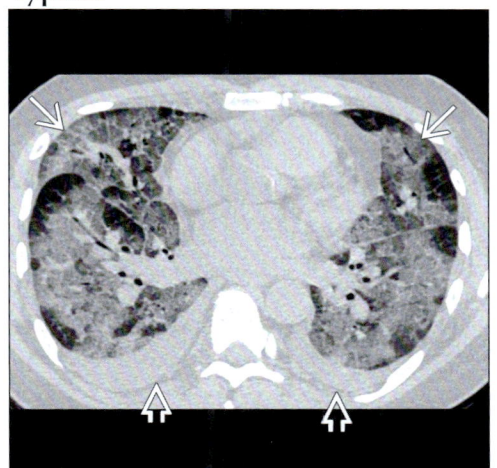
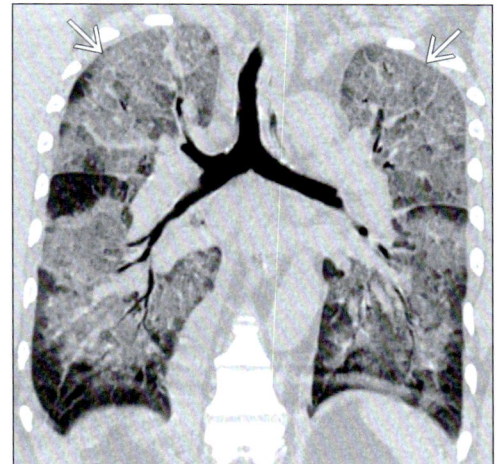

(Left) Axial NECT shows diffuse ground-glass opacities ➡ with geographic sparing in the periphery. Small bilateral pleural effusions ➡. Duration of illness short. *(Right)* Coronal NECT shows extent of ground-glass opacities ➡. Pathology is diffuse and symmetric. Lung volumes preserved. No honeycombing.

Typical

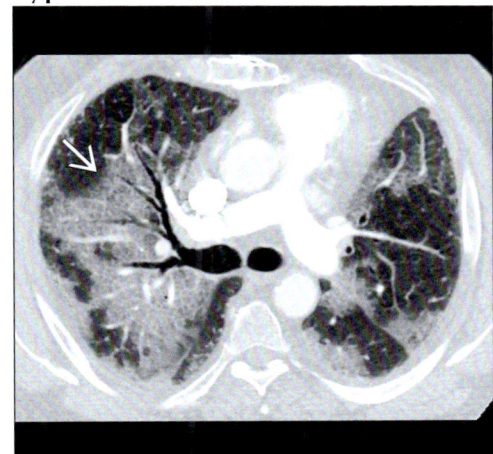
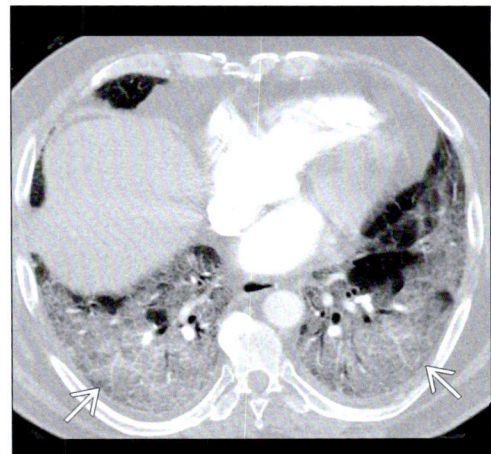

(Left) Axial CECT shows geographic areas of ground-glass opacities containing intralobular reticular lines ➡ (crazy paving pattern). *(Right)* Axial CECT shows bilateral predominant symmetric ground-glass opacities ➡. Most of the lung is abnormal.

Typical

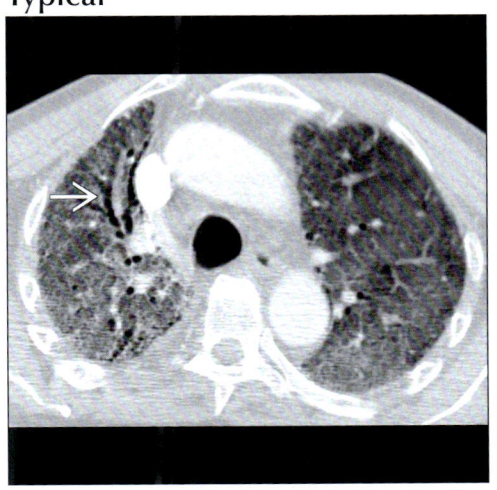
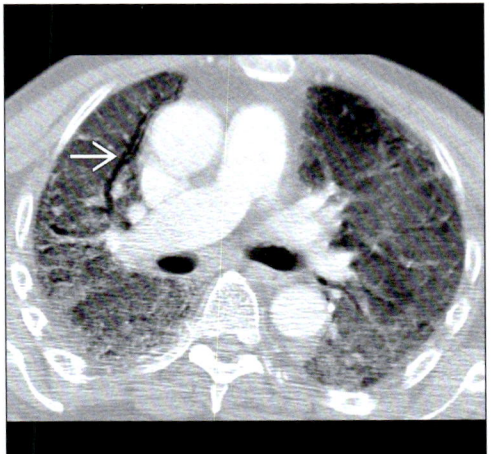

(Left) Axial HRCT shows diffuse, extensive, symmetric, ground-glass opacities. Segmental airways are slightly dilated ➡. *(Right)* Axial HRCT shows diffuse, symmetric, extensive, ground-glass opacities. Central airways are slightly dilated ➡. No known etiology.

ILLICIT DRUG ABUSE, PULMONARY

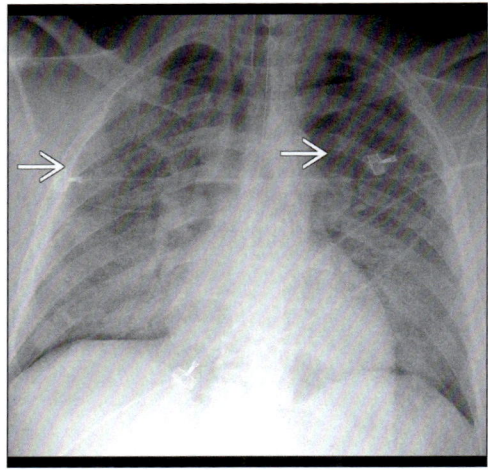

Anteroposterior radiograph shows diffuse consolidation ➡. Intubated and NG in stomach. Crack lung. Edema cleared within 48 hours.

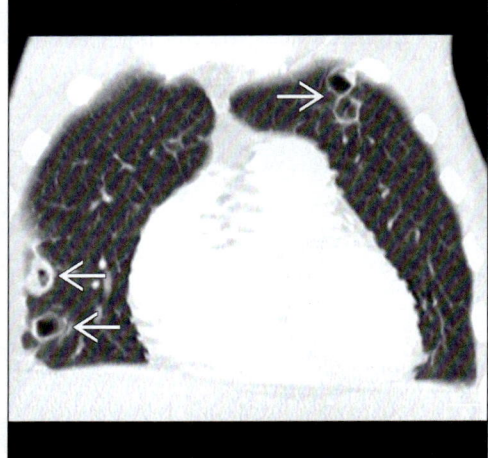

Coronal CECT shows a few small peripheral cavities ➡. Differing wall thicknesses suggest recurrent septic events. Septic emboli.

TERMINOLOGY

Abbreviations and Synonyms
- Intravenous (IV) drug abuse

Definitions
- Pulmonary insults that arise from illicit drug abuse; primarily infection, toxicity of the drug, drug overdose, or toxicity from adulterants added to the drug
- Typical drugs: Heroin, cocaine ("crack"), methamphetamine ("speed"), codeine, methadone, methylphenidate (Ritalin)

IMAGING FINDINGS

General Features
- Best diagnostic clue: Young adult in emergency room with unexplained diffuse or focal lung disease

Radiographic Findings
- Radiography: Multiple radiographic abnormalities none of which are specific for illicit drug abuse

- Lung
  - Atelectasis
    - Variable from subsegmental to lobar
    - Often associated with drug induced respiratory depression and stupor
  - Pneumonia and opportunistic infection
    - Common due to general immunosuppression from nutritional debility or co-existent AIDS
    - Higher risk for tuberculosis
  - Aspiration
    - Obtundation and stupor places at risk, especially from opiates
    - Focal opacities, unilateral or bilateral in gravity dependent lung (especially superior segments lower lobes)
    - May lead to lung abscess
    - Repeated episodes may eventually result in bronchiectasis
  - Pulmonary hemorrhage
    - Severe diffuse alveolar damage (DAD), most common with cocaine and crack
    - Bilateral diffuse nonspecific consolidation, often worse in lower lung zones
    - Pleural effusions uncommon

DDx: Acute Diffuse Disease in Young Adults

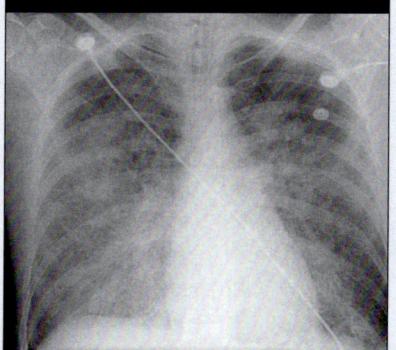

Cardiogenic Pulmonary Edema

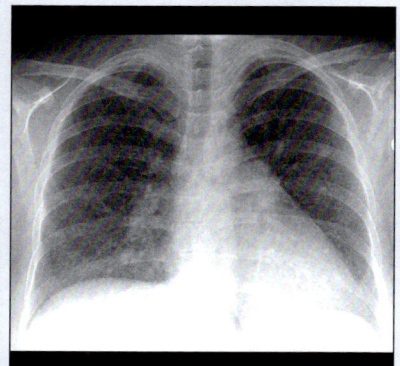

Viral Pneumonia

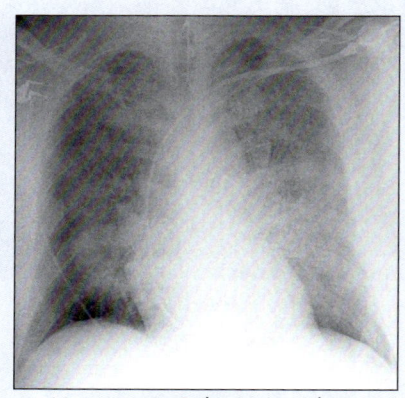

Neurogenic Pulmonary Edema

ILLICIT DRUG ABUSE, PULMONARY

Key Facts

Terminology
- Pulmonary insults that arise from illicit drug abuse; primarily infection, toxicity of the drug, drug overdose, or toxicity from adulterants added to the drug
- Typical drugs: Heroin, cocaine ("crack"), methamphetamine ("speed"), codeine, methadone, methylphenidate (Ritalin)

Imaging Findings
- Best diagnostic clue: Young adult in emergency room with unexplained diffuse or focal lung disease
- Radiography: Multiple radiographic abnormalities none of which are specific for illicit drug abuse

Top Differential Diagnoses
- Pneumonia
- Atypical Edema
- Negative pressure pulmonary edema
- Aspiration
- Contusion Blunt Chest Trauma
- Hypersensitivity Pneumonitis

Pathology
- Most commonly injected drugs: Heroin and cocaine
- Most common complications of IV drug use: Septic emboli, community-acquired pneumonia, tuberculosis

Clinical Issues
- Mortality rate 3-4% per year

Diagnostic Checklist
- Consider IV drug abuse in young adults with unexplained radiographic abnormalities in the ER

- Cardiogenic pulmonary edema
  - Myocardial depression, ischemia, and infarction from vasoconstriction, especially cocaine
  - Small pleural effusions (pleural effusion uncommon in other etiologies)
  - Resolves quickly
- Noncardiac pulmonary edema ("crack lung", heroin lung)
  - Nonspecific consolidation, usually peripheral and bilateral
  - Normal heart size
  - No pleural effusions
  - Etiology: Direct endothelial damage
  - Develops within a few hours of intoxication, resolves over 24-48 hours
  - Methadone may have prolonged resolution over several days (due to prolonged absorption from the GI tract)
- Talcosis
  - Develops slowly over time with chronic IV drug abuse
  - Fine-micronodular pattern, ground-glass opacities, panacinar emphysema
  - Pulmonary artery hypertension
  - Progressive massive fibrosis (PMF) in perihilar regions and of high calcific density (calcific density usually not recognized on radiographs)
- Emphysema
  - Associated with IV drug abuse in younger men (30-40 y)
  - Often paraseptal with large bulla predominantly in upper lung zones from IV cocaine or heroin
  - IV methadone and methylphenidate results in predominantly lower lobe panacinar emphysema
  - Frequency up to 2% of chronic IV drug abuse
- Cryptogenic organizing pneumonia
  - Associated with cocaine inhalation
  - Focal lower lobe chronic air space opacities
- Amyloidosis
  - Secondary to long term drug abuse
  - Multiple pulmonary nodules, may be calcified
- Vascular
  - Septic emboli
    - Multiple pulmonary nodules with rapid cavitation over 24-48 hours, primarily lower lobes
    - Few (mean 15) ill-defined nodules usually < 1 cm in size
    - Etiology: Infected needle, endocarditis, tricuspid valve vegetations, septic thrombophlebitis
  - Pulmonary hypertension
    - Often due to talc granulomatosis
    - Some vasoconstrictive drugs may result in acute hypertension
  - Aortic dissection
    - Acute hypertensive crisis, induced most commonly from cocaine
- Pleural
  - Pneumothorax and pneumomediastinum
    - Direct needle laceration when attempting to access neck veins ("pocket shot")
    - Prolonged Valsalva maneuver leading to barotrauma when inhaling crack cocaine
- Airway
  - Tracheal stenosis
    - Long term sequelae of thermal injury from smoked cocaine abuse
- Skeletal
  - Involvement from septicemia and occasionally direct injury
  - Diskitis and vertebral osteomyelitis
    - Vertebral body collapse and paraspinal mass
  - Costochondritis commonly from Staphylococcus species or fungal organisms such as Aspergillus and Candida
  - Septic arthritis: Predilection sternoclavicular and acromioclavicular joints

Imaging Recommendations
- Best imaging tool
  - Chest radiographs usually suffice for detection and follow-up
  - CT increased sensitivity for pleuro-pulmonary abnormalities

ILLICIT DRUG ABUSE, PULMONARY

DIFFERENTIAL DIAGNOSIS

Pneumonia
- Focal or diffuse due to community-acquired pneumonias
- Most common cause of focal or diffuse opacities in young adult

Atypical Edema
- Neurogenic pulmonary edema
  - Any cause of increased intracranial hypertension
  - Edema slightly more prominent in upper lung zones
- Negative pressure pulmonary edema
  - Neck burns or bruises from suicidal or homicidal insult
  - Edema more prominent in upper lung zones
- Smoke inhalation
  - Skin burns, carbonaceous sputum
  - Edema more prominent in upper lung zones
  - Subglottic edema

Aspiration
- Generally occurs in those obtunded and unable to protect their upper airway
- May have underlying esophageal motility disorder

Contusion Blunt Chest Trauma
- Focal nonsegmental opacity immediately following trauma
- May have associated rib fractures

Hypersensitivity Pneumonitis
- Miliary nodular pattern in mid and lower lung zones
- Air-trapping at expiratory CT in addition to centrilobular nodules
- Detailed exposure history important

PATHOLOGY

General Features
- Etiology
  - Drug effects
    - Cocaine: Sympathomimetic agents increase blood pressure
    - Narcotics: Respiratory depression
  - Septic emboli
    - Source: Subacute bacterial endocarditis and tricuspid vegetations, septic thrombophlebitis, and direct injection of infected fluid
    - Staphylococcus most common organism in septic embolism
  - Emphysema
    - Damage and obliteration of capillary bed may result in bullous emphysema in upper lobes
    - Damage and obliteration of capillary bed may result in panlobular emphysema in lower lobes, primarily with Ritalin
    - Capillary damage may be due to direct drug toxicity or due to intermediate immunologic reaction
- Epidemiology
  - Most commonly injected drugs: Heroin and cocaine
    - Most common complications of IV drug use: Septic emboli, community-acquired pneumonia, tuberculosis
  - More than 1.5 million IV drug users in North America
    - 25% of HIV/AIDS seen in IV drug users
  - Edema common developing in up to 50% of narcotic overdose
- Associated abnormalities: Hepatitis B and C in more than 50% long time IV drug abusers

Microscopic Features
- No specific features for drug induced damage
  - Pulmonary edema may have features of both capillary leak and hydrostatic edema
  - Granulomas from injected fillers such as talc or methylcellulose
  - Birefringent crystals from talc particles
  - Angiothrombosis: Intravascular foreign material mixed with thrombi in various stages of organization

CLINICAL ISSUES

Presentation
- Most common signs/symptoms
  - Hemoptysis common, especially with cocaine abuse
  - Needle tracks: Sclerosed veins and scars at common injection sites
  - Chest pain in cocaine abuse highly associated with myocardial ischemia
- Other signs/symptoms: Toxicologic analysis of blood and urine

Demographics
- Age: Any age but primarily young adults 18-25
- Gender: Males twice more common than females

Natural History & Prognosis
- Morbidity and mortality secondary to: Infection, drug injected, drug overdose, or adulterants added to the drug
- Mortality rate 3-4% per year

Treatment
- Addiction treatment

DIAGNOSTIC CHECKLIST

Consider
- Consider IV drug abuse in young adults with unexplained radiographic abnormalities in the ER
- Consider in young adult presenting with myocardial infarction

SELECTED REFERENCES
1. Wolff AJ et al: Pulmonary effects of illicit drug use. Clin Chest Med. 25(1):203-16, 2004
2. Gotway MB et al: Thoracic complications of illicit drug use: an organ system approach. Radiographics. 22 Spec No:S119-35, 2002

ILLICIT DRUG ABUSE, PULMONARY

IMAGE GALLERY

Typical

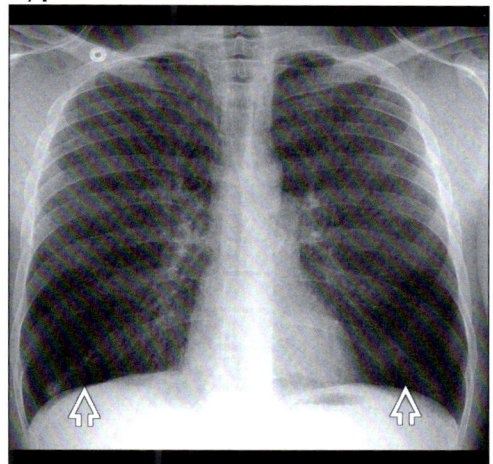
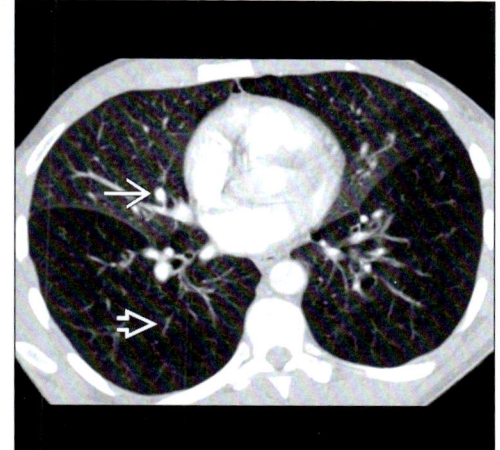

(Left) Frontal radiograph shows hyperinflation and loss of vasculature ➡ in the lower lung zones. Ritalin abuse. *(Right)* Axial CECT shows enlarged pulmonary arteries ➡ in the upper lobes. Lower lobes show marked decrease in vasculature ➡ and decreased density of the lung. Ritalin abuse.

Typical

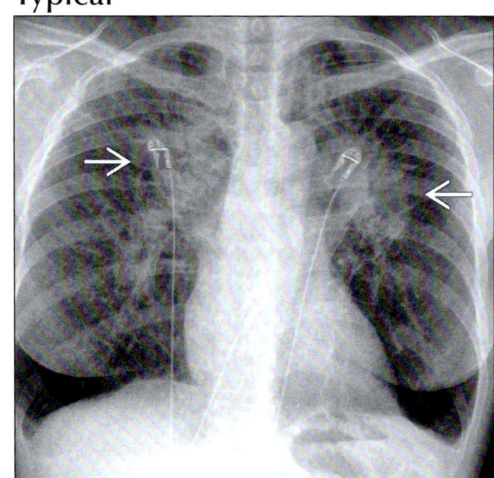
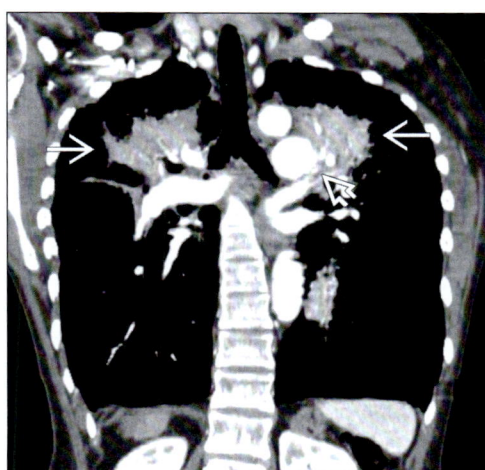

(Left) Frontal radiograph shows progressive massive fibrosis ➡ with volume loss upper lobes. Talcosis. *(Right)* Coronal CECT shows shape and contour of progressive massive fibrosis ➡. Enlarged main pulmonary artery ➡. Talcosis.

Typical

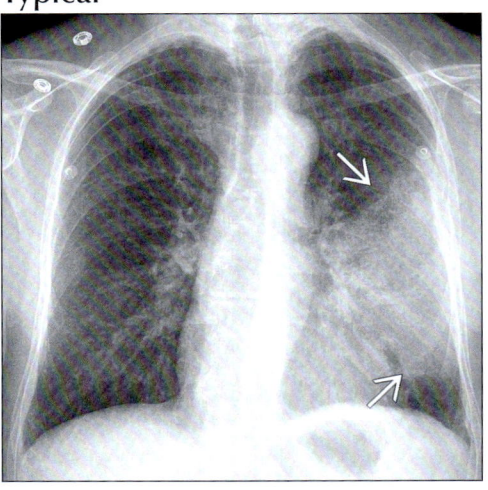
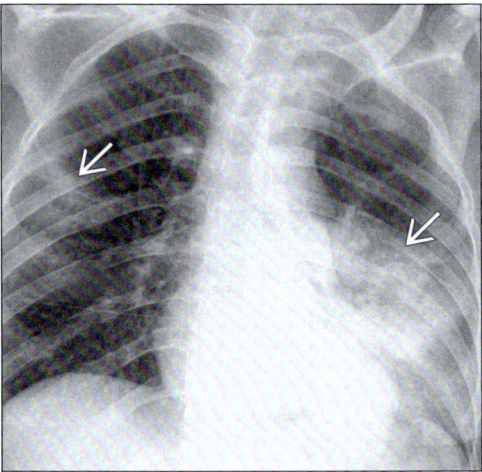

(Left) Frontal radiograph shows lingular lobar pneumonia ➡ in an IV drug abuser. *(Right)* Anteroposterior radiograph shows bilateral, ill-defined, air-space consolidations in the right upper and left lower lobes ➡ from aspiration in narcotic overdose.

TALCOSIS, PULMONARY

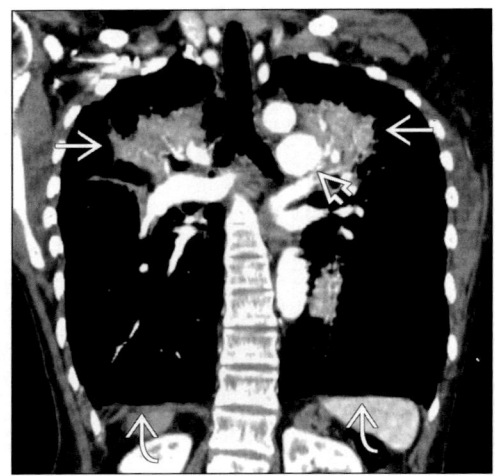

Coronal CECT shows perihilar PMF ➡. Main pulmonary artery enlarged ➡. Lung volumes are increased with flattening hemidiaphragms ➡.

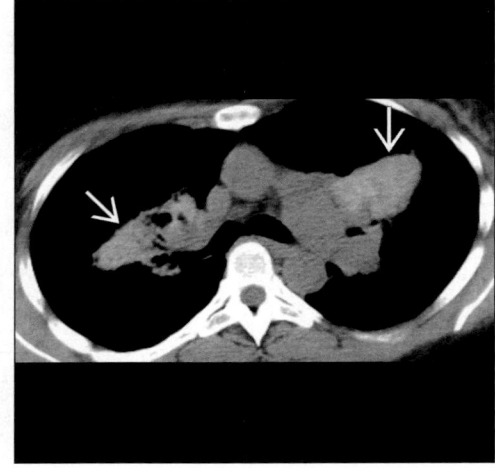

Axial NECT shows perihilar fibrosis to be of high density ➡ from talc. Talcosis from IV drug abuse.

TERMINOLOGY

Abbreviations and Synonyms
- Illicit drug use, simple pneumoconiosis, complicated pneumoconiosis, progressive massive fibrosis

Definitions
- Four forms: 3 inhalational, 1 intravenous
  - Inhalation pure talc (talcosis)
  - Inhalation talc and silica (talco-silicosis)
  - Inhalation talc and asbestos (talco-asbestosis)
  - Intravenous illicit drug use
- Talc also used therapeutically in pleurodesis

IMAGING FINDINGS

General Features
- Best diagnostic clue
  - Diffuse fine-granular nodularity with high attenuation perihilar conglomeration
  - Basilar panlobular emphysema in intravenous Ritalin abusers
- Location
  - Nodularity diffuse
  - Progressive massive fibrosis (PMF) perihilar
  - Emphysema lower lobes
- Size: Pinpoint nodules
- Morphology: Diffuse fine micronodules with perihilar PMF and emphysema

Radiographic Findings
- Radiography
  - Inhalational
    - Multiple small or tiny miliary nodules, International Labor Classification (ILO) type "p"
    - Predominantly upper lung zones
    - May evolve into PMF (may be rapid over 12 months)
    - PMF usually develops closer to hilum as compared to silicosis
    - Lower zone reticular opacities and pleural changes in those with asbestos contamination
    - Enlarged hilar lymph nodes with egg-shell calcification (especially in silico-talcosis)
  - Intravenous
    - Miliary "pinpoint" nodules
    - Occasionally lymphadenopathy

DDx: Talcosis

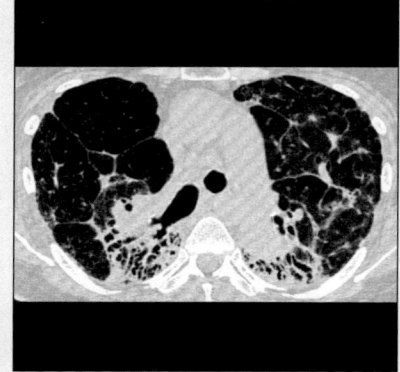
Sarcoidosis

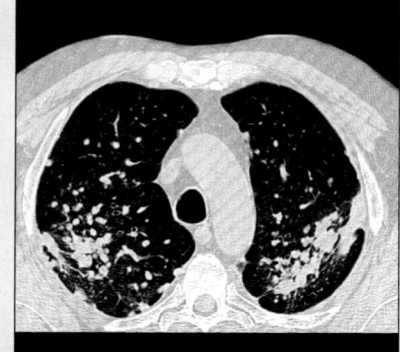
Silicosis

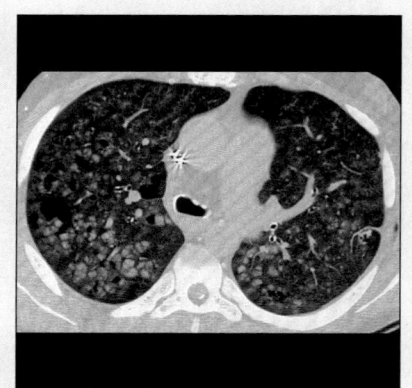
Metastatic Calcification

TALCOSIS, PULMONARY

Key Facts

Terminology
- Four forms: 3 inhalational, 1 intravenous

Imaging Findings
- Miliary "pinpoint" nodules
- Emphysema, either centriacinar (upper lung zones) or panacinar (lower lung zones)
- PMF in perihilar distribution and of high attenuation (highly suggestive of talcosis)

Top Differential Diagnoses
- Sarcoidosis
- Metastatic Pulmonary Calcification
- Silicosis
- Cellulose Granulomatosis
- Amyloidosis
- Neurofibromatosis
- Amiodarone Toxicity

Pathology
- Inhalational: Nodules in lymphatic distribution (centrilobular and subpleural)
- Intravenous: Nodules perivascular distribution (centrilobular) with occasional tree-in-bud opacity
- Crystals birefringent under polarized light

Clinical Issues
- Natural progression from simple nodularity to progressive massive fibrosis similar to silicosis
- No specific treatment for pneumoconiosis available

Diagnostic Checklist
- If PMF of high density, consider talcosis
- Diffuse nodularity, perihilar PMF, and basilar emphysema highly suggestive of Ritalin abuse

---

- PMF in perihilar regions
- Calcification in PMF usually not recognized on radiographs
- Emphysema, either centriacinar (upper lung zones) or panacinar (lower lung zones)
- Pulmonary artery hypertension in severe disease
  ○ Talc pleurodesis
    - Often used for pleurodesis due to the intense inflammation induced by talc
    - Pleural thickened with irregular deposits of calcification in the most dependent lung (dorsal) due to settling of talc in supine position

CT Findings
- NECT
  ○ Progressive massive fibrosis may be of high attenuation
    - Highly suggestive of talcosis
- HRCT
  ○ Inhalational
    - Centrilobular and subpleural nodules, may calcify
    - Aggregation of nodules into PMF (identical to silicosis)
    - Architectural distortion adjacent to PMF
    - Pleural and diaphragmatic plaques identical to those from asbestos
    - Pleural thickening can sometimes be dramatic
  ○ Intravenous
    - Emphysema may be upper lung zone or predominantly lower lung zone (even in the absence of smoking)
    - Methylphenidate (Ritalin) special proclivity for severe lower lobe panacinar emphysema
    - Ritalin may result in severe lower lung zone panacinar emphysema alone without nodularity
    - Centrilobular (fine granular appearance) nodules and tree-in-bud opacities
    - Nodules spare emphysematous lung, but otherwise uniform throughout the lung
    - Nonspecific ground-glass opacities
    - PMF in perihilar distribution and of high attenuation (highly suggestive of talcosis)
    - PMF superimposed on fine-nodular pattern

Imaging Recommendations
- Best imaging tool: HRCT for characterization of interstitial lung disease and detection of high attenuation conglomerate masses

DIFFERENTIAL DIAGNOSIS

Sarcoidosis
- No occupational exposure, PMF less likely
- Nodules usually larger and tend to cluster (galaxy sign)
- Peribronchovascular distribution of nodules
- May have egg-shell calcification lymph nodes, nodules rarely calcify

Metastatic Pulmonary Calcification
- No PMF
- Emphysema if present admixed with ground-glass opacities or consolidation
- Centrilobular nodules larger and mulberry shape and tend to cluster
- Predominantly disease of upper lung zones

Silicosis
- Occupational history
- Nodules tend to be larger than talc
- PMF usually more cephalad and peripheral in upper lung zones and not high in attenuation
- May have egg-shell calcification lymph nodes
- Talc and silica may be admixed together

Cellulose Granulomatosis
- Cellulose filler in oral medications
- Cellulose particles trapped in arterioles leading to granulomatous reaction
- HRCT: Centrilobular nodules and tree-in-bud pattern
- No PMF

Amyloidosis
- Also may be related to IV drug abuse
- Nodular form: Multiple small scattered pulmonary nodules
- May calcify but calcification in small nodules rare

TALCOSIS, PULMONARY

Neurofibromatosis
- Upper lobe bullae
- Lower lobe reticular interstitial fibrosis
- Not nodular
- Cutaneous and skeletal stigmata of neurofibromatosis

Amiodarone Toxicity
- Used to treat tachyarrhythmia
- Accumulates in lung and liver
- Focal areas of consolidation randomly distributed
- Focal lung abnormalities and liver of high attenuation due to drug which contains 3 iodine molecules

PATHOLOGY

General Features
- General path comments
  - Talc: Magnesium silicate
  - Particle size larger in intravenous form
    - Intravenous mean particle diameter 14 ± 9 microns
    - Inhalation mean particle diameter 4 ± 3 microns
  - Talc used in paper, plastics, cosmetic, construction, rubber, and drug industries
  - Less fibrogenic than silica and asbestos particles
- Etiology
  - Inhalational
    - Occupational exposure in mining, milling, packaging of talc
    - Cosmetic use (talcum powder) common but disease from inhalation extremely rare
  - Intravenous
    - Talc (and cellulose) common filler in oral medication; common drugs: Amphetamines, methylphenidate (Ritalin), hydromorphone (Dilaudid), pentazocine (Talwin), propoxyphene (Darvon)
    - Not meant to be ground up and injected intravenously
    - Particles trapped in small arterioles leading to infarction, ischemia, granulomatous inflammation
    - Reduction of the capillary bed may result in panacinar emphysema
- Epidemiology: Latency period 20 years for inhalational form

Gross Pathologic & Surgical Features
- Inhalational: Nodules in lymphatic distribution (centrilobular and subpleural)
- Intravenous: Nodules perivascular distribution (centrilobular) with occasional tree-in-bud opacity
  - Subpleural lung and costophrenic angles tend to be spared

Microscopic Features
- Inhaled and intravenous
  - Granulomatous interstitial inflammation (nonnecrotizing)
  - Needle-shaped crystals both free and in macrophages
  - Crystals birefringent under polarized light
- Inhaled
  - Interstitial fibrosis or poorly-defined fibrotic nodules
  - Difficult to separate talc from contaminants of silica and asbestos

CLINICAL ISSUES

Presentation
- Most common signs/symptoms
  - Inhalational
    - Dry cough and chronic dyspnea progressing to cor pulmonale in end stage disease
  - Intravenous
    - Progressive dyspnea and COPD
- Other signs/symptoms
  - Pulmonary function tests
    - Mixed obstruction (from emphysema) and restriction (from interstitial lung disease)
    - Severe reduction in diffusion capacity
    - End stage obstructive pattern predominates
  - Funduscopic exam: Talc visible in retinal vessels (75%)

Demographics
- Age
  - Middle age and older for inhalational forms
  - Younger for intravenous form
- Gender: Men both for occupational inhalational forms and intravenous drug abuse

Natural History & Prognosis
- Not a known carcinogen
- Natural progression from simple nodularity to progressive massive fibrosis similar to silicosis
- Slow progression even without further inhalational or intravenous exposure

Treatment
- No specific treatment for pneumoconiosis available
- Prevention: Respirators in dusty environments, dust control to reduce ambient dust concentrations
- Removal from work environment or transfer to less dusty environment
- Smoking cessation
- Drug treatment for intravenous abusers

DIAGNOSTIC CHECKLIST

Consider
- If PMF of high density, consider talcosis

Image Interpretation Pearls
- Diffuse nodularity, perihilar PMF, and basilar emphysema highly suggestive of Ritalin abuse

SELECTED REFERENCES
1. Chong S et al: Pneumoconiosis: comparison of imaging and pathologic findings. Radiographics. 26(1):59-77, 2006
2. Marchiori E et al: Inhalational pulmonary talcosis: high-resolution CT findings in 3 patients. J Thorac Imaging. 19(1):41-4, 2004

TALCOSIS, PULMONARY

IMAGE GALLERY

Typical

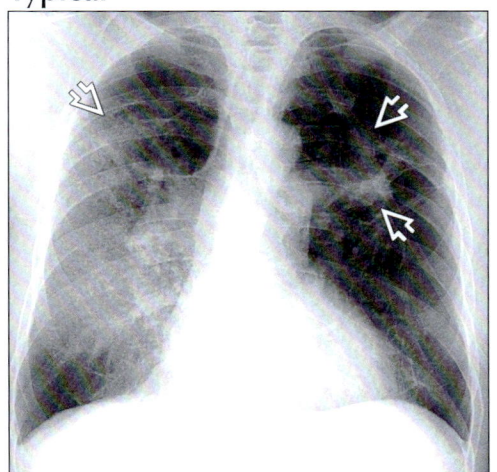
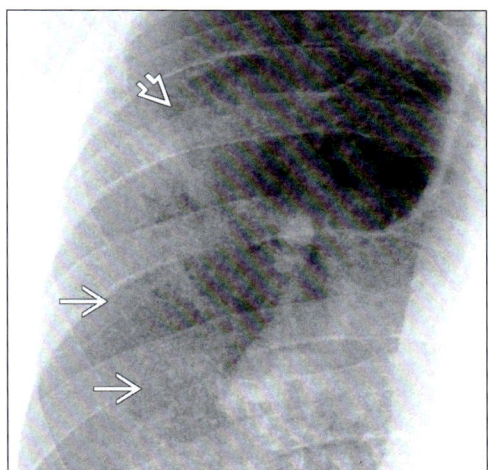

(Left) Frontal radiograph shows large opacities ➡ in a perihilar location. *(Right)* Frontal radiograph magnified view shows a fine miliary pattern ➡ in addition to large opacity ➡. Talcosis from IV drug abuse.

Typical

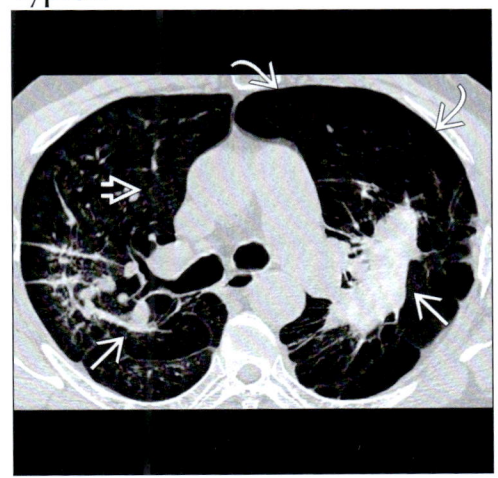
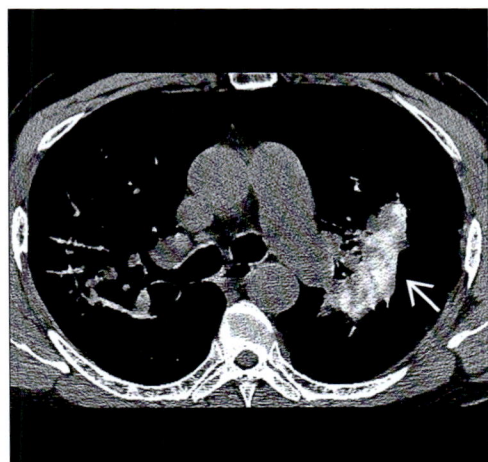

(Left) Axial HRCT show perihilar PMF ➡. Pinpoint micronodules ➡. Large areas of diffuse emphysema ➡. *(Right)* Axial HRCT mediastinal window shows high attenuation in PMF ➡. Talcosis from IV drug abuse.

Typical

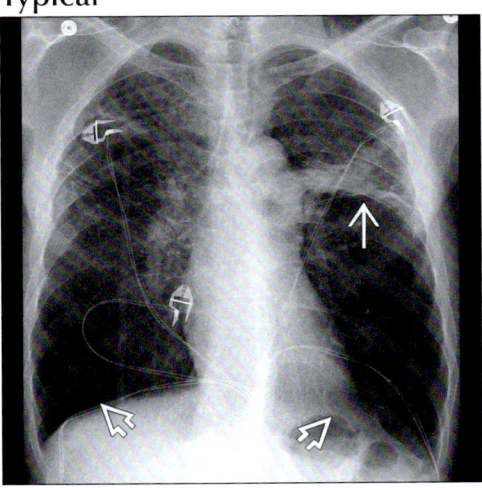
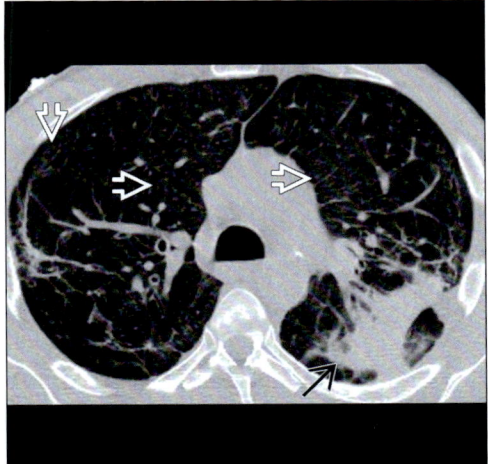

(Left) Frontal radiograph shows basilar emphysema ➡, mild diffuse nodularity in the upper lung zones and perihilar PMF ➡. *(Right)* Axial NECT shows focal peripheral opacity ➡ and ground-glass opacities and micronodules ➡. Talcosis from IV drug abuse.

CHRONIC OBSTRUCTIVE PULMONARY DISEASE

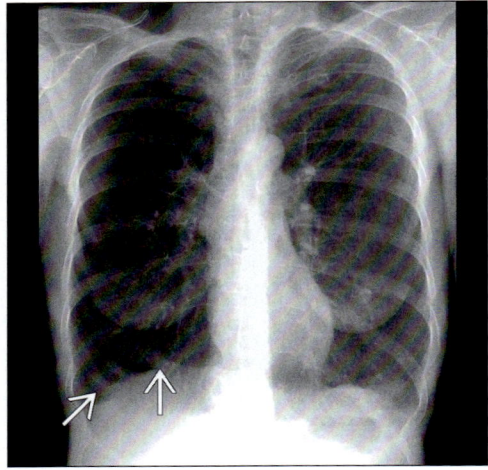

Frontal radiograph shows marked hyperinflation. Flattened hemidiaphragms (diaphragm slips ➡). Peripheral vasculature attenuated.

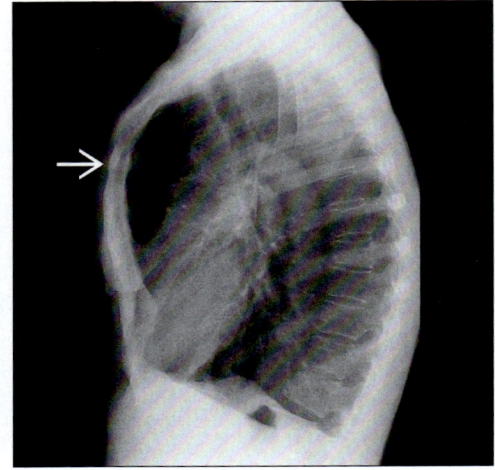

Lateral radiograph shows sternal bulging ➡ with enlarged retrosternal clear space. Hemidiaphragms flattened. Centrilobular emphysema.

TERMINOLOGY

Abbreviations and Synonyms
- Chronic obstructive pulmonary disease (COPD); American Thoracic Society (ATS)

Definitions
- COPD: Presence of airflow obstruction caused by chronic bronchitis or emphysema; the airflow obstruction is generally progressive, may be accompanied by airway hyper reactivity and may be partially reversible
  - Includes asthma, chronic bronchitis, emphysema, and bronchiectasis
- Emphysema types: Centriacinar, panlobular, paraseptal, irregular

IMAGING FINDINGS

General Features
- Best diagnostic clue: Hyperinflation of lungs on chest radiograph

Radiographic Findings
- Utility
  - Sensitivity poor for early disease (25%), rare false positives (specificity 95%)
    - Chest radiograph may be normal
    - Problem is recognition of loss of normal lung
    - Normal lung at chest radiography is 90% air, making detection of slight increases in volume of air nearly impossible
  - Crude correlation between indices of airways obstruction and radiographic findings
  - Exacerbations: Chest radiograph often unchanged (only 20% show new abnormality)
- Signs based on increased lung volumes and parenchymal changes from pathology on airways such as emphysematous destruction of lung: Hyperinflation, parenchymal areas of hypoattenuation, bronchial wall thickening, and pulmonary arterial hypertension
  - Considerable intraobserver and interobserver variation in radiographic signs of emphysema
  - Hyperinflation most reliable sign of COPD
- Hyperinflation

DDx: Hyperinflation

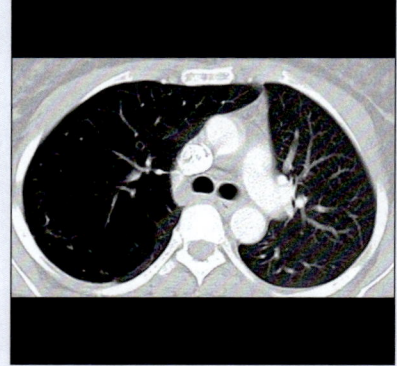

Bronchiolitis Obliterans

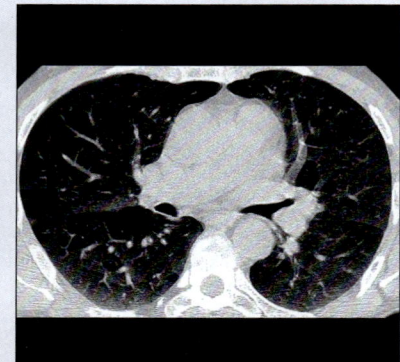

Hypersensitivity Pneumonitis

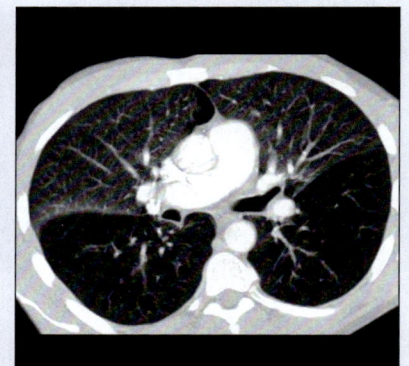

Ritalin Drug Abuse

CHRONIC OBSTRUCTIVE PULMONARY DISEASE

Key Facts

Terminology
- COPD: Presence of airflow obstruction caused by chronic bronchitis or emphysema; the airflow obstruction is generally progressive, may be accompanied by airway hyper reactivity and may be partially reversible

Imaging Findings
- Sensitivity poor for early disease (25%), rare false positives (specificity 95%)
- Exacerbations: Chest radiograph often unchanged (only 20% show new abnormality)
- Hyperinflation most reliable sign of COPD

Top Differential Diagnoses
- Bronchiolitis Obliterans
- Hypersensitivity Pneumonitis

Pathology
- Exacerbations: Related to increased inflammation lower airways from bacteria, viruses, or changes in air quality
- COPD patients have on average 1 to 4 exacerbations a year

Clinical Issues
- Other signs/symptoms: Sputum gram stain and culture usually not helpful
- Progressive decline in ventilatory function and health status punctuated with varying frequency by exacerbations of symptoms
- Exacerbations: In-hospital mortality ~ 10% and 1 year mortality ~ 25-40%

- Difficult to recognize unless extreme, secondary signs include
  - Flat diaphragms
  - Widened retrosternal air space
  - Lung height increased
  - Small narrow heart
- Parenchymal areas of hypoattenuation
  - Inhomogeneous distribution
    - Arterial deficiency, increased branching angle of remaining vessels
  - Bullae
  - "Increased markings" emphysema
    - Not clearly understood, combination of bronchial wall thickening or superimposition of emphysematous walls
- Bronchi
  - Bronchial wall thickening
- Secondary manifestations
  - Pulmonary arterial hypertension
    - Enlarged central pulmonary arteries and peripheral arterial pruning

CT Findings
- HRCT
  - More sensitive than chest radiography
    - False negatives also occur with early disease
  - Emphysematous holes usually have no discernible wall
  - Central artery may remain visible surrounded by destroyed lung
  - Mucus plugging of small airways in asthma and bronchitis
  - Objectively measured by assuming that lung with a threshold HU < -960 is emphysematous lung
  - Paired inspiratory/expiratory scanning
    - May demonstrate air trapping in patients with small airways disease

DIFFERENTIAL DIAGNOSIS

Technical
- Low dose techniques may have false negatives
- Wide windows may cause false negatives

Bronchiolitis Obliterans
- No parenchymal destruction
- Mosaic attenuation pattern at HRCT

Hypersensitivity Pneumonitis
- Granulomatous airway inflammation from allergic reaction to inhaled antigen
- Centrilobular ground-glass nodules
- Hyperinflation of individual secondary pulmonary lobules

Athletic Hyperinflation
- Lungs normal
- Young athletes
- Pulmonary function tests normal

PATHOLOGY

General Features
- General path comments
  - Emphysema: Abnormal enlargement of the airspaces distal to the terminal bronchioles accompanied by destructive changes of the alveolar walls without obvious fibrosis
  - Chronic bronchitis: Chronic cough or mucus production for at least 3 months in 2 successive years
- Etiology
  - Exacerbations: Related to increased inflammation lower airways from bacteria, viruses, or changes in air quality
    - 50% episodes associated with viral infections (majority rhinovirus)
    - 10% episodes due to air pollution
    - 30% episodes unknown
    - 25-50% COPD lower airways colonized by bacteria: Haemophilus influenzae, Streptococcus pneumoniae, Moraxella catarrhalis
  - Emphysema pathogenesis

CHRONIC OBSTRUCTIVE PULMONARY DISEASE

- Approximately 30% of the normal lung must be destroyed before pulmonary function deteriorates
- Pulmonary function tests global summation of airways and lung
- Emphysema usually inhomogeneous
- Pulmonary function usually determined by structural integrity of lower lung zones
- Patients may have anatomic emphysema without alteration of pulmonary function
  - Centriacinar emphysema strongly associated with cigarette smoking
    - Dose and time related
    - Nearly all long term smokers will have anatomic emphysema
- Epidemiology
  - COPD 4th leading cause of death
  - COPD patients have on average 1 to 4 exacerbations a year
    - As disease progresses, intervals between acute exacerbations becomes shorter
- Associated abnormalities: Paraseptal thickening at risk for spontaneous pneumothorax

Gross Pathologic & Surgical Features
- Centriacinar emphysema
  - Dilatation 2nd order respiratory bronchioles in secondary pulmonary lobule
  - Primarily involves upper lung zones
  - Precursor may be respiratory bronchiolitis
- Panlobular emphysema
  - Involves entire secondary pulmonary lobule
  - Primarily involves lower lung zones
  - Seen in senile emphysema and alpha-1-antiprotease deficiency
- Paraseptal emphysema
  - Periphery of the secondary pulmonary lobule
- Irregular emphysema
  - Associated with lung scarring
- Bronchitis
  - Thickened bronchial wall: Mucous glands enlarged, dilatation mucous gland ducts, increase in number of mucous cells, goblet cell hyperplasia
- Bullae
  - Emphysema more than 1 cm in diameter with wall thickness < 1 mm

Staging, Grading or Classification Criteria
- ATS classification of COPD
  - Stage I: FEV_1 > 50% predicted
  - Stage II: FEV_1 35-49% predicted
  - Stage III: FEV_1 < 35% predicted

CLINICAL ISSUES

Presentation
- Most common signs/symptoms
  - Nonspecific: Dyspnea, shortness of breath
  - Exacerbations
    - Type 1: Increased breathlessness, increased sputum volume, and new or increased sputum purulence
    - Type 2: Any 2 of above symptoms
    - Type 3: Any 1 of above symptoms plus 1 additional feature; sore throat or nasal discharge within last 5 days, unexplained fever, increased wheeze, increased cough, or 20% increase in respiratory or heart rate compared with baseline
- Other signs/symptoms: Sputum gram stain and culture usually not helpful
- Pulmonary function tests (ATS criteria for functional emphysema)
  - Obstruction
    - Increased total and residual volumes
    - Residual volume (RV) > 120% predicted
    - Decreased flow volumes
    - Forced expiratory volume one second (FEV_1) < 80% predicted
  - Decreased diffusion capacity, < 80% predicted
- Indications for hospitalization; acute exacerbation
  - Unresponsive to outpatient management
  - Inability to walk between rooms
  - Inability to eat or sleep because of dyspnea
  - Altered mentation
  - Worsening hypoxemia or hypercarbia

Natural History & Prognosis
- Progressive decline in ventilatory function and health status punctuated with varying frequency by exacerbations of symptoms
- Exacerbations: In-hospital mortality ~ 10% and 1 year mortality ~ 25-40%
  - Mortality associated with age, severity of airflow obstruction (FEV_1), severity of hypoxemia, presence of hypercapnia, and marked weight loss

Treatment
- Smoking cessation
  - Pulmonary function will continue to decline
- Exacerbations
  - Supportive: Oxygen
  - Bronchodilators
  - Antibiotics for 5-10 day course
  - Corticosteroids short course systemic therapy
- Vaccinations: Pneumococcal and influenza

DIAGNOSTIC CHECKLIST

Image Interpretation Pearls
- Hyperinflation the most important sign of underlying COPD

SELECTED REFERENCES
1. Sapey E et al: COPD exacerbations. 2: aetiology. Thorax. 61(3):250-8, 2006
2. Vestbo J: Clinical assessment, staging, and epidemiology of chronic obstructive pulmonary disease exacerbations. Proc Am Thorac Soc. 3(3):252-6, 2006
3. Sethi S: Pathogenesis and treatment of acute exacerbations of chronic obstructive pulmonary disease. Semin Respir Crit Care Med. 26(2):192-203, 2005
4. Brunton S et al: Acute exacerbation of chronic bronchitis: a primary care consensus guideline. Am J Manag Care. 10(10):689-96, 2004

CHRONIC OBSTRUCTIVE PULMONARY DISEASE

IMAGE GALLERY

Typical

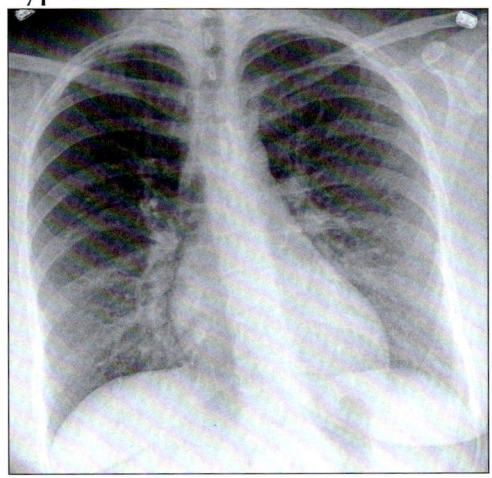
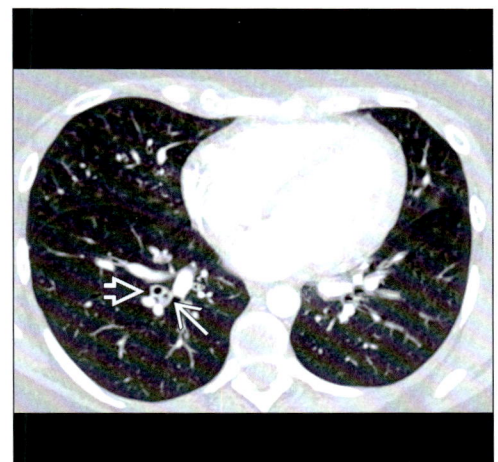

(Left) Frontal radiograph is normal. No hyperinflation. Chronic cough and history of asthma. *(Right)* Axial HRCT shows bronchial wall thickening ➡ and mucus plugs ➡. Note that the distal lung is normal.

Typical

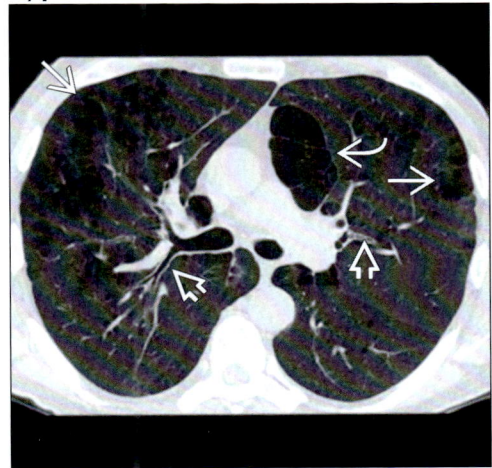
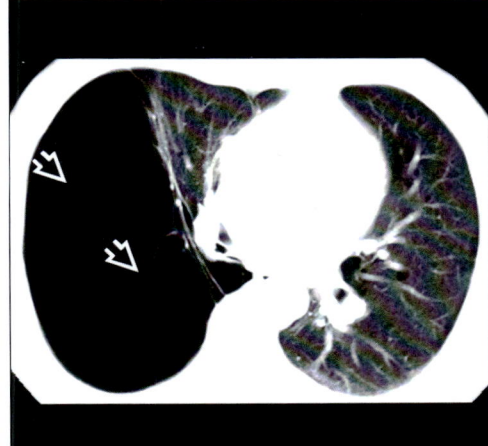

(Left) Axial HRCT shows diffuse bronchial wall thickening ➡ and focal areas of emphysema ➡ and discrete bullae ➡. *(Right)* Axial NECT shows large bulla filling entire right hemithorax with slight shift of the mediastinum to the left. Bulla separated by thin septa ➡.

Typical

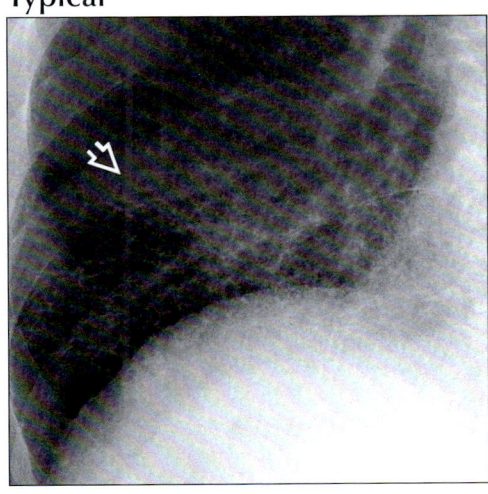
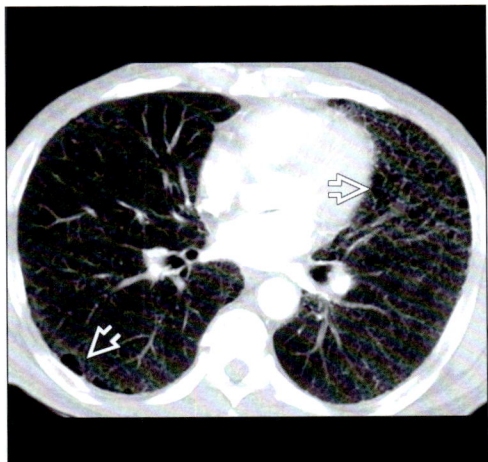

(Left) Frontal radiograph shows diffuse interstitial thickening in the lung base ➡. *(Right)* Axial CECT shows emphysema ➡. "Increased markings" emphysema as a cause of interstitial pattern on chest radiograph.

ASTHMA

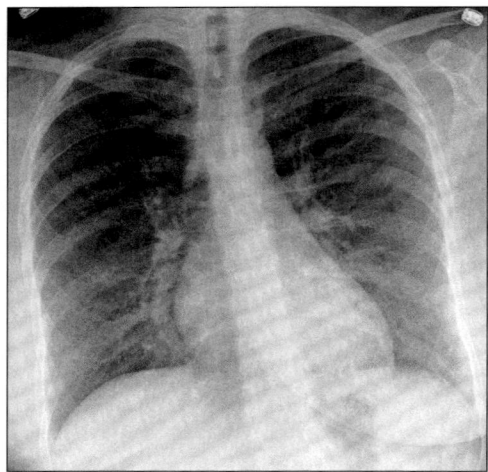

Frontal radiograph is normal. Lung volumes are normal. Acute asthmatic attack.

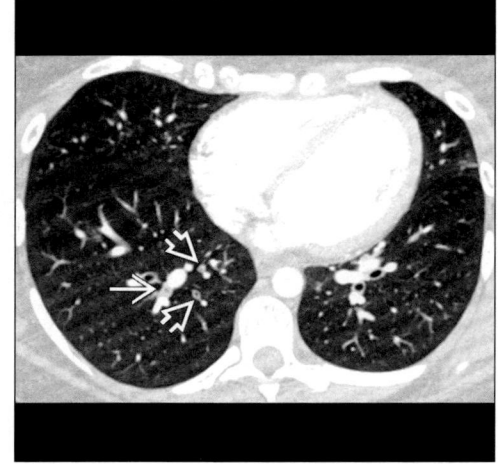

Axial HRCT shows bronchial wall thickening ➡ and mucus plugs ➡.

TERMINOLOGY

Definitions
- Chronic airway inflammation results in reversible airflow obstruction
  - Inflammation may eventually result in airway remodeling and irreversible obstruction
- Status asthmaticus: Medical emergency in which asthmatic attack refractory to bronchodilator therapy

IMAGING FINDINGS

Radiographic Findings
- Limited role in diagnosis, important for complications of and processes that mimic asthma
- In general, the more severe the bronchoconstriction, the more likely the chest radiograph is abnormal
  - Normal radiographs (75%) because
    - Obstruction to airflow nonuniform throughout the lungs
    - Large segments receive a small fraction of each breath (hypoventilated)
    - Small segments receive most of the air (hyperventilated)
    - Summation of hypo and hyperventilated lung often results in normal chest radiography
- Up to 1/3rd of admitted patients will have major abnormalities
  - Focal opacities or diffuse interstitial thickening (presumed pneumonia), enlarged heart, new nodule, pneumothorax, or pulmonary edema
- Nonspecific findings
  - Bronchial wall thickening: More common in chronic asthma
  - Hyperinflation: Flattened diaphragms, deep retrosternal space
  - Atelectasis: Subsegmental to lobar due to airways obstruction from mucus plugs
  - Pulmonary artery hypertension (due to hypoxic vasoconstriction of large portions of the pulmonary vascular bed)
- Acute complications: Pneumomediastinum (5%), pneumothorax (0.3%), pneumonia (up to 2%)
- Status asthmaticus: Paradoxically chest radiograph often normal

DDx: Decreased Lung Attenuation

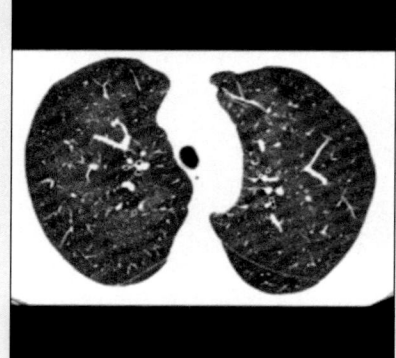

Bronchiolitis Obliterans

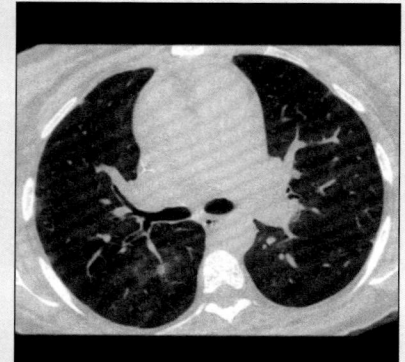

Pulmonary Arterial Hypertension

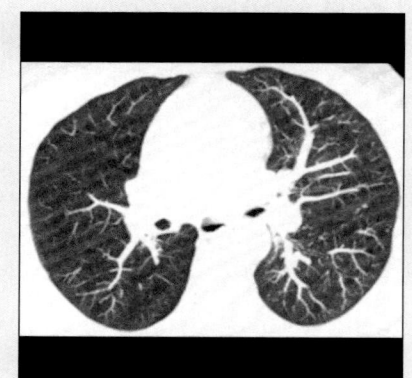

Acute Pulmonary Embolism

ASTHMA

Key Facts

Terminology
- Chronic airway inflammation results in reversible airflow obstruction
- Inflammation may eventually result in airway remodeling and irreversible obstruction

Imaging Findings
- Limited role in diagnosis, important for complications of and processes that mimic asthma
- In general, the more severe the bronchoconstriction, the more likely the chest radiograph is abnormal
- Status asthmaticus: Paradoxically chest radiograph often normal

Top Differential Diagnoses
- Asthma Mimics
- Chronic upper airway obstruction
- Airway foreign bodies
- Cardiac asthma (edema of airway narrows lumen)
- Recurrent pulmonary embolus
- Recurrent aspiration
- Eosinophilic pneumonia
- Polyarteritis nodosa
- Carcinoid syndrome
- Vocal cord dysfunction (factitious asthma)

Clinical Issues
- Mortality 2 deaths per 100,000 (last 2 decades 100% increase in death rate)

Diagnostic Checklist
- The requisition for a patient who wheezes common, consider the asthma mimics

---

- Stage 1: Hyperventilate to maintain oxygenation, lung volumes increased
- Stage 2: Hyperventilate but unable to maintain oxygenation, lung volumes increased
- Stage 3: Fatigue, unable to hyperventilate, PCO_2 normalizes, hypoxic, lung volumes decreased to normal
- Stage 4: Respiratory failure, PCO_2 rises, hypoxia, lung volumes normal

CT Findings
- More sensitive than chest radiography
- Heterogeneous distribution of bronchial and lung parenchymal findings typical
- Airways
  - Bronchial wall thickening (50-90%)
    - Degree of thickening correlates with severity of disease and airflow obstruction
    - Will decrease with treatment
  - Bronchial artery ratio (normal approximately 1:1)
    - 75% of asthmatics (35% of bronchi) have bronchial artery ratio > 1 (but less than 1.5)
  - Bronchial dilatation (30%)
    - Subsegmental bronchi larger than adjacent artery or nontapering airway morphology (typically cylindrical)
    - Bronchiectasis consider: APBA, irreversible airway remodeling, artifactual (from hypoxic vasoconstriction), or physiologic (from ventilation at large lung volumes)
  - Centrilobular micronodules or branching opacities (10-20%)
    - Finding most likely to be seen in patients with near-fatal asthma
- Lung parenchyma
  - Decreased lung attenuation (50%)
  - Air-trapping (total volume > 1 segment) 50%
  - Mosaic lung attenuation
    - Degree of mosaic attenuation correlates with the degree of asthma
  - Emphysema rare
    - Debatable whether secondary to asthma, usually only seen in those who smoke

Imaging Recommendations
- Best imaging tool: HRCT for bronchiectasis
- Protocol advice
  - Choose display window widths > 1,500 HU to avoid artificial bronchial wall thickening
  - Perform expiratory scans to visualize air-trapping

DIFFERENTIAL DIAGNOSIS

Asthma Mimics
- Chronic upper airway obstruction
  - Tracheal stenosis: Wegener, post-intubation stricture, airway tumors
  - Extrinsic: Substernal thyroid or vascular rings
  - Tracheobronchomalacia
- Airway foreign bodies
- Cardiac asthma (edema of airway narrows lumen)
- Recurrent pulmonary embolus
- Recurrent aspiration
- Eosinophilic pneumonia
- Polyarteritis nodosa
- Churg-Strauss vasculitis
- Carcinoid syndrome
- Sarcoidosis
- Bronchocentric granulomatosis
- Vocal cord dysfunction (factitious asthma)
  - Conversion disorder, oxygenation normal, responds to anti-anxiety agents

Bronchiolitis Obliterans
- Mosaic attenuation common
- Decreased lung attenuation sometimes absent (nearly always present in asthma)

PATHOLOGY

General Features
- General path comments: Airway wall inflammation increases smooth muscle tone, increases secretions (mucus plugging)

ASTHMA

- Epidemiology
  - Prevalence of childhood asthma 2-8%
  - Prevalence of adult asthma 3%
- Associated abnormalities: Rhinosinusitis up to 85%

Gross Pathologic & Surgical Features
- Inflammation primarily involves medium-sized and small bronchi

Microscopic Features
- Bronchial wall thickening from edema, increase smooth muscle, size and number of mucous glands, cellular infiltration (eosinophils, lymphocytes, plasma cells)

CLINICAL ISSUES

Presentation
- Most common signs/symptoms
  - Severity of bronchospasm correlates with clinical features
  - Episodic wheezing, chest tightness, breathlessness
    - Symptoms may worsen at night, awakening the patient
  - History of allergic rhinitis or atopic dermatitis
  - Prolonged phase of forced exhalation
  - Increased nasal secretions, mucosal swelling, sinusitis, rhinitis, or nasal polyps
- Other signs/symptoms
  - Peak expiratory flow rate (PEFR)
    - Two or three daily measurements in hospital, at home, or at work
    - Asthma diagnosed when there is greater than 20% diurnal variation on 3 or more days in a week for 2 weeks on a peak flow diary
  - Spirometry
    - Airways obstruction determined by drop of forced expiratory volume in 1 second (FEV_1) below 80% of predicted, or if ratio of FEV_1 to forced vital capacity less than 75%
  - Other lung function tests
    - Flow-volume curves: Can help differentiate between asthma and chronic obstructive pulmonary disease (COPD)
    - Single-breath gas transfer factor: Can be normal in asthma and reduced in COPD
  - Skin prick testing for atopic state
    - May identify potential trigger
    - Lifestyle or workplace modifications for known allergen
  - Measurement of airway hyperresponsiveness
    - FEV_1 measurements during incremental administration of histamine or methacholine
    - Administration stopped once a 20% decrease of FEV_1 reached
    - Result expressed as "provocative dose"
    - Provocative dose reflects degree of airway sensitivity that can reflect asthma severity
  - Sputum examination
    - Sputum eosinophil counts may serve as marker for airway inflammation
    - Rises in sputum eosinophils may predict imminent loss of asthma control
  - Asthma triad: Nasal polyps, urticaria, asthma following aspirin ingestion (up to 10% of asthmatics)
  - Trigger factors
    - Infections: Rhinoviruses, influenza virus, respiratory syncytial virus
    - Exercise: Especially in cold weather
    - Changes in climate: Thunderstorms
    - Pollution: Ozone and sulfur dioxide
    - Occupational factors: Dusty, cold, and wet rooms
    - Drugs: Aspirin, beta-blockers, nonsteroidal anti-inflammatory agents
    - Allergens: Pet allergens, house dust, cockroach allergens, pollens
    - Gastroesophageal reflux
    - Smoking
- Clinical Profile
  - Step 1: Mild and intermittent
    - ≤ 2 days with symptoms per week, 2 < nights with symptoms per week, ≥ 80% peak expiratory flow, < 20% peak expiratory flow variability
  - Step 2: Mild and persistent
    - 3-6 days with symptoms per week, 3-4 nights with symptoms per month, ≥ 80% peak expiratory flow, 20-30% peak expiratory flow variability
  - Step 3: Moderate and persistent
    - Daily symptoms, ≥ 5 nights with symptoms per month, > 60% to < 80% peak expiratory flow, > 30% peak expiratory flow variability
  - Step 4: Severe and persistent
    - Continuous symptoms, frequent nights with symptoms, ≤ 60% peak expiratory flow, > 30% peak expiratory flow variability

Natural History & Prognosis
- Mortality 2 deaths per 100,000 (last 2 decades 100% increase in death rate)

Treatment
- Medical therapy directed towards bronchoconstriction and inflammation of airway wall
  - Bronchodilators: Long-acting β-agonists, theophyllines, corticosteroids
  - Anticholinergic agents: Ipratropium bromide
- Preventive therapies
  - Inhaled corticosteroids
  - Cromoglycate: Mast cell stabilizer
  - Leukotriene modifying agents

DIAGNOSTIC CHECKLIST

Consider
- The requisition for a patient who wheezes common, consider the asthma mimics

SELECTED REFERENCES
1. Sung A et al: The role of chest radiography and computed tomography in the diagnosis and management of asthma. Curr Opin Pulm Med. 13(1):31-6, 2007
2. de Jong PA et al: Computed tomographic imaging of the airways: relationship to structure and function. Eur Respir J. 26(1):140-52, 2005

ASTHMA

IMAGE GALLERY

Typical

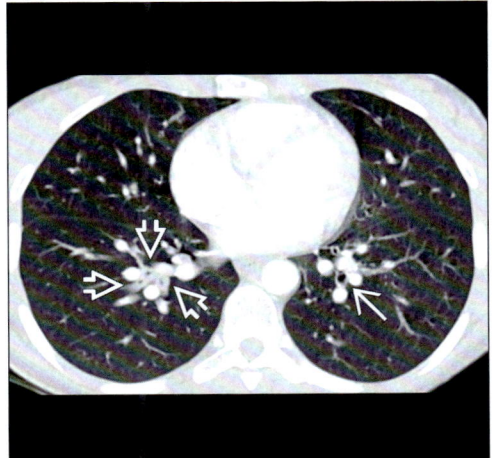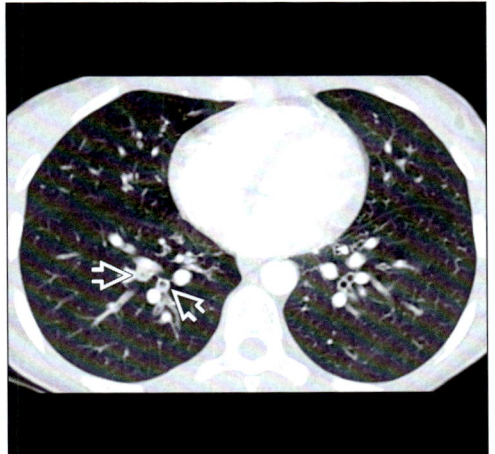

(Left) Axial CECT shows mucus plugs ➡ and narrowing of segmental and subsegmental airways. Other airways are normal ➡. (Right) Axial CECT shows mucus plugs ➡ and narrowing of segmental and subsegmental airways. Note that the lung distal to the mucus plugs is normal.

Typical

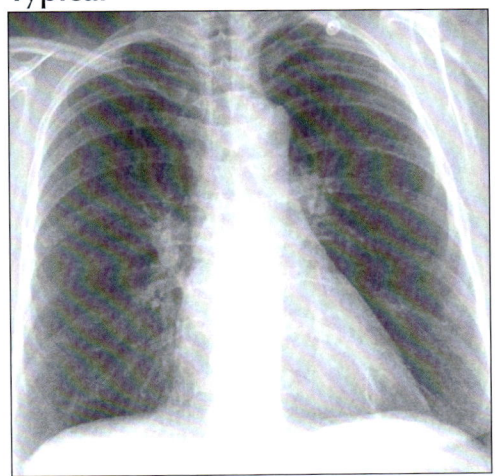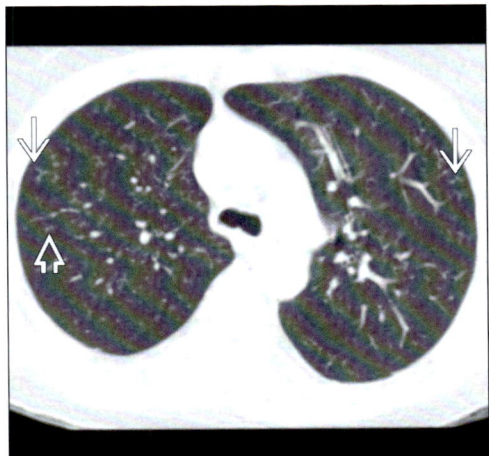

(Left) Frontal radiograph shows increased lung volumes. (Right) Axial HRCT shows centrilobular micronodules ➡ and tree-in-bud opacities ➡ from severe asthmatic attack.

Typical

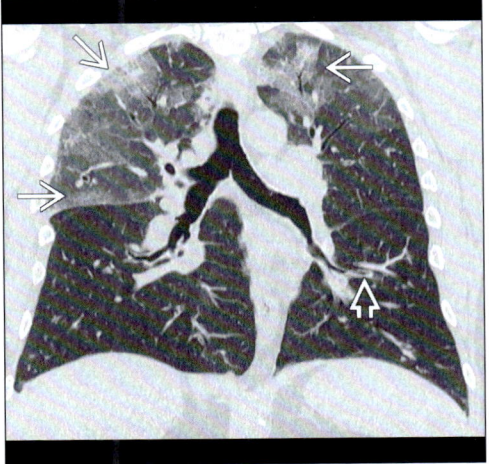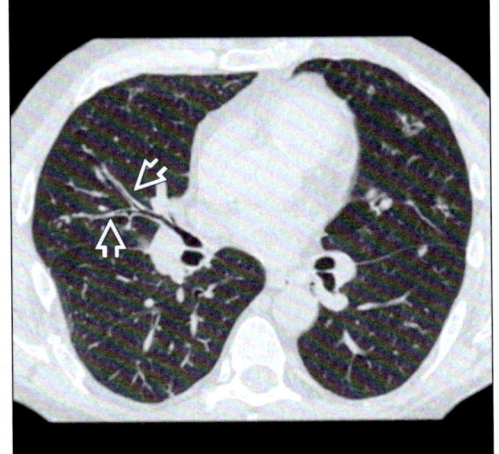

(Left) Coronal HRCT shows lobular ground-glass opacities ➡ predominantly in the upper lobes. Mild diffuse bronchial wall thickening ➡. Lungs hyperinflated. (Right) Axial HRCT shows mild diffuse bronchial wall thickening and mucus plugging ➡. Diagnosis Churg-Strauss vasculitis.

HYPERSENSITIVITY PNEUMONITIS

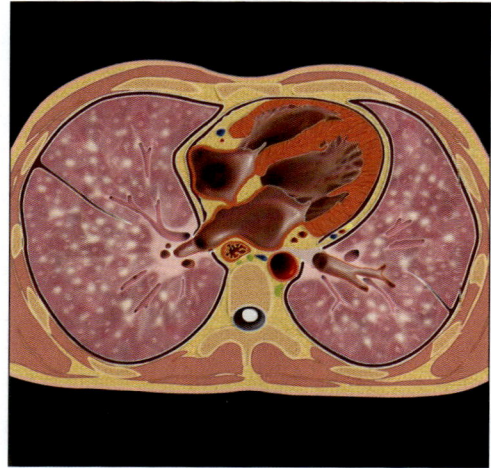

Axial graphic shows typical features of hypersensitivity pneumonitis. Centrilobular ground-glass nodules uniformly distributed throughout the lung.

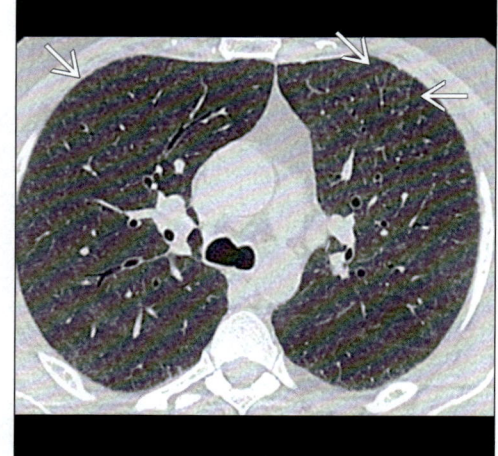

Axial HRCT shows faint centrilobular ground-glass opacities ➔ from hypersensitivity pneumonitis from hot tub lung.

TERMINOLOGY

Abbreviations and Synonyms
- Extrinsic allergic alveolitis, farmer's lung
- Nonspecific interstitial pneumonia (NSIP), usual interstitial pneumonia (UIP), cryptogenic organizing pneumonia (COP)

Definitions
- Diffuse granulomatous interstitial lung disease caused by inhalation of various antigenic particles (microbes, animal proteins and low-molecular weight chemicals)
  - Farmer's lung and bird fancier's lung the most common forms

IMAGING FINDINGS

General Features
- Best diagnostic clue: Ground-glass centrilobular nodules + mosaic perfusion = hypersensitivity pneumonitis (HP)
- Location: Mid-lung most common, spares costophrenic angles
- Morphology: Ground-glass opacities and ground-glass centrilobular nodules

Radiographic Findings
- Radiography
  - Acute stage
    - Chest radiography normal in 90%
    - Fine miliary pattern
    - Consolidation rare
  - Subacute stage
    - Chest radiograph usually abnormal 90%
    - Poorly-defined miliary nodules
    - Diffuse or middle and lower lung increased density
  - Chronic stage
    - Findings of fibrosis: Architectural distortion, volume loss
    - Mid-lung and upper lobes predominate
    - No pleural disease or adenopathy
    - Usually spares or less severe in costophrenic angles
  - Absent: Pleural effusions, cavitation, hilar or mediastinal adenopathy

CT Findings
- CT signs

DDx: Upper Lobe Nodules

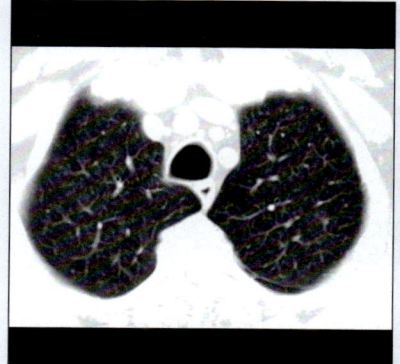

Respiratory Bronchiolitis

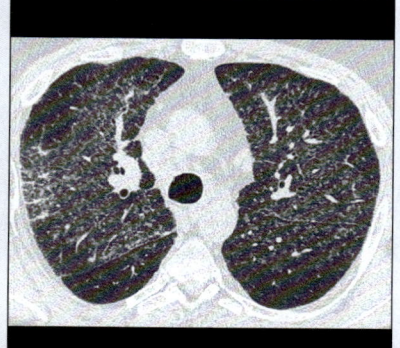

Sarcoidosis

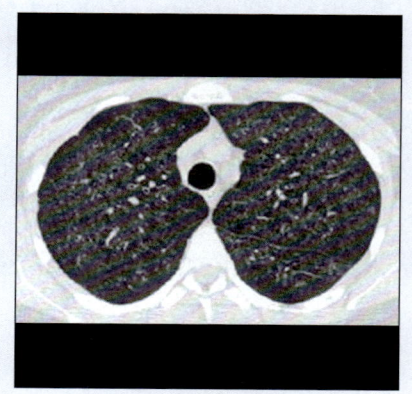

Langerhans Granulomatosis

HYPERSENSITIVITY PNEUMONITIS

Key Facts

Terminology
- Diffuse granulomatous interstitial lung disease caused by inhalation of various antigenic particles (microbes, animal proteins and low-molecular weight chemicals)

Imaging Findings
- Ground-glass centrilobular nodules + mosaic perfusion = hypersensitivity pneumonitis
- Lung cysts (10%)
- Emphysema more common than fibrosis
- Ground-glass opacities, centrilobular nodules, mosaic attenuation and air-trapping may resolve with treatment

Top Differential Diagnoses
- Nonspecific Interstitial Pneumonia
- Respiratory Bronchiolitis
- Langerhans Granulomatosis
- Sarcoidosis

Pathology
- Small particles (< 5 μ diameter) deposit in bronchioles, incite allergic granulomatous reaction
- Histologic features not pathognomonic
- Granulomas may be few and difficult to find, often loosely organized (in contrast to the tightly organized granulomas of sarcoid)

Clinical Issues
- Acute: Sudden onset of a flu-like syndrome (fever, chills, and malaise)
- Subacute: Insidious onset of nonspecific symptoms, malaise, fatigue, weight loss
- Avoid exposure to antigen

- Ground-glass opacities 100%
  - Geographic distribution in central and peripheral portions of the lung
- Faint ill-defined centrilobular nodules (< 5 mm diameter) 70%
  - Pleural surfaces usually spared
- Mosaic perfusion (variable lung attenuation and variable vessel size) 80%
- Air-trapping expiratory scan 95%
- Combined signs
  - Geographic ground-glass attenuation + normal lung + mosaic perfusion + air-trapping = head cheese sign
  - Ground-glass centrilobular nodules + mosaic perfusion = hypersensitivity pneumonitis
- Mediastinal adenopathy 50% (nodes typically < 2 cm short-axis diameter)
- Acute stage
  - Small, ill-defined centrilobular nodules
  - Bilateral airspace ground-glass opacities
  - Mid and lower lung predominance
- Subacute stage
  - Mosaic perfusion
  - Ground-glass opacities (patchy distribution)
  - Small, ill-defined centrilobular nodules
  - Middle and lower lung predominance
  - Lung cysts (10%)
    - Few in number, 3-25 mm diameter, usually associated with ground glass opacities
- Chronic stage
  - Fibrosis: Honeycombing, traction bronchiectasis, and architectural distortion
  - Distribution reticular opacities variable: Peribronchovascular (like NSIP), subpleural (like UIP), or random
    - Middle and upper lung predominance
    - Costophrenic angles less severely involved
  - Superimposed subacute findings: Ground-glass opacities & small, ill-defined, centrilobular nodules
  - Emphysema (not associated with smoking)
    - Emphysema more common than fibrosis
- Resolution

- Ground-glass opacities, centrilobular nodules, mosaic attenuation and air-trapping may resolve with treatment

Imaging Recommendations
- Best imaging tool
  - HRCT: More sensitive for hypersensitivity pneumonitis
  - Inspiratory scans more valuable than expiratory scans

DIFFERENTIAL DIAGNOSIS

Idiopathic Pulmonary Fibrosis
- HRCT: Honeycombing, bibasilar reticular opacities, and traction bronchiectasis
- Typical anatomic distribution: Peripheral, subpleural, and bibasilar
  - Does not spare costophrenic angles, in fact, usually severely involved
- Ground-glass opacities much less than extent of reticular opacities
- Centrilobular nodules uncommon
- Air-trapping not a feature

Nonspecific Interstitial Pneumonia
- Two histologic patterns: Cellular and fibrotic
- HRCT: Ground-glass opacities extent greater than reticular opacities
- Honeycombing absent or minimal
- Peribronchovascular distribution
- Centrilobular nodules uncommon
- Air-trapping not a feature

Respiratory Bronchiolitis
- Smokers (smoking protects from hypersensitivity pneumonitis)
- Centrilobular nodules fewer in number
- Predominantly upper lung zones
- Associated centrilobular emphysema

Langerhans Granulomatosis
- Centrilobular nodules often cavitate

HYPERSENSITIVITY PNEUMONITIS

- Smokers
- Predominantly upper lung zones

Sarcoidosis
- Nodules have soft-tissue attenuation
- Typically bronchovascular and subpleural distribution
  - Subpleural lymphatic deposits rare in HP
- Predominantly upper lung zones

Silicosis
- Occupational history
- Nodules have soft-tissue attenuation
- Typically bronchovascular and subpleural distribution
  - Subpleural lymphatic deposits rare in HP
- May have adenopathy
- Air-trapping not a feature

PATHOLOGY

General Features
- General path comments
  - Allergic reaction to airborne organic particles (1-5 μm)
    - More than 200 different organic antigens from a variety of sources
    - 40% offending agent not identified
  - 95% of cases occurs in nonsmokers
  - Regardless of antigen, < 1% of exposed develop hypersensitivity reaction
- Etiology
  - Microbes: Thermophilic actinomyces grow in moldy hay, principle cause of farmer's lung, bagassosis, and mushroom workers lung
    - Nontuberculous atypical mycobacteria principle cause of hot tub lung
  - Animal proteins: Avian proteins, principle cause of bird fancier's lung
  - Low-molecular weight chemicals: Isocyanates (production of foams, paints) principle cause of occupational asthma and HP
  - Pathophysiology
    - Small particles (< 5 μ diameter) deposit in bronchioles, incite allergic granulomatous reaction
- Epidemiology: Uncommon farmer's lung 2-8%, bird fancier's lung: 1-10%

Gross Pathologic & Surgical Features
- Costophrenic angles less involved

Microscopic Features
- Histologic features not pathognomonic
  - Class triad: Cellular bronchiolitis, lymphocytic interstitial infiltrate, poorly formed nonnecrotizing granulomas
- Acute: Neutrophilic infiltration of respiratory bronchioles and alveoli
- Subacute: Cellular bronchiolitis, noncaseating granulomas, bronchiolocentric interstitial lymphocytic pneumonitis
  - Granulomas may be few and difficult to find, often loosely organized (in contrast to the tightly organized granulomas of sarcoid)
- Chronic: Various fibrotic patterns, 50% NSIP, 40% UIP, 10% COP

CLINICAL ISSUES

Presentation
- Most common signs/symptoms
  - Acute, subacute, chronic forms, considerable overlap
  - Acute: Sudden onset of a flu-like syndrome (fever, chills, and malaise)
    - Pulmonary symptoms: Severe dyspnea, chest tightness, and dry or mildly productive cough
    - Peak intensity of symptoms: 3-6 hours after initial exposure
    - Signs/symptoms gradually clear over 24-48 hours
    - Often mistaken as pneumonia
  - Subacute: Insidious onset of nonspecific symptoms, malaise, fatigue, weight loss
    - Hemoptysis in up to one-fourth
  - Chronic: Dyspnea
    - Indistinguishable from other chronic interstitial lung diseases
- Other signs/symptoms
  - Pulmonary function tests
    - Acute: Restrictive pattern
    - Subacute and chronic: Obstructive pattern

Natural History & Prognosis
- Acute: May completely return to normal
- Subacute/chronic: May progress even after eliminating antigen exposure
- Mortality rates variable: 1-10%

Treatment
- Avoid exposure to antigen
  - Quandary for farmer's whose livelihood at risk
  - Quandary for bird breeder's who develop emotional attachment to birds
- Steroids

DIAGNOSTIC CHECKLIST

Consider
- NSIP should be evaluated for possible hypersensitivity pneumonitis

Image Interpretation Pearls
- Centrilobular nodules and air-trapping in acute-subacute disease
- Subpleural basilar honeycombing with less involvement of costophrenic angles characteristic of chronic hypersensitivity pneumonitis

SELECTED REFERENCES

1. Silva CI et al: Hypersensitivity pneumonitis: spectrum of high-resolution CT and pathologic findings. AJR Am J Roentgenol. 188(2):334-44, 2007
2. Glazer CS et al: Clinical and radiologic manifestations of hypersensitivity pneumonitis. J Thorac Imaging. 17(4):261-72, 2002

HYPERSENSITIVITY PNEUMONITIS

IMAGE GALLERY

Typical

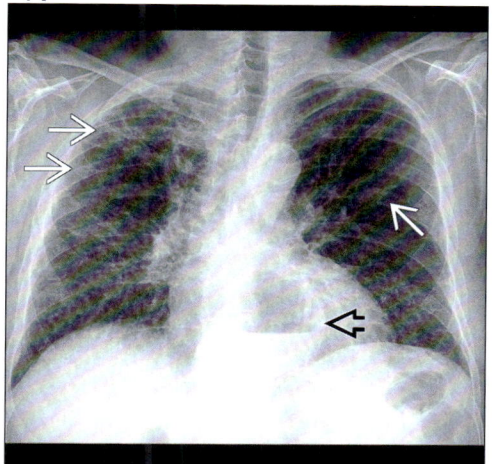
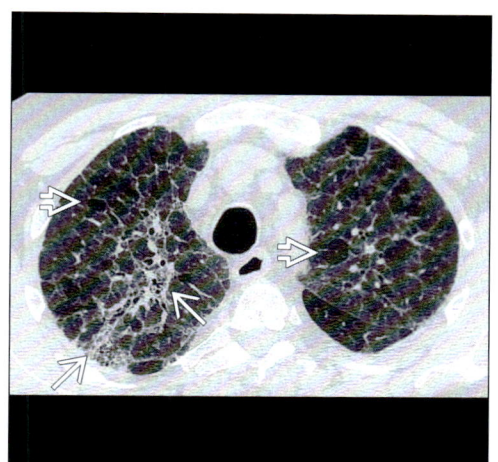

(Left) Frontal radiograph shows ill-defined opacities ➔ in the mid-upper lungs. Large hiatal hernia ⬧. (Right) Axial HRCT shows admixture of linear opacities ➔, hyperinflated lobules ➔ and normal lung (head cheese sign) from chronic hypersensitivity pneumonitis due to farmer's lung.

Typical

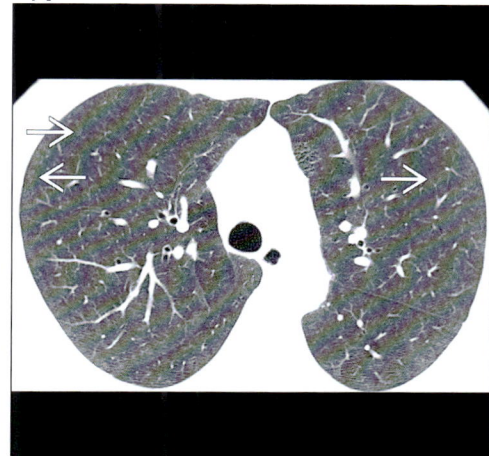
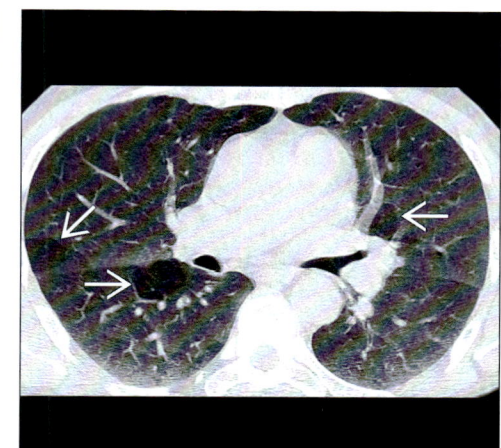

(Left) Axial HRCT shows faint centrilobular ground-glass opacities ➔. Chest radiograph was normal. (Right) Axial HRCT at full expiration shows lobular air-trapping ➔. Hypersensitivity pneumonitis in bird fancier.

Typical

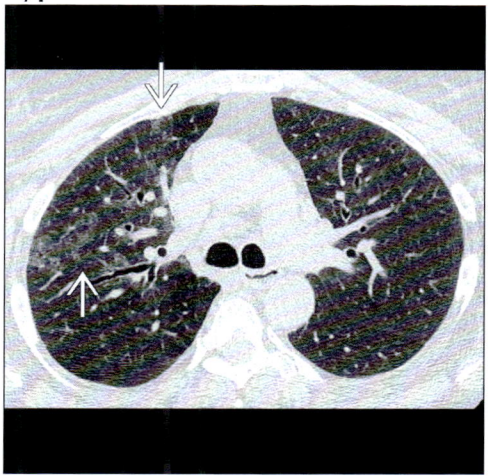
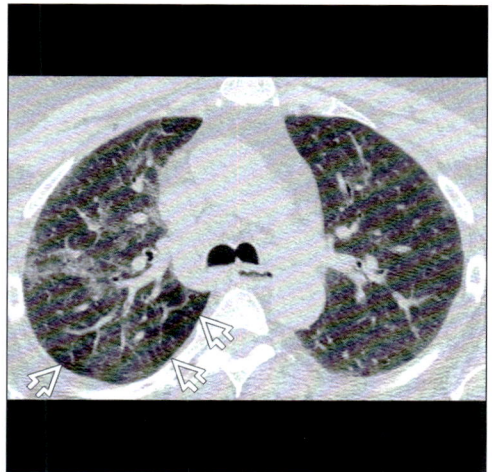

(Left) Axial HRCT shows nonspecific lobular ground-glass opacities ➔. (Right) Axial HRCT at full expiration shows air-trapping ➔. Hypersensitivity pneumonitis. Antigen unknown.

ASPIRATION

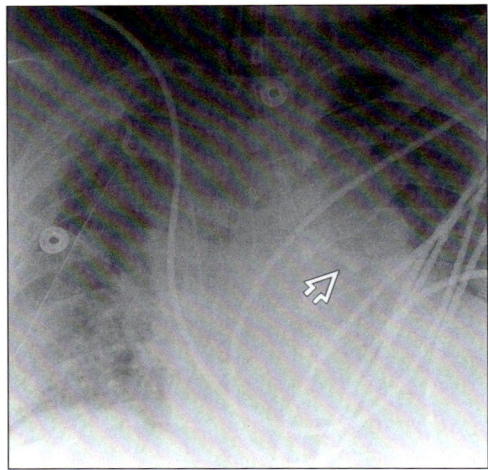

Anteroposterior radiograph shows a tooth ➡ in the left main bronchus. Aspirated tooth happened 10 days into hospitalization for respiratory failure.

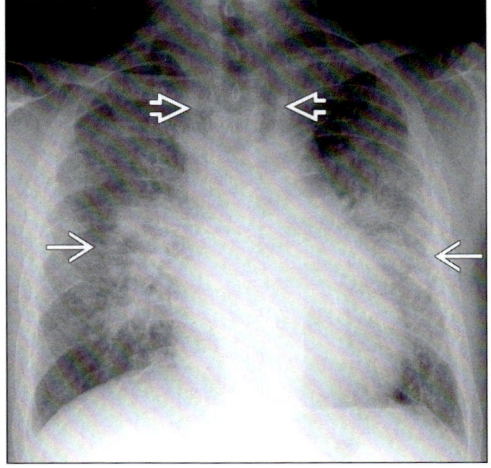

Frontal radiograph shows diffuse central consolidation ➡ from massive aspiration. Dilated esophagus ➡ from achalasia. Pattern is that of pulmonary edema.

TERMINOLOGY

Abbreviations and Synonyms
- Aspiration pneumonia: Pulmonary infection caused by aspiration of colonized oropharyngeal secretions
- Aspiration pneumonitis: Acute lung injury caused by the aspiration of materials toxic to the lungs (gastric acid, milk, mineral oil, and volatile hydrocarbons)

Definitions
- Intake of a variety of solid or liquid materials into the airways and lungs
- Different aspiration syndromes
  - Foreign bodies: Most common endobronchial obstruction in children (toys); food particles (vegetables) and broken fragments of teeth (elderly); main and lobar bronchi, most common location
  - Mendelson syndrome: Aspiration of sterile gastric contents during labor and delivery; can be severe and fatal
  - Exogenous lipoid pneumonia: Repeated aspiration of mineral oil or a related substance; in children, cod liver oil and milk; in adults, oily nose drops and mineral laxatives
  - Hydrocarbon pneumonia: Accidental poisoning in young children (furniture polish); hydrocarbon-containing fluids (petroleum) in fire eaters (fire-eaters pneumonia)
  - Near drowning: Pulmonary edema after acute aspiration of massive amounts of fresh or salt water; pneumonia depending on the water composition
  - Lentil aspiration pneumonia: Granulomatous pneumonitis caused by aspiration of legumes (lentils, beans, and peas)

IMAGING FINDINGS

General Features
- Best diagnostic clue
  - Radiopaque material within the airways (foreign body)
  - Gravity-dependent opacities
- Location: Aspiration syndromes gravity dependent locations: Supine: Superior segments lower lobes & posterior segments upper lobes; upright: Basilar segments lower lobes

DDx: Diffuse Pulmonary Consolidation

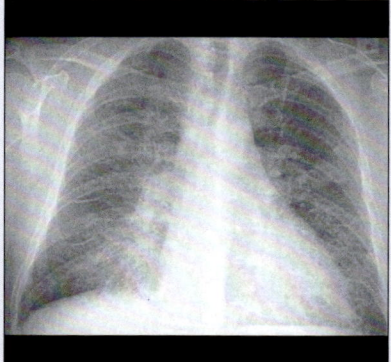

Acute Pulmonary Edema

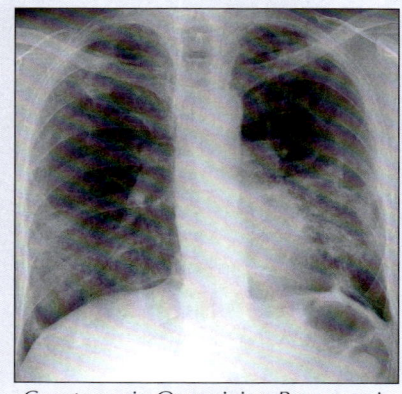

Cryptogenic Organizing Pneumonia

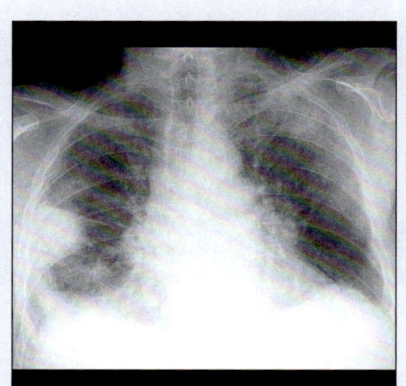

Eosinophilic Pneumonia

ASPIRATION

Key Facts

Terminology
- Aspiration pneumonia: Pulmonary infection caused by aspiration of colonized oropharyngeal secretions
- Aspiration pneumonitis: Acute lung injury caused by the aspiration of materials toxic to the lungs (gastric acid, milk, mineral oil, and volatile hydrocarbons)

Imaging Findings
- **Unilateral** or bilateral air-space consolidation in gravity dependent distribution
- Supine position: Superior segments of the lower lobes and posterior segments of the upper lobes
- Upright position: Basal segments of the lower lobes, R > L
- Decubitus position: Axillary subsegments of the upper lobes
- Even large quantity aspiration syndromes can be unilateral
- Endotracheal or tracheostomy tubes do not protect from aspiration

Top Differential Diagnoses
- Pulmonary embolism
- Pulmonary edema
- Eosinophilic pneumonia

Pathology
- 50% adults aspirate oropharyngeal secretions during sleep

Clinical Issues
- Silent aspiration: 50% of anesthetized patients have no symptoms

Radiographic Findings
- Foreign body
  - Atelectasis: Lung, lobar, or segmental depending of size of foreign body
  - Hyperinflation & air-trapping more common in children
- Aspiration pneumonia & pneumonitis
  - **Unilateral** or bilateral air-space consolidation in gravity dependent distribution
    - Supine position: Superior segments of the lower lobes and posterior segments of the upper lobes
    - Upright position: Basal segments of the lower lobes, R > L
    - Decubitus position: Axillary subsegments of the upper lobes
    - Recurrent aspiration often favors same location due to anatomic drainage patterns
    - Even large quantity aspiration syndromes can be unilateral
  - Diffuse perihilar consolidation more common with pneumonitis
  - Endotracheal or tracheostomy tubes do not protect from aspiration
    - Fluid may accumulate above endotracheal balloon, source of aspiration pneumonia
  - Acute aspiration pneumonitis may quickly evolve into adult respiratory distress syndrome (ARDS)
  - Untreated aspiration pneumonia often leads to necrotizing pneumonia and lung abscess
  - Chronic aspiration syndromes from retained foreign bodies or recurrent aspiration pneumonia (pneumonitis) may lead to bronchiectasis
  - Recurrent: Multiple episodes, sometimes identical in appearance, may wax and wane over time
  - Resolution variable depends on quantity and type of aspirate, nontoxic aspirate will clear within hours

CT Findings
- NECT: More sensitive than chest radiography for complications: Abscess, empyema, and bronchiectasis
- Foreign bodies
  - More useful for radiolucent foreign bodies
- Aspiration pneumonia & pneumonitis
  - Variable patterns, gravitational segmental localization usually better demonstrated
    - Tree-in-bud opacities from aspirated material in small airways, common in lentil aspiration
    - Consolidation from aspirate into airspaces, may evolve into ARDS from acute injury, or may be chronic and mass-like
    - Bronchiectasis from chronic recurrent injury to airways
    - Interstitial fibrosis from chronic injury to airspace
  - Lipoid pneumonia: Low attenuation (fat density) focal consolidation and "crazy-paving" pattern
  - Hydrocarbon pneumonia: Consolidation and **pneumatoceles**
  - Near drowning: "Sand bronchogram" (radiopaque) if sand is aspirated along with water
  - Granulomatous pneumonitis (lentil aspiration pneumonia)
    - Centrilobular ill-defined nodules (foreign body granulomas)
    - Linear and branching structures ("tree-in-bud")

Imaging Recommendations
- Best imaging tool
  - Chest radiography usually sufficient for detection and monitoring
  - CT more sensitive for airspace, airways, and pleural space abnormalities

DIFFERENTIAL DIAGNOSIS

Acute Aspiration
- Pulmonary embolism
  - Common cause of acute respiratory distress in hospitalized patients
  - Infarcts often peripheral and associated with pleural effusion
- Pulmonary edema
  - Cardiomegaly, often with bilateral pleural effusions
  - Kerley B lines uncommon with aspiration
- ARDS

ASPIRATION

  - Identical radiographic findings

Chronic Aspiration
- Endobronchial obstruction
  - Slow-growing endobronchial tumors such as carcinoid or chronic obstructing lesions such as broncholithiasis
- Bronchiectasis and tree-in-bud opacities
  - Mycobacterial opportunistic infections
    - Typically elderly women with chronic cough
    - Bronchiectasis typically middle lobe and lingula, uncommon areas for aspiration

Recurrent Aspiration
- Eosinophilic pneumonia
  - Recurrent consolidation, waxes and wanes over time
- Cryptogenic organizing pneumonia
  - Recurrent focal consolidation, waxes and wanes over time
  - Typically peripheral and basilar in location

PATHOLOGY

General Features
- General path comments
  - Community acquired pneumonia
    - Hemophilus influenza, Streptococcus pneumonia, Staphylococcus pneumonia and Enterobacteria colonize oropharynx and cause community acquired pneumonia
    - Aspiration accounts for 5-15% of community acquired pneumonia
  - Hospitalized aspiration pneumonia
    - Pseudomonas aeruginosa most common cause
    - In contrast to previous notions: Anaerobic organisms rare
- Etiology
  - Predisposing factors: Alcoholism, loss of consciousness, structural abnormalities of the pharynx and esophagus, neuromuscular disorders, and deglutition abnormalities
  - 50% adults aspirate oropharyngeal secretions during sleep
  - Oropharyngeal colonization: Poor dentition increases bacterial load and risk of pneumonia
    - Edentulous patients less likely to develop aspiration pneumonia
    - Cavitary mass in edentulous patients more likely bronchogenic carcinoma than lung abscess
  - Mendelson syndrome: pH < 2.5 and volume of gastric aspirate greater than 25 mL
- Epidemiology
  - 300,000 to 600,000 cases per year in the United States
  - Foreign bodies most common in healthy infants and small children and elderly
  - 10% of patients hospitalized after drug overdose develop aspiration pneumonia
  - 1 in 3,000 anesthetized patients develop aspiration pneumonia
- Associated abnormalities: Hiatal hernia; Zenker diverticulum; gastroesophageal reflux

Gross Pathologic & Surgical Features
- Wide spectrum of injury: Noncardiogenic edema, hemorrhage, bronchopneumonia, bacterial abscesses (acutely): Bronchiectasis and fibrosis (chronically)

CLINICAL ISSUES

Presentation
- Most common signs/symptoms
  - Variable; depends on the amount and type of aspirated material
  - Acute aspiration
    - Cough, wheezing, cyanosis, and tachypnea
    - Abrupt onset: After meat aspiration, mimics myocardial infarction ("cafe coronary syndrome")
  - Chronic or recurrent aspiration
    - May resemble asthma
    - Insidious onset with recurrent pneumonias; usually basilar; may be multifocal (different locations)
  - Silent aspiration: 50% of anesthetized patients have no symptoms

Natural History & Prognosis
- Mortality 1% community acquired aspiration pneumonia, 25% hospitalized acquired aspiration pneumonia
  - Untreated high incidence of lung abscess and empyema
- Mortality 50% for patients who develop ARDS from Mendelson syndrome

Treatment
- Prevention
  - Medications to neutralize gastric pH, elevation of head of bed
  - Gastric suction with nasogastric tube (NG tube should be in fundus, location of pooled gastric contents in supine position)
- Post-aspiration
  - Antibiotics for pneumonia
  - Bronchoscopy to remove foreign bodies
- Surgery for gastroesophageal reflux for those failing medical therapy

DIAGNOSTIC CHECKLIST

Image Interpretation Pearls
- Gravity dependent opacities should think aspiration
- Radiopaque opacity within the airways specific finding

SELECTED REFERENCES
1. Marik PE: Aspiration pneumonitis and aspiration pneumonia. N Engl J Med. 344(9):665-71, 2001
2. Franquet T et al: Aspiration diseases: findings, pitfalls, and differential diagnosis. Radiographics. 20(3):673-85, 2000
3. Marom EM et al: The many faces of pulmonary aspiration. AJR Am J Roentgenol. 172(1):121-8, 1999

ASPIRATION

IMAGE GALLERY

Typical

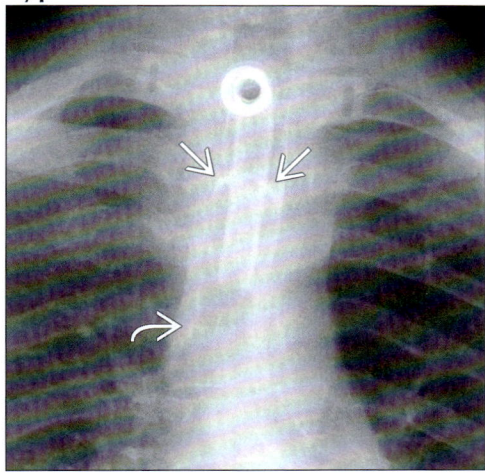
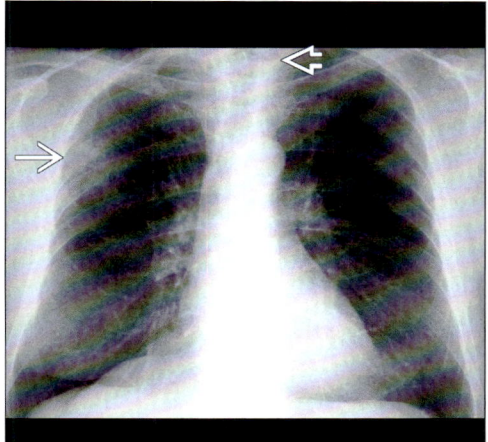

(Left) Frontal radiograph shows tracheostomy tube in normal position above carina. Swallowed barium passes inflated balloon ➡. Barium coats the top of the balloon ➡. Inflated balloon does not prevent aspiration. *(Right)* Frontal radiograph shows focal consolidation in the right upper lobe (axillary segment) ➡ from aspiration. Air-fluid level ➡ just above thoracic inlet from Zenker diverticulum.

Typical

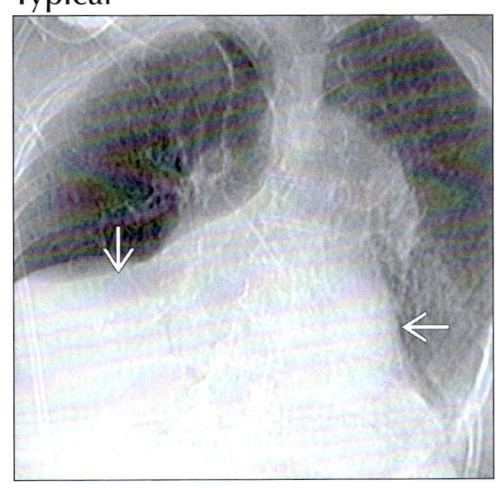
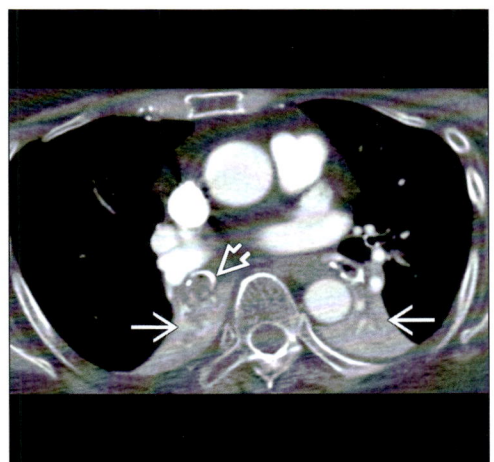

(Left) Frontal radiograph shows sharply-defined, wedge-shaped opacification in both lung bases ➡ from lobar atelectasis. *(Right)* Axial CECT shows atelectasis of both lower lobes ➡. Large airways were filled with aspirated material ➡.

Typical

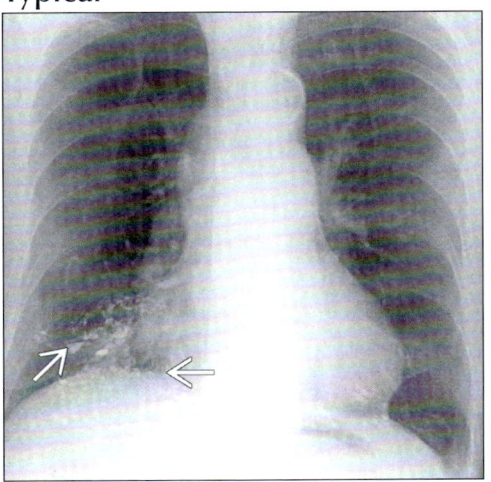
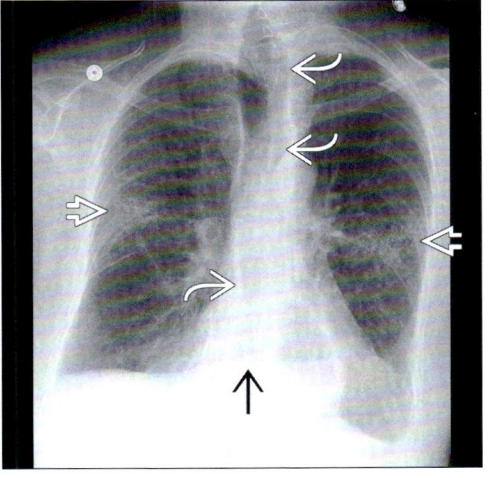

(Left) Frontal radiograph shows aspirated barium ➡ in the lower right lung. Aspiration events may be unilateral or bilateral. *(Right)* Frontal radiograph shows a large hiatal hernia ➡, dilated esophagus ➡ and focal areas of aspiration in the axillary segments of both upper lobes ➡.

MECONIUM ASPIRATION SYNDROME

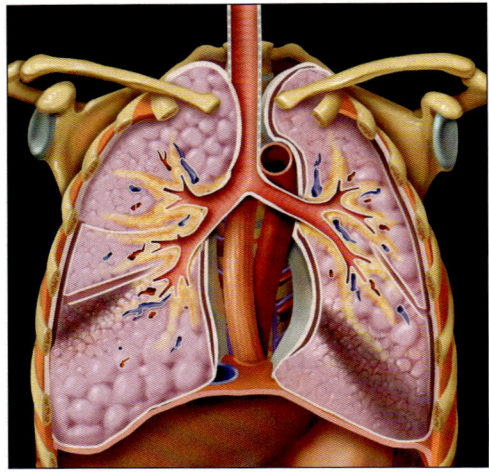

Graphic demonstrates findings: Asymmetric areas of hyperinflation and atelectasis as well as increased, rope-like perihilar densities.

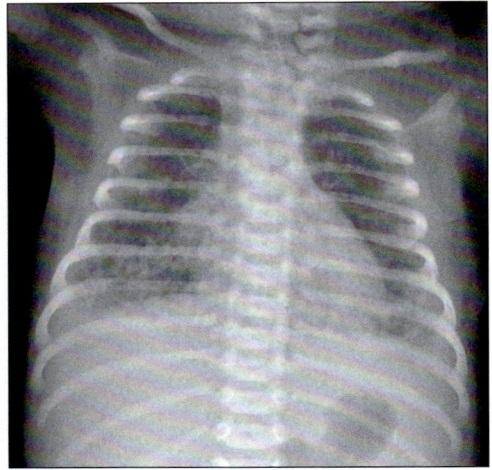

Anteroposterior radiograph shows diffuse bilateral coarse rope-like opacities with greatest involvement at the lung bases.

TERMINOLOGY

Abbreviations and Synonyms
- Meconium aspiration syndrome (MAS)

Definitions
- Respiratory distress that occurs as the result of the aspiration of meconium

IMAGING FINDINGS

General Features
- Best diagnostic clue: Coarse bilateral lung opacities with increased lung volumes in a term infant
- Location
  - Bilateral disease usually in middle two-thirds of the lung
  - Frequently asymmetric
- Morphology: Segmental hyperinflation from air trapping with focal areas of atelectasis

Radiographic Findings
- Radiography
  - Hyperinflated lung volumes
    - Often asymmetric
  - Rope-like perihilar densities
  - Pleural effusion uncommon
  - Chest radiograph useful to assess for complications
    - Air block and leak phenomena
    - Pneumothorax occurs 20-40%
    - Pneumomediastinum and pulmonary interstitial emphysema

CT Findings
- CECT
  - Occasionally obtained for chronic disease
    - Focal areas of lung involvement
    - Focal emphysematous changes
    - For assessing residual disease

Ultrasonographic Findings
- Grayscale Ultrasound
  - In utero ultrasound done to monitor infant fluid and causes of fetal distress
  - Cranial ultrasound done as part of extracorporeal membrane oxygenation (ECMO) work-up
    - Follow-up to assess for intracranial hemorrhage

DDx: Term Infants with Lung Disease

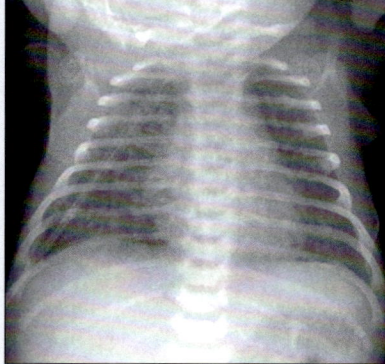

Transient Tachypnea of Newborn

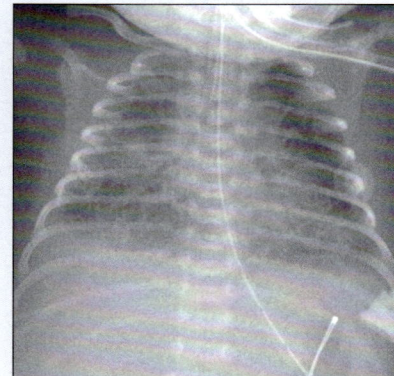

Neonatal Pneumonia

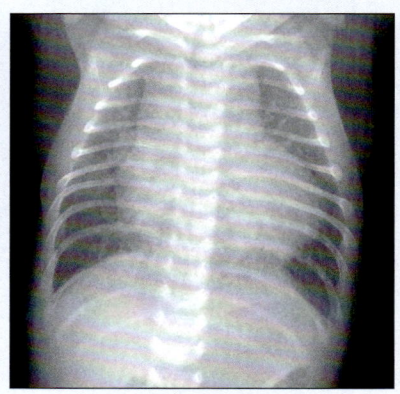

Congenital Heart Disease

MECONIUM ASPIRATION SYNDROME

Key Facts

Terminology
- Respiratory distress that occurs as the result of the aspiration of meconium

Imaging Findings
- Best diagnostic clue: Coarse bilateral lung opacities with increased lung volumes in a term infant
- Pleural effusion uncommon
- Best imaging tool: Chest radiograph

Top Differential Diagnoses
- Congenital Heart Disease (CHD)
- Neonatal Pneumonia
- Transient Tachypnea of the Newborn (TTN)
- Congenital Chest Mass such as Congenital Cystic Adenomatoid Malformation (CCAM)

Pathology
- Meconium is a tenacious, thick and viscous material in neonatal bowel
- Occurs in term infants who have in-utero or intrapartum hypoxia or stress
- Meconium may be detected in amniotic fluid of 10-20% of newborns > 34 weeks gestation
- 25,000-30,000 cases of meconium aspiration yearly in USA

Clinical Issues
- Cyanosis, nasal flaring, intercostal retractions
- Airway obstruction
- Surfactant dysfunction
- Chemical pneumonitis
- Meconium injury contributes to high pulmonary vascular resistance

---

  - Renal ultrasound occasionally done to exclude renal dysplasia associated pulmonary hypoplasia (Potter syndrome)

Imaging Recommendations
- Best imaging tool: Chest radiograph
- Protocol advice: Initial radiographs not predictive of outcome

DIFFERENTIAL DIAGNOSIS

Congenital Heart Disease (CHD)
- Clues to congenital heart disease may be present
  - Abnormal heart size or configuration
  - Right aortic arch or heterotaxy
  - Decreased or increased pulmonary flow
- Echocardiography is gold standard for diagnosis

Neonatal Pneumonia
- Patchy asymmetric perihilar densities and hyperinflation
- More common to see pleural effusion
- Usually no history or presence of meconium aspiration

Transient Tachypnea of the Newborn (TTN)
- Occurs secondary to delayed clearance of fetal pulmonary fluid (often in cesarian section)
- Sometimes pleural effusion or fissural thickening
- Key feature is benign course
- Normal heart size with prominent intersitial markings

Congenital Chest Mass such as Congenital Cystic Adenomatoid Malformation (CCAM)
- Focal areas of parenchymal lung abnormality
- Unilateral, may have mediastinal shift
- Pleural effusions may be present

PATHOLOGY

General Features
- General path comments
  - Meconium is a tenacious, thick and viscous material in neonatal bowel
    - Green-black substance of mucus, vernix, epithelial cells, lanugo, fatty acids, and bile
    - Normal passage of meconium occurs in first 24 hours after birth
- Genetics: No predisposition
- Etiology
  - Intrauterine aspiration
    - When fetus is hypoxic, there is passage of meconium into amniotic fluid which then enters the lung
    - Risk factors include placental insufficiency, maternal hypertension, preeclampsia, oligohydramnios, maternal drug use
  - Aspirated meconium causes injury by several mechanisms
    - Mechanical obstruction of small airways due to tenacious nature with resultant air-trapping and complications such as pneumothorax and pneumomediastinum
    - Chemical pneumonitis causes inflammation of airways and parenchyma
    - Surfactant inactivation strips surfactant from alveolar surface causing diffuse atelectasis
    - Pulmonary hypertension causes pulmonary vasoconstriction which leads to persistent pulmonary hypertension
    - Meconium alters amniotic fluid, increasing risk of bacterial infection
- Epidemiology
  - Occurs in term infants who have in-utero or intrapartum hypoxia or stress
  - Meconium rarely found in amniotic fluid prior to 34 weeks gestation
  - Meconium may be detected in amniotic fluid of 10-20% of newborns > 34 weeks gestation
    - 5% will develop meconium aspiration syndrome
  - 25,000-30,000 cases of meconium aspiration yearly in USA
    - 1,000 deaths annually in US

MECONIUM ASPIRATION SYNDROME

- Associated abnormalities: Secondary effects of air-block and severe pulmonary hypertension

Gross Pathologic & Surgical Features
- Patchy areas of subsegmental atelectasis peripheral to obstructed bronchi
- Compensatory areas of hyperinflation

CLINICAL ISSUES

Presentation
- Most common signs/symptoms
  - Presence of meconium in amniotic fluid
  - Respiratory distress
    - Cyanosis, nasal flaring, intercostal retractions
- Other signs/symptoms
  - Laryngoscopic exam reveals meconium staining on vocal cords
  - Green urine due to excretion of bile acids
  - Overdistention of the chest may be prominent
  - Metabolic acidosis from perinatal stress
  - Respiratory acidosis from parenchymal disease and pulmonary hypertension
  - May be accompanied by inappropriate secretion of antidiuretic hormone (SIADH) or acute renal failure
  - Cyanosis with right to left ductus shunting

Demographics
- Age
  - Usually term infants or post-term
  - Newborn > 34 weeks gestation
- Gender: No gender preference

Natural History & Prognosis
- MAS occurs in term infants who have intrapartum hypoxia or stress
- Meconium directly alters the amniotic fluid
  - Reduces antibacterial activity
  - Irritating to the fetal skin
- Aspiration of meconium into lungs causes three effects
  - Airway obstruction
    - Atelectasis with partial air trapping and hyperdistention of the alveoli
    - May lead to pneumothorax, pneumomediastinum, pneumopericardium
  - Surfactant dysfunction
    - May cause diffuse atelectasis
    - Difficulty ventilating infant
  - Chemical pneumonitis
    - Diffuse pneumonia occurs rapidly after aspiration
- Complications
  - Meconium injury contributes to high pulmonary vascular resistance
  - Severe pulmonary hypertension occurs with resultant persistent fetal circulation with right to left shunting across the patent ductus arteriosus
  - Difficulty ventilating with air block
    - Pneumothorax, pneumomediastinum, pulmonary interstitial emphysema
  - Neurologic damage related to anoxic brain injury
  - Chronic lung disease after prolonged mechanical ventilation
- Outcome of infants depends on degree of aspiration and distress
  - Some recover within 72 hours
  - Up to 25% may develop air-block complications
  - Mortality used to be higher but currently 10%
  - Residual lung disease with abnormal pulmonary function with cough, wheezing, hyperinflation

Treatment
- Before delivery
  - Improved maternal care to reduce risk of meconium aspiration
  - Evidence supporting intrapartum suctioning is conflicting
  - Amnioinfusion of fluid dilutes the meconium but is controversial
- After delivery
  - Meconium stained distressed infant intubated and suctioned immediately
- Therapy directed at treating respiratory distress
  - Ventilator support with conventional or high frequency ventilation
  - Maintain blood pressure, replacement of surfactant
  - Inhaled nitrous oxide may be used for pulmonary vasodilation
  - Steroids to decrease inflammation associated with chemical pneumonitis
  - Antibiotics
- ECMO
  - For severe pulmonary hypertension unresponsive to therapy
  - Delivers oxygen to blood via external oxygenator, reduces barotrauma

DIAGNOSTIC CHECKLIST

Image Interpretation Pearls
- Clinical history of meconium staining is relevant
- Term infants with hyperinflation and coarse bilateral lung disease

SELECTED REFERENCES
1. Gelfand SL et al: Controversies in the treatment of meconium aspiration syndrome. Clin Perinatol. 31(3):445-52, 2004
2. Gelfand SL et al: Meconium stained fluid: approach to the mother and the baby. Pediatr Clin North Am. 51(3):655-67, ix, 2004
3. Wiswell TE: Handling the meconium-stained infant. Semin Neonatol. 6(3):225-31, 2001
4. Niermeyer S et al: International Guidelines for Neonatal Resuscitation: An excerpt from the Guidelines 2000 for Cardiopulmonary Resuscitation and Emergency Cardiovascular Care: International Consensus on Science. Contributors and Reviewers for the Neonatal Resuscitation Guidelines. Pediatrics. 106(3):E29, 2000
5. Cleveland RH. Related Articles et al: A radiologic update on medical diseases of the newborn chest. Pediatr Radiol. 25(8):631-7, 1995

MECONIUM ASPIRATION SYNDROME

IMAGE GALLERY

Typical

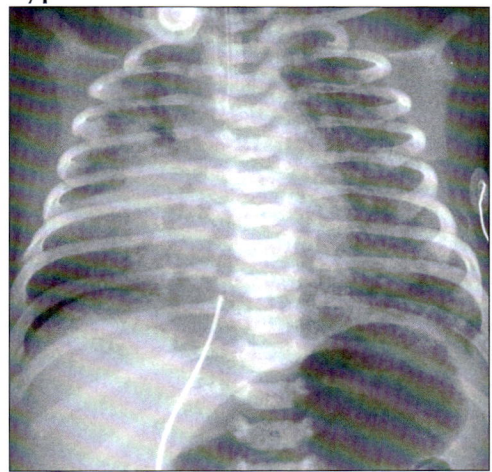
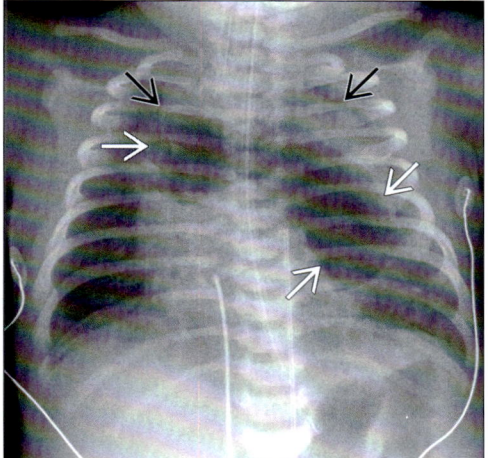

(Left) Anteroposterior radiograph just following delivery shows bilateral coarse rope-like opacities with right middle lobe atelectasis. *(Right)* Anteroposterior radiograph in the same patient on the following day shows hyperlucency, consistent with pneumomediastinum ➡ uplifting the thymic lobe ➡.

Typical

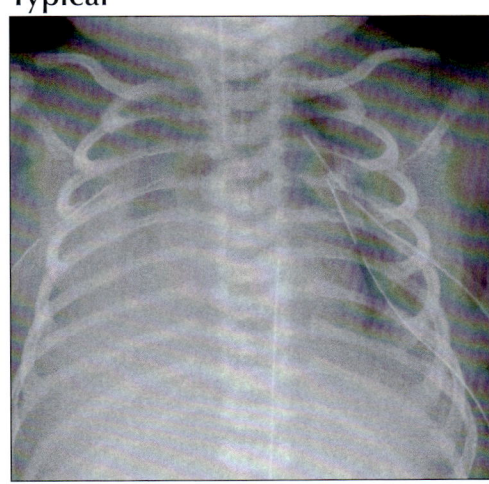
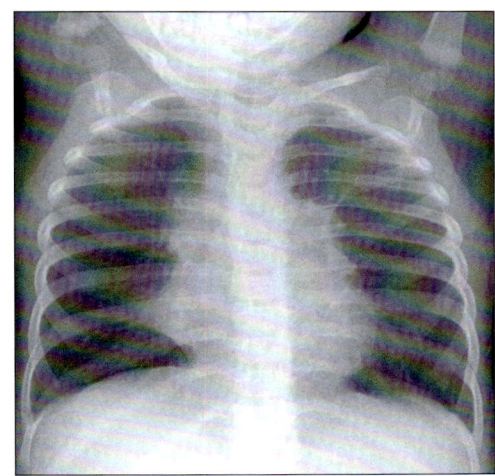

(Left) Anteroposterior radiograph at 2 days of age shows 2 left-sided chest tubes and a residual pneumothorax. The sidehole of the right-sided chest tube is outside the chest wall. *(Right)* Anteroposterior radiograph in the same patient at 16 months of age shows hyperinflation and perihilar linear opacities which has not changed since the child was 1 year old, consistent with scarring and chronic lung change.

Typical

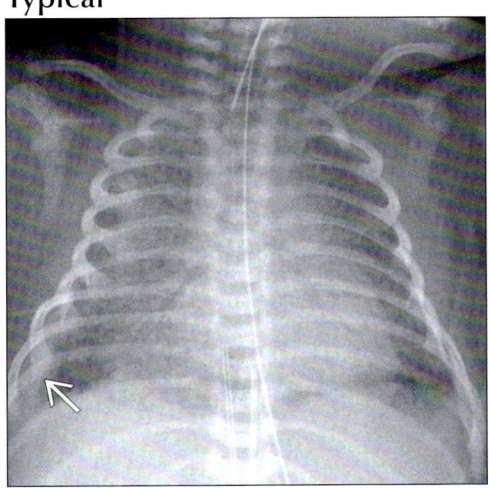
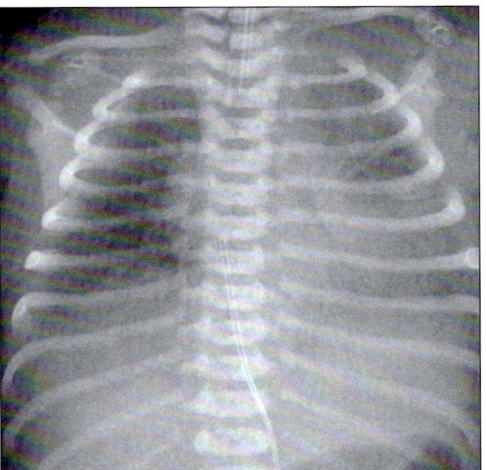

(Left) Anteroposterior radiograph shows diffuse bilateral coarse lung opacities and a small, right-sided, pleural effusion ➡. The endotracheal tube tip is projecting at the thoracic inlet. *(Right)* Anteroposterior radiograph shows asymmetric perihilar rope-like opacities with atelectasis within the left lower lobe.

BRONCHIAL FOREIGN BODY, PEDIATRIC

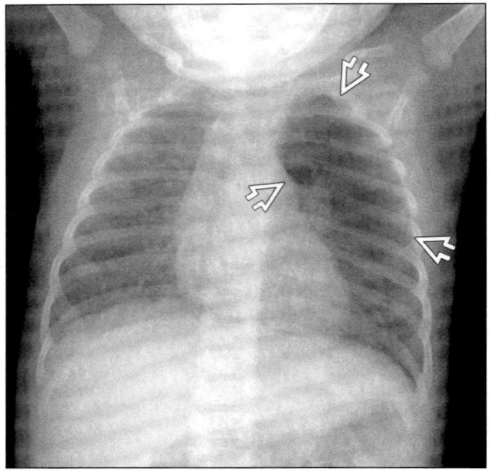

Anteroposterior radiograph in a 1 year old with wheezing shows asymmetric decreased density ➔ in left upper lobe.

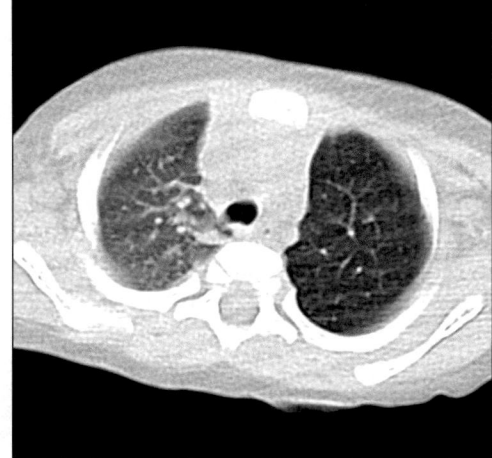

Axial CECT obtained for potential congenital lobar emphysema shows asymmetric hyperlucency and decreased vascularity in left upper lobe. Bronchoscopy showed peanut in left main bronchus.

TERMINOLOGY

Abbreviations and Synonyms
- Lego asthma

Definitions
- Aspiration of a foreign body that lodges in the bronchus leading to bronchial obstruction

IMAGING FINDINGS

General Features
- Best diagnostic clue
  - Static lung volume at different phases of respiratory cycle (need more than inspiratory chest radiograph alone)
    - Alternatives include inspiratory/expiratory radiographs in cooperative patients, fluoroscopy, bilateral decubitus radiographs, radiographs at forced expiration
- Location
  - Bronchial foreign bodies more common than elsewhere
  - Bronchial 76%, laryngeal 6%, tracheal 4%
    - Of bronchial: Right bronchus 58% > left bronchus 42%

Radiographic Findings
- Radiography
  - Static lung volume at different phases of respiratory cycle (need more than inspiratory chest radiograph alone)
  - Volume of affected lung segments can be normal, increased, or decreased
  - Asymmetric lung volumes: Larger lung not always abnormal side
  - Hyperinflation
  - Oligemia
  - Atelectasis
  - Lung consolidation
  - Pneumothorax
  - Pneumomediastinum
  - Rarely aspirated foreign body radiopaque
    - Most are organic
    - Peanut most common

DDx: Hyperinflated Lung

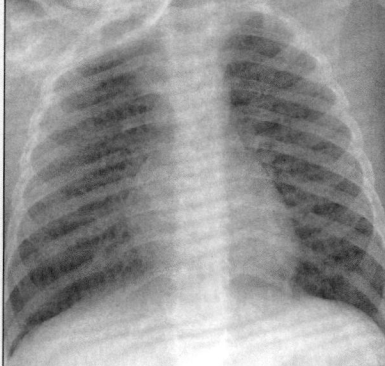

Asthma

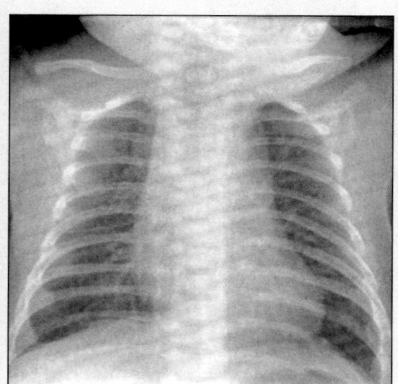

Viral Disease

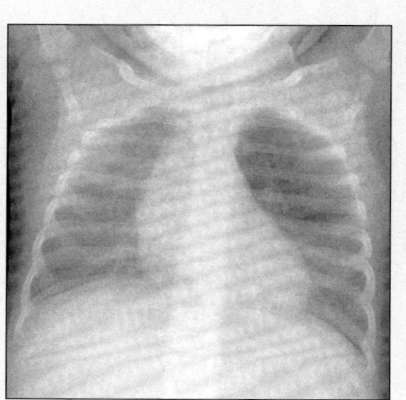

Lobar Emphysema

BRONCHIAL FOREIGN BODY, PEDIATRIC

Key Facts

Imaging Findings
- Static lung volume at different phases of respiratory cycle (need more than inspiratory chest radiograph alone)
- Alternatives include inspiratory/expiratory radiographs in cooperative patients, fluoroscopy, bilateral decubitus radiographs, radiographs at forced expiration
- Bronchial foreign bodies more common than elsewhere
- Bronchial 76%, laryngeal 6%, tracheal 4%
- Volume of affected lung segments can be normal, increased, or decreased
- Reported statistics on presence of findings on static chest radiograph
- Normal: 14-35%

- Obstructive emphysema: 21-43%
- Opacification/atelectasis: 18-29%
- Mediastinal shift: 36.8%
- Radiopaque foreign body: 3-23%

Clinical Issues
- Symptoms may be indolent: Occult presentation (10-25%)
- Typically present with wheezing, cough, sometimes fever
- Typically 8 months to 3 years of age
- 57% between 1 and 2 years of age
- Delay in diagnosis associated with increased risk of major complications

---

  o Normal inspiratory chest radiograph alone does not exclude aspirated foreign body: Must obtain additional image
  o Reported statistics on presence of findings on static chest radiograph
    ▪ Normal: 14-35%
    ▪ Obstructive emphysema: 21-43%
    ▪ Opacification/atelectasis: 18-29%
    ▪ Mediastinal shift: 36.8%
    ▪ Radiopaque foreign body: 3-23%
- Bilateral decubitus radiographs
  o Static lung volume in affected lung when placed in up or down position
  o When hyperinflated, abnormal hyperinflated lung stays same size when that side is placed down
  o Normal non-obstructed lung will decrease in volume when placed down and increase in volume when placed up with decubitus positioning
- Inspiratory/expiratory radiographs
  o In patients who are cooperative, radiographs can be obtained at maximum inspiration and expiration
  o This is minority of patients as most who present with this clinical scenario are between 1 and 2 years of age
  o Lack of change in volume of affected lung with respiratory cycle
- Radiographs with forced expiration
  o Technique has been described where evaluator placed gloved hand on child's abdomen and gently applies pressure immediately prior to and while obtaining radiograph
  o Pressure drives diaphragms superiorly
  o Abnormal side with bronchial obstruction will remain static in volume
  o Normal side will show elevation of the diaphragm as compared to initial neutral radiograph
  o We do not practice or recommend this technique

Fluoroscopic Findings
- Child fluoroscoped in frontal view with child lying on back
- Normally, both diaphragms will move superiorly and inferiorly in synchronous manner
- With obstruction, static lung volume in affected lung with decreased or no motion of ipsilateral diaphragm

CT Findings
- CT not typically advocated in imaging algorithm for suspected foreign body but may be obtained for persistent lung collapse or pneumonia or for work-up of extrinsic airway compression
- Focal hyperinflation or atelectasis
- May see foreign body as filling defect in bronchus
- Some have advocated HRCT in decubitus position to evaluate hyperinflated lung

Imaging Recommendations
- Best imaging tool: Static lung volume at different phases of respiratory cycle
- Protocol advice: Single static radiograph cannot exclude evidence of air trapping
- Imaging recommendations: Dynamic evaluation
  o In order to obtain radiographic images during different phases of respiratory cycle: Inspiratory & expiratory images (in cooperative patients), radiographs with bilateral decubitus positioning, fluoroscopic evaluation of the chest, forced expiratory films (pressure placed on abdomen)
  o Since clinical scenario most common in (uncooperative) infants, decubitus films or fluoroscopic evaluation most commonly used
  o Static lung volume (air trapping) seen as lack of change at different phases of respiratory cycle
  o Normally, lung placed "down" on decubitus films will show some degree of collapse
- However, imaging cannot completely exclude foreign body and if very high clinical suspicion, endoscopic evaluation should be performed even if imaging nonspecific

DIFFERENTIAL DIAGNOSIS

Refractory Asthma
- Much more common than bronchial foreign body
- Increased peribronchial markings

BRONCHIAL FOREIGN BODY, PEDIATRIC

- Lung volumes typically symmetric

Viral Lower Respiratory Tract Infection
- Symmetric lung volume
- More common than foreign body
- Increased peribronchial markings

Pulmonary Sling
- Pulmonary sling is the only vascular ring that results in asymmetric aeration
- Either side may be larger
- Typically presents with respiratory distress at birth
- Often associated with other congenital heart disease

Extrinsic Tracheal Compression by Mass
- Bronchogenic cysts, lymphadenopathy, and other masses may compress bronchi and present with asymmetric aeration

Swyer-James Syndrome
- Bronchiolitis obliterans
- Asymmetric lung hyperlucency
- Affected lucent lung may be smaller than contralateral lung

Congenital Lobar Emphysema
- Asymmetric lung hyperlucency confined to single lobe

PATHOLOGY

General Features
- General path comments
  - Aspirated foreign body lodges in bronchus and leads to partial or intermittent obstruction
  - May have "ball valve" effect leading to
    - Hyperinflation
    - Complete obstruction leading to collapse
- Etiology
  - Young children explore environment with mouth
  - Often put discovered items in mouth

Microscopic Features
- Foreign body lodged in bronchus
- Leukocyte infiltration and edema in surrounding bronchial wall
- Chronic foreign body lead to granuloma formation/granulation tissue

CLINICAL ISSUES

Presentation
- Most common signs/symptoms
  - Aspiration may not be witnessed
  - Symptoms may be indolent: Occult presentation (10-25%)
  - Typically present with wheezing, cough, sometimes fever
  - Wheezing refractory to medical therapy
  - Reported statistics on frequency of presenting symptoms
    - Cough 33%
    - Dyspnea 30%
    - Fever 36%
    - History of choking crisis/other positive history 7-91%

Demographics
- Age
  - Typically 8 months to 3 years of age
  - 57% between 1 and 2 years of age
- Gender
  - Males slightly more common than females
  - M:F = 1.2:1

Natural History & Prognosis
- High degree of suspicion important
- Delay in diagnosis associated with increased risk of major complications
  - Incidence of major complications low if diagnosis rapid
  - Complications: 4% at > 4 days, 91% > 30 days
- Complications of chronic foreign bodies
  - Bronchopulmonary fistula, bronchial rupture, damage to distal lung

Treatment
- Endobronchial removal of foreign body

DIAGNOSTIC CHECKLIST

Image Interpretation Pearls
- Static lung volume at different phases of respiratory cycle (need more than inspiratory chest radiograph alone)

SELECTED REFERENCES

1. Girardi G et al: Two new radiological findings to improve the diagnosis of bronchial foreign-body aspiration in children. Pediatr Pulmonol. 38(3):261-4, 2004
2. Shivakumar AM et al: Bronchial foreign bodies. Indian J Pediatr. 71(9):849-52, 2004
3. Ayed AK et al: Foreign body aspiration in children: diagnosis and treatment. Pediatr Surg Int. 19(6):485-8, 2003
4. Higo R et al: Foreign bodies in the aerodigestive tract in pediatric patients. Auris Nasus Larynx. 30(4):397-401, 2003
5. Shivakumar AM et al: Tracheobronchial foreign bodies. Indian J Pediatr. 70(10):793-7, 2003
6. Schmidt H et al: Foreign body aspiration in children. Surg Endosc. 14(7):644-8, 2000
7. Donnelly LF et al: The multiple presentations of foreign bodies in children. AJR Am J Roentgenol. 170(2):471-7, 1998
8. Messner AH: Pitfalls in the diagnosis of aerodigestive tract foreign bodies. Clin Pediatr (Phila). 37(6):359-65, 1998
9. Wolach B et al: Aspirated foreign bodies in the respiratory tract of children: eleven years experience with 127 patients. Int J Pediatr Otorhinolaryngol. 30(1):1-10, 1994
10. Mu L et al: Inhalation of foreign bodies in Chinese children: a review of 400 cases. Laryngoscope. 101(6 Pt 1):657-60, 1991
11. Mu LC et al: Radiological diagnosis of aspirated foreign bodies in children: review of 343 cases. J Laryngol Otol. 104(10):778-82, 1990
12. Laks Y et al: Foreign body aspiration in childhood. Pediatr Emerg Care. 4(2):102-6, 1988

BRONCHIAL FOREIGN BODY, PEDIATRIC

IMAGE GALLERY

Typical

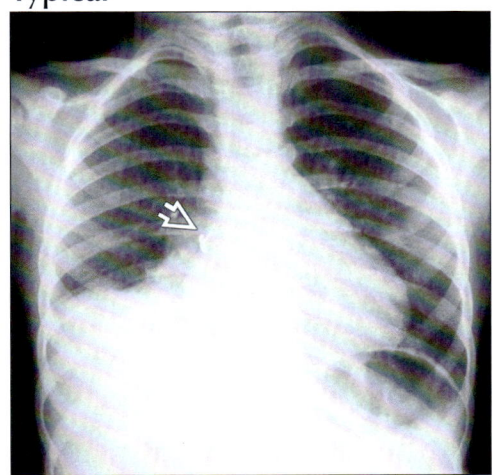
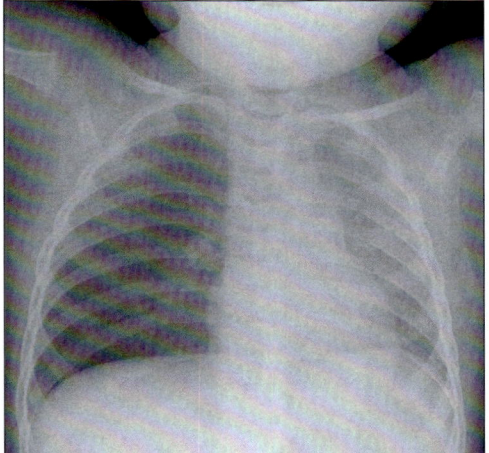

(Left) Anteroposterior radiograph shows radiopaque foreign body ➔ in right main bronchus. There is opacification and volume loss in right middle and right lower lobe. *(Right)* Frontal radiograph shows asymmetric hyperinflation of right lung. Decubitus positioned radiographs were obtained and are shown below.

Typical

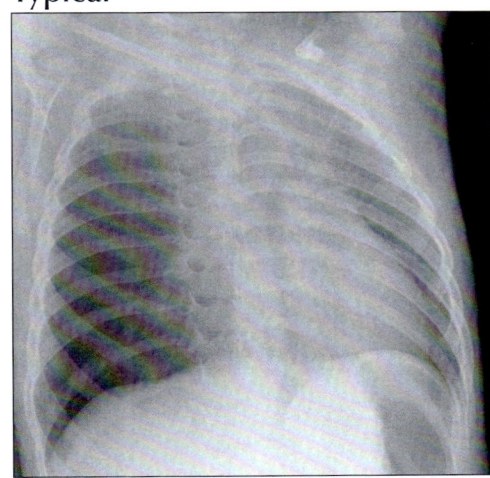
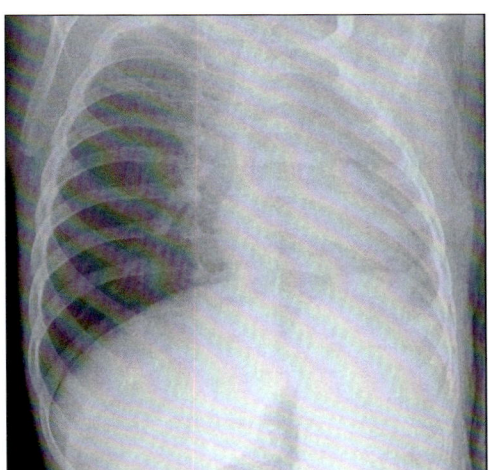

(Left) Decubitus positioned radiograph in same patient as previous image, with right side down shows no change in volume of right lung. Normally, side down should collapse. *(Right)* Decubitus positioned radiograph in same patient as previous image, with left side down shows collapse of left lung, as is normally expected. Bronchoscopy showed peanut in right mainstem bronchus.

Typical

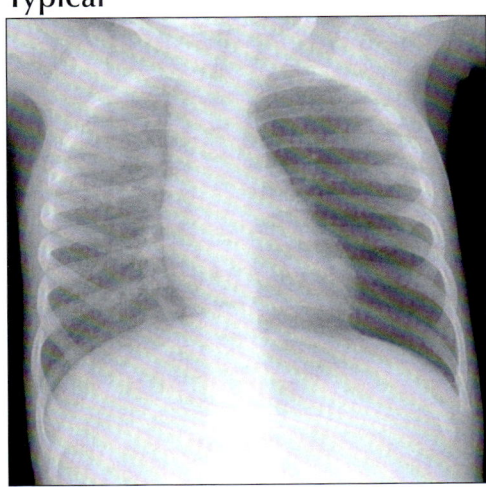
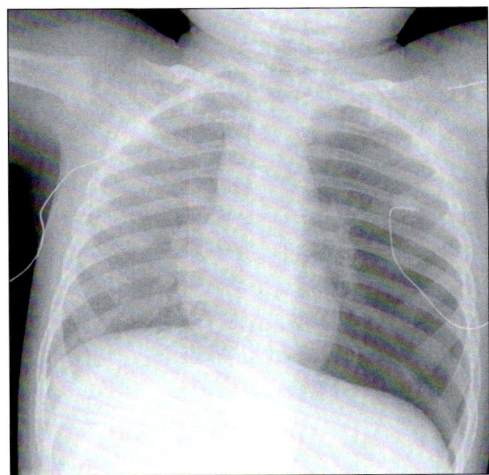

(Left) Frontal radiograph shows asymmetric hyperinflation of left lung compared to right lung. Decubitus radiographs showed left air trapping. Bronchoscopy showed left main bronchus foreign body. *(Right)* Anteroposterior radiograph shows asymmetric lung volumes with hyperlucent left. At endoscopy a peanut was found in the left main stem bronchus.

PULMONARY EMBOLI

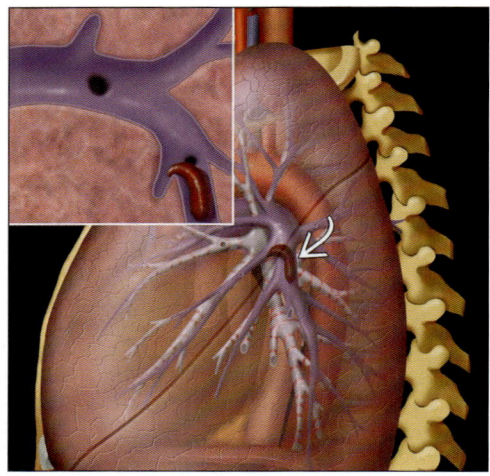

Graphic shows an intravascular embolus in the left interlobar pulmonary artery ➔. Tubular shape from originating vein. Embolus straddles a bifurcation point.

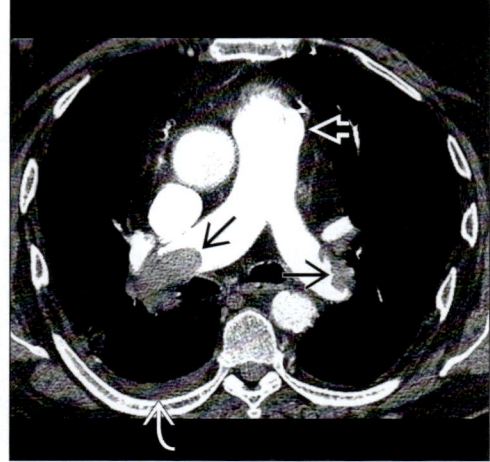

Axial CTA show multiple lobar emboli ➔ and small right pleural effusion ➔. Main pulmonary artery mildly enlarged ➔ from pulmonary hypertension.

TERMINOLOGY

Abbreviations and Synonyms
- Pulmonary embolism (PE), thromboembolism, ventilation perfusion scan (V/Q scan), deep venous thrombosis (DVT), inferior vena cava (IVC), likelihood ratio (LR)

Definitions
- Embolization of thrombi to the pulmonary arteries, usually from deep veins in lower extremities or pelvis

IMAGING FINDINGS

General Features
- Best diagnostic clue: CTA: Clot in pulmonary arteries
- Location: Often straddle bifurcation points (saddle embolus)
- Morphology: Usually tubular casts of veins

Radiographic Findings
- Radiography
  - Chest radiograph: **10% normal**
  - Most abnormalities nonspecific
- Vascular alteration
  - **Westermark sign**: Focal oligemia due to vascular obstruction
  - **Knuckle sign**: Focal enlargement central pulmonary artery (typically right interlobar pulmonary artery) due to physical presence of clot
- Pulmonary infarcts
  - Uncommon; < 10% embolic episodes
    - More common in those with underlying cardiopulmonary disease
  - Any size or shape
    - Usually peripheral in lower lung zones
    - Usually associated with small pleural effusion
    - **Hampton hump**: Pleural-based, cone-shaped opacity pointing toward the hilum
  - Evolution
    - May develop immediately or more commonly delayed 2-3 days following embolus
    - Initially infarct ill-defined, over time becomes sharply defined
    - Infarct "melt": Maintain their initial shape and shrink over time (in contrast, pneumonia and edema "fade" away

DDx: Intravascular Filling Defect

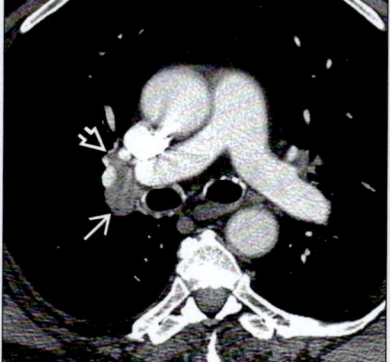

Hilar Lymph Node

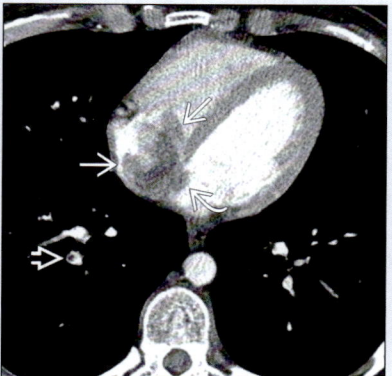

Tumor Emboli

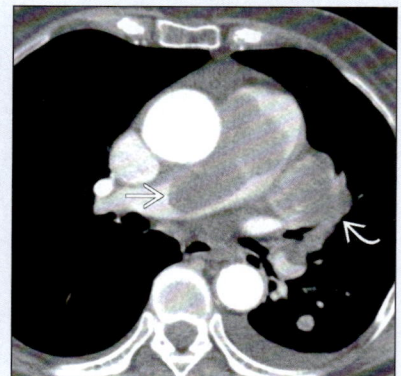

Pulmonary Artery Sarcoma

PULMONARY EMBOLI

Key Facts

Terminology
- Embolization of thrombi to the pulmonary arteries, usually from deep veins in lower extremities or pelvis

Imaging Findings
- Chest radiograph: **10% normal**
- Normal right ventricle (RV)/left ventricle (LV) short axis ratio (at level of tricuspid valve) < 0.9 (severe right ventricular strain if > 1.5)
- Detection of disease other than PE in 70%

Top Differential Diagnoses
- Hilar Lymph Nodes
- Transient Interruption of Contrast
- In Situ Thrombosis
- Pulmonary Artery Sarcoma

Pathology
- Unsuspected incidental pulmonary emboli: 4% of inpatients; 1% of outpatients
- Deep venous clot fragments in right heart, an average of 8 emboli then shower the lung

Clinical Issues
- No telltale signs, symptoms, or laboratory studies that strongly suggest PE (some asymptomatic)
- Because of declining tolerance for diagnostic uncertainty, PE studies now **overutilized**
- + D-Dimer LR 2.0 (1.5-2.5): Little clinical value in altering probability of disease
- Outcome good following negative pulmonary angiograms or CT (< 1% embolic rate)

- Other
  - Subsegmental atelectasis (Fleischner lines), pleural effusions (small to moderate in size), elevated hemidiaphragm(s)

CT Findings
- NECT: Rarely can see intravascular hyperattenuation clot in pulmonary artery
- CTA
  - Directly visualizes intraluminal clot
    - High sensitivity and specificity (> 90%); high inter-observer agreement, [+LR 24, -LR 0.1]
    - Acute PE clot attenuation measures 33 ± 14 HU; chronic clot measures 90 ± 30 HU
  - Acute PE: Partial intraluminal filling defects, sharp interface surrounded by contrast
    - Eccentric or peripheral intraluminal filling defects, form acute angles with vessel wall
    - Total cutoff of vascular enhancement; arterial occlusion may enlarge vessel caliber
  - Clot burden: Miller method
    - Indicates severity of PE, however, poor predictor of mortality (which depends more on the cardiopulmonary status of patient)
    - Right lung 9 segments (RUL 3, RML 2, RLL 4); left lung 7 segments (LUL 2, lingula 2, LLL 3)
    - Clot in artery = 1 point; clot proximal to segmental artery = number of segments arising distally
    - Maximum score for right lung 9, left lung 7, and maximum total score 16
  - **Right ventricular strain**
    - Normal right ventricle (RV)/left ventricle (LV) short axis ratio (at level of tricuspid valve) < 0.9 (severe right ventricular strain if > 1.5)
    - Leftward septal bowing
    - Pulmonary artery diameter > 30 mm (= 20 mm Hg)
    - Increased diameter of superior vena cava or azygos vein
    - Contrast regurgitation into intrahepatic IVC
  - Patent foramen ovale (PFO) or atrial septal defect
    - Prevalence of PFO in normal population 25%
    - Contrast attenuation in aorta (ascending or descending) > or = to attenuation in main pulmonary artery
    - 60% will have indeterminate PE studies
    - If have emboli, at risk for paradoxical embolus
  - Chronic PE: Mural-based, crescent-shaped intraluminal defect
    - Defects form obtuse angles with vessel wall
    - Intimal irregularities, recanalization, webs, bands, flaps or occlusion
    - Stenotic vessels, smaller in caliber than uninvolved same order vessels
    - Enlarged pulmonary and bronchial arteries
    - Pericardial effusion of small to moderate size
- Lung
  - Mosaic perfusion pattern (50%)
    - 50% from vascular occlusion; 50% from air-trapping
  - Infarcts: Pleural-based, wedge-shaped opacities with no contrast-enhancement; may rarely cavitate

MR Findings
- More time consuming and limited role in the critically ill, lack spatial resolution for peripheral emboli

Ultrasonographic Findings
- Lower limb US, low sensitivity, high specificity
- 50% of patients with PE have no DVT

Angiographic Findings
- Once considered "gold standard"
  - 25% false negative for subsegmental emboli
  - Interobserver agreement poor for subsegmental emboli (> 30%)

Nuclear Medicine Findings
- V/Q Scan
  - Indirect indicator of clot; does not directly visualize the clot, only the disruption of vascular perfusion
    - High sensitivity (~ 100%) but poor specificity
    - Normal perfusion scan excludes embolus (LR = 0.05); high probability scan diagnostic of embolus (LR = 18)

PULMONARY EMBOLI

- o Limitation: High percentage of nondiagnostic intermediate probability scans (> 60%)
- o Interobserver agreement poor for low and intermediate V/Q categories (30% agreement)

Imaging Recommendations
- Best imaging tool
  - o CTA: Standard of care for suspected PE; rapid, noninvasive, and readily available
  - o Can be combined with scanning abdomen/pelvis and lower extremities for DVT
  - o Detection of disease other than PE in 70%
  - o Nondiagnostic 3%: Poor contrast bolus, patient motion, obesity, post-partum (high blood volume), right-to-left shunts

DIFFERENTIAL DIAGNOSIS

Hilar Lymph Nodes
- Reformats to show extraluminal location

Transient Interruption of Contrast
- Admixture of nonopacified blood from IVC with deep inspiration
- Lack of opacification seen in multiple vessels at the same level bilaterally
- Presence of unopacified blood in right heart on preceding images

In Situ Thrombosis
- Artery to pneumonectomy stump

Pulmonary Artery Sarcoma
- Lobulated mass that demonstrates enhancement

Tumor Emboli
- Invasion of IVC or hepatic veins from myxoma, renal cell carcinoma, hepatoma, angiosarcoma

PATHOLOGY

General Features
- Etiology
  - o Any hospitalized patient
  - o Venous stasis: Phlebitis, pregnancy, obesity
  - o Hypercoagulable states: Acquired, inherited, malignancy, pregnancy
- Epidemiology
  - o 3rd most common cause of death
  - o Unsuspected incidental pulmonary emboli: 4% of inpatients; 1% of outpatients
- Pathophysiology
  - o Deep venous clot fragments in right heart, an average of 8 emboli then shower the lung
  - o Hemodynamic consequences: > 50% reduction vascular bed, pulmonary hypertension and right heart failure
  - o Airway consequences: Vascular occlusion causes acute airway constriction distal to supplied vascular bed (reflex bronchoconstriction)

CLINICAL ISSUES

Presentation
- Most common signs/symptoms
  - o No telltale signs, symptoms, or laboratory studies that strongly suggest PE (some asymptomatic)
  - o Because of declining tolerance for diagnostic uncertainty, PE studies now **overutilized**
    - Current prevalence of positive PE studies < 3%
    - CT most significant source of radiation exposure in general population
- Well probability estimate [points]
  - o Clinical sign of symptoms of DVT (minimum leg swelling) and pain with palpation of deep veins [3.0]
  - o Alternative diagnosis is less likely than PE [3.0]
  - o Heart rate > 100 [1.5]
  - o Immobilization or surgery in the previous four weeks [1.5]
  - o Previous DVT/PE [1.5]
  - o Hemoptysis [1.0]
  - o Malignancy (on treatment, treated in last 6 months or palliative) [1.0]
  - o Probability scale
    - Low probability: < 2 points (< 4% PE)
    - Moderate probability: 2-6 points (20% PE)
    - High probability: > 6 points (70% PE)
- D-Dimer
  - o Marker for fibrinolysis, 95% sensitive for thrombi
  - o + D-Dimer LR 2.0 (1.5-2.5): Little clinical value in altering probability of disease
  - o - D-Dimer LR 0.1: Usually excludes venous thrombi unless clinical suspicion extremely high

Natural History & Prognosis
- Mortality untreated disease, up to 20%
  - o Outcomes for untreated subsegmental emboli (6% have documented subsegmental emboli only) unknown, however such patients usually have DVT and are at increased risk for further emboli
  - o Outcome good following negative pulmonary angiograms or CT (< 1% embolic rate)
- Outcome: Good outcome with appropriate therapy (mortality < 3%)

Treatment
- Anticoagulation and fibrinolysis
  - o Hemorrhage complications in 2-15%
- IVC filter if contraindications to drug therapy or for recurrent emboli
- Surgical endarterectomy for chronic organizing pulmonary emboli

SELECTED REFERENCES
1. Stein PD et al: Diagnostic Pathways in Acute Pulmonary Embolism: Recommendations of the PIOPED II Investigators. Radiology. 242(1):15-21, 2007
2. Schoepf UJ et al: The Age of CT Pulmonary Angiography. J Thorac Imaging. 20(4):273-9, 2005

PULMONARY EMBOLI

IMAGE GALLERY

Typical

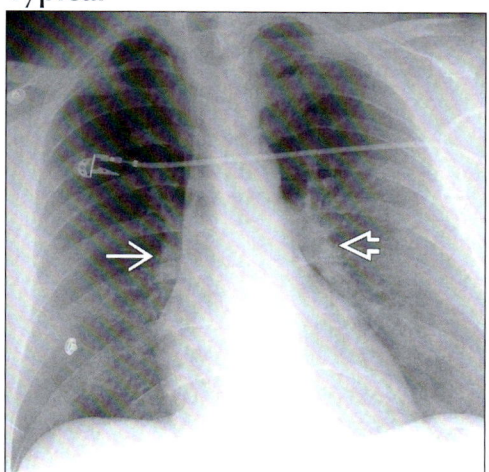 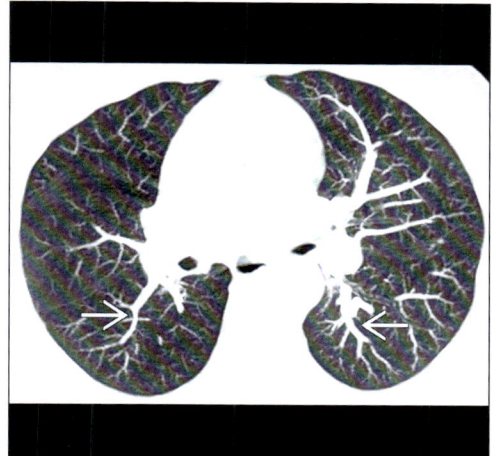

(Left) Anteroposterior radiograph shows hyperlucent right lung (Westermark sign). Right interlobar pulmonary artery ➡ smaller than left pulmonary artery ⇨. *(Right)* Axial CTA MIP shows diminished caliber right pulmonary arteries ➡ compared to the left from central emboli. Lung density decreased on the right compared to the left (Westermark sign).

Typical

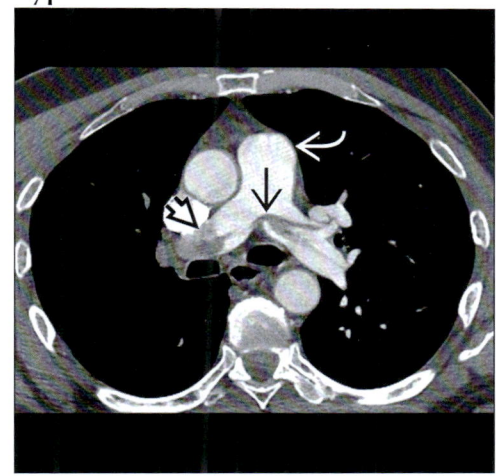 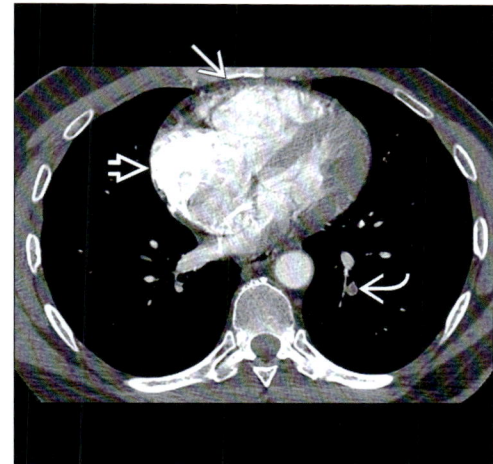

(Left) Axial CTA shows saddle embolus in lobar pulmonary arteries ➡. Large embolus right pulmonary artery ⇨ accounts for the Westermark sign. Main pulmonary artery slightly enlarged ➡. *(Right)* Axial CTA shows right ventricular strain with dilated right ventricle ➡ and dilated right atrium ➡. RV/LV short axis ratio > 1.5. Clot subsegmental artery ➡.

Typical

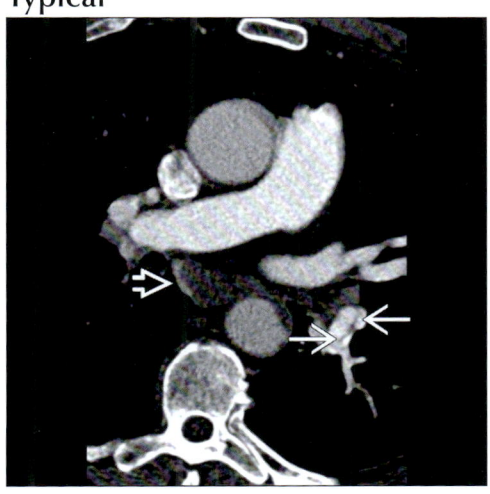 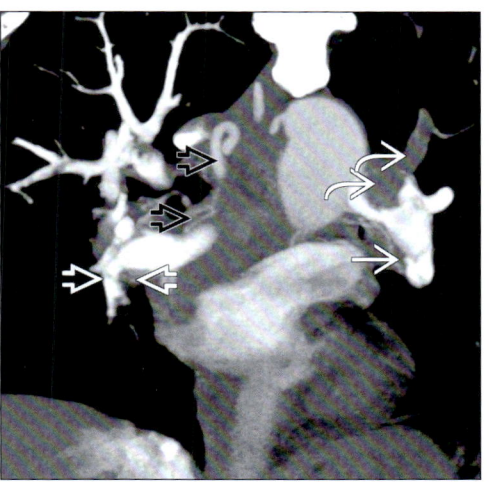

(Left) Axial CECT shows intravascular web ➡ in left lower lobe pulmonary artery from chronic embolus. Bronchial artery ⇨ is hypertrophied. *(Right)* Coronal CECT shows multiple acute emboli ➡ and chronic emboli. Stenosis right interlobar pulmonary artery ⇨ and web in left lower lobe artery ➡. Bronchial arteries ⇨ are hypertrophied.

SEPTIC EMBOLI, PULMONARY

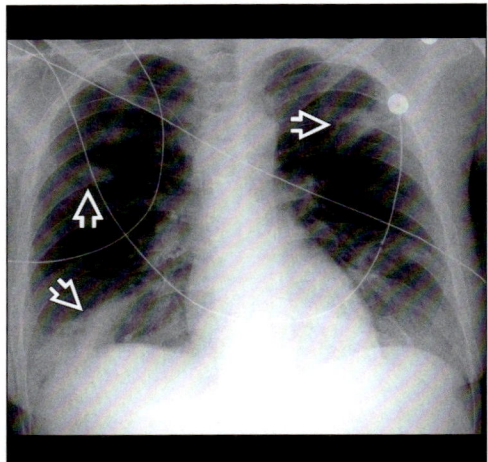

Frontal radiograph shows focal flame shaped opacities with cavities ➡ from septic emboli.

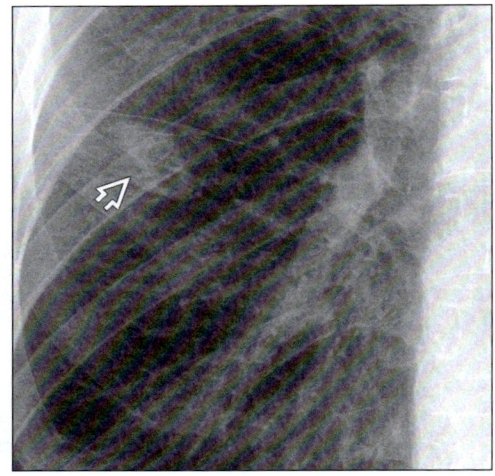

Frontal radiograph shows close-up of flame-shaped focal cavity ➡ from septic emboli.

TERMINOLOGY

Definitions
- Infected embolic material seeding the lung from active extrapulmonary source: Often foreign bodies or infective endocarditis

IMAGING FINDINGS

General Features
- Best diagnostic clue: Multiple nodules or patchy areas of consolidation with rapid cavitation
- Location
  - Primarily lung bases
    - Distribution of blood flow downstream from embolic source determines location
- Size: Usually small (< 3 cm diameter)
- Morphology: Few (mean 15) ill-defined nodules with rapid cavitation

Radiographic Findings
- Radiography
  - Peripheral poorly marginated 1-3 cm diameter nodular or wedge-shaped opacities
    - May change in number or appearance (size or degree of cavitation) from day to day
  - Target sign: Thin-walled cyst with central density
  - Usually basilar (due to gravity and blood flow)
  - Evolve rapidly, cavitation common within 24 hours (50%)
    - Cavity wall often thick
    - Lacks air-fluid level
    - Cavities typically in various stages of evolution
  - Complication
    - Empyema common: Loculated pleural effusions
    - Pneumothorax rare

CT Findings
- CECT
  - Multiple discrete nodules with varying degrees of cavitation (90%)
    - Average number of nodules 15
    - Size 5 mm to 3.5 cm, larger nodules rare
    - Air bronchograms (25%)
    - Cavitation (50%)
    - Peripheral (90%) and bilateral

DDx: Septic Emboli

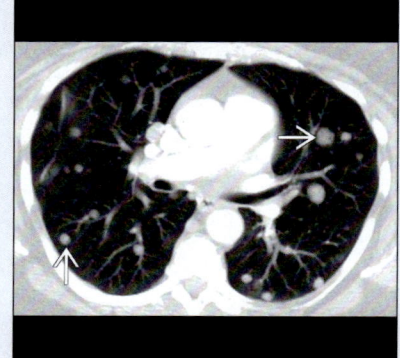

Metastases

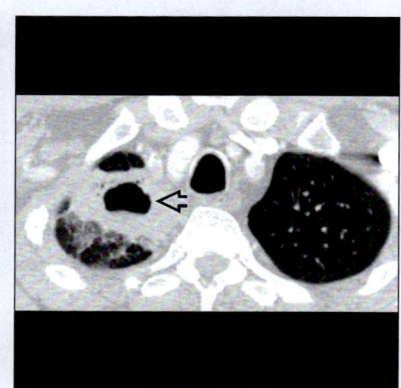

Lung Abscess

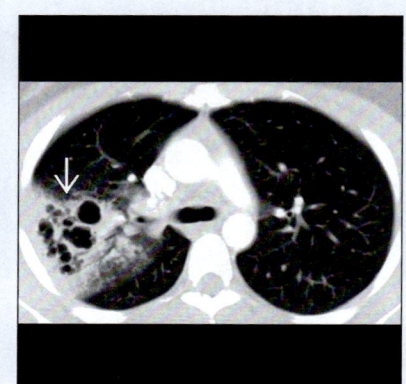

Pneumatoceles Pneumonia

SEPTIC EMBOLI, PULMONARY

Key Facts

Imaging Findings
- Best diagnostic clue: Multiple nodules or patchy areas of consolidation with rapid cavitation
- Distribution of blood flow downstream from embolic source determines location
- Size: Usually small (< 3 cm diameter)
- May change in number or appearance (size or degree of cavitation) from day to day
- Cavity wall often thick
- Lacks air-fluid level
- Empyema common: Loculated pleural effusions
- Average number of nodules 15
- Feeding vessel sign: Vessel may be seen leading directly to nodule or wedge-shaped opacity

Top Differential Diagnoses
- Pulmonary Embolus
- Pneumonia
- Metastases
- Pneumatoceles
- Lung Abscess

Pathology
- Staphylococcus aureus most common organism from foreign bodies and IV drug abuse

Clinical Issues
- Nonspecific: Fever, cough, and hemoptysis (may be massive)
- Radiographic abnormalities may precede positive blood cultures

Diagnostic Checklist
- In any patient with long-term indwelling catheters and new small ill-defined opacities

---

- Central lesions (20%)
  - Subpleural, wedge-shaped areas of increased attenuation with rim-like peripheral enhancement (50%)
  - Cavitation slightly more common in nodules than in wedge-shaped consolidation
  - Cavities in various stages of evolution (thick to thin-walled)
  - Feeding vessel sign: Vessel may be seen leading directly to nodule or wedge-shaped opacity
    - Found in 60-70% of patients with nodules, less common with wedge-shaped opacities
    - Multiplanar reconstructions show that vessel actually courses around the nodules
    - "Feeding vessel" sometimes represents draining vein
  - Mediastinal adenopathy (CT only) in 20%
  - No intravascular clots
  - Pleural effusion, may be loculated in 80%
    - Often evolves into empyema

Echocardiographic Findings
- Useful for valve vegetations

Imaging Recommendations
- Best imaging tool: Chest radiographs usually sufficient for monitoring response to therapy
- Protocol advice: CT: More sensitive than chest radiographs for both lung and pleural disease

DIFFERENTIAL DIAGNOSIS

Pulmonary Embolus
- Infarct: Focal areas of increased opacity from hemorrhage
  - Hampton sign: Pleural-based rounded cone
  - Pulmonary infarction may cavitate, however rare
    - Cavity usually single and large (> 4 cm)
    - Typically location apical segment right upper lobe
  - Infarct evolves from ill-defined consolidation to well-defined infarct
- CTA shows thrombus in pulmonary artery

Pneumonia
- Bacterial or fungal
  - Area of consolidation may be solitary or multiple
    - Not necessarily peripheral in location
  - Cavitation or pneumatoceles common with Staphylococcus, gram-negative organisms, Klebsiella, Tuberculosis
  - Coccidioidomycosis evolves over weeks into thin-walled cyst
  - Associated empyema may also develop

Metastases
- Multiple variable sized pulmonary nodules
  - Tend to be peripheral, 80% within 2 cm of pleural surface
  - Usually sharply marginated in contrast to septic emboli
  - May also have "feeding vessel" sign
  - Indistinct margins in hemorrhagic metastases: Renal cell, choriocarcinoma, melanoma
  - Cavitation common in squamous cell or sarcoma metastases
    - Less common: Primary GI tract adenocarcinomas
- Do not rapidly evolve

Pneumatoceles
- Transient and usually follow known insult (trauma, infection, hydrocarbon ingestion)
- May also evolve rapidly
- Typically thin-walled without air-fluid level

Lung Abscess
- Usually single and unilateral with thick-cavitary wall
- Air-fluid level common
- May be large (up to 10 cm diameter)

Wegener Granulomatosis
- Nodules with varying degrees of cavitation
- Do not rapidly evolve
- May have subglottic stenosis

SEPTIC EMBOLI, PULMONARY

Laryngeal Papillomatosis
- Multiple solid and cystic nodules: Grow extremely slowly
- Perihilar and central in location
- Laryngeal infection with human papilloma virus

PATHOLOGY

General Features
- General path comments: Septic emboli occur from infected embolic material
- Etiology
  - Organisms
    - Staphylococcus aureus most common organism from foreign bodies and IV drug abuse
    - Burn patients: Pseudomonas aeruginosa most common
    - Other organisms include Streptococci, fungi, gram-negative rods (Serratia)
  - Infective endocarditis
    - Tricuspid valve most commonly affected, aortic valve may also be involved
    - Occurs as result of nonbacterial thrombotic endocarditis, with injury to endothelial surface of the heart
    - Transient bacteremia leads to seeding of lesions with adherent bacteria
    - Subsequent infective endocarditis develops
  - Other types of endocarditis
    - Prosthetic valve endocarditis
    - Fungal endocarditis: ICU patients on broad-spectrum antibiotics as well as IV drug users
- Epidemiology
  - Risk factors
    - Indwelling venous catheters
    - Tricuspid valve endocarditis in IV drug abusers
    - Rarely pacemaker wires
    - Immunologic deficiencies, particularly lymphoma, organ transplants
    - Periodontal disease
    - Burns
    - Osteomyelitis (especially in children)

Gross Pathologic & Surgical Features
- Necrotic infected lung
  - Usually sharply demarcated from adjacent normal lung

Microscopic Features
- No specific features; acute inflammatory cells, necrosis, may see colonies of organisms

CLINICAL ISSUES

Presentation
- Most common signs/symptoms
  - Nonspecific: Fever, cough, and hemoptysis (may be massive)
  - Mean duration of symptoms before diagnosis: 18 days
  - Blood cultures often positive
- Other signs/symptoms
  - With endocarditis: Petechiae, splinter hemorrhages (dark red linear lesions in the nailbed)
    - Osler nodes: Tender subcutaneous nodules usually found on distal pads of digits
    - Janeway lesions: Nontender maculae on palms and soles
    - Roth spots: Retinal hemorrhages with small, clear centers
  - Lemierre syndrome
    - Post-anginal sepsis or necrobacillosis, uncommon but potentially life-threatening complication of acute pharyngotonsillitis
    - Septic thrombophlebitis jugular vein from adjacent infection leads to septic emboli
    - Anaerobic infection from gram negative bacillus (Fusobacterium most common)
    - Immunocompetent host
    - Triad: Neck pain, swelling, "cord sign": Palpable thrombosed internal jugular vein

Natural History & Prognosis
- Radiographic abnormalities may precede positive blood cultures
- Often rupture into pleural space and result in empyema

Treatment
- Therapy with broad spectrum antibiotics, long term with endocarditis often 6-8 weeks
- Percutaneous pleural drainage for associated empyema
- Surgery
  - Remove infected source
  - Replace heart valves

DIAGNOSTIC CHECKLIST

Consider
- In any patient with long-term indwelling catheters and new small ill-defined opacities

Image Interpretation Pearls
- Rapid cavitation of nodules

SELECTED REFERENCES

1. Aslam AF et al: Staphylococcus aureus infective endocarditis and septic pulmonary embolism after septic abortion. Int J Cardiol. 105(2):233-5, 2005
2. Cook RJ et al: Septic pulmonary embolism: presenting features and clinical course of 14 patients. Chest. 128(1):162-6, 2005
3. Goldenberg NA et al: Lemierre's and Lemierre's-like syndromes in children: survival and thromboembolic outcomes. Pediatrics. 116(4):e543-8, 2005
4. Parambil JG et al: Causes and presenting features of pulmonary infarctions in 43 cases identified by surgical lung biopsy. Chest. 127(4):1178-83, 2005
5. Gormus N et al: Lemierre's syndrome associated with septic pulmonary embolism: a case report. Ann Vasc Surg. 18(2):243-5, 2004
6. Wittram C et al: CT angiography of pulmonary embolism: diagnostic criteria and causes of misdiagnosis. Radiographics. 24(5):1219-38, 2004

SEPTIC EMBOLI, PULMONARY

IMAGE GALLERY

Typical

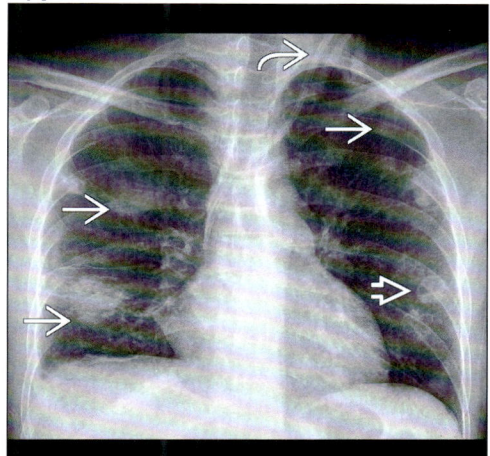
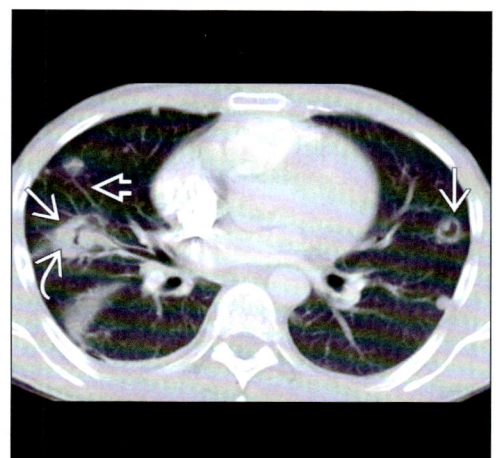

(Left) Frontal radiograph shows multiple variable sized nodules ➡ one of which are cavitated ➡. Hemodialysis catheter ➡ was infected. *(Right)* Axial CECT shows multiple peripheral nodules ➡. Largest nodule is cavitated ➡. Nodules are in various stages of cavitation. Feeding vessel sign ➡.

Typical

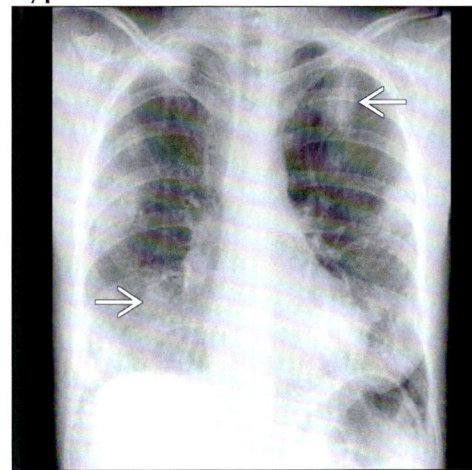
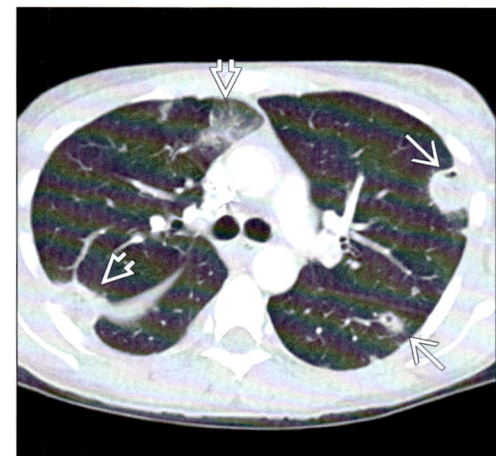

(Left) Frontal radiograph shows abnormal peripheral flame-shaped opacities ➡. *(Right)* Axial CECT shows multiple small peripheral nodules, some of which are cavitated ➡. Some areas are more wedge-shaped ➡.

Typical

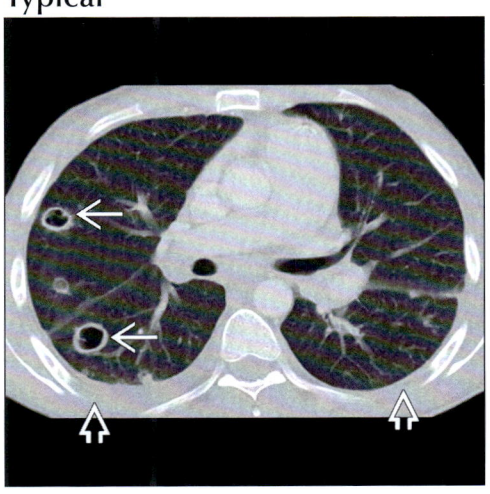
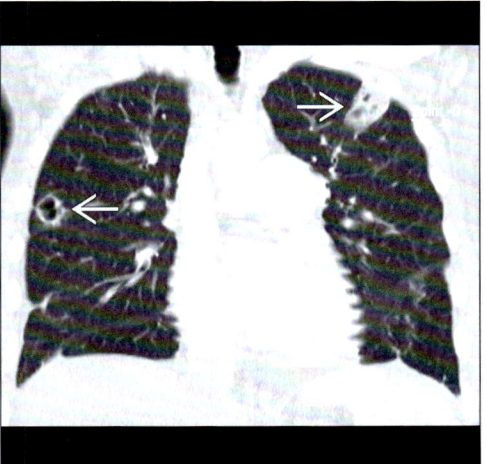

(Left) Transverse CECT shows multiple peripheral thin-walled cavities ➡. Differing wall thicknesses suggest recurrent septic events. Small pleural effusions ➡. *(Right)* Coronal CECT confirm peripheral location and profusion of the cavities ➡. Septic emboli may be either round or wedge-shaped.

AORTIC DISSECTION

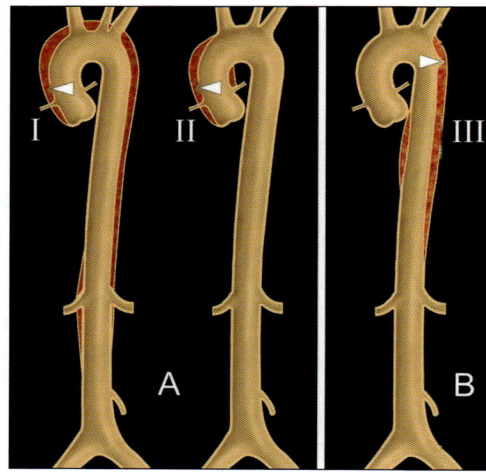

Stanford type A (DeBakey types I & II) involves ascending aorta and requires surgical repair. Type B (type III) involves the descending aorta. Intimal flap (arrowhead).

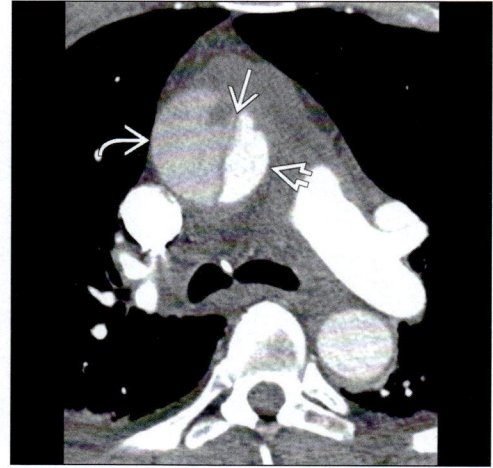

Axial CECT shows intimal flap ➡ separates the true ➡ from false ➡ lumen. Type A dissection. Mediastinal hemorrhage surrounds dissection.

TERMINOLOGY

Abbreviations and Synonyms
- Acute aortic syndrome: Aortic dissection, intramural aortic hematoma, penetrating atherosclerotic ulcer

Definitions
- Aortic dissection: Spontaneous intimal tear with propagation of subintimal hematoma (85% prevalence)
  - Chronic dissection after 2 weeks
- Aortic intramural hematoma: No intimal flap, spontaneous medial hematoma secondary to infarction of the vasa vasorum (10% prevalence)
- Penetrating atherosclerotic ulcer: Atherosclerotic lesion penetrates internal elastic lamina into the media (5% prevalence)

IMAGING FINDINGS

Radiographic Findings
- Radiography
  - Normal in 25%
  - Nonspecific signs
    - Widened superior mediastinum 75%
    - Double aortic knob sign 40%
    - Disparity in size between ascending and descending aorta
    - Progressive aortic enlargement on serial chest radiographs
    - Mediastinal mass effect, left apical cap, cardiomegaly
    - Left pleural effusion suggests aortic rupture
  - Most specific finding
    - Ring sign: Displaced intimal calcification from aortic wall > 1 cm in 5%
    - False positive ring sign due to projection of intimal calcification over aorta at a different location; other processes such as fat may create false aortic wall separated from calcified intima; or aortic wall may be thickened from aortitis

CT Findings
- Aortic dissection, CT nearly 100% accurate
  - Displacement of calcified intima
  - "Double barrel" spirals down the aorta from true and false lumen

DDx: Aortic Dissection

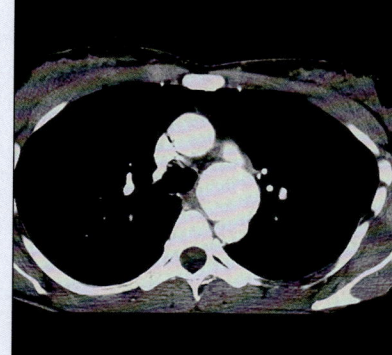

Aortic Transection

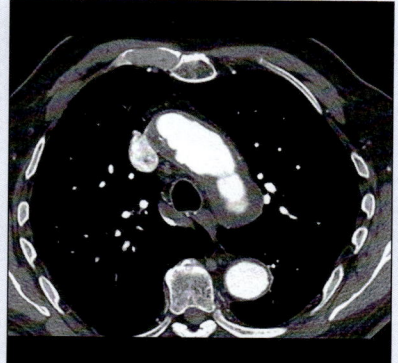

Atherosclerosis

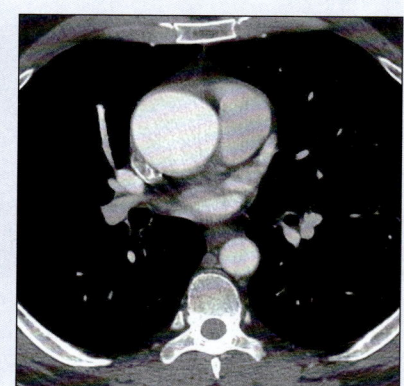

Post-Stenotic Dilatation

AORTIC DISSECTION

Key Facts

Terminology
- Aortic dissection: Spontaneous intimal tear with propagation of subintimal hematoma (85% prevalence)
- Aortic intramural hematoma: No intimal flap, spontaneous medial hematoma secondary to infarction of the vasa vasorum (10% prevalence)
- Penetrating atherosclerotic ulcer: Atherosclerotic lesion penetrates internal elastic lamina into the media (5% prevalence)

Top Differential Diagnoses
- Thoracic Aneurysm
- Tortuosity (Aging) of the Aorta
- Aortic Transection
- Aortic Valve Stenosis
- Mediastinal Germ-Cell Tumors

Pathology
- Greatest hydraulic stress right lateral wall ascending aorta or descending aorta in proximity of ligamentum arteriosum
- Intimal tear spirals with false lumen lying anterior and right in the ascending aorta and posterior and left in the descending aorta
- Stanford classification (preferred classification)
- Type A: Originates in ascending thoracic aorta (60-70%)
- Type B: Originates distal to left subclavian artery (30-40%)

Clinical Issues
- Without treatment mortality rate 1-2% per hour first 48 hours, 75% deaths occur within first 2 weeks

---

- True vs. false lumen?
  - Connect true lumen with non-dissected portion on sequential images
- False lumen
  - Cobwebs: Thin strands crossing lumen
  - Beak sign: Acute angle between the dissected flap and the outer wall, angle may contain thrombus
  - Largest lumen usually the false lumen
  - Delayed contrast passage through false lumen
  - Intraluminal thrombus: Entire lumen may be thrombosed
- Intimo-intimal intussusception: Complete circumferential stripping (360°) inverts the intima like a windsock
  - Tear usually originates near coronary arteries
  - Inner lumen usually the true lumen
- Complications
  - Obstruction aortic branch vessels (left renal artery most common: 25%)
  - Pericardial effusion ominous finding suggests rupture into pericardial sac
- Pitfalls
  - False negatives: Poor contrast-enhancement
  - False positives: Streak artifacts, large calcified atherosclerotic plaques may mimic displaced intima, focal atelectasis adjacent to aortic wall
- Acute intramural hematoma
  - High density crescentic focal or circumferential mass in aortic wall (acute hemorrhage), nonenhanced CT crucial
  - Aortic lumen normal or compressed, intimal calcifications may be displaced
  - May progress to dissection: Predictive findings
    - Type A location
    - Compression true lumen: Ratio of minimum and maximum transverse diameter of true lumen at site of maximal hematoma thickness < 0.75
    - Thickness hematoma (> 15 mm)
    - Pericardial or pleural effusion
- Penetrating aortic ulcer
  - Contrast filled ulcer extends into aortic wall, edges usually jagged
  - Typical location descending aorta
  - Wall usually shows extensive atherosclerotic plaque, wall thickened and may enhance
  - End result saccular aneurysm which may rupture

MR Findings
- T1WI: Cardiac-gated black blood sequence > 95% accurate
- MRA
  - Good for extent of dissection and involvement of branch vessels
  - Useful to quantify aortic regurgitation

Echocardiographic Findings
- Transthoracic echo 60-85% sensitive, transesophageal > 95% accurate
- Highly accurate for demonstrating aortic valve involvement

Imaging Recommendations
- Best imaging tool: Cross-sectional imaging primary acute imaging modality
- Protocol advice: Unenhanced CT prior to CTA useful to detect intramural hematoma

DIFFERENTIAL DIAGNOSIS

Thoracic Aneurysm
- Saccular (20%) or fusiform (80%) dilatation of aorta
- Aneurysmal thrombus difficult to differentiate from thrombosed false lumen
  - Mural thrombus irregular internal border (dissection smooth internal border)
  - Intimal calcification located at periphery of aorta (dissection displaced into lumen)
  - Mural thrombus constant location aortic wall (dissection spirals down aorta)

Tortuosity (Aging) of the Aorta
- Normal aging: Loss of elasticity elongates aorta; because aorta fixed, the aorta buckles with a tortuous course

AORTIC DISSECTION

- No displacement intimal calcification, aorta not dilated

Aortic Transection
- Chronic pseudoaneurysm 5% of aortic transections
- Usual location at aortic isthmus

Aortic Valve Stenosis
- Post-stenotic dilatation involves ascending aorta
- Aortic valve may be calcified

Mediastinal Germ-Cell Tumors
- Rapid enlargement from spontaneous hemorrhage mimics dissection or aneurysm
- Calcification focal, not curvilinear

PATHOLOGY

General Features
- Etiology
  - Hypertension universal risk factor: 60-90% of dissections have elevated blood pressure
  - Collagen disorders: Marfan or Ehlers-Danlos
  - Pregnancy
    - 50% of dissections in women occur during pregnancy
  - Congenital
    - Bicuspid aortic valve
    - Aortic coarctation
    - Polycystic kidney disease
    - Turner syndrome, Noonan syndrome
    - Osteogenesis imperfecta
    - Hypercholesterolemia, homocystinuria
  - Crack cocaine use
  - Trauma rare
- Epidemiology: Incidence 6 cases per 100,000 person-years
- Pathogenesis
  - Greatest hydraulic stress right lateral wall ascending aorta or descending aorta in proximity of ligamentum arteriosum

Gross Pathologic & Surgical Features
- Intimal tear spirals with false lumen lying anterior and right in the ascending aorta and posterior and left in the descending aorta
- Dissection usually stops at an aortic branch vessel or at the level of an atherosclerotic plaque

Microscopic Features
- Cystic medial necrosis from aging, atherosclerosis or inherited disorders (Marfan)

Staging, Grading or Classification Criteria
- Stanford classification (preferred classification)
  - Type A: Originates in ascending thoracic aorta (60-70%)
  - Type B: Originates distal to left subclavian artery (30-40%)
- DeBakey classification
  - Type 1: Ascending and descending thoracic aorta (30-40%)
  - Type 2: Ascending only (10-20%)
  - Type 3: Descending only (40-50%) A: Extends to diaphragm, B: Descends below diaphragm

CLINICAL ISSUES

Presentation
- Most common signs/symptoms
  - Sudden onset chest or back pain 80-90% often described as "ripping"
    - Ischemic heart disease 1,000x more common
    - Anterior, neck, throat, jaw pain suggest involvement anterior aorta
    - Back and abdominal pain suggest involvement descending aorta
- Other signs/symptoms
  - Silent dissections uncommon (10%), more common in Marfan syndrome
  - Neurologic deficits (20%)
  - Hypotension ominous finding, suggests cardiac tamponade or hypovolemia from rupture
  - Occlusion aortic branch vessels
    - Renal failure, mesenteric ischemia; lower extremity ischemia

Demographics
- Age: Peak age 60 years
- Gender: M:F = 3:1
- Ethnicity: More common in blacks

Natural History & Prognosis
- Without treatment mortality rate 1-2% per hour first 48 hours, 75% deaths occur within first 2 weeks
- Long term survival in patients with operative management 50%

Treatment
- Type A: Surgical placement of tubular interposition graft
  - Aortic regurgitation (50%) may require valve replacement
  - Medical treatment mortality rate 60%, surgical treatment mortality 30%
- Type B
  - Control hypertension
  - Surgery if dissecting aneurysm larger than 5 cm or increasing in size by > 1.0 cm per year
  - Medical treatment mortality 10%, surgical mortality 30%
- Aortic intravascular fenestration for end organ ischemia
  - Needle advanced from the true lumen to the false lumen with balloon dilatation of tract
  - Site chosen as close as possible to compromised arteries
- Follow-up examinations
  - 3-6 months for 2 years and then annually

SELECTED REFERENCES
1. Hansen MS et al: Frequency of and inappropriate treatment of misdiagnosis of acute aortic dissection. Am J Cardiol. 99(6):852-6, 2007

AORTIC DISSECTION

IMAGE GALLERY

Typical

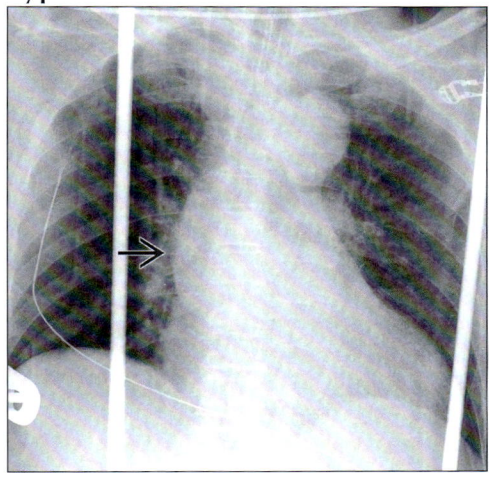
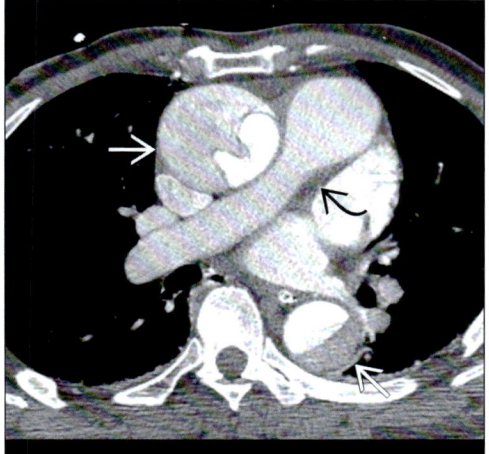

(Left) Anteroposterior radiograph shows tortuous aorta and prominent ascending aorta ➡. *(Right)* Axial CTA shows type A dissection ➡ involving ascending and descending aorta. Ascending aorta dilatation narrows the right pulmonary artery ➡.

Typical

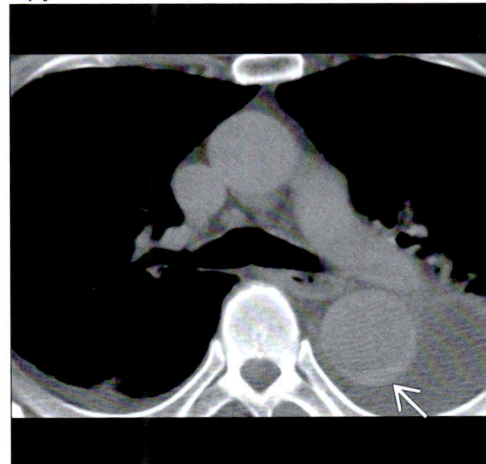
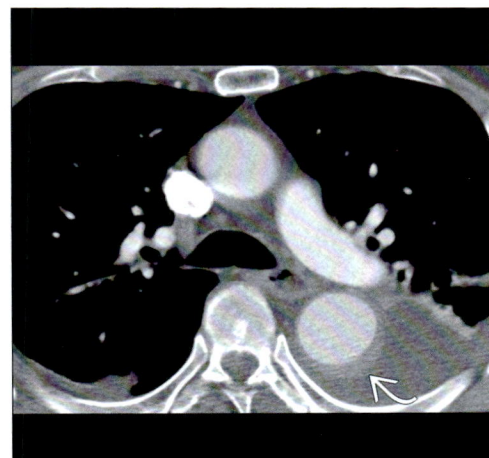

(Left) Axial NECT shows typical type B intramural hematoma ➡. Left pleural effusion suggests possible rupture. *(Right)* Axial CECT shows typical type B aortic dissection and intramural hematoma. Note that the intramural hematoma ➡ is less well demonstrated on the contrast scan. No intimal flap.

Typical

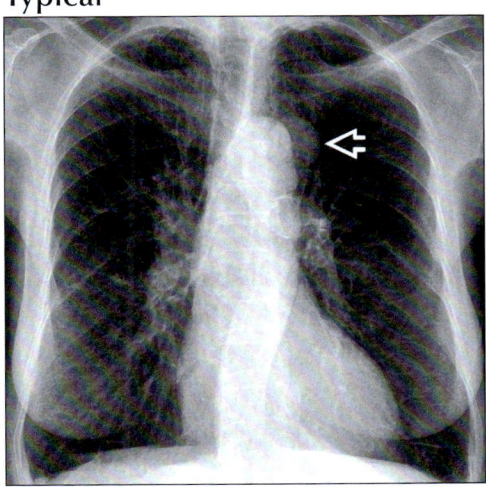
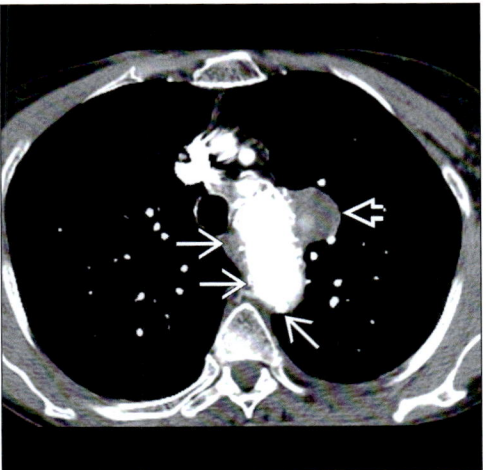

(Left) Frontal radiograph shows sharply defined mediastinal mass ➡ adjacent to the aorta. All mediastinal masses should be viewed as possible aneurysms until proven otherwise. *(Right)* Axial CECT shows focal aneurysm ➡ from penetrating ulcer. Note extensive aortic plaques ➡ elsewhere in aorta.

SVC SYNDROME

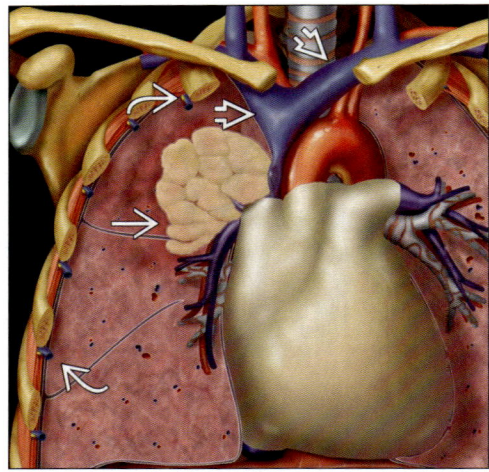

Coronal graphic shows a middle mediastinal mass ➡ causing marked SVC narrowing (and proximal dilatation of the innominate vessels) ➡. There are also prominent right intercostal vein collaterals ➡.

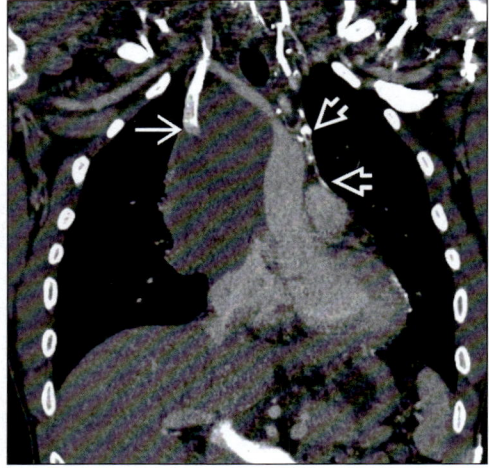

Coronal CECT shows obstruction of SVC from seminoma ➡. Collaterals ➡ along left superior mediastinum. Patient was symptomatic.

TERMINOLOGY

Abbreviations and Synonyms
- Superior vena cava syndrome (SVCS), SVC obstruction

Definitions
- Symptoms from complete or near total obstruction of flow in the superior vena cava due to external compression or intravascular obstruction

IMAGING FINDINGS

General Features
- Best diagnostic clue: Mediastinal widening with enlarged azygos vein and aortic nipple
- Morphology
  ○ SVC 6-8 cm long formed by the junction of the subclavian veins
  ○ Azygous vein loops over the right mainstem bronchus and connects to the posterior wall of the SVC

Radiographic Findings
- Normal chest radiograph 15%
- Abnormal chest radiographs 85%
  ○ Often nonspecific signs
    ▪ Superior mediastinal widening
    ▪ Right upper lobe mass contiguous to mediastinum
  ○ Venous collaterals suggest SVC obstruction
    ▪ Enlargement azygos vein (> 7 mm maximal transverse diameter erect position)
    ▪ Aortic nipple: Dilatation left superior intercostal vein
  ○ Calcification within mass suggests fibrosing mediastinitis
  ○ Pleural effusion suggests underlying malignancy

Fluoroscopic Findings
- Esophagram
  ○ **Downhill varices**
    ▪ Obstruction superior to azygous vein, varices develop in mid-to-upper third of esophagus
    ▪ Obstruction inferior to azygous vein, varices develop the length of esophagus

DDx: Collateral Mimics

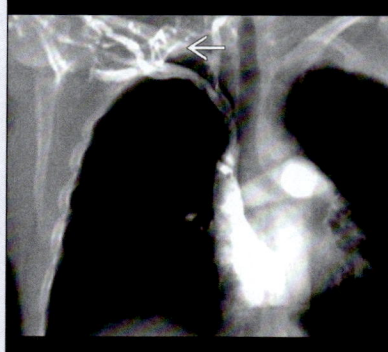
Pseudocollaterals

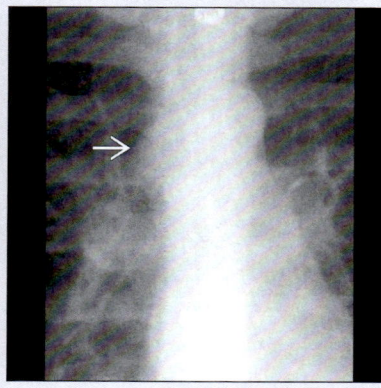
Azygos Continuation

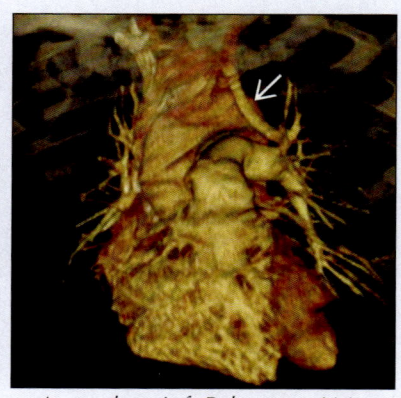
Anomalous Left Pulmonary Vein

SVC SYNDROME

Key Facts

Terminology
- Symptoms from complete or near total obstruction of flow in the superior vena cava due to external compression or intravascular obstruction

Imaging Findings
- Best diagnostic clue: Mediastinal widening with enlarged azygos vein and aortic nipple
- **SVC obstruction diagnosis requires**
- Decrease or absence of opacification of venous blood flow either distal to obstructing lesion or from intraluminal filing defect
- Presence of collaterals
- Best imaging tool: CECT defines cause, exact level of obstruction, extent of disease, maps collateral pathways, and useful in biopsy planning

Top Differential Diagnoses
- Pseudocollaterals
- Interruption of the Inferior Vena Cava with Azygos Continuation
- Partial Anomalous Venous Return

Pathology
- May have radiographic evidence of SVC obstruction without syndrome
- Malignant neoplasms most common cause 60%

Clinical Issues
- Acute onset or change of symptoms suggests superimposed acute thrombosis
- Malignancies invariably symptomatic, in contrast 5% benign etiologies asymptomatic

CT Findings
- SVC obstruction diagnosis requires
  - Decrease or absence of opacification of venous blood flow either distal to obstructing lesion or from intraluminal filing defect
  - Presence of collaterals
    - Acute or rapid obstruction, however, may not allow development of collaterals
- Collateral systems
  - Posterior collateral system
    - Azygous-hemiazygous system
    - Paravertebral system
  - Superior collateral system
    - Periscapular collaterals
    - Anterior jugular venous system
    - External jugular vein
    - Horizontal vein
    - Transverse arch
  - Anterolateral collateral system
    - Anterior intercostal veins
    - Internal mammary veins
    - Long thoracic vein
- False positive findings
  - Mixing opacified blood with unopacified blood flow artifact can be mistaken for thrombus
  - Opacification collateral vessels normal in 5% (due to amount and rate of injection or patient position at time of scanning)

MR Findings
- Similar to CT
- Advantages
  - Does not require contrast administration, useful in patients with contrast allergy
  - Also helpful in patients with no venous access
- Disadvantage
  - Poor demonstration of calcification in fibrosing mediastinitis
  - Longer acquisition time in patients who may not tolerate prolonged recumbency

Other Modality Findings
- Bilateral upper extremity venography can be used to reliably demonstrate obstruction but superseded now by CT
  - May overestimate obstruction size secondary to collateral shunting
  - Usually does not identify cause of obstruction

Imaging Recommendations
- Best imaging tool: CECT defines cause, exact level of obstruction, extent of disease, maps collateral pathways, and useful in biopsy planning

DIFFERENTIAL DIAGNOSIS

Pseudocollaterals
- Hyperabduction of arm may narrow subclavian vein normally
  - Contrast injection may then opacify periscapular veins

Interruption of the Inferior Vena Cava with Azygos Continuation
- No collaterals
- No obstructing mass

Partial Anomalous Venous Return
- Left superior pulmonary vein drains into subclavian vein
- May produce aortic nipple

PATHOLOGY

General Features
- General path comments
  - May have radiographic evidence of SVC obstruction without syndrome
    - More commonly seen with benign etiologies
    - Slower development of obstruction allows more numerous and larger collaterals

SVC SYNDROME

- Etiology
  - Malignant neoplasms most common cause 60%
    - Bronchogenic carcinoma accounts for an overwhelming majority, nearly equally divided between small cell and non-small cell carcinoma
    - Right-sided mass four times more common than left
    - SVCS seen in approximately 2-10% of patients with bronchogenic carcinoma
  - Other malignancies
    - Lymphoma 8%, typically non-Hodgkin
    - Germ cell tumors 3%
    - Others include metastases (especially breast), and thymoma
  - Benign 40%
    - Indwelling intravascular device (catheters, pacemaker wires) 70%
    - Fibrosing mediastinitis 20%
    - Sarcoidosis
    - Radiation fibrosis
    - Syphilitic aneurysms and tuberculosis used to account for 40%, now rare
  - Indwelling catheters
    - 40% develop thrombosis, 10% proceed to SVC syndrome

Gross Pathologic & Surgical Features
- Whether malignant or benign, obstructing mass usually not resectable
- Biopsy and histological confirmation necessary prior to treatment

Staging, Grading or Classification Criteria
- Grade 0: SVC narrowing without SVC syndrome
- Grade 1: Moderate SVC narrowing without collaterals, SVC syndrome
- Grade 2: Severe SVC narrowing azygos primary collateral, SVC syndrome
- Grade 3: SVC obstruction above azygos arch, SVC syndrome
- Grade 4: SVC obstruction at or below azygos arch, SVC syndrome

CLINICAL ISSUES

Presentation
- Most common signs/symptoms
  - Symptoms depend on time course
    - Acute obstruction markedly symptomatic
    - Slowly developing chronic obstruction allows time for collateral development with few or no symptoms
  - Symptoms depend on location relative to azygous vein
    - Obstruction above azygous vein less symptomatic
    - Obstruction below azygous vein more symptomatic
  - Acute onset or change of symptoms suggests superimposed acute thrombosis
  - Dyspnea (50%), cough (50%), face or neck swelling (80%), upper extremity swelling (70%)
  - Malignant etiology: Dyspnea at rest, cough, chest pain
    - Malignancies invariably symptomatic, in contrast 5% benign etiologies asymptomatic

Demographics
- Age
  - Extremely rare in pediatric population
  - Over 40: Malignancy; under 40: Benign etiologies
- Gender
  - More common in males (due to frequency of bronchogenic carcinoma)
  - With benign etiologies, no gender predominance

Natural History & Prognosis
- Depends on underlying etiology
- Prognosis for patients with malignancy is generally less than 6 months

Treatment
- Options, risks, complications: Stent: Migration into heart or pulmonary artery
- Treatment depends on cause of obstruction
- Malignant: Oncologic emergency, treatment aimed at palliation
  - Radiation therapy
    - Tissue diagnosis essential for emergent radiotherapy
    - Symptoms resolve after 1 month
    - Adjuvant chemotherapy and steroid administration may also be helpful
  - Intravascular stents
    - Often more successful (95%) than radiation or chemotherapy
- Benign: Interventional radiology aimed at long term patency
  - Intravascular stents
    - Provides more rapid relief than other modalities
    - Much lower rate of SVCS recurrence compared to radiation or chemotherapy
    - Unclear role for thrombolytics in these patients
    - Stents also beneficial in patients with non-malignant lesions (such as fibrosis)
    - Long term patency unknown
  - Thrombosis-related SVCS
    - Thrombolytics effective for clots five or fewer days old
    - Long term therapy with heparin or Coumadin may be necessary to avoid recurrence
  - Surgery
    - Remove obstructing mass
    - Venous bypass (rarely performed today)

SELECTED REFERENCES

1. Rice TW et al: The superior vena cava syndrome: clinical characteristics and evolving etiology. Medicine (Baltimore). 85(1):37-42, 2006
2. Bolad I et al: Percutaneous treatment of superior vena cava obstruction following transvenous device implantation. Catheter Cardiovasc Interv. 65(1):54-9, 2005
3. Kentos A et al: Long-term remission with surgery for recurrent localized Hodgkin lymphoma. J Thorac Cardiovasc Surg. 129(5):1172, 2005
4. Schifferdecker B et al: Nonmalignant superior vena cava syndrome: Pathophysiology and management. Catheter Cardiovasc Interv. 65(3):416-423, 2005

SVC SYNDROME

IMAGE GALLERY

Typical

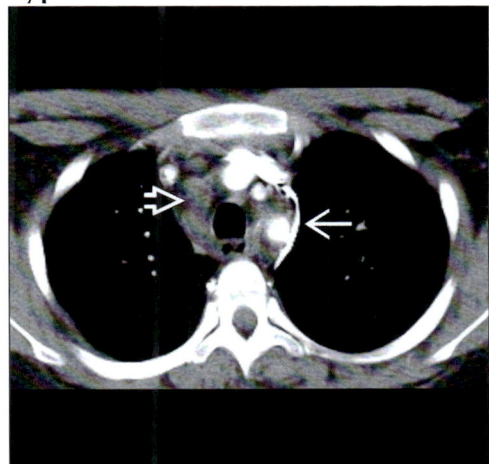
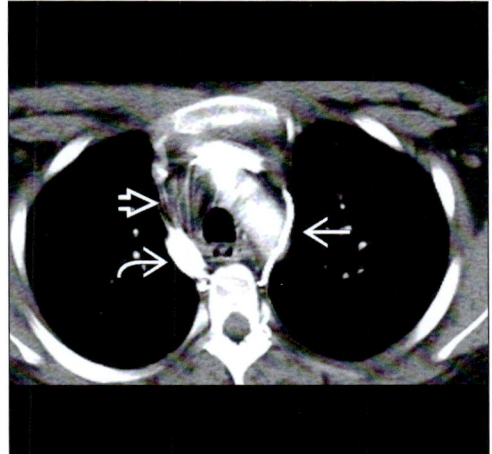

(Left) Axial CECT shows thrombosed SVC ➡ from indwelling catheter. Collateral flow across left superior intercostal vein ➡. (Right) Axial CECT shows thrombosed SVC ➡ and collateral flow across left superior intercostal vein ➡ and azygous vein ➡. Patients usually less symptomatic with azygous vein collateral.

Typical

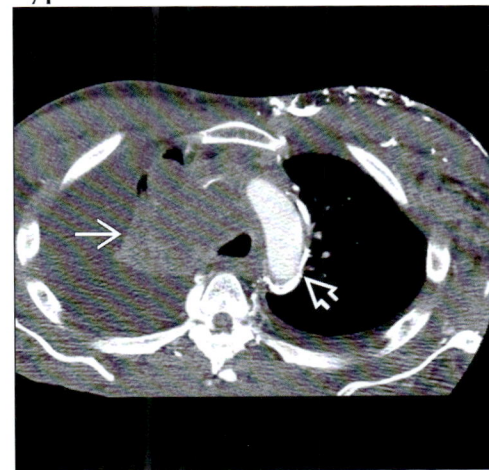
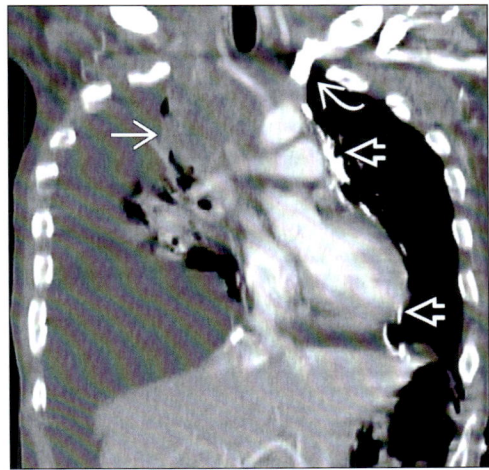

(Left) Axial CECT shows large bronchogenic carcinoma ➡ obstructing superior vena cava. Extensive collaterals in the chest wall and left superior intercostal vein ➡. Large right pleural effusion. (Right) Coronal CECT shows obstructing tumor ➡ and collateral flow through pericardial veins ➡. Left subclavian vein is dilated ➡.

Typical

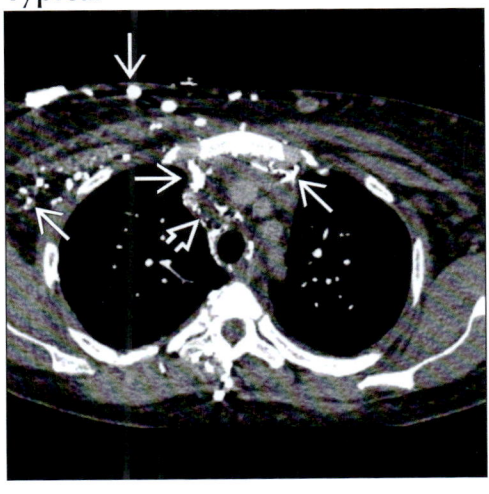
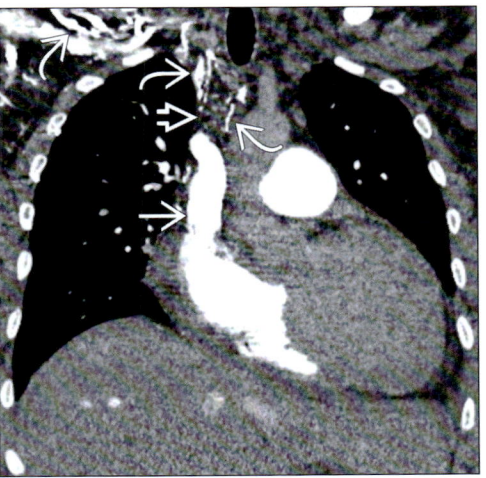

(Left) Axial CECT shows numerous small collaterals in anterior chest wall, mediastinum, and paraspinal pathways ➡. SVC absent and thrombosed ➡. (Right) Coronal CECT shows absence of SVC ➡, SVC patent ➡ below azygos vein. Numerous collaterals in right supraclavicular region and superior mediastinum ➡.

PERICARDIAL TAMPONADE

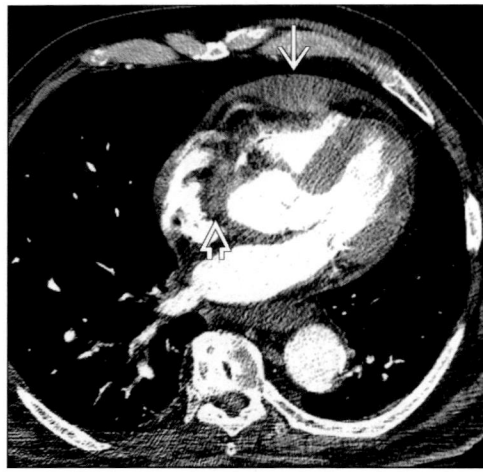

Axial CECT shows pericardial hematoma ➡ compressing the right ventricle from intramural hematoma in ascending aorta ➡.

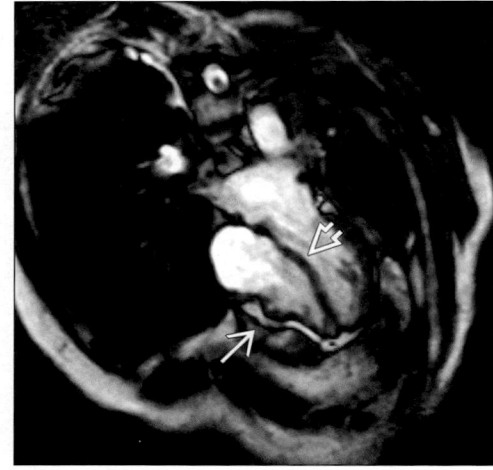

4-Chamber MR cine shows deformed right ventricle from effusive constrictive pericarditis ➡ from previous irradiation. Interventricular bowing ➡.

TERMINOLOGY

Definitions
- Cardiac tamponade: Acute or chronic accumulation of fluid (blood, gas, pus) in pericardial space compressing the heart & equalizing pressures in the cardiac chambers
- Low-pressure tamponade: Tamponade occurring at low diastolic pressures (6-12 mm Hg)
- Regional cardiac tamponade: Cardiac compression by loculated effusion
  - Right atrial tamponade may cause acute right-to-left shunt through patent foramen ovale
- Effusive-constrictive pericarditis: Pre-existing thickened pericardium + pericardial effusion
  - Drainage may have no effect or change the hemodynamics from tamponade to constriction

IMAGING FINDINGS

General Features
- Best diagnostic clue: Cardiomegaly + normal lungs
- Morphology
  - Normal parietal pericardium fibrous structure < 2 mm thick
    - Pericardial space contains 15-50 mL serous fluid
  - Normal pericardium purpose
    - Limits acute cardiac dilatation and enhances mechanical interaction of cardiac chambers
    - Pericardial absence: No known ill effects

Radiographic Findings
- May be normal (especially in acute tamponade)
  - At least 200 mL of pericardial fluid required to enlarge the cardiac silhouette
- Cardiomegaly 90%, most common finding
  - **Water bottle configuration** or shape of Hershey kiss, classic but requires large pericardial effusion
  - Widened subcarinal angle > 75°
  - Rapid increase in cardiac silhouette
  - **Epicardial fat pad sign** (Oreo cookie sign)
    - Separation of retrosternal from the epicardial fat stripe > 2 mm (< 50% sensitivity) on lateral view
  - Differential density sign
    - Increased lucency around the heart margin secondary to effusion, due to different tissue attenuation between blood and saline

DDx: Pericardial Tamponade

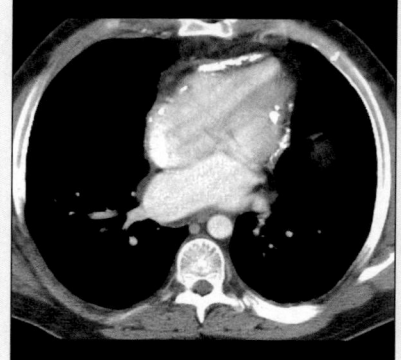

Constrictive Pericarditis

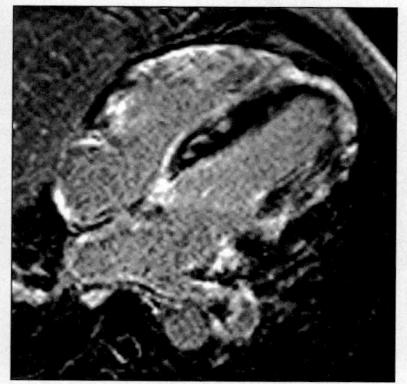

Restrictive Cardiomyopathy

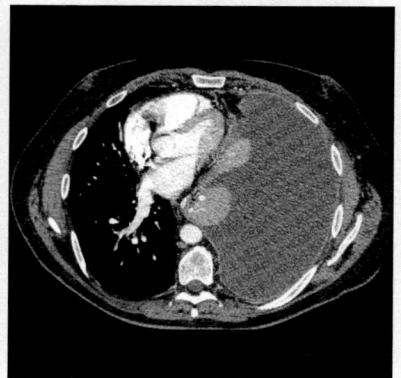

Tension Hydrothorax

PERICARDIAL TAMPONADE

Key Facts

Terminology
- Cardiac tamponade: Acute or chronic accumulation of fluid (blood, gas, pus) in pericardial space compressing the heart & equalizing pressures in the cardiac chambers
- Effusive-constrictive pericarditis: Pre-existing thickened pericardium + pericardial effusion

Imaging Findings
- Best diagnostic clue: Cardiomegaly + normal lungs
- Pericardial space contains 15-50 mL serous fluid
- At least 200 mL of pericardial fluid required to enlarge the cardiac silhouette
- **Water bottle configuration** or shape of Hershey kiss, classic but requires large pericardial effusion
- **Septal bounce:** Septal flattening or leftward septal inversion during early diastole

Top Differential Diagnoses
- Pericardial Constriction
- Restrictive Cardiomyopathy
- Tension Hydrothorax

Pathology
- Normal pericardium: Tamponade develops with acute accumulation of less than 200 mL of fluid
- Chronic pericardial distension: Up to 2 liters of fluid may accumulate without tamponade

Clinical Issues
- Pulsus paradoxus: Inspiratory drop of > 10 mm Hg in systolic blood pressure
- Pericardiocentesis for acute tamponade: Echocardiographic guidance safest

---

- Small heart sign
  - Tension pneumopericardium, heart size returns to normal with evacuation of air
- Lungs often normal, pulmonary edema uncommon
- Pleural effusions either bilateral or left-sided (unilateral right-sided uncommon)

CT Findings
- Pericardium
  - Normal thickness < 2 mm, fluid collects focally in pericardial recesses
  - Pericardial enhancement indicates inflammation (nodularity suggests malignancy)
  - Pericardial effusion
    - Sensitive for as little as 50 mL of fluid
    - Small effusions collect anteriorly
    - Moderate effusions collect laterally, either to the right or left of the surface of the heart
    - Large effusions circumferential around the heart: **Halo sign**
    - Effusion density > 35 Hounsfield units suggestive of hemorrhagic effusion
    - Extravasation of intravenous contrast occasionally seen with perforation
    - Localized collections cause regional tamponade
- Cardiac shape from tamponade
  - Deformed ventricular contour or flattened (in tension pneumopericardium)
  - Angulation of interventricular septum
- Systemic venous hypertension
  - Dilated inferior vena cava and superior vena cava, periportal edema, ascites, contrast reflux into azygous vein
- Mediastinal lymphadenopathy suggestive of tuberculous or neoplastic etiology

MR Findings
- MR Cine
  - **Septal bounce:** Septal flattening or leftward septal inversion during early diastole
  - Inspiratory increase in right ventricular volume limited by size or pressure of pericardial space, increased volume of right ventricle occurs at the expense of left ventricular volume
- Hemorrhage: High signal T1WI and low signal intensity or gradient-recalled echo

Echocardiographic Findings
- Effusions large enough to produce tamponade nearly always circumferential
- Chamber collapse of right ventricle or atria
- Respiratory variation in flow: Septa move leftward, reversing on expiration

Imaging Recommendations
- Best imaging tool
  - Echocardiography demonstrate the presence, size, and hemodynamic consequences
    - Limited by field of view
  - CT or MR provide large field of view of entire pericardium

DIFFERENTIAL DIAGNOSIS

Pericardial Constriction
- Equalization of end-diastolic pressures in all cardiac chambers
- Etiology: Mediastinal radiation, chronic idiopathic pericarditis, following cardiac surgery, tuberculous
- Systemic venous congestion > pulmonary venous congestion
  - Marked jugular venous distension, ascites, peripheral edema: Lungs normal
- Pericardium thickened > 3 mm and often calcified
  - Up to 20% have normal pericardial thickness
- Right ventricular morphology often has a narrow tubular configuration

Restrictive Cardiomyopathy
- Etiology: Amyloid or other infiltrative disease
- Pericardium normal
- Pulmonary hypertension common

PERICARDIAL TAMPONADE

- Ventricular interdependence absent (present in both tamponade and constriction)

Tension Hydrothorax
- May also result in tamponade and right ventricular collapse
- Usually in large malignant effusions
- Occurs even in the absence of pericardium

PATHOLOGY

General Features
- General path comments
  - Volume of most nonhemorrhagic effusions that cause tamponade: 300-600 mL
    - Normal pericardium: Tamponade develops with acute accumulation of less than 200 mL of fluid
    - Chronic pericardial distension: Up to 2 liters of fluid may accumulate without tamponade
- Etiology
  - Acute or chronic idiopathic pericarditis (20%)
  - Iatrogenic effusion (15%)
  - Malignancy (15%)
  - Acute myocardial infarction (8%)
  - Chronic renal disease (5%) or congestive heart failure (5%)
  - Collagen vascular disease (5%)
  - Infection: Tuberculosis, bacterial, or viral (4%)
  - Hemorrhagic
    - Dissecting aortic aneurysm rupture into pericardial space
    - Traumatic or iatrogenic (catheter manipulation)
    - Acute myocardial infarction
    - Neoplastic
  - Effusive constrictive pericarditis most common from pre-existing radiation or neoplasm
- Pathophysiology
  - Compliance (pressure-volume) curve pericardial space limited
    - J-shaped curve exhibits "tipping point" where after asymptomatic accumulation of small amount of fluid, further accumulation causes precipitous rise in pericardial pressure
    - Slow accumulation of fluid allows stretching of pericardium without rise in pressure
  - Ventricular interaction or interdependence
    - Pericardium has fixed volume, when full (due to accumulation of pericardial fluid) any change in the volume of one side of the heart then causes the opposite change in volume of the other side
    - Systemic venous return increases with inspiration, right heart volume increases with bulging of the atrial and ventricular septa into the left atrium and ventricle
    - Physiologic explanation for pulsus paradoxus

Staging, Grading or Classification Criteria
- Incipient tamponade: Pericardial pressure equals right atrial pressure but lower the left atrial pressure
- Mild tamponade: Pericardial pressure equals left atrial pressure
- Moderate tamponade: Pericardial pressure exceeds 10-12 mm Hg, right heart chambers compressed, pulsus paradoxus absent
  - Right atrial compression: Right atrium becomes concave
  - Right ventricular diastolic collapse: Right ventricular free wall indents toward the septum
- Severe tamponade: Pericardial pressure > 25 mm Hg, pulsus paradoxus

CLINICAL ISSUES

Presentation
- Most common signs/symptoms
  - Consider in any patient with shock or pulseless electric activity
  - Symptoms nonspecific: Tachypnea and dyspnea on exertion most common (sensitivity 90%)
  - Signs nonspecific: Tachycardia and jugular venous distension most common
    - Bradycardia consider uremia and hypothyroidism
  - Beck triad (named after thoracic surgeon Claude Schaeffer Beck)
    - Hypotension, increase jugular venous pressure, small-quiet heart
  - Consider tamponade in post cardiac surgery with sudden development of hypotension
- Other signs/symptoms
  - Pulsus paradoxus: Inspiratory drop of > 10 mm Hg in systolic blood pressure
    - Absent with conditions increasing left ventricular diastolic pressure: Atrial septal defect, aortic regurgitation, left ventricular hypertrophy, or in those in severe shock
    - False positive pulsus paradoxus: Severe chronic obstructive pulmonary disease, congestive heart failure, mitral stenosis, massive pulmonary embolism, severe hypovolemic shock, obesity, tense ascites
  - EKG shows
    - Electrical alternation: QRS, T or P wave reverse polarity with each heart beat

Treatment
- Medial treatment usually ineffective: Mechanical ventilation may precipitate sudden drop in blood pressure
- Pericardiocentesis for acute tamponade: Echocardiographic guidance safest
- Pericardial window either from balloon pericardiotomy or surgery

SELECTED REFERENCES
1. Roy CL et al: Does this patient with a pericardial effusion have cardiac tamponade? JAMA. 297(16):1810-8, 2007
2. Little WC et al: Pericardial disease. Circulation. 113(12):1622-32, 2006
3. Goldstein JA: Cardiac tamponade, constrictive pericarditis, and restrictive cardiomyopathy. Curr Probl Cardiol. 29(9):503-67, 2004

PERICARDIAL TAMPONADE

IMAGE GALLERY

Typical

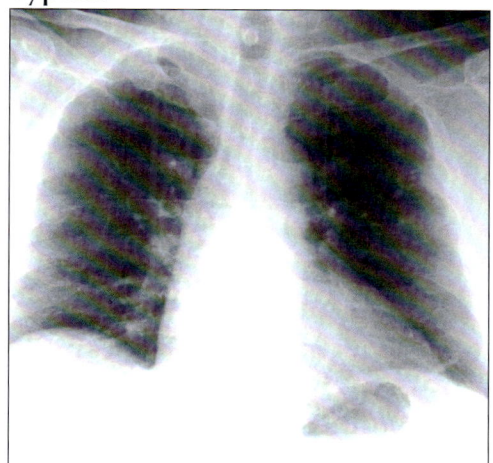
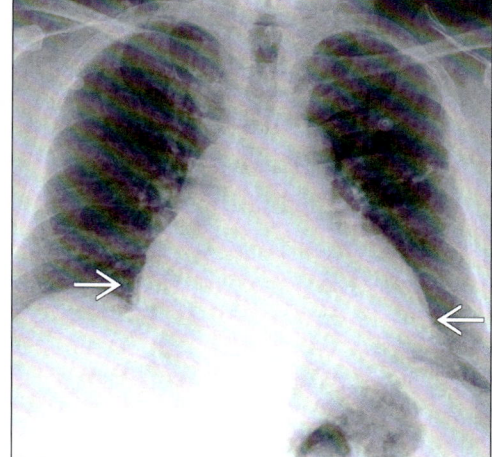

(Left) Frontal radiograph is normal. *(Right)* Frontal radiograph 6 months later shows enlargement of the heart (hint of water bottle shape) ➡. Lungs normal. No effusions.

Typical

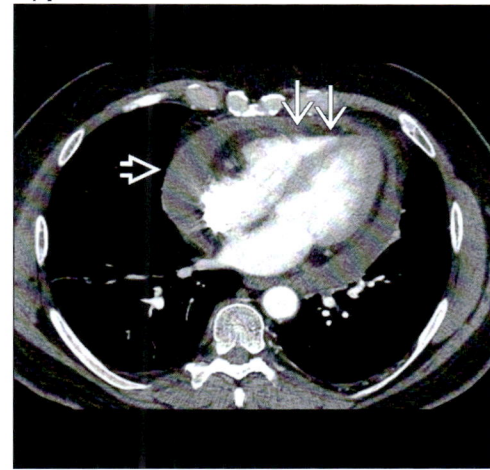
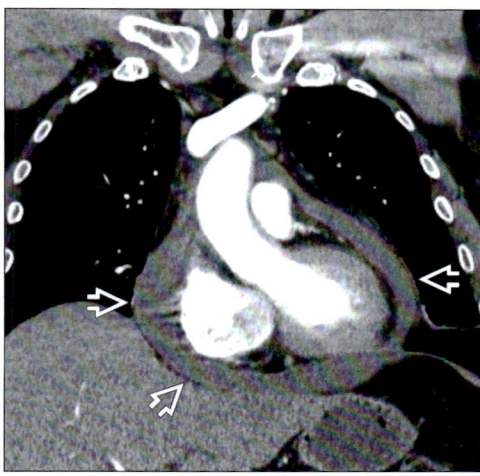

(Left) Axial CECT large pericardial effusion nearly circumferential around the heart ➡. Tubular shape of the right ventricle ➡ suggests tamponade. *(Right)* Coronal CECT shows large pericardial effusion ➡ nearly completely surrounding the heart. Etiology of effusion was idiopathic.

Typical

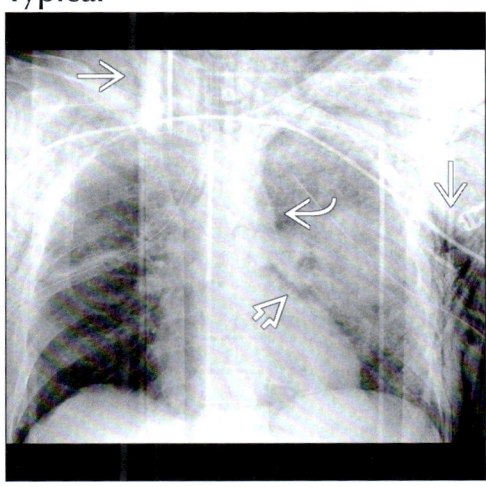
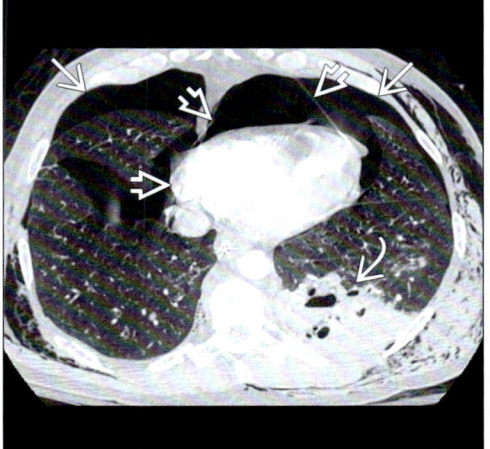

(Left) Anteroposterior radiograph subcutaneous emphysema ➡ and pneumomediastinum ➡. Bilateral chest tubes. Mediastinum is widened and aortic arch is obscured ➡ from aortic transection (not shown). Heart size normal. *(Right)* Axial CECT small heart from tension pneumopericardium ➡. Bilateral pneumothoraces ➡, contusion left base ➡.

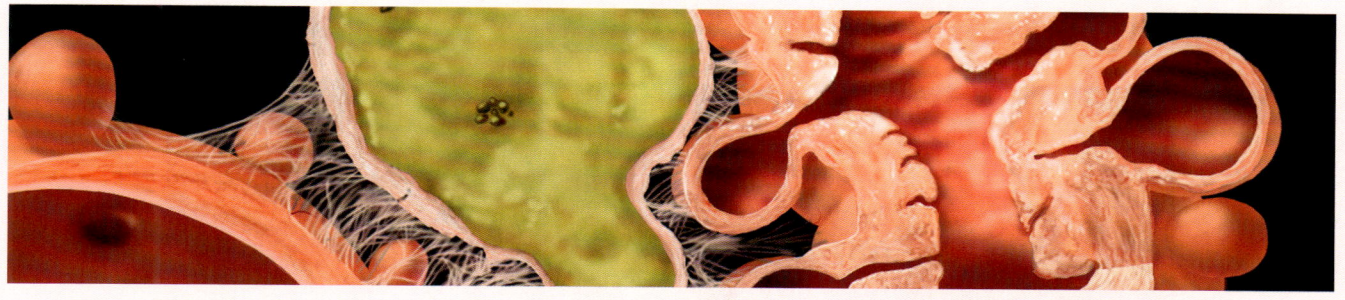

SECTION 3: Abdomen/Pelvis

Introduction and Overview
Abdominal Imaging Issues, Non-Trauma	II-3-2

Abdomen
Abdominal Abscess	II-3-4
Peritonitis	II-3-8
Inguinal Hernia	II-3-12
Femoral Hernia	II-3-16
Paraduodenal Hernia	II-3-20
Transmesenteric Post-Operative Hernia	II-3-24
Duodenal Ulcer	II-3-28
Aorto-Enteric Fistula	II-3-32
Crohn Disease	II-3-34
Pneumatosis of the Intestine	II-3-38
Acute Small Bowel Ischemia	II-3-42
Vasculitis, Small Intestine	II-3-46
Small Bowel Obstruction	II-3-50
Gallstone Ileus	II-3-54
Intussusception	II-3-56
Infectious Colitis	II-3-60
Pseudomembranous Colitis	II-3-64
Typhlitis	II-3-68
Ulcerative Colitis	II-3-70
Toxic Megacolon	II-3-74
Appendicitis	II-3-76
Diverticulitis	II-3-80
Epiploic Appendagitis	II-3-84
Omental Infarct	II-3-88
Ischemic Colitis	II-3-92
Sigmoid Volvulus	II-3-96
Cecal Volvulus	II-3-100
Splenic Infection and Abscess	II-3-102
Splenic Infarction	II-3-106
Hepatic Candidiasis	II-3-110
Hepatic Pyogenic Abscess	II-3-114
Hepatic Amebic Abscess	II-3-118
HELLP Syndrome	II-3-122
Hepatic Infarction	II-3-126
Portal Vein Occlusion	II-3-130
Budd-Chiari Syndrome	II-3-134
Ascending Cholangitis	II-3-138
Recurrent Pyogenic Cholangitis	II-3-140
Choledocholithiasis	II-3-144
Cholecystitis	II-3-148
Acute Pancreatitis	II-3-152
Pyelonephritis	II-3-156
Renal Abscess	II-3-160
Xanthogranulomatous Pyelonephritis	II-3-164
Emphysematous Pyelonephritis	II-3-168
Renal Infarction	II-3-170
Renal Vein Thrombosis	II-3-174
Epididymo-Orchitis	II-3-178
Testicular Torsion	II-3-182
Midgut Volvulus	II-3-186
Duodenal Atresia or Stenosis	II-3-190
Meconium Plug Syndrome	II-3-194
Meconium Ileus	II-3-198
Meconium Peritonitis	II-3-202
Necrotizing Enterocolitis	II-3-206
Hypertrophic Pyloric Stenosis	II-3-210
Gastric Volvulus	II-3-214
Ileocolic Intussusception (Idiopathic)	II-3-218
Meckel Diverticulum	II-3-222
Mesenteric Adenitis	II-3-226
Small Bowel Intussusception, Pediatric	II-3-230

Pelvis
Uterine AVM	II-3-234
Ovarian Torsion	II-3-238
Ovarian Vein Thrombosis	II-3-242
Ovarian Hemorrhage	II-3-246
Pelvic Inflammatory Disease	II-3-250
Ectopic Pregnancy, Tubal	II-3-254

ABDOMINAL IMAGING ISSUES, NON-TRAUMA

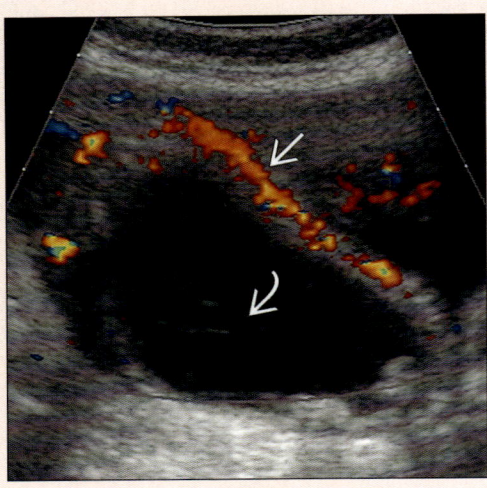

Transverse color Doppler ultrasound of gangrenous cholecystitis reveals marked hypertrophy of cystic artery ➔ and linear membranes in GB lumen ➔ from fibrous strands of pus.

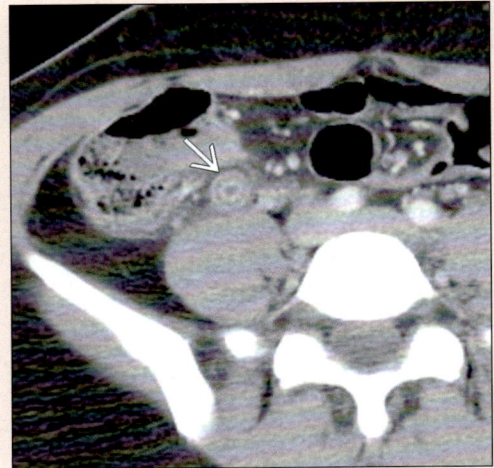

CECT shows early appendicitis with prominent submucosal edema of the appendix. Note target appearance of appendix ➔.

ANATOMY-BASED IMAGING ISSUES

Clinical Overview
- Abdominal pain is a leading cause of non-traumatic emergencies
  - Clinical assessment often limited due to broad overlap of pathology & nonspecific signs/symptoms
- Role of imaging is to rapidly triage patients between medical vs. surgical therapy
- Early imaging is cost-effective; prevents unnecessary surgery, facilitates early discharge of patients without surgical lesions
- For purpose of differential diagnosis, acute abdominal pain is sub-classified according to anatomic location
  - Right upper quadrant (RUQ) pain
  - Right lower quadrant (RLQ) pain
  - Left upper quadrant (LUQ) pain
  - Left lower quadrant (LLQ) pain
  - Midabdominal pain
  - Pelvic pain
  - Flank pain

Imaging Strategy
- RUQ pain
  - US for suspected acute cholecystitis and biliary obstruction
  - HIDA scan if US inconclusive
  - CT for hepatic parenchymal lesion
- RLQ pain
  - US for suspected unruptured appendicitis and complex pericholecystic abscesses
    - Pediatric patients; pregnant patients; thin young adults
  - Contrast-enhanced CT (CECT) if US inconclusive
  - CECT for appendicitis
    - Adults with normal body habitus
    - Patients with suspected ruptured appendicitis or RLQ pain > 72 hours
- LUQ pain
  - CECT
    - Splenic lesions; subphrenic lesions (abscess, hematoma); tail of pancreas lesions
- LLQ pain
  - CECT for suspected diverticulitis, US for possible adnexal mass
- Midabdominal pain
  - CECT
    - Suspected pancreatitis; duodenal ulcer disease; possible bowel infarction or obstruction
- Pelvic pain
  - US with transabdominal & endovaginal probes
    - Ovarian cysts; ovarian torsion; pelvic inflammatory disease (PID); ectopic pregnancy
  - CECT if US inconclusive
- Flank pain
  - NECT for ureteral stones
  - Consider CECT if NECT inconclusive, and for possible pyelonephritis

Imaging Findings
- RUQ pain: Cholecystitis
  - US
    - Gallstones
    - Gallbladder (GB) wall thickness > 3 mm
    - Positive sonographic Murphy sign
  - HIDA scan: Non-filling GB with isotope in duodenum
  - CT: Thick-walled GB with pericholecystic fat stranding and fluid
- RLQ pain: Appendicitis
  - US
    - Distended (> 7 mm) non-compressible appendix
  - CECT
    - Appendix > 7 mm
    - Periappendiceal fat stranding, ± appendicolith
    - Abnormal mural enhancement of appendix
- RLQ pain: Cecal diverticulitis
  - CECT
    - Pericecal fat stranding
    - Mural thickening
    - Inflamed diverticulum
- RLQ pain: Epiploic appendagitis
  - CECT
    - Oval fat-containing appendage with peripheral hyperdense rim

ABDOMINAL IMAGING ISSUES, NON-TRAUMA

Key Facts

Differential Diagnoses
- RUQ pain, R/O cholecystitis: Pancreatitis, peptic ulcer disease (PUD); pyogenic or amebic liver abscess; SBO; right-sided pyelonephritis
- RUQ pain, R/O appendicitis: Mesenteric adenitis; PID; ischemic bowel disease; cecal diverticulitis
- LUQ pain, R/O splenic infarct: Subphrenic abscess; splenic abscess; pancreatitis; splenic rupture
- LLQ pain, R/O diverticulitis: Sigmoid CA; ischemic colitis; pseudomembranous colitis
- Mid-abdominal pain, R/O pancreatitis: Cholecystitis; PUD; SBO; bowel infarction
- Pelvic pain, R/O torsion: PID; ruptured ovarian cyst; ectopic pregnancy; appendicitis
- Flank pain, R/O ureteral stone: Pyelonephritis; renal abscess; renal infarct; ruptured renal tumor; renal cell CA

- "Central dot" sign
- Adjacent fat stranding ± omental edema
- LUQ pain: Splenic infarct
  - CECT
    - Wedge-shaped, linear or peripheral areas of non-enhancement
- LUQ pain: Subphrenic abscess
  - CECT
    - Fluid collection with enhancing rim and mass effect of adjacent structures
    - ± Gas bubbles
- LLQ pain: Sigmoid diverticulitis
  - CECT
    - Mural thickening of sigmoid colon
    - Enhancing wall of inflamed diverticulum
    - Pericolonic fat stranding in sigmoid mesocolon
    - ± Ectopic gas bubbles
    - Free fluid along base of sigmoid mesocolon
    - ± Pelvic abscesses
- Mid-abdominal pain: Acute pancreatitis
  - CECT
    - Pancreatic enlargement
    - ± Areas of focal or diffuse necrosis and/or edema
    - Acute fluid collections in either left anterior pararenal space, lesser sac or transverse mesocolon
    - Peripancreatic fat stranding
- Mid-abdominal pain: Small bowel obstruction (SBO)
  - CECT
    - Distended small bowel loops
    - Transition point between distended & collapsed small bowel loop
- Pelvic pain: Ovarian torsion
  - US
    - Enlarged echogenic ovary
    - Prominent peripheral follicles
    - Absence of central venous flow on spectral Doppler
    - Dampened arterial flow if present at all
- Pelvic pain: PID
  - US
    - Dilated fallopian tube with internal debris (pyosalpinx)
    - "Indefinite" uterus sign as inflammation obscures posterior wall of myometrium
    - Complex solid/cystic adnexal masses (tubo-ovarian abscess)
    - Free fluid with low-level echoes (pus)
- Flank pain
  - NECT
    - Calcified stone in ureter
    - Hydronephrosis
    - Perirenal stranding (forniceal rupture)
    - Nephromegaly

RELATED REFERENCES

1. Ralls PW et al: Real-time sonography in suspected acute cholecystitis. Prospective evaluation of primary and secondary signs. Radiology. 155(3):767-71, 1985

IMAGE GALLERY

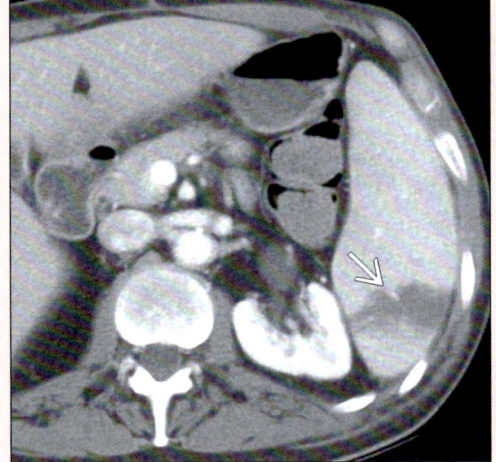
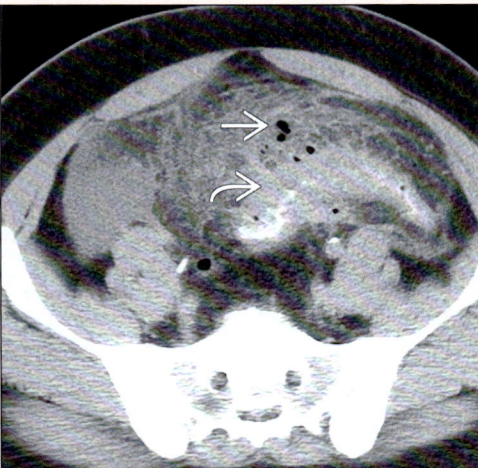

(Left) Axial CECT shows splenomegaly with linear infarct ➡ in lower pole. Note discrete lesion with well-defined linear margins. *(Right)* Axial CECT shows diverticulitis of sigmoid colon. Note extensive pericolonic phlegmon and soft tissue stranding with ectopic gas bubbles ➡ adjacent to thickened sigmoid ➡.

ABDOMINAL ABSCESS

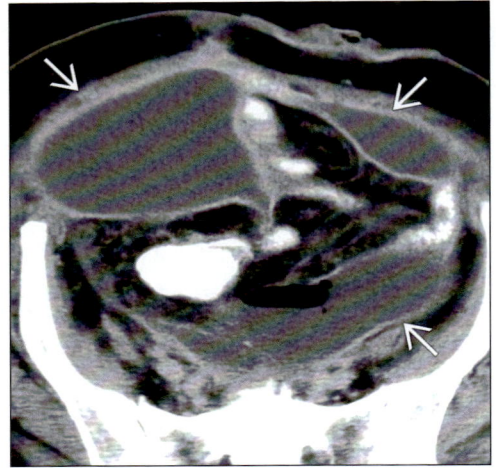 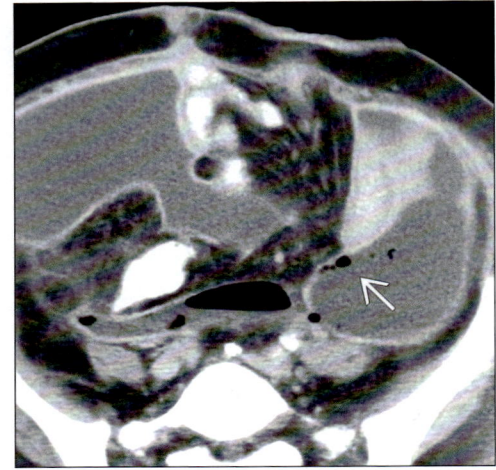

Axial CECT shows multiple post-operative abscesses. Note fluid collections with enhancing rims and mass effect ➔.

Axial CECT (in same patient as left) shows ectopic gas bubbles within abscess in pelvis ➔.

TERMINOLOGY

Definitions
- Localized abdominal collection of pus

IMAGING FINDINGS

General Features
- Best diagnostic clue: Fluid collection with mass effect & enhancing rim with or without gas bubbles or air-fluid level on CECT
- Location: Anywhere within abdominal cavity; intraparenchymal; within intra- or extraperitoneal spaces
- Size: Highly variable; 2-15 cm in diameter; microabscesses < 2 cm
- Morphology: Low density fluid collection with peripheral enhancing rim

Radiographic Findings
- Radiography
  ○ Ectopic gas (50% of cases)
  ○ Air-fluid level
  ○ Soft tissue "mass"
  ○ Focal ileus
  ○ Loss of soft tissue-fat interface
  ○ Subphrenic abscess: Pleural effusion and lower lobe atelectasis

Fluoroscopic Findings
- Abscess sinogram
  ○ Useful after percutaneous drainage to assess degree of residual cavity
  ○ Defines catheter position in dependent portion of abscess
  ○ Identifies fistulas of bowel, pancreas or biliary duct

CT Findings
- NECT: Low attenuation fluid collection, mass effect, gas in 50% of cases
- CECT: Peripheral rim enhancement

MR Findings
- T1WI: Low signal
- T2WI: Intermediate to high signal fluid collection
- T1 C+
  ○ Similar to CECT
  ○ Low signal fluid collection with enhancing rim

DDx: Spectrum of Cystic Abdominal Lesions Mimicking Abscess

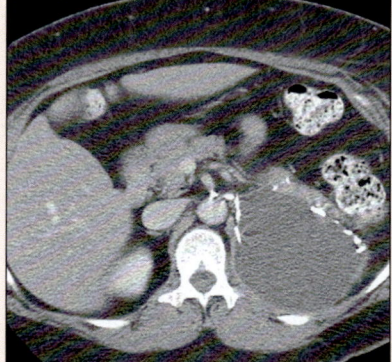 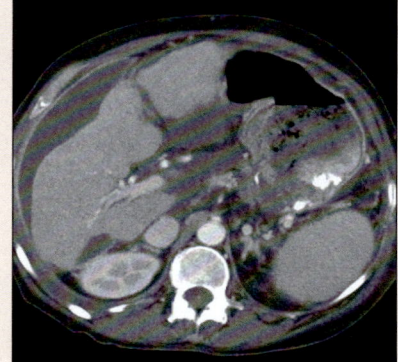 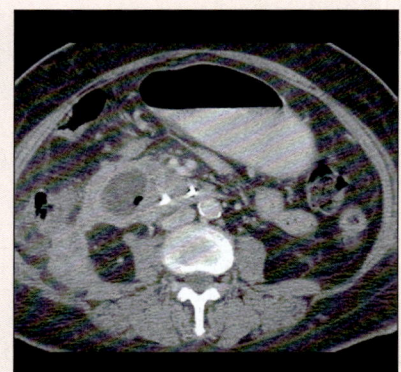

Lymphocele   *Loculated Ascites*   *Pancreatic Pseudocyst*

ABDOMINAL ABSCESS

Key Facts

Terminology
- Localized abdominal collection of pus

Imaging Findings
- Best diagnostic clue: Fluid collection with mass effect & enhancing rim with or without gas bubbles or air-fluid level on CECT
- Location: Anywhere within abdominal cavity; intraparenchymal; within intra- or extraperitoneal spaces
- NECT: Low attenuation fluid collection, mass effect, gas in 50% of cases
- CECT: Peripheral rim enhancement
- Complex fluid collection with internal low level echoes, membranes or septations on US
- Best imaging tool: CECT

Pathology
- General path comments: Pus collection; peripheral fibrocapillary "capsule"; often polymicrobial from enteric organisms
- Enteric perforation

Clinical Issues
- Most common signs/symptoms: Fever, chills; abdominal pain; increased heart rate, decreased blood pressure if septic
- Variable depending on extent of abscess, patient's immune system status; excellent prognosis
- Percutaneous abscess drainage (PAD)

Diagnostic Checklist
- Diagnostic mimics: Biloma, lymphocele, pseudocyst, hematoma

Ultrasonographic Findings
- Grayscale Ultrasound
  - Complex fluid collection with internal low level echoes, membranes or septations on US
  - Dependent echoes representing debris
  - Fluid-fluid level
  - High amplitude linear echoes with reverberation artifacts representing gas bubbles
  - Inflamed fat adjacent to abscess: Echogenic mass
  - Degree of enhanced through sound transmission varies
    - More proteinaceous abscess has relatively little through transmission
- Color Doppler
  - Hypervascular periphery
  - Avascular center of abscess
  - Hyperemic inflamed fat

Nuclear Medicine Findings
- Gallium scan
  - Useful for fever of unknown origin
  - Nonspecific: Positive with tumor such as lymphoma and granulomatous lesions
- WBC scan
  - 73-83% sensitivity
  - False positives with bowel infarct or hematoma
- Newer agents
  - Indium-labeled polyclonal IgG
  - Tc-99m labeled monoclonal antibody

Imaging Recommendations
- Best imaging tool: CECT
- Protocol advice: Oral & IV contrast, 150 mL IV contrast at 2.5 mL/sec

DIFFERENTIAL DIAGNOSIS

Lymphocele
- History of lymph node dissection
- Fluid collections with mass (often bilateral) along lymphatic drainage
- Attenuation values -10 HU to +10 HU

Biloma
- History of biliary or hepatic surgery
- Perihepatic fluid collection commonly in gallbladder fossa or Morison pouch
- Attenuation value 0-15 HU

Loculated Ascites
- Evidence for cirrhosis or chronic liver disease
- Minimal or no mass effect
- Often passively conforms to peritoneal space
- May contain septations on US

Pancreatic Fluid Collection/Pseudocyst
- History of pancreatitis
- Associated pancreatic necrosis on CECT
- Location: Highly variable but most often within pancreatic parenchyma, lesser sac, anterior pararenal space, transverse mesocolon
- Pseudocyst requires several weeks to develop peripheral pseudocapsule

Abdominal Hematoma
- High attenuation clot (> 45 HU) or fluid collection with enhancing rim (> 25 HU)
- Mass effect on bowel or adjacent organs

PATHOLOGY

General Features
- General path comments: Pus collection; peripheral fibrocapillary "capsule"; often polymicrobial from enteric organisms
- Genetics
  - Increased risk if genetically altered immune response
  - Diabetics have increased incidence of gas-forming abscesses
- Etiology
  - Enteric perforation
    - Appendicitis
    - Diverticulitis
    - Crohn disease

ABDOMINAL ABSCESS

- Post-operative
  - Typically intraperitoneal spaces such as cul-de-sac, Morison pouch and subphrenic spaces
- Bacteremia
- Trauma
- Epidemiology
  - Most commonly due to postoperative complication
  - Microabscesses due to fungal infections in immunocompromised patients
  - Higher incidence in diabetics, immunocompromised patients and postoperative patients

Gross Pathologic & Surgical Features
- Often adherent omentum or bowel loops; pus collection
- May or may not have "capsule"

Microscopic Features
- PMN and white cell debris
- Bacteria, fungi detected

Staging, Grading or Classification Criteria
- Organism: Bacterial, fungal amebic
- Related to organ of origin (i.e., liver abscess)
- Intraperitoneal
- Extraperitoneal
- Communicating
  - Underlying fistula to GI tract
  - Connection to biliary tract or pancreatic duct

CLINICAL ISSUES

Presentation
- Most common signs/symptoms: Fever, chills; abdominal pain; increased heart rate, decreased blood pressure if septic
- Clinical Profile: Leukocytosis, + blood cultures and elevated ESR

Demographics
- Age: Any
- Gender: M = F

Natural History & Prognosis
- Variable depending on extent of abscess, patient's immune system status; excellent prognosis

Treatment
- Options, risks, complications
  - Percutaneous abscess drainage (PAD)
    - 80% success rate of percutaneous drainage
    - Patient selection critical for success
    - Best candidates for PAD have well-localized, fluid-filled abscesses > 3 cm with safe catheter access route
  - Contraindications for PAD related to patient
    - Coagulopathy with prothrombin time > 3 sec
    - International normalized ratio > 1.5
    - Platelets < 50,000 µL
  - Contraindications for PAD related to abscess
    - Infected necrosis (i.e., pancreatic abscess)
    - Gas-forming infection such as emphysematous pancreatitis
    - Multiseptated abscess
    - Soft tissue infection (i.e., phlegmon)
    - No safe access route for catheter insertion
  - Surgery indications
    - Extensive intraperitoneal abscesses
    - Debridement of necrotic infected tissue
    - Failed PAD
  - Antibiotic therapy
    - Abscesses < 3 cm

DIAGNOSTIC CHECKLIST

Consider
- Diagnostic mimics: Biloma, lymphocele, pseudocyst, hematoma

Image Interpretation Pearls
- Half of abscesses don't contain gas or air-fluid levels; mass effect & enhancing rim highly suggestive in appropriate clinical context
- Elderly and immunocompromised patients may not have fever or ↑ WBC

SELECTED REFERENCES

1. Benoist S et al: Can failure of percutaneous drainage of postoperative abdominal abscesses be predicted? Am J Surg. 184(2):148-53, 2002
2. Betsch A et al: CT-guided percutaneous drainage of intra-abdominal abscesses: APACHE III score stratification of 1-year results. Acute Physiology, Age, Chronic Health Evaluation. Eur Radiol. 12(12):2883-9, 2002
3. Cinat ME et al: Determinants for successful percutaneous image-guided drainage of intra-abdominal abscess. Arch Surg. 137(7):845-9, 2002
4. Harisinghani MG et al: CT-guided transgluteal drainage of deep pelvic abscesses: indications, technique, procedure-related complications, and clinical outcome. Radiographics. 22(6):1353-67, 2002
5. Lohela P: Ultrasound-guided drainages and sclerotherapy. Eur Radiol. 12(2):288-95, 2002
6. Men S et al: Percutaneous drainage of abdominal abscess. Eur J Radiol. 43(3):204-18, 2002
7. Ralls PW: Inflammatory disease of the liver. Clin Liver Dis. 6(1):203-25, 2002
8. Deck AJ et al: Perinephric abscesses in the neurologically impaired. Spinal Cord. 39(9):477-81, 2001
9. Green BT: Splenic abscess: report of six cases and review of the literature. Am Surg. 67(1):80-5, 2001
10. Jacobs JE et al: Computed tomography evaluation of acute pancreatitis. Semin Roentgenol. 36(2):92-8, 2001
11. Krige JE et al: ABC of diseases of liver, pancreas, and biliary system. BMJ. 322(7285):537-40, 2001
12. Maggard MA et al: Surgical diverticulitis: treatment options. Am Surg. 67(12):1185-9, 2001
13. vanSonnenberg E et al: Percutaneous abscess drainage: update. World J Surg. 25(3):362-9; discussion 370-2, 2001
14. Sirinek KR: Diagnosis and treatment of intra-abdominal abscesses. Surg Infect (Larchmt). 1(1):31-8, 2000
15. Zibari GB et al: Pyogenic liver abscess. Surg Infect (Larchmt). 1(1):15-21, 2000
16. Barakate MS et al: Pyogenic liver abscess: a review of 10 years' experience in management. Aust N Z J Surg. 69(3):205-9, 1999

ABDOMINAL ABSCESS

IMAGE GALLERY

Typical

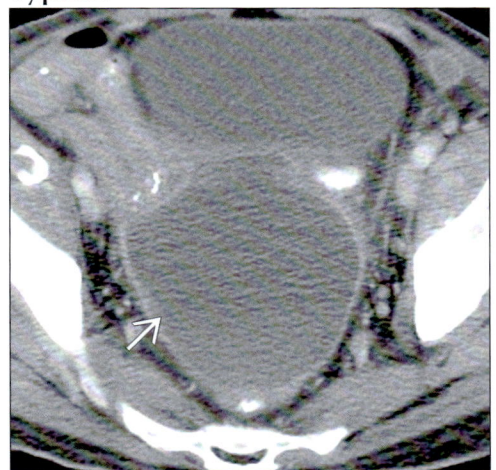
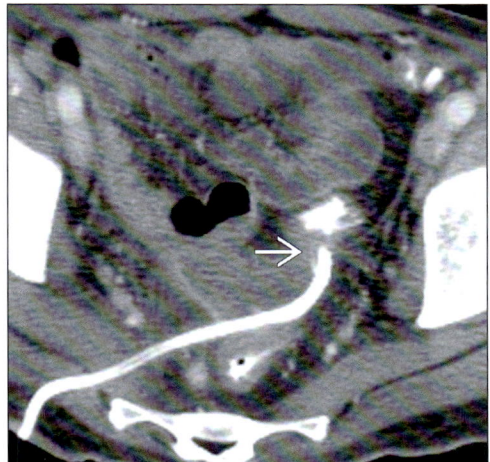

(Left) Axial CECT shows pelvic abscess following hysterectomy. Note large fluid collection with enhancing rim and mass effect ➡. *(Right)* Axial CECT following percutaneous drainage ➡. The abscess has almost completely resolved.

Typical

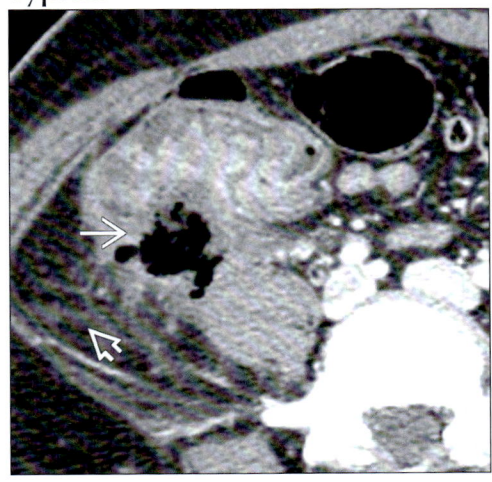
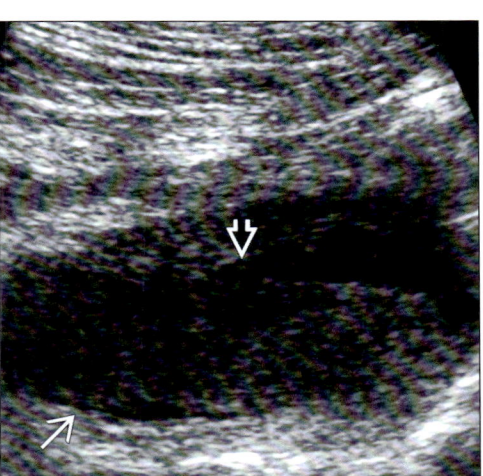

(Left) Axial CECT of gas-forming retrocecal abscess from perforated diverticulum. Note ectopic gas collection from posterior to cecum ➡, cecal thickening, and adjacent fat stranding ➡. *(Right)* Transverse transabdominal ultrasound of post-operative abscess on grayscale image. Note hypoechoic fluid collection ➡ with fluid-fluid level ➡.

Variant

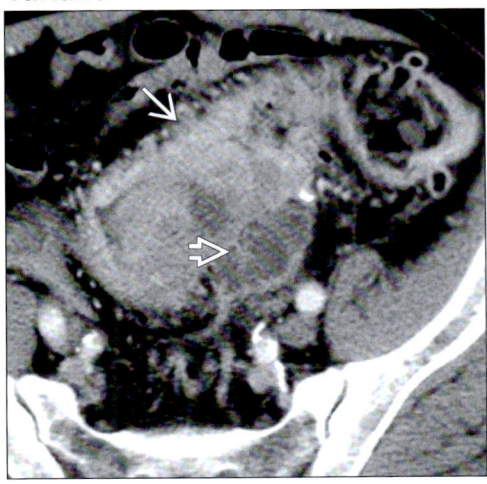
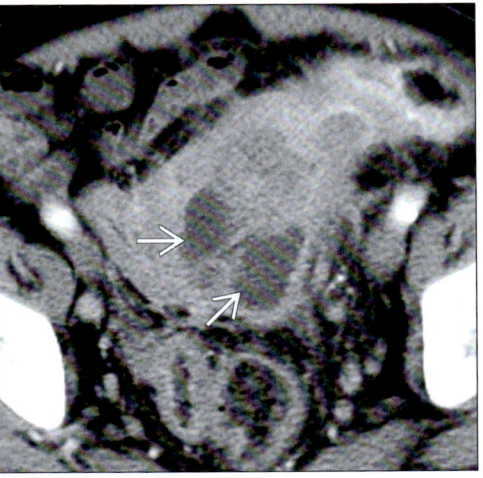

(Left) Axial CECT of intramural abscess of sigmoid from diverticulitis. Note long segment of markedly thickened sigmoid ➡ and ill-defined adjacent fluid collection ➡. *(Right)* Axial CECT (in same patient as previous image) shows more discreet abscess collections on lower plane of section ➡.

PERITONITIS

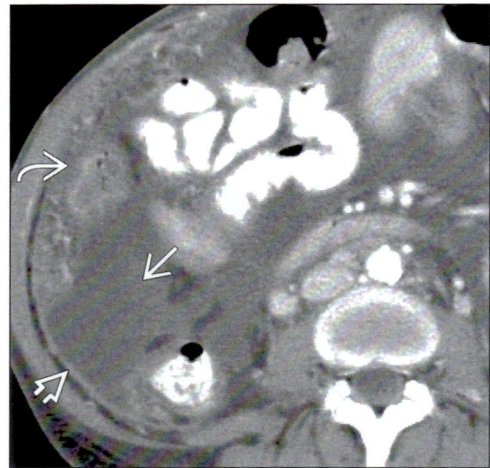

Axial CECT of TB peritonitis. Note large amount of ascites ➡, thickening of parietal peritoneum ➡, and nodular infiltration of omentum ➡.

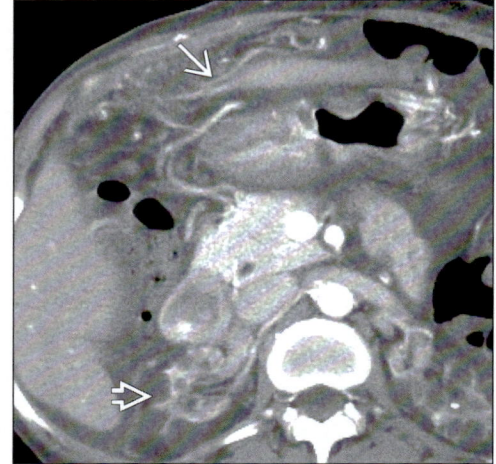

Axial CECT (of same patient as previous image) at more cranial level demonstrates increased vascularity of omentum ➡ and cystic disease of dialysis ➡.

TERMINOLOGY

Definitions
- Infectious or inflammatory process involving peritoneum or peritoneal cavity

IMAGING FINDINGS

General Features
- Best diagnostic clue: Ascites, symmetric enhancement of peritoneum with fat stranding of abdominal fat
- Location: Peritoneal surface, mesentery, omentum
- Size: Variable, may be focal or diffuse
- Morphology: Symmetric thickening of peritoneum

Radiographic Findings
- Radiography
  - Evidence of ascites: More than 500 mL of fluid required for plain film diagnosis
    - Bulging of flanks
    - Indistinct psoas margin
    - Small bowel loops floating centrally
    - Lateral edge of liver displaced medially (Hellmer sign); visible in 80% of patients with significant ascites
    - Pelvic "dog's ear"; present in 90% of patients with significant ascites
    - Medial displacement of cecum and ascending colon; present in 90% of patients with significant ascites
  - +/- Free air
  - Hydropneumoperitoneum
  - Air in lesser sac with perforated gastric ulcer

Fluoroscopic Findings
- Upper GI: Perforated ulcer with contrast leak
- Contrast Enema: Perforation of diverticulum in diverticulitis

CT Findings
- CECT
  - Ascites, enhancing peritoneum with smooth thickening, infiltration & soft tissue stranding of fat within mesentery on CECT
  - +/- Gas bubbles, low attenuation nodes in TB peritonitis on CECT

DDx: Spectrum of Intraperitoneal Fluid

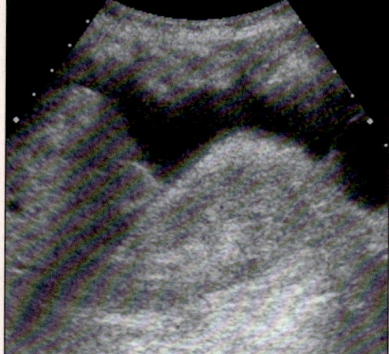

Carcinomatosis

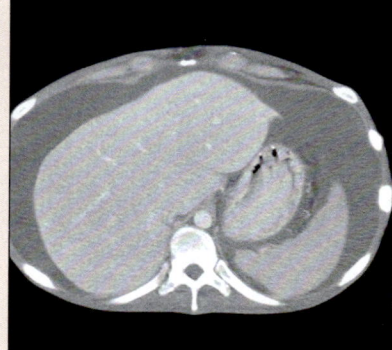

Ascites

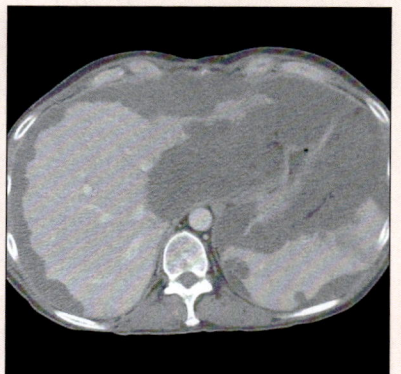

Pseudomyxoma

PERITONITIS

Key Facts

Terminology
- Infectious or inflammatory process involving peritoneum or peritoneal cavity

Imaging Findings
- Best diagnostic clue: Ascites, symmetric enhancement of peritoneum with fat stranding of abdominal fat
- Ascites, enhancing peritoneum with smooth thickening, infiltration & soft tissue stranding of fat within mesentery on CECT
- +/- Gas bubbles, low attenuation nodes in TB peritonitis on CECT
- Peritoneal fluid, septations, thickened echogenic mesentery on grayscale US
- Best imaging tool: CECT

Top Differential Diagnoses
- Peritoneal Carcinomatosis
- Benign Ascites
- Pseudomyxoma Peritonei
- Hemoperitoneum

Pathology
- General path comments: Pus in peritoneal cavity, thickened peritoneum or mesentery

Clinical Issues
- Most common signs/symptoms: Fever, abdominal pain, distension

Diagnostic Checklist
- Peritoneal carcinomatosis
- Symmetric enhancement of thickened peritoneum

MR Findings
- T1WI: Low signal peritoneal fluid
- T2WI: High signal peritoneal fluid
- T1 C+
  - Thickened enhancing peritoneum
  - Low signal peritoneal fluid

Ultrasonographic Findings
- Grayscale Ultrasound
  - Peritoneal fluid, septations, thickened echogenic mesentery on grayscale US
  - Dilated fallopian tube & fluid-debris level (pyosalpinx) in pelvic inflammatory disease (PID)
  - Complex adnexal cystic masses in PID
    - Tubo-ovarian abscesses (TOA)
- Color Doppler
  - Hyperemic thickened echogenic fat
    - Associated with gastrointestinal source of inflammation

Imaging Recommendations
- Best imaging tool: CECT
- Protocol advice
  - Oral and IV contrast (150 mL injected at 2.5 mL/sec)
  - Rectal contrast to distinguish colon from pelvic infection
  - 5 mm collimation, 5 mm reconstruction interval

DIFFERENTIAL DIAGNOSIS

Peritoneal Carcinomatosis
- Nodular implants on peritoneum
- Omental caking
- Ascites
- Mesenteric nodules and adenopathy

Benign Ascites
- Cirrhosis
- Bile leak
  - Due to trauma, surgery, liver biopsy, biliary drainage
- Pancreatic ascites
  - Due to pancreatic duct leakage
- Chylous ascites
- Urine ascites
  - Due to bladder perforation
- Congestive heart failure (CHF), fluid overload

Pseudomyxoma Peritonei
- Massive accumulation of gelatinous ascites in peritoneal cavity
- Scalloping of liver and spleen contour
- Rupture of mucinous tumor of appendix
- Calcified cystic implants
- Cystic masses attached to ligaments such as falciform or gastrohepatic ligament

Hemoperitoneum
- High attenuation intraperitoneal fluid
- Free lysed blood measuring 30-45 HU
- Clotted blood measuring 60 HU
- Active arterial extravasation isodense with adjacent major arterial structures, large surrounding hematoma

PATHOLOGY

General Features
- General path comments: Pus in peritoneal cavity, thickened peritoneum or mesentery
- Etiology
  - Spontaneous
    - Secondary bacterial infection of chronic ascites
  - Bacterial
    - Bowel perforation
    - PID
    - Infected intrauterine device (IUD)
    - Ruptured tubo-ovarian abscess
    - Gastric or duodenal ulcer
    - Ruptured appendicitis
    - Ruptured diverticulitis
  - TB: Ingestion of tuberculous sputum
  - Traumatic
    - Duodenum, jejunum, distal ileum most common sites

PERITONITIS

- Small bowel injury may present 4-6 weeks post-trauma
- Bowel injury from deceleration injury
- Colonic injuries rare, but have rapid clinical onset of peritonitis
  ○ Iatrogenic
    - Inadvertent bowel perforation during laparotomy or diagnostic/therapeutic paracentesis
    - Post-operative anastomotic leak
    - Retained foreign body during surgery
    - Dropped gallstones during laparoscopic cholecystectomy
- Epidemiology
  ○ Increased incidence in patients with chronic ascites
    - Cirrhosis
    - Peritoneal dialysis
  ○ Younger patients have higher incidence of pneumococcal or hemolytic streptococcal infection
  ○ Increased incidence in patients with risk factors for PID
    - IUD
    - Multiple sexual partners

Gross Pathologic & Surgical Features
- Pus in peritoneal cavity
- Inflammatory changes in mesentery
- Inflammatory adhesions
- Hyperemia of adherent omentum or mesentery

Microscopic Features
- > 500 leukocytes per mm^3 indicates infected ascites

Staging, Grading or Classification Criteria
- Localized: Walled off infection
- Diffuse: Multiple peritoneal compartments involved

CLINICAL ISSUES

Presentation
- Most common signs/symptoms: Fever, abdominal pain, distension

Demographics
- Age: Any
- Gender: No predilection for male or female

Natural History & Prognosis
- Sepsis if not treated promptly
- Prognosis determined by primary etiology
  ○ Excellent if localized and no evidence of septicemia
  ○ Poor if generalized peritonitis and gram-negative septicemia

Treatment
- Options, risks, complications
  ○ Etiology of peritonitis determines treatment
  ○ Correct underlying cause (i.e., perforated ulcer)
  ○ Antibiotic therapy
    - Early PID
    - Soft tissue inflammation (phlegmon) from appendicitis or diverticulitis
  ○ Surgery for failed antibiotic therapy
  ○ Surgery for perforated viscus
    - Appendicitis

- Duodenal ulcer
- Diverticulitis

DIAGNOSTIC CHECKLIST

Consider
- Peritoneal carcinomatosis
- Causes of water-attenuation ascitic fluid
  ○ Transudate (e.g., cirrhosis)
  ○ Urine
  ○ Chyle
  ○ Bile
  ○ Pancreatic juice

Image Interpretation Pearls
- Symmetric enhancement of thickened peritoneum
- Inflammatory changes with adjacent fat of mesentery and omentum
- Enlarged fallopian tube with fluid-fluid level & complex adnexal mass in PID

SELECTED REFERENCES

1. Alberti LE et al: Spontaneous bacterial peritonitis in a patient with myxedema ascites. Digestion. 68(2-3):91-3, 2003
2. Brook I: Microbiology and management of intra-abdominal infections in children. Pediatr Int. 45(2):123-9, 2003
3. Cheadle WG et al: The continuing challenge of intra-abdominal infection. Am J Surg. 186(5A):15S-22S; discussion 31S-34S, 2003
4. Chow KM et al: Indication for peritoneal biopsy in tuberculous peritonitis. Am J Surg. 185(6):567-73, 2003
5. Hanbidge AE et al: US of the peritoneum. Radiographics. 23(3):663-84; discussion 684-5, 2003
6. Malangoni MA: Current concepts in peritonitis. Curr Gastroenterol Rep. 5(4):295-301, 2003
7. Marshall JC et al: Intensive care unit management of intra-abdominal infection. Crit Care Med. 31(8):2228-37, 2003
8. Nishie A et al: Fitz-Hugh-Curtis syndrome. Radiologic manifestation. J Comput Assist Tomogr. 27(5):786-91, 2003
9. Reijnen MM et al: Pathophysiology of intra-abdominal adhesion and abscess formation, and the effect of hyaluronan. Br J Surg. 90(5):533-41, 2003
10. Runyon BA: Strips and tubes: improving the diagnosis of spontaneous bacterial peritonitis. Hepatology. 37(4):745-7, 2003
11. Sabri M et al: Pathophysiology and management of pediatric ascites. Curr Gastroenterol Rep. 5(3):240-6, 2003
12. Shetty H et al: Treatment of infections in peritoneal dialysis. Contrib Nephrol. (140):187-94, 2003
13. Sivit CJ et al: Imaging of acute appendicitis in children. Semin Ultrasound CT MR. 24(2):74-82, 2003
14. Troidle L et al: Continuous peritoneal dialysis-associated peritonitis: a review and current concepts. Semin Dial. 16(6):428-37, 2003
15. Veroux M et al: A rare surgical complication of Crohn's diseases: free peritoneal perforation. Minerva Chir. 58(3):351-4, 2003
16. Witte MB et al: Repair of full-thickness bowel injury. Crit Care Med. 31(8 Suppl):S538-46, 2003
17. Yao V et al: Role of peritoneal mesothelial cells in peritonitis. Br J Surg. 90(10):1187-94, 2003

PERITONITIS

IMAGE GALLERY

Typical

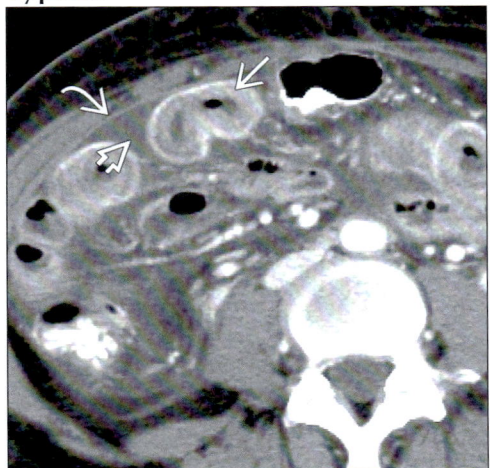
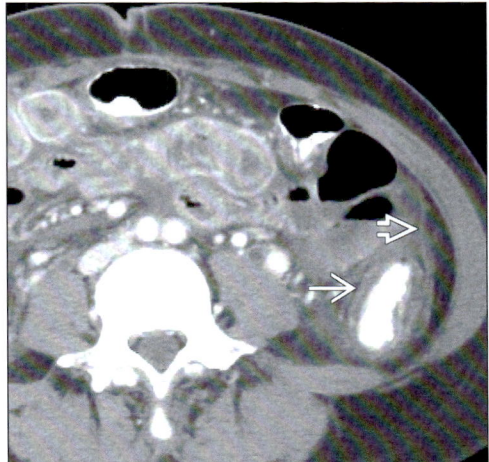

(Left) Axial CECT of acute enteritis & peritonitis from lupus erythematosus: Marked small bowel thickening/prominent submucosal edema ➡, ascites ➡, peritoneal enhancement ➡. *(Right)* Axial CECT at lower level (of same patient as previous image) demonstrates thickening of descending colon ➡ and peritoneal enhancement ➡.

Typical

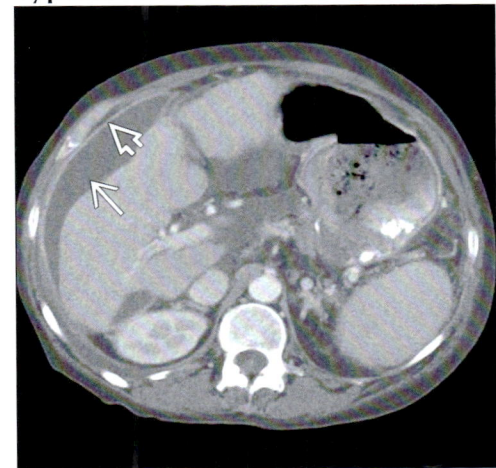
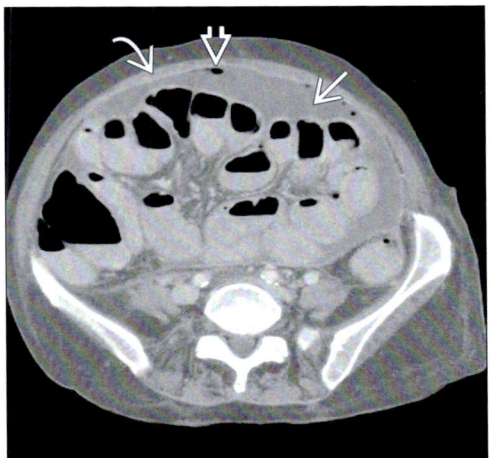

(Left) Axial CECT shows bacterial peritonitis in patient with cirrhosis. Note loculated ascites ➡, thickened & enhancing parietal peritoneum ➡. *(Right)* Axial CECT (in same patient as previous image) shows loculated ascites ➡ and thickened parietal peritoneum ➡. Gas bubble ➡ is also evident within the fluid.

Variant

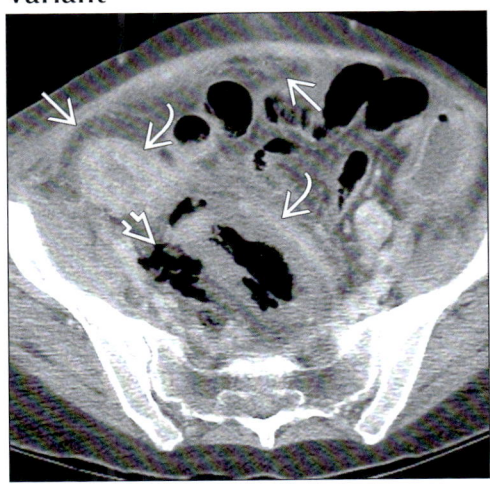
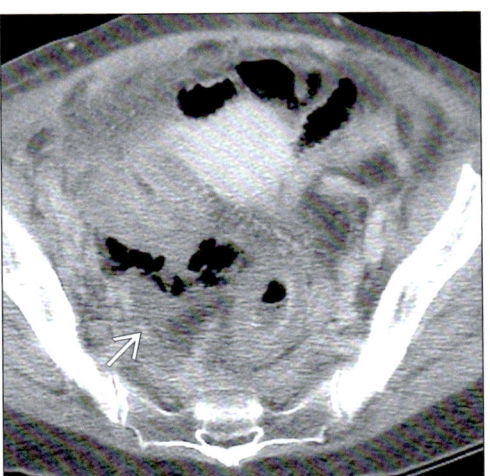

(Left) Axial CECT shows pelvic peritonitis from colonic perforation (pseudomembranous colitis). Diffuse infiltration of soft tissue planes ➡, ectopic gas ➡ adjacent to thickened sigmoid colon ➡. *(Right)* Axial CECT (of same patient as previous image) at more caudal level demonstrates only small amount of free fluid ➡. Diffuse pelvic peritonitis found at surgery.

INGUINAL HERNIA

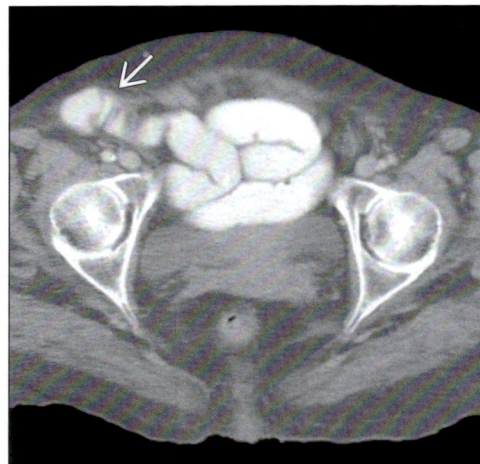

Axial CECT shows hernia sac ➡ lying anterior to right femoral vessels. Contrast-opacified small bowel is present within the hernia, but no sign of bowel obstruction.

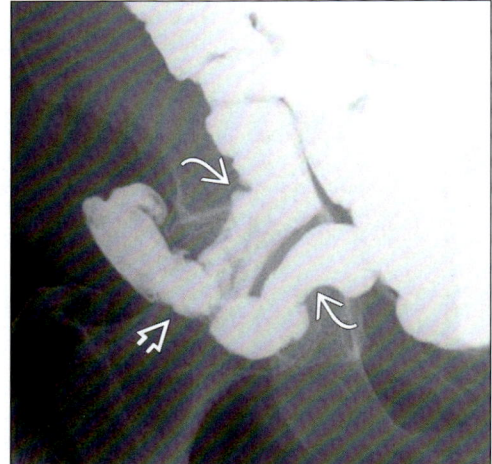

Small bowel follow through shows herniated small bowel ➡. Note constriction of bowel ➡ as it passes through the inguinal ring.

TERMINOLOGY

Abbreviations and Synonyms
- Inguinal hernia (IH)
- Pelvic & groin hernia

Definitions
- External: Abnormal protrusion of intra-abdominal tissue through defect in abdominal or pelvic wall, extending outside abdominal cavity
- Internal (IH): Inguinal location of hernia orifice

IMAGING FINDINGS

General Features
- Location
  - Indirect IH: Passes through internal inguinal ring, down the inguinal canal, emerges at external ring
    - Can extend along spermatic cord into scrotum; complete hernia
    - In females, hernia follows course of round ligament of uterus into labium majus
    - Passes lateral to epigastric vessels (lateral umbilical fold), also known as lateral IH
    - Juxtafunicular: Indirect hernia passes outside spermatic cord
  - Direct IH: Occurs in floor of inguinal canal, through Hesselbach triangle
    - Protrudes medial to inferior epigastric vessels (IEV)
    - Not contained in spermatic cord, generally does not pass into scrotum
    - Medial umbilical fold divides Hesselbach triangle into medial & lateral parts
    - Medial & lateral direct IH
- Morphology
  - Indirect IH within spermatic cord has smooth contour & elongated oblique course
    - Juxtafunicular hernia: More irregular contour; no protrusion into preformed sac
    - Dissect through subcutaneous fat & fibrous tissue
  - Direct IH: Broad, dome-shaped; appears as small bulge in groin; short blunt aperture

Radiographic Findings
- Radiography

DDx: Mass Near Inguinal Ligament

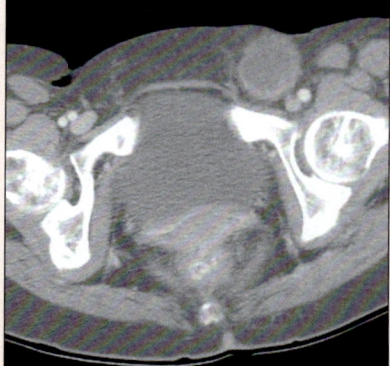

Femoral Hernia

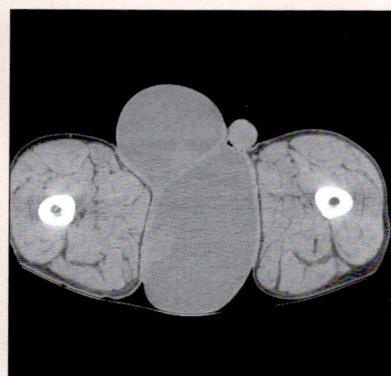

Hydrocele

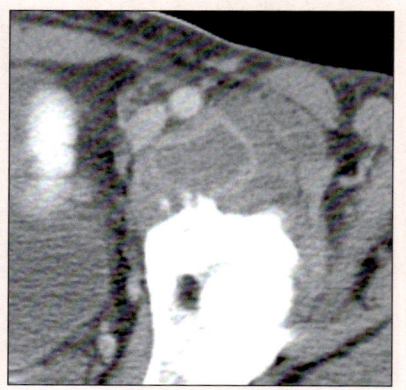

Groin Abscess

INGUINAL HERNIA

Key Facts

Imaging Findings
- Indirect IH: Passes through internal inguinal ring, down the inguinal canal, emerges at external ring
- Direct IH: Occurs in floor of inguinal canal, through Hesselbach triangle
- Indirect IH within spermatic cord has smooth contour & elongated oblique course
- Direct IH: Broad, dome-shaped; appears as small bulge in groin; short blunt aperture
- Indirect IH: May see well-defined ovoid mass in groin
- Collapsed bowel loops & mesenteric fat in hernia sac
- Neck of indirect IH can be demonstrated at deep inguinal ring lateral to IEV
- Direct IH remains medial to IEV throughout

Top Differential Diagnoses
- Femoral Hernia
- Iatrogenic Hematoma
- Lymphadenopathy

Pathology
- 75-80% of all hernias occur in inguinal region
- Indirect 5x more common than direct
- Contents include small bowel loops or mobile colon segments (sigmoid, cecum, appendix)

Clinical Issues
- Diagnosis: History & physical examination
- Indirect IH five to ten times more common in men
- Complications: Incarceration, strangulation

Diagnostic Checklist
- Indirect hernias protrude from lateral inguinal fossa
- Direct hernias are from medial & supravesical fossae

  - Supine abdomen films can indicate incarceration or strangulation
    - Convergence of distended intestinal loops toward inguinal region
    - Soft tissue density or gas-containing mass overlying obturator foramen on affected side
  - Barium examination of small or large bowel
    - Tapered narrowing or obstruction of intestinal segments as it enters hernia orifice
  - Attempt to reduce hernia manually under fluoro
  - Visualize afferent & efferent loops of protruding intestine
- Herniography: Indirect IH; emerges from lateral inguinal fossa, protrudes medially
  - Roughly parallel to superior pubic ramus
  - Persistent processus vaginalis has width of 1-2 mm; may extend into scrotum
    - Communicating hydrocele
  - If length of sac exceeds 4 cm, usually widens abruptly beyond external opening of inguinal canal
  - Widened internal opening of inguinal canal seen as triangular outpouching of lateral inguinal fossa
    - Acute apex directed inferomedially, medial border is concave
  - No plicae or indentations visualized lateral to indirect hernia
  - Open Nuck canal in women; same appearance as patent processus vaginalis in men
- More lateral direct hernia, protruding from medial inguinal fossa; usually dome-shaped with wide neck
- More medially located direct IH; protrudes from supravesical fossa; usually smaller

CT Findings
- Indirect IH: May see well-defined ovoid mass in groin
  - Collapsed bowel loops & mesenteric fat in hernia sac
- Neck of indirect IH can be demonstrated at deep inguinal ring lateral to IEV
  - Direct IH remains medial to IEV throughout
- CT useful if suspicion of another disease process mimicking/precipitating hernia

MR Findings
- Dynamic evaluation in multiple imaging planes may have advantages

Ultrasonographic Findings
- Grayscale Ultrasound
  - Bowel loops may peristalse within hernia
  - Useful when patient presents non-urgently with history suggesting reducible hernia
    - US real-time examination allows patient to stand upright & perform Valsalva maneuver
  - Valsalva maneuver: In direct hernia, distended pampiniform plexus displaced by hernia sac
    - Impaired swelling of pampiniform plexus seen in indirect hernia
- Color Doppler
  - Distinguish among types of groin hernias
    - Demonstrate inferior epigastric artery (origin &/or trunk segment) & relationship with hernia sac

Imaging Recommendations
- Best imaging tool: US; MR for demonstrating acutely strangulated hernia in obese patients
- Protocol advice
  - CT: Oral + IV CECT; axial plane; 5 mm collimation
    - Frequent image reconstructions to show IEV

DIFFERENTIAL DIAGNOSIS

Femoral Hernia
- Medial position within femoral canal posterior to line of inguinal ligament; caudal & posterior to IH
- Frequently has a narrow neck; neck remains below inguinal ligament & lateral to pubic tubercle
- More common in women

Iatrogenic Hematoma
- Arterial puncture following arteriography, needle biopsy or aspiration
  - Hematoma may extend into rectus muscle or lateral abdominal wall muscles

INGUINAL HERNIA

- Blood can track directly from groin along transversalis fascia & transversus abdominis muscle
- CT, US, MR: Appearance of blood; extent of lesion; changes over time
- Pseudoaneurysm: Perivascular, rounded mass; neck + track connecting it with injured artery

Lymphadenopathy
- Appears as mass near inguinal ligament
- CT, US help differentiate hernia contents from other groin & scrotal masses
  - Hydrocele, varix, lipoma of spermatic cord, undescended testicle, abscess, tumor

PATHOLOGY

General Features
- Etiology
  - Indirect IH considered to be congenital defect
    - Patency of processus vaginalis; weakness of crus lateralis at lateral aspect of inguinal canal
  - Direct IH considered acquired lesion
    - Weakness in transversalis fascia of posterior wall of inguinal canal in Hesselbach triangle
- Epidemiology
  - 75-80% of all hernias occur in inguinal region
  - Indirect 5x more common than direct
  - Incidence: IH occurs in 1-3% of all children
    - One-half to 2x greater in premature infants
  - Approximately 5% of men develop IH requiring surgery
  - Bilateral patent processus vaginalis occurs in up to 10% of patients with indirect IH

Gross Pathologic & Surgical Features
- Contents include small bowel loops or mobile colon segments (sigmoid, cecum, appendix)
- Sliding IH: Partially retroperitoneal organs
  - Urinary bladder, distal ureters, ascending or descending colon included in herniation
  - Retroperitoneal structures constitute wall of sac
  - Blood vessels supplying herniated segments, may be injured during surgical repair or trauma
- Littre hernia: Meckel diverticulum in hernia sac
- Richter hernia: Only portion of bowel circumference in sac (antimesenteric)
- Incomplete IH: Sac not extended through external inguinal ring
- Diverticular direct IH: Protrudes from either medial inguinal or supravesical fossa
  - Small opening in otherwise normal transverse fascia
  - Distinct circumscribed neck, usually protrudes more in anterior than inferior direction
- Potential indirect hernias associated with undescended testis or testis in inguinal canal
  - Testicular or spermatic cord hydrocele

CLINICAL ISSUES

Presentation
- Asymptomatic; sudden appearance of lump in groin; intermittently present; ± groin pain; palpable bulge
- Physical exam: Recumbent & upright position; may be reducible; bowel sounds audible; ± tender
  - Indirect hernia lightly touches tip of finger
    - Examining finger placed along spermatic cord at scrotum & passed into external ring along canal
    - During maneuvers that ↑ intra-abdominal pressure
  - Direct hernia causes bulge forward low in canal
- Incarcerated or strangulated hernia: Bowel distension; painful, often tense swelling in groin or scrotum
- Diagnosis: History & physical examination

Demographics
- Age
  - Indirect IH may occur from infancy to old age, generally occur by fifth decade
  - Direct IH increases in occurrence with age
- Gender
  - Indirect IH five to ten times more common in men
  - Direct IH occurs mostly in men

Natural History & Prognosis
- Pediatric IH: Almost always indirect; ↑ risk of incarceration
  - Usually on right (60-75%); often bilateral (10-15%)
- Recurrent hernia: Groin hernias recur after herniorrhaphy in up to 20% of patients
  - Direct IH may develop after repair of indirect hernia
  - Diverticular hernias are a form of recurrence
- Multiple hernias: One is usually direct
  - May obscure smaller clinically significant hernias
- Saddlebag, pantaloon, combined IH: Simultaneous occurrence of direct & indirect IH in same groin
  - Separation of two adjacent hernia sacs by IEV creates bilocular appearance
- Indirect IH accounts for 15% of intestinal obstructions
- Diverticulitis, appendicitis, primary or metastatic tumor may occur within hernia sac
- Complications: Incarceration, strangulation
  - Direct IH rarely becomes incarcerated, less often associated with strangulation

Treatment
- Laparoscopic or open hernia repair

DIAGNOSTIC CHECKLIST

Consider
- Indirect hernias protrude from lateral inguinal fossa
- Direct hernias are from medial & supravesical fossae

SELECTED REFERENCES

1. van den Berg JC: Inguinal hernias: MRI and ultrasound. Semin Ultrasound CT MR. 23(2): 156-73, 2002
2. Shadbolt CL et al: Imaging of groin masses: inguinal anatomy and pathologic conditions revisited. Radiographics. 21 Spec No: S261-71, 2001
3. Zhang GQ et al: Groin hernias in adults: value of color Doppler sonography in their classification. J Clin Ultrasound. 29(8): 429-34, 2001
4. Toms AP et al: Illustrated review of new imaging techniques in the diagnosis of abdominal wall hernias. Br J Surg. 86(10): 1243-9, 1999

INGUINAL HERNIA

IMAGE GALLERY

Typical

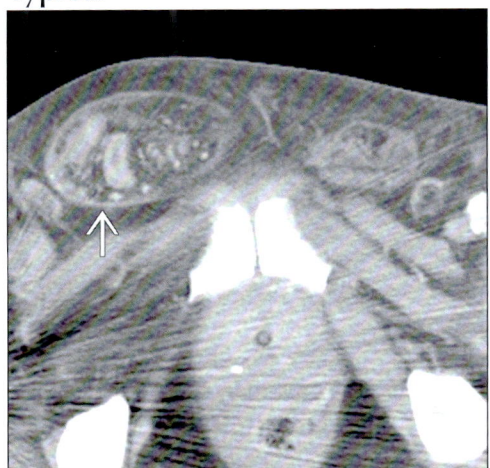
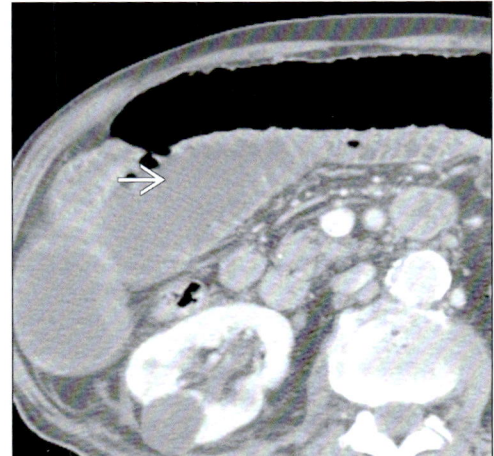

(Left) Axial CECT shows inguinal hernia causing small bowel obstruction. Note entrapped and thickened small bowel in right inguinal hernia sac ➔. *(Right)* Axial CECT at higher level (in same patient as previous image) demonstrates dilated small bowel ➔ from obstruction.

Variant

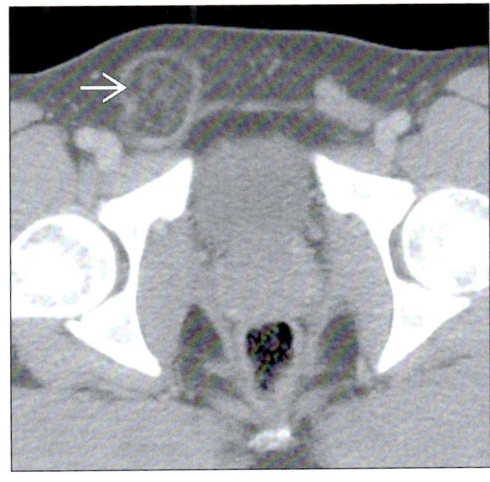
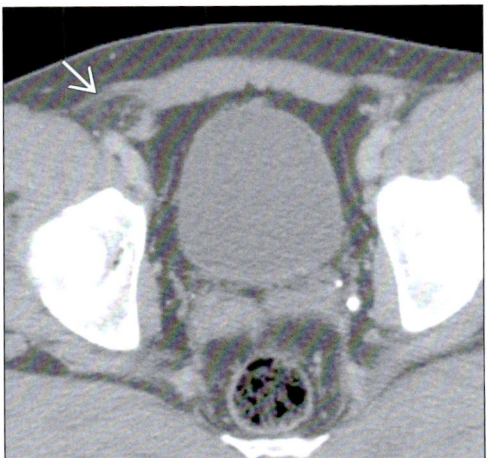

(Left) Axial CECT of right inguinal hernia ➔ containing herniated fat. The fat is somewhat "dirty", or infiltrated, in appearance, suggesting incarceration or ischemia of herniated fat. *(Right)* Axial CECT at higher level (in same patient as previous image) demonstrates abdominal wall defect ➔.

Variant

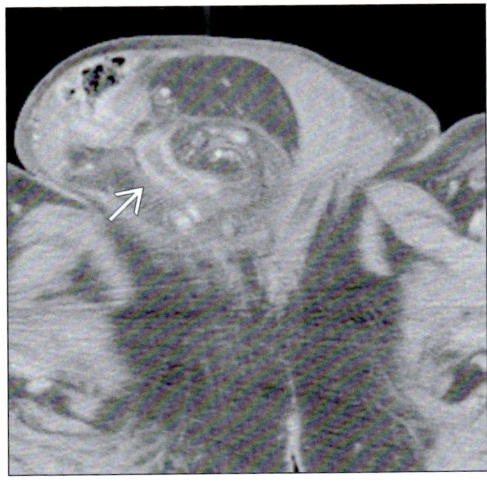
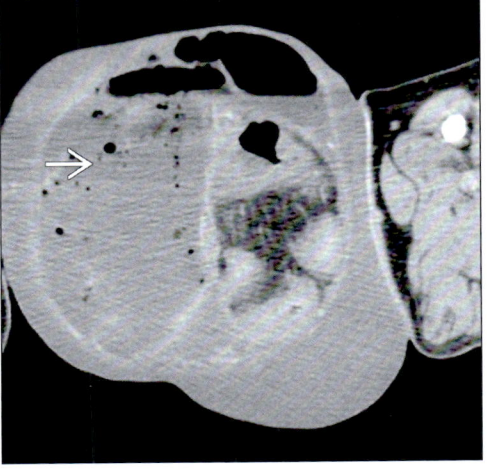

(Left) CECT shows incarcerated small bowel with perforation within inguinal hernia sac. Note thickened small bowel within large hernia sac ➔. *(Right)* CECT at lower level (in same patient as previous image) demonstrates ectopic gas and fluid from perforated small bowel within hernia sac ➔.

FEMORAL HERNIA

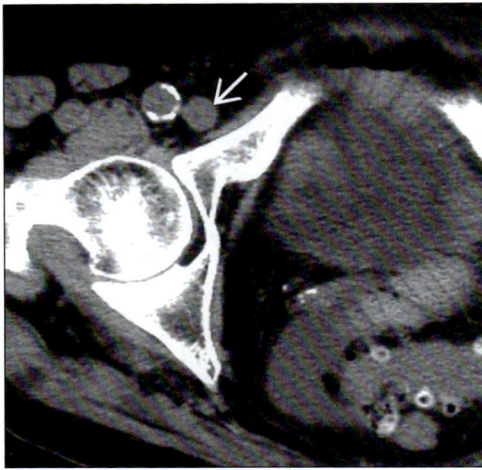

Axial CECT shows femoral hernia with small bowel obstruction. Note loop of bowel entrapped in right femoral canal ➡.

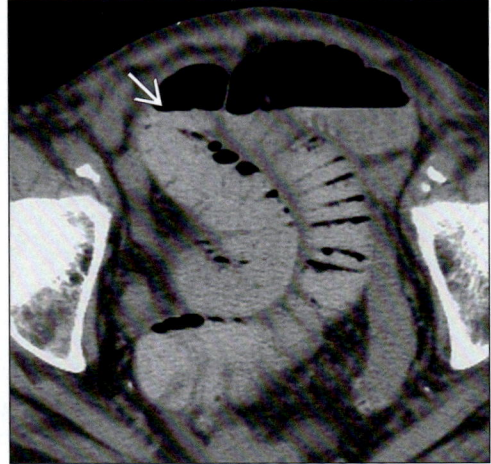

Axial CECT at higher level, in same patient as previous image, reveals a small bowel obstruction ➡.

TERMINOLOGY

Abbreviations and Synonyms
- Femoral hernia (FH)
- Crural hernia; enteromerocele; femorocele

Definitions
- Intra-abdominal contents protruding along femoral sheath in femoral canal medial to femoral vein

IMAGING FINDINGS

General Features
- Best diagnostic clue: History and clinical examination
- Location
  - Protrusion of hernial contents
    - Posteriorly to inguinal ligament
    - Anteriorly to pubic ramus periosteum (Cooper ligament)
    - Medially to femoral vessels
  - FH traverses femoral canal and presents as mass at level of foramen ovale
  - Neck of FH always remains below inguinal ligament & lateral to pubic tubercle
  - Inguinal ligament is not visible on CT as a discrete structure
  - Horizontal plane connecting pubic tubercle defines plane of inguinal ligament
  - Femoral hernia often is recognized posterior to plane of pubic tubercle
- Morphology
  - Protrudes at right angle to inguinal canal
  - Narrow neck and characteristic pear shape

Radiographic Findings
- Herniography: Characteristic posterior "inbulging" due to proximity of symphysis pubis to posterior and medial aspects of hernia

CT Findings
- Omental fat or bowel herniating into femoral canal medial to femoral vein
- Hernia sac lies posterior to horizontal plane of pubic tubercle

DDx: Masses Near Femoral Artery

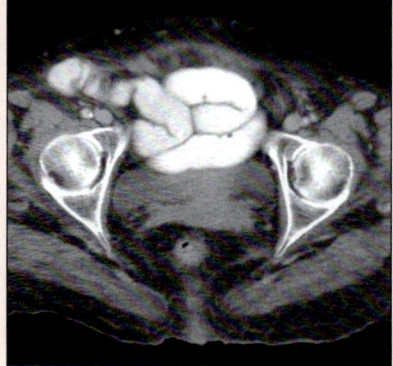

Inguinal Hernia

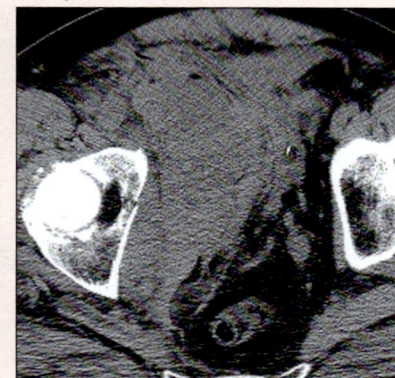

Pelvic Hematoma

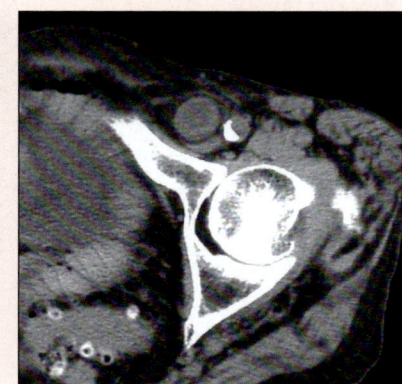

Inguinal Node

FEMORAL HERNIA

Key Facts

Terminology
- Intra-abdominal contents protruding along femoral sheath in femoral canal medial to femoral vein

Imaging Findings
- FH traverses femoral canal and presents as mass at level of foramen ovale
- Neck of FH always remains below inguinal ligament & lateral to pubic tubercle
- Narrow neck and characteristic pear shape
- Best imaging tool: CECT

Top Differential Diagnoses
- Inguinal Hernia
- Iatrogenic Hematoma
- Lymphadenopathy
- Obturator Hernia

Pathology
- May be congenital defect in insertion of transversalis fascia to ileopubic tract

Clinical Issues
- Swelling, with or without pain
- Dragging sensation in groin
- Lump usually felt in top of thigh, below groin crease
- Often difficult to diagnose clinically, especially in obese patients
- Gender: Predominantly women (M:F = 1:3)

Diagnostic Checklist
- Incarcerated hernia if bowel loops are thickened within femoral hernia sac
- Femoral hernia lies posterior to plane of pubic tubercle, medial to femoral vein

Ultrasonographic Findings
- Color Doppler useful to identify hernia sac extending medial to femoral vein
- Identification of inferior epigastric artery aids in determining type of femoral hernia
  - Direct (medial)
  - Indirect (lateral)

Imaging Recommendations
- Best imaging tool: CECT
- Protocol advice
  - MDCT with 150 mL non-ionic contrast 2.5-3 mL/sec with 70 sec scan delay
  - Scan at 5 mm thickness with 1.25 mm collimation, reconstruction interval 1.25-2.5 mm multiplanar reconstruction

DIFFERENTIAL DIAGNOSIS

Inguinal Hernia
- FH differentiated from inguinal hernia by its medial position within femoral canal
  - Posterior to line of inguinal ligament defined by plane of pubic tubercle on CT
- Arises from medial inguinal fossa but protrudes in anterior direction
- Indirect inguinal hernias more prone to bowel obstruction than direct hernias

Iatrogenic Hematoma
- Hematoma following arterial puncture in femoral sheath during arteriography, needle biopsy, etc.
- Appearance of blood and lesion on CT and US
- High attenuation on NECT
- Active arterial extravasation seen on CECT
  - High attenuation focus isodense with major adjacent arteries
  - Active pelvic bleeding may be treated with embolization

Lymphadenopathy
- Common location for enlarged reactive nodes
- Enlarged nodes due to lymphoma or metastatic carcinoma
- Enlarged inguinal nodes, pelvic lymphocele

Obturator Hernia
- Hernia into superior-lateral aspect of obturator canal
- Typically seen in elderly women (80-90%)
- More common on right
- Ileum most often in hernia sac
- Most present with acute symptoms of incarcerated hernia

PATHOLOGY

General Features
- Etiology
  - May be congenital defect in insertion of transversalis fascia to ileopubic tract
    - Forms superior & anterior limit of lacuna vasorum
    - Femoral canal dilates if weakened, resulting in formation of FH
  - Associated with ↑ intra-abdominal pressure
- Epidemiology
  - Approximately 5-10% of groin hernias in adults
  - Approximately one third of groin hernias in women
  - Less than 1% of all groin hernias in children

Gross Pathologic & Surgical Features
- Hernia contents
  - Properitoneal fat
  - Edge of omentum
  - Loop of small bowel
- Richter hernia: Usually in older women with FH
  - Defined as hernia with only one wall of bowel loop within hernia sac

CLINICAL ISSUES

Presentation
- Most common signs/symptoms
  - Swelling, with or without pain

FEMORAL HERNIA

- Dragging sensation in groin
- Lump usually felt in top of thigh, below groin crease
  - Large FH may bulge over inguinal ligament
- Palpable neck lateral and inferior to pubic tubercle
- Other signs/symptoms
  - Nausea, vomiting, severe abdominal pain may occur with strangulated hernia
  - Often difficult to diagnose clinically, especially in obese patients
    - Deep location of femoral canal
    - Abundance of adipose tissue
    - Relatively small size of hernia

Demographics
- Age
  - 36% occur in patients > 80
  - 16% occur in the 7th decade
  - Children are rarely affected
- Gender: Predominantly women (M:F = 1:3)

Natural History & Prognosis
- May displace or narrow femoral vein
- May descend along saphenous vein
- Complications: Incarceration and or strangulation
  - Incarceration: 25-40% are due to narrow neck
  - 8-12x more prone to incarceration and strangulation than inguinal hernia
    - Firm and unyielding margins of femoral ring
  - Rarely may have inflamed appendix in hernia sac
- Morbidity
  - Related to intestinal obstruction
  - Incarceration occurs in 5-20% of femoral hernias
    - Highest rate of incarceration of all groin hernias
- Mortality
  - 1% in 70-79 age group
  - 5% in 80-90 age group
  - Associated with intestinal obstruction

Treatment
- Closure of femoral sheath defect
  - Apposing Cooper ligament and posterior reflection of inguinal ligament
  - Mini-incision, "tension-free" technique, utilizing mesh
  - Floor of inguinal canal is often reinforced using transversalis fascia
  - Laparoscopic approach gaining favor
    - Faster convalescence
    - Mesh plug repair with laparoscopic approach

DIAGNOSTIC CHECKLIST

Consider
- Incarcerated hernia if bowel loops are thickened within femoral hernia sac

Image Interpretation Pearls
- Femoral hernia lies posterior to plane of pubic tubercle, medial to femoral vein

SELECTED REFERENCES

1. Akopian G et al: De Garengeot hernia: appendicitis within a femoral hernia. Am Surg. 71(6):526-7, 2005
2. Bringman S et al: Intestinal obstruction after inguinal and femoral hernia repair: a study of 33,275 operations during 1992-2000 in Sweden. Hernia. 9(2):178-83, 2005
3. Holzheimer RG: Inguinal Hernia: classification, diagnosis and treatment--classic, traumatic and Sportsman's hernia. Eur J Med Res. 10(3):121-34, 2005
4. Ikossi DG et al: Laparoscopic femoral hernia repair using umbilical ligament as plug. J Laparoendosc Adv Surg Tech A. 15(2):197-200, 2005
5. Alvarez JA et al: Incarcerated groin hernias in adults: presentation and outcome. Hernia. 8(2):121-6, 2004
6. Malek S et al: Emergency repair of groin herniae: outcome and implications for elective surgery waiting times. Int J Clin Pract. 58(2):207-9, 2004
7. Hachisuka T: Femoral hernia repair. Surg Clin North Am. 83(5):1189-205, 2003
8. Swarnkar K et al: Sutureless mesh-plug femoral hernioplasty. Am J Surg. 186(2):201-2, 2003
9. Zollinger RM Jr: Classification systems for groin hernias. Surg Clin North Am. 83(5):1053-63, 2003
10. Lau WY: History of treatment of groin hernia. World J Surg. 26(6):748-59, 2002
11. Dieudonne G: Plug repair of groin hernias: a 10-year experience. Hernia. 5(4):189-91, 2001
12. Zhang GQ et al: Groin hernias in adults: value of color Doppler sonography in their classification. J Clin Ultrasound. 29(8):429-34, 2001
13. Ianora AA et al: Abdominal wall hernias: imaging with spiral CT. Eur Radiol. 10(6):914-9, 2000
14. Zissin R et al: CT diagnosis of acute appendicitis in a femoral hernia. Br J Radiol. 73(873):1013-4, 2000
15. Toms AP et al: Illustrated review of new imaging techniques in the diagnosis of abdominal wall hernias. Br J Surg. 86(10): 1243-9, 1999
16. Loftus WK et al: Case report: Femoral hernia causing small bowel obstruction--ultrasound diagnosis. Clin Radiol. 53(8):618-9, 1998
17. Radcliffe G et al: Reappraisal of femoral hernia in children. Br J Surg. 84(1): 58-60, 1997
18. Harrison LA et al: Abdominal wall hernias: review of herniography and correlation with cross-sectional imaging. Radiographics. 15(2):315-32, 1995
19. Chamary VL: Femoral hernia: intestinal obstruction is an unrecognized source of morbidity and mortality. Br J Surg. 80(2): 230-2, 1993
20. Lewin JR: Femoral hernia with upward extension into abdominal wall: CT diagnosis. AJR Am J Roentgenol. 136(1):206-7, 1981

FEMORAL HERNIA

IMAGE GALLERY

Typical

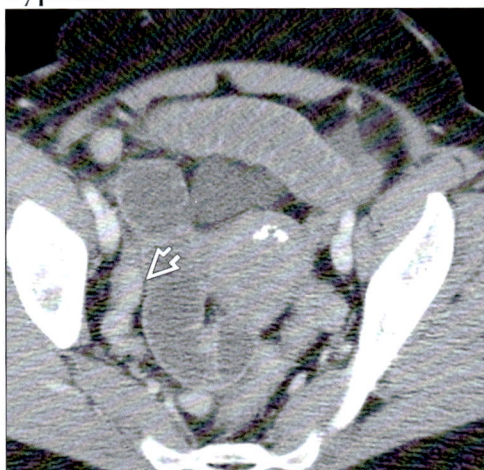
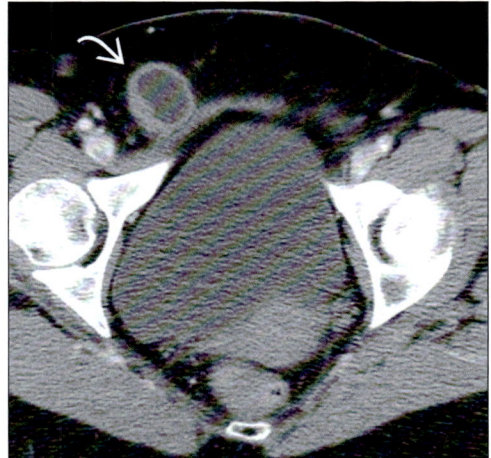

(Left) Axial CECT shows incarcerated femoral hernia in femoral canal. Note decompressed distal small bowel, suggesting small bowel obstruction ➡. *(Right)* Axial CECT (in same patient as previous image) at a lower level identifies the source of obstruction, small bowel trapped in the femoral canal ➡.

Typical

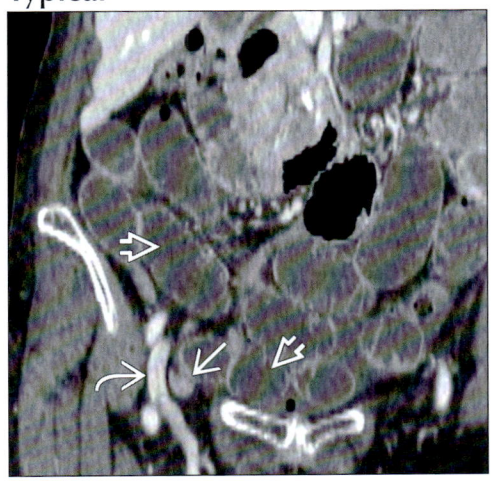
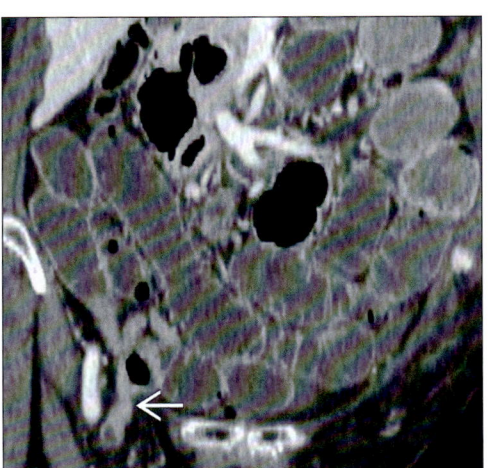

(Left) CECT coronal reformation of femoral hernia causing SBO. Neck of hernia ➡ is medial to femoral vein ➡. Note proximal dilation of small bowel due to obstruction ➡. *(Right)* Coronal reformation (in same patient as previous image) clearly demonstrates herniated small bowel loop ➡.

Variant

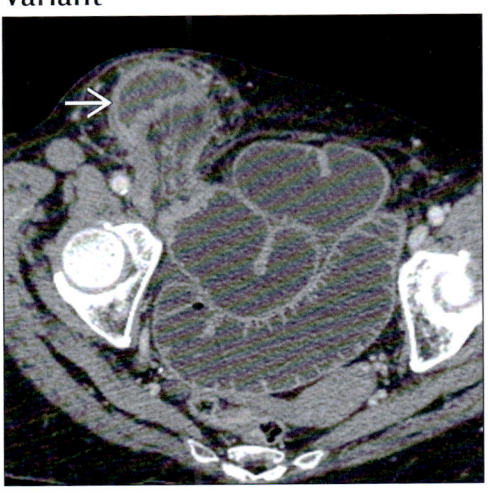
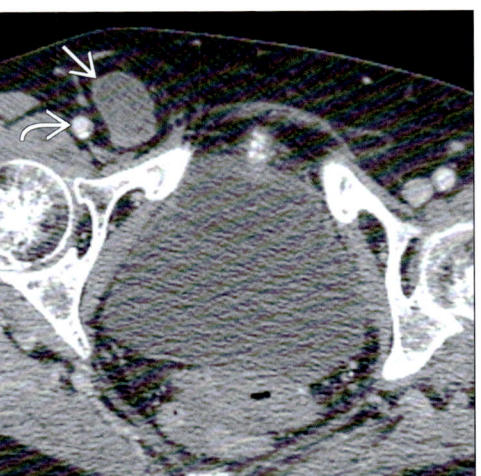

(Left) Axial CECT demonstrates an incarcerated femoral hernia. Note thickened small bowel loops within femoral hernia sac ➡. *(Right)* Axial CECT at lower level demonstrates hernia bowel ➡ medial to femoral vein ➡.

PARADUODENAL HERNIA

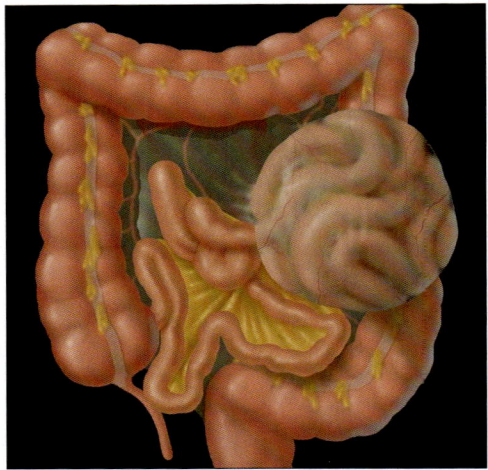

Graphic shows left paraduodenal hernia containing dilated, proximal jejunal loops in a peritoneal "sac".

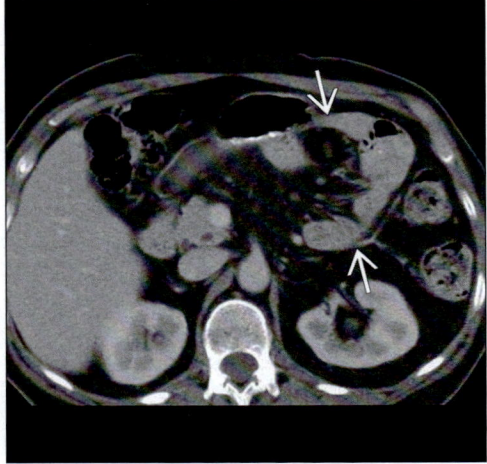

Axial CECT shows cluster of mildly dilated small bowel segments ➡ in LUQ, displacing stomach forward. Mesenteric vessels to herniated bowel segments converge toward center of cluster.

TERMINOLOGY

Definitions
- Protrusion of bowel loops through mesenteric defect within abdominal cavity

IMAGING FINDINGS

General Features
- Best diagnostic clue: CECT: Cluster of dilated bowel loops with distorted mesenteric vessels
- Location
  - Left (75%): Via paraduodenal (lateral to 4th part) mesenteric fossa of Landzert, near ligament of Treitz
  - Right (25%): Via jejunal mesentericoparietal fossa of Waldeyer

Radiographic Findings
- Radiography
  - Supine abdomen
    - "Closed loop": Markedly distended segment of small bowel

Fluoroscopic Findings
- Small bowel follow through (SBFT)
  - Abnormally crowded bowel loops to left or right side of colon; small bowel often absent from pelvis
  - Left: Circumscribed ovoid mass of jejunal loops in LUQ lateral to ascending duodenum
  - Right: Ovoid mass of small bowel loops lateral and inferior to descending duodenum
  - Appear as sac-like mass or with a confining border
  - Point of transition between dilated and non-dilated bowel is common
  - Fixation, stasis and delayed flow of contrast seen in herniated bowel
    - Right side herniated loops more fixed than left
  - Lateral film demonstrates retroperitoneal displacement of herniated bowel loops

CT Findings
- Left
  - Evidence of small bowel obstruction (SBO)
  - Encapsulated, cluster or sac-like mass of small bowel loops between pancreatic body/tail & stomach, left of ligament of Treitz

DDx: Cluster of Dilated Bowel Loops

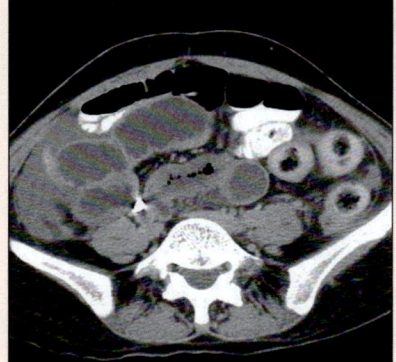

Closed Loop Obstruction

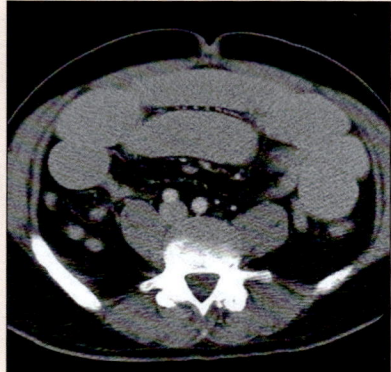

Closed Loop Obstruction

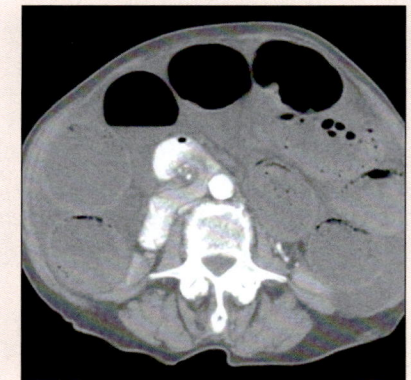

Transmesenteric Internal Hernia

PARADUODENAL HERNIA

Key Facts

Terminology
- Protrusion of bowel loops through mesenteric defect within abdominal cavity

Imaging Findings
- Best diagnostic clue: CECT: Cluster of dilated bowel loops with distorted mesenteric vessels
- Left (75%): Via paraduodenal (lateral to 4th part) mesenteric fossa of Landzert, near ligament of Treitz
- Right (25%): Via jejunal mesentericoparietal fossa of Waldeyer
- Best imaging tool: CECT, SBFT

Top Differential Diagnoses
- Closed Loop Obstruction (SBO)
- Transmesenteric Internal (TMI) Hernia

Pathology
- Congenital or developmental mesenteric anomalies
- Complication of surgery or trauma

Clinical Issues
- Smaller hernias are clinically silent but easily reducible
- Larger hernias: Vague discomfort, abdominal distension, periumbilical colicky pain, palpable mass, localized tenderness

Diagnostic Checklist
- Consider incarceration if bowel loops are thickened
- Cluster of dilated small bowel loops lateral to ascending or descending duodenum with crowded/twisted mesenteric vessels

---

- ○ Bowel loops herniate into sac created by descending & distal transverse mesocolon
- ○ Mass effect on posterior stomach wall; duodeno-jejunal junction inferiorly & medially; transverse colon inferiorly
- ○ Mesenteric vessels crowded & engorged
- Right
  - ○ Clustered or encapsulated small bowel loops lateral and inferior to descending duodenum
  - ○ Superior mesenteric vein rotated anteriorly and to left side
  - ○ Twisted of vascular jejunal branches behind superior mesenteric artery (SMA) and into hernial sac
  - ○ Ascending colon lies lateral to hernia sac
  - ○ Laterally displaced right ureter

Ultrasonographic Findings
- Grayscale Ultrasound: Dilated small bowel loops

Angiographic Findings
- Superior mesenteric arteriogram
  - ○ Normal jejunal branches arise from left margin of main trunk, abruptly turn to right, pass behind to supply herniated loops

Imaging Recommendations
- Best imaging tool: CECT, SBFT

DIFFERENTIAL DIAGNOSIS

Closed Loop Obstruction (SBO)
- Obstruction at two points
- Tends to involve mesentery, prone to produce volvulus
- Usually caused by adhesive band, occasionally by internal or external hernia
- Volvulus: C- or U-shaped or "coffee bean" configuration of bowel loop
- Stretched mesenteric vessels converging toward torsion site
- Collapsed loops adjacent to obstruction
- "Beak sign": Fusiform tapering at point of torsion or obstruction
- "Whirl sign": Due to tightly twisted mesentery with volvulus

Transmesenteric Internal (TMI) Hernia
- Iatrogenic (postoperative)
  - ○ Abdominal surgery: Roux-en-Y gastric bypass (73%)
- Congenital (mesenteric defect)
  - ○ Most common subtype in pediatric age group
  - ○ Near ligament of Treitz, ileocecal valve
  - ○ Mesenteric defect is usually 2-5 cm in diameter
- Herniating loops of small bowel (jejunum and/or ileum)
- Cluster of dilated small bowel loops (right side more common)
- Crowded or twisted mesenteric vessels
- Hepatic flexure displaced inferiorly or posteriorly

PATHOLOGY

General Features
- Etiology
  - ○ Congenital or developmental mesenteric anomalies
    - ■ Anomalies in mesenteric fixation of ascending or descending colon → abnormal openings → hernia
  - ○ Complication of surgery or trauma
    - ■ Abnormal mesenteric defect occurs → abnormal mobility of small bowel & right colon → hernia
  - ○ Left: Herniation via abnormal mesenteric fossa of Landzert
    - ■ Discrete peritoneal opening found in 2% of population
    - ■ Lateral to ascending duodenum
    - ■ Bowel loop herniation into pocket of distal transverse & descending mesocolon, posterior to SMA
  - ○ Right: Herniation via abnormal mesentericoparietal fossa of Waldeyer
    - ■ Jejunal mesentery, immediately behind SMA, inferior to transverse duodenum

PARADUODENAL HERNIA

- Bowel loop herniation into pocket of ascending mesocolon
- Epidemiology
  - Second most common subtype of internal hernia after transmesenteric postoperative hernia
  - Usually congenital or rarely acquired
  - Rare cause of small bowel obstruction

Gross Pathologic & Surgical Features
- Dilated bowel loops herniating via a mesenteric defect

Staging, Grading or Classification Criteria
- Based on anatomic location
  - Internal or intra-abdominal: Herniation of bowel loops via defect within abdominal cavity
  - External: Prolapse of bowel loops via defect in wall of abdomen or pelvis
  - Diaphragmatic: Protrusion of bowel loops via hiatus or congenital defect
- Subclassification of internal hernias
  - Paraduodenal hernia
  - Transmesenteric post-operative hernia
  - Foramen of Winslow, pericecal hernias
  - Intersigmoid and transomental hernias
- Subclassification of paraduodenal based on location
  - Left: 75%; right: 25%

CLINICAL ISSUES

Presentation
- Most common signs/symptoms
  - Smaller hernias are clinically silent but easily reducible
  - Larger hernias: Vague discomfort, abdominal distension, periumbilical colicky pain, palpable mass, localized tenderness

Demographics
- Age: All ages, but typically present between 4th and 6th decades
- Gender: M:F = 3:1

Natural History & Prognosis
- Complications
  - Volvulus, ischemia, strangulation
  - Bowel gangrene, shock & death
- Good prognosis with early surgical correction, poor if surgical correction delayed or complications

Treatment
- Laparotomy: Incision of enclosing mesentery
- Bowel decompression

DIAGNOSTIC CHECKLIST

Consider
- Consider incarceration if bowel loops are thickened

Image Interpretation Pearls
- Cluster of dilated small bowel loops lateral to ascending or descending duodenum with crowded/twisted mesenteric vessels

SELECTED REFERENCES

1. Huang YM et al: Left paraduodenal hernia presenting as recurrent small bowel obstruction. World J Gastroenterol. 11(41):6557-9, 2005
2. Osadchy A et al: Small bowel obstruction related to left-side paraduodenal hernia: CT findings. Abdom Imaging. 30(1):53-5, 2005
3. Ovali GY et al: Transient left paraduodenal hernia. Comput Med Imaging Graph. 29(6):459-61, 2005
4. Tainaka T et al: Left paraduodenal hernia leading to protein-losing enteropathy in childhood. J Pediatr Surg. 40(2):E21-3, 2005
5. Brunner WC et al: Incidental paraduodenal hernia found during laparoscopic colectomy. Hernia. 8(3):268-70, 2004
6. Catalano OA et al: Internal hernia with volvulus and intussusception: case report. Abdom Imaging. 29(2):164-5, 2004
7. Fukunaga M et al: Laparoscopic surgery for left paraduodenal hernia. J Laparoendosc Adv Surg Tech A. 14(2):111-5, 2004
8. Moran JM et al: Paramesocolic hernias: consequences of delayed diagnosis. Report of three new cases. J Pediatr Surg. 39(1):112-6, 2004
9. Papaziogas B et al: Surgical images: soft tissue. Right paraduodenal hernia. Can J Surg. 47(3):195-6, 2004
10. Vyas FL et al: Left paraduodenal hernia: an uncommon cause of chronic abdominal pain. Trop Gastroenterol. 25(4):189-90, 2004
11. Ramachandran P et al: Strangulated left paraduodenal hernia in an infant. Pediatr Surg Int. 19(1-2):120-1, 2003
12. Blachar A et al: Gastrointestinal complications of laparoscopic Roux-en-Y gastric bypass surgery: clinical and imaging findings. Radiology. 223(3): 625-32, 2002
13. Blachar A et al: Internal hernia: an increasingly common cause of small bowel obstruction. Semin Ultrasound CT MR. 23(2): 174-83, 2002
14. Hendrickson RJ et al: Small bowel obstruction due to a paracolonic retroperitoneal hernia. Am Surg. 68(9):756-8, 2002
15. Blachar A et al: Bowel obstruction following liver transplantation: clinical and ct findings in 48 cases with emphasis on internal hernia. Radiology. 218(2): 384-8, 2001
16. Blachar A et al: Internal hernia: clinical and imaging findings in 17 patients with emphasis on CT criteria. Radiology. 218(1): 68-74, 2001
17. Blachar A et al: Radiologist performance in the diagnosis of internal hernia by using specific CT findings with emphasis on transmesenteric hernia. Radiology. 221(2): 422-8, 2001

PARADUODENAL HERNIA

IMAGE GALLERY

Typical

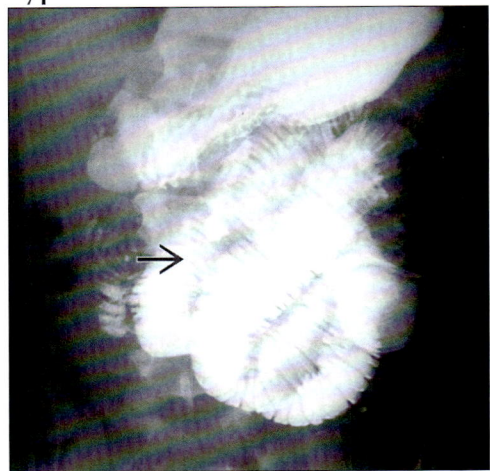
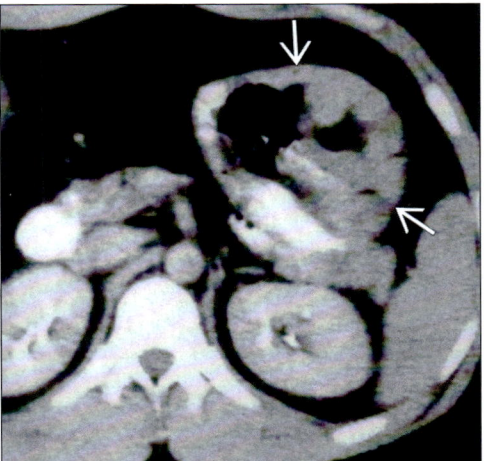

(Left) Delayed film from upper GI series shows tight cluster of dilated jejunal segments ➡ and delayed passage to normal caliber distal small bowel. *(Right)* Axial CECT shows oval cluster of jejunal segments ➡. Note sharply defined outer margin of peritoneal sac around herniated bowel, & mesenteric vessels converging toward sac center.

Typical

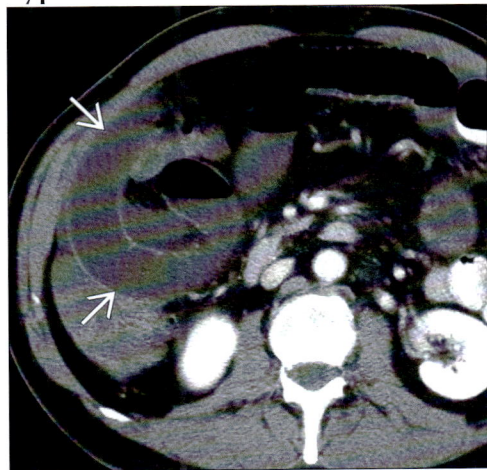
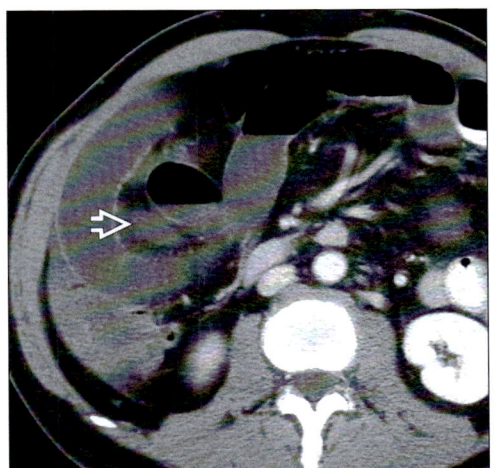

(Left) Axial CECT shows right paraduodenal hernia causing small bowel obstruction. Note U-shaped configuration of bowel loop within right paraduodenal hernia sac ➡. *(Right)* Axial CECT (same patient as previous image, at a higher level) demonstrates edema of mesentery from strangulated obstruction ➡.

Variant

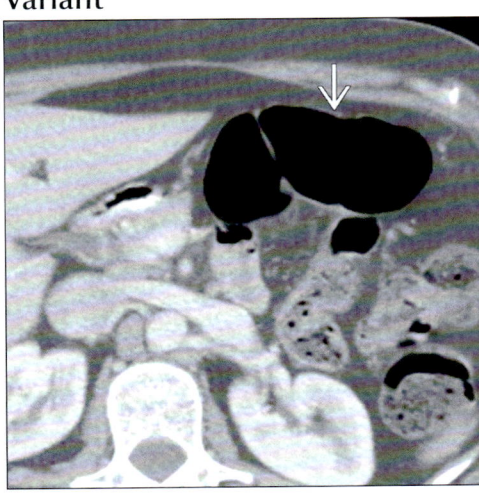
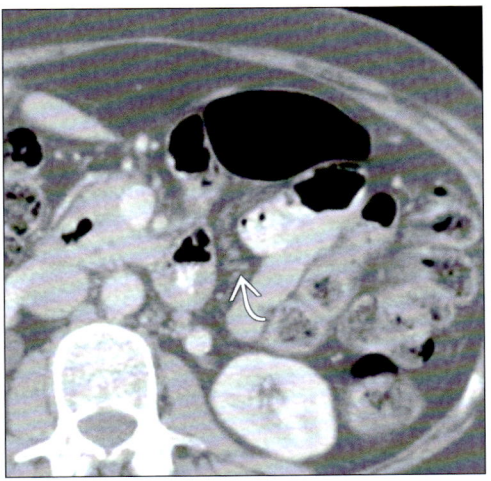

(Left) Axial CECT of LUQ shows cluster of moderately dilated jejunal segments in left upper & mid-abdomen. Note significantly dilated bowel ➡ near pancreatic body, displacing stomach ventrally. *(Right)* Axial CECT again shows clustered jejunal segments in left upper and mid-abdomen. Note subtle crowding and distortion of mesenteric vessels as they enter and leave hernia sac ➡.

TRANSMESENTERIC POST-OPERATIVE HERNIA

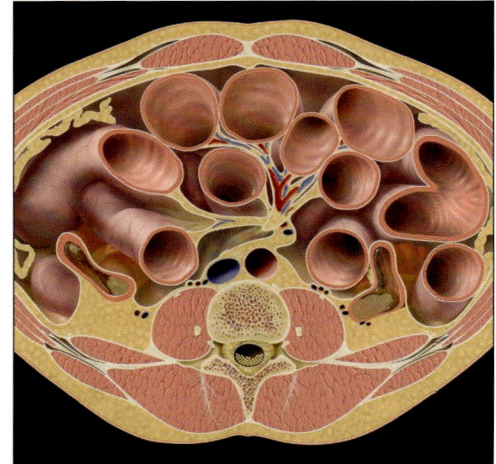

Graphic shows dilated small bowel (SB) that has herniated through a mesenteric defect. Note peripheral position of SB and medial displacement of colon, displaced mesenteric vessels.

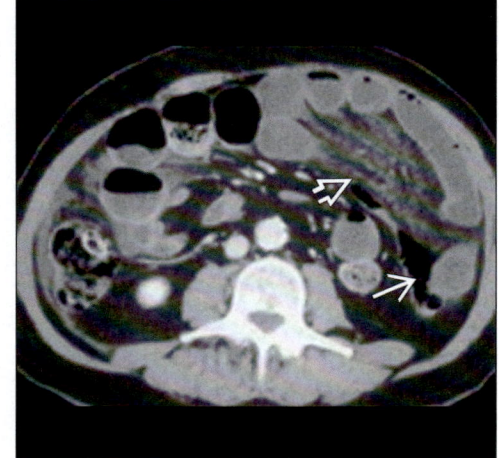

Axial CECT shows clustered dilated segments of small bowel in left mid-abdomen ventral to transverse colon ➡. Mesenteric vessels ➡ supplying herniated bowel are distorted & congested.

TERMINOLOGY

Definitions
- Protrusion of bowel loops through acquired defect of mesentery within abdominal cavity

IMAGING FINDINGS

General Features
- Best diagnostic clue: Cluster of dilated small bowel loops with distorted mesenteric vessels
- Location
  o Abnormal opening in mesentery of small bowel or colon
  o Post-operative hernia from Roux-en-Y gastric bypass surgery
    ▪ Transverse mesocolon (80%)
    ▪ Small bowel mesentery (14%)
    ▪ Behind Roux loop (6%): Peterson-type hernia
  o Hernia post liver transplant
    ▪ Transverse mesocolon (more common)
    ▪ Small bowel mesentery
- Size: Mesenteric defect varies from few millimeters to few centimeters

Radiographic Findings
- Radiography
  o Supine abdomen
    ▪ "Closed loop": Markedly distended segment of small bowel
    ▪ Crowded & dilated small bowel loops in an abnormal location
    ▪ Multiple air fluid levels

Fluoroscopic Findings
- Small bowel follow through
  o Crowding of bowel loops in an abnormal location
    ▪ Right side of abdomen is more common
  o Bowel loops do not appear to be contained in sac or confining border
  o Varying degrees of small bowel obstruction (SBO)
  o Point of transition between dilated & non dilated bowel common
  o Some degree of fixation, stasis & delayed flow of contrast seen in herniated bowel
  o Lateral films useful to demonstrate displacement of herniated bowel loops

DDx: Clustered Dilated Bowel Loops

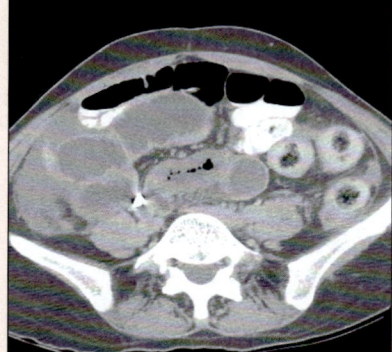

Closed Loop SBO

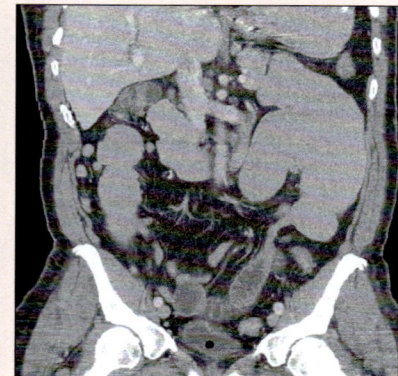

SBO Adhesions

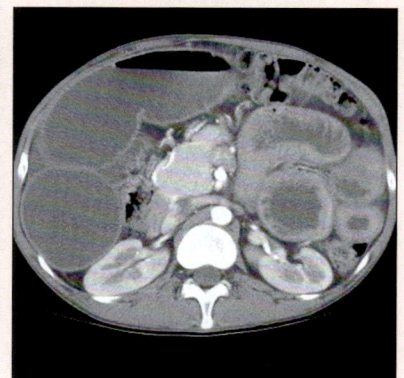

Crohn Stricture

TRANSMESENTERIC POST-OPERATIVE HERNIA

Key Facts

Terminology
- Protrusion of bowel loops through acquired defect of mesentery within abdominal cavity

Imaging Findings
- Best diagnostic clue: Cluster of dilated small bowel loops with distorted mesenteric vessels
- Evidence of small bowel obstruction (100%)
- Transition point dilated-nondilated (100%)
- Usually adjacent to abdominal wall
- Hernia usually not encapsulated or enveloped in a sac
- Mesenteric vessels appear engorged, crowded or twisted
- "Whirl sign": Small bowel volvulus with twisted mesenteric vessels

Top Differential Diagnoses
- Closed Loop Obstruction (SBO)

Pathology
- Roux-en-Y gastric bypass, liver transplantation, small or large bowel surgery
- Abnormal spaces or mesenteric defects are created in prior abdominal surgery

Clinical Issues
- Smaller hernias are clinically silent, easily reducible
- Periumbilical pain, symptoms of bowel obstruction

Diagnostic Checklist
- Cluster of dilated non-encapsulated/non-enveloped small bowel loops adjacent to abdominal wall with crowded/twisted mesenteric vessels

CT Findings
- Cluster of dilated small bowel loops
  - Evidence of small bowel obstruction (100%)
  - Transition point dilated-nondilated (100%)
  - Usually adjacent to abdominal wall
- Hernia usually not encapsulated or enveloped in a sac
- Displacement of overlying omental fat of herniated bowel loop (74%)
- Mesenteric vessels appear engorged, crowded or twisted
- Right or left displacement of main mesenteric trunk
- Colon displacement
  - Hepatic flexure displaced inferiorly & posteriorly
  - Medial displacement of ascending & descending colon is less common
- Thick bowel wall & ascites, particularly in cases with bowel ischemia
- "Whirl sign": Small bowel volvulus with twisted mesenteric vessels
- Smaller transmesenteric hernias after Roux-en-Y surgery (via transverse mesocolon)
  - Small retrogastric cluster of small bowel loops
  - Mass effect on posterior stomach wall
  - Redundant dilated Roux loop
  - No colon or fat displacement

Ultrasonographic Findings
- Grayscale Ultrasound: Dilated small bowel loops in an abnormal location

Angiographic Findings
- Conventional
  - Superior mesenteric arteriogram
    - Abrupt angulation & displacement of visceral branches passing through mesenteric defect to herniated loops

Imaging Recommendations
- Best imaging tool: CECT, small bowel follow through

DIFFERENTIAL DIAGNOSIS

Closed Loop Obstruction (SBO)
- Obstruction of small bowel at two points
- Usually involves mesentery and prone to produce volvulus
  - Most common cause of strangulation
- Most often caused by adhesive band, occasionally by internal or external hernia
- Markedly distended segment of fluid-filled small bowel
- Volvulus: C-, U-shaped, or "coffee bean" configuration of bowel loop
- Stretched mesenteric vessels converging toward site of torsion
- Adjacent collapsed loops at site of obstruction
  - Round, oval or triangular in shape
- "Beak sign": Fusiform tapering at point of torsion or obstruction
- "Whirl sign": Tightly twisted mesentery with volvulus
- May be indistinguishable from transmesenteric hernia, especially if associated with volvulus

PATHOLOGY

General Features
- Etiology
  - Transmesenteric post-operative hernia
    - Roux-en-Y gastric bypass, liver transplantation, small or large bowel surgery
  - Transmesenteric congenital hernia
    - Mesenteric defect located close to ligament of Treitz or ileocecal valve
    - Defect usually 2-5 cm in diameter
  - Pathogenesis & mechanism
    - Abnormal spaces or mesenteric defects are created in prior abdominal surgery
    - Developmental mesenteric anomalies
    - Abnormal mesenteric fixation or defects may lead to abnormal mobility of small bowel loops, facilitating herniation

TRANSMESENTERIC POST-OPERATIVE HERNIA

- Herniating segment of small bowel loops (jejunum/ileum)
- Transient or intermittent herniation
- Epidemiology
  - 0.6-5.8% of small bowel obstruction cases are due to internal hernias in selected populations
    - Transmesenteric post-operative hernia accounts for more than half of these cases
  - Transmesenteric post-operative hernia
    - Accounts for more than 50% of internal hernias
  - Autopsy incidence: Internal hernias: 0.2-0.9%

Gross Pathologic & Surgical Features
- Abnormal opening in mesentery of small bowel or colon
- Dilated small bowel loops herniating through mesenteric defect
- Distorted or twisted mesenteric vessels

Staging, Grading or Classification Criteria
- Classification based on anatomic location
  - Internal or intra-abdominal: Herniation of bowel loops via defect within abdominal cavity
  - External: Prolapse of bowel loops via defect in abdominal or pelvic wall
  - Diaphragmatic: Protrusion of bowel loops via hiatus, congenital or acquired defect
- Subclassification of internal hernias
  - Transmesenteric hernia
  - Paraduodenal hernia
  - Foramen of Winslow, pericecal hernias
  - Intersigmoid and transomental hernias
- Transmesenteric hernia: Two types based on etiology
  - Transmesenteric post-operative hernia (most common subtype of internal hernia in adults)
  - Transmesenteric congenital hernia (most common subtype of internal hernia in children)

CLINICAL ISSUES

Presentation
- Most common signs/symptoms
  - Smaller hernias are clinically silent, easily reducible
  - Larger hernias
    - Vague discomfort, abdominal distension
    - Periumbilical pain, symptoms of bowel obstruction
    - Palpable mass, localized tenderness
  - Small bowel obstruction
    - Chronic & recurrent (low grade) or acute (high grade)
  - Onset usually months after original surgery

Demographics
- Age
  - Transmesenteric post-operative hernias
    - Usually obese adult age group who have had Roux-en-Y gastric bypass surgery
    - Typically between 4th & 6th decade
- Gender: M < F

Natural History & Prognosis
- Complications
  - Volvulus, ischemia, strangulation
  - Bowel gangrene, shock & death
- Prognosis
  - Early surgical correction: Good
  - Delayed surgical correction & complications: Poor

Treatment
- Laparotomy, bowel decompression
- Surgical correction of mesenteric defect

DIAGNOSTIC CHECKLIST

Consider
- Differentiate from other types of internal hernias

Image Interpretation Pearls
- Cluster of dilated non-encapsulated/non-enveloped small bowel loops adjacent to abdominal wall with crowded/twisted mesenteric vessels

SELECTED REFERENCES
1. Agarwal A et al: Internal hernia after pancreas transplantation with enteric drainage: an unusual cause of small bowel obstruction. Transplantation. 80(1):149-52, 2005
2. Hong SS et al: Current diagnostic role of CT in evaluating internal hernia. J Comput Assist Tomogr. 29(5):604-9, 2005
3. Osadchy A et al: Small bowel obstruction due to a paracecal hernia: computerized tomography diagnosis. Emerg Radiol. 11(4):239-41, 2005
4. Catalano OA et al: Internal hernia with volvulus and intussusception: case report. Abdom Imaging, 2004
5. Blachar A et al: Gastrointestinal complications of laparoscopic Roux-en-Y gastric bypass surgery: clinical and imaging findings. Radiology. 223(3): 625-32, 2002
6. Blachar A et al: Internal hernia: an increasingly common cause of small bowel obstruction. Semin Ultrasound CT MR. 23(2): 174-83, 2002
7. Filip JE et al: Internal hernia formation after laparoscopic Roux-en-Y gastric bypass for morbid obesity. Am Surg. 68(7): 640-3, 2002
8. Blachar A et al: Bowel obstruction following liver transplantation: clinical and ct findings in 48 cases with emphasis on internal hernia. Radiology. 218(2): 384-8, 2001
9. Blachar A et al: Internal hernia: clinical and imaging findings in 17 patients with emphasis on CT criteria. Radiology. 218(1): 68-74, 2001
10. Blachar A et al: Radiologist performance in the diagnosis of internal hernia by using specific CT findings with emphasis on transmesenteric hernia. Radiology. 221(2): 422-8, 2001
11. Delabrousse E et al: Strangulated transomental hernia: CT findings. Abdom Imaging. 26(1): 86-8, 2001
12. Huang YC et al: Left paraduodenal hernia presenting as intestinal obstruction: report of one case. Acta Paediatr Taiwan. 42(3): 172-4, 2001
13. Rha SE et al: CT and MR imaging findings of bowel ischemia from various primary causes. Radiographics. 20(1): 29-42, 2000
14. Ha HK et al: Usefulness of CT in patients with intestinal obstruction who have undergone abdominal surgery for malignancy. AJR Am J Roentgenol. 171(6): 1587-93, 1998

TRANSMESENTERIC POST-OPERATIVE HERNIA

IMAGE GALLERY

Typical

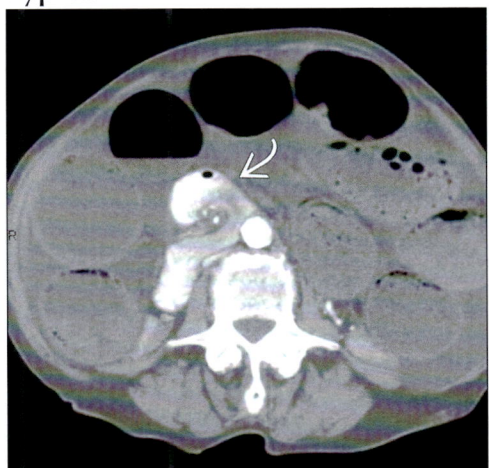
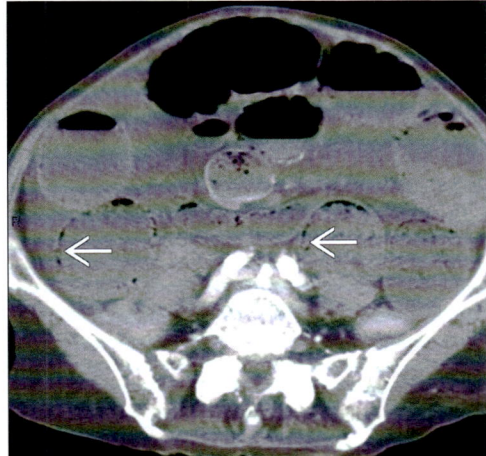

(Left) Axial CECT shows "whirl sign", with twisting of proximal small bowel & mesenteric vessels around their axes ➡. Colon is collapsed & displaced medially by distended small bowel. *(Right)* Axial CECT (same patient as previous image) shows pneumatosis ➡ and ascites, suggesting bowel ischemia. At surgery, small bowel was herniated through mesenteric defect, with extensive infarction.

Typical

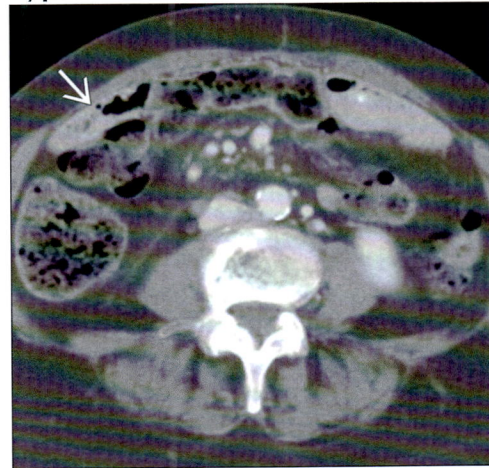
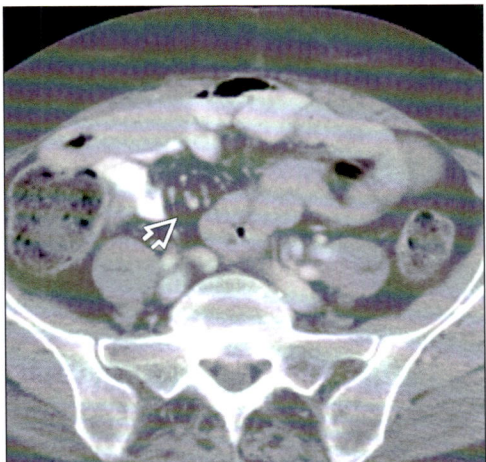

(Left) Axial CECT shows small bowel dilated and displaced against anterior abdominal wall. Note abnormal position of small bowel ➡ ventral to transverse colon. *(Right)* Axial CECT (same patient as previous image) shows that the mesenteric vessels leading to the dilated, displaced segments of bowel ➡ are crowded together and displaced.

Typical

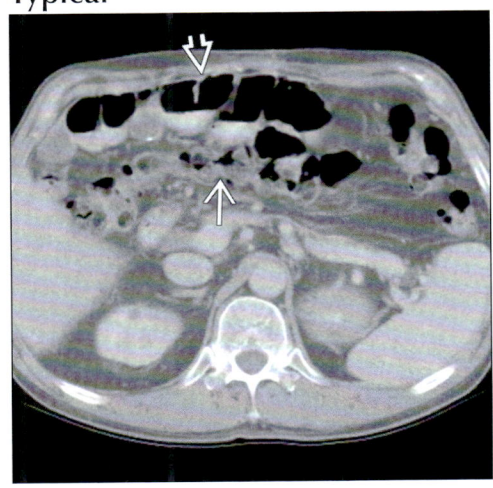
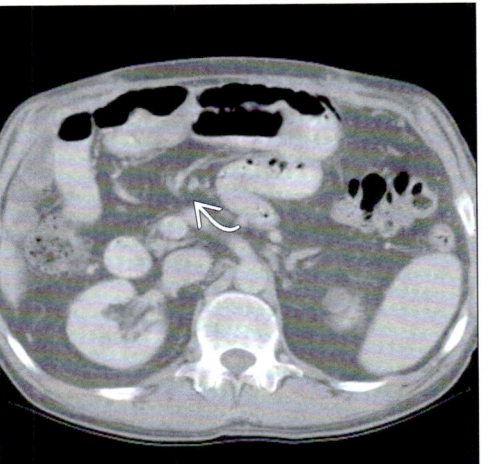

(Left) Axial CECT shows cluster of dilated small bowel loops ➡ pressed against anterior abdominal wall, displacing transverse colon ➡. *(Right)* Axial CECT (same patient as previous image) demonstrates distorted position and course of mesenteric blood vessels ➡ to herniated segments.

DUODENAL ULCER

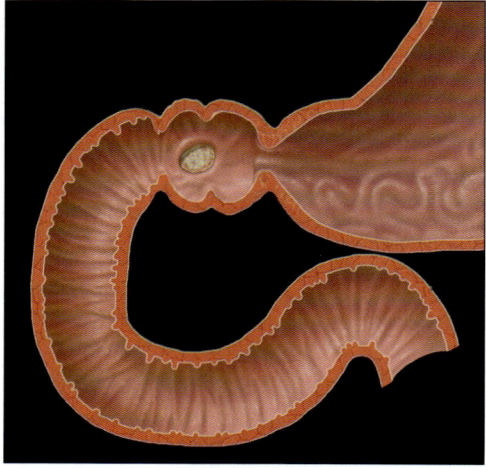

Graphic shows duodenal ulcer with deformed bulb due to converging folds and spasm.

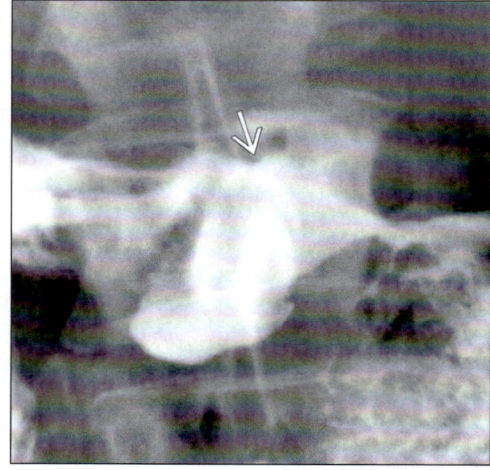

Upper GI shows radiating folds to an ulcer crater ➡ in the duodenal bulb.

TERMINOLOGY

Abbreviations and Synonyms
- Peptic ulcer disease

Definitions
- Mucosal erosion of duodenum

IMAGING FINDINGS

General Features
- Best diagnostic clue: Sharply marginated barium collection with folds radiating to edge of ulcer crater on fluoroscopic-guided double-contrast barium study
- Location
  - 95% duodenal bulbar ulcers; 5% postbulbar ulcers
  - Bulbar ulcers are located at apex, central portion, or base of bulb
  - Postbulbar ulcers located on medial wall of proximal descending duodenum above papilla of Vater
  - 50% of duodenal ulcers located on anterior wall
- Size: Most ulcers are < 1 cm at time of diagnosis
- Morphology
  - Round or ovoid collections of barium
  - 5% of duodenal ulcers have linear configuration

Fluoroscopic Findings
- **Fluoroscopic-guided double-contrast barium studies**
  - Bulbar ulcers
    - Persistent small round, ovoid or linear ulcer niche (barium collection)
    - Smooth, radiolucent ulcer mound of edematous mucosa
    - Radiating folds converge centrally at edge of ulcer crater
    - Ring shadow: Barium coating rim of unfilled anterior wall ulcer crater (air contrast view)
    - Deformity of bulb (edema & spasm/scarring)
    - Residual depression of central portion of scar mimics active ulcer crater
    - Pseudodiverticula balloon out between areas of fibrosis & spasm
    - "Cloverleaf" deformity of pseudodiverticula
  - Postbulbar ulcers
    - Smooth/rounded indentation on lateral wall opposite ulcer crater (edema & spasm)
    - "Ring stricture": Eccentric narrowing (scarring)

DDx: Duodenal Fixed Deformity with/without Contrast Collection

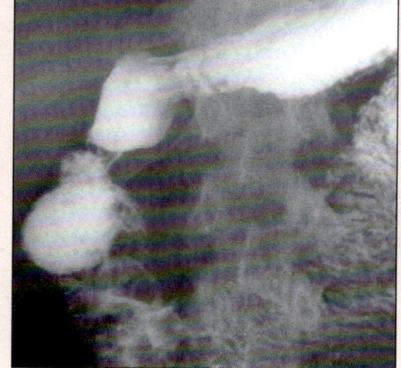

Duodenal Carcinoma

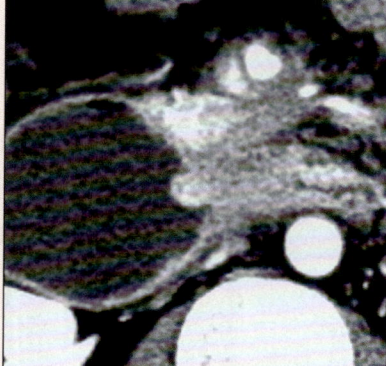

Extrinsic Invasion

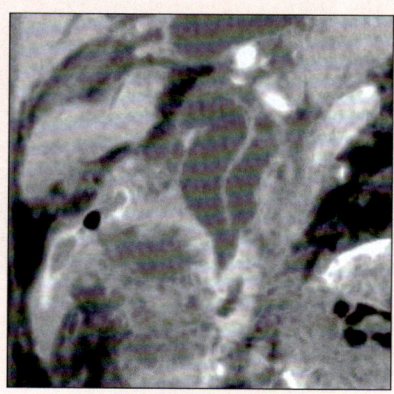

Extrinsic Invasion

DUODENAL ULCER

Key Facts

Terminology
- Mucosal erosion of duodenum

Imaging Findings
- Best diagnostic clue: Sharply marginated barium collection with folds radiating to edge of ulcer crater on fluoroscopic-guided double-contrast barium study
- **Fluoroscopic-guided double-contrast barium studies**
- Persistent small round, ovoid or linear ulcer niche (barium collection)
- Smooth, radiolucent ulcer mound of edematous mucosa
- Radiating folds converge centrally at edge of ulcer crater
- Ring shadow: Barium coating rim of unfilled anterior wall ulcer crater (air contrast view)
- High density barium for views of duodenal bulb
- Protocol advice: Obtain prone compression views of duodenum to observe anterior wall ulcers

Top Differential Diagnoses
- Duodenal Inflammation
- Duodenal Stricture
- Duodenal Carcinoma

Clinical Issues
- Burning, gnawing, or aching pain at epigastrium 2-4 hours after meals; relieved by antacids/food

Diagnostic Checklist
- Eradication of H. pylori is first step of treatment
- Check for duodenal bulb deformity
- Prone compression views necessary to evaluate anterior wall duodenal ulcers

---

- Giant duodenal ulcers (> 2 cm)
  - Always located in duodenal bulb
  - Virtually replaces bulb; mistaken for scarred or normal bulb
  - Fixed or unchanging configuration is key clue
  - Focal narrowing → outlet obstruction (edema & spasm)

CT Findings
- CECT (water/water-soluble oral contrast)
  - Signs of ulcer penetration/perforation
    - Wall thickening or luminal narrowing of duodenum
    - Infiltration of surrounding fat/organs (pancreas)
    - Extraluminal intra- or retroperitoneal gas

Imaging Recommendations
- Best imaging tool
  - Fluoroscopic-guided double-contrast barium studies
  - High density barium for views of duodenal bulb
  - Low density barium: Upright/prone compression views
- Protocol advice: Obtain prone compression views of duodenum to observe anterior wall ulcers

DIFFERENTIAL DIAGNOSIS

Duodenal Inflammation
- Duodenitis: Inflammation without frank ulceration
- Crohn disease
  - Usually with antral involvement
  - Aphthous ulcers are earliest abnormality observed
  - Thickened, nodular folds; cobblestone appearance
  - Asymmetric duodenal narrowing, outward ballooning of duodenal wall between area of fibrosis
  - Smooth, tapered areas of narrowing extend from apical portion of bulb to descending duodenum
  - One or more strictures in second or third portions of duodenum → marked obstruction & proximal dilatation (megaduodenum)
- Tuberculosis
  - Usually with antral involvement
  - Ulcers, thickened folds, narrowing or fistula
  - Enlarged lymph nodes adjacent to duodenum → narrowing or obstruction of lumen

Duodenal Stricture
- Pancreatitis
  - "Inverted 3" sign of Frostberg
    - Central limb of the "3": Point of fixation where pancreatic/common bile ducts insert into papilla
    - Above & below the point reflects edema of major & minor papilla or smooth muscle spasm & edema in duodenal wall
  - Thickened folds associated with medial compression or widening of duodenal sweep
  - Spiculation of mucosal folds (edema/inflammation)
- Gallstone erosion
  - Radiolucent filling defect in duodenum
  - Mucosal inflammation, ulceration, hemorrhage, perforation/obstruction
  - Barium reflux into gallbladder and bile ducts

Duodenal Carcinoma
- < 1% of all gastrointestinal cancers
- Found in postbulbar portion at/distal to papilla of Vater
- Polypoid, ulcerated, or annular lesions
- Narrowed lumen with thickened wall

Duodenal Diverticulum
- 1-5% are incidental findings in barium studies
- Most often located on medial border of descending duodenum in periampullary region
- Smooth, rounded outpouching from medial border of descending duodenum
- Multiple diverticula observed; configuration may change during course of study
- Differentiate from postbulbar ulcers by lack of inflammatory reaction & change in shape

Extrinsic Invasion
- Pancreatic carcinoma
  - Widening of duodenal sweep

DUODENAL ULCER

- Mass effect → double contour effect on medial border of duodenum: Differential filling with interfold spaces along inner aspect containing less barium than corresponding spaces along outer aspect
- Displacement or frank splaying of spikes: Tumor infiltrating duodenal wall with traction & fixation of folds
- Gallbladder carcinoma
  - Compression of bulb or proximal duodenum
- Metastases
  - Widening of duodenal sweep
  - Multiple submucosal masses or "bull's eye" lesion

Duodenal Hematoma
- Radiolucent filling defects from blood clots
- Well-circumscribed intramural masses with discrete margins → stenosis and obstruction
- Diffuse hemorrhage → thickened, spiculated folds or thumbprinting

PATHOLOGY

General Features
- General path comments
  - Multiplicity
    - 15% of patients with duodenal ulcers
    - Ulcers located in duodenal bulb and beyond
    - Suspicious of Zollinger-Ellison syndrome
- Genetics
  - Genetic syndromes
    - Multiple endocrine neoplasia type 1 (MEN 1)
    - Systemic mastocytosis
  - Greater concordance in monozygotic twins
  - Increased incidence with blood type O
- Etiology
  - Two major risk factors: Helicobacter pylori (H. pylori) (95-100%) & NSAIDs
  - Other risk factors: Steroids, tobacco, alcohol, coffee, stress, bile reflux, delayed gastric emptying
  - Less common etiologies
    - Zollinger-Ellison syndrome
    - Hyperparathyroidism
    - Chronic renal failure
    - Chronic obstructive pulmonary disease
  - Pathogenesis
    - H. pylori mediates or facilitates damage to gastric & duodenal mucosa
    - ↑ Gastric acid and ↑ gastric emptying → ↑ acidic exposure in duodenum
- Epidemiology
  - Incidence: 200,000 cases per year
  - 2-3 times more frequent than gastric ulcers

Gross Pathologic & Surgical Features
- Round or oval; sharply punched-out & regular walls; flat adjacent mucosa

Microscopic Features
- Necrotic debris; zone of active inflammation; granulation & scar tissue

CLINICAL ISSUES

Presentation
- Most common signs/symptoms
  - Asymptomatic
  - Burning, gnawing, or aching pain at epigastrium 2-4 hours after meals; relieved by antacids/food
  - Pain that awakens patients from sleep (66%)
  - Other signs/symptoms
    - Pain episodes occurring in clusters of days to weeks followed by longer pain-free intervals
    - Rarely anorexia & weight loss; hyperphagia & weight gain (pain relief through eating)
- Lab data
  - Diagnostic tests (serology or urease breath test) for H. pylori
- Diagnosis: Endoscopy

Demographics
- Age: Adults
- Gender: M = F

Natural History & Prognosis
- Complications
  - Hemorrhage, perforation, obstruction & fistula
  - Giant duodenal ulcers have ↑ risks of complications
- Prognosis: Good with medical treatment/surgery

Treatment
- Ulcer without H. pylori: H2-receptor antagonists (cimetidine, ranitidine, or famotidine) or proton-pump inhibitors (omeprazole or lansoprazole)
- H. pylori treatment: Metronidazole, bismuth and clarithromycin, amoxicillin or tetracycline
- Ulcer with H. pylori: H. pylori treatment and H2-receptor antagonists or proton-pump inhibitors
- Other agent: Sucralfate
- Follow-up: Intractable ulcers & complications

DIAGNOSTIC CHECKLIST

Consider
- Eradication of H. pylori is first step of treatment

Image Interpretation Pearls
- Check for duodenal bulb deformity
- Prone compression views necessary to evaluate anterior wall duodenal ulcers

SELECTED REFERENCES

1. Jayaraman MV et al: CT of the duodenum: an overlooked segment gets its due. Radiographics. 21 Spec No:S147-60, 2001
2. Pattison CP et al: Helicobacter pylori and peptic ulcer disease: Evolution to revolution to resolution. AJR 168: 1415-20, 1997
3. Levine MS et al: The Helicobacter pylori revolution: Radiologic perspective. Radiology 195: 593-6, 1995
4. Jacobs JM: Peptic ulcer disease: CT evaluation. Radiology 178: 745-8, 1991

DUODENAL ULCER

IMAGE GALLERY

Typical

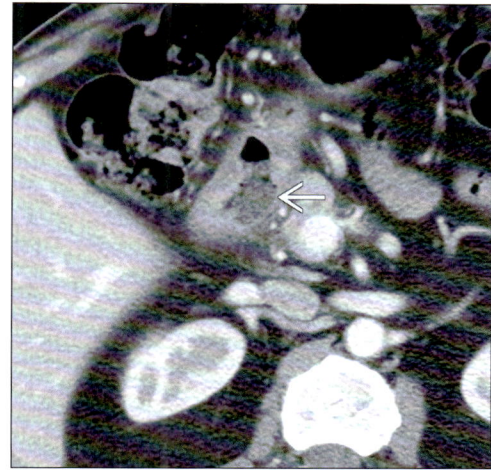
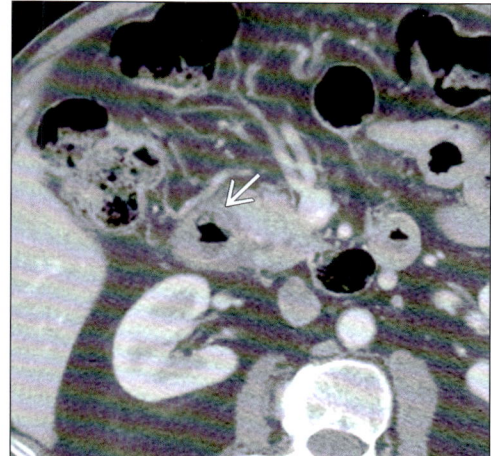

(Left) Axial CECT shows duodenal ulcer. Note large area of penetration into the medial wall of duodenum by ulcer crater ➡. *(Right)* Axial CECT at lower level in same patient as left demonstrates circumferential thickening of duodenum ➡.

Typical

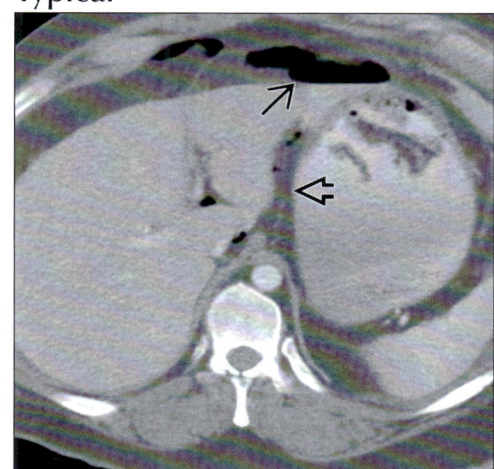
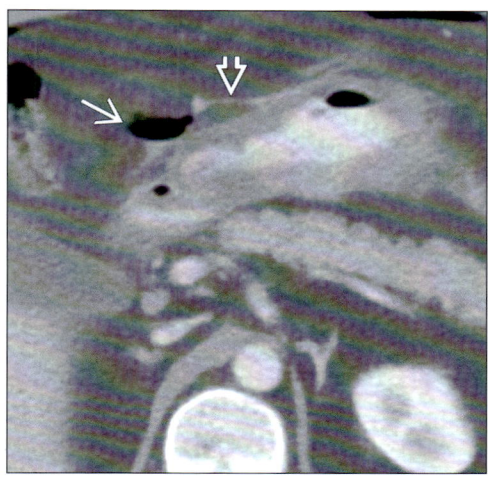

(Left) Axial CECT shows extensive free intraperitoneal gas ➡ in a patient with perforated ulcer. Note thickened gastric wall, probably due to gastritis ➡. *(Right)* Axial CECT in same patient as left shows small collections of extraluminal gas ➡ and oral contrast medium ➡ just ventral to duodenal bulb and antrum, confirming the source of perforation.

Variant

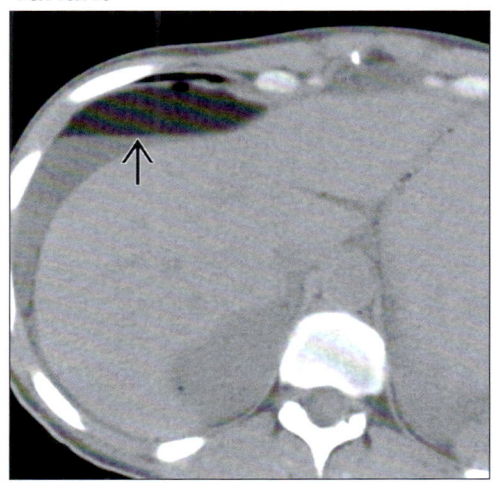
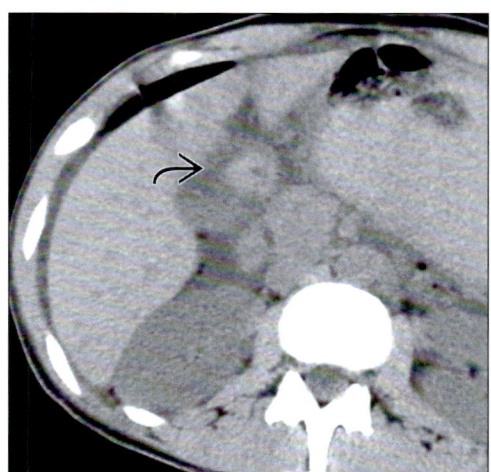

(Left) Axial NECT through the upper abdomen shows air-fat-fluid levels ➡. The fat-density fluid is milk, which extravasated into peritoneal cavity through perforated duodenal ulcer. *(Right)* Axial NECT at lower level in same patient as left shows more free air and fluid. The wall of the duodenum ➡ is thickened.

AORTO-ENTERIC FISTULA

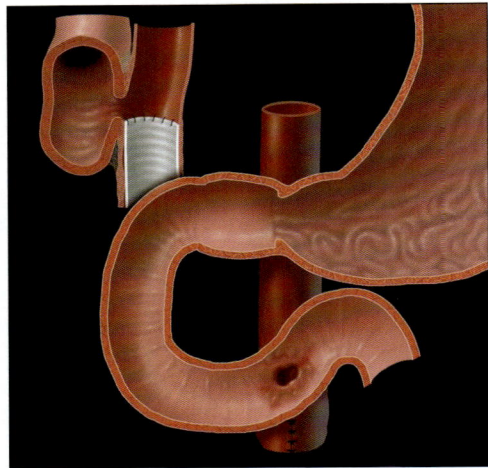

Graphic shows fistula between transverse duodenum and the aorta at the site of graft-aortic suture line.

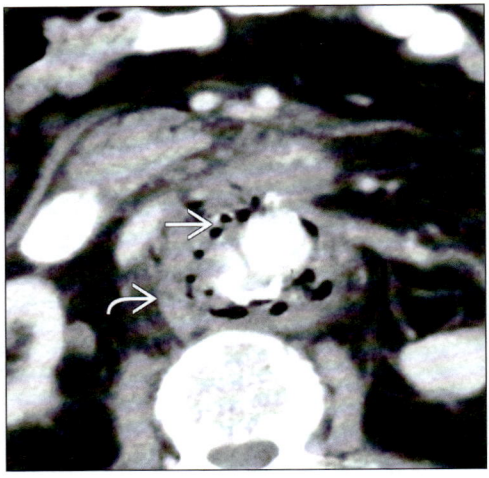

Axial CECT shows aorto-enteric fistula. Note ectopic gas ➡ and abnormal perigraft soft tissue indicating infection ➡. (Courtesy F. Hughes, MD).

TERMINOLOGY

Definitions
- Abnormal communication between aorta & GI tract

IMAGING FINDINGS

General Features
- Best diagnostic clue: Inflammatory stranding and gas between abdominal aorta and third part of duodenum following aneurysm repair
- Location: Duodenum (80%), jejunum and ileum (10-15%), stomach and colon (5%)

CT Findings
- Microbubbles adjacent to aortic graft
- Focal bowel wall thickening and/or perigraft soft tissue thickening > 5 mm
- Pseudoaneurysm, disruption of aneurysmal wrap
- Contrast in pseudoaneurysm on arterial phase
- Arterial phase: ↑ Attenuation of intestinal lumen contents; delayed phase: ↓ Attenuation
- CT-guided needle aspiration: May confirm perigraft infection

Nuclear Medicine Findings
- Tagged RBC within abdominal aorta enters bowel
- White blood cell scan to confirm infection

Imaging Recommendations
- Best imaging tool: CT is 94% sensitive, 85% specific

DIFFERENTIAL DIAGNOSIS

Periaortitis
- Inflammatory perianeurysmal fibrosis
- Soft-tissue attenuation encases aorta, IVC

Retroperitoneal Fibrosis
- Mantle of soft tissue enveloping aorta, IVC, ureters

Post-Operation
- Perigraft fluid may persist for up to 3 months

Post-Endovascular Stent
- Endoleak: Blood flow outside stent, but within aneurysm sac or adjacent vascular segment

DDx: Periaortic Inflammation

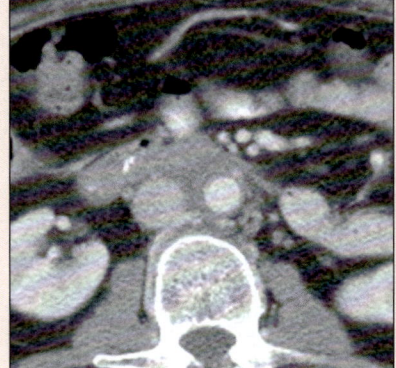
Periaortitis

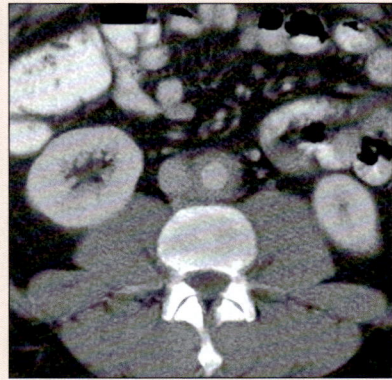
Retroperitoneal Fibrosis

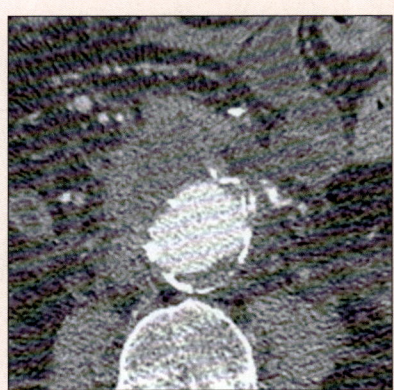
Post-Op Aorta

AORTO-ENTERIC FISTULA

Key Facts

Imaging Findings
- Best diagnostic clue: Inflammatory stranding and gas between abdominal aorta and third part of duodenum following aneurysm repair
- Best imaging tool: CT is 94% sensitive, 85% specific

Top Differential Diagnoses
- Periaortitis
- Post-Operation
- Post-Endovascular Stent

Clinical Issues
- "Herald" GI bleeding, followed hours, days or weeks later by catastrophic hemorrhage

Diagnostic Checklist
- Perigraft infection as evidenced by ectopic gas or perigraft soft tissue raises suspicion of fistula

- Gas bubbles between stent-graft & aortic wall

PATHOLOGY

General Features
- Etiology
  - Primary: Abdominal aortic aneurysms, infectious aortitis, penetrating peptic ulcer, tumor invasion, radiation therapy
  - Secondary: Aortic reconstructive surgery is most common etiology
  - Pathogenesis
    - 3rd portion of duodenum fixed & apposed to anterior wall of aortic aneurysm → pressure necrosis
    - Surgery → blood supply compromised
    - Pseudoaneurysm formation with erosion
    - Graft & suture line infection → anastomotic breakdown
- Epidemiology
  - Incidence: 0.6-1.5% after aortic surgery
  - Onset after surgery: 21 days - 14 years
- Associated abnormalities: Perigraft infection

CLINICAL ISSUES

Presentation
- Most common signs/symptoms
  - "Herald" GI bleeding, followed hours, days or weeks later by catastrophic hemorrhage
  - Abdominal/back pain, palpable & pulsatile mass
  - Intermittent rectal bleeding & recurrent anemia
  - Low grade fever, fatigue, weight loss, leukocytosis

Demographics
- Gender: M:F = 4-5:1
- Age: 55 and older

Natural History & Prognosis
- Very poor prognosis, up to 85% mortality

Treatment
- Percutaneous drainage of infected perigraft fluid may be initial treatment, followed by surgery
- Emergent reconstructive surgery may be required

DIAGNOSTIC CHECKLIST

Image Interpretation Pearls
- Perigraft infection as evidenced by ectopic gas or perigraft soft tissue raises suspicion of fistula

SELECTED REFERENCES

1. Perks FJ et al: Multidetector computed tomography imaging of aortoenteric fistula. J Comput Assist Tomogr. 28(3):343-7, 2004
2. Lenzo NP et al: Aortoenteric fistula on (99m)Tc erythrocyte scintigraphy. AJR Am J Roentgenol. 177(2):477-8, 2001

IMAGE GALLERY

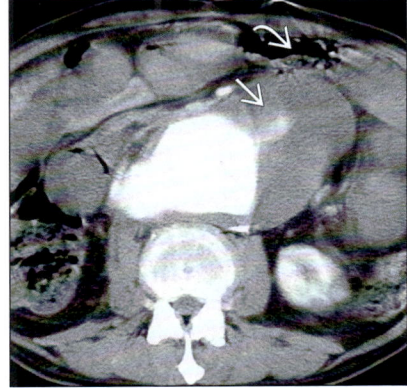 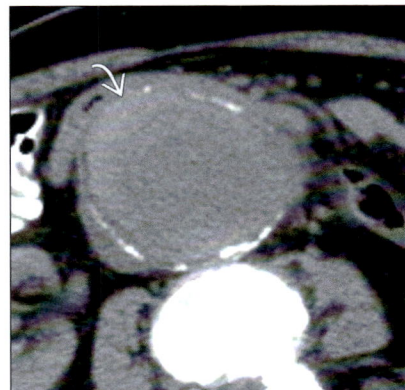 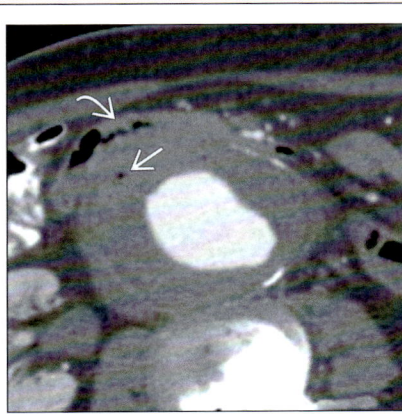

(Left) Axial CECT shows primary aorto-enteric fistula. Note large abdominal aortic aneurysm (AAA) leaking into peri-aortic hematoma. Transverse duodenum is draped over hematoma. (Center) Axial NECT shows large AAA. Note "crescent sign" of higher density between aortic intimal calcification and patent lumen. (Right) Axial CECT in same patient as left shows gas within thrombus, suggesting infection and/or communication to bowel lumen. Third portion of duodenum stretches over and appears to adhere to AAA.

CROHN DISEASE

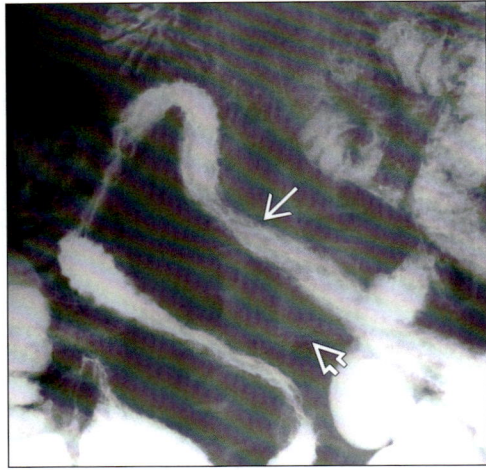

Small bowel follow through shows chronic Crohn disease. Note mucosal cobblestoning ➡ and wide separation of loops from creeping fat ➡.

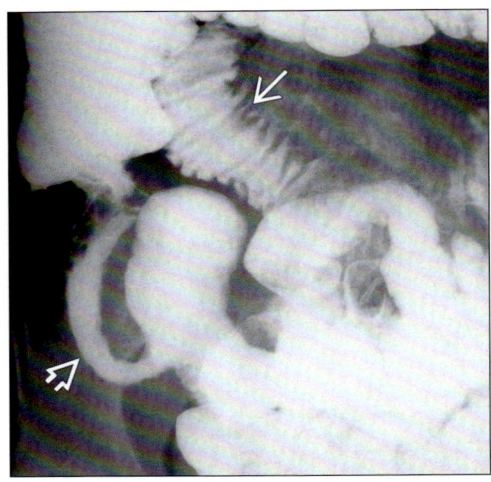

Small bowel follow through shows acute and chronic Crohn disease. Note submucosal thickening of ileum in acute disease ➡ and featureless mucosa of terminal ileum in chronic disease ➡.

TERMINOLOGY

Abbreviations and Synonyms
- Terminal ileitis, regional enteritis, ileocolitis

Definitions
- Chronic, recurrent, segmental, granulomatous inflammatory bowel disease

IMAGING FINDINGS

General Features
- Best diagnostic clue: Segmental areas of ileo-colonic ulceration and wall thickening on barium study
- Location
  - Anywhere along gut from mouth to anus
    - Most common: Terminal ileum & proximal colon
  - Distribution
    - Terminal ileum (95%); colon (22-55%)
    - Rectum (14-50%)
- Morphology
  - Skip lesions (segmental or discontinuous)
  - Transmural, granulomas (noncaseating type)
  - Cobblestone mucosa, fissures & fistulas

Fluoroscopic Findings
- Barium studies
  - Early changes
    - Lymphoid hyperplasia: 1-3 mm mucosal elevations, no ring shadow
    - "Target" or "bull's eye" appearance of aphthoid ulcerations: Punctate shallow central barium collections surrounded by halo of edema
    - Cobblestoning: Combination of longitudinal & transverse ulcers
    - Deep fissuring ulcers
    - Mural thickening: Transmural inflammation, fibrosis
  - Late changes
    - Skip lesions: Segmental/normal intervening areas
    - Sacculations seen on antimesenteric border (↑ luminal pressure)
    - Postinflammatory pseudopolyps, haustral loss, intramural abscess
    - "String sign": Luminal narrowing + ileal stricture
    - Sinus tracts, fissures, fistulas are hallmarks of disease

DDx: Thickened Wall, Narrowed Lumen at Ileocecal Junction

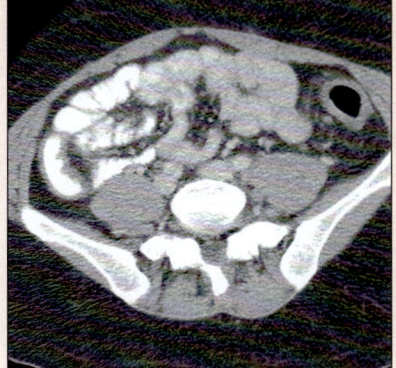

Backwash Ileitis

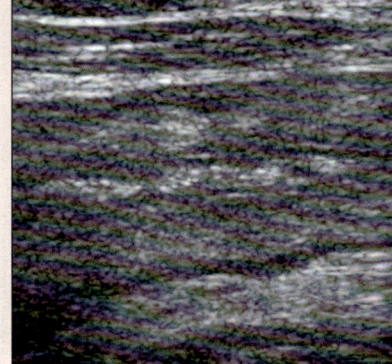

Yersinia Ileitis

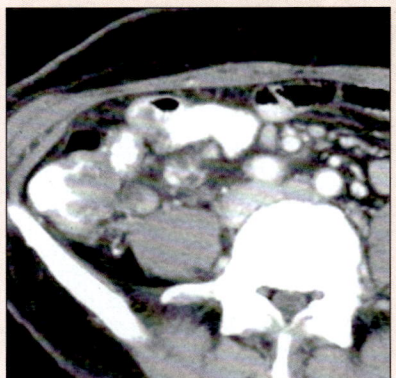

Ileocecal TB

CROHN DISEASE

Key Facts

Terminology
- Terminal ileitis, regional enteritis, ileocolitis
- Chronic, recurrent, segmental, granulomatous inflammatory bowel disease

Imaging Findings
- Best diagnostic clue: Segmental areas of ileo-colonic ulceration and wall thickening on barium study
- Skip lesions (segmental or discontinuous)
- Transmural, granulomas (noncaseating type)
- Cobblestone mucosa, fissures & fistulas

Top Differential Diagnoses
- Ulcerative Colitis ("Backwash" Ileitis)
- Infection
- Ischemia
- Radiation Enteritis
- Metastases & Lymphoma
- Mesenteric Adenitis

Pathology
- Exact etiology unknown
- Immunologic: Antibody & cell-mediated types

Clinical Issues
- Diarrhea, pain, melena, weight loss, fever
- Malabsorption; fissures & fistulas (perianal area)
- Complications: Fistula, sinus, toxic megacolon, obstruction, perforation, malignancy

Diagnostic Checklist
- Associated findings (cholangitis, arthritis)
- Small bowel wall thickening, mesenteric fat proliferation & hyperemia on CECT

- Anorectal lesions: Ulcers, fissures, abscesses, hemorrhoids, stenosis

CT Findings
- Discontinuous & asymmetric bowel wall thickening > 1 cm
- Minimal narrowing in acute or noncicatrizing phase
  - Soft tissue density inner ring (mucosa)
  - Low density middle ring (submucosal edema/fat)
  - Soft tissue density outer ring (muscularis propria-serosa)
  - Proliferation of mesenteric fat ± lymphadenopathy
  - Target or "double halo" sign
    - Intense enhancement of mucosa + muscularis propria
    - ↓ Attenuation in edematous thickened submucosa
- ↑ Luminal narrowing, no target sign in chronic or cicatrizing phase
  - Mural stratification lost: Indistinct mucosa, submucosa, muscularis propria
  - Homogeneous attenuation of thickened bowel wall on CECT
  - Abscesses, fistulas, sinus tracts
  - Mesenteric changes: Abscess, fibrofatty areas, nodes
  - Perianal disease, enlarged mesenteric lymph nodes
  - "Comb" sign: Mesenteric hypervascularity (dilatation, tortuosity, wide spacing)
  - Soft tissue density inner ring (mucosa)

MR Findings
- Breath-holding (FLASH), fat suppression & Gd-DTPA show extent, mural thickening & severity
- Sensitive in detecting fistulas, sinuses & abscesses in perianal Crohn disease

Ultrasonographic Findings
- Grayscale Ultrasound
  - Transrectal sonography
    - Mural thickening, abscesses, fistulas
    - Anal sphincter heterogeneity

Imaging Recommendations
- Best imaging tool
  - Barium enema, enteroclysis
  - MDCT with and without contrast
  - MR for perianal & rectal Crohn disease

DIFFERENTIAL DIAGNOSIS

Ulcerative Colitis ("Backwash" Ileitis)
- 25% of cases have terminal ileal pathology
- Widely patent ileocecal valve, slightly thickened folds
- Mucosa may have nodular or granular pattern
- No strictures/ulcerations; adjacent colonic lesions seen
- Lesions usually continuous, non-transmural, pseudopolyps

Infection
- Yersiniosis: Yersinia enterocolitica
  - Commonly located in terminal ileum
  - Thickened mucosal folds, nodules, aphthous ulcers
  - Lumen narrowing is rare
  - Superficial ulcerations
  - Resolution in 6-8 weeks
- Particularly seen in AIDS patients: Mycobacterial, cryptosporidiosis, CMV
- Typical: Mycobacterium tuberculosis
  - Ileocecal (> common): Transmural, stenosis, fistulas
  - Horizontal ulcers, nodular mucosal thickening
  - Cecal contraction & widely patent ileocecal valve
  - Pericecal lymphadenopathy on CT
- Atypical: Mycobacterium avium-intracellulare (MAI)
  - Small bowel most common site
  - Diffusely thickened folds, micronodular mucosa
  - Mesenteric adenopathy & abscess on CT
- Cryptosporidiosis
  - Most common cause of enteritis in AIDS patients
  - Thickening of folds & bowel wall; ↑ fluid in lumen
  - CT may show small lymph nodes
  - Oocysts in stool & mucosal biopsy
- Cytomegalovirus (CMV)
  - Terminal ileitis indistinguishable from Crohn disease
  - Round intranuclear inclusion bodies

CROHN DISEASE

Ischemia
- Due to vascular insufficiency
- Superior mesenteric artery (SMA) clot or narrowing
  - Pneumatosis: Bubble or "band-like" air in affected small bowel wall, segmental thickening > 3 mm
  - ± Gas in mesenteric or portal vein

Radiation Enteritis
- Due to therapeutic or excessive abdominal irradiation
- Terminal ileum, adjacent colon & rectum
- Thickened bowel wall, narrow pelvic bowel loops
- ± Strictures, sinuses, fistulas simulating Crohn disease

Metastases & Lymphoma
- Non-Hodgkin lymphoma: More common
  - Stomach (51%), small bowel (33%)
  - Nodular, polypoid, infiltrating, invading mesentery
  - Focally infiltrating form of terminal ileum
    - Widened segment devoid of folds
    - Sausage-shaped thickening of affected bowel wall
    - May be indistinguishable from Crohn disease
- Metastases (small bowel)
  - Located along antimesenteric border
  - Malignant melanoma
    - Smoothly polypoid lesions, varied sizes
    - Polypoid lesion with ulcers & radiating folds form typical "spoke-wheel" pattern
  - Bronchogenic carcinoma
    - Single or multiple flat/polypoid intramural lesions, frequently ulcerated, cause narrowing, obstruction
  - Breast carcinoma
    - Highly cellular submucosal masses

Mesenteric Adenitis
- Common cause of right lower quadrant (RLQ) pain in children & adolescents
- Enlarged mesenteric nodes, ileal wall thickening
- Usually resolves spontaneously in 2-4 days

PATHOLOGY

General Features
- General path comments
  - Three stages based on pathology
    - Early: Hyperplasia of lymphoid tissue, obstructive lymphedema in submucosa → shallow mucosal erosions (aphthoid ulcers)
    - Intermediate: Transmural extension in mucosa & submucosa → marked fold thickening
    - Advanced: Transmural extension to serosa & beyond → deep linear clefts of ulceration/fissures
- Genetics
  - Familial disposition
  - Common in monozygotic twins & siblings
  - Polygenic inheritance pattern
- Etiology
  - Exact etiology unknown
  - Possible factors considered
    - Immunologic: Antibody & cell-mediated types
    - Nutritional, hormonal, vascular & traumatic
    - Genetic, environmental, psychologic
- Epidemiology: Four-fold ↑ in incidence with smoking
- Associated abnormalities: Arthritis, gallstones, sclerosing cholangitis, uveitis, ankylosing spondylitis

Gross Pathologic & Surgical Features
- Skip lesions more common in distal ileum
- Edema, inflammation, fibrosis, luminal narrowing
- Adhesions, fistulas, fissures, strictures

Microscopic Features
- Transmural inflammation, lymphoid aggregates, noncaseating granulomas

CLINICAL ISSUES

Presentation
- Most common signs/symptoms
  - Diarrhea, pain, melena, weight loss, fever
  - Malabsorption; fissures & fistulas (perianal area)

Demographics
- Age: Age: 15-25 years (small peak at 50-80 years)
- Gender: M = F
- Ethnicity: More in Caucasians & Jewish

Natural History & Prognosis
- Complications: Fistula, sinus, toxic megacolon, obstruction, perforation, malignancy
- Prognosis
  - 10-20% lead symptom-free lives
  - 30-53% recurrence after surgical resection, usually proximal side of anastomosis

Treatment
- Mucosal biopsy to diagnose
- Medical
  - Steroids, azathioprine, mesalamine
  - Metronidazole, antibody treatment
- Surgical
  - Resection of diseased bowel
  - Strictureplasty, primary fistulotomy

DIAGNOSTIC CHECKLIST

Consider
- Associated findings (cholangitis, arthritis)

Image Interpretation Pearls
- Small bowel wall thickening, mesenteric fat proliferation & hyperemia on CECT

SELECTED REFERENCES
1. Wold PB et al: Assessment of small bowel Crohn disease: noninvasive peroral CT enterography compared with other imaging methods and endoscopy--feasibility study. Radiology. 229(1):275-81, 2003
2. Antes G: Inflammatory disease of the small intestine and colon: Contrast enema and CT. Radiology. 38:41-5, 1998
3. Gore RM et al: CT features of ulcerative colitis and Crohn's disease. AJR. 167:3-15, 1996
4. Hizawa K et al: Crohn disease: early recognition and progress of aphthous lesions. Radiology. 190:451-4, 1994

CROHN DISEASE

IMAGE GALLERY

Typical

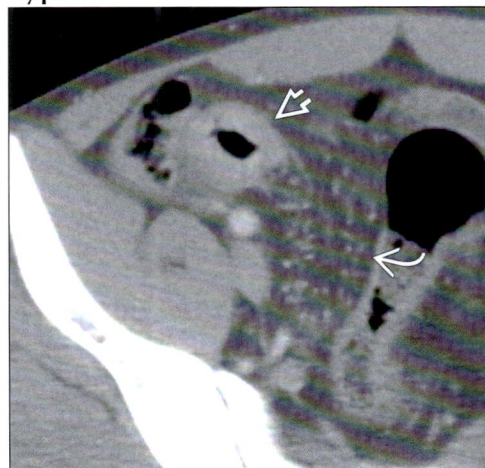
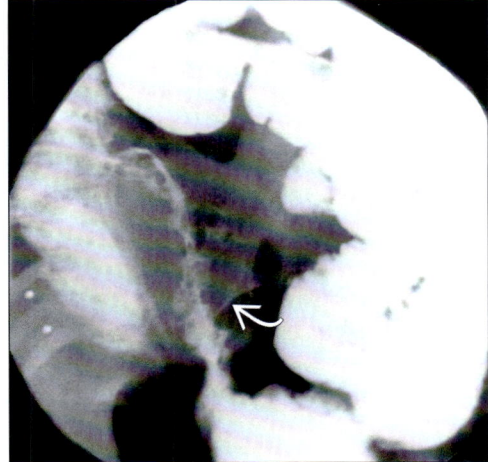

(Left) Axial CECT shows mural thickening of the terminal ileum ➡ and luminal narrowing. Note hyperemia of mesenteric blood vessels supplying inflamed bowel ➡. *(Right)* Small bowel follow through shows longitudinal & transverse ulcerations of ileal mucosa ("cobblestoning") and luminal narrowing. Opacified sinus tract ➡ is also seen.

Typical

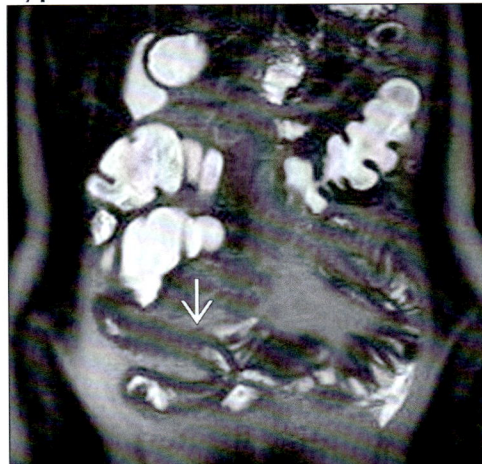
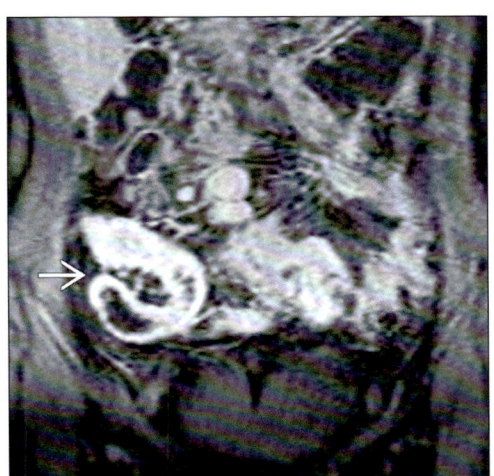

(Left) Coronal T2WI MR shows classic appearance, thickened bowel loop in RLQ, neoterminal ileum ➡. *(Right)* Coronal T1 C+ FS MR (same patient as previous image) shows vivid enhancement of bowel loop post-contrast ➡. Adjacent small bowel and colon do not enhance with same intensity as affected loop.

Typical

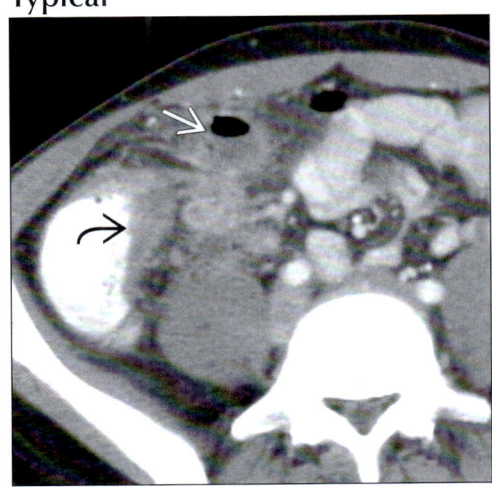
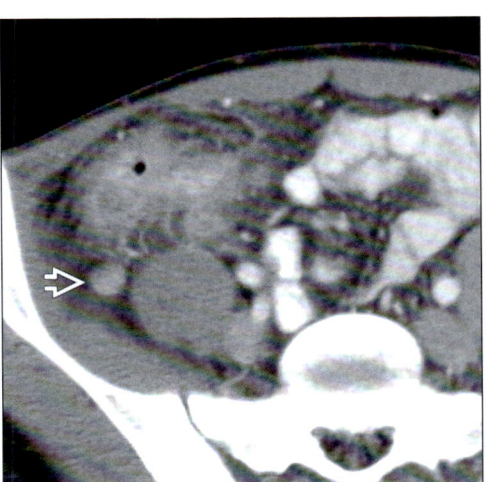

(Left) Axial CECT shows extensive bowel wall thickening ➡ of distal ileum & marked inflammatory infiltration of adjacent mesentery. Note extraluminal bubbles of gas, and presence of small abscess ➡. *(Right)* Axial CECT (same patient as previous image, at lower level) demonstrates enlarged mesenteric nodes ➡.

PNEUMATOSIS OF THE INTESTINE

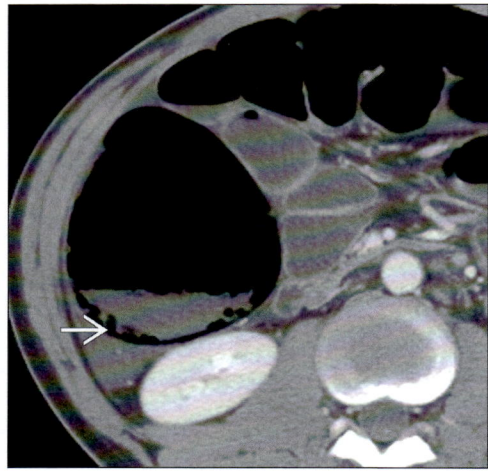

Axial CECT shows cecal pneumatosis due to bowel infarction. Note dilated cecum with intramural air posteriorly ➡.

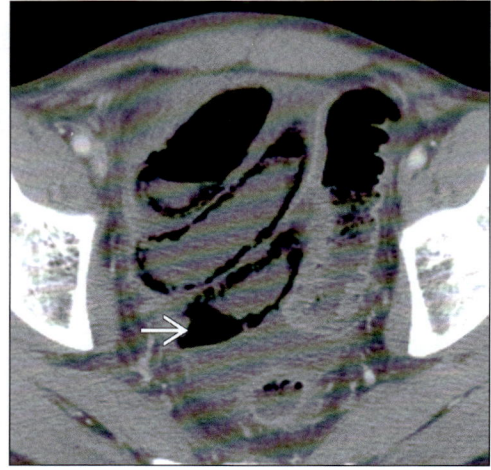

Axial CECT in same patient as left at more caudal level demonstrates extensive pneumatosis of distal ileum ➡.

TERMINOLOGY

Abbreviations and Synonyms
- Pneumatosis cystoides intestinalis; pneumatosis intestinalis; intestinal gas cysts

Definitions
- Cystic or linear collections of gas in subserosal or submucosal layers of gastrointestinal tract wall

IMAGING FINDINGS

General Features
- Best diagnostic clue: Cystic or linear distribution of gas along bowel wall on MDCT
- Classified into primary and secondary pneumatosis intestinalis
  - Primary usually insignificant, asymptomatic, idiopathic
  - Secondary usually due to ischemia, medication or other known etiology
- Pneumatosis intestinalis is a sign, not a disease

Radiographic Findings
- Radiography
  - Primary: Cystic gas collections along wall of colon
  - Secondary: Linear distribution of gas along small bowel or colon, dilated bowel loops

Fluoroscopic Findings
- Barium studies
  - Primary
    - Radiolucent cysts, resembling polyps, clustered along contours of colon
    - Multiple large gas-filled cysts with scalloped defects in bowel wall, resembling inflammatory pseudopolyps
    - Thumbprinting seen with intramural hemorrhage
    - Concentric compression of lumen by cysts
    - Striking lucency of gas-filled cysts
  - Secondary
    - Mottled, bubbly or linear collection of gas in bowel wall; feces-like appearance
    - Dilated bowel loops ± thumbprinting

CT Findings
- CECT

DDx: Pneumatosis of the Small Bowel

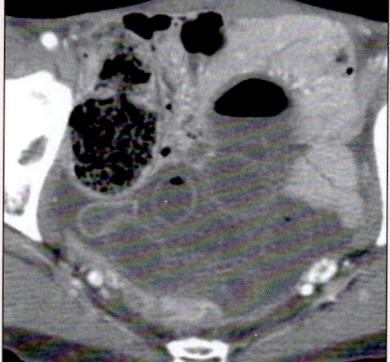

Bowel Necrosis

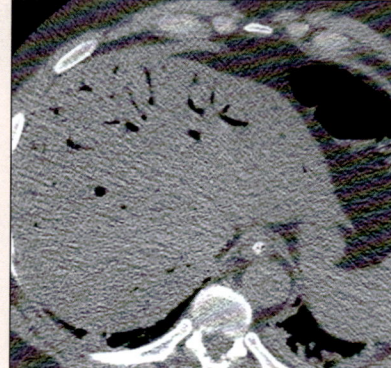

Post-Endoscopy

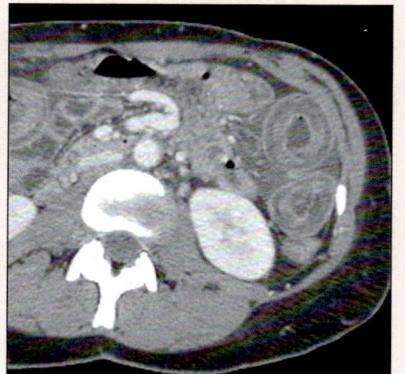

Lupus

PNEUMATOSIS OF THE INTESTINE

Key Facts

Terminology
- Pneumatosis cystoides intestinalis; pneumatosis intestinalis; intestinal gas cysts
- Cystic or linear collections of gas in subserosal or submucosal layers of gastrointestinal tract wall

Imaging Findings
- Best diagnostic clue: Cystic or linear distribution of gas along bowel wall on MDCT
- Pneumatosis intestinalis is a sign, not a disease
- Best imaging tool: MDCT with lung window to detect intramural and venous gas
- Water for oral contrast facilitates CT angiography
- MDCT with IV contrast at 3-4 mL/sec, 1.5-3 mm collimation

Top Differential Diagnoses
- Bowel Necrosis
- Post-Endoscopy
- Post-Operative
- Medication-Induced
- Autoimmune Disease
- Pulmonary Disease

Diagnostic Checklist
- Bowel necrosis is a surgical emergency
- Prognosis depends on underlying cause, not imaging findings
- Other causes of pneumatosis intestinalis usually are asymptomatic; little clinical significance
- Important to recognize pneumatosis intestinalis, but significance depends on etiology and clinical setting

---

- Primary
  - "Bubble-like": Isolated bubbles of air or clusters of cysts in left colonic wall
- Secondary
  - "Band-like": Bands or linear distribution of air in affected bowel wall
  - Linear or curvilinear shape
  - Ischemic etiology: Dilated bowel lumen (ileus), thickened wall, abnormal enhancement
  - ± Pneumoperitoneum or pneumoretroperitoneum
  - ± Mesenteric or portal venous gas (portal venous gas collects in liver periphery; biliary gas collects in central ducts near porta hepatis)
  - ± Mesenteric arterial or venous thrombosis

Imaging Recommendations
- Best imaging tool: MDCT with lung window to detect intramural and venous gas
- Protocol advice
  - Water for oral contrast facilitates CT angiography
  - MDCT with IV contrast at 3-4 mL/sec, 1.5-3 mm collimation
    - 35 second image delay, repeat venous phase after 80 seconds
    - Multiplanar reformation for CT angiography

DIFFERENTIAL DIAGNOSIS

Bowel Necrosis
- Ischemic enteritis, volvulus, necrotizing enterocolitis
- Mucosal damage → entry of bacteria (mainly enteric organisms) into bowel wall → gas in wall
- Necrotizing enterocolitis
  - Ileum and right colon
  - Feces-like appearance in right bowel
  - Premature or debilitated infants
  - Gas in intrahepatic branches of portal vein is catastrophic sign
- Ischemic colitis or enteritis
  - Colonic ischemia often due to hypoperfusion in elderly or debilitated
  - Small bowel infarction often due to embolus, thrombus of large vessels (superior mesenteric artery or vein)
    - Associated mesenteric infiltration
  - Late phase of ischemia → diffuse or localized pneumatosis intestinalis ± mesenteric or portal venous gas
    - Pneumatosis intestinalis can occur with either transmural or partial mural ischemia

Post-Endoscopy
- Mucosal disruption and ↑ pressure → ↑ distension → air dissection into wall

Post-Operative
- Intestinal bypass
- Mucosal disruption and ↑ pressure → ↑ distension → air dissection into wall

Medication-Induced
- Steroids or immunosuppressives
- ↑ Mucosal permeability and ↓ immune system → bacterial gas in wall

Autoimmune Disease
- Systemic lupus erythematosus
- ↑ Mucosal permeability and ↓ immune system → bacterial gas in wall

Pseudopneumatosis
- Gas trapped against mucosal surface of bowel by semisolid feces
- Most common in ascending colon

Pulmonary Disease
- Chronic obstructive pulmonary disease and ventilator (barotrauma)
- Partial bronchial obstruction & coughing → alveolar rupture → air dissection into peribronchial & perivascular tissue planes of mediastinum → hiatus of esophagus & aorta → retroperitoneum → mesentery → subserosa and submucosa of bowel wall

PNEUMATOSIS OF THE INTESTINE

PATHOLOGY

General Features
- General path comments
  - Portal venous gas often accompanies pneumatosis intestinalis
    - Amount of gas does not correlate with etiology, prognosis or need for treatment
    - Not always due to bowel infarction
    - Increased likelihood of transmural infarction from ischemic enteritis versus ischemic colitis
- Etiology
  - 85% of pneumatosis intestinalis is secondary
  - 15% is primary
  - Secondary pneumatosis intestinalis (> 50 reported causes)
    - Bowel necrosis (most common): Necrotizing enterocolitis, bowel infarction, caustic ingestion
    - Mucosal disruption: Endoscopy, ulcers, obstruction, inflammatory bowel disease (IBD, bowel anastomoses
    - Increased mucosal permeability: Steroids, chemotherapy, immunosuppressive therapy, immunodeficiency states
    - Autoimmune: Systemic lupus erythematosus, scleroderma or other collagen vascular diseases
    - Pulmonary: Asthma, chronic obstructive pulmonary disease, positive pressure ventilation, pneumothorax or trauma
  - Portal venous gas
    - Intestinal wall lesions: Ischemia, IBD
    - Bowel distention: Endoscopy, obstruction, trauma
    - Sepsis: Diverticulitis, cholecystitis, appendicitis, colitis including Clostridium difficile infection
  - Pathogenesis
    - Intraluminal gastrointestinal gas: Intramural pressure or mucosal injury → gas entering wall
    - Bacterial gas production: Bacterial invasion → has high tension → gas diffusion
    - Pulmonary gas: Air dissection

Gross Pathologic & Surgical Features
- Primary: Gas cysts in otherwise normal colon
- Secondary: Bowel often abnormal or ischemic

Microscopic Features
- Primary
  - Multiple thin-walled, noncommunicating, gas-filled cysts in subserosal or submucosal layer of bowel
  - Normal muscularis and mucosa
- Secondary
  - Linear streaks of gas parallel to bowel wall
  - Necrotic, inflammatory, ulcerative or ischemic features

CLINICAL ISSUES

Presentation
- Most common signs/symptoms
  - Primary: Asymptomatic; insignificant
  - Secondary: Abdominal pain, distension, melena, fever, vomiting, cough (depends on etiology)

Demographics
- Age
  - Primary: Adults
  - Secondary: Any age
- Gender: M = F

Natural History & Prognosis
- Complications: Spontaneous rupture of pneumatosis → pneumoperitoneum
- Prognosis
  - Primary: Good
  - Secondary: Depends on etiology of gas, not extent
  - Detection of pneumatosis & portomesenteric venous gas
    - Positive on radiography: 75% mortality
    - Positive on CT (more sensitive): 25% mortality
  - Pneumatosis associated with pneumoperitoneum or portal venous gas can be benign, transient
  - Benign or catastrophic prognosis cannot be distinguished by imaging

Treatment
- Primary: No treatment, resolves spontaneously
- Secondary: Dependent on etiology
  - Oxygen may be beneficial: ↓ Gas tension in tissues

DIAGNOSTIC CHECKLIST

Consider
- Bowel necrosis is a surgical emergency
- Prognosis depends on underlying cause, not imaging findings
- Other causes of pneumatosis intestinalis usually are asymptomatic; little clinical significance

Image Interpretation Pearls
- Important to recognize pneumatosis intestinalis, but significance depends on etiology and clinical setting

SELECTED REFERENCES

1. Hou SK et al: Hepatic portal venous gas: clinical significance of computed tomography findings. Am J Emerg Med. 22(3):214-8, 2004
2. See C et al: Images in clinical medicine. Pneumatosis intestinalis and portal venous gas. N Engl J Med. 350(4):e3, 2004
3. Sherman SC et al: Pneumatosis intestinalis and portomesenteric venous gas. J Emerg Med. 26(2):213-5, 2004
4. Taourel P et al: Cecal pneumatosis in patients with obstructive colon cancer: correlation of CT findings with bowel viability. AJR Am J Roentgenol. 183(6):1667-71, 2004
5. Kernagis LY et al: Pneumatosis intestinalis in patients with ischemia: correlation of CT findings with viability of the bowel. AJR Am J Roentgenol. 180(3):733-6, 2003
6. St Peter SD et al: The spectrum of pneumatosis intestinalis. Arch Surg. 138(1):68-75, 2003
7. Sebastia C et al: Portomesenteric vein gas: Pathologic mechanisms, CT findings and prognosis. Radiographics. 20: 1213-24, 2000
8. Pear BL: Pneumatosis intestinalis: A review. Radiology. 207: 13-19, 1998

PNEUMATOSIS OF THE INTESTINE

IMAGE GALLERY

Typical

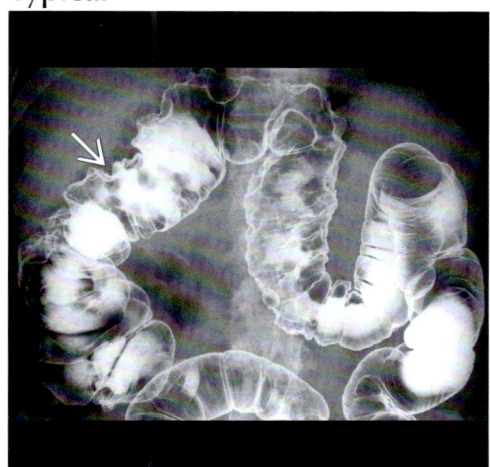
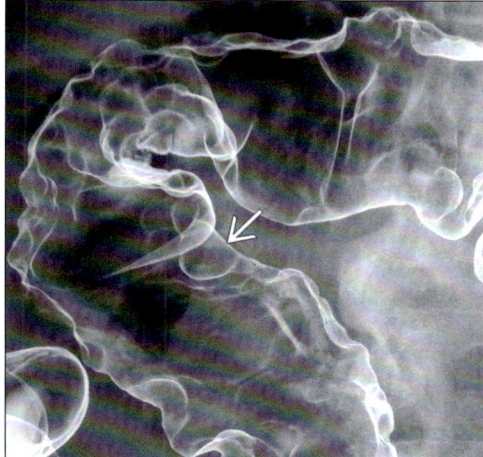

(Left) Frontal contrast enema shows classic benign pneumatosis. Note polypoid lesions ➡ representing gas cysts within colon wall, with barium outlining distortion of mucosal surface. *(Right)* Oblique contrast enema in same patient as left demonstrates submucosal presence of gas density ➡ that allows correct diagnosis.

Typical

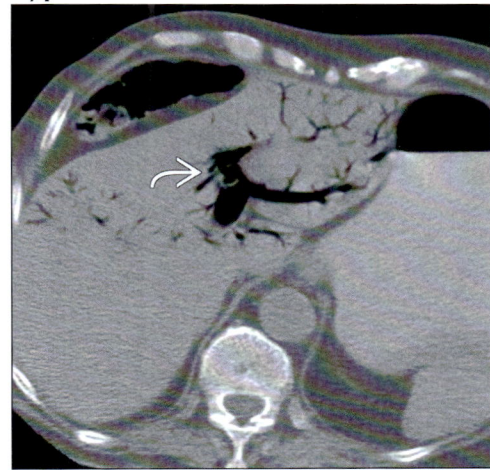
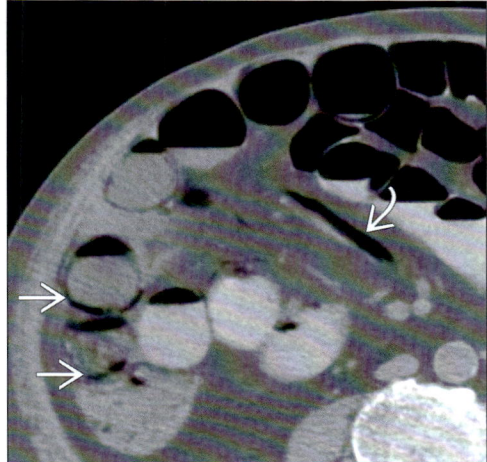

(Left) Axial CECT shows extensive gas within mesenteric veins and intrahepatic portal veins ➡. *(Right)* Axial CECT in same patient as left shows extensive small intestinal pneumatosis ➡ and again demonstrates gas within mesenteric and intrahepatic portal veins ➡.

Variant

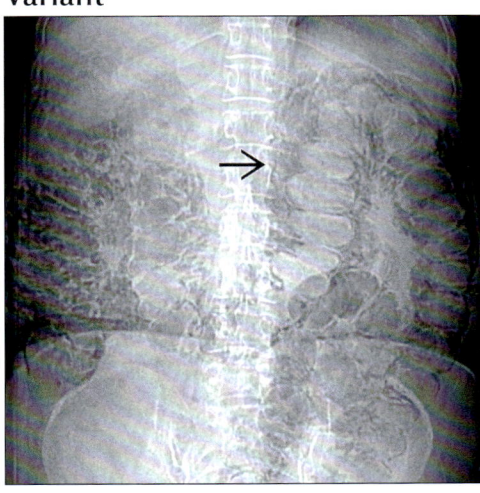
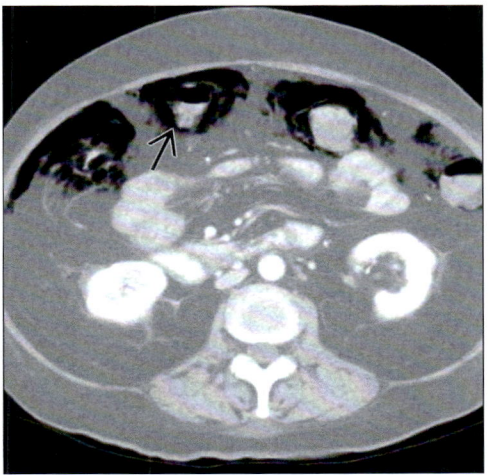

(Left) Frontal radiograph shows extensive pneumatosis ➡ within wall of the colon. Note the absence of ascites or ileus. *(Right)* Axial CECT in same patient as left shows extensive pneumatosis ➡ within colon wall. No clinical/laboratory evidence of ischemia; presumed etiology steroid use/other immunosuppressive medications.

ACUTE SMALL BOWEL ISCHEMIA

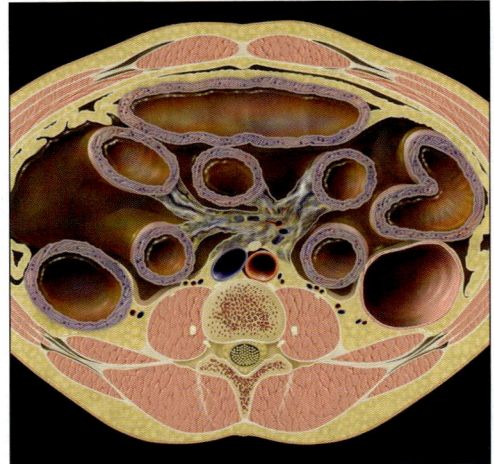

Graphic shows dilated small intestine with thickened wall, ascites, + edematous mesentery; findings seen typically with occlusion of the superior mesenteric vein.

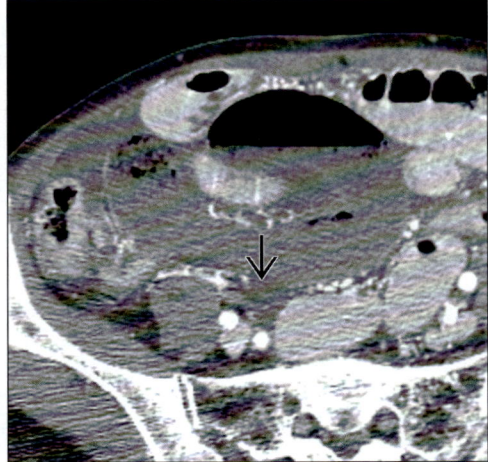

Axial CECT of acute small bowel ischemia due to mesenteric vascular occlusion. Note dilated loop of distal small bowel with lack of bowel wall enhancement ➡.

TERMINOLOGY

Abbreviations and Synonyms
- Acute mesenteric ischemia

Definitions
- Mesenteric arterial or venous narrowing/occlusion leading to inadequate supply of nutrients & oxygen to small intestine

IMAGING FINDINGS

General Features
- Best diagnostic clue: Clot or narrowing of superior mesenteric artery (SMA) or superior mesenteric vein (SMV) with bowel wall thickening
- Other general features
  o Imaging findings vary: Acute vs. chronic; arterial vs. venous thrombosis
  o Late phase ischemia can lead to diffuse or localized pneumatosis intestinalis

Radiographic Findings
- Radiography
  o Multiple air-fluid levels; ileus pattern
  o Thickening of valvulae conniventes
  o Linear distribution of gas (pneumatosis intestinalis)

Fluoroscopic Findings
- Barium studies
  o Thickening of valvulae conniventes
  o "Thumbprinting": Intramural accumulation of blood distending submucosa → focally rounded mesenteric folds, especially along mesenteric border
  o "Stack of coins": Enlarged, smooth, straight, parallel folds perpendicular to longitudinal axis of small bowel (submucosal edema)
  o Strictures often seen with proximal bowel dilation
  o Mottled, frothy, bubbly or linear collections of gas in bowel wall (pneumatosis intestinalis)

CT Findings
- CECT
  o Clot or reduced lumen in SMA, SMV or other mesenteric vessels

DDx: Thickened Bowel Wall with Mesenteric Infiltration

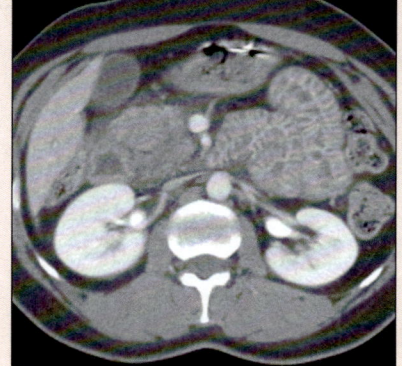

"Shock Bowel"

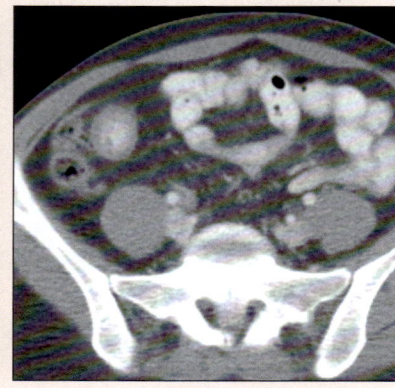

Crohn Disease

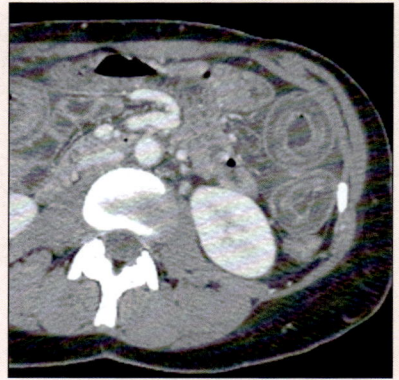

Lupus

ACUTE SMALL BOWEL ISCHEMIA

Key Facts

Terminology
- Acute mesenteric ischemia
- Mesenteric arterial or venous narrowing/occlusion leading to inadequate supply of nutrients & oxygen to small intestine

Imaging Findings
- Best diagnostic clue: Clot or narrowing of superior mesenteric artery (SMA) or superior mesenteric vein (SMV) with bowel wall thickening
- Segmental thickening of bowel wall (> 3 mm); average 8 mm, up to 20 mm

Top Differential Diagnoses
- "Shock Bowel"
- Crohn Disease
- Fibrosing Mesenteritis
- Lupus Enteritis

Pathology
- Vascular occlusion: Embolic events (atrial fibrillation, endocarditis), thrombotic events (atherosclerosis) or mechanical obstruction (strangulation, tumor)

Clinical Issues
- Unremitting abdominal pain disproportionate to physical exam findings
- Intestinal angina: Postprandial abdominal pain subsiding 1-2 hours after meal

Diagnostic Checklist
- Small bowel ischemia is clinico-radiological diagnosis
- Prognosis depends on underlying cause, not imaging
- Gas-filled dilated intestinal loops with multiple air-fluid levels; bowel wall thickening

---

  ○ Segmental thickening of bowel wall (> 3 mm); average 8 mm, up to 20 mm
  ○ Emboli usually observed at origin of SMA or 3-10 cm from SMA distal to middle colic artery
  ○ Lack of mucosal enhancement due to compromised arterial flow
  ○ "Misty mesentery": Mesenteric fat infiltrated by edema; more common with venous thrombosis
  ○ Increased attenuation (venous > arterial thrombosis) due to submucosal hemorrhage or hyperemia
  ○ Pneumatosis intestinalis (venous > arterial thrombus)
    ▪ "Band-like" or "bubble-like" appearance in bowel wall
    ▪ Linear, curvilinear, or cystic gas-filled spaces
    ▪ ± Gas in mesenteric or portal vein
    ▪ Bowel loops partially fluid-filled

Ultrasonographic Findings
- Duplex Doppler
  ○ Mainly used to assess degree of narrowing or occlusion in chronic ischemia
  ○ Narrowed or occluded vessels → ↓ blood flow

Angiographic Findings
- Acute arterial ischemia: Clot or stenosis of SMA or its branches
- Acute venous ischemia: SMV occlusion with collaterals
- Nonocclusive ischemia: Slow flow in SMA
- Chronic ischemia: Narrowing or occlusion of celiac artery, SMA or inferior mesenteric artery
  ○ Increased collateral arteries

Imaging Recommendations
- Best imaging tool
  ○ MDCT with CT angiography
    ▪ More sensitive in assessing strangulation of bowel
    ▪ Lung window setting for pneumatosis intestinalis
  ○ Angiography
    ▪ Diagnostic confirmation and treatment

DIFFERENTIAL DIAGNOSIS

"Shock Bowel"
- Ischemia ± reperfusion of small bowel, usually following trauma or other cause of hypotension
- Intense mucosal enhancement, edema of submucosa and mesentery
- Reversible with resuscitation

Crohn Disease
- Usually affecting distal small bowel
- Asymmetric, discontinuous, thickened bowel wall, proliferation of mesenteric fat
- Persistent fold abnormalities
- Focal, inflammatory, mucosal ulceration & patchy submucosal fibrosis → distortion & interruption of folds

Fibrosing Mesenteritis
- Idiopathic inflammation & fibrosis involving mesenteric fatty tissue
- Bowel wall thickening uncommon, 2° fibrotic constriction of mesenteric veins & lymphatics
- "Misty mesentery" appearance, halo of fat surrounding but not displacing mesenteric vessels
- Mesenteric soft tissue mass (advanced)
- Calcifications seen histologically; rare radiologically

Lupus Enteritis
- Focal bowel wall thickening
- Submucosal edema, "target sign"
- Ascites and peritoneal enhancement

PATHOLOGY

General Features
- General path comments
  ○ Accounts for 1% of acute abdomen
  ○ Arterial > venous occlusive ischemia: 9:1
  ○ 60-70% of acute ischemia due to arterial occlusion, 5-10% due to venous occlusion
  ○ 20-30% of acute ischemia is nonocclusive

ACUTE SMALL BOWEL ISCHEMIA

- Etiology
  - Vascular occlusion: Embolic events (atrial fibrillation, endocarditis), thrombotic events (atherosclerosis) or mechanical obstruction (strangulation, tumor)
  - Closed loop obstruction especially dangerous
  - Hypercoagulable states: Oral contraceptives, protein C deficiency, factor V Leiden deficiency
  - Inflammatory: Pancreatitis, peritonitis or vasculitis
    - Common cause of ischemia in younger patients
    - Systemic lupus erythematosus, polyarteritis nodosa, other collagen vascular diseases
    - Vasculitis may affect kidneys and other organs
    - Angiography may show microaneurysms and occluded vessels
  - Iatrogenic causes: Radiation and chemotherapy, therapeutic drugs (digitalis, dopamine, vasopressin), illicit drugs (heroin, cocaine)
  - Hypoperfusion (more common in ischemic colitis): Low flow states, hypotension, sepsis, heart failure
- Epidemiology: Risk factors of chronic ischemia include hypertension, coronary artery disease, cerebrovascular disease

Gross Pathologic & Surgical Features
- Discolored (purple), infarcted small bowel

Microscopic Features
- Necrotic, inflammatory or ischemic features in small bowel wall

Staging, Grading or Classification Criteria
- Classification
  - Acute occlusive ischemia (arterial or venous)
  - Acute nonocclusive ischemia
  - Chronic ischemia: Older "vasculopaths"

CLINICAL ISSUES

Presentation
- Most common signs/symptoms
  - Acute ischemia
    - Clinical triad: Sudden onset of abdominal pain, diarrhea, vomiting
    - Unremitting abdominal pain disproportionate to physical exam findings
    - Abdominal distention, tenesmus & passage of bloody stool
    - Guarding and rebound (infarction or perforation)
    - Venous ischemia has more gradual onset
  - Chronic ischemia
    - Intestinal angina: Postprandial abdominal pain subsiding 1-2 hours after meal
    - Nausea, vomiting, diarrhea, weight loss
    - Intense pain → fear of eating (sitophobia)
  - Lab data
    - ↑ WBC: 75%; Acidosis: 50%; ↑ amylase: 25%
  - Diagnosis
    - High clinical suspicion key to early diagnosis

Demographics
- Age: Majority > 50 years of age
- Gender: M = F

Natural History & Prognosis
- Complications: Stricture, infarction, necrosis, perforation
- Prognosis
  - Acute ischemia
    - Depends on promptness of diagnosis and amount of salvageable small bowel
    - After surgical resection, results in venous ischemia patients are generally better
    - 50-90% mortality
  - Chronic ischemia
    - Survival dependent on degree of collateral circulation
    - Diagnosis requires occlusion of at least two major mesenteric arteries and narrowing of a third artery
  - Infarction: 69% mortality (in recent series)

Treatment
- Surgical treatment
  - Exploratory laparotomy, bowel resection & mesenteric bypass to re-establish blood flow
  - Main treatment for acute ischemia, chronic ischemia & complications
- Endovascular intervention
  - Intra-arterial thrombolysis, percutaneous transluminal angioplasty ± stent placement
  - Thrombolytics (streptokinase or urokinase)
  - Vasodilators (papaverine) to reduce vasospasm
- Systemic anticoagulation (warfarin or heparin) for venous occlusion

DIAGNOSTIC CHECKLIST

Consider
- Small bowel ischemia is clinico-radiological diagnosis
- Consult referring physician for history, symptoms, key lab values

Image Interpretation Pearls
- Prognosis depends on underlying cause, not imaging
- Gas-filled dilated intestinal loops with multiple air-fluid levels; bowel wall thickening

SELECTED REFERENCES

1. Burns BJ et al: Intestinal ischemia. Gastroenterol Clin North Am. 32(4):1127-43, 2003
2. Chou CK et al: CT of small bowel ischemia. Abdom Imaging, 24-30, 2003
3. Segatto E et al: Acute small bowel ischemia: CT imaging findings. Semin Ultrasound CT MR. 24(5):364-76, 2003
4. Tendler DA: Acute intestinal ischemia and infarction. Semin Gastrointest Dis. 14(2):66-76, 2003
5. Wiesner W et al: CT of acute bowel ischemia. Radiology. 226(3):635-50, 2003
6. Horton KM et al: Computed tomography evaluation of intestinal ischemia. Semin Roentgenol. 36(2):118-25, 2001
7. Horton KM et al: Multi-detector row CT of mesenteric ischemia: can it be done? Radiographics. 21(6):1463-73, 2001
8. Singer A et al: Acute small bowel ischemia: Spectrum of computed tomographic findings. Emer Radiol. 7: 302-307, 2000

ACUTE SMALL BOWEL ISCHEMIA

IMAGE GALLERY

Typical

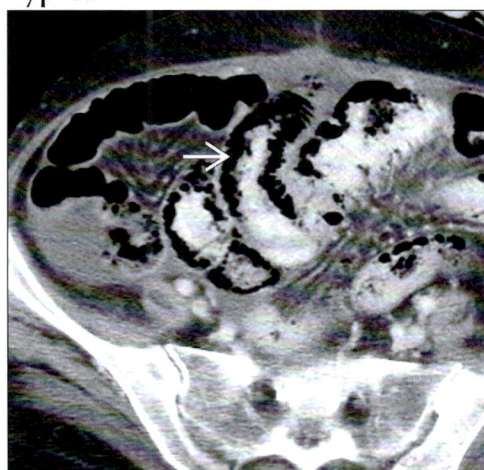
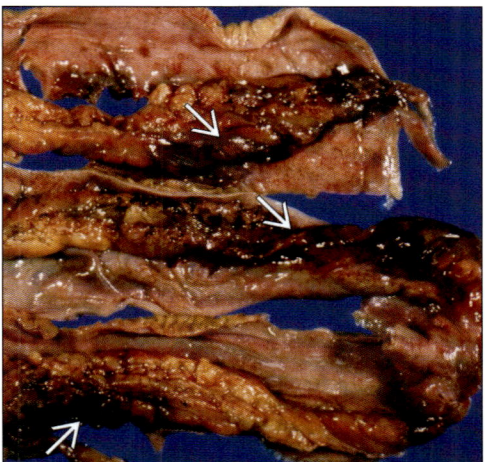

(Left) Axial NECT shows small bowel infarction. Note extensive pneumatosis of distal small bowel ➡. *(Right)* Surgical specimen from patient imaged at left reveals multiple areas of hemorrhagic necrosis ➡.

Typical

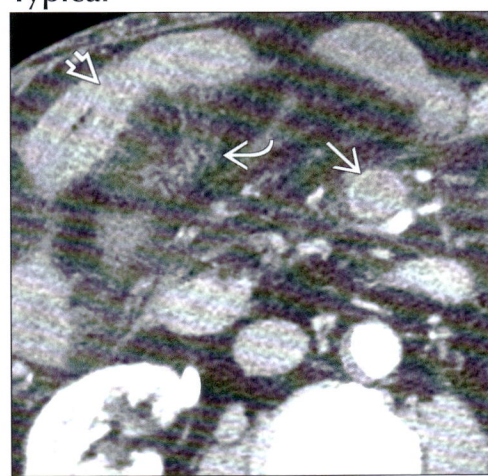
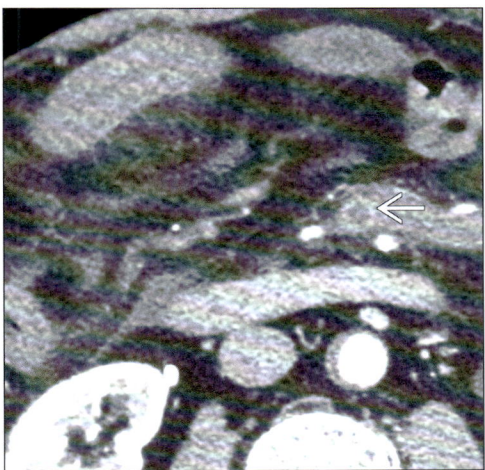

(Left) Axial CECT demonstrates acute mesenteric venous thrombosis. Note distended SMV from acute clot ➡, adjacent mesenteric edema ➡, and bowel wall thickening from ischemia ➡. *(Right)* Axial CECT at more caudal level of same patient as left demonstrates "rim sign" of venous thrombosis ➡.

Variant

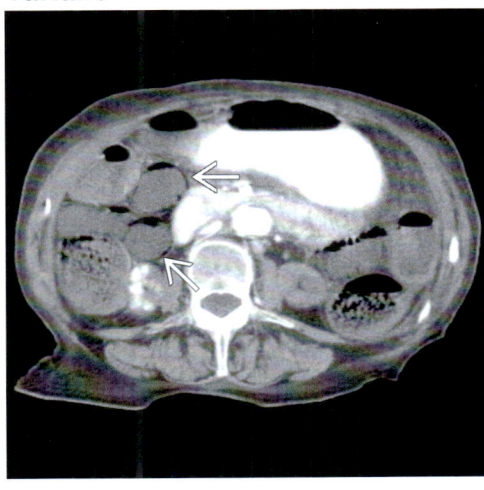
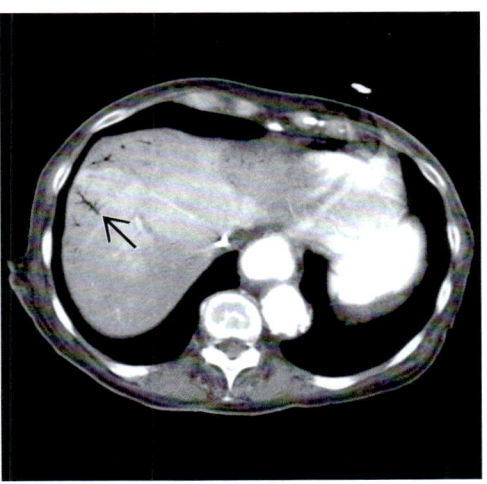

(Left) Axial CECT shows variant pneumatosis with portal venous gas. Note dilated small intestine with gas in wall of small intestine ➡. *(Right)* Axial CECT at higher level in same patient as left shows gas in periphery of liver ➡, compatible with portal venous location. Bowel infarction was confirmed at surgery.

VASCULITIS, SMALL INTESTINE

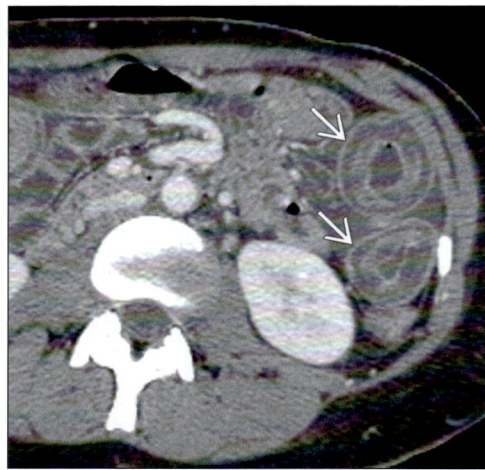

Axial CECT of lupus enteritis. Note marked submucosal edema with "target appearance" due to small vessel vasculitis of small bowel ➡.

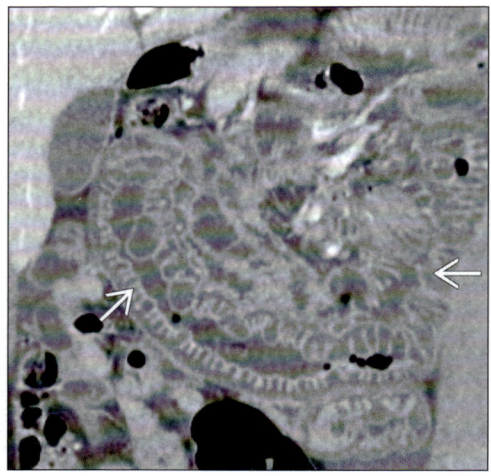

Coronal CECT reformat in same patient as left shows prominent mucosal enhancement of involved small bowel loops ➡.

TERMINOLOGY

Definitions
- Inflammation of the blood vessels of small intestine due to a large group of rare, systemic conditions

IMAGING FINDINGS

General Features
- Best diagnostic clue: Straight thickened folds with luminal dilatation of small bowel
- Different sizes of blood vessels are affected by various systemic conditions, but imaging findings overlap
- Most common systemic conditions
  - Polyarteritis nodosa (small-medium vessel)
  - Henoch-Schönlein purpura (HSP), systemic lupus erythematosus (SLE), Behçet syndrome (small vessel conditions)

Fluoroscopic Findings
- Barium studies
  - Segmental or extensive intestinal involvement
  - Aphthous ulcers
  - Straight, thickened folds ± luminal dilatation
  - Concentric filling defects (submucosal hemorrhage)
  - Ulceration and stricture in small vessel conditions
  - Thumbprinting; pneumatosis intestinalis
  - SLE
    - Nodularity of small bowel folds, motility disorder of lower esophagus, esophagitis, gastritis
  - Behçet syndrome
    - May simulate Crohn disease, involves ileocecal area, especially terminal ileum
    - Narrowing/irregularity of terminal ileum, slight proximal dilatation
    - Large ovoid or irregular ulcers, marked mucosal thickening of surrounding intestinal wall
    - Multiple small discrete "punched-out" ulcers

CT Findings
- Thickened bowel wall ± target sign, bowel wall enhancement, submucosal hemorrhage & edema
- Polyarteritis nodosa
  - Lobulated renal contour & irregular thinning (cortical infarcts)
  - Striated nephrogram: Multiple hypoattenuating bands of kidney (arterial occlusion)

DDx: Thickened Bowel Wall and Ileus

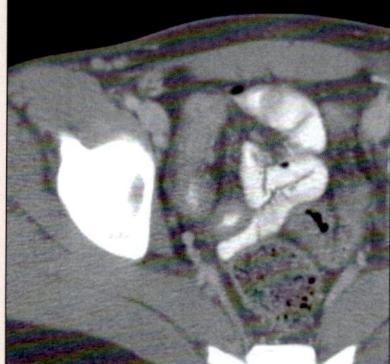

Crohn Disease

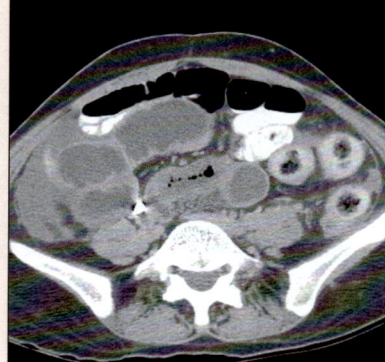

Closed Loop SBO

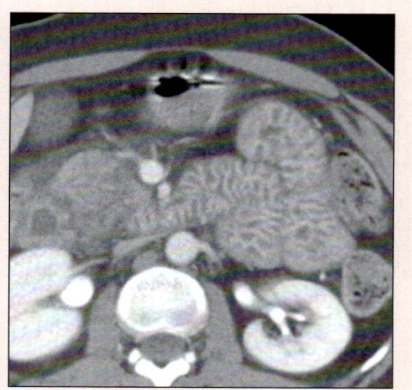

Shock Bowel

VASCULITIS, SMALL INTESTINE

Key Facts

Terminology
- Inflammation of the blood vessels of small intestine due to a large group of rare, systemic conditions

Imaging Findings
- Best diagnostic clue: Straight thickened folds with luminal dilatation of small bowel
- Different sizes of blood vessels are affected by various systemic conditions, but imaging findings overlap
- Best imaging tool: MDCT and angiography

Top Differential Diagnoses
- Ischemic Enteritis
- Crohn Disease
- Small Bowel Obstruction (SBO)
- "Shock Bowel"

Clinical Issues
- Abdominal pain, fever, nausea, vomiting, weight loss, diarrhea or constipation
- Diagnosis: Biopsy of involved tissue may help establish diagnosis
- Prognosis: Good, unless left untreated with complications

Diagnostic Checklist
- Differentiate by extraintestinal pattern of involvement & affected vessel size
- Biopsy, clinical findings essential for diagnosis
- Angiography & other tests essential to definitively diagnosis vasculitis as cause of small bowel disease

---

- SLE
  - Abnormal bowel wall enhancement, dilated bowel
  - "Comb sign": Engorged mesenteric vessels in comb-like arrangement
  - Ascites, lymphadenopathy, hepatomegaly, splenomegaly
  - Striated nephrogram
- Behçet syndrome: Concentric bowel wall thickening or polypoid mass, ± perienteric or pericolonic infiltration

Angiographic Findings
- Aneurysm formation
  - May be seen with polyarteritis nodosa, SLE, Wegener granulomatosis, rheumatoid vasculitis, Churg-Strauss syndrome, drug abuse
- Polyarteritis nodosa visceral involvement
  - Renal (80-90%), GI tract (50-70%), heart (65%), liver (50-60%), spleen (45%), pancreas (25-35%), central nervous system (rare)
  - Small intestine most commonly affected, followed by mesentery and colon
  - Multiple aneurysms (50-60% of cases), typically at branching points
  - 1-5 mm saccular aneurysms (more common) or fusiform aneurysms
  - Arterial stenoses or occlusions

Imaging Recommendations
- Best imaging tool: MDCT and angiography

DIFFERENTIAL DIAGNOSIS

Ischemic Enteritis
- Multiple causes (embolus, thrombosis, volvulus)
- Distinguish by clot or narrowing of SMA, SMV, other mesenteric vessels
- Imaging features usually indistinguishable from vasculitis, especially large-vessel vasculitis

Crohn Disease
- Skip lesions, transmural inflammation, non-caseating granulomas, cobblestone mucosa, fistulas
- Irregular, prominent mural thickening, fused & distorted folds

Small Bowel Obstruction (SBO)
- Closed loop → segmental obstruction & ischemia
- Air-fluid levels; smooth beaking
- Bowel wall thickening
- ± Portal venous gas, pneumatosis intestinalis

"Shock Bowel"
- Ischemia ± reperfusion of small bowel, usually following trauma or other cause of hypotension
- Intense mucosal enhancement, submucosal and mesenteric edema
- Reversible with resuscitation

PATHOLOGY

General Features
- Etiology
  - Large vessel: Giant cell arteritis, Takayasu disease
  - Medium vessel: Polyarteritis nodosa (> 50% involve GI); Kawasaki disease; primary granulomatous central nervous system vasculitis
  - Antineutrophil cytoplasmic autoantibody (ANCA)-associated small-vessel vasculitis
    - Microscopic polyangiitis; Wegener granulomatosis; Churg-Strauss syndrome
  - Immune-complex small-vessel vasculitis
    - HSP (> 50% involve GI); SLE (10-60% involve GI); Behçet syndrome (10-40% involve GI)
    - Cryoglobulinemic vasculitis, rheumatoid vasculitis, Sjögren syndrome
    - Hypocomplementemic urticarial vasculitis
    - Goodpasture syndrome, serum sickness
    - Drug- or infection-induced
  - Paraneoplastic small-vessel vasculitis
    - Lymphoproliferative neoplasm–induced
    - Myeloproliferative neoplasm-induced
    - Carcinoma-induced
  - Inflammatory bowel disease small-vessel vasculitis
  - Risk factors

VASCULITIS, SMALL INTESTINE

- HSP: Bacterial or viral infection, allergies, insect sting, drugs, certain foods
- Associated abnormalities
  - Polyarteritis nodosa: Hepatitis B infection
  - SLE: Hematologic, immunologic & neurologic involvement, photosensitivity, oral ulceration
  - HSP: Renal involvement
  - Behçet syndrome: Neurologic involvement

Gross Pathologic & Surgical Features
- Segmental fibrinoid necrotizing vasculitis
- Nonspecific ulceration or inflammation
- Polyarteritis nodosa: Panmural necrotizing arterial vasculitis; mucoid degeneration
- Behçet syndrome: Discrete "punched-out" ulcers, irregular perforations

Microscopic Features
- Polyarteritis nodosa
  - Acute: Polymorphonuclear cell infiltrate in all layers of arterial wall & perivascular tissue
  - Chronic: Mononuclear cell infiltrate with intimal proliferation, thrombosis, perivascular inflammation
- SLE: Local deposition of antigen-antibody complexes
- HSP: Immunoglobulin A deposits in vessel wall (direct immunofluorescence)
- Behçet syndrome: Immune complex deposits in vessel wall

Staging, Grading or Classification Criteria
- Classification
  - Large vessel: Aorta, main visceral arteries (e.g., SMA)
  - Medium vessel: Main visceral arteries and their branches
  - Small vessel: Arterioles, venules, capillaries

CLINICAL ISSUES

Presentation
- Most common signs/symptoms
  - Abdominal pain, fever, nausea, vomiting, weight loss, diarrhea or constipation
  - Polyarteritis nodosa: Peripheral neuropathies
  - HSP: Palpable purpura, arthritis, GI bleeding
  - SLE: Cough (serositis), oral ulcers, polyarthritis, malar rash, discoid rash
  - Behçet syndrome: Oral and genital ulcers, arthritis, uveitis, erythema nodosum
- Lab data
  - Polyarteritis nodosa: Cryoglobulin, positive for hepatitis B surface antigen
  - HSP: Hematuria, proteinuria
  - SLE: Antinuclear antibody, anti-Smith antibody
- Diagnosis: Biopsy of involved tissue may help establish diagnosis

Demographics
- Age
  - Polyarteritis nodosa: 18-81 years
  - HSP: 3-10 years of age (most common), > 20 years (up to 30% of cases)
  - SLE: 16-41 years
  - Behçet syndrome: 11-30 years
- Gender
  - Polyarteritis nodosa: M:F = 2:1
  - HSP: M:F = 2:1
  - SLE: M:F = 1:10
  - Behçet syndrome: M:F = 2:1

Natural History & Prognosis
- Complications
  - Paralytic ileus, ischemia, hemorrhage, perforation, stricture, fistula, peritonitis, sepsis
  - Polyarteritis nodosa: Renal failure, congestive heart failure, myocardiac infarction, cirrhosis, hepatic carcinoma
  - HSP: Intussusception in children, renal failure
  - SLE: Renal failure
  - Prognosis: Good, unless left untreated with complications

Treatment
- Polyarteritis nodosa: Corticosteroid ± cyclophosphamide
- HSP: Spontaneous resolution
- SLE: Corticosteroid, non-steroid anti-inflammatory drugs, hydroxychloroquine
- Behçet syndrome: Corticosteroid, sulfasalazine

DIAGNOSTIC CHECKLIST

Consider
- Differentiate by extraintestinal pattern of involvement & affected vessel size
- Biopsy, clinical findings essential for diagnosis

Image Interpretation Pearls
- Angiography & other tests essential to definitively diagnose vasculitis as cause of small bowel disease

SELECTED REFERENCES

1. Ha HK et al: Radiologic features of vasculitis involving the gastrointestinal tract. Radiographics. 20(3):779-94, 2000
2. Rha SE et al: CT and MR imaging findings of bowel ischemia from various primary causes. Radiographics. 20(1):29-42, 2000
3. Byun JY et al: CT features of systemic lupus erythematosus in patients with acute abdominal pain: emphasis on ischemic bowel disease. Radiology. 211(1):203-9, 1999
4. Ha HK et al: Intestinal Behcet syndrome: CT features of patients with and patients without complications. Radiology. 209(2):449-54, 1998
5. Jeong YK et al: Gastrointestinal involvement in Henoch-Schonlein syndrome: CT findings. AJR Am J Roentgenol. 168(4):965-8, 1997

VASCULITIS, SMALL INTESTINE

IMAGE GALLERY

Typical

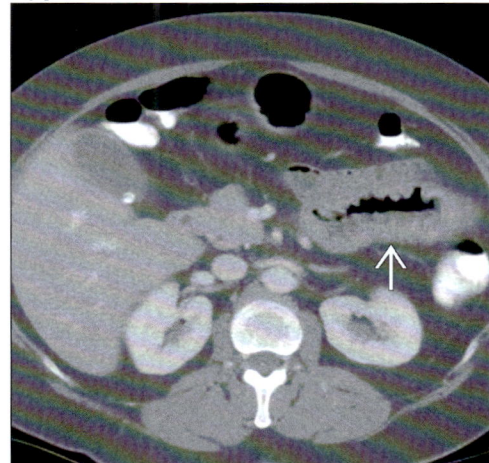 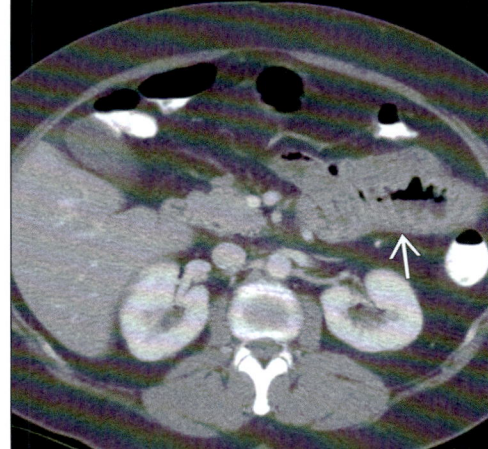

(Left) Axial CECT shows segmental bowel wall thickening 2° intramural hemorrhage. Note marked thickening of proximal jejunum ➡. Lumen is narrowed over length of about 20 cm. *(Right)* Axial CECT in same patient as left again demonstrates segmental bowel wall thickening of proximal jejunum ➡. Remainder of bowel appears normal with no evidence of obstruction.

Typical

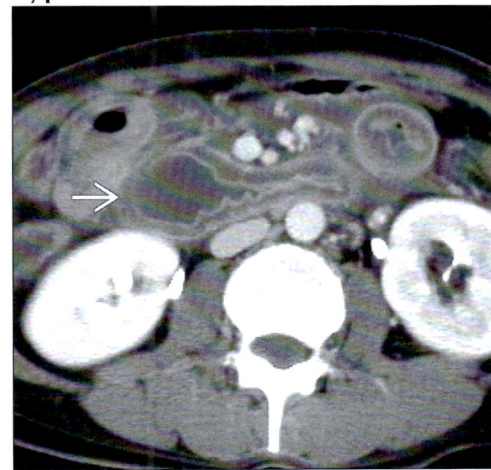 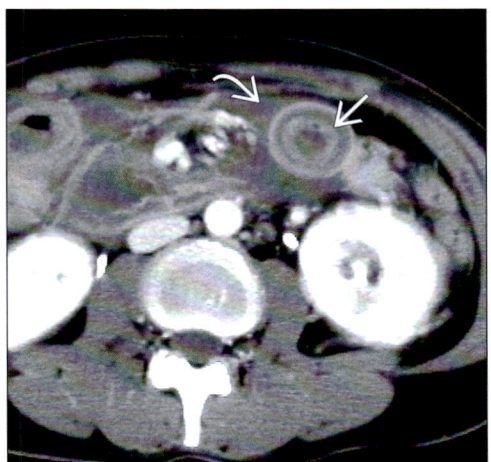

(Left) Axial CECT of duodenal and jejunal vasculitis due to lupus erythematosus. Note marked submucosal edema of transverse duodenum ➡. *(Right)* Axial CECT at more caudal level in same patient as left demonstrates "target sign" of submucosal edema within proximal jejunum ➡ and adjacent ascites ➡.

Variant

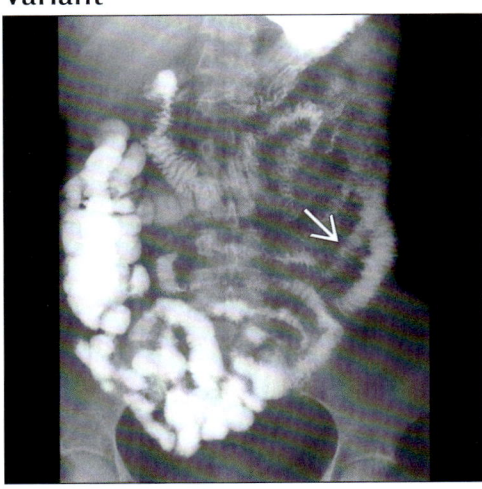 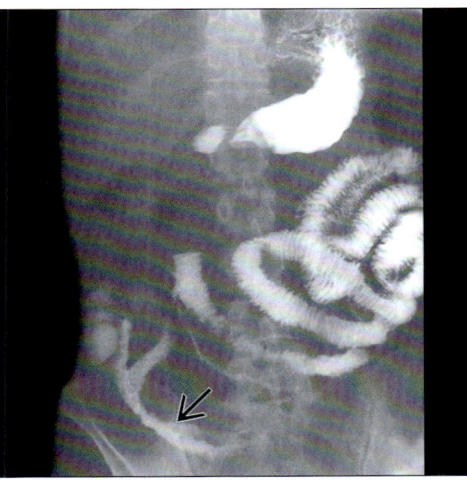

(Left) Anteroposterior small bowel follow through shows diffuse small bowel wall thickening with loop separation and fold thickening ➡. *(Right)* Small bowel follow through in same patient as left shows diffuse small bowel wall thickening, loop separation & fold thickening ➡. Patient history, biopsy, & laboratory analysis diagnosed allergic vasculitis.

SMALL BOWEL OBSTRUCTION

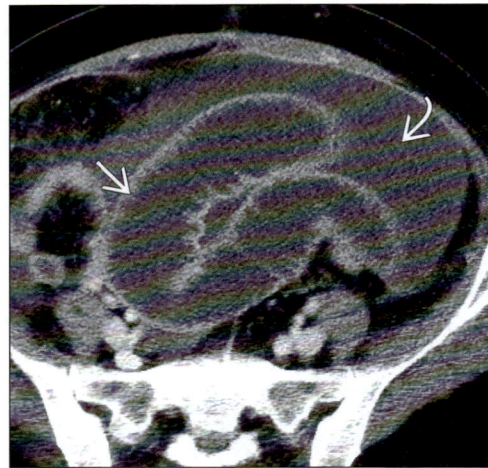 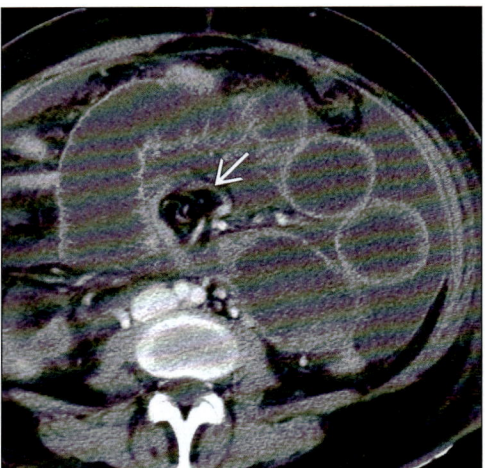

Axial CECT shows closed loop small bowel obstruction. Note U-shaped appearance of dilated ileum ➔ and adjacent intraloop ascites ➔. Bowel wall enhancement suggests viability of bowel.

Axial CECT at more cranial level in same patient as left demonstrates "whirl sign" of mesenteric vessels ➔.

TERMINOLOGY

Abbreviations and Synonyms
- Small bowel obstruction (SBO)

Definitions
- Obstruction or blockage of small bowel loops

IMAGING FINDINGS

General Features
- Best diagnostic clue
  o Dilated small bowel loops with air-fluid levels on upright film
  o Transition zone between normal and abnormal bowel critical to define site and cause of obstruction
- Location: Small bowel, proximal to obstruction
- Size: > 2.5 cm

Radiographic Findings
- Radiography
  o Supine abdomen with upright or decubitus views
  o Dilated proximal small bowel loops, multiple air-fluid levels, collapsed distal bowel
    ■ Pneumoperitoneum: Sign of bowel perforation
  o Can miss SBO (fluid, distended bowel not evident)
  o "String of pearls": Small air bubbles within fluid, distended bowel seen on supine view

Fluoroscopic Findings
- Enteroclysis or small bowel series
  o Incomplete or partial/low grade obstruction
    ■ Sufficient contrast flow through point of obstruction
  o Complete or high grade obstruction
    ■ Stasis or delay in contrast flow beyond point of obstruction
  o Transitions in contrast column can define location & degree of obstruction

CT Findings
- Dilated small bowel loops > 2.5 cm ± air-fluid levels
- "Small bowel feces" sign: Gas bubbles mixed with particulate matter in dilated loops proximal to SBO
- Extrinsic lesions
  o Adhesions

DDx: Small Bowel Distension

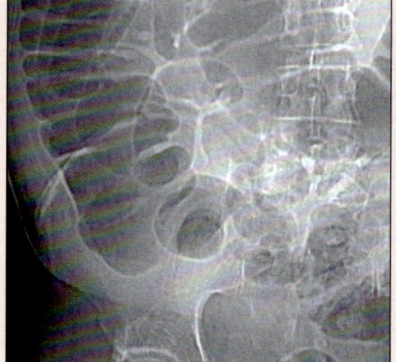
Ileus

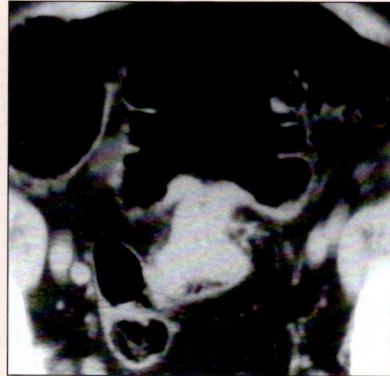
Colonic Obstruction

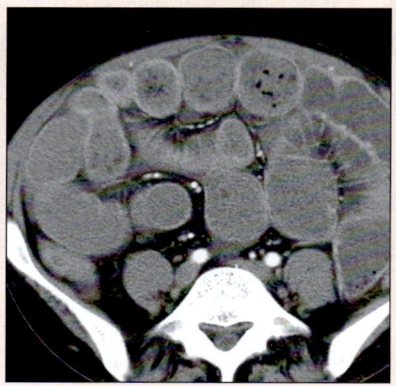
Cystic Fibrosis

SMALL BOWEL OBSTRUCTION

Key Facts

Imaging Findings
- "Small bowel feces" sign: Gas bubbles mixed with particulate matter in dilated loops proximal to SBO
- Dilated fluid-filled small bowel loops > 2.5 cm proximal to collapsed loops
- Gas-filled bowel loops, mesenteric fat, vessels in inguinal canal or other external hernia
- Thickened enhancing wall & luminal narrowing at transition zone
- Intussusception: Target sign; sausage-shaped or reniform mass
- ± Pneumatosis intestinalis; ± portomesenteric venous gas
- Mesenteric vessels: Haziness, obliteration, congestion or hemorrhage; ascites

Top Differential Diagnoses
- Adynamic or Paralytic Ileus
- Aerophagia
- Colonic Obstruction
- Cystic Fibrosis (CF)

Pathology
- Most common: Adhesions (~ 60%), hernias (15%), tumors (~ 15%; metastases > primary tumor)
- Pathogenesis: Obstruction of small bowel → proximal dilatation due to accumulation of GI secretions & swallowed air

Diagnostic Checklist
- CT best to determine presence, site & cause of SBO, any complications

---

- Dilated fluid-filled small bowel loops > 2.5 cm proximal to collapsed loops
- ± Transition zone, minimal mural thickening & enhancement
- Uncomplicated adhesive bands: Typically unidentified on CT (diagnosis of exclusion)
  - Hernia
    - Gas-filled bowel loops, mesenteric fat, vessels in inguinal canal or other external hernia
    - Strangulated hernia: Thickened bowel wall with increased attenuation
    - Internal hernia: Cluster of dilated loops, crowding/twisting of mesenteric vessels
  - Peritoneal carcinomatosis: Omental masses, dilated bowel loops, multiple transition zones
  - Appendicitis: RLQ inflammatory mass, dilated loops, fluid collection, abscess
  - Diverticulitis
    - Complicated: Abscess, peritonitis, obstruction, dilated bowel loops
- Intrinsic lesions: Adenocarcinoma, Crohn, TB, radiation enteropathy
  - Thickened enhancing wall & luminal narrowing at transition zone
  - Fluid & gas-filled dilated bowel loops proximal to collapsed loops
  - Intussusception: Target sign; sausage-shaped or reniform mass
- Intraluminal lesions: Gallstones, foreign bodies, bezoars, ascaris worms
  - Classic triad: Ectopic calcified stone, gas in GB/biliary tree, obstruction = gallstone ileus
  - Bezoar: Intraluminal mass & air in interstices; dilated fluid-filled loops
- Closed loop obstruction: Obstruction at two points, involves mesentery
  - Relatively little dilatation of bowel proximal to closed loop obstruction
  - Stretched mesenteric vessels converging toward site of torsion
  - Fluid-distended bowel, minimal gas
  - "Beak sign": Fusiform tapering at point of torsion/obstruction
  - Volvulus: C-shaped, U-shaped or "coffee bean" bowel loop configuration
    - "Whirl sign" due to tightly twisted mesentery
- Strangulating obstruction: Blocked blood flow to obstructed bowel
  - "Target" or "halo" sign: Circumferentially thickened bowel wall & increased attenuation
  - "Serrated beak sign": Twisting of bowel, mesenteric edema, bowel wall thickening
  - ± Pneumatosis intestinalis; ± portomesenteric venous gas
  - Absence, decreased, or delayed bowel wall enhancement in affected loops
  - Mesenteric vessels: Haziness, obliteration, congestion or hemorrhage; ascites

Imaging Recommendations
- Best imaging tool
  - MDCT: Sensitivity 95%, specificity 96% in high grade SBO
    - Acutely ill patient; suspected ischemia; history of cancer or inflammatory bowel disease
  - Enteroclysis: Intermittent, chronic or low grade SBO
- Protocol advice: Water-soluble contrast agent if perforation suspected

DIFFERENTIAL DIAGNOSIS

Adynamic or Paralytic Ileus
- Common causes: Post-surgery, medications, post-injury, ischemia
- Dilated small & large bowel loops with no transition point, aperistaltic fluid levels
- Absence of obstruction on CT

Aerophagia
- Excessive air swallowing associated with prominent belching, flatulence & abdominal distention
- Dilated small bowel loops simulating SBO
- Gastric & colonic distension without air-fluid levels

SMALL BOWEL OBSTRUCTION

Colonic Obstruction
- Dilation of colon due to mechanical or functional causes
  - Carcinoma, volvulus, diverticulitis are most common mechanical causes
- Acute colonic pseudo-obstruction (Ogilvie syndrome)
  - Multiple causes
  - Decreased parasympathetic tone or excessive sympathetic output
  - Mortality 15%; IV neostigmine may reverse

Cystic Fibrosis (CF)
- Functional obstruction of small bowel possible due to thick, viscous bowel contents
- Fatty replacement of pancreas on CT, often with small bowel feces sign

PATHOLOGY

General Features
- Etiology
  - Most common: Adhesions (~ 60%), hernias (15%), tumors (~ 15%; metastases > primary tumor)
  - Extrinsic lesions: Adhesions; external & internal hernias, tumor, abscess, aneurysm
    - Adhesions: Post-surgery, inflammation, congenital
  - Intrinsic lesions: Tumors, inflammatory, vascular (ischemic), metabolic, radiation enteropathy
  - Intraluminal lesions: Gallstones, bezoars, foreign bodies, ascaris worms
  - Pathogenesis: Obstruction of small bowel → proximal dilatation due to accumulation of GI secretions & swallowed air
    - Bowel dilatation stimulates secretory activity resulting in increased fluid accumulation
- Epidemiology
  - 20% of acute abdomen presentations
  - Mortality: Simple SBO 5-8%; strangulation 20-37%

Gross Pathologic & Surgical Features
- Dilated proximal loop, distal collapsed loop & transition point; (dilated small bowel > 2.5 cm)

Staging, Grading or Classification Criteria
- Classification based on mechanism of obstruction
  - Mechanical: Extrinsic, intrinsic, intraluminal lesions
  - Non-mechanical: Adynamic ileus; dynamic or spastic ileus (due to neuromuscular disturbances)
- Classification based on degree of obstruction
  - Simple
    - Intermittent; incomplete or partial; low grade obstruction
    - Prolonged, complete or high grade obstruction
  - Complicated
    - Closed loop or incarcerated obstruction: Adhesive bands > internal or external hernia
    - Strangulation: Most common cause of closed loop obstruction, indicates vascular compromise

CLINICAL ISSUES

Presentation
- Most common signs/symptoms
  - Variable, mild abdominal pain to vomiting, constipation, fever, signs of acute abdomen
    - Abdominal distention, tenderness, guarding
    - Bowel sounds high pitched or absent (late sign)

Natural History & Prognosis
- Complications
  - Bowel strangulation, infarction, gangrene, perforation, peritonitis & sepsis
- Prognosis
  - Good if simple obstruction, poor if complicated
  - Mortality 25% if surgery postponed > 36 hrs
  - Mortality ↓ to 8% if surgery performed ≤ 36 hrs
  - Mortality 100% for untreated strangulated obstructions

Treatment
- Nasogastric suction, decompression, IV fluids, NPO
- Conservative treatment for incomplete or low grade
- Immediate surgery for complete or high grade

DIAGNOSTIC CHECKLIST

Consider
- CT best to determine presence, site & cause of SBO, any complications
- Difficult to distinguish partial from complete obstruction by imaging alone

Image Interpretation Pearls
- Dilated small bowel loops with small bowel feces sign on CT, string of pearls sign on supine film

SELECTED REFERENCES
1. Mak SY et al: Small bowel obstruction: computed tomography features and pitfalls. Curr Probl Diagn Radiol. 35(2):65-74, 2006
2. Fazel A et al: New solutions to an old problem: acute colonic pseudo-obstruction. J Clin Gastroenterol. 39(1):17-20, 2005
3. Lazarus DE et al: Frequency and relevance of the "small-bowel feces" sign on CT in patients with small-bowel obstruction. AJR Am J Roentgenol. 183(5):1361-6, 2004
4. Khurana B et al: Bowel obstruction revealed by multidetector CT. AJR Am J Roentgenol. 178(5):1139-44, 2002
5. Furukawa A et al: Helical CT in the diagnosis of small bowel obstruction. Radiographics. 21(2):341-55, 2001
6. Maglinte DD et al: Small bowel obstruction: Optimizing radiologic investigation and nonsurgical management. Radiology. 218: 39-46, 2001
7. Caoili EM et al: CT of small bowel obstruction: Another perspective using multiplanar reformations. AJR. 174: 993-8, 2000
8. Nevitt PC: The string of pearls sign. Radiology. 214(1):157-8, 2000
9. Maglinte DD et al: The role of radiology in the diagnosis of small bowel obstruction. AJR. 168: 1171-80, 1997

SMALL BOWEL OBSTRUCTION

IMAGE GALLERY

Typical

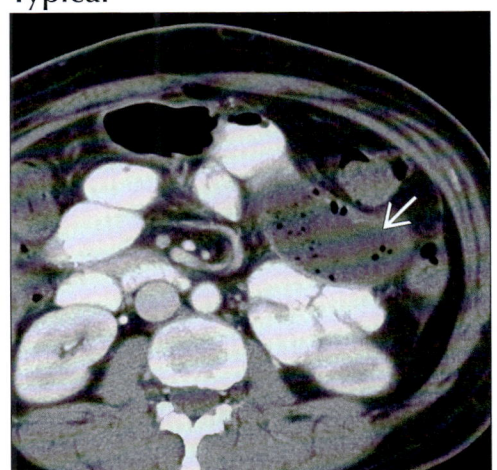
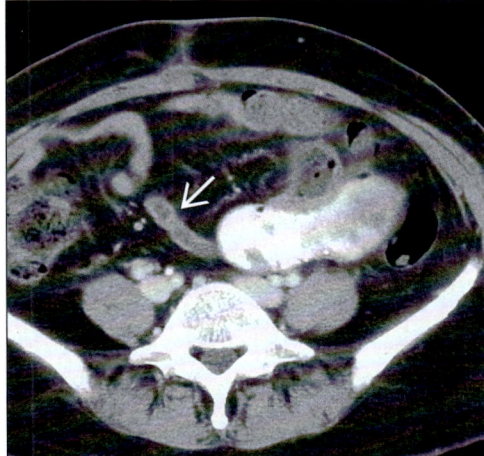

(Left) Axial CECT of SBO. Study performed with oral contrast illustrates dilated unopacified loop with small bowel feces sign ➡. *(Right)* Axial CECT at more caudal level in same patient as left demonstrates collapsed distal bowel loops ➡.

Typical

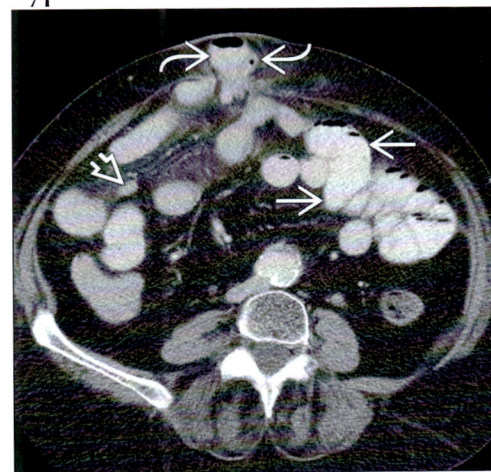
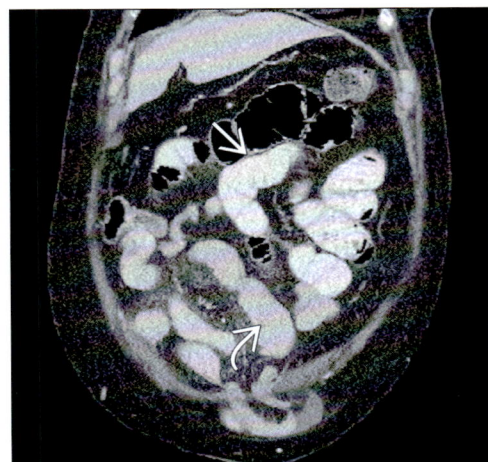

(Left) Axial CECT shows dilated small bowel loops ➡ extending to ventral hernia, incarcerated loops within hernia sac ➡, & decompressed loops ➡ distal to obstruction. *(Right)* Coronal CECT in same patient as left shows denser oral contrast in proximal bowel of LUQ ➡, less dense in distal obstructed segments, reflecting slow transit time & contrast dilution 2° fluid-filled segments in SBO ➡.

Variant

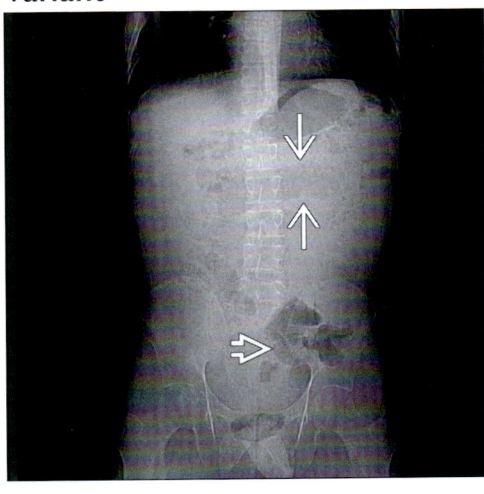
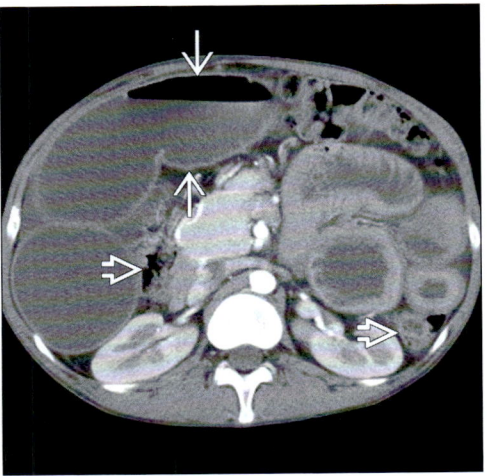

(Left) Frontal scout film from CECT shows dilated small bowel ➡ disproportionate to colon ➡. *(Right)* Axial CECT shows massively dilated fluid-filled small bowel loops ➡; note decompressed colon ➡. At surgery, chronic stricture was resected.

GALLSTONE ILEUS

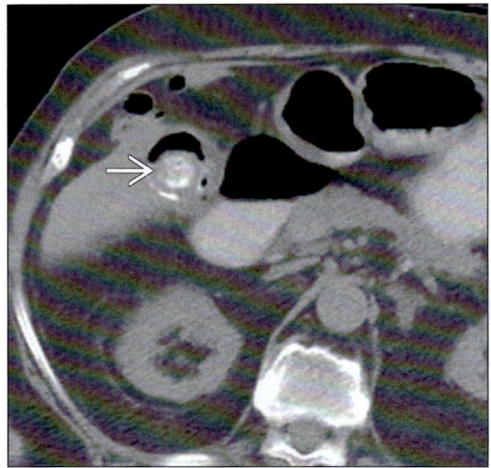

Axial NECT shows gas in gallbladder adjacent to large gallstone ➡.

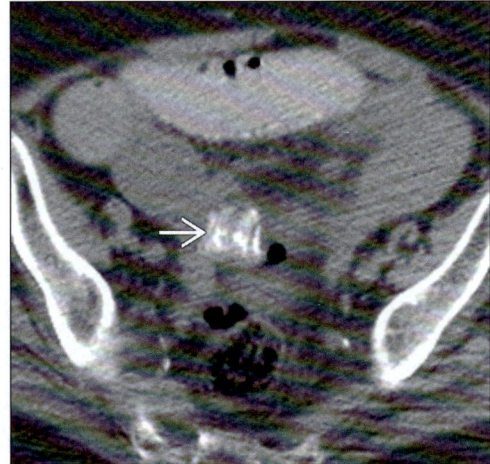

Axial NECT at more caudal level in same patient as left demonstrates calcified gallstone ➡ obstructing distal small bowel.

TERMINOLOGY

Abbreviations and Synonyms
- Gallstone ileus (GSI)

Definitions
- Mechanical bowel obstruction 2° impacted gallstones

IMAGING FINDINGS

General Features
- Best diagnostic clue: Rigler triad: Small bowel (SB) obstruction/gas in biliary tree/ectopic gallstone
- Location: Narrow points of duodenum, ligament of Treitz, ileocecal valve, sigmoid colon
- Size: ≥ 2.5 cm

Radiographic Findings
- Radiography
  - Abdominal films
    - Dilated proximal bowel
    - Gas in shrunken gallbladder (GB) and/or bile ducts
  - Ectopic calcified gallstone (15-25%)
    - Gallstone surrounded by gas in bowel loop
  - Altered position of previously identified gallstone

Fluoroscopic Findings
- UGI or BE
  - Barium-filled collapsed GB, biliary ducts
  - Fistulous communication: Cholecystoduodenal (60%); choledochoduodenal; cholecystocolic

CT Findings
- Gallstone surrounded by gas in bowel loop; cholesterol stones near-water density, often with calcified rim
- Collapsed GB, pneumobilia

DIFFERENTIAL DIAGNOSIS

Intussusception
- "Coiled spring appearance"; sausage-shaped mass

Dropped Gallstone
- Gallstone in peritoneal cavity 2° to laparoscopic cholecystectomy

DDx: Small Bowel Obstruction with Mass

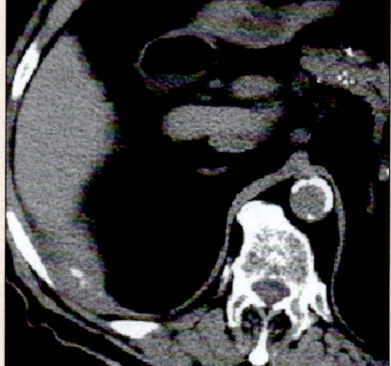

Dropped Gallstone

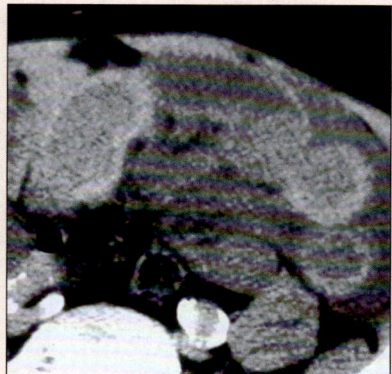

Bowel Ischemia

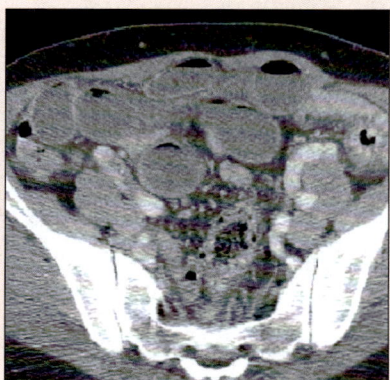

Adhesions

GALLSTONE ILEUS

Key Facts

Terminology
- Mechanical bowel obstruction 2° impacted gallstones

Imaging Findings
- Best diagnostic clue: Rigler triad: Small bowel (SB) obstruction/gas in biliary tree/ectopic gallstone

Top Differential Diagnoses
- Intussusception
- Dropped Gallstone

- Bowel Ischemia

Clinical Issues
- Risk ↑ with age; average 65-75 years
- Gender: 4-7 times more frequent in women than men
- Gallstone erodes inflamed GB wall, passes into GI tract → bowel obstruction

Diagnostic Checklist
- Identify biliary-enteric fistula on barium studies

Bowel Ischemia
- Thickened wall, dilated proximal bowel, SB obstruction
- Transition zone from dilated to nondilated SB
- No mass/calcified stone obstruction point

PATHOLOGY

General Features
- Etiology
  - Occurs with chronic cholecystitis
  - Delayed (up to 2 months) complication of ERCP
  - Complication of endoscopic sphincterotomy
  - Diagnosis frequently delayed or missed
- Epidemiology
  - 0.4-5% of all intestinal obstructions
  - In < 1% of patients with cholelithiasis

CLINICAL ISSUES

Presentation
- Most common signs/symptoms: Intermittent acute colicky abdominal pain (20-30%), nausea, vomiting, fever, distension, obstipation

Demographics
- Age
  - Risk ↑ with age; average 65-75 years
  - Elderly females: Can be underlying condition at site of colon obstruction
- Gender: 4-7 times more frequent in women than men

Natural History & Prognosis
- Gallstone erodes inflamed GB wall, passes into GI tract → bowel obstruction
- Large stones can pass into duodenum after unsuccessful sphincterotomy
- Recurrence: 5-10% (additional silent proximal calculi)
- Operative mortality 19%

Treatment
- Surgical therapy to relieve bowel obstruction
- Cholecystectomy & biliary fistula excision
- Staged laparoscopic management of GSI & associated cholecystoduodenal fistula

DIAGNOSTIC CHECKLIST

Consider
- Elderly female, recurrent RUQ pain, recently more severe & prolonged vomiting
- Identify biliary-enteric fistula on barium studies

SELECTED REFERENCES
1. Vaidya JS et al: Gallstone ileus. Lancet. 362(9390):1105, 2003
2. Lyburn ID et al: Gall-stone ileus: imaging features. Hosp Med. 63(7):434-5, 2002

IMAGE GALLERY

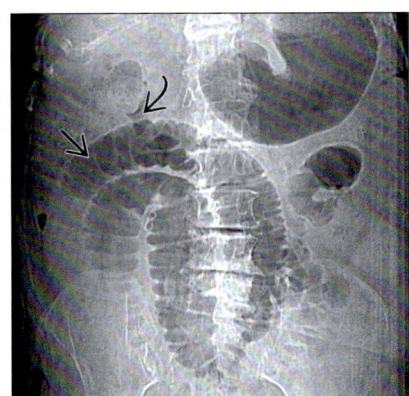 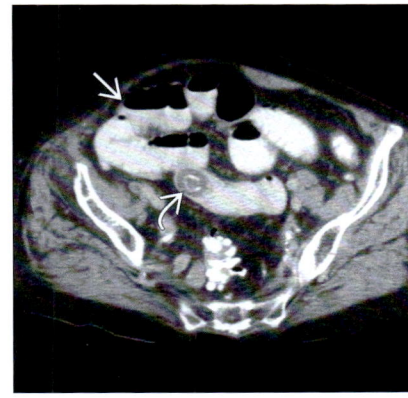 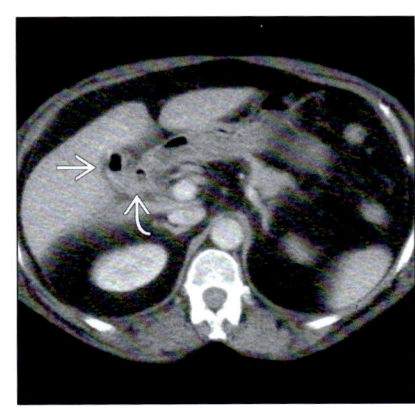

(Left) Anteroposterior radiograph shows dilated small bowel ➡ confirming obstruction, and gas in gallbladder ➡. *(Center)* Axial CECT shows dilated proximal small bowel ➡ and laminated filling defect ➡ at transition point, which proved to represent an obstructing gallstone. *(Right)* Axial CECT shows cholecystoduodenal fistula from prior episode of GSI. Note gas in GB ➡ and close proximity of GB to duodenum ➡.

INTUSSUSCEPTION

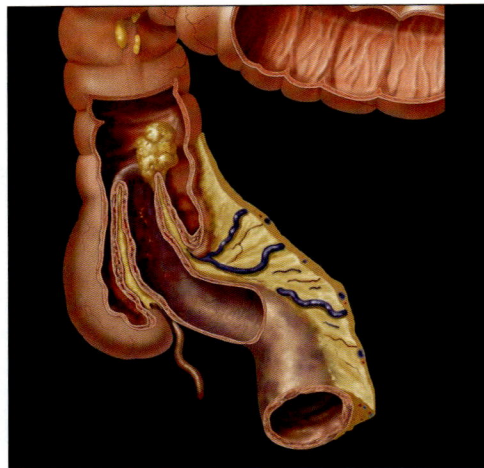

Graphic shows ileocolic intussusception with a tumor in the bowel wall as the "lead mass". Note vascular compromise and ischemia.

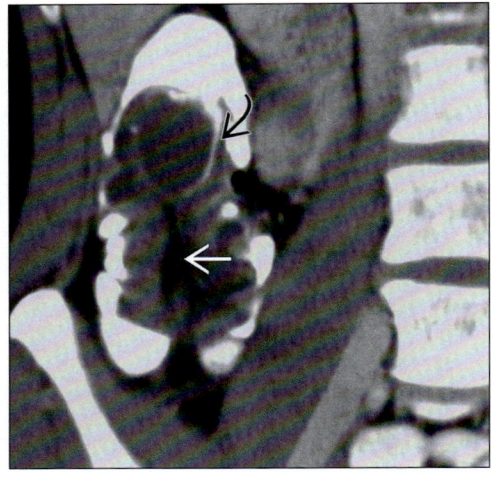

Coronal CECT reformat shows mesenteric fat associated with intussusceptum ➡ within the cecum. Calcified wall of appendiceal cystadenoma ➡ is also evident. (Courtesy M. Hollett, MD).

TERMINOLOGY

Definitions
- Invagination or telescoping of proximal segment of bowel (intussusceptum) into lumen of distal segment (intussuscipiens)

IMAGING FINDINGS

General Features
- Best diagnostic clue: Bowel within bowel, "coiled spring" appearance
- Location
  - Ileoileal > ileocolic > colocolic
  - Usually small bowel in adults, ileocolic in children
  - Colon: Malignant tumors more common than benign
  - Small bowel: Benign tumors more common than malignant

Radiographic Findings
- Radiography: Air-fluid levels, proximal bowel dilatation, absence of gas in distal collapsed bowel

Fluoroscopic Findings
- Fluoroscopic-guided barium study
  - Classic "coiled spring" appearance
    - Trapping of contrast between folds of intussusceptum & intussuscipiens
  - Bowel obstruction, proximal dilatation, distal collapsed loops

CT Findings
- "Target" sign on CT: Earliest stage
  - Outer layer represents intussuscipiens, inner layer represents intussusceptum
- Sausage-shaped mass on CT: Layering pattern (later phase)
  - Alternating layers of low attenuation mesenteric fat & high attenuation bowel wall
  - Enhancing mesenteric vessels
- Reniform mass on CT: Edema or mural thickening (vascular compromise)
  - Vascular compromise seen in returning wall of intussusceptum as hypodense layer in middle of inner thickened bowel wall, crescent-shaped fluid or gas collections
- Features of intestinal obstruction

DDx: Bowel Obstruction with Mass

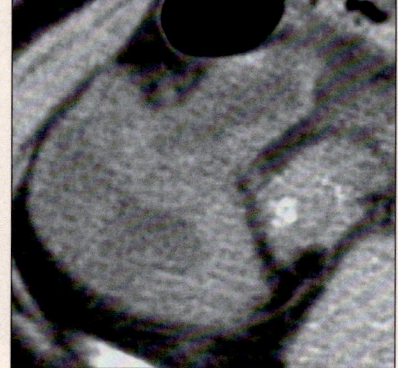
Cecal Carcinoma

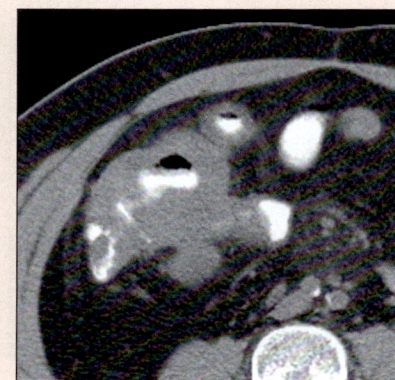
Lymphoma

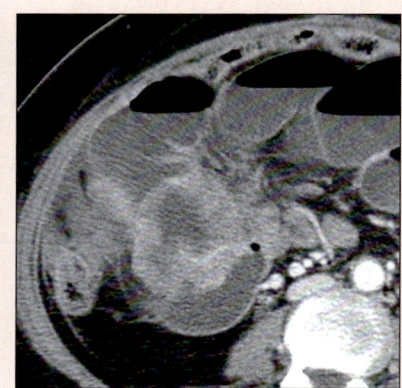
Melanoma

INTUSSUSCEPTION

Key Facts

Terminology
- Invagination or telescoping of proximal segment of bowel (intussusceptum) into lumen of distal segment (intussuscipiens)

Imaging Findings
- Best diagnostic clue: Bowel within bowel, "coiled spring" appearance
- Ileoileal > ileocolic > colocolic
- Usually small bowel in adults, ileocolic in children
- "Target" sign on CT: Earliest stage
- Sausage-shaped mass on CT: Layering pattern (later phase)
- Reniform mass on CT: Edema or mural thickening (vascular compromise)
- Transverse US: Target, doughnut or "bull's eye" sign
- Longitudinal US: "Pseudokidney" or hay fork sign

Top Differential Diagnoses
- Primary Bowel Tumor
- Metastases & Lymphoma
- Endometrial Implant
- Meckel Diverticulum

Pathology
- Most adult intussusceptions are short segment, transient, non-obstructing, not associated with lead tumor mass

Diagnostic Checklist
- Short segment, non-obstructing intussusceptions are common in adults; require no therapy
- "Coiled spring" appearance due to trapped barium
- Lead point: Lobulated mass etched in white

---

  o Air-fluid levels, proximal bowel distension

MR Findings
- Bowel-within-bowel or coiled-spring appearance
- Best seen on turbo spin-echo T2WI

Ultrasonographic Findings
- Grayscale Ultrasound
  o Transverse US: Target, doughnut or "bull's eye" sign
    - Peripheral hypoechoic halo: Edematous wall of intussuscipiens
    - Intermediate hyperechoic area: Space between intussuscipiens & intussusceptum
    - Internal hypoechoic ring
  o Longitudinal US: "Pseudokidney" or hay fork sign
    - Multiple, thin, parallel, hypoechoic & echogenic stripes
- Color Doppler: Mesenteric vessels dragged between entering & returning wall of intussusceptum

Imaging Recommendations
- Best imaging tool
  o Depends on patient age/presentation
  o MDCT, barium studies, US

DIFFERENTIAL DIAGNOSIS

Primary Bowel Tumor
- Carcinoid tumor, adenocarcinoma, stromal tumor, lipoma, adenoma
- Enteroclysis: Best for detecting mass

Metastases & Lymphoma
- Non-Hodgkin lymphoma (more common)
  o Distribution: Stomach (51%), small-bowel (33%)
  o Nodular, polypoid, infiltrating, invading mesentery
  o Sausage-shaped thickening of affected bowel wall simulating intussusception
  o May cause intussusception
- Metastases (small bowel): Malignant melanoma, lung & breast cancer
  o Location: Antimesenteric border
  o Malignant melanoma
    - Smoothly polypoid lesions of different sizes
    - "Spoke-wheel" pattern: Polypoid lesion with ulcers, radiating folds
  o Bronchogenic carcinoma
    - Single/multiple intramural lesions (flat/polypoid), frequently ulcerated, narrowing and obstruction
  o Breast carcinoma
    - Highly cellular submucosal masses
    - Multiple strictures, intervening bowel dilatation
    - Intussusception of ulcerated mural lesions

Endometrial Implant
- Endometrial tissue outside myometrium
- Common location: Pelvic organs; bowel involved in 37% of cases
- Crenulation of folds, plaque-like deformities
- High grade or low grade small bowel obstruction, usually due to fibrosis, rarely intussusception

Meckel Diverticulum
- Most frequent congenital anomaly of GI tract
- Ileal outpouching (2 feet from ileocecal valve)
- Causes of small bowel obstruction
  o Torsion associated with a persistent vitelline band
  o Extrusion of diverticulum into an inguinal hernia (hernia of Littre)
  o Intussusception of an inverted diverticulum

PATHOLOGY

General Features
- Etiology
  o Most adult intussusceptions are short segment, transient, non-obstructing, not associated with lead tumor mass
  o Tumor related lead point: Benign & malignant
    - Benign: Polyp, leiomyoma, lipoma, adenoma of appendix, appendiceal stump granuloma (more common in small bowel)
    - Malignant: Primary (more common in colon), metastases and lymphoma (more common in small bowel)

INTUSSUSCEPTION

- Postoperative risk factors (more common in small bowel)
  - Suture lines, ostomy closure sites
  - Adhesions, long intestinal tubes
  - Bypassed intestinal segments, submucosal edema
  - Abnormal bowel motility, electrolyte imbalance
  - Chronic dilated loop
- Meckel diverticulum; celiac & Whipple disease
- Colitis (eosinophilic & pseudomembranous)
- Epiploic appendagitis
• Epidemiology
  - Uncommon in adults, more common in children
    - 95% of all intussusceptions in children, idiopathic in 90% of cases (lymphoid hyperplasia)
    - 2nd most common cause of acute abdomen in children

Gross Pathologic & Surgical Features
• Three layers are seen
  - Intussusceptum: Entering or inner tube and returning or middle tube
  - Intussuscipiens: Sheath or outer tube

Microscopic Features
• Early: Inflammatory changes; late ischemic necrosis, mucosal sloughing

Staging, Grading or Classification Criteria
• Short segment, non-obstructing intussusception
  - Usually self-limited without lead mass
• Long segment, obstruction intussusception: Mass

CLINICAL ISSUES

Presentation
• Most common signs/symptoms
  - Children: Acute pain, palpable oblong abdominal mass, "red currant jelly" stools
  - Adults: Intermittent pain, vomiting, red blood in stool

Demographics
• Age: Any age group, children more common than adults
• Gender: M = F

Natural History & Prognosis
• Complications: Obstruction, infarction necrosis, hemorrhage, perforation, peritonitis
• Prognosis
  - Early: Good after reduction or surgical resection; recurrence very rare
  - Late: Poor, due to risk of severe vascular compromise, gangrene, perforation

Treatment
• None for transient, non-obstructing
• Resection for ileocolic, ileocecocolic & colocolic
• Children: Hydrostatic or pneumatic reduction; surgical reduction or resection

DIAGNOSTIC CHECKLIST

Consider
• Short segment, non-obstructing intussusceptions are common in adults; require no therapy

Image Interpretation Pearls
• Lumen of intussusceptum as narrow, tubular structure lined by twisted mucosal folds
• "Coiled spring" appearance due to trapped barium
• Lead point: Lobulated mass etched in white

SELECTED REFERENCES

1. El Fortia M et al: Tetra-layered sign of adult intussusception (new ultrasound approach). Ultrasound Med Biol. 32(4):479-82, 2006
2. Henry MC et al: The appendix sign: a radiographic marker for irreducible intussusception. J Pediatr Surg. 41(3):487-9, 2006
3. Mateen MA et al: Transient small bowel intussusceptions: ultrasound findings and clinical significance. Abdom Imaging. 2006
4. Grosfeld JL: Intussusception then and now: a historical vignette. J Am Coll Surg. 201(6):830-3, 2005
5. Kim KH et al: Intussusception after gastric surgery. Endoscopy. 37(12):1237-43, 2005
6. Ouyang EC et al: Ileocolonic intussusception. MedGenMed. 7(3):15, 2005
7. Huang BY et al: Adult intussusception: diagnosis and clinical relevance. Radiol Clin North Am. 41(6):1137-51, 2003
8. Lvoff N et al: Distinguishing features of self-limiting adult small-bowel intussusception identified at CT. Radiology. 227(1):68-72, 2003
9. Saenz De Ormijana J et al: Idiopathic enteroenteric intussusceptions in adults. Abdom Imaging. 28(1):8-11, 2003
10. Gayer G et al: Pictorial review: adult intussusception--a CT diagnosis. Br J Radiol. 75(890):185-90, 2002
11. Fujimoto T et al: Unenhanced CT findings of vascular compromise in association with intussusceptions in adults. AJR Am J Roentgenol. 176(5):1167-71, 2001
12. Warshauer DM et al: Adult intussusception detected at CT or MR imaging: clinical-imaging correlation. Radiology. 212(3):853-60, 1999
13. Catalano O: Transient small bowel intussusception: CT findings in adults. Br J Radiol. 70(836):805-8, 1997
14. Lorigan JG et al: The computed tomographic appearances and clinical significance of intussusception in adults with malignant neoplasms. Br J Radiol. 63(748):257-62, 1990
15. Merine D et al: Enteroenteric intussusception: CT findings in nine patients. AJR Am J Roentgenol. 148(6):1129-32, 1987

INTUSSUSCEPTION

IMAGE GALLERY

Typical

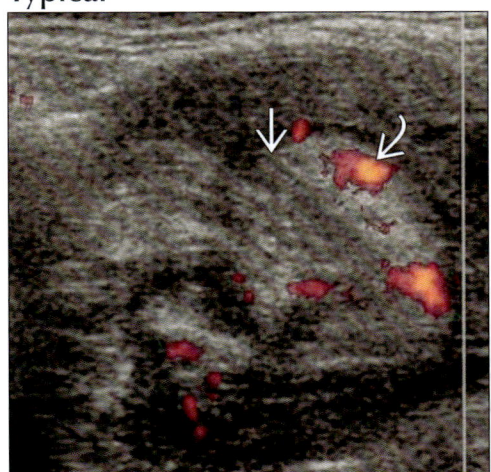
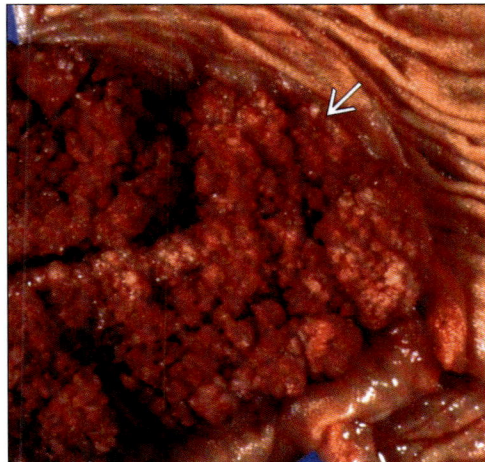

(Left) Transverse power Doppler ultrasound shows colo-colonic intussusception from ileocecal carcinoma. Note echogenic mass representing invaginated mesenteric fat ➔ with accompanying vasculature ➔. *(Right)* Pathology specimen of same patient as left reveals large ileocecal carcinoma ➔.

Typical

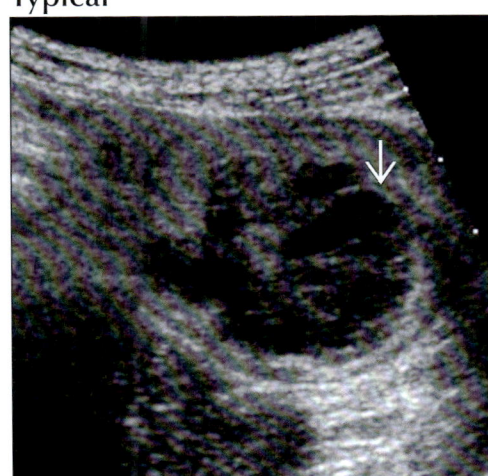
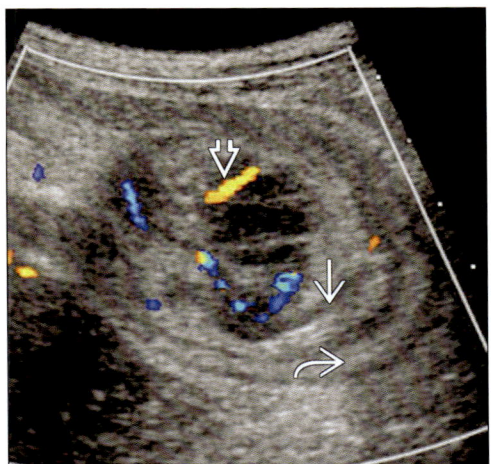

(Left) Transverse grayscale sonogram shows small bowel intussusception from metastatic melanoma. Sonographic imaging of LUQ reveals hypoechoic mass involving small bowel ➔. *(Right)* Transverse color Doppler ultrasound in same patient as left demonstrates echogenic submucosal bowel wall layer of intussusceptum ➔ and intussuscipiens ➔. Note invaginated mesenteric vessels ➔.

Variant

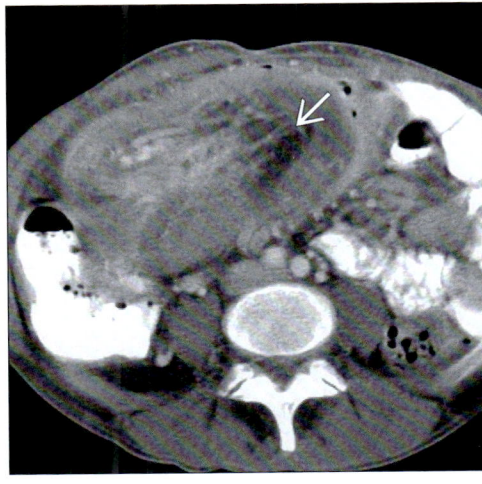
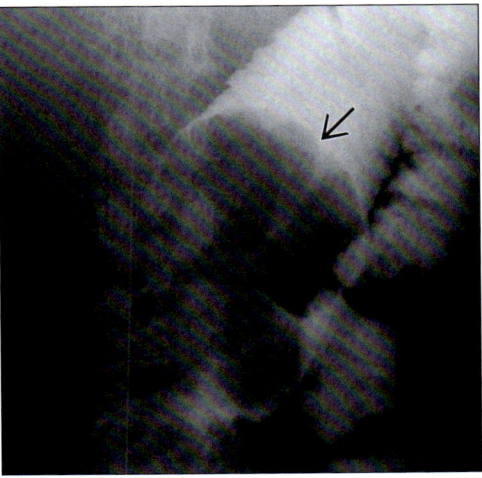

(Left) Axial CECT shows ileo-cecal intussusception from cystic fibrosis. Note invaginated mass with mesenteric fat ➔. *(Right)* Anteroposterior single contrast barium enema demonstrates obstructing mass from intussusception within transverse colon ➔. At surgery, lead mass was due to inspissated mucoid material within terminal ileum.

INFECTIOUS COLITIS

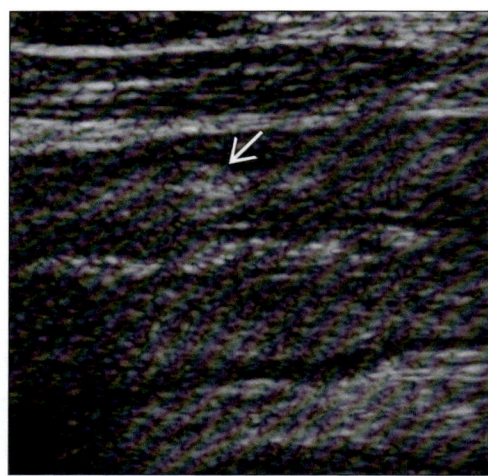

Longitudinal grayscale sonography of infectious ileocolitis due to Campylobacter. Scan of terminal ileum demonstrates mural thickening with echogenic submucosa due to edema ➔.

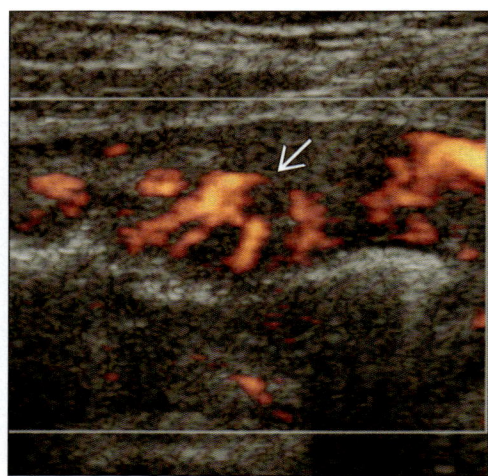

Longitudinal power Doppler ultrasound of cecum in same patient as left reveals marked hyperemia ➔.

TERMINOLOGY

Definitions
- Colonic inflammation due to bacterial, viral, fungal, or parasitic infections

IMAGING FINDINGS

General Features
- Best diagnostic clue: Focal or diffuse colonic wall thickening with mucosal ulcerations
- Location
  - Dependent on etiology
    - Typhoid fever (Salmonellosis): Cecum or right colon, invariably in ileum
    - Shigellosis: Predominantly in left colon
    - Campylobacteriosis: Small bowel & colon
    - Yersinia enterocolitis: Predominantly right colon, occasionally left; invariably in terminal ileum
    - E. coli colitis: Transverse colon; extends to right, left or both sides of colon
    - Tuberculosis (TB): Right & proximal transverse colon, involves ileum
    - Actinomycosis: Rectosigmoid colon (intrauterine devices), ileocecal region (appendectomy)
    - Gonorrheal, Chlamydia, Herpes virus colitis: Rectosigmoid colon
    - Cytomegalovirus (CMV) colitis: Cecum & proximal colon, extends to distal ileum
    - Histoplasmosis: Ileocecal region
    - Mucormycosis: Right colon
    - Anisakiasis: Occasionally in right colon, rarely in transverse colon
    - Amebiasis: Right colon, terminal ileum spread
    - Schistosomiasis: Left or sigmoid colon

Fluoroscopic Findings
- Contrast Enema
  - Narrowed lumen, loss of haustra (edema/spasm)
  - Thickened folds & colonic wall; ulceration → mucosal irregularity; superficial or deep "collar button" ulcers
  - Discrete punctate, aphthous or large oval ulcers; may simulate Crohn disease
  - ± Small nodules or inflammatory polyps, ± diffuse mucosal granularity; may simulate ulcerative colitis

DDx: Long Segment Wall Thickening

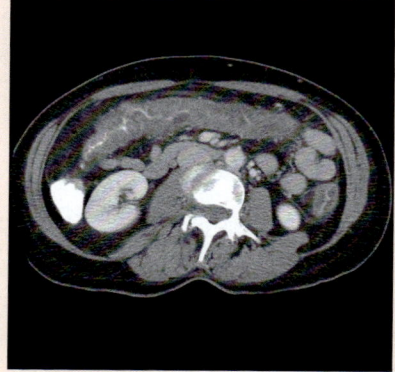

Pseudomembranous Colitis

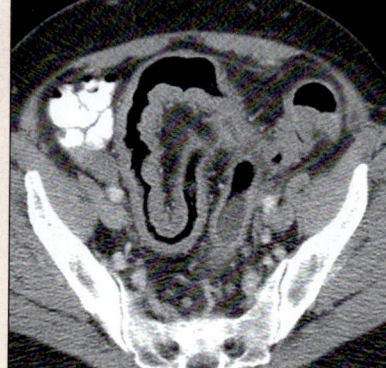

Ulcerative Colitis

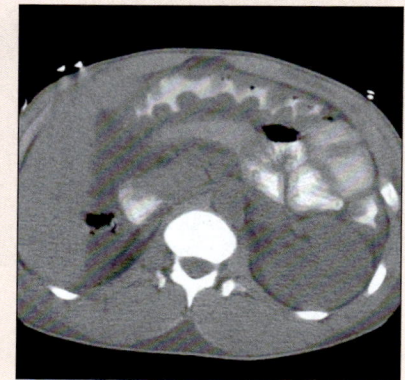

Ischemic Colitis

INFECTIOUS COLITIS

Key Facts

Terminology
- Colonic inflammation due to bacterial, viral, fungal, or parasitic infections

Imaging Findings
- Best diagnostic clue: Focal or diffuse colonic wall thickening with mucosal ulcerations
- E. coli colitis: Transverse colon; extends to right, left or both sides of colon
- Narrowed lumen, loss of haustra (edema/spasm)
- Discrete punctate, aphthous or large oval ulcers; may simulate Crohn disease
- ± Small nodules or inflammatory polyps, ± diffuse mucosal granularity; may simulate ulcerative colitis
- ± Thumbprinting, may simulate ischemic colitis; ± fistulas or sinus tracts
- Best imaging tool: Fluoroscopic-guided barium enema

Top Differential Diagnoses
- Pseudomembranous Colitis
- Granulomatous Colitis (Crohn Disease)
- Ulcerative Colitis
- Ischemic Colitis

Clinical Issues
- Usually acute in onset, except TB (chronic)
- Watery or bloody diarrhea, crampy abdominal pain & tenderness, palpable abdominal mass
- Diagnosis: Stool cultures, blood cultures, endoscopic biopsy, serology studies

Diagnostic Checklist
- Diagnosis by clinical presentation; lab tests
- Barium enema or CT detects colitis; need clinical confirmation of specific type

---

- ± Extrinsic mass with inflammatory changes → distortion, short strictures; may simulate carcinoma
- ± Thumbprinting, may simulate ischemic colitis; ± fistulas or sinus tracts
- Typhoid fever findings: Ileal fold thickening & ulceration
- Shigellosis findings: Mucosal granularity of rectum
- TB findings
  - Oval/circumferential, transverse ulcers, loss of ileum & right colon anatomic demarcation
  - Fleischner sign: Right-angle intersection between ileum & cecum, marked ileocecal valve hypertrophy
  - Exuberant mural thickening > than Crohn disease
  - "Apple core" colonic stricture; indistinguishable from carcinoma
- Histoplasmosis findings: Rectal polyps, pericecal masses; may simulate appendicitis
- Mucormycosis findings: Polypoid mass
- Amebiasis findings
  - Skip lesions that may simulate granulomatous colitis
  - Ameboma: Marked granulation in short segments of right colon
  - Discrete ulcers appearing as marginal effects or granularity with barium flecks
- Schistosomiasis findings: Inflammatory polyps, granulation response to eggs deposited in bowel wall
- Trichuriasis findings
  - Clumping/granularity of barium due to excessive mucus
  - Wavy, linear 3-5 cm lucencies, occasionally terminates in ring shape with central barium collection (worm)

CT Findings
- Wall thickening, low attenuation, mucosal & serosal enhancement, ascites
- Multiple air-fluid levels, inflammatory pericolic fat
- Salmonellosis: ± Small bowel thickening & effacement
- TB: Marked low-density enlargement of lymph nodes; changes in lungs (usually from ingestion)
- Actinomycosis: Large inflammatory masses
- CMV colitis: Deep ulcers & marked wall thickening if advanced; mucosal & serosal enhancement, hypodense thickening of intervening bowel wall; increased wall attenuation due to hemorrhage
- Histoplasmosis: Mesenteric adenopathy, hepatosplenomegaly ± calcifications
- Mucormycosis: Sinus, lung & central nervous system changes
- Schistosomiasis: Changes in mesenteric or hemorrhoidal vein, urinary tract, terminal ileum; ± calcification of bowel wall or liver

Imaging Recommendations
- Best imaging tool: Fluoroscopic-guided barium enema

DIFFERENTIAL DIAGNOSIS

Pseudomembranous Colitis
- Colonic wall thickening, nodularity
- "Accordion sign" on CT: Trapped oral contrast between thickened colonic haustral folds
- Usually more colonic wall thickening than other colitides

Granulomatous Colitis (Crohn Disease)
- Concurrent small bowel (distal ileum) disease
- Barium enema
  - Cobblestoning: Longitudinal & transverse ulcerations produce a paving-stone appearance
  - Transmural, skip lesions, sinuses, fistulas

Ulcerative Colitis
- Barium enema
  - Pancolitis with ↓ haustration & multiple ulcerations
  - "Mucosal islands" or inflammatory pseudopolyps
  - Diffuse & symmetric thickening of colon wall
  - Chronic phase → "lead-pipe" colon

Ischemic Colitis
- Usually located in watershed areas; focal or diffuse
- Barium enema: Thumbprinting, ulcerations (1-3 weeks after onset); strictures (later)

INFECTIOUS COLITIS

- CT: ± Pneumatosis, portomesenteric venous gas; ± thrombus within splanchnic vessels

PATHOLOGY

General Features
- Etiology
  - Bacterial organisms (most common in Western countries): Salmonella, Shigella, Campylobacter, Yersinia, Staphylococcus, E. coli (O157:H7), M. tuberculosis, Actinomyces, Chlamydia trachomatis, C. gonorrhea
    - Chlamydia is causative agent for lymphogranuloma venereum
  - Viral organisms: Herpes virus, CMV, Norwalk virus, Rotavirus
  - Fungal organisms: Histoplasma, Mucor
  - Parasitic organisms (most common in underdeveloped countries): Anisakis, Amoeba, Schistosoma, Strongyloides, Trichuriasis
  - Risk factors
    - Salmonella, Shigella: Outbreaks, warm weather
    - E. coli: Travel, nursing homes (O157:H7)
    - TB, CMV: AIDS
    - Actinomycosis: Intrauterine devices, appendectomy
    - Histoplasma, Mucor: Chronic debilitation or immunosuppression
    - Strongyloides: Severe debilitation
  - Pathogenesis
    - Ingestion of pathogenic organisms (often fecal-oral route)
    - Chlamydia, gonorrhea, Herpes virus: Direct inoculation of rectum (anal intercourse)

Gross Pathologic & Surgical Features
- Varies based on etiology

Microscopic Features
- Varies based on etiology

CLINICAL ISSUES

Presentation
- Most common signs/symptoms
  - Usually acute in onset, except TB (chronic)
  - Watery or bloody diarrhea, crampy abdominal pain & tenderness, palpable abdominal mass
  - Fever, headache, nausea, vomiting, weight loss, anemia, malaise, rash
  - Arthritis, pneumonitis, seizures, peripheral neuropathy, microangiopathy
  - E. coli colitis: Traveler's diarrhea, hemolytic-uremic syndrome (O157:H7)
  - Schistosomiasis: Hepatosplenomegaly → portal hypertension
- Lab data
  - Bacterial organisms: ↑ Neutrophilic count
  - Viral organisms: ↑ Lymphocytes (↓ in AIDS)
  - Fungal, parasitic organisms: Eosinophilia
- Diagnosis: Stool cultures, blood cultures, endoscopic biopsy, serology studies

Demographics
- Age: All ages, but incidence ↑ with age
- Gender: M = F

Natural History & Prognosis
- Complications
  - Hemorrhage, perforation, obstruction, toxic megacolon, bacteremia, sepsis, death
  - Yersinia enterocolitis: Hepatic abscess
  - E. coli colitis: Hemolytic-uremic syndrome
  - Amebiasis: Liver and lung abscesses
- Prognosis
  - Usually very good with treatment
  - Campylobacteriosis: 25% recurrence if untreated
  - E. coli O157:H7 colitis: ↑ Morbidity, 33% mortality
  - CMV colitis: Hemorrhage & ischemia can be fatal
  - Mucormycosis, Strongyloidiasis: Fatal

Treatment
- Bacterial organisms: Mostly self-limiting; last 1-2 weeks, up to 1 month
  - Salmonellosis: Parenteral cephalosporins if severe
  - Shigellosis: Ampicillin in severe cases
  - Yersinia enterocolitis: Lasts several months; no treatment available
  - E. coli O157:H7 colitis: Supportive treatment, isolation procedures
  - TB: Antituberculosis drugs, no steroids
- Viral organisms: Mostly self-limiting
  - CMV: Treat underlying AIDS
- Parasitic organisms: Antihelminthic drugs
  - Anisakiasis: Mostly self-limiting, last 7-10 days
- Fungal organisms: Antifungal drugs

DIAGNOSTIC CHECKLIST

Consider
- Diagnosis by clinical presentation; lab tests

Image Interpretation Pearls
- Barium enema or CT detects colitis; need clinical confirmation of specific type

SELECTED REFERENCES

1. Thielman NM et al: Clinical practice. Acute infectious diarrhea. N Engl J Med. 350(1):38-47, 2004
2. Horton KM et al: CT evaluation of the colon: inflammatory disease. Radiographics. 20(2):399-418, 2000
3. Philpotts LE et al: Colitis: use of CT findings in differential diagnosis. Radiology. 190(2):445-9, 1994
4. Schmitt SL et al: Bacterial, fungal, parasitic, and viral colitis. Surg Clin North Am. 73(5):1055-62, 1993
5. Wall SD et al: Gastrointestinal tract in the immunocompromised host: opportunistic infections and other complications. Radiology. 185(2):327-35, 1992

INFECTIOUS COLITIS

IMAGE GALLERY

Typical

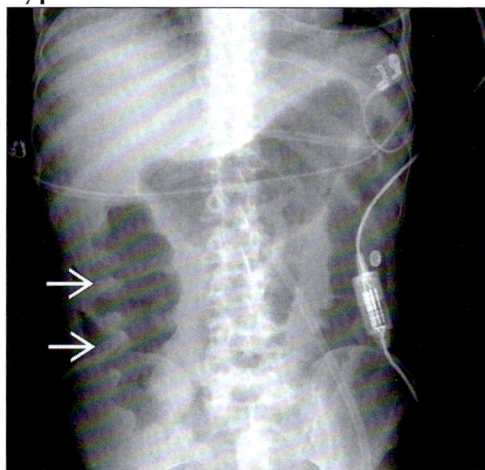 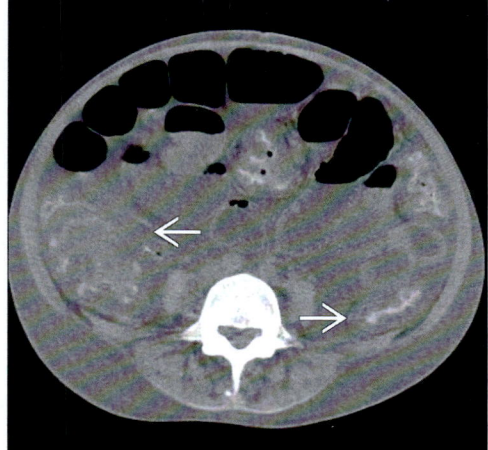

(Left) Supine radiograph shows massive thickening of colonic haustra with a thumbprinted appearance ➡. *(Right)* Axial CECT in same patient as left shows anasarca, ascites, & dilation of small bowel lumen. Entire colonic wall ➡ is massively thickened. Biopsy showed CMV infiltrating colonic wall & inducing hemorrhagic necrosis.

Typical

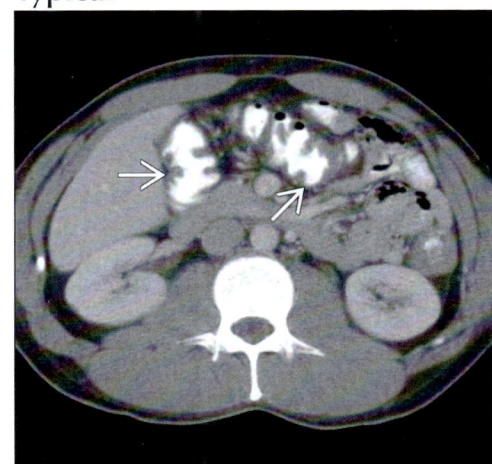 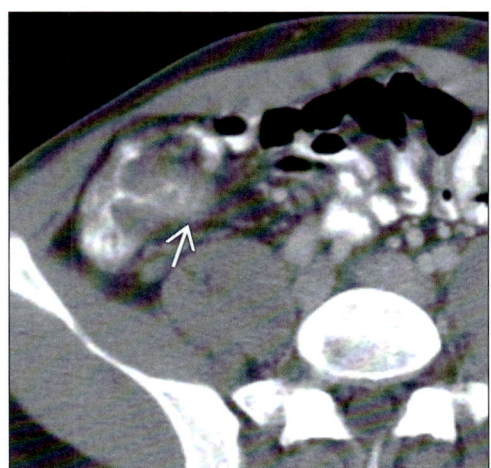

(Left) Axial CECT shows mural thickening of ascending transverse colon ➡. *(Right)* Axial CECT in same patient as left shows mural thickening of terminal ileum ➡. Yersinia tends to involve right colon preferentially, and almost always involves terminal ileum, unlike most causes of acute infectious colitis.

Variant

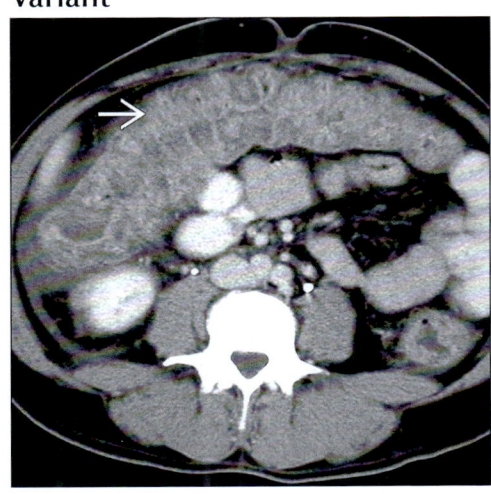 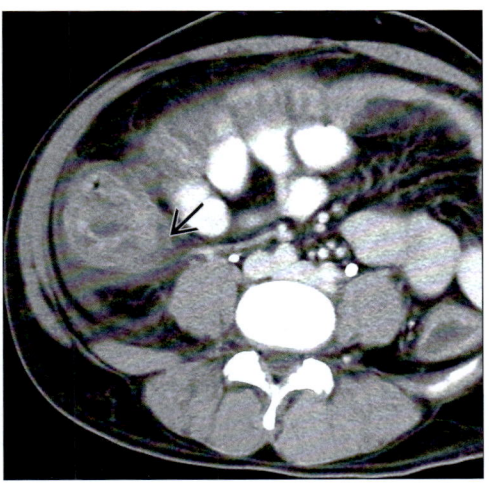

(Left) Axial CECT of CMV colitis in AIDS patient mimics pseudomembranous colitis. Note marked haustral edema ➡ of transverse colon. *(Right)* Axial CECT at more caudal level in same patient as left reveals marked submucosal edema of cecum ➡.

PSEUDOMEMBRANOUS COLITIS

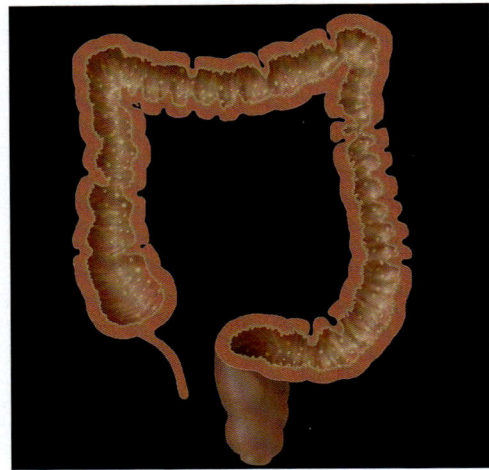

Graphic shows pancolitis with marked mural thickening with multiple elevated yellow-white plaques (pseudomembranes).

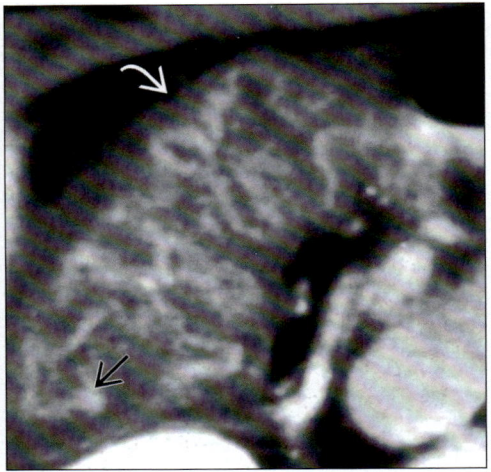

Axial CECT of pseudomembranous colitis demonstrates marked mucosal hyperemia ➔ and submucosal edema ➔ of hepatic flexure.

TERMINOLOGY

Abbreviations and Synonyms
- Pseudomembranous colitis (PMC)
- Antibiotic colitis, Clostridium difficile colitis

Definitions
- Acute inflammation of colon caused by toxins produced by Clostridium difficile bacteria

IMAGING FINDINGS

General Features
- Best diagnostic clue: Marked submucosal edema over long segment of colon
- Location
  - Usually entire colon (pancolitis)
  - Rectum & sigmoid colon (typically involved in 80-90% of cases)
  - Confined to more proximal colon (10% of cases)
- Morphology: Plaque-like adhesions of fibrinopurulent necrotic debris & mucus on damaged colonic mucosa with submucosal edema

Radiographic Findings
- Radiography
  - Colonic ± small bowel ileus
  - Gaseous distension of colon + nodular haustral thickening
  - Thumbprinting
    - Unusual, wide, transverse bands due to haustral fold thickening
    - Most prominent in transverse colon
  - Severe cases: Polypoid mucosal thickening
    - Represent pseudomembranous plaques protruding into air-containing lumen
  - Fulminant cases
    - Toxic megacolon
    - Pneumoperitoneum

Fluoroscopic Findings
- Contrast enema studies
  - Marked mural thickening, wide haustral folds due to intramural edema
  - Findings vary depending on severity, extent of disease
  - Contraindicated in severe PMC (due to ↑ risk of perforation)

DDx: Other Causes of Colitis

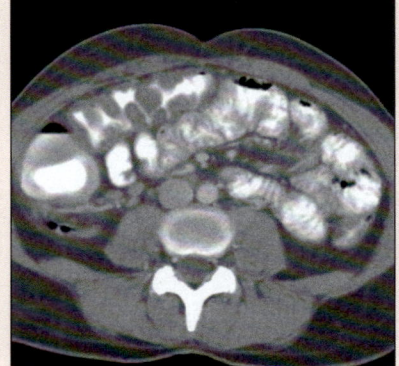

Campylobacter

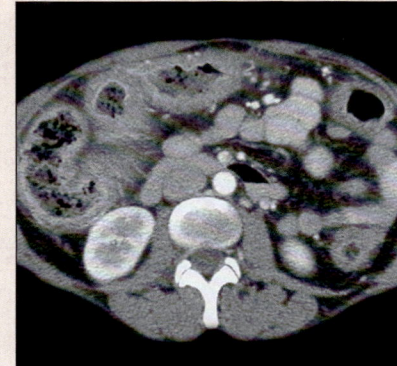

Ulcerative Colitis

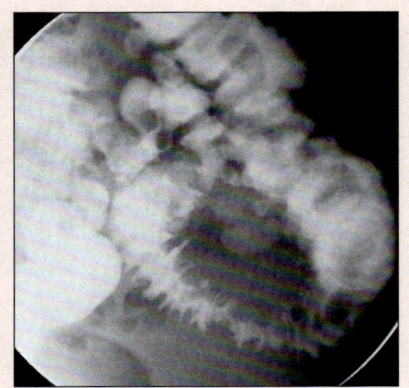

Ischemic Colitis

PSEUDOMEMBRANOUS COLITIS

Key Facts

Terminology
- Pseudomembranous colitis (PMC)
- Antibiotic colitis, Clostridium difficile colitis
- Acute inflammation of colon caused by toxins produced by Clostridium difficile bacteria

Imaging Findings
- Best diagnostic clue: Marked submucosal edema over long segment of colon
- Usually entire colon (pancolitis)
- Rectum & sigmoid colon (typically involved in 80-90% of cases)
- "Accordion sign": Trapped enteric contrast between thickened colonic haustral folds
- Pericolonic stranding
- Ascites common

Top Differential Diagnoses
- Other Infectious Colitis
- Granulomatous Colitis (Crohn Disease)
- Ulcerative Colitis
- Ischemic Colitis
- Neutropenic Enterocolitis

Clinical Issues
- Clinical Profile: Patient with history of watery diarrhea after antibiotic use or hospitalization
- Age: Elderly are at higher risk for developing PMC & recurrent PMC than young

Diagnostic Checklist
- Check history of antibiotic use or debilitating diseases
- Suspect in any hospitalized patient with acute colitis

  ○ Limited role in PMC diagnosis

CT Findings
- CECT with oral contrast
  ○ Colonic wall thickening & nodularity
    ▪ More irregular & shaggy thickening compared to Crohn disease
  ○ "Accordion sign": Trapped enteric contrast between thickened colonic haustral folds
    ▪ Alternating bands of high attenuation (contrast) + low attenuation (edematous haustra)
    ▪ Usually seen in advanced cases, highly suggestive of PMC
    ▪ Non-specific: May be seen in other colonic infections & other causes of colonic edema
  ○ "Target sign"
    ▪ Intense mucosal enhancement (hyperemia)
    ▪ Thickened, non-enhancing submucosa, ↓ HU (edema)
  ○ Pericolonic stranding
    ▪ Usually mild 2° to primary mucosal & submucosal nature of PMC
    ▪ Relative paucity of pericolonic inflammation + marked colonic wall thickening differentiates PMC from other colitides
  ○ Ascites common
  ○ ± Pneumatosis coli or air in intrahepatic portal vein
  ○ Small pleural effusions & subcutaneous edema
    ▪ May be due to primary disease or debilitated state

Imaging Recommendations
- Best imaging tool: CECT with oral contrast
- Protocol advice: 150 mL IV contrast @ 2.5 mL/sec with 5 mm collimation & 5 mm reconstruction interval

DIFFERENTIAL DIAGNOSIS

Other Infectious Colitis
- Campylobacter, cytomegalovirus, etc.
- Often have less severe colonic wall thickening
- May be indistinguishable from PMC

Granulomatous Colitis (Crohn Disease)
- Usually concurrent small bowel disease (distal ileum)
- Cobblestoning: Longitudinal & transverse ulcerations produce paving stone appearance
- Segmental distribution
- Transmural, skip lesions, sinuses, fissures, fistulas
- Fibrofatty proliferation of mesentery & enlarged mesenteric lymph nodes on CT

Ulcerative Colitis
- Pancolitis with decreased haustration & multiple ulcerations on barium enema
- Colorectal narrowing; ↑ presacral space > 1.5 cm
- Mucosal islands or inflammatory pseudopolyps
- Diffuse & symmetric colonic wall thickening
- Backwash ileitis: Distal ileum involvement (10-40%)
- Chronic phase: Right colon with loss of haustra ("lead pipe" colon)

Ischemic Colitis
- Usually seen in watershed areas; focal or diffuse
  ○ Left side colon: Typical in elderly (hypoperfusion)
    ▪ Splenic flexure: Junction of SMA & IMA
  ○ Right side colon: Younger patients
    ▪ Due to decreased collateral blood supply
- Barium findings
  ○ Thumbprinting: Submucosal edema or hemorrhage
  ○ Ulceration: 1-3 weeks after onset of disease
  ○ Stricture: Seen in late phase
- CT findings
  ○ Bowel wall thickening ± luminal dilatation
  ○ ± Pneumatosis, portomesenteric venous gas
  ○ ± Thrombus within splanchnic vessels
- Less wall thickening than PMC

Neutropenic Enterocolitis
- Clinical history of neutropenia & immunosuppression
- Usually focal disease in right colon & cecum
- Mural thickening limited to right colon & distal ileum
- Thumbprinting, luminal narrowing, ulceration
- Immunocompromised with PMC mimics neutropenic colitis when localized to cecum & right colon

PSEUDOMEMBRANOUS COLITIS

PATHOLOGY

General Features
- Etiology
  - C. difficile infection responsible for virtually all cases of PMC
    - C. difficile infection of colon follows insult to gut by antibiotic or chemotherapy
  - Other causes
    - Abdominal surgery, colonic obstruction, uremia, prolonged hypotension or hypoperfusion of bowel
    - Severe debilitating diseases (e.g., lymphoma, leukemia, AIDS)
  - Pathogenesis
    - Antibiotic therapy (clindamycin) usually within 2 days to 2 weeks, rarely up to 6 months
    - Clindamycin most common
    - Ampicillin, tetracycline, erythromycin, penicillin (less common)
    - Inhibits & alters normal intestinal microflora
    - Overgrowth of resistant enteric C. difficile
    - Enterotoxin (toxin A) & cytotoxin (toxin B) → mucosal damage
- Epidemiology
  - 1-10 cases per 1,000 patient discharges from hospital
  - 1 case per 10,000 antibiotic prescriptions written outside hospital

Gross Pathologic & Surgical Features
- Erythematous & inflamed colonic mucosa with multiple elevated, yellow-white plaques (pseudomembranes) on endoscopy

Microscopic Features
- Colonization of colon by C. difficile
- Mild-early
  - Focal necrosis of surface epithelial cells in glandular crypts
  - Neutrophilic infiltration, fibrin plugging of capillaries in lamina propria
  - Mucus hypersecretion in adjacent crypts
- Moderate: Crypt abscesses
- Severe-late: Necrosis & denudation of mucosa with thrombosis of submucosal venules

CLINICAL ISSUES

Presentation
- Most common signs/symptoms
  - Mild: Watery diarrhea
  - Severe: Acute abdomen
    - Fever, abdominal pain & tenderness, tachycardia
    - Dehydration, leukocytosis, sepsis
- Clinical Profile: Patient with history of watery diarrhea after antibiotic use or hospitalization
- Diagnosis
  - Demonstration of C. difficile toxins in stool
    - Typically takes 48 hours to confirm
  - Proctosigmoidoscopy or colonoscopy
    - Adherent yellow plaques 2-10 mm in diameter

Demographics
- Age: Elderly are at higher risk for developing PMC & recurrent PMC than young
- Gender: M = F

Natural History & Prognosis
- Complications
  - Range from watery diarrhea to toxic megacolon, sepsis, perforation & death
- Prognosis
  - If treated early, full recovery expected
  - Recurrence rate higher in women & elderly
  - Severe cases may need colectomy
  - Untreated cases can lead to perforation, acute abdomen & death (mortality rate 1.1-3.5%)

Treatment
- Mild cases: Discontinue offending antibiotic therapy
- Severe cases
  - Metronidazole (drug of choice) or oral vancomycin
  - Fulminant & toxic megacolon: Colectomy

DIAGNOSTIC CHECKLIST

Consider
- Check history of antibiotic use or debilitating diseases
- Suspect in any hospitalized patient with acute colitis

Image Interpretation Pearls
- Marked submucosal edema over long segment of colon
- "Accordion sign": Trapped oral contrast between thickened colonic haustral folds
- Usually pancolitis; rectum & sigmoid colon involved in 80-90% of cases

SELECTED REFERENCES
1. Gore RM et al: Inflammatory conditions of the colon. Semin Roentgenol. 36(2):126-37, 2001
2. Kirkpatrick ID et al: Evaluating the CT diagnosis of Clostridium difficile colitis: should CT guide therapy? AJR Am J Roentgenol. 176(3):635-9, 2001
3. Horton KM et al: CT evaluation of the colon: inflammatory disease. Radiographics. 20(2):399-418, 2000
4. Kawamoto S et al: Pseudomembranous colitis: can CT predict which patients will need surgical intervention? J Comput Assist Tomogr. 23(1):79-85, 1999
5. Kawamoto S et al: Pseudomembranous colitis: spectrum of imaging findings with clinical and pathologic correlation. Radiographics. 19(4):887-97, 1999
6. Macari M et al: The accordion sign at CT: a nonspecific finding in patients with colonic edema. Radiology. 211(3):743-6, 1999
7. O'Sullivan SG: The accordion sign. Radiology. 206(1):177-8, 1998
8. Ros PR et al: Pseudomembranous colitis. Radiology. 198(1):1-9, 1996
9. Gore RM et al: Radiologic investigation of acute inflammatory and infectious bowel disease. Gastroenterol Clin North Am. 24(2):353-84, 1995
10. Fishman EK et al: Pseudomembranous colitis: CT evaluation of 26 cases. Radiology. 180(1):57-60, 1991
11. Rubesin SE et al: Pseudomembranous colitis with rectosigmoid sparing on barium studies. Radiology. 170(3 Pt 1):811-3, 1989

PSEUDOMEMBRANOUS COLITIS

IMAGE GALLERY

Typical

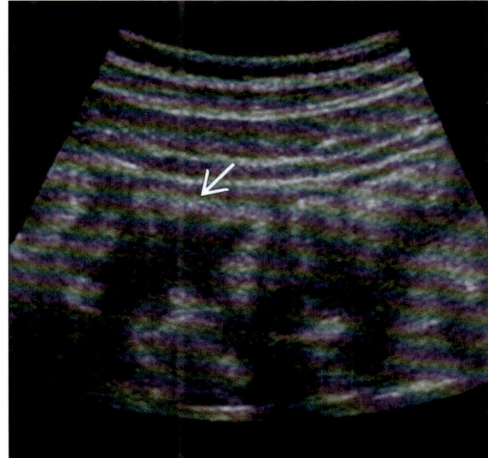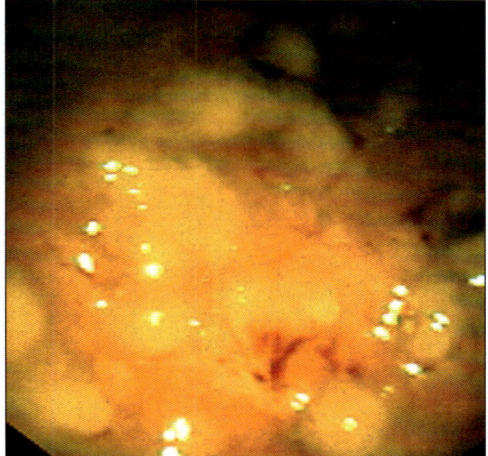

(Left) Longitudinal grayscale ultrasound of right colon in PMC. Note mural thickening with sticking echogenicity of submucosal layer indicating edema ➔. *(Right)* Endoscopic image of right colon in same patient as left shows characteristic features of PMC with mucosal edema and yellowish exudate.

Typical

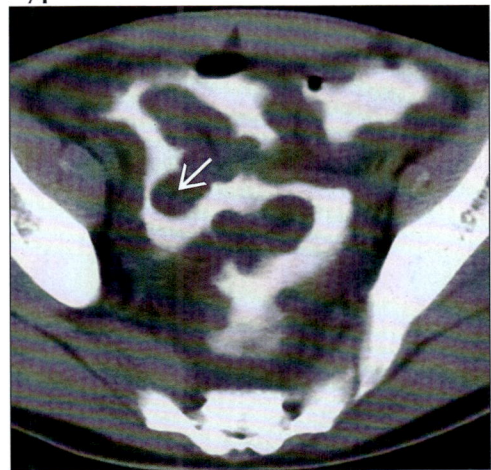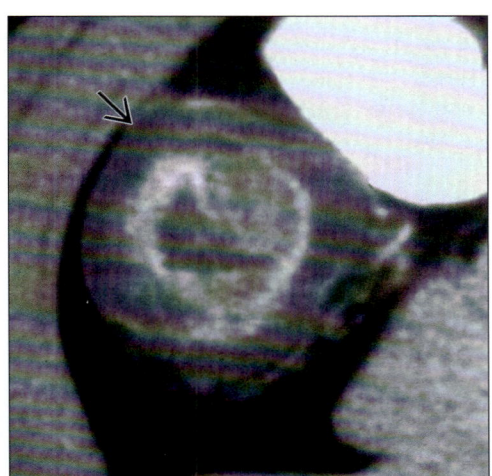

(Left) Axial CT with rectal contrast of PMC. Note marked mural thickening of rectosigmoid colon with "thumbprinting" pattern of haustral edema ➔. *(Right)* Axial CECT of PMC of right colon. Note extensive submucosal edema ➔.

Variant

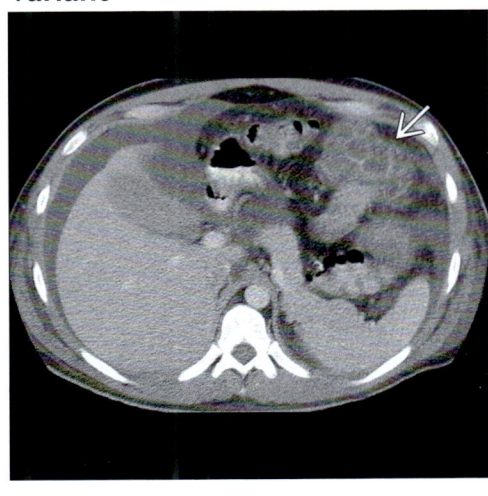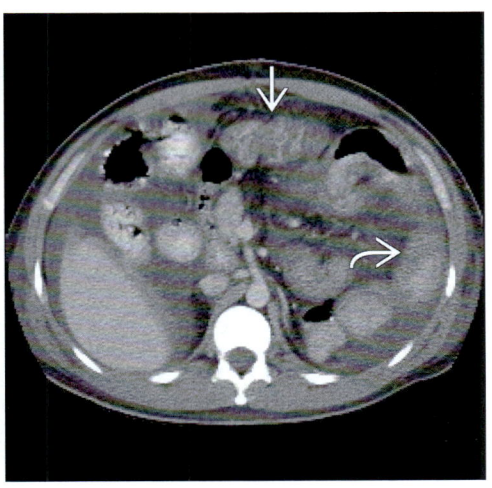

(Left) Axial CECT shows pseudomembranous colitis with small bowel involvement. Note evidence of bowel wall thickening of colon ➔. *(Right)* Axial CECT in same patient as left shows thickening of both colon ➔ and small bowel ➔. While PMC typically involves only the colon, small bowel involvement is known to occur.

TYPHLITIS

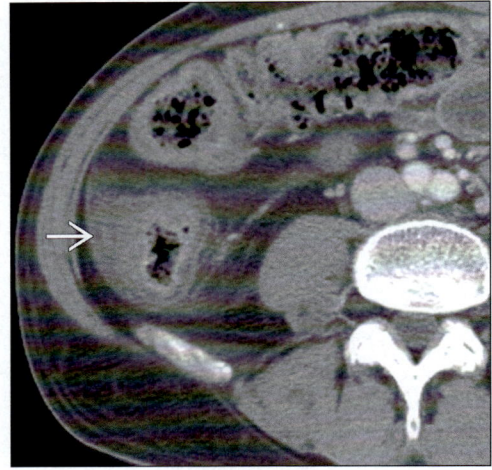
Axial CECT of typhlitis following bone marrow transplantation shows marked mural thickening of cecum ➡.

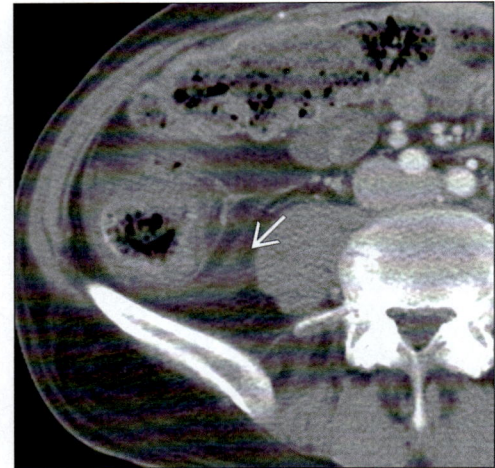
Axial CECT at more caudal level in same patient as left demonstrates pericecal edema ➡.

TERMINOLOGY

Abbreviations and Synonyms
- Neutropenic colitis, ileocecal syndrome, cecitis, necrotizing enteropathy

Definitions
- Inflammatory or necrotizing process involving cecum, ascending colon, occasionally distal ileum/appendix

IMAGING FINDINGS

General Features
- Best diagnostic clue: Massive mural thickening of cecal ± ascending colon wall
- Location: Cecum, ascending colon (more common)
- Morphology: Dilated/narrowed lumen, thickened wall

Radiographic Findings
- Radiography
  - Ileocecal dilatation with air-fluid levels
  - RLQ soft tissue mass; thumbprinting 2° edema
  - ± Pneumatosis: Speckled or linear pattern

CT Findings
- NECT
  - Circumferential wall thickening of cecum ± ascending colon & distal ileum
  - ↓ Bowel wall attenuation due to edema
  - Pericecal fat stranding, thickened fascial planes
  - ± Pneumatosis, pneumoperitoneum
  - ± Dilated adjacent bowel loops (paralytic ileus)
- CECT: Heterogeneous bowel wall enhancement

Ultrasonographic Findings
- Grayscale Ultrasound
  - Hypoechoic or hyperechoic thickened bowel wall
  - Anechoic free fluid; ± mixed echoic abscess

Imaging Recommendations
- Best imaging tool: MDCT with water-soluble contrast

DIFFERENTIAL DIAGNOSIS

Appendicitis
- Thickened cecal wall adjacent to inflamed appendix

DDx: Fold Thickening, Contraction of Cecum

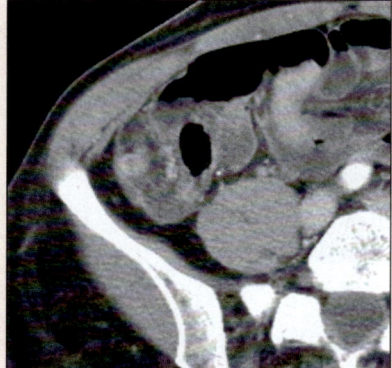
Appendicitis

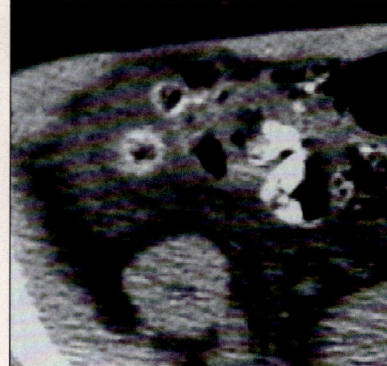
Cecal Diverticulitis

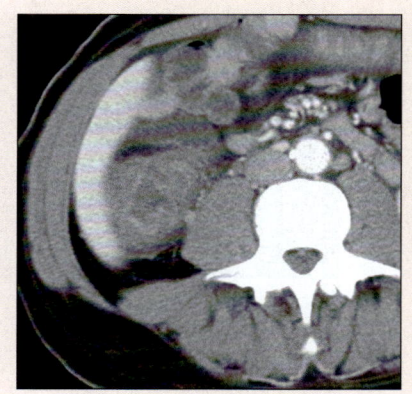
Pseudomembranous Colitis

TYPHLITIS

Key Facts

Imaging Findings
- Best diagnostic clue: Massive mural thickening of cecal ± ascending colon wall
- Pericecal fat stranding, thickened fascial planes
- CECT: Heterogeneous bowel wall enhancement
- Best imaging tool: MDCT with water-soluble contrast

Top Differential Diagnoses
- Appendicitis
- Cecal Diverticulitis
- Pseudomembranous Colitis

Pathology
- Hemorrhagic, thick, boggy cecum & adjacent colon

Clinical Issues
- Complications: Abscess, necrosis, perforation, sepsis

Diagnostic Checklist
- Consider history of chemotherapy for leukemia or bone marrow transplantation

Cecal Diverticulitis
- Bowel wall thickening, fat stranding, free fluid/air, cecal outpouching

Pseudomembranous Colitis
- Due to C. difficile bacteria, usually pancolitis

PATHOLOGY

General Features
- Etiology
  - Severely neutropenic patients
    - Post chemotherapy, transplant patients
    - AIDS; viral, bacterial & fungal infections
    - Idiopathic, aplastic anemia, ischemia, antibiotics
  - Chemotherapy/antibiotics → immunosuppression → neutropenia → infection → typhlitis

Gross Pathologic & Surgical Features
- Hemorrhagic, thick, boggy cecum & adjacent colon

Microscopic Features
- Inflammatory, ischemic, necrotic, ulcerative changes

CLINICAL ISSUES

Presentation
- Most common signs/symptoms
  - Fever, RLQ tenderness in immunosuppressed patient
  - Watery diarrhea, ± hematochezia

Demographics
- Age: Children > adults
- Gender: M = F

Natural History & Prognosis
- Complications: Abscess, necrosis, perforation, sepsis
- Prognosis: Early stage good; late stage poor

Treatment
- Medical: High doses of antibiotics & IV fluids
- Complicated case: Granulocyte transfusions; surgical resection if CT sign of perforation

DIAGNOSTIC CHECKLIST

Consider
- Consider history of chemotherapy for leukemia or bone marrow transplantation

Image Interpretation Pearls
- Cecal wall thickening, pericolonic inflammation

SELECTED REFERENCES
1. Horton KM et al: CT evaluation of the colon: Inflammatory disease. RadioGraphics. 20: 399-418, 2000
2. Adams GW et al: CT detection of typhlitis. Journal of Computed Assisted Tomography. 9: 363-5, 1985
3. Frick MP et al: Computed tomography of neutropenic colitis. AJR. 143: 763-5, 1984

IMAGE GALLERY

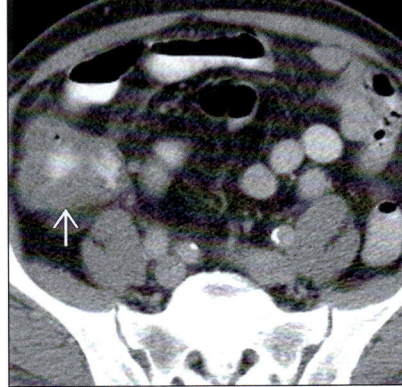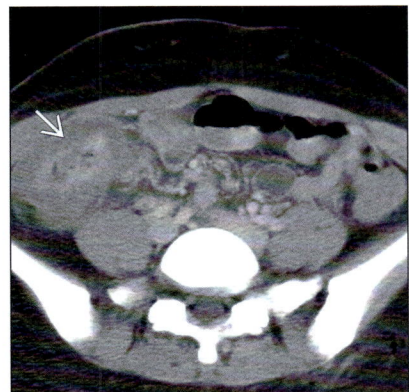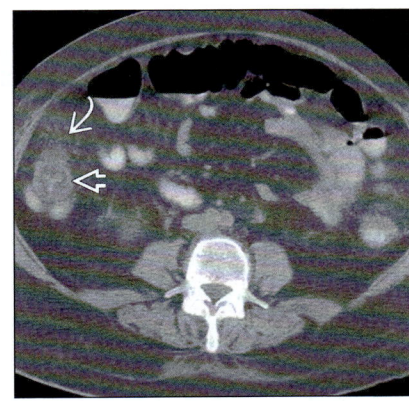

(Left) Axial CECT shows typical appearance of typhlitis. Note marked circumferential inflammation of right colon & cecum, decreased wall attenuation and sparing of remaining colon ➔. *(Center)* Axial CECT shows diffuse wall thickening & edema confined to right colon ➔. Remaining colon and small bowel are normal. *(Right)* Axial CECT shows thick-walled cecum ➔ with inflammatory stranding in adjacent fat ➔.

ULCERATIVE COLITIS

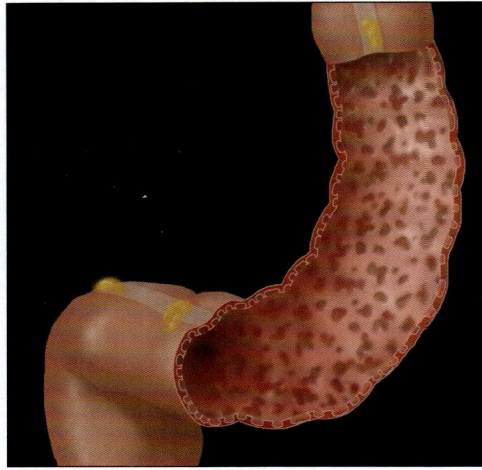

Graphic shows innumerable "collar button" ulcers and loss of haustra throughout descending and sigmoid colon.

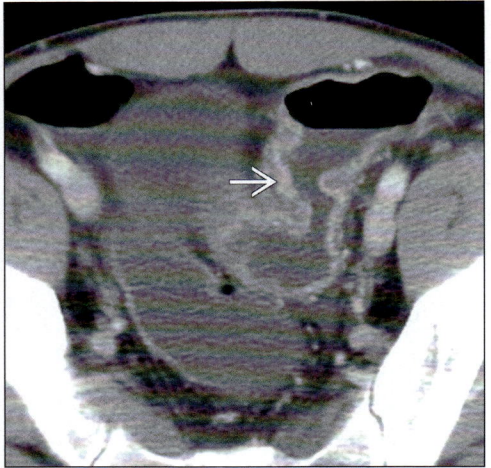

Axial CECT demonstrates mucosal hyperemia ➡ in acute rectosigmoid UC.

TERMINOLOGY

Abbreviations and Synonyms
- Ulcerative colitis (UC)

Definitions
- Chronic, idiopathic diffuse inflammatory disease primarily involving colorectal mucosa & submucosa

IMAGING FINDINGS

General Features
- Best diagnostic clue: Pancolitis, decreased haustration, multiple ulcerations on barium enema
- Location: Rectum (30%); rectum + colon (40%); pancolitis (30%); limited to mucosa & submucosa
- Morphology
  ○ Narrow lumen, superficial ulcers, pseudopolyps
  ○ "Lead-pipe" colon & lack of haustra (chronic phase)

Fluoroscopic Findings
- Barium enema
  ○ Acute
    ▪ Colorectal narrowing, incomplete filling (spasm + irritability)
    ▪ Fine mucosal granular pattern (edema/hyperemia)
    ▪ Mucosal stippling: Punctate barium collections and ulcers due to erosion of crypt abscesses
    ▪ Thickened & edematous haustra
    ▪ Flask-shaped "collar button" ulcers: Ulcers enlarge → configuration lost → mucosal islands & polyps
    ▪ Inflammatory & postinflammatory pseudopolyps
  ○ Chronic
    ▪ Shortened colon, depressed flexures (reversible)
    ▪ "Lead-pipe" colon
    ▪ Blunted or complete haustral loss
    ▪ Backwash ileitis: Inflamed distal 5-25 cm of ileum
    ▪ Luminal narrowing & widened presacral space > 1.5 cm
    ▪ Benign strictures: Local sequelae of UC
  ○ Rectal valve abnormalities (double-contrast study)
    ▪ Lateral rectal view: At least one rectal valve should be visible
    ▪ Fold usually seen at level of S3 & S4 (< 5 mm thick)
    ▪ Proctitis: Valve thickness > 6.5 mm or absent

DDx: Ulceration, Wall Thickening of Colon

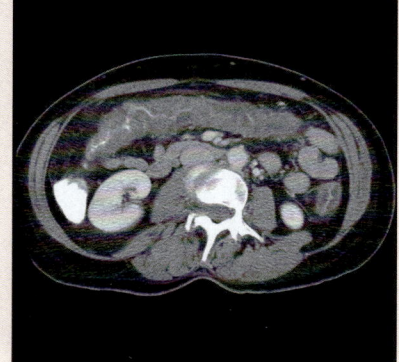

Pseudomembranosus Colitis

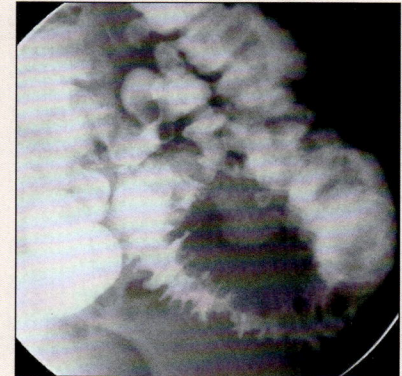

Ischemic Colitis

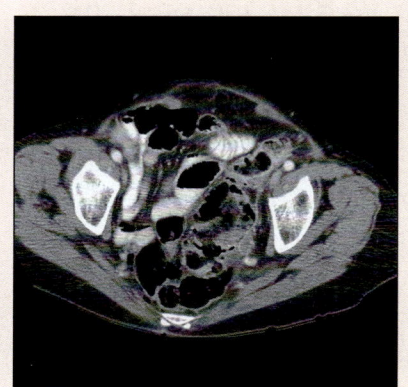

Sigmoid Diverticulitis

ULCERATIVE COLITIS

Key Facts

Terminology
- Chronic, idiopathic diffuse inflammatory disease primarily involving colorectal mucosa & submucosa

Imaging Findings
- Best diagnostic clue: Pancolitis, decreased haustration, multiple ulcerations on barium enema
- Location: Rectum (30%); rectum + colon (40%); pancolitis (30%); limited to mucosa & submucosa
- Fine mucosal granular pattern (edema/hyperemia)
- Mucosal stippling: Punctate barium collections and ulcers due to erosion of crypt abscesses
- Thickened & edematous haustra
- Flask-shaped "collar button" ulcers: Ulcers enlarge → configuration lost → mucosal islands & polyps
- Inflammatory & postinflammatory pseudopolyps
- "Lead-pipe" colon
- Backwash ileitis: Inflamed distal 5-25 cm of ileum
- Diffuse, symmetric colonic wall thickening < 10 mm

Top Differential Diagnoses
- Granulomatous Colitis (Crohn Disease)
- Pseudomembranous Colitis (PMC)
- Ischemic Colitis
- Neutropenic Enterocolitis
- Diverticulitis

Diagnostic Checklist
- Colorectal narrowing, punctate & "collar button" ulcers
- Continuous concentric & symmetric involvement
- "Lead-pipe" colon & haustral loss
- Consider UC in any patient with sclerosing cholangitis

CT Findings
- NECT
  - Colorectal narrowing & widening of presacral space > 1.5 cm
  - Diffuse, symmetric colonic wall thickening < 10 mm
  - Mural thickening & luminal narrowing in subacute or chronic cases
- CECT
  - "Target" or "halo" sign
    - Enhancing inner ring of bowel wall (mucosa)
    - Nonenhancing middle ring of bowel wall (submucosa)
    - Enhancing outer ring of bowel wall (muscularis propria)
  - Enhancement of mucosal islands or inflammatory pseudopolyps; inflammatory pericolonic stranding

Imaging Recommendations
- Best imaging tool: Barium enema (single- & double-contrast); MDCT with/without contrast

DIFFERENTIAL DIAGNOSIS

Granulomatous Colitis (Crohn Disease)
- Barium enema
  - Aphthae: Punctate central collections of barium
  - Cobblestoning: Longitudinal & transverse ulcerations with paving-stone appearance
  - Segmental distribution: Colon & small bowel (60% of cases); isolated to colon (20% of cases)
  - Transmural, skip lesions, sinuses, fissures, fistulas
  - Indistinguishable from ulcerative colitis (late stage)
- CT
  - Bowel wall thickening (1-2 cm), "creeping fat" or fibrofatty mesenteric proliferation
  - Enlarged mesenteric lymph nodes
  - "Comb" sign: Mesenteric hypervascularity indicates active disease

Pseudomembranous Colitis (PMC)
- Antibiotic colitis or Clostridium difficile colitis
- Usually involves entire colon
- Colonic wall thickening & nodularity
- "Accordion" sign: Contrast trapped between thickened colonic folds
- Ascites common in PMC, unusual in other inflammatory bowel diseases (IBD)

Ischemic Colitis
- Usually seen in watershed areas; focal or diffuse
- Left side colon: Elderly patients due to hypoperfusion
  - Splenic flexure: Junction of SMA & IMA
- Right-side colon: Young patients due to decreased collateral blood supply
- Barium enema
  - Thumbprinting: Submucosal edema or hemorrhage
  - Ulceration 1-3 weeks after onset; stricture (late phase)
- CT
  - Bowel wall thickening, ± luminal dilatation
  - ± Pneumatosis, portomesenteric venous gas
  - ± Thrombus within splanchnic vessels

Cathartic Colon
- Long-term use/abuse of laxatives & cathartics
- Ahaustral "rigid" colon simulates UC

Neutropenic Enterocolitis
- Neutropenia & immunosuppression
- Usually located in right colon & cecum
- Mural thickening limited to right colon ± distal ileum
- Thumbprinting, luminal narrowing
- Shallow or deep ulcerations ± pneumatosis

Diverticulitis
- Most common in sigmoid colon
- Bowel wall & fascial thickening, fat stranding, free fluid/air
- Pericolic inflammatory changes: Abscess, sinuses, fistulas
- "Arrowhead" sign: Edema of diverticular orifice
- Focal area of eccentric luminal narrowing
- Uncommon in patients with UC

ULCERATIVE COLITIS

PATHOLOGY

General Features
- Genetics
  - Increased incidence in monozygotic twins
  - HLA B5, BW52 & DR2 linked to UC
- Etiology
  - Genetic, familial, environmental, neural, hormonal
  - Infectious, nutritional, immunological, vascular
  - Traumatic, psychological & stress factors
- Epidemiology: First-degree relatives 30-100 times greater incidence than general population
- Associated abnormalities
  - Primary sclerosing cholangitis, uveitis
  - Ankylosing spondylitis, rheumatoid arthritis
  - Pyoderma gangrenosum, sacroiliitis
  - Greater risk of colorectal cancer in UC than Crohn colitis
    - Annual incidence: 10% after first decade of UC
    - Pancolitis in 75-80% of colon cancer patients
    - Multiple carcinomas in 25% of UC cases

Gross Pathologic & Surgical Features
- Continuous concentric & symmetric colonic involvement; pseudopolyps

Microscopic Features
- Inflammatory infiltrate, crypt microabscesses
- Limited to mucosa & submucosa

CLINICAL ISSUES

Presentation
- Most common signs/symptoms
  - Relapsing bloody mucus diarrhea
  - Fever, weight loss, abdominal pain & cramps
- Lab data: Blood & mucus in stool
- Diagnosis: Mucosal biopsy & histology

Demographics
- Age: Initial onset 15-25 years of age (small peak at 55-65 years)
- Gender: M < F
- Ethnicity: More common in Caucasians & Jews

Natural History & Prognosis
- Begins in rectum with proximal extension to part or all of colon
- Backwash ileitis: Inflamed distal ileum in 10-40% of chronic UC patients
- Complications
  - Toxic megacolon, colorectal cancer, strictures
  - Increased incidence of colon carcinoma (up to 50%) after 25 years of disease
- Prognosis
  - Improves with diagnosis & management

Treatment
- Medical
  - Sulfasalazine, steroids, azathioprine
  - Methotrexate, LTB4 inhibitors
- Surgical: Total or proctocolectomy, Brooke or continent ileostomy (Kock pouch)

DIAGNOSTIC CHECKLIST

Consider
- Rule out other inflammatory diseases of colon

Image Interpretation Pearls
- Colorectal narrowing, punctate & "collar button" ulcers
- Continuous concentric & symmetric involvement
- "Lead-pipe" colon & haustral loss
- Consider UC in any patient with sclerosing cholangitis

SELECTED REFERENCES

1. Haboubi N: Small bowel inflammation in ulcerative colitis. Colorectal Dis. 8(4):245-6, 2006
2. Hanauer SB: New lessons: classic treatments, expanding options in ulcerative colitis. Colorectal Dis. 8 Suppl 1:20-4, 2006
3. Hancock L et al: Inflammatory bowel disease: the view of the surgeon. Colorectal Dis. 8 Suppl 1:10-4, 2006
4. Rutter MD et al: Thirty-year analysis of a colonoscopic surveillance program for neoplasia in ulcerative colitis. Gastroenterology. 130(4):1030-8, 2006
5. Sandborn WJ: What's new: innovative concepts in inflammatory bowel disease. Colorectal Dis. 8 Suppl 1:3-9, 2006
6. Carucci LR et al: Radiographic imaging of inflammatory bowel disease. Gastroenterol Clin North Am. 31(1):93-117, ix, 2002
7. Horton KM et al: CT evaluation of the colon: inflammatory disease. Radiographics. 20(2):399-418, 2000
8. Balthazar EJ et al: Ischemic colitis: CT evaluation of 54 cases. Radiology. 211(2):381-8, 1999
9. Kawamoto S et al: Pseudomembranous colitis: spectrum of imaging findings with clinical and pathologic correlation. Radiographics. 19(4):887-97, 1999
10. Antes G: Inflammatory disease of the small intestine and colon: Contrast enema and CT. Radiology. 38: 41-5, 1998
11. Gore RM et al: CT features of ulcerative colitis and Crohn's disease. AJR. 167: 3-15, 1996
12. Jacobs JE et al: CT of inflammatory disease of the colon. Semin Ultrasound CT MR. 16(2):91-101, 1995
13. Gore RM et al: CT findings in ulcerative, granulomatous, and indeterminate colitis. AJR Am J Roentgenol. 143(2):279-84, 1984
14. Kelvin FM et al: Double contrast barium enema in Crohn's disease and ulcerative colitis. AJR Am J Roentgenol. 131(2):207-13, 1978
15. Laufer I et al: The radiological differentiation between ulcerative and granulomatous colitis by double contrast radiology. Am J Gastroenterol. 66(3):259-69, 1976

ULCERATIVE COLITIS

IMAGE GALLERY

Typical

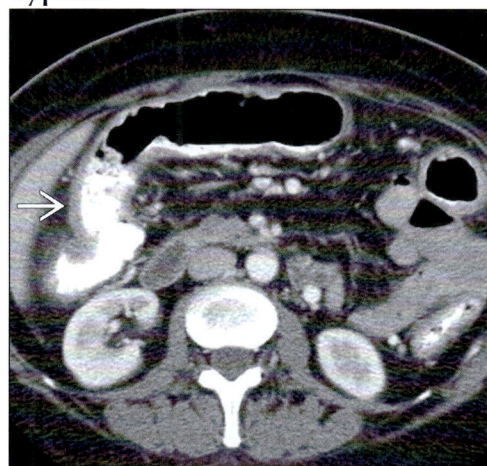
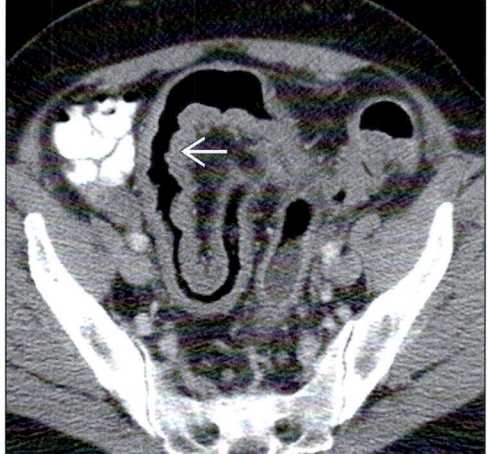

(Left) Axial CECT shows diffuse right colonic wall thickening without significant hyper-enhancement of mucosa ➡, a typical appearance of long-standing UC with fibrosis. *(Right)* Axial CECT in same patient as left demonstrates thumbprinting and subtle mucosal hyper-enhancement of sigmoid colon, suggesting active inflammation ➡.

Typical

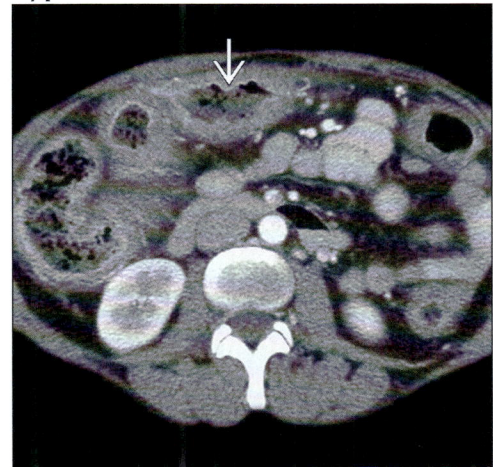
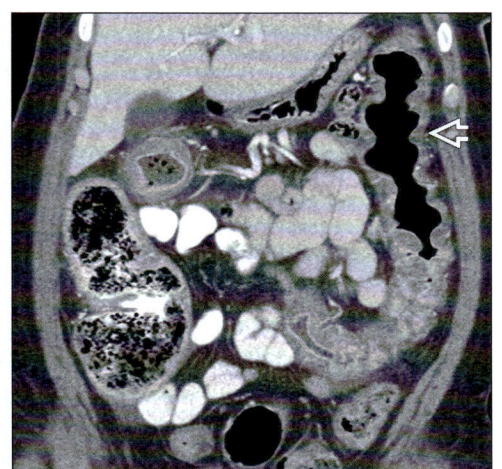

(Left) Axial CECT shows acute UC flare. Note marked diffuse colonic wall thickening with hyper-enhancement of mucosa ➡. The low attenuation in bowel wall is due to submucosal edema. *(Right)* Coronal CECT in same patient as left shows thumbprinting of bowel wall from submucosal edema ➡.

Typical

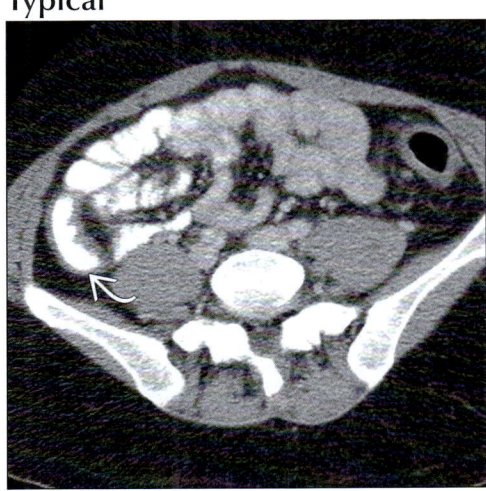
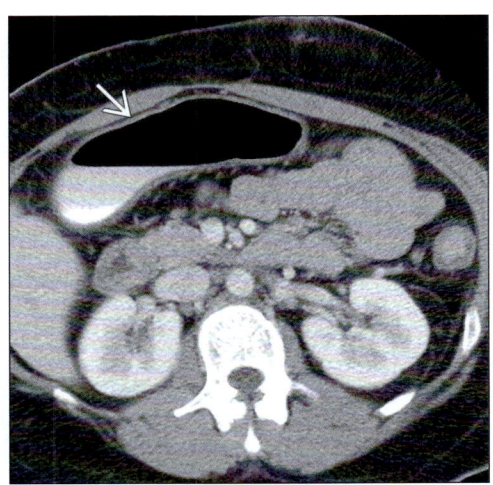

(Left) Axial CECT shows thickening of distal terminal ileum, known as backwash ileitis ➡. Patient had known primary sclerosing cholangitis, one of the abnormalities associated with UC. *(Right)* Axial CECT in same patient as left shows diffuse colonic fibrosis & haustral blunting, classic "lead pipe" appearance ➡. Homogeneous low attenuation of thickened colonic wall suggests long-standing disease.

TOXIC MEGACOLON

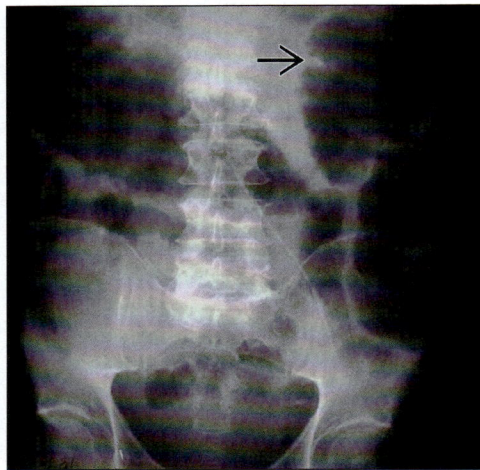

Anteroposterior radiograph shows typical appearance of toxic megacolon with diffuse colonic distention, especially transverse & descending, and suggestion of wall thickening ⇒ due to subserosal & omental edema.

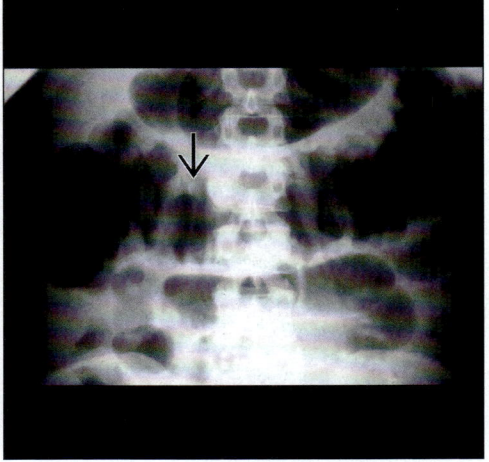

Anteroposterior radiograph shows severe & classic toxic megacolon. Note colonic distention, especially transverse, and suggestion of pseudopolyps ⇒.

TERMINOLOGY

Definitions
- Acute transmural fulminant colitis with neuromuscular degeneration & colonic dilatation

IMAGING FINDINGS

General Features
- Best diagnostic clue: Dilated ahaustral colon with pseudopolyps & air-fluid levels
- Location: Transverse colon
- Other general features
  - Most severe, life-threatening complication of inflammatory bowel disease
  - Most common cause of death directly related to ulcerative colitis (UC)

Radiographic Findings
- Radiography
  - Hallmark: Marked colonic dilatation
    - Transverse colon most common
    - Increased colon caliber on serial radiographs
    - Mean diameters of dilated segments 8.2-9.2 cm
  - Mucosal islands or pseudopolyps
  - Thickened bowel wall (subserosal & omental edema)
  - Pericolic fat line: Radiolucent stripe parallel to colon
  - Haustral loss 2° profound inflammation & ulceration
  - Pneumatosis coli ± pneumoperitoneum

CT Findings
- Distended colon filled with air, fluid, blood
- Distorted or absent haustral pattern
- Irregular nodular contour of colonic wall
- Intramural air ± blood
- ± Mesenteric abscess or pneumoperitoneum

Imaging Recommendations
- Best imaging tool
  - Supine & lateral decubitus abdominal radiographs
  - NECT

DIFFERENTIAL DIAGNOSIS

Colonic Obstruction
- Gas- and stool-filled colon to point of obstruction

DDx: Dilated Transverse Colon

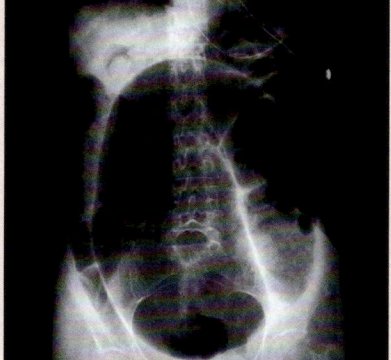

Sigmoid Volvulus

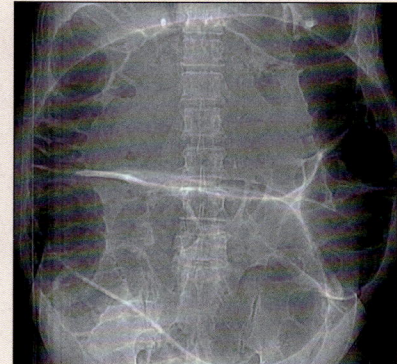

Sigmoid Volvulus

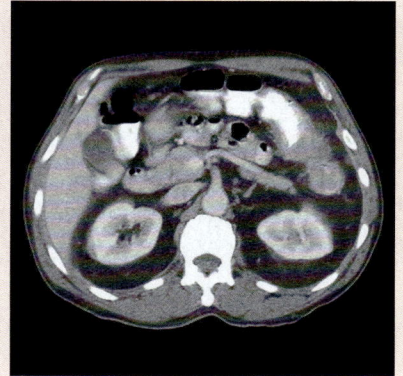

Colon Carcinoma

TOXIC MEGACOLON

Terminology
- Acute transmural fulminant colitis with neuromuscular degeneration & colonic dilatation

Imaging Findings
- Best diagnostic clue: Dilated ahaustral colon with pseudopolyps & air-fluid levels

Top Differential Diagnoses
- Colonic Obstruction

Key Facts
- Adynamic or Paralytic Ileus

Pathology
- UC (most common), other colitides

Diagnostic Checklist
- Prior history of underlying colonic pathology
- Extensive ahaustral colonic dilatation, air-fluid levels, mucosal islands or pseudopolyps

---

- Retained haustral pattern excludes toxic megacolon

Adynamic or Paralytic Ileus
- Dilated small & large bowel loops up to rectum
- Normal haustral pattern excludes toxic megacolon

PATHOLOGY

General Features
- Etiology
  - UC (most common), other colitides
  - Amebiasis, strongyloidiasis, bacillary dysentery
  - Typhoid fever, cholera, Behcet syndrome
- Epidemiology
  - Seen in 1.6-13% of ulcerative colitis cases
  - Medical & surgical mortality: 21.5%

Gross Pathologic & Surgical Features
- Grossly dilated colon + air & fluid; mucosal ulceration
- Absence of haustral pattern (thin bowel wall 2-3 mm)

Microscopic Features
- Transmural inflammation, large areas of denuded mucosa + edema, fissuring ulcers extending to serosa

CLINICAL ISSUES

Presentation
- Most common signs/symptoms: Fever, pain, tenderness, abdominal distension, bloody diarrhea
- Lab data: ↑ WBC; ↑ ESR; + fecal occult blood test

Demographics
- Age: 20-35 years
- Gender: M < F

Natural History & Prognosis
- Endoscopy; use of opiates & anticholinergic drugs
- Progressive metabolic alkalosis; aerophagia
- Complications: Perforation, abscess, peritonitis
- Prognosis: Good if colectomy without complications, poor if perforation & complications

Treatment
- Colectomy; treat complications

DIAGNOSTIC CHECKLIST

Consider
- Prior history of underlying colonic pathology

Image Interpretation Pearls
- Extensive ahaustral colonic dilatation, air-fluid levels, mucosal islands or pseudopolyps

SELECTED REFERENCES
1. Halpert RD: Toxic dilatation of the colon. Radiologic Clinics of North America 25: 147-155, 1987
2. Truelove SC et al: Toxic megacolon: Part I. Pathogenesis, diagnosis & treatment. Clinical Gastroenterology 10: 107: 114, 1981

IMAGE GALLERY

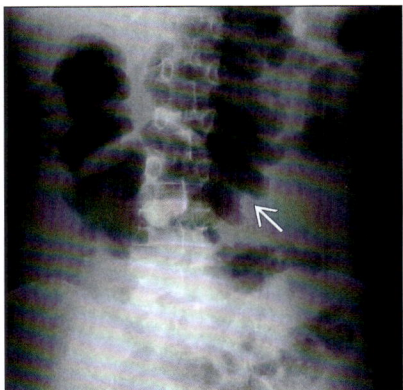
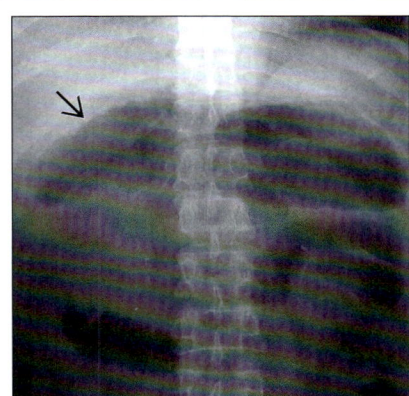
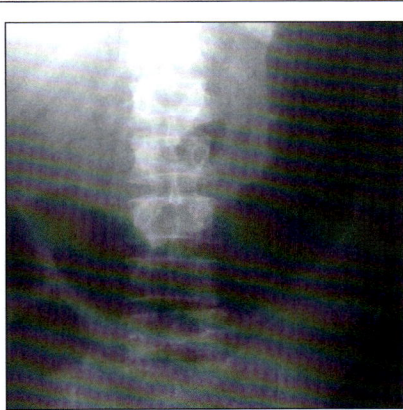

(Left) Anteroposterior CECT demonstrates typical appearance of toxic megacolon on plain film. Note diffuse colonic dilatation with marked thumbprinting ➡. *(Center)* Anteroposterior radiograph of supine abdomen demonstrates marked dilatation of transverse colon with scalloped contour ➡ indicating edematous mucosa. *(Right)* Anteroposterior radiograph of transverse colon in ulcerative colitis shows variant appearance of toxic megacolon. The colon is ahaustral but without pseudopolyps typically seen in toxic megacolon.

APPENDICITIS

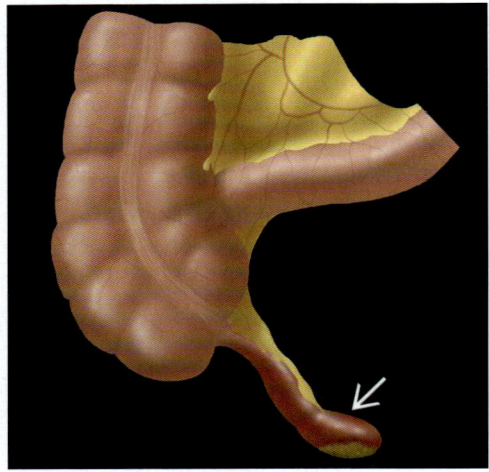

Graphic of acute appendicitis. Note enlarged, inflamed appendix ➡.

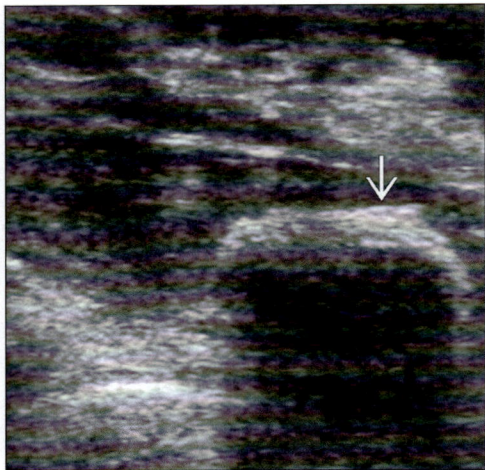

Transverse grayscale sonogram of acute appendicitis. Note dilated noncompressible appendix with large appendicolith ➡.

TERMINOLOGY

Definitions
- Acute appendiceal inflammation due to luminal obstruction and superimposed infection

IMAGING FINDINGS

General Features
- Best diagnostic clue
  - Distended noncompressible appendix (≥ 7 mm) on US or CECT
  - Abnormal mural enhancement of appendix on CECT
  - Periappendiceal fat stranding on CECT
- Location: Cecal tip
- Size
  - Noncompressible appendix > 6 mm has sensitivity of 100%, but specificity of only 64%
  - Noncompressible appendix > 7 mm has sensitivity of 94% and specificity of 88%
  - Noncompressible appendix 6-7 mm equivocal size; increased flow on color Doppler in appendix indicates positive study
- Morphology: Tip of appendix is often first site of inflammation and appendiceal perforation

Radiographic Findings
- Radiography
  - Appendicolith in 5-10% of patients
  - Air-fluid levels within bowel in RLQ
  - Splinting
  - Loss of right psoas margin
  - Free peritoneal air very uncommon
  - With perforation
    - Small bowel obstruction
    - RLQ extraluminal gas
    - Displacement of bowel loops from RLQ

Fluoroscopic Findings
- Barium enema
  - Non-filling of appendix (normal in 1/3 of patients)
  - Focal mural thickening of medial wall of cecum ("arrowhead deformity")

DDx: Mimics of Appendicitis

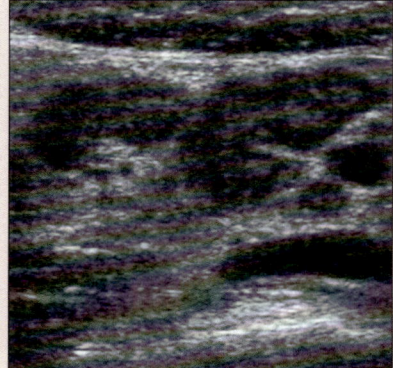

Mesenteric Adenitis

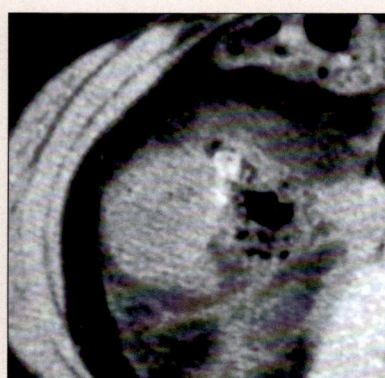

Cecal Diverticulitis

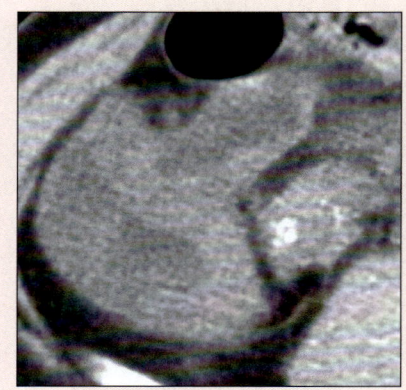

Cecal Carcinoma

APPENDICITIS

Key Facts

Terminology
- Acute appendiceal inflammation due to luminal obstruction and superimposed infection

Imaging Findings
- Dilated appendix ≥ 7 mm; abnormal enhancement of appendiceal wall on CECT; appendicolith may or may not be present; focal bowel wall thickening of cecal tip
- In pediatric patients, thin young adults & pregnant patients: US first imaging method, to avoid excessive radiation
- CT performed for patients with inconclusive US, if perforation suspected or if obese

Top Differential Diagnoses
- Mesenteric Adenitis
- Ileocolitis
- Pelvic Inflammatory Disease
- Cecal Diverticulitis

Pathology
- General path comments: Obstructed appendiceal lumen: Appendicolith or hypertrophied Peyer patches; pus-filled lumen; thickened appendiceal wall with infiltration by inflammatory cells

Clinical Issues
- Periumbilical pain migrating to RLQ; peritoneal irritation at McBurney point; atypical signs in a third of patients
- Nonspecific presentation more common in young children

CT Findings
- NECT
  - Dilated appendix ≥ 7 mm
  - Periappendiceal fat stranding
  - Appendicolith
    - May be incidental finding
    - Seen much more frequently on CT than on radiography
  - With perforation
    - Small bowel obstruction
    - Inflammatory fluid collections demonstrating mass effect, most commonly in RLQ or dependent pelvis (cul-de-sac)
- CECT
  - Dilated appendix ≥ 7 mm; abnormal enhancement of appendiceal wall on CECT; appendicolith may or may not be present; focal bowel wall thickening of cecal tip
    - Sensitivity 95%, specificity 95%

Ultrasonographic Findings
- Grayscale Ultrasound
  - Noncompressible appendix ≥ 7mm
  - Sonographic "McBurney sign" with focal pain over appendix
  - Shadowing, echogenic appendicolith
  - RLQ fluid, phlegmon, abscess
- Color Doppler
  - Flow within wall of appendix is abnormal, indicating inflammation
    - Sensitivity 85%, specificity 90%

Imaging Recommendations
- Best imaging tool
  - In pediatric patients, thin young adults & pregnant patients: US first imaging method, to avoid excessive radiation
  - CT performed for patients with inconclusive US, if perforation suspected or if obese
  - CT procedure of choice for
    - Elderly: Consider cecal or appendiceal tumor
    - Subacute symptoms or palpable mass
    - Differentiation of inflammation, abscess, tumor
- Protocol advice
  - Oral contrast alone or rectal contrast alone may be given
  - NECT may be performed in patients with ample intraperitoneal fat
  - CECT
    - Visualize early appendicitis (abnormal mural enhancement)
    - Diagnose perforation with nonenhancement of appendix & surrounding inflammation or abscess

DIFFERENTIAL DIAGNOSIS

Mesenteric Adenitis
- Enlarged and clustered lymphadenopathy in mesentery and RLQ
- Normal appendix
- May have ileal wall thickening due to GI involvement
- Pain when pressure applied with US transducer over nodes
- Dx of exclusion as appendicitis (especially perforated appendicitis) may have enlarged mesenteric nodes

Ileocolitis
- Crohn disease or infectious (e.g., Yersinia)
- US: Mural thickening of cecum and terminal ileum; increased mural flow on color Doppler
- CECT: Submucosal edema of cecum and terminal ileum; surrounding cecal inflammation

Pelvic Inflammatory Disease
- Complex adnexal mass
- Dilated fallopian tube with fluid-fluid level (pyosalpinx)
- "Indefinite uterus" sign with obscuration of posterior wall of myometrium

Cecal Diverticulitis
- Cecal diverticulum with mural thickening
- Pericecal inflammatory changes
- Thickening of lateral conal fascia

APPENDICITIS

- Abscess in anterior pararenal space

Appendiceal Tumor
- Soft tissue density mass infiltrating and/or obstructing appendix
- Usually little surrounding infiltration
- Carcinoma; lymphoma; carcinoid

Cecal Carcinoma
- May obstruct appendiceal orifice
- Appendix is dilated but no periappendiceal inflammation
- Circumferential cecal mass and lymphadenopathy suggest tumor rather than appendicitis

PATHOLOGY

General Features
- General path comments: Obstructed appendiceal lumen: Appendicolith or hypertrophied Peyer patches; pus-filled lumen; thickened appendiceal wall with infiltration by inflammatory cells
- Etiology: Obstruction of appendiceal lumen by appendicolith or Peyer patches
- Epidemiology: 7% of all individuals in Western world develop appendicitis during their lifetime

Gross Pathologic & Surgical Features
- Distended appendix with or without appendicolith
- Surrounding adhesions

Microscopic Features
- Pus in lumen
- Leukocyte infiltration of appendiceal wall
- Mucosal ulceration
- Necrosis if gangrenous

Staging, Grading or Classification Criteria
- Nonperforated
  - No evidence for necrosis and/or perforation
- Perforated
  - May have surrounding periappendiceal abscess or soft tissue inflammation of mesentery and omentum

CLINICAL ISSUES

Presentation
- Most common signs/symptoms
  - Periumbilical pain migrating to RLQ; peritoneal irritation at McBurney point; atypical signs in a third of patients
  - Other signs/symptoms
    - Anorexia, nausea, vomiting, diarrhea, possible fever
    - Nonspecific presentation more common in young children
- Clinical Profile
  - Highly variable and not reliable
  - WBC may or may not be elevated

Demographics
- Age: All ages affected
- Gender: M = F

Natural History & Prognosis
- Treatment
  - Surgery if non-perforated or minimal perforation
  - Percutaneous drainage if well-localized abscess > 3 cm
  - Antibiotic therapy if periappendiceal soft tissue inflammation and no abscess
- Complications
  - Gangrene and perforation; abscess formation
  - Peritonitis; septicemia; liver abscess
  - Pyelophlebitis
- Prognosis
  - Excellent with early surgery

DIAGNOSTIC CHECKLIST

Consider
- Mesenteric adenitis if appendix normal and nodes enlarged

Image Interpretation Pearls
- Distended non-compressible appendix ≥ 7 mm
- May or may not have appendicolith
- Periappendiceal fat stranding on contrast enhancement

SELECTED REFERENCES

1. Andersson RE: Meta-analysis of the clinical and laboratory diagnosis of appendicitis. Br J Surg. 91(1):28-37, 2004
2. Rosendahl K et al: Imaging strategies in children with suspected appendicitis. Eur Radiol, 2004
3. Horrow MM et al: Differentiation of perforated from nonperforated appendicitis at CT. Radiology. 227(1):46-51, 2003
4. Jacobs JE et al: CT imaging in acute appendicitis: techniques and controversies. Semin Ultrasound CT MR. 24(2):96-100, 2003
5. Lee JH: Sonography of acute appendicitis. Semin Ultrasound CT MR. 24(2):83-90, 2003
6. Macari M et al: The acute right lower quadrant: CT evaluation. Radiol Clin North Am. 41(6):1117-36, 2003
7. Neumayer L et al: Imaging in appendicitis: a review with special emphasis on the treatment of women. Obstet Gynecol. 102(6):1404-9, 2003
8. O'Malley ME et al: US of gastrointestinal tract abnormalities with CT correlation. Radiographics. 23(1):59-72, 2003
9. Paulson EK et al: Clinical practice. Suspected appendicitis. N Engl J Med. 348(3):236-42, 2003
10. Puylaert JB: Ultrasonography of the acute abdomen: gastrointestinal conditions. Radiol Clin North Am. 41(6):1227-42, vii, 2003
11. Wijetunga R et al: The CT diagnosis of acute appendicitis. Semin Ultrasound CT MR. 24(2):101-6, 2003
12. Bendeck SE et al: Imaging for suspected appendicitis: negative appendectomy and perforation rates. Radiology. 225(1):131-6, 2002
13. Raman SS et al: Accuracy of nonfocused helical CT for the diagnosis of acute appendicitis: a 5-year review. AJR Am J Roentgenol. 178(6):1319-25, 2002
14. Jones PF: Suspected acute appendicitis: trends in management over 30 years. Br J Surg. 88(12):1570-7, 2001
15. van Breda Vriesman AC et al: Epiploic appendagitis and omental infarction. Eur J Surg. 167(10):723-7, 2001

APPENDICITIS

IMAGE GALLERY

Typical

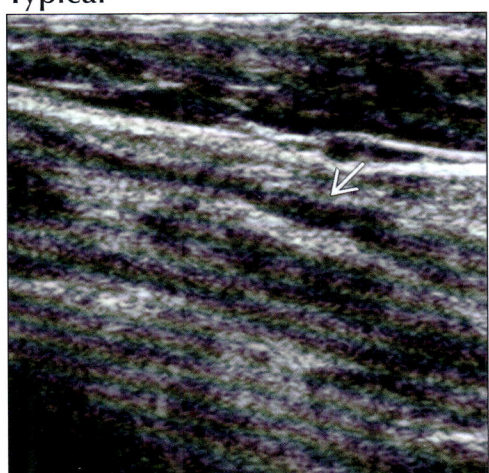
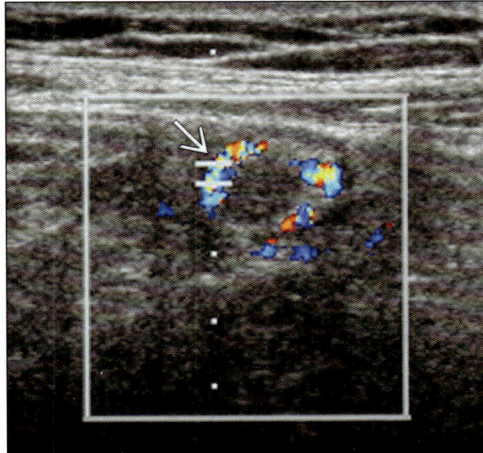

(Left) longitudinal grayscale sonogram in early appendicitis. Note noncompressible 7 mm appendix with well-preserved submucosal layer ➡. *(Right)* Color Doppler ultrasound in same patient as left image demonstrates increased mural flow ➡.

Typical

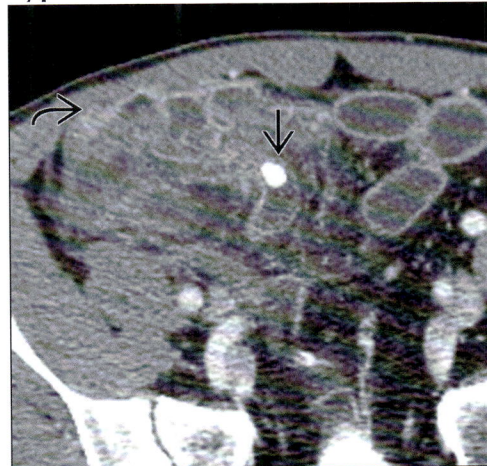
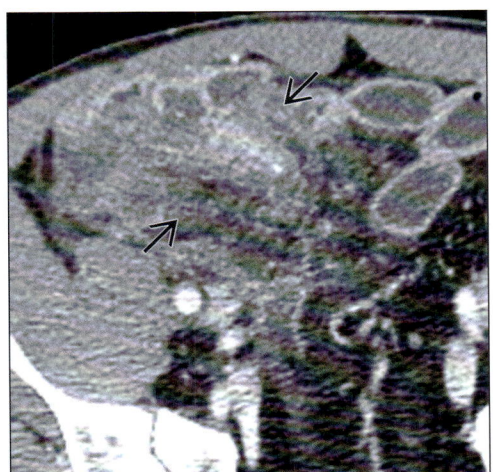

(Left) Axial CECT shows perforated appendicitis. Note appendicolith ➡ and cecal wall thickening ➡. *(Right)* Axial CECT peri-appendiceal fat stranding ➡ is evident from perforation of same patient as left.

Variant

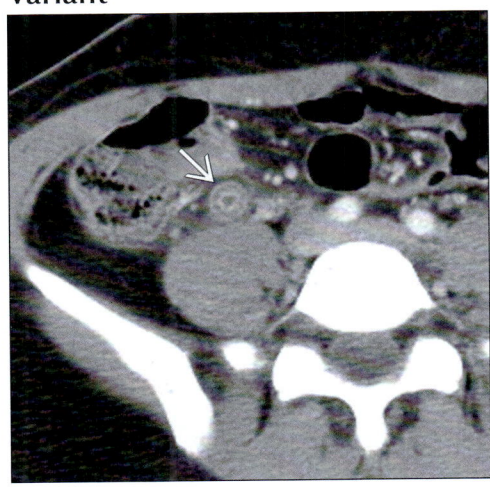
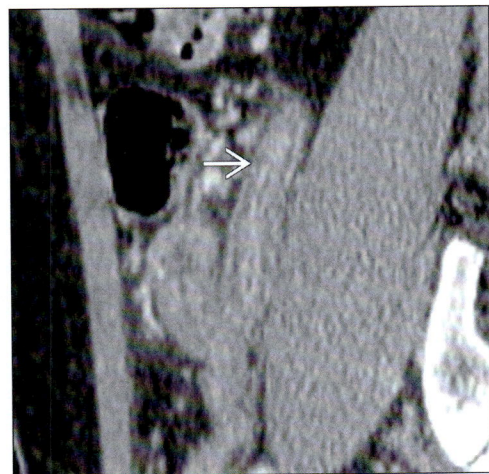

(Left) Axial CECT shows early appendicitis with prominent submucosal edema of the appendix. Note target appearance of appendix ➡. *(Right)* Sagittal reformation in same patient as left demonstrates long retrocecal appendix ➡ extending along psoas muscle.

DIVERTICULITIS

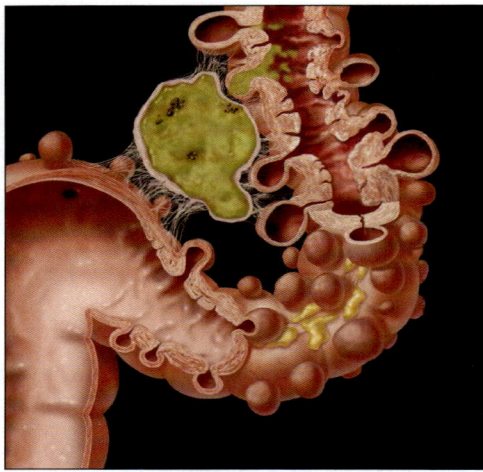

Graphic shows sigmoid diverticula, luminal narrowing + wall thickening (circular muscle hypertrophy). Pericolic abscess due to perforated diverticulum. Rectum spared.

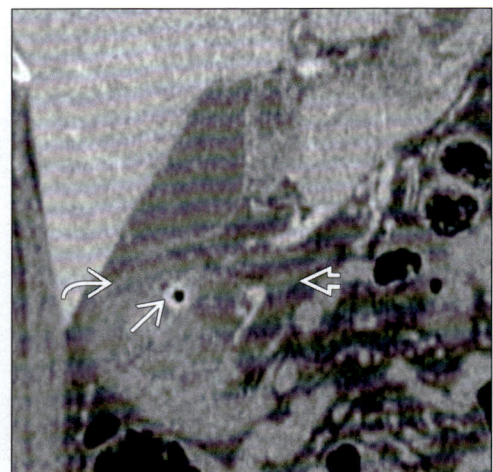

Coronal CECT reformat of diverticulitis mimicking acute cholecystitis. Note calcified enterolith within hepatic flexure diverticulum ➡, adjacent mural thickening ➡, & pericolonic inflammatory changes ➡.

TERMINOLOGY

Definitions
- Inflammation or perforation of colonic diverticula, which are acquired herniations of mucosa & submucosa through muscular layers of bowel wall

IMAGING FINDINGS

General Features
- Best diagnostic clue: Small colonic outpouchings with irregular wall thickening & pericolic fat stranding
- Location
  ○ Most common in sigmoid colon
  ○ Diverticula occur mainly where vasa recta vessels pierce muscularis propria, between mesenteric & antimesenteric taeniae
- Size: Diverticula usually 0.5-1.0 cm
- Morphology: Saccular outpouchings of colon with perforation, inflammation & abscess formation
- Other general features
  ○ Colonic diverticula are pseudodiverticula
    ▪ Mucosa + submucosa; no muscularis propria

Fluoroscopic Findings
- Single contrast barium enema
  ○ Immature diverticula
    ▪ Resemble punctate ulcer en face; conical or triangular (1-2 mm high) in profile
  ○ Mature diverticula: Shape varies by angle & degree of barium fill
    ▪ En face: Ring shadow or round barium collection
    ▪ Profile: Flask-like protrusion, long or large neck
    ▪ Diverticulum with long & narrow neck mimics pedunculated polyp on air-contrast enema
    ▪ Diverticulum with large neck mimics sessile polyp
    ▪ "Bowler hat sign": Dome of hat points away from bowel wall (diverticulum); toward lumen (polyp)
  ○ Progressive disease: Irregular diverticula, narrowed lumen with serrated or "cog wheel" appearance

CT Findings
- Diverticulosis
  ○ Mural thickening of colon, 4-15 mm
  ○ Multiple air-, contrast- or stool-filled outpouchings (diverticula)
- Diverticulitis
  ○ CT more than 95% accurate in diagnosis

DDx: Wall Thickening with Pericolonic Infiltration

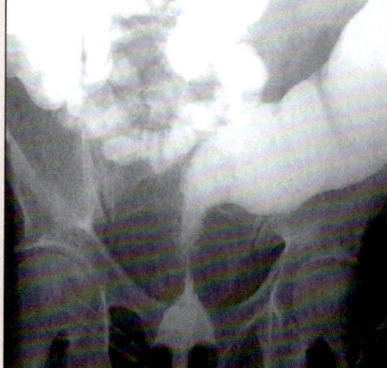

Radiation Colitis

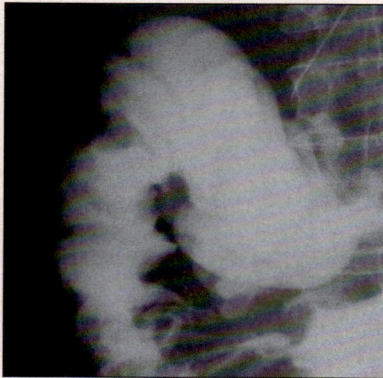

Ischemic Colitis

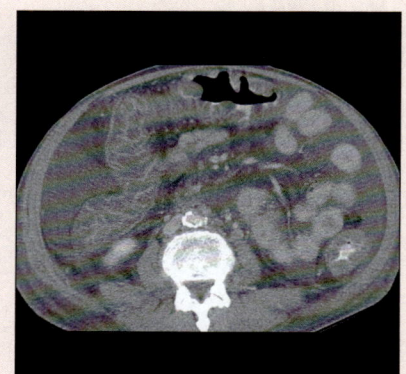

Pseudomembranous Colitis

DIVERTICULITIS

Key Facts

Terminology
- Inflammation or perforation of colonic diverticula, which are acquired herniations of mucosa & submucosa through muscular layers of bowel wall

Imaging Findings
- Best diagnostic clue: Small colonic outpouchings with irregular wall thickening & pericolic fat stranding
- Most common in sigmoid colon
- CT more than 95% accurate in diagnosis
- MDCT: Oral & IV ± rectal contrast for acutely ill

Top Differential Diagnoses
- Colon Carcinoma
- Radiation Colitis
- Ischemic Colitis
- Pseudomembranous Colitis (PMC)

Pathology
- Rare in less developed countries (less processed food, higher fiber diet)

Clinical Issues
- Percutaneous abscess drainage can obviate surgery or allow elective one-step procedure in most cases

Diagnostic Checklist
- Bowel wall thickening, pericolic infiltration & fat stranding affecting sigmoid colon
- Long segment colonic involvement, extensive inflammatory changes & absence of nodes or metastases favors diverticulitis over colon cancer

---

  - Bowel wall thickening, fat stranding, thickened base of sigmoid mesocolon, free fluid
  - Long segment (> 10 cm) of colonic involvement
  - Pericolic abscess, sinus tracts, fistulas, intramural or abdomino-pelvic abscess
  - "Arrowhead" sign: Edema at orifice of inflamed diverticulum
  - Inflammation usually localized to pericolonic area
  - ± Gas or thrombus in mesenteric & portal veins following course of interior mesenteric vein
  - ± Liver abscesses
  - Free air + peritonitis (less common)
    - Omentum acts to "wall off" and limit spread of pericolonic abscess

Ultrasonographic Findings
- Grayscale Ultrasound
  - Diverticulosis
    - Thickened bowel wall (> 4 mm)
    - Diverticula: Round or oval hypo-/hyperechoic foci protruding from colonic wall, focal disruption of normal layer ± acoustic shadows
  - Diverticulitis
    - Pericolic inflammation: Increased echogenicity ± ill-defined hypoechoic areas
    - Pericolic abscess: Hypoechoic ± internal echoes
    - Mural thickening
- Color and Power Doppler
  - Hyperemia of pericolonic fat

Imaging Recommendations
- Best imaging tool
  - MDCT: Oral & IV ± rectal contrast for acutely ill
  - Single-contrast barium enema for diverticulosis

DIFFERENTIAL DIAGNOSIS

Colon Carcinoma
- Asymmetric bowel wall thickening ± irregular surface
- Wall thickening, fat stranding & pericolonic infiltration mimics diverticulitis
- CT findings: Short segment involvement (< 10 cm), wall thickness > 2 cm, mesenteric lymphadenopathy, metastases

Radiation Colitis
- Barium enema
  - Acute radiation colitis/proctitis
    - Disrupted/distorted mucosal pattern (edema or hemorrhage)
  - Chronic radiation colitis/proctitis
    - Diffuse or focal narrowing with tapered margins
    - Colonic stricture or fistula
    - Widened presacral space
- CT
  - More uniform wall thickening + luminal narrowing, less pericolonic inflammation than diverticulitis
  - Colonic luminal narrowing or stricture; ± sinuses or fistulas
- Diagnosis: History of radiation therapy

Ischemic Colitis
- Usual sites: Splenic flexure more frequently than rectosigmoid junction
- Barium enema
  - Thumbprinting (usually within 24 hrs) due to submucosal edema or hemorrhage
  - Ulceration: Sloughing of mucosa, usually 1-3 weeks after onset
- CT
  - More uniform, extensive wall thickening, less pericolonic infiltration than diverticulitis
  - Hypoattenuated bowel wall: Submucosal or diffuse edema
  - Hyperattenuated bowel wall: Submucosal or diffuse bleeding
  - ± Pneumatosis & portomesenteric venous gas
- Diagnosis: History of nonocclusive vascular disease; hypoperfusion in elderly (CHF, arrhythmia, shock, drugs)

Pseudomembranous Colitis (PMC)
- Massive wall thickening, usually pancolonic
- Often transmural with pericolonic infiltration

DIVERTICULITIS

- "Accordion sign": Trapped enteric contrast between thickened colonic folds

PATHOLOGY

General Features
- General path comments
  - Most common complication of diverticulosis, in 30% of patients with moderate diverticulosis
  - Diverticulitis occurs in sigmoid colon in 95% of patients
- Etiology
  - Fecal impaction at mouth of diverticulum with subsequent perforation
  - Contributing factors to development of diverticula
    - Pressure gradient between lumen & serosa (sigmoid): Narrowest portion of colon + increased pressure + dehydrated stool
    - Bowel wall weakness between mesenteric & antimesenteric taeniae
- Epidemiology
  - Incidence
    - 33-50% of cases over 50 years old have diverticulosis
    - More than 50% have diverticulosis after 80 years
    - Can occur in young adults (< 30 years old)
  - Most common colonic disease in Western world
  - Rare in less developed countries (less processed food, higher fiber diet)
- Associated abnormalities: Liver abscesses

Gross Pathologic & Surgical Features
- Inflamed outpouchings from sigmoid colon between taenia coli

Microscopic Features
- Diverticula: Mucosal herniation through defect in circular layer of muscle
- Diverticulitis: Perforation with inflammation & micro-/macroabscess

CLINICAL ISSUES

Presentation
- Most common signs/symptoms
  - Diverticulitis
    - LLQ colicky pain, tenderness, palpable mass
    - Fever, altered bowel habits
  - Diverticulosis
    - Asymptomatic; pain & rectal bleeding (30% cases)
    - Alternating constipation & diarrhea due to luminal narrowing
  - Lab-data: ↑ WBC count; anemia; ± blood in stool

Demographics
- Age: 5th-8th decade (peak), though frequently occurs in younger patients
- Gender: M = F

Natural History & Prognosis
- Diverticular disease of colon is a sequence of events
  - Prediverticular phase: Circular muscular thickening of colonic wall
  - Diverticulosis: Frank outpouchings (diverticula)
  - Diverticulitis: Perforation & localized pericolic inflammation or abscess
- Complications
  - Perforation, pericolonic abscess, vesicocolonic fistula, sinus
  - Obstruction, hemorrhage
  - Pylephlebitis (portal vein thrombus); liver abscesses
  - Immunocompromised at ↑ risk for peritonitis, sepsis
- Prognosis: Good if early stage or with surgery

Treatment
- High-fiber diet (preventive)
- Antibiotics, IV fluids, bowel rest
- Emergent surgery for fecal peritonitis
- Percutaneous abscess drainage can obviate surgery or allow elective one-step procedure in most cases

DIAGNOSTIC CHECKLIST

Image Interpretation Pearls
- Bowel wall thickening, pericolic infiltration & fat stranding affecting sigmoid colon
- Long segment colonic involvement, extensive inflammatory changes & absence of nodes or metastases favors diverticulitis over colon cancer

SELECTED REFERENCES
1. Janes SE et al: Management of diverticulitis. BMJ. 332(7536):271-5, 2006
2. Blake MF et al: Laparoscopic sigmoid colectomy for chronic diverticular disease. JSLS. 9(4):382-5, 2005
3. Salzman H et al: Diverticular disease: diagnosis and treatment. Am Fam Physician. 72(7):1229-34, 2005
4. Tack D et al: Suspected acute colon diverticulitis: imaging with low-dose unenhanced multi-detector row CT. Radiology. 237(1):189-96, 2005
5. Gore RM et al: Helical CT in the evaluation of the acute abdomen. AJR 174: 901-13, 2000
6. Horton KM et al: CT evaluation of the colon: inflammatory disease. Radiographics. 20(2):399-418, 2000
7. Jang HJ et al: Acute diverticulitis of the cecum and ascending colon: the value of thin-section helical CT findings in excluding colonic carcinoma. AJR Am J Roentgenol. 174(5):1397-402, 2000
8. Chintapalli KN et al: Diverticulitis versus colon cancer: differentiation with helical CT findings. Radiology. 210(2):429-35, 1999
9. Rao PM et al: Colonic diverticulitis: evaluation of the arrowhead sign and the inflamed diverticulum for CT diagnosis. Radiology. 209(3):775-9, 1998
10. Padidar AM et al: Differentiating sigmoid diverticulitis from carcinoma on CT scans: mesenteric inflammation suggests diverticulitis. AJR Am J Roentgenol. 163(1):81-3, 1994

DIVERTICULITIS

IMAGE GALLERY

Typical

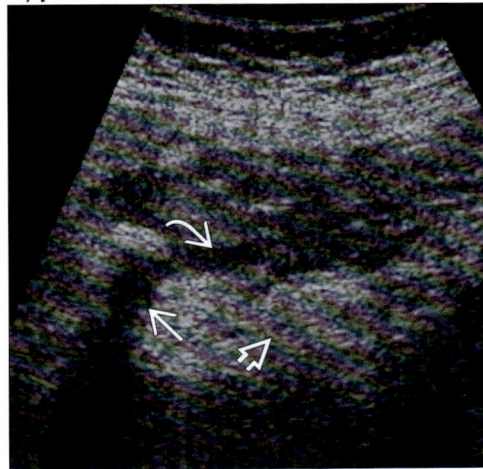
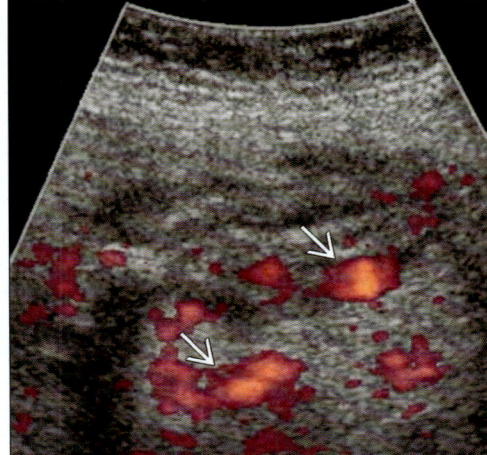

(Left) Transverse grayscale sonography of hepatic flexure in ascending colon diverticulitis shows focal shadowing from inflamed diverticulum ➡, mural thickening ➡, & echogenic pericolonic fat ➡. (Right) Transverse power Doppler ultrasound in same patient as left demonstrates hyperemia with inflamed pericolonic fat ➡.

Typical

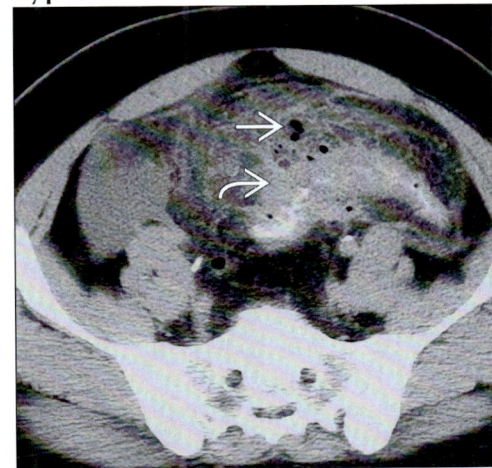
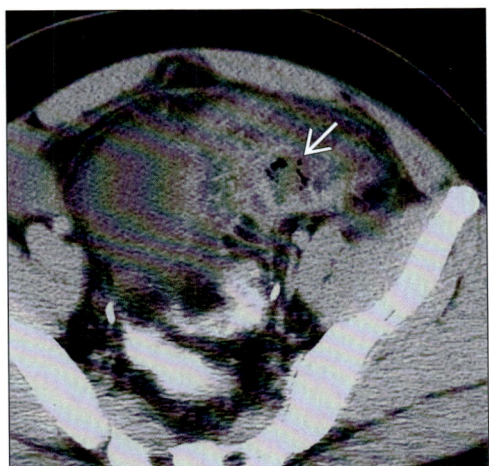

(Left) Axial CECT shows diverticulitis of sigmoid colon. Note extensive pericolonic phlegmon with ectopic gas bubbles ➡ adjacent to thickened sigmoid ➡. (Right) Axial CECT at more caudal level in same patient as left demonstrates intramural abscess with gas ➡.

Variant

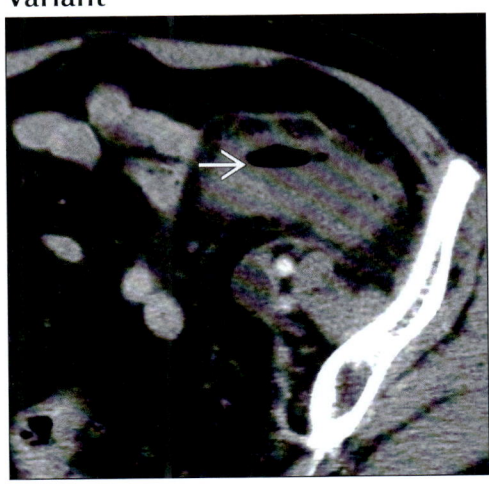
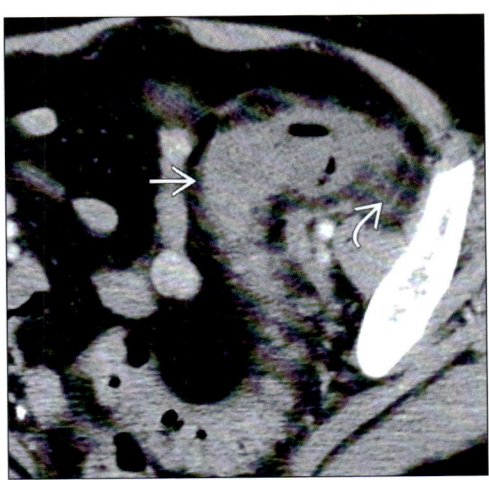

(Left) Axial CECT of sigmoid diverticulitis. Note intramural abscess within sigmoid colon with air/fluid level ➡. (Right) Axial CECT at more caudal level in same patient as left demonstrates colonic thickening ➡ and minimal pericolonic stranding ➡.

EPIPLOIC APPENDAGITIS

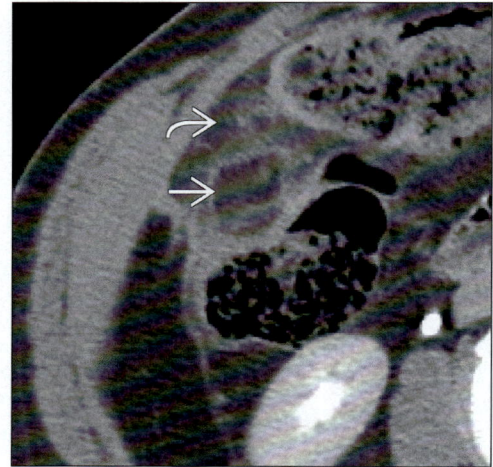

Axial CECT shows epiploic appendagitis. Note fat density mass anterior to cecum ➔ with surrounding edematous changes in pericecal fat ➔.

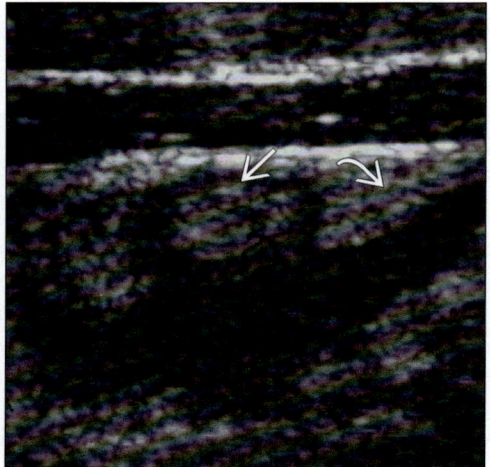

Transverse ultrasound in same patient as left demonstrates edematous appendage as an echogenic mass ➔ with adjacent hypoechoic thickening of cecal wall ➔.

TERMINOLOGY

Abbreviations and Synonyms
- Epiploic appendagitis (EA)

Definitions
- Acute inflammation or infarction of epiploic appendages

IMAGING FINDINGS

General Features
- Best diagnostic clue: Small oval pericolonic fatty nodule with hyperdense ring & surrounding inflammation
- Location
  o LLQ > RLQ
    ▪ Rectosigmoid junction (57%); ileocecal (26%); ascending colon (9%)
    ▪ Transverse colon (6%); descending colon (2%); occasionally appendix
- Morphology: Epiploic appendages: Small adipose structures protruding from serosal surface of colon
- Other general features
  o Rarely diagnosed clinically but highly characteristic CT features
  o Potential misdiagnosis of EA on CT as diverticulitis or appendicitis

CT Findings
- Normal epiploic appendages
  o Small lobulated masses of pericolonic fat, most evident in rectosigmoid
  o Seen on CT only when outlined by ascites
- 1-4 cm, ovoid, fat-density paracolic lesion with adjacent fat stranding
- Thickened & compressed bowel wall, thickened visceral & parietal peritoneum
- ± Central increased attenuation "dot" within inflamed appendage (thrombosed vein)
- Hyperattenuating ring sign: Characteristic postcontrast finding
  o Pericolonic round fat-containing mass with thin hyperattenuating ring
  o Ring: Thickened visceral peritoneum of inflamed epiploic appendage
  o May calcify when infarcted

DDx: Pericolonic Infiltration

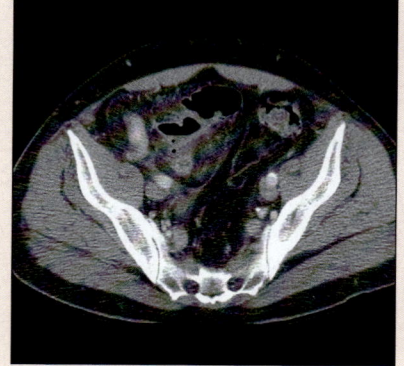

Diverticulitis

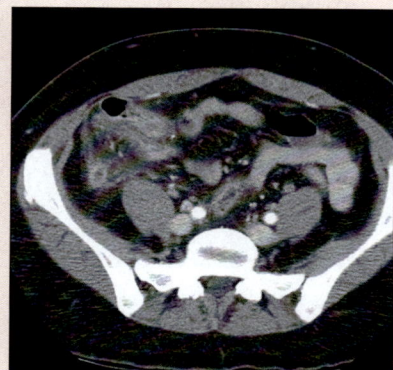

Appendicitis

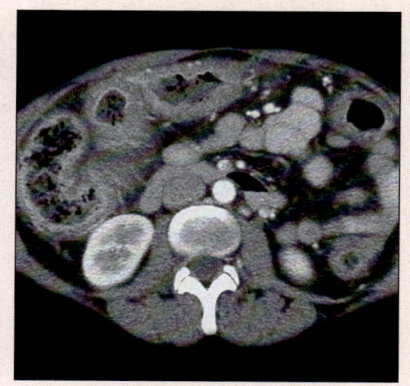

Ulcerative Colitis

EPIPLOIC APPENDAGITIS

Key Facts

Terminology
- Acute inflammation or infarction of epiploic appendages

Imaging Findings
- Best diagnostic clue: Small oval pericolonic fatty nodule with hyperdense ring & surrounding inflammation
- LLQ > RLQ
- ± Central increased attenuation "dot" within inflamed appendage (thrombosed vein)
- Pericolonic round fat-containing mass with thin hyperattenuating ring
- Infarcted EA: May explain smooth calcified "stones" occasionally found in dependent peritoneal recesses

Top Differential Diagnoses
- Diverticulitis
- Appendicitis
- Pseudomembranous Colitis (PMC)
- Ulcerative Colitis

Pathology
- Small pouches of peritoneum protruding from serosal surface of colon filled with fat & small vessels

Diagnostic Checklist
- Differentiate epiploic appendagitis from diverticulitis (LLQ) & appendicitis (RLQ)
- Pericolonic ovoid fatty mass (1-4 cm) with hyperdense rim (most common in rectosigmoid area)
- Not limited to left colon or elderly

- Infarcted EA: May explain smooth calcified "stones" occasionally found in dependent peritoneal recesses

MR Findings
- T1 & T2WI breathheld spoiled gradient echo (SGE) images
  - Increased signal lesion, hypointense central dot, thin hypointense ring
- T1 C+ fat-suppressed gradient echo image
  - Increased ring enhancement

Ultrasonographic Findings
- Grayscale Ultrasound: Solid hyperechoic noncompressible ovoid mass adherent to colonic wall surrounded by hypoechoic ring corresponding to ↑ HU ring on CT

Imaging Recommendations
- Best imaging tool: MDCT

DIFFERENTIAL DIAGNOSIS

Diverticulitis
- Barium enema
  - Focal eccentric luminal narrowing; marked thickening & distortion of haustral folds
  - Colonic obstruction with zone of transition; intramural fistulous tract ("double-track")
- CT
  - Most common in sigmoid colon
  - Bowel wall & fascial thickening, luminal narrowing; pericolonic fat stranding, free fluid & air
  - Pericolic inflammatory changes: Abscess, sinuses, fistulas
  - Diverticular orifice edema ("arrowhead" sign)

Appendicitis
- CT
  - Appendicolith (usually calcified) within distended tubular appendix
  - Distended enhancing appendix with surrounding inflammation (fat stranding)
  - Wall thickening of cecum or terminal ileum, RLQ lymphadenopathy
  - Perforation: Fluid collection in RLQ or dependent pelvis (cul-de-sac); abscess, small bowel obstruction
- Ultrasound
  - Echogenic appendicolith with posterior shadowing; fluid or abscess collection in RLQ
  - Noncompressible blind-ending tubular structure > 7 mm diameter

Pseudomembranous Colitis (PMC)
- Antibiotic colitis or C. difficile colitis
- Usually pancolitis
- CT
  - Colonic wall thickening, nodularity, thumbprinting; ascites common
  - "Accordion" sign: Trapped enteric contrast between thickened colonic folds

Ulcerative Colitis
- Continuous, not transmural, pseudopolyps, crypt microabscesses
- Classic appearance: Pancolitis with decreased haustration & multiple ulcerations on barium enema
- Colorectal narrowing; ↑ presacral space > 1.5 cm; diffuse & symmetric colonic wall thickening
- Mucosal islands or inflammatory pseudopolyps
- Distal ileum involvement in backwash ileitis
- "Lead-pipe" colon: Rigid colon with loss of haustra; chronic phase

PATHOLOGY

General Features
- General path comments
  - Small pouches of peritoneum protruding from serosal surface of colon filled with fat & small vessels
    - Seen along free tenia & tenia omentalis between cecum & sigmoid colon
- Etiology
  - Torsion & venous thrombosis of appendages

EPIPLOIC APPENDAGITIS

- ○ Spontaneous venous thrombosis of draining appendageal vein
- ○ Predisposing factors for torsion & infarction of epiploic appendages
  - ▪ Precarious blood supply from colic arterial branches
  - ▪ Pedunculated morphology; ↑ mobility & obesity
- Epidemiology
  - ○ Uncommon inflammatory & ischemic condition, uncommon cause of acute abdomen; not as rare as assumed
  - ○ Seen in 2.3-7.1% of clinically suspected colonic diverticulitis cases
  - ○ Reported in 1% of suspected appendicitis cases

Gross Pathologic & Surgical Features
- Round, fat-containing paracolic lesion; fat stranding; thickened wall

Microscopic Features
- Visceral peritoneal lining of inflamed epiploic appendage covered with fibrinoleukocytic exudates
- Fat necrosis within appendage

CLINICAL ISSUES

Presentation
- Most common signs/symptoms
  - ○ Sudden onset of focal abdominal pain, usually LLQ or RLQ
  - ○ Increased pain with coughing, deep breathing, abdominal stretching
  - ○ Symptoms usually subside within one week of onset
  - ○ Physical exam: Localized tenderness, no rigidity, some guarding
  - ○ Lab data
    - ▪ WBC count normal or slightly ↑ in most cases

Demographics
- Age: Typically seen in obese people in 2nd-5th decades of life, can occur in children
- Gender: M = F

Natural History & Prognosis
- Complications
  - ○ Intraperitoneal loose bodies
  - ○ Infarction
  - ○ Recurrent inflammatory episodes (unusual)
- Prognosis
  - ○ Benign self-limiting process; spontaneous resolution within 1 week
  - ○ Good prognosis after medical or surgical treatment

Treatment
- Conservative treatment with analgesics
- Simple ligation & excision of infarcted epiploic appendage; rarely required if accurately diagnosed

DIAGNOSTIC CHECKLIST

Consider
- Differentiate epiploic appendagitis from diverticulitis (LLQ) & appendicitis (RLQ)

Image Interpretation Pearls
- Pericolonic ovoid fatty mass (1-4 cm) with hyperdense rim (most common in rectosigmoid area)
- Not limited to left colon or elderly

SELECTED REFERENCES

1. Ng KS et al: CT features of primary epiploic appendagitis. Eur J Radiol. 2006
2. Pereira JM et al: CT and MR imaging of extrahepatic fatty masses of the abdomen and pelvis: techniques, diagnosis, differential diagnosis, and pitfalls. Radiographics. 25(1):69-85, 2005
3. Singh AK et al: Acute epiploic appendagitis and its mimics. Radiographics. 25(6):1521-34, 2005
4. Sandrasegaran K et al: Primary epiploic appendagitis: CT diagnosis. Emerg Radiol. 11(1):9-14, 2004
5. Singh AK et al: CT appearance of acute appendicitis. AJR Am J Roentgenol. 183(5):1303-7, 2004
6. Chowbey PK et al: Torsion of appendices epiploicae presenting as acute abdomen: laparoscopic diagnosis and therapy. Indian J Gastroenterol. 22(2):68-9, 2003
7. Ghosh BC et al: Primary epiploic appendagitis: diagnosis, management, and natural course of the disease. Mil Med. 168(4):346-7, 2003
8. van Breda Vriesman AC: The hyperattenuating ring sign. Radiology. 226(2):556-7, 2003
9. Chung SP et al: Primary epiploic appendagitis. Am J Emerg Med. 20(1):62, 2002
10. Hollerweger A et al: Primary epiploic appendagitis: sonographic findings with CT correlation. J Clin Ultrasound. 30(8):481-95, 2002
11. Legome EL et al: Epiploic appendagitis: the emergency department presentation. J Emerg Med. 22(1):9-13, 2002
12. Sirvanci M et al: Primary epiploic appendagitis: MRI findings. Magn Reson Imaging. 20(1):137-9, 2002
13. Son HJ et al: Clinical diagnosis of primary epiploic appendagitis: differentiation from acute diverticulitis. J Clin Gastroenterol. 34(4):435-8, 2002
14. van Breda Vriesman AC et al: Epiploic appendagitis and omental infarction: pitfalls and look-alikes. Abdom Imaging. 27(1):20-8, 2002
15. Horton KM et al: CT evaluation of the colon: inflammatory disease. Radiographics. 20(2):399-418, 2000
16. Rao PM et al: Case 6: primary epiploic appendagitis. Radiology. 210(1):145-8, 1999
17. Habib FA et al: Laparoscopic approach to the management of incarcerated hernia of appendices epiploicae: report of two cases and review of the literature. Surg Laparosc Endosc. 8(6):425-8, 1998
18. Rao PM et al: Misdiagnosis of primary epiploic appendagitis. Am J Surg. 176(1):81-5, 1998
19. Rao PM et al: Primary epiploic appendagitis: evolutionary changes in CT appearance. Radiology. 204(3):713-7, 1997
20. Rioux M et al: Primary epiploic appendagitis: clinical, US, and CT findings in 14 cases. Radiology. 191(2):523-6, 1994

EPIPLOIC APPENDAGITIS

IMAGE GALLERY

Typical

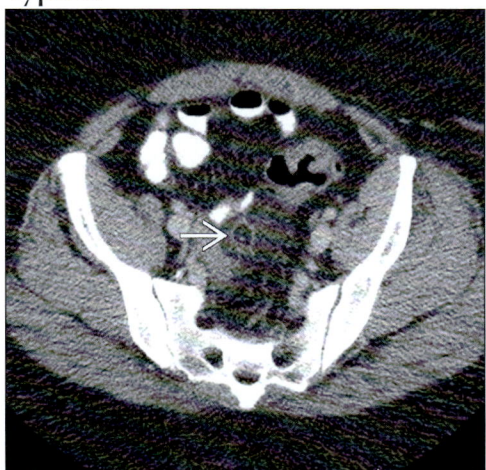
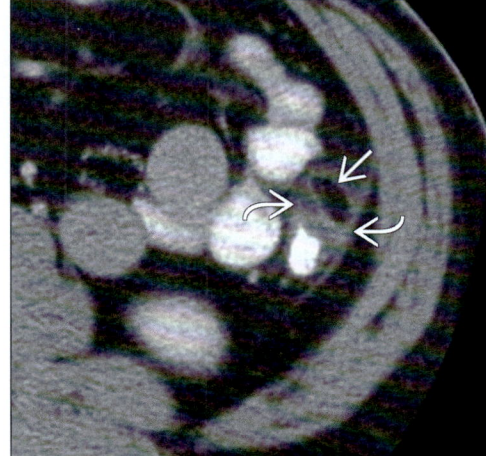

(Left) Axial CECT of classic EA. Small oval foci of fat surrounded by hyperdense rim & sigmoid mesenteric stranding is caused by torsion & infarction of epiploic appendage ➡. *(Right)* Axial CECT shows characteristic fatty appendage ➡ surrounded by acute inflammatory changes ➡. There is inflammatory thickening of adjacent descending colon.

Typical

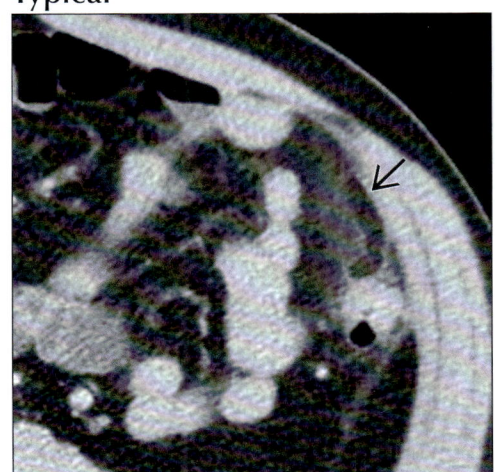
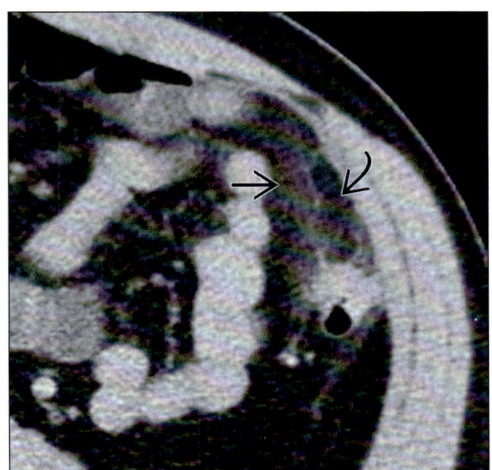

(Left) Axial CECT shows EA of descending colon. Note elongated inflamed appendage ➡ with peripheral enhancement. *(Right)* Axial CECT at more superior level in same patient as left demonstrates soft tissue stranding ➡ adjacent to inflamed appendage ➡.

Variant

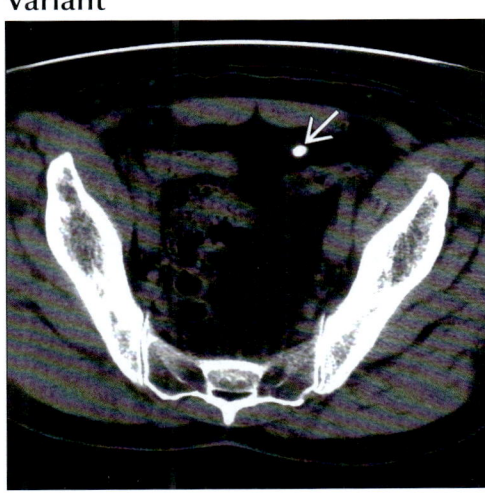
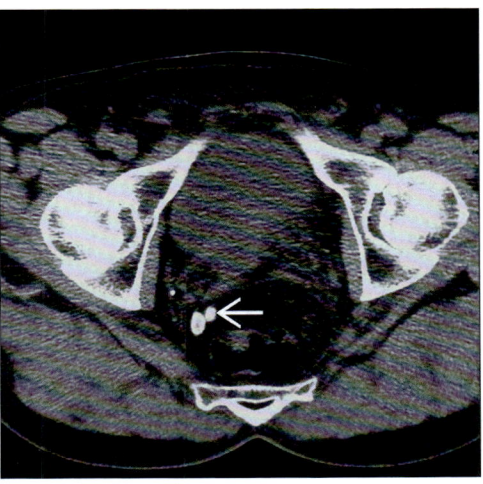

(Left) Axial NECT demonstrates a small oval calcified mass ➡ in the left pelvis. *(Right)* Axial NECT of same patient as left on a different day demonstrates same calcified mass ➡ now in right inferior pelvis. Chronic torsion & infarction of epiploic appendage may result in small calcified mass migrating to different locations within peritoneal space.

OMENTAL INFARCT

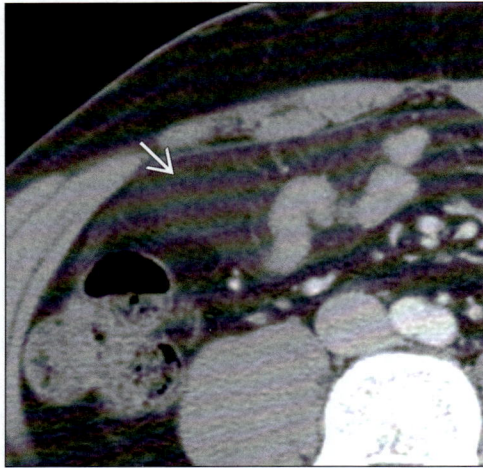

Axial CECT shows omental infarct. Note edematous changes within omental fat anterior to right colon ➡.

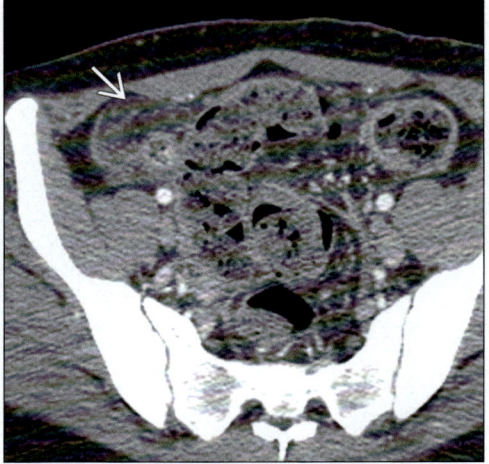

Axial CECT shows omental infarct. Note rounded mass-like area of edematous fat in right lower quadrant ➡.

TERMINOLOGY

Definitions
- Necrosis caused by interruption of arterial blood supply to omentum

IMAGING FINDINGS

General Features
- Best diagnostic clue: Focal mass of heterogeneous density within omental fat
- Size: Varies from 3.5-15.0 cm
- Morphology
  ○ Inflamed omental fat with or without hemorrhage
  ○ Triangular, ovoid or cake-like in shape

CT Findings
- Heterogeneous fatty mass with hyperattenuated streaks located between anterior abdominal wall and colon
- Pericolonic inflammatory changes
  ○ Colonic wall thickening less common
- Adherence to colon or parietal peritoneum
- Free fluid may be visualized
- Peripheral hyperdense rim typical of omental infarction following surgery
- Fatty mass with "whirled pattern" of vessels
- Thickening of overlying abdominal wall (rare)

Ultrasonographic Findings
- Grayscale Ultrasound
  ○ Hyperechoic, non-mobile, non-compressible fixed mass
  ○ Free fluid may be seen
  ○ Focal tenderness with graded compression
- Color Doppler: Decreased or absent flow within echogenic mass

Imaging Recommendations
- Best imaging tool: CECT
- Protocol advice: MDCT with IV and/or oral contrast, 2.5 mm collimation and 5 mm reconstruction

DIFFERENTIAL DIAGNOSIS

Acute Appendicitis
- Periappendiceal soft tissue stranding

DDx: Omental Infarct

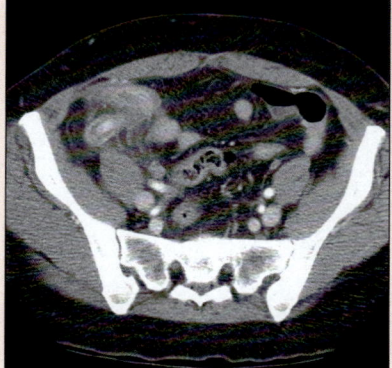

Acute Appendicitis

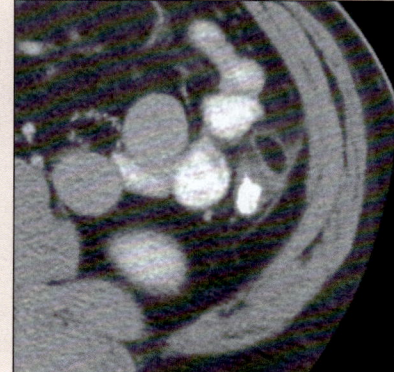

Epiploic Appendagitis

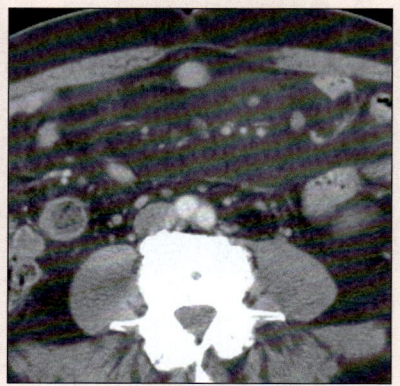

Mesenteritis

OMENTAL INFARCT

Key Facts

Imaging Findings
- Best diagnostic clue: Focal mass of heterogeneous density within omental fat
- Pericolonic inflammatory changes
- Adherence to colon or parietal peritoneum
- Best imaging tool: CECT
- Protocol advice: MDCT with IV and/or oral contrast, 2.5 mm collimation and 5 mm reconstruction

Top Differential Diagnoses
- Acute Appendicitis
- Epiploic Appendagitis
- Omental Torsion
- Pancreatitis
- Fibrosing Sclerosing Mesenteritis

Clinical Issues
- Acute abdominal pain
- Right-sided in 90% of cases
- Fever, with or without palpable mass in right lower quadrant
- Benign, self-limited disorder
- Rebound tenderness in right lower quadrant with palpable mass
- Elderly obese people (85% of cases)

Diagnostic Checklist
- Omental infarct in case of acute abdominal pain with absence of constitutional symptoms or increased WBC
- CT: Fatty mass with hyperattenuated streaks between abdominal wall & colon on right side

---

- Wall thickening of cecum or terminal ileum
- Right lower quadrant fluid or abscess
- Appendicolith may be seen in 10-15% of cases

Epiploic Appendagitis
- Paracolic fatty mass with hyperattenuating ring
- Location: More common in left lower quadrant (rectosigmoid)
- Pericolonic fat stranding
- Thickened peritoneum and/or bowel
- Primary caused by torsion or thrombosis
- Secondary caused by adjacent inflammation
  - Diverticulitis
  - Appendicitis
  - Cholecystitis
- Benign and self-limited disorder

Omental Torsion
- Due to omental cysts, hernias, tumors, adhesions
- Fibrous and fatty folds converging towards torsion
- Primary omental torsion due to anomaly
  - Bifid
  - Accessory omental tissue
- Secondary omental torsion
  - More common than primary omental torsion
  - Postoperative adhesions and/or hernias
  - Cysts
  - Tumors

Pancreatitis
- Focal or diffuse enlargement of pancreas
- Fluid collections
- Infiltration of peripancreatic fat
- Abscess, pseudocyst, gallstones
- Chest: Pleural effusion & basal atelectasis
- Extent of necrosis is best predictor of clinical outcome

Fibrosing Sclerosing Mesenteritis
- Soft tissue mass of fibrous tissue
  - Usually found in root of small bowel mesentery
- Thickening, infiltration, displacement, narrowing of bowel loops
- Calcification within spiculated mesenteric fibrosis mimics mesenteric carcinoid

PATHOLOGY

General Features
- General path comments
  - Hemorrhagic infarction with fat necrosis
  - Followed by inflammatory infiltrate
  - Fibrosis & retraction → healing or autoamputation
- Etiology
  - Half of cases are idiopathic, half are secondary to abdominal surgery
    - Right epiploic vessels involved in 90% of cases
  - Precipitating factors
    - Obesity
    - Vascular congestion
    - Kinking of vessels
    - Increase in intra-abdominal pressure
  - Kinking or pressure on omental veins may be caused by sudden positional change
- Epidemiology: Adults (85%), children (15%)

Gross Pathologic & Surgical Features
- Infarcted omentum often adherent to parietal peritoneum or colon
- Serosanguineous fluid in peritoneal cavity

Microscopic Features
- Inflammatory infiltrate
  - Predominantly plasmocytic, lymphocytic and histiocytic cells
- Fat necrosis
- Collagenous scarring in chronic cases

CLINICAL ISSUES

Presentation
- Most common signs/symptoms
  - Mimics acute appendicitis or rarely acute cholecystitis

OMENTAL INFARCT

- Acute abdominal pain
  - Right-sided in 90% of cases
- Fever, with or without palpable mass in right lower quadrant
- Rarely nausea, vomiting, diarrhea
  - Symptoms seen particularly in children
- Benign, self-limited disorder
- Other signs/symptoms
  - Lab data
    - WBC and ESR normal or mildly elevated
  - Physical examination
    - Rebound tenderness in right lower quadrant with palpable mass

Demographics
- Age
  - Elderly obese people (85% of cases)
  - Less common in children (15% of cases)
    - Primary infarction occurs more often in young patients compared to secondary infarction
- Gender
  - M > F
  - Predisposing factors
    - Obesity
    - Digitalis
    - Blunt trauma
    - Abdominal surgery
    - Heart failure
    - Vigorous activity
    - Rarely superior mesenteric artery occlusion

Natural History & Prognosis
- Complications
  - Abscess
  - Adhesions
  - Bowel obstruction
- Prognosis
  - Usually self limiting
  - Usually resolves spontaneously in one to four months
- Surgery can be avoided, especially when normal appendix is identified

Treatment
- Conservative management
- Laparoscopic excision
  - Omental infarct may be missed at laparoscopy unless there is careful evaluation of omentum

DIAGNOSTIC CHECKLIST

Consider
- Omental infarct in case of acute abdominal pain with absence of constitutional symptoms or increased WBC

Image Interpretation Pearls
- CT: Fatty mass with hyperattenuated streaks between abdominal wall & colon on right side

SELECTED REFERENCES

1. Coulier B: Segmental omental infarction in childhood: a typical case diagnosed by CT allowing successful conservative treatment. Pediatr Radiol. 36(2):141-3, 2006
2. Hirano Y et al: Left-sided omental torsion with inguinal hernia. World J Gastroenterol. 12(4):662-4, 2006
3. Singh AK et al: Omental infarct: CT imaging features. Abdom Imaging. 2006
4. Bachar GN et al: Sonographic diagnosis of right segmental omental infarction. J Clin Ultrasound. 33(2):76-9, 2005
5. Feo CF et al: Primary torsion of the greater omentum: a difficult diagnosis. Dig Dis Sci. 50(7):1283-4, 2005
6. Kerem M et al: Torsion of the greater omentum: preoperative computed tomographic diagnosis and therapeutic laparoscopy. JSLS. 9(4):494-6, 2005
7. Loh MH et al: Omental infarction--a mimicker of acute appendicitis in children. J Pediatr Surg. 40(8):1224-6, 2005
8. Singh AK et al: Acute epiploic appendagitis and its mimics. Radiographics. 25(6):1521-34, 2005
9. van Breda Vriesman AC et al: Omental infarction: a self-limiting disease. AJR Am J Roentgenol. 185(1):280; author reply 280-1, 2005
10. Abadir JS et al: Accurate diagnosis of infarction of omentum and appendices epiploicae by computed tomography. Am Surg. 70(10):854-7, 2004
11. Pereira JM et al: Disproportionate fat stranding: a helpful CT sign in patients with acute abdominal pain. Radiographics. 24(3):703-15, 2004
12. Singh AK et al: Omental infarct: an unusual CT appearance after superior mesenteric artery occlusion. Emerg Radiol. 10(5):276-8, 2004
13. Macari M et al: The acute right lower quadrant: CT evaluation. Radiologic clinics of North America. 14(6):1117-36, 2003
14. Paroz A et al: Idiopathic segmental infarction of the greater omentum: a rare cause of acute abdomen. J Gastrointest Surg. 7(6):805-8, 2003
15. Varjavandi V et al: Omental infarction: risk factors in children. J Pediatr Surg. 38(2):233-5, 2003
16. Grattan-Smith JD et al: Omental infarction in pediatric patients: sonographic and CT findings. AJR Am J Roentgenol. 178(6):1537-9, 2002
17. McClure MJ et al: Radiological features of epiploic appendagitis and segmental omental infarction. Clin Radiol. 56(10):819-27, 2001
18. Amin Z et al: A case of acute right-sided abdominal pain. Br J Radiol. 72(856):421-2, 1999
19. Schlesinger AE et al: Sonographic appearance of omental infarction in children. Pediatr Radiol. 29(8):598-601, 1999

OMENTAL INFARCT

IMAGE GALLERY

Typical

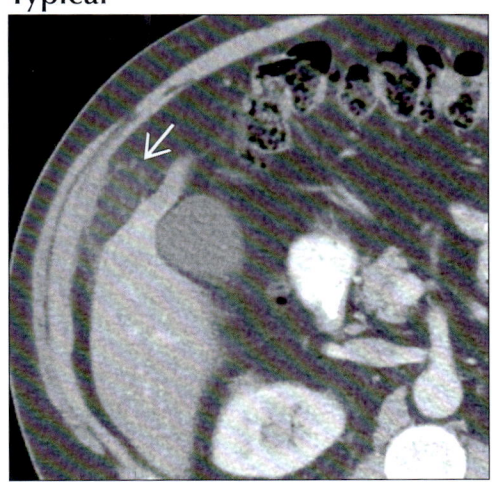
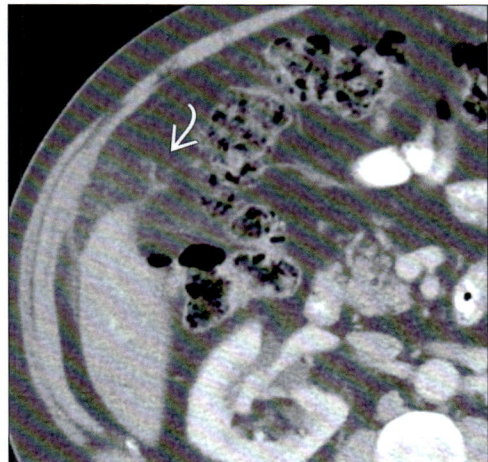

(Left) Axial CECT shows classic right side omental infarct. Note oval encapsulated fat-containing lesion ➡ within omentum overlying hepatic flexure. This is the typical site and appearance for spontaneous omental infarction. *(Right)* Axial CECT in same patient as previous image shows slightly infiltrated fat within lesion and within some of the surrounding omentum ➡.

Typical

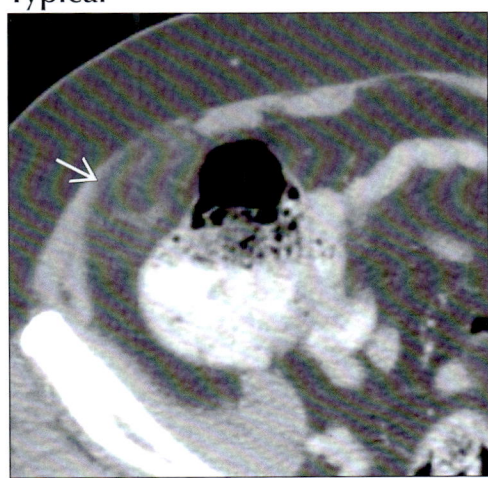
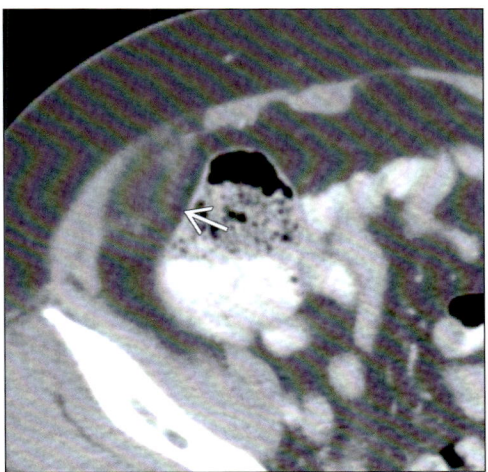

(Left) Axial CECT shows classic presentation & appearance of spontaneous omental infarction. Note infiltrated ovoid fatty mass, which appears to be encapsulated ➡, overlying ascending colon. *(Right)* Axial CECT in same patient as previous image demonstrates subtle mass effect on cecum ➡.

Variant

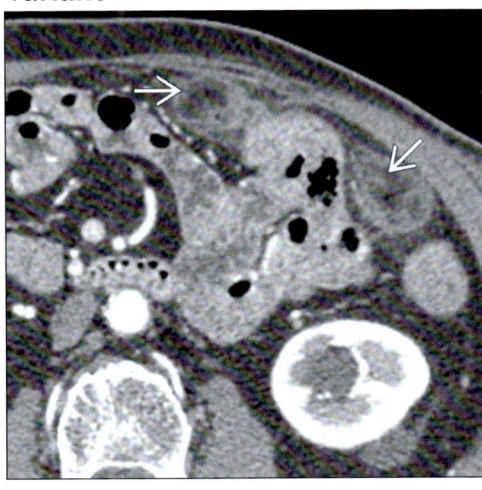
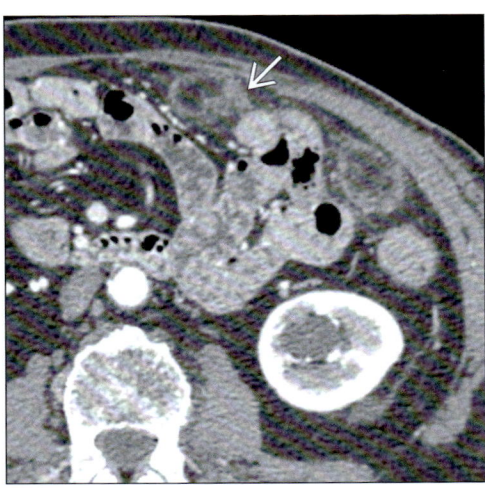

(Left) Axial CECT shows postoperative fat necrosis and omental infarction following gastric surgery. Note two areas of edematous fat within left omentum ➡. *(Right)* Axial CECT in higher plane (of same patient as previous image) demonstrates soft tissue infiltration around areas of fat necrosis ➡.

ISCHEMIC COLITIS

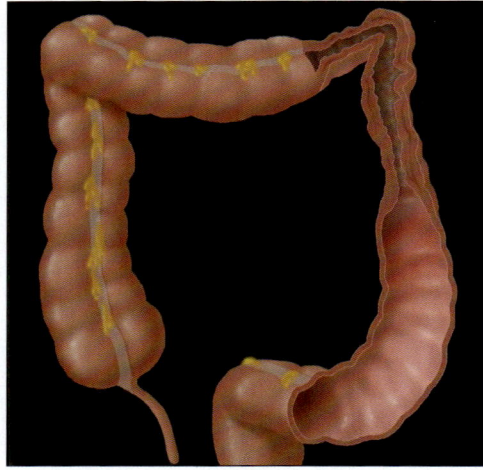

Graphic shows luminal narrowing and wall thickening near the splenic flexure, the "watershed" area between the vascular distribution of the SMA and IMA.

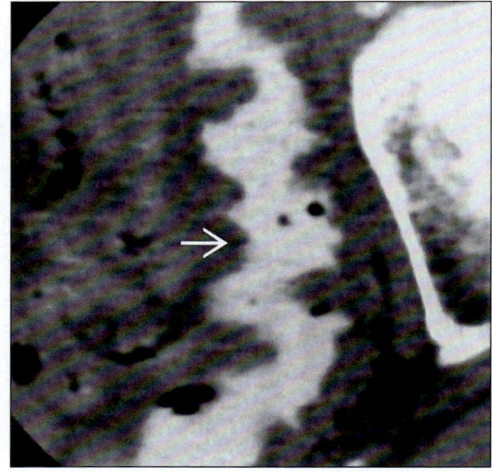

Axial NECT with rectal contrast shows ischemic colitis of sigmoid colon. Note prominent thumbprinting ➡ due to submucosal hemorrhage.

TERMINOLOGY

Definitions
- Compromise of mesenteric blood supply leading to colonic injury

IMAGING FINDINGS

General Features
- Best diagnostic clue: Pneumatosis, mesenteric venous gas, symmetric bowel wall thickening or thumbprinting on CT
- Location
  ○ Watershed segments of colon
    ▪ Splenic flexure: Junction of superior mesenteric artery (SMA) & inferior mesenteric artery (IMA) (Griffith point)
    ▪ Rectosigmoid: Junction of IMA & hypogastric artery (Sudeck point)
    ▪ Left colon: Typical in elderly with decreased perfusion
    ▪ Right colon: Young patients due to decreased collateral blood supply; chronic renal failure patients

Radiographic Findings
- Radiography
  ○ Supine abdominal films
    ▪ Normal or nonspecific ileus
    ▪ Thumbprinting (submucosal edema or bleed)
    ▪ Luminal narrowing or transverse ridging (spasm)
    ▪ Rarely ahaustral loops

Fluoroscopic Findings
- Barium enema
  ○ Hallmark: Serial change on studies performed over days, weeks or months
  ○ Thumbprinting
    ▪ Usually within 24 hrs after onset
    ▪ Smooth, round, polypoid scalloped filling defects along lumen (submucosal edema or hemorrhage)
    ▪ Most consistent & characteristic finding (75% of cases)
  ○ Ulceration: Mucosal sloughing (46-60% of cases)
    ▪ Usually 1-3 weeks after onset
    ▪ Longitudinal/discrete; superficial/deep; small/large

DDx: Wall Thickening and Pericolonic Infiltration

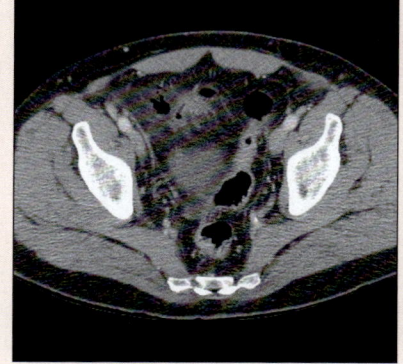

Diverticulitis

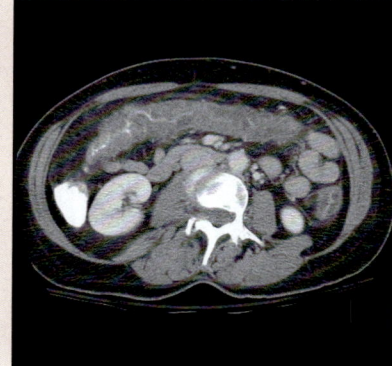

Pseudomembranous Colitis

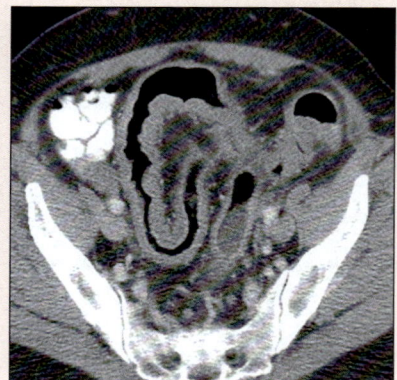

Ulcerative Colitis

ISCHEMIC COLITIS

Key Facts

Terminology
- Compromise of mesenteric blood supply leading to colonic injury

Imaging Findings
- Best diagnostic clue: Pneumatosis, mesenteric venous gas, symmetric bowel wall thickening or thumbprinting on CT
- Watershed segments of colon
- Hypoattenuation of bowel wall: Submucosal or diffuse edema
- Hyperattenuation of bowel wall: Submucosal or diffuse bleeding
- ± Circumferential or band-like pneumatosis
- ± Portomesenteric venous gas in liver periphery

Top Differential Diagnoses
- Diverticulitis
- Pseudomembranous Colitis (PMC)
- Ulcerative Colitis (UC)
- Granulomatous Colitis (Crohn Disease)
- Colon Carcinoma

Pathology
- Hypoperfusion: Predisposing factors
- Hypotensive episodes: Hemorrhagic, cardiogenic or septic shock
- CHF, arrhythmia, drugs (e.g. digitalis), trauma

Diagnostic Checklist
- Consider history of cardiac, bowel, renal problems & hypotensive medication use in elderly

---

- Transverse ridging: Less common finding (13% of cases)
  - Parallel, symmetric thickened folds perpendicular to bowel lumen
  - Early finding, usually resolves rapidly
- Stricture: 12% of cases heal with stricture formation
- Intramural barium rarely, due to sloughing of necrotic wall

CT Findings
- NECT
  - Circumferential, symmetric wall thickening ± thumbprinting
  - Hypoattenuation of bowel wall: Submucosal or diffuse edema
  - Hyperattenuation of bowel wall: Submucosal or diffuse bleeding
  - Heterogeneous bowel wall: Outer serosa & muscular layers
  - ± Luminal narrowing, dilatation & air-fluid levels
  - Loss of haustral pattern (rare); pericolic streakiness; paracolic fluid collections
  - ± Circumferential or band-like pneumatosis
  - ± Portomesenteric venous gas in liver periphery
- CECT
  - Double halo or target sign: Concentric layers of low & high attenuation
    - Mucosal & serosal enhancement (hyperemia or hyperperfusion during recovery)
    - Nonenhancement of submucosa (submucosal edema or hemorrhage)
  - ± Thrombus within splanchnic vessels

Ultrasonographic Findings
- Color Doppler
  - Hypoechoic bowel wall thickening
  - Absent arterial flow in colon wall

Imaging Recommendations
- Best imaging tool
  - MDCT with/without contrast, supine abdominal films
  - Single-contrast barium enema for chronic disease

DIFFERENTIAL DIAGNOSIS

Diverticulitis
- Barium enema
  - Focal eccentric luminal narrowing
  - Marked thickening & distortion of haustral folds
  - Colonic obstruction with zone of transition
  - "Double-tracking": Longitudinal intramural fistulous tract
- CT
  - Most common in sigmoid colon
  - Bowel wall & fascial thickening; fat stranding; free fluid/air
  - Pericolic inflammatory changes (abscess, sinuses, fistulas)
  - "Arrowhead" sign: Diverticular orifice edema
  - Focal area of eccentric luminal narrowing

Pseudomembranous Colitis (PMC)
- Antibiotic colitis or C. difficile colitis
- Usually pancolitis
- Barium enema (contraindicated in acutely ill)
  - Small, irregular plaques on mucosal surface (pseudomembranes)
  - Small, subtle elevated, round nodules
  - Single-contrast study: Thumbprinting indistinguishable from ischemic colitis
- CT
  - Colonic wall thickening & nodularity
  - "Accordion" sign: Trapped enteric contrast between thickened colonic folds
  - Ascites common

Ulcerative Colitis (UC)
- Continuous, nontransmural, pseudopolyps, crypt microabscesses
- Pancolitis, decreased haustration, multiple ulcerations on barium enema
- Colorectal narrowing; ↑ presacral space > 1.5 cm
- "Mucosal islands" or "inflammatory pseudopolyps"
- Diffuse & symmetric colonic wall thickening
- Backwash ileitis: Distal ileum involvement

ISCHEMIC COLITIS

- "Lead-pipe" colon: Rigid colon with haustral loss (chronic phase)

Granulomatous Colitis (Crohn Disease)
- Barium enema
  - Cobblestoning: Paving-stone appearance of longitudinal & transverse ulcerations
  - Transmural, skip lesions, sinuses, fissures, fistulas
  - Segmental distribution
    - Both colon & small bowel (60% of cases)
    - Isolated to colon (20% of cases)
- CT
  - Bowel wall thickening (1-2 cm)
  - "Creeping fat" or mesenteric fibrofatty proliferation
  - Enlarged mesenteric lymph nodes
  - "Comb" sign: Hypervascularity (active disease)

Colon Carcinoma
- Asymmetric mural thickening, irregular surface
- Classic annular "apple core" lesion
  - Circumferential bowel narrowing, mucosal destruction with shelf-like, overhanging borders
  - High grade obstruction + ischemia: Proximal bowel dilatation with thumbprinting
- Extracolonic tumor extension
  - Soft tissue stranding: Serosal surface → pericolic fat
  - Loss of fat planes between colon & adjacent muscles

PATHOLOGY

General Features
- Etiology
  - Most common vascular disorder of GI tract, most common form is segmental (90%) or pancolitis
  - Hypoperfusion: Predisposing factors
    - Hypotensive episodes: Hemorrhagic, cardiogenic or septic shock
    - CHF, arrhythmia, drugs (e.g. digitalis), trauma
    - Arteriosclerotic disease, chronic renal failure
    - Vasculitis, colonic obstruction
  - 20% colonic ischemia are proximal to obstruction
    - Colon cancer, volvulus, closed loop obstruction
- Epidemiology
  - Major predisposing cause in elderly: Nonocclusive vascular disease (hypoperfusion)
  - Most common cause of colitis in elderly, often self-limiting
  - Mortality rate 7%

Gross Pathologic & Surgical Features
- Segmental or focal; localized or diffuse
- Thickened bowel wall; dark red or purple
  - Edematous, hemorrhagic, ulcerated

Microscopic Features
- Mucosal erosions, ulceration, necrosis; submucosal edema, hemorrhage

CLINICAL ISSUES

Presentation
- Most common signs/symptoms
  - Rectal bleeding, bloody diarrhea, hypotension
  - Mild or severe abdominal pain
- Lab data
  - Increased leukocytosis; positive guaiac stool test
  - Negative blood cultures; EKG changes may be seen

Demographics
- Age: Usually elderly (> 50 years)
- Gender: M = F

Natural History & Prognosis
- Complications
  - Reversible or transient ischemic colitis frequent
  - Colonic stricture, gangrene of colon, perforation
  - Transmural bowel infarction → perforation → death
- Prognosis
  - Partial mural ischemia: Good
  - Transmural infarction: Poor

Treatment
- Partial mural ischemia (nonocclusive): Conservative medical treatment
- Transmural infarction: Surgical resection

DIAGNOSTIC CHECKLIST

Consider
- Consider history of cardiac, bowel, renal problems & hypotensive medication use in elderly

Image Interpretation Pearls
- Segmental bowel wall thickening in watershed areas, thumbprinting, pneumatosis, portal venous gas

SELECTED REFERENCES

1. Green BT et al: Ischemic colitis: a clinical review. South Med J. 98(2):217-22, 2005
2. Korotinski S et al: Chronic ischaemic bowel diseases in the aged--go with the flow. Age Ageing. 34(1):10-6, 2005
3. Ripolles T et al: Sonographic findings in ischemic colitis in 58 patients. AJR Am J Roentgenol. 184(3):777-85, 2005
4. Sreenarasimhaiah J: Diagnosis and management of ischemic colitis. Curr Gastroenterol Rep. 7(5):421-6, 2005
5. Wiesner W et al: CT of acute bowel ischemia. Radiology. 226(3):635-50, 2003
6. Horton KM et al: Volume-rendered 3D CT of the mesenteric vasculature: normal anatomy, anatomic variants, and pathologic conditions. Radiographics. 22(1):161-72, 2002
7. Horton KM et al: Multi-detector row CT of mesenteric ischemia: can it be done? Radiographics. 21(6):1463-73, 2001
8. Horton KM et al: CT evaluation of the colon: inflammatory disease. Radiographics. 20(2):399-418, 2000
9. Balthazar EJ et al: Ischemic colitis: CT evaluation of 54 cases. Radiology. 211(2):381-8, 1999
10. Iida M et al: Ischemic colitis: serial changes in double-contrast barium enema examination. Radiology. 159(2):337-41, 1986

ISCHEMIC COLITIS

IMAGE GALLERY

Typical

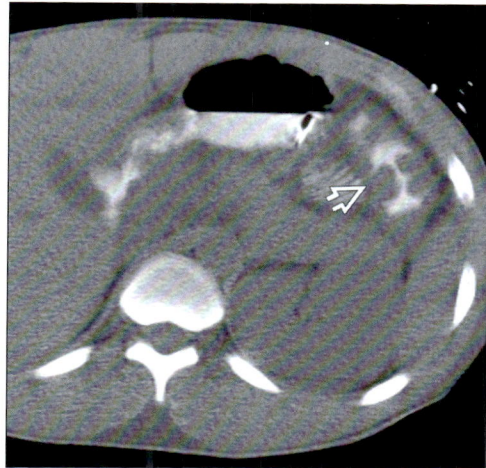
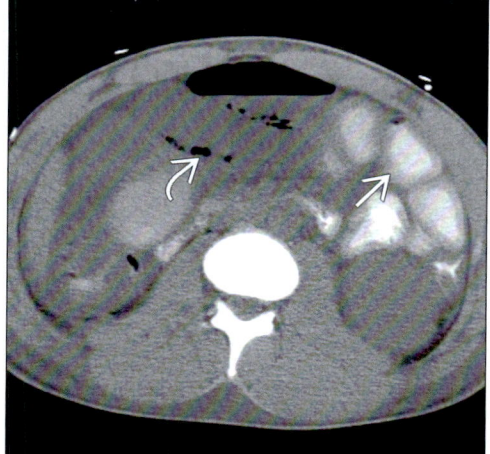

(Left) Axial CECT of bowel ischemia shows thickened wall of colon, with thumbprinting appearance ➡. *(Right)* Axial CECT in same patient as left demonstrates thickening of small intestine wall ➡ and focal pneumatosis ➡.

Typical

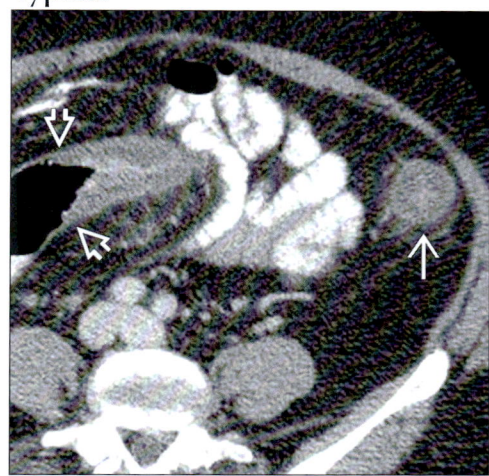
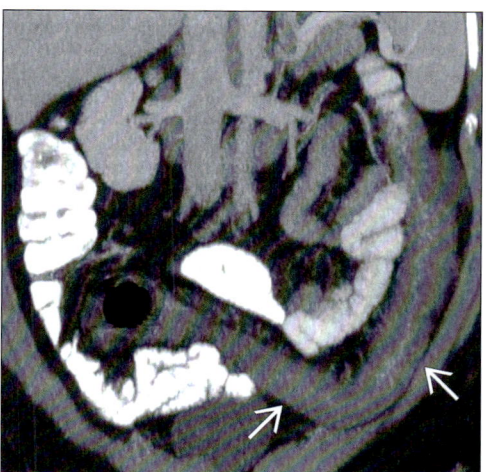

(Left) Axial CECT shows acute IMA ischemia. Descending & sigmoid colon are thick-walled with small amount of pericolonic infiltration ➡. Note abrupt transition to normal sigmoid colon ➡. *(Right)* Coronal reformatted image in same patient as left better depicts extent of disease, which corresponds to inferior mesenteric artery vascular distribution ➡. Ischemia was confirmed endoscopically.

Variant

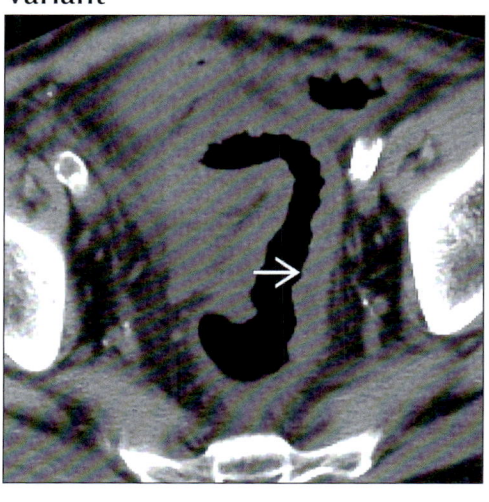
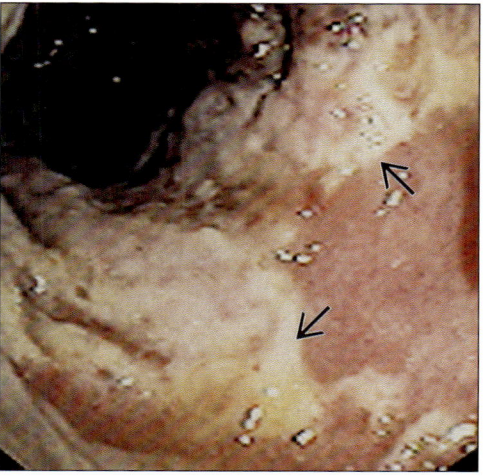

(Left) Axial NECT shows chronic ischemic colitis. Note marked mural thickening of sigmoid colon ➡. *(Right)* Endoscopic image of sigmoid colon in same patient as left demonstrates extensive areas of denuded mucosa ➡.

SIGMOID VOLVULUS

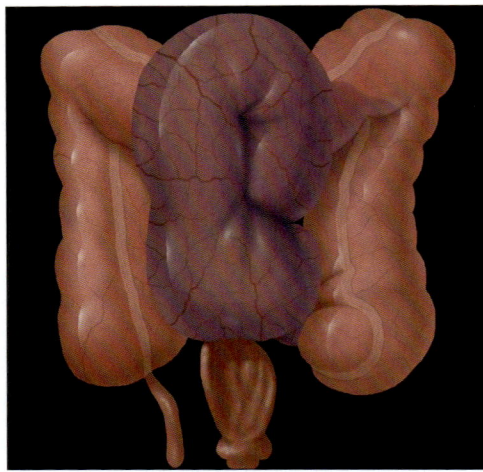

Graphic shows dilated, twisted, elongated sigmoid colon with venous engorgement + colonic obstruction.

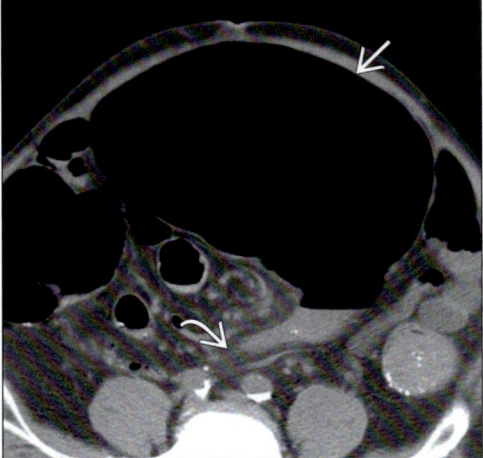

Axial NECT demonstrates sigmoid volvulus. Note massive dilatation of sigmoid colon with beaking at site of volvulus.

TERMINOLOGY

Definitions
- Torsion or twisting of sigmoid colon around its mesenteric axis

IMAGING FINDINGS

General Features
- Best diagnostic clue: Dilated sigmoid colon with inverted-U configuration and absent haustra
- Location: Midline; directed toward RUQ or LUQ; elevation of hemidiaphragm

Radiographic Findings
- Radiography
  ○ Sigmoid volvulus
    ▪ Diagnostic in 75% of cases
    ▪ Vertical dense white line: Apposed inner walls of sigmoid colon pointing toward pelvis
    ▪ Closed loop obstruction: Segment of bowel obstructed at two points
    ▪ Gas in proximal small intestine and colon; absence of gas in rectum
    ▪ Absent rectal gas in spite of prone or decubitus views
    ▪ Inverted-U shape with absent haustra
    ▪ "Northern exposure" sign: Dilated, twisted sigmoid colon projects above transverse colon on supine radiograph
    ▪ Apex above T10 vertebra and under left hemidiaphragm; directed toward right shoulder
  ○ Compound volvulus
    ▪ Dilated sigmoid loop in mid-abdomen extending to RLQ with distended small bowel
    ▪ Medially deviated distal left colon

Fluoroscopic Findings
- Water-soluble contrast enema
  ○ Can use low pressure barium enema without balloon inflation
  ○ "Beaking": Smooth, tapered narrowing or point of torsion at rectosigmoid junction
  ○ Mucosal folds often show corkscrew pattern at point of torsion

DDx: Dilated Colon

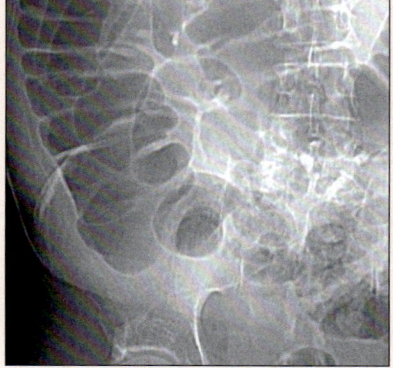
Ileus

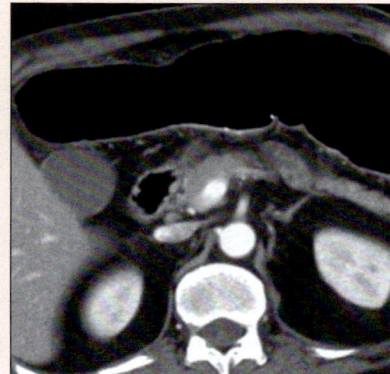
Toxic Megacolon

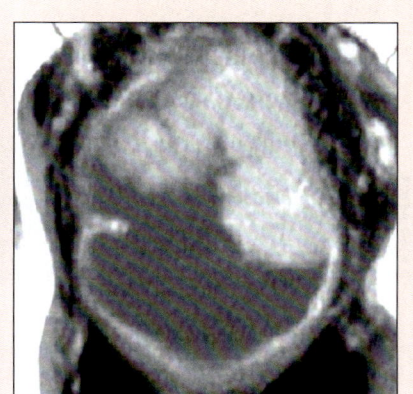
Colon Carcinoma

SIGMOID VOLVULUS

Key Facts

Terminology
- Torsion or twisting of sigmoid colon around its mesenteric axis

Imaging Findings
- Best diagnostic clue: Dilated sigmoid colon with inverted-U configuration and absent haustra
- Location: Midline; directed toward RUQ or LUQ; elevation of hemidiaphragm
- Gas in proximal small intestine and colon; absence of gas in rectum
- "Northern exposure" sign: Dilated, twisted sigmoid colon projects above transverse colon on supine radiograph
- "Whirl" sign: Tightly twisted mesentery & bowel
- Abdominal radiography, water-soluble contrast enema, MDCT are best imaging tools

Top Differential Diagnoses
- Acute Ileus
- Functional Megacolon
- Toxic Megacolon
- Distal Colon Obstruction

Clinical Issues
- Acute or insidious onset
- Abdominal pain (< 33%), vomiting, distension, obstipation

Diagnostic Checklist
- Acute abdomen; rule out other causes of obstruction
- Dilated sigmoid colon in inverted-U configuration; absent haustra; "beaking"; "whirl" sign, "northern exposure" sign

---

  - Shouldering: Localized wall thickening at site of twist (chronic)

CT Findings
- CECT
  - "Beaking": Progressive tapering of afferent & efferent limbs leading into twist
  - "Whirl" sign: Tightly twisted mesentery & bowel
  - Compound volvulus: Medial deviation of distal left colon with pointed appearance of medial border

Imaging Recommendations
- Best imaging tool
  - Abdominal radiography, water-soluble contrast enema, MDCT are best imaging tools
    - Supine, upright, prone and decubitus views of abdomen

DIFFERENTIAL DIAGNOSIS

Acute Ileus
- Post-op, medication, post-traumatic injury, ischemia
- Dilated large and small bowel with no transition point
- Air-fluid levels without peristalsis
- No colonic obstruction

Functional Megacolon
- Gross constipation without organic cause
- Markedly dilated, ahaustral, air- or stool-filled colon
- Ogilvie syndrome: Nonobstructive dilation of colon

Toxic Megacolon
- Dilated ahaustral transverse colon in patient with known ulcerative colitis
- Thumbprinting due to edematous mucosa

Distal Colon Obstruction
- Change in stool caliber over several months
- Gas-filled intestinal loops proximal to obstruction; no distal gas
- Abrupt transition at site of obstruction
- Malignancy
  - Most common cause of colonic obstruction (55%)
  - Insidious onset
  - Weakness, weight loss, anorexia, rectal bleeding
  - "Apple-core" configuration, mucosal destruction
  - Positive fecal occult blood test highly suggestive of colon cancer
- Stricture secondary to diverticulitis
  - Second most common cause of colonic obstruction (12%)
  - History of recurrent diverticulitis
  - Other diverticula present

PATHOLOGY

General Features
- Etiology
  - Major predisposing factors
    - Diet: Fiber increase → increased bulk of stool, elongation and dilatation of colon
    - Chronic constipation & obtundation from medications → gaseous distension
  - Compound volvulus (ileosigmoid knot)
    - Hyperactive ileum winding around narrow pedicle of passive sigmoid colon
  - Etiology in children
    - Malrotation and other mesenteric attachment abnormalities
    - Constipation (mental retardation, Hirschsprung disease, cystic fibrosis, aerophagia)
- Epidemiology
  - Third most common cause of colonic obstruction (10%)
  - 60-75% of cases of colonic volvulus involve sigmoid colon
  - 1-2% of intestinal obstructions in U.S.
  - Increased incidence in elderly men & residents of nursing homes and/or mental hospitals (constipation & obtundation)
  - Significant increase in South America and Africa (increased fiber in diet leads to bulkier stool, dilating colon)

SIGMOID VOLVULUS

- Associated abnormalities: Comorbid disease: 30% with psychiatric disease; 13% are institutionalized at time of diagnosis

Gross Pathologic & Surgical Features
- Twisted narrow segment with marked proximally dilated bowel loop

Microscopic Features
- Localized thickening of mucosal folds; ischemic and necrotic changes

CLINICAL ISSUES

Presentation
- Most common signs/symptoms
  - Acute or insidious onset
  - Abdominal pain (< 33%), vomiting, distension, obstipation
  - Compound volvulus
    - Rapid deterioration (greater than other colonic volvulus)
    - Pain disproportionate to physical findings; absolute constipation
  - Diagnosis: Radiography in 75% of cases

Demographics
- Age: 60-70 years

Natural History & Prognosis
- Complications
  - Closed loop obstruction → strangulation
  - Ischemia, necrosis (15-20%) and perforation
  - Ileosigmoid knot → strangulation and gangrene of small bowel within hours
- Prognosis
  - Uncomplicated: Good
  - Complicated: Poor
  - 40-50% recurrence after nonoperative reduction
  - Degree of rotation relative to chance of nonsurgical decompression: 180°:35%; 360°:50%; 540°:10%
    - Twist > 360° does not resolve spontaneously
  - 3% recurrence after nonoperative and operative reduction

Treatment
- Nonoperative
  - Proctoscopic/colonoscopic decompression of obstruction ± stabilization via rectal tube insertion
  - 70-80% success rate
- Nonoperative + operative
  - Decompression, mechanical cleansing & elective sigmoid resection
- Complicated cases
  - Surgical emergency
- Follow-up
  - Water-soluble contrast enema to rule out underlying colon cancer

DIAGNOSTIC CHECKLIST

Consider
- Acute abdomen; rule out other causes of obstruction

Image Interpretation Pearls
- Dilated sigmoid colon in inverted-U configuration; absent haustra; "beaking"; "whirl" sign, "northern exposure" sign

SELECTED REFERENCES

1. Hirao K et al: Sigmoid volvulus showing "a whirl sign" on CT. Intern Med. 45(5):331-2, 2006
2. Tiah L et al: Sigmoid volvulus: diagnostic twists and turns. Eur J Emerg Med. 13(2):84-7, 2006
3. Agaoglu N et al: Surgical treatment of the sigmoid volvulus. Acta Chir Belg. 105(4):365-8, 2005
4. Chandrasekaran TV et al: Minimally invasive stapled surgical approach to the management of sigmoid volvulus. Ann R Coll Surg Engl. 87(5):381-2, 2005
5. Matsumoto S et al: Computed tomographic imaging of abdominal volvulus: pictorial essay. Can Assoc Radiol J. 55(5):297-303, 2004
6. Chiu HH et al: Recurrent sigmoid volvulus. Gastrointest Endosc. 56(3):419-20, 2002
7. Kuzu MA et al: Emergent resection for acute sigmoid volvulus: results of 106 consecutive cases. Dis Colon Rectum. 45(8):1085-90, 2002
8. Chirdan LB et al: Sigmoid volvulus and ileosigmoid knotting in children. Pediatr Surg Int. 17(8):636-7, 2001
9. Moore CJ et al: CT of cecal volvulus: unraveling the image. AJR Am J Roentgenol. 177(1):95-8, 2001
10. Daniels IR et al: Recurrent sigmoid volvulus treated by percutaneous endoscopic colostomy. Br J Surg. 87(10):1419, 2000
11. Dulger M et al: Management of sigmoid colon volvulus. Hepatogastroenterology. 47(35):1280-3, 2000
12. Lee SH et al: The ileosigmoid knot: CT findings. AJR Am J Roentgenol. 174(3):685-7, 2000
13. Madiba TE et al: The management of sigmoid volvulus. J R Coll Surg Edinb. 45(2):74-80, 2000
14. Chung YF et al: Minimizing recurrence after sigmoid volvulus. Br J Surg. 86(2):231-3, 1999
15. Javors BR et al: The northern exposure sign: A newly described finding in sigmoid volvulus. AJR 173:571-574, 1999
16. Choi D et al: Endoscopic sigmoidopexy: a safer way to treat sigmoid volvulus? J R Coll Surg Edinb. 43(1):64, 1998
17. Catalano O: Computed tomographic appearance of sigmoid volvulus. Abdominal Imaging 21:314-317, 1996
18. Frizelle FA et al: Colonic volvulus. Adv Surg. 29:131-9, 1996
19. Forde KA: Therapeutic colonoscopy. World J Surg. 16(6):1048-53, 1992
20. Gibney EJ: Volvulus of the sigmoid colon. Surg Gynecol Obstet. 173(3):243-55, 1991

SIGMOID VOLVULUS

IMAGE GALLERY

Typical

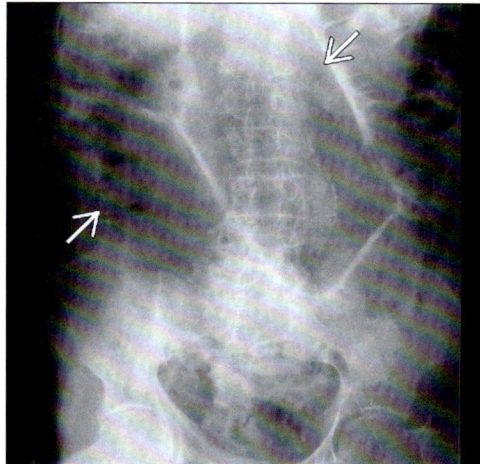
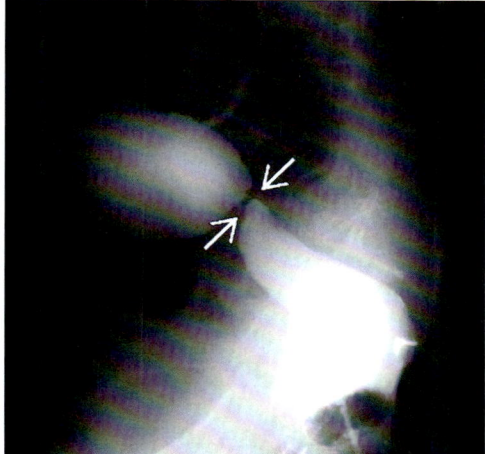

(Left) Frontal radiograph shows classic case of sigmoid volvulus. Note classic inverted-U shaped massively dilated sigmoid colon directed toward right hemidiaphragm ➡. *(Right)* Lateral contrast enema in same patient as left shows contrast-filled rectum and "bird's beak" sign ➡, corresponding to luminal narrowing at site of sigmoid obstruction.

Typical

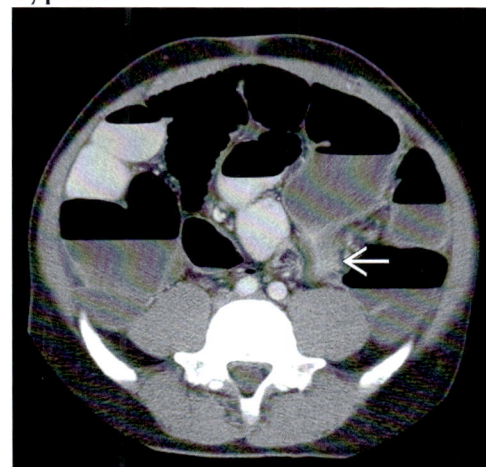
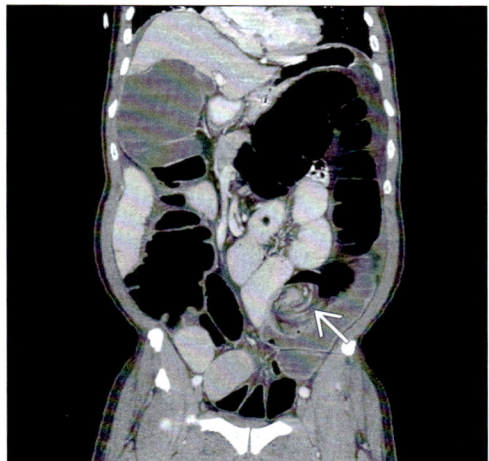

(Left) Axial CECT shows massive colonic redundancy and distention of large & small bowel. Sigmoid volvulus is evident in LLQ by "beaked" appearance of descending loop ➡ of twisted sigmoid colon. *(Right)* Coronal CECT in same patient as left demonstrates classic swirled appearance of mesenteric pedicle at site of sigmoid volvulus ➡.

Variant

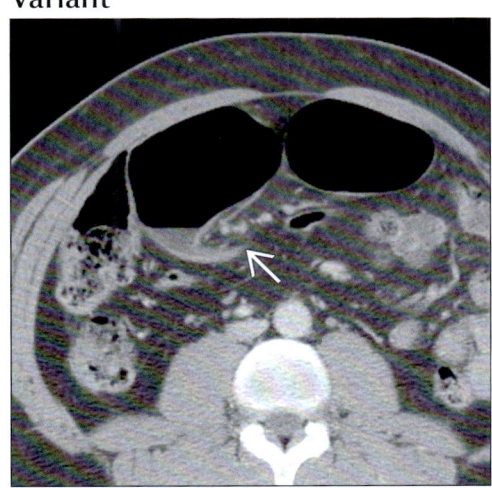
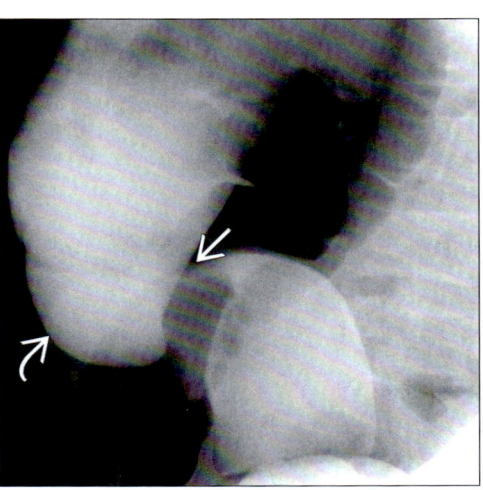

(Left) Axial NECT shows partially obstructing sigmoid volvulus. Note beaking of sigmoid at site of twist ➡. *(Right)* Oblique water-soluble contrast enema of sigmoid colon in same patient as left reveals beaking at site of volvulus ➡ and distal filling of dilated colon ➡ due to partial obstruction.

CECAL VOLVULUS

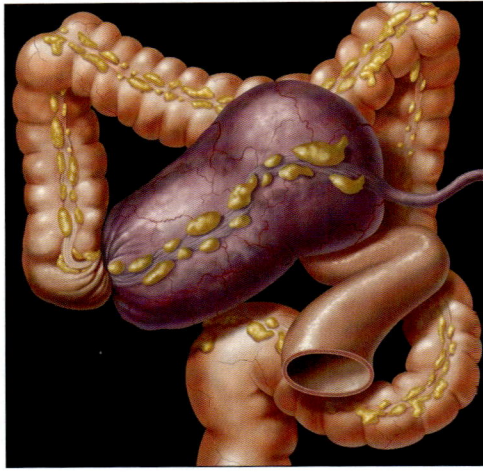

Graphic shows twist (volvulus) of ascending colon, obstructing lumen and blood supply. Cecum, on a mesentery, dilated + displaced toward left upper quadrant.

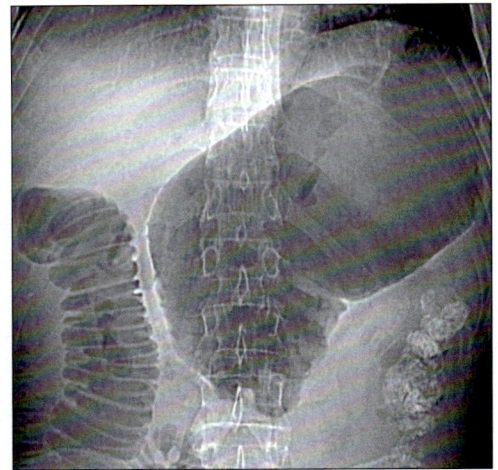

Anteroposterior radiograph in supine view of cecal volvulus. Note markedly dilated cecum in LUQ and distended small bowel in right mid-abdomen from associated small bowel obstruction.

TERMINOLOGY

Abbreviations and Synonyms
- Volvulus of cecum, ascending colon

Definitions
- Rotational twist of right colon on its axis

IMAGING FINDINGS

General Features
- Best diagnostic clue: Dilated, twisted cecum with tip pointing to LUQ

Radiographic Findings
- Radiography
  - Dilated air-filled cecum in LUQ
  - Single, long air-fluid level
  - Medially placed ileocecal valve → soft tissue indentation → kidney or coffee bean-shaped gas-filled cecum
  - Markedly distended gas or fluid-filled small bowel (SB); little gas in distal colon

Fluoroscopic Findings
- Water-soluble contrast enema: Point of torsion at mid-ascending colon ("beaking")

CT Findings
- CECT
  - "Beaking": Progressive tapering of afferent & efferent limbs leading into twist
  - "Whirl" sign: Tightly twisted mesenteric vessels

Imaging Recommendations
- Best imaging tool: Contrast enema or CT

DIFFERENTIAL DIAGNOSIS

Sigmoid Volvulus
- Dilated, ahaustral sigmoid loop, inverted U configuration

Acute Ileus
- Dilated colon to rectum with haustra pattern

Distal Colon Obstruction
- Gas- and stool-filled colon

DDx: Marked Colonic Distention

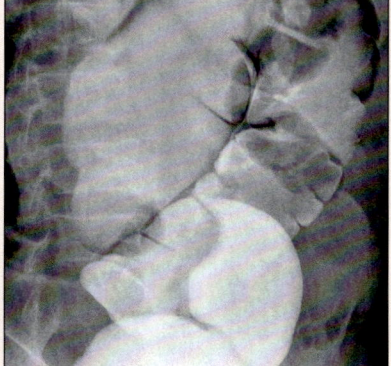

Sigmoid Volvulus

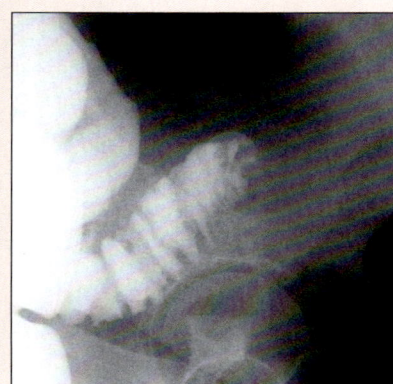

Colonic Obstruction

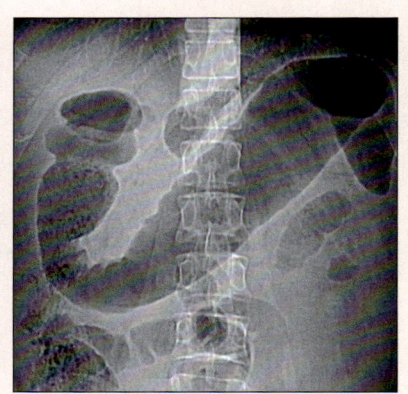

Toxic Megacolon

CECAL VOLVULUS

Key Facts

Imaging Findings
- Best diagnostic clue: Dilated, twisted cecum with tip pointing to LUQ
- Single, long air-fluid level
- Medially placed ileocecal valve → soft tissue indentation → kidney or coffee bean-shaped gas-filled cecum
- Markedly distended gas or fluid-filled small bowel (SB); little gas in distal colon

Top Differential Diagnoses
- Sigmoid Volvulus
- Acute Ileus

Clinical Issues
- Most common signs/symptoms: Acute or insidious onset; abdominal pain, distension & vomiting

Diagnostic Checklist
- Rule out ileus, Ogilvie syndrome

Toxic Megacolon
- Markedly dilated, ahaustral transverse colon

Ogilvie Syndrome
- Colonic pseudo-obstruction without mechanical cause

PATHOLOGY

General Features
- General path comments
  - Cecal bascule
    - Anterior folding of cecum at mid-abdomen
  - Embryology-anatomy
    - Right colon incompletely fused to posterior parietal peritoneum
- Etiology
  - Congenital defect in right colon attachment
  - Postpartum ligamentous laxity, mobile cecum
  - Colon distension (pseudo-obstruction, distal tumor, endoscopy, enema, post-operative ileus)
  - Chronic constipation, laxative use
- Epidemiology: 1/3rd of colonic volvulus cases, 2-3% of colonic obstructions
- Associated abnormalities: Malrotation, long mesentery

Gross Pathologic & Surgical Features
- Twisted, markedly dilated segment

Microscopic Features
- Localized mucosal ischemic & necrotic changes

CLINICAL ISSUES

Presentation
- Most common signs/symptoms: Acute or insidious onset; abdominal pain, distension & vomiting

Natural History & Prognosis
- Complications: Ischemia, necrosis, perforation
- Prognosis: Good if uncomplicated, poor if complicated

Treatment
- Colonoscopy to reduce volvulus
- Complicated cases: Surgery (cecopexy, cecostomy, resection)

DIAGNOSTIC CHECKLIST

Consider
- Rule out ileus, Ogilvie syndrome

Image Interpretation Pearls
- Massively dilated cecum at mid-abdomen, "beaking"

SELECTED REFERENCES
1. Moore CJ et al: CT of cecal volvulus. AJR. 177:95-98, 2001
2. Hemingway AP: Cecal volvulus: A new twist to the barium enema. British Journal Radiol. 53:806-807, 1980

IMAGE GALLERY

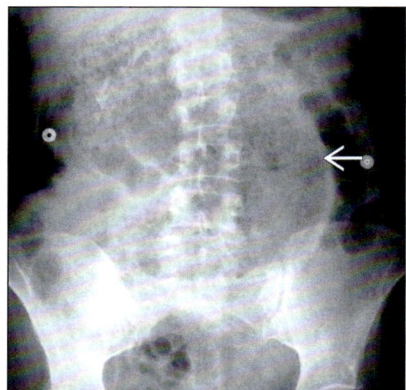 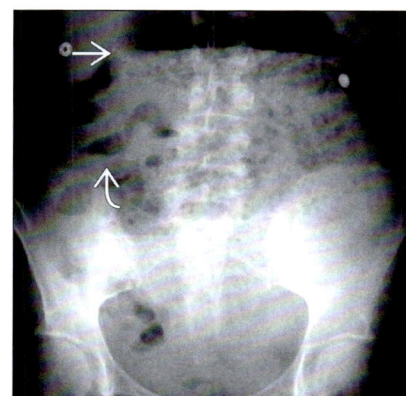 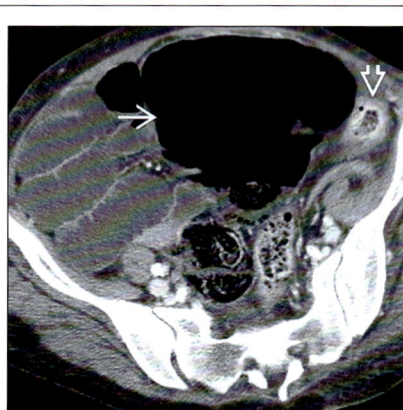

(Left) Anteroposterior radiograph shows typical appearance of cecal volvulus. Supine radiograph shows large fluid- and debris-filled structure in mid-abdomen, displacing SB loops ➔. (Center) Anteroposterior radiograph in upright view (same patient as left) shows single, long air-fluid level in LUQ, representing twisted cecum ➔. Note displaced prominent SB loops in RUQ with air-fluid levels ➔. (Right) Axial CECT shows multiple dilated cecum in left mid-abdomen ➔ and compressed, stool-filled sigmoid colon ➔ deviated by dilated cecum.

SPLENIC INFECTION AND ABSCESS

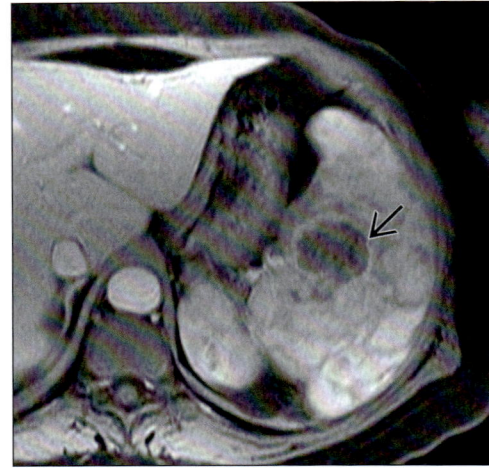 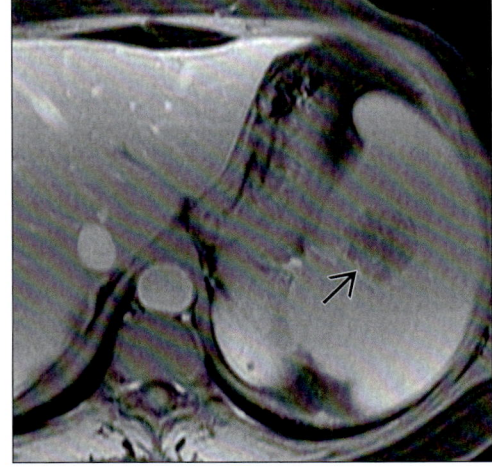

Axial gadolinium-enhanced MRI of pyogenic splenic abscess. Early-phase spoiled GRASS MRI reveals rim enhancement around low-signal abscess ➔.

Axial gadolinium-enhanced MRI at later phase in same patient as left shows multi-septated abscess ➔.

TERMINOLOGY

Abbreviations and Synonyms
- Collection of liquified pus within splenic parenchyma

IMAGING FINDINGS

General Features
- Best diagnostic clue: Rounded low attenuation complex fluid collection with mass effect
- Location: Variable; may be located anywhere within splenic parenchyma
- Size: Variable; typically 3-5 cm for pyogenic abscesses; microabscesses (often fungal) < 1.5 cm
- Morphology
  o Rounded or with irregular borders
  o May have multiple locules similar to hepatic "cluster sign" of pyogenic abscess
  o Mass effect on splenic capsule
  o Internal septations common

Radiographic Findings
- Radiography
  o Rarely gas bubbles within abscess
  o Associated with left lower lobe atelectasis and left pleural effusion on chest x-ray

CT Findings
- NECT
  o Low attenuation ill-defined lesion within splenic parenchyma
  o May rarely contain gas bubbles or air-fluid levels
- CECT
  o Low attenuation, nonenhancing complex fluid collection
    ▪ May extend to subcapsular location
    ▪ Rarely causes splenic rupture with generalized peritonitis
  o May have enhancing peripheral rim

MR Findings
- T1WI: Low or intermediate signal lesion
- T2WI: High signal lesion
- T1 C+: Low signal lesion with peripheral enhancement

Ultrasonographic Findings
- Grayscale Ultrasound
  o Typical pyogenic abscess

DDx: Splenic Lesions Mimicking Infection

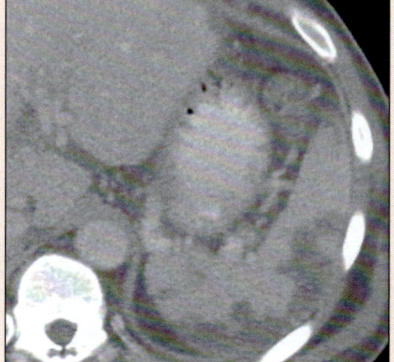 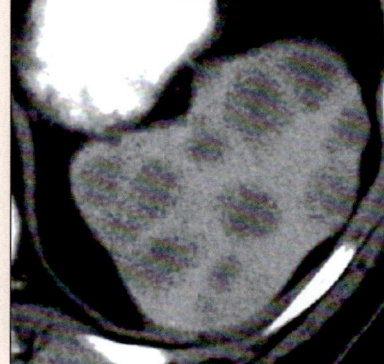 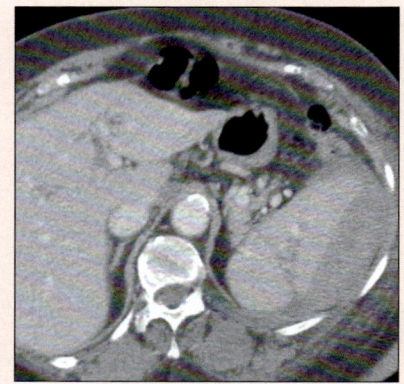

Splenic Infarct   *Splenic Lymphoma*   *Splenic Trauma*

SPLENIC INFECTION AND ABSCESS

Key Facts

Terminology
- Collection of liquified pus within splenic parenchyma

Imaging Findings
- Best diagnostic clue: Rounded low attenuation complex fluid collection with mass effect
- Protocol advice: 150 mL IV contrast injected at 2.5 mL/sec; 5 mm slice thickness & 5 mm reconstruction interval

Top Differential Diagnoses
- Splenic Infarct
- Splenic Tumor
- Splenic Trauma
- Infiltrating Disorders

Pathology
- General path comments: Liquified pus, splenomegaly
- Genetics: Hemoglobinopathies (sickle-cell) predispose

Clinical Issues
- Most common signs/symptoms: Fever (92%), chills, LUQ pain (77%), splenomegaly
- Percutaneous drainage for unilocular unruptured abscesses
- Splenectomy for multiple pyogenic abscesses and/or abscess rupture

Diagnostic Checklist
- Consider infarct; necrotic or cystic mets; lymphoma
- Single or multiple low attenuation lesions in febrile patient

---

- Hypoechoic with internal septations, low-level echoes representing pus or debris
- May have little distal acoustic enhancement
  - Atypical pyogenic abscess
    - Reverberation artifacts from gas
    - Rarely echogenic
    - 90% sensitivity for pyogenic abscess
  - Microabscesses
    - Target or "bull's eye" appearance similar to hepatic microabscesses
- Color Doppler
  - Typical pyogenic abscess shows no internal flow
  - Hypoechoic nodular avascular microabscesses

Nuclear Medicine Findings
- PET: Increased isotope uptake from hypermetabolic focus
- WBC Scan
  - Increased isotope uptake

Imaging Recommendations
- Best imaging tool: CECT, US
- Protocol advice: 150 mL IV contrast injected at 2.5 mL/sec; 5 mm slice thickness & 5 mm reconstruction interval

DIFFERENTIAL DIAGNOSIS

Splenic Infarct
- Wedge-shaped, occasionally rounded in configuration
- Low attenuation
- Peripheral location
- Nonenhancement with contrast

Splenic Tumor
- Single or multiple lesions
- Solid: Lymphoma, melanoma
- Cystic: Ovarian carcinoma, germ cell tumors or sarcoma
- Benign: Lymphangioma, hemangioma
- Rounded with variable enhancement

Splenic Trauma
- History of blunt injury
- Associated with perisplenic hematoma and hemoperitoneum
- May have active arterial extravasation with high-attenuation areas isodense with major arteries
- Arterial clot adjacent to spleen in small lacerations

Infiltrating Disorders
- Sarcoid
  - Multiple low attenuation lesions
- Gaucher disease
  - Multiple low attenuation lesions

PATHOLOGY

General Features
- General path comments: Liquified pus, splenomegaly
- Genetics: Hemoglobinopathies (sickle-cell) predispose
- Etiology
  - Generalized septicemia
  - Septic emboli
    - Endocarditis
  - Immunosuppression
    - Fungal microabscesses
  - Secondary infection of traumatic splenic hematoma or infarct
  - Hematologic disorders
- Epidemiology
  - Rare: 0.2% of reported autopsies
  - 25% are immunocompromised patients
- Associated abnormalities
  - Post-operative state
  - Endocarditis with mitral and/or aortic valve vegetations
  - Immunocompromised state
  - Pancreatitis, colon cancer
  - Remote infection
  - Diabetes

SPLENIC INFECTION AND ABSCESS

Gross Pathologic & Surgical Features
- Necrotic areas of liquified pus

Microscopic Features
- Liquefactive necrosis
- Pus with leukocyte debris
- Gram stain for pyogenic abscess
  - Fungal stain for mycotic organism
  - TB stains for tuberculous abscesses
  - Pyogenic: 57% aerobic
    - Staphylococcus
    - Strep E. coli
    - Salmonella
  - Fungal
    - Candida most common
    - Aspergillus and cryptococcus
    - Tuberculosis (TB) and mycobacterium avium intracellulari (MAI) in AIDS patient

Staging, Grading or Classification Criteria
- Pyogenic
  - Unilocular (65%)
  - Multilocular or multiple (20%)
  - Gram-negative organisms in 55%, Klebsiella pneumoniae most common pathogen
- Fungal
  - Microabscesses < 1.5 cm (25%)
- Parasitic
  - Echinococus granulosa

CLINICAL ISSUES

Presentation
- Most common signs/symptoms: Fever (92%), chills, LUQ pain (77%), splenomegaly
- Other signs/symptoms
  - Lab data
    - Leukocytosis (66%)
    - Positive blood cultures
    - May mimic pneumonia, ulcer disease or pancreatitis

Demographics
- Age: Adult patients with predisposing factors
- Gender: M = F
- Ethnicity: No known predilection

Natural History & Prognosis
- Variable
- Excellent prognosis for pyogenic abscesses in immunocompetent patient
- Guarded prognosis in immunocompromised patients with fungal microabscesses

Treatment
- Options, risks, complications
  - Antibiotics alone may be curative in 75% of small pyogenic abscesses (< 4 cm)
  - Percutaneous drainage for unilocular unruptured abscesses
    - Reported success rate of 67-100%
  - Splenectomy for multiple pyogenic abscesses and/cr abscess rupture
  - Mortality post-splenectomy 6%

DIAGNOSTIC CHECKLIST

Consider
- Consider infarct; necrotic or cystic mets; lymphoma

Image Interpretation Pearls
- Single or multiple low attenuation lesions in febrile patient
- Morphology variable

SELECTED REFERENCES

1. Tasar M et al: Computed tomography-guided percutaneous drainage of splenic abscesses. Clin Imaging. 28(1):44-8, 2004
2. Chiang IS et al: Splenic abscesses: review of 29 cases. Kaohsiung J Med Sci. 19(10):510-5, 2003
3. Kaushik R et al: Splenic abscess. Trop Doct. 32(4):246-7, 2002
4. Ng KK et al: Splenic abscess: diagnosis and management. Hepatogastroenterology. 49(44):567-71, 2002
5. Thanos L et al: Percutaneous CT-guided drainage of splenic abscess. AJR Am J Roentgenol. 179(3):629-32, 2002
6. Green BT: Splenic abscess: report of six cases and review of the literature. Am Surg. 67(1):80-5, 2001
7. Loualidi A et al: Splenic abscess caused by Peptostreptococcus species, diagnosed with the aid of abdominal computerized tomography and treated with percutaneous drainage and antibiotics: a case report. Neth J Med. 59(6):280-5, 2001
8. Drevelengas A: The spleen in infectious disorders. JBR-BTR. 83(4):208-10, 2000
9. Frumiento C et al: Complications of splenic injuries: expansion of the nonoperative theorem. J Pediatr Surg. 35(5):788-91, 2000
10. Mehanna D et al: Cat scratch disease presenting as splenic abscess. Aust N Z J Surg. 70(8):622-4, 2000
11. Murray AW et al: A case of multiple splenic abscesses managed non-operatively. J R Coll Surg Edinb. 45(3):189-91, 2000
12. Poggi SH et al: Puerperal splenic abscess. Obstet Gynecol. 96(5 Pt 2):842, 2000
13. Smyrniotis V et al: Splenic abscess. An old disease with new interest. Dig Surg. 17(4):354-7, 2000
14. Bernabeu-Wittel M et al: Etiology, clinical features and outcome of splenic microabscesses in HIV-infected patients with prolonged fever. Eur J Clin Microbiol Infect Dis. 18(5):324-9, 1999
15. Duggal RK et al: Splenic abscess as a complication of acute pancreatitis. J Assoc Physicians India. 47(3):338-9, 1999
16. Nakao A et al: Portal venous gas associated with splenic abscess secondary to colon cancer. Anticancer Res. 19(6C):5641-4, 1999
17. Al-Salem AH et al: Splenic abscess and sickle cell disease. Am J Hematol. 58(2):100-4, 1998
18. Alterman P et al: Splenic abscess in geriatric care. J Am Geriatr Soc. 46(11):1481-3, 1998
19. de Bree E et al: Splenic abscess: a diagnostic and therapeutic challenge. Acta Chir Belg. 98(5):199-202, 1998
20. Wang Y et al: CT findings in splenic tuberculosis. J Belge Radiol. 81(2):90-1, 1998

SPLENIC INFECTION AND ABSCESS

IMAGE GALLERY

Typical

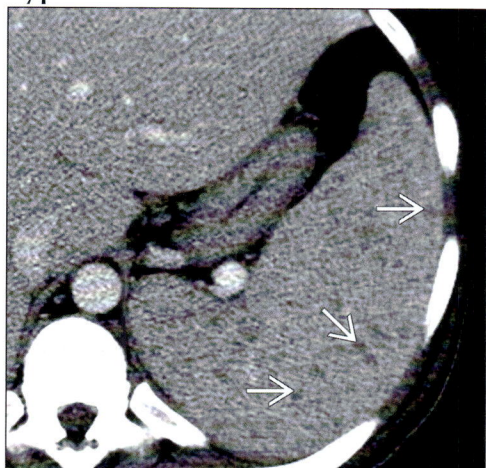
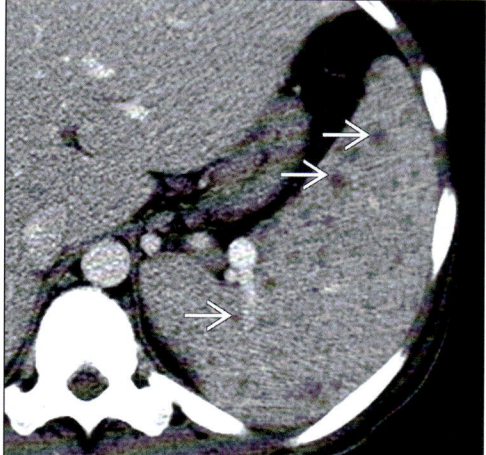

(Left) Axial CECT of patient with AML and splenic microabscesses from Candida shows innumerable low-attenuation lesions ➔. *(Right)* Axial CECT at lower level in same patient as left shows additional fungal microabscesses ➔.

Variant

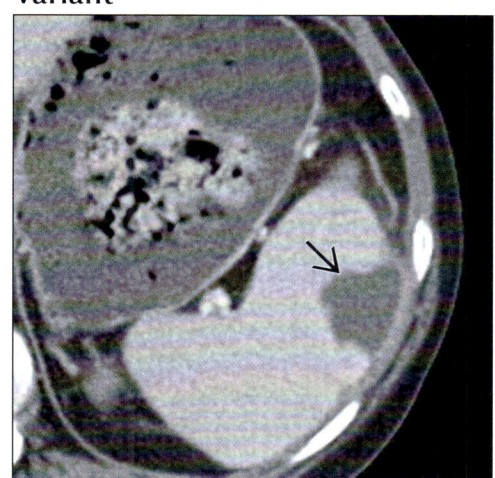
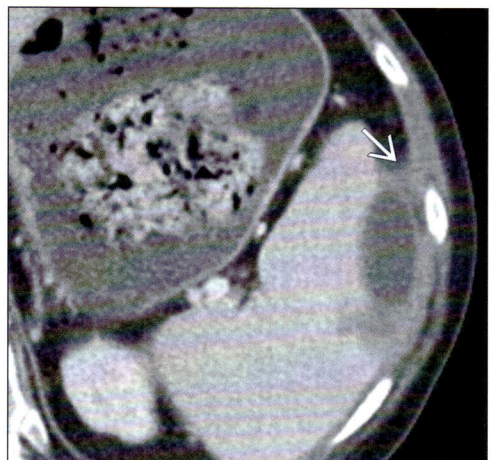

(Left) Axial CECT of pyogenic splenic abscess in patient with endocarditis shows peripheral low-attenuation lesion ➔. *(Right)* Axial CECT at more caudal level in same patient as left demonstrates subcapsular extension of abscess ➔.

Typical

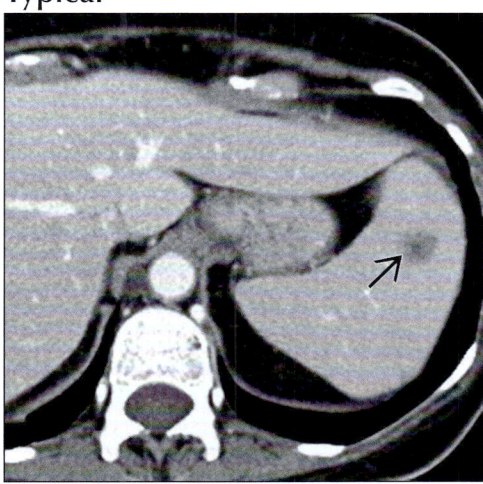
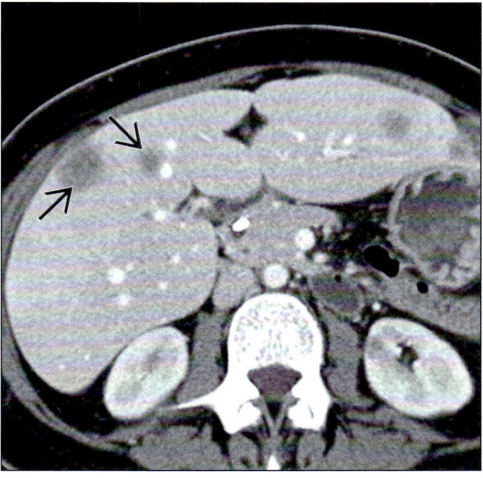

(Left) Axial CECT shows unusually large fungal abscess in spleen. Leukemic patient with candida sepsis demonstrates hypodense splenic abscess ➔ larger than typical fungal microabscesses. *(Right)* Axial CECT at more caudal level in same patient as left demonstrates multiple hepatic fungal abscesses ➔.

SPLENIC INFARCTION

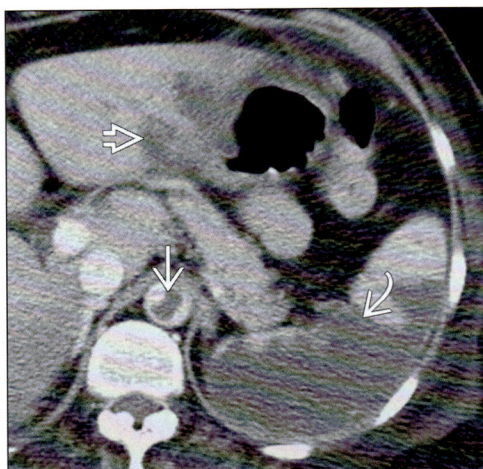
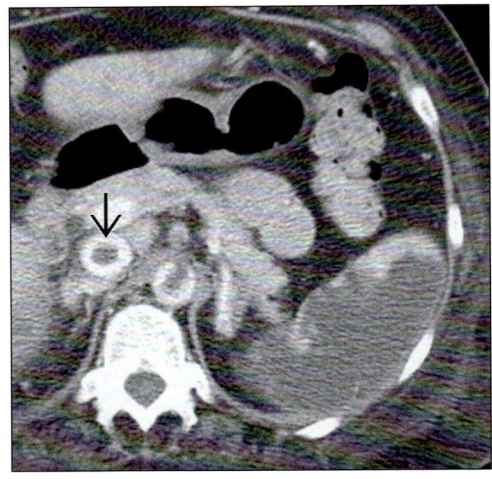

Axial CECT shows thrombus in aorta ➡ and extensive area of nonenhancement due to splenic infarction ➡. Note also left lobe hepatic infarction ➡.

Axial CECT at more caudal level in same patient as left reveals additional finding of thrombus in inferior vena cava ➡.

TERMINOLOGY

Definitions
- Global or segmental parenchymal splenic ischemia & necrosis caused by vascular occlusion

IMAGING FINDINGS

General Features
- Best diagnostic clue: Peripheral, wedge-shaped, nonenhancing areas within splenic parenchyma on CECT in patient with LUQ pain
- Location: Entire spleen may be infarcted or more commonly segmental areas
- Size
  - Variable; global or segmental
  - Spleen may or may not demonstrate splenomegaly
- Morphology
  - Most commonly wedge-shaped when segmental
  - Straight margins indicate vascular lesion
  - May be rounded (atypical)

Radiographic Findings
- Radiography: May be associated with left lower lobe atelectasis and pleural effusion on chest x-ray

CT Findings
- CECT
  - Segmental: Wedge-shaped or rounded low attenuation area on CECT
  - Global: Complete nonenhancement of spleen with or without "cortical rim sign" on CECT

MR Findings
- T1WI
  - Recent onset: High signal areas of hemorrhagic infarction
  - Chronic: Low signal
- T2WI: High signal within area of infarct
- T1 C+: Wedge-shaped area of low signal

Ultrasonographic Findings
- Grayscale Ultrasound: Hypoechoic or anechoic wedge-shaped or rounded parenchymal defect
- Color Doppler: Absent flow in areas of infarction

DDx: Splenic Lesions Mimicking Infarction

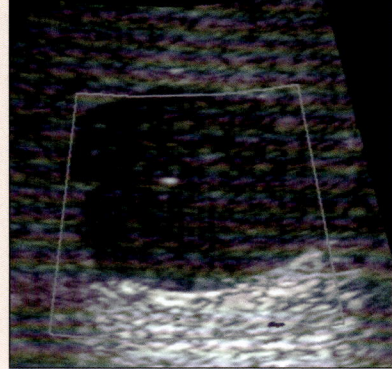
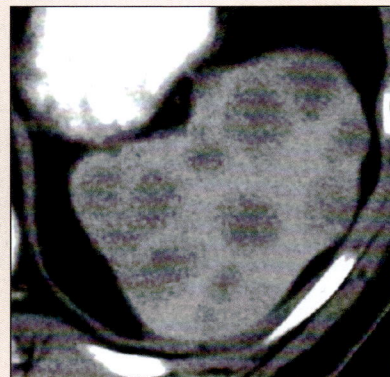
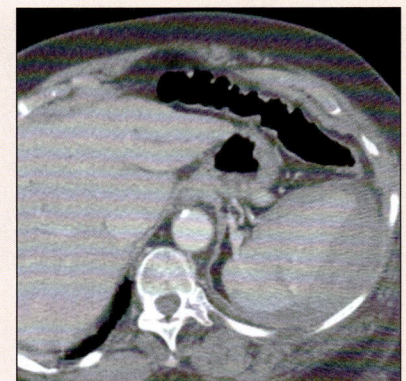

Splenic Abscess | Splenic Lymphoma | Splenic Laceration

SPLENIC INFARCTION

Key Facts

Terminology
- Global or segmental parenchymal splenic ischemia & necrosis caused by vascular occlusion

Imaging Findings
- Best diagnostic clue: Peripheral, wedge-shaped, nonenhancing areas within splenic parenchyma on CECT in patient with LUQ pain
- Segmental: Wedge-shaped or rounded low attenuation area on CECT
- Global: Complete nonenhancement of spleen with or without "cortical rim sign" on CECT
- Protocol advice: 150 mL IV contrast at 2.5 mL/sec; 5 mm collimation & 5 mm reconstruction interval

Top Differential Diagnoses
- Splenic Abscess
- Splenic Tumor
- Splenic Laceration

Pathology
- Genetics: Predisposition among some hematologic causes such as sickle-cell disease, sickle-cell trait

Clinical Issues
- LUQ pain, chills, fever, malaise
- Complications: Abscess, rupture, subcapsular hematoma, hemorrhage, pseudocyst formation
- Asymptomatic: No treatment
- Symptomatic: Splenectomy for increasing pain or splenic rupture

Diagnostic Checklist
- Consider splenic abscess or tumor

Angiographic Findings
- Conventional: Main splenic artery occlusion or segmental emboli

Imaging Recommendations
- Best imaging tool: CECT
- Protocol advice: 150 mL IV contrast at 2.5 mL/sec; 5 mm collimation & 5 mm reconstruction interval

DIFFERENTIAL DIAGNOSIS

Splenic Abscess
- Complex fluid collection, internal septations, debris
- Low level echoes on sonography
- Multiple gas bubbles
- Rounded, mass effect
- Multiple small lesions (microabscesses) in fungal infections in immunocompromised patients

Splenic Tumor
- Primary malignant
  - Angiosarcoma
  - Hypervascular lesions with prominent areas of necrosis
- Primary benign
  - Hemangioma
  - May have contrast-enhancement pattern similar to hepatic hemangiomas
- Secondary
  - Lymphoma, melanoma, ovarian carcinoma
  - Often complex cystic masses
  - May have perisplenic cystic implants

Splenic Laceration
- History of trauma
- Associated hemoperitoneum
- May have high attenuation active arterial extravasation on CECT
- High attenuation perisplenic hematoma
- Intra-parenchymal low attenuation hematoma on CECT

Splenic Cyst
- Non-neoplastic cysts divided into two categories
  - True epithelial cysts ("primary")
  - "Pseudocysts" or "secondary cysts" lacking an epithelial lining
- Epidermoid cysts are 10-25% of all splenic cysts
- Secondary cysts most often due to infection, infarction or trauma
- Primary cysts may be due to parasitic infection (echinococcal) or epidermoid cysts
- Calcification of cyst wall in 14% of primary cysts, 50% of secondary cysts
- Low-level echoes and thin septations on US in both primary and secondary cysts

PATHOLOGY

General Features
- General path comments: Liquefactive necrosis
- Genetics: Predisposition among some hematologic causes such as sickle-cell disease, sickle-cell trait
- Etiology
  - Embolic
    - Atrial fibrillation
    - Aortic atherosclerotic disease with embolization to splenic artery
    - Aortic valve emboli from subacute bacterial endocarditis
  - Hematologic
    - Sickle hemoglobinopathies
    - Myelofibrosis
    - Hypercoagulable states
    - Leukemia and lymphoma
    - Any cause of hypersplenism
  - Anatomic causes
    - Splenic torsion, torsion due to wandering spleen
  - Miscellaneous
    - Pancreatic disease, pseudocysts
    - Collagen vascular disease
    - Gastric tumors invading gastro-splenic ligament
    - Torsion of "wandering spleen"

SPLENIC INFARCTION

- Epidemiology
  - Embolic
    - Elderly cardiac patients with atrial fibrillation
  - Hematologic
    - Younger patients with sickle hemoglobinopathy or myeloproliferative disease

Gross Pathologic & Surgical Features
- Acute infarction
  - Hemorrhagic or bland necrosis
- Chronic infarction
  - Fibrous scar
  - Rarely calcification

Microscopic Features
- Coagulative necrosis, hemorrhage

Staging, Grading or Classification Criteria
- Segmental
  - Wedge-shaped or round segmental lesion
  - Straight margins typical
- Global
  - Entire spleen is avascular
  - May demonstrate "cortical rim" sign

CLINICAL ISSUES

Presentation
- Most common signs/symptoms
  - LUQ pain, chills, fever, malaise
  - 69% of patients have fever in embolic infarction
  - Associated with renal and bowel infarcts in patients with cardiac source of emboli
- Lab data
  - Anemia in 53% of patients
  - Leukocytosis in 41% of patients
  - Elevated platelet count in 7% of patients

Demographics
- Age: 2-87 yrs, mean age 54
- Gender: M = F

Natural History & Prognosis
- Highly variable
  - May require no treatment
  - Surgery for increased pain or rupture
- Morbidity 36%
- Complications: Abscess, rupture, subcapsular hematoma, hemorrhage, pseudocyst formation

Treatment
- Options, risks, complications
  - Asymptomatic: No treatment
  - Symptomatic: Splenectomy for increasing pain or splenic rupture

DIAGNOSTIC CHECKLIST

Consider
- Consider splenic abscess or tumor

Image Interpretation Pearls
- Wedge-shaped peripheral area of nonenhancement

SELECTED REFERENCES

1. Gorg C et al: Chronic recurring infarction of the spleen: sonographic patterns and complications. Ultraschall Med. 24(4):245-9, 2003
2. Romero JR et al: Wandering spleen: a rare cause of abdominal pain. Pediatr Emerg Care. 19(6):412-4, 2003
3. Sodhi KS et al: Torsion of a wandering spleen: acute abdominal presentation. J Emerg Med. 25(2):133-7, 2003
4. Wilkinson NW et al: Splenic infarction following laparoscopic Nissen fundoplication: management strategies. JSLS. 7(4):359-65, 2003
5. Hatipoglu AR et al: A rare cause of acute abdomen: splenic infarction. Hepatogastroenterology. 48(41):1333-6, 2001
6. Andrews MW: Ultrasound of the spleen. World J Surg. 24(2):183-7, 2000
7. Barzilai M et al: Noninfectious gas accumulation in an infarcted spleen. Dig Surg. 17(4):402-4, 2000
8. Toth PP et al: Spontaneous splenic infarction secondary to diabetes-induced microvascular disease. Arch Fam Med. 9(2):195-7, 2000
9. Nores M et al: The clinical spectrum of splenic infarction. Am Surg. 64(2):182-8, 1998
10. Argiris A: Splenic and renal infarctions complicating atrial fibrillation. Mt Sinai J Med. 64(4-5):342-9, 1997
11. Rypens F et al: Splenic parenchymal complications of pancreatitis: CT findings and natural history. J Comput Assist Tomogr. 21(1):89-93, 1997
12. Beeson MS: Splenic infarct presenting as acute abdominal pain in an older patient. J Emerg Med. 14(3):319-22, 1996
13. Frippiat F et al: Splenic infarction: report of three cases of atherosclerotic embolization originating in the aorta and retrospective study of 64 cases. Acta Clin Belg. 51(6):395-402, 1996
14. Collie DA et al: Case report: computed tomography features of complete splenic infarction, cavitation and spontaneous decompression complicating pancreatitis. Br J Radiol. 68(810):662-4, 1995
15. Chin JK et al: Liver/spleen scintigraphy for diagnosis of splenic infarction in cirrhotic patients. Postgrad Med J. 69(815):715-7, 1993
16. Valentine RJ et al: Splenic infarction after splenorenal arterial bypass. J Vasc Surg. 17(3):602-6, 1993
17. Orringer EP et al: Case report: splenic infarction and acute splenic sequestration in adults with hemoglobin SC disease. Am J Med Sci. 302(6):374-9, 1991
18. Goerg C et al: Splenic infarction: sonographic patterns, diagnosis, follow-up, and complications. Radiology. 174(3 Pt 1):803-7, 1990
19. Ting W et al: Splenic septic emboli in endocarditis. Circulation. 82(5 Suppl):IV105-9, 1990

SPLENIC INFARCTION

IMAGE GALLERY

Typical

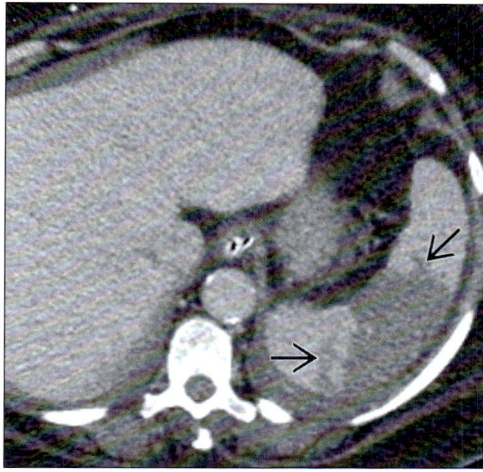
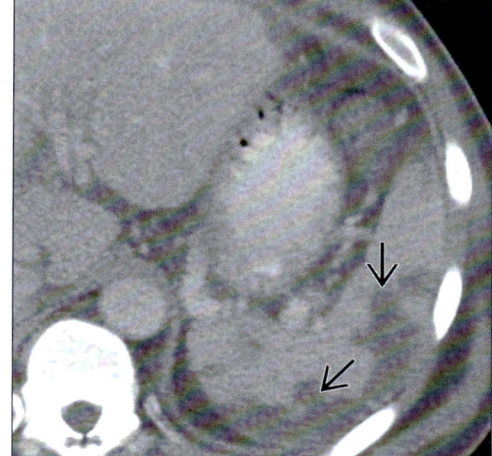

(Left) Axial CECT shows typical signs of acute infarction. Note segmental foci of nonenhancing splenic tissue ➔. The absence of capsular retraction (volume loss) confirms acute nature of infarcts. *(Right)* Axial CECT shows acute segmental infarction in patient with recent transplantation. Note multiple segmental, wedge-shaped foci of nonenhancement within spleen ➔.

Typical

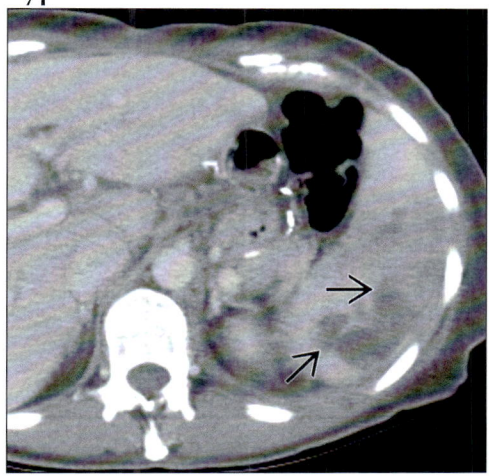
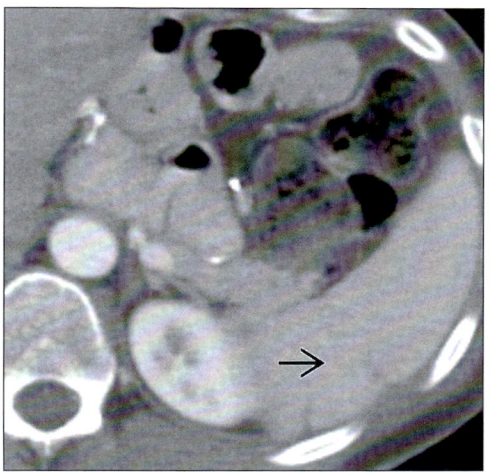

(Left) Axial CECT performed soon after surgery shows irregular wedge-shaped foci ➔ of nonenhancing spleen, characteristic of acute infarction. *(Right)* Axial CECT of same patient as left repeated 7 months later shows only small residual scars ➔ as sequelae of infarcted tissue.

Typical

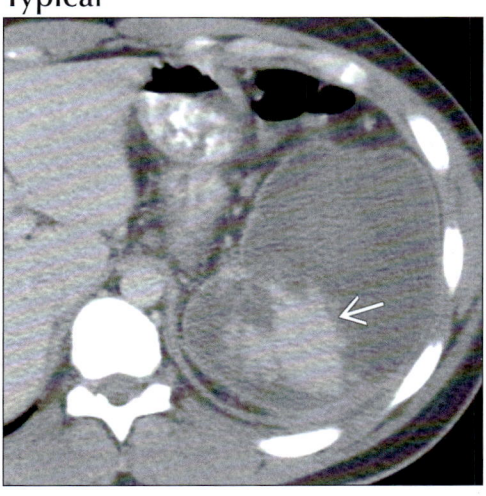
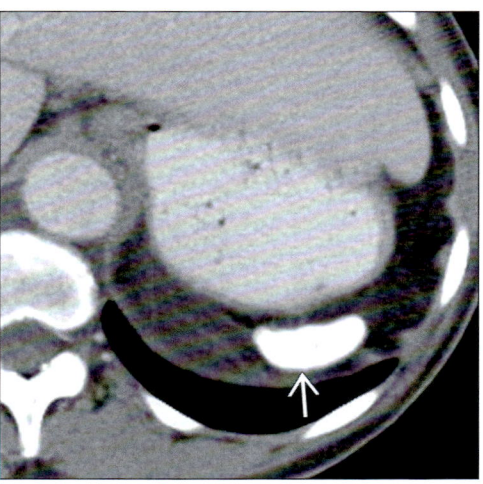

(Left) Axial CECT shows acute infarction in patient with enlarged spleen due to mononucleosis. Most of the spleen is nonenhancing and infarcted, with only scattered islands of viable tissue ➔. *(Right)* Axial CECT shows classic signs of sickle cell disease, including "autosplenectomy". The spleen is very small and densely calcified ➔ and would be nonfunctional, or "autosplenectomy".

HEPATIC CANDIDIASIS

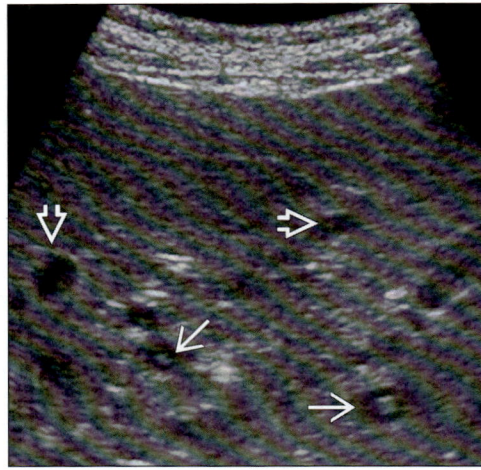

Transverse grayscale sonogram of hepatic candidiasis. Note multiple small target lesions ➡ as well as hypoechoic abscesses ➡.

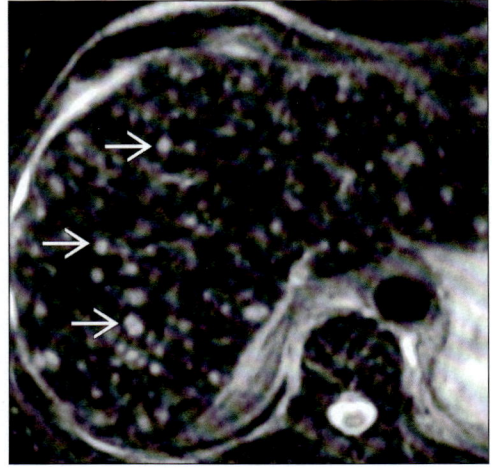

Axial T2-weighted MRI in same patient as left reveals innumerable high-signal fungal abscesses ➡.

TERMINOLOGY

Definitions
- Systemic fungal infection (Candida albicans) often affecting abdominal viscera

IMAGING FINDINGS

General Features
- Best diagnostic clue: Multiple well-defined, rounded microabscesses in liver
- Location
  ○ Both lobes of liver
  ○ Chronic disseminated candidiasis
    ▪ Involvement of several organs
- Size: Microabscesses less than 1 cm

CT Findings
- NECT
  ○ Multiple small hypodense lesions
  ○ ± Periportal areas of increased attenuation (fibrosis)
  ○ ± Scattered areas of calcific density (healing phase)
- CECT
  ○ Biphasic CT may be more accurate than venous phase only
  ○ Nonenhancing hypodense areas
  ○ ± Peripheral enhancement
  ○ Central or eccentric "dot" felt to represent hyphae
  ○ Rarely may demonstrate unusual central enhancement on arterial phase with double peripheral rim

MR Findings
- T1WI: Hypointense
- T2WI: Hyperintense
- STIR: Short T1 inversion recovery (STIR): Hyperintense
- T1 C+: Nonenhancing hypointense lesions
- Contrast-enhanced FLASH (fast low-angle shot) images
  ○ Detect more lesions

Ultrasonographic Findings
- Grayscale Ultrasound
  ○ Four major patterns of hepatic Candidiasis
    ▪ "Wheel within a wheel": Peripheral zone surrounds inner echogenic wheel, which surrounds central hypoechoic nidus (early stage)

DDx: Extensive Hypodense Liver Lesions

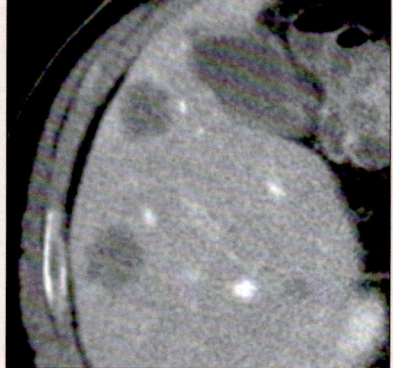

Metastases

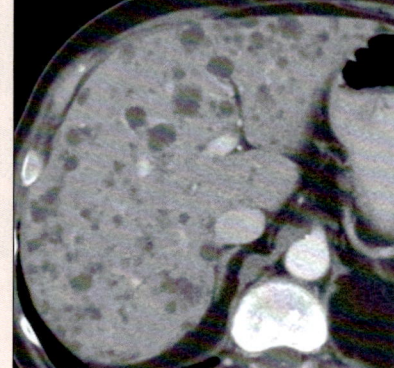

Biliary Hamartoma

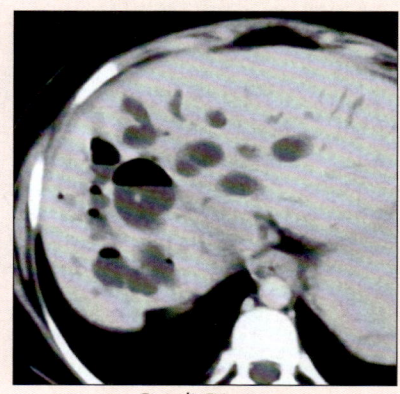

Caroli Disease

HEPATIC CANDIDIASIS

Key Facts

Terminology
- Systemic fungal infection (Candida albicans) often affecting abdominal viscera

Imaging Findings
- Best diagnostic clue: Multiple well-defined, rounded microabscesses in liver
- Both lobes of liver
- Size: Microabscesses less than 1 cm

Top Differential Diagnoses
- Metastases
- Lymphomatous/Leukemic Foci in Liver
- Biliary Hamartomas
- Caroli Disease

Pathology
- Originates from intestinal seeding of portal & venous circulation
- Candida albicans

Clinical Issues
- Asymptomatic or abdominal pain & fever
- Erythematous papules on skin
- Immunocompromised patient recovering from neutropenia
- Antifungal therapy (amphotericin B & fluconazole) in large doses required for disseminated form

Diagnostic Checklist
- Rule out other "innumerable hypodense liver lesions"
- Biopsy specimen for histology/microbiology

- "Bull's eye": 1-4 mm lesion with hyperechoic center surrounded by hypoechoic rim (neutrophil count returns to normal)
- "Uniformly hypoechoic": Most common appearance (fibrosis & debris)
- "Echogenic": Scar formation
- After antifungal therapy: Lesions increase in echogenicity, decrease in size, often disappearing altogether

Nuclear Medicine Findings
- Candida microabscesses
  - Cold lesions on technetium sulfur colloid (decreased uptake)
  - Cold lesions on gallium scan (diminished uptake)

Imaging Recommendations
- Best imaging tool: MDCT, MRI
- Protocol advice
  - MDCT: IV contrast at 2.5 mL/sec with 5 mm collimation and 5 mm reconstruction interval
  - MR: FLASH sequences
  - Gadolinium enhancement required to detect very small lesions

DIFFERENTIAL DIAGNOSIS

Metastases
- Less numerous, larger, usually do not affect spleen
- Epithelial metastases: Rim enhancement
- Can be cystic or calcified

Lymphomatous/Leukemic Foci in Liver
- Less well-defined; less numerous; larger
- Usually foci can also be seen in spleen

Biliary Hamartomas
- Rare benign congenital malformation of bile ducts
- Intraparenchymal or subcapsular
- Innumerable subcentimeter nodules in both lobes
- Diagnosis: Biopsy & histologic exam

Caroli Disease
- "Central dot" sign: Enhancing tiny dot (portal radicle) within dilated cystic intrahepatic ducts on CECT is best clue
- Two types: Simple & periportal
  - Simple: Cystic dilatation of bile ducts without periportal fibrosis
  - Periportal: Ductal dilatation, cysts & periportal fibrosis

PATHOLOGY

General Features
- Etiology
  - Originates from intestinal seeding of portal & venous circulation
  - Candida albicans
    - Most common cause of Candidiasis
  - Candida tropicalis
    - Accounts for 1/3 of visceral candidiasis cases
    - Usually in tropical countries
- Epidemiology
  - Most common fungal infection in immunocompromised patients
  - More common in patients with
    - Acquired immunodeficiency syndrome (AIDS)
    - Intensive chemotherapy
    - Acute leukemia (50-70%) recovering from profound neutropenia
    - Renal transplant
    - Chronic granulomatous disease of childhood
    - Lymphoma (50%) at time of autopsy
- Associated abnormalities
  - AIDS, leukemia, lymphoma, underlying malignancy
  - Neutropenia due to other causes
    - Chemotherapy, post-radiation therapy, organ transplant

Gross Pathologic & Surgical Features
- Multiple microabscesses of liver

HEPATIC CANDIDIASIS

Microscopic Features
- Simple media: Oval, budding cells
- Special culture
  - Hyphae: Elongated branching (pseudohyphae)
- In serum
  - Germ tubes: Thick-walled spores (chlamydospores)

CLINICAL ISSUES

Presentation
- Most common signs/symptoms
  - Asymptomatic or abdominal pain & fever
  - Erythematous papules on skin
    - Acute candidemia (neutropenic patients)
  - Rarely hepatomegaly
  - Fever in neutropenic patients whose WBC count is returning to normal
- Clinical Profile
  - Immunocompromised patient recovering from neutropenia
  - High incidence in transplant patients with fungal colonization
- Lab data: Increased alkaline phosphatase
- Diagnosis: Histologic section of biopsy specimens
  - Pseudohyphae in central necrotic portion of lesion
  - Blood cultures positive in only 50% of affected patients
- Post-transplantation risk factors
  - Epstein-Barr virus
  - Fungal colonization

Demographics
- Age: Any age group
- Gender: M = F

Natural History & Prognosis
- Systemic fungal infection
- Origin: Intestinal seeding
- Liver lesions via portal & venous circulation
- Prognosis usually good with prompt diagnosis & treatment
- Complications (rare)
  - Microabscess rupture
  - Cholangitis due to candidiasis of biliary tract

Treatment
- Liver microabscesses
  - Antifungal therapy (amphotericin B & fluconazole) in large doses required for disseminated form
    - Lesions may disappear on CT and US during neutropenia and antifungal therapy
    - Therapy should not be discontinued on basis of imaging alone
  - Very rarely surgical or percutaneous drainage

DIAGNOSTIC CHECKLIST

Consider
- Rule out other "innumerable hypodense liver lesions"
- Biopsy specimen for histology/microbiology

Image Interpretation Pearls
- Multiple small rounded lesions on CT and MR (FLASH) sequences

SELECTED REFERENCES

1. Masood A et al: Chronic disseminated candidiasis in patients with acute leukemia: emphasis on diagnostic definition and treatment. Leuk Res. 29(5):493-501, 2005
2. Rudolph J et al: Unusual enhancement pattern of liver lesions in hepatosplenic candidiasis. Acta Radiol. 45(5):499-503, 2004
3. Hanninen EL et al: Detection of focal liver lesions at biphasic spiral CT: randomized double-blind study of the effect of iodine concentration in contrast materials. Radiology. 216(2):403-9, 2000
4. Wig JD et al: Cholangitis due to candidiasis of the extra-hepatic biliary tract. HPB Surg. 11(1):51-4, 1998
5. Pestalozzi BC et al: Hepatic lesions of chronic disseminated candidiasis may become invisible during neutropenia. Blood. 90(10):3858-64, 1997
6. Semelka RC et al: Hepatosplenic fungal disease: Diagnostic accuracy and spectrum of appearances on MR imaging. AJR 169:1311-6, 1997
7. Giamarellou H et al: Epidemiology, diagnosis, and therapy of fungal infections in surgery. Infect Control Hosp Epidemiol. 17(8):558-64, 1996
8. van Leeuwen MS et al: Focal liver lesions: characterization with triphasic spiral CT. Radiology. 201(2):327-36, 1996
9. Lamminen AE et al: Infectious liver foci in leukemia: Comparison of short-inversion-time inversion-recovery, T1-weighted spin-echo, and dynamic gadolinium-enhanced MR imaging. Radiology. 191:539-43, 1994
10. Olcott EW et al: Polyarteritis nodosa mimicking hepatic candidiasis on postcontrast CT. J Comput Assist Tomogr. 18(2):305-7, 1994
11. Semelka RC et al: Detection of acute and treated lesions of hepatosplenic candidiasis: comparison of dynamic contrast-enhanced CT and MR imaging. J Magn Reson Imaging. 2(3):341-5, 1992
12. Meunier F: Candidiasis. Eur J Clin Microbiol Infect Dis. 8(5):438-47, 1989
13. Cunha BA: Systemic infections affecting the liver. Some cause jaundice, some do not. Postgrad Med. 84(5):148-58, 161-3, 166-8, 1988
14. Maxwell AJ et al: Fungal liver abscesses in acute leukaemia--a report of two cases. Clin Radiol. 39(2):197-201, 1988
15. Pastakia B et al: Hepatosplenic candidiasis: Wheels within wheels. Radiology. 166:417-21, 1988
16. Thaler M et al: Hepatic candidiasis in cancer patients: the evolving picture of the syndrome. Ann Intern Med. 108(1):88-100, 1988
17. Itai Y et al: Hepatic scar in a case of healed candidiasis showing prolonged enhancement on CT. Radiat Med. 5(4):101-3, 1987
18. Shirkhoda A: CT findings in hepatosplenic and renal candidiasis. J Comput Assist Tomogr. 11(5):795-8, 1987
19. Shirkhoda A et al: Hepatosplenic fungal infection: CT and pathologic evaluation after treatment with liposomal amphotericin B. Radiology. 159(2):349-53, 1986
20. Tashjian LS et al: Focal hepatic candidiasis: a distinct clinical variant of candidiasis in immunocompromised patients. Rev Infect Dis. 6(5):689-703, 1984

HEPATIC CANDIDIASIS

IMAGE GALLERY

Typical

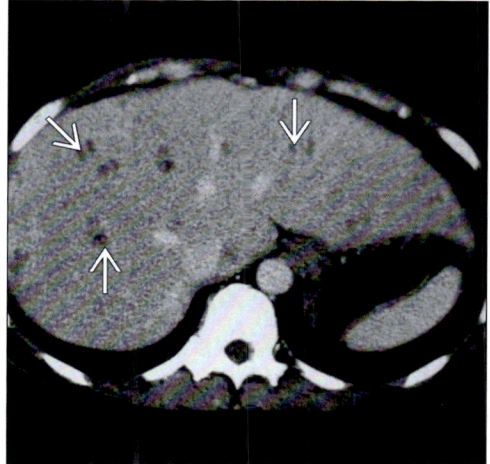
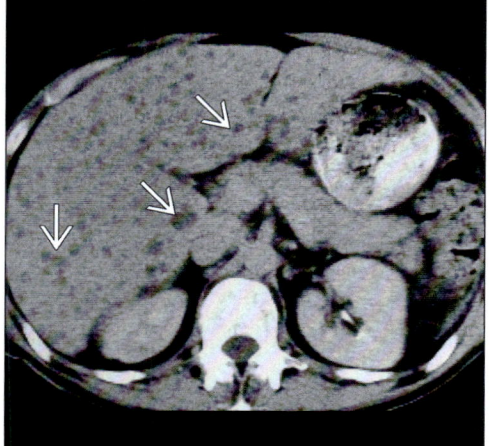

(**Left**) Axial CECT shows multiple small hypodense lesions ➡ throughout liver in patient with fungal sepsis. Lesions vary in size, but all are < 2 cm. Splenic involvement was not radiographically visible. (**Right**) Axial CECT shows fungal abscesses due to candida in patient with leukemia. Note multiple small lesions ➡, all < 1 cm, in all lobes of liver.

Typical

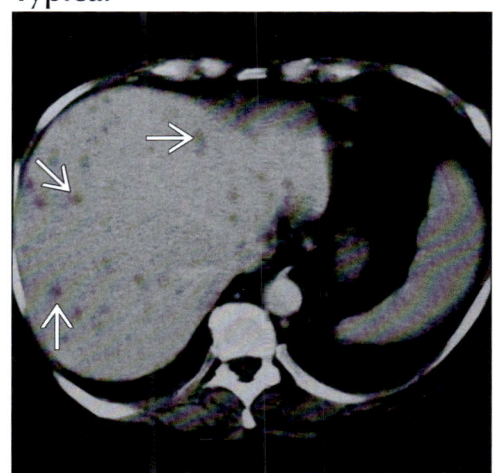
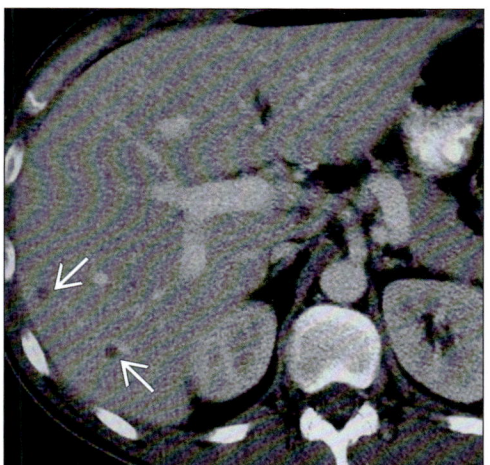

(**Left**) Axial CECT shows multiple poorly defined low density lesions < 1 cm in size ➡ within liver parenchyma in patient on chemotherapy for breast cancer. Biopsy confirmed candidiasis and anti-fungal therapy was instituted. (**Right**) Axial CECT shows acute lymphocytic leukemia. Note several small sub-centimeter hepatic lesions ➡, classical appearance of microabscesses due to fungal or bacterial organisms.

Typical

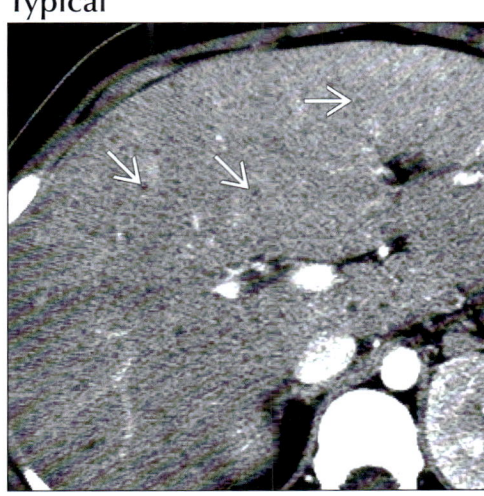
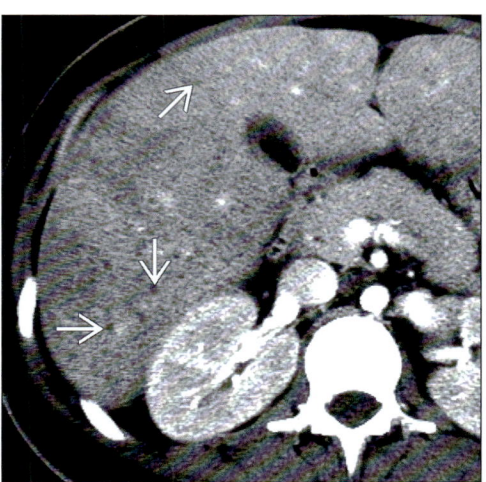

(**Left**) Axial CECT shows early hepatic candidiasis. Note innumerable tiny hypodense lesions ➡. (**Right**) Axial CECT at lower level in same patient as left shows demonstrates additional lesions ➡.

HEPATIC PYOGENIC ABSCESS

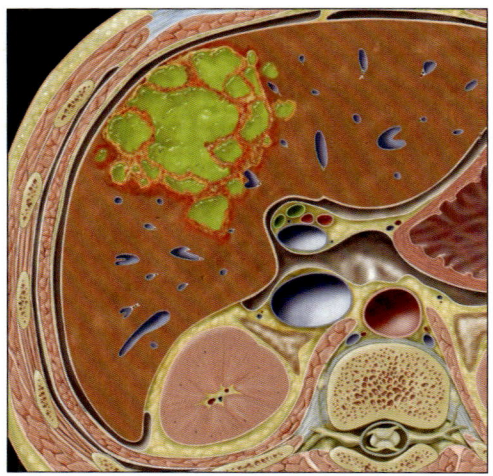

Graphic shows peripheral multiloculated collections of pus with surrounding inflamed liver.

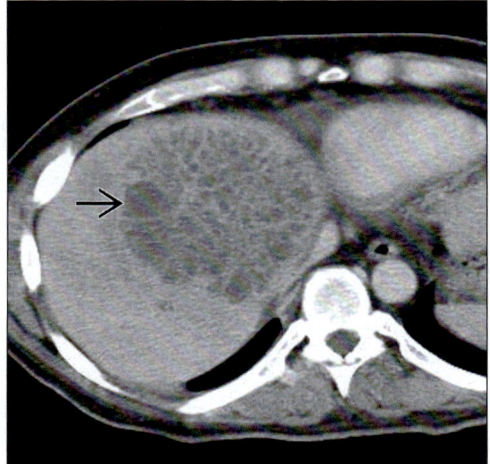

Axial CECT shows multiloculated pyogenic liver abscess ➔ with innumerable septations and contents slightly higher than water-density. Abscess resolved slowly over several months.

TERMINOLOGY

Definitions
- Localized collection of pus in liver due to bacterial infectious process with destruction of hepatic parenchyma & stroma

IMAGING FINDINGS

General Features
- Best diagnostic clue: "Cluster" sign - small pyogenic abscesses coalesce into a single large cavity
- Location
  - Based on origin
    - Biliary tract: 90% involve both lobes
    - Portal: Right lobe (65%); left lobe (12%); both lobes (23%)
- Size
  - Varies from few mm to 10 cm, may be single or multiple
    - Biliary tract origin: Multiple small abscesses
    - Portal origin: Usually solitary larger abscess
    - Direct extension & trauma: Solitary large abscess

Radiographic Findings
- Radiography
  - Chest radiograph
    - Elevation of right hemidiaphragm
    - Right lower lobe (RLL) atelectasis
    - Infiltrative lesions, right pleural effusion
  - Abdominal radiograph
    - Hepatomegaly, intrahepatic gas, air-fluid level

Fluoroscopic Findings
- Contrast studies of gut and urinary tract
  - May show cause of abscess
    - Diverticulitis
    - Perforated ulcer
    - Renal abscess
- ERCP
  - Accurate definition of level & cause of biliary obstruction

CT Findings
- NECT
  - Simple abscess
    - Well-defined, round, hypodense mass (0-45 HU)
  - "Cluster" sign

DDx: Cystic Liver Lesion with/without Gas

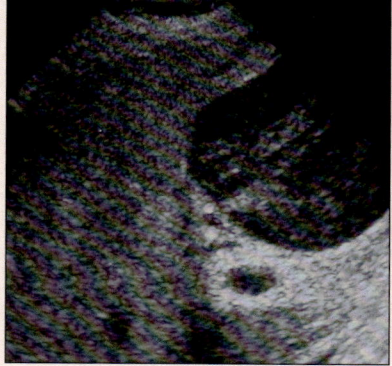

Cystic Metastases

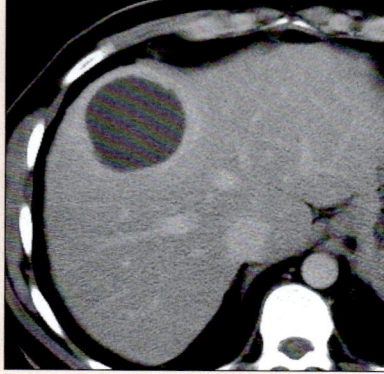

Amebic Abscess

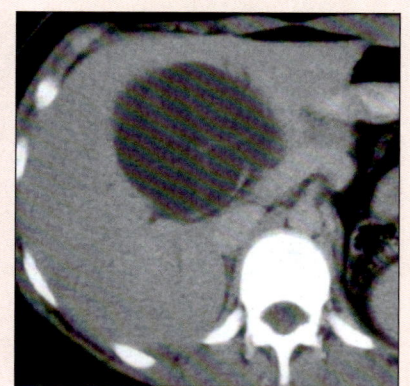

Biliary Cystadenocarcinoma

HEPATIC PYOGENIC ABSCESS

Key Facts

Terminology
- Localized collection of pus in liver due to bacterial infectious process with destruction of hepatic parenchyma & stroma

Imaging Findings
- Best diagnostic clue: "Cluster" sign - small pyogenic abscesses coalesce into a single large cavity
- Biliary tract: 90% involve both lobes
- Portal: Right lobe (65%); left lobe (12%); both lobes (23%)
- Right lower lobe (RLL) atelectasis

Top Differential Diagnoses
- Post-Treatment Metastases
- Hepatic Amebic Abscess
- Infarction in Liver Transplant (OLT)
- Hepatic Hydatid Cyst
- Biliary Cystadenocarcinoma

Pathology
- E. coli (adults) & S. aureus (children)
- Diverticulitis, appendicitis

Clinical Issues
- Clinical Profile: Middle-aged/elderly patient with history of fever, RUQ & LLQ pain, tender hepatomegaly & increased WBC count

Diagnostic Checklist
- Rule out amebic or fungal liver abscesses, cystic tumors
- Check for history of transplantation or ablation/chemotherapy for liver tumor

---

- Small abscesses coalesce into single large cavity, usually septated
  - Complex abscess: "Target" lesion
    - Isodense periphery
  - Abscess with central gas (seen in less than 20% of cases)
    - Seen as air bubbles or air-fluid level
  - Large air-fluid or fluid-debris level
    - Often associated with gut communication or necrotic tissue
- CECT
  - Sharply-defined, round, hypodense mass
  - Rim/capsule enhancement & septal enhancement
  - RLL atelectasis, pleural effusion
  - Non-liquified infection may simulate hypervascular tumor

MR Findings
- T1WI: Hypointense
- T2WI
  - Hyperintense mass
  - High signal intensity perilesional edema
- T1 C+
  - Hypointense mass
  - Rim or capsule enhancement
  - Small abscesses less than 1 cm
    - May show homogeneous enhancement, mimic hemangiomas
- MRCP
  - Highly specific in detecting obstructive biliary pathology
    - Leading cause of cholangitis → pyogenic abscess

Ultrasonographic Findings
- Grayscale Ultrasound
  - Variable shape & echogenicity
  - Usually spherical or ovoid
  - Irregular hypoechoic/mildly echogenic wall
  - Echogenicity of abscesses
    - Anechoic (50%), hyperechoic (25%), hypoechoic (25%)
  - ± Septa or fluid level within abscess
  - ± Debris & posterior enhancement
  - Early lesions tend to be echogenic & poorly demarcated
  - May evolve into well-demarcated, nearly anechoic lesions
  - Gas seen as brightly echogenic foci with posterior artifact

Nuclear Medicine Findings
- Hepatobiliary & sulfur colloid scans
  - Rounded, cold areas
  - Occasionally communication between abscess cavity & biliary system
- Gallium scan (Gallium citrate Ga-67)
  - Hot lesions
  - Mixed lesion: Cold center, hot rim
- WBC Scan
  - Hot lesions (WBC accumulation)
  - Highly specific compared to nuclear or cross-sectional imaging

Imaging Recommendations
- Best imaging tool: CECT
- Protocol advice: CT-guided aspiration

DIFFERENTIAL DIAGNOSIS

Post-Treatment Metastases
- Usually does not appear as cluster or septated cystic mass
- No elevation of diaphragm or atelectasis
- No fever or ↑ WBC
- Treated necrotic metastases may be indistinguishable from abscess

Hepatic Amebic Abscess
- Usually peripheral, round or ovoid
- Sharply defined hypoechoic or low attenuation abscess
- Most often solitary (85%)
- Affects right lobe more than left (72% vs. 13%)
- Abuts liver capsule
  - Homogeneous echoes + distal enhancement on US

HEPATIC PYOGENIC ABSCESS

- More common in recent immigrants, institutionalized, homosexuals

Infarction in Liver Transplant (OLT)
- Hepatic artery thrombosis (HAT) → hepatic & biliary necrosis
- Indistinguishable from pyogenic abscess

Hepatic Hydatid Cyst
- Large cystic liver mass with peripheral daughter cysts
- ± Curvilinear or ring-like pericyst calcification
- ± Dilated intrahepatic bile ducts due to mass effect and/or rupture into bile ducts

Biliary Cystadenocarcinoma
- Rare, multiseptated, water-density cystic mass
- No surrounding inflammatory changes

PATHOLOGY

General Features
- General path comments
  - Pyogenic abscess can develop via five major routes
  - Biliary: Ascending cholangitis
    - Choledocholithiasis
    - Benign or malignant biliary obstruction
  - Portal vein: Pylephlebitis
    - Appendicitis, diverticulitis, proctitis, inflammatory bowel disease
    - Right colon infection spread: Superior mesenteric vein → portal vein → liver
    - Left colon infection spread: Inferior mesenteric vein → splenic vein → portal vein → liver
  - Hepatic artery: Septicemia
    - Bacterial endocarditis, pneumonitis, osteomyelitis
  - Direct extension
    - Perforated gastric or duodenal ulcer
    - Subphrenic abscess, pyelonephritis
  - Traumatic: Blunt or penetrating injuries
- Etiology
  - Western countries
    - Diverticulitis or ascending cholangitis; infection of infarcted tissue (post-liver transplantation, necrotic tumor)
    - Infection of infarcted tissue (post-liver transplantation, necrotic tumor)
  - Developing countries
    - Mostly due to parasitic infections (Amebic, echinococcal or other protozoal/helminthic)
  - Most common bacterial organisms
    - E. coli (adults) & S. aureus (children)
- Epidemiology
  - Accounts for 88% of all liver abscesses
  - Increasing incidence in Western countries due to ascending cholangitis & diverticulitis
- Associated abnormalities
  - Diverticulitis, appendicitis
  - Benign or malignant biliary obstruction
  - Perforated gastric or duodenal ulcer
  - Bacterial endocarditis, pneumonitis, osteomyelitis

Gross Pathologic & Surgical Features
- Multiple or solitary lesions

CLINICAL ISSUES

Presentation
- Most common signs/symptoms
  - Fever, RUQ pain, rigors, malaise
  - Nausea, vomiting, weight loss, tender hepatomegaly
  - If subphrenic, atelectasis and pleural effusion possible
- Clinical Profile: Middle-aged/elderly patient with history of fever, RUQ & LLQ pain, tender hepatomegaly & increased WBC count
- Lab data
  - Increased leukocytes & serum alkaline phosphatase
- Diagnosis: Fine-needle aspiration cytology (FNAC)

Demographics
- Age: Middle age to elderly

Natural History & Prognosis
- Complications
  - Spread of infection to subphrenic space
    - Atelectasis & pleural effusion
- Prognosis
  - Good with medical therapy & aspiration
  - Catheter drainage failure rate: 8.4%
  - Recurrent abscess rate: 8%

Treatment
- Antibiotics
- Percutaneous aspiration + parenteral antibiotics
- Percutaneous catheter drainage
- Surgical drainage

DIAGNOSTIC CHECKLIST

Consider
- Rule out amebic or fungal liver abscesses, cystic tumors
- Check for history of transplantation or ablation/chemotherapy for liver tumor

Image Interpretation Pearls
- "Cluster" sign, presence of central gas or fluid level
- Elevation of right hemidiaphragm
- RLL atelectasis & pleural effusion

SELECTED REFERENCES

1. Lederman ER et al: Pyogenic liver abscess with a focus on Klebsiella pneumoniae as a primary pathogen: an emerging disease with unique clinical characteristics. Am J Gastroenterol. 100(2):322-31, 2005
2. Kurland JE et al: Pyogenic and amebic liver abscesses. Curr Gastroenterol Rep. 6(4):273-9, 2004
3. Johannsen EC et al: Pyogenic liver abscesses. Infect Dis Clin North Am. 14(3):547-63, vii, 2000
4. Giorgio A et al: Pyogenic liver abscesses: 13 years of experience in percutaneous needle aspiration with US guidance. Radiology. 195: 122-4, 1995
5. Mendez RZ et al: Hepatic abscesses: MR imaging findings. Radiology. 190: 431-6, 1994
6. Jeffrey RB et al: CT small pyogenic hepatic abscesses: The cluster sign. AJR. 151(3): 487-9, 1988

HEPATIC PYOGENIC ABSCESS

IMAGE GALLERY

Typical

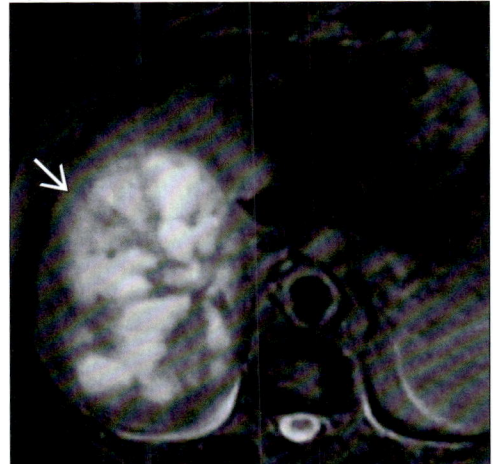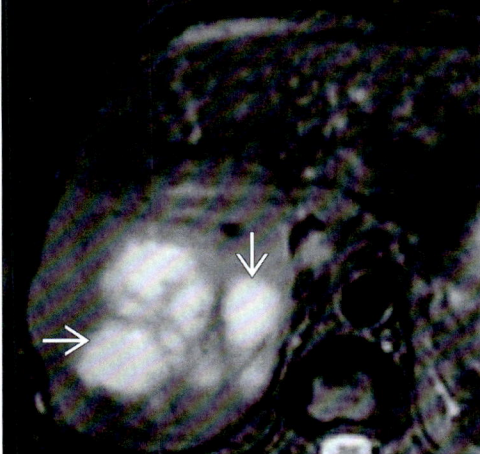

(Left) Axial T2WI FS MR of pyogenic liver abscess shows multiple locules of high-signal fluid representing clustering of multiseptated abscess ➡. *(Right)* Axial T2WI FS MR at more caudal level in same patient as left demonstrates more discrete abscess pockets ➡.

Typical

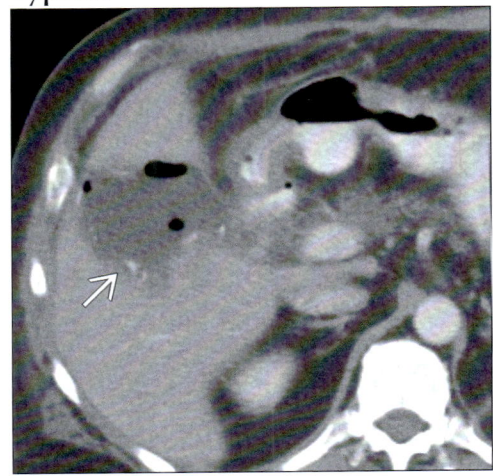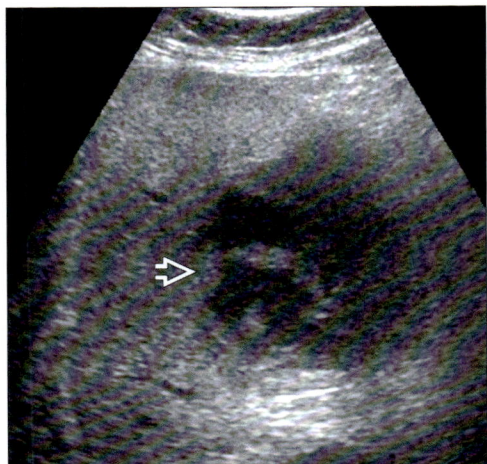

(Left) Axial CECT shows pyogenic abscess ➡ containing gas fluid in liver and gallbladder bed. *(Right)* Transverse ultrasound in same patient as left shows complex fluid collection ➡. Patient underwent ultrasound-guided catheter drainage with rapid clinical improvement.

Typical

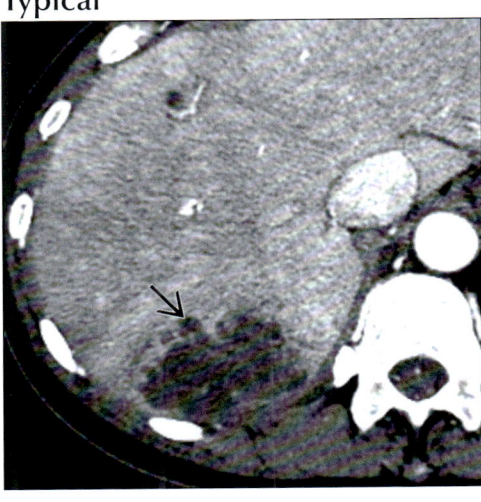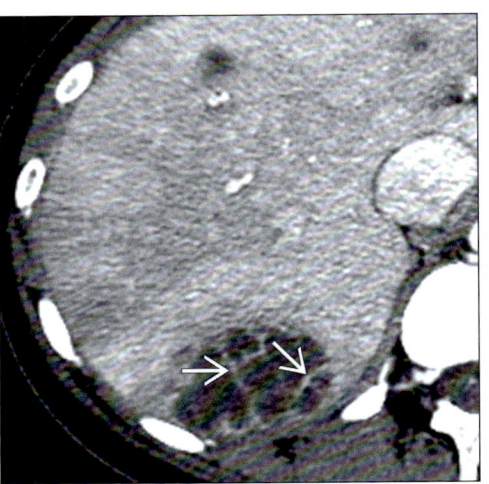

(Left) Axial CECT of pyogenic liver abscess shows low-density lesion ➡ with irregular contours in segment 6. *(Right)* Axial CECT at more caudal level in same patient as left shows multiple septations within abscess cavity ➡.

HEPATIC AMEBIC ABSCESS

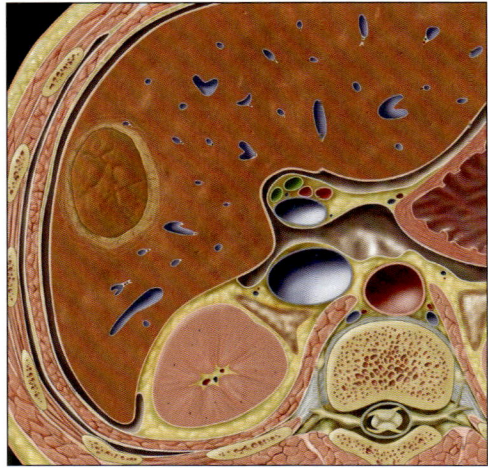

Graphic shows unilocular encapsulated mass with "anchovy paste" contents.

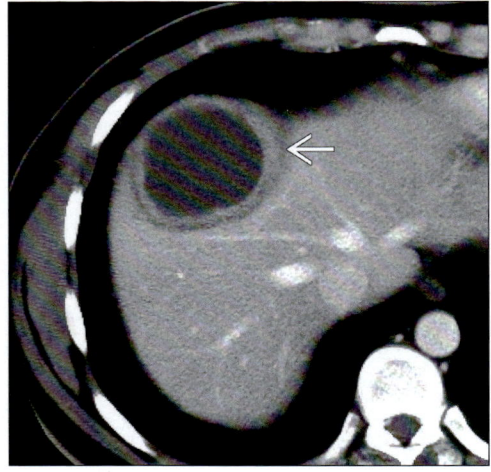

Axial CECT of amebic abscess shows low-attenuation rim of edema ➡ surrounding abscess.

TERMINOLOGY

Definitions
- Localized collection of pus in liver due to entamoeba histolytica with destruction of hepatic parenchyma & stroma

IMAGING FINDINGS

General Features
- Best diagnostic clue: Peripherally located, sharply defined, round, hypodense mass with enhancing capsule
- Location
  - Right lobe (72%) or left lobe (13%)
  - Usually peripheral
- Size: Few mm - several cm

Radiographic Findings
- Radiography
  - Elevation of right hemidiaphragm
  - Right lower lobe (RLL) atelectasis or infiltrate
  - Right pleural effusion
  - Ruptured amebic abscess into chest
    - Lung abscess, cavity, hydropneumothorax, pericardial effusion

Fluoroscopic Findings
- Contrast enema often shows changes of amebic colitis

CT Findings
- NECT: Peripheral, round or oval hypodense mass (10-20 HU)
- CECT
  - Unilocular or multilocular lesions
  - Low-attenuation enhancement of peripheral rim or capsule (edema)
  - May demonstrate nodularity of margins
  - Extrahepatic abnormalities
    - RLL atelectasis, right pleural effusion, colonic changes
    - Rarely gastric changes

MR Findings
- T1WI: Hypointense abscess
- T2WI
  - Hyperintense abscess
  - Perilesional edema: High signal intensity

DDx: Complex Cystic Mass

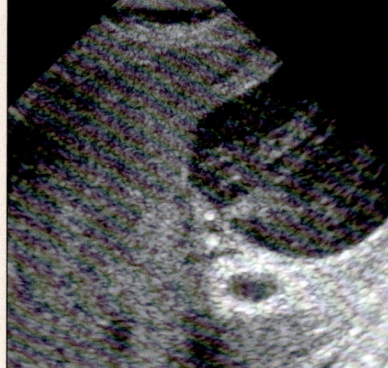

Cystic Metastases

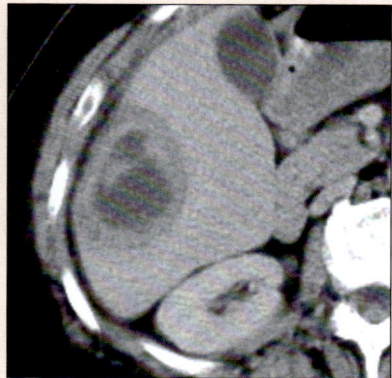

Pyogenic Abscess

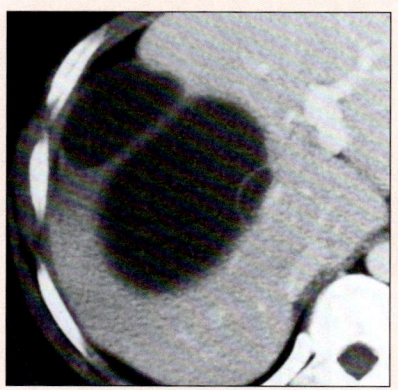

Hydatid Cyst

HEPATIC AMEBIC ABSCESS

Key Facts

Terminology
- Localized collection of pus in liver due to entamoeba histolytica with destruction of hepatic parenchyma & stroma

Imaging Findings
- Best diagnostic clue: Peripherally located, sharply defined, round, hypodense mass with enhancing capsule
- Elevation of right hemidiaphragm
- Right lower lobe (RLL) atelectasis or infiltrate
- Unilocular or multilocular lesions
- Low-attenuation enhancement of peripheral rim or capsule (edema)

Top Differential Diagnoses
- Post-Treatment Metastases (Cystic or Necrotic)
- Hepatic Pyogenic Abscess
- Infarcted Liver After Transplantation (OLT)
- Hepatic Hydatid Cyst
- Biliary Cystadenocarcinoma

Pathology
- Entamoeba histolytica

Clinical Issues
- Most common signs/symptoms: RUQ pain, tender hepatomegaly, diarrhea with mucus
- Indirect hemagglutination positive in 90% of cases

Diagnostic Checklist
- Rule out pyogenic or fungal abscess, cystic lesions
- Check for history of transplantation & ablation or chemotherapy for liver tumor or metastasis

---

- T1 C+
  - Abscess contents: No enhancement
  - Enhancement of rim or capsule

Ultrasonographic Findings
- Grayscale Ultrasound
  - Round or oval, sharply-defined hypoechoic mass
  - Abuts liver capsule with homogeneous echoes & distal enhancement

Nuclear Medicine Findings
- Hepatobiliary scan (HIDA): Cold lesion with hot periphery
- Technetium sulfur colloid: Cold defects
- WBC Scan: Cold center, hot rim

Imaging Recommendations
- Best imaging tool: CECT
- Protocol advice: Scan to include lung bases through pelvis

DIFFERENTIAL DIAGNOSIS

Post-Treatment Metastases (Cystic or Necrotic)
- May be indistinguishable from amebic abscess
- Usually no elevation of diaphragm or atelectasis
- No fever or increased WBC

Hepatic Pyogenic Abscess
- Simple pyogenic abscess
  - Well-defined round, hypodense mass (0-45 HU)
  - "Cluster" sign: Small abscesses coalesce into single septated cavity
- Abscess with central gas (air bubbles or air-fluid level)

Infarcted Liver After Transplantation (OLT)
- Hepatic artery thrombosis (HAT) causes biliary & hepatic necrosis
- Can look exactly like abscess with or without gas

Hepatic Hydatid Cyst
- Large well-defined cystic liver mass
- Numerous peripheral daughter cysts
- May show curvilinear or ring-like pericyst calcification
- Intrahepatic duct dilatation may be seen

Biliary Cystadenocarcinoma
- Rare, multiseptated, water-density cystic mass
- No surrounding inflammatory changes

PATHOLOGY

General Features
- Etiology
  - Entamoeba histolytica
  - Primary source of infection: Human carriers pass amebic cysts into stool
  - May become secondarily infected with pyogenic bacteria
- Epidemiology
  - Most common extraintestinal manifestation of amebic infestation
  - Approximately 10% of world population infected with E. histolytica
- Associated abnormalities: Amebic colitis

Gross Pathologic & Surgical Features
- Usually solitary abscess with dark, reddish-brown fluid consistency of "anchovy paste"

Microscopic Features
- Blood, destroyed hepatocytes
- Necrotic tissue & rarely trophozoites

CLINICAL ISSUES

Presentation
- Most common signs/symptoms: RUQ pain, tender hepatomegaly, diarrhea with mucus
- Clinical presentation mimics pyogenic liver abscess
- Lab data
  - Stool exam: Usually nonspecific or negative
  - Indirect hemagglutination positive in 90% of cases

HEPATIC AMEBIC ABSCESS

Demographics
- Age: More common in 3rd-5th decade, but can occur in any age group
- Gender: M:F = 4:1
- Most common in developing countries
- High risk groups in Western countries
  - Recent immigrants, institutionalized & homosexuals

Natural History & Prognosis
- Cystic form of E. histolytica gains access via contaminated water
- Mature cysts resistant to gastric acid, pass unchanged into intestine
- Cyst wall digested by trypsin, invasive trophozoites released
- Trophozoites enter mesenteric venules & lymphatics
- Spread from colon to liver via portal vein & lymphatics
- Rarely direct spread
  - Colonic wall to peritoneum
  - Peritoneum to liver capsule & liver
- Complications
  - Pleuropulmonary amebiasis (20-35%)
    - Pulmonary consolidation or abscess
    - Effusion, empyema or hepatobronchial fistula
  - Peritoneal amebiasis (2-7.5%), mortality 2.4% if peritonitis
  - Rupture of liver abscess and/or rupture of amebic colitis
  - Pericardial or renal amebiasis
- Prognosis
  - Good with amebicidal therapy
  - Poor if complications
  - Mortality rate in United States is < 3%
    - < 1% when confined to liver
    - 6% if extension into chest
    - 30% if extension into pericardium
    - Second leading cause of death due to parasite in developing world

Treatment
- 90% respond to antimicrobial therapy
  - Metronidazole or chloroquine
- 10% require aspiration & drainage

DIAGNOSTIC CHECKLIST

Consider
- Rule out pyogenic or fungal abscess, cystic lesions
- Check for history of transplantation & ablation or chemotherapy for liver tumor or metastasis

Image Interpretation Pearls
- Peripheral, round/ovoid hypodense mass with rim or capsule enhancement on CT
- Lesion abutting liver capsule with homogeneous echoes & distal enhancement on US

SELECTED REFERENCES
1. Balci NC et al: MR imaging of infective liver lesions. Magn Reson Imaging Clin N Am. 10(1):121-35, vii, 2002
2. Ralls PW: Inflammatory disease of the liver. Clin Liver Dis. 6(1):203-25, 2002
3. Sharma MP et al: Management of amebic and pyogenic liver abscess. Indian J Gastroenterol. 20 Suppl 1:C33-6, 2001
4. Hughes MA et al: Amebic liver abscess. Infect Dis Clin North Am. 14(3):565-82, viii, 2000
5. Natarajan A et al: Ruptured liver abscess with fulminant amoebic colitis: case report with review. Trop Gastroenterol. 21(4):201-3, 2000
6. Das P et al: Molecular mechanisms of pathogenesis in amebiasis. Indian J Gastroenterol. 18(4):161-6, 1999
7. Rajak CL et al: Percutaneous treatment of liver abscesses: needle aspiration versus catheter drainage. AJR Am J Roentgenol. 170(4):1035-9, 1998
8. Ralls PW: Focal inflammatory disease of the liver. Radiol Clin North Am. 36(2):377-89, 1998
9. Kimura K et al: Amebiasis: modern diagnostic imaging with pathological and clinical correlation. Semin Roentgenol. 32(4):250-75, 1997
10. Fujihara T et al: Amebic liver abscess. J Gastroenterol. 31(5):659-63, 1996
11. Takhtani D et al: Intrapericardial rupture of amebic liver abscess managed with percutaneous drainage of liver abscess alone. Am J Gastroenterol. 91(7):1460-2, 1996
12. Giorgio A et al: Pyogenic liver abscesses: 13 years of experience in percutaneous needle aspiration with US guidance. Radiology. 195: 122-124, 1995
13. Mendez RZ et al: Hepatic abscesses: MR imaging findings. Radiology. 190: 431-436, 1994
14. Van Allan RJ et al: Uncomplicated amebic liver abscess: prospective evaluation of percutaneous therapeutic aspiration. Radiology. 183(3):827-30, 1992
15. Gibney EJ: Amoebic liver abscess. Br J Surg. 77(8):843-4, 1990
16. Frey CF et al: Liver abscesses. Surg Clin North Am. 69(2):259-71, 1989
17. Ken JG et al: Perforated amebic liver abscesses: successful percutaneous treatment. Radiology. 170(1 Pt 1):195-7, 1989
18. Rustgi AK et al: Pyogenic and amebic liver abscess. Med Clin North Am. 73(4):847-58, 1989
19. Jeffrey RB et al: CT small pyogenic hepatic abscesses: The cluster sign. AJR. 151(3): 487-9, 1988

HEPATIC AMEBIC ABSCESS

IMAGE GALLERY

Typical

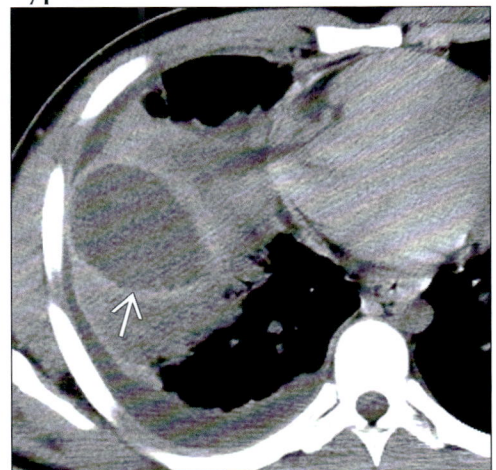
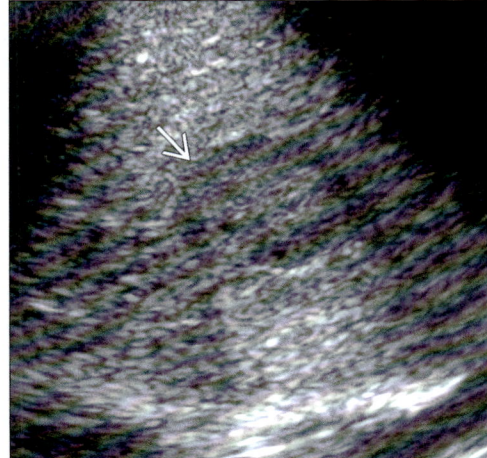

(Left) Axial CECT shows low-density mass ➡ in dome of liver. (Right) Sagittal oblique sonogram in same patient as left shows low echogenicity mass ➡ just below the diaphragm, causing lifted or "splinted" diaphragm, with associated pleural effusion & atelectasis.

Typical

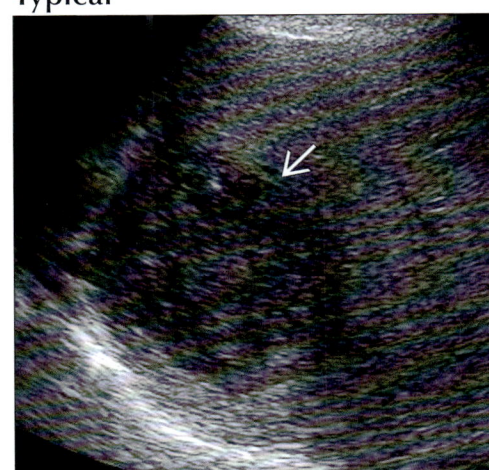
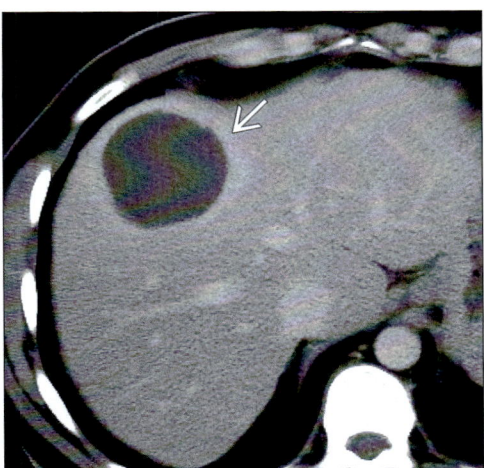

(Left) Sagittal grayscale sonogram of hepatic amebic abscess. Note lesion of mixed echogenicity ➡ adjacent to right hemidiaphragm with little distal enhanced through-sound transmission. (Right) Axial CECT during late portal venous phase in same patient as left reveals enhancing rim around abscess ➡.

Variant

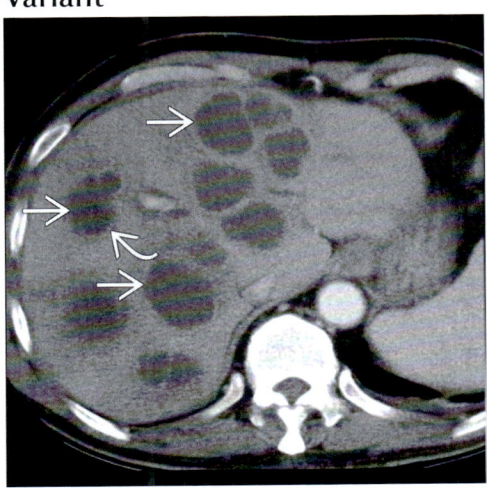
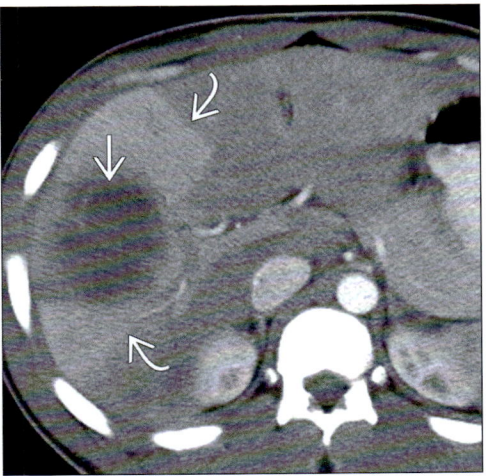

(Left) Axial CECT shows multiple large and small low-density intrahepatic lesions ➡. Note rim enhancement in several lesions ➡. (Right) Axial CECT shows shaggy cystic mass ➡ with nonenhancing contents, representing typical amebic abscess. Note hyperperfusion of anterior right lobe of liver ➡, result of ↑ arterial blood flow.

HELLP SYNDROME

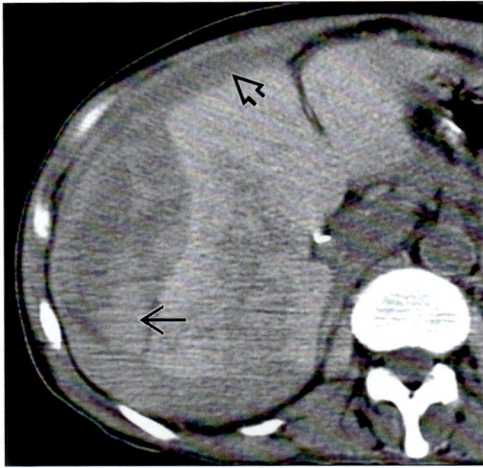

Axial NECT of HELLP syndrome shows high-attenuation subcapsular hematoma that has ruptured into perihepatic peritoneal cavity.

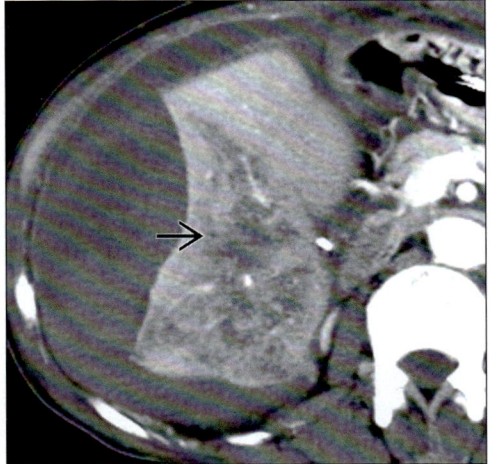

Axial CECT in same patient as left reveals large areas of low-attenuation fatty liver adjacent to subcapsular hematoma.

TERMINOLOGY

Abbreviations and Synonyms
- Hemolysis, elevated liver enzymes, low platelets (HELLP)

Definitions
- Severe variant of preeclampsia

IMAGING FINDINGS

General Features
- Best diagnostic clue: Intrahepatic or subcapsular fluid collection (hematoma) on US or CT
- Location: Subcapsular or intraparenchymal liver

CT Findings
- Liver hematomas
  - Well-defined hyperdense or hypodense
  - Nonenhancing
  - Acute: Hyperattenuating (24-72 hours)
  - Chronic: Decreased attenuation after 72 hours
- Liver infarction
  - Small or large areas of low attenuation, usually peripheral & wedge-shaped
- Occasionally active contrast extravasation or ascites

MR Findings
- T1WI & T2WI
  - Varied signal intensity
    - Degree & age of hemorrhage or infarct
    - Degree of necrosis & steatosis
- Greater degree of edema & cellular necrosis
- T1WI: Low signal intensity
- T2WI: High signal intensity

Ultrasonographic Findings
- Grayscale Ultrasound
  - Irregular or wedge-shaped liver hemorrhage or infarct with increased echogenicity; usually peripheral
  - Periportal halo sign: Hyperechoic thickening of periportal area
  - Subcapsular hematoma: Complex echogenic fluid collection
  - Enlarged liver (predominantly right lobe)
  - Occasionally ascites

DDx: Diffuse or Focal Liver Lesion with Hemorrhage

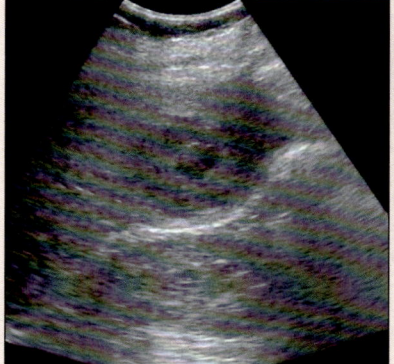

Hepatocellular Carcinoma

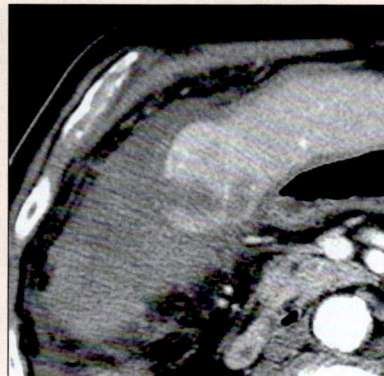

Ruptured HCC

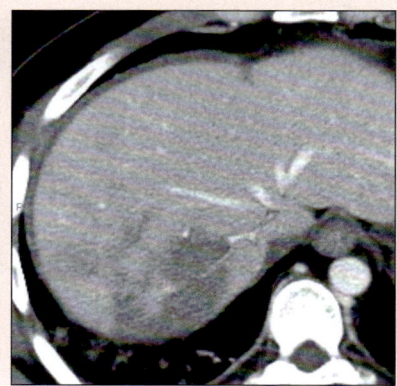

Hepatic Trauma

HELLP SYNDROME

Key Facts

Terminology
- Hemolysis, elevated liver enzymes, low platelets (HELLP)
- Severe variant of preeclampsia

Imaging Findings
- Best diagnostic clue: Intrahepatic or subcapsular fluid collection (hematoma) on US or CT
- Acute: Hyperattenuating (24-72 hours)
- Chronic: Decreased attenuation after 72 hours

Top Differential Diagnoses
- Bleeding Hepatic Tumor (Adenoma or HCC)
- Spontaneous Bleed (Coagulopathy)
- Hepatic Trauma

Clinical Issues
- Acute epigastric & RUQ pain
- Clinical Profile: African-American female, primigravida with features of preeclampsia & lab data showing findings of hemolysis, elevated liver enzymes & low platelets
- Age: 2nd & 3rd decades
- Supportive treatment for most cases
- Standard treatment: Expeditious delivery of fetus
- Surgery & selective embolization for hepatic rupture & intra-abdominal hemorrhage

Diagnostic Checklist
- Rule out bleeding liver tumor, other liver pathologies
- Look for heterogeneous enhancing spherical liver tumors

- US features may be seen before increase in biological markers (41% of cases)

Imaging Recommendations
- Best imaging tool: Ultrasonography
- Protocol advice: CT not recommended due to radiation exposure to fetus

DIFFERENTIAL DIAGNOSIS

Bleeding Hepatic Tumor (Adenoma or HCC)
- Intraparenchymal or subcapsular fluid collection on US or CT; may bleed
- Enhancing heterogeneous spherical hepatic mass
- Indistinguishable from HELLP syndrome

Spontaneous Bleed (Coagulopathy)
- Subcapsular or intrahepatic blood collection, occasionally active extravasation
- History of bleeding disorder
- Lab data: Abnormal bleeding time, clotting time, prothrombin time & partial thromboplastin time
- Indistinguishable from HELLP syndrome without history

Hepatic Trauma
- History of liver injury
- Intraparenchymal or subcapsular hematoma
- Lacerations, wedge-shaped areas of infarction
- Areas of active hemorrhage isodense with vessels
- Hemoperitoneum & pseudoaneurysm

Acute Fatty Liver of Pregnancy
- Usually diffuse increase echogenicity of liver on US
- No intraparenchymal or subcapsular fluid collection (no hemorrhage)

PATHOLOGY

General Features
- General path comments
  - Pathophysiology of HELLP syndrome: Begins in placental bed
    - Arteriolar vasospasm → endothelial damage → fibrin deposition
    - Platelet deposition on fibrin aggregates → decrease number of circulating platelets
  - RBC destruction by fibrin aggregates (hemolytic anemia)
    - Abnormal cells in peripheral smear (burr cells & schistocytes)
    - Elevated indirect bilirubin levels & anemia
  - Hepatocyte destruction due to hepatic microemboli (↑ LFT levels)
    - Distention of liver due to impeded blood flow (RUQ pain)
    - Liver rupture & subcapsular hematoma in severe cases
  - Pathophysiology of preeclampsia
    - Primary site: Increased size of glomerular endothelial cells
    - Abnormal vasoconstriction + hyperactive vascular smooth muscle
    - Hypertension → proteinuria → edema
- Etiology
  - Variant of severe preeclampsia & occasionally eclampsia
  - Preeclampsia & eclampsia etiology
    - Coagulation abnormalities, hormonal factors, uteroplacental ischemia, immune mechanisms
- Epidemiology
  - Preeclampsia: Leading cause of maternal death in USA & Europe
  - Prevalence of HELLP
    - 4-12% of patients with severe preeclampsia
    - 1 per 150 live births
    - Toxemia in 6% of pregnancies
  - Maternal mortality rate (MMR) in severe preeclampsia due to HELLP syndrome is 3.5%

Gross Pathologic & Surgical Features
- Enlarged liver, subcapsular hematoma; parenchymal hemorrhage or infarct

HELLP SYNDROME

Microscopic Features
- Periportal necrosis, microthrombi; fibrin deposits in sinusoids & portal veins

Staging, Grading or Classification Criteria
- Based on classification of American college of Obstetricians/Gynecologists
  - Bilirubin: More than 1.2 mg/dL
  - Lactate dehydrogenase: More than 600 U/L
  - Aspartate aminotransferase: More than 70 U/L
  - Platelet count: Less than 100,000/mm³

CLINICAL ISSUES

Presentation
- Most common signs/symptoms
  - Acute epigastric & RUQ pain
  - Preeclampsia: Classic triad
    - Hypertension, proteinuria & edema
  - Eclampsia: Classic triad of preeclampsia
    - Associated with convulsions & coma
  - Clinical differential diagnoses
    - Viral hepatitis, gallstones, peptic ulcer
    - Pancreatitis, acute fatty liver
    - Hemolytic uremic syndrome
    - Idiopathic thrombocytopenic purpura (ITP)
- Other signs/symptoms
  - Malaise, nausea, vomiting, weight gain
  - Edema, headache, visual impairment, jaundice
- Clinical Profile: African-American female, primigravida with features of preeclampsia & lab data showing findings of hemolysis, elevated liver enzymes & low platelets
- Lab data
  - Hemoglobin: Less than 11 g/dL
  - Bilirubin: More than 1.2 mg/dL
  - Lactate dehydrogenase: More than 600 U/L
  - Aspartate aminotransferase: More than 70 U/L
  - Platelet count: Less than 100,000/mm³

Demographics
- Age: 2nd & 3rd decades
- Gender: Females
- Ethnicity: More frequent in African-Americans

Natural History & Prognosis
- Variant of toxemia in primigravidas
  - Usually preeclampsia & occasionally eclampsia
  - Usually 3rd trimester onset
  - Occasionally postpartum onset
  - Rarely seen in multiparous patients
- Usually seen in primigravidas with preeclampsia, occasionally seen in eclampsia patients
- Maternal risk factors
  - Nulliparity, young age, African-American females, familial
  - Underlying diseases
    - Hypertension, diabetes, renal disease
- Complications
  - Rupture of subcapsular hematoma
  - Hepatic necrosis, pulmonary edema, hypoglycemia
  - Disseminated intravascular coagulation (DIC)
  - Abruptio placenta & renal failure
  - Maternal mortality rate: 3.5% if delayed diagnosis & treatment

Treatment
- Supportive treatment for most cases
- Standard treatment: Expeditious delivery of fetus
- Surgery & selective embolization for hepatic rupture & intra-abdominal hemorrhage

DIAGNOSTIC CHECKLIST

Consider
- Rule out bleeding liver tumor, other liver pathologies

Image Interpretation Pearls
- Look for heterogeneous enhancing spherical liver tumors

SELECTED REFERENCES

1. Araujo AC et al: Characteristics and treatment of hepatic rupture caused by HELLP syndrome. Am J Obstet Gynecol. 2006
2. Nunes JO et al: Abdominal imaging features of HELLP syndrome: a 10-year retrospective review. AJR Am J Roentgenol. 185(5):1205-10, 2005
3. Di Salvo DN: Sonographic imaging of maternal complications of pregnancy. J Ultrasound Med. 22(1):69-89, 2003
4. Suarez B et al: Abdominal pain and preeclampsia: sonographic findings in the maternal liver. J Ultrasound Med. 21(10):1077-83; quiz 1085-6, 2002
5. Casillas VJ et al: Imaging of nontraumatic hemorrhagic hepatic lesions. Radiographics. 20(2):367-78, 2000
6. Haddad B et al: HELLP (hemolysis, elevated liver enzymes, and low platelet count) syndrome versus severe preeclampsia: onset at < or =28.0 weeks' gestation. Am J Obstet Gynecol. 183(6):1475-9, 2000
7. Chan AD et al: Imaging of subcapsular hepatic and renal hematomas in pregnancy complicated by preeclampsia and the HELLP syndrome. J Clin Ultrasound. 27(1):35-40, 1999
8. Risseeuw JJ et al: Liver rupture postpartum associated with preeclampsia and HELLP syndrome. J Matern Fetal Med. 8(1):32-5, 1999
9. van Pampus MG et al: Maternal and perinatal outcome after expectant management of the HELLP syndrome compared with pre-eclampsia without HELLP syndrome. Eur J Obstet Gynecol Reprod Biol. 76(1):31-6, 1998
10. Barton JR et al: Hepatic imaging in HELLP syndrome (hemolysis, elevated liver enzymes, and low platelet count). Am J Obstet Gynecol. 174(6):1820-5; discussion 1825-7, 1996
11. Sibai BM et al: Pregnancies complicated by HELLP syndrome (hemolysis, elevated liver enzymes, and low platelets): subsequent pregnancy outcome and long-term prognosis. Am J Obstet Gynecol. 172(1 Pt 1):125-9, 1995
12. Peitz U et al: Sonographic findings of liver and gallbladder in early hemolysis, elevated liver enzymes, and low platelet count syndrome. J Clin Ultrasound. 21(8):557-60, 1993
13. Reubinoff BE et al: HELLP syndrome--a syndrome of hemolysis, elevated liver enzymes and low platelet count--complicating preeclampsia-eclampsia. Int J Gynaecol Obstet. 36(2):95-102, 1991
14. Kronthal AJ et al: Hepatic infarction in preeclampsia. Radiology. 177(3):726-8, 1990

HELLP SYNDROME

IMAGE GALLERY

Typical

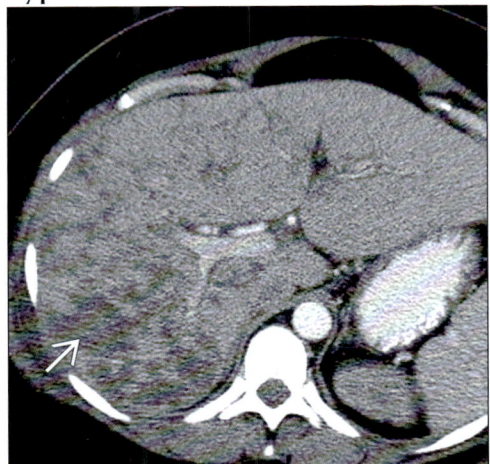
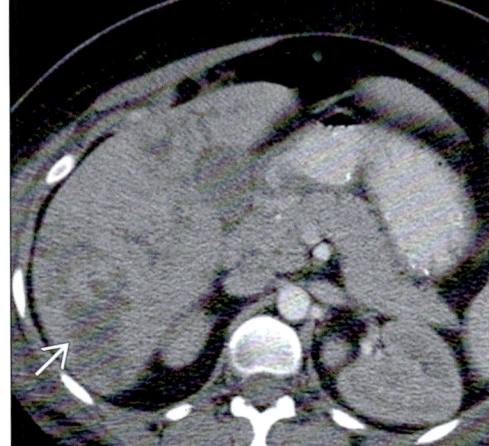

(Left) Axial CECT shows areas of low density ➡ in liver due to fatty infiltration. In HELLP syndrome, liver can undergo fatty infiltration (such as in this patient) or areas of infarction or hemorrhage. *(Right)* Axial CECT in same patient as left shows further evidence of low density in liver ➡.

Typical

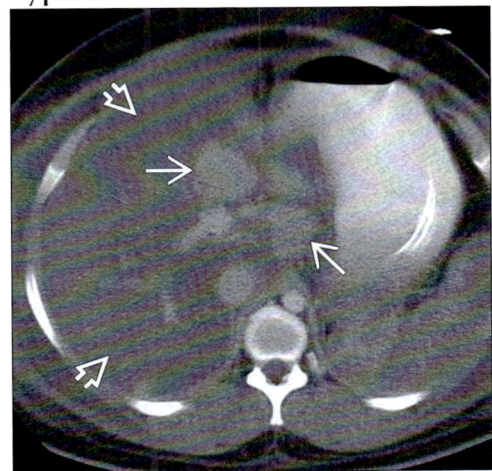
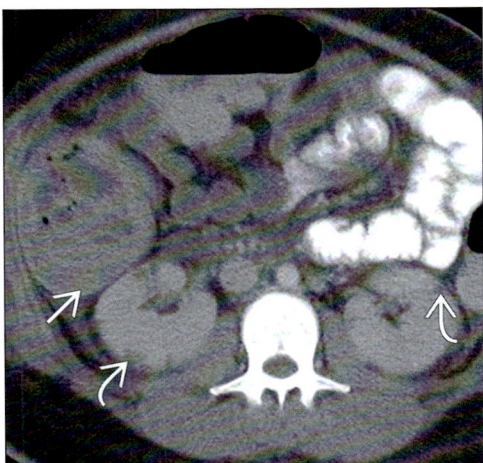

(Left) Axial CECT in patient with HELLP syndrome shows diffuse fatty infiltration of liver ➡ with areas of spared liver ➡. *(Right)* Axial CECT in same patient as left shows right colonic wall thickening due to intramural hemorrhage ➡, as well as areas of renal infarction ➡.

Typical

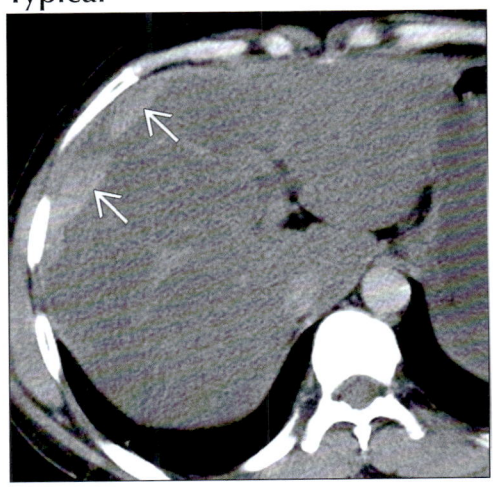
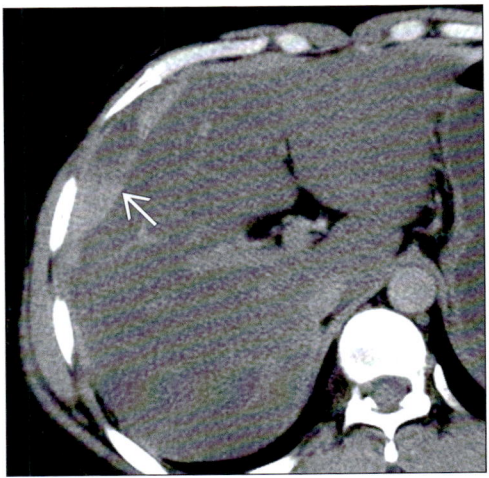

(Left) Axial NECT of subcapsular hematoma in HELLP syndrome shows high-density clot ➡ compressing liver. *(Right)* Axial NECT at more caudal level in same patient as left demonstrates hematoma ➡ confined to subcapsular space.

HEPATIC INFARCTION

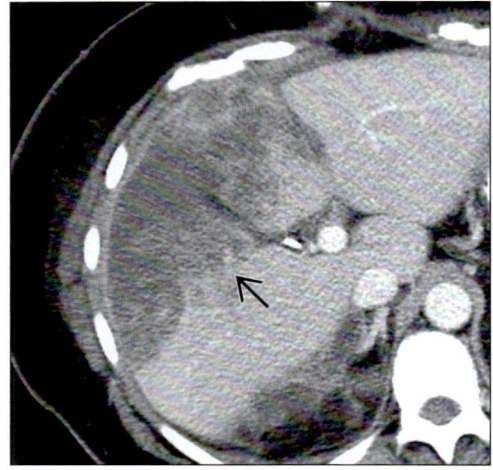

Axial CECT of hepatic infarct following liver transplantation shows large peripheral wedge-shaped area →.

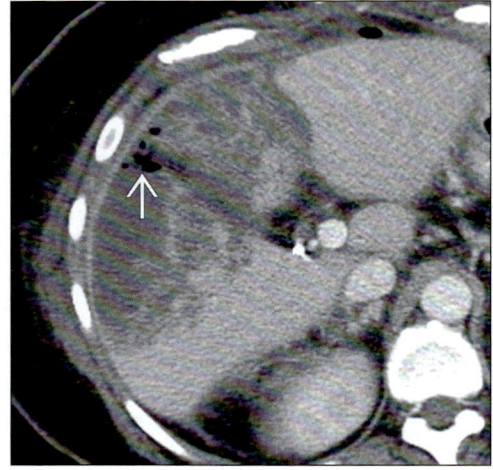

Axial CECT at more caudal level in same patient as left demonstrates gas bubbles within infarcted area →. There was no clinical evidence for infection.

TERMINOLOGY

Abbreviations and Synonyms
- Liver infarction

Definitions
- Area of coagulation necrosis 2° local ischemia resulting from obstruction of circulation, most commonly by thrombus or embolus

IMAGING FINDINGS

General Features
- Best diagnostic clue: Peripheral wedge-shaped, low-attenuation areas with absent or heterogeneous enhancement
- Location: Peripheral & wedge-shaped, but can present more central & rounded
- Size: Variable: Few mm - cm

CT Findings
- NECT
  - Wedge-shaped, rounded, ovoid or irregularly shaped low-attenuation areas paralleling bile ducts
    - Acute: Poorly demarcated low-density lesions
    - Subacute: Confluent, more distinct margins
  - ± Gas formation within sterile or infected infarcts
  - Bile lakes seen as late sequela
- CECT
  - Lesions may have geographic segmental distribution with straight margins
  - Lesions more conspicuous after enhancement (perfusion defects)
  - Heterogeneous patchy enhancement; zones of enhancement = liver parenchyma
  - Lesion remain hypodense on arterial, portal venous & delayed phases
    - Necrotic tissue, hemorrhage or fibrous tissue with no/minimum revascularization on histology
  - Lesions isoenhance with surrounding liver parenchyma on portal venous phase
    - Retained viable tissue or fibrotic tissue with revascularization

MR Findings
- T1WI

DDx: Segmental/Lobar Hypodensity or Decreased Enhancement

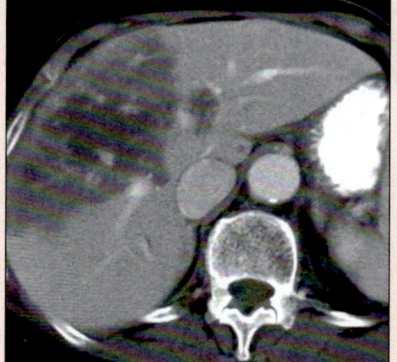

Focal Steatosis

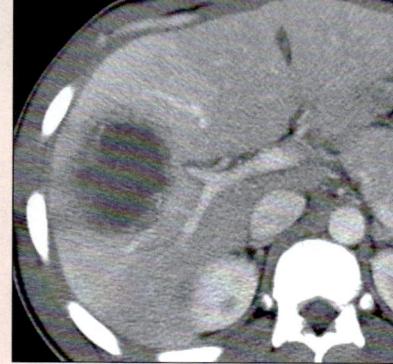

Hepatic Abscess

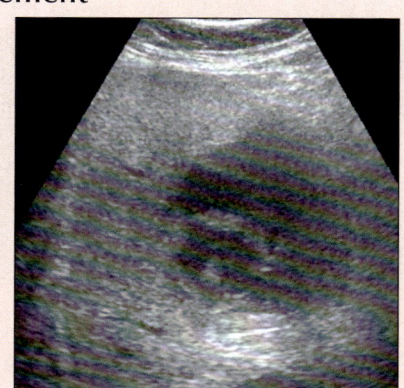

Hepatic Abscess

HEPATIC INFARCTION

Key Facts

Imaging Findings
- Best diagnostic clue: Peripheral wedge-shaped, low-attenuation areas with absent or heterogeneous enhancement
- Lesions may have geographic segmental distribution with straight margins
- Lesions more conspicuous after enhancement (perfusion defects)
- CT/MR angiography can be diagnostic
- Catheter angiography may be necessary for diagnosis and treatment

Top Differential Diagnoses
- Focal Steatosis
- Hepatic Abscess

Pathology
- Rarity of hepatic infarction due to dual blood supply from hepatic artery & portal vein, extensive collateral pathways

Clinical Issues
- Serious complication of liver transplantation; significant morbidity & mortality often requiring re-transplantation

Diagnostic Checklist
- Preservation of portal tracts helps differentiate infarction from abscess, biloma or post-biopsy hematoma
- New focal liver lesion with branching pattern in transplant patient with deteriorating function suggests infarction

---

  - Small, relatively well-defined, hypointense
  - Edema of infarction shows lower signal intensity
- T2WI
  - Heterogeneous appearance of liver parenchyma
  - Edema of infarction shows higher signal intensity
- T1 C+
  - Heterogeneous parenchymal enhancement & perfusion area defect
  - Necrotic areas predominantly hypointense compared with enhancing parenchyma in arterial, portal venous & delayed phases

Ultrasonographic Findings
- Grayscale Ultrasound
  - Native liver
    - Early: Hypoechoic lesion with indistinct margins (sufficient edema & round cell infiltration)
    - Small bile duct cysts; large bile duct lakes (necrotic tissue resorption)
  - Liver transplant
    - Geographic areas hypoechoic, preservation of portal tracts (early sign of ischemia)
    - Transient small hyperechoic lesions (progression to true infarction)
- Color Doppler
  - Hepatic artery thrombosis: Absence of normal hepatic artery signal
    - Much more common than portal vein thrombosis
  - Transplant vasculature or portal vein thrombosis
  - Porto-systemic shunting, collateral supply

Angiographic Findings
- Conventional: Confirm hepatic artery occlusion

Nuclear Medicine Findings
- Hepatobiliary scan
  - Peripheral, wedge-shaped, sharply defined lesion
  - Communication with bile lakes in post-transplantation infarcts
- Technetium sulfur colloid: Photopenic area
- Cholescintigraphy: Communication with bile lakes in post-transplantation infarcts

Imaging Recommendations
- Best imaging tool
  - Real-time B-mode & Doppler US: Evaluate allograft dysfunction, post-operative complications
  - Triphasic MDCT with CT angiography
  - CT/MR angiography can be diagnostic
- Protocol advice
  - CECT + CTA
  - Dynamic contrast-enhanced gradient-echo & contrast-enhanced T1-weighted spin-echo images with MRA
  - Catheter angiography may be necessary for diagnosis and treatment

DIFFERENTIAL DIAGNOSIS

Focal Steatosis
- May be geographic, wedge-shaped
- Preserved patent enhancing vessels within "lesion"
- Characteristic suppression of signal on opposed-phased GRE MR

Hepatic Abscess
- Usually spherical, often septated
- Central nonenhancing contents, enhancing rim

Hepatic Trauma
- Jagged low-attenuation areas of laceration
- Subcapsular hematoma compresses lateral contour

PATHOLOGY

General Features
- General path comments
  - Rarity of hepatic infarction due to dual blood supply from hepatic artery & portal vein, extensive collateral pathways
  - Portal thrombosis superimposes on hepatic arterial occlusion, resulting in chronic insufficiency & infarction

HEPATIC INFARCTION

- o Infarcted regenerative cirrhotic nodules 2° hypoperfusion of liver, followed by ischemic nodular necrosis vulnerable to hypoxia
- o Hepatic artery thrombosis in liver allograft more likely to lead to infarction (collateral supply severed during transplant)
- Etiology
  - o Iatrogenic
    - Cholecystectomy, hepatobiliary surgery, intrahepatic chemoembolization
    - Transjugular intrahepatic portosystemic shunt (TIPS) procedure
  - o Liver transplantation: Hepatic artery stenosis or thrombosis
  - o Blunt trauma: Hepatic artery, portal vein lacerations
  - o Hypercoagulable states
    - Sickle cell/antiphospholipid antibody syndrome
  - o Vasculitis: Polyarteritis, lupus, etc.
  - o Infection: Rare emphysematous hepatitis; following sepsis & shock
- Epidemiology
  - o Hepatic infarction uncommon
  - o Hepatic artery thrombosis following transplant reported in 3% of adults, 12% of children
- Diagnosed by laparotomy, autopsy or imaging

Gross Pathologic & Surgical Features
- Liver at autopsy: Atrophic, hard & irregularly surfaced
- Multiple focal necrotic areas, peripheral collapse of parenchymal tissue with fibrosis

Microscopic Features
- Central congestion & centrilobular necrosis surrounded by hemorrhagic rims
- Infarcted nodules have central core of amorphous eosinophilic material (remnants of necrotic hepatocytes)
  - o Cells with foamy cytoplasm (macrophages) surround necrotic core
  - o Ultimate replacement by fibrovascular tissue

CLINICAL ISSUES

Presentation
- Most common signs/symptoms
  - o Asymptomatic, nonspecific: RUQ or back pain, fever
  - o Massive infarction: Jaundice, ascites
- Other signs/symptoms: In pregnancy associated with hemolytic anemia with elevated liver enzymes & low platelets (HELLP), pre-eclampsia, eclampsia
- May be complication of hepatic artery angiography or embolization
- Lab data: Leukocytosis, abnormal liver function tests

Demographics
- Age: Any age group
- Gender: M = F

Natural History & Prognosis
- Parenchymal atrophy & scarring, progressive liquefaction; affects center of hepatic lobule most prominently, relative sparing of portal end
- Serious complication of liver transplantation; significant morbidity & mortality often requiring re-transplantation
- Complications
  - o Native liver: Liver failure, fibrosis
  - o Transplanted liver: Biliary strictures, bilomas, abscess
  - o Renal failure, coma

Treatment
- Revascularization, re-transplantation, spontaneous resolution

DIAGNOSTIC CHECKLIST

Consider
- Pre-TIPS evaluation of arterial supply to liver by Doppler/angiography
- Post-TIPS: If pain develops in right upper quadrant, fever, shock & disseminated intravascular coagulation
- Recognize infarction as separate entity among spectrum of pregnancy-related liver disorders to avoid delay in diagnosis & treatment
- Ischemia alone may show sonographic features of infarction; may be reversible with early diagnosis

Image Interpretation Pearls
- Preservation of portal tracts helps differentiate infarction from abscess, biloma or post-biopsy hematoma
- New focal liver lesion with branching pattern in transplant patient with deteriorating function suggests infarction

SELECTED REFERENCES
1. Giovine S et al: Retrospective study of 23 cases of hepatic infarction: CT findings and pathological correlations. Radiol Med (Torino). 111(1):11-21, 2006
2. Fujiwara H et al: Hepatic infarction following abdominal interventional procedures. Acta Med Okayama. 58(2):97-106, 2004
3. Hou SK et al: Hepatic portal venous gas: clinical significance of computed tomography findings. Am J Emerg Med. 22(3):214-8, 2004
4. Blachar A et al: Acute fulminant hepatic infection causing fatal "emphysematous hepatitis": case report. Abdom Imaging. 27(2):188-90, 2002
5. Mayan H et al: Fatal liver infarction after transjugular intrahepatic portosystemic shunt procedure. Liver. 21(5):361-4, 2001
6. Quiroga S et al: Complications of orthotopic liver transplantation: spectrum of findings with helical CT. Radiographics. 21(5):1085-102, 2001
7. Kim T et al: Infarcted regenerative nodules in cirrhosis: CT and MR imaging findings with pathologic correlation. AJR Am J Roentgenol. 175(4):1121-5, 2000
8. Wallace S et al: Hepatic chemoembolization: clinical and experimental correlation. Acta Gastroenterol Belg. 63(2):169-73, 2000
9. Smith GS et al: Hepatic infarction secondary to arterial insufficiency in native livers: CT findings in 10 patients. Radiology. 208(1):223-9, 1998
10. Holbert BL et al: Hepatic infarction caused by arterial insufficiency: spectrum and evolution of CT findings. AJR Am J Roentgenol. 166(4):815-20, 1996

HEPATIC INFARCTION

IMAGE GALLERY

Typical

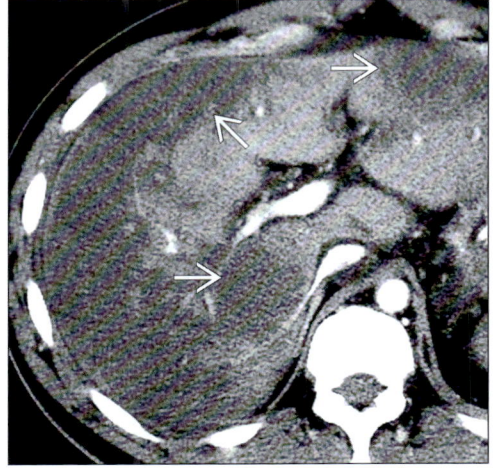
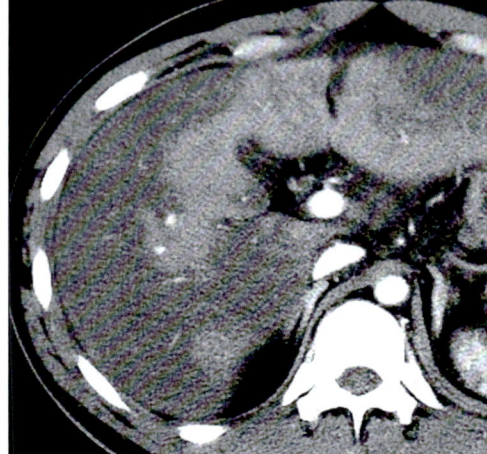

(Left) Axial CECT of extensive hepatic infarct following cardiac arrest shows large geographic areas of low attenuation in periphery of liver ➡. *(Right)* Axial CECT at lower level in same patient as left demonstrates absence of enhancing vessels within infarcted areas.

Typical

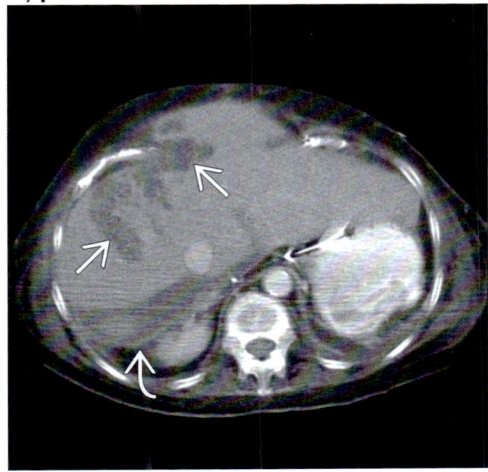
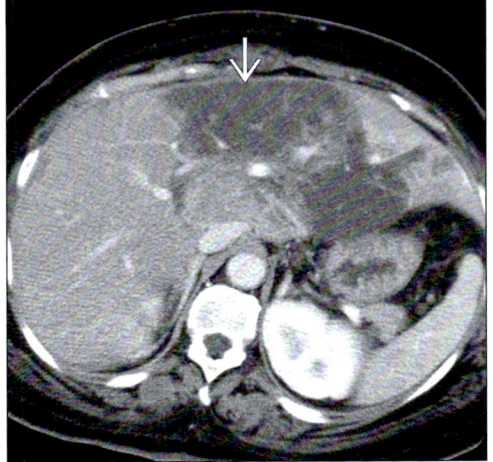

(Left) Axial CECT illustrates hepatic infarction. Note geographic & peripheral areas of decreased enhancement ➡, as well as perihepatic hematoma ➡, a common post-transplantation finding. *(Right)* Axial CECT shows hepatic infarction due to surgical disruption of hepatic arterial flow. Note wedge-shaped hypoattenuation of left lobe of liver with linear, geographic distribution ➡.

Variant

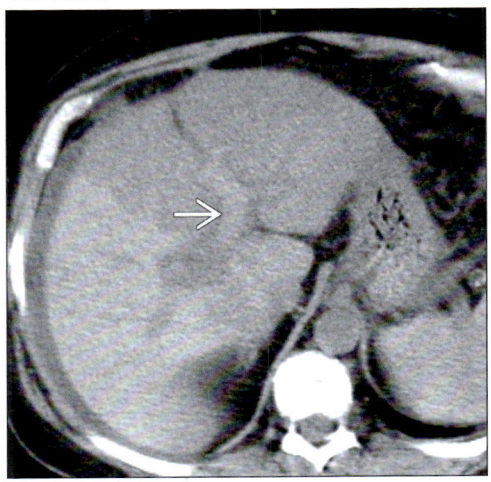
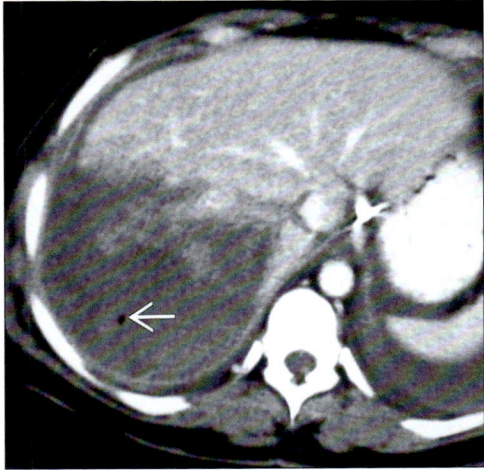

(Left) Axial NECT shows extensive portal vein thrombosis & liver infarction. Hyperdense thrombus ➡ within left portal vein is denser than flowing blood in other vessels. *(Right)* Axial CECT shows hepatic infarction. Note lack of perfusion of right lobe, with straight line of demarcation from normally perfused left lobe. Gas bubble ➡ within infarcted lobe is 2° release of gas by infarcted tissue, rather than infection.

PORTAL VEIN OCCLUSION

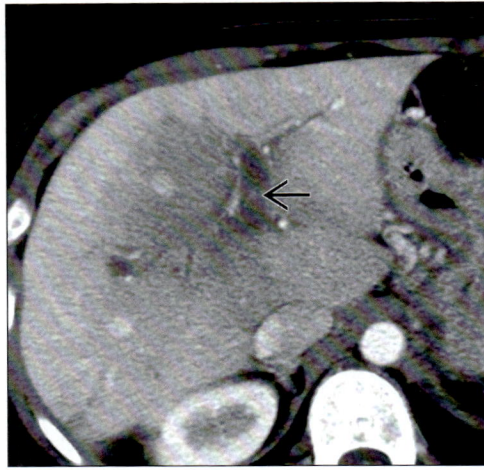

Axial CECT shows acute PV thrombosis secondary to pancreatitis. Note low attenuation thrombus in left portal vein ➞.

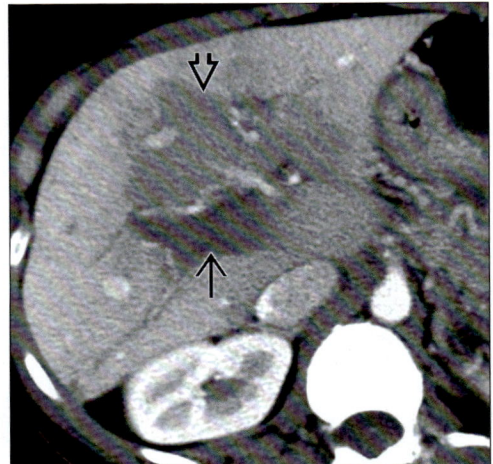

Axial CECT in lower plane of section in same patient as previous image reveals acute clot distending right portal vein ➞. Note regional flow disturbance, diminished hepatic central flow ➞.

TERMINOLOGY

Definitions
- Acute, chronic or neoplastic occlusion of the portal vein (PV) due to thrombosis or tumor invasion
- Chronic portal venous occlusion with numerous periportal collaterals, referred to as "cavernous transformation"

IMAGING FINDINGS

General Features
- Best diagnostic clue
  - Low attenuation thrombus in PV on CECT
  - Absence of blood flow or flow void in PV on MR and power Doppler
  - Non-visualization of PV (chronic occlusion) on MR and power Doppler
  - Cavernous transformation of PV (collateralization in porta hepatis) on MR and power Doppler
- Location: May involve any portion of intra- or extrahepatic PV
- Morphology: Acute thrombosis results in distension of PV

CT Findings
- CECT of acute thrombosis
  - Arterial phase (25-40 seconds post bolus injection)
    - High attenuation within involved lobe or segment due to arterio-portal shunting
  - Venous phase (60-70 seconds post bolus injection)
    - Equilibration of contrast-enhancement
    - Visualization of low density thrombus
    - Enhancement of PV walls from vasa vasorum, i.e., "rim sign"
  - Non-occlusive thrombosis: Low density thrombus partially filling patent PV
  - Occlusive thrombosis: Low density thrombus filling dilated PV
    - Extent variable: May include major intrahepatic branches, splenic vein, superior mesenteric vein (SMV)
    - Congested (non-occluded) mesenteric veins distal to thrombus, mesenteric edema, bowel wall thickening from venous congestion

DDx: Lesions Mimicking Portal Vein Thrombosis

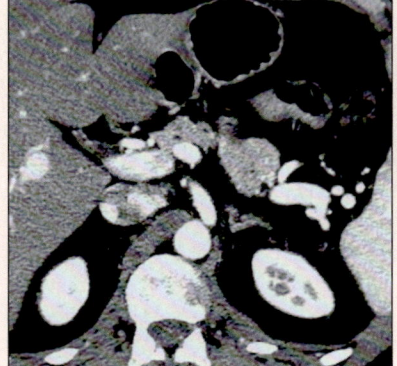

Streaming Artifact

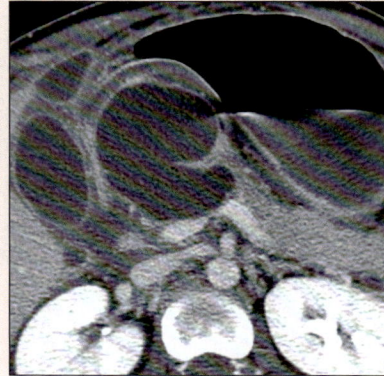

Extrinsic Compression

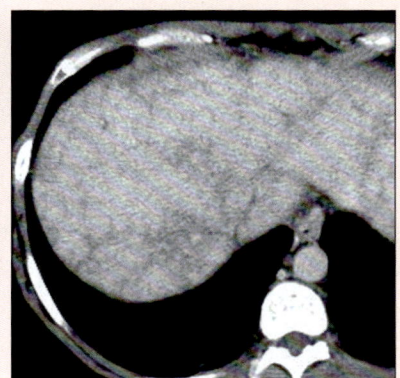

Budd-Chiari Syndrome

PORTAL VEIN OCCLUSION

Key Facts

Terminology
- Acute, chronic or neoplastic occlusion of the portal vein (PV) due to thrombosis or tumor invasion

Imaging Findings
- Low attenuation thrombus in PV on CECT
- Absence of blood flow or flow void in PV on MR and power Doppler
- Non-visualization of PV (chronic occlusion) on MR and power Doppler
- Cavernous transformation of PV (collateralization in porta hepatis) on MR and power Doppler

Top Differential Diagnoses
- Streaming Artifact
- Extrinsic Compression
- Budd-Chiari Syndrome

Pathology
- PV occlusion is uncommon
- Most often associated with hepatic cirrhosis and pancreatitis

Clinical Issues
- Liver dysfunction
- Abdominal pain (from bowel congestion, ileus, rare venous infarction)
- Clinical Profile: Presentation varies from acute symptoms to clinically unrecognized

Diagnostic Checklist
- Neoplastic invasion of PV if thrombus enhances
- Distension of PV more likely with acute clot

- Ileus, ascites and splenomegaly are all possible associated findings
- CECT of chronic PV thrombosis
    - Chronic occlusion (cavernous transformation) of PV
        - Numerous periportal collaterals along the usual course of PV
        - Peripancreatic, GB and/or splenic varices may be identified
    - Non-visualization of PV and/or splenic vein
        - Thrombosed vein becomes fibrotic "cord" not visible on imaging studies
    - Well-developed portosystemic collaterals, as in portal hypertension
    - Associated findings
        - Splenomegaly
        - Atrophy/nodular regeneration of ischemic liver segments
        - Increased hepatic artery size and/or flow
- CECT of PV tumor invasion
    - Similar to acute thrombosis
    - Variable degree of contrast enhancement of intraluminal tumor thrombus
        - Often linear enhancement "threads and streaks" sign: Best seen on arterial phase of biphasic MDCT
        - Primary tumor usually visible in hepatic parenchyma or pancreas, often in direct contiguity with thrombus
        - Commonly seen in hepatocellular carcinoma
        - Less common in pancreatic carcinoma, cholangiocarcinoma, islet cell tumor of pancreas, metastases

MR Findings
- T1WI: High signal filling defect
- T2WI: High signal acute clot
- T2* GRE: PV tumor enhances avidly, especially on GRE sequences
- T1 C+ FS
    - Liver parenchyma supplied by thrombosed veins may enhance avidly in arterial phase, due to increased hepatic artery flow
    - Subacute thrombus hyperintense on T1 and T2 due to methemoglobin
    - Acute thrombus: Low signal flow void in PV
    - Analogous to CT findings
- MRA: Contrast-enhanced MRA more accurate than time of flight and phase contrast

Ultrasonographic Findings
- Grayscale Ultrasound
    - Acute
        - Echogenic or anechoic clot
    - Subacute
        - Isoechoic clot
- Color Doppler
    - Tumor vessels usually visible within tumor thrombus
    - Partial thrombosis
        - Filling defect
    - Cavernous transformation
        - Numerous venous collaterals in porta hepatis
    - Neoplastic invasion of portal vein
        - Pulsatile arterial waveforms with reversed flow

Angiographic Findings
- Conventional
    - Venous phase of selective superior mesenteric artery (SMA) injection
        - Periportal collaterals in chronic occlusion (cavernous transformation)
        - Filling defect (clot) in partial occlusion

Imaging Recommendations
- Best imaging tool
    - US initially: Highly accurate and cost effective
    - Contrast CT for comprehensive evaluation/search for cause (MR as alternative for CT)

DIFFERENTIAL DIAGNOSIS

Streaming Artifact
- Low attenuation "pseudothrombus" 2° uneven mixing of blood during PV inflow
- PV fills during later scans (equilibrium)

PORTAL VEIN OCCLUSION

Extrinsic Compression
- Mass effect on PV from porta hepatis nodes
- Primary tumor, pseudocyst, hematoma most common

Budd-Chiari Syndrome
- Acute or chronic thrombus of hepatic veins and/or intrahepatic IVC
- Acute abdominal pain, tender hepatomegaly and ascites
- Idiopathic is most common cause, also hypercoagulable states and neoplasms
- Severe centrilobular congestion
- CECT
  - Hypertrophied hyperdense caudate lobe 2° separate venous drainage into IVC
  - Peripheral decreased attenuation
  - Clots in hepatic veins

PATHOLOGY

General Features
- General path comments
  - PV occlusion is uncommon
    - Most often associated with hepatic cirrhosis and pancreatitis
  - Anatomy
    - Venous flow from bowel/spleen normally traverses PV
    - PV occlusion = extensive portosystemic collateral network
    - Increased size and flow of hepatic artery due to decreased PV flow
- Etiology
  - Thrombosis
    - Stasis from cirrhosis-related sinusoidal obstruction
    - Acute pancreatitis
    - Seeding of PV by infected material (acute appendicitis, intraperitoneal abscess, inflammatory bowel disease)
    - Hypercoagulable states (primary or tumor-related)
  - Tumor invasion
    - Hepatocellular carcinoma (HCC) most common
    - Pancreatic carcinoma
    - Liver metastases

CLINICAL ISSUES

Presentation
- Most common signs/symptoms
  - Liver dysfunction
  - Abdominal pain (from bowel congestion, ileus, rare venous infarction)
- Other signs/symptoms
  - Possible ascites
  - Incidental finding on imaging study: Common in advanced cirrhosis
    - Also seen in healthy, non-cirrhotic individual with unrecognized, previous PV thrombosis (e.g., acute pancreatitis, now resolved)
- Clinical Profile: Presentation varies from acute symptoms to clinically unrecognized

Demographics
- Age: May occur at any age
- Gender: M = F

Natural History & Prognosis
- Non-occlusive PV thrombosis may lyse with no residual or minor PV scarring
- Occlusive PV thrombosis = permanent PV occlusion
  - Portal hypertension morbidity (gastrointestinal hemorrhage) from splenic varices
  - Reduced hepatic blood flow, possible tissue death, regeneration
- PV tumor invasion associated with poor clinical outcome

Treatment
- Supportive therapy only
- Anticoagulation for acute thrombosis (if liver function permits)

DIAGNOSTIC CHECKLIST

Consider
- Neoplastic invasion of PV if thrombus enhances

Image Interpretation Pearls
- Distension of PV more likely with acute clot

SELECTED REFERENCES

1. Gonzalez F et al: Extensive portal vein thrombosis related to abdominal trauma. Gastroenterol Clin Biol. 30(2):314-6, 2006
2. Hidajat N et al: Imaging and radiological interventions of portal vein thrombosis. Acta Radiol. 46(4):336-43, 2005
3. Okada T et al: Postoperative portal and splenic vein thrombosis in children: identification of risk factors. Pediatr Surg Int. 21(11):918-21, 2005
4. Wang JT et al: Portal vein thrombosis. Hepatobiliary Pancreat Dis Int. 4(4):515-8, 2005
5. Bradbury MS et al: Noninvasive assessment of portomesenteric venous thrombosis: current concepts and imaging strategies. J Comput Assist Tomogr. 26(3):392-404, 2002
6. Gallego C et al: Congenital and acquired anomalies of the portal venous system. Radiographics. 22(1):141-59, 2002
7. Kreft B et al: Detection of thrombosis in the portal venous system: comparison of contrast-enhanced MRA with intraarterial DSA. Radiology. 216:86-92, 2000
8. Sheen CL et al: Clinical features, diagnosis and outcome of acute portal vein thrombosis. QJM. 93(8):531-4, 2000
9. Bach AM et al: Portal vein evaluation with US: comparison to angiography combined with CT arterial portography. Radiology. 201(1):149-154, 1996

PORTAL VEIN OCCLUSION

IMAGE GALLERY

Typical

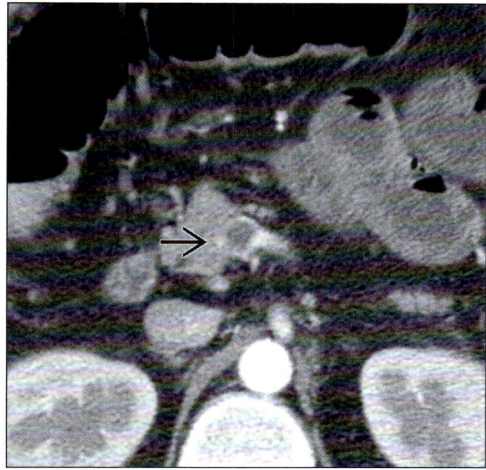 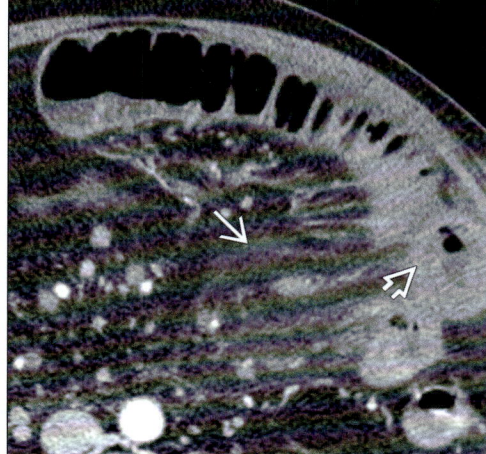

(Left) Axial CECT shows acute PV occlusion. Note low attenuation thrombus ➡ at confluence of PV and SMV. *(Right)* Axial CECT at more caudal level in same patient as left demonstrates mesenteric edema ➡ and focal thickening of small bowel loops ➡.

Typical

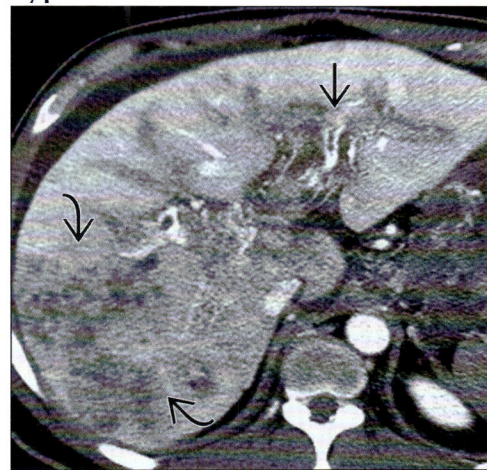 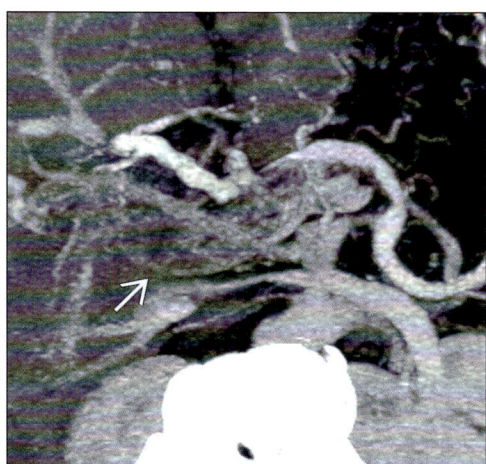

(Left) Tumor invasion of PV by HCC on CECT. Note linear enhancement of neovascularity from tumor thrombus in left PV ➡ and multiple low attenuation areas within liver 2° multifocal HCC ➡. *(Right)* Thin slab MIP in same patient as previous image demonstrates extension of tumor thrombus into extrahepatic portal vein ➡.

Variant

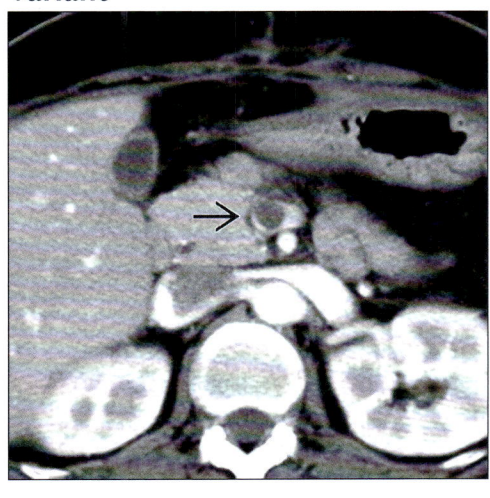 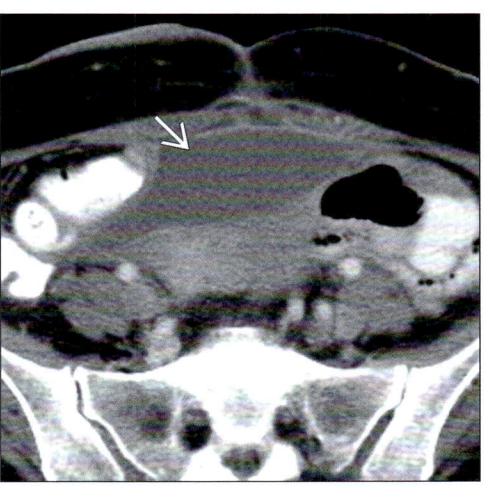

(Left) Axial CECT shows septic thrombosis of PV. Note low attenuation thrombus at spleno-portal confluence ➡. *(Right)* Axial CECT shows postoperative pelvic abscess ➡ at lower level (in same patient as previous image).

BUDD-CHIARI SYNDROME

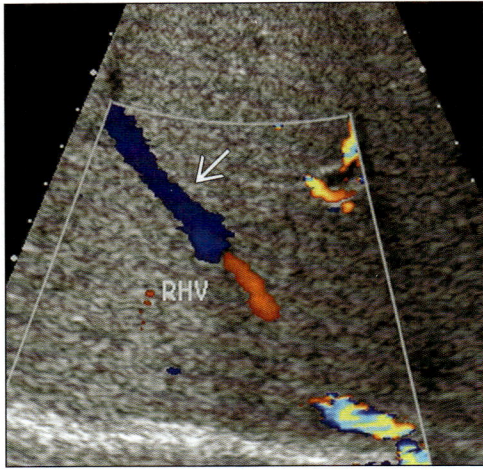

Transverse color Doppler ultrasound of acute Budd-Chiari syndrome. Note reversal of flow in right hepatic vein ➡.

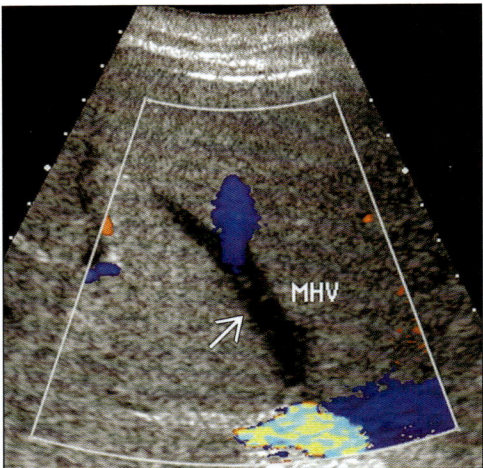

Transverse color Doppler ultrasound of middle hepatic vein (in same patient as previous image) demonstrates acute thrombosis with absence of flow ➡.

TERMINOLOGY

Abbreviations and Synonyms
- Hepatic venous outflow obstruction

Definitions
- Global or segmental hepatic venous outflow obstruction (at level of large hepatic veins or suprahepatic segment of IVC)

IMAGING FINDINGS

General Features
- Best diagnostic clue: "Bicolored" hepatic veins (due to intrahepatic collateral pathways) on color Doppler US
- Location: Hepatic veins, IVC or centrilobar veins
- Key concepts
  ○ Characteristic finding: Nodular regenerative hyperplasia in dysmorphic liver

CT Findings
- NECT
  ○ Acute phase
    ▪ Diffusely hypodense enlarged liver
    ▪ Narrowed IVC + hepatic veins & ascites
    ▪ Hyperdense IVC & hepatic veins (due to ↑ attenuation of thrombus)
  ○ Chronic phase
    ▪ Diffusely hypodense liver
    ▪ Non-visualization of IVC & hepatic veins
    ▪ Hypertrophy of caudate lobe
    ▪ Atrophy of peripheral segments
    ▪ Ratio of caudate width to right lobe: ≥ 0.55:1
- CECT
  ○ Acute phase
    ▪ Classic "flip-flop" pattern is seen
    ▪ Early enhancement of caudate lobe & central portion around IVC, ↓ peripheral liver enhancement
    ▪ Later decreased enhancement centrally with increased enhancement peripherally
    ▪ Narrowed hypodense hepatic veins & IVC with hyperdense walls
  ○ Chronic phase
    ▪ Total obliteration of IVC & hepatic veins
    ▪ "Large regenerative nodules": Nodular regenerative hyperplasia

DDx: Dysmorphic Liver with Lobular Contour

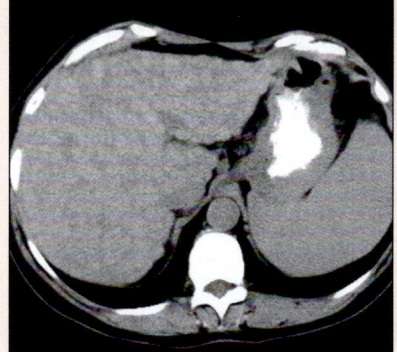

Hepatic Cirrhosis

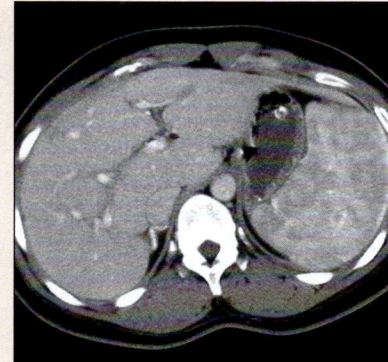

Primary Sclerosing Cholangitis

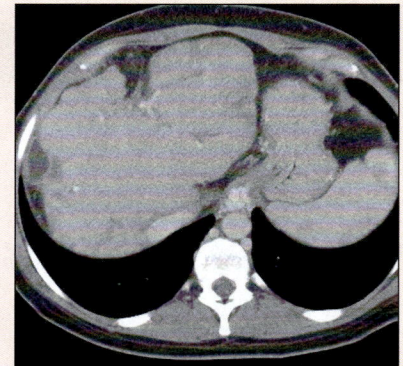

Primary Sclerosing Cholangitis

BUDD-CHIARI SYNDROME

Key Facts

Terminology
- Hepatic venous outflow obstruction
- Global or segmental hepatic venous outflow obstruction (at level of large hepatic veins or suprahepatic segment of IVC)

Imaging Findings
- Best diagnostic clue: "Bicolored" hepatic veins (due to intrahepatic collateral pathways) on color Doppler US
- Non-visualization of IVC & hepatic veins
- "Spider web" pattern of hepatic venous collaterals

Top Differential Diagnoses
- Hepatic Cirrhosis
- Primary Sclerosing Cholangitis (PSC)

Pathology
- Primary: Venous outflow membranous obstruction
- Secondary: Thrombotic, rarely nonthrombotic
- Type I: Occlusion of IVC ± hepatic veins
- Type II: Occlusion of major hepatic veins ± IVC
- Type III: Occlusion of small centrilobar veins ("veno-occlusive disease")

Diagnostic Checklist
- Rule out cirrhosis & primary sclerosing cholangitis
- Absent, reversed or flat flow in hepatic veins, reversed flow in IVC on color Doppler US
- Characteristic large benign regenerative nodules
- Check for hypercoagulable conditions, prior chemotherapy or bone marrow transplant

---

- Enhancing 1-4 cm hyperdense nodules ± hypodense ring
- CTA: Hepatic venous outflow obstruction

MR Findings
- T1WI
  - Increased intensity of liver centrally with peripheral heterogeneity
  - Narrowed or absent hepatic veins & IVC
  - Hyperintense nodules & enlarged caudate lobe
- T2WI
  - Non-visualized hepatic veins & IVC
  - Isointense or hypointense regenerative nodules
- T2* GRE: No demonstrable flow in hepatic veins or IVC
- T1 C+
  - Tumor thrombus (rare cause) may show contrast enhancement
  - Acute phase
    - Involved parenchyma enhances less than surrounding liver
  - Congested liver with ↑ water content
    - Peripheral liver enhances less than central liver 2° ↑ parenchymal pressure & decreased blood supply
  - Chronic phase
    - Enhancement is more variable, may be increased
    - Nodules: Intense homogeneous enhancement
- MRA: Depicts thrombus & level of venous obstruction

Ultrasonographic Findings
- Grayscale Ultrasound: Hepatic veins narrowed, non-visualized, or filled with thrombus, hypertrophied caudate vein
- Color Doppler
  - Hepatic veins & IVC
    - Absent or flat flow in hepatic veins
    - Reversed flow in hepatic veins or IVC
    - "Bicolored" hepatic veins due to intrahepatic collateral pathways
    - Sensitivity: 87.5%
  - Portal vein
    - Slow hepatofugal flow: < 11 cm/sec
    - Congestion index: > 0.1
  - Hepatic artery: Resistive index ≥ 0.75

Angiographic Findings
- Inferior venacavography or hepatic venacavography
  - "Spider web" pattern of hepatic venous collaterals
  - Thrombus in hepatic veins or IVC
  - Long segmental compression of IVC
    - Acute phase: Due to diffuse hepatomegaly
    - Chronic phase: Hypertrophy of caudate lobe
  - Hepatic arteries
    - Acute phase: Narrowing, stretching, bowing
    - Chronic phase: Dilated & arterioportal shunts

Imaging Recommendations
- Best imaging tool: Color Doppler sonography or angiography

DIFFERENTIAL DIAGNOSIS

Hepatic Cirrhosis
- Hypertrophy: Caudate & lateral segment of left lobe
- Atrophy: Right lobe & medial segment of left lobe
- Varices, ascites, splenomegaly
- Patent hepatic veins & IVC
- Regenerative nodules
  - Usually small in size compared to Budd-Chiari
  - Cirrhotic nodules often have increased iron
    - Usually hypovascular, decreased signal on T2WI

Primary Sclerosing Cholangitis (PSC)
- Chronic cholestatic disease of unknown cause
- 70% of cases associated with ulcerative colitis
- Bile ducts on cholangiography: Segmental strictures, beading, pruning, nodular thickening, skip dilatations
- Atrophy/hypertrophy of lobes, ± cirrhotic changes

PATHOLOGY

General Features
- General path comments
  - Embryology/anatomy

BUDD-CHIARI SYNDROME

- Primary type: Total or incomplete membranous obstruction of hepatic venous outflow
  - Deviations of complex embryologic process of IVC
- Etiology
  - Primary: Venous outflow membranous obstruction
    - Controversial etiology
    - Congenital, injury or infection
  - Secondary: Thrombotic, rarely nonthrombotic
    - Obstruction of central & sublobular veins: Chemotherapy & radiation
    - Obstruction of major hepatic veins: Hypercoagulable states (oral contraceptives, polycythemia, protein C deficiency)
    - Obstruction of small centrilobular veins (veno-occlusive disease): Bone marrow transplantation, antineoplastic drugs
    - Nonthrombotic: Hepatic & extrahepatic masses
- Epidemiology
  - Primary (congenital-membranous): Common in Japan, India, Israel, South Africa
  - Secondary (thrombotic): Most common in Western countries, usually due to hypercoagulable state
  - Secondary (nonthrombotic): 2nd most common in Western countries

Gross Pathologic & Surgical Features
- Acute phase
  - Liver enlarged, congested, occlusion of hepatic veins & IVC
- Chronic phase
  - Shrunken, nodular liver, may be cirrhotic, hypertrophied caudate lobe, atrophy of other lobes

Microscopic Features
- Centrilobular congestion, dilated sinusoids
- Fibrosis, necrosis & cell atrophy

Staging, Grading or Classification Criteria
- Three classifications, based on location
  - Type I: Occlusion of IVC ± hepatic veins
  - Type II: Occlusion of major hepatic veins ± IVC
  - Type III: Occlusion of small centrilobar veins ("veno-occlusive disease")

CLINICAL ISSUES

Presentation
- Most common signs/symptoms
  - Acute phase: Rapid onset RUQ pain, tender liver, hypotension
  - Chronic phase: RUQ pain, hepatomegaly, splenomegaly, jaundice, ascites, varices
- Lab data
  - Acute
    - Liver function tests: Mild to markedly increased
    - Clotting factors: Decreased
  - Chronic
    - Transaminases: Normal or moderately increased
    - Albumin & clotting factors: Decreased

Demographics
- Age: Any age group
- Gender: F > M

Natural History & Prognosis
- Complications
  - Acute: Liver failure, emboli from IVC thrombus
  - Chronic: Variceal bleeding (cirrhosis), portal HTN
  - Membranous obstruction of IVC
    - Complicated by hepatocellular carcinoma in 20-40% cases in Japan & South Africa
- Prognosis
  - Based on rate/degree of hepatic outflow obstruction
    - Mild-moderate obstruction: Good
    - Severe obstruction: Poor
  - Acute early phase (good), acute late phase (poor)
  - Chronic phase: Poor (with or without treatment)
  - Veno-occlusive disease: Varies from mild with complete recovery to fulminant failure and death

Treatment
- Medical management: Steroids, nutritional therapy, anticoagulants
- Balloon angioplasty, lasers, stent insertion for membranous occlusion of IVC & hepatic veins
- TIPS (transjugular intrahepatic portosystemic shunt)
- Surgical alternatives: Membranotomy, membranectomy, cavoplasty, liver transplantation

DIAGNOSTIC CHECKLIST

Consider
- Rule out cirrhosis & primary sclerosing cholangitis

Image Interpretation Pearls
- Absent, reversed or flat flow in hepatic veins, reversed flow in IVC on color Doppler US
- Characteristic large benign regenerative nodules
- Check for hypercoagulable conditions, prior chemotherapy or bone marrow transplant

SELECTED REFERENCES

1. Chaubal N et al: Sonography in Budd-Chiari syndrome. J Ultrasound Med. 25(3):373-9, 2006
2. Lee BB et al: Primary Budd-Chiari syndrome: outcome of endovascular management for suprahepatic venous obstruction. J Vasc Surg. 43(1):101-8, 2006
3. Brancatelli G et al: Benign regenerative nodules in Budd-Chiari syndrome and other vascular disorders of the liver: radiologic-pathologic and clinical correlation. RadioGraphics. 22:847-62, 2002
4. Vilgrain V et al: Hepatic nodules in Budd-Chiari syndrome: imaging features. Radiology. 210:443-50, 1999
5. Kane R et al: Diagnosis of Budd-Chiari syndrome: comparison between sonography and MR angiography. Radiology. 195(1):117-21, 1995
6. Millener P et al: Color Doppler imaging findings in patients with Budd-Chiari syndrome: correlation with venographic findings. AJR Am J Roentgenol. 161(2):307-12, 1993

BUDD-CHIARI SYNDROME

IMAGE GALLERY

Typical

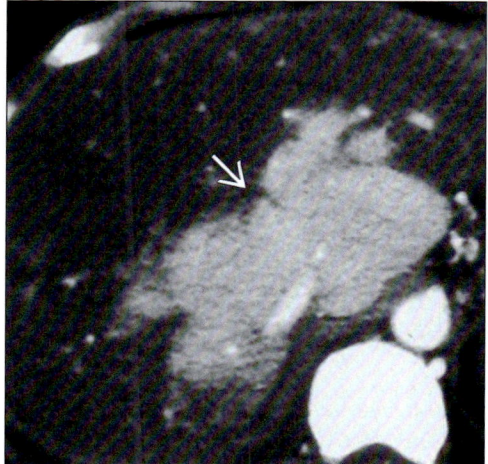
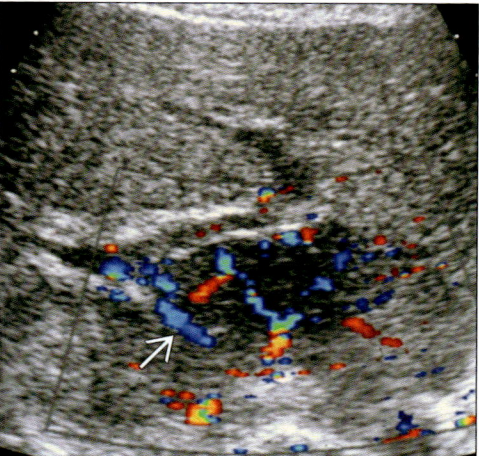

(Left) Axial CECT of Budd-Chiari syndrome shows marked enhancement of hypertrophied caudate lobe with diminished peripheral flow ➔. *(Right)* Color Doppler ultrasound (in same patient as previous image) reveals prominent caudate lobe collaterals ➔.

Typical

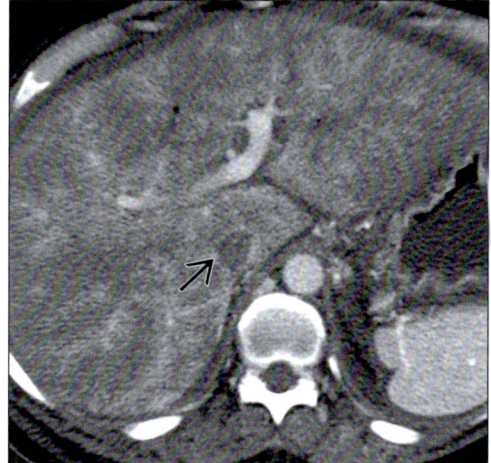
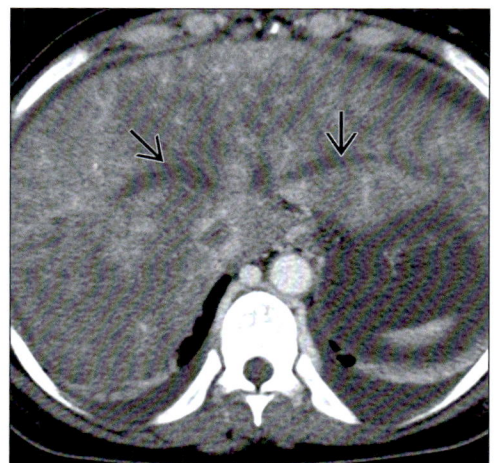

(Left) Axial CECT shows acute Budd-Chiari due to polycythemia vera. Note thrombosis of IVC ➔ and mottled enhancement of liver. *(Right)* Axial CECT (in same patient as previous image). Note the level of confluence of the hepatic veins demonstrating low density thrombus in right and left hepatic veins ➔.

Variant

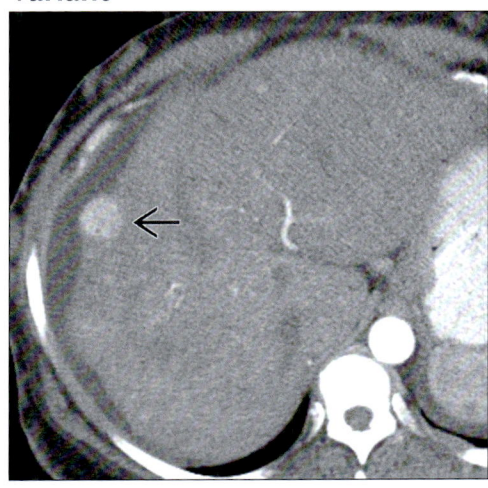
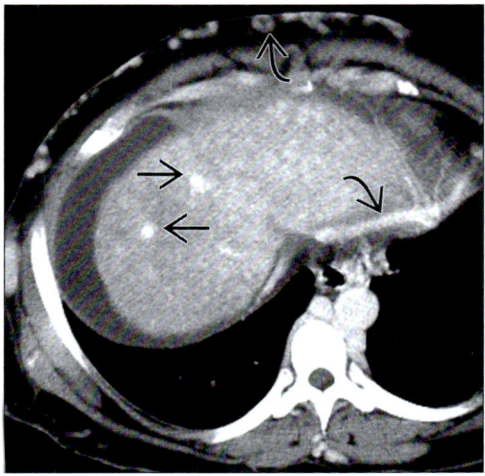

(Left) Axial CECT shows large hypervascular mass (regenerative nodule) ➔ within heterogeneously enhancing dysmorphic liver. *(Right)* Axial CECT on portal venous phase shows multiple hyperdense regenerative nodules ➔ with extensive subcutaneous and intrahepatic collaterals ➔.

ASCENDING CHOLANGITIS

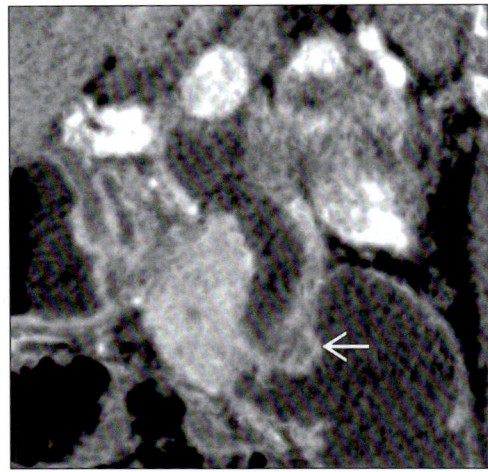

Coronal CECT minimum-intensity image of ascending cholangitis related to obstructing common duct stone. Note dilatation of common duct from an impacted stone ➔.

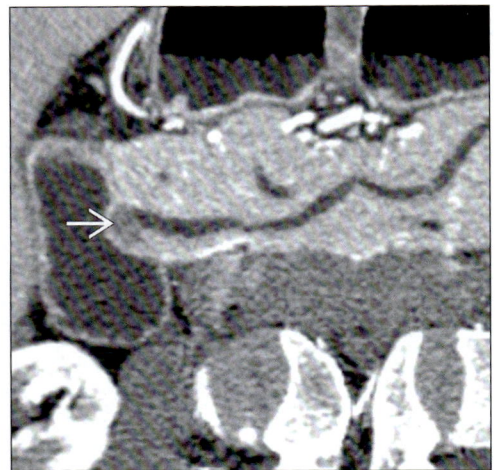

CECT curved planar reformation of pancreatic duct in same patient as left reveals impacted ampullary stone ➔ causing mild dilatation of pancreatic duct.

TERMINOLOGY

Abbreviations and Synonyms
- Bacterial cholangitis

Definitions
- Inflammation of intra-/extrahepatic bile duct walls due to ductal obstruction and infection

IMAGING FINDINGS

General Features
- Best diagnostic clue: Irregular contour, branching pattern, bile duct dilatation

CT Findings
- Dilatation of intra-/extrahepatic bile ducts
- High density intraductal material (purulent bile)
- Calcific/soft-tissue/water-density obstructing stone
- "Bull's eye" sign: Rim of bile surrounding stone
- Communicating small hepatic abscesses possible

MR Findings
- T1WI
  - Dilatation, stricture, thickening of bile duct walls
  - Hypointense stones and bile
- T2WI: Hypointense stones, hyperintense bile
- MRCP
  - Irregular strictures, proximal bile duct dilatation
  - Low-signal filling defects (stones) within ↑ signal (bile)

Fluoroscopic Findings
- Cholangiography
  - Irregular thick bile duct lumen/wall
  - Ductal stricture, obstruction & proximal dilatation
  - Radiolucent filling defect (stone)
  - Intrahepatic bile duct may show communicating hepatic abscesses

Ultrasonographic Findings
- Grayscale Ultrasound
  - Dilatation, stenosis & thickening of bile duct walls
  - Intraluminal echogenic material (purulent bile)
  - Thickened gallbladder wall with or without calculi

Imaging Recommendations
- Best imaging tool: US, MRCP, cholangiography

DDx: Irregularly Dilated Bile Ducts

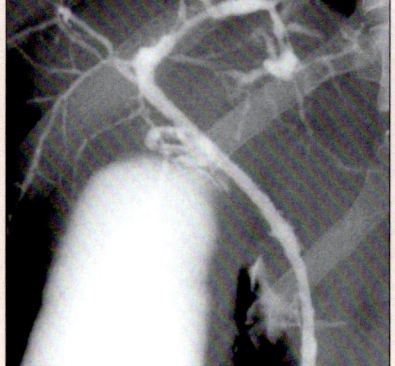

Sclerosing Cholangitis

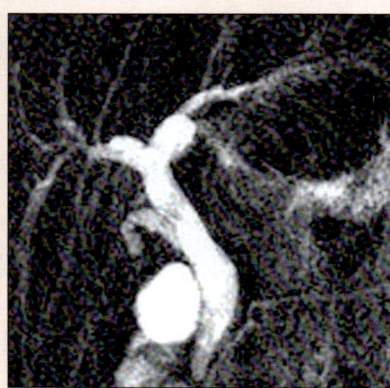

AIDS Cholangitis

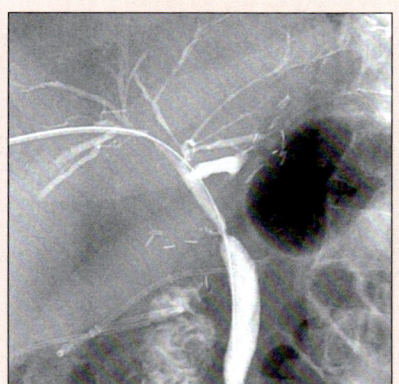

Chemotherapy Cholangitis

ASCENDING CHOLANGITIS

Key Facts

Terminology
- Bacterial cholangitis

Imaging Findings
- Best diagnostic clue: Irregular contour, branching pattern, bile duct dilatation
- High density intraductal material (purulent bile)
- "Bull's eye" sign: Rim of bile surrounding stone
- Communicating small hepatic abscesses possible

Top Differential Diagnoses
- Primary Sclerosing Cholangitis (PSC)
- Recurrent Pyogenic (RPC), AIDS, Chemotherapy Cholangitis

Diagnostic Checklist
- Correlate with clinical & lab data for accurate cholangiographic interpretation
- Cholangiography: Strictures, dilatations, intraluminal filling defects

DIFFERENTIAL DIAGNOSIS

Primary Sclerosing Cholangitis (PSC)
- Segmental strictures, beaded and pruned ducts
- Involves intra- & extrahepatic ducts
- End-stage: Lobular liver, hypertrophy & atrophy

Recurrent Pyogenic (RPC), AIDS, Chemotherapy Cholangitis
- Clinical setting supports diagnosis

PATHOLOGY

General Features
- Etiology
  - Bile duct calculi, stricture & papillary stenosis
  - Pathogenesis: Stone/obstruction/bile stasis/infection
- Epidemiology
  - Most common cholangitis in Western countries
  - Usually due to poor nutrition & parasitic infestation in developing countries

CLINICAL ISSUES

Presentation
- Most common signs/symptoms: Charcot triad: Pain, fever, jaundice
- Lab data: ↑ WBC count, ↑ bilirubin, ↑ alkaline phosphatase; positive blood cultures (toxic phase)

Demographics
- Age: 20-50 years
- Gender: M = F

Natural History & Prognosis
- Complications: Liver abscesses, sepsis
- Prognosis: 100% mortality if not decompressed

Treatment
- Antibiotics to treat gram-negative organisms
- Interventional management of stones/strictures

DIAGNOSTIC CHECKLIST

Consider
- Correlate with clinical & lab data for accurate cholangiographic interpretation

Image Interpretation Pearls
- Cholangiography: Strictures, dilatations, intraluminal filling defects

SELECTED REFERENCES

1. Arai K et al: Dynamic CT of acute cholangitis: early inhomogeneous enhancement of the liver. AJR Am J Roentgenol. 181(1):115-8, 2003
2. Song HH et al: Eosinophilic cholangitis: US, CT, and cholangiography findings. J Comput Assist Tomogr. 21(2):251-3, 1997

IMAGE GALLERY

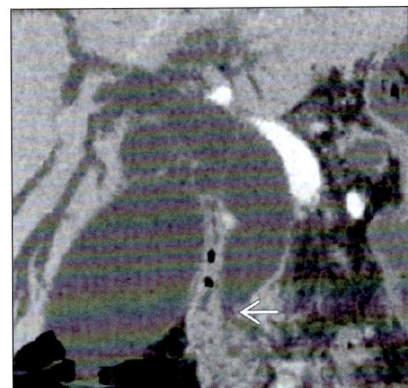 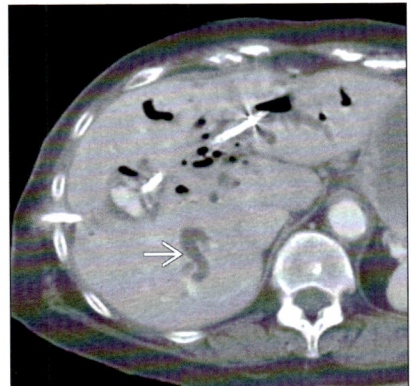 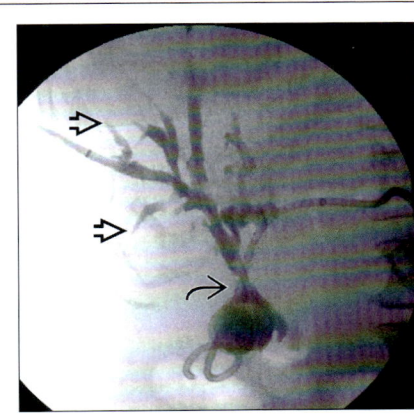

(Left) Coronal CECT shows cholangitis from obstructing pancreatic carcinoma. Minimum intensity projection demonstrates intra- and extrahepatic dilatation from pancreatic head carcinoma ➡. (Center) Axial CECT shows transhepatic biliary stents & dilated intrahepatic bile ducts ➡. Ducts contain gas 2° stents & duct-enteric anastomosis. (Right) Frontal transhepatic cholangiography in same patient as left shows anastomosis ➢ & ductal dilation. Note irregular arborization of ducts & abrupt "arrowhead" terminations ➢ characteristic of cholangitis.

RECURRENT PYOGENIC CHOLANGITIS

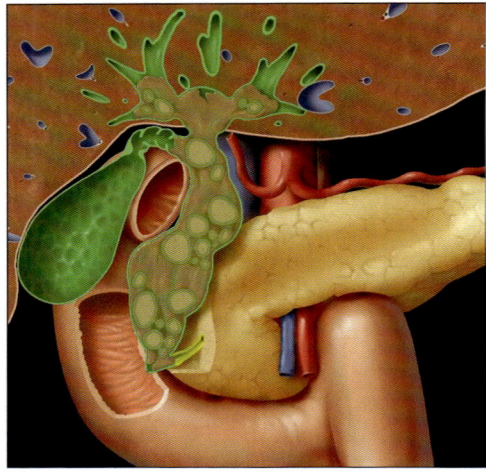

Graphic demonstrates marked dilation of intrahepatic bile ducts with multiple common bile duct and intrahepatic stones.

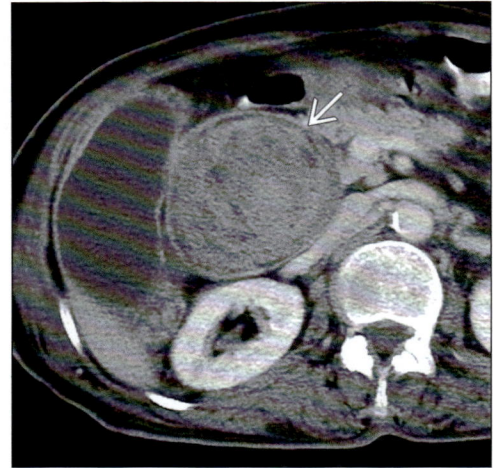

Axial CECT shows massive dilatation of common duct from pigment stone in RPC. Note soft-tissue density stone within markedly distended intra-pancreatic portion of duct ➔.

TERMINOLOGY

Abbreviations and Synonyms
- Recurrent pyogenic cholangitis (RPC), oriental cholangitis, oriental cholangiohepatitis

Definitions
- Intra- and extrahepatic biliary pigment stones occurring in patients and immigrants from SE Asia

IMAGING FINDINGS

General Features
- Best diagnostic clue: Intra- and extrahepatic biliary stones without stones in gallbladder (GB)
- Location: Confined to left lobe (often lateral segment), or involving all biliary ductal segments & common bile duct (CBD)
- Size: Stones typically 1-4 cm in size
- Morphology: Combination of pigment stones and biliary sludge

Fluoroscopic Findings
- ERCP
  - Dilated intra- and extrahepatic bile ducts
  - Common duct stones and intrahepatic duct stones without stones in gallbladder
  - Rapid tapering of dilated intrahepatic ducts with "arrowhead" configuration
  - Non-filling of biliary ductal segments due to strictures of intrahepatic ducts

CT Findings
- NECT: Biliary stones may be high attenuation or isodense to liver
- CECT
  - Dilated intra- and extrahepatic biliary ducts within involved segments on CECT
  - CBD may be markedly enlarged
  - May be associated with low-attenuation pyogenic liver abscesses, fatty liver atrophy of segments with chronic biliary obstruction

MR Findings
- T1WI: Hypointense dilated ducts and intermediate intensity biliary calculi; may have hyperintense rim

DDx: Spectrum of Biliary Lesions Mimicking RPC

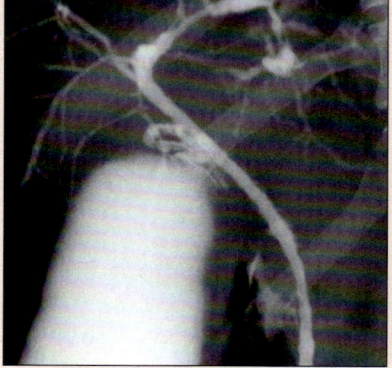

Sclerosing Cholangitis

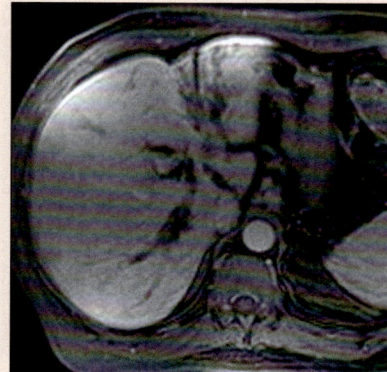

Cholangiocarcinoma

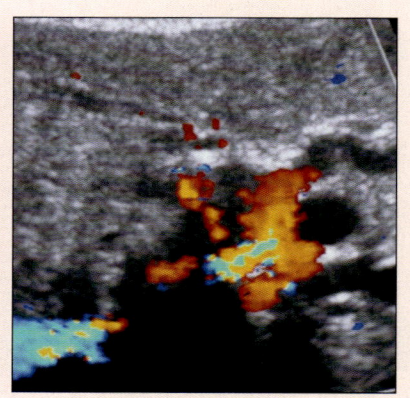

Cholangiocarcinoma

RECURRENT PYOGENIC CHOLANGITIS

Key Facts

Terminology
- Intra- and extrahepatic biliary pigment stones occurring in patients and immigrants from SE Asia

Imaging Findings
- Best diagnostic clue: Intra- and extrahepatic biliary stones without stones in gallbladder (GB)
- Location: Confined to left lobe (often lateral segment), or involving all biliary ductal segments & common bile duct (CBD)
- Dilated intra- and extrahepatic biliary ducts within involved segments on CECT

Top Differential Diagnoses
- Intrahepatic Stones Secondary to Biliary Stricture
- Sclerosing Cholangitis
- Bacterial Cholangitis
- Cholangiocarcinoma

Pathology
- Intraductal pigment calculi within intra- and extrahepatic ducts, proliferative fibrosis of CBD walls, periductal abscesses
- Associated with biliary parasitic infection from Clonorchis sinensis and/or ascaris lumbricoides

Clinical Issues
- RUQ pain, recurrent fevers, jaundice
- Leukocytosis, elevated alkaline phosphatase and bilirubin

Diagnostic Checklist
- Intra- & extrahepatic bile duct dilatation/stones in SE Asian patients

---

- T2WI: Hyperintense bile within obstructed ducts and low-signal calculi
- T1 C+: Hypointense dilated bile ducts with low- to intermediate-signal biliary calculi
- MRCP
  - Dilated intra- and extrahepatic ducts with low-signal filling defects (stones)
  - Rapidly tapering intrahepatic ducts ("arrowhead sign")

Ultrasonographic Findings
- Grayscale Ultrasound: Dilated intrahepatic ducts with echogenic debris; calculi may/may not cause acoustic shadowing
- Color Doppler: No flow within dilated bile ducts

Nuclear Medicine Findings
- WBC Scan
  - Positive for cholangitic liver abscesses

Other Modality Findings
- Cholangiographic findings: Dilated intra- and extrahepatic ducts with filling defects (stones)
  - "Arrowhead" deformity of rapidly tapering intrahepatic ducts
  - Similar to ERCP

Imaging Recommendations
- Best imaging tool: CECT
- Protocol advice
  - 150 mL IV contrast at 2.5 mL/sec with 5 mm collimation and 5 mm reconstruction intervals
  - Heavily T2WI/MRCP and gadolinium-enhanced breathheld GRE

DIFFERENTIAL DIAGNOSIS

Intrahepatic Stones Secondary to Biliary Stricture
- Non-Asian patient
- Stricture may be due to prior surgery, trauma or chemotherapy
- Similar clinical presentation: RUQ pain, fever, chills

Sclerosing Cholangitis
- Diffuse CBD thickening
- Multiple intrahepatic strictures
- Stones form distal to strictures
- Associated with inflammatory bowel disease

Bacterial Cholangitis
- Dilated intra- and extrahepatic ducts
- Stones, sludge and pus in bile ducts
- Intra- or extrahepatic strictures

Cholangiocarcinoma
- Associated with sclerosing cholangitis, choledochal cyst, RPC, clonorchiasis
- Infiltrative type at confluence of right and left ducts most common
- Ductal dilatation of involved segments with or without parenchymal mass
- CECT shows delayed enhancement within parenchymal mass components

PATHOLOGY

General Features
- General path comments
  - Intraductal pigment calculi within intra- and extrahepatic ducts, proliferative fibrosis of CBD walls, periductal abscesses
  - End-stage biliary cirrhosis
- Etiology
  - Associated with biliary parasitic infection from Clonorchis sinensis and/or ascaris lumbricoides
  - Associated with E. coli infection of bile ducts
    - Bacterial production of beta-glucuronidase
    - Leads to hydrolysis of bilirubin, development of calcium bilirubinate stones within intra- & extrahepatic bile ducts
  - Associated with poor general nutrition

RECURRENT PYOGENIC CHOLANGITIS

- Epidemiology: Endemic in SE Asian patients & immigrants from SE Asia (China, Vietnam, Philippines)
- Associated abnormalities: Poor nutrition

Gross Pathologic & Surgical Features
- Dilated bile ducts with brown mud-like pigment stones, pus
- May have parasitic infection in biliary ducts (Clonorchis or ascaris)

Microscopic Features
- Periductal inflammatory changes
- Infiltration of periportal spaces with inflammatory cells
  - Periductal fibrosis, biliary cirrhosis
- Localized segmental hepatic atrophy
- Fatty changes in liver

Staging, Grading or Classification Criteria
- Classification based on distribution of affected biliary segment
  - Isolated to left lobe, particularly lateral segment
  - Involving all biliary segments and CBD

CLINICAL ISSUES

Presentation
- Most common signs/symptoms
  - RUQ pain, recurrent fevers, jaundice
  - Other signs/symptoms
    - Hypotension, shaking, chills
    - Related to gram-negative septicemia
- Clinical Profile
  - Leukocytosis, elevated alkaline phosphatase and bilirubin
  - Diagnosis by CT, US or cholangiography

Demographics
- Age: Over 40
- Gender: Affects males and females equally
- Ethnicity: Chinese and SE Asian population

Natural History & Prognosis
- Repeated episodes of cholangitis
- Complications
  - Liver abscesses, biliary stricture and biliary stones
    - Long-term repeated episodes of cholangitis & stricture formation lead to biliary cirrhosis
  - Cholangiocarcinoma

Treatment
- Options, risks, complications
  - Endoscopic sphincterotomy
  - Surgical
    - Biliary drainage with hepatico-jejunostomy
    - Subcutaneous jejunal ostomy (biliary access)
    - Left hepatic lobe resection if isolated left lobe disease
  - Interventional radiology
    - Percutaneous biliary drainage of affected segments
    - Basket removal of pigment stones
    - Balloon dilation of biliary strictures
    - Repeated percutaneous procedures to clear stones & debris
  - Medical therapy
    - Long-term suppressive antibiotic therapy

DIAGNOSTIC CHECKLIST

Image Interpretation Pearls
- Intra- & extrahepatic bile duct dilatation/stones in SE Asian patients
- Massive CBD dilatation
- Rapid tapering of intrahepatic ducts ("arrowhead" sign)

SELECTED REFERENCES

1. Lee WJ et al: Radiologic spectrum of cholangiocarcinoma: emphasis on unusual manifestations and differential diagnoses. Radiographics. 21 Spec No:S97-S116, 2001
2. Park MS et al: Recurrent pyogenic cholangitis: comparison between MR cholangiography and direct cholangiography. Radiology. 220(3):677-82, 2001
3. Cosenza CA et al: Current management of recurrent pyogenic cholangitis. Am Surg. 65(10):939-43, 1999
4. Kim MJ et al: MR imaging findings in recurrent pyogenic cholangitis. AJR Am J Roentgenol. 173(6):1545-9, 1999
5. Harris HW et al: Recurrent pyogenic cholangitis. Am J Surg. 176(1):34-7, 1998
6. Leow CK et al: Re: Biliary access procedure in the management of oriental cholangiohepatitis. Am Surg. 64(1):99, 1998
7. Lee DW et al: Biliary infection. Baillieres Clin Gastroenterol. 11(4):707-24, 1997
8. Lo CM et al: The changing epidemiology of recurrent pyogenic cholangitis. HKMJ. 3(3):302-4, 1997
9. Sperling RM et al: Recurrent pyogenic cholangitis in Asian immigrants to the United States: natural history and role of therapeutic ERCP. Dig Dis Sci. 42(4):865-71, 1997
10. Kirby CL et al: US case of the day. Oriental cholangiohepatitis. Radiographics. 15(6):1503-6, 1995
11. Mack E: Pathogenesis and Clinical Presentation of Bile Duct Calculi. Semin Laparosc Surg. 2(2):76-84, 1995
12. Reynolds WR et al: Oriental cholangiohepatitis. Mil Med. 159(2):158-60, 1994
13. Enriquez G et al: Intrahepatic biliary stones in children. Pediatr Radiol. 22(4):283-6, 1992
14. Kusano S et al: Oriental cholangiohepatitis: correlation between portal vein occlusion and hepatic atrophy. AJR Am J Roentgenol. 158(5):1011-4, 1992
15. Goldberg HI et al: Diagnostic and interventional procedures for the biliary tract. Curr Opin Radiol. 3(3):453-62, 1991
16. Lim JH: Oriental cholangiohepatitis: pathologic, clinical, and radiologic features. AJR Am J Roentgenol. 157(1):1-8, 1991
17. Schulte SJ et al: CT of the extrahepatic bile ducts: wall thickness and contrast enhancement in normal and abnormal ducts. AJR Am J Roentgenol. 154(1):79-85, 1990
18. Kashi H et al: Recurrent pyogenic cholangiohepatitis. Ann R Coll Surg Engl. 71(6):387-9, 1989
19. vanSonnenberg E et al: Oriental cholangiohepatitis: diagnostic imaging and interventional management. AJR Am J Roentgenol. 146(2):327-31, 1986
20. Federle MP et al: Recurrent pyogenic cholangitis in Asian immigrants. Use of ultrasonography, computed tomography, and cholangiography. Radiology. 143(1):151-6, 1982

RECURRENT PYOGENIC CHOLANGITIS

IMAGE GALLERY

Typical

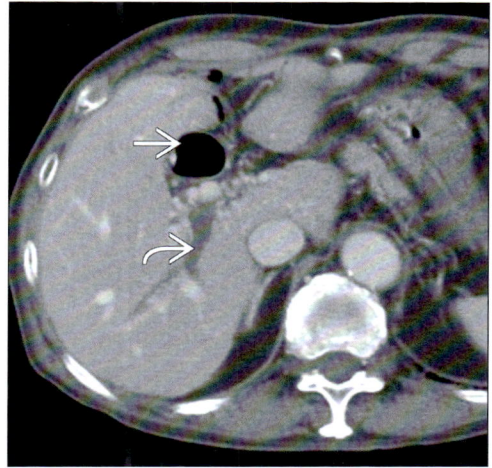
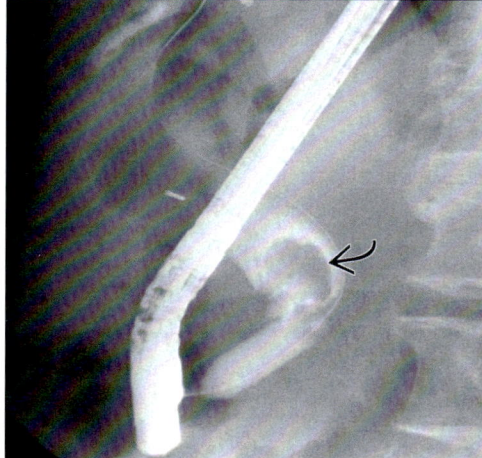

(Left) Axial CECT shows gross dilation of the intra- and extrahepatic bile ducts ➡, with gas in nondependent portions and fluid in dependent ducts ➡. *(Right)* Frontal ERCP in same patient as left confirms ductal dilation and pneumobilia. Note presence of large "soft" stones within bile duct ➡, later cleared by basket sweep of the duct.

Typical

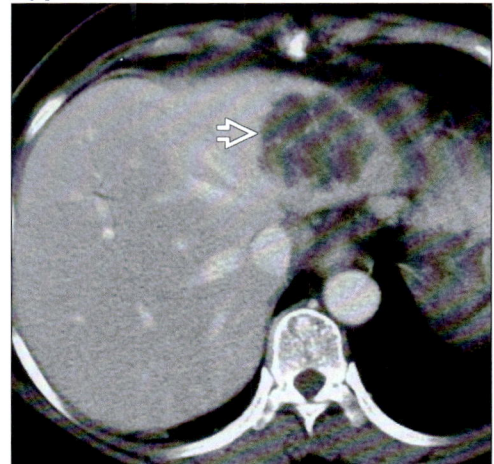
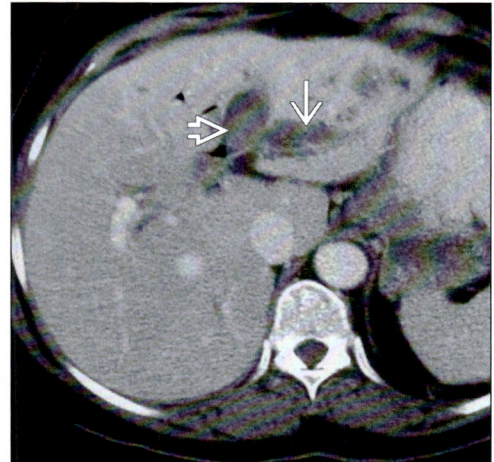

(Left) Axial CECT shows focal abscess in lateral segment of left lobe ➡. *(Right)* Axial CECT in same patient as left shows predominantly intrahepatic bile duct dilatation ➡ involving left ductal system & filling defect due to pigment calculus ➡.

Typical

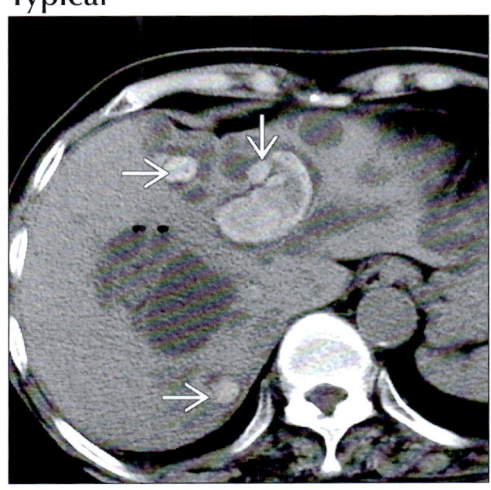
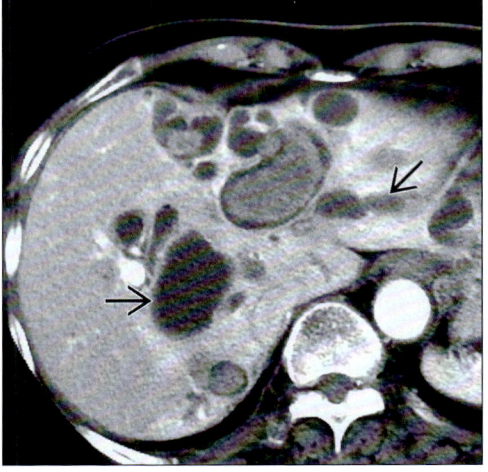

(Left) Axial NECT of intrahepatic pigment stones in RPC. Note multiple high-attenuation stones within left and right hepatic lobes ➡. *(Right)* Axial CECT in same patient as left depicts dilated intrahepatic ducts to better advantage ➡.

CHOLEDOCHOLITHIASIS

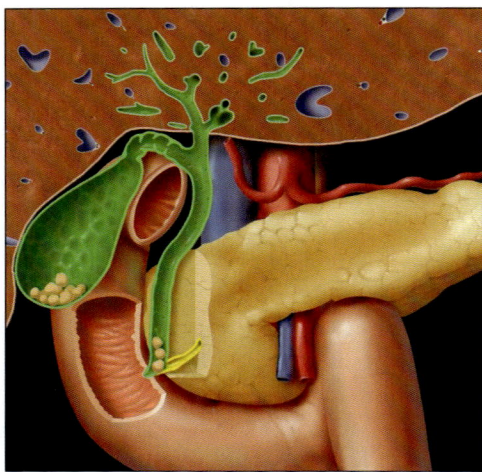

Coronal graphic shows multiple small nonobstructive stones in distal CBD and gallbladder.

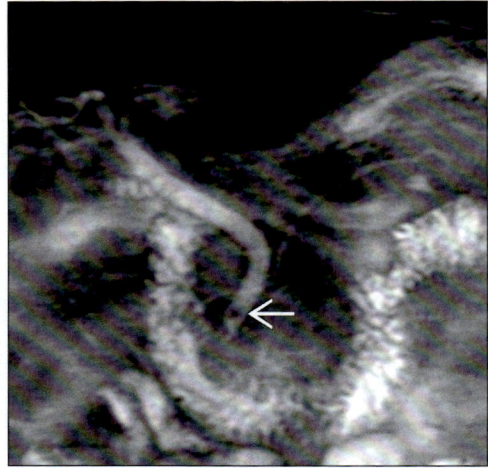

Coronal MRCP shows low-signal filling defect ➡ representing stone in CBD.

TERMINOLOGY

Abbreviations and Synonyms
- Cholangiolithiasis or biliary calculi

Definitions
- Intra- and/or extrahepatic stones or calculi

IMAGING FINDINGS

General Features
- Best diagnostic clue: Discrete low-signal filling defects within bile ducts on MR cholangiography
- Location
  - Intra- & extrahepatic bile ducts (more common in CBD)
  - Secondary stones: Within CBD anywhere between porta hepatis and ampulla of Vater
- Size: Varies from 1-15 mm

Fluoroscopic Findings
- ERCP (diagnostic and/or therapeutic)
  - Opacification of extra- & intrahepatic duct system + pancreatic duct
  - Stones seen as radiolucent filling defects
- Intra-operative & post-operative (T-tube) cholangiography
  - Direct tests for CBD stone detection
  - Meniscus of contrast material clearly outlines margins of stones

CT Findings
- NECT
  - Attenuation of calculi varies
    - Less than water density
    - Soft-tissue density
    - Dense calcification
  - Mixed stones: Predominantly cholesterol & calcium bilirubinate (usually calcified rim or central nidus)
    - Increased attenuation (75-85% stones due to sufficient Ca++ bilirubinate)
    - "Bull's eye" sign (60-80% sensitive): Rim of bile surrounding duct stone
    - Thin meniscus of water-density bile around stone posteriorly
    - Some stones isodense to soft tissue

DDx: Obstruction of Common Bile Duct

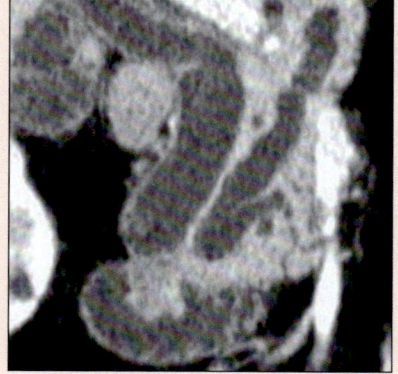
Ampullary Carcinoma

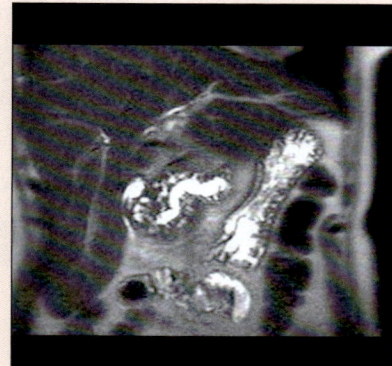
Chronic Pancreatitis

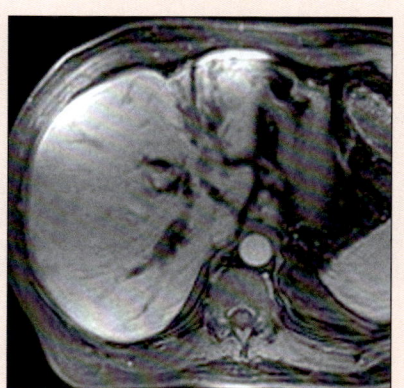
Cholangiocarcinoma

CHOLEDOCHOLITHIASIS

Key Facts

Terminology
- Intra- and/or extrahepatic stones or calculi

Imaging Findings
- Best diagnostic clue: Discrete low-signal filling defects within bile ducts on MR cholangiography
- "Bull's eye" sign (60-80% sensitive): Rim of bile surrounding duct stone
- Thin meniscus of water-density bile around stone posteriorly

Top Differential Diagnoses
- Pancreatic or Ampullary Cancer
- Chronic Pancreatitis
- Cholangiocarcinoma
- Papillary Stenosis or Dysfunction
- Primary Sclerosing Cholangitis (PSC)

Pathology
- Obstruction, dilatation, sclerosis, stricture
- Bile stasis/infection: Bilirubinate stone formation
- Secondary duct stones: Gallstones into CBD
- Approximately 25 million Americans have gallstones, 15% also have CBD stones
- Associated abnormalities: Gallstones

Clinical Issues
- Acute RUQ pain, pruritus, jaundice, pancreatitis
- Increased alkaline phosphatase & direct bilirubin
- Gender: M < F

Diagnostic Checklist
- Rule out other causes of CBD obstruction
- MRC & ERCP: Discrete filling defects or obstruction & prestenotic dilatation of CBD/IHBD

- Rarely pure cholesterol stones
  - Isodense with bile (indistinguishable)
- Abrupt termination of CBD: Complete obstruction by large stone
  - Stone isodense to bile or pancreas
  - Less accurate than "bull's eye" sign
- CBD and/or intrahepatic bile duct dilatation (IHBD) varies
  - Stone size, degree & duration of obstruction
  - Water-density tubular branching structures

MR Findings
- MR cholangiography (MRC)
  - Bile: Very bright signal
  - Ductal stones: Decreased signal intensity foci
  - Low-signal filling defects within increased-signal intensity bile

Ultrasonographic Findings
- Grayscale Ultrasound
  - Echogenic focus with posterior acoustic shadowing: Stone within CBD
  - 10% of stones produce no acoustic shadow
    - Small size, soft & porous composition
  - CBD/IHBD based on stone size, degree & duration of obstruction
    - CBD: 4-6 mm (normal); 6-7 mm (equivocal); > 8 mm (dilatation)
    - Common hepatic duct: 4-5 mm (normal)
    - IHBD: 1-2 mm (usually not visible)

Nuclear Medicine Findings
- Hepatobiliary scan (HIDA)
  - Diagnose early, low-grade obstruction
  - Stones with intermittent obstruction: Retention & delayed passage of isotope

Imaging Recommendations
- Best imaging tool
  - ERCP: Gold standard for CBD stone detection in absence of T-tube
  - MRC: Sensitivity 81-100%; specificity 85-100%
- Protocol advice
  - MRC: Two techniques
    - RARE: Single-slab rapid acquisition with relaxation enhancement
    - HASTE: Multislice half-Fourier acquisition single-shot turbo spin-echo
  - MDCT without contrast: Thin sections (≤ 5 mm) have sensitivity of 75-85%

DIFFERENTIAL DIAGNOSIS

Pancreatic or Ampullary Cancer
- Hypodense mass in head of pancreas or ampulla
- "Double duct" sign: Obstruction & dilatation of pancreatic duct/CBD
- Heterogeneous poorly enhancing mass
- Contiguous organ invasion may be seen in duodenum, stomach, mesenteric root
- Duodenal distention with water is helpful for CT visualization

Chronic Pancreatitis
- Focal or diffuse atrophy of gland; enlarged head
- Dilated main pancreatic duct with ductal calculi
- Distal CBD long stricture causes prestenotic dilatation
- Thickening of peripancreatic fascia & fat necrosis

Cholangiocarcinoma
- Extrahepatic CBD growth (stricture or polypoid mass)
- Obstruction & dilatation of CBD/IHBD
- ERCP depicts stricture or intraductal tumor mass

Papillary Stenosis or Dysfunction
- Dilatation of CBD & intrahepatic bile ducts
- No mass or filling defect

Primary Sclerosing Cholangitis (PSC)
- Idiopathic or autoimmune reaction, or genetic
- CBD always involved; IHBD & extrahepatic in 68-89% of cases
- ERCP: Classic "beaded appearance"
  - Alternating segments of dilatation & focal strictures

CHOLEDOCHOLITHIASIS

PATHOLOGY

General Features
- General path comments
  - Mechanism of stones in CBD & IHBD
    - Obstruction, dilatation, sclerosis, stricture
    - Bile stasis/infection: Bilirubinate stone formation
    - Infection: E. coli, Klebsiella, other gram-negative organisms with β-glucuronidase activity
- Etiology
  - Primary duct stones: Form within bile ducts, composed largely of pigment
    - Chronic hemolytic disease, recurrent cholangitis
    - Congenital anomalies of bile ducts (e.g. Caroli disease)
    - Motor disorder of sphincter of Oddi
    - Low fat/protein diet
    - Foreign body (e.g. suture material)
    - Parasites: Clonorchis sinensis & ascaris (major causes in Asia)
  - Secondary duct stones: Gallstones into CBD
    - Obesity, Crohn disease, ileal resection
    - Hemolytic anemias (sickle cell anemia, hereditary spherocytosis)
    - Increased triglycerides, hyperalimentation
    - Major composition: Cholesterol 70-80%, pigment 20-30% in Western countries; calcium bilirubinate in Eastern countries
    - 12-15% of cholecystectomy patients have choledocholithiasis
- Epidemiology
  - Most frequent cause of biliary obstruction without ductal dilatation
  - Approximately 25 million Americans have gallstones, 15% also have CBD stones
  - Primary stones account for 5% of cases in USA
  - Secondary duct stones account for 95% of cases in USA
    - 95% of patients with CBD stones have or have had gallstones
    - 15-25% acute calculous cholecystitis patients have CBD stones
- Associated abnormalities: Gallstones

Staging, Grading or Classification Criteria
- Classified into two types based on etiology
  - Primary duct stones
  - Secondary duct stones

CLINICAL ISSUES

Presentation
- Most common signs/symptoms
  - Acute RUQ pain, pruritus, jaundice, pancreatitis
  - Small stones spontaneously pass with/without pain
- Clinical Profile: Obese female in 4th decade with history of acute or intermittent RUQ pain & jaundice
- Lab data
  - Increased alkaline phosphatase & direct bilirubin
  - Late phase: Increased AST & ALT levels
- Diagnosis: MRC, ERCP, intra-operative/post-operative T-tube cholangiography

Demographics
- Age: 4th decade, but can be seen in any age group
- Gender: M < F
- Ethnicity: Native Americans (secondary stones)

Natural History & Prognosis
- Complications: Cholangitis, obstructive jaundice, pancreatitis, secondary biliary cirrhosis
- Undetected duct stones left behind in 1-5% of cholecystectomy patients
- Prognosis

Treatment
- Stones < 3 mm usually pass spontaneously
- Stones 3-10 mm: Endoscopic sphincterotomy
  - Stone retrieval balloon to sweep duct, basket to snare stones
- Stones > 10-15 mm: Lithotripsy required

DIAGNOSTIC CHECKLIST

Consider
- Rule out other causes of CBD obstruction

Image Interpretation Pearls
- MRC & ERCP: Discrete filling defects or obstruction & prestenotic dilatation of CBD/IHBD

SELECTED REFERENCES

1. Dalton SJ et al: Routine magnetic resonance cholangiopancreatography and intra-operative cholangiogram in the evaluation of common bile duct stones. Ann R Coll Surg Engl. 87(6):469-70, 2005
2. Kim YJ et al: Preoperative evaluation of common bile duct stones in patients with gallstone disease. AJR Am J Roentgenol. 184(6):1854-9, 2005
3. Kondo S et al: Detection of common bile duct stones: comparison between endoscopic ultrasonography, magnetic resonance cholangiography, and helical-computed-tomographic cholangiography. Eur J Radiol. 54(2):271-5, 2005
4. Shanmugam V et al: Is magnetic resonance cholangiopancreatography the new gold standard in biliary imaging? Br J Radiol. 78(934):888-93, 2005
5. Kim TK et al: Diagnosis of intrahepatic stones: superiority of MR cholangiopancreatography over endoscopic retrograde cholangiopancreatography. AJR Am J Roentgenol. 179(2):429-34, 2002
6. Soto JA et al: Detection of choledocholithiasis with MR cholangiography: comparison of three-dimensional fast spin-echo and single- and multisection half-Fourier rapid acquisition with relaxation enhancement sequences. Radiology. 215(3):737-45, 2000
7. Vitellas KM et al: MR cholangiopancreatography of bile and pancreatic duct abnormalities with emphasis on the single-shot fast spin-echo technique. RadioGraphics. 20: 939-957, 2000
8. Fulcher AS et al: MR cholangiography: technical advances and clinical applications. Radiographics. 19(1):25-41; discussion 41-4, 1999
9. Varghese JC et al: The diagnostic accuracy of magnetic resonance cholangiopancreatography and ultrasound compared with direct cholangiography in the detection of choledocholithiasis. Clin Radiol. 54(9):604-14, 1999

CHOLEDOCHOLITHIASIS

IMAGE GALLERY

Typical

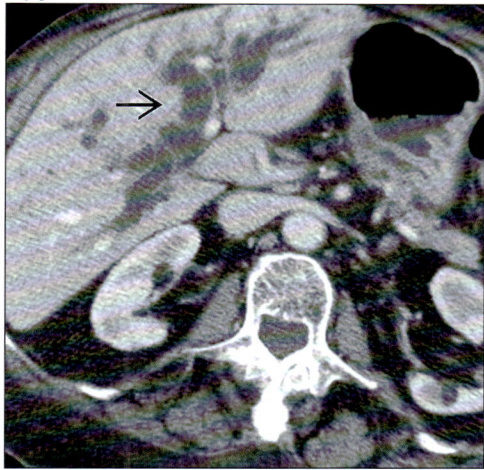
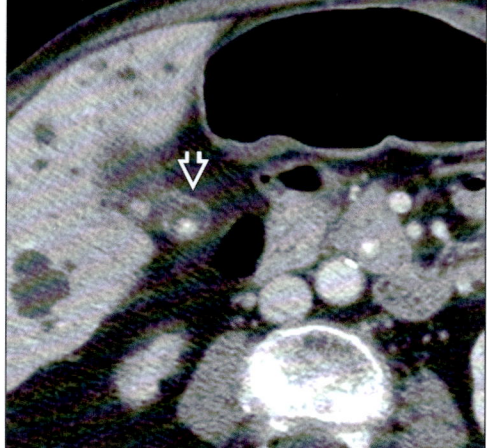

(Left) Axial CECT of extreme biliary ductal dilatation caused by choledocholith, demonstrated by marked IHBD ➡. *(Right)* Axial CECT at more caudal level in same patient as left identifies stone in distal CBD ➡. Patient went on to ERCP for sphincterotomy and basket extraction of stone.

Typical

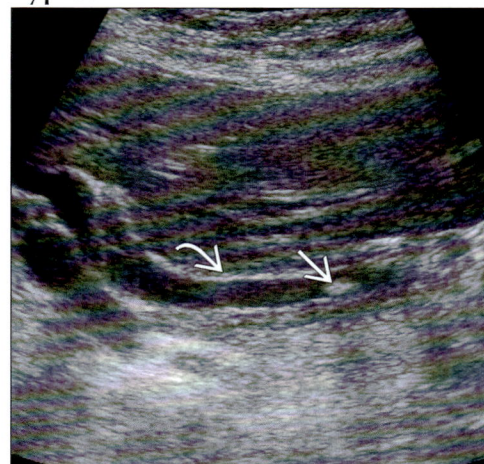
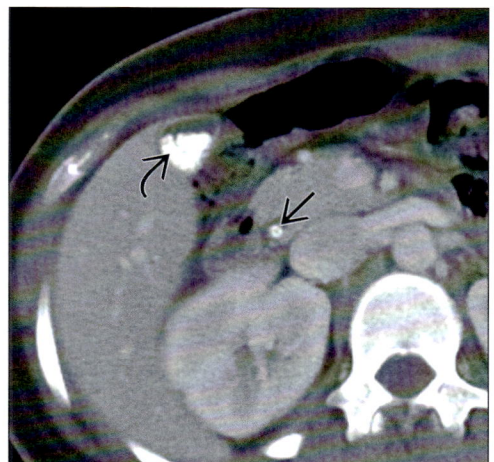

(Left) Sagittal grayscale sonogram of common duct stone. Note small echogenic stone ➡ with normal-sized duct ➡. *(Right)* Axial CECT in same patient as left confirms small stone in distal duct ➡, as well as calcified cholelithiasis ➡.

Typical

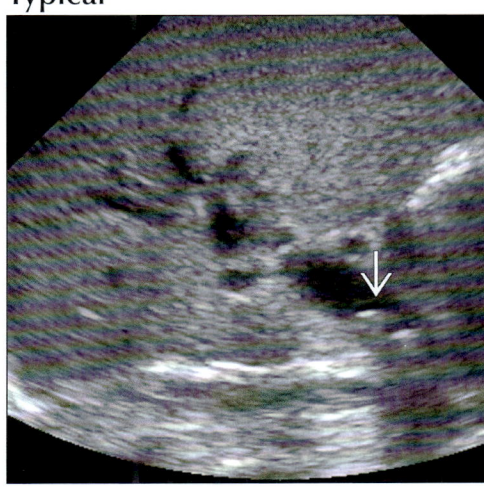
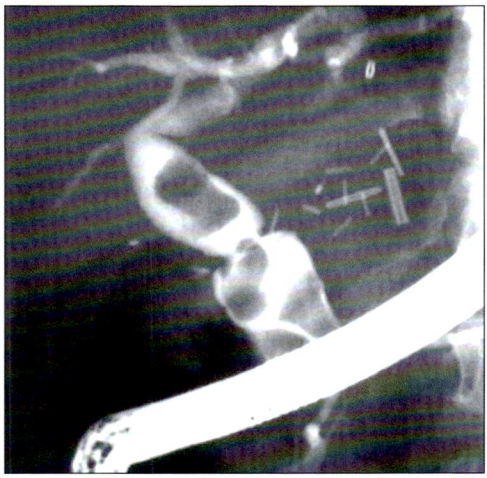

(Left) Transverse transabdominal ultrasound of choledocholithiasis demonstrates echogenic foci with posterior acoustic shadowing in CBD ➡ and dilatation of CBD. *(Right)* Anteroposterior ERCP confirms multiple CBD stones in patient status-post orthotopic liver transplant.

CHOLECYSTITIS

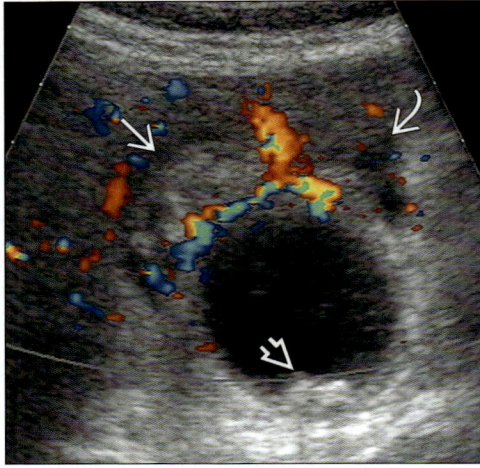
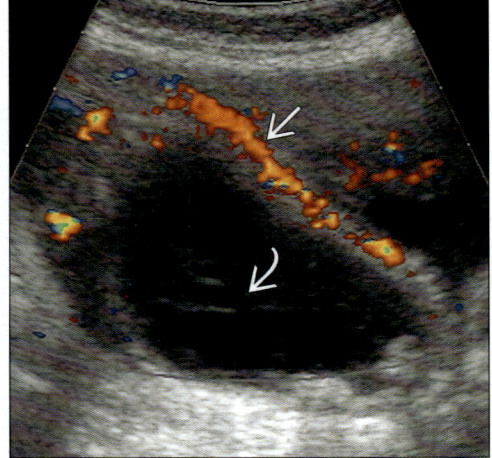

Transverse color Doppler ultrasound of gangrenous cholecystitis demonstrates hyperemia of omental fat at fundus of GB ➡, small amount of pericholecystic fluid ➡ and small gallstones ➡.

Sagittal color Doppler ultrasound of same patient as left reveals marked hypertrophy of cystic artery ➡ and linear membranes in GB lumen ➡ from fibrous strands of pus.

TERMINOLOGY

Abbreviations and Synonyms
- Acute calculous cholecystitis, acute acalculous cholecystitis

Definitions
- Acute inflammation of gallbladder (GB)

IMAGING FINDINGS

General Features
- Best diagnostic clue
  - Impacted gallstone in cystic duct
  - Positive sonographic Murphy sign
  - GB wall thickening
- Location: Stone impacted in GB neck or cystic duct
- Size: Distended GB (> 5 cm transverse diameter)
- Morphology: Distended GB more rounded than normal "pear-shaped" configuration

Fluoroscopic Findings
- ERCP
  - No filling of GB
  - May document common bile duct (CBD) stones in patients with associated cholangitis

CT Findings
- NECT
  - Distended GB
  - Edematous pericholecystic fat with stranding
  - Calcified gallstones (15% of cases)
- CECT
  - Uncomplicated cholecystitis
    - GB wall thickening
    - Increased mural enhancement
    - Pericholecystic fat stranding
    - Cholesterol stones typically not visible
  - Complicated cholecystitis
    - Intramural or pericholecystic abscesses leading to asymmetric GB wall thickening
    - Gas in lumen and/or wall of GB
    - High-attenuation GB hemorrhage
    - Focal interruption of GB wall due to necrosis
    - Adherent omentum

MR Findings
- T2WI

DDx: Spectrum of Diseases Mimicking Cholecystitis

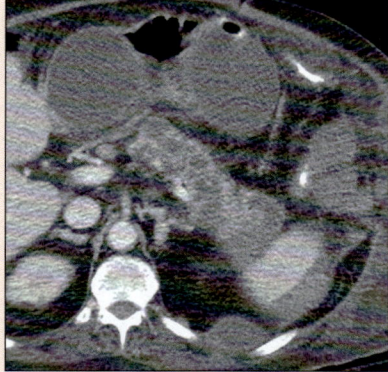
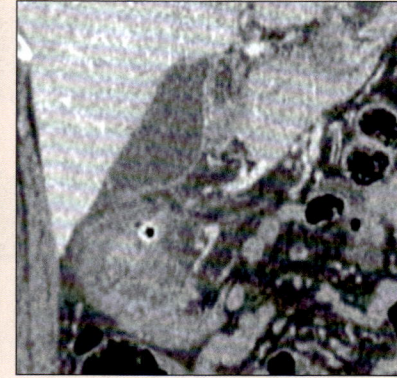
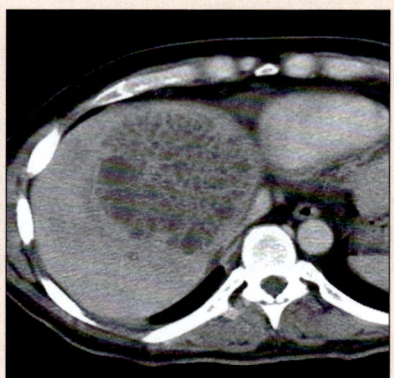

Pancreatitis

Hepatic Flexure Diverticulitis

Hepatic Abscess

CHOLECYSTITIS

Key Facts

Terminology
- Acute inflammation of gallbladder (GB)

Imaging Findings
- Uncomplicated: Positive sonographic Murphy sign; gallstone impacted in neck of GB or cystic duct; thickened GB wall (> 4 cm) on US
- Complicated: Gallstones; pericholecystic fluid/abscess; intraluminal membranes; gas in GB wall/lumen; sonographic Murphy sign absent in 1/3 of patients; asymmetric wall thickening on US
- Best imaging tool: US or biliary scintigraphy
- Protocol advice: Longitudinal and transverse images of GB, parasagittal images of GB neck region & cystic duct in LPO position to detect impacted gallstones (i.e., immobile)

Clinical Issues
- Most common signs/symptoms: Acute RUQ pain, fever
- Other signs/symptoms: Calcified stones in only 15-20% of patients with cholecystitis
- May progress to gangrenous cholecystitis and perforation if untreated
- Excellent prognosis in uncomplicated cases or with prompt surgery

Diagnostic Checklist
- Perforated ulcer or pancreatitis with secondary GB wall thickening
- Stone impacted in cystic duct
- Sonographic Murphy sign must be unequivocal to be considered positive

---

- o Distended GB with stones
- o High-signal pericholecystic fat
- T1 C+
  - o "Rim sign" of increased hepatic enhancement in patient with gangrenous cholecystitis
  - o Focal interruption of enhancement

Ultrasonographic Findings
- Grayscale Ultrasound
  - o Uncomplicated: Positive sonographic Murphy sign; gallstone impacted in neck of GB or cystic duct; thickened GB wall (> 4 cm) on US
  - o Complicated: Gallstones; pericholecystic fluid/abscess; intraluminal membranes; gas in GB wall/lumen; sonographic Murphy sign absent in 1/3 of patients; asymmetric wall thickening on US

Nuclear Medicine Findings
- Hepatobiliary Scintigraphy
  - o Tc-99m iminodiacetic acid derivatives
  - o Non-visualization of GB at 4 hours has 99% specificity
  - o Increased uptake in GB fossa during arterial phase due to hyperemia in 80% of patients
  - o "Rim sign" seen in 34% of patients is due to increased uptake in GB fossa
    - Positive predictive value of 57% for gangrenous cholecystitis

Imaging Recommendations
- Best imaging tool: US or biliary scintigraphy
- Protocol advice: Longitudinal and transverse images of GB, parasagittal images of GB neck region & cystic duct in LPO position to detect impacted gallstones (i.e., immobile)

DIFFERENTIAL DIAGNOSIS

Peptic Ulcer Disease (PUD)
- Thickened duodenum
- Ectopic gas if perforation
- Periduodenal inflammatory changes in anterior pararenal space
- Secondary GB wall thickening

Acute Pancreatitis
- Enlarged pancreas
- Peripancreatic fluid or inflammatory changes
- Nonenhancing areas of necrosis

Hepatic Flexure Diverticulitis
- Colonic diverticula
- Pericolonic inflammation
- Fecalith

Liver Abscess
- CECT
  - o "Cluster sign" of multiloculated pyogenic abscesses
  - o Air-fluid level from gas-forming organism
- US
  - o Irregular, hypoechoic mass
  - o Little enhancement through transmission

PATHOLOGY

General Features
- General path comments
  - o Distended GB
  - o Thickened, inflamed GB wall
  - o Pericholecystic adhesions to omentum
- Genetics
  - o Increased incidence of gallstones in selected population
    - Hispanics, Pima Indians
- Etiology
  - o 95% calculous
    - Obstructing stone in cystic duct
  - o 5% acalculous
    - Ischemia with secondary inflammation/infection
    - AIDS patients have opportunistic GB infection
- Epidemiology
  - o Incidence parallels prevalence of gallstones
    - 25 million Americans have gallstones

CHOLECYSTITIS

Gross Pathologic & Surgical Features
- Gallstones in GB neck or cystic duct
- Thickened GB wall with hyperemia of wall
- Omental adhesions

Microscopic Features
- Lumen: Gallstones, sludge
- GB mucosa: Ulcerations
- GB wall: Acute polymorphonuclear (PMN) infiltration
- Bacterial cultures positive in 40-70% of patients

Staging, Grading or Classification Criteria
- Non-perforated
  - GB wall intact on CT and/or US
- Gangrenous
  - US: Pericholecystic fluid, intraluminal membranes, asymmetric GB wall thickening
- Perforated
  - CECT: Pericholecystic abscess, GB wall necrosis with lack of enhancement

CLINICAL ISSUES

Presentation
- Most common signs/symptoms: Acute RUQ pain, fever
- Other signs/symptoms: Calcified stones in only 15-20% of patients with cholecystitis
- Lab data
  - Increased WBC
  - May have mild elevation in liver enzymes

Demographics
- Age: Typically > 25 years of age
- Gender: M:F = 1:3

Natural History & Prognosis
- May progress to gangrenous cholecystitis and perforation if untreated
- Excellent prognosis in uncomplicated cases or with prompt surgery
- Complications
  - Mirizzi syndrome and Bouveret syndrome (gallstone erodes into duodenum causing obstruction)

Treatment
- Prompt cholecystectomy
  - Laparoscopic surgery for uncomplicated cases
- Percutaneous cholecystectomy
  - Useful for poor operative risk patients with GB empyema
- Percutaneous drainage
  - Well-defined, well-localized pericholecystic abscesses

DIAGNOSTIC CHECKLIST

Consider
- Perforated ulcer or pancreatitis with secondary GB wall thickening

Image Interpretation Pearls
- Stone impacted in cystic duct
- Sonographic Murphy sign must be unequivocal to be considered positive

SELECTED REFERENCES

1. Barie PS et al: Acute acalculous cholecystitis. Curr Gastroenterol Rep. 5(4):302-9, 2003
2. Bennett GL et al: Ultrasound and CT evaluation of emergent gallbladder pathology. Radiol Clin North Am. 41(6):1203-16, 2003
3. Browning JD et al: Gallstone disease and its complications. Semin Gastrointest Dis. 14(4):165-77, 2003
4. Cheema S et al: Timing of laparoscopic cholecystectomy in acute cholecystitis. Ir J Med Sci. 172(3):128-31, 2003
5. Fayad LM et al: Functional magnetic resonance cholangiography (fMRC) of the gallbladder and biliary tree with contrast-enhanced magnetic resonance cholangiography. J Magn Reson Imaging. 18(4):449-60, 2003
6. Gandolfi L et al: The role of ultrasound in biliary and pancreatic diseases. Eur J Ultrasound. 16(3):141-59, 2003
7. Ko CW et al: Gastrointestinal disorders of the critically ill. Biliary sludge and cholecystitis. Best Pract Res Clin Gastroenterol. 17(3):383-96, 2003
8. Oh KY et al: Limited abdominal MRI in the evaluation of acute right upper quadrant pain. Abdom Imaging. 28(5):643-51, 2003
9. Ozaras R et al: Acute viral cholecystitis due to hepatitis A virus infection. J Clin Gastroenterol. 37(1):79-81, 2003
10. Pazzi P et al: Biliary sludge: the sluggish gallbladder. Dig Liver Dis. 35 Suppl 3:S39-45, 2003
11. Pedrosa I et al: The interrupted rim sign in acute cholecystitis: a method to identify the gangrenous form with MRI. J Magn Reson Imaging. 18(3):360-3, 2003
12. Roth T et al: Acute acalculous cholecystitis associated with aortic dissection: report of a case. Surg Today. 33(8):633-5, 2003
13. Trowbridge RL et al: Does this patient have acute cholecystitis? JAMA. 289(1):80-6, 2003
14. Yusoff IF et al: Diagnosis and management of cholecystitis and cholangitis. Gastroenterol Clin North Am. 32(4):1145-68, 2003
15. Abou-Saif A et al: Complications of gallstone disease: Mirizzi syndrome, cholecystocholedochal fistula, and gallstone ileus. Am J Gastroenterol. 97(2):249-54, 2002
16. Adusumilli S et al: MR imaging of the gallbladder. Magn Reson Imaging Clin N Am. 10(1):165-84, 2002
17. Bingener-Casey J et al: Reasons for conversion from laparoscopic to open cholecystectomy: a 10-year review. J Gastrointest Surg. 6(6):800-5, 2002
18. Gore RM et al: Imaging benign and malignant disease of the gallbladder. Radiol Clin North Am. 40(6):1307-23, vi, 2002
19. Indar AA et al: Acute cholecystitis. BMJ. 325(7365):639-43, 2002
20. Kitano S et al: Laparoscopic cholecystectomy for acute cholecystitis. J Hepatobiliary Pancreat Surg. 9(5):534-7, 2002

CHOLECYSTITIS

IMAGE GALLERY

Typical

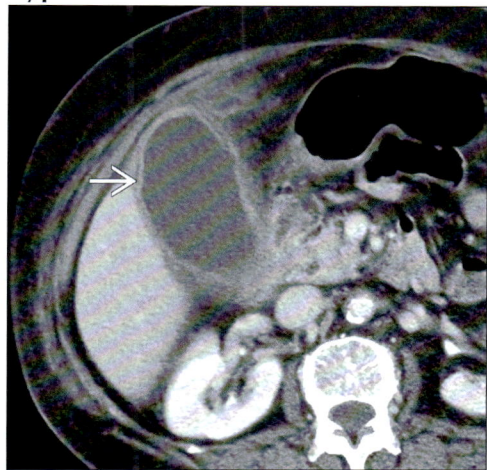 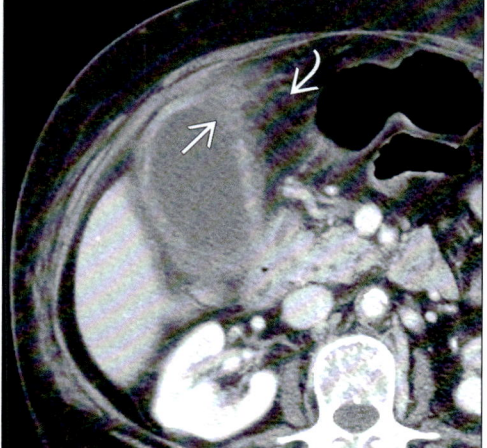

(Left) Axial CECT shows acute gangrenous cholecystitis. Note distended GB with thickened wall ➔. *(Right)* Axial CECT at more caudal level in same patient demonstrates focal necrosis of GB wall with lack of contrast enhancement ➔. Note adjacent inflammatory changes in omental fat ➔.

Typical

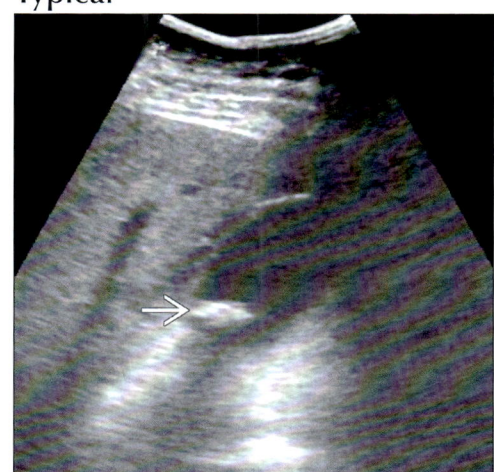 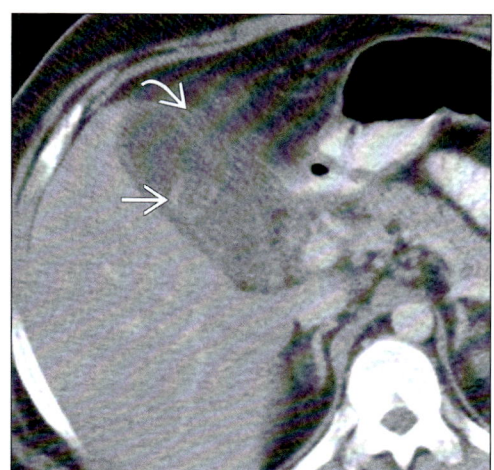

(Left) Sagittal ultrasound shows gallstones ➔, but GB wall was judged to be of normal thickness & patient was not very tender over GB. *(Right)* Axial CECT in same patient as left, performed immediately after US, shows gallstone ➔, as well as mural thickening & pericholecystic inflammation ➔. Acute cholecystitis was confirmed at surgery.

Variant

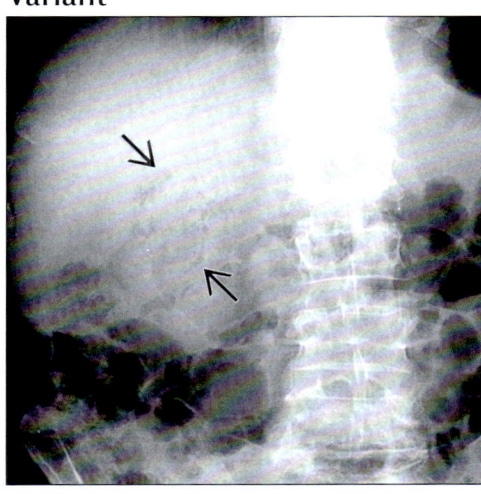 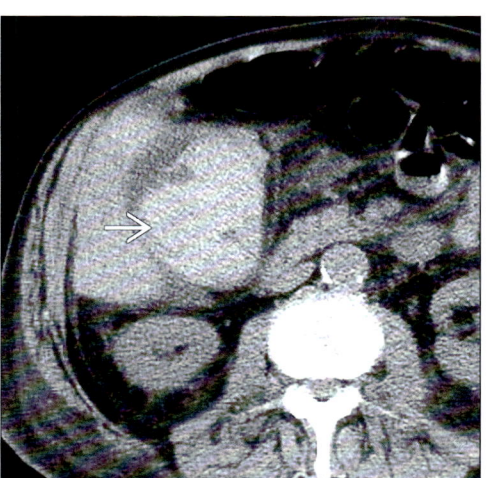

(Left) Anteroposterior radiograph shows classic appearance of emphysematous cholecystitis, an infection of GB wall caused by gas-forming organisms. Note air in oval configuration in expected location of GB ➔. *(Right)* Axial NECT of acute hemorrhagic cholecystitis shows high attenuation clot in GB ➔.

ACUTE PANCREATITIS

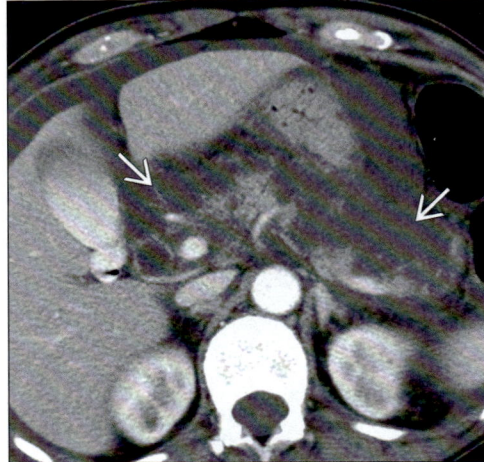

Axial CECT of necrotizing pancreatitis following ERCP. Note extensive areas of non-enhancement indicating necrosis ➡ of body and tail of pancreas.

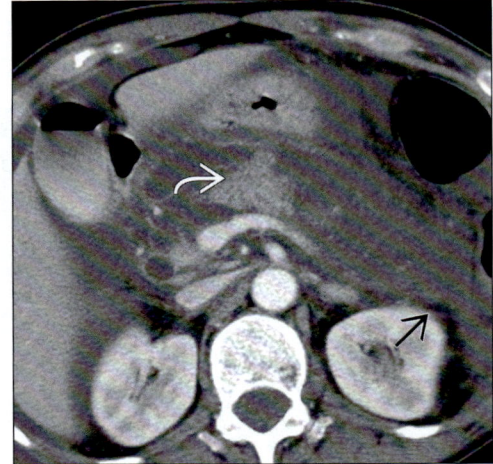

Axial CECT at level of splenic vein in same patient as left shows acute fluid collection in anterior pararenal space ➡ with only small area of residual normally enhancing pancreas ➡.

TERMINOLOGY

Definitions
- Acute inflammatory process of pancreas with variable involvement of other regional tissues or remote organ systems

IMAGING FINDINGS

General Features
- Best diagnostic clue: Enlarged pancreas, fluid collections & obliteration of fat planes
- Location: Pancreatic & peripancreatic
- Size: Pancreas increased in size (focal or diffuse)

Radiographic Findings
- Radiography
  - Duodenal ileus
  - Sentinel loop
    - Mildly dilated, gas-filled segment of small bowel with or without air-fluid levels
  - "Colon cutoff" sign
    - Markedly distended transverse colon with air
    - Absence of gas distal to splenic flexure due to functional colonic spasm (spread of pancreatic inflammation to proximal descending colon)

Fluoroscopic Findings
- ERCP
  - Dilated or normal main pancreatic duct (MPD)
  - Communication of pseudocyst with MPD (acutely)
  - May show narrowed & tapered distal common bile duct (CBD) with prestenotic biliary dilatation

CT Findings
- Focal or diffuse pancreatic enlargement
- Heterogeneous enhancement; nonenhancing necrotic areas
- Rim enhancement of acute fluid collections, abscesses and pseudocysts
- Infiltration of peripancreatic fat; gallstones
- Pseudoaneurysm: May simulate pseudocyst; isodense to adjacent blood vessels
- Pleural effusions, basal atelectasis

MR Findings
- T1WI
  - Gradient-echo image

DDx: Peripancreatic Infiltration

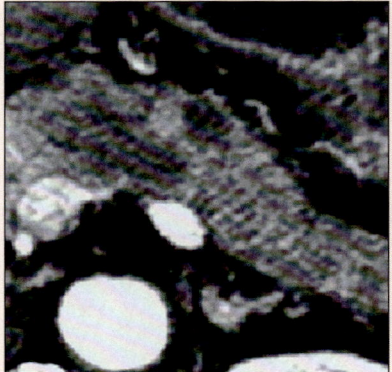

Infiltrating Carcinoma

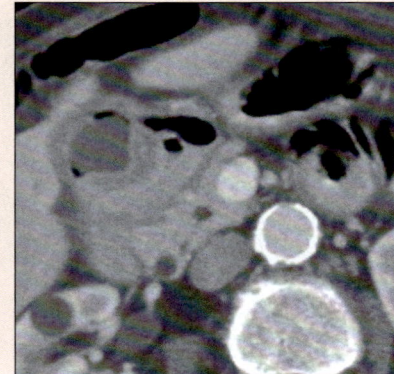

Perforated Duodenal Ulcer

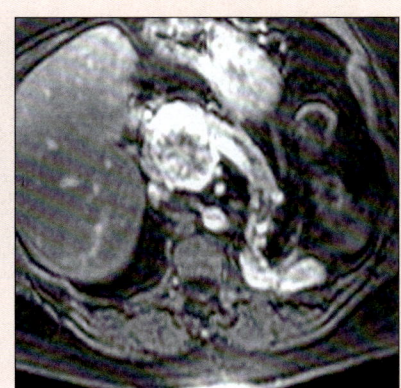

Pancreatic Metastases

ACUTE PANCREATITIS

Key Facts

Terminology
- Acute inflammatory process of pancreas with variable involvement of other regional tissues or remote organ systems

Imaging Findings
- Best diagnostic clue: Enlarged pancreas, fluid collections & obliteration of fat planes
- Heterogeneous enhancement; nonenhancing necrotic areas
- Pseudoaneurysm: May simulate pseudocyst; isodense to adjacent blood vessels

Top Differential Diagnoses
- Infiltrating Pancreatic Carcinoma
- Perforated Duodenal Ulcer
- "Shock" Pancreas
- Lymphoma & Metastases

Pathology
- Alcohol, gallstones, metabolic, infection, trauma, drugs
- Pathogenesis: Reflux of pancreatic enzymes, bile, duodenal contents & increased ductal pressure

Clinical Issues
- Clinical Profile: Patient with history of alcoholism, fever & severe mid-epigastric pain radiating to back
- Increased serum amylase & lipase
- Leukocytosis, hypocalcemia (poor prognostic sign)

Diagnostic Checklist
- Bulky, irregularly enlarged pancreas with obliteration of peripancreatic fat planes, fluid collections, pseudocyst or abscess formation

---

- - Variable decreased signal intensity & enlarged gland
- T2WI FS
  - Fluid collections, pseudocyst, necrotic areas: Hyperintense
  - Gallstones or intraductal calculi: Hypointense
- T1 C+
  - Heterogeneous enhancement pattern
    - Nonenhancing decreased signal areas (necrosis, fluid collection and/or pseudocyst)
    - Pancreatic pseudocyst contiguous with main pancreatic duct (MPD)
    - Vascular occlusions
- MRCP
  - All fluid-containing structures: Hyperintense
  - Dilated or normal MPD
  - Pseudocyst contiguous with MPD

Ultrasonographic Findings
- Grayscale Ultrasound: Enlarged hypoechoic gland, fluid collection, abscess and/or pseudocyst

Angiographic Findings
- Conventional
  - Performed when pseudoaneurysm is suspected
  - Useful when pancreatitis is due to vascular cause
    - Vasculitis, polyarteritis nodosum, lupus
    - Postaortic aneurysm resection

Imaging Recommendations
- Best imaging tool: MDCT with & without contrast; T2 WI with fat suppression; MRCP; ERCP

DIFFERENTIAL DIAGNOSIS

Infiltrating Pancreatic Carcinoma
- Irregular, heterogeneous, poorly enhancing mass
- Abrupt obstruction & dilatation of pancreatic duct
- Obliteration of retropancreatic fat
- No hemorrhage, calcium very rare
- Local tumor extension to splenic hilum & porta hepatis
- Contiguous organ invasion (duodenum, stomach, mesenteric root)
- ERCP of MPD
  - Irregular, nodular, rat-tailed eccentric obstruction
  - Prestenotic dilatation
- Angiography: Hypovascular mass encasing vessels

Perforated Duodenal Ulcer
- May infiltrate anterior pararenal space
- Fewer than 50% of cases show extraluminal gas or contrast medium collections
- Pancreatic head may be involved

"Shock" Pancreas
- Infiltration of peripancreatic & mesenteric fat planes following hypotensive episode
- Pancreas looks normal or diffusely enlarged
- Usually presents with "shock bowel" appearance of mucosal enhancement & submucosal edema
- Quickly resolves following resuscitation

Lymphoma & Metastases
- Nodular, bulky, enlarged pancreas due to infiltration
- Retroperitoneal adenopathy
- MPD & side branches
  - Extrinsic mass effect & ductal draping
    - Smooth ductal splaying or some narrowing
  - Lack of communication with tumor
- Peripancreatic infiltration (obliteration of fat planes)
- Primary may be seen in case of metastatic infiltration

PATHOLOGY

General Features
- General path comments
  - Embryology-anatomy
    - Congenital anomalies may cause pancreatitis
    - Annular pancreas: Failure of migration of ventral bud to contact dorsal bud
    - Pancreas divisum: Ventral & dorsal pancreatic buds fail to fuse; relative block at minor papilla
- Genetics

ACUTE PANCREATITIS

- ○ Hereditary pancreatitis
  - ▪ Autosomal dominant & incomplete penetrance
- Etiology
  - ○ Alcohol, gallstones, metabolic, infection, trauma, drugs
  - ○ Pathogenesis: Reflux of pancreatic enzymes, bile, duodenal contents & increased ductal pressure
    - ▪ MPD or terminal duct blockage
    - ▪ Edema, spasm, incompetence of sphincter of Oddi
    - ▪ Periduodenal diverticulum or tumor
- Epidemiology
  - ○ USA: Urban & VA hospitals (alcohol); suburban & rural (gallstones)
  - ○ Incidence in USA: 0.005-0.01% of general population

Gross Pathologic & Surgical Features
- Bulky pancreas, necrosis, fluid collection, pseudocyst

Microscopic Features
- Acute edematous pancreatitis
  - ○ Edema, congestion, leukocytic infiltrates
- Acute hemorrhagic pancreatitis
  - ○ Tissue destruction, fat necrosis, hemorrhage
- Dilated ducts & protein plugs may be seen

Staging, Grading or Classification Criteria
- CT classification: Five grades based on severity
  - ○ Grade A: Normal pancreas
  - ○ Grade B
    - ▪ Focal or diffuse enlargement of gland
    - ▪ Contour irregularities & heterogeneous attenuation
    - ▪ No peripancreatic inflammation
  - ○ Grade C
    - ▪ Intrinsic pancreatic abnormalities
    - ▪ Associated inflammatory changes in peripancreatic fat
  - ○ Grade D
    - ▪ Small, usually single, ill-defined fluid collection
  - ○ Grade E
    - ▪ Two or more large fluid collections
    - ▪ Presence of gas in pancreas or retroperitoneum
- Most important criterion: Presence & extent of necrotizing pancreatitis (nonenhancing parenchyma)

CLINICAL ISSUES

Presentation
- Most common signs/symptoms
  - ○ Epigastric pain, often radiating to back
  - ○ Tenderness, fever, nausea, vomiting
  - ○ Grey Turner sign: Bluish discoloration of flanks
  - ○ Cullen sign: Periumbilical discoloration
- Clinical Profile: Patient with history of alcoholism, fever & severe mid-epigastric pain radiating to back
- Lab data
  - ○ Increased serum amylase & lipase
  - ○ Hyperglycemia, increased lactate dehydrogenase
  - ○ Leukocytosis, hypocalcemia (poor prognostic sign)
  - ○ Fall in hematocrit, rise in blood urea nitrogen (BUN)

Demographics
- Age
  - ○ Usually young & middle age group
  - ○ Can be seen in any age group
- Gender: M > F

Natural History & Prognosis
- Complications
  - ○ Pancreatic: Fluid collections, pseudocyst, necrosis, abscess
  - ○ Gastrointestinal: Hemorrhage, infarction, obstruction, ileus
  - ○ Biliary: Obstructive jaundice
  - ○ Vascular: Pseudoaneurysm, porto-splenic vein thrombosis, hemorrhage
  - ○ Disseminated intravascular coagulation (DIC)
  - ○ Shock due to pulmonary & renal failure
  - ○ Cardiac, CNS & metabolic complications
- Prognosis
  - ○ Early detection with minor complications: Good
  - ○ Late detection with major complications: Poor
  - ○ Infected pancreatic necrosis: Near 50% mortality even with surgical debridement

Treatment
- Conservative: NPO, gastric tube, atropine, analgesics, antibiotics
- Drainage of infected or obstructing pseudocysts
- Infected necrosis requires surgery

DIAGNOSTIC CHECKLIST

Consider
- Underlying carcinoma obstructing pancreatic duct

Image Interpretation Pearls
- Bulky, irregularly enlarged pancreas with obliteration of peripancreatic fat planes, fluid collections, pseudocyst or abscess formation

SELECTED REFERENCES

1. Balthazar EJ: Acute pancreatitis: assessment of severity with clinical and CT evaluation. Radiology. 223(3):603-13, 2002
2. Balthazar EJ: Complications of acute pancreatitis: clinical and CT evaluation. Radiol Clin North Am. 40(6):1211-27, 2002
3. Balthazar EJ: Staging of acute pancreatitis. Radiol Clin North Am. 40(6):1199-209, 2002
4. Piironen A: Severe acute pancreatitis: contrast-enhanced CT and MRI features. Abdom Imaging. 26(3):225-33, 2001
5. Lecesne R et al: Acute pancreatitis: interobserver agreement and correlation of CT and MR cholangiopancreatography with outcome. Radiology. 211(3):727-35, 1999
6. Sica GT et al: Comparison of endoscopic retrograde cholangiopancreatography with MR cholangiopancreatography in patients with pancreatitis. Radiology. 210: 605-10, 1999
7. Vitellas KM et al: Pancreatitis complicated by gland necrosis: evolution of findings on contrast-enhanced CT. J Comput Assist Tomogr. 23(6):898-905, 1999

ACUTE PANCREATITIS

IMAGE GALLERY

Typical

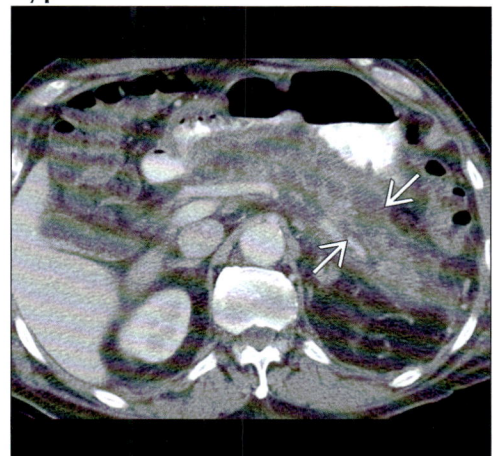
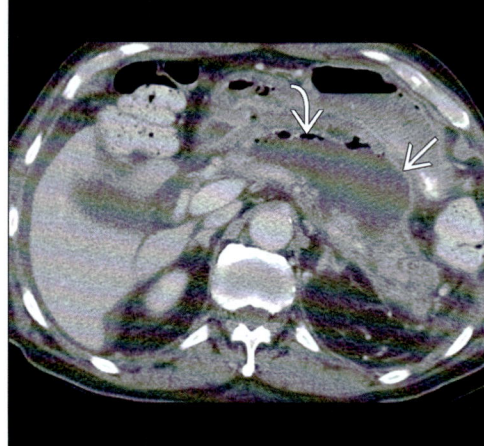

(**Left**) Axial CECT shows acute necrotizing pancreatitis. Note heterogeneous & diminished enhancement of pancreas ➡. (**Right**) Axial CECT four weeks later in same patient as left shows organized pancreatic necrosis ➡ or pseudocyst within body of pancreas. Foci of gas within this area ➡ likely represents superimposed infection.

Typical

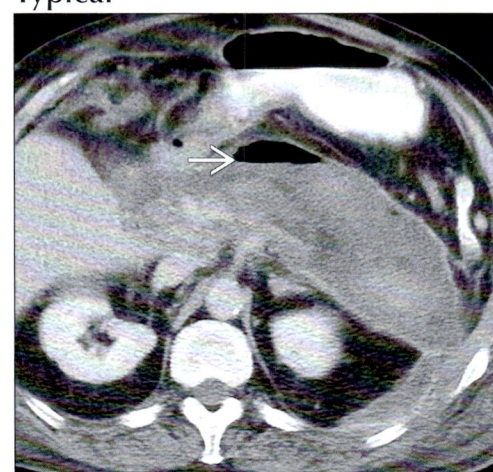
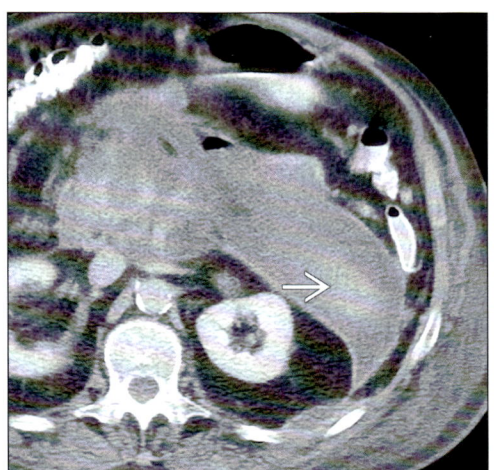

(**Left**) Axial CECT of necrotizing & hemorrhagic pancreatitis complicated by infection. Note extensive pancreatic necrosis with air-fluid level ➡ indicating gas-forming infection. (**Right**) Axial CECT at more caudal level in same patient as left reveals high-attenuation fluid (hematoma) ➡ extending into left anterior pararenal space.

Variant

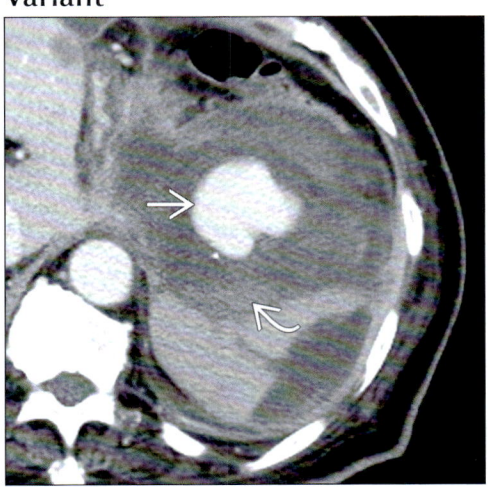
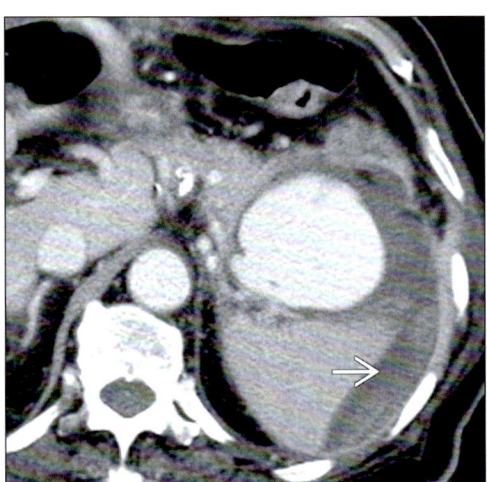

(**Left**) Axial CECT of life-threatening bleed from ruptured pseudoaneurysm (PA) of splenic artery from pancreatitis. Note high-attenuation PA ➡ with surrounding hemorrhage ➡. (**Right**) Axial CECT at more caudal level in same patient as left demonstrates extension of hematoma into splenic subcapsular space ➡.

PYELONEPHRITIS

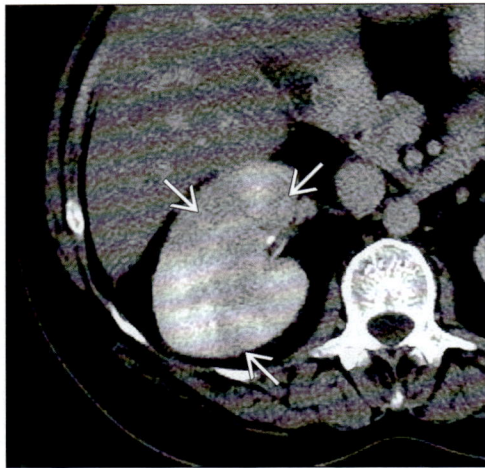

Axial CECT of acute pyelonephritis shows multiple wedge-shaped areas of decreased enhancement ➡ within right kidney.

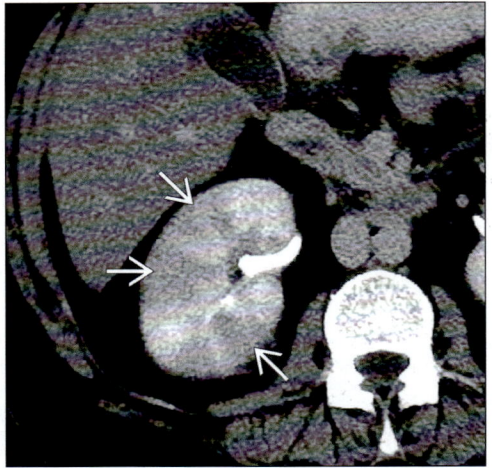

Axial CECT at more caudal level in same patient as previous image reveals additional areas of low-attenuation infection ➡.

TERMINOLOGY

Abbreviations and Synonyms
- Acute lobar nephronia, focal bacterial nephritis

Definitions
- Acute infection of renal parenchyma

IMAGING FINDINGS

General Features
- Best diagnostic clue: Focal swelling, decreased enhancement of affected parenchyma on CECT
- Morphology: Typically wedge-shaped, can be rounded & mass-like

Radiographic Findings
- IVP
  ○ Striated nephrogram
  ○ Seldom performed in pediatric patients

CT Findings
- CECT
  ○ Wedge-shaped or rounded areas of poor or streaky enhancement
    ■ Best identified on excretory phase (2 minutes post-injection)
    ■ Small areas of pyelonephritis may be missed on corticomedullary-phase images
  ○ Inflammatory changes in perirenal fat
  ○ Occasionally mass-like, may distort normal renal contour
  ○ May have contralateral asymptomatic areas of infection
  ○ Very delayed scans show minimal enhancement unlike infarction, which has no enhancement
  ○ Unlike infarction, no cortical rim sign

MR Findings
- T2WI
  ○ High-signal intensity in affected areas of renal parenchyma 2° increased water content
  ○ Inflammatory changes in perirenal fat

Ultrasonographic Findings
- Grayscale Ultrasound
  ○ Poor corticomedullary differentiation & focal areas of ↑ or ↓ echogenicity

DDx: Striated or Wedge-Shaped Defects

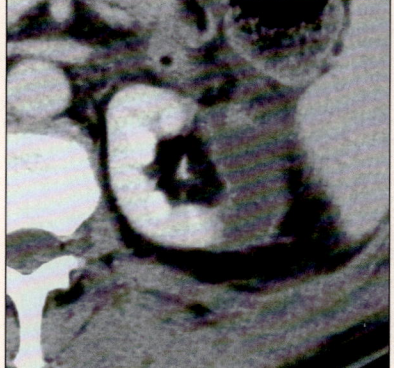

Renal Infarction

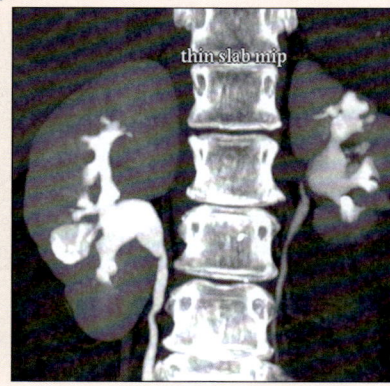

Renal Scarring

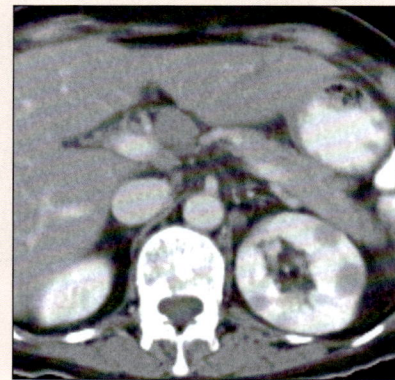

Renal Lymphoma

PYELONEPHRITIS

Key Facts

Terminology
- Acute infection of renal parenchyma

Imaging Findings
- Best diagnostic clue: Focal swelling, decreased enhancement of affected parenchyma on CECT
- Wedge-shaped or rounded areas of poor or streaky enhancement
- Poor corticomedullary differentiation & focal areas of ↑ or ↓ echogenicity
- Color Doppler: ↓ Perfusion in areas of pyelonephritis
- ↓ Accumulation of renal cortical agents in wedge-shaped distribution pointing toward renal hilum

Top Differential Diagnoses
- Renal Infarction
- Renal Scarring
- Renal Mass

Pathology
- Associated with vesicoureteral reflux in approximately 25-40% of cases

Clinical Issues
- Most common signs/symptoms: Often nonspecific: Malaise, irritability, fever, abdominal pain, change in urinary habits/enuresis, flank pain, vomiting, hematuria, dysuria

Diagnostic Checklist
- Simulates infarction, but no cortical rim sign & some degree of enhancement on delayed images

---

- Localized or generalized swelling
- Unilateral renal enlargement may be only indicator
- Rounded or mass-like areas of altered echotexture
- Color Doppler: ↓ Perfusion in areas of pyelonephritis
- Power Doppler: ↓ Perfusion in areas of pyelonephritis

Nuclear Medicine Findings
- Nuclear Scintigraphic Findings
  - ↓ Accumulation of renal cortical agents in wedge-shaped distribution pointing toward renal hilum
  - Findings persist up to 6 weeks after acute infection
  - Pinhole collimation, SPECT imaging improve diagnostic sensitivity & accuracy
  - Tc-99m DMSA or glucoheptonate are both used

Imaging Recommendations
- Best imaging tool
  - Doppler US, nuclear renal cortical scans, CT, MR
  - US for associated complications, congenital anomalies, hydronephrosis

DIFFERENTIAL DIAGNOSIS

Renal Infarction
- Wedge-shaped pattern of absent perfusion
- "Cortical rim sign" on CECT due to enhancement from capsular artery
  - Emboli, vasculitis, trauma, aortic dissection, atherosclerosis

Renal Scarring
- Scarring usually more superficial than pyelonephritis
- Typically related to ascending infection from reflux nephropathy

Renal Mass
- Wilm tumor, nephroblastomatosis, lymphoma
- Renal cell carcinoma
  - Invades perirenal space & renal vein
  - Periaortic adenopathy
- Large transitional cell carcinoma invades renal parenchyma

- Focal, mass-like swelling of renal cortex

PATHOLOGY

General Features
- General path comments
  - Patchy interstitial suppurative inflammation & tubular necrosis
  - Infection may occur via ascending route, vesicoureteral reflux, hematogenous spread, or related to instrumentation
- Etiology: Vast majority of urine cultures grow gram-negative bacilli, normal inhabitants of intestinal tract (E. coli most common)
- Epidemiology
  - Associated with vesicoureteral reflux in approximately 25-40% of cases
  - Higher incidence in obstruction, duplicated kidneys, other anomalies

Gross Pathologic & Surgical Features
- Suppurative abscesses visible on cortical surface

Microscopic Features
- Abundant neutrophilic infiltrate
- Focal necrosis (acute phase)
- Fibrous depressions on cortex with tubular atrophy (scarring)

CLINICAL ISSUES

Presentation
- Most common signs/symptoms: Often nonspecific: Malaise, irritability, fever, abdominal pain, change in urinary habits/enuresis, flank pain, vomiting, hematuria, dysuria
- Other signs/symptoms
  - Strong-smelling urine in any age
  - Newborn with jaundice, failure to thrive
- Laboratory studies
  - Urine dipstick for nitrite, leukocyte esterase

PYELONEPHRITIS

- Associated with higher likelihood of positive urine culture
  - Urine for gram stain
    - E. coli is causative agent in > 80% of first-time urinary tract infection (UTI)
  - Leukocytosis, occasionally positive blood cultures
  - Positive urine culture
    - \> 1,000 colony forming units/mL for suprapubic aspirate
    - \> 10,000 cfu/mL for catheter specimen
    - \> 100,000 cfu/mL for clean-catch midstream specimen
- Complications
  - Perirenal abscess, necrotizing papillitis, pyonephrosis (obstruction), cortical scarring
  - Recurrent infections, subsequent scarring lead to end-stage renal disease
  - Permanent scarring more likely complication in children < 2 years old

Demographics
- Gender: M:F = 1:2
- Ethnicity: Less common in African-Americans

Natural History & Prognosis
- Generally excellent unless complications or recurrent infections
- Potential sequelae of renal scarring, chronic renal failure, hypertension & pregnancy-related complications drive aggressive imaging work-up & treatment regimens

Treatment
- Seven- to fourteen-day course of antimicrobial therapy
- Imaging work-up of intravenous pyelogram (IVP) & voiding cystourethrogram (VCUG) for vesicoureteral reflux & congenital abnormalities
- Prophylactic antibiotics for vesicoureteral reflux, other predisposing conditions

DIAGNOSTIC CHECKLIST

Consider
- Reflux nephropathy as underlying cause
- Underlying congenital anomaly
- Associated pyonephrosis if ureteral obstruction & dilatation of collecting system

Image Interpretation Pearls
- Simulates infarction, but no cortical rim sign & some degree of enhancement on delayed images
- Pitfall: Lesion may be poorly visualized if scanned too early (corticomedullary phase); best imaged during excretory phase of CECT

SELECTED REFERENCES

1. Cox AR et al: Emphysematous pyelonephritis: a case report and review of the literature. Can J Urol. 13(2):3039-43, 2006
2. Piccoli GB et al: Development of kidney scars after acute uncomplicated pyelonephritis: relationship with clinical, laboratory and imaging data at diagnosis. World J Urol. 24(1):66-73, 2006
3. Gonzalez E et al: Impact of vesicoureteral reflux on the size of renal lesions after an episode of acute pyelonephritis. J Urol. 173(2):571-4; discussion 574-5, 2005
4. Larcombe J: Urinary tract infection in children. Clin Evid. (14):429-40, 2005
5. Ramakrishnan K et al: Diagnosis and management of acute pyelonephritis in adults. Am Fam Physician. 71(5):933-42, 2005
6. Sheffield JS et al: Urinary tract infection in women. Obstet Gynecol. 106(5 Pt 1):1085-92, 2005
7. Wang YT et al: Correlation of renal ultrasonographic findings with inflammatory volume from dimercaptosuccinic acid renal scans in children with acute pyelonephritis. J Urol. 173(1):190-4; discussion 194, 2005
8. Fanos V et al: Antibiotics or surgery for vesicoureteric reflux in children. Lancet. 364(9446):1720-2, 2004
9. Hoberman A et al: Imaging studies after a first febrile urinary tract infection in young children. N Engl J Med. 348(3):195-202, 2003
10. Lin KY et al: Acute pyelonephritis and sequelae of renal scar in pediatric first febrile urinary tract infection. Pediatr Nephrol. 18(4):362-5, 2003
11. Maturen KE et al: Computed tomographic diagnosis of unsuspected pyelonephritis in children. Can Assoc Radiol J. 53(5):279-83, 2002
12. Kraus SJ: Genitourinary imaging in children. Pediatr Clin North Am. 48(6):1381-424, 2001
13. Majd M et al: Acute pyelonephritis: comparison of diagnosis with 99mTc-DMSA, SPECT, spiral CT, MR imaging, and power Doppler US in an experimental pig model. Radiology. 218(1):101-8, 2001
14. Wennerstrom M et al: Ambulatory blood pressure 16-26 years after the first urinary tract infection in childhood. J Hypertens. 18(4):485-91, 2000
15. No authors listed: Practice parameter: the diagnosis, treatment, and evaluation of the initial urinary tract infection in febrile infants and young children. American Academy of Pediatrics. Committee on Quality Improvement. Subcommittee on Urinary Tract Infection. Pediatrics. 103(4 Pt 1):843-52, 1999
16. Roberts KB: A synopsis of the American Academy of Pediatrics' practice parameter on the diagnosis, treatment, and evaluation of the initial urinary tract infection in febrile infants and young children. Pediatr Rev. 20(10):344-7, 1999
17. Yen TC et al: Identification of new renal scarring in repeated episodes of acute pyelonephritis using Tc-99m DMSA renal SPECT. Clin Nucl Med. 23(12):828-31, 1998
18. Dacher JN et al: Power Doppler sonographic pattern of acute pyelonephritis in children: comparison with CT. AJR Am J Roentgenol. 166(6):1451-5, 1996
19. Winters WD: Power Doppler sonographic evaluation of acute pyelonephritis in children. J Ultrasound Med. 15(2):91-6; quiz 97-8, 1996
20. Martinell J et al: Pregnancies in women with and without renal scarring after urinary infections in childhood. BMJ. 300(6728):840-4, 1990

PYELONEPHRITIS

IMAGE GALLERY

Typical

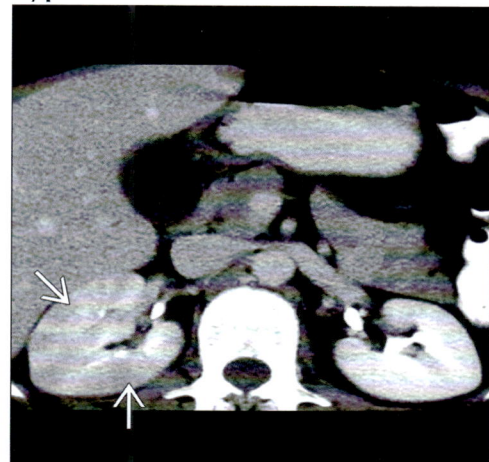 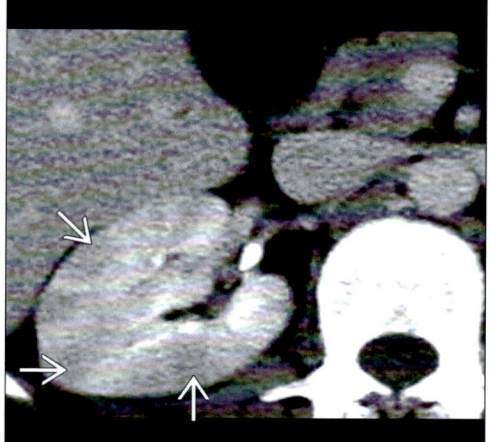

(Left) Axial CECT shows patchy areas of low density in right kidney ➡. *(Right)* Axial CECT magnified image in same patient as previous image shows patchy low-density regions in greater detail ➡.

Typical

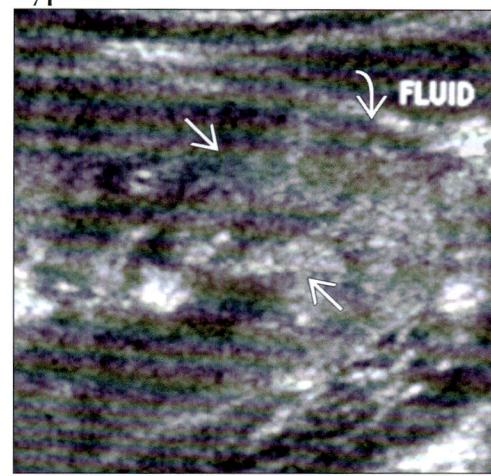 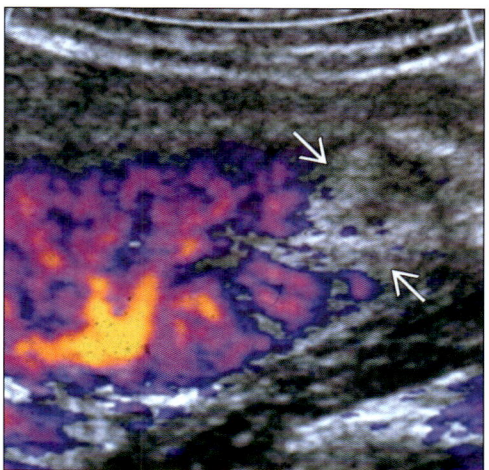

(Left) Sagittal grayscale sonogram of acute hemorrhagic pyelonephritis. Note wedge-shaped area of increased echogenicity within lower pole ➡ & thin rim of adjacent perinephric fluid ➡. *(Right)* Sagittal power Doppler ultrasound in same patient as previous image demonstrates absence of flow in area of pyelonephritis ➡.

Variant

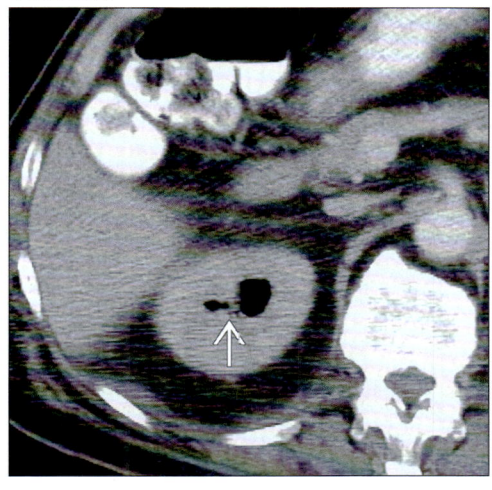 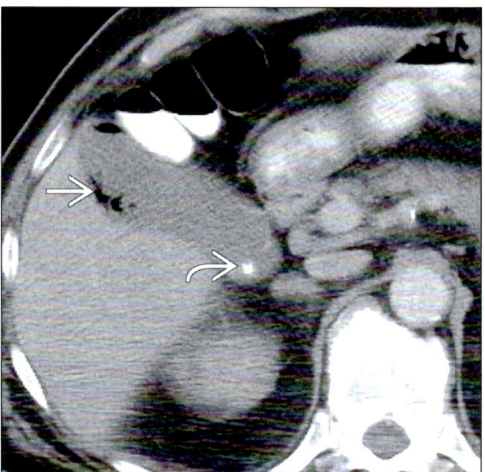

(Left) Axial CECT of diabetic patient with both emphysematous pyelonephritis and emphysematous cholecystitis. Note gas within renal collecting system of right kidney ➡. *(Right)* Axial CECT at level of gallbladder in same patient as previous image reveals gas in gallbladder lumen ➡ and calcified stone ➡.

RENAL ABSCESS

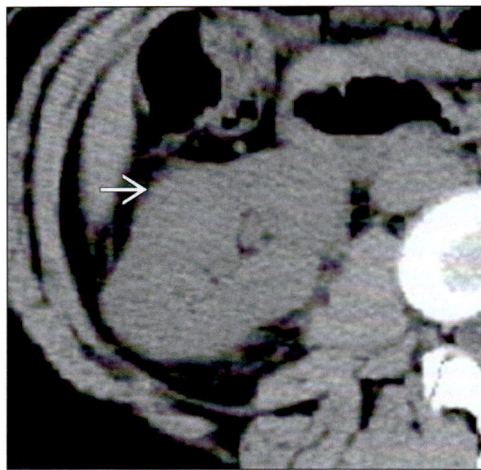

Axial NECT of renal abscess. Note slight bulge to right lateral renal contour ➡. Abscess cavity is not visible on NECT.

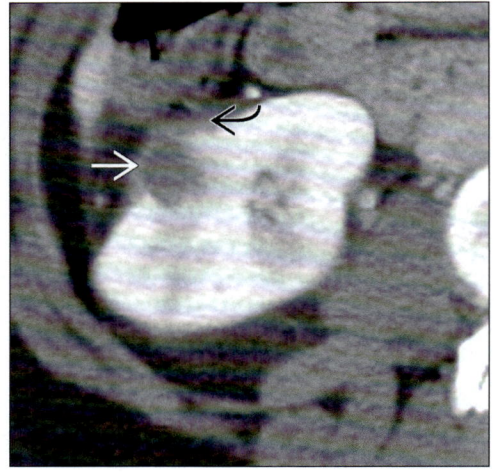

Axial CECT of same patient as left clearly reveals low-attenuation abscess ➡ with minimal perinephric extension ➡.

TERMINOLOGY

Definitions
- Localized collection of pus due to suppurative necrosis in kidney

IMAGING FINDINGS

General Features
- Best diagnostic clue: Spherical nonenhancing renal mass with perinephric stranding on CECT

Fluoroscopic Findings
- IVP
  - Impaired excretion
    - Delayed appearance time, decreased contrast density, decreased nephrogram
    - ± Absence of nephrogram and calyceal opacification
  - Heterogeneous nephrogram
  - Single or multiple, well-defined, round or irregular lucent mass
  - Calyceal or pelvic effacement
  - ± Calyceal, pelvic or ureteral dilatation

CT Findings
- NECT
  - Single (more common) or multiple; unilateral or bilateral
  - Round, well-marginated, low-attenuation masses
  - ± Gas within collection
- CECT
  - Enlarged kidney with focal areas of hypoattenuation (acute)
  - "Rim" or "ring" sign: Enhancement of abscess wall (subacute or chronic)
  - No central enhancement of lesion; enhancement of normal renal tissue
  - Obliteration of renal sinus or calyceal effacement
  - Thickened walls, mild dilatation of renal pelvis & ureter
  - Perinephric reaction or extension
    - Altered renal contour, indistinct renal outline, renal displacement
    - Edema or obliteration of perinephric fat
    - Thickened Gerota fascia and perinephric septa

DDx: Thick-Walled Cystic or Necrotic Lesion

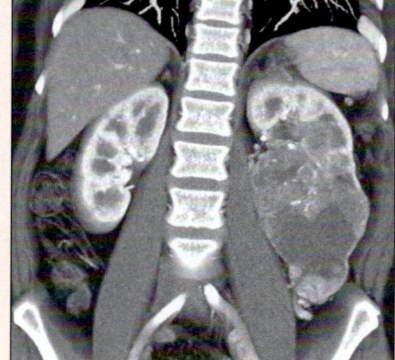

Renal Cell Carcinoma

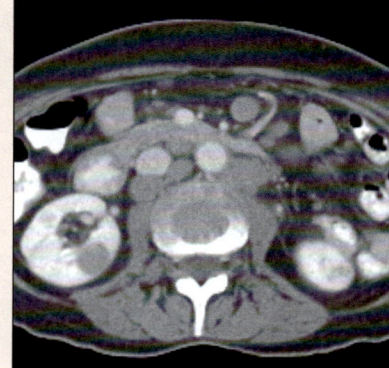

Renal Lymphoma

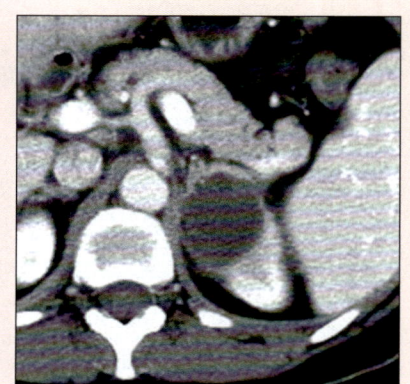

Infected Cyst

RENAL ABSCESS

Key Facts

Terminology
- Localized collection of pus due to suppurative necrosis in kidney

Imaging Findings
- Best diagnostic clue: Spherical nonenhancing renal mass with perinephric stranding on CECT
- ± Gas within collection
- "Rim" or "ring" sign: Enhancement of abscess wall (subacute or chronic)
- No central enhancement of lesion; enhancement of normal renal tissue

Top Differential Diagnoses
- Renal Cell Carcinoma (RCC)
- Metastases and Lymphoma
- Infected or Hemorrhagic Cyst

Pathology
- Accounts for 2% of all renal masses
- Sequelae of acute renal infections
- Acute pyelonephritis or focal bacterial nephritis
- Usually seen 1-2 weeks after infection
- Urinary tract infection → ascends to kidney → acute pyelonephritis or acute focal bacterial nephritis → liquefaction → sequestration → renal abscess

Clinical Issues
- Fever, flank or abdominal pain, chills, dysuria
- Antibiotic therapy

Diagnostic Checklist
- "Rim" sign; absence of lesion enhancement; perinephric stranding

MR Findings
- T1WI: Hypointense mass
- T2WI: Hyperintense mass, increased signal surrounding mass (perilesional edema)
- T1 C+: Rim enhancement (lesion < 1 cm enhances homogeneously)

Ultrasonographic Findings
- Grayscale Ultrasound
  o Anechoic or hypoechoic to echogenic fluid collection that blends with normal echogenic fat within Gerota fascia
  o Mass within or displacing kidney
  o Round, thick- or smooth-walled complex mass
  o Low-level internal echoes move with change of position (internal debris)
  o "Comet sign": Internal echogenic foci (gas within abscess)
    ▪ Associated posterior "dirty" shadowing
  o ± Internal septations or loculations

Angiographic Findings
- Conventional: Peripheral distribution, fine neovascular pattern

Nuclear Medicine Findings
- WBC Scan
  o ↑ Uptake of indium-111 labeled leukocytes noted within renal ± perinephric abscess
  o Possible false-negative leukocyte scans: Prior antibiotic therapy, walled-off abscesses, poorly developed inflammatory response
  o More sensitive or specific in early detection of renal ± perinephric infection

Imaging Recommendations
- Best imaging tool
  o MDCT with and without contrast
    ▪ Distinguish abscess from tumor

DIFFERENTIAL DIAGNOSIS

Renal Cell Carcinoma (RCC)
- CT enhancement of solitary mass
- Angiography: Hypervascularity
- Symptoms rare, usually asymptomatic
- 25-40% are diagnosed by incidental findings on CT or US
- 25-30% are present with metastases (lung, mediastinum, bone, liver)
- Clinical history and urinalysis can differentiate

Metastases and Lymphoma
- Metastases (lung, breast, gastrointestinal, malignant melanoma)
  o Almost all develop via hematogenous spread
  o Lung, breast & colon carcinoma are occasionally large & solitary; difficult to differentiate from RCC
  o Multifocal, small, enhancing (5-30 HU) nodules on CT; widespread nonrenal metastases
  o Angiography: Hypovascular pattern
  o Asymptomatic (most common), or flank pain & hematuria
  o CT- or US-guided biopsy for pathologic confirmation
- Lymphoma
  o CT: Multiple distinct masses (45%); direct invasion from enlarged retroperitoneal nodes (25%); solitary mass (15%); diffuse infiltration (10%); predominantly perinephric involvement (5%)
  o Asymptomatic (most common); fever, weight loss, flank pain, hematuria, renal failure

Infected or Hemorrhagic Cyst
- Solitary, nonenhancing lesion
- CT: Absence of perinephric stranding, "rim" sign, shaggy wall, hyperintense mass
- May be indistinguishable on imaging

RENAL ABSCESS

PATHOLOGY

General Features
- General path comments
  - Accounts for 2% of all renal masses
  - Sequelae of acute renal infections
    - Acute pyelonephritis or focal bacterial nephritis
    - Usually seen 1-2 weeks after infection
- Etiology
  - Ascending urinary tract infections (80%)
    - Calculi, obstruction, renal anomalies, urinary reflux (diabetes or pregnancy)
    - Iatrogenic intervention (catheterization)
    - Gram-negative organisms (E. coli, Proteus species, Klebsiella species)
    - Abscesses likely form at corticomedullary junction
  - Hematogenous spread (20%)
    - IV drug users and skin infection
    - Hematogenous seeding from other infected sites (valvular heart disease, prosthesis)
    - Iatrogenic intervention (cyst aspiration, embolization of kidney vessels)
    - Gram-positive and gram-negative organisms (Staphylococcus aureus, Streptococcus species or Enterobacteriaceae family)
    - Abscesses likely form at renal cortex
  - Risk factors: Diabetes mellitus, long-term hemodialysis, IV drug users
  - Pathogenesis
    - Urinary tract infection → ascends to kidney → acute pyelonephritis or acute focal bacterial nephritis → liquefaction → sequestration → renal abscess
- Epidemiology: Incidence: Renal abscess (0.2%); perinephric abscess (0.02%)
- Associated abnormalities: 20-60% of patients with renal or perinephric abscess have urolithiasis

Gross Pathologic & Surgical Features
- Well-defined, round, thick- or smooth-walled mass

Microscopic Features
- Infected and necrotic tissue; ± gas

CLINICAL ISSUES

Presentation
- Most common signs/symptoms
  - Fever, flank or abdominal pain, chills, dysuria
  - Symptoms longer than 2 weeks
  - Costovertebral angle tenderness, palpable flank mass
- Lab data
  - Urinalysis: Elevated WBC (75%), positive bacterial culture (33%)
  - Blood tests: Elevated erythrocyte sedimentation rate (ESR), positive bacterial culture (50%)

Demographics
- Age: All ages
- Gender: M = F

Natural History & Prognosis
- Complications
  - Rupture into perinephric space (perinephric abscess) → beyond Gerota fascia (paranephric abscess) → psoas or transversalis muscles → anterior peritoneal cavity → subdiaphragmatic or pelvic abscess
  - Rupture → renal collecting system → pyonephrosis
  - Compression or obstruction → hydronephrosis → renal atrophy
  - Necrosis and cavitation
- Prognosis
  - Good if early diagnosis and treatment
  - Poor if delayed diagnosis and treatment

Treatment
- Antibiotic therapy
  - If causative organisms are known, use specific antibiotics
  - If unknown, treat empirically with broad-spectrum antibiotics (ampicillin or vancomycin with aminoglycoside or third-generation cephalosporin)
- If abscess not resolved within 48 hours post antibiotics, percutaneous aspiration & drainage under CT or US
  - Well-defined mass on CT or fluid-filled mass on US indicates "ripe" abscess for drainage
- If abscess still not resolved, open surgical drainage or nephrectomy
- Follow-up
  - Imaging to confirm resolution of abscess
  - Evaluate for underlying urinary tract abnormalities

DIAGNOSTIC CHECKLIST

Consider
- Clinical history & urinalysis to diagnose & differentiate from malignancy

Image Interpretation Pearls
- "Rim" sign; absence of lesion enhancement; perinephric stranding

SELECTED REFERENCES

1. Dalla Palma L et al: Medical treatment of renal and perirenal abscesses: CT evaluation. Clin Radiol. 54(12):792-7, 1999
2. Yen DH et al: Renal abscess: early diagnosis and treatment. Am J Emerg Med. 17(2):192-7, 1999
3. Davidson AJ et al: Radiologic assessment of renal masses: Implications for patient care. Radiology 202: 297-305, 1997
4. Kawashima A et al: CT of renal inflammatory disease. Radiographics. 17: 851-866, 1997
5. Brown ED et al: Renal abscesses: appearance on gadolinium-enhanced magnetic resonance images. Abdom Imaging. 21(2):172-6, 1996
6. Rinder MR: Renal abscess: an illustrative case and review of the literature. Md Med J. 45(10):839-43, 1996
7. Siegel JF et al: Minimally invasive treatment of renal abscess. J Urol. 155(1):52-5, 1996
8. Talner LB et al: Acute pyelonephritis: can we agree on terminology? Radiology 192: 297-305, 1994
9. Goldman SM et al: Upper urinary tract infection: the current role of CT, ultrasound, and MRI. Semin Ultrasound CT MR. 12(4):335-60, 1991
10. Jeffrey RB et al: CT and ultrasonography of acute renal abnormalities. Radiol Clin North Am. 21(3):515-25, 1983

RENAL ABSCESS

IMAGE GALLERY

Typical

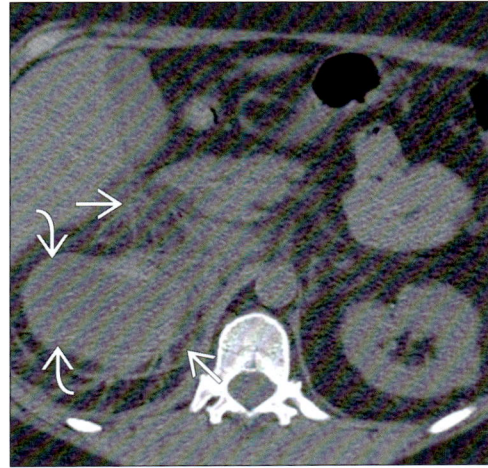
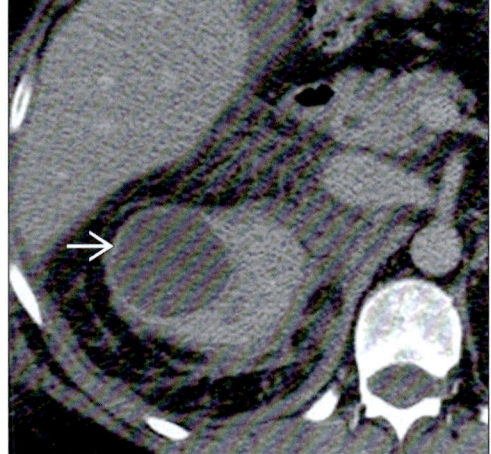

(Left) Axial NECT shows significant perinephric fat stranding around right kidney ➡, with exophytic, high-attenuation, mass-like collection ➡ in right kidney. *(Right)* Axial CECT in same patient as left several days post-antibiotic treatment. Follow-up examination was performed & shows smaller, organized & well-capsulated cystic mass ➡, which was drained via US guidance.

Variant

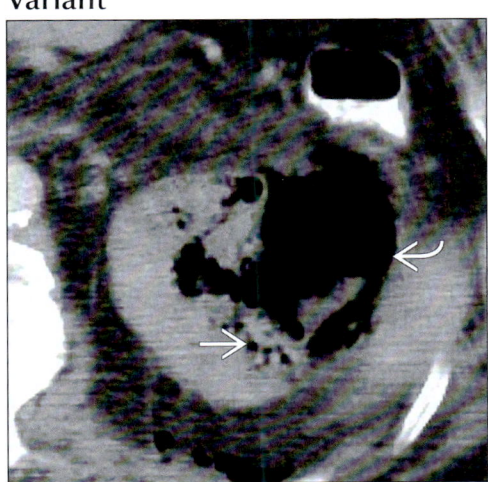
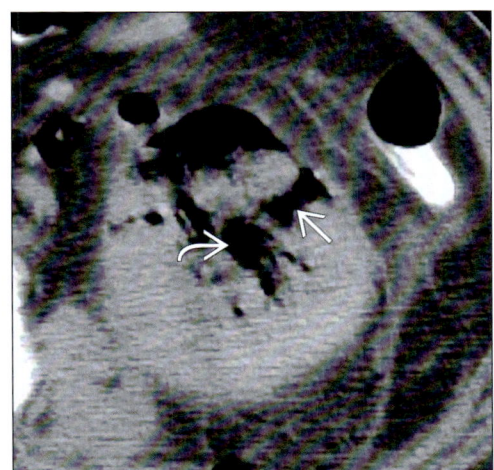

(Left) Axial NECT of gas-forming renal & perirenal abscess in diabetic patient. Note extensive gas collection ➡ within renal parenchyma with perinephric extension ➡. *(Right)* Axial NECT at lower level in same patient as left reveals parenchymal gas ➡ and gas in central collection system ➡.

Typical

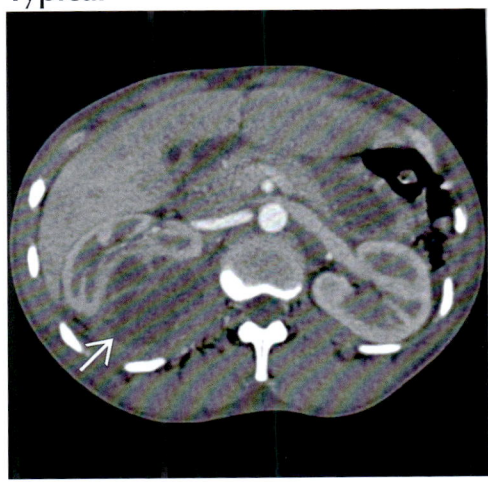
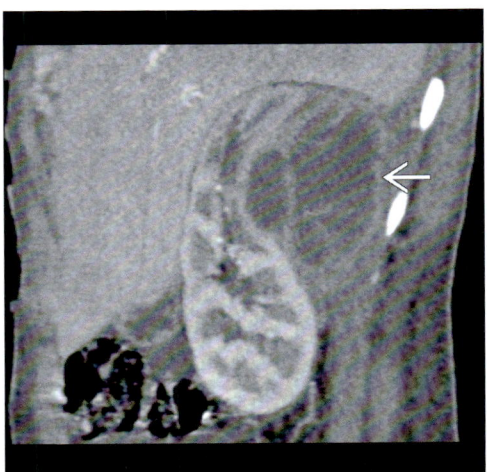

(Left) Axial CECT shows renal & perirenal abscess. Corticomedullary phase shows large mass ➡ deforming & displacing upper pole of right kidney. *(Right)* Sagittal CECT reformatted image in same patient as left demonstrates relationship of mass to upper pole of right kidney. Abscess ➡ is multi-septated & replaces part of upper pole.

XANTHOGRANULOMATOUS PYELONEPHRITIS

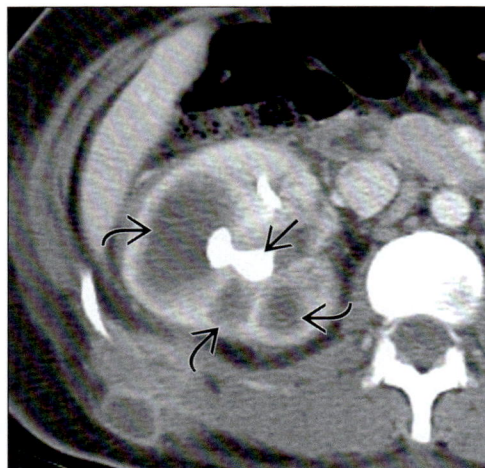 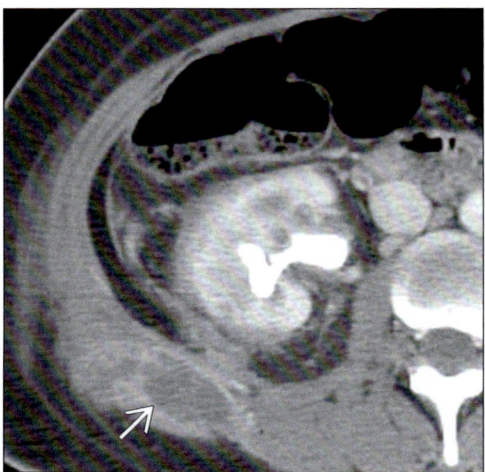

Axial CECT of XGP with flank abscess. Non-functioning right kidney demonstrates staghorn calculus ➔ and extensive low-attenuation areas of necrotic tissue within parenchyma ➔.

Axial CECT at lower level in same patient as left reveals associated flank abscess ➔.

TERMINOLOGY

Abbreviations and Synonyms
- Xanthogranulomatous pyelonephritis (XGP) or (XGPN)

Definitions
- Chronic infection of kidney & surrounding tissues characterized by destruction of renal parenchyma & replacement by lipid-laden macrophages

IMAGING FINDINGS

General Features
- Best diagnostic clue: Obstructing calculus, atrophic or nonfunctioning kidney, perirenal fibrofatty proliferation
- Location
  - Two forms of XGP
    - Diffuse (83-90%): Involves entire kidney
    - Segmental or focal (10-17%): Tumefactive due to obstructed single infundibulum; one moiety of duplex system
  - Most often unilateral
- Size: 2.5-5.8 cm; mean 3.8 cm
- Morphology: Well-circumscribed mass with global or focal renal enlargement

Fluoroscopic Findings
- IVP
  - Diffuse or focally absent nephrogram
  - Contracted pelvis; dilated calices
  - Centrally obstructing calculus; staghorn (75%)
- Retrograde pyelography
  - Complete obstruction at ureteropelvic junction; infundibulum; proximal ureter
  - Contracted renal pelvis; dilated deformed calices with nodular filling defects
  - Irregular parenchymal masses with cavitation

CT Findings
- Multiple, focal, low-attenuation (-10 to +30 HU) masses scattered throughout kidney
  - Dilated, debris-filled calyces & xanthoma collections
- Bright enhancement of rims of xanthoma collections due to inflammatory hypervascularity
  - No enhancement of collections

DDx: Decreased Renal Function and Mass

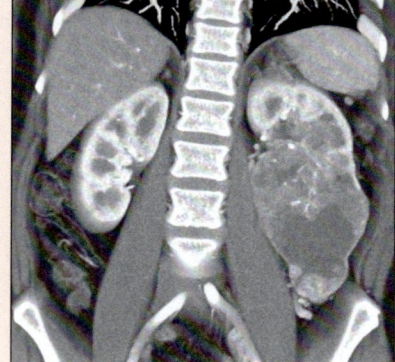 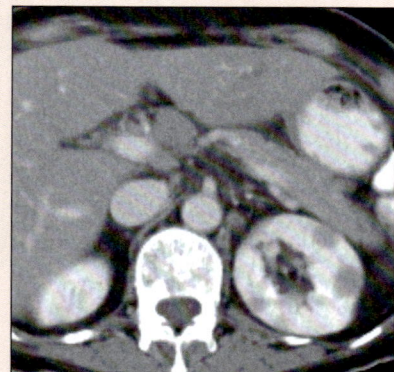 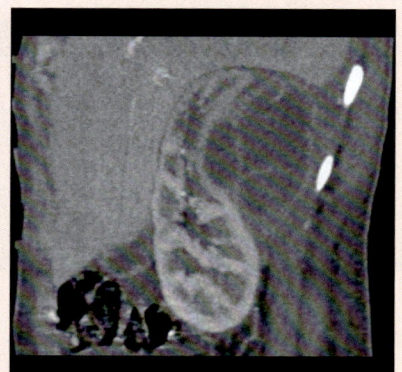

Renal Cell Carcinoma   *Non-Hodgkin Lymphoma*   *Perirenal Abscess*

XANTHOGRANULOMATOUS PYELONEPHRITIS

Key Facts

Terminology
- Chronic infection of kidney & surrounding tissues characterized by destruction of renal parenchyma & replacement by lipid-laden macrophages

Imaging Findings
- Best diagnostic clue: Obstructing calculus, atrophic or nonfunctioning kidney, perirenal fibrofatty proliferation

Top Differential Diagnoses
- Renal Cell Carcinoma
- Transitional Cell Carcinoma
- Renal Metastases and Lymphoma
- Renal Abscess
- Hydronephrosis/Pyonephrosis

Pathology
- Accumulation of lipid-laden "foamy" macrophages (xanthoma cells) & granulomatous infiltrate

Clinical Issues
- Antibiotic treatment prior to surgical intervention
- Nephrectomy usually required: Radical in complete XGP, partial in focal XGP

Diagnostic Checklist
- Some variation possible (small kidney, lack of calculi); difficult to distinguish XGP from other infections or neoplasms
- Histologic diagnosis required, not based solely on imaging studies
- Poor or absent contrast excretion from kidney; staghorn calculi

---

- Poor or absent excretion of contrast into collecting system (nonfunctioning kidney)
- Obliterated renal sinus fat (inflammation)
- Perinephric extension (14%)
  - Perirenal space, pararenal space, ipsilateral psoas muscle, colon, spleen, diaphragm, posterior abdominal wall, skin
- Large central calculus, often staghorn
- Gas seen rarely

MR Findings
- Thin renal parenchymal rim
- Loss of corticomedullary differentiation
- T1 & T2WI: Intermediate to high signal intensity of dilated collecting system & surrounding renal parenchyma
  - Increased fat content in macrophages
- T2WI: Negative defects within dilated collecting system (renal calculi)

Ultrasonographic Findings
- Grayscale Ultrasound
  - Multiple anechoic or hypoechoic masses replacing normal corticomedullary differentiation & contracted pelvis
  - Peripelvic fibrosis may obscure acoustic shadowing from central staghorn calculus
  - Parenchymal thinning & hydronephrosis
  - Echoes in dilated collecting system
  - Perinephric fluid collection

Angiographic Findings
- Conventional
  - Stretching of segmental or interlobar arteries around large avascular masses
  - Hypervascularity/blush around mass periphery in late arterial phase (granulation tissue)
  - Venous encasement with occlusion

Imaging Recommendations
- Best imaging tool: MDCT

DIFFERENTIAL DIAGNOSIS

Renal Cell Carcinoma
- Solitary, soft tissue density mass (30-50 HU) with central necrosis
- Hypervascular mass at renal cortex

Transitional Cell Carcinoma
- Renal infiltration → calyceal invasion, renal enlargement, poorly defined margins without change in shape
- Renal pelvic filling defect, irregular narrowing of collecting system
- Encasing pelvicaliceal system → hypovascular tumor

Renal Metastases and Lymphoma
- Metastases: Lung, breast, colon, malignant melanoma
  - Usually hypovascular with infiltrative growth
- Lymphoma
  - Usually multiple or bilateral with infiltrative growth
  - Hypoechoic, hypovascular, solitary, intrarenal mass ± adenopathy

Renal Abscess
- Solitary or multiple, round, well-marginated, low-attenuation mass
- Wall enhancement without central enhancement
- Perinephric stranding
- ± Presence of gas

Hydronephrosis/Pyonephrosis
- Pus-filled collecting system may simulate XGP

PATHOLOGY

General Features
- General path comments
  - Usually found with chronic obstruction (calculus, stricture, carcinoma)
  - Renal pelvis often less dilated than expected for high-grade chronic obstruction
- Etiology

XANTHOGRANULOMATOUS PYELONEPHRITIS

- ○ Escherichia coli
- ○ Proteus mirabilis
- ○ Staphylococcus aureus
- ○ Klebsiella species
- ○ Pseudomonas species
- ○ Enterobacter species
- ○ Risk factors
  - Recurrent or chronic urinary tract infections
  - Diabetes mellitus in immunocompromised patients
  - Abnormal lipid metabolism
- ○ Pathogenesis
  - Chronic renal obstruction & infection with failure of local host immunity
- Epidemiology: Incidence: 1% of all renal infections
- Associated abnormalities: Urolithiasis

Gross Pathologic & Surgical Features

- Diffuse
  - ○ Renal enlargement, indurated or thickened perinephric fat
  - ○ Dilated renal pelvis with staghorn calculus
  - ○ Replacement of corticomedullary junction with soft yellow nodules; pus- and debris-filled calices
- Focal
  - ○ Yellowish-white, solid or semisolid renal mass

Microscopic Features

- Accumulation of lipid-laden "foamy" macrophages (xanthoma cells) & granulomatous infiltrate
- Foam cells contain neutral fat & cholesterol (ester granules); positive for periodic acid-Schiff (PAS) stain
- Diffuse infiltration by plasma cells & histiocytes

Staging, Grading or Classification Criteria

- Three stages of XGP
  - ○ Stage 1: Confined to kidney
  - ○ Stage 2: Extension to perirenal space
  - ○ Stage 3: Spread to pararenal spaces ± abdominal wall

CLINICAL ISSUES

Presentation

- Most common signs/symptoms
  - ○ Dull or persistent flank pain, fever
  - ○ Palpable mass, weight loss
- Lab data
  - ○ Urinalysis: Microscopic hematuria, proteinuria, pyuria
  - ○ Urine culture: Specific bacterial species
  - ○ Elevated liver function tests
  - ○ Elevated erythrocyte sedimentation rate (ESR)

Demographics

- Age
  - ○ 45-65 years of age most common
  - ○ Very rare in childhood; focal form more common in children
- Gender: M:F = 1:3-4

Natural History & Prognosis

- Symptomatic 6 months prior to diagnosis (40% of cases)
- Complications
  - ○ Hepatic dysfunction (reversible)
  - ○ Extrarenal extension
  - ○ Fistulas (pyelocutaneous, ureterocutaneous)
  - ○ Hemorrhage
- Prognosis good
- Rare mortality, but morbidity can be substantial

Treatment

- Antibiotic treatment prior to surgical intervention
- Nephrectomy usually required: Radical in complete XGP, partial in focal XGP

DIAGNOSTIC CHECKLIST

Consider

- Some variation possible (small kidney, lack of calculi); difficult to distinguish XGP from other infections or neoplasms
- Histologic diagnosis required, not based solely on imaging studies

Image Interpretation Pearls

- Poor or absent contrast excretion from kidney; staghorn calculi

SELECTED REFERENCES

1. Kim J: Ultrasonographic features of focal xanthogranulomatous pyelonephritis. J Ultrasound Med. 23(3):409-16, 2004
2. Cakmakci H et al: Pediatric focal xanthogranulomatous pyelonephritis: dynamic contrast-enhanced MRI findings. Clin Imaging. 26(3):183-6, 2002
3. Kim JC: US and CT findings of xanthogranulomatous pyelonephritis. Clin Imaging. 25(2):118-21, 2001
4. Tiu CM et al: Sonographic features of xanthogranulomatous pyelonephritis. J Clin Ultrasound. 29(5):279-85, 2001
5. Verswijvel G et al: Xanthogranulomatous pyelonephritis: MRI findings in the diffuse and the focal type. Eur Radiol. 10(4):586-9, 2000
6. Fan CM et al: Xanthogranulomatous pyelonephritis. AJR Am J Roentgenol. 165(4):1008, 1995
7. Eastham J et al: Xanthogranulomatous pyelonephritis: clinical findings and surgical considerations. Urology. 43(3):295-9, 1994
8. Rabushka LS et al: Pictorial review: computed tomography of renal inflammatory disease. Urology. 44(4):473-80, 1994
9. Chuang CK et al: Xanthogranulomatous pyelonephritis: experience in 36 cases. J Urol. 147(2):333-6, 1992
10. Hayes WS et al: From the Archives of the AFIP. Xanthogranulomatous pyelonephritis. Radiographics. 11(3):485-98, 1991
11. Mulopulos GP et al: MR imaging of xanthogranulomatous pyelonephritis. J Comput Assist Tomogr. 10(1):154-6, 1986
12. Goldman SM et al: CT of xanthogranulomatous pyelonephritis: radiologic-pathologic correlation. AJR Am J Roentgenol. 142(5):963-9, 1984
13. Bissada NK et al: Preoperative diagnosis of xanthogranulomatous pyelonephritis. Urology. 7(2):228-30, 1976
14. Cha EM et al: Xanthogranulomatous pyelonephritis. Angiographic evaluation. Urology. 3(2):159-62, 1974
15. Vinik M et al: Xanthogranulomatous pyelonephritis: angiographic considerations. Radiology. 92(3):537-40, 1969

XANTHOGRANULOMATOUS PYELONEPHRITIS

IMAGE GALLERY

Typical

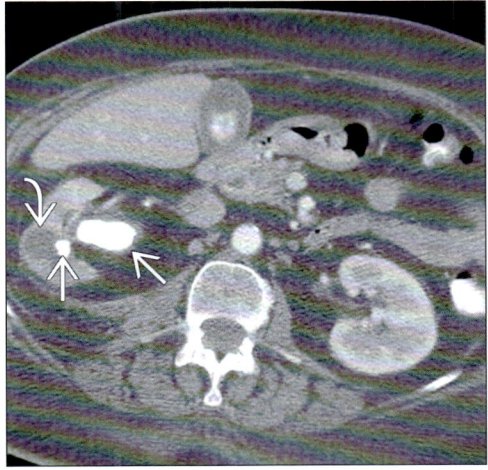
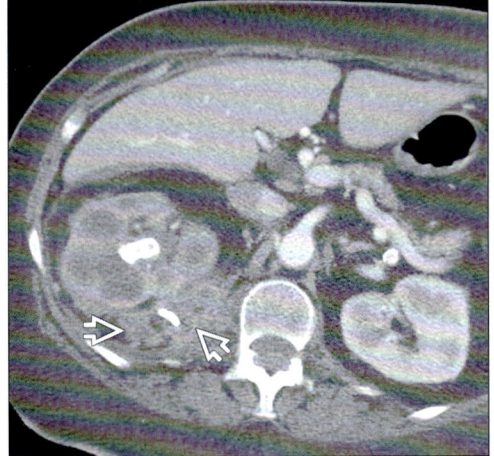

(Left) Axial CECT shows XGP with perirenal abscess. Large central staghorn calculi ⮕ cause replacement of right kidney with low-density substance 2° chronic obstruction ⮕. *(Right)* Axial CECT in same patient as left demonstrates additional finding of perirenal fluid collections ⮕, indicating perirenal extension of infection.

Typical

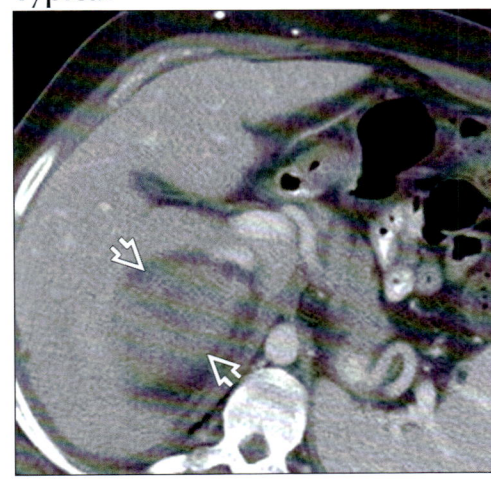
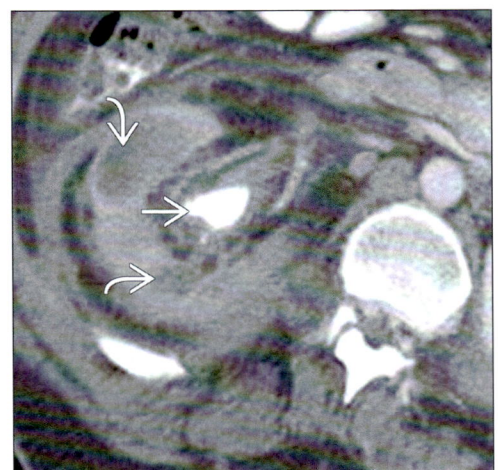

(Left) Axial CECT shows inflammatory changes in right perinephric region ⮕ due to xanthogranulomatous nephritis. *(Right)* Axial CECT in same patient as left shows central large staghorn calculus ⮕ as well as low-density regions ⮕, due to chronic inflammatory tissue replacing kidney.

Variant

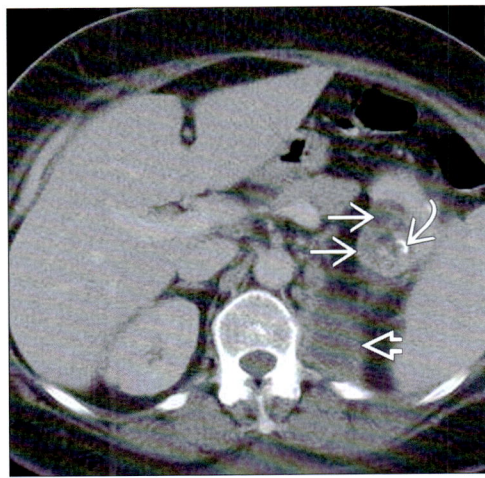
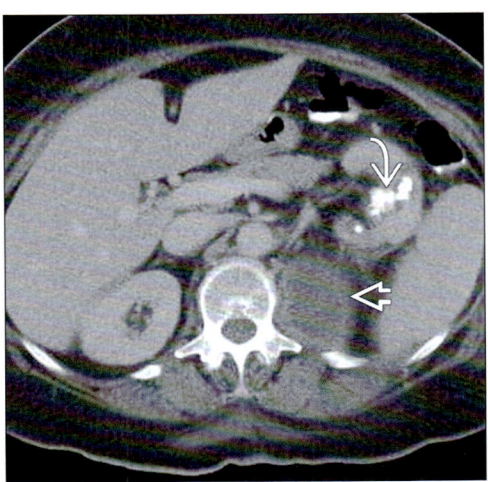

(Left) Axial CECT shows focal areas of low density in posterior aspect of upper pole of left kidney, extending centrally ⮕ due to focal XGP. Note calculi ⮕ & large paraspinal/posterior pararenal abscess ⮕. *(Right)* Axial CECT in same patient as left again demonstrates calculi ⮕ and abscess ⮕.

EMPHYSEMATOUS PYELONEPHRITIS

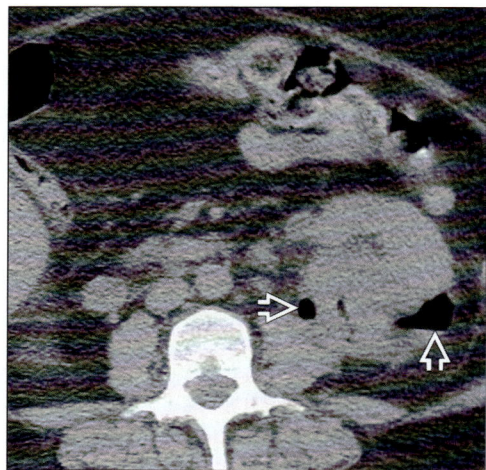

Axial NECT shows large gas collections in left renal parenchyma ➡.

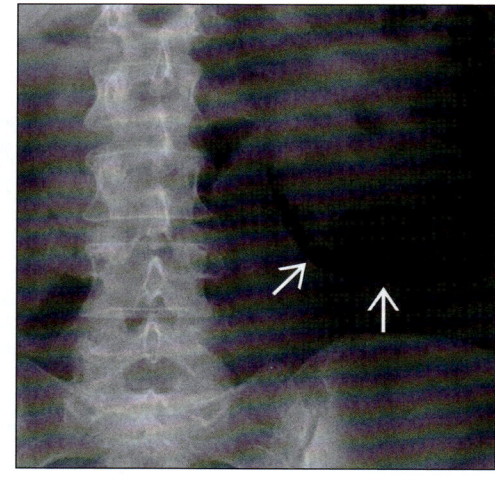

Anteroposterior radiograph in same patient as left demonstrates curvilinear gas collection ➡ outlining lower pole of left kidney.

TERMINOLOGY

Abbreviations and Synonyms
- Emphysematous pyelonephritis (EPN)

Definitions
- Gas-forming renal infection

IMAGING FINDINGS

General Features
- Best diagnostic clue: Gas in renal parenchyma on CT

Radiographic Findings
- Radiography: Gas in parenchyma ± perinephric space

CT Findings
- CECT
  - Type I: Parenchymal destruction without fluid; streaky/mottled gas radiating from medulla to cortex; ± crescent of subcapsular or perinephric gas
  - Type II: Renal or perirenal fluid abscesses; bubbly gas pattern; ± gas within renal pelvis
  - Mottled areas of ↓ attenuation
  - Intraparenchymal, intracaliceal, intrapelvic gas

Ultrasonographic Findings
- Grayscale Ultrasound
  - Highly echogenic areas within renal sinus & parenchyma with "dirty" shadowing
  - Ring-down artifacts: Air bubbles trapped in fluid

Imaging Recommendations
- Best imaging tool: MDCT

DIFFERENTIAL DIAGNOSIS

Emphysematous Pyelitis
- Gas in renal pelvis & calices, not parenchyma
- 50% diabetics; less grave prognosis than EPN

Perforated Duodenal Ulcer
- Occasionally gas "outlines" kidney

Iatrogenic
- Retrograde pyelography, nephrostomy
- Chemoembolization/ablation of renal tumor

DDx: Gas in or Around Kidney

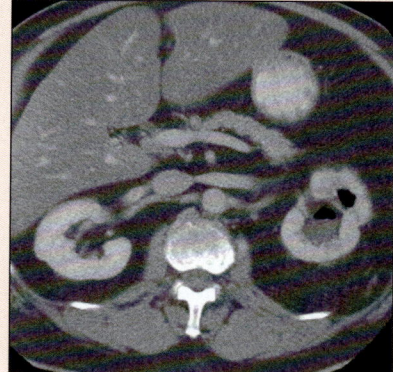

Emphysematous Pyelitis

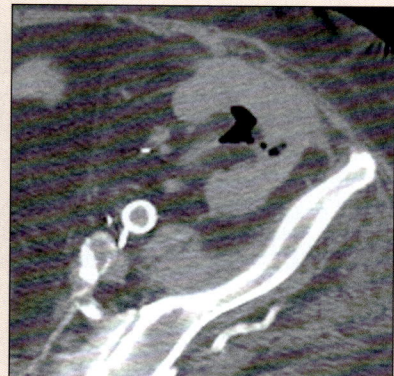

Emphysematous Pyelitis

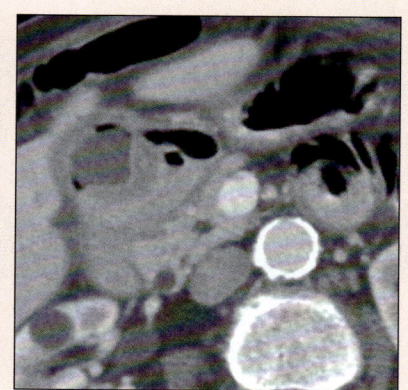

Perforated Duodenal Ulcer

EMPHYSEMATOUS PYELONEPHRITIS

Key Facts

Imaging Findings
- Best diagnostic clue: Gas in renal parenchyma on CT
- Type I: Parenchymal destruction without fluid; streaky/mottled gas radiating from medulla to cortex; ± crescent of subcapsular or perinephric gas
- Type II: Renal or perirenal fluid abscesses; bubbly gas pattern; ± gas within renal pelvis

Top Differential Diagnoses
- Emphysematous Pyelitis
- Perforated Duodenal Ulcer
- Iatrogenic

Clinical Issues
- Poor prognosis: Mortality 66% with type 1, 60-75% with antibiotic therapy, 80% if perinephric extension

Diagnostic Checklist
- Exclude EPN in diabetics with pyelonephritis

PATHOLOGY

General Features
- Etiology
  - Single or mixed organism infection
    - E. coli (68%), Klebsiella pneumoniae (9%)
  - Risk factors
    - Recurrent or chronic UTI
    - Immunocompromised diabetics (87-97%)
    - Ureteral obstruction (20-40%): Calculi, stenosis
  - Pathogenesis: Pyelonephritis → ischemia & low oxygen tension → facultative anaerobes proliferation in anaerobic environment → CO_2 production

Gross Pathologic & Surgical Features
- Suppurative necrotizing renal parenchyma & perirenal tissue, multiple cortical abscesses

Staging, Grading or Classification Criteria
- Type I: "True" EPN (33% of cases)
  - Parenchymal destruction without fluid; streaky or mottled gas radiating from medulla to cortex
- Type II (66% of cases)
  - Renal or perirenal fluid abscesses with bubbly gas

CLINICAL ISSUES

Presentation
- Most common signs/symptoms
  - Fever, chills, flank pain, lethargy, confusion
  - Nausea, vomiting, dyspnea, crepitant mass
- Lab data: Hyperglycemia, acidosis, electrolyte imbalance, thrombocytopenia; positive blood, urine, and/or aspiration cultures

Demographics
- Age: 19-81 years of age; mean 54 years
- Gender: M:F = 1:2-6

Natural History & Prognosis
- Complications: Sepsis
- Poor prognosis: Mortality 66% with type 1, 60-75% with antibiotic therapy, 80% if perinephric extension

Treatment
- Antibiotic therapy; nephrectomy for type I
- CT-guided drainage (type II): 70% success rate

DIAGNOSTIC CHECKLIST

Consider
- Exclude EPN in diabetics with pyelonephritis

SELECTED REFERENCES
1. Grayson DE et al: Emphysematous infections of the abdomen and pelvis: a pictorial review. Radiographics. 22(3):543-61, 2002
2. Wan YL et al: Acute gas-producing bacterial renal infection: correlation between imaging findings and clinical outcome. Radiology. 198(2):433-8, 1996

IMAGE GALLERY

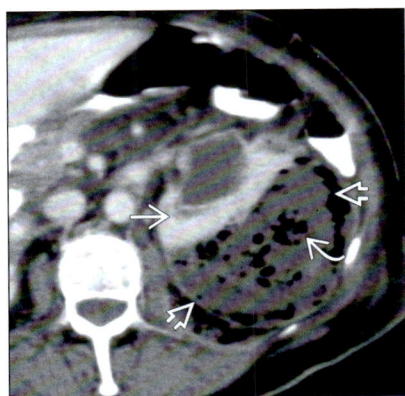 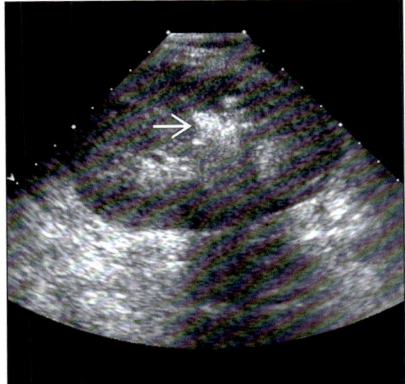 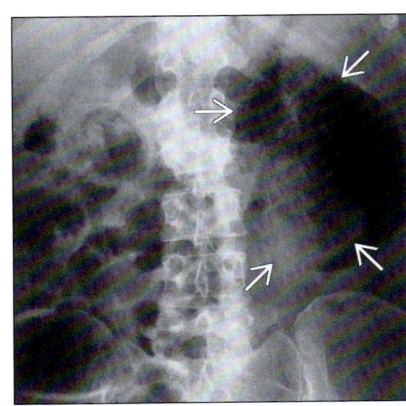

(Left) Axial CECT shows large left perinephric fluid collection ➔ containing gas bubbles ➔; note compressed left kidney ➔. (Center) Transverse ultrasound shows echogenic foci with shadowing ➔, indicative of parenchymal gas. This patient expired before surgery could be considered. (Right) Frontal radiograph shows typical radiographic appearance of emphysematous pyelonephritis. Mottled lucency in left retroperitoneum ➔ corresponds to kidney infected by gas-forming organism.

RENAL INFARCTION

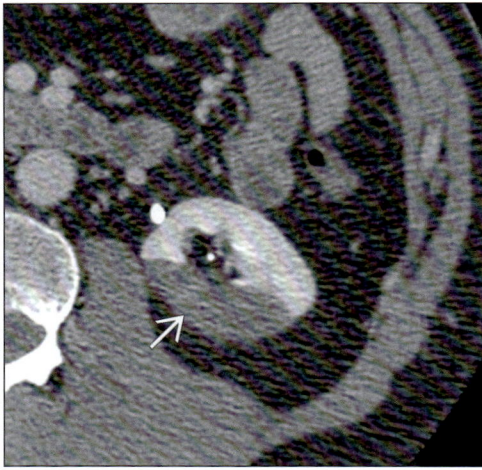

Axial CECT of acute left renal infarction. Note wedge-shaped area of nonenhancement within posterior left kidney ➡.

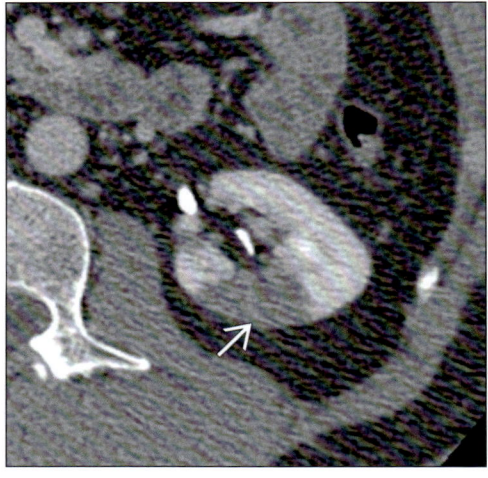

Axial CECT at more cranial level in same patient as left demonstrates area of infarction ➡.

TERMINOLOGY

Definitions
- Localized or global area of ischemic necrosis in kidney, resulting most often from sudden occlusion of renal artery (RA) supply

IMAGING FINDINGS

General Features
- Best diagnostic clue: Nonenhancing wedge-shaped area with enhancing cortical rim

Fluoroscopic Findings
- IVP
  ○ Segmental or subsegmental infarction
    ▪ Focal absent or decreased nephrogram
  ○ Global infarction
    ▪ Complete absence of nephrogram & excretion

CT Findings
- Variable based on etiology
  ○ Embolic: Multifocal & bilateral
  ○ Traumatic & thrombotic: Segmental or global & unilateral
- Focal subsegmental infarction
  ○ Small, sharply demarcated, wedge-shaped area of decreased or poor contrast enhancement
  ○ Base of wedge pointed towards renal capsule, apex towards hilum
- Focal segmental infarction
  ○ Sharply demarcated, dorsal or ventral segmental area of decreased enhancement
  ○ Straight-line demarcation between normal enhancing & abnormal nonenhancing parenchyma
    ▪ Strongly suggestive of ischemia
- Global infarction
  ○ Total absence of renal enhancement, no excretion, no perinephric hematoma (RA thrombosis)
    ▪ Renal outline preserved
  ○ Total absence of enhancement, large perinephric hematoma (RA avulsion)
  ○ ± Medullary striations: "Spoke-wheel" enhancement (collateral circulation)
- Acute infarction
  ○ Normal or enlarged kidney; smooth contour; ± subcapsular fluid collection

DDx: Striated, Wedge or Global Nonenhancement

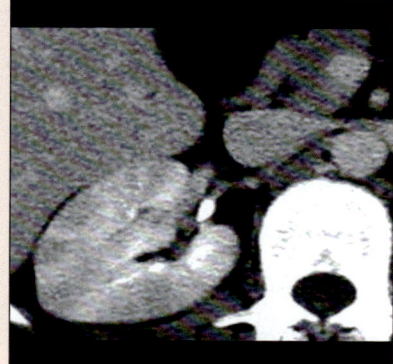

Pyelonephritis

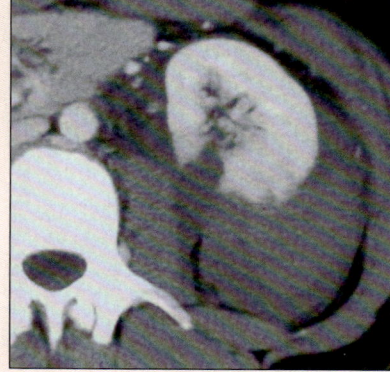

Renal Trauma

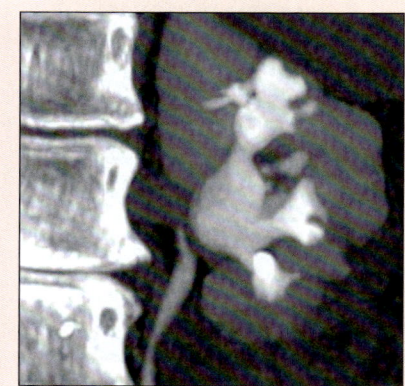

Renal Tuberculosis

RENAL INFARCTION

Key Facts

Terminology
- Localized or global area of ischemic necrosis in kidney, resulting most often from sudden occlusion of renal artery (RA) supply

Imaging Findings
- Best diagnostic clue: Nonenhancing wedge-shaped area with enhancing cortical rim
- Total absence of renal enhancement, no excretion, no perinephric hematoma (RA thrombosis)
- Total absence of enhancement, large perinephric hematoma (RA avulsion)
- "Cortical rim" sign: Subacute infarction

Top Differential Diagnoses
- Pyelonephritis
- Vasculitis
- Renal Trauma
- Renal Tuberculosis (TB)

Pathology
- Cardiac embolism is most common etiology
- Thrombosis
- Trauma

Clinical Issues
- Complications: Necrosis, infection, abscess formation

Diagnostic Checklist
- Correlate with history: Trauma, cardiac, aortic disease
- Pyelonephritis & acute infarction may have similar appearance
- Straight line demarcation & cortical rim sign favor infarction
- Perinephric stranding favors pyelonephritis

  - Absent or decreased nephrogram
  - "Cortical rim" sign: Subacute infarction
    - Preserved capsular or subcapsular enhancement
    - Usually seen 6-8 hrs after infarction
    - Seen in 50% cases of infarction (intact collateral circulation)
- Chronic infarction
  - Small kidney with smooth or irregular contour
  - Absent or diminished enhancement; no cortical rim sign

MR Findings
- T1WI: Low-signal intensity lesion
- T2WI: Low-signal intensity lesion
- T1 C+: Sharply demarcates nonenhanced infarction from densely enhancing noninfarcted tissue

Ultrasonographic Findings
- Color Doppler: May show focal or global absence of blood flow in affected kidney

Angiographic Findings
- Conventional
  - Confirm diagnosis of renal infarction with selective renal arteriography
    - Focal segmental infarction: Nonopacification of focal cortical area
    - Global infarction: Total absence of renal enhancement

Nuclear Medicine Findings
- SPECT imaging with Tc-99m DMSA
  - Acute infarction: Photon-deficient area

Imaging Recommendations
- Best imaging tool: MDCT with contrast; color Doppler sonography; selective renal angiography

DIFFERENTIAL DIAGNOSIS

Pyelonephritis
- Acute
  - Cortical wedge-shaped or striated nephrogram
    - May simulate focal segmental or subsegmental infarction
  - Loss of normal corticomedullary differentiation
  - Renal enlargement, focal swelling
  - Thickening of Gerota fascia & perinephric stranding
  - Calyceal effacement, dilated renal pelvis & ureter
- Chronic
  - Small kidney with cortical scarring over dilated calices
  - Unilateral with compensatory hypertrophy of contralateral kidney

Vasculitis
- Polyarteritis nodosa; SLE; scleroderma; drug abuse
- Wedge-shaped or striated nephrogram, usually bilateral & diffuse
- Parenchymal scarring, capsular retraction (may be same pathology as infarction)
- Microaneurysmal dilatation of small vessels

Renal Trauma
- Irregular linear or segmental nonenhancing tissue & subcapsular or perinephric hematoma
- Lacerations: Irregular or linear hypodense areas
- "Shattered kidney"
  - RA avulsion
    - Global infarction & perinephric hematoma
  - RA thrombosis
    - Global infarction + no perinephric hematoma
- Segmental infarction: Nonenhancing wedge-shaped areas

Renal Tuberculosis (TB)
- Multiple cortical scars
- Parenchymal calcification
- Strictures of collecting system and ureter
  - "Putty kidney" of end-stage calcification

PATHOLOGY

General Features
- Etiology

RENAL INFARCTION

- ○ Cardiac embolism is most common etiology
  - ▪ Rheumatic, arrhythmias, MI, prosthetic valve, SBE
- ○ Thrombosis
  - ▪ Atherosclerosis, polyarteritis nodosa
  - ▪ Aneurysm or dissection (aorta, RA)
  - ▪ Sickle cell disease, thrombotic thrombocytopenic purpura, thromboangiitis obliterans
- ○ Trauma
  - ▪ Blunt or penetrating
  - ▪ Surgery, interventional procedures
- Associated abnormalities: Cardiac abnormalities, hypercoagulable state, aortic aneurysm or dissection

Gross Pathologic & Surgical Features
- Wedge-shaped infarct, white or pale in color
- RA thrombus or traumatic avulsion
- Large or small kidney with smooth or irregular contour

Microscopic Features
- Focal or global renal ischemic changes
- Necrosis & scarring

Staging, Grading or Classification Criteria
- Classification based on onset
  - ○ Acute, subacute & chronic
- Classification based on anatomy & vascular distribution
  - ○ Focal: Segmental or subsegmental (cortex ± medulla)
  - ○ Global
- Focal traumatic segmental or subsegmental renal infarct (more common)
  - ○ Grade I & II renal injuries
  - ○ Thrombosis or laceration of segmental RA branch
  - ○ Solitary or multiple, frequently associated with other renal injuries
  - ○ Results in renal scar
- Global traumatic renal infarct
  - ○ Grade III renal injury
  - ○ Thrombosis, transection or avulsion of main RA

CLINICAL ISSUES

Presentation
- Most common signs/symptoms
  - ○ Asymptomatic, flank pain, tenderness (traumatic), hematuria
  - ○ Hypertension in chronic infarction

Demographics
- Age: Any age group
- Gender: M = F

Natural History & Prognosis
- Complications: Necrosis, infection, abscess formation
- Prognosis
  - ○ Focal infarction: Good
  - ○ Global infarction: Poor

Treatment
- Medical
  - ○ Antithrombolytics, anticoagulants, antihypertensives
- Surgery or angioplasty for atherosclerosis RA stenosis
- Nephrectomy for irreversible traumatic global infarction

DIAGNOSTIC CHECKLIST

Consider
- Correlate with history: Trauma, cardiac, aortic disease

Image Interpretation Pearls
- Pyelonephritis & acute infarction may have similar appearance
- Straight line demarcation & cortical rim sign favor infarction
- Perinephric stranding favors pyelonephritis

SELECTED REFERENCES

1. Kawashima A et al: Imaging evaluation of posttraumatic renal injuries. Abdom Imaging. 27(2):199-213, 2002
2. Schreyer HH et al: Helical CT of the urinary organs. Eur Radiol. 12(3):575-91, 2002
3. Suzer O et al: CT features of renal infarction. Eur J Radiol. 44(1):59-64, 2002
4. Kaushik S et al: Abdominal thrombotic and ischemic manifestations of the antiphospholipid antibody syndrome: CT findings in 42 patients. Radiology. 218(3):768-71, 2001
5. Kawashima A et al: Imaging of renal trauma: a comprehensive review. Radiographics. 21(3):557-74, 2001
6. Kawashima A et al: CT evaluation of renovascular disease. Radiographics. 20(5):1321-40, 2000
7. Carey HB et al: Bilateral renal infarction secondary to paradoxical embolism. Am J Kidney Dis. 34(4):752-5, 1999
8. Dalla-Palma L et al: Delayed CT in acute renal infection. Semin Ultrasound CT MR. 18(2):122-8, 1997
9. Kawashima A et al: CT of renal inflammatory disease. Radiographics. 17(4):851-66; discussion 867-8, 1997
10. Kamel IR et al: Assessment of the cortical rim sign in posttraumatic renal infarction. J Comput Assist Tomogr. 20(5):803-6, 1996
11. Krinsky G: Unenhanced helical CT in patients with acute flank pain and renal infarction: the need for contrast material in selected cases. AJR Am J Roentgenol. 167(1):282-3, 1996
12. Nunez D Jr et al: Traumatic occlusion of the renal artery: helical CT diagnosis. AJR Am J Roentgenol. 167(3):777-80, 1996
13. Saunders HS et al: The CT nephrogram: implications for evaluation of urinary tract disease. Radiographics. 15(5):1069-85; discussion 1086-8, 1995
14. Levine E: Acute renal and urinary tract disease. Radiol Clin North Am. 32(5):989-1004, 1994
15. Fanney DR et al: CT in the diagnosis of renal trauma. Radiographics. 10(1):29-40, 1990
16. Sant GR et al: Computed tomography in evaluation of blunt renal trauma. Potential for misdiagnosis of renal infarction. Urol Int. 43(6):321-3, 1988
17. Bankoff MS et al: Computed tomography differentiation of pyelonephritis and renal infarction. J Comput Tomogr. 8(3):239-43, 1984
18. Wong WS et al: Renal infarction: CT diagnosis and correlation between CT findings and etiologies. Radiology. 150(1):201-5, 1984
19. Haaga JR et al: CT appearance of renal infarct. J Comput Assist Tomogr. 4(2):246-7, 1980

RENAL INFARCTION

IMAGE GALLERY

Typical

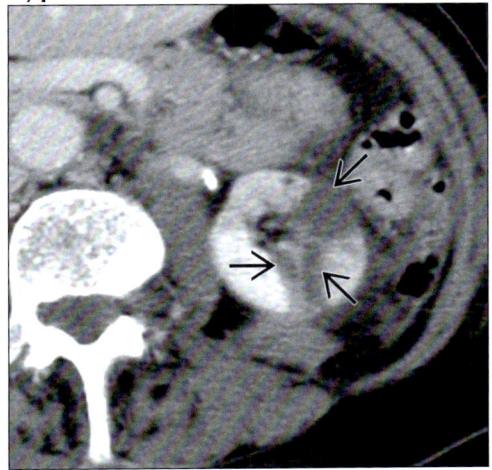
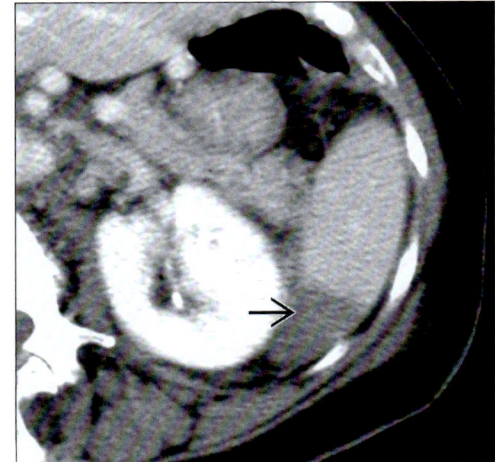

(Left) Axial CECT of endocarditis with renal & splenic infarcts. Note multiple wedge-shaped renal infarcts ➔ in lower pole of left kidney. *(Right)* Axial CECT at level of spleen in same patient as previous image reveals lower pole splenic infarct ➔.

Typical

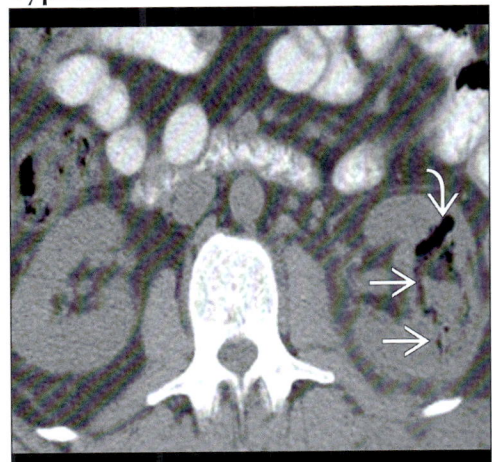
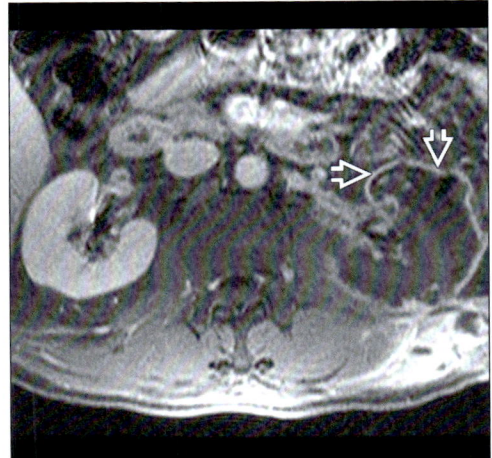

(Left) Axial NECT shows gas bubbles ➔ within left kidney at site of partial nephrectomy ➔ due to post-operative change & "Oxycel", placed to prevent hemorrhage. *(Right)* Axial T1 C+ FS MR after gadolinium enhancement in same patient as left shows cortical rim sign ➔ with no parenchymal perfusion. At nephrectomy, renal infarction 2° RA thrombus was confirmed.

Typical

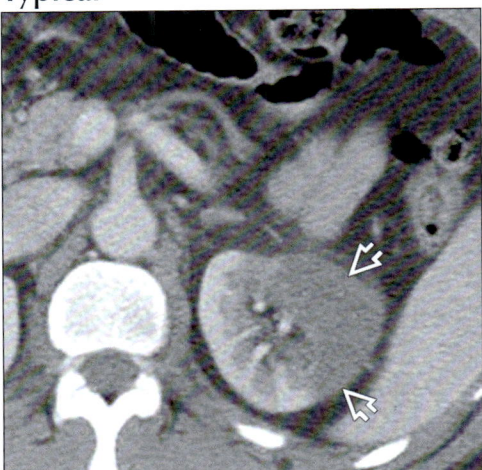
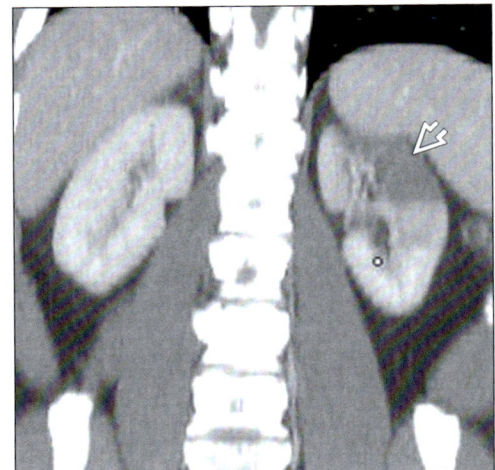

(Left) Axial CECT shows large area of decreased perfusion ➔ in upper pole of left kidney due to renal infarct. No local renal vascular causes such as renal artery or renal vein occlusion were detected. *(Right)* Coronal CECT in same patient as left again shows large area of decreased perfusion ➔ in upper pole of left kidney, presumed to be due to small vessel disease in patient with suspected vasculitis.

RENAL VEIN THROMBOSIS

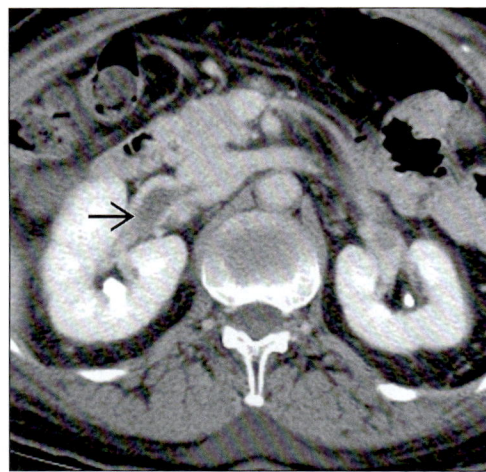

Axial CECT of bilateral acute renal vein thrombosis in patient with lupus erythematosus. Note low-attenuation thrombosis seen as filling defect in right renal vein ➔.

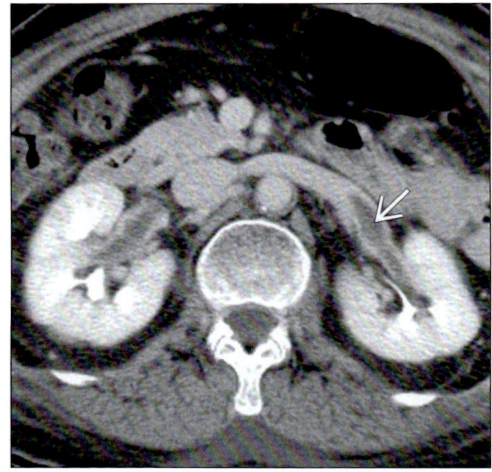

Axial CECT at lower level in same patient as left reveals clot in left renal vein ➔.

TERMINOLOGY

Abbreviations and Synonyms
- Renal vein thrombosis (RVT)

Definitions
- Obstruction of renal vein by thrombus

IMAGING FINDINGS

General Features
- Best diagnostic clue: Renal vein mass with renal enlargement & delayed renal function
- Location
  o Unilateral > bilateral
    ▪ Bilateral more common in children
  o Left > right
- Size
  o Renal enlargement (75% of cases)
  o Small shrunken kidney (rare)
- Morphology: Mass in renal vein ± extension to inferior vena cava (IVC) ± right atrium

Fluoroscopic Findings
- IVP
  o Dense, prolonged nephrogram (partial)
  o Little or no nephrographic opacification (complete)
  o ↓ Amount of opaque urine in renal calyces, infundibula & pelvis
  o Opacified veins in perinephric space
  o Venous notching or ureteral indentation by tortuous collateral veins
  o Rarely alternating radiopaque & radiolucent striations in renal cortex

CT Findings
- CECT
  o Low-attenuation filling defect within renal vein
  o ↓ Nephrographic attenuation
  o Persistent parenchymal opacification
  o No corticomedullary differentiation
  o Delayed corticomedullary junction time, contrast excretion into renal calyces & pelvis
  o Renal vein attenuation & enlargement; most visible on left
  o Thickened Gerota fascia & perinephric "whiskering" (edema or hemorrhage)

DDx: Enlarged Kidney Delayed Function

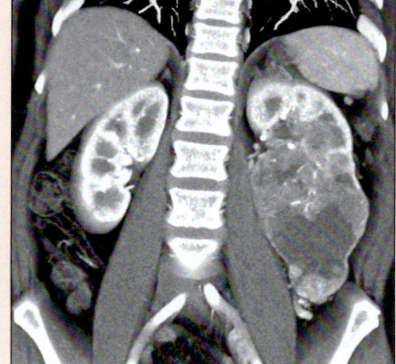

Renal Cell Carcinoma

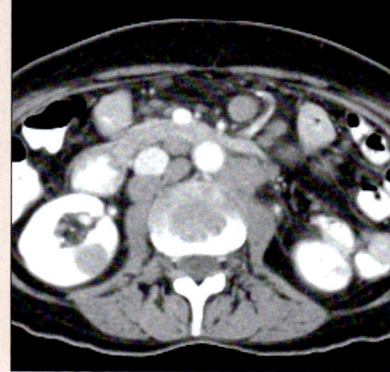

Lymphoma

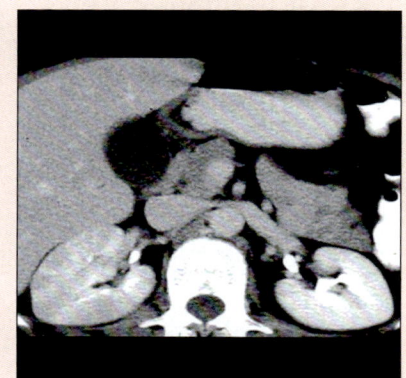

Pyelonephritis

RENAL VEIN THROMBOSIS

Key Facts

Terminology
- Obstruction of renal vein by thrombus

Imaging Findings
- Best diagnostic clue: Renal vein mass with renal enlargement & delayed renal function
- Morphology: Mass in renal vein ± extension to inferior vena cava (IVC) ± right atrium
- Low-attenuation filling defect within renal vein
- No corticomedullary differentiation
- Venous collateralization
- Best imaging tool: US followed by MDCT or MR

Top Differential Diagnoses
- Ureteral Obstruction
- Infiltrating Tumor
- Pyelonephritis

Pathology
- Most commonly associated with nephrotic syndrome in adults
- Most commonly associated with dehydration and sepsis in children

Clinical Issues
- Asymptomatic or thromboembolic disease; fever, edema
- Age: More common in adults, also seen < 2 years of age
- Anticoagulation therapy

Diagnostic Checklist
- Adequate return of renal circulation may prevent renal function deterioration
- Filling defect within renal vein; venous collaterals

  - Opacified periureteral & perinephric collaterals ("cobwebs")
- CTA
  - Tortuous & dilated collateral veins close to ureters
  - Venous collateralization
  - Retrograde flow in dilated superficial epigastric veins

MR Findings
- T1WI: No corticomedullary differentiation
- MRA: High contrast between flowing blood, vascular walls & surrounding tissue
- T1WI, T2WI
  - Filling defect in renal vein
  - Prolonged relations times of renal cortex and medulla → low-signal intensity
  - Low-signal intensity band in outer medulla
  - Obliteration of renal sinus fat, compression of renal collecting systems
  - ↑ Attenuation of renal veins
  - Multiple perinephric collateral veins
  - Gonadal vein dilatation

Ultrasonographic Findings
- Grayscale Ultrasound
  - Renal edema
  - ↓ Echogenicity (acute), ↑ after 10-14 days
  - ± Corticomedullary differentiation
  - Thrombus or tumor in IVC (≤ 20%)
  - Intraluminal echoes with renal vein dilatation proximal to occlusion; more visible on left
- Color Doppler
  - Renal artery & proximal branches
    - Peaked, sudden decreased systolic-frequency shifts
    - Retrograde plateau-like shifts during diastole
  - Absent venous signal
  - Increased blood velocity & turbulence (partial)
  - No blood flow (complete)
  - Anechoic or hypoechoic clot (acute)
  - Echogenic thrombus (chronic)

Angiographic Findings
- Conventional
  - Renal vein reflux

  - Venous collateralization

Nuclear Medicine Findings
- Delayed or absent renal perfusion

Imaging Recommendations
- Best imaging tool: US followed by MDCT or MR
- Protocol advice: CTA: Corticomedullary phase best; second acquisition performed 90-120 seconds

DIFFERENTIAL DIAGNOSIS

Ureteral Obstruction
- Filling defect & irregular ureteral narrowing
- Decreased contrast density in collecting system
- Hydronephrosis; hydroureter; perinephric or periureteral stranding

Infiltrating Tumor
- Transitional cell carcinoma, renal cell carcinoma, renal metastases, lymphoma
- Poorly defined margins without change in shape
- Heterogeneous mass ± calcification
- Enhancing mass with soft tissue attenuation

Pyelonephritis
- Multiple necrotic masses with renal enlargement
- Differentiate by clinical history and urinalysis

PATHOLOGY

General Features
- General path comments
  - Most commonly associated with nephrotic syndrome in adults
  - Most commonly associated with dehydration and sepsis in children
- Genetics: Inherited hypercoagulable states (antithrombin III, protein S, protein C deficiency)
- Etiology
  - Nephrotic syndrome
    - Membranous glomerulonephritis

RENAL VEIN THROMBOSIS

- Membranoproliferative glomerulonephritis
- Focal sclerosis, amyloidosis, lipoid nephrosis
○ Other primary renal disease
- Other glomerulonephritis
- Pyelonephritis, vasculitis
○ Renal hypoperfusion by hypovolemia or vascular stasis
- Dehydration, sepsis, hemorrhage
- Gastrointestinal fluid loss
- Congestive heart failure, aortic insufficiency
- Constrictive pericarditis
○ Tumor extension
- Renal cell carcinoma, renal angiomyolipoma
- Wilms tumor, transitional cell carcinoma
- Metastasis (adrenal, gonadal carcinoma)
○ Iatrogenic
- Drugs (oral contraceptive pills, estrogens)
- Abdominal surgery, renal transplant rejection
○ Other hypercoagulable states
- Pregnancy, septic abortion
- Disseminated malignancy, genetics
○ Abdominal trauma
○ Thrombus extension
- Left ovarian vein thrombosis
- Deep vein thrombosis (leg, pelvic)
- Retrograde IVC extension
○ Other systemic disease
- Polyarteritis nodosa, sickle cell anemia
- Diabetes mellitus (maternal diabetes, glomerulosclerosis)
- Systemic lupus erythematosus
○ Mechanical compression
- Pregnancy, retroperitoneal fibrosis
- Tumor (lymphoma, carcinoma of pancreatic tail), urinoma
- Abscess, lymphocele, hematoma (adrenal)
- Aberrant arteries, arterial aneurysms
- Epidemiology
○ Incidence
- Nephrotic syndrome: 16-42% of patients

Gross Pathologic & Surgical Features
- Renal fibrosis, hemorrhage, necrosis, calcification

CLINICAL ISSUES

Presentation
- Most common signs/symptoms
○ Acute (more common in children)
- Flank pain, nausea, vomiting, palpable kidney, hypertension
○ Chronic
- Asymptomatic or thromboembolic disease; fever, edema
- Lab data
○ Acute: Gross or microscopic hematuria on urinalysis
○ Chronic: Proteinuria on urinalysis

Demographics
- Age: More common in adults, also seen < 2 years of age

Natural History & Prognosis
- Effects of RVT depend on site of origin, time to occlusion, collateral veins & extent of recanalization
- Complications: Pulmonary embolism is most common
○ Widespread thrombosis; renal hemorrhage, atrophy & failure
- Prognosis: Good, with frequent spontaneous recovery

Treatment
- Anticoagulation therapy
○ IV heparin, then oral warfarin
- Thrombolytic therapy: Bilateral RVT, RVT extension into IVC, massive clot, pulmonary emboli, severe flank pain or failed anticoagulation therapy
- Steroids or other immunosuppressive medications: Autoimmune disease
- Suprarenal vena cava filter: Thrombus extending into IVC
- Surgical thrombectomy or nephrectomy for failed medical treatment, tumor thrombus

DIAGNOSTIC CHECKLIST

Consider
- Adequate return of renal circulation may prevent renal function deterioration

Image Interpretation Pearls
- Filling defect within renal vein; venous collaterals

SELECTED REFERENCES

1. Akbar SA et al: Complications of renal transplantation. Radiographics. 25(5):1335-56, 2005
2. Goldenberg NA: Long-term outcomes of venous thrombosis in children. Curr Opin Hematol. 12(5):370-6, 2005
3. Noble VE et al: Renal ultrasound. Emerg Med Clin North Am. 22(3):641-59, 2004
4. Butty S et al: Body MR venography. Radiol Clin North Am. 40(4):899-919, 2002
5. Urban BA et al: Three-dimensional volume-rendered CT angiography of the renal arteries and veins: normal anatomy, variants, and clinical applications. Radiographics. 21(2):373-86; questionnaire 549-55, 2001
6. Kawashima A et al: CT evaluation of renovascular disease. Radiographics. 20(5):1321-40, 2000
7. Tempany CM et al: MRI of the renal veins: assessment of nonneoplastic venous thrombosis. J Comput Assist Tomogr. 16(6):929-34, 1992
8. Gatewood OM et al: Renal vein thrombosis in patients with nephrotic syndrome: CT diagnosis. Radiology. 159(1):117-22, 1986
9. Glazer GM et al: Computed tomography of renal vein thrombosis. J Comput Assist Tomogr. 8(2):288-93, 1984
10. Jeffrey RB et al: CT and ultrasonography of acute renal abnormalities. Radiol Clin North Am. 21(3):515-25, 1983
11. Bradley WG Jr et al: Renal vein thrombosis: occurrence in membranous glomerulonephropathy and lupus nephritis. Radiology. 139(3):571-6, 1981
12. Chait A et al: Renal vein thrombosis. Radiology. 90(5):886-96, 1968

RENAL VEIN THROMBOSIS

IMAGE GALLERY

Typical

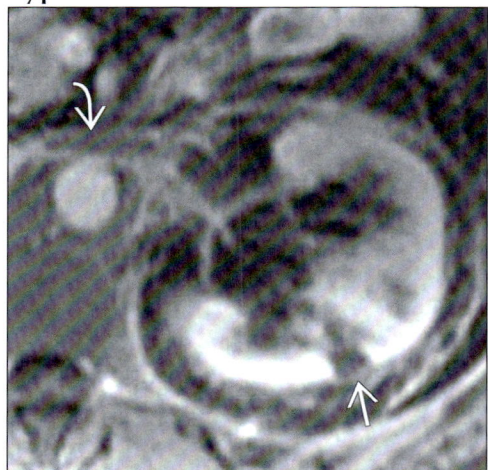
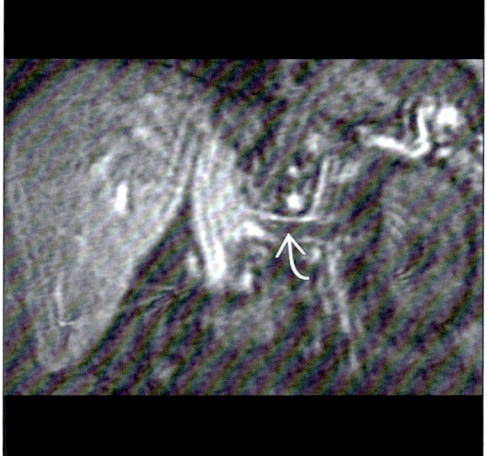

(Left) Axial T1 C+ FS MR with gadolinium contrast reveals renal parenchymal swelling due to parenchymal hematoma with areas of focal infarction ➔ and filling defects in left renal vein ➔. *(Right)* Coronal T1 C+ FS MR in same patient as left again demonstrates filling defects in left renal vein ➔.

Typical

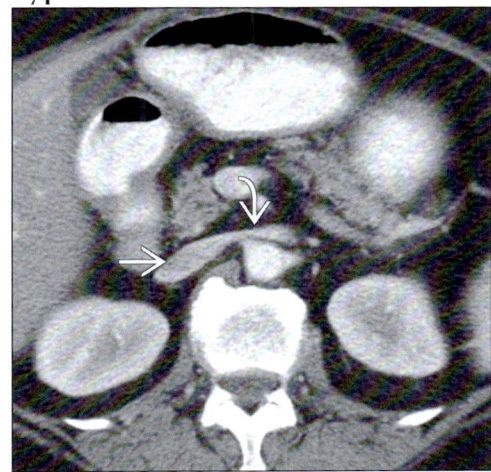
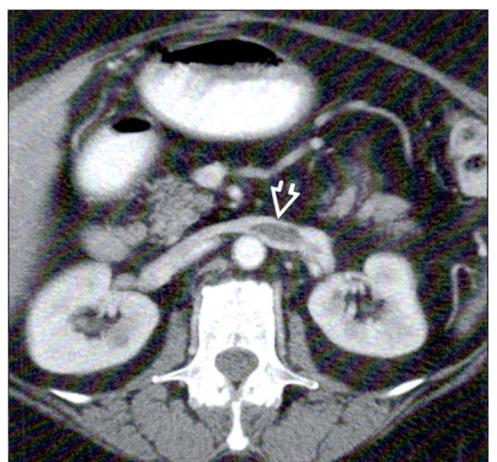

(Left) Axial CECT shows patent inferior vena cava ➔ & distal left renal vein ➔. *(Right)* Axial CECT in same patient as left reveals thrombus ➔ occupying part of left renal vein lumen. Note contrast opacifying remainder of renal vein lumen.

Variant

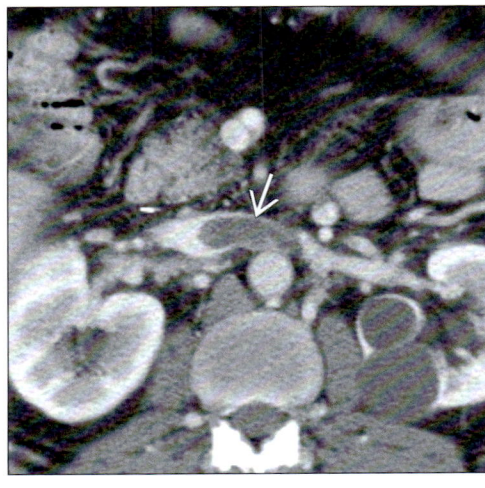
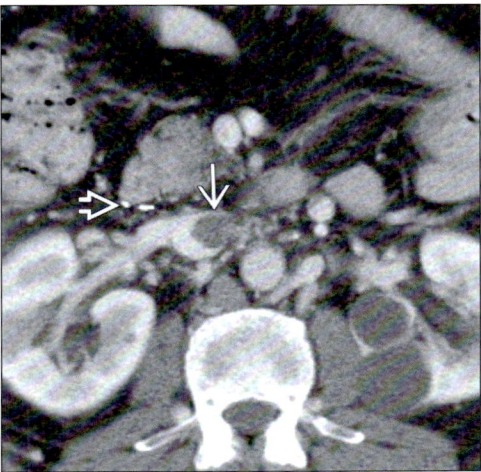

(Left) Axial CECT shows thrombus within IVC & left renal vein ➔. *(Right)* Axial CECT in same patient as left again shows thrombus in IVC & left renal vein ➔, as well as surgical clips ➔ from prior resection of tumor in vena cava.

EPIDIDYMO-ORCHITIS

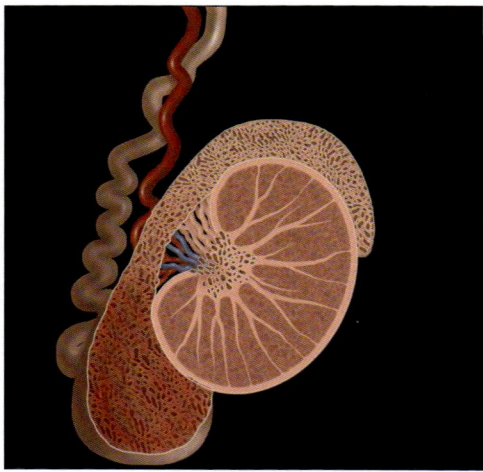

Graphic of acute epididymo-orchitis. Note swollen and inflamed tail of the epididymis with adjacent normal testis.

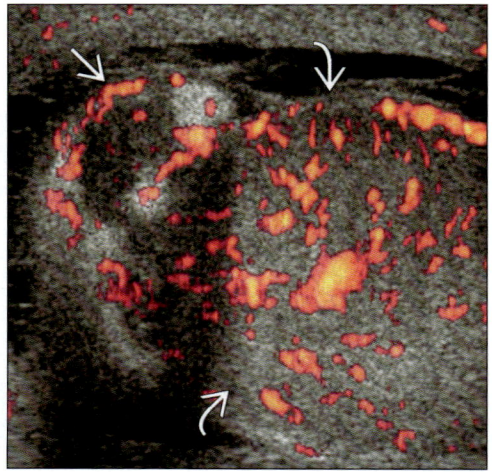

Sagittal power Doppler ultrasound of epididymo-orchitis. Note thickened & hyperemic epididymis ➔ & marked increased flow to testis ➔.

TERMINOLOGY

Abbreviations and Synonyms
- Acute scrotum, orchitis, epididymitis

Definitions
- Infectious inflammation of epididymis/testicle

IMAGING FINDINGS

General Features
- Best diagnostic clue: Enlarged, hyperemic epididymis/testicle on color Doppler US
- Location: Tail of epididymis (early)
- Size: 2-3 times larger than normal

Ultrasonographic Findings
- Grayscale Ultrasound
  - Enlarged, thickened epididymis initially involving tail
    - Often associated with complex hydrocele
  - Echogenicity may be coarse or predominantly hypoechoic due to edema &/or hemorrhage
  - Testis may have relatively normal appearance, or heterogeneous hypoechoic areas & linear striations along centripetal vessels due to septal edema
  - Areas of abscess formation within epididymis or testis are typically hypoechoic
- Color Doppler
  - Enlarged epididymis with hyperemia on both color & power Doppler
  - Increased flow within capsular & centripetal arteries of testis

Nuclear Medicine Findings
- Tc-99m
  - Differentiate torsion from epididymo-orchitis
  - Increased flow within testicular vessels & vas deferens

Imaging Recommendations
- Best imaging tool: Grayscale & color Doppler US with high-frequency transducers ≥ 10 mHz
- Protocol advice: Contralateral testicle comparison of echogenicity & vascularity

DDx: Testicular Lesions Mimicking Epididymo-Orchitis

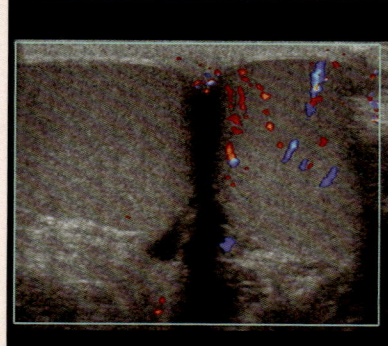

Testicular Torsion

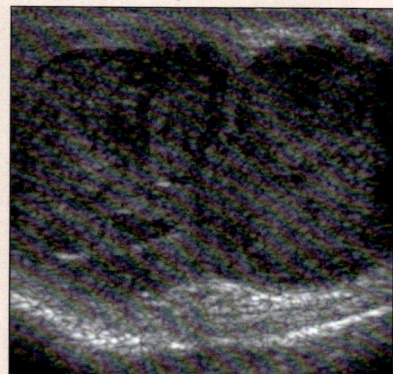

Testicular Tumor

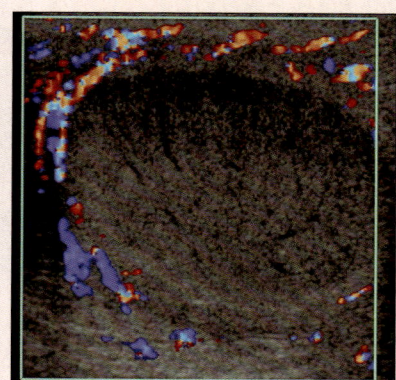

Testicular Infarct

EPIDIDYMO-ORCHITIS

Key Facts

Terminology
- Acute scrotum, orchitis, epididymitis
- Infectious inflammation of epididymis/testicle

Imaging Findings
- Best diagnostic clue: Enlarged, hyperemic epididymis/testicle on color Doppler US
- Echogenicity may be coarse or predominantly hypoechoic due to edema &/or hemorrhage
- Testis may have relatively normal appearance, or heterogeneous hypoechoic areas & linear striations along centripetal vessels due to septal edema
- Areas of abscess formation within epididymis or testis are typically hypoechoic
- Best imaging tool: Grayscale & color Doppler US with high-frequency transducers ≥ 10 mHz
- Protocol advice: Contralateral testicle comparison of echogenicity & vascularity

Top Differential Diagnoses
- Testicular Torsion
- Testicular Tumor
- Segmental Infarct
- Torsion Appendix Testis
- Testicular Trauma

Clinical Issues
- Acutely painful scrotum; scrotal swelling, erythema; fever; dysuria, urethral discharge
- Excellent prognosis with early antibiotics

Diagnostic Checklist
- Consider torsion if low flow to testicle

DIFFERENTIAL DIAGNOSIS

Testicular Torsion
- 20% of all acute scrotal pathology
- Absent or diminished flow
- Epididymis may be enlarged but not hyperemic
- Bell-clapper deformity
  - Congenital anomaly (tunica vaginalis completely surrounds testis & epididymis)
  - Predisposes to intravaginal-type torsion
- Extravaginal torsion
  - Occurs in newborns without bell-clapper deformity
  - Due to poor attachment of testis to scrotal wall
- US findings
  - Grayscale images of testis may be normal in first 6 hours
  - After 6 hours, testis becomes heterogeneous with hypoechoic areas
  - Spermatic cord twisted above testis (whirlpool sign)
  - Epididymis often enlarged & heterogeneous due to edema & hemorrhage
  - Color & power Doppler with low-volume flow settings most often demonstrate decreased flow to affected testicle
    - Sensitivity 80-98%
  - Rarely color Doppler is normal if torsion < 180°
  - Testicular infarction if torsion > 540°
- Testicular salvage rate 80-100% in first 5-7 hours of onset of pain

Testicular Tumor
- Focal mass, abnormal vessels
- 65-94% of patients present with painless unilateral mass
- Classification
  - Germ-cell tumors most common
    - Seminoma, non-seminomatous germ-cell tumors
  - Stromal tumor
  - Mixed germ-cell/stromal tumor
  - Metastatic tumor
- US findings
  - 98% sensitive for detection
  - Solid hypoechoic mass
    - May be well- or ill-defined within testis
  - Typically increased color Doppler flow if > 1.5 cm
  - Calcification in "burned-out" germ-cell tumors, embryonal cell carcinoma & teratomatous lesions
  - Bilateral involvement in lymphoma, leukemia

Segmental Infarct
- Acute pain
- No trauma history
- Focal hypoechoic avascular area
- Increased incidence in patients with hypercoagulable states or advanced atherosclerosis

Torsion Appendix Testis
- Acute scrotal pain in children or adolescents
- Clinically evident as "blue dot sign"
- May appear as hypoechoic or echogenic mass adjacent to normally perfused testis on US
- Slight increase in color Doppler flow adjacent to torsed appendix testis
- May lie adjacent to head of epididymis & upper pole of testis

Testicular Trauma
- US findings
  - Complex fluid in tunica vaginalis = hematocele
  - Heterogeneous echotexture
  - Discrete fracture plane in only 17%
- Cold flow confirms avascular areas of hematoma
- Early surgery key to salvage rate of testis
- 90% salvage rate if surgery within 72 hours of trauma

PATHOLOGY

General Features
- General path comments
  - Infectious inflammatory response
  - Risk of abscess if untreated
- Etiology
  - Inflammation/infection first starts in epididymis (typically tail of epididymis)

EPIDIDYMO-ORCHITIS

- Spreads by direct extension to testis in 20% of cases
- Bacterial seeding in genitourinary (GU) anomalies; common organisms include
  - E. coli pseudomonas & Klebsiella, which cause lower urinary tract infection
  - Sexually transmitted organisms such as Chlamydia & gonococcus, which cause urethritis
  - Rare organisms such as varicella, TB, viruses (mumps) & syphilis
- Sexually-transmitted ascending GU tract infection
- Epidemiology
  - Most common in sexually active young men
  - Epididymitis is most common cause of acute scrotal pain in adult males
    - Represents 75% of all scrotal inflammatory processes

Microscopic Features
- Inflammatory infiltrate of testis & epididymis

Staging, Grading or Classification Criteria
- Isolated epididymitis
- Isolated orchitis (boys with mumps)
- Combined epididymitis & orchitis

CLINICAL ISSUES

Presentation
- Most common signs/symptoms
  - Acutely painful scrotum; scrotal swelling, erythema; fever; dysuria, urethral discharge
    - Scrotal pain is often insidious for 1-2 days
- Clinical Profile
  - Positive urinalysis for WBC & bacteria
  - May have increased WBC count

Demographics
- Age: 15-35 years; peak incidence at 40-50 years
- Gender: Male

Natural History & Prognosis
- Excellent prognosis with early antibiotics
- Complications
  - Abscess formation
  - Testicular ischemia (entrapment of testicular artery & inflammation)
- Recurrent cases may lead to long-term fertility problems

Treatment
- Antibiotic therapy
- Follow-up scans to exclude abscess if not improved
- Work-up for GU anomalies in younger children and recurrent cases
- Surgery if abscess formation

DIAGNOSTIC CHECKLIST

Consider
- Consider torsion if low flow to testicle

Image Interpretation Pearls
- Hyperemic, enlarged epididymis and/or testis

SELECTED REFERENCES

1. Wittenberg AF et al: Sonography of the acute scrotum: the four T's of testicular imaging. Curr Probl Diagn Radiol. 35(1):12-21, 2006
2. Haecker FM et al: Acute epididymitis in children: a 4-year retrospective study. Eur J Pediatr Surg. 15(3):180-6, 2005
3. Akin EA et al: Ultrasound of the scrotum. Ultrasound Q. 20(4):181-200, 2004
4. Blaivas M et al: Testicular ultrasound. Emerg Med Clin North Am. 22(3):723-48, ix, 2004
5. Cole FL et al: The acute, nontraumatic scrotum: assessment, diagnosis, and management. J Am Acad Nurse Pract. 16(2):50-6, 2004
6. Dogra V et al: Acute painful scrotum. Radiol Clin North Am. 42(2):349-63, 2004
7. Hagley M: Epididymo-orchitis and epididymitis: a review of causes and management of unusual forms. Int J STD AIDS. 14(6):372-7; quiz 378, 2003
8. Mushtaq I et al: Retrospective review of paediatric patients with acute scrotum. ANZ J Surg. 73(1-2):55-8, 2003
9. Corbett HJ et al: Management of the acute scrotum in children. ANZ J Surg. 72(3):226-8, 2002
10. McAndrew HF et al: The incidence and investigation of acute scrotal problems in children. Pediatr Surg Int. 18(5-6):435-7, 2002
11. Blaivas M et al: Emergency evaluation of patients presenting with acute scrotum using bedside ultrasonography. Acad Emerg Med. 8(1):90-3, 2001
12. Lefort C et al: [Ischemic orchiditis: review of 5 cases diagnosed by color Doppler ultrasonography] J Radiol. 82(7):839-42, 2001
13. Kashiwagi B et al: Acute epididymo-orchitis with abscess formation due to Pseudomonas aeruginosa: report of 3 cases. Hinyokika Kiyo. 46(12):915-8, 2000
14. Izawa JI et al: Tuberculous epididymo-orchitis: a case report. Can J Urol. 6(2):751-756, 1999
15. Dubinsky TJ et al: Color-flow and power Doppler imaging of the testes. World J Urol. 16(1):35-40, 1998
16. Jenkin GA et al: Candidal epididymo-orchitis: case report and review. Clin Infect Dis. 26(4):942-5, 1998
17. Junnila J et al: Testicular masses. Am Fam Physician. 57(4):685-92, 1998
18. Pannek J et al: Orchitis due to vasculitis in autoimmune diseases. Scand J Rheumatol. 26(3):151-4, 1997
19. Sidler D et al: A 25-year review of the acute scrotum in children. S Afr Med J. 87(12):1696-8, 1997
20. Horstman WG et al: Color Doppler US of the scrotum. Radiographics. 11(6):941-57; discussion 958, 1991

EPIDIDYMO-ORCHITIS

IMAGE GALLERY

Typical

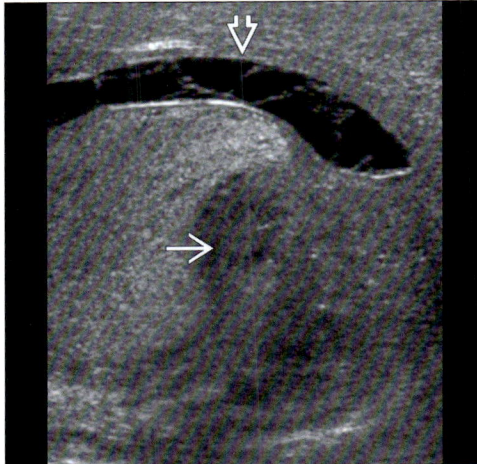
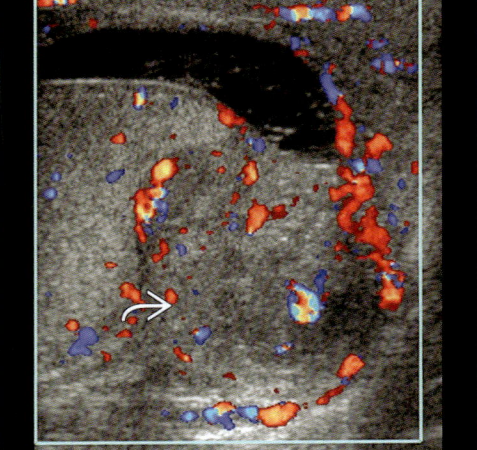

(Left) Transverse ultrasound shows inflammation, edema, and enlargement of epididymal head ➡, which is hypoechoic. Note septated irregular fluid collection representing reactive hydrocele ➡. (Right) Transverse color Doppler ultrasound of same patient as left shows increased flow to the epididymis ➡, hallmark sign of epididymitis.

Typical

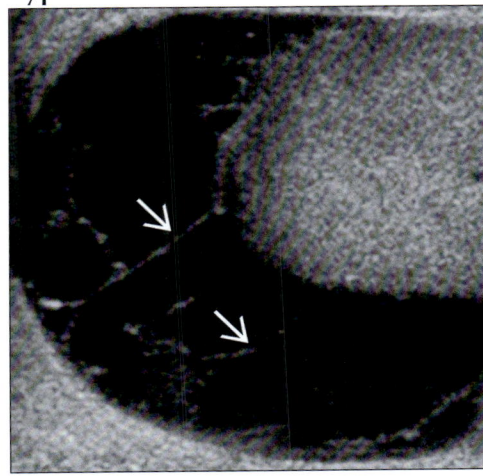
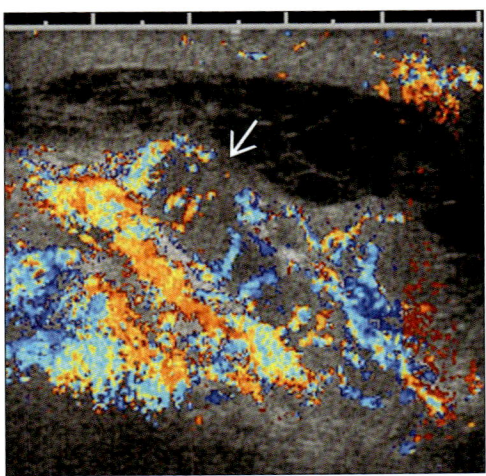

(Left) Longitudinal ultrasound of reactive hydrocele in epididymo-orchitis. Note multiple linear septations ➡ within hydrocele. (Right) Longitudinal color Doppler ultrasound in same patient as left demonstrates thickening & hyperemia of epididymis ➡.

Typical

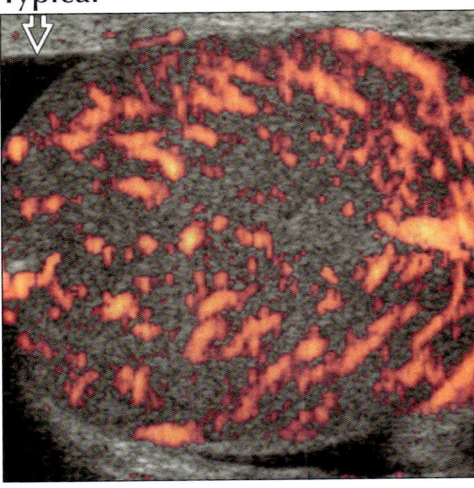
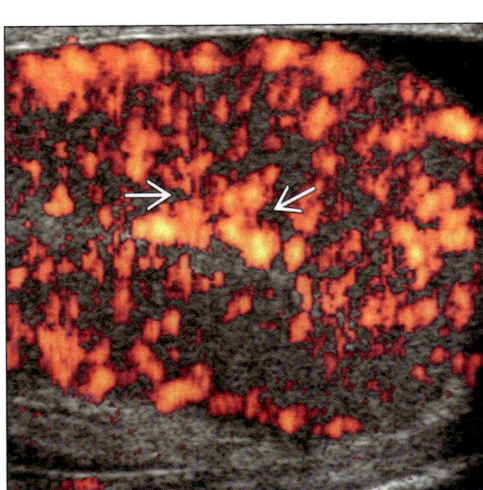

(Left) Transverse power Doppler ultrasound of mumps orchitis in 11-year-old boy demonstrates marked hyperemia with small surrounding hydrocele ➡. (Right) Longitudinal power Doppler ultrasound in same patient as left reveals hypertrophied centripetal arteries ➡ due to hyperemia.

TESTICULAR TORSION

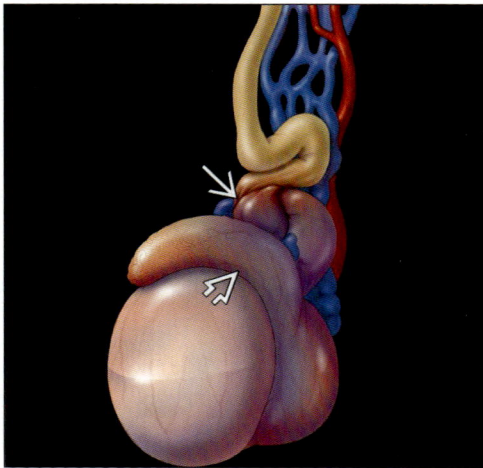

Anatomic drawing of testicular torsion. Note twisted cord ➔ and enlarged epididymis ➔.

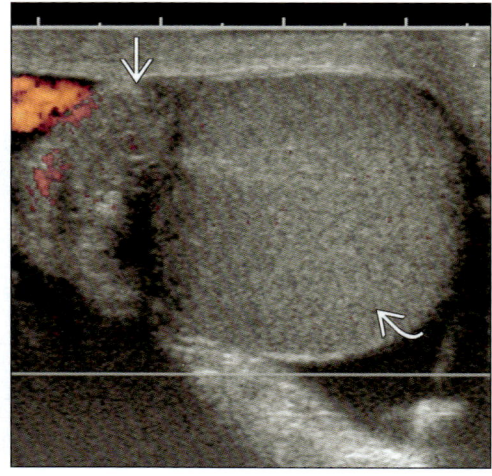

Longitudinal color Doppler ultrasound of acute testicular torsion demonstrates twisted cord & epididymis ➔ & absent flow to testis ➔.

TERMINOLOGY

Abbreviations and Synonyms
- Spermatic cord torsion

Definitions
- Spontaneous/traumatic twisting of testis & spermatic cord within scrotum, resulting in vascular occlusion/infarction

IMAGING FINDINGS

General Features
- Best diagnostic clue
  - Decreased or absent testicular blood flow on color Doppler US
  - "Whirlpool sign" of twisted cord superior to testis or in inguinal canal
- Location: Unilateral in 95% of patients
- Size
  - Normal testicular volume
    - 1 cc in newborn
    - 15-20 cc in post-pubertal males

Ultrasonographic Findings
- Grayscale Ultrasound
  - Testicular parenchyma may be entirely normal, especially in cases of very recent torsion
  - Horizontally oriented testis
  - Enlarged testicle & epididymis, heterogeneous echotexture or hypoechoic testicle more often found
  - Intratesticular necrosis, hemorrhage or fragmentation seen if delayed diagnosis
  - "Spiral" twist of spermatic cord from inguinal canal to testis ("whirlpool sign")
    - Snail shell-shaped mass measuring 11-33 mm
  - Reactive or secondary hydrocele
- Color Doppler
  - Absent or decreased blood flow to testicle
  - Sensitivity 80-90%
  - Sensitivity 86%, specificity 100%, accuracy 97% when presence of identifiable intratesticular flow is sole criterion
  - Small percentage of patients with early or partial torsion have normal exam

Nuclear Medicine Findings
- Tc-99m pertechnetate

DDx: Testicular Lesions Mimicking Torsion

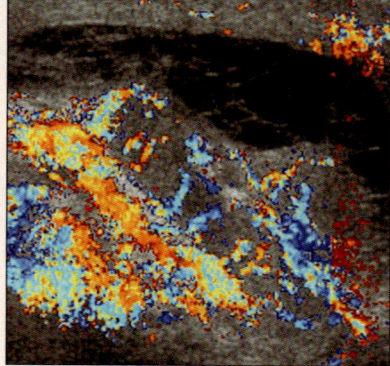

Epididymo-Orchitis

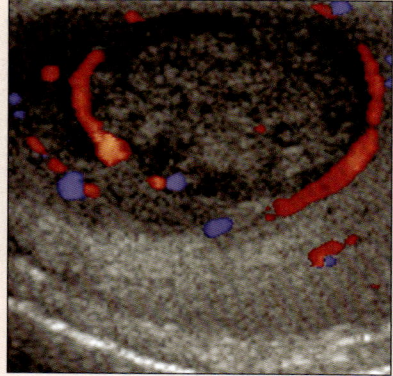

Testicular Carcinoma

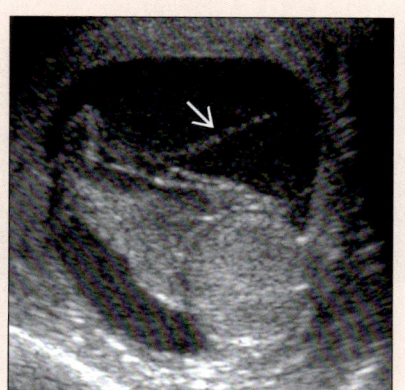

Testicular Trauma

TESTICULAR TORSION

Key Facts

Terminology
- Spontaneous/traumatic twisting of testis & spermatic cord within scrotum, resulting in vascular occlusion/infarction

Imaging Findings
- Decreased or absent testicular blood flow on color Doppler US
- "Whirlpool sign" of twisted cord superior to testis or in inguinal canal
- Best imaging tool: US with high-frequency linear transducer & color Doppler; power Doppler helpful in neonates, young boys

Top Differential Diagnoses
- Epididymo-Orchitis or Orchitis
- Torsion of Testicular Appendage or Appendix Epididymis
- Testicular Tumor
- Testicular Trauma
- Hernia Complications

Clinical Issues
- Clinical Profile: Male child with acute scrotal pain
- Surgical emergency: Testicular infarction if not treated promptly
- Surgical exploration; de-torsion; bilateral orchidopexy if viable testicle
- Risk of testicular loss nearly 80% in patients with intermittent torsion

Diagnostic Checklist
- Normal US does not exclude early or partial torsion

- Dynamic flow imaging at 2-5 second intervals for 1 minute (vascular phase)
- 5 minute intervals for tissue phase
- Pinhole collimation useful, especially in young patients
- Sensitivity 80-90%
- Penis positioned out of field of view, usually secured to anterior abdominal wall
- Scrotum supported symmetrically on towels
- Decreased perfusion to symptomatic testis on dynamic flow image
- Photopenia of affected testis on static images

Imaging Recommendations
- Best imaging tool: US with high-frequency linear transducer & color Doppler; power Doppler helpful in neonates, young boys
- Protocol advice: Power Doppler with comparison to contralateral testis

DIFFERENTIAL DIAGNOSIS

Epididymo-Orchitis or Orchitis
- Enlarged hypoechoic epididymis
- Increased color Doppler flow

Torsion of Testicular Appendage or Appendix Epididymis
- Devascularized, enlarged appendix testis or appendix epididymis
- Diffuse increase in scrotum on scintigraphy

Testicular Tumor
- Focal mass on US
- Abnormal flow within tumor

Testicular Trauma
- Hematocele, echogenic clot
- Irregular testicular contours
- Heterogeneous parenchymal echogenicity
- Focal area of hypoechoic hematoma

Hernia Complications
- Incarcerated hernia, torsion of hernia sac

PATHOLOGY

General Features
- General path comments: Varying degrees of ischemic necrosis & fibrosis depending on duration of symptoms
- Etiology: Most occur spontaneously; occasionally traumatic
- Epidemiology
  - Infant & adolescent boys most often affected
  - Incidence 1 in 4000 males
  - Increased incidence in December, January
- Associated abnormalities
  - Abnormally high attachment of tunica vaginalis results in "bell clapper" deformity
    - "Intra-vaginal" torsion
    - Testicle rotates freely within scrotum, twists spermatic cord, occluding venous & arterial flow
    - Present in 12% of male population
  - Torsion of spermatic cord proximal to attachments of tunica vaginalis
    - "Extra-vaginal" torsion
    - More common in neonates
    - Only 5% of all testicular torsion cases
    - Bilateral in 20% of cases

Gross Pathologic & Surgical Features
- Purple, edematous, ischemic testicle, may rapidly re-perfuse when manually untwisted

Microscopic Features
- Hemorrhage, interstitial edema, necrosis

Staging, Grading or Classification Criteria
- Acute, subacute, or delayed based on duration of symptoms
  - Duration of symptoms not always predictive of salvage rate, especially in partial or intermittent torsion

TESTICULAR TORSION

- Salvage rates
  - 80-100% if patients present within 6 hours of pain
  - Virtually 0% after 12 hours

CLINICAL ISSUES

Presentation
- Most common signs/symptoms
  - Acute scrotal and/or inguinal pain
  - Swollen, erythematous hemiscrotum, no known trauma
  - Physical findings
    - Elevation & transverse position of affected testicle
    - Anterior rotation of epididymis, absence of cremasteric reflex
    - Pain relief with manual de-torsion
  - In neonates, purple discoloration of swollen scrotum
    - More common in high birth-weight babies
    - Can be confused with scrotal hematoma due to birth trauma
- Other signs/symptoms
  - Nausea, vomiting
  - Low-grade torsion may be tolerated for long periods
  - History of similar spontaneously resolved symptoms in 50% of patients
    - Spontaneous torsion & detorsion
- Clinical Profile: Male child with acute scrotal pain

Demographics
- Age
  - Bimodal peak
    - 14 years
    - Neonates
- Gender: Male

Natural History & Prognosis
- Surgical emergency: Testicular infarction if not treated promptly
- Viability depends on
  - Degree of torsion, > 540° worse
  - Duration of symptoms
  - Time to surgical intervention
- Unilateral testicular loss typically does not lead to infertility problems

Treatment
- Testicle twists medially in 2/3, manual de-torsion laterally is more likely to be effective
  - Direction of manual detorsion described as "opening a book"
- Surgical exploration; de-torsion; bilateral orchidopexy if viable testicle
  - Non-viable testicle usually removed; anti-sperm antibody theory
  - Higher risk of subsequent torsion on contralateral side
  - Orchiopexy does not guarantee against future torsion
- Bilateral pexy advocated in children with intermittent scrotal pain
  - Risk of testicular loss nearly 80% in patients with intermittent torsion

DIAGNOSTIC CHECKLIST

Consider
- Normal US does not exclude early or partial torsion

Image Interpretation Pearls
- Decreased or absent flow on power and pulsed Doppler US

SELECTED REFERENCES

1. Vijayaraghavan SB: Sonographic Differential Diagnosis of Acute Scrotum: Real-time Whirlpool Sign, a Key Sign of Torsion. J Ultrasound Med. 25(5):563-74, 2006
2. Akin EA et al: Ultrasound of the scrotum. Ultrasound Q. 20(4):181-200, 2004
3. Ciftci AO et al: Clinical predictors for differential diagnosis of acute scrotum. Eur J Pediatr Surg. 14(5):333-8, 2004
4. Dogra V et al: Acute painful scrotum. Radiol Clin North Am. 42(2):349-63, 2004
5. Dogra VS et al: Torsion and beyond: new twists in spectral Doppler evaluation of the scrotum. J Ultrasound Med. 23(8):1077-85, 2004
6. Hormann M et al: Imaging of the scrotum in children. Eur Radiol. 14(6):974-83, 2004
7. Kalfa N et al: Ultrasonography of the spermatic cord in children with testicular torsion: impact on the surgical strategy. J Urol. 172(4 Pt 2):1692-5; discussion 1695, 2004
8. Kwong Y et al: A case of traumatic testicular torsion associated with a ruptured epididymis. Int J Urol. 11(5):349-51, 2004
9. Matsumoto A et al: Torsion of the hernia sac within a hydrocele of the scrotum in a child. Int J Urol. 11(9):789-91, 2004
10. Mernagh JR et al: Testicular torsion revisited. Curr Probl Diagn Radiol. 33(2):60-73, 2004
11. Sorensen MD et al: Prenatal bilateral extravaginal testicular torsion--a case presentation. Pediatr Surg Int. 20(11-12):892-3, 2004
12. Candocia FJ et al: An infant with testicular torsion in the inguinal canal. Pediatr Radiol. 33(10):722-4, 2003
13. Diamond DA et al: Neonatal scrotal haematoma: mimicker of neonatal testicular torsion. BJU Int. 91(7):675-7, 2003
14. Dogra V: Bell-clapper deformity. AJR Am J Roentgenol. 180(4):1176; author reply 1176-7, 2003
15. Dogra VS et al: Sonography of the scrotum. Radiology. 227(1):18-36, 2003
16. Kamaledeen S et al: Intermittent testicular pain: fix the testes. BJU Int. 91(4):406-8, 2003
17. Nelson CP et al: The cremasteric reflex: a useful but imperfect sign in testicular torsion. J Pediatr Surg. 38(8):1248-9, 2003
18. Sessions AE et al: Testicular torsion: direction, degree, duration and disinformation. J Urol. 169(2):663-5, 2003
19. Stehr M et al: Critical validation of colour Doppler ultrasound in diagnostics of acute scrotum in children. Eur J Pediatr Surg. 13(6):386-92, 2003
20. Traubici J et al: Original report. Testicular torsion in neonates and infants: sonographic features in 30 patients. AJR Am J Roentgenol. 180(4):1143-5, 2003
21. Williams CR et al: Testicular torsion: is there a seasonal predilection for occurrence? Urology. 61(3):638-41; discussion 641, 2003
22. Lrhorfi H et al: Trauma induced testicular torsion. J Urol. 168(6):2548, 2002
23. Kravchick S et al: Color Doppler sonography: its real role in the evaluation of children with highly suspected testicular torsion. Eur Radiol. 11(6):1000-5, 2001

TESTICULAR TORSION

IMAGE GALLERY

Typical

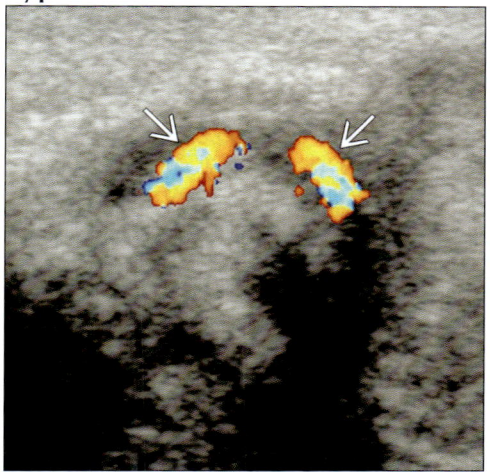
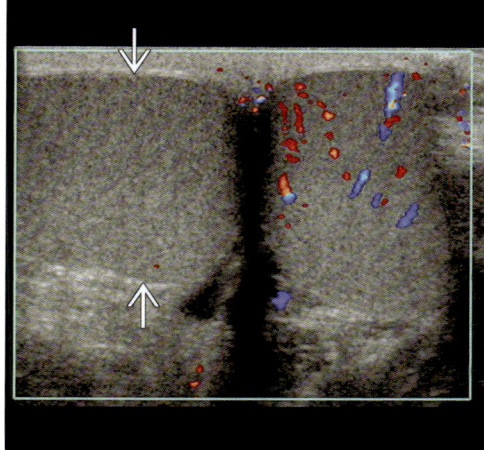

(Left) Transverse color Doppler ultrasound shows whirlpool sign of testicular torsion. Twisted cord superior to testis reveals arcing of vessels due to torsion ➡. *(Right)* Coronal color Doppler ultrasound of right & left testicle demonstrates absence of flow in right testicle ➡ & normal flow in left testicle.

Typical

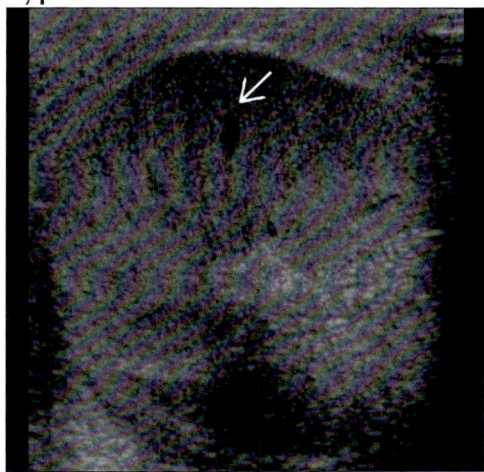
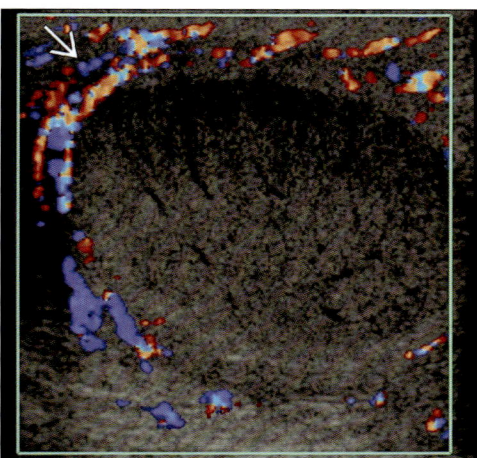

(Left) Transverse ultrasound shows typical appearance of infarcted left testicle. Left testicle appears heterogeneous in echotexture with linear bands of hypoechogenicity throughout ➡. *(Right)* Longitudinal color Doppler ultrasound in same patient as left demonstrates absent blood flow within testicle & marked hyperemia in paratesticular tissue ➡.

Variant

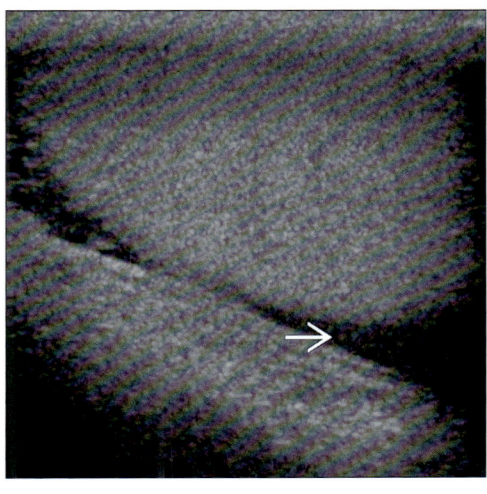
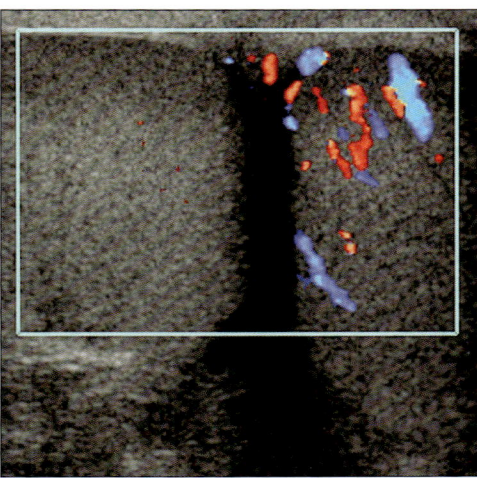

(Left) Longitudinal ultrasound of testis does not reveal any discreet abnormalities in testis except hydrocele ➡. *(Right)* Axial color Doppler ultrasound in same patient as left demonstrates no significant flow within affected testis. This case underscores importance of comparison of contralateral testis.

MIDGUT VOLVULUS

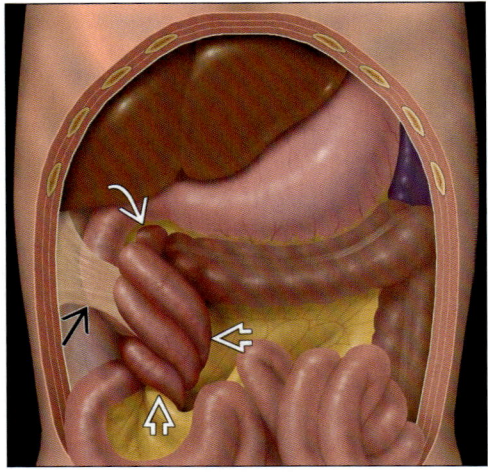

Graphic shows volvulus with twisted loops of proximal small bowel ⇨ and Ladd band ➔. The cecum ➔ is malpositioned within the right upper quadrant.

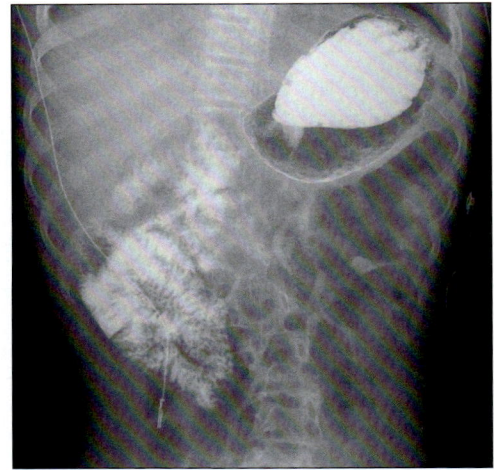

Frontal upper GI shows malrotation with all of proximal small bowel in right abdomen. Note duodenum does not pass to left abdomen.

TERMINOLOGY

Definitions
- Malrotation: Abnormal fixation of small bowel mesentery resulting in short mesenteric base that is prone to twisting
- Volvulus: Abnormal twisting of small bowel about the superior mesenteric artery that can result in bowel obstruction and bowel ischemia/necrosis
- Ligament of Treitz: Duodenojejunal junction (DJJ), where duodenum passes through transverse mesocolon and becomes jejunum
- Ladd bands: Abnormal fibrous peritoneal bands that can cause duodenal obstruction
- Bilious vomiting: Green/yellow vomit typically from obstruction of duodenum distal to ampulla of Vater

IMAGING FINDINGS

General Features
- Best diagnostic clue
  ○ Malrotation: Abnormal position of duodenojejunal junction
    ■ Abnormal position of cecum by small bowel follow through or barium enema
  ○ Volvulus: Cork screw or "Z"-shaped appearance of the duodenum which does not cross to the left of midline
- Morphology
  ○ Twisting of the mesentery occurs about the superior mesenteric artery which can cause venous obstruction, bowel wall ischemia and necrosis
  ○ Ladd band may cause duodenal obstruction

Radiographic Findings
- Radiography
  ○ May be normal
  ○ May show distended stomach and proximal duodenum
    ■ Duodenal bulb should not be markedly enlarged with acute volvulus
    ■ Markedly enlarged bulb indicative of long-standing obstruction as seen in duodenal atresia or in-utero volvulus
  ○ May show diffuse bowel distention from ischemia/necrosis
    ■ Such children will be extremely ill

DDx: Vomiting Infant

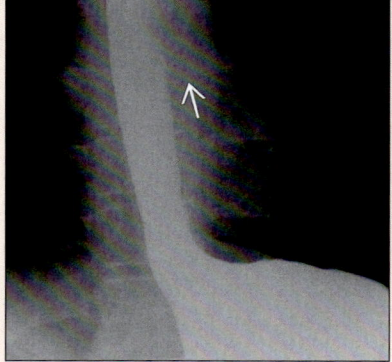

Gastroesophageal Reflux

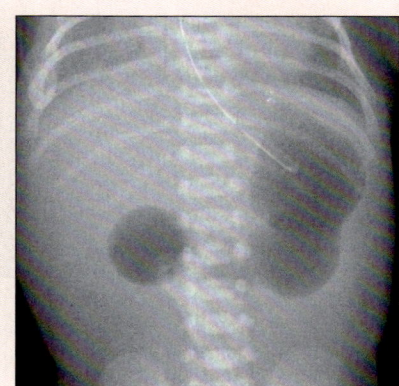

Duodenal Atresia

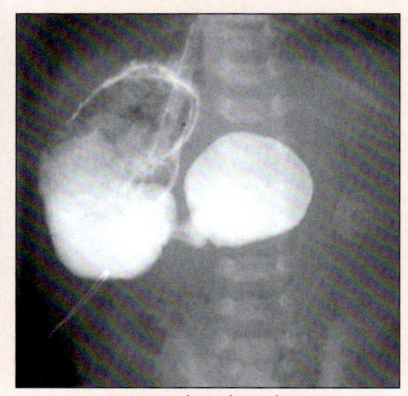

Duodenal Web

MIDGUT VOLVULUS

Key Facts

Terminology
- Malrotation: Abnormal fixation of small bowel mesentery resulting in short mesenteric base that is prone to twisting
- Volvulus: Abnormal twisting of small bowel about the superior mesenteric artery that can result in bowel obstruction and bowel ischemia/necrosis

Imaging Findings
- Abnormal position of cecum by small bowel follow through or barium enema
- Volvulus: Cork screw or "Z"-shaped appearance of the duodenum which does not cross to the left of midline
- Diagnosis of malrotation made on upper GI when criteria for normal position of DJJ (ligament of Treitz) are not met
- DJJ is at the same level or more superior than duodenal bulb
- On lateral view, duodenum typically courses posteriorly, then inferiorly

Pathology
- With normal embryonic rotation, both the duodenojejunal and ileocolic portions of the bowel rotate counterclockwise 270° around the axis of the omphalomesenteric vessels
- Etiology: Development anomaly resulting in narrow mesenteric pedicle secondary to abnormal fixation and rotation of bowel

Clinical Issues
- Most common signs/symptoms: Classic presentation: Bilious vomiting

---

   o Pneumatosis, portal venous gas, free peritoneal air

Fluoroscopic Findings
- Upper GI
  o Diagnosis of malrotation made on upper GI when criteria for normal position of DJJ (ligament of Treitz) are not met
  o Criteria for normal DJJ
    ▪ AP supine positioning
    ▪ DJJ: Where 4th portion of duodenum turns left and becomes jejunum
    ▪ DJJ is to the left of the spine
    ▪ DJJ is at the same level or more superior than duodenal bulb
  o Obvious cases: Duodenum coursing into RUQ; never crossing spine
  o In borderline cases, small bowel follow through is often helpful to document position of cecum
  o With near normal DJJ and RLQ cecum, probably not at risk for volvulus (long small bowel mesentery)
  o DJJ is mobile in children and can be "factitiously" moved into normal or abnormal position by distended bowel, masses, or indwelling NJ tube
  o On lateral view, duodenum typically courses posteriorly, then inferiorly
    ▪ With malrotation, may not initially course posteriorly
  o Goal of upper GI in neonate with bilious vomiting is to exclude or demonstrate findings of malrotation (not necessarily with volvulus)
  o In an infant with bilious vomiting, findings of malrotation considered a surgical emergency, even if radiographic findings of volvulus not identified
  o Volvulus: Duodenum and jejunum appear as corkscrew or as complete duodenal obstruction
  o Malrotation may be an incidental finding
- Contrast enema
  o Cecum not in right lower quadrant
  o Cecal location in RUQ or LUQ has greatest prognostic implication for volvulus/obstruction

CT Findings
- CECT
  o Relationship of superior mesenteric vein (SMV) and artery (SMA)
    ▪ Normally SMV to right of SMA
    ▪ SMA: Smaller, rounder, surrounded by fat
    ▪ SMV: Larger, thinner walled
  o With malrotation, often SMV to left of SMA
    ▪ Finding is not specific or sensitive
    ▪ Abnormal relationship can be seen with normal rotation and vice versa
  o With volvulus, swirling pattern of bowel about SMA
  o May have small bowel distention
  o Pneumatosis, portal venous gas and free peritoneal air may be present

Ultrasonographic Findings
- If US done to exclude hypertrophic pyloric stenosis (HPS) and HPS not identified, look for findings of malrotation/volvulus
  o US not done in cases of suspected malrotation, UGI performed
- SMV/SMA relationship and other findings as on CT
- Proximal duodenum may be persistently fluid-filled

Imaging Recommendations
- Best imaging tool
  o Infant with bilious vomiting indication for emergency upper GI
  o Small bowel follow through (SBFT) or barium enema (BE) for borderline DJJ to document position of cecum
- Protocol advice: Imaging of first pass of barium helpful to avoid DJJ being obscured by contrast in antrum or jejunum

DIFFERENTIAL DIAGNOSIS

Prominent Gastroesophageal Reflux (GER)
- Non-bilious vomiting
- Very common and clinical finding leading to most UGI performed in infants

MIDGUT VOLVULUS

Spectrum of Congenital Duodenum Obstruction
- Spectrum of related abnormalities: Duodenal atresia, duodenal stenosis, annular pancreas, duodenal web
- Tend to have distention of proximal duodenum 2nd to chronic obstruction

PATHOLOGY

General Features
- General path comments
  - With normal embryonic rotation, both the duodenojejunal and ileocolic portions of the bowel rotate counterclockwise 270° around the axis of the omphalomesenteric vessels
  - Understanding of the embryogenesis is emphasized, but an understanding of the results is more important
  - With normal rotation, duodenojejunal junction positioned in left upper quadrant and cecum positioned in right lower quadrant
    - Result in long, fixed base between ligament of Treitz and cecum that keeps mesentery from twisting
  - If duodenojejunal and ileocecal junctions not in normal positions (malrotation), base of small bowel mesentery may be short and predisposed to twisting (volvulus)
  - Malrotation may also be associated with duodenal obstruction from
    - Ladd bands (abnormal fibrous peritoneal bands)
    - Paraduodenal hernias
- Etiology: Development anomaly resulting in narrow mesenteric pedicle secondary to abnormal fixation and rotation of bowel
- Epidemiology
  - 2.86/10,000 new births
  - Incidence inversely proportional to maternal age
- Associated abnormalities
  - Entities associated with malrotation
    - Congenital diaphragmatic hernia
    - Abdominal wall defects: Gastroschisis, omphalocele
    - Abdominal heterotaxies

Microscopic Features
- Ischemic or necrotic bowel

CLINICAL ISSUES

Presentation
- Most common signs/symptoms: Classic presentation: Bilious vomiting
- Other signs/symptoms
  - Acute abdominal pain
  - Vomiting, crampy abdominal pain
  - Failure to thrive
  - Patients may be asymptomatic, have atypical or chronic symptoms

Demographics
- Age
  - 39% present within first 10 days of life
  - > 90% present within first 3 months of life
  - Can occur at any age
- Gender: Slightly higher incidence in boys
- Ethnicity: > In Asian populations

Natural History & Prognosis
- Potential volvulus leading to bowel necrosis
- Possible midgut volvulus is one of few true emergencies in pediatric GI

Treatment
- Surgical emergency
- Ladd procedure: Reduction of volvulus, resect nonviable bowel, transect Ladd bands (if present), place small bowel in right and colon in left abdomen

DIAGNOSTIC CHECKLIST

Consider
- Delay in diagnosis can result in diffuse bowel necrosis or death
- Infant with bilious vomiting indication for emergency upper GI
- Borderline cases of DJJ location, SBFT or BE should be performed to document the location of the cecum

Image Interpretation Pearls
- DJJ should be at the same level or more superior than duodenal bulb
- On lateral view, duodenum typically courses posterior then inferiorly

SELECTED REFERENCES
1. Patino MO et al: Utility of the sonographic whirlpool sign in diagnosing midgut volvulus in patients with atypical clinical presentations. J Ultrasound Med. 23(3):397-401, 2004
2. Strouse PJ: Disorders of intestinal rotation and fixation ("malrotation"). Pediatr Radiol. 34(11):837-51, 2004
3. Millar AJ et al: Malrotation and volvulus in infancy and childhood. Semin Pediatr Surg. 12(4):229-36, 2003
4. Buonomo C: Neonatal gastrointestinal emergencies. Radiol Clin North Am. 35(4):845-64, 1997
5. Long FR et al: Radiographic patterns of intestinal malrotation in children. Radiographics. 16(3):547-56; discussion 556-60, 1996
6. Berdon WE et al: Midgut malrotation and volvulus. Which films ar most helpful? Radiology. 96(2):375-84, 1970

MIDGUT VOLVULUS

IMAGE GALLERY

Variant

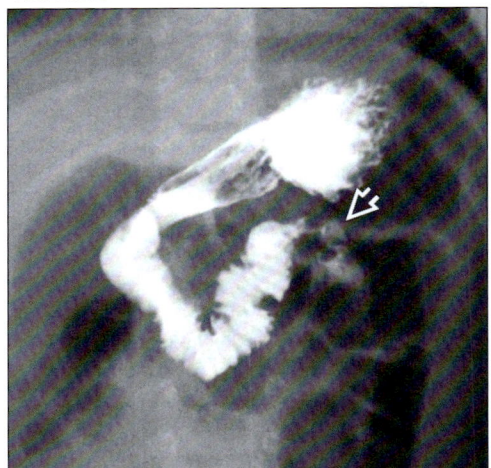
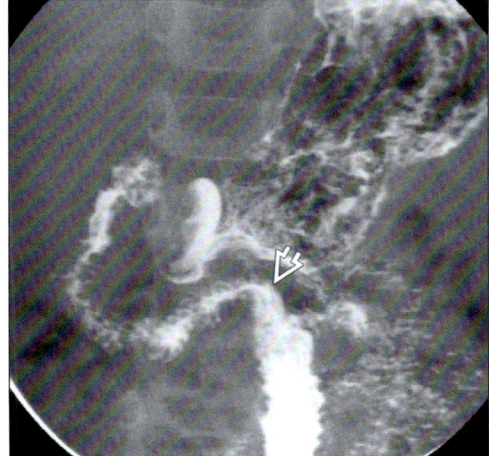

(Left) Frontal upper GI shows normal position of the duodenojejunal junction ➔ on first pass of contrast with DJJ left of the spine, and at the same superior to inferior level as duodenal bulb. *(Right)* Frontal upper GI shows borderline abnormal DJJ ➔ positioned not quite to left of the spine and more inferior than the duodenal bulb. Patient did have malrotation.

Typical

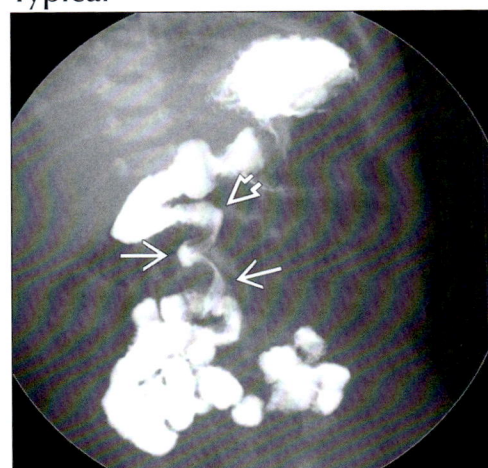
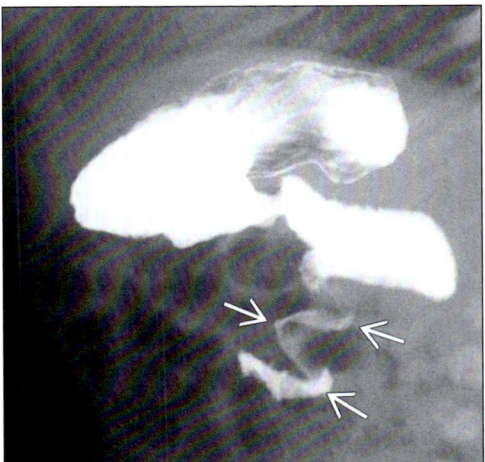

(Left) Frontal upper GI shows malrotation and volvulus. Note DJJ ➔ below the level of the duodenal bulb, corkscrew appearance ➔ of the proximal jejunum c/w volvulus. *(Right)* Lateral upper GI shows duodenum not to be retroperitoneal in course and corkscrew appearance ➔ of the volvulus. Proximal duodenum is slightly fluid-filled.

Typical

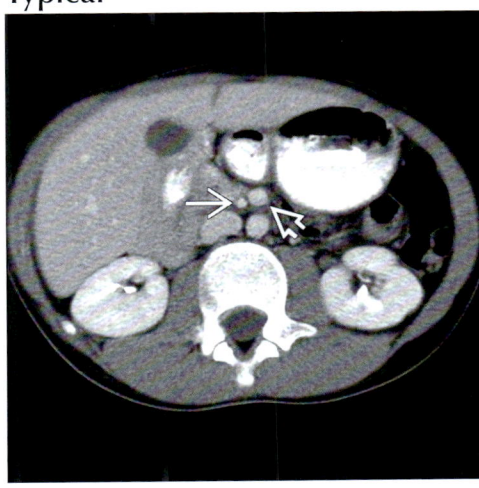
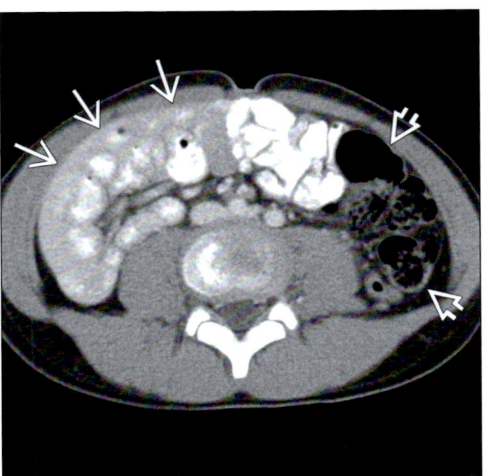

(Left) Axial CECT shows findings suggestive of malrotation with reversal of normal SMA/SMV anatomic relationship: SMA ➔ to right of SMA ➔. *(Right)* Axial CECT in the same patient as left with malrotation shows small bowel in the right abdomen ➔ and colon ➔ in the left abdomen.

DUODENAL ATRESIA OR STENOSIS

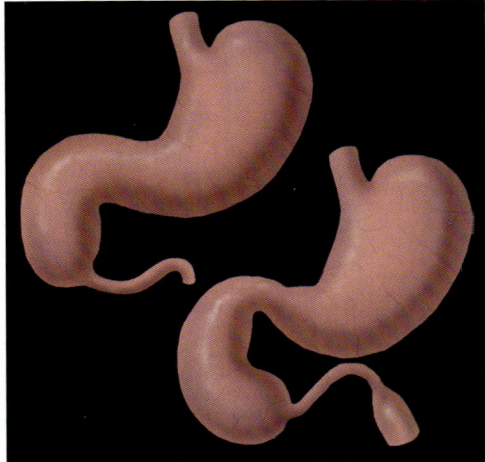

Graphic shows dilation of the stomach and duodenum to the level of duodenal atresia (left) and to the level of duodenal stenosis (right).

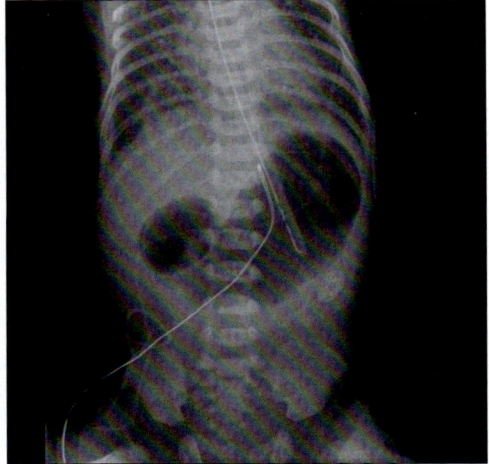

Frontal radiograph of a 1 day old neonate shows dilated stomach and duodenum, the "double bubble" of duodenal atresia. There was also an endocardial cushion defect on echocardiogram.

TERMINOLOGY

Abbreviations and Synonyms
- Duodenal atresia (DA), duodenal stenosis (DS)

Definitions
- Congenital atresia/stenosis of the duodenum
- Duodenal maldevelopment not an ischemic insult
- Most common upper bowel obstruction in neonate

IMAGING FINDINGS

General Features
- Best diagnostic clue: "Double bubble"
- Location
  - 2nd or 3rd portion of the duodenum
  - In the region of the Ampulla of Vater
- Size: Large stomach and duodenum
- Morphology: Dilated stomach and duodenum proximal to atresia

Radiographic Findings
- Radiography
  - Gas distending stomach and proximal duodenum
    - Dilated duodenum implies chronic obstruction
  - Atresia: No distal gas
  - Stenosis: Distal gas; **must exclude** midgut volvulus by UGI

Fluoroscopic Findings
- Not usually performed for DA, plain films diagnostic
- If upper gastrointestinal (UGI) performed, either
  - Duodenal obstruction
  - Partial duodenal obstruction
  - **Must see duodenal jejunal junction (DJJ) to exclude volvulus**
- If DA with pancreas divisum, distal contrast possible
  - Bile duct drains on either side of atretic segment

MR Findings
- T1WI: Fetal: Low signal in dilated stomach and duodenum
- T2WI: Fetal: High signal in dilated stomach and duodenum

Ultrasonographic Findings
- Grayscale Ultrasound

DDx: Duodenal Obstruction

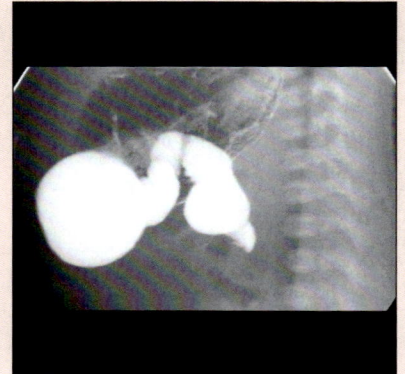

Midgut Volvulus

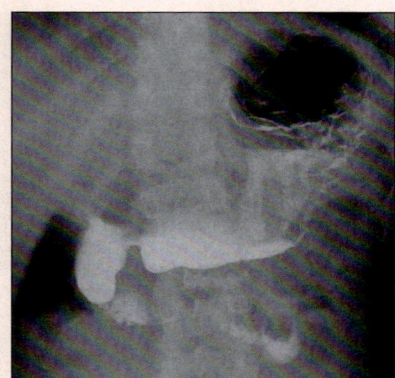

Duodenal Web

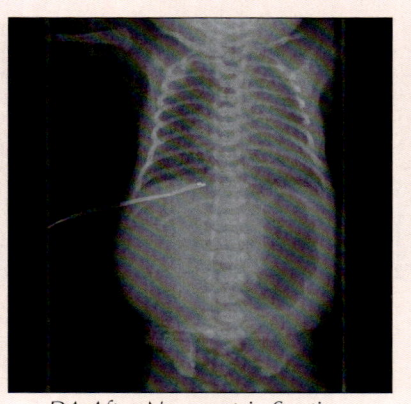

DA After Nasogastric Suction

DUODENAL ATRESIA OR STENOSIS

Key Facts

Terminology
- Most common upper bowel obstruction in neonate

Imaging Findings
- Best diagnostic clue: "Double bubble"
- In the region of the Ampulla of Vater
- Duodenal obstruction
- **Must see duodenal jejunal junction (DJJ) to exclude volvulus**
- If "double bubble" on x-ray, no further study required
- If distal gas, upper GI

Top Differential Diagnoses
- Malrotation and Midgut Volvulus: Extrinsic
- Duodenal Web or Diaphragm: Intrinsic
- Other Anomalies Associated with Intrinsic Duodenum Obstruction
- Annular pancreas in 33%
- Preduodenal portal vein

Pathology
- Failure of vacuolization (recanalization)
- 30% with DA have Down syndrome (trisomy 21)
- Malrotation: 28%
- Annular pancreas: 33%
- Other associated anomalies: Intestinal atresias; congenital heart disease; anorectal, biliary, renal anomalies; absence of gallbladder; situs anomalies, preduodenal portal vein
- Type I: Most common in DA

Clinical Issues
- Onset of vomiting within hours of birth
- Duodenoduodenostomy most common operation

- Anechoic, dilated, fluid-filled stomach and duodenum
- Associated abdominal findings that can be seen
  - Annular pancreas, preduodenal portal vein, biliary anomalies
- Prenatal sonography
  - Dilated stomach and duodenum
  - Polyhydramnios in 40%
  - Gastric duplication may mimic DA in utero

Echocardiographic Findings
- Echocardiogram
  - Associated congenital heart disease
  - If Down syndrome
    - Atrial septal defect (ASD)
    - Ventriculoseptal defect (VSD)
    - Patent ductus arteriosis (PDA)
    - Atrioventricular (AV) canal

Imaging Recommendations
- Best imaging tool
  - Plain film radiography for atresia
  - UGI if distal gas
- Protocol advice
  - If "double bubble" on x-ray, no further study required
  - If distal gas, upper GI
  - Use barium by nasogastric tube for pre-op upper GI
    - Aspirate stomach, then inject barium
    - Puff air to advance barium
  - ± Enema to exclude other atresias pre-operatively
  - Post-op upper GI; isotonic water-soluble contrast
    - To exclude post-op leak

DIFFERENTIAL DIAGNOSIS

Extrinsic vs. Intrinsic Considerations
- May often be differentiated only at surgery

Malrotation and Midgut Volvulus: Extrinsic
- Proximal duodenum is typically not dilated in acute volvulus
- In-utero volvulus may cause duodenal dilation
- Upper GI: Malpositioned DJJ, corkscrew appearance of duodenum/jejunum
- May involve Ladd bands

Duplication Cyst: Extrinsic
- Sonography may show diagnostic double ring sign
- "Gut signature" (hyperechoic inner, hypoechoic outer wall)

Duodenal Web or Diaphragm: Intrinsic
- Later presentation
- Windsock appearance

Other Anomalies Associated with Intrinsic Duodenum Obstruction
- Annular pancreas in 33%
- Preduodenal portal vein

PATHOLOGY

General Features
- General path comments
  - 2 theories of duodenal maldevelopment
    - Failure of vacuolization (recanalization)
    - Inadequate endodermal proliferation
  - Most DA is the membranous type
  - Spectrum of disease
    - No canalization, blind ending: DA
    - Partial canalization: DS or duodenal web
  - Duodenum most common site of intestinal atresia
- Genetics
  - Several reports of familial occurrence
  - Strong association with Down syndrome
  - Feingold syndrome
    - Combination of hand and foot anomalies, microcephaly, tracheo-esophageal fistula, esophageal/duodenal atresia, short palpebral fissures and developmental delay
  - Partial monosomy 10q with partial trisomy 11q
  - 2q24.3: Quarter deletion
  - Of 265 fetal karyotypes, 43% with DA abnormal

DUODENAL ATRESIA OR STENOSIS

- Etiology
  - Unknown
  - 50% associated with other malformations
  - Developmental error in early period of gestation
  - Different from other atresias which are due to vascular accidents late in development
- Epidemiology: Incidence 1:7,500 to 1:40,000 live births
- Associated abnormalities
  - 50% of patients with DA
  - 30% with DA have Down syndrome (trisomy 21)
    - 11 pairs of ribs, macroglossia, flat acetabular angles, cardiomegaly with shunt vascularity (ASD, VSD, PDA, AV canal)
  - Malrotation: 28%
  - Annular pancreas: 33%
  - Other associated anomalies: Intestinal atresias; congenital heart disease; anorectal, biliary, renal anomalies; absence of gallbladder; situs anomalies, preduodenal portal vein

Gross Pathologic & Surgical Features
- Dilated duodenum with an otherwise intact wall
- Usually well perfused, not ischemic at operation

Staging, Grading or Classification Criteria
- Type I: Most common in DA
  - Intact intestinal wall and mesentery
  - Septal or membranous luminal obstruction
  - Diameter proximal >> distal segment
- Type II
  - Intestinal segments separated by fibrous cord
- Type III
  - Two blind ends without intervening cord
  - With wedge-shaped mesenteric defect

CLINICAL ISSUES

Presentation
- Most common signs/symptoms
  - DA/DS present in the newborn
  - Onset of vomiting within hours of birth
    - 85% bilious
    - 15% nonbilious: Proximal to ampulla of Vater
  - Scaphoid abdomen
  - Feeding intolerance
- Other signs/symptoms: Dehydration, weight loss, electrolyte imbalance, bile-stained aspirates from orogastric tube

Demographics
- Age
  - Newborn in DA/DS
  - 46% were premature in large series

Natural History & Prognosis
- Untreated, dehydration, severe electrolyte abnormalities, death
- With surgical treatment, survival rate > 90%

Treatment
- Surgical repair
  - If radiographically diagnostic of DA surgical repair urgent but not emergent unless clinically warranted
  - Partial duodenal obstructions possibly malrotated treated emergently
- Duodenoduodenostomy most common operation
  - Side-to-side vs. diamond-shaped technique
- Contraindications to immediate surgical repair
  - Electrolyte or fluid balance disturbances
  - Severe cardiac defects repaired first
  - Severe respiratory insufficiency

DIAGNOSTIC CHECKLIST

Consider
- Presence or absence of distal bowel gas
- Associated anomalies
- Rare causes of distal gas

Image Interpretation Pearls
- "Double bubble" on radiography/sonography
- If distal gas, think possible volvulus

SELECTED REFERENCES

1. Forrester MB et al: Population-based study of small intestinal atresia and stenosis, Hawaii, 1986-2000. Public Health. 118(6):434-8, 2004
2. Sugimoto T et al: Choledochal cyst and duodenal atresia: a rare combination of malformations. Pediatr Surg Int. 20(9):724-6, 2004
3. Doray B et al: Esophageal and duodenal atresia in a girl with a 12q24.3-qter deletion. Clin Genet. 61:468-71, 2002
4. Haeusler MC et al: Prenatal ultrasonographic detection of gastrointestinal obstruction: results from 18 European congenital anomaly registries. Prenat Diagn. 22(7):616-23, 2002
5. Mordehai J et al: Preduodenal portal vein causing duodenal obstruction associated with situs inversus, intestinal malrotation, and polysplenia: A case report. J Pediatr Surg. 37(4):E5, 2002
6. Pumberger W et al: Duodeno-jejunal atresia with volvulus, absent dorsal mesentery, and absent superior mesenteric artery: a hereditary compound structure in duodenal atresia? Am J Med Genet. 109(1):52-5, 2002
7. Rothenberg SS: Laparoscopic duodenoduodenostomy for duodenal obstruction in infants and children. J Pediatr Surg. 37(7):1088-9, 2002
8. Sencan A et al: Symptomatic annular pancreas in newborns. Med Sci Monit. 8(6):CR434-7, 2002
9. Maruyama K et al: Partial monosomy 10q with partial trisomy 11q due to paternal balanced translocation. J Paediatr Child Health. 37(2):198-200, 2001
10. Dalla Vecchia LK et al: Intestinal atresia and stenosis: a 25-year experience with 277 cases. Arch Surg. 133(5):490-6; discussion 496-7, 1998
11. Grosfeld JL: Jejunoileal atresia and stenosis. In: O'neal JA, Rowe MI, Grosfeld JL, eds. Pediatric Surgery, 3rd ed. St Louis: Mosby. 1145-58, 1998
12. Buonomo C: Neonatal gastrointestinal emergencies. Radiol Clin North Am. 35:845-64, 1997
13. Courtens W et al: Feingold syndrome: report of a new family and review. Am J Med Genet. 73(1):55-60, 1997
14. Lemire EG et al: A familial disorder with duodenal atresia and tetralogy of Fallot. Am J Med Genet. 66(1):39-44, 1996
15. Long FR et al: Intestinal malrotation in children: tutorial on radiographic diagnosis in difficult cases. Radiology. 198:775-80, 1996

DUODENAL ATRESIA OR STENOSIS

IMAGE GALLERY

Typical

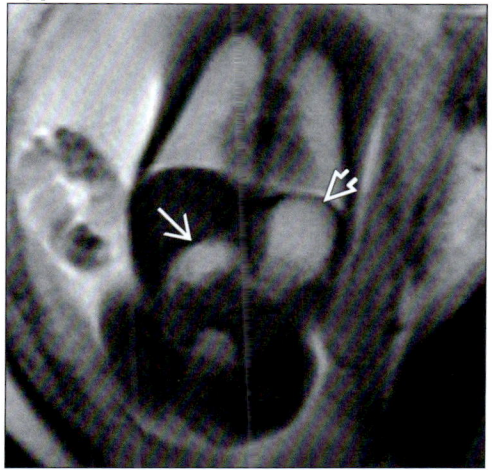
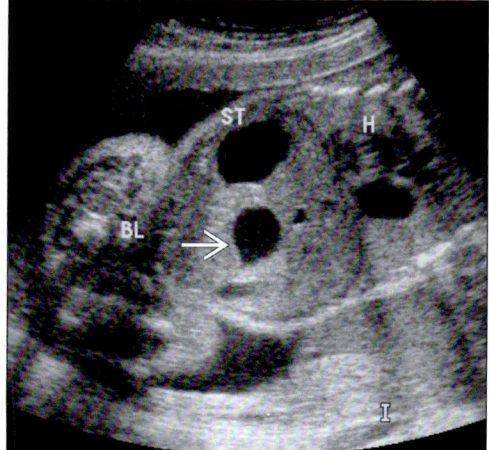

(Left) Coronal T2WI MR of a fetus with duodenal atresia shows high signal of the fluid within the stomach ➡ and obstructed duodenum ➡. *(Right)* Coronal ultrasound performed prenatally on the same patient as previous image (done concurrently) also shows distended stomach (ST) and dilated duodenum ➡ of duodenal atresia.

Typical

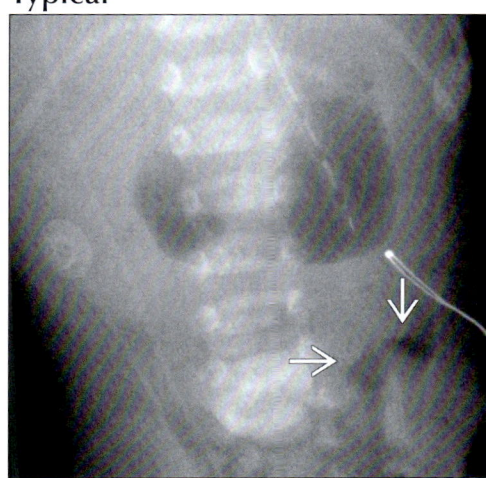
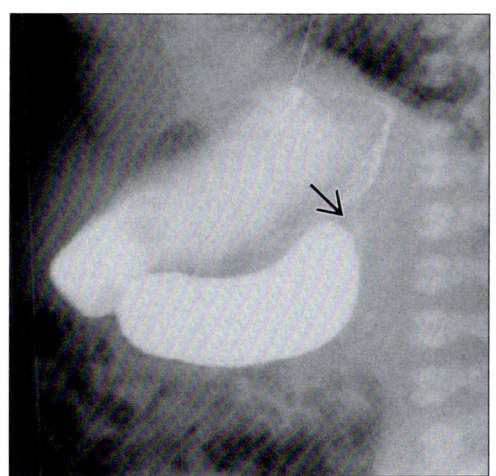

(Left) Frontal radiograph prior to upper GI shows air-filled stomach and duodenum with a small amount of distal gas ➡. Differential considerations must include malrotation and midgut volvulus. *(Right)* Lateral upper GI of the same patient as previous image shows dilated duodenum and a tiny opening ➡ in the duodenum at the end of the dilated segment, consistent with duodenal stenosis.

Variant

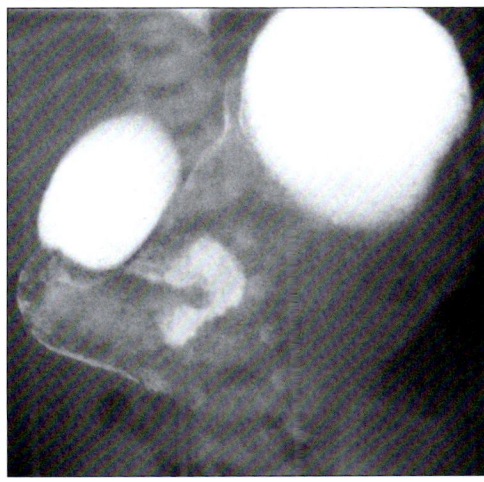
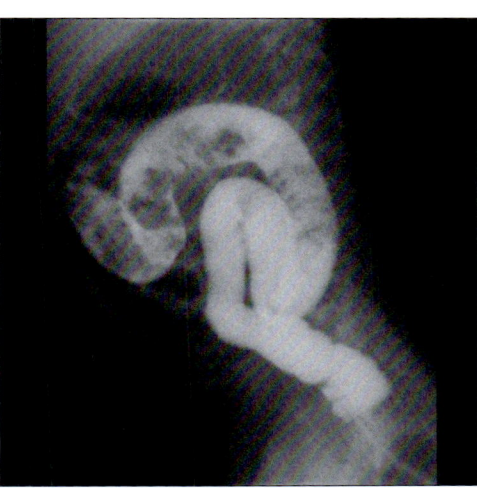

(Left) Frontal upper GI in a patient with duodenal stenosis shows midline position of the duodenal-jejunal junction, findings of malrotation which are not uncommon in patients with duodenal atresia or stenosis. *(Right)* Lateral contrast enema in patient with DA and Down syndrome shows abnormally small colon at least to the transverse colon. There is an increased incidence of Hirschsprung disease in Down syndrome.

MECONIUM PLUG SYNDROME

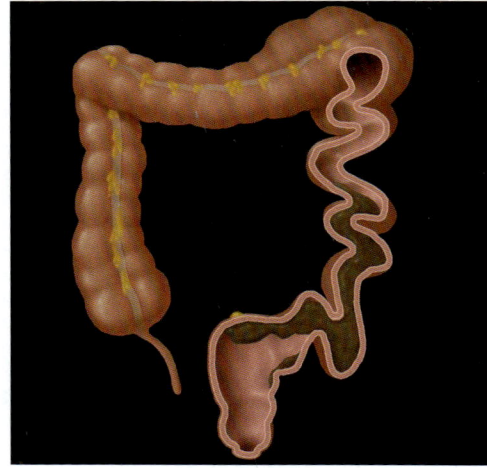

Anteroposterior graphic shows meconium plug (small left colon) syndrome, also known as functional immaturity of the colon. Note small left colon with plugs of meconium, usually to splenic flexure.

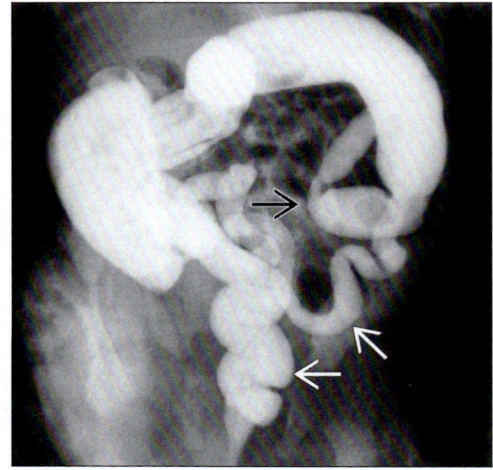

Anteroposterior contrast enema shows typical findings of MPS with a normal rectosigmoid ratio ➔, small left colon, and a transition zone to dilated colon at the level of the splenic flexure ➔.

TERMINOLOGY

Abbreviations and Synonyms
- Meconium plug syndrome (MPS), small left colon syndrome (SLCS), functional immaturity of the colon (FIC)

Definitions
- Transient functional obstruction of the newborn colon
- Common cause of distal neonatal bowel obstruction

IMAGING FINDINGS

General Features
- Best diagnostic clue
  - Multiple dilated bowel loops in neonate
  - Contrast enema findings include
    - Normal recto-sigmoid (R/S) ratio: Usually
    - Small left colon to the splenic flexure
    - Abrupt zone of transition to dilated proximal colon at the splenic flexure
    - Multiple meconium plugs in the colon
- Location: Left colon
- Size: Small left colon with transition to dilated proximal bowel at splenic flexure
- Morphology: Small but otherwise normal left colon

Radiographic Findings
- Radiography
  - Multiple dilated loops of bowel
  - Cannot differentiate dilated large from small bowel loops in neonates
  - Findings nonspecific, cannot differentiate from other causes of distal bowel

Fluoroscopic Findings
- Contrast enema
  - Recto-sigmoid ratio usually > 1
  - Small caliber left colon to the splenic flexure
  - Abrupt transition to dilated proximal colon
  - Multiple filling defects may fill left colon, but not required
  - Frequently pass meconium plugs during enema

Other Modality Findings
- Contrast enema
  - R/S ratio usually > 1
  - Descending and sigmoid colon small in caliber

DDx: Neonatal Distal Bowel Obstruction

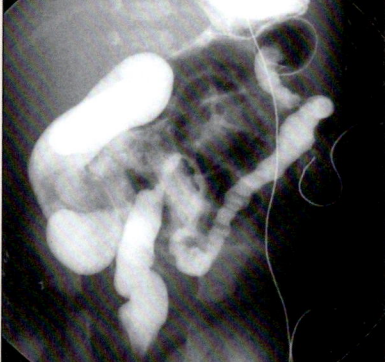

Total Colonic Hirschsprung Disease

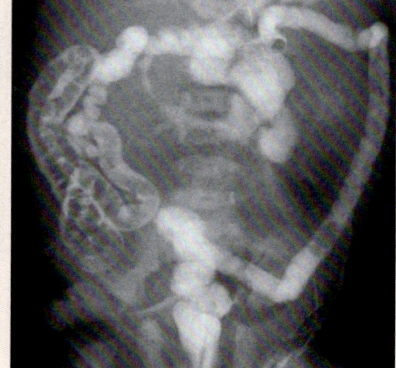

Meconium Ileus

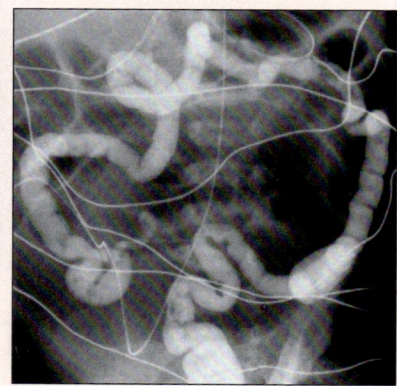

Ileal Atresia

MECONIUM PLUG SYNDROME

Key Facts

Terminology
- Meconium plug syndrome (MPS), small left colon syndrome (SLCS), functional immaturity of the colon (FIC)
- Transient functional obstruction of the newborn colon
- Common cause of distal neonatal bowel obstruction

Imaging Findings
- Multiple dilated bowel loops in neonate
- Small left colon to the splenic flexure
- Abrupt zone of transition to dilated proximal colon at the splenic flexure
- Multiple filling defects may fill left colon, but not required
- Differential diagnosis long segment Hirschsprung disease
- Best imaging tool: Water-soluble contrast enema

Pathology
- Distal colon spastic and narrowed, causes functional obstruction usually at splenic flexure
- Genetics: No association with cystic fibrosis
- Etiology: Probably immaturity of ganglion cells or hormonal receptors
- Associated abnormalities: Most with MPS do not have associated abnormalities

Clinical Issues
- Abdominal distention
- Delayed or failed passage of meconium (> 24-48 hours)
- Bilious emesis
- Condition resolves over time, hastened by enemas

- Abrupt zone of caliber transition in region of splenic flexure
- ± Filling defects (meconium plugs) within colon
- Ascending and transverse colon increased in caliber
- Differential diagnosis long segment Hirschsprung disease
- Enema often therapeutic; pass meconium plugs during or just after enema

Imaging Recommendations
- Best imaging tool: Water-soluble contrast enema
- In neonate with abdominal distention, failure to pass meconium, bilious emesis
  - Abdominal radiograph: 2 views
    - If multiple dilated loops: Suspect distal bowel obstruction
    - If distal obstruction: Water-soluble contrast enema
  - Enema
    - Non-balloon tipped catheter
    - Ionic, water-soluble agents, isosmotic to body fluids
    - Barium avoided in neonate; etiology of obstruction unknown
    - Initial lateral image: Filled rectum through splenic flexure
    - If enema shows normal colon (rare) but dilated small bowel loops then perform upper gastrointestinal (GI) to exclude midgut volvulus (malrotation)

DIFFERENTIAL DIAGNOSIS

Hirschsprung Disease
- Rectum smaller than sigmoid diameter, serrated mucosa
- Differential diagnosis meconium plug syndrome
- Broad cone-like zone of transition if near splenic flexure

Ileal Atresia
- Microcolon
- Portions of ileum opacified are collapsed and blind ends
- Cannot opacify dilated loops (proximal to atresia)

Meconium Ileus
- Microcolon
- Distal ileum filled with meconium pellets
- Small bowel proximal to meconium filled segment is dilated
- Nearly all have cystic fibrosis

Colonic Atresia
- Microcolon to level of atresia
- Very rare
- Distal obstruction with a single disproportionately dilated loop

Midgut Volvulus
- Normal caliber colon on enema: Perform upper GI
- Mimics distal obstruction: Late presentation
- Dilated bowel loops due to ischemia not obstruction
- Upper GI shows
  - Abnormal duodenal jejunal junction
  - Obstruction at 2nd to 3rd portion duodenum
  - Corkscrew, spiral appearance

PATHOLOGY

General Features
- General path comments
  - Transient functional disorder of the colon
  - No pathologic or laboratory abnormality
  - Clinical and radiographic disorder only
  - Distal colon spastic and narrowed, causes functional obstruction usually at splenic flexure
- Genetics: No association with cystic fibrosis
- Etiology: Probably immaturity of ganglion cells or hormonal receptors
- Epidemiology
  - Predisposing factors: Infants of
    - Mothers with diabetes

MECONIUM PLUG SYNDROME

- Mothers treated with magnesium sulfate for preeclampsia
- Associated abnormalities: Most with MPS do not have associated abnormalities

Gross Pathologic & Surgical Features
- Not a pathologic or surgical abnormality

CLINICAL ISSUES

Presentation
- Most common signs/symptoms
  - Abdominal distention
  - Delayed or failed passage of meconium (> 24-48 hours)
  - Bilious emesis
- Other signs/symptoms: Otherwise well infant
- Most frequent encountered diagnosis in neonates who fail to pass meconium
- Increased incidence of meconium plug syndrome
  - Infants of mothers with diabetes
  - Infants of mothers who receive magnesium sulfate for eclampsia
- Meconium plug syndrome and meconium ileus (cystic fibrosis) are distinct entities not to be confused
  - Meconium plug syndrome: Zone of transition splenic flexure of colon
  - Meconium ileus: Microcolon with obstructing meconium plugs in terminal ileum

Demographics
- Age: Neonates
- Gender: No gender predilection
- Ethnicity: No known ethnicity predilection

Natural History & Prognosis
- Temporary phenomenon: Usually resolves; benign course
- Prognosis excellent
- Potential complications: Rare
  - Perforation due to unresolved obstruction
  - If hypertonic water-soluble contrast used for enema
    - Rapid fluid shift into colon causing potentially severe, life-threatening hypotension
    - Electrolyte imbalance

Treatment
- Condition resolves over time, hastened by enemas
- Often resolves after diagnostic water-soluble contrast enema
- Suction rectal biopsy to exclude Hirschsprung disease, especially if persistent symptoms

DIAGNOSTIC CHECKLIST

Consider
- Hirschsprung disease
- Immature colon if premature infant

Image Interpretation Pearls
- Normal R/S ratio (> 1)
- Small left colon ± meconium plugs
- Transition point to dilated bowel at splenic flexure

SELECTED REFERENCES

1. Burge D et al: Meconium plug obstruction. Pediatr Surg Int. 20(2):108-10, 2004
2. Hajivassiliou CA: Intestinal obstruction in neonatal/pediatric surgery. Semin Pediatr Surg. 12(4):241-53, 2003
3. De Backer AI et al: Radiographic manifestations of intestinal obstruction in the newborn. JBR-BTR. 82(4):159-66, 1999
4. Lassmann G et al: Transient functional obstruction of the colon in neonates: examination of its development by manometry and biopsies. Prog Pediatr Surg. 24:202-16, 1989
5. Hall SL et al: Neonatal intussusception associated with neonatal small left colon syndrome. Clin Pediatr (Phila). 26(4):191-3, 1987
6. Amodio J et al: Microcolon of prematurity: a form of functional obstruction. AJR Am J Roentgenol. 146(2):239-44, 1986
7. Ellerbroek C et al: Neonatal small left colon in an infant with cystic fibrosis. Pediatr Radiol. 16(2):162-3, 1986
8. Johnson JF et al: Localized bowel distension in the newborn: a review of the plain film analysis and differential diagnosis. Pediatrics. 73(2):206-15, 1984
9. Rosenfield NS et al: Hirschsprung disease: accuracy of the barium enema examination. Radiology. 150(2):393-400, 1984
10. Cohen MD et al: Neonatal small left colon syndrome in twins. Gastrointest Radiol. 7(3):283-6, 1982
11. Dunn V et al: Infants of diabetic mothers: radiographic manifestations. AJR Am J Roentgenol. 137(1):123-8, 1981
12. Rangecroft L: Neonatal small left colon syndrome. Arch Dis Child. 54(8):635-7, 1979
13. Berdon WE et al: Neonatal small left colon syndrome: its relationship to aganglionosis and meconium plug syndrome. Radiology. 125(2):457-62, 1977
14. Ferrara TP et al: The radiology corner. Neonatal small left colon syndrome. Am J Gastroenterol. 68(6):608-12, 1977
15. Stewart DR et al: Neonatal small left colon syndrome. Ann Surg. 186(6):741-5, 1977
16. Davis WS et al: Neonatal small left colon syndrome. Occurrence in asymptomatic infants of diabetic mothers. Am J Dis Child. 129(9):1024-7, 1975
17. Davis WS et al: Neonatal small left colon syndrome. Am J Roentgenol Radium Ther Nucl Med. 120(2):322-9, 1974
18. Berdon WE et al: Microcolon in newborn infants with intestinal obstruction. Its correlation with the level and time of onset of obstruction. Radiology. 90(5):878-85, 1968

MECONIUM PLUG SYNDROME

IMAGE GALLERY

Typical

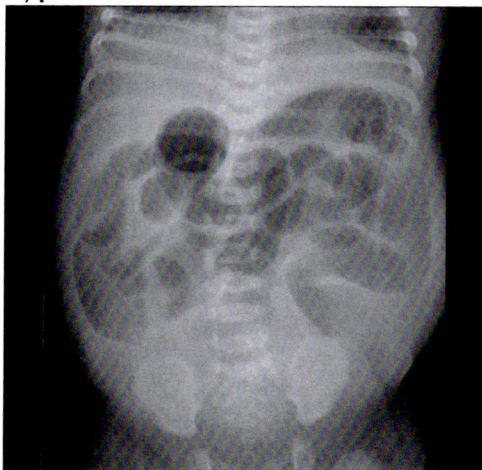
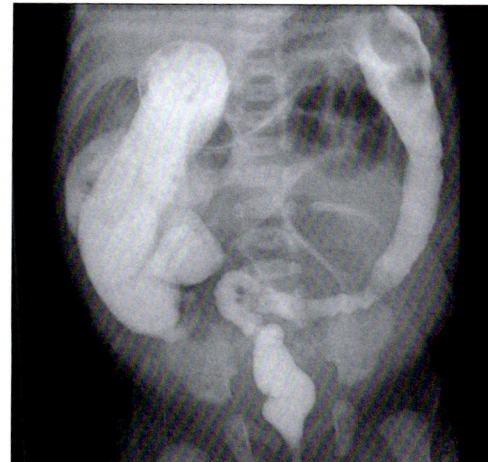

(Left) Anteroposterior radiograph of a 2-day-old, full term infant from a diabetic mother, shows multiple dilated loops of bowel characteristic of neonatal distal bowel obstruction. Clinically, the patient was otherwise healthy. *(Right)* Anteroposterior contrast enema in the same patient as previous image, shows a small left colon to the level of the splenic flexure with a normal rectosigmoid ratio. Rectal biopsy showed normal ganglion cells.

Typical

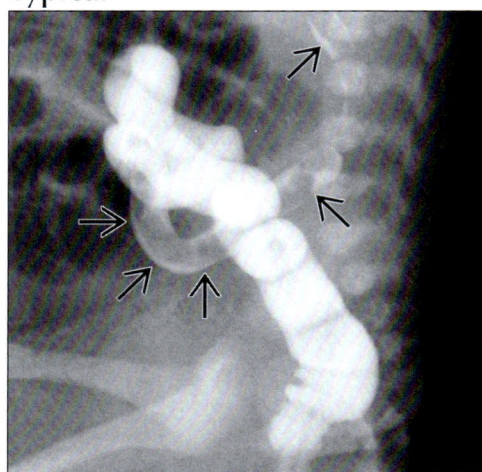
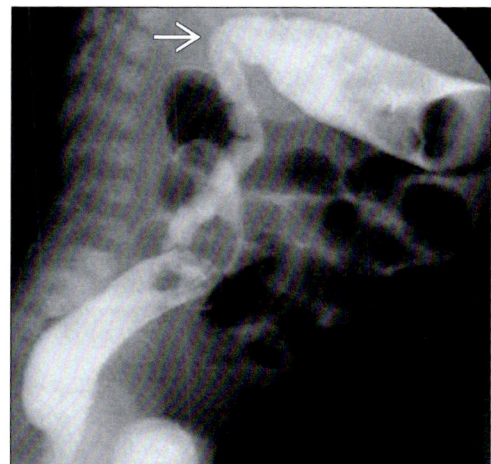

(Left) Lateral contrast enema shows a tubular plug of meconium ➡ within the sigmoid colon in this 2 day old infant whose mother was treated for pre-eclampsia with Magnesium sulfate. Rectosigmoid ratio was normal. *(Right)* Lateral contrast enema in this 1 1/2 day old male full-term infant, shows small left colon with abrupt transition zone to dilated bowel at the splenic flexure ➡. Meconium plug is seen in small left colon.

Typical

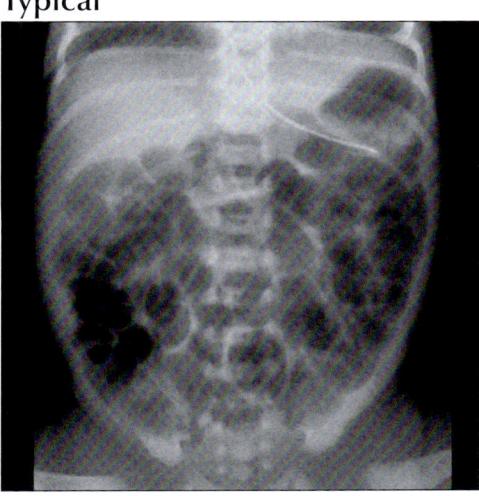
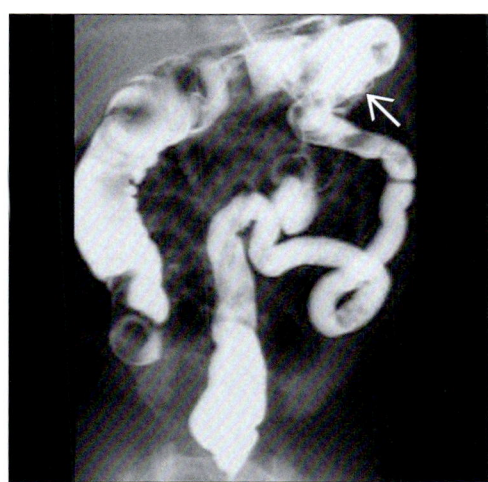

(Left) Anteroposterior radiograph in a 2 day old infant who failed to pass meconium, shows findings of distal bowel obstruction. No free air or abnormal calcifications to suggest complication. *(Right)* Anteroposterior contrast enema in the same patient as previous image, shows a small left colon with transition zone at the splenic flexure ➡. Differential diagnosis includes meconium plug syndrome and Hirschsprung disease.

MECONIUM ILEUS

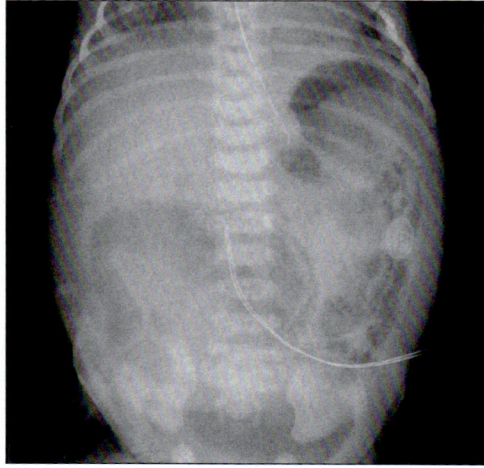

Anteroposterior radiograph at 2 days of age shows distended loops of bowel with mottled density overlying loops, probably meconium and not pneumatosis. Decubitus showed no free air or fluid levels.

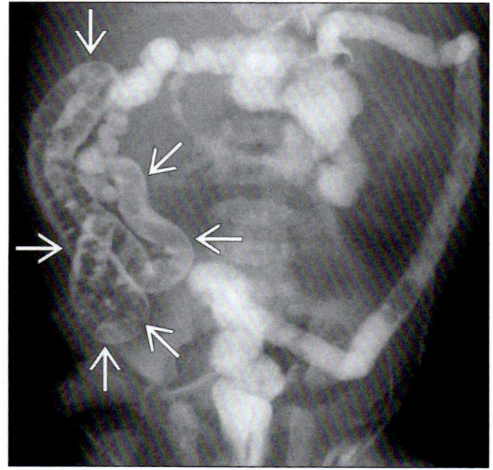

Anteroposterior contrast enema in same patient as previous image shows microcolon with terminal ileum filled with meconium plug and pellets like "pearls on a string" ➡, consistent with meconium ileus.

TERMINOLOGY

Abbreviations and Synonyms
- Meconium ileus (MI)

Definitions
- Neonatal obstruction of the distal ileum due to abnormally thick, tenacious meconium
  - Essentially all patients with MI have cystic fibrosis (CF)
  - Presenting illness in approximately 15% of CF patients

IMAGING FINDINGS

General Features
- Best diagnostic clue: Distal bowel obstruction with microcolon and meconium-filled terminal ileum (TI) on enema
- Location: Terminal ileum obstruction
- Size: Microcolon (dis-use), small TI, dilated proximal small bowel
- Morphology: Small but morphologically normal TI and colon

Radiographic Findings
- Radiography
  - Difficult to distinguish neonatal large vs. small bowel
  - Uncomplicated MI
    - Multiple dilated bowel loops
    - ± Bubbly lucencies right lower quadrant (RLQ)
    - Few, if any air-fluid levels (sticky meconium)
    - Contrast enema to diagnose cause of obstruction
  - Complicated MI
    - Soft tissue mass or gasless abdomen
    - ± Intrauterine perforation and peritonitis
    - Curvilinear calcifications on peritoneal surface or lining pseudocyst
    - Enemas for treatment usually fail, microcolon suggests diagnosis
    - Almost all eventually require surgical treatment

Fluoroscopic Findings
- Water-soluble contrast enema
  - Smallest of microcolons
  - Reflux contrast into TI

DDx: Neonatal Distal Bowel Obstruction: Microcolon

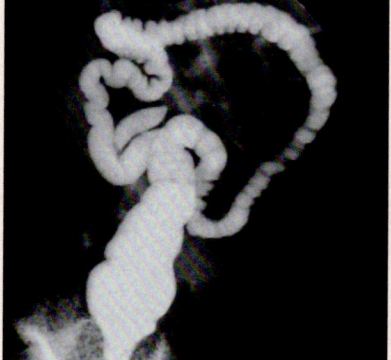

Ileal Atresia

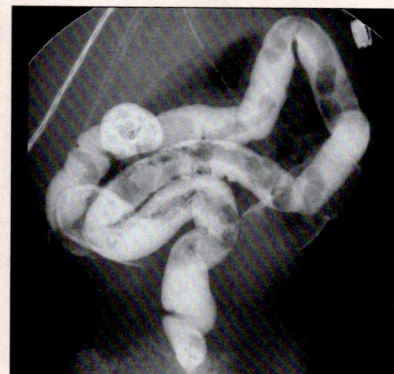

Immature Colon in Premie

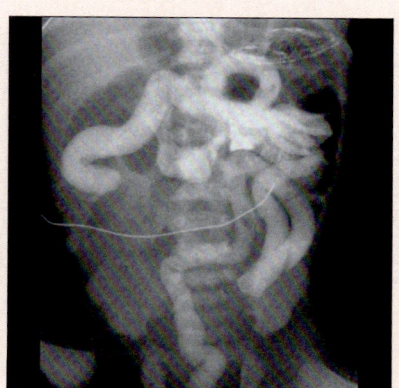

Total Colonic Hirschsprung

MECONIUM ILEUS

Key Facts

Terminology
- Neonatal obstruction of the distal ileum due to abnormally thick tenacious meconium
- Essentially all patients with MI have cystic fibrosis (CF)

Imaging Findings
- Best diagnostic clue: Distal bowel obstruction with microcolon and meconium-filled terminal ileum (TI) on enema
- Multiple dilated bowel loops
- ± Bubbly lucencies right lower quadrant (RLQ)
- Few, if any air-fluid levels (sticky meconium)
- Soft tissue mass or gasless abdomen
- Curvilinear calcifications on peritoneal surface or lining pseudocyst
- Smallest of microcolons
- Dilated, thick-walled, echogenic bowel loops
- Best imaging tool: Water-soluble enema

Top Differential Diagnoses
- Ileal Atresia
- Total Colonic Hirschsprung Disease (HD)

Pathology
- Mutations in CFTCRG, faulty electrolyte transport across epithelium

Clinical Issues
- Most common signs/symptoms: Failure to pass meconium, abdominal distention, bilious emesis
- Uncomplicated MI: Serial hyperosmotic, water-soluble enemas vs. surgery
- Complicated MI: Surgery

   - Meconium pellets in TI; not much in colon
   - Can be therapeutic in uncomplicated MI

Ultrasonographic Findings
- Grayscale Ultrasound
   - Dilated, thick-walled, echogenic bowel loops
   - If perforation: Echogenic ascites or pseudocyst, calcification
- Prenatal ultrasound
   - Dilated echogenic bowel especially RLQ, peritoneal calcifications, pseudocyst

Imaging Recommendations
- Best imaging tool: Water-soluble enema
- If distal bowel obstruction on radiographs: Contrast enema
- Enemas performed with non-balloon tip catheter
- Dilute, ionic, water-soluble agents
- Much debate concerning optimal contrast used
- Meglumine diatrizoate (Gastrografin): High osmolar agent for treatment of MI
   - Controversial
   - Full-strength dangerous secondary to fluid shifts
- If enema shows no abnormalities (rare), upper gastrointestinal (GI)
   - Exclude midgut volvulus with diffuse ischemia

DIFFERENTIAL DIAGNOSIS

Ileal Atresia
- Microcolon
- Portions of ileum opacified normal
- Cannot opacify bowel proximal to atresia

Total Colonic Hirschsprung Disease (HD)
- Microcolon
- Meconium plugs in colon ± TI
- Abnormal rectosigmoid index, smallish colon, serrated mucosa
- Very rare

Meconium Plug Syndrome (Small Left Colon Syndrome)
- No microcolon; small colon distal to splenic flexure
- Not closely associated with cystic fibrosis
- Meconium plugs in colon not TI
- Enema usually curative

PATHOLOGY

General Features
- General path comments
   - Cystic fibrosis gene (chromosome 7) results in failure of cell membrane chloride pump
   - This failure results in abnormally thick, tenacious meconium
      - Occludes distal ileum and results in bowel obstruction
   - Obstruction can also result in perforation, meconium peritonitis
   - Twisting of meconium-filled loops: In utero bowel volvulus and atresia
- Genetics
   - Autosomal recessive, chromosome 7
   - Mutation of cystic fibrosis transmembrane conductance regulator gene (CFTCRG)
- Etiology
   - Mutations in CFTCRG, faulty electrolyte transport across epithelium
      - Dehydration of luminal contents; obstruction of glands and ducts
      - Pancreas, intestine and lung are organs most affected
- Epidemiology
   - 15% of CF present with MI
   - CF: 1:3,000 live births
   - Caucasian children
- Associated abnormalities
   - Lung disease: Upper lobe predominance
      - Bronchiectasis
      - Mucous plugging

MECONIUM ILEUS

- Pneumonia atypical pathogens
- Exocrine pancreas failure: Enzyme deficiency
- Biliary disease: Obstruction, cholangitis
- Concurrent GI manifestations: 50% with MI
  - Meconium peritonitis, small intestinal atresia/stenoses, duplication, segmental volvulus, mesenteric bands or adhesions

Gross Pathologic & Surgical Features
- Uncomplicated: Distal small bowel obstruction, obstructing meconium in TI
- Complicated
  - Meconium peritonitis
  - Giant cystic meconium peritonitis
  - Volvulus of dilated bowel segment
  - Atresia in region of segmental volvulus or perforation
  - Obstructing mesenteric bands

Staging, Grading or Classification Criteria
- Uncomplicated MI: 50%
- Complicated MI: 50%
  - Perforation
    - Ascites with diffuse peritonitis
    - Giant cystic meconium peritonitis
    - Calcification: Speckled or curvilinear
  - Segmental volvulus
  - Atresia

CLINICAL ISSUES

Presentation
- Most common signs/symptoms: Failure to pass meconium, abdominal distention, bilious emesis

Demographics
- Age
  - Newborn; sometimes premature newborns
    - Immature colon can mimic MI
- Gender: Male = female
- Ethnicity: Predominantly Caucasian disease

Natural History & Prognosis
- Poor prognosis if obstruction not treated
- MI associated with worst survival and lung disease outcomes in CF
- 1 year survival in patients with MI: 1993 data
  - Uncomplicated: 92%
  - Complicated: 89%
- Estimated probability of long term survival for patients with CF
  - Without MI: 62% ± 14%
  - With MI: 32% ± 18%

Treatment
- Uncomplicated MI: Serial hyperosmotic, water-soluble enemas vs. surgery
  - Success 70-80% (with experience)
  - Perforation rate of enema 1-3%
    - Greatest with injection and use of rectal balloon
  - Surgical if patient decompensates, enemas fail, or perforation
    - Enterotomy, remove meconium, primary closure
- Complicated MI: Surgery
  - Resect abnormal bowel, remove meconium, primary anastomosis
  - If giant meconium cyst: Enterostomy, delayed takedown
- Testing for cystic fibrosis

DIAGNOSTIC CHECKLIST

Consider
- Causes of distal obstruction and microcolon
- Hyperosmolar water-soluble enema if presumed uncomplicated MI
- Enema rarely curative in complicated MI

SELECTED REFERENCES

1. Lai HJ et al: Association between initial disease presentation, lung disease outcomes, and survival in patients with cystic fibrosis. Am J Epidemiol. 159(6):537-46, 2004
2. Eckoldt F et al: Meconium peritonitis and pseudo-cyst formation: prenatal diagnosis and post-natal course. Prenat Diagn. 23(11):904-8, 2003
3. Hajivassiliou CA: Intestinal obstruction in neonatal/pediatric surgery. Semin Pediatr Surg. 12(4):241-53, 2003
4. Burke MS et al: New strategies in nonoperative management of meconium ileus. J Pediatr Surg. 37(5):760-4, 2002
5. Oliveira MC et al: Effect of meconium ileus on the clinical prognosis of patients with cystic fibrosis. Braz J Med Biol Res. 35(1):31-8, 2002
6. Berrocal T et al: Congenital anomalies of the small intestine, colon, and rectum. Radiographics. 19(5):1219-36, 1999
7. De Backer AI et al: Radiographic manifestations of intestinal obstruction in the newborn. JBR-BTR. 82(4):159-66, 1999
8. Feingold J et al: Genetic comparisons of patients with cystic fibrosis with or without meconium ileus. Clinical Centers of the French CF Registry. Ann Genet. 42(3):147-50, 1999
9. Mushtaq I et al: Meconium ileus secondary to cystic fibrosis. The East London experience. Pediatr Surg Int. 13(5-6):365-9, 1998
10. Buonomo C: Neonatal gastrointestinal emergencies. Radiol Clin North Am. 35(4):845-64, 1997
11. Murshed R et al: Meconium ileus: a ten-year review of thirty-six patients. Eur J Pediatr Surg. 7(5):275-7, 1997
12. Neal MR et al: Neonatal ultrasonography to distinguish between meconium ileus and ileal atresia. J Ultrasound Med. 16(4):263-6; quiz 267-8, 1997
13. Kao SC et al: Nonoperative treatment of simple meconium ileus: a survey of the Society for Pediatric Radiology. Pediatr Radiol. 25(2):97-100, 1995
14. Stringer MD et al: Meconium ileus due to extensive intestinal aganglionosis. J Pediatr Surg. 29(4):501-3, 1994
15. Docherty JG et al: Meconium ileus: a review 1972-1990. Br J Surg. 79(6):571-3, 1992
16. Leonidas JC et al: Meconium ileus and its complications. A reappraisal of plain film roentgen diagnostic criteria. Am J Roentgenol Radium Ther Nucl Med. 108(3):598-609, 1970
17. Berdon WE et al: Microcolon in newborn infants with intestinal obstruction. Its correlation with the level and time of onset of obstruction. Radiology. 90(5):878-85, 1968

MECONIUM ILEUS

IMAGE GALLERY

Variant

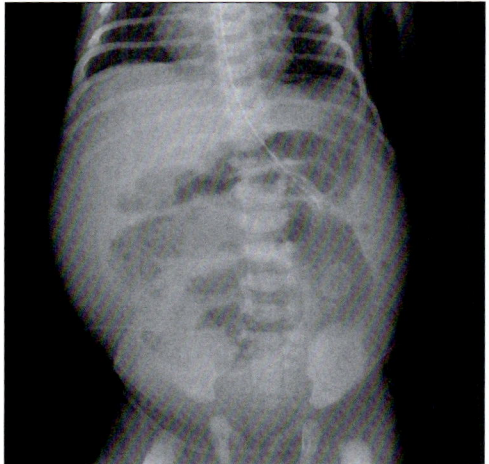
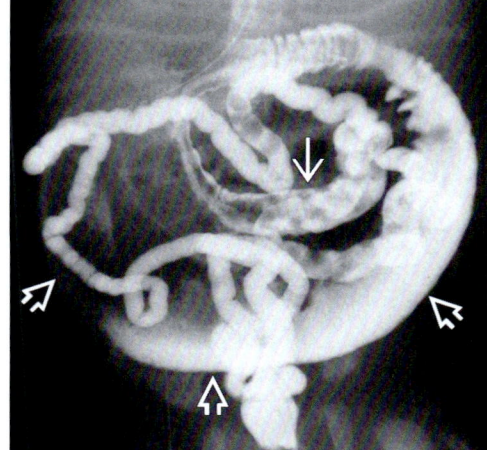

(Left) Lateral radiograph in a neonate shows no free air or air fluid levels but dilated loops of bowel suggestive of distal bowel obstruction. No calcifications to suggest perforation. *(Right)* Posteroanterior contrast enema in prone patient at left shows microcolon with terminal ileal meconium obstruction ➡ and contrast in dilated loops proximally ➡, the goal of therapeutic enema.

Variant

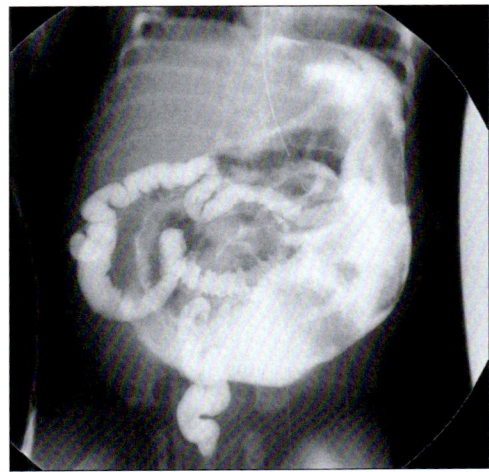
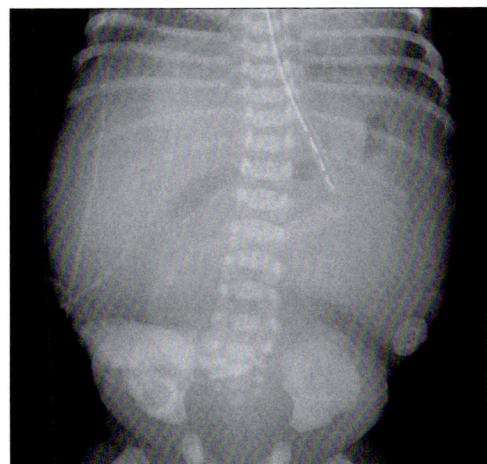

(Left) Anteroposterior contrast enema on the following day compared to above right shows persistent dilated loop of contrast-filled bowel with extravasation of contrast, perforation likely due to ischemic loop of bowel. *(Right)* Anteroposterior radiograph in 2 day old neonate shows relatively gasless abdomen with round, rim calcification indicative of pseudocyst formation, probably in utero perforation.

Variant

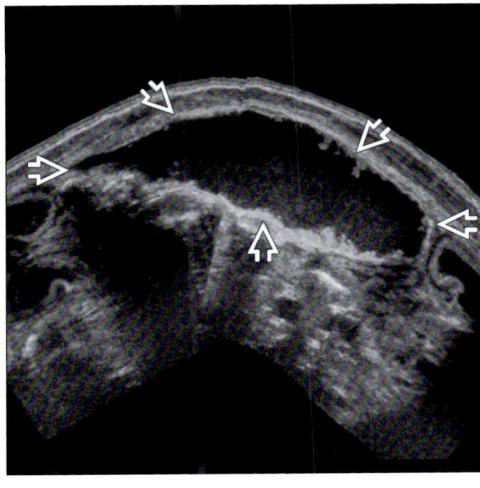
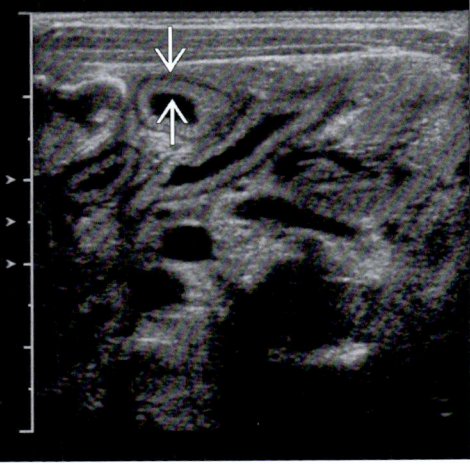

(Left) Transverse ultrasound with extended view feature in same patient as previous image shows thick-walled, meconium-filled pseudocyst ➡ consistent with meconium peritonitis, similar to plain image. *(Right)* Transverse ultrasound in the same patient as previous image, shows thick, echogenic bowel ➡, a nonspecific finding but in the context of perforation is frequently seen in patients with complicated meconium ileus.

MECONIUM PERITONITIS

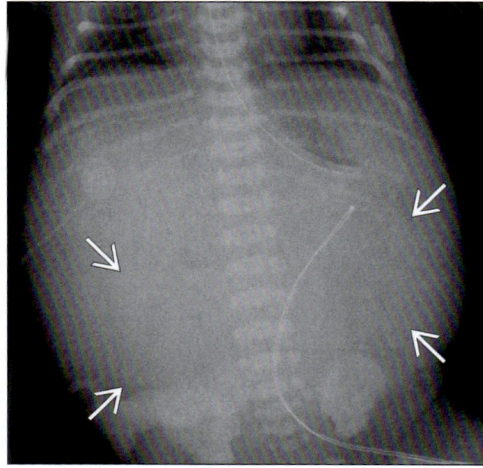

AP radiograph on day of life #1 shows an almost gasless abdomen with faint curvilinear calcification lining a meconium pseudocyst ➔, indicative of in utero perforation and meconium peritonitis.

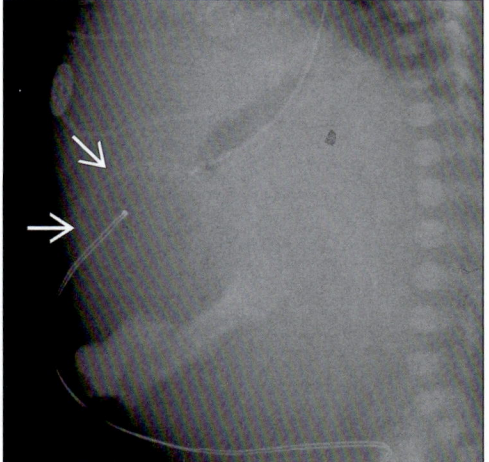

Cross-Table lateral radiograph shows the curvilinear calcifications ➔ to better advantage, a diagnostic sign suggestive of in utero perforation.

TERMINOLOGY

Definitions
- Chemical peritonitis with associated inflammatory response from in utero bowel perforation and peritoneal leakage of sterile meconium

IMAGING FINDINGS

General Features
- Best diagnostic clue
  - Abdomen radiograph showing linear, curvilinear, or punctate peritoneal calcifications
    - 86% of fetuses with meconium peritonitis
    - Takes 1 to 8 days after meconium spillage to perceive calcification
  - Ultrasound showing peritoneal calcifications and/or pseudocyst ± rim calcification
- Location: Peritoneal reflections of the abdomen or pelvis including the scrotum
- Morphology: Follows contour of the peritoneal lining

Radiographic Findings
- Radiography
  - Soft tissue mass
  - Punctate or curvilinear calcifications
  - Ascites
  - Dilated bowel

Fluoroscopic Findings
- Upper GI
  - Normal or duodenal malrotation
  - ± Small bowel obstruction
- Contrast Enema
  - Microcolon (small colon)
    - Suggests distal small bowel obstruction
    - Abrupt obstruction to reflux of contrast in terminal ileum (TI) suggests ileal atresia
    - Abundant meconium pellets in TI suggests meconium ileus
    - Intraluminal calcification suggests total colonic Hirschsprung, anorectal malformation or small bowel atresias
  - Normal colon
    - Possible proximal small bowel obstruction
  - Colonic transition very rare

DDx: Meconium Peritonitis

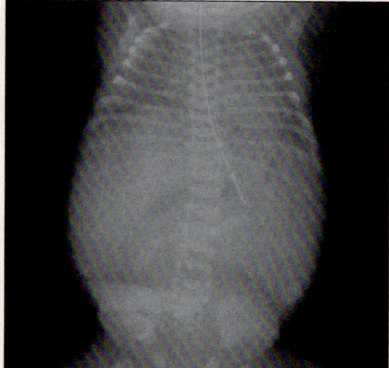

Complicated Meconium Ileus

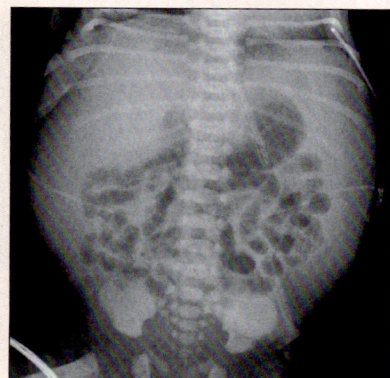

Ileal Atresia and Perforation

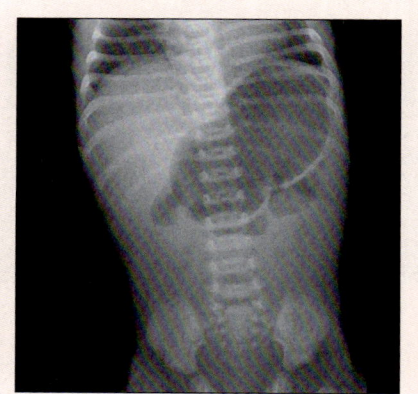

Midgut Volvulus

MECONIUM PERITONITIS

Key Facts

Terminology
- Chemical peritonitis with associated inflammatory response from in utero bowel perforation and peritoneal leakage of sterile meconium

Imaging Findings
- Abdomen radiograph showing linear, curvilinear, or punctate peritoneal calcifications
- Ultrasound showing peritoneal calcifications and/or pseudocyst ± rim calcification
- Calcifications; punctate or linear
- If prenatal US suggestive, post-natal abdomen x-ray
- Contrast fluoroscopic study to limit differential diagnosis

Top Differential Diagnoses
- Cystic Fibrosis: Meconium Ileus
- Intestinal atresia
- Malrotation with midgut volvulus
- Intussusception
- Mesenteric/internal bowel hernias
- Congenital bands
- Viral Infections

Clinical Issues
- Peritoneal calcifications on prenatal or neonatal imaging
- Abdominal distention
- Failure to pass meconium after birth

MR Findings
- Calcifications; punctate or linear
- ± Polyhydramnios
- Fetal ascites
- Bowel distention
- Heterogeneous abdominal mass with calcified wall

Ultrasonographic Findings
- Grayscale Ultrasound
  - Hyperechoic punctate echoes ± shadowing
  - ± Polyhydramnios
  - Fetal ascites
  - Bowel distention
  - Heterogeneous mass with calcified wall

Imaging Recommendations
- Best imaging tool
  - Prenatal and post-natal sonography
  - Radiography in the neonate
- Protocol advice
  - If prenatal US suggestive, post-natal abdomen x-ray
  - Contrast fluoroscopic study to limit differential diagnosis

DIFFERENTIAL DIAGNOSIS

Cystic Fibrosis: Meconium Ileus
- Microcolon
- Complicated form of meconium ileus
- Linear peritoneal calcifications

Intrauterine Vascular Insufficiency Associated with Mechanical Obstruction
- Intestinal atresia
  - Microcolon if distal ileum
  - May be multiple small bowel
- Malrotation with midgut volvulus
  - Proximal obstruction
  - Bilious emesis
- Intussusception
  - Rarely can occur in utero
  - Polyp
  - Meckel diverticulum
- Mesenteric/internal bowel hernias
  - Very rare
- Congenital bands
  - Commonly associated with malrotation

Viral Infections
- Cytomegalovirus
- Parvovirus B-19

PATHOLOGY

General Features
- Etiology
  - In utero intestinal perforation
  - Meconium and digestive enzymes leak into peritoneal cavity
  - Intense chemical peritonitis and inflammatory response
  - Granulomatous response and calcification within days
- Epidemiology
  - 1:35,000 live births
  - 15-40% have meconium ileus and CF
- Associated abnormalities
  - Meconium ileus
    - Complicated by perforation due to secondary ileal atresia, segmental volvulus
  - Congenital bowel obstruction
  - In-utero midgut volvulus
    - Secondary bowel ischemia and perforation
  - Intrauterine vascular insufficiency
    - Resulting in atresia and perforation

Gross Pathologic & Surgical Features
- Organized peritonitis
- Fibrosis/adhesions
- Calcification
- ± Pseudocyst
- Meconium periorchitis in males with patent processus vaginalis

MECONIUM PERITONITIS

Microscopic Features
- Peritoneal squames
- Bile pigment
- Fibrosis
- Calcification
- Chronic inflammation

CLINICAL ISSUES

Presentation
- Most common signs/symptoms
  - Peritoneal calcifications on prenatal or neonatal imaging
  - Abdominal distension
  - Failure to pass meconium after birth
- Other signs/symptoms
  - Prenatal sonographic findings
    - Pseudocyst
    - Ascites
    - Calcifications
    - Polyhydramnios
  - Meconium periorchitis

Demographics
- Age: 2nd trimester gestational age through birth
- Gender: No predilection

Natural History & Prognosis
- In utero perforation
  - Generalized meconium peritonitis - minority of cases
  - Pseudocyst formation
  - Bowel distension/obstruction
- 75% survival if treated appropriately

Treatment
- Almost always surgical

DIAGNOSTIC CHECKLIST

Consider
- Most common causes of in utero perforation
  - Complicated meconium ileus (CF)
    - Sweat test
    - Chromosomal markers for CF
  - Intestinal atresia

Image Interpretation Pearls
- Ascites and peritoneal calcifications on prenatal sonography is suggestive
- Curvilinear or peritoneal calcifications on post-natal radiography
- Post-natal sonography
  - Ascites
  - Fluid-filled mass lined by calcification, likely pseudocyst

SELECTED REFERENCES

1. Eckoldt F et al: Meconium peritonitis and pseudo-cyst formation: prenatal diagnosis and post-natal course. Prenat Diagn. 23(11):904-8, 2003
2. Ekinci S et al: Inguinal hernia as a rare manifestation of meconium peritonitis: report of a case. Surg Today. 32(8):758-60, 2002
3. Park WH et al: Congenital gastric teratoma with gastric perforation mimicking meconium peritonitis. J Pediatr Surg. 37(5):E11, 2002
4. Su WH et al: Fetal meconium peritonitis in the infant of a woman with fulminant hepatitis B. A case report. J Reprod Med. 47(11):952-4, 2002
5. Han SJ et al: Biliary atresia associated with meconium peritonitis caused by perforation of small bowel atresia. J Pediatr Surg. 36(9):1390-3, 2001
6. Hu MX et al: An unusual case of neonatal peritoneal calcifications associated with hydrometrocolpos. Pediatr Radiol. 31(10):742-4, 2001
7. Agarwal N et al: Idiopathic origin of meconium peritonitis. Indian J Pediatr. 67(11):845-6, 2000
8. Kamata S et al: Meconium peritonitis in utero. Pediatr Surg Int. 16(5-6):377-9, 2000
9. Khadaroo RG et al: Fetus-in-fetu presenting as cystic meconium peritonitis: diagnosis, pathology, and surgical management. J Pediatr Surg. 35(5):721-3, 2000
10. Reynolds E et al: Meconium peritonitis. J Perinatol. 20(3):193-5, 2000
11. Shimotake T et al: Ultrasonographic detection of intrauterine intussusception resulting in ileal atresia complicated by meconium peritonitis. Pediatr Surg Int. 16(1-2):43-4, 2000
12. Varkonyi I et al: Meconium periorchitis: case report and literature review. Eur J Pediatr Surg. 10(6):404-7, 2000
13. Berrocal T et al: Congenital anomalies of the small intestine, colon, and rectum. Radiographics. 19(5):1219-36, 1999
14. Kolker SE et al: Disseminated intravascular meconium in a newborn with meconium peritonitis. Hum Pathol. 30(5):592-4, 1999
15. McDuffie RS Jr et al: Fetal meconium peritonitis after maternal hepatitis A. Am J Obstet Gynecol. 180(4):1031-2, 1999
16. Niramis R et al: Meconium peritonitis. J Med Assoc Thai. 82(11):1063-70, 1999
17. Ramesh JC et al: Meconium peritonitis: prenatal diagnosis and postnatal management--a case report. Med J Malaysia. 54(4):528-30, 1999
18. Salman AB et al: Abdominal, scrotal, and thoracic calcifications owing to healed meconium peritonitis. J Pediatr Surg. 34(9):1415-6, 1999
19. Tatekawa Y et al: The mechanism of focal intestinal perforations in neonates with low birth weight. Pediatr Surg Int. 15(8):549-52, 1999
20. Patton WL et al: Systemic spread of meconium peritonitis. Pediatr Radiol. 28(9):714-6, 1998
21. Tseng CW et al: Color Doppler energy in prenatal diagnosis of meconium peritonitis: a case report. Changgeng Yi Xue Za Zhi. 20(1):58-61, 1997
22. Ali SW et al: Meconium peritonitis--a leading cause of neonatal peritonitis in Kashmir. Indian J Pediatr. 63(2):229-32, 1996
23. Dirkes K et al: The natural history of meconium peritonitis diagnosed in utero. J Pediatr Surg. 30(7):979-82, 1995
24. DuBois JJ et al: Inflammatory pseudocyst associated with trisomy 21 and Hirschsprung's disease. Mil Med. 160(9):477-9, 1995
25. Konje JC et al: Antenatal diagnosis and management of meconium peritonitis: a case report and review of the literature. Ultrasound Obstet Gynecol. 6(1):66-9, 1995

MECONIUM PERITONITIS

IMAGE GALLERY

Typical

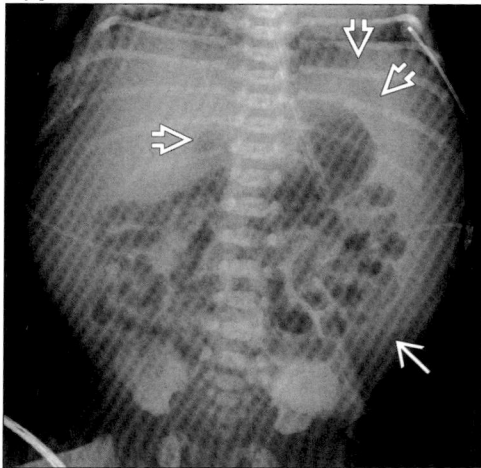
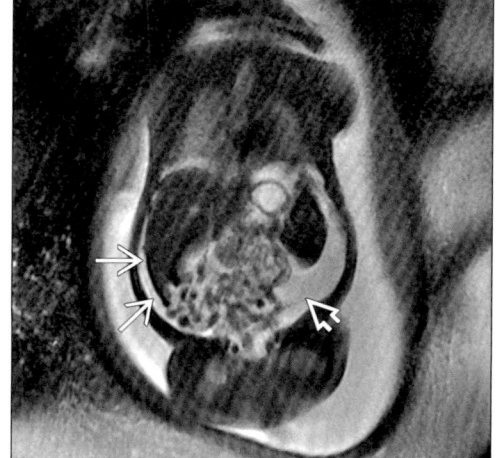

(Left) Anteroposterior radiograph of a neonate shows linear peritoneal calcification along the left flank ➡ as well as free air ➡ in this patient with meconium peritonitis. *(Right)* Coronal T2WI MR performed prenatally in patient at left shows decreased signal along the liver surface ➡ consistent with peritoneal calcification. The fetus also has ascites ➡ throughout the abdomen.

Typical

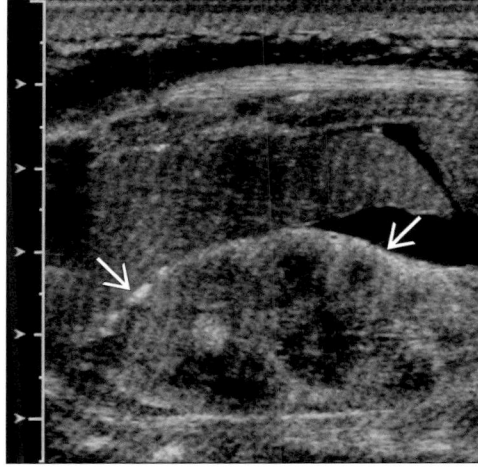
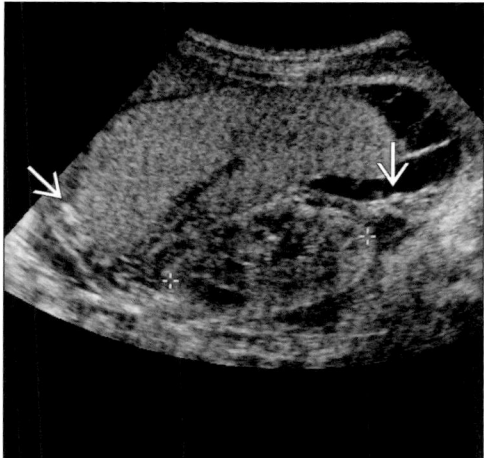

(Left) Longitudinal ultrasound in the hepatorenal region in a patient with meconium peritonitis shows calcification along the surface of the kidney ➡, a peritoneal reflection. *(Right)* Longitudinal ultrasound of the spleen and left kidney of the same patient as previous image shows perisplenic and perirenal calcification ➡ of meconium peritonitis.

Typical

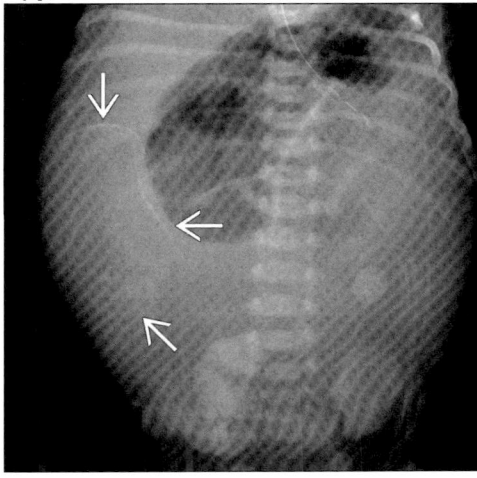
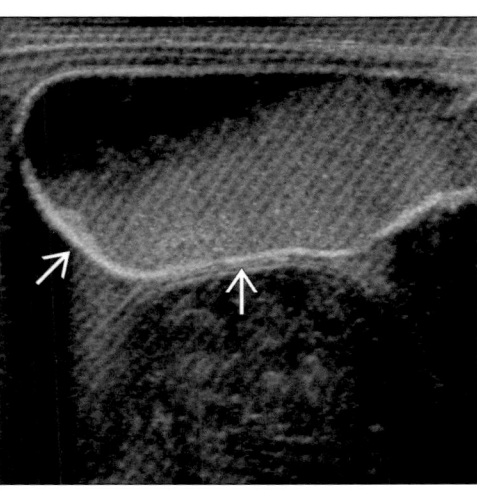

(Left) Anteroposterior radiograph of the abdomen in a neonate shows curvilinear calcification in the right abdomen ➡ with dilated bowel suggestive of bowel obstruction. This appearance suggests meconium pseudocyst. *(Right)* Longitudinal transabdominal ultrasound of the patient at left shows rim-calcified cyst ➡ filled with echogenic material, likely meconium.

NECROTIZING ENTEROCOLITIS

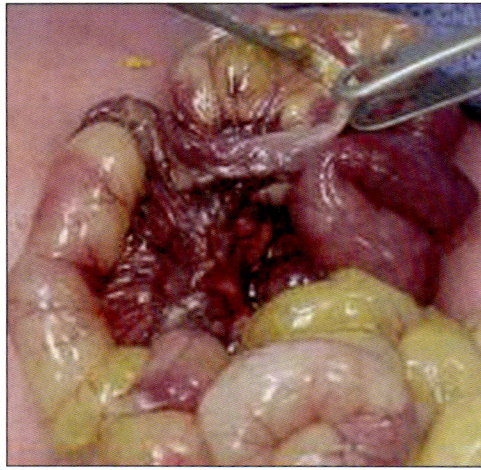

Surgical photograph shows multiple loops of ischemic/necrotic bowel. The entire bowel from duodenum to terminal ileum was necrotic. The patient died several days later.

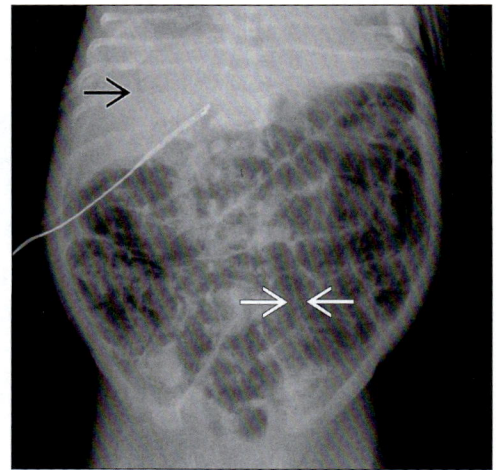

Anteroposterior radiograph performed prior to surgical photo (see previous image) shows bowel distention, pneumatosis, portal venous gas ➔, and Rigler sign of free air ➔ in premie with NEC.

TERMINOLOGY

Abbreviations and Synonyms
- Necrotizing enterocolitis (NEC)

Definitions
- Idiopathic enterocolitis in very low birth weight premature infants most likely related to some combination of infection and ischemia characterized by coagulative and hemorrhagic necrosis and inflammation of portions of the small and large intestine

IMAGING FINDINGS

General Features
- Best diagnostic clue: Pneumatosis
- Location: Most common right colon and terminal ileum; can occur anywhere in gastrointestinal (GI) tract
- Morphology
  - Acutely either normal caliber or dilated bowel
  - Chronically may be narrow caliber or stricture, single or multiple

Radiographic Findings
- Radiography
  - Findings: Nonspecific to suggestive to diagnostic
  - Suggestive findings
    - Asymmetric bowel dilation
    - Featureless "unfolded" bowel loops
    - Separation of bowel loops
    - Fixed configuration of bowel loop(s) over serial films
  - Definitive finding: Pneumatosis (50-75% of patients)
    - Can occur anywhere in bowel
    - Bubble-like (submucosal) or curvilinear (serosal) lucencies
    - Mimics meconium or stool (not typically seen in nonfed infants)
  - Definitive finding: Portal venous gas (PVG)
    - Branching lucencies over the liver
    - More peripheral extension than biliary gas
  - Definitive finding: Free intraperitoneal air
    - Triangles of anterior lucency, X-table lateral X-ray

DDx: Signs Mimicking Necrotizing Enterocolitis

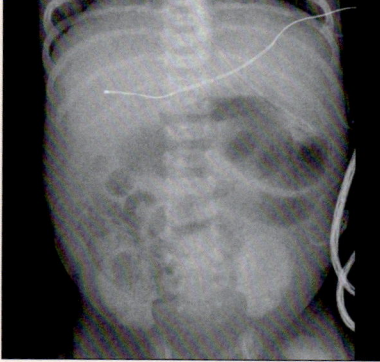

Pneumatosis: Cocaine Use in Mother

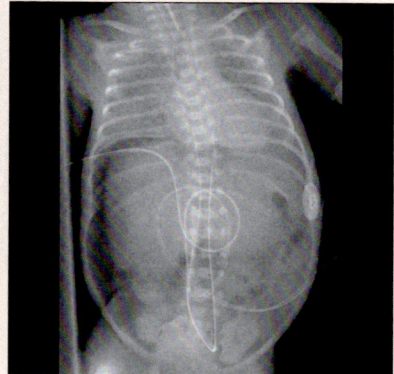

Gastric Perforation by NG Tube

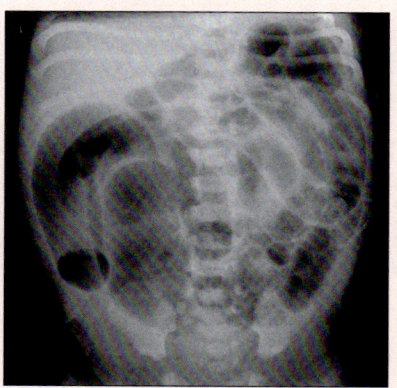

Premie with Hirschsprung

NECROTIZING ENTEROCOLITIS

Key Facts

Terminology
- Idiopathic enterocolitis in very low birth weight premature infants most likely related to some combination of infection and ischemia characterized by coagulative and hemorrhagic necrosis and inflammation of portions of the small and large intestine

Imaging Findings
- Best diagnostic clue: Pneumatosis
- Best imaging tool: Radiography +/- sonography
- Suspected acute NEC: Serial abdominal radiographs
- Question ischemic bowel: Sonography with color Doppler

Pathology
- Multifactorial etiology

- Incidence: 0.3-2.4 cases per 1,000 live births
- Increased; more premature babies surviving

Clinical Issues
- Most common signs/symptoms: Abdominal distention, bloody stools, diarrhea, feeding intolerance, increased gastric aspirates, sepsis, apnea and bradycardia, lethargy, temperature instability
- 1-3 week old premature infant; often with (HMD)
- 10% are term babies
- Overall mortality 20-30%

Diagnostic Checklist
- Asymmetric bowel distention
- Pneumatosis may be linear or bubbly
- PVG closer to the liver capsule than biliary gas

- Lucency adjacent to liver, left lateral decubitus X-ray
- Overall increased lucency, supine radiographs
- Air on both sides of bowel wall (Rigler sign)
- Outline of falciform ligament (football sign)

Fluoroscopic Findings
- Enema contraindicated in presumed acute NEC
- Mucosa permeable to water-soluble contrast and excreted into kidneys
- Stricture: Single or multiple, small bowel or colon

CT Findings
- Not typically used for diagnosis
- Bowel wall thickening with increased or decreased enhancement
- Pneumatosis, free air, PVG, ascites

Ultrasonographic Findings
- Grayscale Ultrasound
  - Thickened and/or dilated bowel wall loops
  - Ascites; simple or complex
- Color Doppler: Increased (inflamed) or decreased (ischemic) vascularity

Imaging Recommendations
- Best imaging tool: Radiography +/- sonography
- Protocol advice
  - Suspected acute NEC: Serial abdominal radiographs
    - Anteroposterior supine ± left decubitus or X-table lateral
  - Question ischemic bowel: Sonography with color Doppler
    - Ultrasound with color Doppler
  - Children with suspected NEC-related stricture after acute episode
    - Anteroposterior supine radiograph
    - Multiple dilated loops: Enema
    - Non obstructive pattern: Upper gastrointestinal (UGI) and small bowel follow-through

DIFFERENTIAL DIAGNOSIS

Bowel Obstruction
- Immature (premature) colon
- Hirschsprung disease

Bowel Perforation
- Idiopathic or idiosyncratic most common

Enterocolitis of Term Infants
- Infants of cocaine users
- Allergic: Usually milk allergy
- Infants with cyanotic heart disease

Nonspecific Gaseous Distention
- Bag ventilation at intubation

PATHOLOGY

General Features
- General path comments
  - Combination of infection and ischemia
  - Inflammation: Mucosal to full thickness
  - Necrosis leads to perforation
- Etiology
  - Multifactorial etiology
  - Intestinal ischemia: Reduced splanchnic and/or systemic perfusion, hypoxia, intestinal gaseous distention
  - Bacterial colonization: Not primarily infectious process; no specific organism
    - Inflammatory mediators induced by bacterial toxins
  - Oral milk feedings: Bacterial flora proliferate; may affect perfusion
  - Prematurity
- Epidemiology
  - Frequency
    - Varies by nursery
    - Not seasonal or geographic
    - Outbreaks frequently follow epidemic pattern but no infectious agent known

NECROTIZING ENTEROCOLITIS

- Incidence: 0.3-2.4 cases per 1,000 live births
  - Increased; more premature babies surviving
- Associated abnormalities
  - Hyaline membrane disease (HMD)
  - Cyanotic CHD
  - Left to right shunts especially patent ductus arteriosus

Gross Pathologic & Surgical Features
- Dilated, gray, hemorrhagic, friable bowel

Microscopic Features
- Mucosal coagulation, ulceration, submucosal hemorrhage, submucosal or subserosal gas (pneumatosis intestinalis), PVG, mesenteric gas

Staging, Grading or Classification Criteria
- Bell classification
  - Stage I: Early or suspected NEC
    - Nonspecific
    - Scalloping/separation/unfolding bowel loops
    - Asymmetric bowel distention
  - Stage II: Definite NEC
    - Pneumatosis intestinalis: Mucosal, serosal; not always correlating with clinical symptoms/signs
  - Stage III: Advanced disease (perforation or impending perforation)
    - PVG, free intraperitoneal air, persistent loop sign, ascites

CLINICAL ISSUES

Presentation
- Most common signs/symptoms: Abdominal distention, bloody stools, diarrhea, feeding intolerance, increased gastric aspirates, sepsis, apnea and bradycardia, lethargy, temperature instability
- Other signs/symptoms
  - 1/3 fulminant course with bowel perforation
  - 1/3 have septic shock
- Most commonly in infants < 1,000 g at birth
- Typically in the intensive care unit
- More common in infants being fed enterally
- Can occur in older infants under extreme stress
  - Cardiac surgery, infants of mothers using cocaine

Demographics
- Age
  - 1-3 week old premature infant; often with (HMD)
  - Age of incidence inversely related to birth weight and gestational age
    - Infants < 1,000 g have highest incidence
  - 10% are term babies
    - NEC occurs earlier; 1-3 days of life
    - Systemically ill: Birth asphyxia, respiratory distress, CHD, metabolic abnormalities
    - Placental insufficiency, maternal cocaine abuse
- Gender: M = F
- Ethnicity: No proven race predilection

Natural History & Prognosis
- Death secondary to sepsis from bowel perforation
- Delayed bowel strictures in 10-20% of survivors
- Short gut syndrome
- Overall mortality 20-30%
  - Infants < 1,500 g 10-44%
  - Infants > 2,500 g 0-20%

Treatment
- When NEC suspected
  - IV nutrition + antibiotics
- Indication for surgery: Clinical ± radiologic findings
  - Free air considered absolute indication

DIAGNOSTIC CHECKLIST

Consider
- Gestational age of premature infant
- NEC in full term babies at risk
- Bowel distention, pneumatosis, PVG, free air

Image Interpretation Pearls
- Asymmetric bowel distention
- Pneumatosis may be linear or bubbly
- PVG closer to the liver capsule than biliary gas

SELECTED REFERENCES

1. DE Plaen IG et al: Inhibition of Nuclear Factor-kappaB Ameliorates Bowel Injury and Prolongs Survival in a Neonatal Rat Model of Necrotizing Enterocolitis. Pediatr Res. 2007
2. Epelman M et al: Necrotizing enterocolitis: review of state-of-the-art imaging findings with pathologic correlation. Radiographics. 27(2):285-305, 2007
3. Lambert DK et al: Necrotizing enterocolitis in term neonates: data from a multihospital health-care system. J Perinatol. 2007
4. Sharma R et al: Neonatal gut barrier and multiple organ failure: role of endotoxin and proinflammatory cytokines in sepsis and necrotizing enterocolitis. J Pediatr Surg. 42(3):454-61, 2007
5. Upperman JS et al: Mathematical modeling in necrotizing enterocolitis--a new look at an ongoing problem. J Pediatr Surg. 42(3):445-53, 2007
6. Warner BB et al: Ontogeny of salivary epidermal growth factor and necrotizing enterocolitis. J Pediatr. 150(4):358-63, 2007
7. Hall N et al: Necrotizing enterocolitis. Hosp Med. 65(4):220-5, 2004
8. Henry MC et al: Current issues in the management of necrotizing enterocolitis. Semin Perinatol. 28(3):221-33, 2004
9. Maayan-Metzger A et al: Necrotizing enterocolitis in full-term infants: case-control study and review of the literature. J Perinatol. 24(8):494-9, 2004
10. Updegrove K: Necrotizing enterocolitis: the evidence for use of human milk in prevention and treatment. J Hum Lact. 20(3):335-9, 2004
11. Hsueh W et al: Neonatal necrotizing enterocolitis: clinical considerations and pathogenetic concepts. Pediatr Dev Pathol. 6(1):6-23, 2003
12. Kafetzis DA et al: Neonatal necrotizing enterocolitis: an overview. Curr Opin Infect Dis. 16(4):349-55, 2003
13. Noerr B: Current controversies in the understanding of necrotizing enterocolitis. Part 1. Adv Neonatal Care. 3(3):107-20, 2003
14. Pierro A et al: Surgical treatments of infants with necrotizing enterocolitis. Semin Neonatol. 8(3):223-32, 2003

NECROTIZING ENTEROCOLITIS

IMAGE GALLERY

Variant

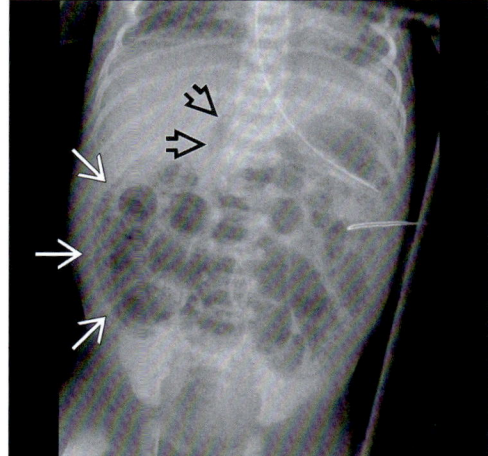
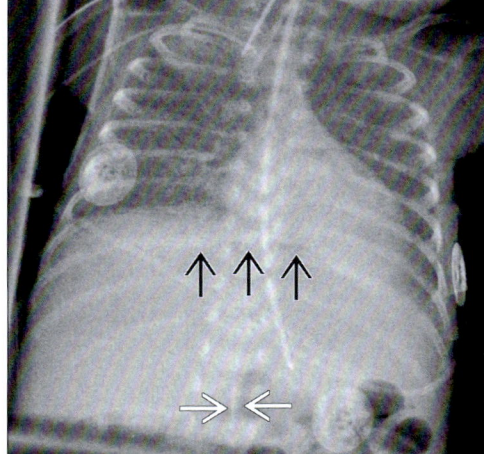

(Left) Anteroposterior radiograph of premature infant with clinical findings worrisome for NEC shows pneumatosis in the right abdomen ➡ and free air ⇨ in the upper paraspinal region. *(Right)* Anteroposterior radiograph of the chest in patient with NEC shows continuous diaphragm sign ➡, falciform ligament sign ➡, and diffuse lucency over upper abdomen, signs of free air.

Typical

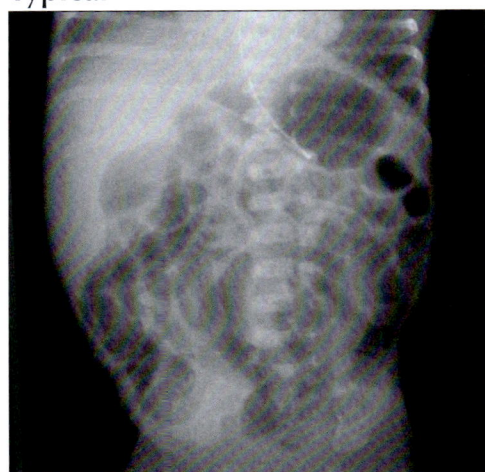
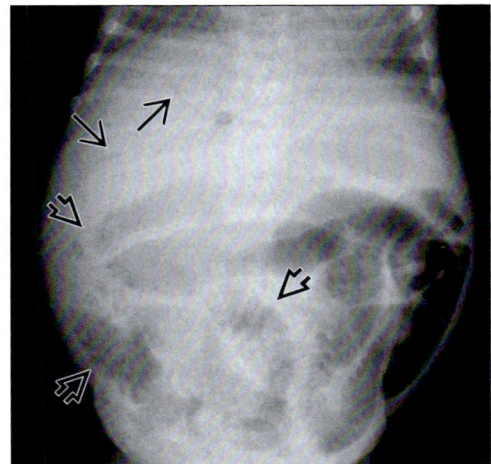

(Left) Anteroposterior radiograph in a premature infant with bloody stools shows asymmetric bowel distention and unfolding of bowel loops, a nonspecific finding, but could represent early NEC. *(Right)* Anteroposterior radiograph in a premature infant shows signs of NEC, but no free air. Note the portal venous gas overlying the liver ➡ and the pneumatosis ⇨ in the mid and right abdomen.

Typical

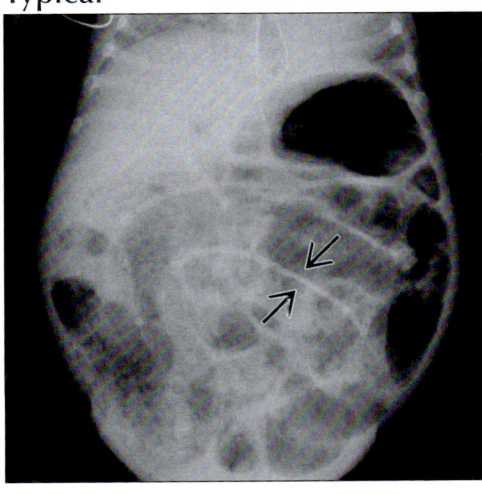
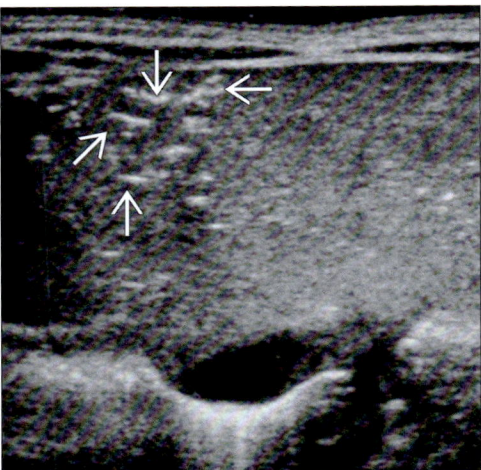

(Left) Anteroposterior radiograph performed hours later in the same patient as previous image shows air on both sides of the bowel loops ➡, Rigler sign of free air. At operation, there was extensive NEC. *(Right)* Transverse ultrasound of the liver in a premie with pneumatosis shows linear echogenicities near the non-dependent surface of the liver consistent with portal venous gas ➡.

HYPERTROPHIC PYLORIC STENOSIS

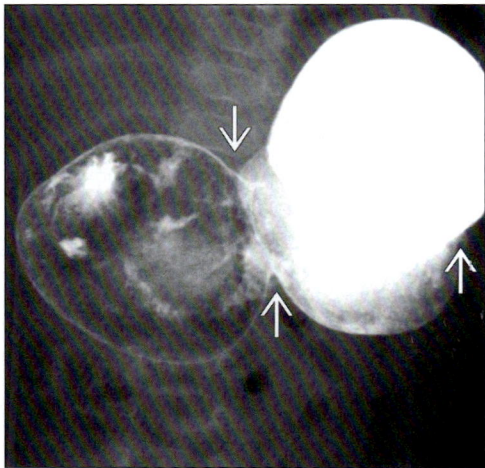

Anteroposterior upper GI shows caterpillar stomach or hyperperistalsis caused by muscular contractions ➡ attempting to push the oral contrast through the hypertrophied pylorus.

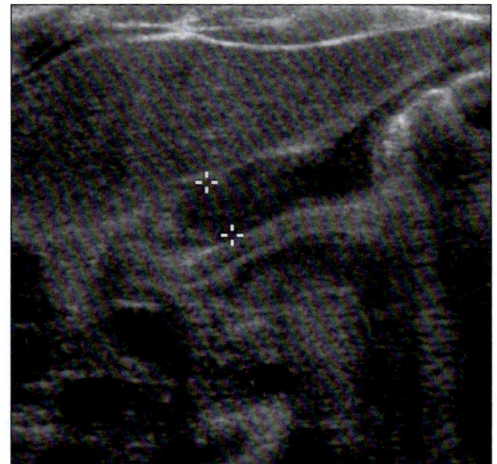

Transverse transabdominal ultrasound shows thickening of the hypoechoic pyloric muscle (calipers), measuring 6 mm in this infant with HPS. The pyloric channel length measured 19 mm.

TERMINOLOGY

Abbreviations and Synonyms
- Pyloric stenosis, hypertrophic pyloric stenosis (HPS)

Definitions
- Idiopathic pyloric muscle thickening which can lead to progressive gastric outlet obstruction
- Typically seen in 2-12 week old infants with progressive non-bilious projective vomiting
- HPS is the cause of vomiting in 1 of every 5 infants referred for imaging
- Incidence of 2.5-3 per 1,000 live births

IMAGING FINDINGS

General Features
- Best diagnostic clue
  o Near complete gastric outlet obstruction due to enlarged and thickened pyloric muscle
  o Ultrasound reveals hypertrophied muscle and decreased gastric emptying on dynamic exam
  o Upper GI shows minimal barium traversing pyloric channel with mass effect on the antrum and duodenal bulb from a thickened pyloric muscle
- Location: Near the gallbladder by US

Radiographic Findings
- Radiography
  o Overdistended stomach and decreased bowel gas distally
  o Stomach may be collapsed if infant has recently vomited

Fluoroscopic Findings
- Overdistended stomach
- Caterpillar stomach: Exaggerated gastric motility
- Tram track or string sign of barium within the narrowed channel
- Shoulders of pyloric muscle create an impression on distal antrum
- Teat or beak where the peristaltic wave encounters the thickened pyloric muscle
- Mushroom sign of hypertrophied muscle indenting the base of duodenal bulb

DDx: Other Causes of Vomiting

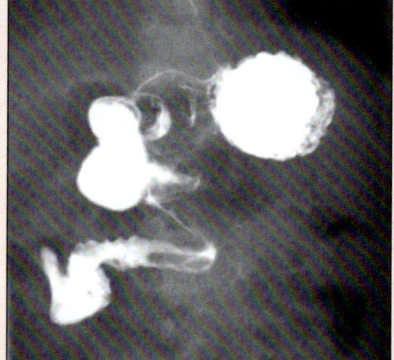

Midgut Volvulus

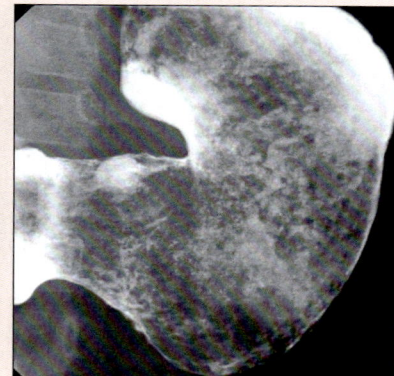

Trichobezoar

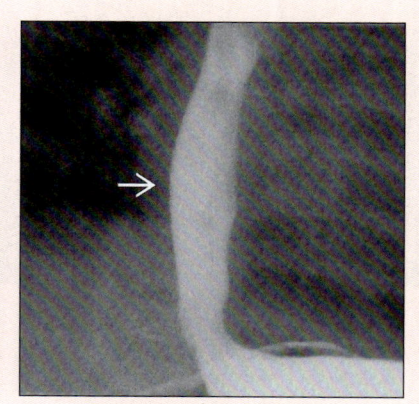

Gastroesophageal Reflux

HYPERTROPHIC PYLORIC STENOSIS

Terminology
- Idiopathic pyloric muscle thickening which can lead to progressive gastric outlet obstruction
- Typically seen in 2-12 week old infants with progressive non-bilious projective vomiting
- Incidence of 2.5-3 per 1,000 live births

Imaging Findings
- Caterpillar stomach: Exaggerated gastric motility
- Tram track or string sign of barium within the narrowed channel
- Shoulders of pyloric muscle create an impression on distal antrum
- Teat or beak where the peristaltic wave encounters the thickened pyloric muscle
- Mushroom sign of hypertrophied muscle indenting the base of duodenal bulb

Key Facts
- Commonly accepted threshold values for HPS
- Single wall thickness of pylorus > 3 mm
- Pyloric channel length > 16 mm
- Pyloric diameter > 15 mm

Top Differential Diagnoses
- Pylorospasm
- Gastroesophageal (GE) Reflux
- Malrotation with Midgut Volvulus

Clinical Issues
- Gender: M:F = 4-5:1
- Surgical: Pyloromyotomy
- Nonsurgical: Atropine and frequent small feedings are an alternative to surgery

Diagnostic Checklist
- Pylorospasm mimics HPS, but is typically transient

CT Findings
- CECT: Consider pylorospasm as CT does not provide dynamic evaluation of gastric emptying

Ultrasonographic Findings
- Grayscale Ultrasound
  - Threshold for abnormal measurements of pyloric muscle and channel length vary by author
  - In general, higher threshold measurements increase specificity but decrease sensitivity
  - Commonly accepted threshold values for HPS
    - Single wall thickness of pylorus > 3 mm
    - Pyloric channel length > 16 mm
    - Pyloric diameter > 15 mm
  - Echogenic mucosal lining also tends to hypertrophy, becomes redundant
  - Gastric hyperperistalsis and obliterated pyloric lumen on dynamic exam
  - Feeding glucose water or formula helpful to assess gastric emptying, define the pyloric channel
  - When duodenal bulb is easily identified distended with fluid, diagnosis of HPS is unlikely
- Color Doppler: Increased flow has been demonstrated in both the muscle and mucosa of infants with HPS

Imaging Recommendations
- Best imaging tool
  - Ultrasound is exam of choice when HPS is suspected
  - Barium UGI used when history atypical or if emesis is bilious
- Protocol advice
  - Begin the ultrasound scan with the patient rolled onto their right side in order to pool gastric fluids in the antrum
  - Administer glucose water in small amounts, as overdistending the stomach may displaced the pyloric channel posteriorly or into the right lower quadrant
  - Watch for gastric peristaltic waves to propel fluid through the pyloric channel
  - Gastric contractions which are vigorous in the body and antrum, but do not open the pylorus suggest the diagnosis of HPS
  - Formula or glucose water will "swirl" against the thickened pylorus with each wave of gastric peristalsis in HPS

DIFFERENTIAL DIAGNOSIS

Pylorospasm
- Typically seen in irritable infants, resolves with time, wait and re-image

Gastroesophageal (GE) Reflux
- Cause of vomiting in 2/3 of all infants referred to radiology
- Presumed diagnosis when ultrasound is normal

Malrotation with Midgut Volvulus
- Surgical emergency, best diagnosed by UGI
- Emesis is classically greenish from bile

Gastric Bezoar
- Caused by accumulation of undigested matter in stomach
  - Trichobezoar: Composed of hair and sometimes nails
  - Phytobezoar: Composed of plant or vegetable fiber

Other Causes of Gastric Outlet Obstruction
- Duodenal stenosis or antral web
- Antral polyps, annular pancreas, choledochocele, right upper quadrant mass

PATHOLOGY

General Features
- General path comments
  - Idiopathic hypertrophy of circular muscle bundles in pylorus
    - Gradually progressive and spontaneously remits after many weeks

HYPERTROPHIC PYLORIC STENOSIS

- Abnormal muscle tone/electrophysiology of the gastroduodenal junction shown in HPS
- Associated with erythromycin exposure prenatally and postnatally via breast milk
- Higher incidence of HPS in patients with cystic fibrosis
- Genetics
  - Tends to run in families, not truly inherited
  - Discordant incidence among monozygotic twins favors environmental factors over genetic predisposition
- Etiology: Unclear: Idiopathic, prostaglandin induced, neural mediated, familial
- Associated abnormalities: Eosinophilic gastritis, prostaglandin induced antral mucosal hyperplasia, hypergastrinemia, nasoenteric tubes, erythromycin

Gross Pathologic & Surgical Features

- Hypertrophy of muscular layers of pylorus
- Thickening of mucosa in antrum and pylorus, to approximately 1/3 diameter of pylorus

CLINICAL ISSUES

Presentation
- Most common signs/symptoms
  - Progressive vomiting in an infant who previously tolerated feedings
  - Palpable "olive" is 97% specific in experienced hands
- Other signs/symptoms: Weight loss

Demographics
- Age: 2-12 weeks or even later in premature infants
- Gender: M:F = 4-5:1
- Ethnicity: Slightly more common in Caucasians

Natural History & Prognosis
- Weight loss and parental concerns typically prompt imaging
- Excellent prognosis following surgery or conservative medical management
  - No significant GI disturbances seen in German study of infants treated surgically or medically 16-26 years after diagnosis

Treatment
- Surgical: Pyloromyotomy
  - Pyloromyotomy splits the thickened muscle longitudinally and reapproximates edges transversely thereby opening the channel
  - Laparoscopic pyloromyotomy does not appear to offer significant advantages over the open procedure
- Nonsurgical: Atropine and frequent small feedings are an alternative to surgery
  - Treatment takes several weeks before resuming normal feeding without medications

DIAGNOSTIC CHECKLIST

Image Interpretation Pearls
- Pylorospasm mimics HPS, but is typically transient

SELECTED REFERENCES

1. Cohen HL et al: The sonographic double-track sign: not pathognomonic for hypertrophic pyloric stenosis; can be seen in pylorospasm. J Ultrasound Med. 23(5):641-6, 2004
2. Hall NJ et al: Meta-analysis of laparoscopic versus open pyloromyotomy. Ann Surg. 240(5):774-8, 2004
3. Helton KJ et al: The impact of a clinical guideline on imaging children with hypertrophic pyloric stenosis. Pediatr Radiol. 34(9):733-6, 2004
4. Huang YC et al: Medical treatment with atropine sulfate for hypertrophic pyloric stenosis. Acta Paediatr Taiwan. 45(3):136-40, 2004
5. Yagmurlu A et al: Comparison of the incidence of complications in open and laparoscopic pyloromyotomy: a concurrent single institution series. J Pediatr Surg. 39(3):292-6; discussion 292-6, 2004
6. Hernanz-Schulman M et al: Hypertrophic pyloric stenosis in infants: US evaluation of vascularity of the pyloric canal. Radiology. 229(2):389-93, 2003
7. Hernanz-Schulman M: Infantile hypertrophic pyloric stenosis. Radiology. 227(2):319-31, 2003
8. Sorensen HT et al: Risk of infantile hypertrophic pyloric stenosis after maternal postnatal use of macrolides. Scand J Infect Dis. 35(2):104-6, 2003
9. Kakish KS: Cystic fibrosis and infantile hypertrophic pyloric stenosis: is there an association? Pediatr Pulmonol. 33(5):404-5, 2002
10. Hernanz-Schulman M et al: In vivo visualization of pyloric mucosal hypertrophy in infants with hypertrophic pyloric stenosis: is there an etiologic role? AJR Am J Roentgenol. 177(4):843-8, 2001
11. Kawahara H et al: Motor abnormality in the gastroduodenal junction in patients with infantile hypertrophic pyloric stenosis. J Pediatr Surg. 36(11):1641-5, 2001
12. Kobayashi H et al: Pyloric stenosis: new histopathologic perspective using confocal laser scanning. J Pediatr Surg. 36(8):1277-9, 2001
13. Cohen HL et al: Vomiting in infants up to 3 months of age. American College of Radiology. ACR Appropriateness Criteria. Radiology. 215 Suppl:779-86, 2000
14. Aktug T et al: Analyzing the diagnostic efficiency of olive palpation for hypertrophic pyloric stenosis. J Pediatr Surg. 34(10):1585-6, 1999
15. Callahan MJ et al: The development of hypertrophic pyloric stenosis in a patient with prostaglandin-induced foveolar hyperplasia. Pediatr Radiol. 29(10):748-51, 1999
16. Bisset GS 3rd et al: Pediatric imaging perspective: the vomiting infant. J Pediatr. 133(2):306-7, 1998
17. Rohrschneider WK et al: Pyloric muscle in asymptomatic infants: sonographic evaluation and discrimination from idiopathic hypertrophic pyloric stenosis. Pediatr Radiol. 28(6):429-34, 1998
18. Yamamoto A et al: Ultrasonographic follow-up of the healing process of medically treated hypertrophic pyloric stenosis. Pediatr Radiol. 28(3):177-8, 1998
19. Schechter R et al: The epidemiology of infantile hypertrophic pyloric stenosis. Paediatr Perinat Epidemiol. 11(4):407-27, 1997
20. Babyn P et al: Radiologic features of gastric outlet obstruction in infants after long-term prostaglandin administration. Pediatr Radiol. 25(1):41-3; discussion 44, 1995
21. Hernanz-Schulman M et al: Hypertrophic pyloric stenosis in the infant without a palpable olive: accuracy of sonographic diagnosis. Radiology. 193(3):771-6, 1994
22. Ludtke FE et al: Gastric emptying 16 to 26 years after treatment of infantile hypertrophic pyloric stenosis. J Pediatr Surg. 29(4):523-6, 1994

HYPERTROPHIC PYLORIC STENOSIS

IMAGE GALLERY

Typical

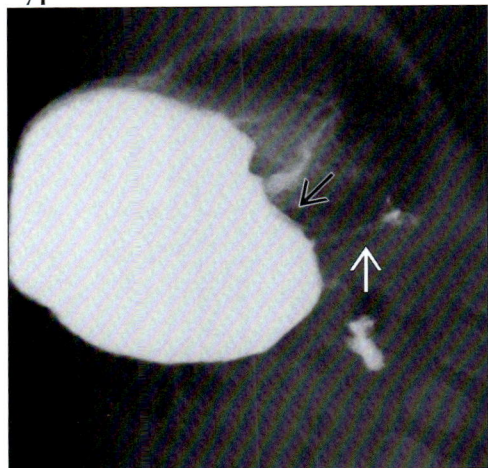
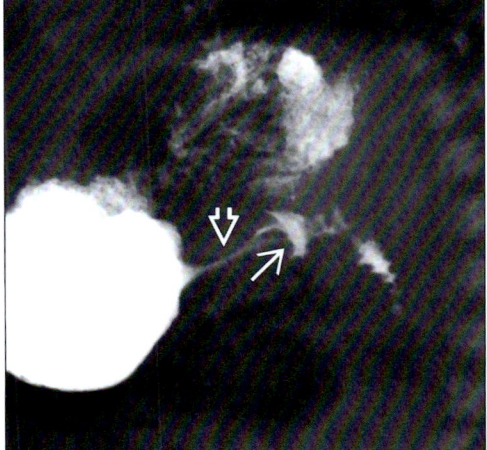

(Left) Lateral upper GI shows tram track or string sign of barium ➡ within an elongated pyloric channel. Note the mild impression on the distal antrum ➡ caused by the hypertrophied pyloric muscle. *(Right)* Lateral upper GI shows impression on the underside of the duodenal bulb ➡ or mushroom sign caused by the hypertrophied pyloric muscle. Note the string sign ➡ from the narrowed elongated pyloric channel in this patient with HPS.

Typical

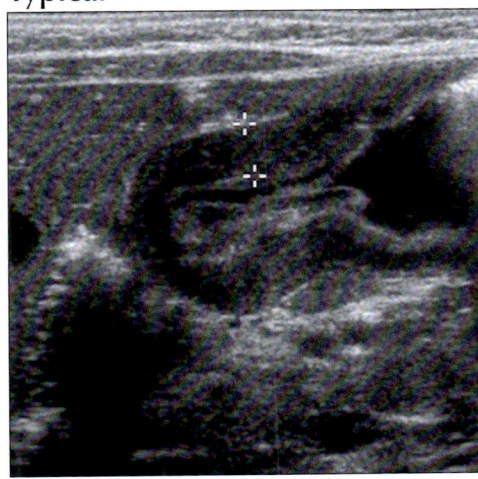
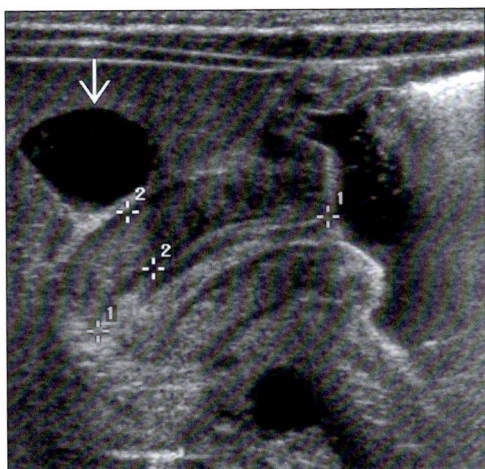

(Left) Transverse transabdominal ultrasound shows thickening of the hypoechoic pyloric muscle (calipers), measuring 5 mm in this patient with HPS. *(Right)* Transverse transabdominal ultrasound shows thickening of the pyloric muscle (caliper #2) of 5 mm and elongation of the pyloric channel (caliper #1) of 22 mm in this patient with HPS. Notice the close proximity of the gallbladder ➡.

Typical

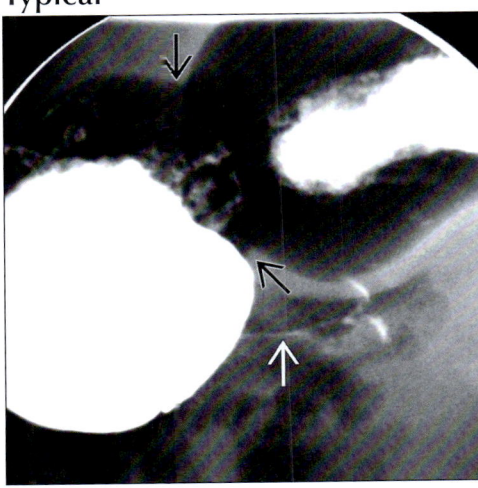
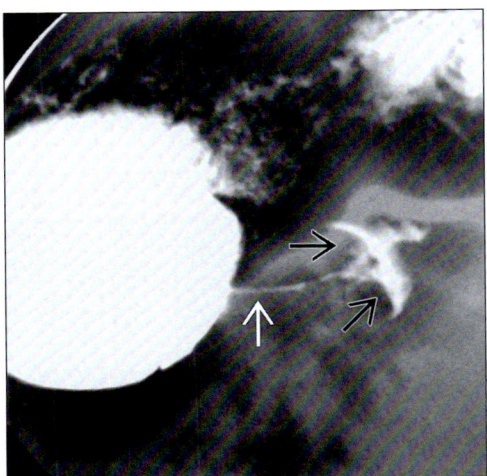

(Left) Lateral upper GI shows elongated & narrowed pyloric channel or string sign ➡ in this patient with HPS. Note the prominent gastric muscle contractions ➡ in attempt to pass oral contrast through thickened pyloric muscle. *(Right)* Lateral upper GI in the same patient shows a string sign ➡ of barium within an elongated & narrowed pyloric channel. Note impression of duodenal bulb ➡ or mushroom sign caused by hypertrophied pyloric muscle.

GASTRIC VOLVULUS

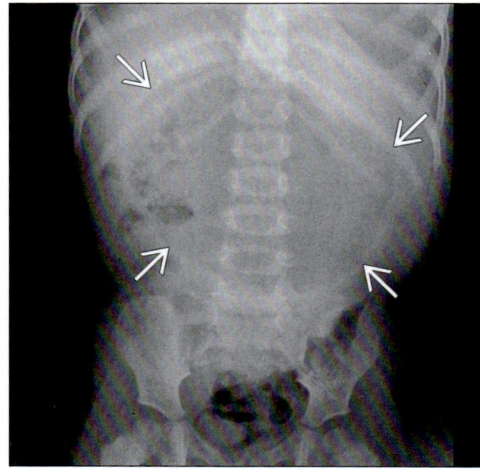

Anteroposterior radiograph in an 18 month old infant shows massive gastric distention ➡ with a paucity of distal gas. Patient was vomiting and dehydrated and was found to have gastric volvulus.

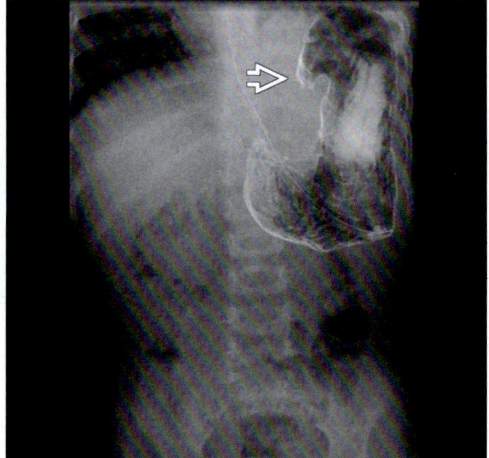

Anteroposterior upper GI through nasoenteric tube shows contrast in the stomach which is positioned with duodenum in left upper quadrant ➡, suggestive of mesoaxial gastric volvulus.

TERMINOLOGY

Abbreviations and Synonyms
- Gastric volvulus (GV), organoaxial volvulus (OAV), mesenteroaxial volvulus (MAV)

Definitions
- Rotation of all or part of stomach > 180°, +/- closed-loop obstruction, +/- strangulation
  ○ It is rotation, not obstruction which defines presence of GV

IMAGING FINDINGS

General Features
- Best diagnostic clue
  ○ Mesenteroaxial volvulus
    ▪ Spherical, distended stomach, 2 air-fluid levels (inferior fundus and superior antrum)
    ▪ Beak-like, inferior gastroesophageal junction (GEJ)
  ○ Organoaxial volvulus
    ▪ Difficult diagnosis on radiography
    ▪ Paucity of gas beyond stomach
    ▪ Low GEJ, marked gastric dilation, slow passage barium
- Location: Predominantly left upper abdomen
- Types of GV: Organoaxial (most common); mesenteroaxial; mixed
  ○ Organoaxial (OAV): Rotation about longitudinal axis (most common)
    ▪ Axis extending from cardia to pylorus
    ▪ Stomach twists anteriorly or posteriorly
    ▪ Antrum moves inferior to superior
  ○ Mesenteroaxial (MAV): Rotation about mesenteric axis
    ▪ Axis across stomach right angles to lesser & greater curves
    ▪ Rotation right to left or left to right about gastrohepatic omentum
  ○ Mixed volvulus: Combination of OAV & MAV

Radiographic Findings
- Radiography
  ○ Abdominal X-ray; patient upright
    ▪ Double air-fluid level
    ▪ Distended stomach; viscus displaced up to left
    ▪ Elevation of diaphragm

DDx: Gastric Malposition

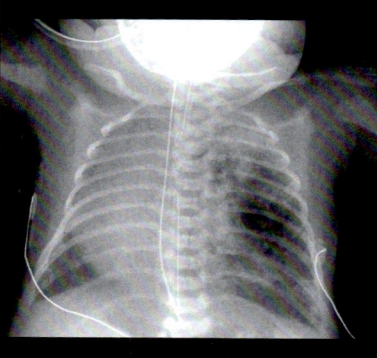
Congenital Diaphramatic Hernia

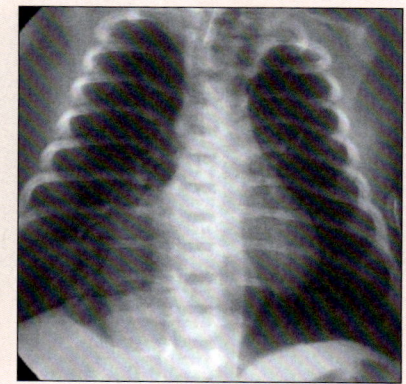
Hiatal Hernia

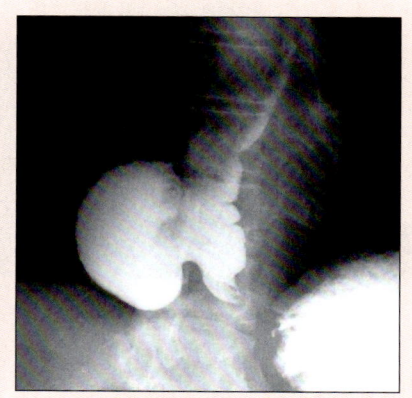
Epiphrenic Diverticulum

GASTRIC VOLVULUS

Key Facts

Terminology
- Rotation of all or part of stomach > 180°, +/- closed-loop obstruction, +/- strangulation

Imaging Findings
- Organoaxial (OAV): Rotation about longitudinal axis (most common)
- Axis extending from cardia to pylorus
- Mesenteroaxial (MAV): Rotation about mesenteric axis
- Axis across stomach right angles to lesser & greater curves
- Double air-fluid level
- Inversion of stomach
- Greater curve above lesser
- Cardia & pylorus at same level
- Downward pointing pylorus & duodenum
- Incomplete/absent entrance or exit of contrast to/from stomach

Top Differential Diagnoses
- Hiatal Hernia
- Post-Operative

Pathology
- Large esophageal or paraesophageal hernia
- Diaphragmatic eventration or paralysis

Clinical Issues
- Complications: Intramural emphysema; perforation
- Mortality rate: 30%
- Detorse stomach
- Repair of associated defects
- Prevent recurrence

- Paucity distal gas
- +/- Intramural emphysema gastric wall
- Chest X-ray: Intrathoracic up-side down stomach
  - Retrocardiac fluid level; 2 air-fluid levels different heights
  - Fluid levels above & below diaphragm

Fluoroscopic Findings
- Massive stomach left upper quadrant +/- into chest
- Inversion of stomach
  - Greater curve above lesser
  - Cardia & pylorus at same level
  - Downward pointing pylorus & duodenum
- +/- "Beaking" at point of twist
- OAV: 2 points of twist; luminal obstruction
- Incomplete/absent entrance or exit of contrast to/from stomach
- Gastric outlet obstruction
- MAV: Antrum & pylorus above gastric fundus

CT Findings
- Not generally performed for GV
- Incidental finding
- CT appearance variable
  - Depends on extent of gastric herniation, points of torsion, position of stomach
  - +/- Linear septum within gastric lumen (torsion)
- CT chest & abdomen
  - Associated malformation or malposition
  - Unattached herniated peritoneal sac
  - Hiatal hernia accompanied by partial GV
  - "Pseudothrombosis" of inferior vena cava
- False positives/negatives
  - Paraesophageal hernia without torsion

MR Findings
- Similar to CT
  - 2 different signal intensities reflect point of torsion

Angiographic Findings
- Acute upper gastrointestinal hemorrhage
- Gastric vascular supply displaced

Imaging Recommendations
- Best imaging tool
  - Fluoroscopic upper gastrointestinal (UGI)
    - Demonstrate volvulus, anatomic detail
  - Fluoroscopic guidance to advance feeding tube into obstructed stomach
    - Attempt decompression; stabilize patient
  - CT; complementary role

DIFFERENTIAL DIAGNOSIS

Hiatal Hernia
- Stomach enters thorax through esophageal hiatus
- GEJ above diaphragmatic hiatus (type I, sliding)
- GE junction below diaphragm (type II; paraesophageal)
  - Herniation of fundus through hiatus
- Giant paraesophageal hernia: Up to 1/3 of stomach in chest
  - +/- Herniation of small bowel/colon
- Traction or torsion of stomach at or near level of hiatus (volvulus)

Post-Operative
- Esophagectomy with gastric pull through
  - Complete mobilization of stomach, resection of lower esophagus, pyloroplasty, transhiatal dissection
  - Intrathoracic stomach

Epiphrenic Diverticulum
- Retrocardiac mass +/- air-fluid level

PATHOLOGY

General Features
- General path comments
  - Point of anatomic fixation: Second portion of duodenum, retroperitoneal
  - Ligaments normally anchor stomach

GASTRIC VOLVULUS

- Gastrohepatic, gastrosplenic, gastrocolic, gastrophrenic
- Gastrolienal ligaments contribute to fixation
○ Torsion of stomach + significant degree of herniation
○ Predisposing factors: Bands, adhesions
- Rapid changes intraabdominal pressure; ↑ size of esophageal hiatus
- Unusually long gastrohepatic + gastrocolic mesenteries
• Etiology
○ Primary GV: Stabilizing ligaments are lax
- Absence of tethering gastric ligaments
- One third of cases
○ Secondary GV: Paraesophageal hernia
- Congenital or acquired diaphragmatic defects
- Children; Morgagni hernia
○ Idiopathic; no apparent cause
• Epidemiology
○ Children, MAV most common; associated anatomic defects
○ 5 cases of combined organomesenteroaxial GV in children in world literature
• Associated abnormalities
○ Large esophageal or paraesophageal hernia
- Part or all stomach intrathoracic
○ Diaphragmatic eventration or paralysis
○ Wandering spleen: Absence of gastrosplenic attachments
○ Hernia of colonic transverse loop with anterior OAV
- Sliding hernia

Gross Pathologic & Surgical Features
• Partial or complete volvulus
• "Gastric volvulus" used by some to identify gastric malposition without obstruction
○ "Upside-down stomach"; gastric displacement through hernias
• "True volvulus"; term used only when obstruction

CLINICAL ISSUES

Presentation
• Most common signs/symptoms
○ Classic clinical triad (Borchardt triad)
- Violent retching with little vomitus
- Constant severe epigastric pain
- Difficulty advancing nasogastric tube into stomach
• Other signs/symptoms: Bleeding and anemia, distention

Demographics
• Age
○ Pediatric & adult patients
○ Primarily after fourth decade of life

Natural History & Prognosis
• GV can be asymptomatic
• Small herniations, proximal stomach enters hernia sac first
○ Obstruction/strangulation almost never at this stage

- As herniation progresses; body & variable portion antrum above diaphragm
○ Stomach can become entirely intrathoracic; prone to volvulus
• Obstruction can occur at points of torsion or twisting
○ Stomach re-descends through hiatus
○ 180° twisting +/- obstruction/strangulation
○ > 180°; obstruction & acute abdomen
○ OAV: +/- Obstruct; not usually strangulation
○ MAV: +/- Occlude gastric vessels; strangulation
• "Upside-down stomach"
○ Typically sliding hernia & (180° OAV)
- Enlarged esophageal hiatus or Bochdalek defect
○ Bleeding & anemia; not usually obstruction or strangulation
• Acute volvulus; associated interference of blood supply
○ Vascular occlusion, necrosis, shock
○ Surgical emergency
• Chronic GV: Chronic or recurrent form
○ Frequently not recognized early
○ Vague symptoms; causes delay in diagnosis
○ Incidentally noted on CT or MR
• Complications: Intramural emphysema; perforation
○ Strangulation, mucosal ischemia
○ Focal necrosis; gas to dissect into gastric wall
○ Perforation from full-thickness necrosis
• Prognosis: GV is potentially catastrophic condition
• Mortality rate: 30%

Treatment
• Goals: Early recognition/surgical repair
○ Detorse stomach
○ Repair of associated defects
○ Prevent recurrence
• Laparoscopic detorsion & percutaneous endoscopic gastropexy
• Gastric resection; for strangulation & necrosis
• Upside-down stomach: Balloon repositioning; percutaneous fixation

DIAGNOSTIC CHECKLIST

Consider
• If suspicious for GV, UGI
• Identification of GV as incidental finding on CT
• Whenever stomach is malpositioned

SELECTED REFERENCES
1. Shivanand G et al: Gastric volvulus: acute and chronic presentation. Clin Imaging. 27(4):265-8, 2003
2. Tabo T et al: Balloon repositioning of intrathoracic upside-down stomach and fixation by percutaneous endoscopic gastrostomy. J Am Coll Surg. 197(5):868-71, 2003
3. Godshall D et al: Gastric volvulus: case report and review of the literature. J Emerg Med. 17(5):837-40, 1999
4. Schaefer DC et al: Gastric volvulus: an old disease process with some new twists. Gastroenterologist. 5(1):41-5, 1997
5. Chiechi MV et al: Gastric herniation and volvulus: CT and MR appearance. Gastrointest Radiol. 17(2):99-101, 1992
6. Miller DL et al: Gastric volvulus in the pediatric population. Arch Surg. 126(9):1146-9, 1991

GASTRIC VOLVULUS

IMAGE GALLERY

Typical

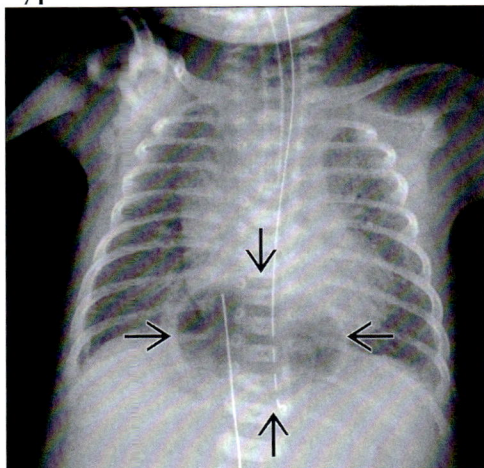
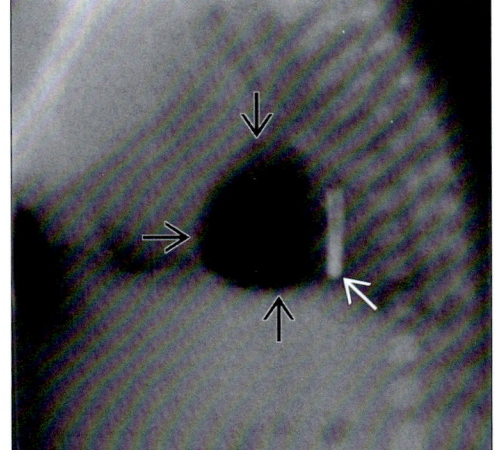

(Left) Anteroposterior radiograph of the chest; to the right is lateral view of the same premature neonate shows stomach in the midline above the diaphragm ➔ consistent with hiatal hernia, most having volvulus. *(Right)* Lateral radiograph of patient at left shows that the lucency in the midline is the stomach ➔ with enteric tube ➔ within it.

Variant

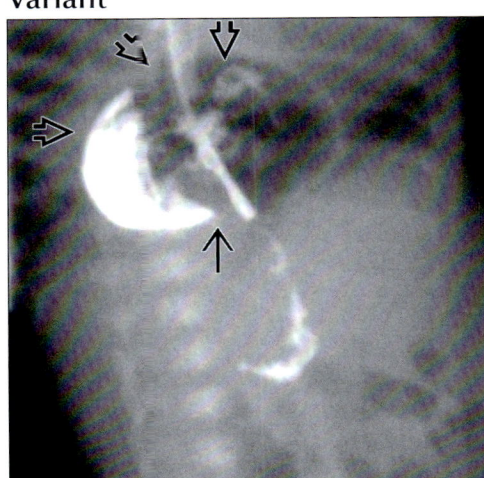
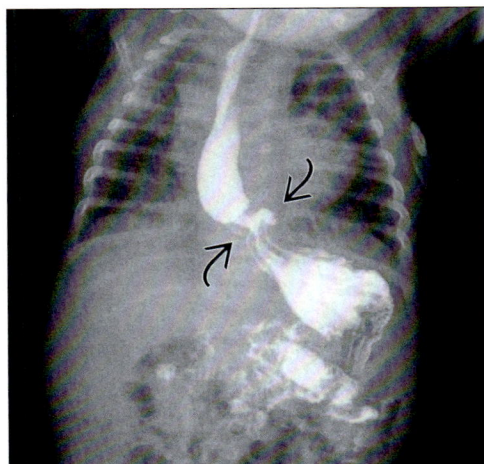

(Left) Oblique upper GI shows superior location of the greater curve ➔ of the stomach consistent with organoaxial volvulus. Even the gastric outlet ➔ is above the diaphragm. *(Right)* Anteroposterior upper GI after repair shows residual sliding hiatal hernia ➔ with GE reflux to upper esophagus on this post-UGI radiograph.

Typical

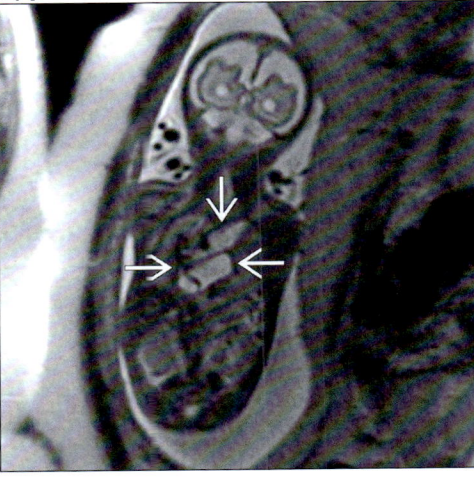
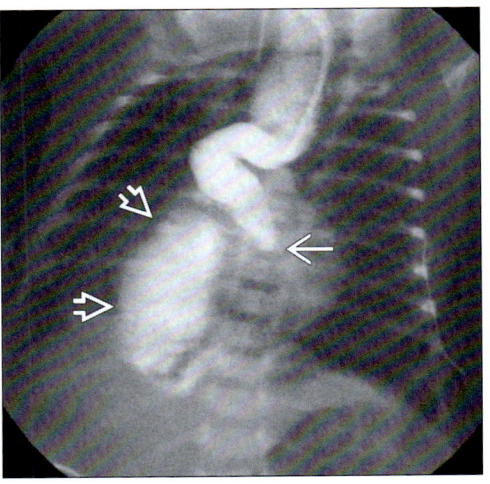

(Left) Coronal T2WI MR (fetal) shows stomach and other bowel in thorax ➔ with superior position of greater curvature, similar to upper GI study in previous image, showing hiatal hernia with gastric volvulus. *(Right)* Anteroposterior upper GI shows a small amount of contrast entering the stomach at the gastroesophageal junction ➔. The greater curve of the stomach ➔ is on the right in this hiatal hernia with organoaxial gastric volvulus.

ILEOCOLIC INTUSSUSCEPTION (IDIOPATHIC)

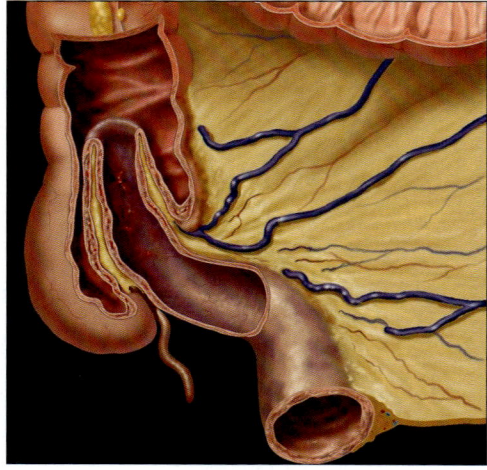

Graphic shows intussusception with terminal ileum invaginating into cecum and ascending colon. Note vascular congestion of intussusceptum.

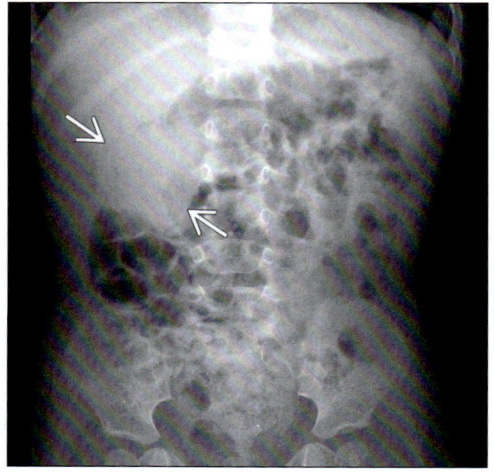

Anteroposterior radiograph shows typical case of idiopathic intussusception with a right upper quadrant soft tissue mass ➡ overlying hepatic flexure.

TERMINOLOGY

Definitions
- Intussusception: Forward peristalsis results in invagination of more proximal bowel (the intussusceptum) into lumen of more distal bowel (the intussuscipiens) in a telescope-like manner

IMAGING FINDINGS

General Features
- Best diagnostic clue: Radiography: Meniscus of soft tissue mass outlined in air-filled colon
- Location
  ○ Most common site: Terminal ileum/ileocecal valve
  ○ 90% ileocolic
- Size
  ○ May involve small segment of terminal ileum and ileocecal valve
  ○ May progress to involve a large segment of ileum with extension into the transverse or descending colon
  ○ Invagination may begin with telescoping of ileum into distal ileum and then into cecum or ascending colon, ileo-ileocolic intussusception

Radiographic Findings
- Radiography
  ○ Rarely completely normal
  ○ Paucity of right lower quadrant (RLQ) gas
  ○ Non-visualization of air-filled cecum
  ○ Left-side-down decubitus/prone views can be helpful in showing lack of air-filled cecum
  ○ Meniscus of soft tissue mass outlined in air-filled colon
  ○ Small bowel obstruction

Fluoroscopic Findings
- Air contrast enema
  ○ Intussusception easily recognized as round mass that moves retrograde with increased pressure
  ○ Reflux of gas into small bowel and resolution of soft tissue mass denotes successful reduction
- Liquid contrast enema
  ○ Similar findings as with air enema but with positive contrast

DDx: Abdominal Pain in a Child

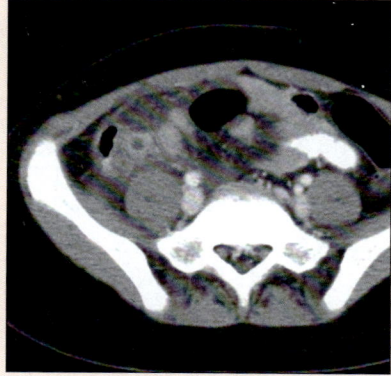

Appendicitis

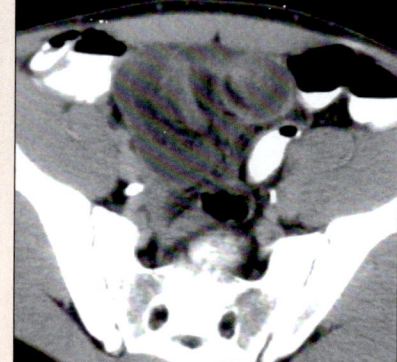

Meckel

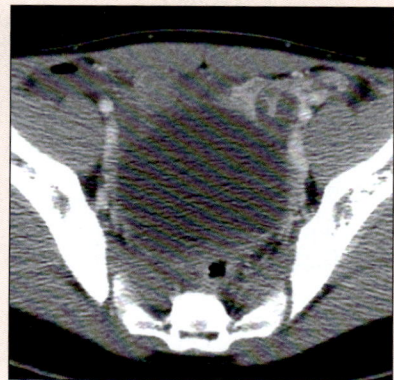

Ovarian Pathology

ILEOCOLIC INTUSSUSCEPTION (IDIOPATHIC)

Key Facts

Terminology
- Intussusception: Forward peristalsis results in invagination of more proximal bowel (the intussusceptum) into lumen of more distal bowel (the intussuscipiens) in a telescope-like manner

Imaging Findings
- Best diagnostic clue: Radiography: Meniscus of soft tissue mass outlined in air-filled colon
- Most common site: Terminal ileum/ileocecal valve

Pathology
- Bowel wall congestion from venous obstruction may lead to bowel ischemia and necrosis
- Seasonal occurrence (winter, spring) with viral illnesses

Clinical Issues
- Alternating lethargy and irritability
- Colic
- Most common between 3 months-1 year of age
- Surgery reserved for cases of reduction failure
- Success rates 80-90% with air reduction
- Risk of perforation 0.5%

Diagnostic Checklist
- Left-side-down decubitus/prone views can be helpful in showing lack of air-filled cecum
- CT: Colonic mass with alternating rings of high and low attenuation
- May not be located in RLQ if intussusception has progressed distally

CT Findings
- CECT
  - Not advocated as diagnostic tool for suspected intussusception but intussusception may be encountered on abdominal CT performed for nonspecific abdominal pain
  - Colonic mass with alternating rings of high and low attenuation
  - May be able to appreciate continuity with adjacent mesenteric fat and areas of low attenuation within the bowel lumen
  - May not be located in RLQ if intussusception has progressed distal

Ultrasonographic Findings
- Grayscale Ultrasound
  - Can be used in cases in which radiographs or history are inconclusive
  - Mass with alternating rings of hyper- and hypoechogenicity
  - "Pseudo-kidney" appearance on longitudinal images
  - May not be located in RLQ if intussusception has progressed distal
    - Need to scan entire left and right abdomen

Imaging Recommendations
- Best imaging tool: Radiography and ultrasound
- Protocol advice
  - Radiography for initial evaluation of abdominal pain
  - Ultrasound for cases with equivocal history or radiographic findings
  - Reduction enema: Used to both confirm and treat intussusception

DIFFERENTIAL DIAGNOSIS

Normal Position of Sigmoid Colon
- In infants and young children, sigmoid colon may be in right lower quadrant of abdomen 43% of time
- May be misinterpreted as air in cecum and falsely exclude intussusception

Appendicitis
- May present with similar symptoms of abdominal pain, typically older age group
- Identification of appendicolith is helpful
- In cases of perforation, there may be extrinsic mass effect on the cecum mimicking soft tissue mass

Gastroenteritis
- Plain film typically shows multiple air fluid levels within mildly distended bowel loops
- Air fluid levels in colon support gastroenteritis and make intussusception unlikely

Ovarian Pathology
- May present as fussiness or pain in young child

Meckel Diverticulum
- May serve as lead point for intussusception, cause gastrointestinal (GI) bleeding, or abdominal pain

PATHOLOGY

General Features
- General path comments
  - Bowel wall congestion from venous obstruction may lead to bowel ischemia and necrosis
  - Bowel perforation may occur during reduction attempt
- Etiology
  - 90% idiopathic variety (2nd to lymphoid hyperplasia)
  - May be preceded by viral illness
- Epidemiology
  - Relatively common cause of abdominal pain in children 3 months to 1 year of age
  - Seasonal occurrence (winter, spring) with viral illnesses
  - If > 3 years of age, think pathologic lead point, such as lymphoma, Meckel diverticulum, Henoch-Schönlein purpura (wall hematoma)

ILEOCOLIC INTUSSUSCEPTION (IDIOPATHIC)

Gross Pathologic & Surgical Features
- Telescoping to terminal ileum and ileocecal valve into the cecum or ascending colon

CLINICAL ISSUES

Presentation
- Most common signs/symptoms
  - Alternating lethargy and irritability
  - Colic
  - Palpable right-sided abdominal mass
  - May have empty RLQ, Dance sign
- Other signs/symptoms
  - Bloody diarrhea, ("currant jelly") stools
  - Crampy abdominal pain
  - Vomiting, may be bilious

Demographics
- Age
  - Most common between 3 months-1 year of age
  - If greater than 3 years: Pathologic lead point?
- Gender: M < F

Natural History & Prognosis
- Medical urgency: Can infarct bowel if not reduced
- If bowel necrosis, perforation can occur leading to peritonitis, shock and even death
- In a small number there may be spontaneous reduction
- Intussusception recurs after successful reduction in 5-10%
- Most recurrences within first 72 hours

Treatment
- Imaging guided pressure reduction is treatment of choice
- Surgery reserved for cases of reduction failure
- Air insufflation or liquid contrast with fluoroscopic guidance most common methods
- Hydrostatic reduction under ultrasound guidance
- Contraindications: Peritonitis - exam, free peritoneal air - radiography (rare)
- Findings associated with decreased success rate but not contraindications
  - Small bowel obstruction
  - Prolonged history of symptoms (days)
  - Poor clinical condition: Lethargy
- Preparation guidelines: Adequate hydration, IV access, physical examination, pediatric surgery consultation (in case of perforation)
- If child appears not well (lethargic), good idea to have surgery present at time of reduction
- Guidelines: Good rectal seal, 120 mmHg maximal pressure at rest but can be greater during crying/Valsalva, typically three attempts during any one sitting, after rest period additional attempts can be made
- Intussusception encountered as round mass that moves retrograde with increased pressure
- Success: Reflux of gas into small bowel, resolution of soft tissue mass
- Mass most likely to "get stuck" at ileocecal valve
- If initial progression of mass on initial attempts but not able to reduce beyond ileocecal valve, a period of an hour may allow for edema to decrease and increased chance of success
- May be difficult at times to differentiate edematous ileocecal valve from persistent intussusception: Follow clinically
  - Edematous ileocecal valve may predispose to recurrence
- Success rates 80-90% with air reduction
- Risk of perforation 0.5%
- Recurrences can be treated on up to three occurrences prior to considering surgical exploration for potential pathological lead point

DIAGNOSTIC CHECKLIST

Image Interpretation Pearls
- Left-side-down decubitus/prone views can be helpful in showing lack of air-filled cecum
- CT: Colonic mass with alternating rings of high and low attenuation
- US: Mass with alternating rings of hyper- and hypoechogenicity, "pseudo-kidney" appearance on longitudinal image
- May not be located in RLQ if intussusception has progressed distally

SELECTED REFERENCES
1. Daneman A et al: Intussusception. Part 2: An update on the evolution of management. Pediatr Radiol. 34(2):97-108; quiz 187, 2004
2. Navarro O et al: Intussusception. Part 3: Diagnosis and management of those with an identifiable or predisposing cause and those that reduce spontaneously. Pediatr Radiol. 34(4):305-12; quiz 369, 2004
3. Daneman A et al: Intussusception. Part 1: a review of diagnostic approaches. Pediatr Radiol. 33(2):79-85, 2003
4. Melcher ML et al: Ileocolic intussusception in an adult. J Am Coll Surg. 197(3):518, 2003
5. Strouse PJ et al: Transient small-bowel intussusception in children on CT. Pediatr Radiol. 33(5):316-20, 2003
6. Khong PL et al: Ultrasound-guided hydrostatic reduction of childhood intussusception: technique and demonstration. Radiographics. 20(5):E1, 2000
7. Kornecki A et al: Spontaneous reduction of intussusception: clinical spectrum, management and outcome. Pediatr Radiol. 30(1):58-63, 2000
8. Peh WC et al: Ileoileocolic intussusception in children: diagnosis and significance. Br J Radiol. 70(837):891-6, 1997
9. Strouse PJ et al: Ileocolic intussusception presenting with bilious vomiting due to extrinsic duodenal obstruction. Pediatr Radiol. 25 Suppl 1:S167-8, 1995
10. Shiels WE 2nd et al: Air enema for diagnosis and reduction of intussusception: clinical experience and pressure correlates. Radiology. 181(1):169-72, 1991
11. Eklof O et al: Reliability of the abdominal plain film diagnosis in pediatric patients with suspected intussusception. Pediatr Radiol. 9(4):199-206, 1980

ILEOCOLIC INTUSSUSCEPTION (IDIOPATHIC)

IMAGE GALLERY

Typical

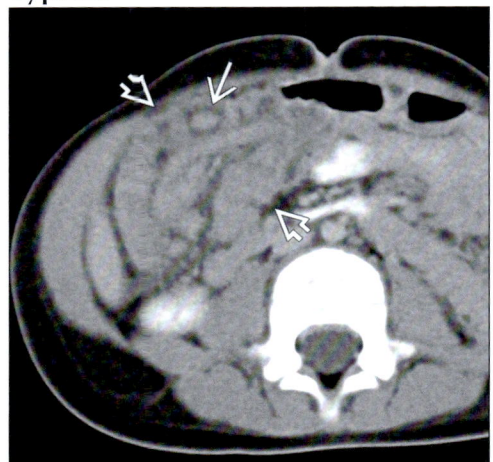
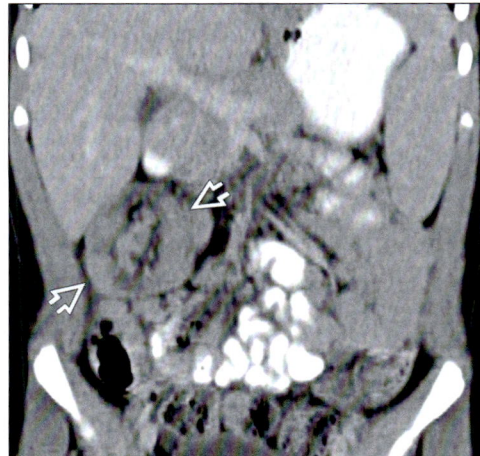

(Left) Axial CECT from a 2-year-old who had abdominal pain after a fall shows RLQ intussusception ➲ as mass with alternating high/low attenuation areas. Note lymph node ➜. *(Right)* Coronal CECT of same patient as previous image, better shows intussusception ➲ with soft tissue and fat attenuation in alternating rings.

Typical

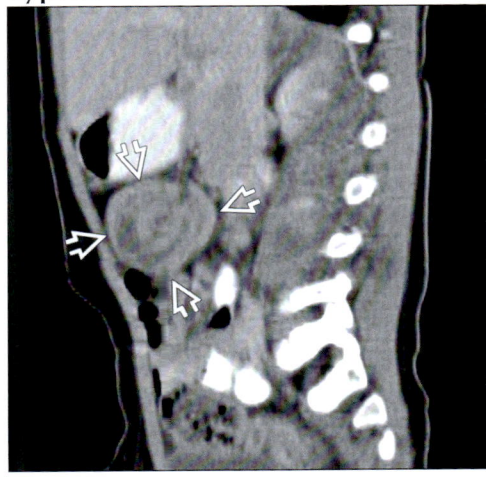
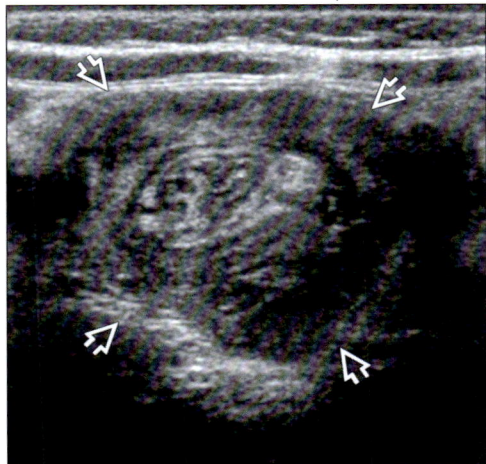

(Left) Sagittal CECT of same patient as previous image, again shows intussusception ➲. *(Right)* Ultrasound in same patient as previous image performed after transfer to tertiary center shows persistence of intussusception ➲ with alternating rings of high and low echogenicity.

Typical

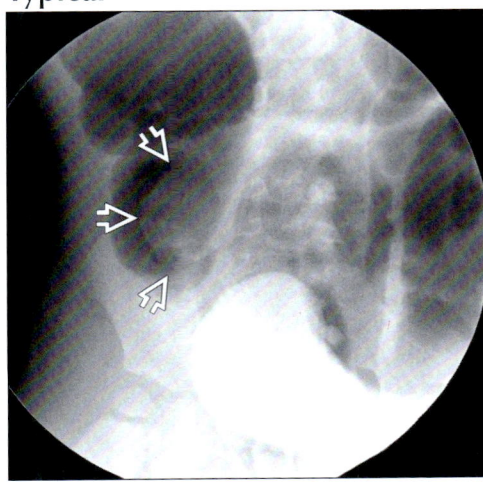
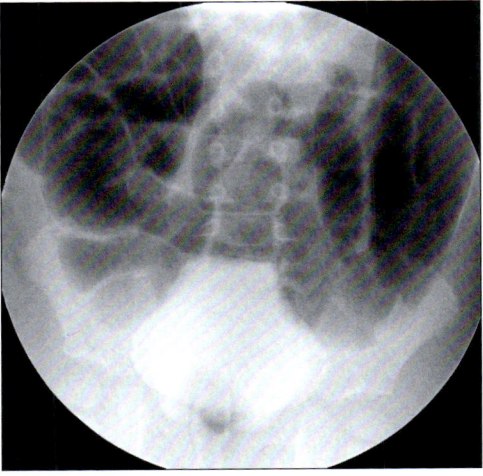

(Left) Frontal image from air enema in same patient as previous image, shows intussusception ➲ as soft tissue mass moved to region of ileocecal valve. *(Right)* Frontal image from air enema (same patient as previous) moments later, shows resolution of soft tissue mass and reflux of gas into small bowel, consistent with resolution of intussusception.

MECKEL DIVERTICULUM

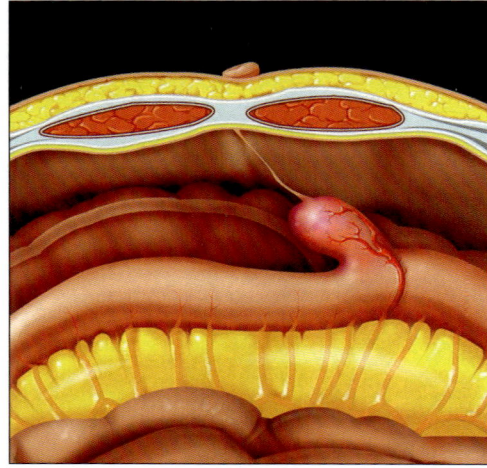

Graphic shows an inflamed Meckel diverticulum growing off the antimesenteric border of the intestine with the obliterated remnant of the omphalomesenteric duct extending from its tip.

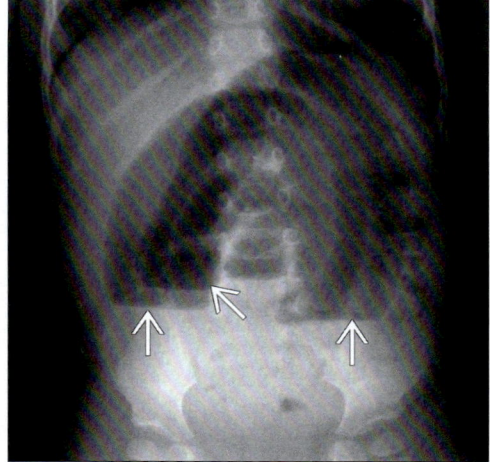

Anteroposterior radiograph shows dilated small bowel containing differential air fluid levels ➔ with the same segment consistent with small bowel obstruction caused by an omphalomesenteric duct band.

TERMINOLOGY

Definitions
- Remnant of the omphalomesenteric duct, can cause bleeding (when contains ectopic gastric mucosa), intussusception, bowel obstruction or perforation
- Rule of 2s: Incidence 2% of general population, found within 2 feet of ileocecal valve, most have clinical symptoms before age 2 years

IMAGING FINDINGS

General Features
- Best diagnostic clue
  - Classic imaging appearance on nuclear pertechnetate scan is focal accumulation in right lower quadrant that is coincident with, and as intense as, gastric uptake, and increases in visibility with time
  - Nuclear scintigraphy is most accurate: Radiographs, sonography, CT scan or barium studies show nonspecific signs of a right lower quadrant inflammatory process
- Location
  - Within 2 feet of ileocecal valve
  - Right lower quadrant or midline/periumbilical in location
- Size: 5-6 cm in length, though inflammatory mass may be much larger

Radiographic Findings
- Radiography
  - Abdominal films may show a right lower quadrant mass or displacement of bowel loops, obstruction, or be normal
  - Enteroliths are occasionally reported in Meckel diverticulum

Fluoroscopic Findings
- Often normal
- Barium studies show indirect evidence of mass and inflammatory changes in adjacent bowel

CT Findings
- CECT
  - Findings very similar to appendicitis; thick-walled blind ending structure near cecum with surrounding inflammation

DDx: Clinical Mimickers of Meckel Diverticulum

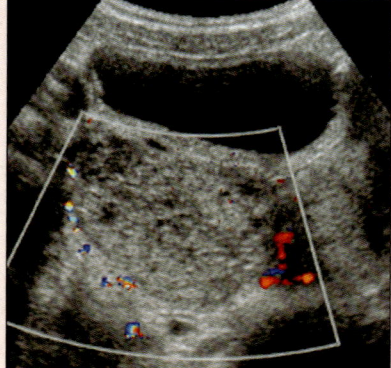

Ovarian Torsion

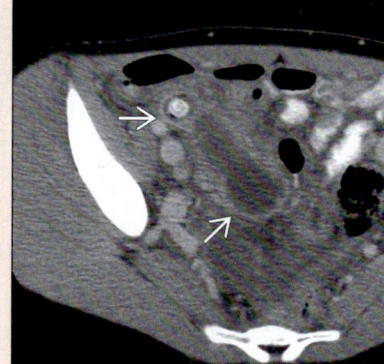

Acute Appendicitis

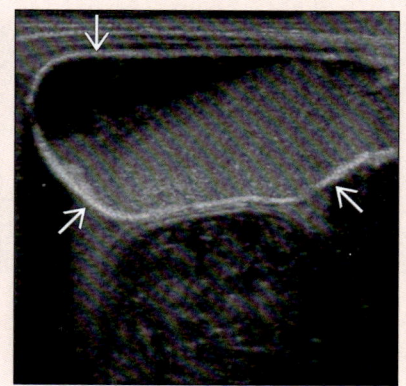

Meconium Pseudocyst

MECKEL DIVERTICULUM

Key Facts

Terminology
- Remnant of the omphalomesenteric duct, can cause bleeding (when contains ectopic gastric mucosa), intussusception, bowel obstruction or perforation
- Rule of 2s: Incidence 2% of general population, found within 2 feet of ileocecal valve, most have clinical symptoms before age 2 years

Imaging Findings
- Classic imaging appearance on nuclear pertechnetate scan is focal accumulation in right lower quadrant that is coincident with, and as intense as, gastric uptake, and increases in visibility with time
- Nuclear scintigraphy is most accurate: Radiographs, sonography, CT scan or barium studies show nonspecific signs of a right lower quadrant inflammatory process
- Size: 5-6 cm in length, though inflammatory mass may be much larger
- Findings very similar to appendicitis; thick-walled blind ending structure near cecum with surrounding inflammation

Top Differential Diagnoses
- Appendicitis
- Intestinal Duplication Containing Gastric Mucosa
- Hemangioma
- Inflammatory Bowel Disease
- Ovarian Pathology
- Meconium Pseudocyst

Pathology
- Enteroliths are found in the lumen in some cases

  - If perforated may see abscess and free air
  - CT is more accurate in diagnosing Meckel diverticulum than arteriography when presenting symptom is gastrointestinal bleeding in pediatric patients
  - Non-inflamed Meckel diverticula can move slightly with the bowel in the lower abdomen on sequential imaging

Ultrasonographic Findings
- Grayscale Ultrasound
  - Heterogeneous echotexture mass in right lower quadrant, may mimic appendicitis
  - Thick-walled tubular structure or hyperemic bowel loops in right lower quadrant
  - Inflamed Meckel diverticulum may present as a cyst, but with mucosal layer more irregular than typically found in an intestinal duplication
- Color Doppler: Hyperemia related to inflammatory process

Nuclear Medicine Findings
- Tc-99m pertechnetate scan
  - Most specific test for Meckel diverticulum: Accuracy ~ 90%
  - Pertechnetate accumulates in mucous cells when they are in an acidic environment, in this case in ectopic gastric mucosa
  - Diverticulum typically does not communicate with the bowel lumen, so radiotracer does not appear to move downstream in bowel unless there is active bleeding
  - Pharmacologic enhancement of pertechnetate scans by using subcutaneous pentagastrin, oral or intravenous ranitidine or cimetidine, and IM glucagon is advocated by some
  - However, given the high sensitivity of unenhanced scans, additional medications may be reserved for repeat studies in patients with high clinical suspicion of Meckel diverticular disease and normal initial scans
  - False negative pertechnetate scans
    - Lack of any or sufficient gastric mucosa to localize radiotracer
    - Secondary ischemia due to volvulus or intussusception

Imaging Recommendations
- Best imaging tool: Tc-99m pertechnetate scan

DIFFERENTIAL DIAGNOSIS

Appendicitis
- Hyperemia may cause early increase in pertechnetate activity at the lesion

Intestinal Duplication Containing Gastric Mucosa
- Also common in right lower quadrant, also need to be surgically removed

Hemangioma
- Hemangioma can also cause bleeding, obstruction, or intussusception

Inflammatory Bowel Disease
- Hyperemia causes mildly increased accumulation of pertechnetate

Ovarian Pathology
- Negative on pertechnetate scans, but in the same lower quadrant on other imaging studies

Meconium Pseudocyst
- Negative on pertechnetate scans, but in the same lower quadrant on other imaging studies

PATHOLOGY

General Features
- General path comments
  - Remnant of the omphalomesenteric duct found in 2-3% of autopsy series

MECKEL DIVERTICULUM

- Small percentage of Meckel become symptomatic, typically due to the presence of ectopic gastric mucosa
- Rarely, the diverticulum contains rests of pancreatic tissue
- Embryology-anatomy
  - Omphalomesenteric duct was the connection between the yolk sac and primitive digestive tract in early fetal life
  - Meckel diverticulum is the most common end result of the spectrum of omphalomesenteric duct anomalies, which also include umbilicoileal fistula, umbilical sinus, umbilical cyst, and a fibrous cord connecting the ileum to the umbilicus

Gross Pathologic & Surgical Features
- Typically 5-6 cm in length, positioned within 2 feet proximal to the ileocecal valve
- Enteroliths are found in the lumen in some cases

Microscopic Features
- Composed of same layers as adjacent small bowel but with the addition of heterotopic gastric or pancreatic rests

CLINICAL ISSUES

Presentation
- Most common signs/symptoms: Gastrointestinal (GI) bleeding, ulceration, abdominal pain, or mass
- Other signs/symptoms
  - May present as intermittent abdominal pain, occult fecal blood, frank blood in stool, small bowel obstruction, intussusception, volvulus, or perforation
  - Perforation of Meckel diverticulum with hemoperitoneum in children is a rare and serious complication
  - Torsion of a Meckel diverticulum may present with nonspecific abdominal pain and mass

Demographics
- Age
  - Most often become symptomatic before two years of age
  - 60% of patients come to medical attention before 10 years of age, with the remainder of cases manifesting in adolescence and adulthood
  - Older patients more likely to present with intussusception or small bowel obstruction than with GI bleeding
- Gender
  - Males = females in true incidence
  - Bleeding and other symptoms/complications are more common in males

Treatment
- Surgical resection, incidental appendectomy usually also performed
- Meckel diverticula are generally removed when found incidentally on imaging or in the operating room

DIAGNOSTIC CHECKLIST

Image Interpretation Pearls
- Tc-99m pertechnetate scan
  - Positive in only those Meckel diverticula containing gastric mucosa

SELECTED REFERENCES

1. Baldisserotto M: Color Doppler sonographic findings of inflamed and perforated Meckel diverticulum. J Ultrasound Med. 23(6):843-8, 2004
2. Bennett GL et al: CT of Meckel's diverticulitis in 11 patients. AJR Am J Roentgenol. 182(3):625-9, 2004
3. Levy AD et al: From the archives of the AFIP. Meckel diverticulum: radiologic features with pathologic Correlation. Radiographics. 24(2):565-87, 2004
4. Ojha S et al: Meckel's diverticulum with segmental dilatation of the ileum: radiographic diagnosis in a neonate. Pediatr Radiol. 34(8):649-51, 2004
5. Rerksuppaphol S et al: Ranitidine-enhanced 99mtechnetium pertechnetate imaging in children improves the sensitivity of identifying heterotopic gastric mucosa in Meckel's diverticulum. Pediatr Surg Int. 20(5):323-5, 2004
6. Segal SD et al: Rare mesenteric location of Meckel's diverticulum, a forgotten entity: a case study aboard USS Kitty Hawk. Am Surg. 70(11):985-8, 2004
7. Singh MV et al: A fading Meckel's diverticulum: an unusual scintigraphic appearance in a child. Pediatr Radiol. 34(3):274-6, 2004
8. Adams BK et al: A moving Meckel's diverticulum on Tc-99m pertechnetate imaging in a patient with lower gastrointestinal bleeding. Clin Nucl Med. 28(11):908-10, 2003
9. Baldisserotto M et al: Sonographic findings of Meckel's diverticulitis in children. AJR Am J Roentgenol. 180(2):425-8, 2003
10. Danzer D et al: Bleeding Meckel's diverticulum diagnosis: an unusual indication for computed tomography. Abdom Imaging. 28(5):631-3, 2003
11. Onen A et al: When to resect and when not to resect an asymptomatic Meckel's diverticulum: an ongoing challenge. Pediatr Surg Int. 19(1-2):57-61, 2003
12. Jelenc F et al: Meckel's diverticulum perforation with intraabdominal hemorrhage. J Pediatr Surg. 37(6):E18, 2002
13. Mortele KJ et al: Giant Meckel's diverticulum containing enteroliths: typical CT imaging findings. Eur Radiol. 12(1):82-4, 2002
14. Sy ED et al: Meckel's diverticulum associated with ileal volvulus in a neonate. Pediatr Surg Int. 18(5-6):529-31, 2002
15. Farris SL et al: Axial torsion of Meckel's diverticulum presenting as a pelvic mass. Pediatr Radiol. 31(12):886-8, 2001
16. Neidlinger NA et al: Meckel's diverticulum causing cecal volvulus. Am Surg. 67(1):41-3, 2001
17. Oguzkurt P et al: Cystic Meckel's diverticulum: A rare cause of cystic pelvic mass presenting with urinary symptoms. J Pediatr Surg. 36(12):1855-8, 2001
18. O'Hara SM: Pediatric gastrointestinal nuclear imaging. Radiol Clin North Am. 34(4):845-62, 1996
19. Wilton G et al: The "false-negative" Meckel's scan. Clin Nucl Med. 7(10):441-3, 1982
20. Sfakianakis GN et al: Detection of ectopic gastric mucosa in Meckel's diverticulum and in other aberrations by scintigraphy: I. Pathophysiology and 10-year clinical experience. J Nucl Med. 22(7):647-54, 1981

MECKEL DIVERTICULUM

IMAGE GALLERY

Typical

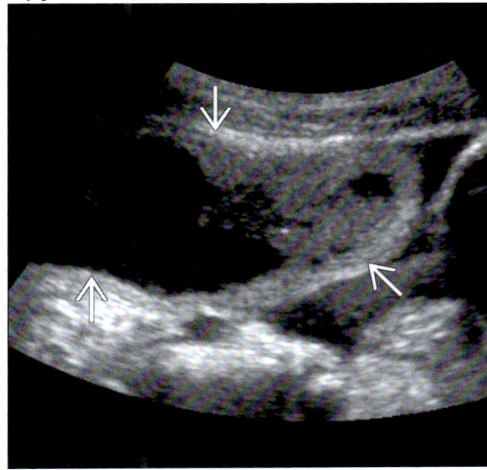
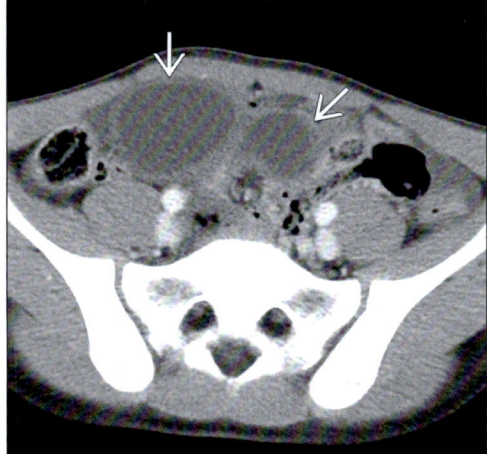

(Left) Longitudinal ultrasound shows a cystic mass ➡ containing debris within the right lower quadrant. *(Right)* Axial CECT in the same patient as previous image, shows a cystic mass ➡, Meckel diverticulum with adjacent small amount of free fluid.

Typical

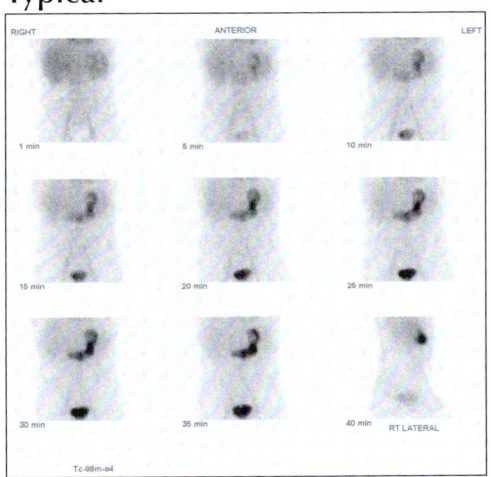
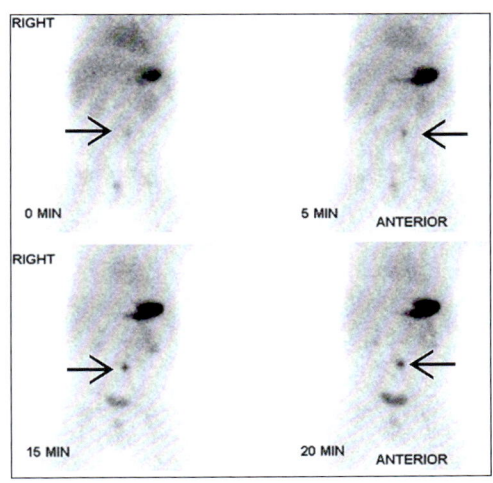

(Left) Anterior images from Tc-99m pertechnetate scan show normal distribution of the radioisotope within the abdomen. *(Right)* Anterior images from Tc-99m pertechnetate scan show progressive intense, focal radioisotope accumulation in the lower abdominal ➡ Meckel diverticulum.

Typical

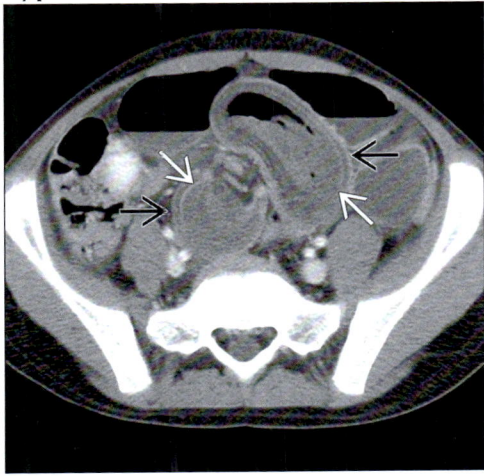
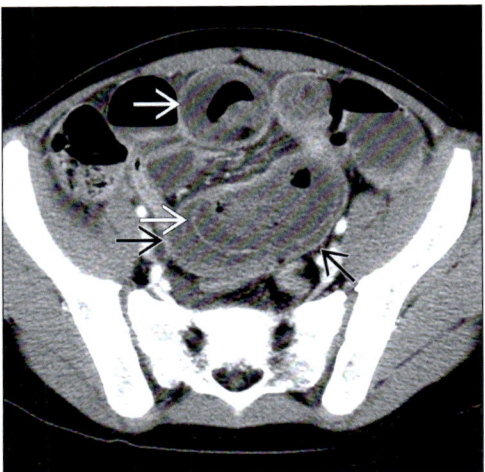

(Left) Axial CECT shows a cystic mass ➡ with a double wall caused from invaginating or intussuscepting of the cystic mass into distal small bowel ➡. *(Right)* Axial CECT shows the Meckel diverticulum ➡ intussuscepting into a distal small bowel segment ➡.

MESENTERIC ADENITIS

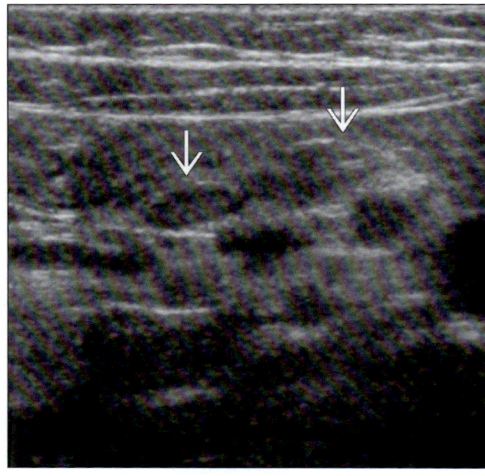

Transverse ultrasound shows numerous, enlarged, right lower quadrant lymph nodes ➔ anterior to the right iliac vessels.

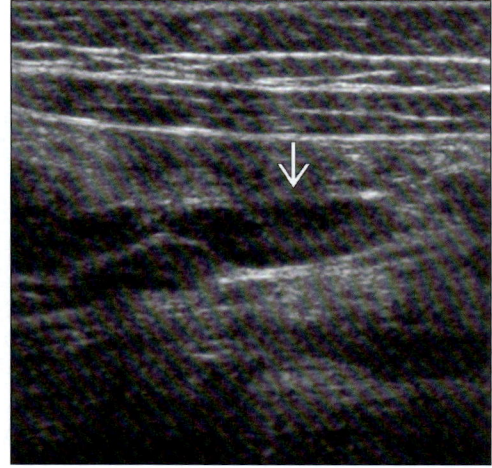

Oblique ultrasound shows an enlarged hypoechoic lymph node ➔ within the right lower quadrant.

TERMINOLOGY

Abbreviations and Synonyms
- Mesenteric lymphadenitis

Definitions
- Self-limiting benign inflammation of lymph nodes in the bowel mesentery
- Diagnosis of exclusion

IMAGING FINDINGS

General Features
- Best diagnostic clue
  - 3 or more clustered lymph nodes that measure ≥ 5 mm in short axis diameter
  - Normal appendix
- Location: Mesentery: Diffuse or focal right lower quadrant (RLQ)
- Size
  - ≥ 5 mm in size
  - Cluster of ≥ 3 enlarged lymph nodes
- Mimics appendicitis: Similar presenting signs & symptoms
- Most frequent alternative diagnosis at surgery for appendicitis

Radiographic Findings
- Radiography
  - Typically normal
  - May have focal bowel wall thickening &/or regional ileus RLQ

CT Findings
- Cluster of ≥ 3 lymph nodes in RLQ mesentery
  - ≥ 5 mm in short axis diameter
  - Most commonly anterior to right psoas muscle
  - 1/2 in small bowel mesentery
  - Appendicitis also associated with RLQ lymph nodal enlargement (40-82%)
    - Average: 9 mm
    - Average: 11 mm in mesenteric adenitis
    - More numerous lymph nodes throughout the mesentery in mesenteric adenitis
- Normal appendix
- Ileal wall thickening (up to 33%)
  - More common < 5 year olds

DDx: Right Lower Quadrant Pain

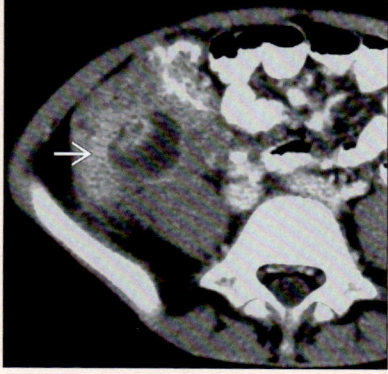

Appendicitis

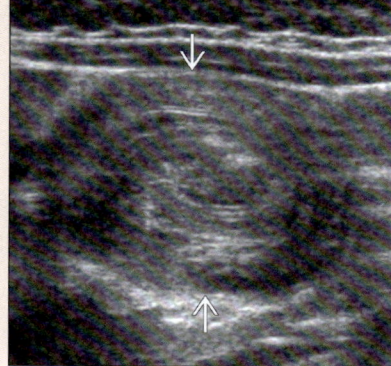

Intussusception

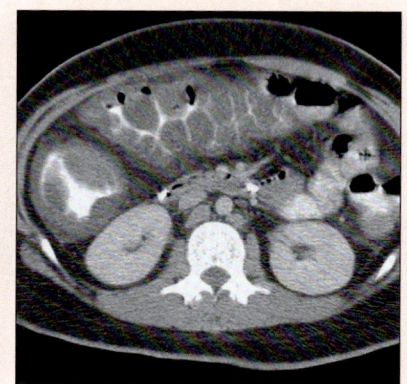

Pseudomembranous Colitis

MESENTERIC ADENITIS

Key Facts

Terminology
- Self-limiting benign inflammation of lymph nodes in the bowel mesentery

Imaging Findings
- 3 or more clustered lymph nodes that measure ≥ 5 mm in short axis diameter
- Normal appendix
- ≥ 5 mm in size
- Cluster of ≥ 3 enlarged lymph nodes
- Mimics appendicitis: Similar presenting signs & symptoms
- Appendicitis also associated with RLQ lymph nodal enlargement (40-82%)
- More numerous lymph nodes throughout the mesentery in mesenteric adenitis
- **Graded compression US**
  - Preferred due to radiation exposure of CECT

Top Differential Diagnoses
- Appendicitis
- Infectious Enteritis
- Crohn Disease
- Intussusception

Clinical Issues
- Most common signs/symptoms: Diffuse or focal RLQ tenderness & pain ± rebound
- Children & young adults

Diagnostic Checklist
- When appendix is normal & a cluster of 3 or more enlarged RLQ lymph nodes

---

  - ≥ 3 mm over at least 5 cm
- Colonic wall thickening (up to 18%)
  - More common < 5 year olds

Ultrasonographic Findings
- Graded compression procedure of choice of ultrasound (US)
- May have RLQ pain with compression
- Numerous RLQ or diffuse mesenteric enlarged lymph nodes (≥ 5 mm)
- Normal appendix (< 7 mm & compressible)
- ± Ileal or ileocolonic wall thickening
- No abscess or phlegmon

Imaging Recommendations
- Best imaging tool
  - Graded compression US
    - Preferred due to radiation exposure of CECT
    - Normal appendix can be seen
    - Numerous enlarged lymph nodes in the RLQ or diffusely in the small bowel mesentery

DIFFERENTIAL DIAGNOSIS

Appendicitis
- Dilated appendix
  - ≥ 7 mm in diameter
  - Noncompressible on US
- Abscesses or phlegmon common
- Also causes ileal or colonic wall thickening
- Less numerous lymph nodes

Infectious Enteritis
- Yersinia: Typically terminal ileum (TI)
- TB: Narrowed cecum & TI
- Others: Salmonella (colon), amebiasis, shigella (distal colon), CMV, herpes & fungal

Crohn Disease
- Entire GI tract
  - From mouth to anus, segmental & skip lesions
- Transmural, eccentric, sinuses, fissures, fistulas
- Aphthoid ulcers (mucosa) to deep ulcers (submucosa)
  - Cobblestoning: Longitudinal & transverse ulcers
- US & CECT
  - Mural thickening of cecum & TI
  - Average: 11 mm

Intussusception
- Invagination of one segment of bowel into another
- Idiopathic (typical)
- 2 months → 3 years
  - Younger & older patient consider pathologic lead point
- Mostly ileocolic
- US: Pseudokidney sign
  - Hypoechoic layers with echogenic internal mesenteric fat
- "Coiled spring" sign: Bowel invaginating into bowel
- Also can follow upper respiratory infection (URI) or gastroenteritis
- May have blood in stool, "currant jelly" stool

Pseudomembranous Colitis
- Usually related to antibiotic therapy & overgrowth of clostridium difficile bacteria
- Pancolitis (typical)
- CECT
  - "Accordion sign": Trapped enteric contrast between thickened large bowel folds
  - "Target sign": Intensely enhancing mucosa surrounded by diminished attenuation mural thickening

Ulcerative Colitis
- Chronic, idiopathic inflammatory disease that primarily involves the colorectal mucosa & submucosa
- Diffuse, continuous, concentric & symmetric wall thickening of the colon
- "Collar button" ulcers
- "Lead-pipe" colon
  - Shortened, rigid & symmetric narrowing of the lumen
- Backwash ileitis
  - Distal 5-25 cm of ileum is inflamed (10-40%)

MESENTERIC ADENITIS

Pelvic Inflammatory Disease
- Complex adnexal mass
- Sexually active girls
- Common bacteria
  - Neisseria gonorrhea
  - Chlamydia trachomatis
- Laboratory findings
  - Leukocytosis with a left shift
  - ↑ Erythrocyte sedimentation rate
- Cervical motion tenderness
- Lower abdominal &/or pelvic pain

Epiploic Appendagitis
- Acute
  - Infarction: Torsion or venous thrombosis
  - Inflammation of the epiploic appendages
- Hyperdense ring surrounding an internal hypodense (fat) nodule
- Left > right
- Older age group
  - Typically 2nd decade or later
- Symptoms usually spontaneously resolve by 1 week

PATHOLOGY

General Features
- Etiology
  - Yersinia enterocolitica (most common)
    - Yersinia infections: Meat, milk & water contamination
  - Yersinia pseudotuberculosis, Helicobacter jejuni, Salmonella, Shigella, Campylobacter, Staphylococcal
  - Viral: Coxsackievirus & adenovirus
  - Following Streptococcal URI
- Epidemiology: Most frequent alternative diagnosis to appendicitis
- Associated abnormalities: Streptococcal URI (25%)

Microscopic Features
- Hyperplastic cortical & paracortical pulp with dilated sinuses
- ↑ Plasma cells & immunoblasts

CLINICAL ISSUES

Presentation
- Most common signs/symptoms: Diffuse or focal RLQ tenderness & pain ± rebound
- Other signs/symptoms
  - Nausea, vomiting, diarrhea
  - Laboratory: Leukocytosis (50%)
  - During or following URI
    - Cervical adenopathy (20%)

Demographics
- Age
  - Children & young adults
  - Most common < 15 years old
  - Ileocolitis usually < 5 years old
- Gender: Yersinia more common in boys

Natural History & Prognosis
- Symptoms typically resolve by 2 weeks
- Diagnosis sometimes not made until after surgery

Treatment
- Conservative, self-limiting

DIAGNOSTIC CHECKLIST

Consider
- When appendix is normal & a cluster of 3 or more enlarged RLQ lymph nodes
- Diagnosis of exclusion

SELECTED REFERENCES

1. Lee CC et al: Mesenteric adenitis caused by Salmonella enterica serovar Enteritidis. J Formos Med Assoc. 103(6):463-6, 2004
2. Burke BB et al: Mesenteric Adenitis. eMedicine. Apr, 2003
3. Likitnukul S et al: Appendicitis-like syndrome owing to mesenteric adenitis caused by Salmonella typhi. Ann Trop Paediatr. 22(1):97-9, 2002
4. Macari M et al: Mesenteric adenitis: CT diagnosis of primary versus secondary causes, incidence, and clinical significance in pediatric and adult patients. AJR Am J Roentgenol. 178(4):853-8, 2002
5. Lamps LW et al: The role of Yersinia enterocolitica and Yersinia pseudotuberculosis in granulomatous appendicitis: a histologic and molecular study. Am J Surg Pathol. 25(4):508-15, 2001
6. Lee JH et al: The etiology and clinical characteristics of mesenteric adenitis in Korean adults. J Korean Med Sci. 12(2):105-10, 1997
7. Rao PM et al: CT diagnosis of mesenteric adenitis. Radiology. 202(1):145-9, 1997
8. Rao PM et al: Sensitivity and specificity of the individual CT signs of appendicitis: experience with 200 helical appendiceal CT examinations. J Comput Assist Tomogr. 21(5):686-92, 1997
9. Van Noyen R et al: Causative role of Yersinia and other enteric pathogens in the appendicular syndrome. Eur J Clin Microbiol Infect Dis. 10(9):735-41, 1991
10. Tertti R et al: Clinical manifestations of Yersinia pseudotuberculosis infection in children. Eur J Clin Microbiol Infect Dis. 8(7):587-91, 1989
11. Black RE et al: Yersinia enterocolitica. Infect Dis Clin North Am. 2(3):625-41, 1988
12. Puylaert JB: Mesenteric adenitis and acute terminal ileitis: US evaluation using graded compression. Radiology. 161(3):691-5, 1986
13. Marriott DJ et al: Yersinia enterocolitica infection in children. Med J Aust. 143(11):489-92, 1985
14. Saebo A: The Yersinia enterocolitica infection in acute abdominal surgery. A clinical study with a 5-year follow-up period. Ann Surg. 198(6):760-5, 1983
15. Constantinides CG et al: Suppurative mesenteric lymphadenitis in children. Case reports. S Afr Med J. 60(16):629-31, 1981
16. Schapers RF et al: Mesenteric lymphadenitis due to Yersinia enterocolitica. Virchows Arch A Pathol Anat Histol. 390(2):127-38, 1981
17. Kohl S: Yersinia enterocolitica infections in children. Pediatr Clin North Am. 26(2):433-43, 1979
18. Gilmore OJ et al: Appendicitis and mimicking conditions. A prospective study. Lancet. 2(7932):421-4, 1975

MESENTERIC ADENITIS

IMAGE GALLERY

Typical

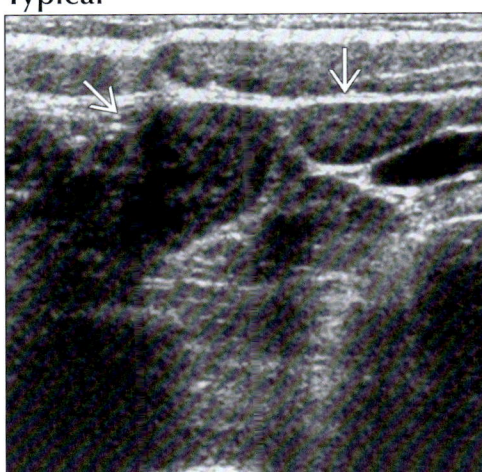 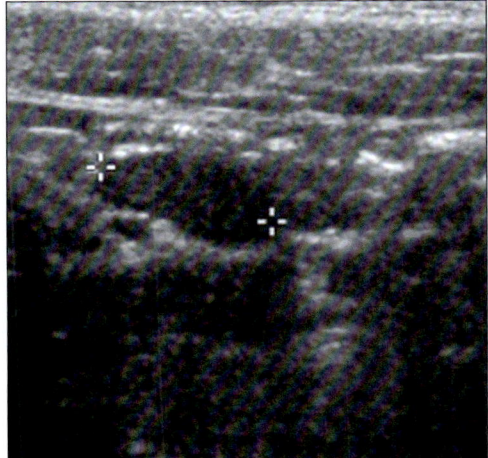

(Left) Transverse ultrasound shows numerous enlarged lymph nodes ➡ within the right lower quadrant. *(Right)* Transverse ultrasound in the same patient as previous image, shows an enlarged, right lower quadrant, hypodense mass, lymph node (cursors), measuring 1.7 cm.

Typical

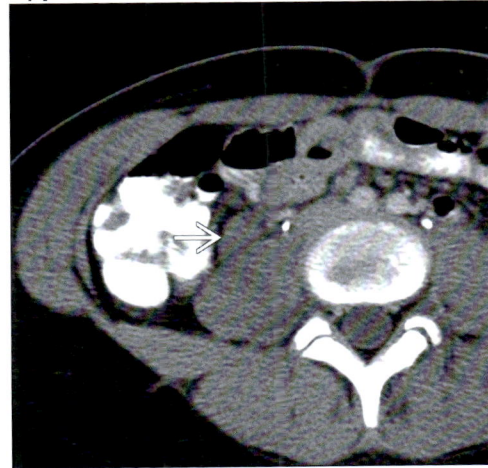 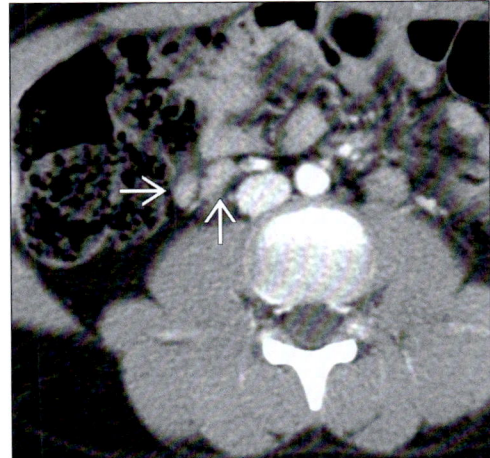

(Left) Axial CECT shows an enlarged lymph node ➡ within the right lower quadrant lateral to contrast in the right ureter and anterior to the right psoas muscle. *(Right)* Axial CECT shows enlarged lymph nodes ➡ lateral to the inferior vena cava and anterior to the right psoas muscle.

Typical

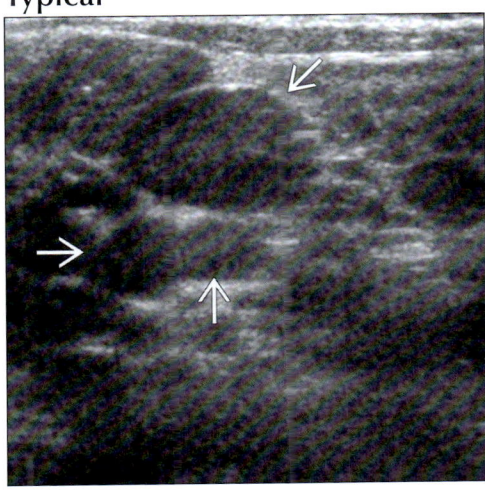 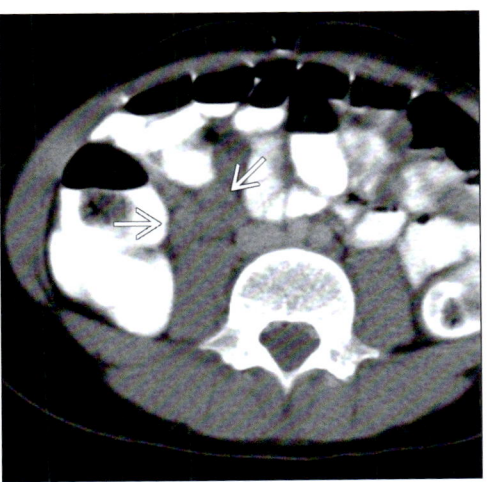

(Left) Transverse ultrasound shows numerous right lower quadrant lymph nodes ➡. *(Right)* Transverse CECT shows numerous, right lower quadrant, hypodense masses ➡, lymph nodes in presumed mesenteric adenitis.

SMALL BOWEL INTUSSUSCEPTION, PEDIATRIC

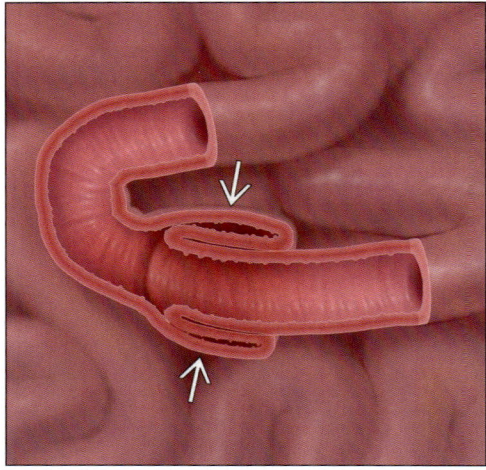

Graphic shows SB-SB intussusception. Note small bowel invaginating ➔ into more distal bowel in direction of peristalsis.

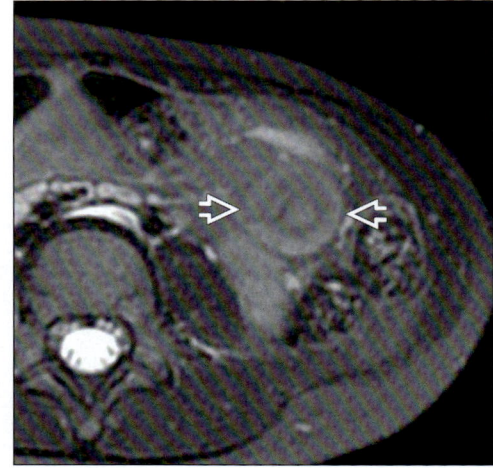

Axial T2WI MR shows a "target" sign of an intussusception ➔, in this case SB-SB.

TERMINOLOGY

Abbreviations and Synonyms
- Enteroenteric intussusceptions [small bowel-small bowel (SB-SB)]

Definitions
- Telescoping or invagination of proximal bowel (intussusceptum) into a contiguous bowel segment (intussuscipiens)

IMAGING FINDINGS

General Features
- Best diagnostic clue
  - "Target" sign
    - Internal mesenteric fat with vessels surrounded by higher attenuation bowel wall
  - "Layered" appearance
    - Alternating high attenuation (enhancing bowel wall) & lower attenuation (mesenteric fat)
- Location
  - Enteroenteric (SB-SB) uncommon
    - Ileoileal most common in adults
    - SB-SB: Up to 40% of intussusceptions in adults
  - Ileocolic (90%), ileoileocolic 2nd most common
- Size
  - SB-SB: Size smaller than ileocolic intussusceptions
  - Average: 2 cm
    - Length important in determining self-limiting verses surgical (< 3.5 cm)
- Morphology
  - SB-SB intussusceptions
    - Transient in children
    - Adults more likely pathologic lead point (benign > malignant)
    - Usually detected as an incidental finding when CECT performed for other reasons
  - Intussusceptions (ileocolic)
    - Children account for the majority of intussusceptions (90-95%)
    - Idiopathic (90-95%)
    - Possibly related to lymphoid hyperplasia

Fluoroscopic Findings
- Air Enema: Mostly normal

DDx: Other Causes of Intussusception

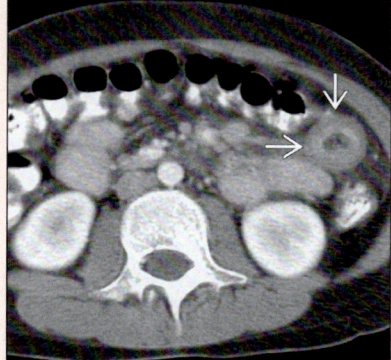

Henoch-Schönlein Purpura

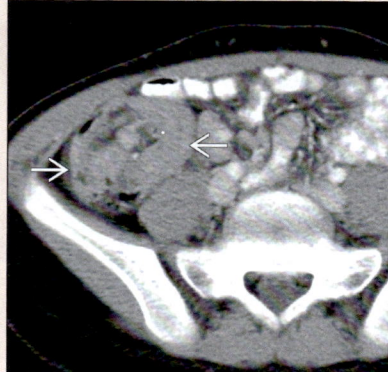

Ileocolic

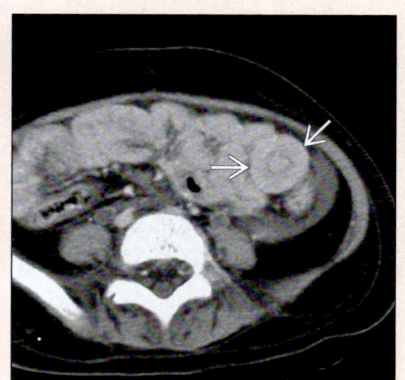

Pancreatitis

SMALL BOWEL INTUSSUSCEPTION, PEDIATRIC

Key Facts

Terminology
- Telescoping or invagination of proximal bowel (intussusceptum) into a contiguous bowel segment (intussuscipiens)

Imaging Findings
- Enteroenteric (SB-SB) uncommon
- Length important in determining self-limiting verses surgical (< 3.5 cm)
- "Target" or "bull's eye" sign
- "Pseudokidney" sign
- SB-SB: Smaller than ileocolic intussusceptions
- Small size, (-) wall edema, short segment, preserved wall motion

Top Differential Diagnoses
- Ileocolic Intussusception
- Meckel Diverticulum
- Henoch-Schönlein Purpura (HSP)
- Duplication Cyst
- Intraabdominal Inflammation
- Cystic Fibrosis
- Malabsorption Syndromes
- Lymphoma
- Non-Hodgkin lymphoma most common

Pathology
- Adults higher incidence of lead point than children
- SB-SB: Uncommon

Clinical Issues
- 2-20 years in children
- Average age 11 years
- Gender: M > F

CT Findings
- Intussusceptions: (General)
  - "Target" sign: Early
    - Mass with internal mesenteric fat & blood vessels
  - Crescent of gas or fluid may insinuate between intussusceptum and intussuscipiens
  - Rim of enteric contrast between the intussusceptum & intussuscipiens
  - Long axis image, sausage shaped mass (later stage)
    - "Layered" appearance
    - Alternating bands of high (enhancing bowel wall) & low (mesenteric fat & blood vessels) attenuation
  - Reniform mass
    - Bowel wall thickening or edema
  - Small bowel obstruction and ascites: Uncommon
    - More frequent in surgical cases

Ultrasonographic Findings
- Intussusceptions: (General)
  - "Target" or "bull's eye" sign
    - Alternating hypoechoic & hyperechoic concentric rings
    - Hypoechoic outer edematous wall of intussuscipiens
    - Hyperechoic middle ring of mesenteric fat
    - Hypoechoic inner ring of the intussusceptum
  - "Pseudokidney" sign
    - Hypoechoic bowel segment on each side of echogenic central mesenteric fat
  - SB-SB: Smaller than ileocolic intussusceptions
    - Small size, (-) wall edema, short segment, preserved wall motion

Imaging Recommendations
- Best imaging tool: Ultrasound (US) or CECT performed for abdominal pain or for some other indication

DIFFERENTIAL DIAGNOSIS

Ileocolic Intussusception
- 2 months → 3 year olds
- Larger than enteroenteric intussusceptions
- Idiopathic, ileocolic (90%)
- Intermittent abdominal pain, vomiting or diarrhea
- Currant jelly stool
- US for diagnosis (no radiation)
- Air contrast enema for diagnosis & therapy (barium contrast enema studies also)

Meckel Diverticulum
- Remnant of omphalomesenteric duct
- Rule of 2s
  - 2% of population, 2 feet from ileocecal valve, presents < 2 years old, length 2 inches
- 15% contain gastric mucosa
- Complications (20%): Obstruction, bleeding, perforation & intussusception
- Mass with fluid attenuation surrounded by collar of soft tissue
- Tc-99m pertechnetate: For diagnosis in those containing gastric mucosa
- Mostly asymptomatic

Henoch-Schönlein Purpura (HSP)
- Systemic hypersensitivity reaction with a small vessel vasculitis
- Purpuric rash on legs or extensor surface of arms
- Abdominal pain &/or bloody diarrhea may precede rash
- Mural bleed predisposes to intussusceptions
- Complications: Bowel infarction, perforation or intussusceptions (3%)

Duplication Cyst
- Most common terminal ileum & ileocecal area
- Contain both mucosa & muscular layers ("double wall" sign on US)
- Complication: Bleeding, intussusception & volvulus

Intraabdominal Inflammation
- Any diffuse abdominal process that causes inflammation of the bowel wall
  - Diverticulitis, gastroenteritis, pancreatitis, etc.

SMALL BOWEL INTUSSUSCEPTION, PEDIATRIC

Cystic Fibrosis
- Autosomal recessive, ↑ Caucasian
- 1% incidence of intussusception
- Meconium ileus
- Distal intestinal obstruction syndrome = meconium ileus equivalent

Malabsorption Syndromes
- Celiac disease ↑ incidence
  - Nontropical sprue, gluten enteropathy
  - Diarrhea (hallmark of disease): 90%
  - Reversal of jejunum & ileal fold pattern

Lymphoma
- Non-Hodgkin lymphoma most common
- Must consider in children > typical age for ileocolic intussusceptions
- Aneurysmal dilation of bowel
- Nodular, polypoid mucosa, infiltrating mass with adenopathy

PATHOLOGY

General Features
- Etiology
  - Abnormal peristalsis leading to invagination of bowel segment with mesenteric fat into a contiguous bowel segment
  - Most adult intussusceptions are transient, non-obstructing & no lead point
    - Adults higher incidence of lead point than children
  - Most children intussusceptions are ileocolic & idiopathic
    - SB-SB: Uncommon, self-limiting, idiopathic & no lead point
  - Meckel diverticulum, Henoch-Schönlein purpura, duplication cyst, inflammatory process, malabsorption syndromes, cystic fibrosis, adhesions, polyps, intramural hematoma, foreign body, lipoma, neurofibroma
  - Post-operative abdominal surgery
    - Small bowel more common
  - Gastrojejunal enteric tubes
- Epidemiology
  - SB-SB: Uncommon
  - Intussusception (general)
    - Children > > adults
    - Idiopathic: 85-90% (most commonly lymphoid hyperplasia)
    - Children: Ileocolic & ileoileocolic comprise 90% of intussusceptions

Gross Pathologic & Surgical Features
- 3 layers
  - Intussuscipiens: Receiving the intussusception (outer loop)
  - Intussusceptum: 2 layers, entering & exiting bowel segment
- If lead point specific pathology for that diagnosis

CLINICAL ISSUES

Presentation
- Most common signs/symptoms
  - Most commonly asymptomatic, > 1/2
  - Irritability, abdominal distension, pain, vomiting
- Other signs/symptoms: Intermittent abdominal pain

Demographics
- Age
  - 2-20 years in children
    - Average age 11 years
- Gender: M > F

Natural History & Prognosis
- SB-SB
  - Transient
  - Majority resolve
  - Recurrent, multiple or persistent
    - Further evaluation
    - Repeat US to assure resolution
    - Small bowel follow through or enteroclysis to evaluate for lead point
    - Surgical referral

Treatment
- SB-SB
  - Conservative
  - Usually resolve without treatment

SELECTED REFERENCES

1. Munden MM et al: Sonography of Pediatric Small-Bowel Intussusception: Differentiating Surgical from Nonsurgical Cases. AJR. 188(1):275-79, 2007
2. Kim JH: US features of transient small bowel intussusception in pediatric patients. Korean J Radiol. 5(3):178-84, 2004
3. Sandrasegaran K et al: Proximal small bowel intussusceptions in adults: CT appearance and clinical significance. Abdom Imaging. 29(6):653-7, 2004
4. Lvoff N et al: Distinguishing features of self-limiting adult small-bowel intussusception identified at CT. Radiology. 227(1):68-72, 2003
5. Strouse PJ et al: Transient small-bowel intussusception in children on CT. Pediatr Radiol. 33(5):316-20, 2003
6. Gayer G et al: Pictorial review: adult intussusception--a CT diagnosis. Br J Radiol. 75(890):185-90, 2002
7. Harris JP et al: Sonographic diagnosis of multiple small-bowel intussusceptions in Peutz-Jeghers syndrome: a case report. Pediatr Radiol. 32(9):681-3, 2002
8. Ko SF et al: Small bowel intussusception in symptomatic pediatric patients: experiences with 19 surgically proven cases. World J Surg. 26(4):438-43, 2002
9. Hughes UM et al: Further report of small-bowel intussusceptions related to gastrojejunostomy tubes. Pediatr Radiol. 30(9):614-7, 2000
10. Kornecki A et al: Spontaneous reduction of intussusception: clinical spectrum, management and outcome. Pediatr Radiol. 30(1):58-63, 2000
11. Mushtaq N et al: Small bowel intussusception in celiac disease. J Pediatr Surg. 34(12):1833-5, 1999
12. Catalano O: Transient small bowel intussusception: CT findings in adults. Br J Radiol. 70(836):805-8, 1997
13. Merine D et al: Enteroenteric intussusception: CT findings in nine patients. AJR Am J Roentgenol. 148(6):1129-32, 1987

SMALL BOWEL INTUSSUSCEPTION, PEDIATRIC

IMAGE GALLERY

Typical

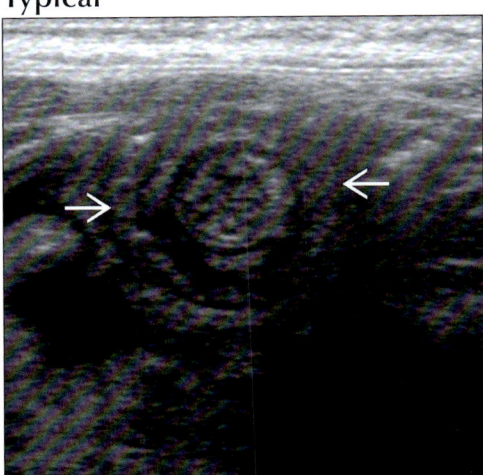
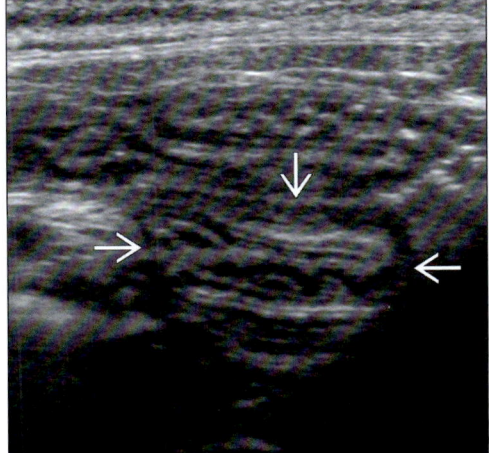

(Left) Axial ultrasound shows "bull's eye" sign of an intussusception ➡, small bowel. *(Right)* Longitudinal ultrasound in the same patient shows "pseudokidney" or hay fork sign ➡ of a small bowel intussusception that measured 1.5 cm in length. Patient was imaged 30 minutes later and the intussusception resolved.

Typical

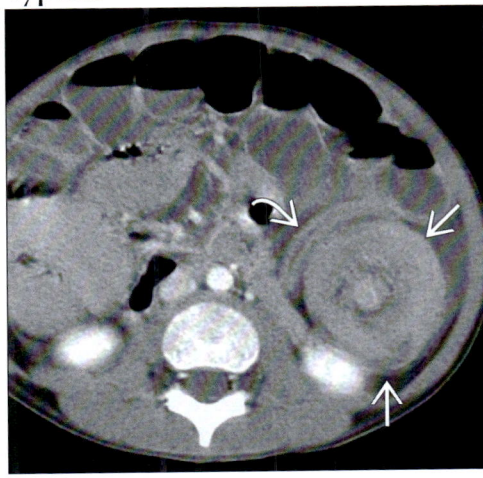
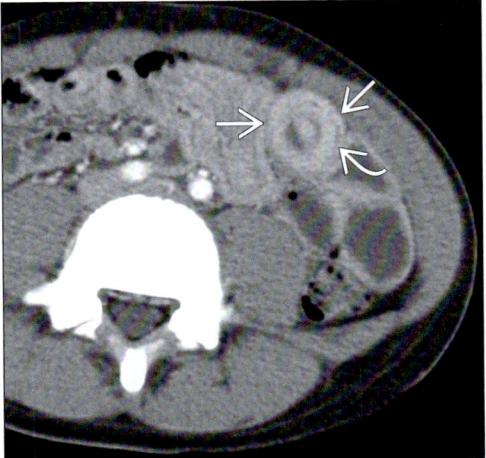

(Left) Axial CECT shows a pathologic lead point (lymphoma) in this SB-SB intussusception ➡ with a layered coiled-spring appearance ➡ & small bowel obstruction. The SB-SB intussusception measured > 3.5 cm in length. *(Right)* Axial CECT shows a typical small sized, SB-SB intussusception ➡, in this patient with Crohn disease. Notice the small amount of fluid ➡ trapped between the layered appearance of the intussusception.

Typical

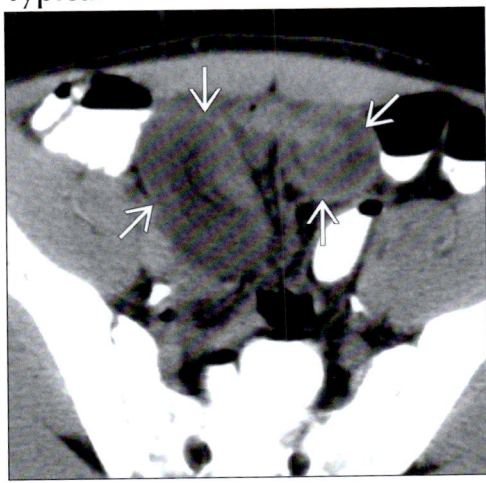
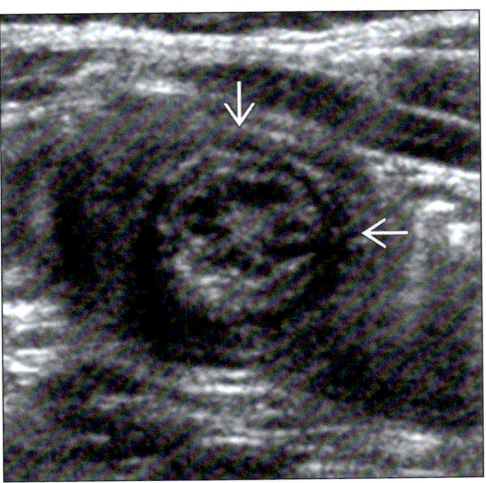

(Left) Axial CECT shows a large (> 3.5 cm) SB-SB intussusception ➡, on more cephalad images the 2 masses are contiguous. Notice fluid within the intussusception. A large Meckel diverticulum was found at surgery. *(Right)* Axial ultrasound shows a small SB-SB intussusception ➡. This resolved without treatment.

UTERINE AVM

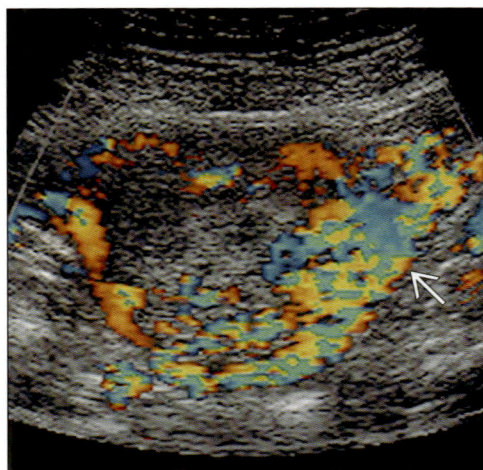

Transverse color Doppler ultrasound of uterine AVM after multiple D&Cs demonstrates marked hypervascularity of uterus with aliasing due to turbulent flow ➔.

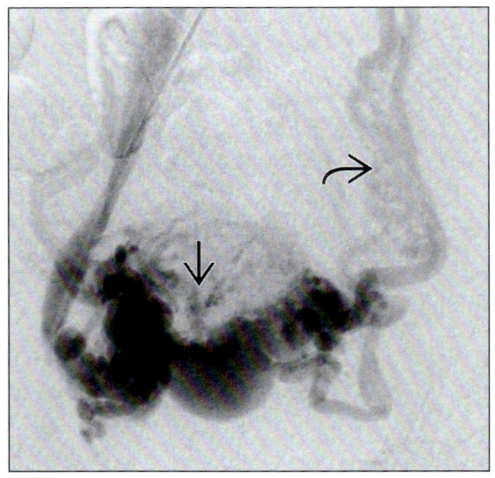

Anteroposterior selective uterine artery arteriogram reveals uterine AVM ➔ with early draining veins ➔.

TERMINOLOGY

Abbreviations and Synonyms
- Uterine arteriovenous malformation (AVM)
- Uterine arteriovenous (AV) fistula

Definitions
- Multiple small AV fistulas between intramural arterial branches & myometrial venous plexus without intervening capillary network

IMAGING FINDINGS

General Features
- Best diagnostic clue
  - US: Serpiginous anechoic structures within myometrium demonstrate high-velocity systolic & diastolic flow on color Doppler
  - Low-resistance, high-velocity flow patterns on Doppler US
  - MR: Areas of flow-related signal void in myometrium
- Size: Prominent parametrial vessels

MR Findings
- T2WI (SE/FSE) and T1WI (SE)
  - Multiple serpiginous, flow-related signal voids within lesion
  - Involved portion appears bulky
  - Distortion of uterine zonal anatomy on T2WI
- 2D or 3D spoiled-gradient echo: Typical flow-related signal voids often absent
- CEMR/MRA
  - Findings parallel angiography

Ultrasonographic Findings
- Grayscale Ultrasound
  - Variable appearance, may be nonspecific
  - Echogenic clot in endometrial cavity
  - Multiple tubular anechoic spaces within myometrium resulting in "spongy" myometrial echotexture
  - Subtle myometrial inhomogeneity
  - Focal intramural mass resembling leiomyoma or endometrial mass mimicking endometrial polyp (uncommon findings)
- Color Doppler
  - Critical for making diagnosis

DDx: Lesions Mimicking Uterine AVM

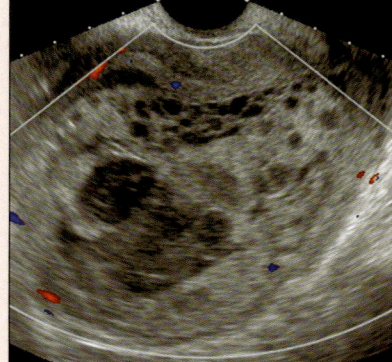

Gestational Trophoblastic Disease

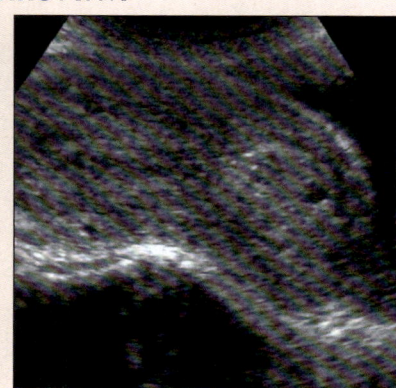

Retained Products of Conception

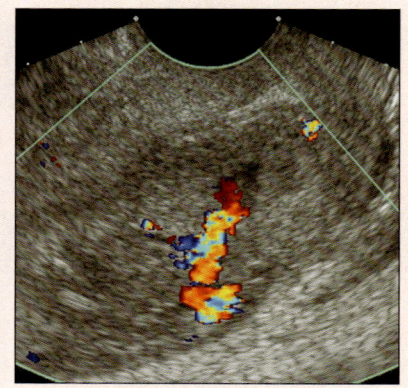

Retained Products of Conception

UTERINE AVM

Key Facts

Terminology
- Uterine arteriovenous malformation (AVM)
- Multiple small AV fistulas between intramural arterial branches & myometrial venous plexus without intervening capillary network

Imaging Findings
- MR: Areas of flow-related signal void in myometrium
- Apparent flow reversal of juxtaposed reds & blues indicating vessels of varying orientation with different flow directions on color Doppler
- Color aliasing with different flow velocities due to turbulence on color Doppler
- Pseudoaneurysms demonstrate swirling arterial flow on color Doppler
- Spectral Doppler:
- Low resistance (RI: 0.20-0.55; PI: 0.3-0.6)
- High PSV: > 60 cm/sec, may be lower: 20-100 cm/sec

Top Differential Diagnoses
- Gestational Trophoblastic Disease (GTD)
- Retained Products of Conception (RPC)
- Pelvic Varicosities

Pathology
- Acquired (traumatic): Previous dilatation & curettage (D&C) for spontaneous/therapeutic abortion, GTD or endometrial carcinoma; uterine surgery; cervical AVM associated with diethylstilbestrol exposure; no nidus present

Clinical Issues
- Negative serum β-hCG
- Avoid diagnostic D&C: May precipitate massive hemorrhage

---

  o Apparent flow reversal of juxtaposed reds & blues indicating vessels of varying orientation with different flow directions on color Doppler
  o Color aliasing with different flow velocities due to turbulence on color Doppler
  o Pseudoaneurysms demonstrate swirling arterial flow on color Doppler
- Spectral Doppler:
  o Low resistance (RI: 0.20-0.55; PI: 0.3-0.6)
  o High PSV: > 60 cm/sec, may be lower: 20-100 cm/sec
  o Low pulsatility arterial spectral waveform
  o Pulsatile high-velocity venous waveform, little variation in systolic-diastolic velocities

Angiographic Findings
- Conventional
  o Standard of reference
  o Complex tangle of vessels with enlarged feeding arteries
  o Early venous drainage during arterial phase
  o Stasis of contrast medium within abnormal vasculature
  o Acquired: Single or bilateral feeding uterine arteries

Imaging Recommendations
- Best imaging tool
  o Doppler US; also preferred for follow-up
  o MRI with contrast-enhanced T1WI/MRA to confirm diagnosis & determine disease extent
  o Doppler US with MR imaging can replace diagnostic angiography
  o Angiography to delineate feeding arteries & draining veins for treatment planning

DIFFERENTIAL DIAGNOSIS

Gestational Trophoblastic Disease (GTD)
- Spectrum of trophoblastic disorders
  o Molar pregnancy
  o Invasive mole
  o Choriocarcinoma
  o Placenta-site trophoblastic tumor
- Echogenic mass filling endometrial cavity with multiple cystic spaces (hydropic villi)
- Markedly elevated β-hCG levels
- Most common form is complete hydatidiform mole
  o Occurs in 1:1000 pregnancies in North America
- Partial molar pregnancy contains anomalous (triploid) fetal tissue typically growth retarded with fetal demise
- Associated with bilateral theca-luteal cysts

Retained Products of Conception (RPC)
- Echogenic mass within endometrial cavity
- Positive β-hCG suggests retained products
- False positives occur with echogenic clot
- Areas of strong color Doppler signs may be due to focal percreta

Pelvic Varicosities
- Prominent parametrial vessels, normal venous spectral waveforms on color Doppler sonography
- Associated with multiparous women

PATHOLOGY

General Features
- General path comments
  o Tangles of vessels of different sizes, histologic characteristics of both arteries & veins, no intervening capillary network
  o Acquired AVM: Single or bilateral feeding uterine arteries without supply from extrauterine arteries
  o Congenital AVM: Multiple feeding arteries & draining veins
- Etiology
  o Incidence rare; most are acquired
  o Acquired (traumatic): Previous dilatation & curettage (D&C) for spontaneous/therapeutic abortion, GTD or endometrial carcinoma; uterine surgery; cervical AVM associated with diethylstilbestrol exposure; no nidus present
  o Congenital
    ▪ Anomalous differentiation in primitive capillary plexus

UTERINE AVM

- Usually multiple; nidus present

Gross Pathologic & Surgical Features
- Markedly dilated & tortuous uterine arteries & veins within area of AVM

CLINICAL ISSUES

Presentation
- Most common signs/symptoms: Extensive vaginal bleeding
- Other signs/symptoms
  - Menorrhagia
  - Menometrorrhagia
    - Blood transfusion required in 30% of cases
- Clinical Profile: Multiple D&Cs
- Lab data
  - Negative serum β-hCG
  - Falling HCT if significant bleeding

Demographics
- Gender: Female

Natural History & Prognosis
- May cause life-threatening vaginal bleeding
- Preservation of fertility after embolization of both uterine arteries

Treatment
- Usually conservative
  - Transcatheter arterial embolization in women desiring to maintain fertility
  - Successful pregnancies have been reported post-embolization
- Hysterectomy
- Avoid diagnostic D&C: May precipitate massive hemorrhage

DIAGNOSTIC CHECKLIST

Image Interpretation Pearls
- Always use color Doppler to assess uterine abnormalities in patient with vaginal bleeding
- Adnexal varices in multiparous patients have only venous waveforms

SELECTED REFERENCES

1. Delotte J et al: Pregnancy after embolization therapy for uterine arteriovenous malformation. Fertil Steril. 85(1):228, 2006
2. Grivell RM et al: Uterine arteriovenous malformations: a review of the current literature. Obstet Gynecol Surv. 60(11):761-7, 2005
3. Chan CC et al: Treating a recurrent uterine arteriovenous malformation with uterine artery embolization. A case report. J Reprod Med. 48(11):905-7, 2003
4. Ghai S et al: Efficacy of embolization in traumatic uterine vascular malformations. J Vasc Interv Radiol. 14(11):1401-8, 2003
5. Gopal M et al: Embolization of a uterine arteriovenous malformation followed by a twin pregnancy. Obstet Gynecol. 102(4):696-8, 2003
6. Kelly SM et al: Arteriovenous malformation of the uterus associated with secondary postpartum hemorrhage. Ultrasound Obstet Gynecol. 21(6):602-5, 2003
7. Kido A et al: Retained products of conception masquerading as acquired arteriovenous malformation. J Comput Assist Tomogr. 27(1):88-92, 2003
8. Timmerman D et al: Color Doppler imaging is a valuable tool for the diagnosis and management of uterine vascular malformations. Ultrasound Obstet Gynecol. 21(6):570-7, 2003
9. Kwon JH et al: Obstetric iatrogenic arterial injuries of the uterus: diagnosis with US and treatment with transcatheter arterial embolization. Radiographics. 22(1):35-46, 2002
10. Nasu K et al: Uterine arteriovenous malformation: ultrasonographic, magnetic resonance and radiological findings. Gynecol Obstet Invest. 53(3):191-4, 2002
11. Polat P et al: Color Doppler US in the evaluation of uterine vascular abnormalities. Radiographics. 22(1):47-53, 2002
12. Van den Bosch T et al: Color Doppler and gray-scale ultrasound evaluation of the postpartum uterus. Ultrasound Obstet Gynecol. 20(6):586-91, 2002
13. Timmerman D et al: Vascular malformations in the uterus: ultrasonographic diagnosis and conservative management. Eur J Obstet Gynecol Reprod Biol. 92(1):171-8, 2000
14. Valenzano M et al: Color Doppler sonography of uterine arteriovenous malformation. J Clin Ultrasound. 28(3):146-9, 2000
15. Huang MW et al: Uterine arteriovenous malformations: gray-scale and Doppler US features with MR imaging correlation. Radiology. 206(1):115-23, 1998
16. Arredondo-Soberon F et al: Uterine arteriovenous malformation in a patient with recurrent pregnancy loss and a bicornuate uterus. A case report. J Reprod Med. 42(4):239-43, 1997
17. Mungen E et al: Color Doppler sonographic features of uterine arteriovenous malformations: report of two cases. Ultrasound Obstet Gynecol. 10(3):215-9, 1997
18. Manolitsas T et al: Uterine arteriovenous malformation--a rare cause of uterine haemorrhage. Aust N Z J Obstet Gynaecol. 34(2):197-9, 1994
19. Jain KA et al: Gynecologic vascular abnormalities: diagnosis with Doppler US. Radiology. 178(2):549-51, 1991

UTERINE AVM

IMAGE GALLERY

Typical

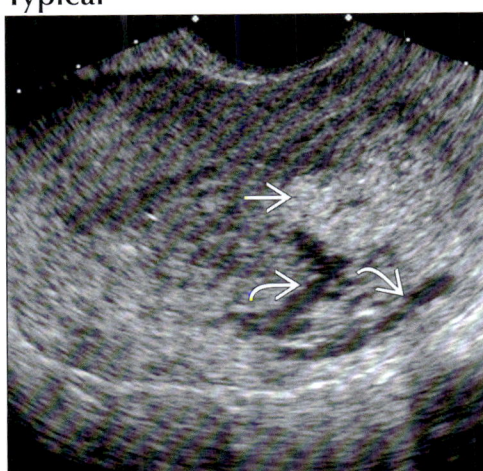
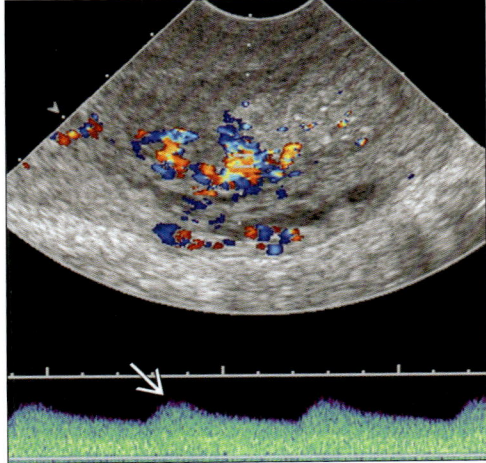

(Left) Sagittal endovaginal sonogram of uterine AVM demonstrates echogenic clot in endometrial cavity ➡ as well as hypoechoic dilated vessels posteriorly within myometrium ➡. (Right) Sagittal endovaginal color Doppler sonogram of same patient as left reveals typical high systolic & high diastolic flow of AVM ➡.

Typical

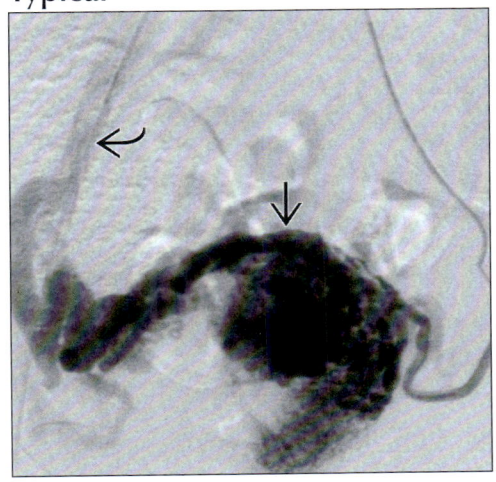
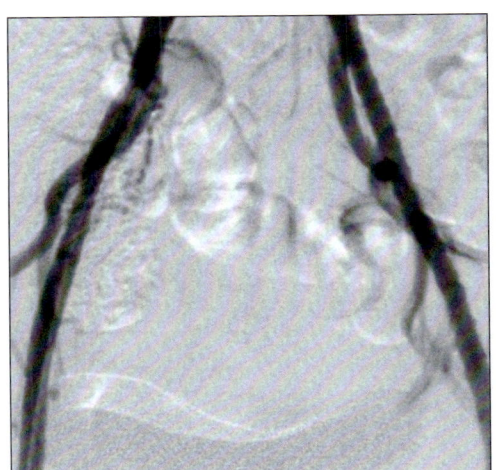

(Left) Anteroposterior selective left uterine artery arteriography of uterine AVM demonstrates marked uterine hypervascularity ➡ with early draining veins ➡. (Right) Anteroposterior arteriography post-embolization in same patient as left reveals complete occlusion of AVM.

Variant

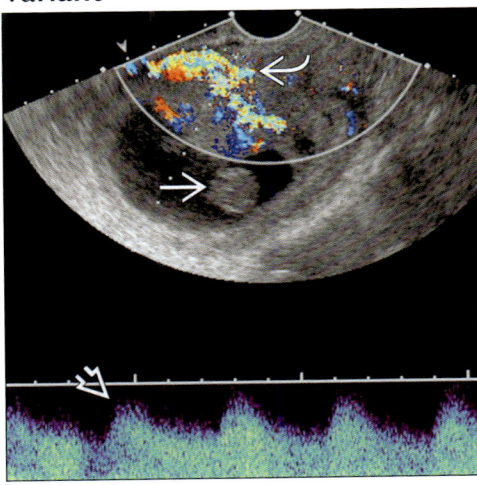
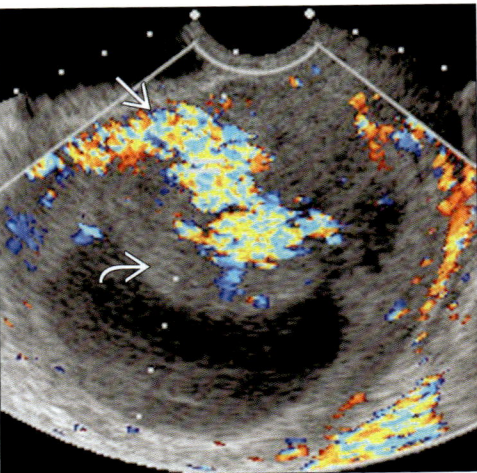

(Left) Sagittal endovaginal sonogram with color Doppler of retroplacental AVM during pregnancy reveals fetal pole ➡, uterine hypervascularity ➡, and spectral Doppler tracing of high-flow AVM ➡. (Right) Sagittal endovaginal color Doppler sonogram in same patient as left reveals retroplacental location of AVM ➡. (➡ = placenta).

OVARIAN TORSION

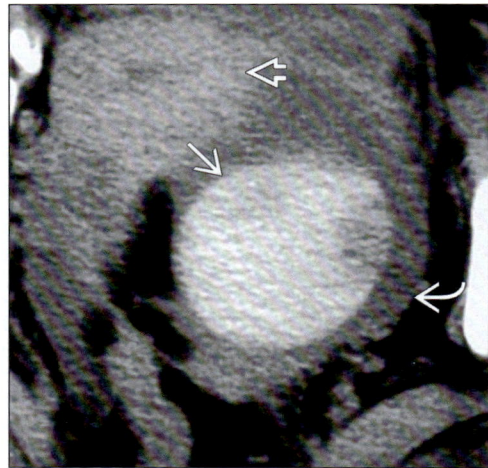
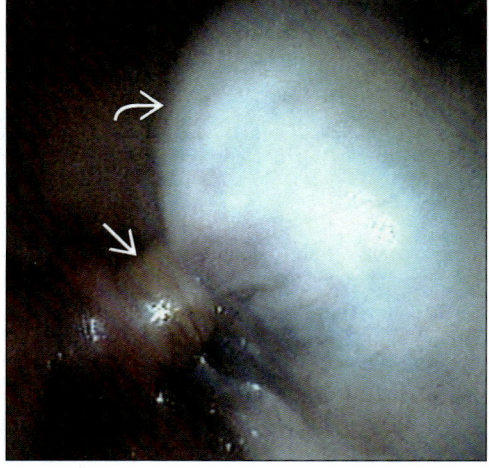

Axial NECT of acute ovarian torsion due to hemorrhagic cyst. Note high attenuation clot ➡ in left adnexal mass with associated hemoperitoneum ⇗; ⇨ = uterus.

Laparoscopic image in same patient as left demonstrates twisted ovarian pedicle ➡ and large bluish hemorrhagic cyst ⇨.

TERMINOLOGY

Definitions
- Rotation of ovary on its vascular pedicle resulting in venous congestion & ultimately infarction of ovary

IMAGING FINDINGS

General Features
- Best diagnostic clue
  - Enlarged echogenic ovary with prominent peripheral follicles & absent venous flow on endovaginal color Doppler sonography
  - Twisted vascular pedicle sign
- Location: Torsed ovary/tube often located midline cranial or anterior to uterine fundus
- Size: Enlarged ovary; normal size 10 cm³ volume

CT Findings
- CECT
  - Hemorrhagic fallopian tube/vascular pedicle > 50 HU
  - Hemorrhagic cyst > 50 HU

MR Findings
- T1WI
  - Hyperintense fallopian tube/vascular pedicle (hemorrhage)
  - Hyperintense hemorrhagic cyst content or wall in adults
  - ± Enhancing ovary/mass
- T2WI
  - Hyperintense hemorrhagic fallopian tube/vascular pedicle
  - Concentric or eccentric (edematous ovarian tissue) along cyst wall
  - ± Enhancing ovary/mass

Ultrasonographic Findings
- Grayscale Ultrasound
  - Most common finding: Enlarged, echogenic, edematous, ovarian stroma
  - Multiple small peripheral fluid-filled follicles displaced due to edematous stroma and/or mass
  - Pelvic free fluid; low-level echoes indicates hemoperitoneum
  - Twisted vascular pedicle (broad ligament, fallopian tube, ovarian vessels)

DDx: Lesions Mimicking Ovarian Torsion

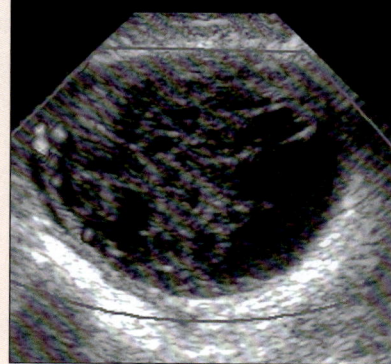
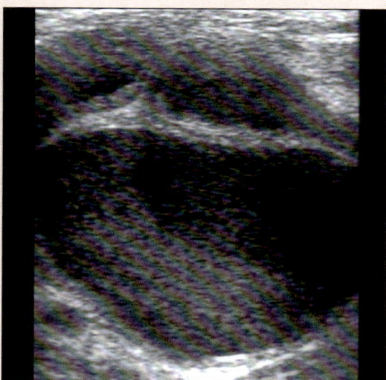
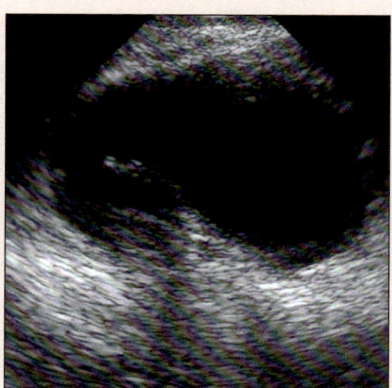

Hemorrhagic Cyst — *Tubo-Ovarian Abscess* — *Hydrosalpinx*

OVARIAN TORSION

Key Facts

Terminology
- Rotation of ovary on its vascular pedicle resulting in venous congestion & ultimately infarction of ovary

Imaging Findings
- Enlarged echogenic ovary with prominent peripheral follicles & absent venous flow on endovaginal color Doppler sonography
- Twisted vascular pedicle sign
- Endovaginal US with both grayscale & color Doppler is best initial imaging examination
- CT/MR more likely to show torsed pedicle, high attenuation (> 35 HU) hemorrhage within ovary

Top Differential Diagnoses
- Ruptured Functional Hemorrhagic Cyst
- Pelvic Inflammatory Disease (PID)
- Hydrosalpinx
- Ruptured Tubal Ectopic

Pathology
- Most common risk factor: Prior pelvic or abdominal surgery
- Earliest pathologic changes include edema, stromal & microscopic hemorrhage within ovary

Clinical Issues
- Severe unremitting acute pelvic pain is most common symptom
- Adnexal mass may or may not be palpable
- Surgical untwisting in non-infarcted adnexa either with laparoscopy or open surgery

Diagnostic Checklist
- Consider ruptured ectopic in pregnant patient

- Round hyperechoic structure, multiple hypoechoic concentric stripes ("target sign"): Twisted vascular pedicle
- Beaked structure: Twisted fallopian tube
- Heterogeneous tubular structure: Edematous fallopian tube
- Coiled twisted pedicle ("whirlpool sign")
  - Lack of vascularity more common with nonviable ovary
- Color Doppler
  - Early changes with spectral Doppler include absence of venous flow
  - Due to dual arterial blood supply to ovary, arterial flow (with elevated resistive index) may be preserved in early torsion
  - Late torsion with infarcted ovary: Absent venous & arterial flow

Imaging Recommendations
- Best imaging tool
  - Endovaginal US with both grayscale & color Doppler is best initial imaging examination
  - CT/MR more likely to show torsed pedicle, high attenuation (> 35 HU) hemorrhage within ovary

DIFFERENTIAL DIAGNOSIS

Ruptured Functional Hemorrhagic Cyst
- Collapsing hemorrhagic cyst in normal-sized ovary
- Clotted blood in pelvis
- Endovaginal sonography
  - "Fish net" sign of fibrinous strands
  - Retracting clot sign
  - Fluid-fluid level
  - Diffuse low-level echoes (ground glass appearance)
- Endovaginal grayscale color Doppler: Avascular; no internal flow

Pelvic Inflammatory Disease (PID)
- Uniformly thickened & dilated fallopian tubes
- Pyosalpinx
- Contains low-level echoes or fluid-filled level
- ± Enlarged ovaries 2° oophoritis
  - Normal flow pattern on color Doppler
- ± Tubo-ovarian abscess
  - Complex cystic/solid masses
- "Indefinite uterus sign" with obscuration of posterior margin of myometrium by inflammation

Hydrosalpinx
- Dilated fallopian tube with bulbous ampullary segment
- May contain low-level echoes

Ruptured Tubal Ectopic
- Positive β-hCG
- No evidence of intrauterine pregnancy on endovaginal sonography
- Extra-ovarian echogenic mass
- "Adnexal ring sign": Echogenic ring with thick (> 4 mm) wall
- Visualization of embryo or yolk sac within tubal gestational sac
- Free fluid in pelvis & Morrison pouch from hemoperitoneum

PATHOLOGY

General Features
- General path comments
  - Ovarian torsion, tubal torsion (most often both)
  - Torsed ovary may/may not show vascularity
  - Swollen hemorrhagic adnexa ± infarction
  - Isolated torsed fallopian tube possible
  - Calcified mass in chronic cases
- Etiology
  - In adults, 50-80% have associated ovarian tumors, usually benign
    - Dermoid, paraovarian cysts most common causes
  - Infants & children rarely have associated mass
    - Hypermobility due to long mesosalpinx
  - Sequential venous, lymphatic, & arterial obstruction
  - Most common risk factor: Prior pelvic or abdominal surgery

OVARIAN TORSION

  - Ovarian hyperstimulation syndrome in 9% of patients
- Epidemiology
  - Most common in first three decades
  - More common during pregnancy
  - 2.7% of all gynecologic emergencies
  - 47% of patients have no known risk factors

Gross Pathologic & Surgical Features
- Earliest pathologic changes include edema, stromal & microscopic hemorrhage within ovary
- Prominent fluid-filled peripheral follicles
- Late findings include hemorrhagic infarction
  - Cystic spaces filled with blood & associated hemoperitoneum
- Surgical findings vary due to degree of torsion & ovarian ischemia
  - May or may not have associated ovarian mass
    - Functional cyst, dermoid, etc.
    - Associated masses nearly always benign
- Pathology may reveal torsion of "normal ovary" & adnexal structures or underlying benign mass in < 1% of cases
  - Functional cyst, dermoid or cystadenoma

CLINICAL ISSUES

Presentation
- Most common signs/symptoms
  - Severe unremitting acute pelvic pain is most common symptom
  - Adnexal mass may or may not be palpable
  - Vomiting
  - Fever if ovary infarcted

Demographics
- Age: First three decades
- Gender: Female

Natural History & Prognosis
- Spontaneous detorsion common, can recur
- Early diagnosis prevents irreversible damage

Treatment
- Surgical untwisting in non-infarcted adnexa either with laparoscopy or open surgery
  - Preservation of ovary possible if normal blood flow restored after de-torsing ovary
- Salpingo-oophorectomy in infarcted ovary
- Adnexal sparing surgery in 20%

DIAGNOSTIC CHECKLIST

Consider
- Consider ruptured ectopic in pregnant patient
- Enlarged ovary due to oophoritis in PID has normal venous flow

Image Interpretation Pearls
- Absent venous flow in enlarged echogenic ovary with prominent peripheral follicles is earliest reliable sign

SELECTED REFERENCES

1. Breech LL et al: Adnexal torsion in pediatric and adolescent girls. Curr Opin Obstet Gynecol. 17(5):483-9, 2005
2. Cass DL: Ovarian torsion. Semin Pediatr Surg. 14(2):86-92, 2005
3. Ogburn T et al: Adnexal torsion: experience at a single university center. J Reprod Med. 50(8):591-4, 2005
4. Schultz KA et al: Pediatric ovarian tumors: a review of 67 cases. Pediatr Blood Cancer. 44(2):167-73, 2005
5. White M et al: Ovarian torsion: 10-year perspective. Emerg Med Australas. 17(3):231-7, 2005
6. Gittleman AM et al: Ovarian torsion: CT findings in a child. J Pediatr Surg. 39(8):1270-2, 2004
7. Lambert MJ et al: Gynecologic ultrasound in emergency medicine. Emerg Med Clin North Am. 22(3):683-96, 2004
8. Ratani RS et al: Pediatric gynecologic ultrasound. Ultrasound Q. 20(3):127-39, 2004
9. Webb EM et al: Adnexal mass with pelvic pain. Radiol Clin North Am. 42(2):329-48, 2004
10. Crouch NS et al: Ovarian torsion: to pex or not to pex? Case report and review of the literature. J Pediatr Adolesc Gynecol. 16(6):381-4, 2004
11. Ignacio EA et al: Ultrasound of the acute female pelvis. Ultrasound Q. 19(2):86-98; quiz 108-10, 2003
12. Nishino M et al: Magnetic resonance imaging findings in gynecologic emergencies. J Comput Assist Tomogr. 27(4):564-70, 2003
13. Ozcan C et al: Adnexal torsion in children may have a catastrophic sequel: asynchronous bilateral torsion. J Pediatr Surg. 37(11):1617-20, 2002
14. Promecene PA: Laparoscopy in gynecologic emergencies. Semin Laparosc Surg. 9(1):64-75, 2002
15. Rha SE et al: CT and MR imaging features of adnexal torsion. Radiographics 22:283-94, 2002
16. Tseng D et al: Minimally invasive management of the prenatally torsed ovarian cyst. J Pediatr Surg. 37(10):1467-9, 2002
17. Derchi LE et al: Ultrasound in gynecology. Eur Radiol. 11(11):2137-55, 2001
18. Garel L et al: US of the pediatric female pelvis: a clinical perspective. Radiographics. 21(6):1393-407, 2001
19. Bau A et al: Acute female pelvic pain: Ultrasound evaluation. Semin Ultrasound CT MR 21:78-93, 2000
20. Lee EJ et al: Diagnosis of ovarian torsion with color Doppler sonography: Depiction of twisted vascular pedicle. J Ultrasound Med 17:83-9, 1998

OVARIAN TORSION

IMAGE GALLERY

Typical

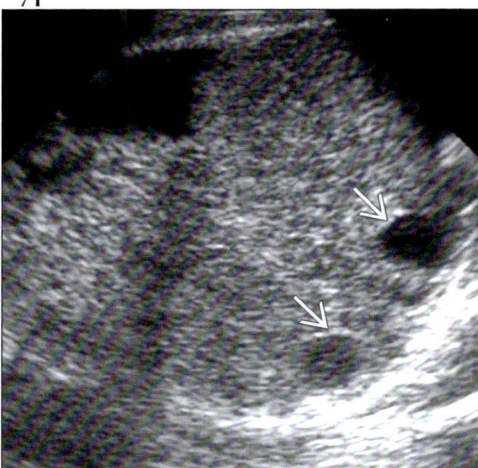
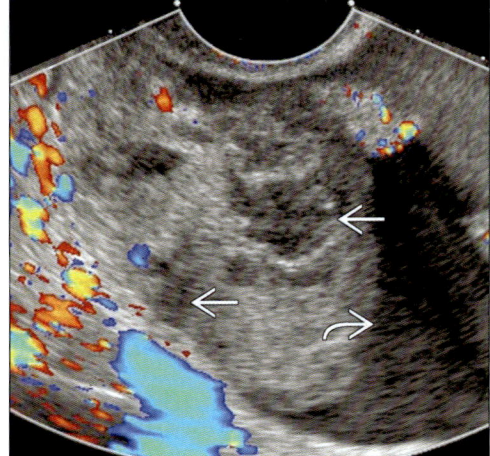

(Left) Sagittal grayscale endovaginal sonogram of ovarian torsion demonstrates enlarged ovary with prominent peripheral follicles ➡. (Right) Lateral color Doppler ultrasound reveals cystic spaces ➡ within infarcted ovary representing areas of cystic necrosis. Note adjacent echogenic fluid (hemoperitoneum) ➡.

Typical

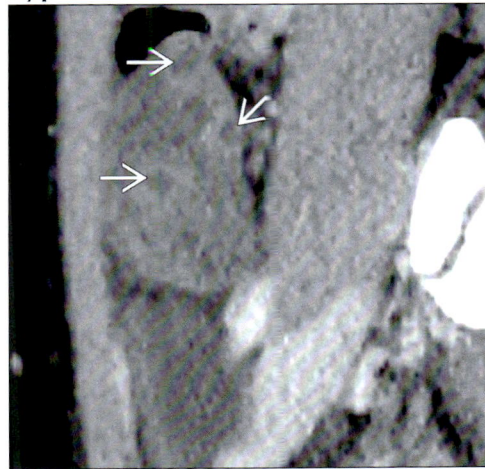
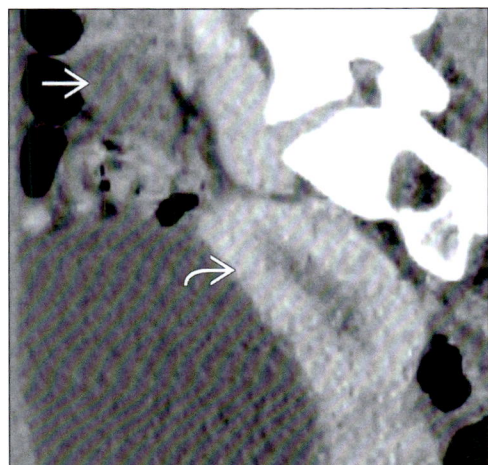

(Left) Sagittal CECT reformation of ovarian torsion demonstrates enlarged edematous ovary with peripheral follicles ➡. (Right) CECT at more midline view in same patient as left reveals ectopic location of torsed ovary ➡ above the uterus ➡.

Variant

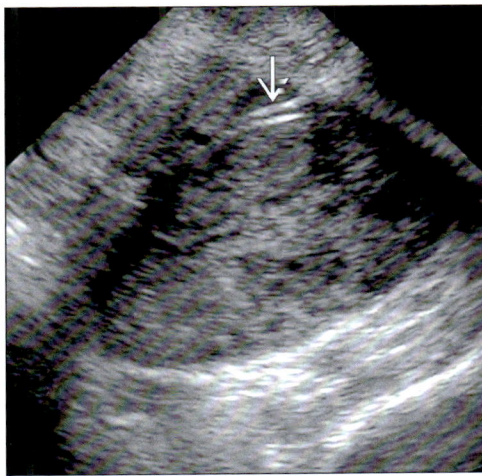
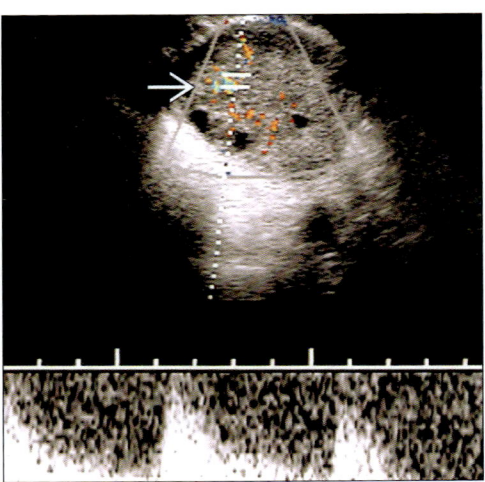

(Left) Sagittal grayscale sonogram of ovarian torsion with preserved arterial flow. Note enlarged echogenic left ovary ➡. (Right) Sagittal endovaginal color Doppler sonogram in same patient as left reveals areas of preserved arterial flow ➡.

OVARIAN VEIN THROMBOSIS

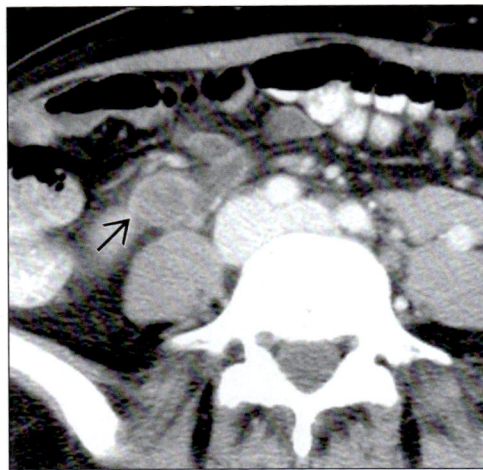

Axial CECT of OVT. Note distended clot-filled ovarian vein adjacent to right psoas muscle ➔.

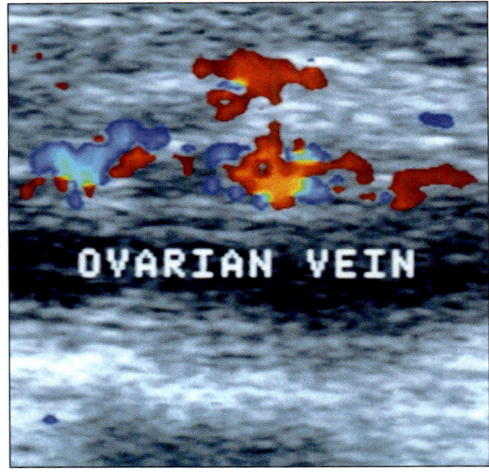

Sagittal color Doppler ultrasound along psoas muscle reveals tubular clotted ovarian vein with absent color flow.

TERMINOLOGY

Abbreviations and Synonyms
- Ovarian vein thrombosis (OVT), gonadal vein thrombosis

Definitions
- Rare complication associated with postpartum ascending ovarian vein thrombophlebitis
  - Incidence 1-2% following cesarean section complicated by endometritis
  - Incidence < 0.2% following vaginal delivery

IMAGING FINDINGS

General Features
- Best diagnostic clue: Enlarged, well-defined, tubular retroperitoneal mass extending from pelvis to infrarenal inferior vena cava (IVC) along ovarian vein without demonstrable flow
- Location: Right ovarian vein involved more than left
- Size: Vein often distended to twice its normal size

CT Findings
- NECT: Hyperdense to isodense clot relative to venous wall & psoas muscle
- CECT
  - Enlarged ovarian vein
  - Low-attenuation central lumen (filling defect)
  - Sharply-defined enhancing wall
  - Perivascular inflammation, abdominal/pelvic mass
  - Imaging pitfall: Right ovarian vein pseudothrombosis due to flow artifact
    - Asymmetric ovarian vein opacification: Left > right
    - Etiology: Early reflux of contrast down left ovarian vein

MR Findings
- T1WI
  - Intermediate to high signal intensity intraluminal clot
  - Occasional low signal intensity center due to retracting clot
- T2WI: High signal intensity intraluminal clot
- CEMR: Signal-void central lumen with sharply-defined enhancing wall

DDx: Lesions Mimicking Ovarian Vein Thrombosis

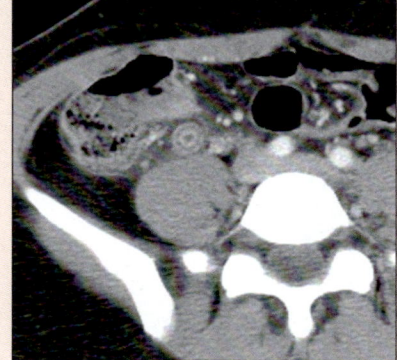

Appendicitis

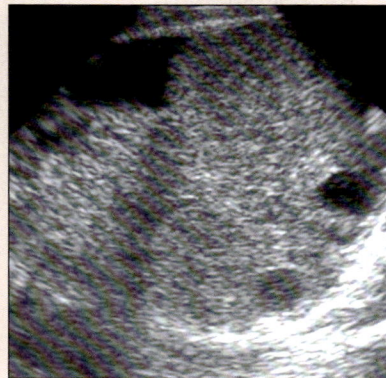

Ovarian Torsion

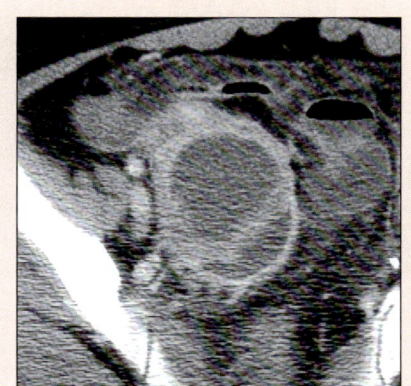

Tubo-Ovarian Abscess

OVARIAN VEIN THROMBOSIS

Key Facts

Terminology
- Ovarian vein thrombosis (OVT), gonadal vein thrombosis
- Rare complication associated with postpartum ascending ovarian vein thrombophlebitis
- Incidence 1-2% following cesarean section complicated by endometritis
- Incidence < 0.2% following vaginal delivery

Imaging Findings
- Best diagnostic clue: Enlarged, well-defined, tubular retroperitoneal mass extending from pelvis to infrarenal inferior vena cava (IVC) along ovarian vein without demonstrable flow
- Imaging pitfall: Right ovarian vein pseudothrombosis due to flow artifact

- Etiology: Early reflux of contrast down left ovarian vein

Top Differential Diagnoses
- Appendicitis
- Adnexal Torsion
- Tubo-Ovarian Abscess (TOA)/Pelvic Inflammatory Disease (PID)

Clinical Issues
- May result in septic pulmonary emboli, ureteral obstruction
- Antibiotics for at least 1 week (+/- anticoagulation for up to 3 weeks)
- Surgical intervention (thrombectomy &/or vein interruption/ligation) if failed medical therapy with progression of thrombus into IVC

  ○ Perivascular inflammation; abdominal/pelvic mass

Ultrasonographic Findings
- Grayscale Ultrasound
  ○ May be obscured by overlying bowel gas
  ○ Variable echogenicity intraluminal clot (can extend to IVC) on two-dimensional US
  ○ Tubular hypoechoic structure anterior to psoas muscle
- Color Doppler: Partial or absent flow within vein
- Power Doppler: Partial or absent flow within vein
- Less sensitive than CT or MR for diagnosis

Imaging Recommendations
- Best imaging tool: CECT; CEMR in patients with contraindication to CT
- Protocol advice: 150 mL IV contrast injected @ 2.5 mL/sec; 5 mm collimation & 5 mm reconstruction interval

DIFFERENTIAL DIAGNOSIS

Appendicitis
- Initial midepigastric pain moving to RLQ
- Dilated non-compressible appendix > 7 mm in A-P diameter on grayscale US
- Dilated appendix with inflammatory changes in mesoappendix on CECT

Adnexal Torsion
- Enlarged echogenic ovary with prominent peripheral follicles
- Absent venous flow
- Absent arterial flow with infarcted ovary

Tubo-Ovarian Abscess (TOA)/Pelvic Inflammatory Disease (PID)
- Complex solid/cystic mass in adnexa
- Associated with dilated pus-filled fallopian tube (pyosalpinx)
- Indefinite uterus sign due to pelvic peritonitis

- Peritoneal enhancement around edge of right lobe of liver (Fitz-Hugh-Curtis syndrome)

PATHOLOGY

General Features
- General path comments
  ○ Delivery provides infectious agent to initiate ascending thrombophlebitis
  ○ Right ovarian vein affected 5 times more frequently than left
    ▪ Compression of right vein at pelvic rim by enlarged uterus
    ▪ Retrograde flow in left vein protects against ascending infection
- Etiology
  ○ Early in puerperium; typically within 10 days of delivery
  ○ Related to Virchow Triad
    ▪ Hypercoagulability (pregnancy & puerperium associated with increased levels of factors I, II, VII, IX & X)
    ▪ Alterations in vein wall (high estrogen levels, surgical insult, bacterial insult to endothelium)
    ▪ Stasis of blood flow (postpartum venous velocity drops sharply)
  ○ Malignancy (neoplasm- and/or chemotherapy-induced thrombosis)
  ○ Post-gynecologic surgery (hysterectomy, oophorectomy)
  ○ Pelvic inflammatory disease, post-abortion infection
  ○ Acute gastrointestinal inflammation (men & women)
  ○ Risk factors
    ▪ Postpartum endometritis
    ▪ Pelvic inflammatory disease
    ▪ Pelvic abscess
    ▪ Diverticulitis or appendicitis
    ▪ Ovarian Cancer
- Epidemiology
  ○ 1/600-2000 births; 0.15-0.18% of puerperia

OVARIAN VEIN THROMBOSIS

  - More common following cesarean sections complicated by endometritis

CLINICAL ISSUES

Presentation
- Most common signs/symptoms
  - RLQ abdominal or flank pain; enigmatic or refractory fever; tender, right-sided, elongated mass coursing superiorly
  - May be asymptomatic
  - If left sided, pain and mass manifest on left
- Other signs/symptoms: Rarely signs of pulmonary embolism if thrombus extends to inferior vena cava (IVC)
- Clinical Profile: Postpartum patient with RLQ pain & fever, or patient with pelvic abscess (diverticulitis, appendicitis, etc.)

Demographics
- Gender: Female

Natural History & Prognosis
- Overall prognosis: Good
- Spontaneous resolution may be seen in some patients
- May result in septic pulmonary emboli, ureteral obstruction
- Mortality: 18/1,000,000 pregnancies

Treatment
- Antibiotics for at least 1 week (+/- anticoagulation for up to 3 weeks)
- Surgical intervention (thrombectomy &/or vein interruption/ligation) if failed medical therapy with progression of thrombus into IVC

DIAGNOSTIC CHECKLIST

Consider
- Clinically mimics appendicitis with acute onset of RLQ pain & fever

Image Interpretation Pearls
- Distended clot-filled vein anterior to psoas muscle on CECT or MR
- Look for extension into IVC

SELECTED REFERENCES

1. Sinha D et al: Postpartum inferior vena cava and ovarian vein thrombosis--a case report and literature review. J Obstet Gynaecol. 25(3):312-3, 2005
2. Umeoka S et al: Vascular dilatation in the pelvis: identification with CT and MR imaging. Radiographics. 24(1):193-208, 2004
3. Van Gerpen R et al: Thromboembolic disorders in cancer. Clin J Oncol Nurs. 8(3):289-99, 2004
4. Al-toma A et al: Postpartum ovarian vein thrombosis: report of a case and review of literature. Neth J Med. 61(10):334-6, 2003
5. Dessole S et al: Postpartum ovarian vein thrombosis: an unpredictable event: two case reports and review of the literature. Arch Gynecol Obstet. 267(4):242-6, 2003
6. Scialpi M et al: Postpartum ovarian vein thrombosis with simultaneous pyelocaliectasis: diagnosis and follow-up by MR imaging. Case report and literature review. Emerg Radiol. 10(1):60-3, 2003
7. Kubik-Huch RA et al: Role of duplex color Doppler ultrasound, computed tomography, and MR angiography in the diagnosis of septic puerperal ovarian vein thrombosis. Abdom Imaging 24:85-91, 1999
8. Johnson SC et al: Sonography of postpartum ovarian vein thrombophlebitis. J Clin Ultrasound. 26(3):143-9, 1998
9. Twickler DM et al: Imaging of puerperal septic thrombophlebitis: Prospective comparison of MR imaging, CT, and sonography. Am J Roentgenol 164:1039-43, 1997
10. Zuckerman J et al: Imaging of postpartum complications. Am J Roentgenol 170:1395-6, 1997
11. Witlin AG et al: Septic pelvic thrombophlebitis or refractory postpartum fever of undetermined etiology. J Matern Fetal Med. 5(6):355-8, 1996
12. Van Hoe L et al: Abdominal pain in the postpartum: role of imaging. J Belge Radiol. 78(3):186-9, 1995
13. Witlin AG et al: Postpartum ovarian vein thrombosis after vaginal delivery: a report of 11 cases. Obstet Gynecol. 85(5 Pt 1):775-80, 1995
14. Simons GR et al: Ovarian vein thrombosis. Am Heart J. 126(3 Pt 1):641-7, 1993
15. Toland KC et al: Postpartum ovarian vein thrombosis presenting as ureteral obstruction: a case report and review of the literature. J Urol. 149(6):1538-40, 1993
16. Bahnson RR et al: Renal vein thrombosis following puerperal ovarian vein thrombophlebitis. Am J Obstet Gynecol. 152(3):290-1, 1985
17. Duff P et al: Pelvic vein thrombophlebitis: diagnostic dilemma and therapeutic challenge. Obstet Gynecol Surv. 38(6):365-73, 1983
18. Allan TR et al: Postpartum and Postabortal Ovarian Vein Thrombophlebitis. Obstet Gynecol. 47(5):525-8, 1976
19. Nasser N et al: Ovarian vein thrombosis. A rare cause of pelvic pain. Report of a case and review of the literature. J Lancet. 88(11):306-8, 1968
20. Lotze EC et al: Postpartum ovarian vein thrombophlebitis. Obstet Gynecol Surv. 21(6):853-70, 1966

OVARIAN VEIN THROMBOSIS

IMAGE GALLERY

Typical

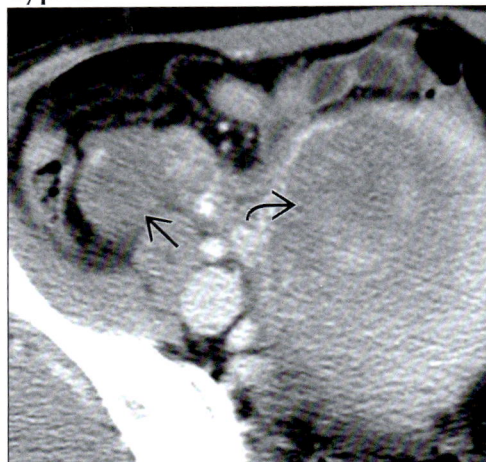
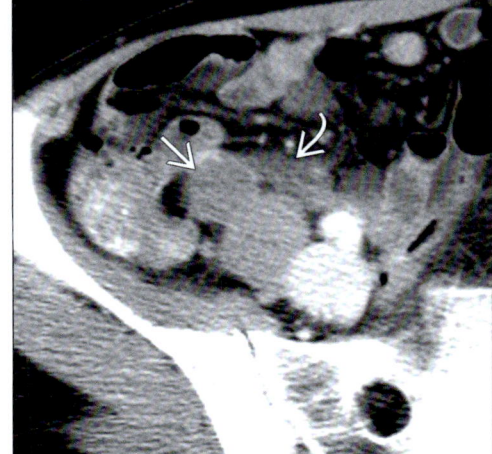

(Left) Axial CECT of postpartum patient with OVT. Note enlarged right ovary ➡ and postpartum uterus ➡. *(Right)* Axial CECT at higher level in same patient as left demonstrates OVT anterior to psoas muscle ➡. Note surrounding fluid from septic thrombophlebitis ➡.

Typical

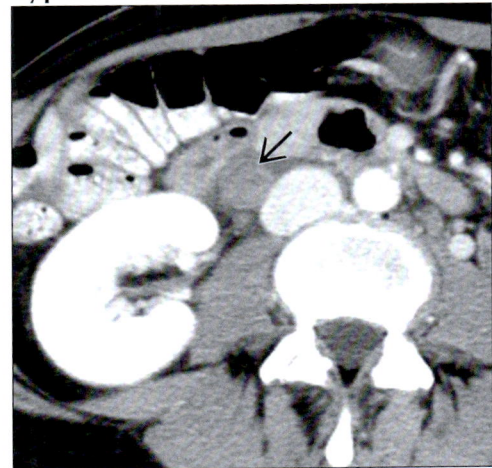
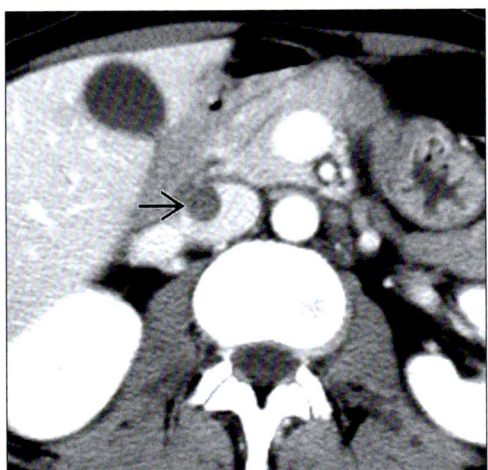

(Left) Axial CECT of OVT extension to IVC. Note OVT adjacent to IVC ➡. *(Right)* Axial CECT at higher level in same patient as left reveals clot extending into IVC ➡.

Variant

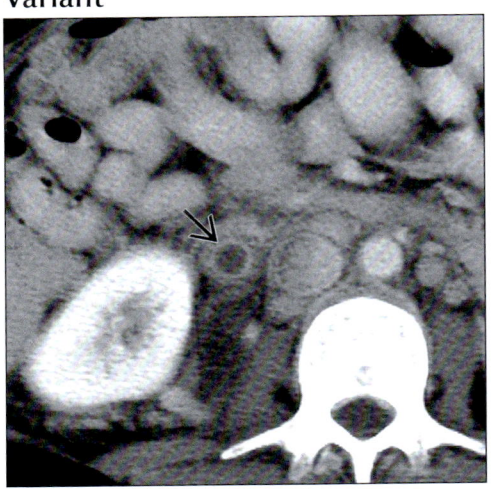
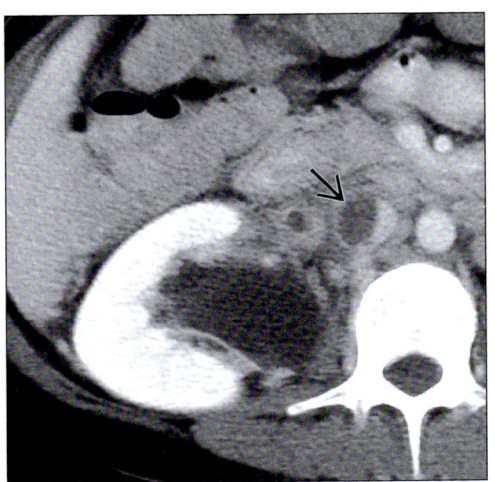

(Left) Axial CECT shows rim sign of clot within ovarian vein ➡. *(Right)* Axial CECT at higher level in same patient as left reveals extension of clot into IVC ➡.

OVARIAN HEMORRHAGE

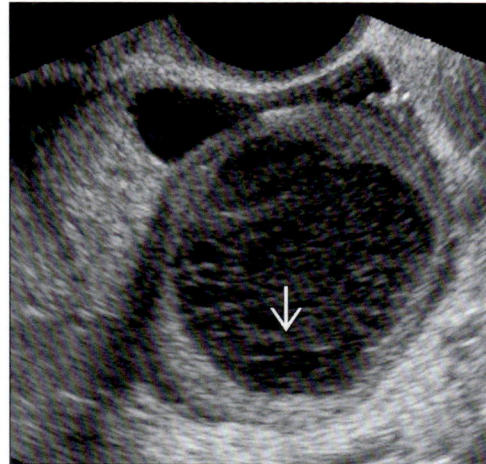

Sagittal transvaginal ultrasound of HC demonstrates hypoechoic mass with low-level echoes & linear echoes (fishnet sign) ➡.

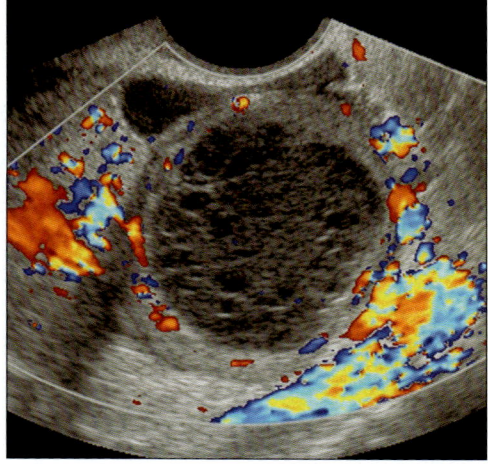

Sagittal transvaginal color Doppler sonogram in same patient as left reveals no flow within hemorrhagic cyst.

TERMINOLOGY

Abbreviations and Synonyms
- Hemorrhagic ovarian cyst (HC)

Definitions
- Functional cyst with internal hemorrhage

IMAGING FINDINGS

General Features
- Best diagnostic clue
  - Acute: Cystic mass with echogenic blood, ± fluid-fluid level
  - Subacute: Diffuse low-level echoes (ground-glass appearance); intersecting linear strands (fishnet sign)
  - Echogenic retracting clot with concave or straight margin
  - Avascular on color Doppler
- Location: Ovary
- Size: Variable; 3-10 cm
- Morphology: Rounded cyst with linear or low-level echoes, echogenic clot

CT Findings
- NECT
  - Adnexal cyst containing high-attenuation fluid
    - Typically > 30 HU
  - May have associated hemoperitoneum
    - Typically > 25 HU
- CECT: No internal enhancement of cyst

MR Findings
- T1WI: High signal within adnexal cyst
- T1WI FS: Signal does not decrease with fat saturation
- T2WI: High signal within adnexal cyst

Ultrasonographic Findings
- Specific US appearance in 90% of cases
  - Intersecting linear strands
  - Echogenic retracting clot with concave or straight margin
  - Avascular on endovaginal color Doppler
  - Absence of true septations or mural nodularity
    - Helpful in distinguishing from malignancy

DDx: Mimics of Ovarian Hemorrhage

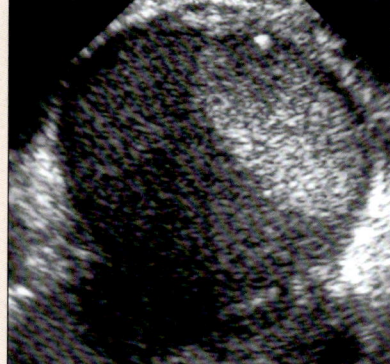

Endometrioma

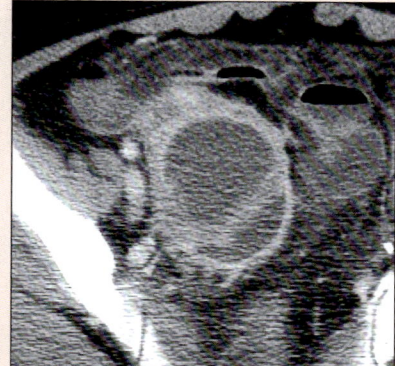

Tubo-Ovarian Abscess

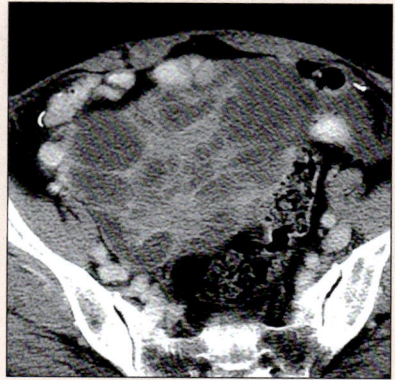

Ovarian Carcinoma

OVARIAN HEMORRHAGE

Key Facts

Terminology
- Hemorrhagic ovarian cyst (HC)
- Functional cyst with internal hemorrhage

Imaging Findings
- Acute: Cystic mass with echogenic blood, ± fluid-fluid level
- Subacute: Diffuse low-level echoes (ground-glass appearance); intersecting linear strands (fishnet sign)
- Echogenic retracting clot with concave or straight margin
- Avascular on color Doppler
- Best imaging tool: US with color Doppler
- Protocol advice: Endovaginal US

Top Differential Diagnoses
- Endometrioma
- Tubo-Ovarian Abscess
- Ovarian Cancer
- Adnexal Torsion
- Dermoid Cyst (Cystic Teratoma)

Clinical Issues
- Acute pelvic pain
- Palpable adnexal mass
- negative β-hCG
- No evidence of fever or increased WBC count
- Age: 14-50 years (pre-menopausal)
- May require surgery if rupture & significant hemoperitoneum

Diagnostic Checklist
- Consider endometrioma if lesion is unchanged after 6-8 weeks

Imaging Recommendations
- Best imaging tool: US with color Doppler
- Protocol advice: Endovaginal US

DIFFERENTIAL DIAGNOSIS

Endometrioma
- Extrauterine functional endometrial tissue involving ovary (endometriosis)
- Hemorrhagic ovarian cyst ("chocolate cyst")
- Bilateral in 15 to 20% of cases
- US
  - Unilocular or multilocular cystic mass with diffuse low-level echoes ("ground-glass" appearance)
  - Fluid-fluid level with echogenic clot layering dependently on US
  - Peripheral echogenic foci within wall of cyst, due to cholesterol deposits
  - May have "solid" mural nodules that are avascular
- MR
  - T1 high-signal cystic mass
  - T2 high signal does not suppress signal with fat saturation
  - "Shadowing" on T2 images with loss of signal within cyst
- CT
  - Attenuation values in cyst > 25 HU
- Unlike functional HC, tends to persist over many menstrual cycles with little change
- Associated with infertility, unlike HC

Tubo-Ovarian Abscess
- Complex septic mass involving fallopian tube, ovary & loculated peritoneal abscess
- Hyperemic wall of cystic mass on color Doppler
- Inflamed echogenic fat surrounding mass on US
- Associated with dilated fallopian tube with low-level echoes (pyosalpinx) & perihepatic inflammatory changes (Fitz-Hugh-Curtis syndrome)

Ovarian Cancer
- Complex cystic mass containing mural &/or septal nodules with color Doppler flow with low resistive indices
- Solid mural components with color flow
- Associated with omental & peritoneal implants, ascites

Adnexal Torsion
- Twisted pedicle sign
- Normal to diminished vascularity of adnexa
- High-signal intensity of T1WI & T2WI, with layering on T2WI
- Enlarged echogenic ovary with prominent peripheral follicles
- Absent venous flow
- Absent arterial flow with infarcted ovary

Dermoid Cyst (Cystic Teratoma)
- Most common ovarian neoplasm
  - 15-25% of all neoplasms
- 10-15% bilateral
- Comprised of derivatives of three germ layers with predominance of ectodermal elements
- Can occur at any age, but most common during reproductive years
- Complications: Torsion & rupture with chemical peritonitis
- US findings
  - "Tip of iceberg" sign: Shadowing from hair & sebum
  - Dermoid mesh due to linear intersecting strands of hair
  - Echogenic mural nodule (dermoid plug contains hair, teeth, and/or fat) frequently has distal acoustic shadowing
  - Fat-fluid level
  - Calcifications
  - Echogenic mass
  - Typically avascular on color Doppler sonography, except in cases with vascularized ectopic thyroid tissue (struma ovarii)

OVARIAN HEMORRHAGE

PATHOLOGY

General Features
- Etiology: Unknown
- Associated abnormalities
  - Rupture
  - Hemoperitoneum
  - Ovarian torsion

Gross Pathologic & Surgical Features
- Thin-walled cyst with clot & serosanguineous fluid
- May have associated hemoperitoneum

Microscopic Features
- Benign epithelial cyst with internal hemorrhage

CLINICAL ISSUES

Presentation
- Most common signs/symptoms
  - Acute pelvic pain
    - Unlike endometriosis, which is chronic & associated with painful menstrual periods
- Other signs/symptoms
  - Palpable adnexal mass
  - negative β-hCG
  - No evidence of fever or increased WBC count

Demographics
- Age: 14-50 years (pre-menopausal)
- Gender: Female

Natural History & Prognosis
- Most resolve or decrease in size within 8 weeks

Treatment
- Observation if resolving on follow-up exam
- May require surgery if rupture & significant hemoperitoneum

DIAGNOSTIC CHECKLIST

Consider
- Consider endometrioma if lesion is unchanged after 6-8 weeks

Image Interpretation Pearls
- Linear intersecting strands of fibrin (fishnet sign)
- Retracting echogenic clot
- Avascular on color Doppler sonography

SELECTED REFERENCES

1. Kurioka H et al: Hemorrhagic ovarian cyst without peritoneal bleeding in a patient with ovarian hyperstimulation syndrome: case report. Chin Med J (Engl). 118(18):1577-81, 2005
2. Patel MD et al: The likelihood ratio of sonographic findings for the diagnosis of hemorrhagic ovarian cysts. J Ultrasound Med. 24(5):607-14; quiz 615, 2005
3. Kives SL et al: Ruptured hemorrhagic cyst in an undescended ovary. J Pediatr Surg. 39(11):e4-6, 2004
4. Swire MN et al: Various sonographic appearances of the hemorrhagic corpus luteum cyst. Ultrasound Q. 20(2):45-58, 2004
5. Huang PH et al: Hemorrhagic corpus luteum cyst torsion in term pregnancy: a case report. Kaohsiung J Med Sci. 19(2):75-8, 2003
6. Nemoto Y et al: Ultrasonographic and clinical appearance of hemorrhagic ovarian cyst diagnosed by transvaginal scan. J Nippon Med Sch. 70(3):243-9, 2003
7. Teng SW et al: Comparison of laparoscopy and laparotomy in managing hemodynamically stable patients with ruptured corpus luteum with hemoperitoneum. J Am Assoc Gynecol Laparosc. 10(4):474-7, 2003
8. Jain KA: Sonographic spectrum of hemorrhagic ovarian cysts. J Ultrasound Med. 21(8):879-86, 2002
9. Weinstein AS et al: Case 7.Hemorrhagic ovarian cyst. J Ultrasound Med. 21(5):594, 611-2, 2002
10. Yilmaz E et al: Sonographic and MRI findings in prepubertal adnexal hemorrhagic cyst with torsion. J Clin Ultrasound. 29(3):200-2, 2001
11. Hertzberg BS et al: Adnexal ring sign and hemoperitoneum caused by hemorrhagic ovarian cyst: pitfall in the sonographic diagnosis of ectopic pregnancy. AJR Am J Roentgenol. 173(5):1301-2, 1999
12. Hertzberg BS et al: Ovarian cyst rupture causing hemoperitoneum: imaging features and the potential for misdiagnosis. Abdom Imaging. 24(3):304-8, 1999
13. Quint EH et al: Ovarian surgery in premenarchal girls. J Pediatr Adolesc Gynecol. 12(1):27-9, 1999
14. Merz E et al: A new sonomorphologic scoring system (Mainz Score) for the assessment of ovarian tumors using transvaginal ultrasonography. Part I: A comparison between the scoring-system and the assessment by an experienced sonographer. Ultraschall Med. 19(3):99-107, 1998
15. Ishihara K et al: Sonographic appearance of hemorrhagic ovarian cyst with acute abdomen by transvaginal scan. Nippon Ika Daigaku Zasshi. 64(5):411-5, 1997
16. Ou CS: Vascular complications following laparoscopy: two unusual cases. JSLS. 1(2):159-61, 1997
17. Kayaba H et al: Hemorrhagic ovarian cyst in childhood: a case report. J Pediatr Surg. 31(7):978-9, 1996
18. O'Brien PM et al: Management of an acute hemorrhagic ovarian cyst in a female patient with hemophilia A. J Pediatr Hematol Oncol. 18(2):233-6, 1996
19. Sarihan H et al: Massive haemoperitoneum due to spontaneous rupture of ovarian cyst in children. A report of 2 cases. S Afr J Surg. 34(1):44-6, 1996
20. Quillin SP et al: Transabdominal color Doppler ultrasonography of the painful adolescent ovary. J Ultrasound Med. 13(7):549-55, 1994

OVARIAN HEMORRHAGE

IMAGE GALLERY

Typical

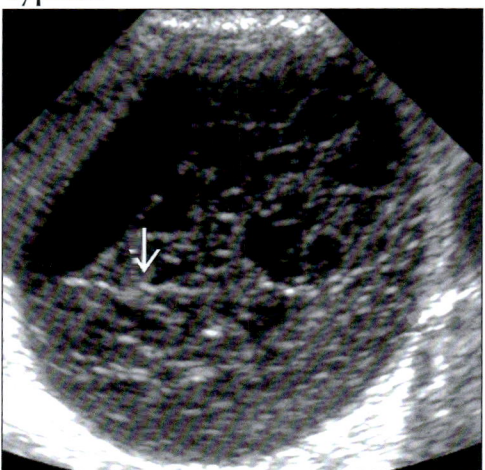
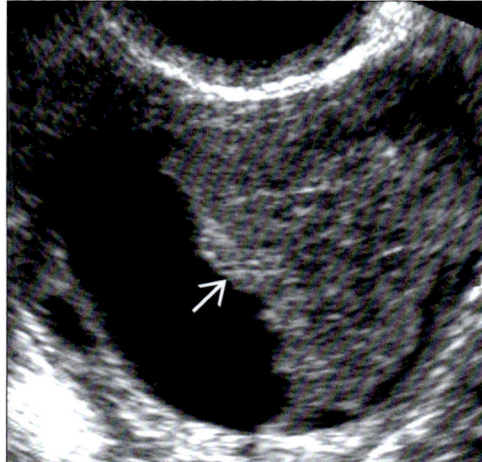

(Left) Sagittal transvaginal ultrasound of HC demonstrates "fishnet sign" of multiple intersecting linear strands of fibrin ➔. *(Right)* Sagittal endovaginal grayscale sonogram of retracting clot sign. Note straight margin of clot within HC ➔.

Typical

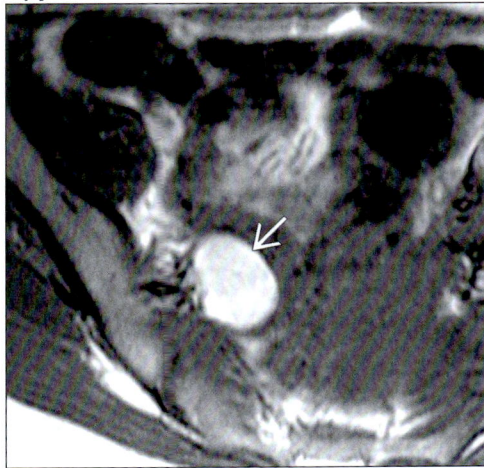
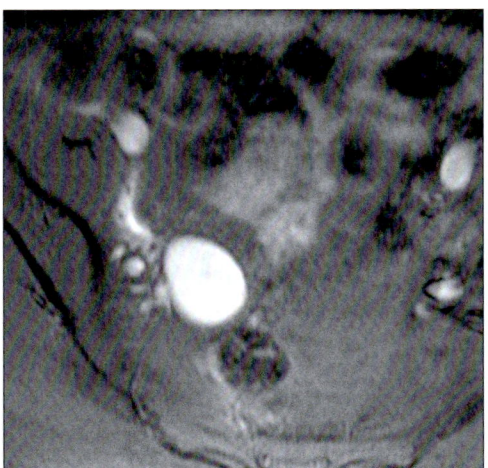

(Left) Axial T1WI MR of hemorrhagic cyst reveals high signal cystic mass in right ovary ➔. *(Right)* Axial T1WI FS MR in same patient as left shows no loss of signal, indicating hemorrhagic cyst.

Variant

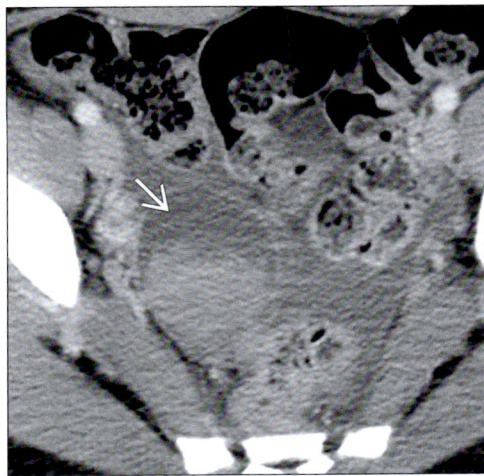
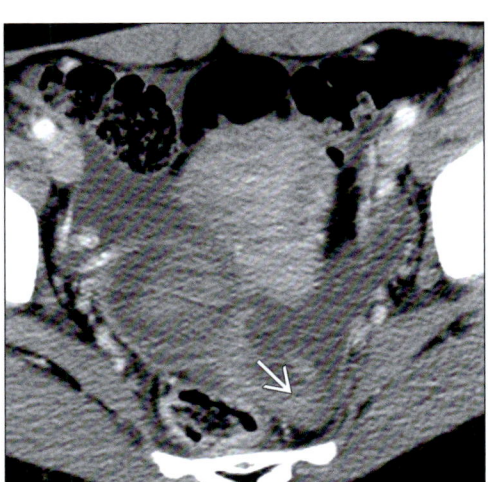

(Left) Axial CECT of ruptured HC with hemoperitoneum. Note high attenuation clot (HU = 48) within right adnexal cyst ➔. *(Right)* Axial CECT at more caudal level in same patient as left reveals high attenuation fluid (HU = 35), representing hemoperitoneum ➔.

PELVIC INFLAMMATORY DISEASE

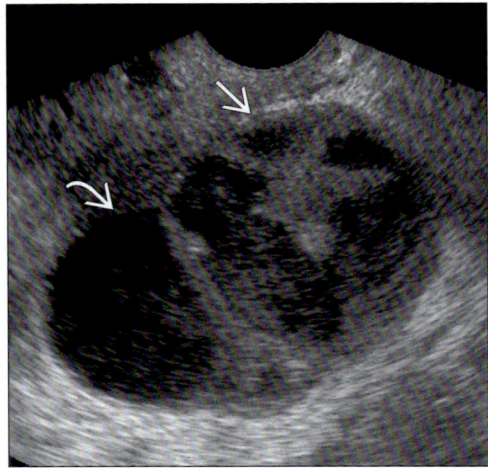
Sagittal grayscale sonography of oophoritis in early PID. Endovaginal scan demonstrates marked enlargement of ovary ➡ with prominent cystic areas within ovarian parenchyma ➡.

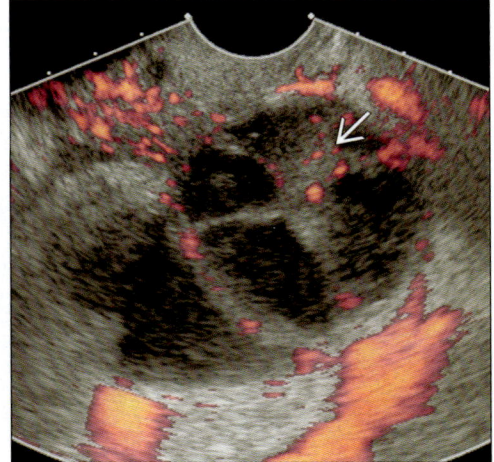
Power Doppler endovaginal sonogram of same patient as left reveals ovarian hyperemia ➡.

TERMINOLOGY

Abbreviations and Synonyms
- Acute pyogenic pelvic inflammatory disease (PID)
  o Includes salpingitis, pyosalpinx, oophoritis, tubo-ovarian abscesses (TOA), pelvic abscesses

Definitions
- Infection of upper female genital tract including endometrium, fallopian tubes, ovaries, peritoneal cavity

IMAGING FINDINGS

General Features
- Best diagnostic clue
  o Endometritis with endometrial fluid and/or gas
  o Dilated fallopian tube with low-level echoes (pyosalpinx)
  o Multiple pelvic abscesses in cul-de-sac
  o Obscuration of pelvic fat planes
  o Tubo-ovarian abscess: Complex cystic/solid mass with septations & irregular margins
- Location: Adnexal areas, cul-de-sac
- Morphology: Tubular (pyosalpinx)

CT Findings
- CECT
  o Early
    ▪ Abnormal endometrial enhancement
    ▪ Ovarian enlargement
    ▪ Free fluid in pelvis
    ▪ Obscuration of pelvic fat planes
  o Late
    ▪ Multiple pelvic abscesses in adnexa & cul-de-sac
    ▪ Dilated fallopian tubes
    ▪ Peritoneal enhancement & fluid around right lobe of liver (Fitz-Hugh-Curtis syndrome)

MR Findings
- T1WI
  o Fluid contents: Hypointense to intermediate signal intensity
  o Abscess wall: 1-3 mm hyperintense inner rim (granulation tissue)
- T2WI: Fluid contents: Intermediate to high signal intensity

DDx: Lesions Mimicking Pelvic Inflammatory Disease

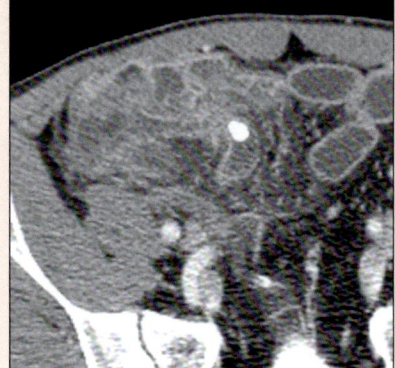
Perforated Appendicitis

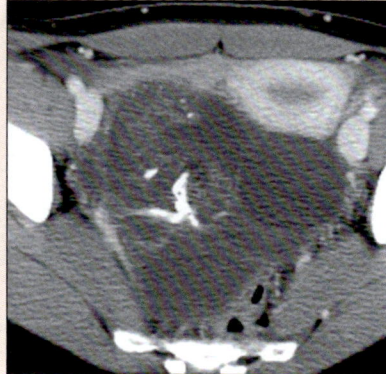
Ruptured Dermoid

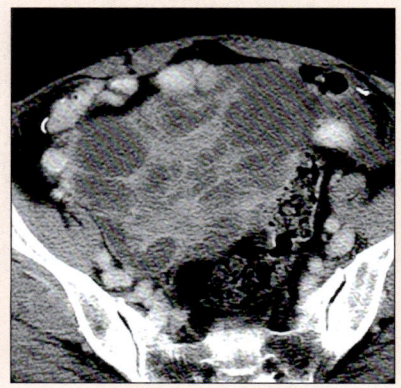
Ovarian Carcinoma

PELVIC INFLAMMATORY DISEASE

Key Facts

Terminology
- Acute pyogenic pelvic inflammatory disease (PID)
- Infection of upper female genital tract including endometrium, fallopian tubes, ovaries, peritoneal cavity

Imaging Findings
- Endometritis with endometrial fluid and/or gas
- Dilated fallopian tube with low-level echoes (pyosalpinx)
- Multiple pelvic abscesses in cul-de-sac
- Obscuration of pelvic fat planes
- Tubo-ovarian abscess: Complex cystic/solid mass with septations & irregular margins
- US for initial evaluation & follow-up, guidance for abscess/pyosalpinx drainage
- CT for complicated PID, guidance for abscess drainage
- MR for differentiation between multicystic mass & abnormal fallopian tube

Top Differential Diagnoses
- Perforated Appendicitis
- Ruptured Dermoid
- Ovarian Neoplasm
- Adnexal Torsion

Clinical Issues
- Laparoscopy & endometrial sampling for diagnosis
- Antibiotic therapy ± image-guided or surgical drainage of pelvic abscess

Ultrasonographic Findings
- Grayscale Ultrasound
  - Early PID
    - Increased echogenicity of pelvic fat
    - Fallopian tube thickening ± distention with simple fluid
    - Enlarged ovaries with indistinct margins, multiple cysts
    - May be normal
  - Advanced PID
    - Pyosalpinx: Cogwheel sign/incomplete septa; fallopian tube wall thickening > 5 mm & increased echogenicity
    - Tubo-ovarian/pelvic abscess: Multilocular/unilocular, complex, thick-walled, cystic adnexal mass

Imaging Recommendations
- Best imaging tool
  - US for initial evaluation & follow-up, guidance for abscess/pyosalpinx drainage
  - CT for complicated PID, guidance for abscess drainage
  - MR for differentiation between multicystic mass & abnormal fallopian tube

DIFFERENTIAL DIAGNOSIS

Perforated Appendicitis
- Dilated appendix > 7 mm ± appendicolith
- Soft tissue stranding in mesoappendix & periappendiceal fat
- Multiple complex fluid collections in pelvis (abscesses)

Ruptured Dermoid
- Cystic adnexal mass containing fat ± calcifications or bone
- Soft tissue inflammatory changes in pelvis
- Ectopic location of mass suggests torsion of adnexa

Ovarian Neoplasm
- Vascular solid component within cystic mass
- Thick vascular septations
- Large amount of free fluid
- No inflammation of fat

Adnexal Torsion
- Twisted pedicle sign
- Normal to diminished vascularity of adnexa
- High signal intensity of T1WI & T2WI, with layering on T2WI

PATHOLOGY

General Features
- Etiology
  - Sexually transmitted diseases
    - Most commonly Neisseria gonorrhoeae or Chlamydia trachomatis (30-40% polymicrobial)
    - Additional organisms include gram negative rods & Mycoplasma genitalium
- Epidemiology
  - Affects 1 million women annually in US
    - 275,000 require hospitalization

Gross Pathologic & Surgical Features
- Surgical findings
  - Dense fibroses and adhesions encompassing tubes, ovaries & uterus
  - Requires total abdominal hysterectomy & bilateral salpingo-oophorectomy
    - Inability to dissect ovary from tubes & uterus

Microscopic Features
- Fibrosis, acute & chronic inflammatory changes

Staging, Grading or Classification Criteria
- Early
  - Mild pelvic edema
    - Haziness/stranding of pelvic fat, obscuring of fascial planes
  - Mild salpingitis: Mural thickening of fallopian tube > 5 mm with low-level echoes
  - Mild oophoritis: Enlarged, heterogeneously enhancing ovaries ± polycystic appearance of ovaries

PELVIC INFLAMMATORY DISEASE

- Abnormal endometrial/endocervical enhancement with fluid in cavity
- Enhanced peritoneum on CECT
* Advanced
    - Pyosalpinx
        - Greater degree of wall thickening, enhancement
        - Filled with complex fluid, fluid-debris level
    - Tubo-ovarian or pelvic abscess
        - Complex fluid collection ± internal septa
        - Thick-walled with ill-defined outer borders
        - Inner borders may be irregular
        - Inflamed echogenic fat surrounding enlarged ovary
* Involvement of adjacent structures
    - Small or large bowel ileus/obstruction
    - Thickening of small/large bowel wall, bladder wall
    - Ureteropelvicaliectasis: Functional or mechanical obstruction
    - Fitz-Hugh and Curtis syndrome: Inflammation of RUQ peritoneal surfaces, thick gallbladder wall, heterogeneous liver enhancement

CLINICAL ISSUES

Presentation
* Most common signs/symptoms
    - Acute
        - Pelvic pain, fever, vaginal discharge
    - Subacute
        - Symptoms of bowel obstruction due to adhesions
        - RUQ pain from adhesions (Fitz-Hugh-Curtis syndrome)
* Clinical Profile: Sexually active patient with multiple partners

Demographics
* Age: Sexually active women
* Gender: Female

Natural History & Prognosis
* Can lead to infertility and ectopic pregnancies if not diagnosed & treated in early stages due to tubal scarring
* Risk factors
    - Multiple sex partners
    - Intrauterine device
    - Prior uterine procedure (e.g., D&C, biopsy)

Treatment
* Laparoscopy & endometrial sampling for diagnosis
* Antibiotic therapy ± image-guided or surgical drainage of pelvic abscess
* In severe cases, total abdominal hysterectomy & bilateral salpingo-oophorectomy is required, due to inability to dissect ovary from tubes & uterus

DIAGNOSTIC CHECKLIST

Consider
* Consider perforated appendix with pelvic abscess if appendicolith present

Image Interpretation Pearls
* Low-level echoes in dilated fallopian tube = pyosalpinx

SELECTED REFERENCES

1. Latthe P et al: Factors predisposing women to chronic pelvic pain: systematic review. BMJ. 332(7544):749-55, 2006
2. Banikarim C et al: Pelvic inflammatory disease in adolescents. Semin Pediatr Infect Dis. 16(3):175-80, 2005
3. Barrett S et al: A review on pelvic inflammatory disease. Int J STD AIDS. 16(11):715-20; quiz 721, 2005
4. Faro S: Postpartum endometritis. Clin Perinatol. 32(3):803-14, 2005
5. Risser WL et al: The epidemiology of sexually transmitted infections in adolescents. Semin Pediatr Infect Dis. 16(3):160-7, 2005
6. Ross J: Pelvic inflammatory disease. Clin Evid. (13):2031-7, 2005
7. Banikarim C et al: Pelvic inflammatory disease in adolescents. Adolesc Med Clin. 15(2):273-85, viii, 2004
8. French LM et al: Antibiotic regimens for endometritis after delivery. Cochrane Database Syst Rev. (4):CD001067, 2004
9. Horrow MM: Ultrasound of pelvic inflammatory disease. Ultrasound Q. 20(4):171-9, 2004
10. Krivak TC et al: Tubo-ovarian abscess: diagnosis, medical and surgical management. Compr Ther. 30(2):93-100, 2004
11. Lambert MJ et al: Gynecologic ultrasound in emergency medicine. Emerg Med Clin North Am. 22(3):683-96, 2004
12. Patel DR: Management of pelvic inflammatory disease in adolescents. Indian J Pediatr. 71(9):845-7, 2004
13. Bennett GL et al: CT of the acute abdomen: gynecologic etiologies. Abdom Imaging. 28(3):416-32, 2003
14. Bennett GL et al: Gynecologic causes of acute pelvic pain: spectrum of CT findings. Radiographics. 22(4):785-801, 2002
15. Sam JW et al: Spectrum of CT findings in acute pyogenic pelvic inflammatory disease. Radiographics 22:1327-34, 2002
16. Bau A et al: Acute female pelvic pain: Ultrasound evaluation. Seminars in Ultrasound, CT, and MRI 21:78-93, 2000
17. Witlin AG et al: Septic pelvic thrombophlebitis or refractory postpartum fever of undetermined etiology. J Matern Fetal Med. 5(6):355-8, 1996
18. Taourel P et al: Role of CT in the acute nontraumatic abdomen. Semin Ultrasound CT MR. 16(2):151-64, 1995
19. McCormack WM: Pelvic inflammatory disease. NEJM 330:115-19, 1994
20. Dobrin PB et al: Radiologic diagnosis of an intra-abdominal abscess. Do multiple tests help? Arch Surg. 121(1):41-6, 1986

PELVIC INFLAMMATORY DISEASE

IMAGE GALLERY

Typical

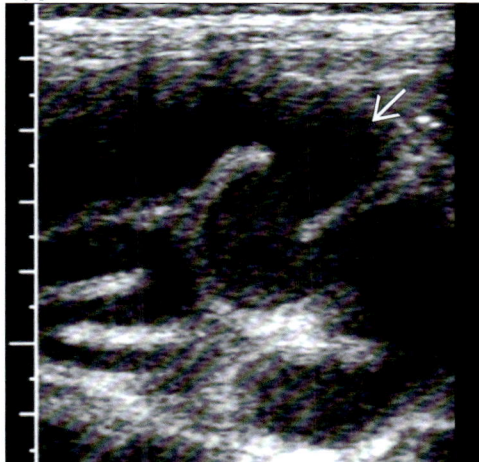
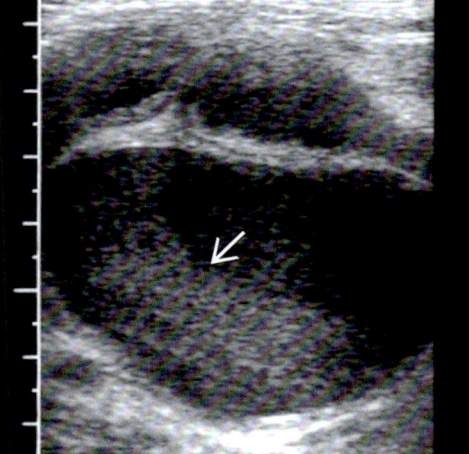

(Left) Transverse ultrasound of PID. Right adnexa demonstrates dilated fallopian tube ➔ with low-level echoes, consistent with pyosalpinx. *(Right)* Transverse ultrasound of ampullary portion of fallopian tube in same patient as left reveals rounded complex fluid collection with fluid-fluid level ➔ from TOA.

Typical

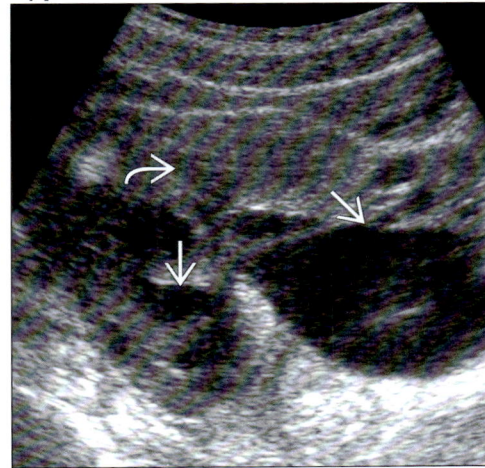
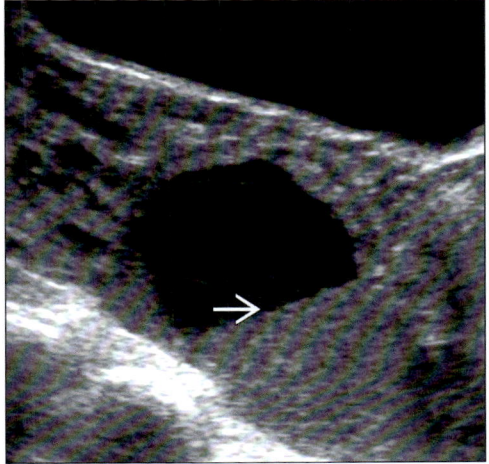

(Left) Transverse grayscale sonogram of pelvic abscesses from PID reveals bilateral complex fluid collections ➔ in cul-de-sac with loss of definition of posterior uterus ➔ (indefinite uterus sign). *(Right)* Sagittal ultrasound of pelvic abscess from PID reveals fluid collection with fluid-fluid level ➔.

Typical

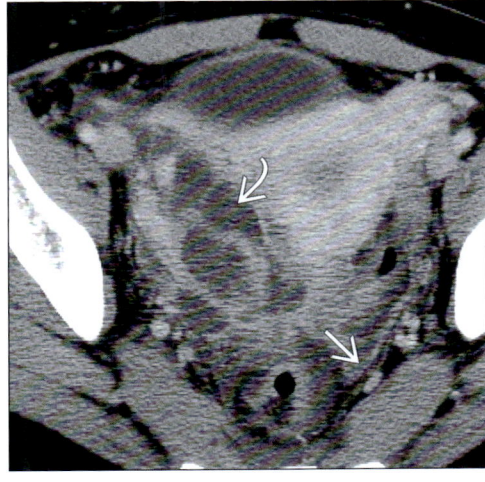
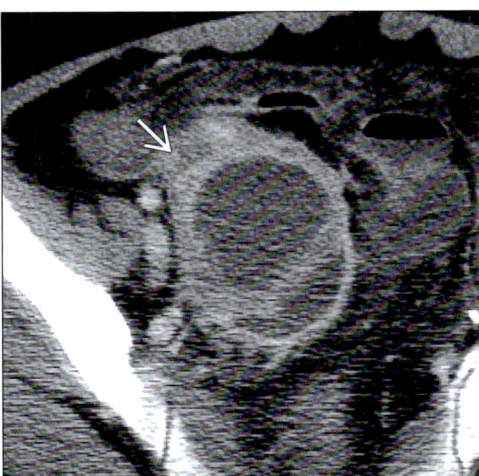

(Left) Axial CECT of acute PID with multiple abscess. Note enhancing peritoneum from peritonitis ➔ and multiple right adnexal abscesses ➔. *(Right)* Axial CECT of TOA. Note complex right adnexal cystic mass with surrounding induration of soft tissue planes ➔.

ECTOPIC PREGNANCY, TUBAL

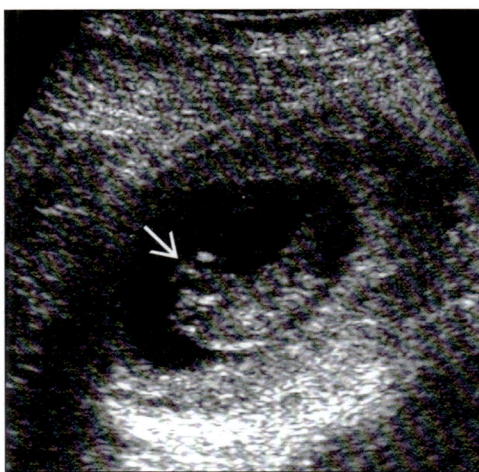

Transverse transabdominal grayscale sonography demonstrates ectopic pregnancy ➔ in right adnexa.

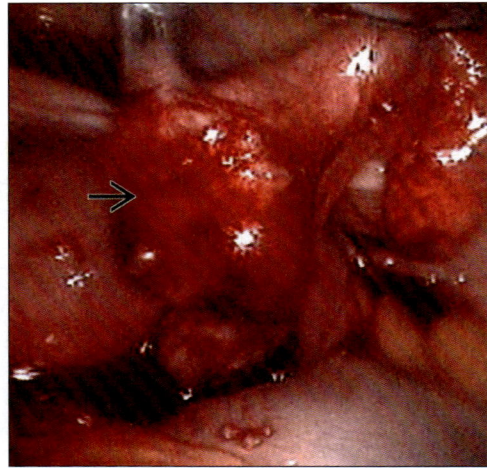

Laparoscopic image of ectopic pregnancy in same patient as left. Note acute hemorrhage from dilated right fallopian tube due to ectopic pregnancy ➔.

TERMINOLOGY

Abbreviations and Synonyms
- Ectopic pregnancy (EP)
- Extrauterine pregnancy
- Tubal pregnancy

Definitions
- Tubal implantation of gestational sac

IMAGING FINDINGS

General Features
- Best diagnostic clue: No intrauterine pregnancy (IUP), and embryo or yolk sac present within echogenic tubal ring (gestational sac in adnexa on endovaginal US)
- Location
  - 80% of EP are within ampullary portion of tube
  - 5% are in the fimbrial end of tube
  - 10-15% are cornual or interstitial
  - 0.5% are within ovary
  - Abdominal & cervical EP exceptionally rare
- Size: EP usually ruptures at 6-8 weeks with gestational sac < 4 cm
- Morphology: Rounded; echogenic tubal ring

Ultrasonographic Findings
- Uterus
  - Empty endometrial cavity
  - Intrauterine fluid collection surrounded by single decidual layer
    - Decidual cast or pseudogestational sac
    - Unlike early IUP, which has double layer of decidual reaction
- Adnexa
  - Live EP in approximately 15-25% of all EP
  - Echogenic tubal ring
    - Present in 49% of all patients with EP, 68% of patients with unruptured EP
    - Extra-ovarian in location, unlike corpus luteal cyst
    - Wall of EP ring is more echogenic than corpus luteal cyst; wall is typically more echogenic than endometrium
    - Both echogenic tubal ring and corpus luteal cyst may have prominent peripheral flow on color Doppler

DDx: Lesions Mimicking Tubal Ectopic Pregnancy

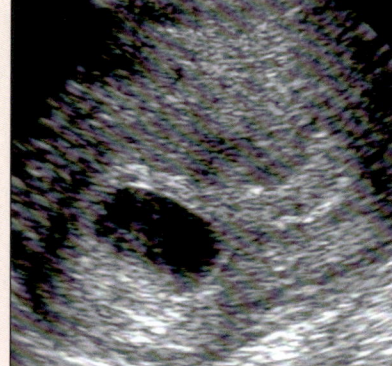
Cornual Ectopic

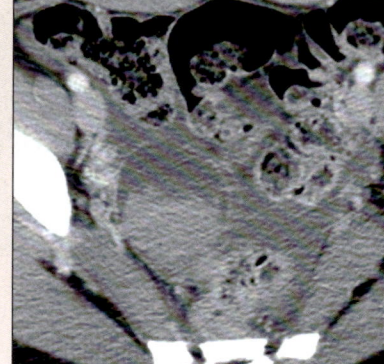
Ruptured Functional Cyst

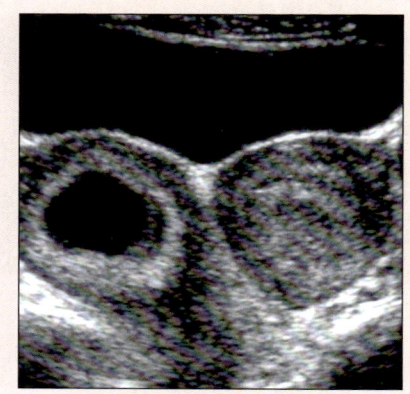
Didelphys Intrauterine Pregnancy

ECTOPIC PREGNANCY, TUBAL

Key Facts

Terminology
- Tubal implantation of gestational sac

Imaging Findings
- Best diagnostic clue: No intrauterine pregnancy (IUP), and embryo or yolk sac present within echogenic tubal ring (gestational sac in adnexa on endovaginal US)
- 80% of EP are within ampullary portion of tube
- Size: EP usually ruptures at 6-8 weeks with gestational sac < 4 cm
- Begin scanning Morrison pouch in RUQ with 3.5-6 MHz transducer to evaluate for hemoperitoneum
- Scan pelvis transabdominally if bladder full
- If bladder empty, do endovaginal scan with 5-7 MHz transducer

Top Differential Diagnoses
- Cornual Ectopic
- Ruptured Hemorrhagic Cyst
- Didelphys IUP
- Corpus Luteal Cyst
- Adnexal Torsion

Clinical Issues
- Classic clinical triad of pelvic pain, vaginal bleeding & palpable adnexal mass is present in only 65%
- Positive β-hCG with amenorrhea

Diagnostic Checklist
- Consider rupture of hemorrhagic cyst if β-hCG is negative & significant hemoperitoneum in cul-de-sac or right paracolic gutter

---

  - May or may not have yolk sac visible within echogenic ring
- Echogenic extra-ovarian adnexal mass
  - Combination of hematosalpinx & hemoperitoneum
- Echogenic clot in cul-de-sac and/or peritoneum
  - Often similar echogenicity to uterus
- Free fluid in cul-de-sac
  - Low-level echoes indicate complex fluid = hemoperitoneum

Imaging Recommendations
- Best imaging tool: US
- Protocol advice
  - Begin scanning Morrison pouch in RUQ with 3.5-6 MHz transducer to evaluate for hemoperitoneum
  - Scan pelvis transabdominally if bladder full
  - If bladder empty, do endovaginal scan with 5-7 MHz transducer
  - Use color Doppler to evaluate adnexal mass

DIFFERENTIAL DIAGNOSIS

Cornual Ectopic
- Implantation of gestation sac within interstitial (intramural) portion of fallopian tube
- Interstitial line sign on endovaginal US
  - Thin echogenic line extending from endometrial canal to cornual sac
  - Seen in 92% of cornual EP
- Ruptures later than tubal ectopic
  - Typically at 10-12 weeks
  - Associated with catastrophic hemorrhage

Ruptured Hemorrhagic Cyst
- Endovaginal US
  - Fishnet sign of intersecting strands of fibrin; avascular on color Doppler
  - Retracting clot sign with concave or linear margin
- Hemoperitoneum
  - Echogenic clot on US
  - Free fluid with low-level echoes on US
  - CT attenuation values > 30 HU

Didelphys IUP
- Uterine duplication with IUP in one horn
- Widely separated endometrial cavities with deep notch & indentation at fundus
- Associated with renal anomalies such as agenesis

Corpus Luteal Cyst
- Ovarian cyst with wall echogenicity ≤ endometrium
- Tubal ring sign of EP is typically more echogenic than endometrial cavity
- Both may demonstrate prominent peripheral flow on color Doppler

Adnexal Torsion
- β-hCG negative
- Acute severe pelvic pain; pain may subside if de-torsion occurs
- Enlarged echogenic ovary with prominent peripheral follicles on grayscale US
- Color Doppler sonography
  - Absent venous flow
  - Arterial flow may be present due to dual arterial supply to ovary

PATHOLOGY

General Features
- Etiology
  - Risk factors
    - Prior pelvic inflammatory disease (PID), particularly if inadequately treated
    - Prior tubal ectopic pregnancy
    - Tubal reconstructive surgery
    - Intrauterine device
    - Infertility treatment with in vitro fertilization
    - Increased age, smoking
- Epidemiology
  - Incidence increasing
    - EP rate increased threefold in USA from 1970-1987 (from 4.5 to 16.8/1,000 pregnancies), due to increased incidence of PID & infertility programs

ECTOPIC PREGNANCY, TUBAL

- Current EP rate is approximately 20/1,000 pregnancies & appears stable

Gross Pathologic & Surgical Features
- Unruptured tubal EP
  - Dilated fallopian tube with gestational sac
- Ruptured EP
  - Tubal perforation
  - Areas of necrosis
  - Varying degrees of hemoperitoneum

CLINICAL ISSUES

Presentation
- Most common signs/symptoms
  - Classic clinical triad of pelvic pain, vaginal bleeding & palpable adnexal mass is present in only 65%
  - Positive β-hCG with amenorrhea
- Lab data
  - Serum β-hCG > 1500 mIU with no IUP seen on endovaginal US strongly suggests EP
  - Half of all women with EP have β-hCG < 2000 mIU

Demographics
- Age: Reproductive years, 14-50 years of age
- Gender: Female

Natural History & Prognosis
- Excellent response to medical therapy (methotrexate) if early unruptured EP
- EP accounts for 15% of all maternal deaths

Treatment
- Expectant treatment if β-hCG is low (< 1000 mIU) & falling on serial follow-up, adnexal mass < 3 cm & no fetal heartbeat
- Medical treatment with methotrexate (folic acid antagonist) with unruptured EP
  - Single or serial injections if persistent EP
  - Single methotrexate has 88% success rate compared to 93% with multiple injections
- Surgical treatment for ruptured ectopic & hemoperitoneum
  - Usually involves salpingectomy if fallopian tube damage
  - Laparoscopy with salpingostomy preferred over salpingectomy in early EP
  - Conception rate 77% after surgery

DIAGNOSTIC CHECKLIST

Consider
- Consider rupture of hemorrhagic cyst if β-hCG is negative & significant hemoperitoneum in cul-de-sac or right paracolic gutter

Image Interpretation Pearls
- Pseudogestational sac mimics IUP & has only one echogenic layer around it
- Normal endovaginal US does not exclude unruptured EP

SELECTED REFERENCES
1. Kirk E et al: The non-surgical management of ectopic pregnancy. Ultrasound Obstet Gynecol. 27(1):91-100, 2006
2. Seeber BE et al: Suspected ectopic pregnancy. Obstet Gynecol. 107(2 Pt 1):399-413, 2006
3. Farquhar CM: Ectopic pregnancy. Lancet. 366(9485):583-91, 2005
4. Latchaw G et al: Risk factors associated with the rupture of tubal ectopic pregnancy. Gynecol Obstet Invest. 60(3):177-80, 2005
5. Lozeau AM et al: Diagnosis and management of ectopic pregnancy. Am Fam Physician. 72(9):1707-14, 2005
6. Murray H et al: Diagnosis and treatment of ectopic pregnancy. CMAJ. 173(8):905-12, 2005
7. Bazian Ltd: Ectopic pregnancy. Clin Evid. (11):1833-9, 2004
8. Dialani V et al: Ectopic pregnancy: a review. Ultrasound Q. 20(3):105-17, 2004
9. Fernandez H et al: Ectopic pregnancies after infertility treatment: modern diagnosis and therapeutic strategy. Hum Reprod Update. 10(6):503-13, 2004
10. Kirk E et al: Ectopic pregnancy deaths: what should we be doing? Hosp Med. 65(11):657-60, 2004
11. Luciano DE et al: Ectopic pregnancy--from surgical emergency to medical management. J Am Assoc Gynecol Laparosc. 11(1):107-21, quiz 122, 2004
12. Paspulati RM et al: Sonographic evaluation of first-trimester bleeding. Radiol Clin North Am. 42(2):297-314, 2004
13. Schollmeyer T et al: Experience of laparoscopic tubal surgery at the department of obstetrics and gynecology, University of Kiel, from 1999 through 2000. JSLS. 8(4):334-8, 2004
14. Shannon C et al: Ectopic pregnancy and medical abortion. Obstet Gynecol. 104(1):161-7, 2004
15. Sowter MC et al: Ectopic pregnancy: an update. Curr Opin Obstet Gynecol. 16(4):289-93, 2004
16. Stein MW et al: Sonographic comparison of the tubal ring of ectopic pregnancy with the corpus luteum. J Ultrasound Med. 23(1):57-62, 2004
17. Webb EM et al: Adnexal mass with pelvic pain. Radiol Clin North Am. 42(2):329-48, 2004
18. Ignacio EA et al: Ultrasound of the acute female pelvis. Ultrasound Q. 19(2):86-98; quiz 108-10, 2003
19. Olagundoye V et al: Laparoscopic surgical management of ectopic pregnancy: a district general hospital experience. J Obstet Gynaecol. 20(6):620-3, 2000
20. Akrong E et al: Ectopic pregnancy - laparoscopic management in a district general hospital. J Obstet Gynaecol. 19(6):636-9, 1999

ECTOPIC PREGNANCY, TUBAL

IMAGE GALLERY

Typical

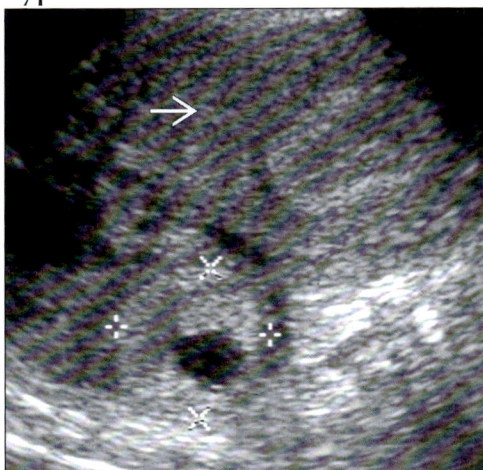 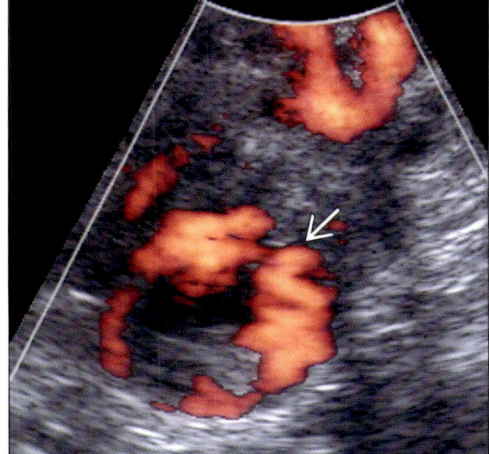

(Left) Coronal endovaginal grayscale sonography of tubal ring sign of ectopic pregnancy. Image demonstrates right adnexal echogenic ring (calipers) representing tubal EP adjacent to uterus ➔. *(Right)* Coronal endovaginal power Doppler US reveals prominent peritrophoblastic flow on periphery of tubal EP ➔.

Typical

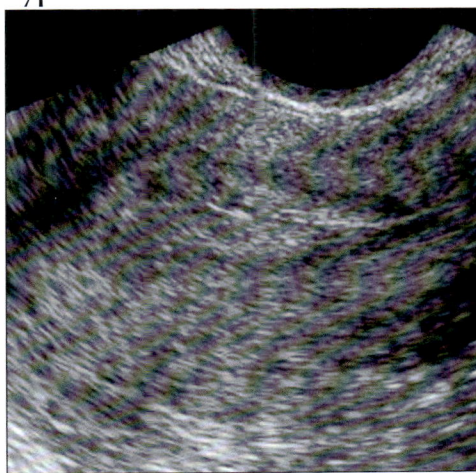 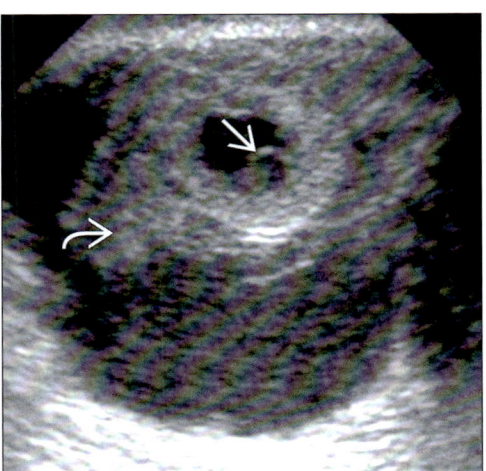

(Left) Sagittal endovaginal grayscale US of ruptured EP. Scan of uterine cavity reveals no evidence of intrauterine pregnancy. *(Right)* Coronal endovaginal grayscale US of same patient as left demonstrates tubal ectopic with visible yolk sac ➔. Note surrounding echogenic hemoperitoneum ➔.

Typical

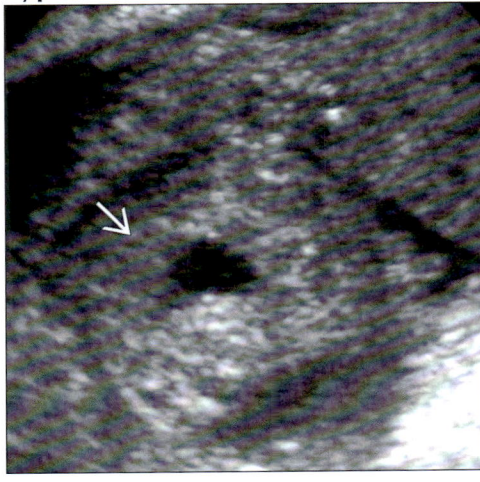 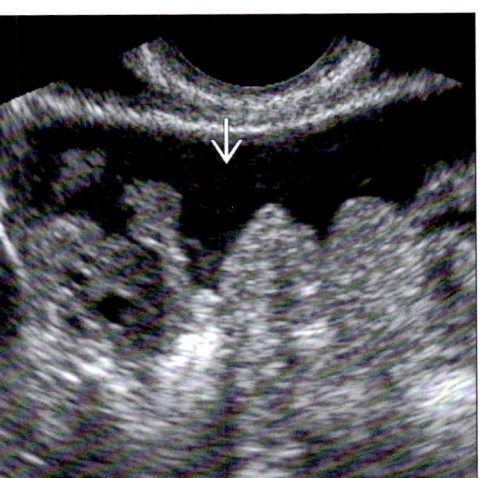

(Left) Coronal endovaginal grayscale US of ruptured EP. Scan reveals echogenic tubal ring ➔ in right adnexa. *(Right)* Sagittal transabdominal US of right flank in same patient as left reveals free fluid ➔ with low-level echoes representing hemoperitoneum.

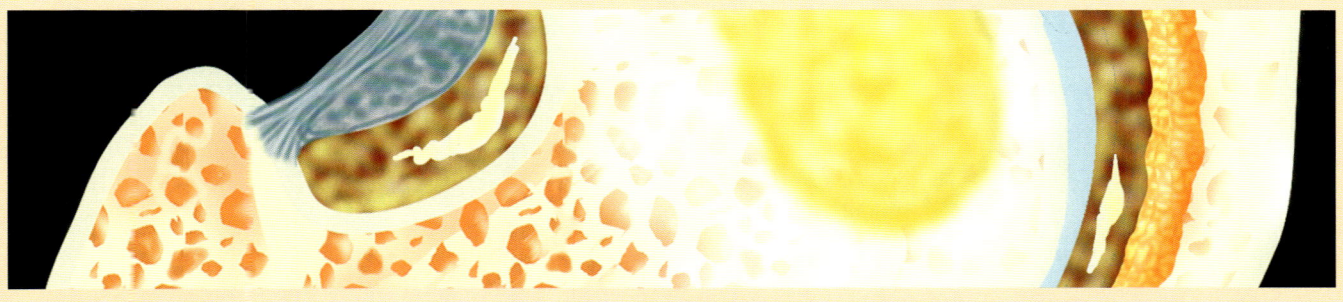

SECTION 4: Musculoskeletal

Introduction and Overview
Musculoskeletal Imaging Issues, Non-Trauma   **II**-4-2

Infection
Soft Tissue Abscess   **II**-4-4
Osteomyelitis, Adult   **II**-4-6
Osteomyelitis, Pediatric   **II**-4-10
Septic Joint   **II**-4-14
Diabetes: MSK Complications   **II**-4-18

Acute Arthritic Flares
Gout   **II**-4-22
Pyrophosphate Arthropathy   **II**-4-26
Calcific Periarthritis   **II**-4-30

Joint Swelling
Pigmented Villonodular Synovitis (PVNS)   **II**-4-34
Synovial Osteochondromatosis   **II**-4-38
Charcot, Neuropathic   **II**-4-42

Osteonecrosis
Transient Bone Marrow Edema   **II**-4-46
Osteonecrosis, Hip   **II**-4-48
Osteonecrosis, Wrist (Scaphoid & Lunate)   **II**-4-52
Osteochondritis Dissecans   **II**-4-54

Orthopedic Hardware Complications
Arthroplasty Loosening & Dislocation   **II**-4-58
Arthroplasty Hardware/Periprosthetic Fx   **II**-4-62
Arthroplasty Component Wear/Particle Disease   **II**-4-66

Miscellaneous, Systemic Diseases
Sickle Cell Anemia: MSK Complications   **II**-4-70
HIV-AIDS: MSK Complications   **II**-4-74
Hemophilia: MSK Complications   **II**-4-78

MUSCULOSKELETAL IMAGING ISSUES, NON-TRAUMA

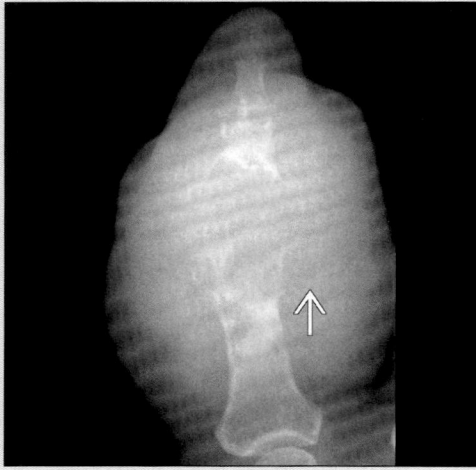

Radiograph shows a large mass which might initially suggest tumor. However, careful analysis shows it to be an articular process, with an "overhanging edge" ➔, leading to diagnosis of gout. No further workup needed.

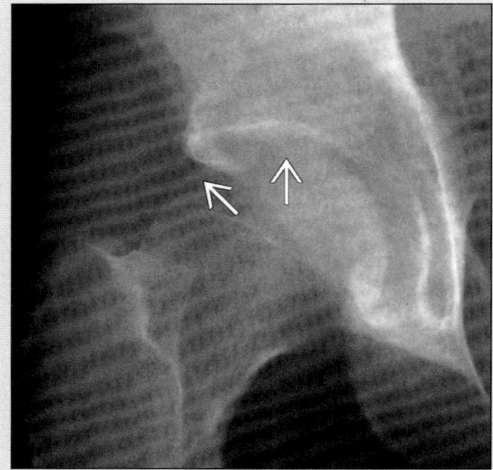

Radiograph shows osteopenia, effusion, & cortical bone destruction ➔. Septic hip must be presumed & the hip must be aspirated immediately. Further imaging would only delay this important diagnosis.

CLINICAL IMPLICATIONS

Clinical Importance
- Musculoskeletal pain is a leading cause of ER visits
- Imaging is effectively used to rapidly triage patients
  - Surgical vs. non-surgical
  - Some patients may be easily diagnosed, immediately treated, & discharged
  - Some patients require further imaging to define the disease process
    - Of these, some cases will be urgent enough to require emergent imaging (CT, MR, US)
    - Others will not need emergent imaging, but should be sent to subspecialty clinics for the work-up
- Special consideration should be made for patients with a "mass"
  - Unless abscess is suspected, further work-up is likely not emergent
  - Radiographs may help elucidate the nature of the "mass"
    - Calcification within the mass may lead to a diagnosis of myositis ossificans
    - Evidence of trauma may make the diagnosis of hematoma likely
    - Location of "mass" may identify it as an articular process
    - Destructive process may be centered on joint, making it an articular process & less likely neoplastic
  - Examples of "masses" frequently sent unnecessarily to the oncologic orthopedist
    - Sequelae of soft-tissue trauma (hematoma, myositis ossificans)
    - Arthritis & rheumatologic disorders
    - Fibroxanthoma (nonossifying fibroma)
    - Muscle inflammation & infection
    - Osteonecrosis (avascular necrosis)
    - Stress fracture & stress reaction
    - Synovial recesses & bursae
  - If there is a true mass present, referral to orthopedic oncologist is appropriate, without further immediate imaging
    - Orthopedic oncologists are more aware of the sequence & appropriateness of further imaging
    - Any biopsy should be performed by either the orthopedic oncologist or the radiologist, in conjunction with the surgeon
    - Location & direction of any biopsy or resection must be considered carefully to account for any required reconstructive surgery & performed only by those specifically trained for this

TYPES OF NON-TRAUMATIC MSK ABNORMALITIES COMMONLY SEEN IN EMERGENCY ROOM

Common Systemic Diseases Causing Acute Pain
- Diabetes: Musculoskeletal complications
  - Infection is the most important, requiring emergent diagnosis
    - If radiograph is not diagnostic, MR may be required
    - In the presence of Charcot foot, MR may not be able to unequivocally differentiate sequelae of Charcot joint from osteomyelitis & abscess
  - Fracture, Charcot joint should be diagnosed by radiograph
- Hemophilia: Musculoskeletal complications
  - Hemarthrosis: Radiographic & clinical diagnosis
  - Pseudotumor: Radiographic diagnosis; MR may be useful to fully define, but generally not emergently
- HIV-AIDS: Musculoskeletal complications
  - Infection is the most emergent; generally radiograph is suggestive
    - MR may be required for definitive diagnosis & full evaluation
  - Less emergent diagnoses: Avascular necrosis, lymphoma

MUSCULOSKELETAL IMAGING ISSUES, NON-TRAUMA

Key Facts

Imaging Used to Triage MSK Patients
- "Mass" requires special consideration
  - Unless abscess is suspected, further work-up is likely not emergent
  - Radiographs may help elucidate the nature of the "mass"
  - If there is a true mass present, refer to orthopedic oncologist, without further immediate imaging
- Infectious processes
  - Often require MR, but not emergently
- Sickle cell anemia: Musculoskeletal complications
  - Infection is most important emergent complication
    - Because of underlying infarcts, infection may be difficult to diagnose by radiograph; MR may be needed emergently
  - Less emergent diagnoses: Avascular necrosis, bone infarct
    - Often require MR, but not emergently

Joint Swelling Which May Be of Rapid Onset or Painful Enough for ER Visit
- Pyrophosphate arthropathy
  - Clinically may simulate infection ("pseudogout")
  - Radiographic appearance usually quite specific
  - Send aspirate for crystals as well as septic evaluation
- Gout: Generally classic radiographic appearance
  - Occasionally non-classic: Remember to have a high degree of suspicion
- Calcific periarthritis: May be acutely painful as calcification extrudes from tendon into bursa
  - Watch for distribution of calcific densities on radiographs

Other Monoarticular Processes Which May Be Acutely Painful
- Osteonecrosis or transient bone marrow edema: If advanced, diagnosed by radiograph
  - MR needed if not apparent on radiograph; urgent, but not emergent
  - Radiograph may be suggestive, but not acutely
  - MR may be helpful & may be needed emergently
  - Diagnosis established by needle aspiration; fluoroscopic, US, or CT may be needed for localization
- Complications of arthroplasty
  - Radiograph is generally diagnostic of all complications except infection
  - If infection is suspected, aspiration must be performed

- PVNS, synovial osteochondromatosis, osteochondritis dissecans
  - Generally suggested by radiograph
  - MR may be necessary for diagnosis: Not emergent

Infections Processes: Septic Joint, Osteomyelitis, Abscess
- Radiograph may be suggestive, but only subacutely
- MR may be helpful & may be needed emergently
- Aspiration is diagnostic; imaging with fluoroscopy, US or CT may be useful in confirming position of needle in difficult joints

Complications of Arthroplasty
- Radiograph is generally diagnostic of all complications except infection
  - Watch especially for periprosthetic fracture, which is often non-displaced
  - Dislocation & other hardware failure should be diagnosed by radiograph & high index of suspicion
- If infection is suspected, aspiration must be performed
- CT may be useful for evaluation of prosthetic loosening or particle disease with osteolysis; not emergent

RELATED REFERENCES
1. Stacy GS et al: Pitfalls in MR image interpretation prompting referrals to an orthopedic oncology clinic. Radiographics. 27:805-28, 2007

IMAGE GALLERY

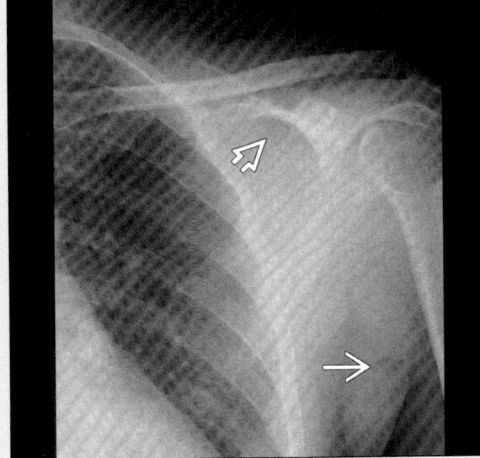
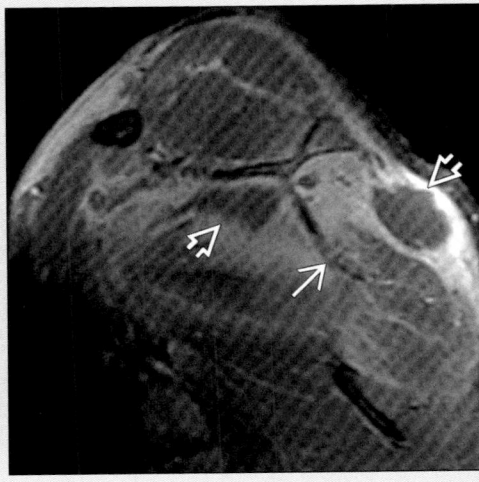

(Left) Radiograph shows air in the soft tissues ➡ & suspected osseous destruction ➡. Infection is suspected. MR is needed urgently to evaluate for osteomyelitis and/or abscess formation. (Right) Sagittal T1 C+ FS MR shows abscess formation on either side of the body of scapula ➡, with osseous destruction of the body itself ➡. MR easily confirms the diagnosis of osteomyelitis & allows early & correct triage of this patient to appropriate management. Note that CT would likely allow incomplete analysis & should not be the first choice of examination.

SOFT TISSUE ABSCESS

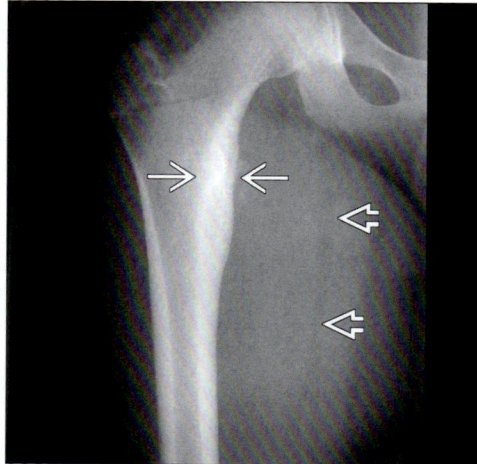

AP radiograph shows near complete obliteration of fat planes ➡. There is thick periosteal reactive bone formation ➡. The appearance is typical of soft tissue abscess with adjacent osseous reaction.

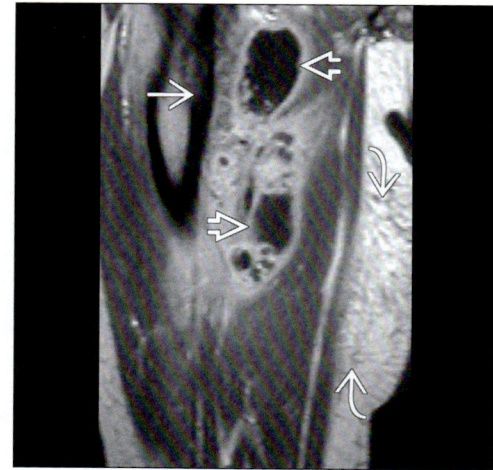

Coronal T1 C+ MR confirms multiloculated abscess ➡. Note that the bone marrow is normal, but the cortex is thickened in reaction to the adjacent abscess ➡. There is subcutaneous swelling & stranding ➡.

IMAGING FINDINGS

General Features
- Best diagnostic clue: Subtle radiographic findings, confirmed by CT, MR, or US

Radiographic Findings
- Nonspecific & subtle radiographic findings
  - Soft tissue swelling
  - Obliteration of fat plane definition
    - Tumor displaces but does not obliterate fat planes, which may help differentiate from abscess
  - Stranding in adjacent fat tissue
  - Adjacent reactive bone formation
  - Adjacent sympathetic joint effusion
- Gas in soft tissues: Rare

CT Findings
- Fluid attenuation collection by CT
- Abscess walls & internal septa enhance with CT
- Associated cellulitis
- CT can be useful for chest wall, pelvis, & thigh because of prominent fat planes
- Regions with less prominent fat planes (arm, forearm, leg) less easily diagnosed by CT

MR Findings
- Low SI T1, high SI T2 soft tissue collection by MR
- Thick enhancing rim and septa by MR
- Associated cellulitis
- Adjacent reactive bone formation
  - Periosteal/endosteal reaction
  - Patchy intermediate signal in bone; reactive vs. osteomyelitis
- +/- Saucerization of adjacent cortex & extension as osteomyelitis

Ultrasonographic Findings
- Well-defined fluid collection
- Hyperechoic rim
- +/- Debris

Imaging Recommendations
- Best imaging tool
  - MR most sensitive for deep abscess; image to define disease extent & complications
  - Aspirate/drain under US or CT control, depending on depth & accessibility

DDx: Soft Tissue Abscess

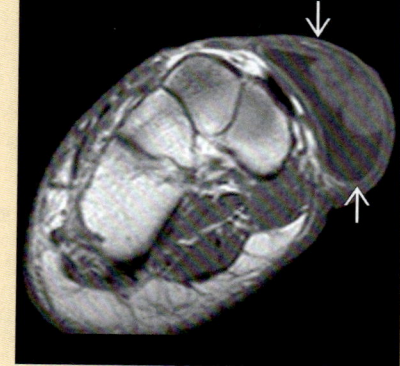
Tumor: Intact Fat Planes

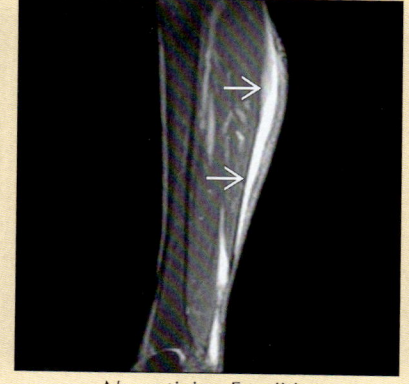
Necrotizing Fasciitis

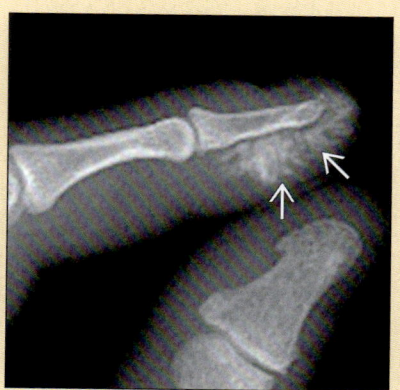
Foreign Body: Paint Gun Injury

SOFT TISSUE ABSCESS

Key Facts

Imaging Findings
- Nonspecific & subtle radiographic findings
- Obliteration of fat plane definition
- Tumor displaces but does not obliterate fat planes, which may help differentiate from abscess
- Adjacent reactive bone formation
- Fluid attenuation collection by CT
- Abscess walls & internal septa enhance with CT
- Low SI T1, high SI T2 soft tissue collection by MR
- Thick enhancing rim and septa by MR
- +/- Saucerization of adjacent cortex & extension as osteomyelitis
- MR most sensitive for deep abscess; image to define disease extent & complications

Top Differential Diagnoses
- Cellulitis
- Necrotizing Fasciitis

DIFFERENTIAL DIAGNOSIS

Cellulitis
- Usually a clinical diagnosis; image to rule out abscess or complications
- CT or MR: ↑ Attenuation or signal (respectively) with enhancement in subcutaneous fat

Necrotizing Fasciitis
- Fluid extending along fascial planes

PATHOLOGY

General Features
- Epidemiology
  - Direct inoculation
    - Trauma
    - IV drug abusers
  - Patients at risk for infection: Diabetics, end stage renal disease, steroid users

CLINICAL ISSUES

Presentation
- Most common signs/symptoms: Pain, soft tissue swelling, redness

Natural History & Prognosis
- Complications
  - May progress to severe systemic sepsis
  - Septic arthritis
  - Tenosynovitis
  - Osteomyelitis
  - Soft tissue ulceration
  - Fistula formation

Treatment
- Drainage: Either incision or percutaneous, depending on extent & location
- Appropriate antibiotics

DIAGNOSTIC CHECKLIST

Consider
- Watch for adjacent involvement of bone
- Use character of fat plane displacement/obliteration to suggest tumor vs. abscess

Image Interpretation Pearls
- Adjacent bone may show patchy increased signal as reaction & not be truly infected
- Condensed regions of low signal within marrow on T1 imaging makes osteomyelitis more likely than simple osseous reaction

SELECTED REFERENCES
1. Johnson C et al: Imaging features of soft tissue infections & other complications in drug users after direct subcutaneous injection ("skin popping"). AJR. 182:1195-202, 2004

IMAGE GALLERY

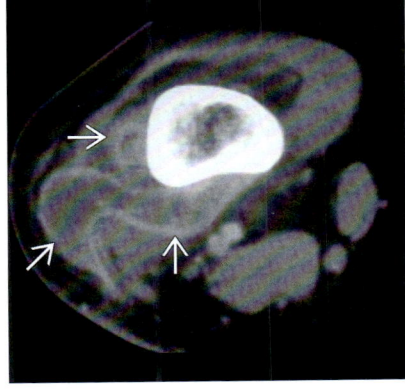 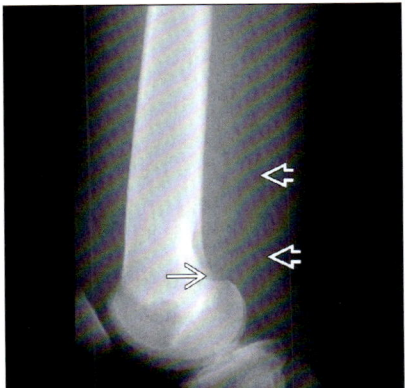 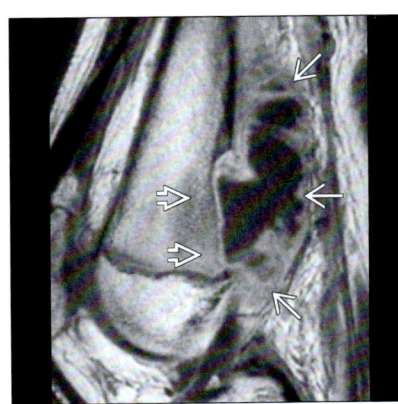

(Left) Axial CECT shows multiloculated thigh abscess, with a thick enhancing rim ➡. CT is not as ideal as MR for identifying abscess, but in the thigh where there are prominent soft tissue fat planes, it is easier than in the leg or forearm. **(Center)** Radiograph in a different patient shows obliteration of fat planes ➡ & faint scalloping of posterior cortex ➡. **(Right)** Sagittal T1 C+ MR shows large abscess ➡, with adjacent invasion of cortex & focal osteomyelitis ➡. The patient had been camping near Reno & had cervical & mediastinal adenopathy; proven Yersinia pestis.

OSTEOMYELITIS, ADULT

AP radiograph shows a multiloculated lytic lesion ➔ with dense surrounding osseous reactive bone ➔ in this middle-aged, non-English speaking patient. The appearance is highly suspicious for osteomyelitis.

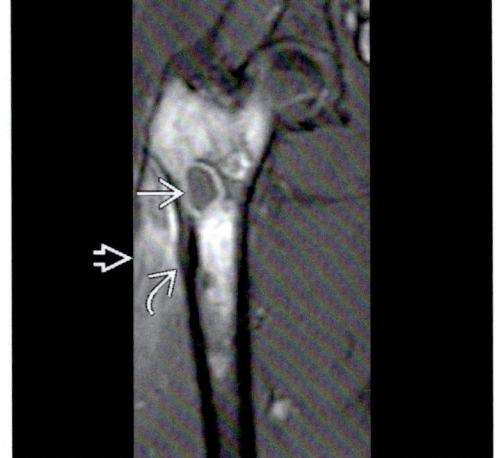

Coronal T1 C+ FS MR is confirmatory, with regions of marrow enhancement surrounding rim-enhancing fluid ➔, & cortical/endosteal reactive bone ➔. Adjacent soft tissue enhancement is without abscess ➔.

IMAGING FINDINGS

General Features
- Best diagnostic clue: Lytic destructive osseous change, often with osseous reaction
- Location
  - Long bones: With hematogenous spread, location of infection relates to vascular anatomy
    - In infants up to 12 months of age, some of metaphyseal vessels penetrate the physis & anastomose with epiphyseal vessels
    - Infections in infants therefore involve the metaphysis, epiphysis, and joint
    - Related to epiphyseal infection, infants may develop slipped epiphyses & growth deformities
    - In toddlers & older children, blood vessels terminate in loops within the metaphysis
    - Blood flow is sluggish in these terminal loops; children develop osteomyelitis in the metaphyses
    - In adults, terminal metaphyseal & epiphyseal vessels anastomose across the physeal scar
    - Adult osteomyelitis therefore may involve the joint more frequently than in a child
  - Infection rarely may be located in the cortex
  - With direct inoculation, may be diaphyseal
- Morphology
  - Destructive pattern of osteomyelitis has wide range
    - May appear as aggressive as a round cell tumor
    - May be geographic, with a sclerotic margin

Radiographic Findings
- Soft tissue abnormalities
  - ± Cellulitis, soft tissue mass
    - Mass may blur or obliterate fat planes
    - Obliteration of fat planes differentiates infectious mass from tumor, which cleanly distorts fat planes
  - Rarely, air seen in sinus tract
- Osseous abnormalities
  - No osseous change for 1-2 weeks
  - Earliest osseous change is indistinctness of cortex
  - Subacute osseous change
    - Permeative osseous destruction; may have a serpiginous, branching pattern
    - Endosteal scalloping or osseous reaction
    - Periosteal reaction
  - Late osseous change: Sequestrum & involucrum
    - Sequestrum: Necrotic bone, surrounded by purulent material or granulation tissue

Other Cases of Osteomyelitis

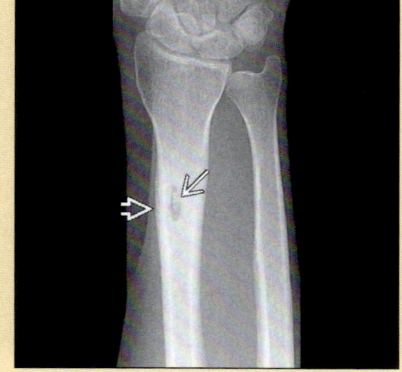
Sequestrum & Reactive Bone

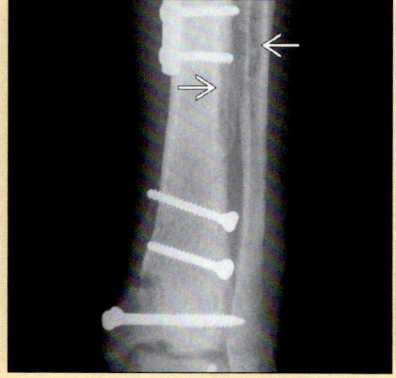
Serpiginous Tracking

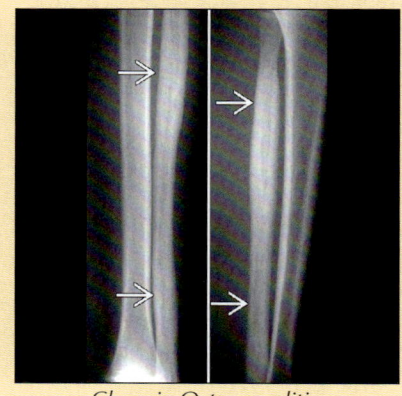
Chronic Osteomyelitis

OSTEOMYELITIS, ADULT

Key Facts

Imaging Findings
- Long bones: With hematogenous spread, location of infection relates to vascular anatomy
- Destructive pattern of osteomyelitis has wide range
- Obliteration of fat planes differentiates infectious mass from tumor, which cleanly distorts fat planes
- Earliest osseous change is indistinctness of cortex
- Permeative osseous destruction; may have a serpiginous, branching pattern
- Periosteal reaction
- Late osseous change: Sequestrum & involucrum
- Sequestrum: Necrotic bone, surrounded by purulent material or granulation tissue
- Sequestrum may harbor bacteria, serving as a source for chronic osteomyelitis
- Late osseous change: Brodie abscess

- T1: Confluent region of low signal intensity
- Fluid sensitive sequences: ↑ Signal within bone & soft tissue abscess; overly sensitive for osteomyelitis when interpreted independently of corresponding T1 MR
- Even with MR, differentiating osteomyelitis from abnormalities in Charcot foot is extremely difficult

Clinical Issues
- Pain, fever, chills
- Elevated sedimentation rate, white cell count
- May present without systemic symptoms or abnormal laboratory values
- Reactivation may be difficult to diagnose since changes of chronic osteomyelitis may mask it
- Chronic osteomyelitis with draining sinus tract may develop squamous cell carcinoma

---

- Sequestrum is usually normal density (due to loss of blood supply), with surrounding osteopenia
- Sequestrum may harbor bacteria, serving as a source for chronic osteomyelitis
- Involucrum: Bone shell surrounding purulent material & sequestrum
- Cloaca: Cortical & periosteal defect through which pus drains from infected medullary cavity
  - Late osseous change: Brodie abscess
    - Lytic, generally oval lesion with sclerotic, well-marginated rim
    - Surrounding osseous sclerosis
    - Dense, regular periosteal reaction
    - Less aggressive appearance than acute osteomyelitis
    - Generally in a child, and metaphyseal
    - May be found in the epiphysis of a very young child (differential of chondroblastoma and Langerhans cell histiocytosis)
    - May not have associated fever or laboratory abnormalities (↑ sedimentation rate or WBC)

CT Findings
- Osseous lytic destructive change, often with serpiginous tracking
- Reactive bone formation
  - Central, endosteal, or periosteal
- Obliteration of soft tissue planes
- Enhancing rim around bone or soft tissue abscess

MR Findings
- Highly sensitive & specific when contrast is utilized
- Air may be seen in soft tissue ulcer/sinus tract: Low signal on all sequences
- T1: Confluent region of low signal intensity
  - Unequivocal confluence of decreased signal increases specificity of MR
  - Differentiated from the hazy reticulated pattern seen with bone reaction to adjacent soft tissue infection
- Fluid sensitive sequences: ↑ Signal within bone & soft tissue abscess; overly sensitive for osteomyelitis when interpreted independently of corresponding T1 MR
- Subcutaneous edema common

- Contrast shows enhancing rim around abscess & within bone
  - Remember that tumor necrosis may show central low signal with surrounding enhancement
- Even with MR, differentiating osteomyelitis from abnormalities in Charcot foot is extremely difficult

Nuclear Medicine Findings
- Multiphase Tc-99m bone scanning shows ↑ tracer uptake on all phases in acute osteomyelitis
- Osteomyelitis may be "cold" on delayed images of bone scan, especially in children in early acute phase
- Gallium-67 nearly 100% sensitive for osteomyelitis, but nonspecific
- Combined WBC imaging & complementary bone marrow imaging with Tc-99m sulfur colloid 90% accurate for diagnosing osteomyelitis
- Recent meta-analysis suggests high accuracy of FDG PET to diagnose chronic osteomyelitis

Imaging Recommendations
- Best imaging tool
  - Radiograph is appropriately the first-line test; relatively insensitive; MR is gold standard
  - Even MR may be nonspecific for osteomyelitis in the presence of Charcot joint changes
- Protocol advice
  - T1 imaging in at least 2 planes is useful to differentiate osseous changes due to osteomyelitis from those due to reactive bone change
  - Post contrast imaging is mandatory

DIFFERENTIAL DIAGNOSIS

Round Cell Tumor
- Round cell tumor (Ewing sarcoma, lymphoma): Same degree of aggressiveness as osteomyelitis
- In children, metastatic neuroblastoma shows same degree of aggressiveness
- Langerhans cell histiocytosis: May occasionally be as aggressive as osteomyelitis

OSTEOMYELITIS, ADULT

Cortical Osteomyelitis: Osteoid Osteoma or Stress Fracture with Reaction
- Osteoid osteoma may show a rounded central lucency; however, this nidus may be masked by reactive bone
- Stress fracture may show a linear pattern of sclerosis

Diabetic Foot: Charcot Changes vs. Osteomyelitis in the Presence of Charcot
- Charcot foot may have large fluid collections with enhancing rim, even in absence of sepsis
- Charcot foot may have soft tissue ulceration
- Charcot foot may show reactive bone changes: Decreased T1 signal, increased signal on fluid sensitive sequences, enhancement, even without sepsis
- Factors which help to differentiate the two
  - Confluent T1 signal seen in bone with osteomyelitis; reticulated hazy signal in reactive bone
  - Osseous fragments more likely to be seen in Charcot fluid collections than abscess from infection
  - Sinus tracts & soft tissue fat replacement more common with infection
  - Diffuse joint fluid enhancement more common in infection; thin rim-enhancement in Charcot

PATHOLOGY

General Features
- Etiology
  - Hematogenous spread is most frequent
    - Neonates: Staphylococcus aureus, group B Streptococcus, Escherichia coli
    - Normal child: Staphylococcus aureus most common
    - Children & adults with sickle cell disease: Staphylococcus predominates, but Salmonella has higher incidence than normal
    - Normal adults: Staphylococcus most frequent; enteric pathogens also seen
    - IV drug users: Often gram negative species (Pseudomonas, Klebsiella)
  - Soft tissue ulceration & contiguous spread
  - Soft tissue infection of hand or foot spreads along fascial planes & tendon sheaths
    - Site of osteomyelitis may be distant from the initial soft tissue injury
  - Hand bones at risk from infection from human bite (particularly if skin broken from punching mouth)
  - Stubbed toe with hematoma beneath nail bed (nail bed is adjacent to periosteum)
  - Direct blow with hematoma formation
  - Systemic diseases may increase risk of osteomyelitis
    - Diabetic patients
    - HIV-AIDS patients
    - Sickle cell anemia patients
  - Tuberculosis or fungal osteomyelitis
    - Slower course than bacterial osteomyelitis
    - Demonstrate less host reaction than pyogenic osteomyelitis
    - May be first seen as dactylitis in child
  - Syphilis osteomyelitis
    - Congenital: Metaphyseal irregularity & periostitis
    - Acquired: Chronic osteomyelitis with periostitis & enlarged, bowed bone ("saber shin" tibia)
  - Chronic recurrent multifocal osteomyelitis (plasma cell osteomyelitis)
    - Children & adolescents
    - Repeated episodes of pain & soft tissue swelling
    - Infectious organism identified only by biopsy (or may never be identified)
    - Radiographs often normal; diagnosed by MR

CLINICAL ISSUES

Presentation
- Most common signs/symptoms
  - Pain, fever, chills
  - Elevated sedimentation rate, white cell count
  - May present without systemic symptoms or abnormal laboratory values

Natural History & Prognosis
- Acute osteomyelitis
  - If untreated may progress to aggressive destruction & abscess formation
  - If untreated may be walled off by reactive bone & progress to chronic osteomyelitis
- Chronic osteomyelitis
  - May appear unchanged for years, then reactivate
  - Reactivation may be difficult to diagnose since changes of chronic osteomyelitis may mask it
  - Serial imaging may show new destruction
  - If no radiographic progression, bone scanning and/or tagged leukocyte nuclear medicine scanning may improve specificity
  - Chronic osteomyelitis with draining sinus tract may develop squamous cell carcinoma
    - Generally after several years of drainage
    - New pain & bone destruction in the setting of chronic drainage should suggest the diagnosis
    - Generally difficult to treat; high mortality rate

DIAGNOSTIC CHECKLIST

Consider
- Time course of destructive changes in osteomyelitis is faster than tumor
  - Exception is Langerhans cell histiocytosis, which rarely may show extremely rapid destruction

SELECTED REFERENCES

1. Ahmadi ME et al: Neuropathic arthropathy of the foot with and without superimposed osteomyelitis: MR imaging characteristics. Radiology. 238(2):622-31, 2006
2. Palestro CJ et al: Combined labeled leukocyte and technetium 99m sulfur colloid bone marrow imaging for diagnosing musculoskeletal infection. Radiographics. 26(3):859-70, 2006
3. Collins MS et al: T1-weighted MRI characteristics of pedal osteomyelitis. AJR Am J Roentgenol. 185(2):386-93, 2005
4. Termaat MF et al: The accuracy of diagnostic imaging for the assessment of chronic osteomyelitis: a systematic review and meta-analysis. J Bone Joint Surg Am. 87(11):2464-71, 2005

OSTEOMYELITIS, ADULT

IMAGE GALLERY

Typical

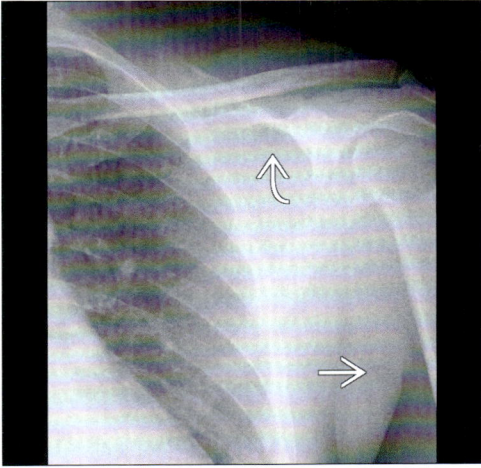
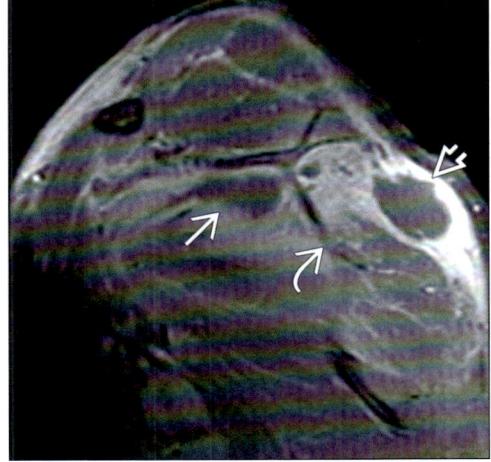

(Left) This patient recently arrived from Africa with shoulder pain & swelling. The radiograph shows air within the soft tissues ➡, as well as a lytic lesion in the scapula ➡. *(Right)* Sagittal T1 C+ FS MR confirms osteomyelitis, with destructive change seen within the scapula ➡, & abscesses within the subscapularis ➡ and infraspinatus ➡ muscles. The aspirate cultured out Staphylococcus.

Typical

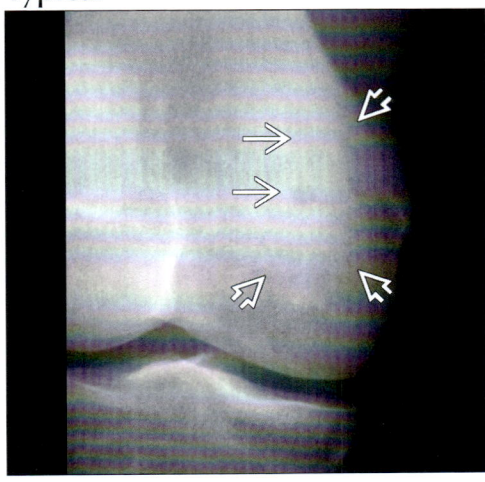
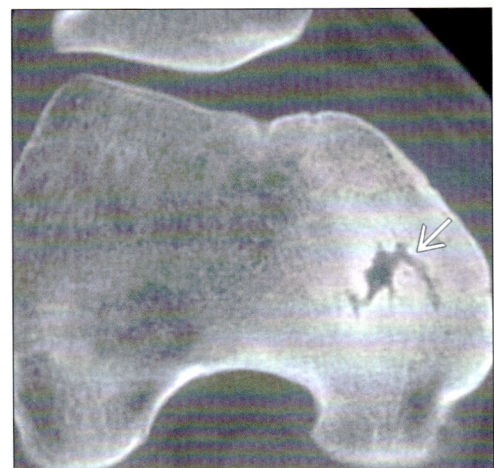

(Left) Anteroposterior radiograph shows classic findings for osteomyelitis. There is a permeative lucency in the medial femoral condyle ➡, surrounded by fairly dense reactive bone formation ➡, which is typically seen. *(Right)* Axial bone CT confirms the permeative pattern of bone destruction, which actually involves this entire cross-section, but also has the focal lytic region noted on radiograph ➡, with serpiginous branching.

Typical

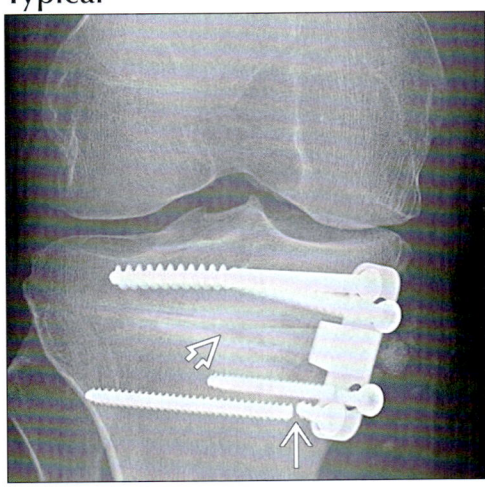
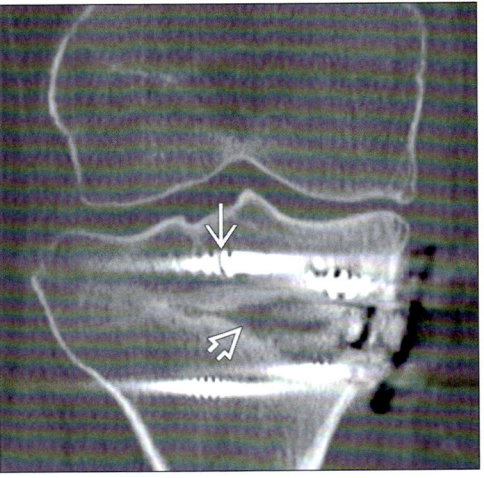

(Left) AP radiograph shows screw fracture ➡ in high tibial osteotomy, & resorption/irregularity of the host bone ➡. This is highly suspicious for failure due to osteomyelitis. *(Right)* Coronal bone CT confirms a 2nd fractured screw ➡. The host bone adjacent to the bone graft shows resorption as well as dense bone reaction ➡. This is more typical of destructive change related to osteomyelitis (culture proven) than resorption & bone bridging.

OSTEOMYELITIS, PEDIATRIC

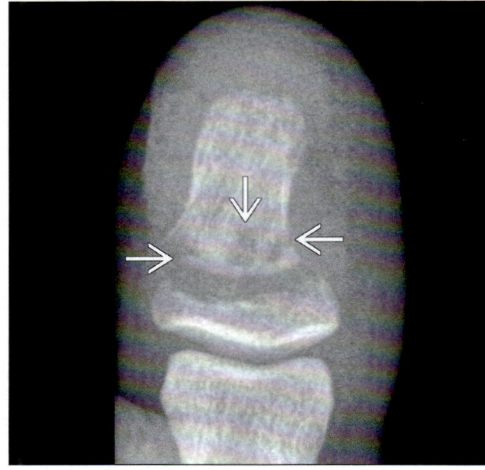

Anteroposterior radiograph shows areas of osteomyelitis ➡ in toe distal phalanx 12 days after a Salter-Harris type II fracture, an injury that is often an open/compound fracture.

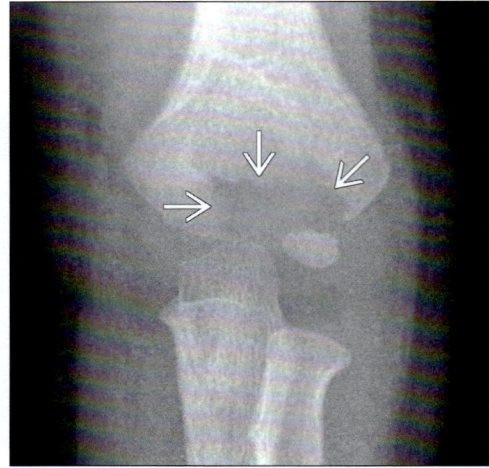

Anteroposterior radiograph shows osteomyelitis ➡ due to Streptococcus, type A, in the distal humerus of a 3 year old.

TERMINOLOGY

Definitions
- Bone and bone marrow inflammation usually due to an infectious agent: Bacterial mostly; fungal, viral, parasitic occasionally

IMAGING FINDINGS

General Features
- Best diagnostic clue: Aggressive destructive lesion in metaphysis of child < 5 years old
- Location
  - Long-bone metaphyses 70% (femur > tibia > humerus > fibula), short bones 6%, pelvis 5%, spine 2%
  - Calvaria
    - Potts puffy tumor of scalp: Subgaleal abscess forms over osteomyelitis; usually due to frontal sinusitis
    - Infected cephalohematoma
  - Mandible
    - Primary chronic osteomyelitis: Nonsuppurative, noninfectious
    - Actinomycosis
  - Cervical spine
    - Adenoidectomy a cause of osteomyelitis
  - Pelvis: Symptoms mimic urinary tract infection, septic hip, acute abdomen, radiculitis
  - Calcaneus
    - Puncture through sole: Inferior cortex, Pseudomonas (P) aeruginosa
    - Hematogenous: Posterior half near apophysis
  - Great toe
    - Stubbing → hyperflexion → distal phalanx physeal distraction fracture → nail bed disruption → distal phalanx osteomyelitis

Radiographic Findings
- Radiography
  - Absence of findings does not exclude osteomyelitis
  - Earliest finding: Soft tissue swelling next to bone
  - Displacement or obliteration of fat planes
  - Bony destruction 7-14 days (or longer) after onset
    - Vague lucency → permeation → destruction
  - Periosteal reaction seen at 7-10 days

DDx: Osteolytic Lesions

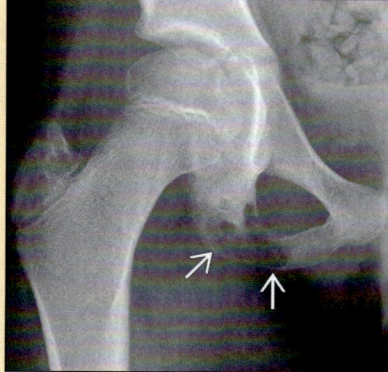

Langerhans Cell Histiocytosis

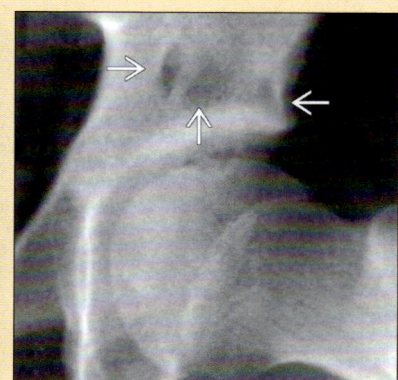

Ewing Sarcoma

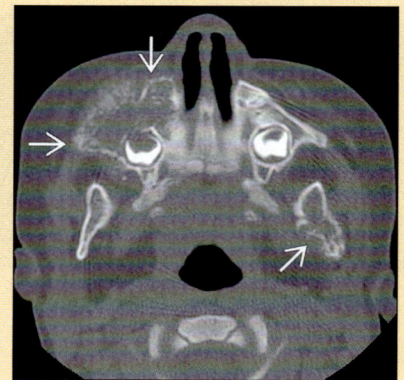

Neuroblastoma Metastases

OSTEOMYELITIS, PEDIATRIC

Key Facts

Imaging Findings
- Best diagnostic clue: Aggressive destructive lesion in metaphysis of child < 5 years old
- Long-bone metaphyses 70% (femur > tibia > humerus > fibula), short bones 6%, pelvis 5%, spine 2%
- Pelvis: Symptoms mimic urinary tract infection, septic hip, acute abdomen, radiculitis
- Earliest finding: Soft tissue swelling next to bone
- CT: Bone destruction, intramedullary gas and fat-fluid level, periosteal reaction, sequestrum, involucrum
- Well-defined areas that do not enhance with gadolinium: Suspect necrosis or abscess formation
- Grayscale Ultrasound: Excludes/includes pyarthrosis, shows soft tissue swelling, also periosteal thickening, hyperemia and elevation due to subperiosteal abscess
- Bone scan: Positive 24-72 hours, demonstrates multiple sites
- Best imaging tool: MR best choice when abscess recognition will dictate need for surgery

Pathology
- Tendency to occur in metaphyses or metaphyseal equivalents (bone next to cartilage, e.g., calcaneal apophysis and acetabulum)
- Staphylococcus (S) aureus commonest (43%), then β-hemolytic streptococcus (S) (10%) and S. pneumoniae (10%)

Clinical Issues
- Incidence 1-3:1,000 in neonatal intensive care

  - Chronic osteomyelitis: Sclerosis or mixed sclerotic/lucent; lucent tract extending through cortex; sequestrum (radiodense)

CT Findings
- NECT
  - CT: Bone destruction, intramedullary gas and fat-fluid level, periosteal reaction, sequestrum, involucrum
  - CT: Increased attenuation of involved marrow
- CECT: Rim-enhancement of intra- and extraosseous abscesses
- Bony destruction/sclerosis
- Surrounding soft tissue swelling
- CT may be performed to better delineate bony changes
  - Lucent tract through cortex
  - Bony sequestrum

MR Findings
- T1WI: Marrow edema: Hypointense signal
- T2WI
  - Marrow edema: Hyperintense signal
  - Cellulitis and sinus tracts: Hyperintense signal
  - Extramedullary fat-fluid level
    - Cortical perforation allows marrow fat to leak outside bone
- STIR: Marrow edema: Hyperintense signal
- T1 C+
  - Enhancement: Marrow and periosteal inflammation
  - Abscess: Peripheral enhancement/central nonenhancement
- Usually large areas of surrounding edema in soft tissue/marrow
- Well-defined areas that do not enhance with gadolinium: Suspect necrosis or abscess formation

Ultrasonographic Findings
- Grayscale Ultrasound: Excludes/includes pyarthrosis, shows soft tissue swelling, also periosteal thickening, hyperemia and elevation due to subperiosteal abscess

Nuclear Medicine Findings
- Bone Scan
  - Increased uptake in angiographic, blood-pool, and delayed phases; sensitivity 82%
    - Central photopenia if intraosseous infarct or abscess
  - Bone scan: Positive 24-72 hours, demonstrates multiple sites

Other Modality Findings
- Brodie abscess
  - Intramedullary, lytic on CT, target appearance on MR, geographic destruction, well-defined edges, marginal sclerosis, no bone enlargement
  - Metadiaphysis of tubular bones: 63% lower extremities

Imaging Recommendations
- Best imaging tool: MR best choice when abscess recognition will dictate need for surgery
- Protocol advice: T1, T2 FS, STIR, T1 C+
- If suspicious of focal area based on symptoms or radiographic findings: MR
- If area of involvement not clear or multiple areas suspected: Bone scintigraphy
- If further evaluating sclerotic bone lesion: CT

DIFFERENTIAL DIAGNOSIS

Permeative Bone Lesion in Child < 5 Years
- Osteomyelitis
- Langerhans cell histiocytosis (LCH)
- Neuroblastoma metastasis

Permeative Bone Lesion in Child > 5 Years
- Ewing sarcoma
- Lymphoma
- Leukemia
- Osteomyelitis
- Langerhans cell histiocytosis

OSTEOMYELITIS, PEDIATRIC

PATHOLOGY

General Features
- General path comments
  - Tendency to occur in metaphyses or metaphyseal equivalents (bone next to cartilage, e.g., calcaneal apophysis and acetabulum)
    - Thought related to rich but slow-moving blood supply to these regions
- Etiology
  - Staphylococcus (S) aureus commonest (43%), then β-hemolytic streptococcus (S) (10%) and S. pneumoniae (10%)
    - Penetrating trauma: P. aeruginosa
    - Sickle cell disease: Salmonella
  - SAPHO syndrome: Synovitis, acne, pustulosis, hyperostosis, osteitis
    - Recurrent multifocal osteomyelitis of long-bone metaphyses and medial clavicles
  - CRMO: Chronic recurrent multifocal osteomyelitis
    - Non-pyogenic, unknown cause, prolonged or recurrent course, children and adolescents
- Epidemiology
  - 1/5,000 children < 13 years in USA; 1:800-1:10,000 elsewhere
  - Three routes of infection: Hematogenous, contiguous, direct implantation
  - Neonates at highest risk
    - Immature host-defense system
    - Transphyseal sinusoids connect metaphyseal and epiphyseal blood vessels allowing metaphyseal-epiphyseal infection spread: Increased incidence of epiphyseal damage
    - Newborn intensive care babies: Umbilical catheter a risk factor
    - Most common: S. aureus, β streptococcus, Candida (C) albicans

Gross Pathologic & Surgical Features
- Inflammation: Inflammatory cellular response
  - Myelitis
    - Involvement of fat and hematopoietic tissue
    - Abscess if ischemia (increased intraosseous pressure), infarct, necrosis, and liquefaction
  - Osteitis
    - Involvement of cortical and trabecular bone
    - If bone necrosis and resorption: Cortex porous/fenestrated exposing subperiosteal space to infection
    - Sequestrum if large volume necrotic; subsequently extruded, surgically removed, or dissolved by osteoclasts
  - Periostitis
    - Subperiosteal abscess
    - Periosteal elevation: Cortical bone infarct due to interrupted blood supply
    - Subperiosteal new bone formation

CLINICAL ISSUES

Presentation
- Most common signs/symptoms: Fever, pain, tenderness
- Neonatal osteomyelitis
  - Nonspecific: Lethargy, irritability, poor feeding, unstable temperature
  - Specific: Limited movement or discomfort with movement, tenderness, pseudoparalysis, swelling, warmth, erythema
  - Hematogenous origin
  - Commonest: Humerus, femur, tibia, fibula
  - Accompanying septic arthritis frequent
- Because of young age, presentation typically nonspecific and diagnosis delayed
- May present with fever of unknown origin, sepsis, chronic irritability
- Sickle cell disease: Osteomyelitis frequently due to salmonella as well as S. aureus
- Erythrocyte sedimentation rate elevated in vast majority

Demographics
- Age
  - Primarily a disease of infants and young children
    - 1/3 cases occur before 2 years of age
    - 1/2 cases occur before 5 years of age
  - Incidence 1-3:1,000 in neonatal intensive care
  - Vertebral osteomyelitis: Age 8-20 years
  - Vertebral diskitis: Age < 5 years

Natural History & Prognosis
- Neonatal osteomyelitis: 40% have later extremity shortening/deformity due to physeal injury
- Adjacent septic arthritis common when age < 1

Treatment
- Identify infectious agent: Imaging-guided needle aspiration or open surgical biopsy
- Antibiotics, pain management
- Surgery/intervention
  - Abscess (intraosseous, subperiosteal, parosteal) drainage, sequestrectomy, management of sinus tracts and pathological fractures

SELECTED REFERENCES
1. Pineda C et al: Imaging of osteomyelitis: current concepts. Infect Dis Clin North Am. 20(4):789-825, 2006
2. Saigal G et al: Imaging of osteomyelitis with special reference to children. Semin Musculoskelet Radiol. 8(3):255-65, 2004
3. Ibia EO et al: Group A beta-hemolytic streptococcal osteomyelitis in children. Pediatrics. 112(1 Pt 1):e22-6, 2003
4. Studler U et al: Widening of the greater trochanteric physis in the immature skeleton: a radiographic sign of femoral osteomyelitis (2003:6b). Eur Radiol. 13(9):2238-40, 2003
5. Kleinman PK: A regional approach to osteomyelitis of the lower extremities in children. Radiol Clin North Am. 40(5):1033-59, 2002
6. Oudjhane K et al: Imaging of osteomyelitis in children. Radiol Clin North Am. 39(2):251-66, 2001

OSTEOMYELITIS, PEDIATRIC

IMAGE GALLERY

Typical

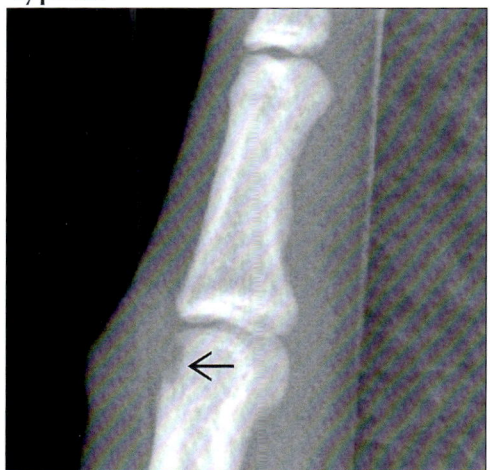 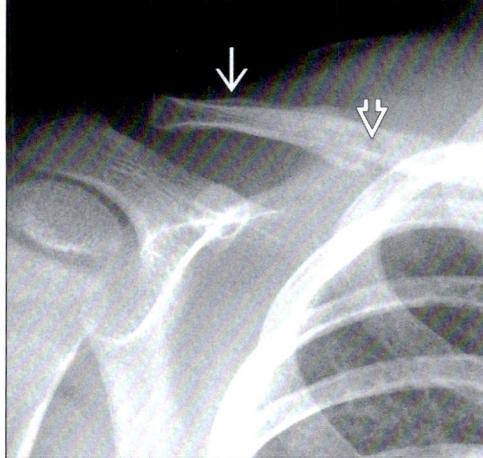

(Left) Lateral radiograph shows an area of osteomyelitis ➡ in the cortex of index finger's proximal phalanx 32 days after accidental laceration by opponent's teeth during a basketball game. *(Right)* Anteroposterior radiograph shows periosteal reaction ➡ and focal bone destruction ➡ due to Staphylococcus aureus osteomyelitis of the clavicle.

Typical

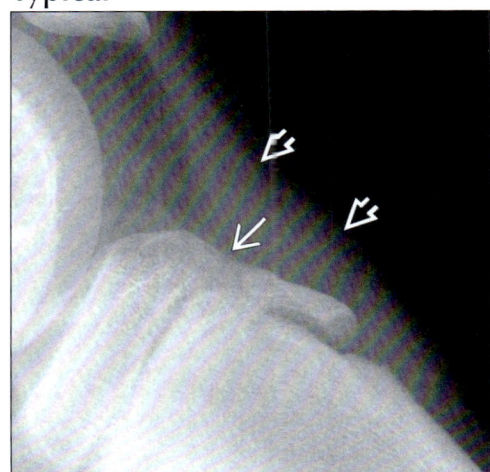 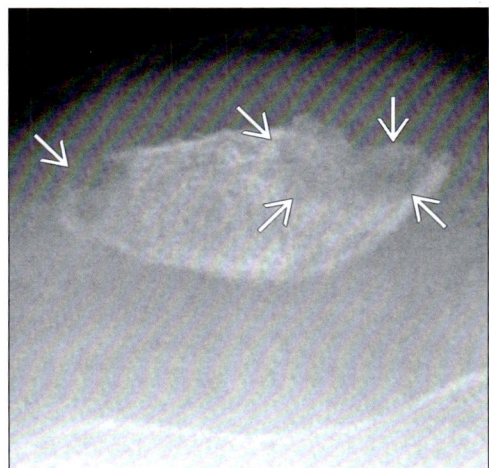

(Left) Lateral radiograph shows focal cortical destruction ➡ in tibial epiphysis osteomyelitis with inflammation extending into patellar tendon ➡. *(Right)* Sunrise radiograph shows areas of patellar osteomyelitis ➡ due to Staphylococcus aureus.

Typical

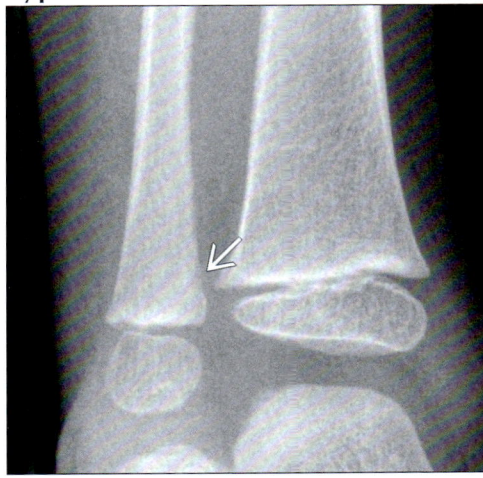 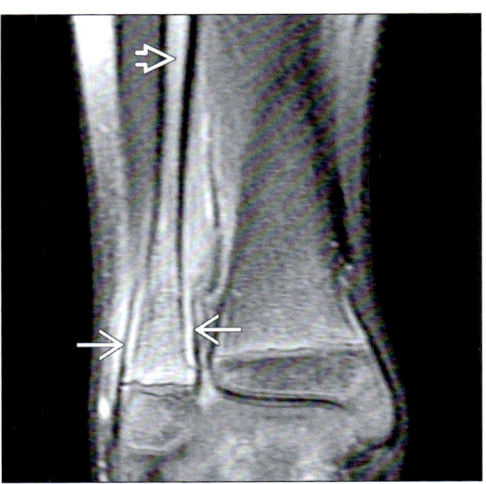

(Left) Oblique radiograph shows subtle bone loss ➡ in the fibular cortex. *(Right)* Coronal T1 C+ FS MR shows fibular osteomyelitis with elevated periosteum ➡ and marrow enhancement ➡ in the same child as previous image.

SEPTIC JOINT

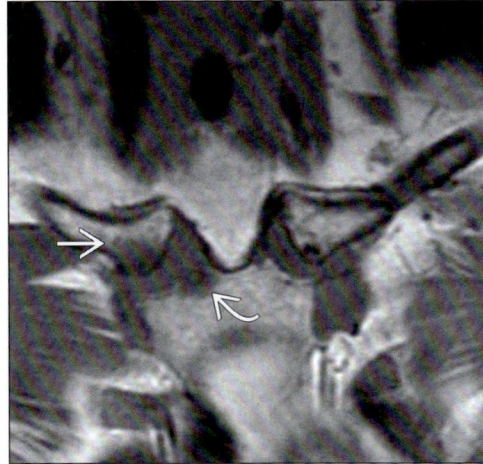

Angled coronal T1WI MR shows decreased signal intensity in the clavicle ➡ & adjacent manubrium ➡ in a 65 year old woman. The elderly are at particular risk for developing septic arthritis at this site.

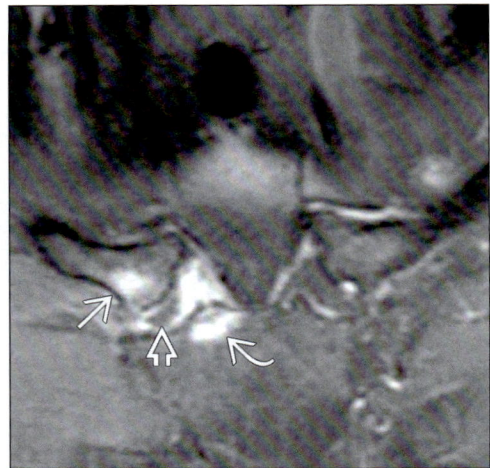

Angled coronal T2WI FS MR shows ↑ signal in the clavicle ➡, adjacent manubrium ➡, & fluid within the joint (⇨ shows the disk in the joint). Note how well the joint is depicted with this angulation.

TERMINOLOGY

Abbreviations and Synonyms
- Infectious arthritis; pyogenic arthritis, bacterial arthritis, nonpyogenic arthritis, nonbacterial arthritis

IMAGING FINDINGS

General Features
- Best diagnostic clue: Effusion seen by radiograph or ultrasound; may be associated with decreased joint space (cartilage destruction), osteopenia, & osseous destruction
- Location
  ○ Any joint is at risk; knee most common in adults
  ○ Hip especially at risk in children
  ○ Sacroiliac joint & sternoclavicular joint at particular risk in diabetics, HIV-AIDS, IV drug abusers

Radiographic Findings
- Early in process, radiographs are normal
- With progression, nonspecific findings
- First sign: Joint effusion
  ○ Bulging fat planes
  ○ Radiographic signs of hip effusion
    ■ Requires perfect AP pelvis with hips in internal rotation
    ■ Fat planes: Obturator, gluteal, iliopsoas
    ■ Increased distance between radiographic teardrop and femoral metaphysis, compared to contralateral hip
    ■ Air arthrogram with traction on hip rules out effusion
  ○ Radiographic signs of knee effusion
    ■ Suprapatellar effusion
    ■ Obliteration of Hoffa fat pad
  ○ Radiographic signs of ankle effusion
    ■ Bulging anterior fat pad at tibiotalar joint
    ■ Dorsiflexion of tibiotalar joint: False positive
  ○ Radiographic signs of shoulder effusion
    ■ None; glenohumeral joint is large & can decompress into subscapularis bursa
  ○ Radiographic signs of elbow effusion
    ■ Bulging anterior fat pad (sail sign)
    ■ Presence of posterior fat pad
  ○ Radiographic signs of wrist effusion
    ■ Bulging pronator fat pad

Other Septic Joints: Radiographic Findings

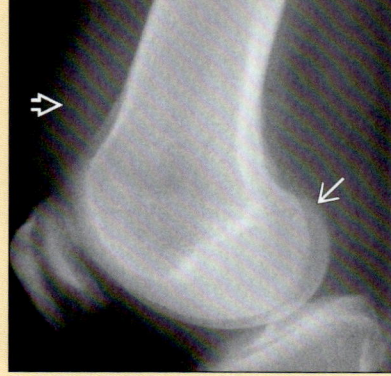

Effusion + Deossification

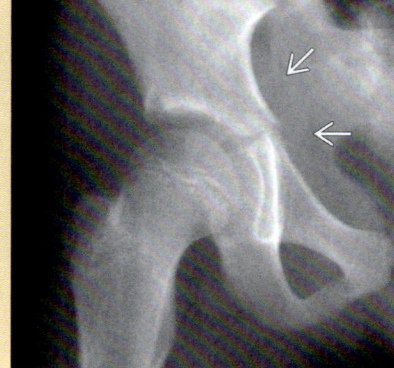

Obturator Fat Pad = Effusion

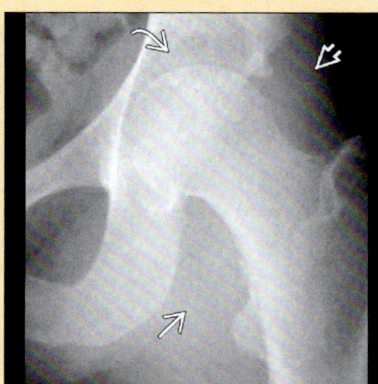

Effusion + Cortical Destruction

SEPTIC JOINT

Key Facts

Imaging Findings
- Any joint is at risk; knee most common in adults
- Hip especially at risk in children
- Sacroiliac joint & sternoclavicular joint at particular risk in diabetics, HIV-AIDS, IV drug abusers
- First sign: Joint effusion
- Hyperemia leads to periarticular osteoporosis
- Cartilage destruction (joint space narrowing)
- Cortical bone becomes indistinct
- Marginal erosions
- Sclerotic host reaction if septic joint is bacterial
- MR sensitive (100%) & more specific (77%) than other imaging; abnormal within 24 hours of onset
- Synovial enhancement 98%
- Marrow abnormal T2 signal 84% & abnormal enhancement 81%
- Perisynovial edema 84%
- Joint effusion 70% (almost 1/3 lack an effusion; joints of hand or foot predominate)
- Radiograph may show signs of effusion & early destruction; insensitive early & nonspecific later
- With clinical suspicion, aspiration required
- MR shows nonspecific abnormalities; useful in situations of clinical uncertainty
- Suspicion of septic hip in child should be evaluated with ultrasound
- Protocol advice: MR evaluation must include post contrast sequences

Clinical Issues
- Patients who are symptomatic for > 7 days prior to diagnosis & treatment have more severe damage

---

- Hyperemia leads to periarticular osteoporosis
- Cartilage destruction (joint space narrowing)
- Cortical bone becomes indistinct
- Marginal erosions
- Osteomyelitis may develop
- Sclerotic host reaction if septic joint is bacterial
- Eventual ankylosis (rare; more frequent in tuberculous than pyogenic arthritis)
- Arthroplasties
  - Generally no abnormality seen
  - Rarely, serpiginous osseous destruction & periosteal reaction
  - Fluffy periarticular bone formation is suggestive

CT Findings
- Rarely used with suspicion of septic joint
- Findings similar to those of radiographs: Soft tissue swelling, joint effusion, joint space narrowing, bone & cartilage erosions
- May show erosions or sclerosis in joints which are difficult to evaluate (sacroiliac & sternoclavicular)
- Guide difficult aspirations (sternoclavicular, sacroiliac)

MR Findings
- MR sensitive (100%) & more specific (77%) than other imaging; abnormal within 24 hours of onset
- T1 weighted sequence: Low signal within subchondral bone on both sides of joint
- Fluid sensitive sequences: Hyperintense effusion; hyperintense subchondral bone; perisynovial soft tissue enhancement
- Post-contrast T1 fat-saturated imaging: Synovial thickening surrounding effusion; subchondral bone enhancement; occasional adjacent soft tissue abscess
- Frequency of findings
  - Synovial enhancement 98%
  - Marrow bare area changes 86%
  - Marrow abnormal T2 signal 84% & abnormal enhancement 81%
  - Marrow abnormal T1 signal 66%
  - Perisynovial edema 84%
  - Joint effusion 70% (almost 1/3 lack an effusion; joints of hand or foot predominate)

Ultrasonographic Findings
- Highly sensitive for joint fluid if the joint is superficial enough to evaluate
- Not specific for type of effusion
- US is diagnostic method of choice for hip effusion in children; also guides aspiration

Non-Vascular Interventions
- Aspiration required with suspicion of septic joint
  - Sterile technique
  - Positioning may be difficult due to painful joint, often held in flexion
  - Large bore needle required since purulent material may be thick (18 gauge)
  - Local anesthetic; try to avoid injecting into joint (lidocaine is weakly bacteriostatic)
  - If aspiration yields no fluid, inject non-bacteriostatic saline & then re-aspirate
  - If need to confirm intraarticular location, inject a small amount of radiographic contrast (contrast is weakly bacteriostatic)
  - Send fluid for gram stain, culture (with appropriate sensitivities), glucose, leukocyte count/differential

Nuclear Medicine Findings
- Bone Scan
  - Sensitive (90-100%), but not specific (75%), for septic arthritis
  - Blood flow and blood pool images show increased activity on both sides of joint
  - Delayed phase shows continued increase in activity if septic joint has progressed to osteomyelitis
- Ga-67 Scintigraphy: Increased specificity, but has a significant false positive rate
- Labeled Leukocyte Scintigraphy: Increased specificity, but still has a significant false positive rate
- Arthroplasties are particularly problematic
  - Increased uptake with all nuclear medicine studies for a variable amount of time following surgery

Imaging Recommendations
- Best imaging tool

SEPTIC JOINT

- Radiograph may show signs of effusion & early destruction; insensitive early & nonspecific later
- With clinical suspicion, aspiration required
- MR shows nonspecific abnormalities; useful in situations of clinical uncertainty
- Suspicion of septic hip in child should be evaluated with ultrasound
- Protocol advice: MR evaluation must include post contrast sequences

DIFFERENTIAL DIAGNOSIS

Non-Septic Effusion
- Inflammatory arthritis
- Viral synovitis

PATHOLOGY

General Features
- Etiology
  - Hematogenous spread most common
    - From distant source such as pneumonia, wound infection, endocarditis
  - Direct seeding through trauma or surgery
  - Spread from contiguous infection (osteomyelitis or cellulitis)
  - Pyogenic: Staphylococcus aureus most frequent (64% in one series)
    - Other organisms include Streptococcus pneumoniae (20%), group B streptococci, Gonococcus (2%), Escherichia coli (10%), Haemophilus, Klebsiella, Pseudomonas (4%)
  - IV drug abusers often have unusual organisms: Mycobacterium avium, Pseudomonas aeruginosa, Enterobacter species
  - Septic hip in child: Common
    - Osteomyelitis develops in proximal femoral metaphysis
    - Metaphysis is within the hip joint capsule
    - Extension from osteomyelitis to septic joint is common because of this anatomic arrangement
  - Nonpyogenic: Tuberculous or fungal septic arthritis
    - More chronic processes than bacterial
    - Elicit little or no host bone reaction
    - Cartilage destruction is slower (joint width remains normal for some time)
    - Osteoporosis
    - Erosions develop late; once seen they may be well-delineated
    - Phemister triad: Peripheral osseous erosions, juxtaarticular osteoporosis, gradual narrowing of joint space
    - Most common sites: Hip > knee > wrist

Gross Pathologic & Surgical Features
- Infection of synovial membrane: Edema/hypertrophy
- Exudative fluid produced by synovium
- Cartilage destroyed via release of proteolytic enzymes
- Process eventually extends to underlying bone, resulting in erosion and osteomyelitis

CLINICAL ISSUES

Presentation
- Most common signs/symptoms
  - Traditionally a clinical diagnosis, but findings are not specific; deep joint sepsis is particularly challenging
  - Warm, swollen joint, decreased range of motion
  - ± Fever, chills
  - Monoarticular in 90%
  - Blood cultures positive in 50%
- Other signs/symptoms: Gonococcal arthritis: 66% have associated dermatitis; 25% have associated genitourinary symptoms

Demographics
- Age
  - Septic hip in children generally < 3 years of age
  - Septic joints increase in incidence in teenagers
  - Elderly most at risk due to prevalence of arthroplasties & chronic diseases
- Populations at increased risk:
  - Chronic illness
  - Rheumatoid arthritis
  - Diabetes, end stage renal disease
  - IV drug use
  - HIV-AIDS
  - Steroids
  - Joint prostheses
  - Joint surgery

Natural History & Prognosis
- With appropriate treatment 60% recover completely
- Remainder have permanent damage to joint, resulting in deformity or mechanical arthritis
- Patients who are symptomatic for > 7 days prior to diagnosis & treatment have more severe damage
- S. aureus & gram-negative tend to be more destructive

Treatment
- Antibiotics, appropriate to infecting organism
- Drainage; needle aspiration or open drainage, depending on site
- Arthroplasty is special case
  - Remove components plus all cement; anything remaining serves as a nidus for continued infection
  - Antibiotic-impregnated cement often placed at defect for several weeks
  - Joint must be evaluated for continued infection prior to placement of revision prosthesis

DIAGNOSTIC CHECKLIST

Consider
- Septic hip is clinical emergency; immediate aspiration

SELECTED REFERENCES

1. Mathews CJ et al: Management of septic arthritis: a systematic review. Ann Rheum Dis. 66(4):440-5, 2007
2. Karchevsky M et al: MRI findings of septic arthritis and associated osteomyelitis in adults. AJR Am J Roentgenol. 182(1):119-22, 2004

SEPTIC JOINT

IMAGE GALLERY

Typical

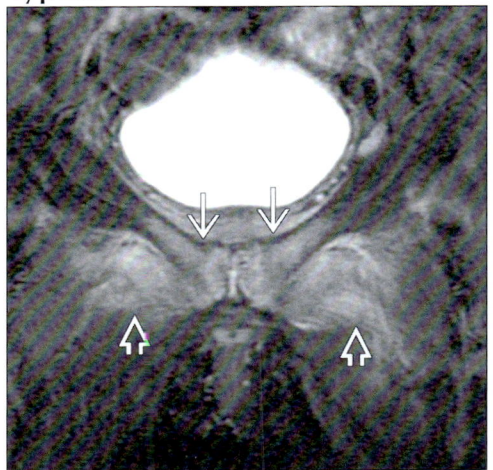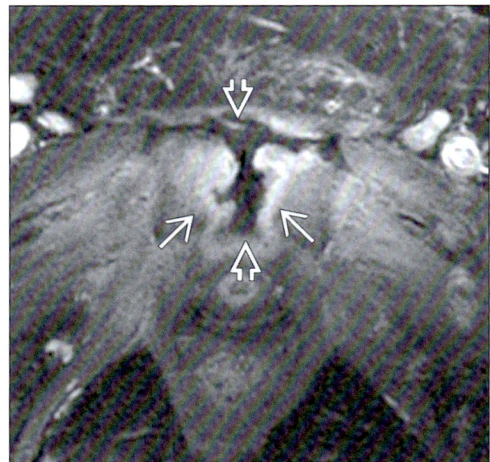

(Left) Coronal T2WI FS MR shows ↑ signal intensity within superior & inferior pubic rami bilaterally ➡; fluid is seen within the symphysis. Abnormally high signal is seen within the adjacent adductor muscles bilaterally ➡. *(Right)* Axial T1 C+ FS MR confirms septic arthritis, with enhancement of the adjacent bones of the pubic symphysis ➡. There is fluid within the joint ➡. This joint is at risk in patients with unusual infectious risk factors; this patient has end stage renal disease.

Typical

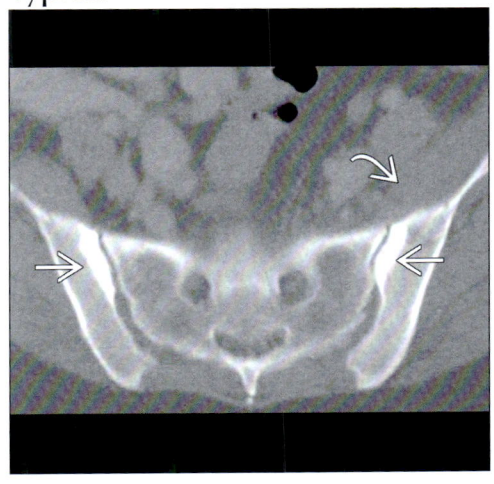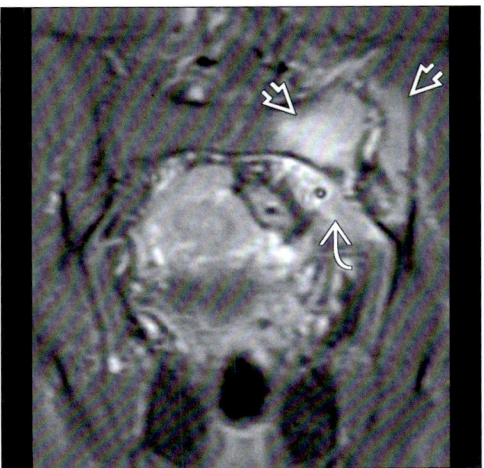

(Left) Axial bone CT shows classic bilateral osteitis condensans ilei ➡. However, there is also thickening of the left iliacus ➡. This patient is an IV drug abuser, and SI joint infection must be strongly considered. *(Right)* Coronal STIR MR confirms septic joint, with high signal in the iliac wing and adjacent sacral ala ➡ and fluid within the joint. The swollen iliacus is well seen ➡. Remember that patients at increased risk for septic arthritis often seed this joint.

Typical

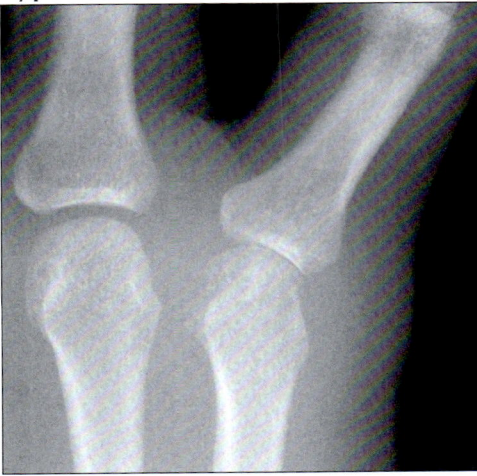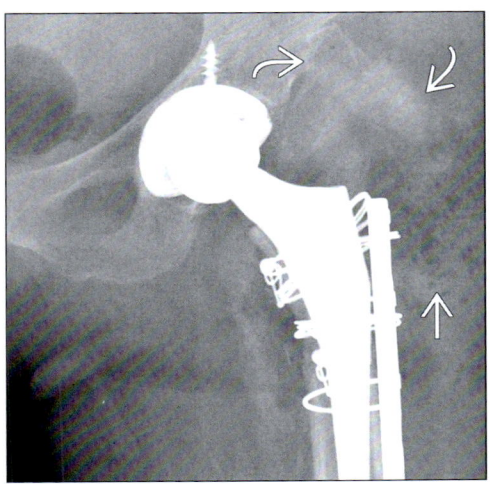

(Left) Anteroposterior radiograph shows cartilage loss and deossification at the 5th MCP in a prisoner. This appearance at this location should alert one to the possibility of septic joint from punching an opponent in the mouth; oral bacteria are particularly virulent. *(Right)* AP radiograph shows air in the soft tissues ➡ around a 5-year hip arthroplasty. There is fluffy heterotopic ossification present ➡. This combination of findings is typical for infection of an arthroplasty.

DIABETES: MSK COMPLICATIONS

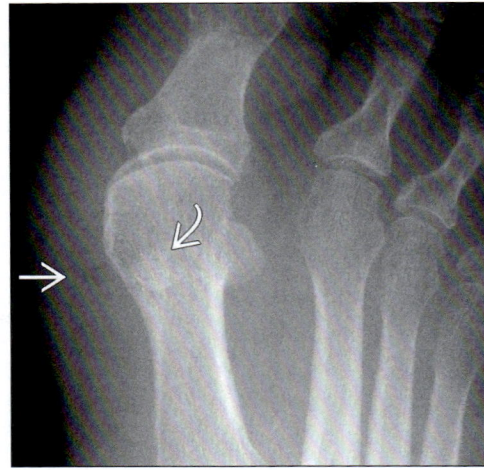
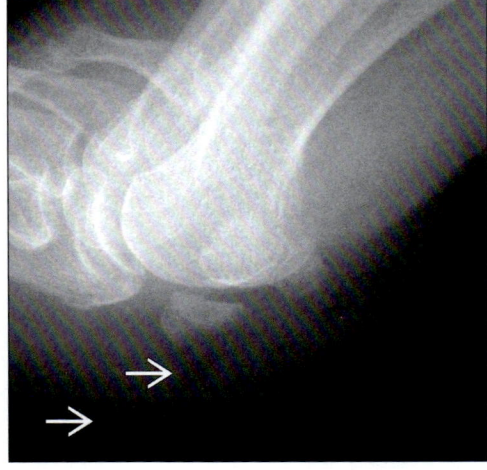

AP radiograph in this diabetic patient shows soft tissue swelling and air ➡ adjacent to an abnormal appearing medial sesamoid ⤴. This is a highly suspicious combination suggesting osteomyelitis.

Lateral radiograph confirms that the air in the soft tissues continues in a sinus tract ➡ from the plantar ulcer to the destroyed sesamoid. One does not often find this combination of obvious sinus tract & osteomyelitis.

TERMINOLOGY

Abbreviations and Synonyms
- End stage renal disease (ESRD)
- Charcot = neuropathic joint

IMAGING FINDINGS

General Features
- Best diagnostic clue
  - Osteopenia/insufficiency fracture: Radiograph
  - Infection
    - Osteomyelitis: Air in soft tissues with adjacent osseous destruction
    - Septic joint: Effusion & intraarticular de-ossification in appropriate setting
  - Neuropathic (Charcot) joint
    - 5 Ds: Normal bone Density, joint Distension, bony Debris, joint Disorganization, Dislocation
  - Muscle infarction: Hyperintense muscle swelling on MR, particularly thigh; adjacent soft tissue reaction
  - Renal osteodystrophy: Altered bone density & various resorptive patterns
  - Crystal deposition: Nodular soft tissue density, generally periarticular
- Location
  - Insufficiency fracture: Posterior tuberosity of calcaneus most frequent
  - Osteomyelitis: Particularly foot, at sites of pressure such as 1st or 5th MTP, 1st distal phalanx, or heel
  - Septic joint
    - Particularly in foot (1/3 of patients with pedal osteomyelitis have adjacent septic joints)
    - Any joint at risk, particularly sacroiliac & hip
  - Neuropathic (Charcot) joint
    - Charcot foot: Lisfranc (TMT) > talonavicular > Chopart (hindfoot-midfoot) > intertarsal joints
  - Renal osteodystrophy: All bones, but particularly notable in hands, cranium, distal clavicles
  - Diabetic muscle infarction: Thigh in ≥ 80%; calf is second most common site
    - Within the thigh, vasti complex most frequently involved
    - Often more than one compartment
    - Bilateral in 40%

Other MSK Complications of Diabetes

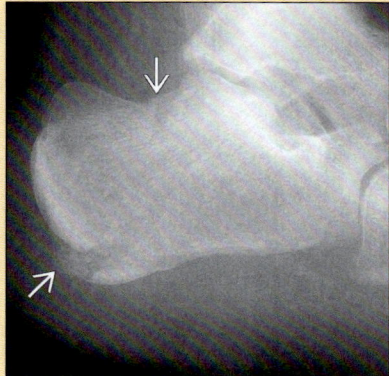
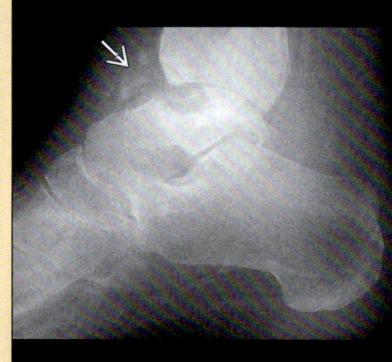
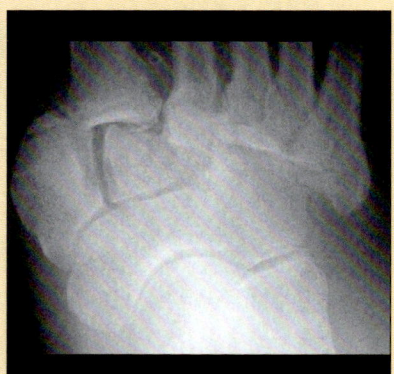

Calcaneal Insufficiency Avulsion Fx | Talonavicular Charcot Joint | Lisfranc Charcot Joint

DIABETES: MSK COMPLICATIONS

Key Facts

Imaging Findings
- Insufficiency fracture: Posterior tuberosity of calcaneus most frequent
- Osteomyelitis: Particularly foot, at sites of pressure such as 1st or 5th MTP, 1st distal phalanx, or heel
- Charcot foot: Lisfranc (TMT) > talonavicular > Chopart (hindfoot-midfoot) > intertarsal joints
- Renal osteodystrophy: All bones, but particularly notable in hands, cranium, distal clavicles
- Diabetic muscle infarction: Thigh in ≥ 80%; calf is second most common site

Pathology
- 15% of diabetics in US have neuropathic arthropathy
- Diabetic muscle infarction: Poorly controlled diabetic with severe ESRD

Clinical Issues
- Note: Septic hip should be considered an emergency; needs immediate aspiration & treatment

Diagnostic Checklist
- Diabetic muscle infarct when severity of pain seems disproportionate, in a poorly controlled diabetic
- **Osteomyelitis & osseous reaction to Charcot joints may be indistinguishable by MR**
- Both show hyperintense enhancing osseous signal
- Both may have associated fluid collections
- Presence of sinus tract leading to osseous destruction can define the abnormality as osteomyelitis
- Character of T1 regions of hypointensity (confluent vs. reticulated) may help differentiate the two

Radiographic Findings
- Calcaneal insufficiency avulsion (CIA fracture)
  - Posterior tuberosity of calcaneus
  - Extraarticular, with proximal displacement of the large tongue of posterior tuberosity by the Achilles
- Osteomyelitis
  - Air in sinus tract
  - Osseous destruction or periosteal reaction
- Septic joint
  - Some joints demonstrate effusion by displacement of fat pads (particularly hip & elbow)
  - De-ossification of subarticular cortex may be seen earlier than frank osseous destruction
- Neuropathic (Charcot) joint
  - Large effusion
  - Debris (hypertrophic); debris may resorb (atrophic)
  - Subluxation/dislocation
- Renal osteodystrophy
  - Generalized osteopenia, often with regions of sclerosis (vertebral body endplates)
  - Various resorptive patterns
    - Subperiosteal: Particularly radial aspect of middle phalanges & medial cortex of proximal metaphyses of long bones
    - Subligamentous: Particularly distal inferior clavicle & ischial tuberosity
    - Subchondral: Particularly distal clavicle, sacroiliac joint, subchondral regions of phalanges
    - Endosteal: Particularly small bones of hand
    - Trabecular: "Salt and pepper" pattern on skull
- Crystal deposition
  - Soft tissue mass; gouty tophus may have ↑ density
  - May erode adjacent bone
- Radiography unlikely to show abnormality with diabetic muscle infarction

MR Findings
- Calcaneal insufficiency avulsion
  - Low signal fracture line on T1 with displacement of posterior tuberosity fragment
  - High signal fracture line with surrounding edema on fluid sensitive sequences
- Osteomyelitis
  - Air in soft tissue sinus tracts, leading to osseous destruction
  - T1: Areas of confluent low signal in bone
  - Fluid sensitive sequences: Hyperintense regions of bone with adjacent & subcutaneous edema
  - Diffuse enhancement following contrast administration; may have adjacent abscess
- Septic joint: Nonspecific findings
  - Effusion
  - Thickening of synovium with contrast enhancement
  - Aspiration required to confirm diagnosis
- Neuropathic (Charcot) joint
  - Large effusion, often containing debris
  - Disruption of joint, with osseous reaction
    - T1: Subcortical bone shows finely reticulated low signal regions
    - Fluid sensitive sequences: Hyperintense regions of bone, particularly adjacent to disrupted regions
    - Enhancement in areas of osseous reaction
- Renal osteodystrophy: Patchy nonspecific osseous signal
- Crystal deposition
  - Mass generally is low signal on both T1 and fluid sensitive sequences (inhomogeneous in latter)
  - Mass generally shows inhomogeneous enhancement
- Diabetic muscle infarction
  - Acute: Marked muscle swelling
    - T1: Isointense compared with skeletal muscle
    - Fluid sensitive sequences: Hyperintense
    - Diffuse enhancement following contrast administration; may have foci with only rim-enhancement, indicating necrosis
    - Diffuse subcutaneous edema
    - Fascial fluid frequently seen
  - Chronic: Atrophic muscles, not hyperintense

Imaging Recommendations
- Best imaging tool: Begin with radiograph; often progress to MR
- Protocol advice: If attempting to differentiate osteomyelitis from osseous reaction in Charcot joint, obtain T1 in at least 2 planes

DIABETES: MSK COMPLICATIONS

DIFFERENTIAL DIAGNOSIS

Differential for Pedal Osteomyelitis
- Charcot joint: Osseous reaction can be virtually indistinguishable from osteomyelitis on MR

Differential for Septic Arthritis
- Non-infectious inflammation: Reactive or arthritic

Differential for Diabetic Muscle Infarction
- Soft tissue abscess
- Pyomyositis
- Necrotizing fasciitis
- Other causes of myositis (dermatomyositis, nodular myositis, proliferative myositis)
- Diagnosis relies on combined clinical & imaging findings; may require histologic confirmation

PATHOLOGY

General Features
- Etiology
  - Pedal osteomyelitis results almost exclusively from contiguous soft tissue ulcer or skin defect
    - Foot ulceration results from combination of peripheral neuropathy, peripheral arterial disease, & susceptibility to infection
  - Neuropathic (Charcot) joint
    - ↓ Proprioception → recurrent trauma → progressive destruction → disorganization of joint
  - Renal osteodystrophy: Combination of osteomalacia & secondary hyperparathyroidism
  - Crystal deposition: Generally sodium urate (gout) or amyloid; may also be hydroxyapatite or pyrophosphate crystals
  - Diabetic muscle infarction: Extensive thrombosis of medium & small arterioles
- Epidemiology
  - 15% of diabetics in US have neuropathic arthropathy
  - Diabetic muscle infarction: Poorly controlled diabetic with severe ESRD

Gross Pathologic & Surgical Features
- Neuropathic joint: Cartilaginous & osseous debris within synovial membrane
- Diabetic muscle infarction
  - Areas of muscle infarction with zonal necrosis, foci of hemorrhage, & fatty infiltration
  - Muscle fibers in various stages of degeneration & regeneration
  - Atherosclerotic calcifications within medium-sized arteries

CLINICAL ISSUES

Presentation
- Most common signs/symptoms
  - Calcaneal insufficiency avulsion
    - May be painful, but proprioception likely reduced
    - Deformity of posterior heel, with bulbous osseous prominence at usual site of distal Achilles
  - Osteomyelitis: Deep ulceration
  - Septic joint: Swelling, decreased range of motion
  - Neuropathic joint: Swollen, warm, deformed joint
  - Diabetic muscle infarction
    - Sudden onset of severe pain & tenderness, with or without palpable mass
    - Pain more severe than in other etiologies of myositis
    - Bilateral in approximately 40%

Natural History & Prognosis
- Calcaneal insufficiency avulsion
  - Shows progressive displacement
  - Healing slow & poor, whether treated with cast or surgically
- Osteomyelitis: Progressive destruction
- Septic joint: Progressive destruction
- Neuropathic: Progressive destruction & deformity
- Diabetic muscle infarction
  - Symptoms resolve over several weeks
  - Patients often have other complications of diabetes & have a near-term high rate of mortality

Treatment
- Osteomyelitis: Incision & drainage; often amputation; antibiotics
- Septic joint: Incision & washing out; antibiotics
  - Note: Septic hip should be considered an emergency; needs immediate aspiration & treatment

DIAGNOSTIC CHECKLIST

Consider
- Diabetic muscle infarct when severity of pain seems disproportionate, in a poorly controlled diabetic

Image Interpretation Pearls
- Osteomyelitis & osseous reaction to Charcot joints may be indistinguishable by MR
  - Both show hyperintense enhancing osseous signal
  - Both may have associated fluid collections
  - Presence of sinus tract leading to osseous destruction can define the abnormality as osteomyelitis
  - Character of T1 regions of hypointensity (confluent vs. reticulated) may help differentiate the two
  - Presence of osseous debris more suggestive of neuropathic joint than osteomyelitis

SELECTED REFERENCES

1. Ahmadi ME et al: Neuropathic arthropathy of the foot with and without superimposed osteomyelitis: MR imaging characteristics. Radiology. 238(2):622-31, 2006
2. Collins MS et al: T1-weighted MRI characteristics of pedal osteomyelitis. AJR Am J Roentgenol. 185(2):386-93, 2005
3. Ledermann HP et al: MR image analysis of pedal osteomyelitis: distribution, patterns of spread, and frequency of associated ulceration and septic arthritis. Radiology. 223(3):747-55, 2002
4. Jelinek JS et al: Muscle infarction in patients with diabetes mellitus: MR imaging findings. Radiology. 211(1):241-7, 1999

DIABETES: MSK COMPLICATIONS

IMAGE GALLERY

Typical

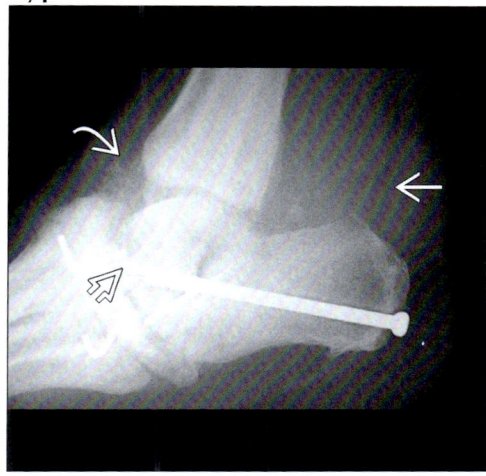 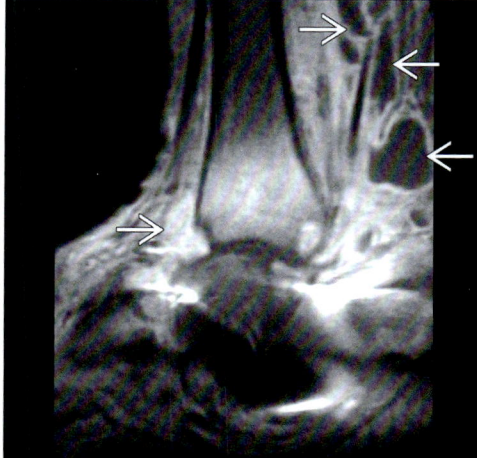

(Left) Lateral radiograph shows a failed triple arthrodesis ⇨ in a diabetic. There is tremendous soft tissue swelling ⇨ & destruction of the tibiotalar joint, with debris seen anteriorly ⇨, indicating Charcot joint. (Right) Sagittal T1 C+ FS MR shows (despite metal artifact) soft tissue fluid collections ⇨, some containing debris, along with high signal in the tibia. These abnormalities are typical of Charcot joint, & in its presence should not be misinterpreted as infection.

Typical

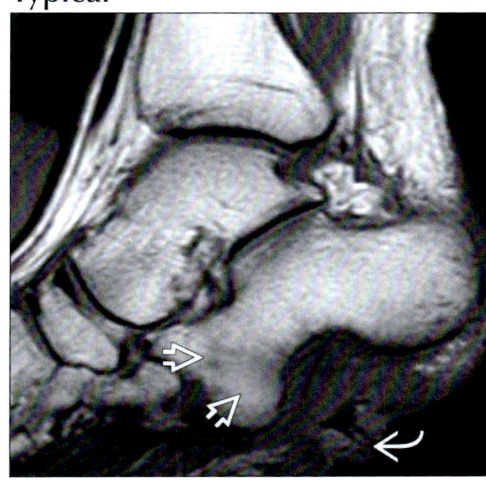 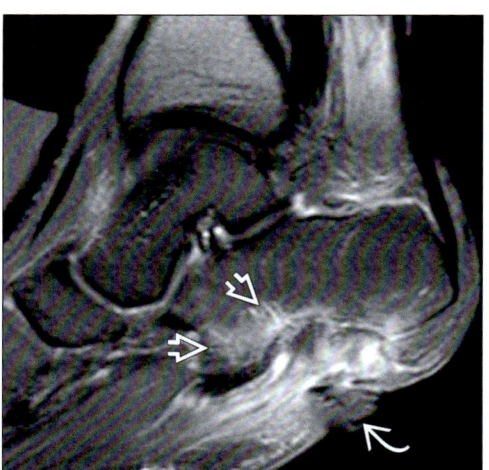

(Left) Sagittal T1WI MR shows plantar ulceration ⇨, with air approaching a morphologically abnormal calcaneus. There is a fine reticulated pattern of abnormal T1 signal ⇨, which usually does not represent osteomyelitis. (Right) Sagittal T1 C+ FS MR shows the same ulceration ⇨ and surrounding soft tissue infection. The calcaneus shows high signal ⇨, but this proved to be reactive bone rather than osteomyelitis.

Typical

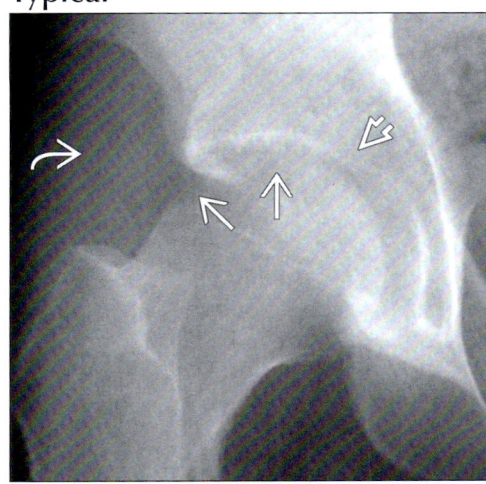 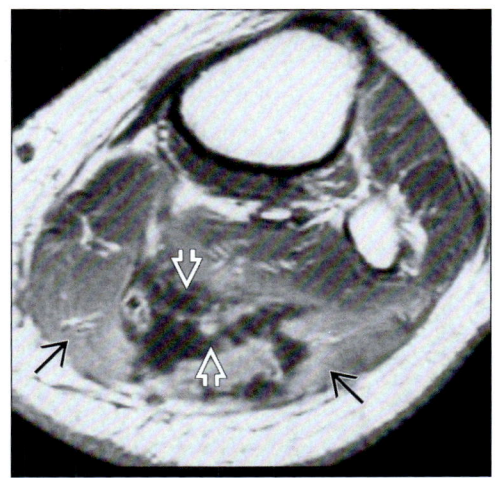

(Left) AP radiograph shows a hip effusion (note the distended gluteal fat pad ⇨). There is deossification of the acetabular cortex ⇨ & destruction of the femoral head cortex ⇨. Findings are classic for septic hip. (Right) Axial T1WI post Gd shows diffuse muscle enhancement ⇨, with central necrosis ⇨; the low signal region is thought to be necrotic rather than abscess because there is no enhancing rim. The vessels are diminutive. Findings are of diabetic muscle infarct.

GOUT

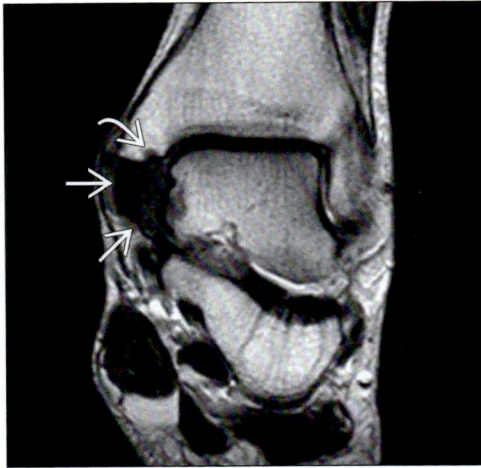

Coronal T2WI MR shows a low signal mass surrounding the distal medial malleolus ➔. There is a tiny erosion ➔, which was not seen on radiograph. The low T2 signal is highly suggestive of gout.

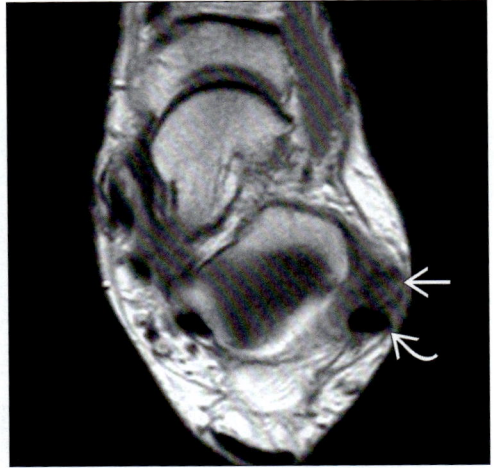

Axial PD/Intermediate MR of the same ankle shows a second low signal mass ➔, immediately distal to the lateral malleolus and displacing the peroneal tendons posteriorly ➔. This confirms the diagnosis of gout.

TERMINOLOGY

Definitions
- Hyperuricemia, resulting in sodium urate crystal deposition in soft tissues & joints

IMAGING FINDINGS

General Features
- Best diagnostic clue: Dense tophi, juxtaarticular erosions with overhanging edges
- Location
  - 1st metatarsal phalangeal (MTP) most frequent site
  - Lower extremity > upper extremity
  - Small joints > large joints
  - Any musculoskeletal site can be involved!
  - Usually oligoarticular but may be polyarticular; generally not symmetric
- Size: Tophi & erosive disease may be small and discrete (few millimeters), or several centimeters in size
- Morphology: Overhanging edge said to be characteristic: Excrescence of juxtaarticular erosion extending vertically from underlying bone

Imaging Recommendations
- Best imaging tool
  - Radiographs usually diagnostic
  - If presentation is soft tissue mass without characteristic tophaceous density, MR is useful

Radiographic Findings
- Radiographs usually normal first 7-10 yrs disease activity
- Classic radiographic features
  - Normal bone density maintained, even after onset of radiographic abnormality
  - Cartilage damage occurs only late in disease
  - Erosions are well-circumscribed + sclerotic margins
    - Erosion edge may end with an "overhanging edge"
    - Erosions often intraarticular, but classically are juxtaarticular as well
  - Tophi: Dense nodules
    - Density is usually cloudy, amorphous
    - Tophi occasionally contain distinct calcifications
    - Eccentric, not necessarily associated with joint
- Unusual, late radiographic features
  - Rare intraosseous calcifications
    - Simulate appearance of enchondroma or infarct

DDx: Gout

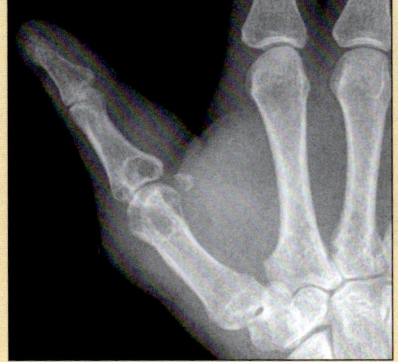

Giant Cell Tumor Tendon Sheath

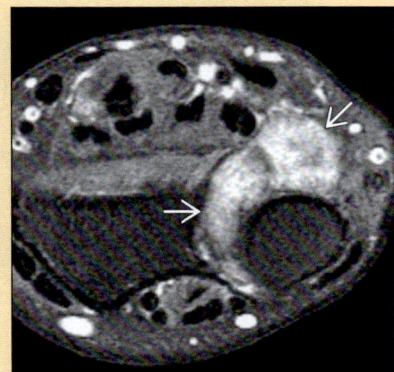

Pigmented Villonodular Synovitis

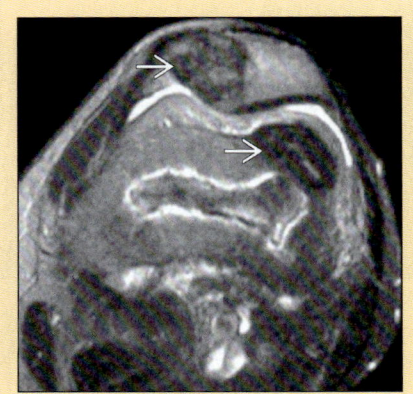

Brown Tumors, ESRD

GOUT

Key Facts

Terminology
- Hyperuricemia, resulting in sodium urate crystal deposition in soft tissues & joints

Imaging Findings
- Best diagnostic clue: Dense tophi, juxtaarticular erosions with overhanging edges
- 1st metatarsal phalangeal (MTP) most frequent site
- Lower extremity > upper extremity
- Gouty tophus has constant T1 MR appearance: Intermediate homogeneous signal intensity
- Gouty tophus appears variably on T2 & other fluid sensitive sequences: Mixed low and high signal
- Gouty tophus enhances with contrast

Clinical Issues
- Gender: M:F = 20:1
- Ethnicity: Pacific Islanders (Maori, Polynesians) > Caucasians > African Americans

Diagnostic Checklist
- Radiograph usually diagnostic; obviates need for MR
- MR of a mass should not be interpreted without corresponding radiograph
- Septic arthritis & crystal-induced arthropathy can occur simultaneously; aspirated fluid should be evaluated for both
- A good adage to remember: Gout can look like anything & present anywhere in the musculoskeletal system!
- Location of disease may be atypical
- Soft tissue tophus may mimic an infectious or neoplastic process
- Gout is common; maintain a high index of suspicion!

- Related to intraosseous penetration of crystals
- Usually long-standing gout + severe renal disease
- Distal aspect of 1st metatarsal most frequent site; may have adjacent soft tissue calcification
- Tophus may be so large & osseous destruction so severe that tumor is suspected
  - Look for any sign that the process may be articular; destructive articular tumors are rare
  - Look for other joint involvement

MR Findings
- Effusion: Low T1 and high T2 signal; seen in 50%
- Synovial pannus: Thickened synovium, low signal T1 & T2 which has peripheral enhancement
- Erosion (intraarticular or juxtaarticular)
- Adjacent soft tissue and/or bone marrow edema: Low signal T1, high signal T2
- Characteristics of gouty tophi
  - Gouty tophus has constant T1 MR appearance: Intermediate homogeneous signal intensity
  - Gouty tophus appears variably on T2 & other fluid sensitive sequences: Mixed low and high signal
    - Similar variability whether tophus is soft tissue or intraosseous
    - Variability related to amount of calcium present
    - Most common appearance on fluid sensitive sequences: Intermediate to low signal, heterogeneous
  - Gouty tophus enhances with contrast
    - Likely related to hypervascular synovium & granulation tissue surrounding tophus

DIFFERENTIAL DIAGNOSIS

Inflammatory Arthrides (RA, CPPD)
- Any single erosive site may have similar appearance
- Thickened hypervascular pannus/synovium

Amyloid Deposition
- Intraarticular & extraarticular deposition has similar MR signal characteristics to gout
- May cause erosions

PVNS & Giant Cell Tumor Tendon Sheath
- Nodular mass has similar MR signal characteristics to gout, but may bloom with gradient echo
- Erosions/subchondral cysts may be prominent

Synovial Osteochondromatosis
- May form a conglomerate, nodular-appearing mass which may have similar MR signal characteristics
- May cause erosions

Brown Tumor of Hyperthyroidism
- Subchondral location may simulate erosion or subchondral cyst
- Low signal intensity on both T1 & T2 MR imaging simulates that of intraosseous gout
- With treatment, brown tumor may hyperossify over time, differentiating it from deposition diseases
- Patients with end stage renal disease are at risk for brown tumor formation, gout, & amyloid

Xanthofibroma, Benign Fibroblastic Tumor
- Soft tissue mass which may have similar MR signal characteristics to gout because of predominance of fibrous tissue

PATHOLOGY

General Features
- Etiology
  - Biochemical derangement: Hyperuricemia → deposition of urate crystals in soft tissue → penetration of cartilage → penetration into bone → inflammatory response & destruction
    - Minority of patients with elevated serum urate level develop an acute attack of gouty arthritis
    - Tophaceous gout: Chronic phase of disease (rarely, tophi noted at time of first attack)
  - Majority of cases are idiopathic; may be familial
  - Minority of cases seen in patients with chronic disease or high rate of cellular turnover such as end stage renal disease, psoriasis, treated widespread tumor

GOUT

- Epidemiology
  - < 0.5% of US population
  - 5% of all patients with arthritis
  - < 5% of patients with hyperuricemia
  - In families affected by gout, incidence range: 6-80%
- Associated abnormalities: May cause gouty nephropathy: Crystals impair renal function (pyelonephritis, urinary obstruction)

Microscopic Features
- Tophus: Mass of urates
  - Either crystalline or amorphous
  - Surrounded by vascular inflammatory reaction (macrophages, lymphocytes, fibroblasts)
- Synovial fluid
  - Negative birefringent needle-shaped crystals under polarized light microscopy
  - White blood cell count 7,000-10,000

CLINICAL ISSUES

Presentation
- Most common signs/symptoms
  - Patients usually have had gout 10-12 years before tophi are seen radiographically or on physical exam
  - Classic presentation is sudden onset of pain at 1st MTP, often at night (podagra)
  - Clinical presentation of soft tissue tophus may be atypical of gout
    - Occasionally presents without erosive or articular process, with swelling & erythema
    - Clinical consideration of painful mass may be infection or neoplasm
    - Rare presentation as nerve compression by tophus

Demographics
- Age: 30-60 years of age at onset, unless patient has predisposing factor
- Gender: M:F = 20:1
- Ethnicity: Pacific Islanders (Maori, Polynesians) > Caucasians > African Americans
- Other predisposing factors
  - Metabolic syndrome (obesity, hypertension, hyperlipidemia, diabetes, prothrombotic state, proinflammatory state) has a remarkably high prevalence of gout
  - Use of thiazide diuretics
  - Lead toxicity (particularly from home-made stills for alcohol production)
  - Heavy alcohol consumption
  - End stage renal disease
  - Tumor lysis syndrome (rapid increase in uric acid with rapid response to oncologic therapy)
  - Innate immune system may relate to response to hyperuricemia

Natural History & Prognosis
- If untreated, causes significant episodic pain
- Over time, progressively destructive arthritic disease

Treatment
- Acute attacks: Nonsteroidal anti-inflammatory medications, particularly indomethacin
- Long-term control
  - Probenecid: Enhances uric acid excretion
  - Allopurinol: Inhibits uric acid production
  - Various forms of uricase: Catalyses conversion of uric acid to more readily excreted allantoin
    - Difficulty with antigenicity; new forms being produced; may be used as induction agent
- Dietary & alcohol consumption modifications
- Consider the strong association of metabolic syndrome & gout; recognize & treat comorbidities
- Studies are currently underway to show the efficacy of MR, CT, & US to monitor pharmacological treatment

DIAGNOSTIC CHECKLIST

Consider
- Radiograph usually diagnostic; obviates need for MR
- MR of a mass should not be interpreted without corresponding radiograph
- Septic arthritis & crystal-induced arthropathy can occur simultaneously; aspirated fluid should be evaluated for both

Image Interpretation Pearls
- A good adage to remember: Gout can look like anything & present anywhere in the musculoskeletal system!
  - Location of disease may be atypical
  - Soft tissue tophus may mimic an infectious or neoplastic process
  - Gout is common; maintain a high index of suspicion!

SELECTED REFERENCES

1. Cammalleri L et al: Rasburicase represents a new tool for hyperuricemia in tumor lysis syndrome and in gout. Int J Med Sci. 4(2):83-93, 2007
2. Centers for Disease Control and Prevention (CDC): Projected state-specific increases in self-reported doctor-diagnosed arthritis and arthritis-attributable activity limitations--United States, 2005-2030. MMWR Morb Mortal Wkly Rep. 56(17):423-5, 2007
3. Choi HK et al: Prevalence of the metabolic syndrome in patients with gout: the Third National Health and Nutrition Examination Survey. Arthritis Rheum. 57(1):109-15, 2007
4. Keith MP et al: Updates in the management of gout. Am J Med. 120(3):221-4, 2007
5. Pascual E et al: Therapeutic advances in gout. Curr Opin Rheumatol. 19(2):122-7, 2007
6. Perez-Ruiz F et al: Imaging modalities and monitoring measures of gout. Curr Opin Rheumatol. 19(2):128-33, 2007
7. Reginato AM et al: Genetics and experimental models of crystal-induced arthritis. Lessons learned from mice and men: is it crystal clear? Curr Opin Rheumatol. 19(2):134-45, 2007
8. Shah K et al: Does the presence of crystal arthritis rule out septic arthritis? J Emerg Med. 32(1):23-6, 2007
9. Stamp LK et al: Emerging therapies in the long-term management of hyperuricaemia and gout. Intern Med J. 37(4):258-66, 2007
10. Wise CM: Crystal-associated arthritis in the elderly. Rheum Dis Clin North Am. 33(1):33-55, 2007

GOUT

IMAGE GALLERY

Typical

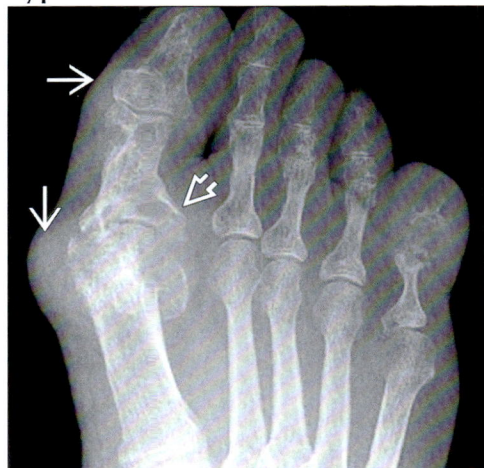
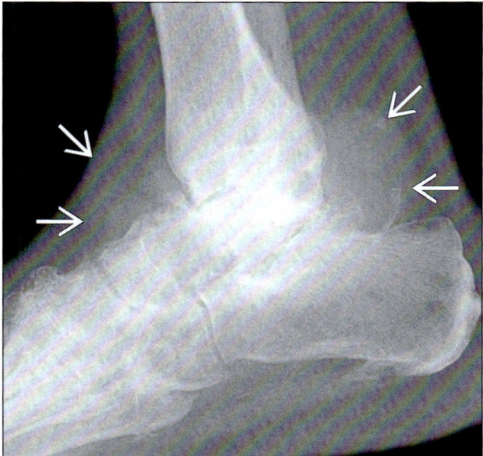

(Left) Anteroposterior radiograph shows classic signs of gout. There are dense soft tissue tophi at several sites ➔, along with multiple well-defined erosions. There is an overhanging edge seen at one marginal erosion ➔. (Right) Lateral radiograph shows erosions within the distal tibia. There is a very large and dense soft tissue mass outlining the tibiotalar joint ➔. This represents crystal deposition within the tophus.

Typical

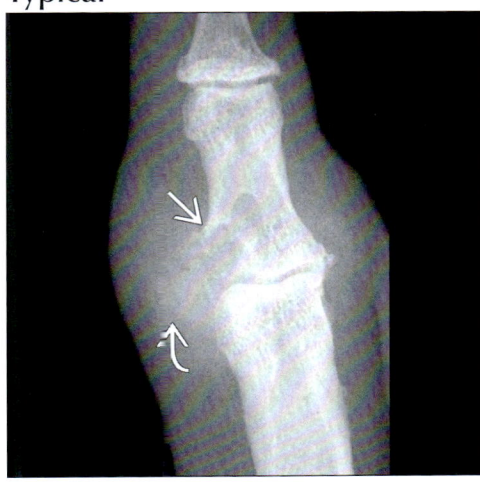
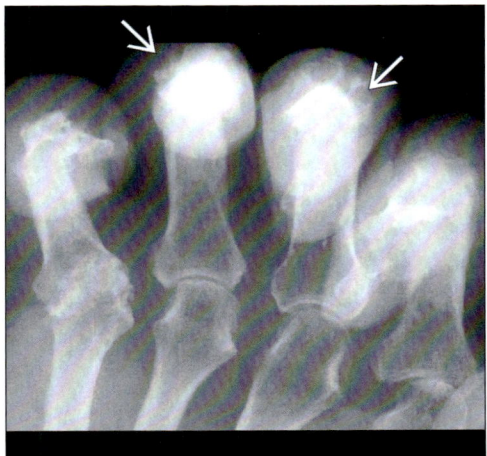

(Left) PA radiograph shows a typical appearance of advanced gout, with a moderately well-defined juxtaarticular erosion ➔ developing an overhanging edge, and prominent dense soft tissue tophus ➔. (Right) PA radiograph of the hand shows the bizarre appearance which can be found in advanced, untreated gout. There are multiple deep, destructive erosions at all of the PIP joints ➔. Gout does not always follow the expected distribution.

Typical

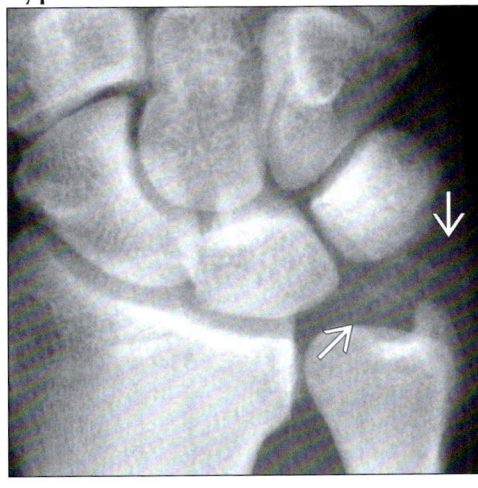
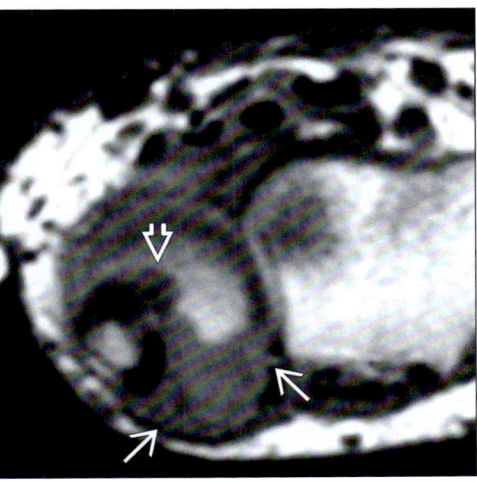

(Left) Posteroanterior radiograph shows abnormal calcific density in the region of the DRUJ ➔ in a 25 year old male. (Right) Axial T1WI MR shows that the low signal mass is within the DRUJ ➔, and has eroded the distal ulna ➔. The mass maintained low signal intensity on all sequences, and is typical for gout. This case serves as a reminder that gout can occur in young patients with risk factors; in this instance the risk was the patient's Polynesian ancestry.

PYROPHOSPHATE ARTHROPATHY

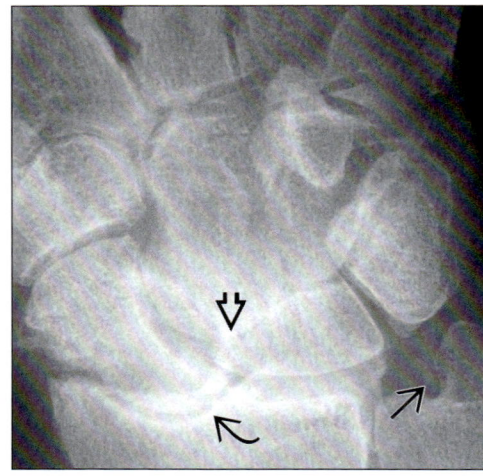

AP radiograph shows chondrocalcinosis ➡, in the presence of radiocarpal arthritic change ➡, with cartilage narrowing. A SLAC wrist deformity is developing, with capitate migrating proximally ➡.

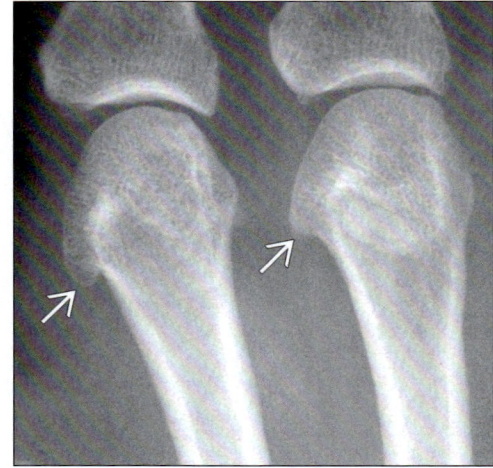

AP radiograph of the 2nd and 3rd MCP joints shows cartilage narrowing and hook-like osteophytes ➡. The other MCPs were normal. This disease distribution is typical of pyrophosphate arthropathy.

TERMINOLOGY

Abbreviations and Synonyms
- Calcium pyrophosphate dihydrate (CPPD) crystal deposition disease; pseudogout; chondrocalcinosis

Definitions
- Terminology has been confusing since terms have been used interchangeably though they are not synonymous
- Chondrocalcinosis: General term for cartilage calcification (pathologically or radiologically apparent)
  - May or may not result in an arthropathy
  - Calcification may be within hyaline or fibrocartilage (menisci, TFCC)
  - Calcification may be deposition of: Pyrophosphate, calcium hydroxyapatite, or dicalcium phosphate dihydrate crystals (or combinations)
- Pyrophosphate arthropathy: Specific pattern of structural joint damage that occurs from CPPD crystal deposition in intra-articular & para-articular locations
- Pseudogout: Gout-like clinical syndrome produced by CPPD crystal deposition; NOT a radiologic diagnosis

IMAGING FINDINGS

General Features
- Best diagnostic clue: Knee or hand with chondrocalcinosis + radiocarpal, metacarpophalangeal (MCP), or patellofemoral arthropathy
- Location
  - Usually polyarticular
  - Usually symmetric (2/3)
  - Chondrocalcinosis: Knee > symphysis pubis > wrist > hip (acetabular labrum) > shoulder > elbow
  - Arthropathy: Knee > wrist > hand > shoulder, hip, elbow
  - Knee: Patellofemoral shows isolated or greater involvement than medial or lateral compartments
  - Wrist: Radiocarpal joint
  - Hand: Metacarpals, particularly 2nd & 3rd
  - Rare pseudorheumatoid location, involving interphalangeal as well as MCPs
- Morphology: SLAC (scapholunate advanced collapse) is common associated wrist deformity

Imaging Recommendations
- Best imaging tool: Radiographic diagnosis

DDx: Pyrophosphate Arthropathy

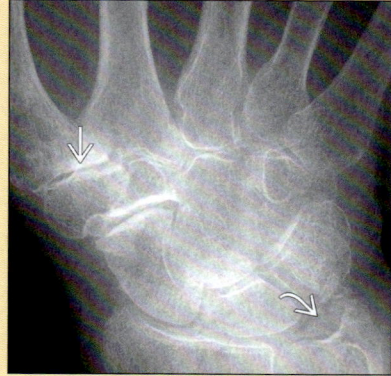

OA with Chondrocalcinosis

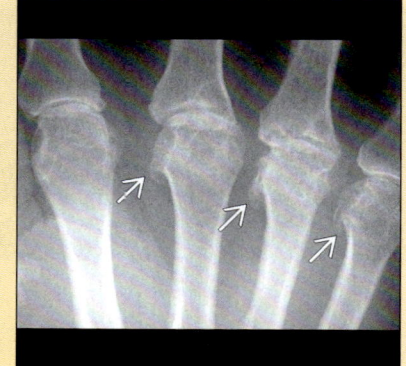

Hemochromatosis

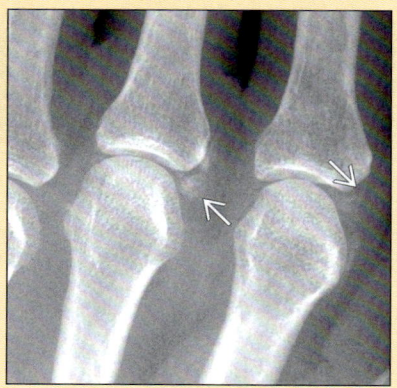

Hydroxyapatite Deposition Disease

PYROPHOSPHATE ARTHROPATHY

Key Facts

Terminology
- Terminology has been confusing since terms have been used interchangeably though they are not synonymous
- Chondrocalcinosis: General term for cartilage calcification (pathologically or radiologically apparent)
- Pyrophosphate arthropathy: Specific pattern of structural joint damage that occurs from CPPD crystal deposition in intra-articular & para-articular locations
- Pseudogout: Gout-like clinical syndrome produced by CPPD crystal deposition; NOT a radiologic diagnosis

Top Differential Diagnoses
- Septic Arthritis
- Hemochromatosis
- Giant Cell Tumor (GCT)

Diagnostic Checklist
- Remember that chondrocalcinosis need not be present to diagnose pyrophosphate arthropathy
- If appearance is "OA with an unusual distribution", consider pyrophosphate arthropathy
- Distribution of arthropathy is most suggestive of dx
- Very specific joint distribution within wrist & hand (radiocarpal & MCPs)
- Specific compartment distribution within knee (patellofemoral > medial or lateral)
- MR of chondrocalcinosis can be confusing
- Sensitivity & specificity for diagnosis of meniscal tear is adversely affected by chondrocalcinosis

Radiographic Findings
- Chondrocalcinosis (usually, not invariably, present)
  - Need not be present radiographically for arthropathy to develop
  - May line hyaline cartilage
    - In knee, particularly along femoral condyles
    - In wrist, particularly at lunate-triquetral articulation
  - May be easiest to see in fibrocartilage
    - Triangular shape in menisci
    - Triangular or amorphous shape in TFCC (triangular fibrocartilage complex)
  - Less frequently seen in synovium & joint capsule
- Arthropathy appearance
  - Arthropathy is generally productive
    - "Hook-like" or "drooping" osteophytes are distinctive at metacarpal heads
  - Early arthropathy may be mixed or even purely erosive (1/8 will show an erosion)
  - Rare pseudoneuropathic appearance, with fragmentation & severe destruction
- Arthropathy location: Quite specific
  - Hand & wrist: Radiocarpal & MCP (2nd & 3rd > others)
  - Knee: Patellofemoral compartment significantly more affected than medial or lateral
- Cartilage narrowing
- Normal bone density maintained
- Sclerosis, loose bodies later in disease
- Subchondral cysts: Common
  - Well-delineated, with sclerotic margin
  - May be large, simulating neoplasm
- Malalignment
  - Radial deviation MCPs is common
  - SLAC (scapholunate advanced collapse) is common
    - Separation of scaphoid and lunate, with capitate migrating proximally, forcing itself between them
    - Scaphoid erodes into distal radial articular surface

CT Findings
- Mirrors findings on radiographs; may be more conspicuous
- Particularly noted in spine
  - Lobulated calcified mass in ligamentum flavum or joint capsule
  - Disk calcifications
  - Pressure erosions, subchondral cysts
  - Occasional fracture (usually odontoid)

MR Findings
- ± Chondrocalcinosis
  - May not be conspicuous on MR
  - Meniscus may appear enlarged
  - Chondrocalcinosis may be low or high signal on either T1 or fluid sensitive sequences
    - Signal alterations from chondrocalcinosis significantly decreases sensitivity & specificity for diagnosis of meniscal tears
    - Interpretation in conjunction with radiograph helps prevent false positive diagnosis of tear
- Arthropathy: Findings nonspecific except by distinctive location
  - Inflammatory changes, granulation tissue, fibrosis

DIFFERENTIAL DIAGNOSIS

Septic Arthritis
- Clinical presentation very similar (red, swollen)
- Septic arthritis may show de-ossification
- Aspirate should be analyzed for crystals + infection

Hemochromatosis
- Younger males may develop an arthropathy identical to pyrophosphate arthropathy
  - Arthropathy develops in up to 50% of those with hemochromatosis
- "Hook-like" character of MCP osteophytes is said to be more prominent in hemochromatosis
- Primary hemochromatosis: Increased gastrointestinal absorption of iron
- Secondary hemochromatosis: Blood transfusions, alcoholism, excess iron ingestion

PYROPHOSPHATE ARTHROPATHY

Giant Cell Tumor (GCT)
- Subchondral cysts of pyrophosphate arthropathy can be so large as to simulate a subchondral GCT
- Differentiate by presence of chondrocalcinosis & multiplicity of cysts in pyrophosphate arthropathy
- GCT generally has areas of low signal intensity on T2, whereas subchondral cyst is uniformly high signal

Chondrosarcoma
- Amorphous chondrocalcinosis can be misdiagnosed as matrix in temporomandibular joint & spine
- Lobulated calcified mass of chondrocalcinosis causes adjacent erosion

PATHOLOGY

General Features
- Genetics: Mutations in gene AKNH shown to have effect on regulation of intra- & extracellular levels of pyrophosphate
- Etiology
  - Enzyme or saturation abnormalities allow formation of excess pyrophosphate
  - Pyrophosphate deposits in cartilage, resulting in an inflammatory cascade
  - Amplification loop hypothesis: Aging cartilage may predispose to crystal deposition because of changes in concentration of proteoglycan
- Epidemiology: 5% of adults
- Associated abnormalities
  - CPPD crystal deposition can be seen in association with several metabolic abnormalities
    - Hemochromatosis
    - Wilson disease
    - Hyperparathyroidism
  - CPPD crystal deposition can be associated with OA
    - May be synchronous & unrelated, or may be due to repetitive microtrauma

Gross Pathologic & Surgical Features
- Chondrocalcinosis: Calcified sheet over the articular surface (extruded calcium pyrophosphate)

CLINICAL ISSUES

Presentation
- Most common signs/symptoms
  - Pseudogout: Acute self-limited attacks simulating gout or septic arthritis (10-20%)
  - Pseudo-RA: More continuous acute attacks simulating RA clinically & in distribution (2-6%)
  - Pseudo-OA: Chronic degenerative joint changes without acute exacerbations (35-60%)
  - Pseudoneuropathic arthropathy: Rapidly destructive form of arthritis (< 2%)
  - May be asymptomatic (10-20%)
  - Diagnosis proven by joint aspiration
- Other signs/symptoms
  - Pain, swelling, fever, elevated erythrocyte sedimentation rates
    - May accompany pseudogout attacks
    - Simulate infection

Demographics
- Age: Rare before age 30, then increases significantly in the elderly (27-50% in patients aged 85-90)
- Gender: No gender predilection

Natural History & Prognosis
- Progressive pain & disability

Treatment
- Based on prevention of crystal formation, dissolution of crystals, & decreasing the biologic consequences
- Lavage of joints, intra-articular injection of hyaluronan
- Nonsteroidal antiinflammatory medication, corticosteroids, low doses of colchicine

DIAGNOSTIC CHECKLIST

Consider
- Remember that chondrocalcinosis need not be present to diagnose pyrophosphate arthropathy
- If appearance is "OA with an unusual distribution", consider pyrophosphate arthropathy
  - MCP osteophytes with normal interphalangeal joints virtually never occurs in OA
  - OA of shoulder or elbow is rare in the absence of trauma or occupational injury
- Distribution of arthropathy is most suggestive of dx
  - Very specific joint distribution within wrist & hand (radiocarpal & MCPs)
  - Specific compartment distribution within knee (patellofemoral > medial or lateral)
- If septic joint is suspected clinically in a joint showing chondrocalcinosis
  - Remember that pyrophosphate arthropathy often has a similar clinical presentation (pseudogout)
  - Look for signs of arthropathy to confirm diagnosis of pyrophosphate arthropathy
  - Send aspirate for crystal analysis as well as microbiology

Image Interpretation Pearls
- MR of chondrocalcinosis can be confusing
  - Chondrocalcinosis can be high signal on T1 & fluid sensitive sequences
  - Sensitivity & specificity for diagnosis of meniscal tear is adversely affected by chondrocalcinosis

SELECTED REFERENCES
1. Wise CM: Crystal-associated arthritis in the elderly. Rheum Dis Clin North Am. 33(1):33-55, 2007
2. Zaka R et al: Genetics of chondrocalcinosis. Osteoarthritis Cartilage. 13(9):745-50, 2005
3. Marsot-Dupuch K et al: Massive calcium pyrophosphate dihydrate crystal deposition disease: a cause of pain of the temporomandibular joint. AJNR. 25(5):876-9, 2004
4. Kaushik S et al: Effect of chondrocalcinosis on the MR imaging of knee menisci. Am J Roent. 177(4):905-9, 2001
5. Steinbach LS et al: Calcium pyrophosphate dihydrate crystal deposition disease revisited. Radiology. 200(1):1-9, 1996

PYROPHOSPHATE ARTHROPATHY

IMAGE GALLERY

Typical

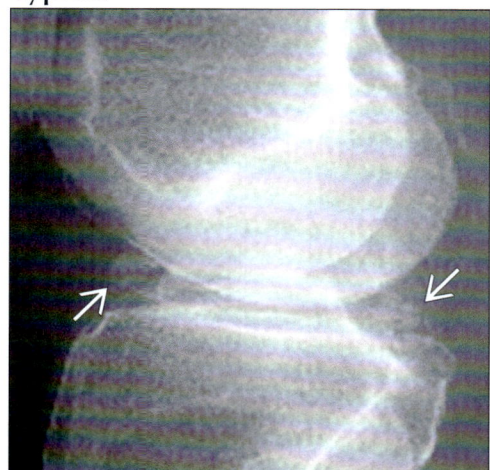
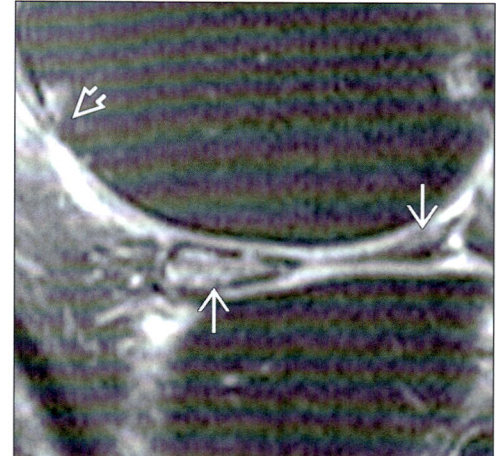

(Left) Lateral radiograph shows prominent chondrocalcinosis within the menisci ➡. *(Right)* Sagittal PD/Intermediate FS MR shows the chondrocalcinosis is high signal ➡, and enlarges the anterior horn. Additionally, there is patellofemoral arthropathy, with cartilage erosion & early osseous change ➡. The combination of predominant patellofemoral arthropathy & chondrocalcinosis is typical of pyrophosphate arthropathy.

Typical

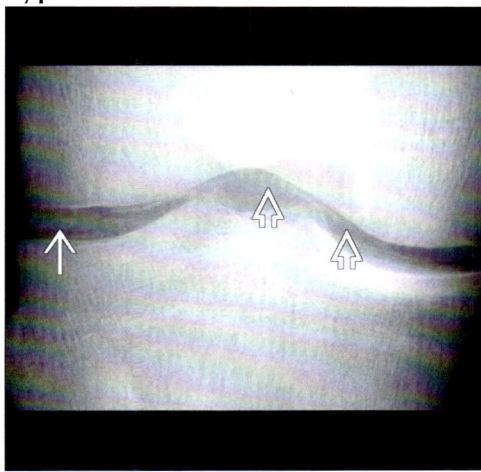
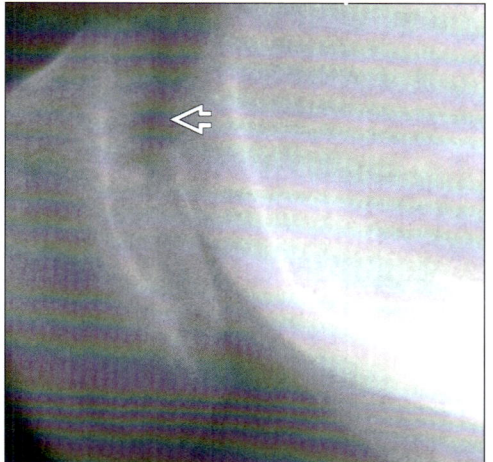

(Left) AP shows early pyrophosphate arthropathy, with chondrocalcinosis in the fibrocartilage ➡ & hyaline cartilage ➡. Note that there is no joint space narrowing in the medial or lateral compartments, & no osteophyte formation. *(Right)* Lateral shows early arthritic disease of the patellofemoral joint, primarily erosive ➡. The location & chondrocalcinosis fits the pyrophosphate arthropathy profile perfectly, & erosions may be seen early in the disease.

Typical

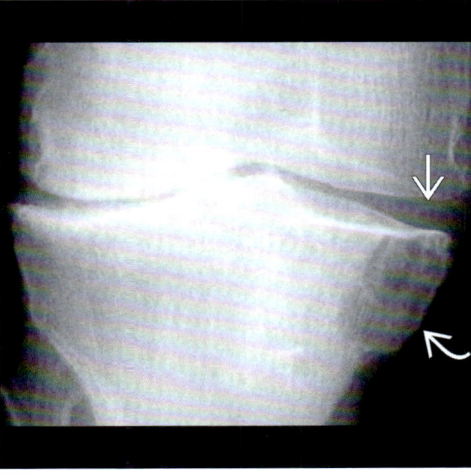
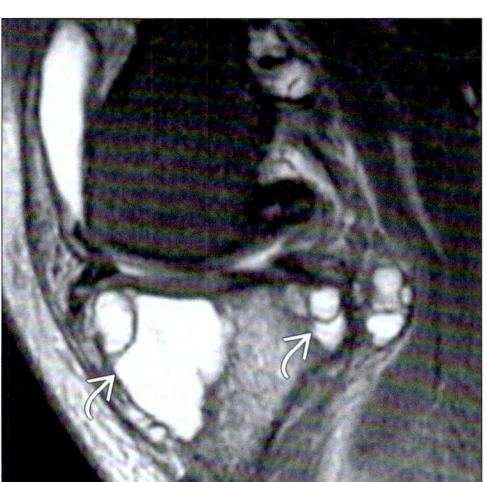

(Left) AP radiograph shows a large lytic lesion in the medial proximal tibia ➡. This might be considered a tumor; however, chondrocalcinosis ➡ & cartilage narrowing is also seen. *(Right)* Sagittal T2WI MR shows an effusion, as well as several multiloculated subchondral cysts ➡. Such cysts can be a prominent finding in pyrophosphate arthropathy. They should not be allowed to distract from the correct diagnosis.

CALCIFIC PERIARTHRITIS

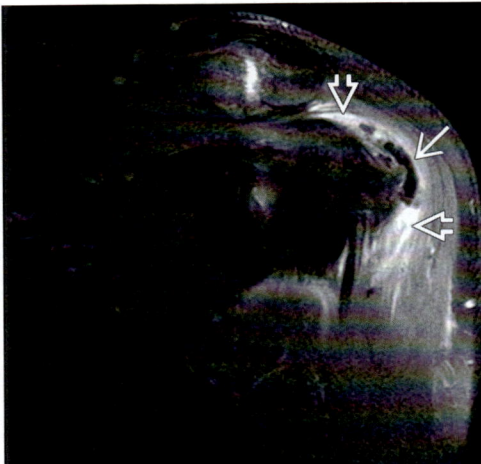

Coronal PD/Intermediate FS MR shows hypointense calcific deposit ➔ in the supraspinatus tendon. There is hyperintense subacromial bursitis ➔.

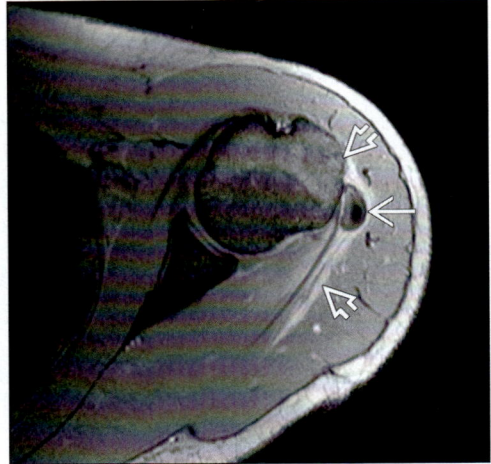

Axial T2 GRE MR shows hypointense calcific deposit in the infraspinatus tendon ➔. There is extension into the subdeltoid bursa in the mechanical phase with hyperintense subdeltoid bursitis ➔.*

TERMINOLOGY

Abbreviations and Synonyms
- Calcific tendonitis, calcium hydroxyapatite deposition disease (HADD), peritendinitis

Definitions
- Calcification within tendons and periarticular soft tissues

IMAGING FINDINGS

General Features
- Best diagnostic clue
  - Calcific deposits: Increased density on radiographs and CT
  - Decreased signal intensity on all pulse sequences on MR
- Location
  - Tendon: Any tendon in the body can be involved
    - Shoulder: Rotator cuff tendons most frequently affected (SST > ISP > TM > SSC)
    - Elbow: Adjacent to medial and lateral epicondyles, insertion of triceps tendon
    - Wrist: Flexor carpi ulnaris (most common), flexor carpi radialis, extensor carpi ulnaris
    - Hip and pelvis: Gluteal insertions, rectus femoris, quadriceps
    - Knee: Adjacent to femoral condyles, fibular head, prepatellar soft tissues
    - Foot and ankle: Flexor hallucis longus and brevis
    - Neck: Longus colli
  - Periarticular soft tissues
    - Capsule
    - Bursa: Subacromial-subdeltoid bursa (shoulder), olecranon bursa (elbow)
    - Ligaments: Collateral ligaments (elbow)
- Size: From small (mm) to large (cm)
- Morphology
  - Homogeneous, well-defined
  - Diffuse, heterogeneous, fluffy, ill-defined

Radiographic Findings
- Calcification within tendons and peritendinous soft tissues

DDx: Calcific Periarthritis

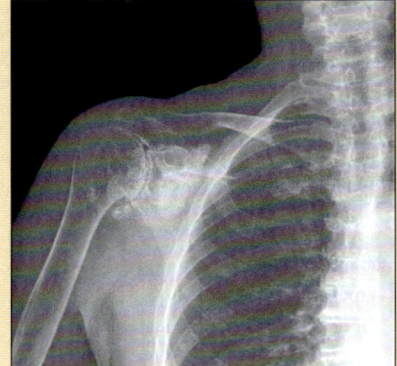

Osteochondromatosis

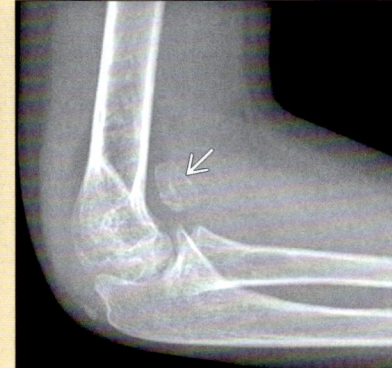

Loose Body

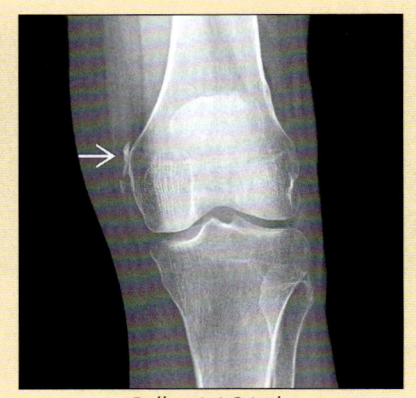

Pellegrini Stieda

CALCIFIC PERIARTHRITIS

Key Facts

Terminology
- Calcification within tendons and periarticular soft tissues

Imaging Findings
- Calcific deposits: Increased density on radiographs and CT
- Decreased signal intensity on all pulse sequences on MR
- Tendon: Any tendon in the body can be involved

Top Differential Diagnoses
- Dystrophic Calcification
- Loose Bodies
- Osteochondromatosis
- Trauma
- Neoplasm

Pathology
- Calcification can lead to mechanical block if large enough

Clinical Issues
- Acute: Pain, tenderness on pressure
- Chronic: Mild pain
- Can resolve and heal spontaneously
- Can progress, causing symptoms, require therapy
- Needling, aspiration and lavage (more successful in resorptive phase)
- Extracorporeal shock wave therapy

Diagnostic Checklist
- Can look aggressive on MR, CT
- T2*GRE most sensitive for detection of calcific deposits

- Acute: Calcific deposits thin, cloud-like, fluffy, ill-defined
- Chronic: Calcific deposits dense, homogeneous, well-defined
  - Underlying bone: Normal, osteoporosis, reactive sclerosis, cysts
- Calcific deposits can change size, shape and location (i.e. extrusion from tendon into bursa)
- Calcific deposits can decrease in size, disappear
- Cortical erosions: Most common associated with gluteal and pectoralis major insertion
- Periosteal reaction: Non-aggressive (solid) > aggressive (lamellated)

CT Findings
- Calcific deposit: Increased density
  - Flame-shaped, comet tail
  - Solid, stippled, amorphous
- Best modality to evaluate cortical erosions

MR Findings
- T1WI
  - Hypointense homogeneous signal of calcific deposit
  - ± Thickening of adjacent tendon
- T2WI: Hypointense signal of calcific deposit
- PD/Intermediate FS
  - Hypointense signal of calcific deposit
  - Hyperintense edema surrounding calcific deposit
  - Hyperintense subacromial-subdeltoid fluid in shoulder
  - Calcific deposit can be heterogeneous in inflammatory phase
- T2* GRE
  - Most sensitive sequence for detection of calcific deposits
    - Calcification may bloom due to susceptibility artifact
- T1 C+: Perilesional edema may enhance
- Calcific deposits: Decreased signal on all pulse sequences
- Calcific deposits may be occult on MR

Ultrasonographic Findings
- Can be more sensitive than radiographs/CT to detect calcific deposits
  - Requires experienced ultrasound technologist
- Increased echogenicity mass with shadowing

Nuclear Medicine Findings
- Bone Scan: Calcific deposits may take up radiotracer

Imaging Recommendations
- Best imaging tool: CT
- Protocol advice: MR: T2* GRE, PD FSE FS

DIFFERENTIAL DIAGNOSIS

Dystrophic Calcification
- Dystrophic calcification usually smaller
- Different chemical composition
- Older age group
- Occur in necrotic tissue

Loose Bodies
- Calcified lesion within the joint
- Hypointense on all pulse sequences

Osteochondromatosis
- Synovial metaplasia
- Cartilage/osseous bodies
- Intra-articular loose bodies

Metastatic Calcification
- Disturbance of calcium and phosphorus metabolism
- Renal osteodystrophy, hypoparathyroidism, hypervitaminosis D
- Calcific deposits in periarticular and other soft tissues
- Often bilateral, symmetric

Trauma
- Medial collateral ligament of the knee (Pellegrini Stieda)
- Coracoclavicular ligament

CALCIFIC PERIARTHRITIS

Neoplasm
- Cortical erosion, periosteal reaction can mimic juxtacortical sarcoma
- Marrow edema on MR can look aggressive

PATHOLOGY

General Features
- General path comments
  - Calcification can lead to mechanical block if large enough
  - Often asymptomatic
- Genetics: Possible genetic predisposition: Associated with HLA-A1, HLA-A2, HLA-BW35
- Etiology
  - Avascular change
  - Repetitive trauma
  - Abnormal mineral metabolism
- Epidemiology
  - 3% of adults
  - 3-20% of painless shoulders, 40-45% of painful shoulders in some series

Gross Pathologic & Surgical Features
- Macroscopic clumps of calcification often surrounded by indurated inflamed tendon
  - Calcific deposits: Milky, cheesy, chalk-like
- Intraosseous extension of calcific deposits

Microscopic Features
- Crystalline hydroxyapatite in tendon
- Tendon often edematous with influx of inflammatory cells
- Macrophages, multinuclear giant cells present during resorptive phase
- Fibroblasts in post-calcific phase

Staging, Grading or Classification Criteria
- Moseley classification (shoulder)
  - Silent phase: Deposition of calcium in substance of tendon, may be asymptomatic
  - Mechanical phase: Increase in size of deposits, mass effect upon the subacromial bursa - painful
    - Subbursal rupture: Partial extrusion of deposits from tendon under floor of bursa
    - Intrabursal rupture: Complete rupture of deposits into bursa (painful)
  - Adhesive periarthritic phase: Calcific deposits and adhesive bursitis
- Radiographic-pathologic staging system
  - Formative phase
    - Fibrocartilaginous transformation of tendon
    - Calcification of transformed tissue
    - Calcific deposit resembles chalk
  - Resting phase
    - May cause mechanical symptoms
    - ± Pain
  - Resorptive phase
    - Macrophages, multinuclear giant cells absorb calcific deposits
    - Calcific deposits resemble toothpaste
    - Can leak into bursa
    - May be very painful
  - Postcalcific phase
    - Fibroblasts reconstitute tendon integrity

CLINICAL ISSUES

Presentation
- Most common signs/symptoms
  - Acute: Pain, tenderness on pressure
    - Edema, swelling
    - Restricted motion
  - Chronic: Mild pain
    - Often asymptomatic
    - Mechanical symptoms if calcific deposit is large
- Other signs/symptoms: ESR and WBC can be elevated, fever

Demographics
- Age: 40-70 years
- Gender: F > M

Natural History & Prognosis
- Can resolve and heal spontaneously
- Can progress, causing symptoms, require therapy
- Acute symptoms usually resolve within 3 weeks
- Chronic symptoms often resolve within months-years
- Can recur after treatment (16-18%)

Treatment
- Needling, aspiration and lavage (more successful in resorptive phase)
- Extracorporeal shock wave therapy
- Steroid injection
- Surgical resection
- NSAIDs

DIAGNOSTIC CHECKLIST

Consider
- Can look aggressive on MR, CT

Image Interpretation Pearls
- T2*GRE most sensitive for detection of calcific deposits
  - Increases conspicuity of calcification relative to surrounding soft tissues

SELECTED REFERENCES
1. Cacchio A et al: Effectiveness of radial shock-wave therapy for calcific tendinitis of the shoulder: single-blind, randomized clinical study. Phys Ther. 86(5):672-82, 2006
2. Chung CB et al: Calcific tendinosis and periarthritis: classic magnetic resonance imaging appearance and associated findings. J Comput Assist Tomogr. 28(3):390-6, 2004
3. Flemming DJ et al: Osseous involvement in calcific tendinitis: a retrospective review of 50 cases. AJR Am J Roentgenol. 181(4):965-72, 2003
4. Garcia GM et al: Hydroxyapatite crystal deposition disease. Semin Musculoskelet Radiol. 7(3):187-93, 2003
5. Hurt G et al: Calcific tendinitis of the shoulder. Orthop Clin North Am. 34(4):567-75, 2003

CALCIFIC PERIARTHRITIS

IMAGE GALLERY

Typical

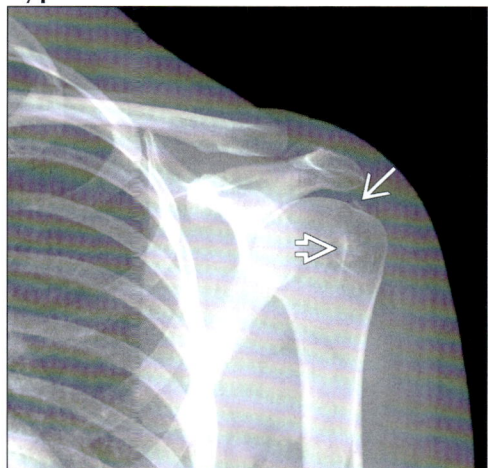 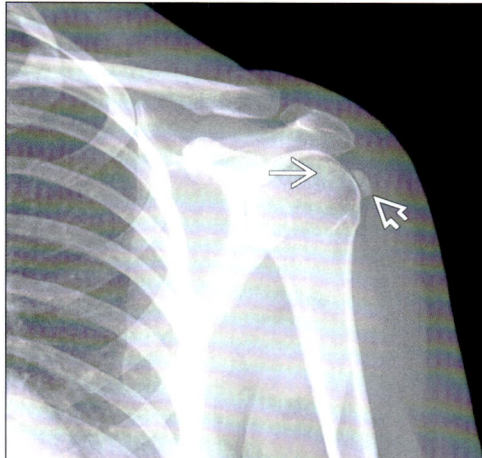

(Left) Anteroposterior radiograph in external rotation shows calcific deposit in the supraspinatus ➡ adjacent to the greater tuberosity. Infraspinatus deposit ➡ overlies the greater tuberosity. *(Right)* Anteroposterior radiograph in internal rotation shows calcific deposit of the infraspinatus ➡ lateral to the greater tuberosity. Supraspinatus deposit ➡ is located more medially.

Typical

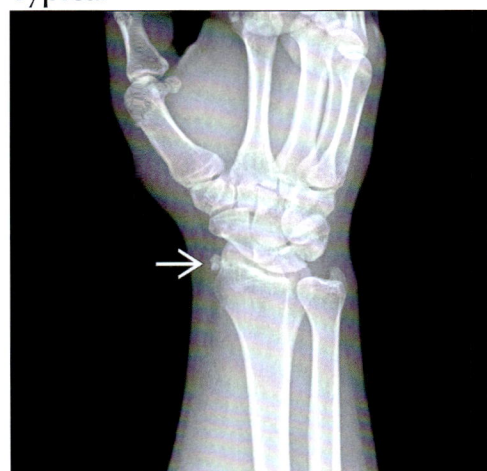 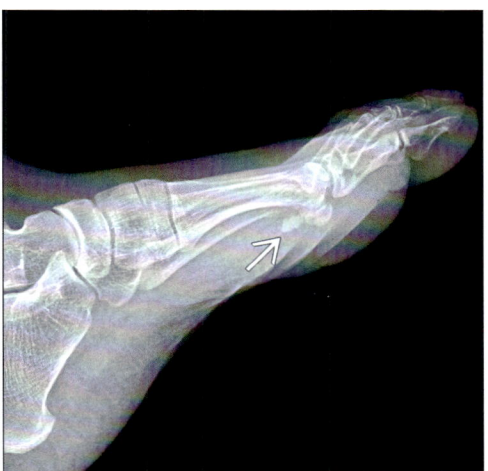

(Left) Anteroposterior radiograph shows calcific deposit ➡ at the radial aspect of the wrist in the location of the flexor carpi radialis. *(Right)* Lateral radiograph shows calcification ➡ in the location of the flexor hallucis longus.

Typical

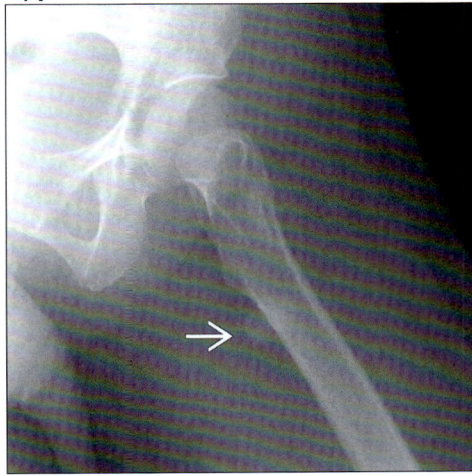 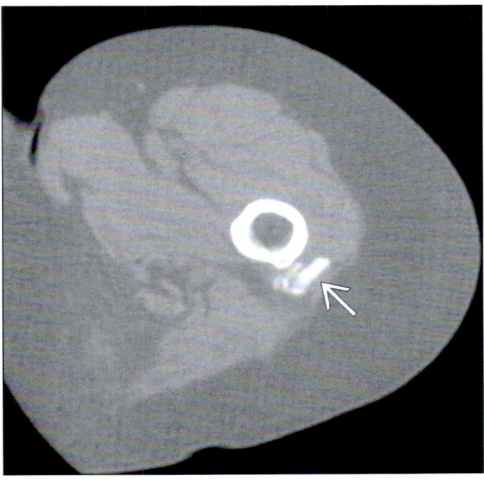

(Left) Anteroposterior radiograph shows calcific deposits ➡ adjacent to the gluteal tuberosity of the femur in the expected location of the gluteus maximus tendon. *(Right)* Axial bone CT shows elongated calcification ➡ at the gluteus maximus insertion. Note the character of the calcification; it has more of a "toothpaste" appearance than either osseous or chondroid matrix.

PIGMENTED VILLONODULAR SYNOVITIS (PVNS)

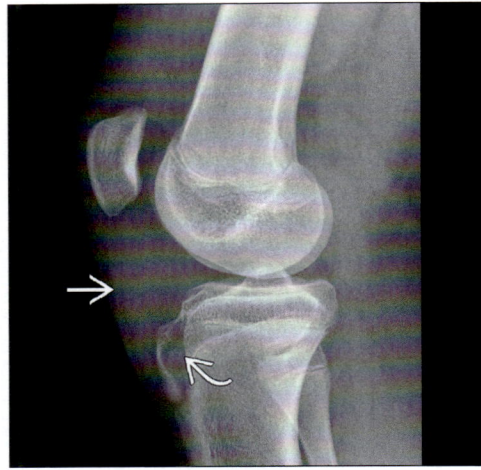

Lateral radiograph shows mass occupying the region of Hoffa fat pad ➔, displacing the inferior patellar tendon anteriorly. The mass has eroded the adjacent tibial apophysis, resulting in an apparent lytic lesion ➔.

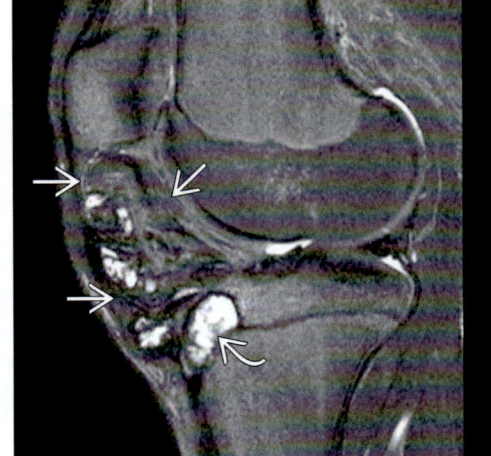

Sagittal T2WI FS MR shows the mass to contain several areas of low signal, with variable regions of high and intermediate signal ➔. The erosion contains low signal nodular regions ➔; findings are of PVNS.

TERMINOLOGY

Abbreviations and Synonyms
- Pigmented villonodular synovitis (PVNS), giant cell tumor of tendon sheath (not illustrated in this section); benign synovioma; nodular tenosynovitis

Definitions
- Monoarticular proliferation of hemorrhagic synovium
- Occurs in joint, bursa, tendon sheath
- PVNS: Diffuse, articular form
- Giant cell tumor of the tendon sheath: Localized, extra-articular form

IMAGING FINDINGS

General Features
- Best diagnostic clue
  - Radiograph: Large effusion ± associated erosions & subchondral cysts
  - MR: Effusion with synovial proliferation, low signal on all sequences & blooms on gradient echo
- Location
  - Monostotic; joints, bursae, tendon sheathes
  - PVNS (intraarticular): 80% occur in knee
    - Knee > ankle > hip > shoulder > elbow
  - Giant cell tumor of the tendon sheath
    - Hand & wrist (65-89%): Volar aspect of digits
    - Foot & ankle
- Size
  - Begins as a small focal mass attached to synovium
  - May enlarge to involve entire joint, lining entire synovial surface
- Morphology
  - May be focal nodular mass
  - May be diffuse, with villonodular proliferation of entire synovium & in all potential joint recesses
    - In knee, can extend down popliteus tendon sheath & into the posterolateral compartment, coronary recess, meniscofemoral recess, into popliteal cyst, into intercondylar notch, & even along collateral ligaments

Imaging Recommendations
- Best imaging tool: MR demonstrates extent; characteristic but not pathognomonic (diagnostic in 95%)

DDx: Pigmented Villonodular Synovitis

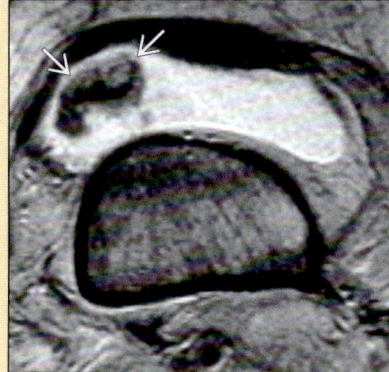

Synovial Osteochondromatosis

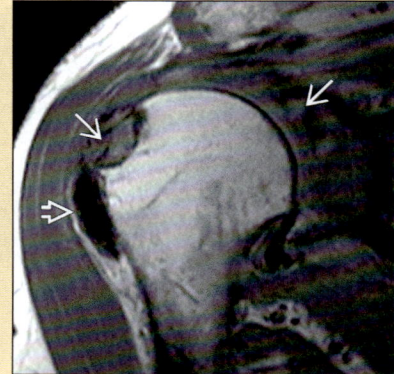

Hemophilia

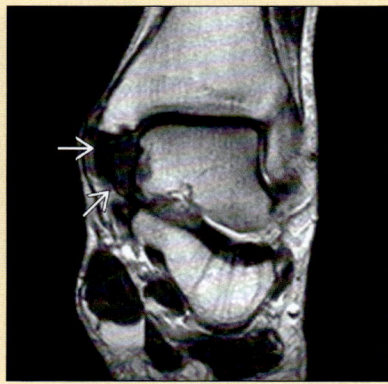

Gout

PIGMENTED VILLONODULAR SYNOVITIS (PVNS)

Key Facts

Terminology
- Monoarticular proliferation of hemorrhagic synovium
- Occurs in joint, bursa, tendon sheath
- PVNS: Diffuse, articular form
- Giant cell tumor of the tendon sheath: Localized, extra-articular form

Imaging Findings
- Radiograph: Large effusion ± associated erosions & subchondral cysts
- MR: Effusion with synovial proliferation, low signal on all sequences & blooms on gradient echo
- PVNS (intraarticular): 80% occur in knee
- Knee > ankle > hip > shoulder > elbow
- Hand & wrist (65-89%): Volar aspect of digits
- May be focal nodular mass
- May be diffuse, with villonodular proliferation of entire synovium & in all potential joint recesses
- Best imaging tool: MR demonstrates extent; characteristic but not pathognomonic (diagnostic in 95%)
- Protocol advice: Gradient echo imaging shows blooming phenomenon of hemosiderin-laden nodules

Diagnostic Checklist
- If suspicious of PVNS, use gradient echo sequence to elicit blooming
- Blooming on gradient echo is not pathognomonic for PVNS; hemophilia is other major consideration
- Search carefully for all regions of involvement, including all recesses, to achieve complete resection

---

- Protocol advice: Gradient echo imaging shows blooming phenomenon of hemosiderin-laden nodules

Radiographic Findings
- Intraarticular PVNS
  - Large effusion
    - Rarely, after repeated bleeding, may appear dense
  - Normal bone density
  - Cartilage preserved until late in process
  - ± Erosion; occurs in 50%
  - ± Large, well-marginated subchondral cyst
  - Secondary degenerative changes late in process
    - Cartilage narrowing, osteophyte formation
  - Very rarely & late, may show dystrophic calcification
- Giant cell tumor of the tendon sheath
  - Soft tissue mass, generally on volar side of finger
  - Pressure erosions of underlying bone: 15%
  - Rare dystrophic calcifications

CT Findings
- Nonspecific, but may be suggestive if subchondral cysts are large
- Effusion, soft tissue mass
  - May have increased attenuation, related to hemosiderin deposits
  - Post-contrast, synovium enhances
- Well-defined erosions, sclerotic margins

MR Findings
- Effusion, generally large
- Erosions (may be subtle)
- Synovial-based masses
  - May be solitary nodular mass
  - May thicken synovium throughout most of joint, with nodularity
  - May extend through capsular defects along juxta-articular ligaments
  - T1 MR: Low signal, homogeneous
    - Rare foci of high signal: Lipid laden macrophages
  - T2 & other fluid sensitive sequences: Variably low signal & inhomogeneous
    - Majority of mass is usually low signal on fluid sensitive sequences
    - Variability relates to variable amounts of fat, fibrous tissue, blood products, & edema present
  - Gradient echo sequence: "Blooms", relating to presence of hemosiderin
  - Post-contrast imaging: Moderate to intense enhancement, with inhomogeneity
    - May add conspicuity for evaluation of extent of lesion, but not required for diagnosis

DIFFERENTIAL DIAGNOSIS

Gout
- Low signal intensity nodular lesions on T1
- T2: Low/inhomogeneously mixed signal intensity
- Juxta-articular location (if present) makes gout more likely than PVNS

Amyloid
- Similar to gout, with low signal intensity T1 & T2 articular & juxta-articular mass
- Enhances with contrast, but no blooming with gradient echo
- Generally has a predisposing disease process

Hemophilic Arthropathy
- Effusion with low signal synovial proliferation on T1 & T2, as PVNS
- Enhances with contrast
- Blooms on gradient echo, as PVNS
- Erosions of adjacent bone, as PVNS
- Morphology, with overgrowth of epiphyses/metaphyses should differentiate hemophilic arthropathy from PVNS
- Familial (X-linked), so found only in males

Synovial Chondromatosis
- Generally bodies are seen as separate entities, often following signal of bone or cartilage
- Usually bodies are seen on radiograph, making differentiation of the diagnoses simple

PIGMENTED VILLONODULAR SYNOVITIS (PVNS)

- Occasional conglomerate low signal mass in synovial chondromatosis, not seen on radiograph, may be confused for PVNS
  - Does not bloom with gradient echo imaging

PATHOLOGY

General Features
- Genetics
  - Clonal chromosomal aberrations, aneuploidy
  - Gene & protein expression patterns suggest the ongoing proliferation is sustained by apoptosis resistance
- Etiology
  - Unknown etiology; reactive inflammatory process
  - Treated as a low grade, locally aggressive neoplasm
  - Abnormal synovium is prone to hemorrhage with minor trauma
    - Repeated hemorrhagic effusions result in iron deposition in the synovium & nodules
  - With proliferation of the abnormal synovium, focal erosions & subchondral cysts develop
- Epidemiology
  - 5% of all primary soft tissue tumors
  - Giant cell tumor of tendon sheath: Second most common soft tissue mass of hand

Gross Pathologic & Surgical Features
- Intraarticular PVNS
  - Joint filled with unclotted dark brown blood
  - Villonodular frond-like proliferation of synovial membrane
    - Cut surface: Yellow-brown (iron deposition)
- Giant cell tumor of tendon sheath
  - Small rubbery encapsulated multinodular mass
  - Yellow-brown in color: Deposition of lipid & hemosiderin

Microscopic Features
- Synovial proliferation
  - Multinucleated giant cells, hemosiderin-laden macrophages
  - Intra- and extracellular hemosiderin

CLINICAL ISSUES

Presentation
- Most common signs/symptoms
  - Painful swollen joint; insidious onset
  - Limited, painful range of motion
  - Sharp & sudden increase of pain if nodule is torsed
  - Monoarticular
  - Effusion is often grossly a chocolate brown color
  - Rapid re-accumulation of effusion
  - Rare pathologic fx into a large subchondral cyst

Demographics
- Age
  - Intraarticular PVNS
    - Wide age range; adolescents to elderly
    - Most frequent: 30-40 years
  - Giant cell tumor of tendon sheath: 30-50 years
- Gender
  - Intraarticular PVNS M:F = 1:2
  - Giant cell tumor of tendon sheath: M = F

Natural History & Prognosis
- Benign, locally aggressive lesion
- If untreated, repeated bleeding & proliferation leads to joint destruction

Treatment
- Resection with synovectomy
- Incomplete resection has high recurrence rate
  - Overall recurrence of intraarticular PVNS: 20-50% (the higher rate related to incomplete synovectomy)
- Arthroscopic synovectomy unlikely to have complete access to some lesions & open procedure required
  - Posterior to cruciate ligaments
  - Superior to femoral condyles
  - Inferior to tibial plateau
- Radiation synovectomy occasionally is used following recurrence
- Refractory cases with severe osteoarthritis require arthroplasty or arthrodesis

DIAGNOSTIC CHECKLIST

Consider
- If suspicious of PVNS, use gradient echo sequence to elicit blooming

Image Interpretation Pearls
- Blooming on gradient echo is not pathognomonic for PVNS; hemophilia is other major consideration
- Search carefully for all regions of involvement, including all recesses, to achieve complete resection

SELECTED REFERENCES

1. Berger B et al: External beam radiotherapy as postoperative treatment of diffuse pigmented villonodular synovitis. Int J Radiat Oncol Biol Phys. 67(4):1130-4, 2007
2. Ward WG Sr et al: Diffuse pigmented villonodular synovitis: preliminary results with intralesional resection and p32 synoviorthesis. Clin Orthop Relat Res. 454:186-91, 2007
3. Wu CC et al: Two incision synovectomy and radiation treatment for diffuse pigmented villonodular synovitis of the knee with extra-articular component. Knee. 14(2):99-106, 2007
4. Chiari C et al: What affects the recurrence and clinical outcome of pigmented villonodular synovitis? Clin Orthop Relat Res. 450:172-8, 2006
5. Finis K et al: Analysis of pigmented villonodular synovitis with genome-wide complementary DNA microarray and tissue array technology reveals insight into potential novel therapeutic approaches. Arthritis Rheum. 54(3):1009-19, 2006
6. Mendenhall WM et al: Pigmented villonodular synovitis. Am J Clin Oncol. 29(6):548-50, 2006
7. Tyler WK et al: Pigmented villonodular synovitis. J Am Acad Orthop Surg. 14(6):376-85, 2006
8. Stubbs AJ et al: Pigmented villonodular synovitis of the knee: disease of the popliteus tendon and posterolateral compartment. Arthroscopy. 21(7):893, 2005

PIGMENTED VILLONODULAR SYNOVITIS (PVNS)

IMAGE GALLERY

Typical

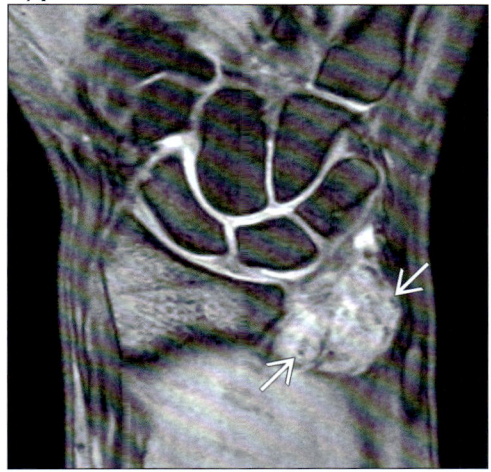 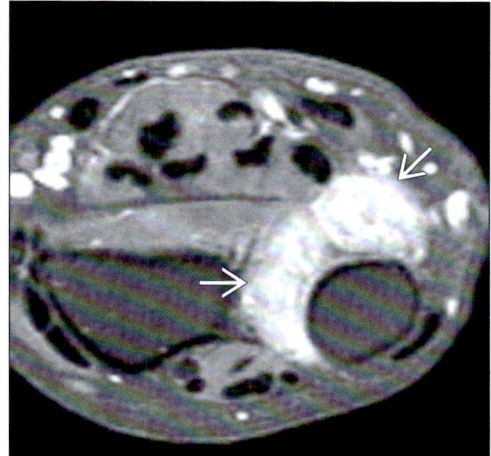

(Left) Coronal T2* GRE MR shows blooming of low signal nodules ➔ within a mass located in the DRUJ. The nodules remained low signal, but were less apparent on T1 and T2 sequences. The blooming results from hemosiderin deposits within the nodules. *(Right)* Axial T1 C+ FS MR of the same case shows enhancement. The DRUJ is quite distended ➔. It is typical for PVNS to show low signal in the nodules on all sequences, but intense enhancement with contrast.

Typical

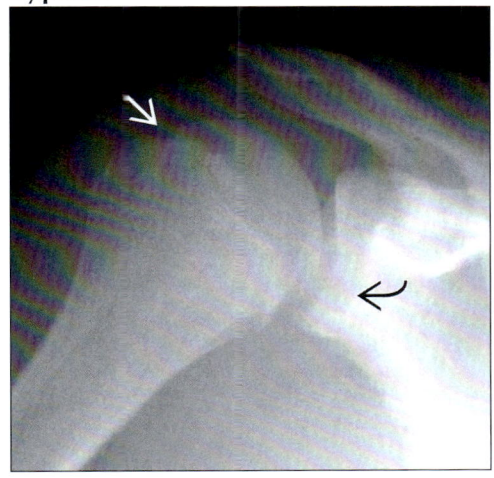 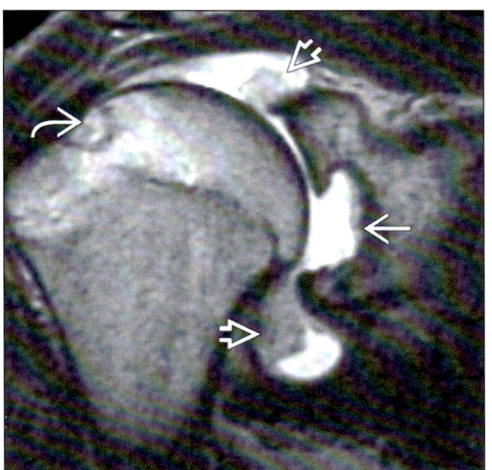

(Left) Radiograph in internal rotation shows a marginal erosion at the posterolateral humeral head ➔, as well as a large erosion centrally within the glenoid ➔. Large erosions should suggest the diagnosis of PVNS. *(Right)* Coronal T2WI MR confirms the glenoid ➔ and humeral head ➔ erosions. Note also the thick nodular low signal intensity masses lining the synovium ➔. The combination is typical of PVNS in a young patient with monoarticular disease.

Typical

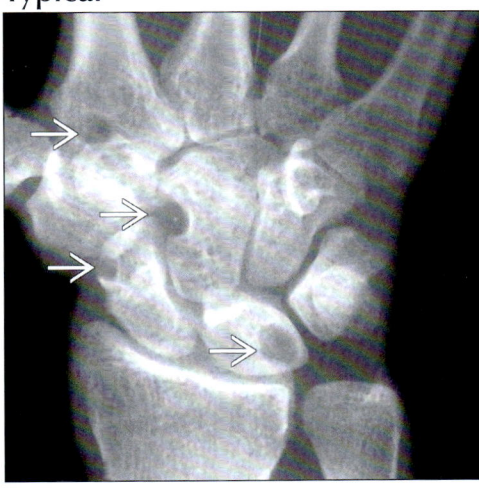 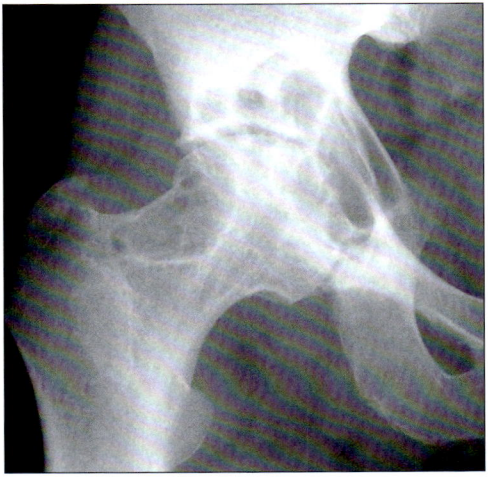

(Left) AP radiograph shows multiple, well-defined cysts in the midcarpal joint, including the scaphoid, lunate, capitate, and base of 2nd MC ➔. Since the other joints are normal, one should consider PVNS in this monoarticular process. *(Right)* AP radiograph in another patient shows a monoarticular process characterized by large, well-marginated erosions, proven to be PVNS. PVNS does not invariably affect the bone, but such erosions or cysts can be prominent.

SYNOVIAL OSTEOCHONDROMATOSIS

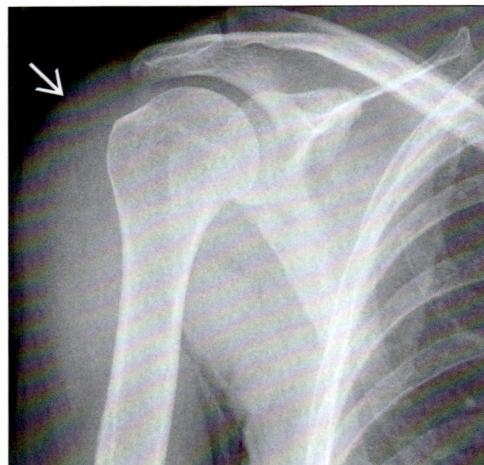

AP radiograph shows a soft tissue mass outlined by the deltoid muscle ➡. There are no other defining characteristics (calcifications/erosions). However, the location should suggest that it is bursal or articular.

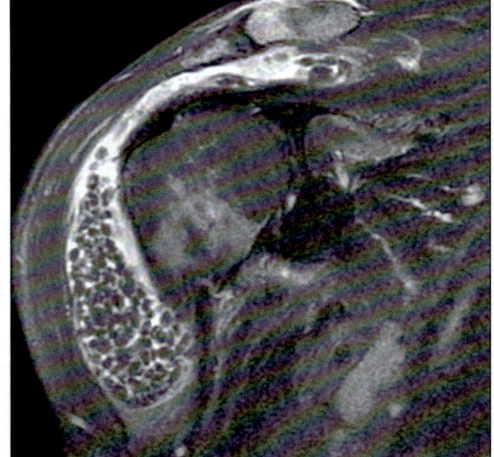

Coronal T2WI FS MR shows that the "mass" is indeed bursal, and filled with innumerable low signal bodies. Synovial osteochondromatosis may be bursal, and has a variety of expected signal characteristics of the bodies.

TERMINOLOGY

Abbreviations and Synonyms
- Synovial chondromatosis, primary synovial chondromatosis (PSC)

Definitions
- Synovial disorder, with synovial membrane proliferation & formation of cartilaginous or osseous bodies
  - May be within joint, bursa, or tenosynovial structures

IMAGING FINDINGS

General Features
- Best diagnostic clue
  - Multiple, round, similar-sized calcified bodies seen on radiograph
    - 85% calcified sufficiently for detection by radiograph
  - Detection & evaluation by MR for those which are not calcified
- Location
  - Generally monoarticular (not invariably)
  - Intraarticular, particularly in large joints
    - Knee > shoulder > elbow > hip
  - Bursal locations: Subdeltoid, popliteal most common
  - Tenosynovial chondromatosis: Hands & feet most common
  - Extracapsular spread through usual sites of joint decompression
    - Across rotator cuff tear into subacromial/subdeltoid bursa
    - From hip into iliopsoas bursa
  - Rare extension into adjacent muscle & fascial tissue
- Size: Ranges from millimeter to > 2 centimeter bodies
- Morphology
  - Rounded bodies, generally of similar size throughout
  - Bodies may appear lamellated, with concentric rings of calcification
  - Occasionally will form a conglomerate mass within joint, or extend into extracapsular tissues

Imaging Recommendations
- Best imaging tool: Radiograph, MR

DDx: Synovial Osteochondromatosis

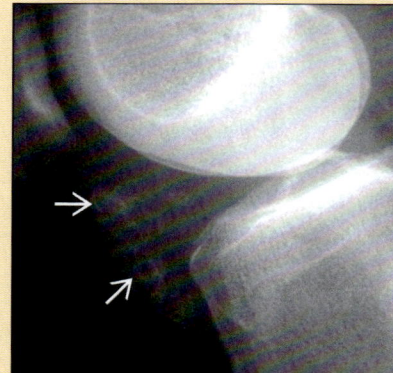

Intraarticular Chondroma

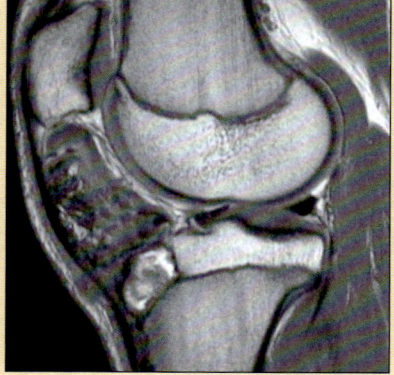

Pigmented Villonodular Synovitis

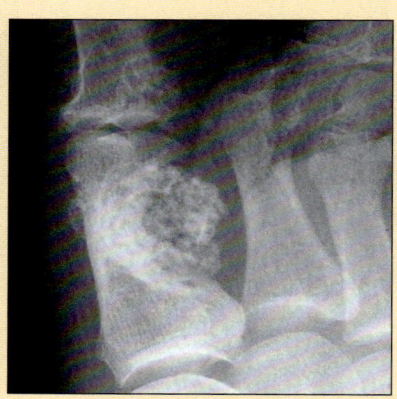

Juxtacortical Chondroma

SYNOVIAL OSTEOCHONDROMATOSIS

Key Facts

Terminology
- Synovial disorder, with synovial membrane proliferation & formation of cartilaginous or osseous bodies

Imaging Findings
- 85% calcified sufficiently for detection by radiograph
- Generally monoarticular (not invariably)
- Intraarticular, particularly in large joints
- Knee > shoulder > elbow > hip
- Bursal locations: Subdeltoid, popliteal most common
- Tenosynovial chondromatosis: Hands & feet most common
- Extracapsular spread through usual sites of joint decompression
- Rounded bodies, generally of similar size throughout
- Occasionally will form a conglomerate mass within joint, or extend into extracapsular tissues
- Occasionally, bodies not calcified & only mass with occasional erosion is seen radiographically
- 80% have erosions detectable by MR
- Bodies are of variable MR signal, depending on proportion of calcium, chondroid, and mature ossific tissue
- May follow signal of either mature bone or cartilage throughout all sequences, or may be less determinate

Diagnostic Checklist
- Consider diagnosis with radiograph showing monoarticular osteopenic joint with erosions
- Calcification/ossification of bodies absent in 15%; MR makes diagnosis
- Consider diagnosis in extraarticular locations

Radiographic Findings
- Multiple round bodies of similar size & variable calcification
  - Range from tiny speckled calcifications to large round, lamellated cartilage or ossified bodies
  - Bodies may be formed in a conglomerate mass rather than free-floating
  - Degree of calcification highly variable
- Associated erosions not uncommon
  - Caused by saucerization; well-marginated
- Occasionally, bodies not calcified & only mass with occasional erosion is seen radiographically
- Extraarticular form: Generally hands or feet
  - Calcifications in location of tendon sheaths or bursae
  - May cause saucerization of adjacent bone

CT Findings
- Multiple bodies with similar calcific appearance to that of radiograph
- May not demonstrate full extent of disease

MR Findings
- 80% have erosions detectable by MR
- Large effusion (hyperintense on fluid sensitive sequences, low signal on T1)
- Bodies are of variable MR signal, depending on proportion of calcium, chondroid, and mature ossific tissue
  - May follow signal of either mature bone or cartilage throughout all sequences, or may be less determinate
    - Ranges from low signal bodies on all sequences to marrow signal bodies on all sequences
  - Bodies are round, multifaceted
  - Bodies may be loose & dependent in joint
  - Bodies may be conglomerate, appearing as a "mass" within the joint
- Contrast with T1 FS imaging shows hyperplastic synovium as enhancing, surrounding low signal effusion & bodies (often obscured)
- Malignant transformation: Extremely rare & no reliable distinguishing feature
  - Watch for "snowstorm" appearance of calcification which has a different appearance from that of the chondromatosis
  - Watch for associated soft tissue mass or osseous destruction

DIFFERENTIAL DIAGNOSIS

Intraarticular Chondroma
- Most frequently located in Hoffa fat pad
- Calcification can mimic the nodular mass-like presentation of PSC

Synovial Chondrosarcoma
- Significantly more rare than PSC
- PSC which has transformed to chondrosarcoma may not be differentiated by imaging
  - Snowstorm appearance of calcified cartilage, with different overall appearance than other PSC bodies may be suggestive

Pigmented Villonodular Synovitis (PVNS)
- May be confusing if only MR is available or if bodies of PSC are not calcified
- Intraarticular nodularity which causes extrinsic erosions, similar to PSC
- Low signal on both T1 & T2, with blooming on gradient echo sequences demonstrates hemosiderin in PVNS

Secondary Synovial Osteochondromatosis
- Loose bodies in osteoarthritis
- Generally bodies are of different size

Juxtacortical Chondroma/Chondroma of Soft Parts
- May be confusing in hands & feet
- Cartilaginous calcification causing extrinsic scalloping of underlying bone

SYNOVIAL OSTEOCHONDROMATOSIS

- May not be able to differentiate from tenosynovial chondromatosis

PATHOLOGY

General Features
- Genetics
  - Chromosome 6 abnormalities common in PSC
    - Suggests a neoplastic rather than metaplastic origin
  - Dysregulation of hedgehog signaling seems to play an important role in PSC
    - Feature of several other benign cartilage tumors
- Etiology
  - Etiology unknown; genetic relationship is likely
  - Once formed, nodules grow
    - If remain attached to synovium, develop a blood supply and may become osseous
    - If loose within joint, nourished by synovial fluid & become cartilaginous
  - Articular cartilage destruction is likely of mechanical origin; not inflammatory

Gross Pathologic & Surgical Features
- Tenosynovial chondromatosis
  - Multinodular cartilaginous proliferation
  - Involves tenosynovium and/or subsynovial connective tissue
  - Mild or moderate atypia is frequent; relates to high local recurrence rate

Microscopic Features
- Cell cultures from PSC are enriched with osteoprogenitors
  - Differentiate along osteogenic & chondrogenic lineages
  - Distinct from cell cultures established from osteoarthritis or normal synovium

CLINICAL ISSUES

Presentation
- Most common signs/symptoms
  - Mass, generally centered on joint
  - Generally painful, but may be asymptomatic
    - Pain often of several years duration
  - Occasional clicking, locking
- Other signs/symptoms: Occasionally present with monoarticular osteopenia & restrictive capsulitis

Demographics
- Age
  - 3rd-5th decades most frequent
  - Wide range, with less frequent cases seen in adolescents & elderly
- Gender: Male > female

Natural History & Prognosis
- Generally slow enlargement
- Progresses to osteoarthritis
- Rare progression to chondrosarcoma
  - In long-standing disease
  - Generally following multiple attempts at resection

Treatment
- Resection of bodies, along with synovectomy
- Extensive disease has high recurrence rate, even with synovectomy
- Tenosynovial chondromatosis has a particularly high recurrence rate
- After multiple recurrences, radiation therapy has been successfully used

DIAGNOSTIC CHECKLIST

Image Interpretation Pearls
- Consider diagnosis with radiograph showing monoarticular osteopenic joint with erosions
  - Calcification/ossification of bodies absent in 15%; MR makes diagnosis
- Consider diagnosis in extraarticular locations
  - Bursae
  - Tendon sheaths, especially hands & feet

SELECTED REFERENCES

1. Chong CC et al: Radiotherapy in the management of recurrent synovial chondromatosis. Australas Radiol. 51(1):95-8, 2007
2. Crawford A et al: A case of chondromatosis indicates a synovial stem cell aetiology. Rheumatology (Oxford). 45(12):1529-33, 2006
3. Jbara M et al: MR imaging: Arthropathies and infectious conditions of the elbow, wrist, and hand. Radiol Clin North Am. 44(4):625-42, ix, 2006
4. Lim SJ et al: Operative treatment of primary synovial osteochondromatosis of the hip. J Bone Joint Surg Am. 88(11):2456-64, 2006
5. Butt SH et al: Primary synovial osteochondromatosis presenting as constrictive capsulitis. Skeletal Radiol. 34(11):707-13, 2005
6. Chillemi C et al: Primary synovial chondromatosis of the shoulder: clinical, arthroscopic and histopathological aspects. Knee Surg Sports Traumatol Arthrosc. 13(6):483-8, 2005
7. Hopyan S et al: Dysregulation of hedgehog signalling predisposes to synovial chondromatosis. J Pathol. 206(2):143-50, 2005
8. Ryan RS et al: Synovial osteochondromatosis: the spectrum of imaging findings. Australas Radiol. 49(2):95-100, 2005
9. Sheldon PJ et al: Imaging of intraarticular masses. Radiographics. 25(1):105-19, 2005
10. Chan WL et al: Tenosynovial osteochondromatosis of both flexor and extensor tendons. Hand Surg. 9(1):89-95, 2004
11. Robinson P et al: Primary synovial osteochondromatosis of the hip: extracapsular patterns of spread. Skeletal Radiol. 33(4):210-5, 2004
12. Buddingh EP et al: Chromosome 6 abnormalities are recurrent in synovial chondromatosis. Cancer Genet Cytogenet. 140(1):18-22, 2003
13. Fetsch JF et al: Tenosynovial (extraarticular) chondromatosis: an analysis of 37 cases of an underrecognized clinicopathologic entity with a strong predilection for the hands and feet and a high local recurrence rate. Am J Surg Pathol. 27(9):1260-8, 2003
14. Wittkop B et al: Primary synovial chondromatosis and synovial chondrosarcoma: a pictorial review. Eur Radiol. 12(8):2112-9, 2002

SYNOVIAL OSTEOCHONDROMATOSIS

IMAGE GALLERY

Typical

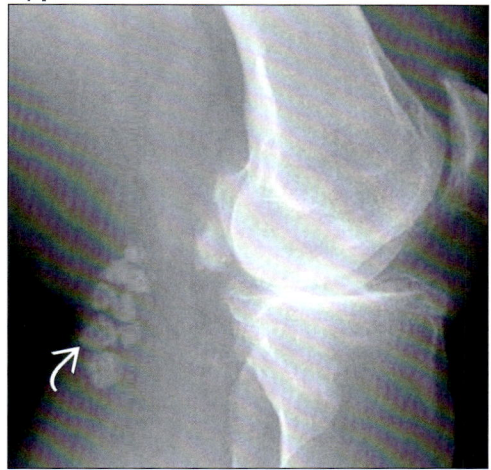
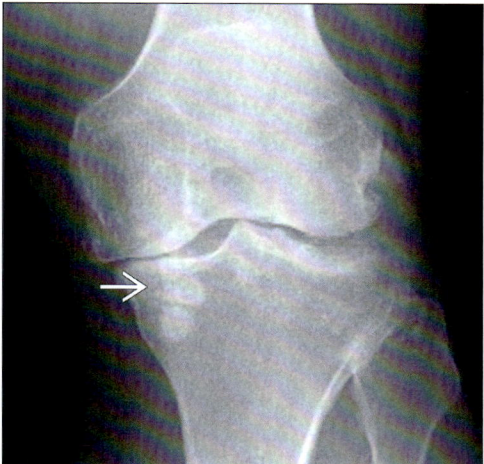

(Left) Lateral radiograph shows multiple round bodies of similar size and appearance located posterior to the knee joint. Note the lamellated appearance of the bodies ➡. *(Right)* Anteroposterior radiograph localizes the bodies to the medial side of the joint ➡. They must be contained within the semimembranosus gastrocnemius (popliteal) bursa. The appearance is typical of bursal synovial osteochondromatosis.

Typical

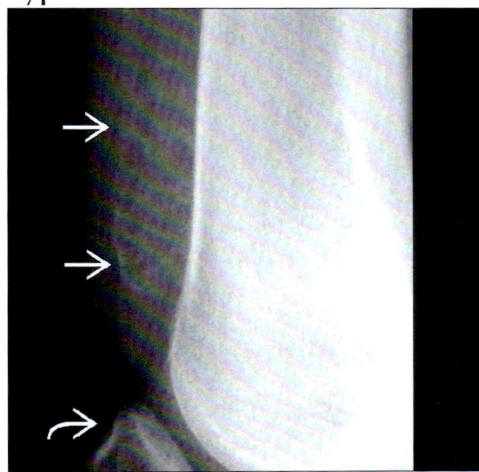
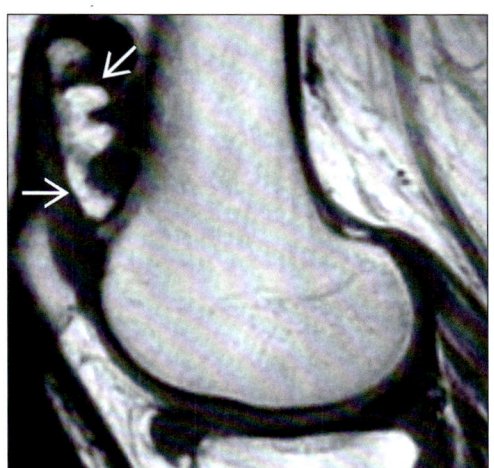

(Left) Lateral radiograph shows calcified bodies, seen as faint calcifications with a curvilinear outline around the inferior portion ➡ (note the superior portion of the patella as an aid to orientation ➡). *(Right)* Sagittal T1WI MR shows that even though the mass was only faintly calcified on the radiographs, it assumes the bright signal of marrow ➡, which also matched marrow on other sequences. Synovial chondromatosis occasionally presents as a conglomerate mass, as in this case.

Typical

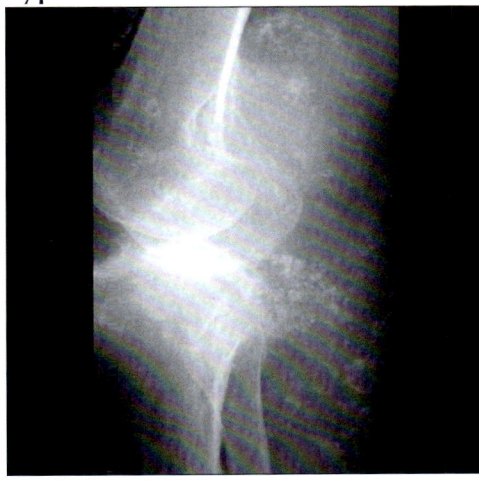
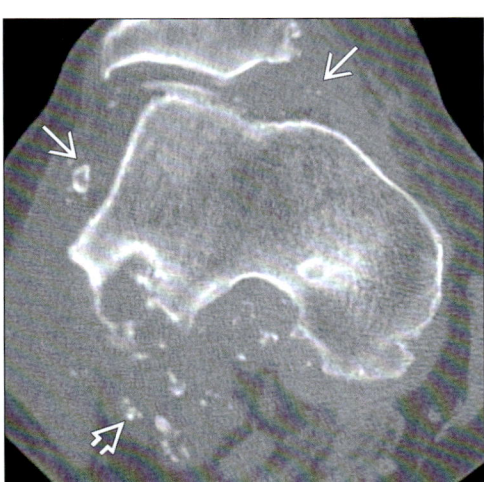

(Left) Lateral radiograph shows a snowstorm appearance of punctate calcifications surrounding the knee joint & its extraarticular soft tissues. *(Right)* Axial bone CT shows that many of the bodies are intraarticular ➡. However, others have extended extraarticularly ➡ and have eroded the adjacent bone. While this is concerning for transformation to chondrosarcoma, at surgery this proved to be synovial chondromatosis with extraarticular extension.

CHARCOT, NEUROPATHIC

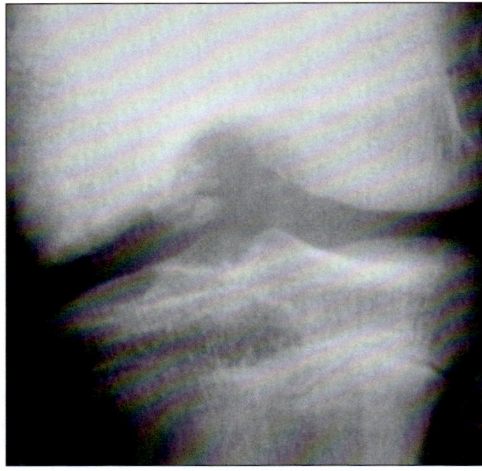

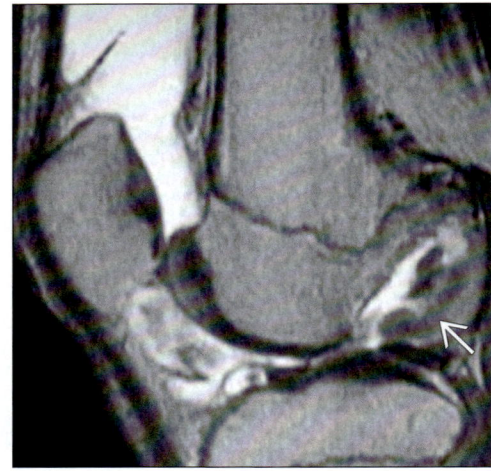

AP radiograph shows fragmentation of the lateral femoral condyle, with debris contained within the joint. Similar abnormalities were found in the contralateral knee, as well as scars on his hands & corneas.

T2 sagittal MR shows a huge effusion & fragmentation replacing the posterior lateral femoral condyle ➡. The findings are typical of Charcot joint; the scarring makes the diagnosis of congenital insensitivity to pain.

TERMINOLOGY

Abbreviations and Synonyms
- Charcot = neuropathic joint

Definitions
- Severely & rapidly destructive joint process, with etiology often suggested by location

IMAGING FINDINGS

General Features
- Best diagnostic clue
  - "5 D's"
    - Normal bone **density** for patient
    - Joint **distention**
    - Bony **debris**
    - Cartilage **destruction**
    - Joint **disorganization** (or **dislocation** or **deformity**)
- Location
  - **Location is strongly suggestive of etiology**
  - Shoulder: Syringomyelia
  - Wrist: Diabetes, syringomyelia
  - Spine: Spinal cord injury, tabes, diabetes
    - Mobile segments caudad to a stabilized segment of spine in paraplegic are at risk
  - Hip: Alcohol, tabes
  - Knee: Tabes, congenital indifference or insensitivity to pain, steroid injection
  - Ankle/foot: Diabetes
    - Lisfranc (tarsal-metatarsal) > talonavicular > intertarsal > Chopart (hindfoot-midfoot), tibiotalar, subtalar
- Morphology
  - Hypertrophic (prominent bony debris): 20%, particularly seen in knees
  - Atrophic (bony debris mostly resorbed): 40%, particularly seen in diabetic ankle/foot
  - Combined hypertrophic & atrophic: 40%

Radiographic Findings
- Rate of destruction can be extremely fast, rivaling that of septic joint
- All Charcot joints have large effusions
  - Effusions can be so tense that they may present as a "mass"

Other Charcot Joints

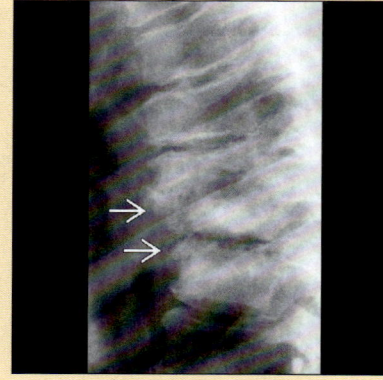

Charcot Spine: Paraplegic

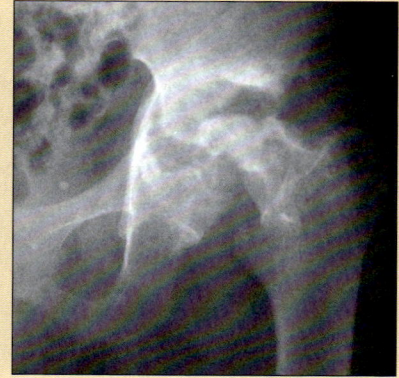

Charcot Hip: Tabes

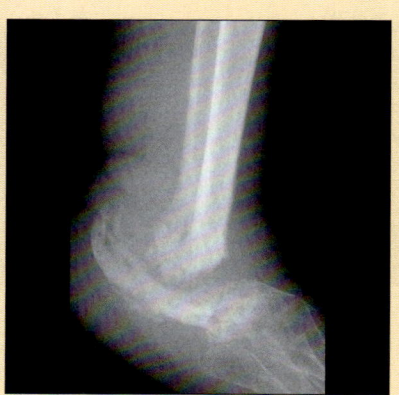

Congenital Indifference to Pain

CHARCOT, NEUROPATHIC

Key Facts

Imaging Findings
- "5 D's"
- Normal bone **density** for patient
- Joint **distention**
- Bony **debris**
- Cartilage **destruction**
- Joint **disorganization** (or **dislocation** or **deformity**)
- **Location is strongly suggestive of etiology**
- Shoulder: Syringomyelia
- Wrist: Diabetes, syringomyelia
- Spine: Spinal cord injury, tabes, diabetes
- Hip: Alcohol, tabes
- Knee: Tabes, congenital indifference or insensitivity to pain, steroid injection
- Ankle/foot: Diabetes

Pathology
- Likely an initial alteration in sympathetic nerve control of osseous blood flow →
- Hyperemia & active bone resorption
- **Secondary neurotraumatic mechanism resulting in a destructive cycle**
- Blunted pain sensation & proprioception →
- Relaxation of skeletal supporting structures →
- Chronic instability →
- Recurrent injury by normal biomechanical stresses but abnormal joint loading →
- Osseous fragmentation & joint disorganization

Diagnostic Checklist
- Even though debris & other findings may be distant from joint, establish that the primary process is articular; this makes the diagnosis

---

- Massive effusions in shoulder often extend from glenohumeral joint across a rotator cuff tear to the subacromial/subdeltoid bursa
  ○ Large effusions can decompress, carrying osseous debris away from the joint
    ▪ This is seen particularly in the knee, with debris dissecting down fascial planes of the leg
  ○ Large fluid collections around a Charcot joint in foot or ankle may be mistaken for abscess
  ○ Paraspinous fluid collections in Charcot spine
- Bony debris (whether prominent in hypertrophic form or minimal in atrophic form)
  ○ Density is osseous, not chondroid or calcific
  ○ Debris floats within the large effusions, so may be placed several centimeters away from the joint
  ○ Debris may decompress along with effusions and dissect away from joint
- Density of bone is typically normal, unless the underlying density is decreased as in elderly or diabetic patient
- Early cartilage destruction
- Mixed erosive & productive osseous changes
  ○ Shoulder Charcot can be significantly atrophic, resorbing nearly the entire humeral head & neck: May have the appearance of a surgical resection
- Ligamentous laxity, with joint subluxation/dislocation
  ○ Judge subluxation at Lisfranc joint on AP for 1st & 2nd TMT joints, on oblique for 3rd-5th TMT joints

CT Findings
- Generally not utilized for this diagnosis
- Shows articular destruction
- Shows distended joint space containing osseous debris
  ○ Because of tremendous distension, this debris within an apparent "mass" may appear several centimeters distant from the joint
  ○ Be careful not to misinterpret this appearance as a mass containing matrix (i.e., chondrosarcoma)
- Reformats show disorganization of joint

MR Findings
- MR can be used to problem-solve
- MR establishes the articular nature of the process
- T1 sequence
  ○ Osseous destruction of both sides of joint
  ○ Adjacent bone may show reactive low signal
    ▪ If the low signal is hazy & reticulated, it is likely to be reactive
    ▪ If the low signal is confluent & prominent, it is more likely osteomyelitis
  ○ Surrounding low signal effusion
- Fluid sensitive sequences
  ○ Shows huge effusion distending the joint
  ○ May show effusion decompressed into adjacent bursa or fascial planes
  ○ Debris located within fluid collection
  ○ Osseous destruction on both sides of joint, outlined by effusion
  ○ Adjacent bone may show reactive hyperintense signal; difficult to differentiate from osteomyelitis
- Contrast enhanced sequences
  ○ High signal rim surrounds fluid collections, either effusions or decompressed pockets of fluid
  ○ Osseous enhancement adjacent to destroyed articular bone
    ▪ This enhancement may be seen simply as reactive bone & need not imply osteomyelitis

Imaging Recommendations
- Best imaging tool
  ○ Diagnosis usually made by radiograph
  ○ If shoulder arthropathy is determined to be neuropathic, MR of cervical spine should be obtained to evaluate for syrinx
  ○ MR of joint is used for problem-solving
    ▪ May help in differentiation of Charcot foot from osteomyelitis in Charcot foot, but significant overlap exists
- Protocol advice
  ○ MR must include T1 sequence in at least 2 planes to help differentiate Charcot from osteomyelitis
  ○ MR must include post contrast sequences

CHARCOT, NEUROPATHIC

DIFFERENTIAL DIAGNOSIS

Ankle/Foot: Osteomyelitis or Septic Joint
- Neuropathic & septic joint may coexist
- Both can have large effusions/fluid collections
- Both diagnoses can have enhancement of bone
- There are a few factors which may favor infection
  - Abnormal T1 signal in bone is more confluent than hazy/reticular in infection
  - Fluid collections have less bony debris in cases of infection
  - Air in sinus tract leading to abnormal bone diagnoses infection
  - Fat replacement by abnormal signal suggests infection rather than Charcot process

Shoulder: Chondrosarcoma
- Surprisingly, even though the two lesions are distinctively different, Charcot joint is often misdiagnosed on radiograph as chondrosarcoma
- Mass in chondrosarcoma is not intraarticular
- Matrix in chondrosarcoma is chondroid, rather than the bony debris seen in Charcot shoulder

Osteoarthritis or Inflammatory Arthritis
- Early stage osteoarthritis resembles early Charcot
- Osseous debris generally less prominent
- Joint dislocation should not be seen in arthritis
- Effusions generally smaller in arthritis

Spine: Diskitis
- Both diskitis & Charcot spine may have paraspinal soft tissue mass/fluid collections
- Both show disk & endplate destruction, with debris
- Both may show subluxation
- Patients with spinal cord injury or diabetes are at risk for both diskitis & Charcot spine
- Presence of prominent debris, subluxation, vacuum disk, & facet involvement makes Charcot more likely
- Many cases will require aspiration to prove diagnosis

PATHOLOGY

General Features
- Etiology
  - Primary pathogenesis uncertain
  - Likely an initial alteration in sympathetic nerve control of osseous blood flow →
  - Hyperemia & active bone resorption
  - **Secondary neurotraumatic mechanism resulting in a destructive cycle**
    - Blunted pain sensation & proprioception →
    - Relaxation of skeletal supporting structures →
    - Chronic instability →
    - Recurrent injury by normal biomechanical stresses but abnormal joint loading →
    - Osseous fragmentation & joint disorganization
  - Diabetes: Mostly affects peripheral joints (foot, hand)
  - Tabes dorsalis: Affects spine, knee > hip, ankle/foot
  - Syringomyelia: Shoulder, wrist
  - Spinal cord injury: Spine, more caudad than site of injury (unprotected motion)
  - Active paraplegic patients (weight lifting, wheelchair athletics) put the non-stabilized portion of their spinal column at risk
  - Congenital insensitivity/indifference to pain: Lower extremity (knee, ankle)
  - Intraarticular steroid use: Knee most common
  - Alcoholism: Hip, metatarsophalangeal, IP joints
  - Amyloidosis: Knee & ankle
  - Leprosy: IP joints of hand, MTP joints of foot
  - Multiple sclerosis
  - Meningomyelocele: Ankle & intertarsal joints
  - Neurologic conditions: Charcot-Marie-Tooth, Riley-Day syndrome (dysautonomia)
- Epidemiology
  - 15% of diabetics develop Charcot joints
  - 20% syringomyelia patients develop Charcot joints
  - World-wide, 10-20% of patients with tabes dorsalis develop Charcot joints

Gross Pathologic & Surgical Features
- Significant amount of cartilaginous & osseous debris within the synovial membrane

CLINICAL ISSUES

Presentation
- Most common signs/symptoms
  - Swollen, unstable joint
  - Up to 30% have near normal proprioception
    - Careful exam needed to elicit neurological abnormality
    - Response to deep pain & proprioception may be ↓

Demographics
- Age
  - Relates to underlying etiology
    - Age of onset of diabetes
    - Congenital pain insensitivity/indifference: Teens

Natural History & Prognosis
- Rapidly progressive destruction
- With worsening alignment, at risk for skin ulceration & eventual osteomyelitis

Treatment
- If conservative treatment fails, needs reconstruction
- Arthrodesis difficult to achieve; 25% recur or have significant complications

DIAGNOSTIC CHECKLIST

Image Interpretation Pearls
- Even though debris & other findings may be distant from joint, establish that the primary process is articular; this makes the diagnosis

SELECTED REFERENCES
1. Rose DM et al: Charcot spinal arthropathy in a paraplegic weight lifter: case report. Spine. 31(11):E339-41, 2006
2. Schwarz RJ et al: Results of arthrodesis in neuropathic feet. J Bone Joint Surg Br. 88(6):747-50, 2006

CHARCOT, NEUROPATHIC

IMAGE GALLERY

Typical

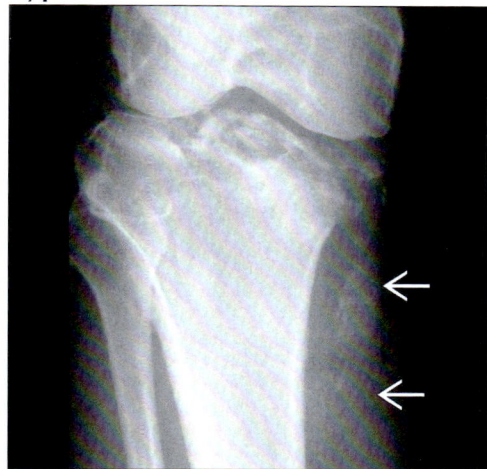
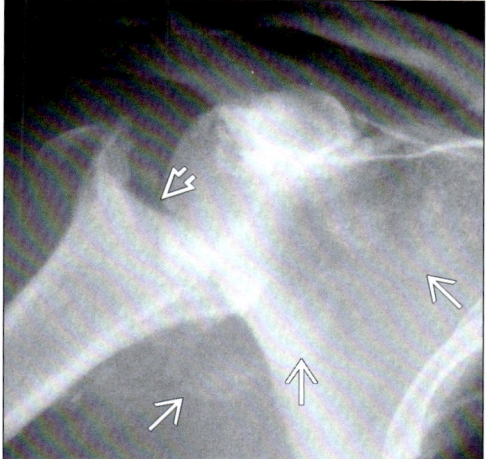

(Left) AP radiograph shows fragmentation & a tense effusion, which decompressed down fascial planes of the leg. This decompression carried bony debris distal to the joint ➡. This is a typical Charcot knee in a patient with acquired syphilis. (Right) AP shoulder shows severe destructive change, with a cut-off of the dislocated humeral head ➡. The large effusion contains bony debris within the joint space ➡. This is a typical Charcot shoulder; cervical spine MR showed a syrinx.

Typical

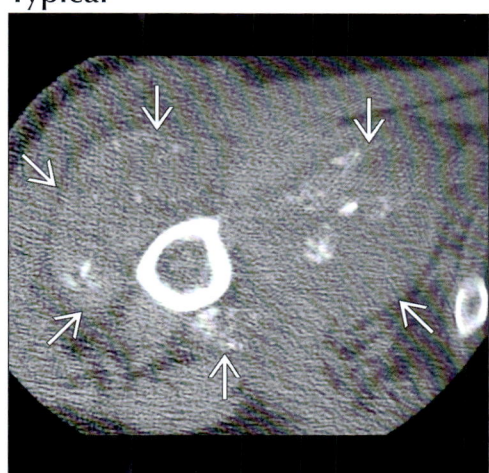
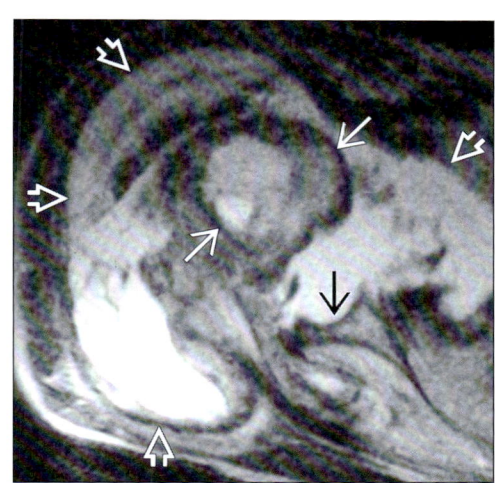

(Left) Axial CT shows an enormous effusion extending from the shoulder down around the proximal shaft of the humerus ➡. The fluid contains abundant osseous debris. (Right) Axial T2WI MR shows the remnant of glenoid ➡ & humeral head ➡, with surrounding huge effusion (glenohumeral joint, extending into subdeltoid bursa) ➡. The MR proves the abnormality to be articular. This is a classic Charcot shoulder; the patient had syringomyelia as the etiology.

Typical

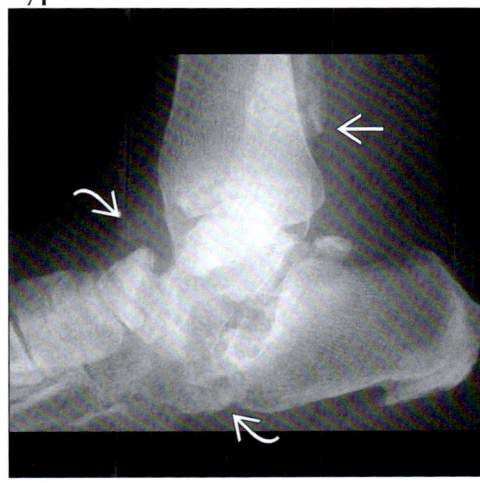
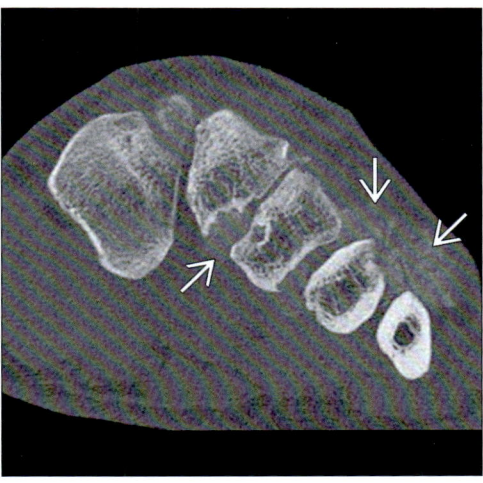

(Left) Sagittal radiograph shows Charcot foot, with disorganization of the Chopart (hindfoot-midfoot) joint ➡. The patient is diabetic, & little debris is seen in this atrophic joint. There was a clinically unsuspected subacute fibular fracture ➡ as well. (Right) Axial CT in a different diabetic patient, located at the Lisfranc (TMT) joint, shows large effusions which contain fine osseous debris ➡. Radiographs were normal. The CT proves early Lisfranc Charcot joint.

TRANSIENT BONE MARROW EDEMA

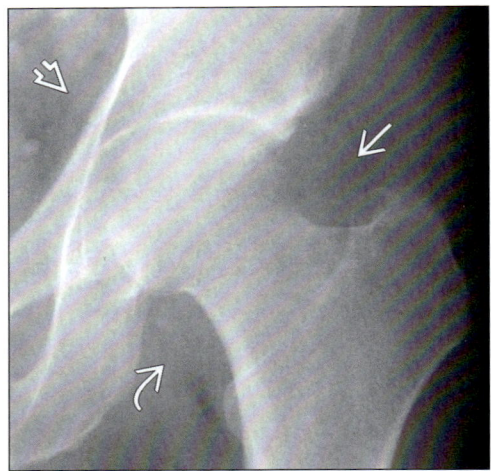 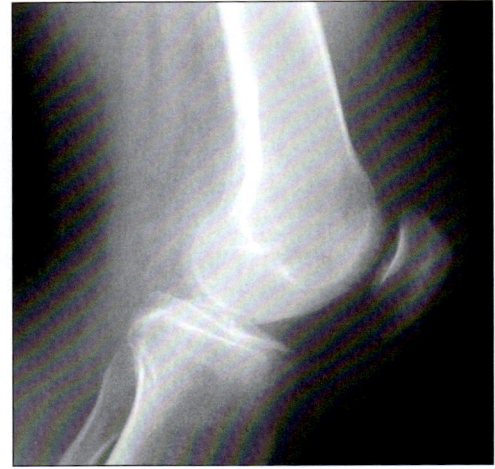

AP shows osteopenia of the femoral head, neck, & acetabulum. There is an effusion, with bulging fat pads (gluteal ➡, iliopsoas ➡, & obturator ➡). With negative aspirate, diagnosis is bone marrow edema.

Radiograph of the knee in the same patient, 10 months earlier, shows effusion & osteoporosis. Diagnosis is transient migratory bone marrow edema. Both imaging & symptoms returned to normal over several months.

TERMINOLOGY

Abbreviations and Synonyms
- Transient regional osteoporosis; transient osteoporosis of the hip; regional migratory osteoporosis

Definitions
- Transient, painful, osteoporosis; usually involving hip

IMAGING FINDINGS

General Features
- Best diagnostic clue
  - Radiograph: Joint effusion & osteoporosis (ideally, but not often, involving both sides of joint)
  - MR: Edema pattern; highly sensitive
- Location
  - Hip most frequent; occasionally other large joints, particularly lower extremity
    - Usually entire femoral head, extending to neck
- Morphology
  - Edema & osteoporosis; no cartilage loss
  - In hip, edema involves entire head & much of neck

Imaging Recommendations
- Often need to aspirate to rule out septic joint
- May need to re-image after several weeks to differentiate bone marrow edema from early AVN

Radiographic Findings
- Effusion (in hip, bulging fat pads)
- Osteoporosis
  - Watch for diminished bone density, thin trabeculae
  - Also watch for loss of cortical density & "crispness"
  - Ideally, seen on both sides of joint, but usually not
- Cartilage intact
- No erosive or contour changes of bone

MR Findings
- T1: Decreased signal, typical of bone edema
- T2: Effusion, hyperintense signal, typical of edema
- Post-contrast: Enhancement of edematous region
- No subchondral fracture or double line sign
- Delayed peak enhancement on perfusion imaging

Nuclear Medicine Findings
- Bone Scan: Increased uptake; non-specific

DDx: Transient Bone Marrow Edema

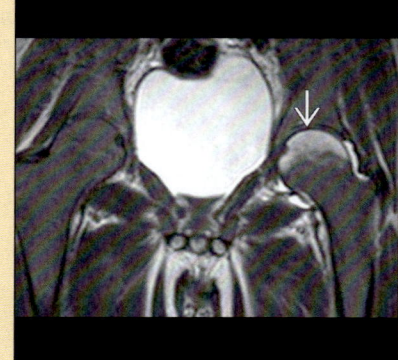 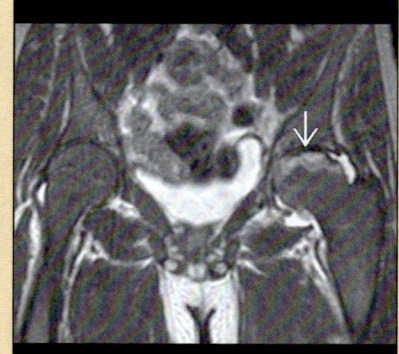 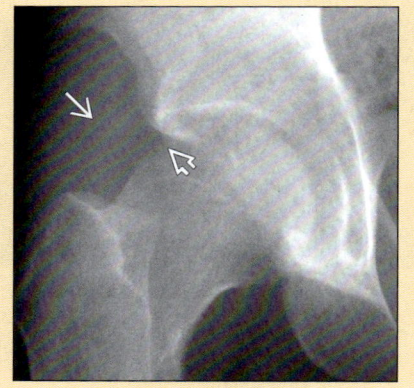

Sickle Cell with Edema — *7 Months Later: AVN* — *Septic Hip, Diabetic*

TRANSIENT BONE MARROW EDEMA

Key Facts

Terminology
- Transient, painful, osteoporosis, usually hip

Imaging Findings
- Edema & osteoporosis; no cartilage loss
- In hip, edema involves entire head & much of neck
- Often need to aspirate to rule out septic joint
- May need to re-image after several weeks to differentiate bone marrow edema from early AVN

Top Differential Diagnoses
- **Septic Joint**
- Presents initially as osteoporosis & effusion, not differentiated from transient bone marrow edema
- If advanced, cartilage is destroyed; bony erosions
- Aspiration required to differentiate from transient bone marrow edema
- **Avascular Necrosis**
- Marrow edema & effusion may be first manifestation

DIFFERENTIAL DIAGNOSIS

Septic Joint
- Presents initially as osteoporosis & effusion, not differentiated from transient bone marrow edema
- If advanced, cartilage is destroyed; bony erosions
- Aspiration required to differentiate from transient bone marrow edema

Avascular Necrosis
- Marrow edema & effusion may be first manifestation
- Important to differentiate in follow-up, since AVN may require early intervention to preserve joint integrity

PATHOLOGY

General Features
- Etiology: Unknown; self-limited

Gross Pathologic & Surgical Features
- Elevated pressure within bone marrow
- Normal articular cartilage & cortex
- Effusion & synovial inflammation

CLINICAL ISSUES

Presentation
- Most common signs/symptoms: Sudden severe pain

Demographics
- Age: 2nd, 3rd decades
- Gender
  - Males > females
  - Described in pregnant females (usually left hip)

Natural History & Prognosis
- Self-limited, usually reversing after several months; imaging returns to normal
- Occasionally is migratory, moving to involve another joint (usually hip or knee)

Treatment
- Conservative; protected weight-bearing
- Bisphosphonate therapy suggested by some
- For debilitating pain, core decompression has been suggested; shown to shorten the course of disease

DIAGNOSTIC CHECKLIST

Consider
- Septic joint must be ruled out, usually by aspiration
- Bone marrow edema may be earliest form of AVN

SELECTED REFERENCES

1. Hofmann S: The painful bone marrow edema syndrome of the hip joint. Wien Klin Wochenschr. 117(4):111-20, 2005
2. Malizos KN et al: MR imaging findings in transient osteoporosis of the hip. Eur J Radiol. 50(3):238-44, 2004

IMAGE GALLERY

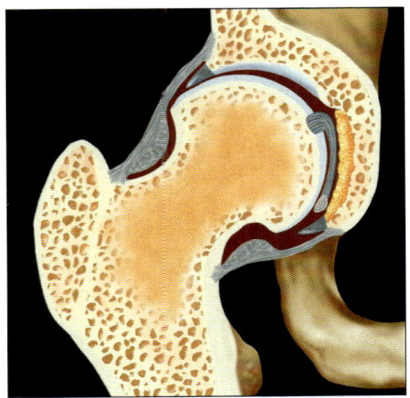 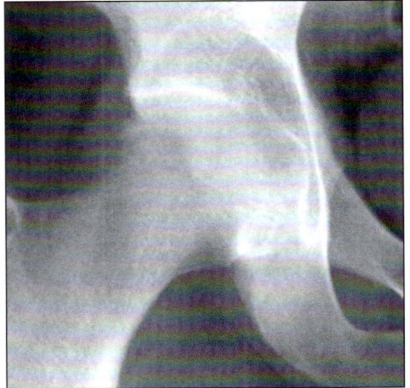 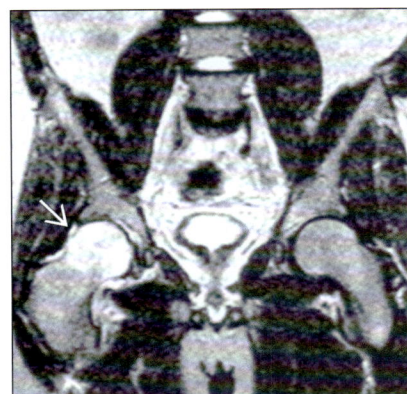

(Left) Graphic shows the usual distribution of transient bone marrow edema of the hip. *(Center)* Anteroposterior radiograph shows relative osteopenia of the femoral head & neck. Note particularly the lack of distinctness of the femoral head cortex. *(Right)* Coronal T2WI MR shows focal marrow edema within the right femoral head ➡. Aspirate yielded normal synovial fluid; diagnosis is transient bone marrow edema. The patient's symptoms, as well as the imaging abnormalities, resolved over the following several months.

OSTEONECROSIS, HIP

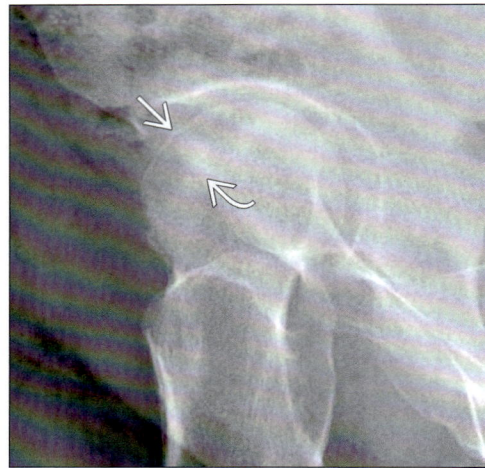

False profile view of the hip shows subtle sclerosis within the anterior superior weight-bearing portion of the femoral head ➡. There is also slight flattening ➡, typical of early avascular necrosis.

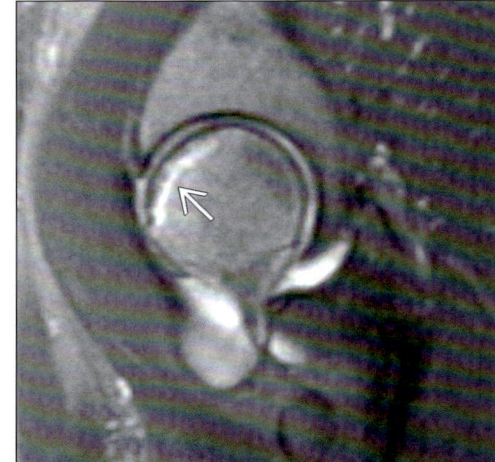

Sagittal T2WI FS MR shows the classic double line sign at the site of the subchondral fracture ➡, confirming the diagnosis of AVN. Note the anterosuperior position, 9 to 12 o'clock, typical initial site of involvement.

TERMINOLOGY

Abbreviations and Synonyms
- Ischemic necrosis, osteonecrosis, aseptic necrosis, AVN

Definitions
- Necrosis of cellular elements of bone, related to increased marrow pressure with impeded venous drainage or intraluminal vascular obstruction

IMAGING FINDINGS

General Features
- Best diagnostic clue
  - Early radiograph: Sclerosis femoral head
  - Late radiograph: Flattening, subchondral fracture; intact cartilage & acetabulum
  - MR: Double line sign in femoral head, ± significant edema
- Location
  - Anterior weight-bearing femoral head early
  - Atraumatic AVN common bilaterally (30-70% at time of presentation), but progresses asymmetrically
- Size: Small focus early, may extend to occupy entire superior half of femoral head
- Morphology
  - Early: Rounded femoral head is retained
  - Later: Flattening weight-bearing portion of head
  - Infarct itself is generally wedge-shaped

Imaging Recommendations
- Best imaging tool: MR is most sensitive & specific
- Protocol advice
  - Surgeons need complete information regarding extent of involvement
    - Use "face of clock" descriptive terminology
    - Image with MR in both coronal & sagittal planes to fully demonstrate extent

Radiographic Findings
- Early AVN: Relative sclerosis femoral head
  - Resorption of calcium around focus of ischemic bone, which itself retains normal density
- Subchondral fracture line & flattening of head
  - Linear lucency in weight-bearing portion, beneath & paralleling subchondral cortex; "crescent sign"
  - Best seen on frog lateral or false profile lateral view
- Late: Collapse femoral head

Etiologies of AVN of Hip

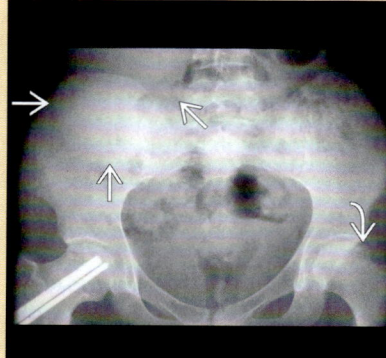

Gaucher Disease, Hepatomegaly

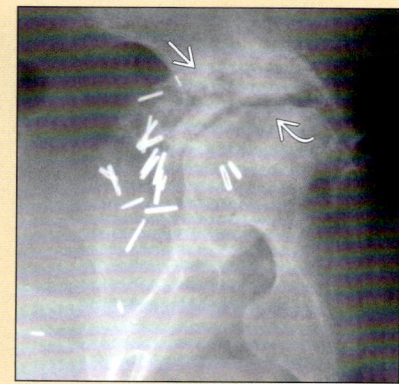

Radiation Necrosis

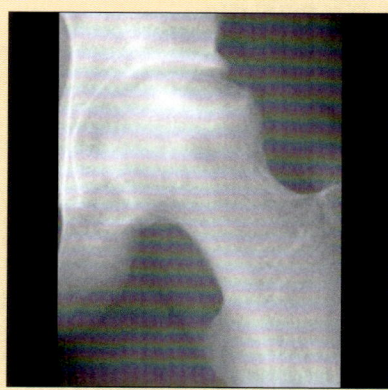

Sickle Cell Anemia; Patchy Sclerosis

OSTEONECROSIS, HIP

Key Facts

Imaging Findings
- Surgeons need complete information regarding extent of involvement
- Use "face of clock" descriptive terminology
- Image with MR in both coronal & sagittal planes to fully demonstrate extent
- Early AVN: Relative sclerosis femoral head
- Subchondral fracture line & flattening of head
- Linear lucency in weight-bearing portion, beneath & paralleling subchondral cortex; "crescent sign"
- Note: Until secondary osteoarthritis occurs, joint (acetabulum & cartilage width) remains intact; AVN is not a primary articular process
- May see abnormalities on an abdominal or pelvic radiograph which suggest an etiology for hip AVN
- Earliest, nonspecific MR abnormality: Marrow edema
- Fluid sensitive sequences: Double line sign in 80% (hyperintense inner border parallel to hypointense periphery)
- MR is 98% sensitive; 85% specific for AVN

Pathology
- 15,000 cases hip AVN in US per year
- Steroid use responsible for 30-40% of cases of nontraumatic AVN
- Alcoholism responsible for 20-40%

Diagnostic Checklist
- Edema in femoral head/neck in presence of AVN appears to relate to significant pain
- Watch for contralateral side involvement (may be clinically silent)

- Mixed lucent & sclerotic bone: Sclerosis due to new bone formation along reactive interface with retained ischemic bone
- Note: Until secondary osteoarthritis occurs, joint (acetabulum & cartilage width) remains intact; AVN is not a primary articular process
- May see abnormalities on an abdominal or pelvic radiograph which suggest an etiology for hip AVN
  - Sickle cell anemia
    - Patchy bone sclerosis (diffuse infarcts)
    - Autosplenectomy, gallstones
  - Renal transplant: Reniform mass, clips in iliac fossa
  - Trauma from dislocation: Acetabular fixation
  - Gaucher: Hepatosplenomegaly
  - Alcoholism: Pancreatic calcifications
  - Cushing (endogenous steroids): 12th rib resection from adrenalectomies
  - Radiation necrosis: Port-like configuration

CT Findings
- Bone CT
  - Osteoporosis & distortion of bony "asterisk" of femoral head trabeculae
  - Reformats: Subchondral fracture & flattening
  - Not as sensitive (55%) or accurate as MR

MR Findings
- Earliest, nonspecific MR abnormality: Marrow edema
  - Hypointense on T1, hyperintense on fluid sequences
  - Edema throughout femoral head & proximal neck
  - Identical to MR appearance of transient bone marrow edema (transient osteoporosis)
- Specific appearance for AVN
  - T1WI: Hypointense peripheral band outlining central region of bone marrow (reactive interface between necrotic & reparative zones)
    - Hypointense joint effusion
    - ± Flattening femoral head
  - Fluid sensitive sequences: Double line sign in 80% (hyperintense inner border parallel to hypointense periphery)
    - ± Edema in remaining femoral head & neck (hyperintense T2, fairly uniform)
    - Hyperintense effusion
    - Subchondral fx line may be obscured by edema
    - ± Flattening femoral head
  - T1 C+: Decreased enhancement in early AVN; later, no enhancement of nonviable segments
- Use both coronal & sagittal to evaluate extent of abnormality, using face of clock analogy
- Edema in presence of AVN appears highly correlated with severe pain
  - Edema found in 48% of patients with AVN
  - 72% of cases with edema occur in Steinberg stage III disease (AVN with subchondral lucency)
  - May presage collapse of head & suggest the latest point where core decompression may be efficacious
- MR is 98% sensitive; 85% specific for AVN

Nuclear Medicine Findings
- Bone Scan
  - Very early: Photopenic
  - Later: Increased activity: Revascularization & repair
  - May be more sensitive than radiograph (85% sensitivity on SPECT), but significantly less than MR

DIFFERENTIAL DIAGNOSIS

Transient Bone Marrow Edema (Transient Osteoporosis)
- Identical marrow edema pattern + effusion to earliest signs of AVN
- Self-limited; does not progress to collapse

PATHOLOGY

General Features
- General path comments: Bones that are mostly covered with articular cartilage (such as femoral head) are particularly at risk for AVN because of tenuous blood supply
- Etiology
  - Post-traumatic: Disrupted blood supply

OSTEONECROSIS, HIP

- Hip dislocation: If not reduced within 12 hours, 50% develop AVN
- Subcapital fracture: 30% displaced femoral fractures develop AVN
- Corticosteroid use: Enlargement of intramedullary fat cells → increased pressure
  - Of all patients on steroids, 2% develop AVN
  - Risk greater for patients treated for short duration (6 weeks) with high doses (> 20 mg); 5-25% of these patients develop AVN
  - Risk greater in renal transplant patients on steroids (40% develop AVN), with underlying osteodystrophy
  - 10% of long term survivors of bone marrow transplantation who received high doses of steroids develop AVN
- Alcohol abuse: Likely due to fat emboli from liver
- Sickle cell anemia: Thrombosis in microvasculature by sickled cells at low oxygen tension
- Gaucher disease: Marrow packing → increased pressure
- Systemic lupus erythematosus (SLE): Vasculitis + steroids; 5-40% develop AVN
- Caisson disease: Nitrogen air embolization from dysbaric phenomena
- Radiation: Vasculitis results in osteonecrosis
- HIV/AIDS: May relate to antiretroviral therapy or hyperlipidemia
- SCFE (slipped capital femoral epiphysis) & DDH (developmental dysplasia hip) both at risk for AVN
- Etiology of pain related to AVN is not well understood
  - AVN does not always produce pain; 6% of patients with renal transplant (treated with steroids) who had AVN diagnosed by MR were asymptomatic
  - Presence of marrow edema is extremely highly correlated with degree of pain
  - Relief of pressure by core decompression relieves pain promptly
  - Development of fracture may exacerbate pain
  - Joint effusion appears to not be significantly related to pain
- Epidemiology
  - 15,000 cases hip AVN in US per year
  - Steroid use responsible for 30-40% of cases of nontraumatic AVN
  - Alcoholism responsible for 20-40%
  - 10% of hip arthroplasties performed for AVN

Gross Pathologic & Surgical Features
- Softened necrotic cancellous bone at interface with viable bone
- Necrotic bone extends to subarticular surface

Staging, Grading or Classification Criteria
- Steinberg classification
  - Stage I: Normal radiographs
  - Stage II: Cystic or sclerotic change
  - Stage III: Subchondral lucency or crescent sign
  - Stage IV: Flattening of femoral head
  - Stage V: Joint space narrowing
  - Stage VI: Advanced degenerative disease

CLINICAL ISSUES

Presentation
- Most common signs/symptoms
  - Hip, groin, or referred pain to thigh
  - Decreased range of motion
  - Check for associated history of trauma, steroid use, alcohol abuse, SLE, or sickle cell anemia

Demographics
- Age: 3rd through 6th decades
- Gender: M:F = 4:1

Natural History & Prognosis
- Rarely may revascularize without progression
- Generally → flattening → collapse femoral head → OA

Treatment
- Treatment decisions of early disease not always straightforward
  - Some cases of renal transplant with MR-diagnosed AVN are asymptomatic & spontaneously resolve
  - Pain occasionally lessens spontaneously with conservative management; generally follows resolution of marrow edema
  - Core decompression generally relieves pain promptly (average duration of symptoms ↓)
    - Likely mechanism is relieving marrow edema & intraosseous hypertension
    - May be particularly useful in stage III patients (without significant collapse) with marrow edema (correlates with severe pain)
    - May continue on to collapse
  - Core decompression with vascularized fibular grafting is unproven as more efficacious than core decompression alone
- Treatment of later disease: Required in 50% of patients within 3 years of diagnosis
  - Varus & anterior angulated osteotomy rarely used to alter weightbearing portion of femoral head
  - Collapse prior to development of OA: Endoprosthesis (retaining native acetabulum)
  - Once significant OA has developed, total hip arthroplasty may be only effective treatment

DIAGNOSTIC CHECKLIST

Consider
- Edema in femoral head/neck in presence of AVN appears to relate to significant pain
- Watch for contralateral side involvement (may be clinically silent)

SELECTED REFERENCES
1. Ito H et al: Relationship between bone marrow edema and development of symptoms in patients with osteonecrosis of the femoral head. AJR Am J Roentgenol. 186(6):1761-70, 2006
2. Thomas J et al: HIV infection--a risk factor for osteoporosis. J Acquir Immune Defic Syndr. 33(3):281-91, 2003
3. Scribner AN et al: Osteonecrosis in HIV: a case-control study. J Acquir Immune Defic Syndr. 25(1):19-25, 2000

OSTEONECROSIS, HIP

IMAGE GALLERY

Typical

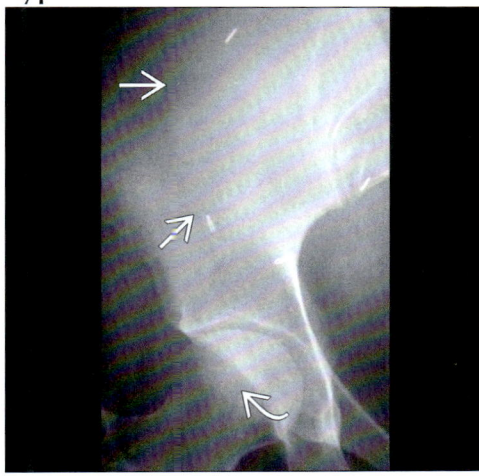
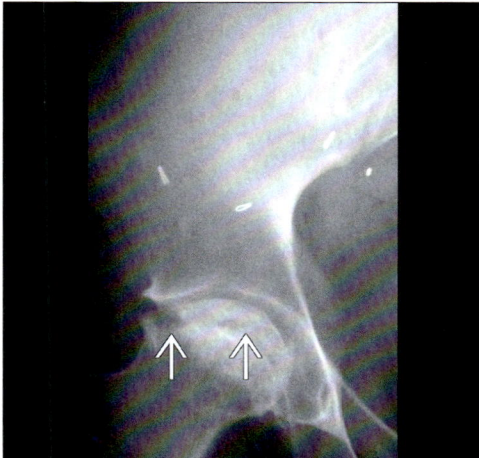

(Left) AP shows relative sclerosis within the femoral head ➡. This patient has a reniform soft tissue mass overlying the iliac wing ➡. This is a renal transplant; the patient has AVN related to steroid use. *(Right)* Radiograph obtained 6 months later shows severe AVN, with subchondral fracture ➡ and flattening. It is too late at this point for effective therapy; remember that relative sclerosis of the femoral head is an early sign of AVN, particularly in a setting of high risk.

Typical

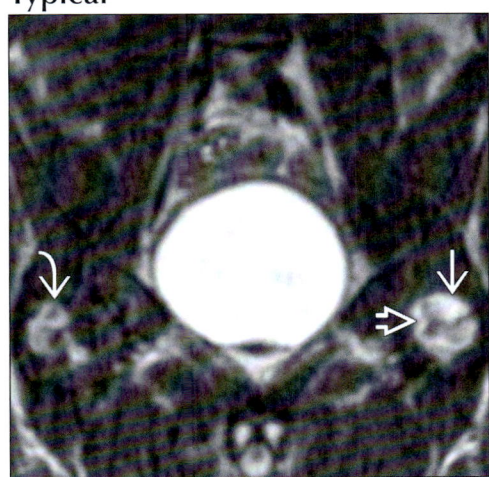
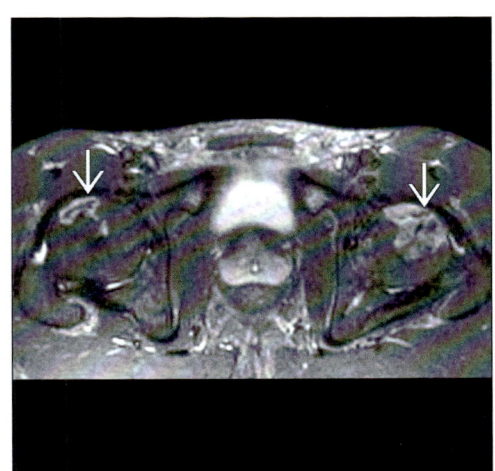

(Left) Coronal T2WI MR shows diffuse low signal within the bones typical of marrow conversion in a sickle cell patient. There is also marrow edema in the left femoral head ➡, as well as the double line sign indicating AVN ➡. Finally, there is a double line indicating an infarct within the greater trochanter on the right ➡. *(Right)* Axial STIR MR confirms bilateral AVN of the femoral heads ➡. Note the anterior position of the AVN within the head, which is typical.

Typical

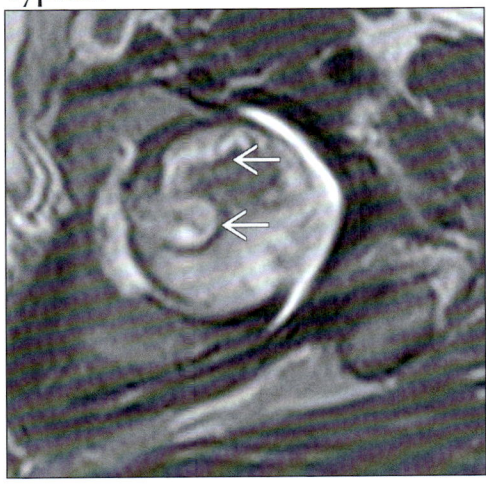
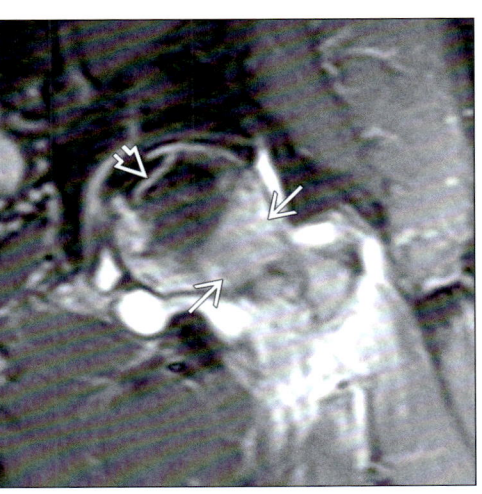

(Left) Axial T2WI FS MR shows the serpiginous double line sign ➡ which is typically seen on fluid sensitive sequences in avascular necrosis. Note the anterior location, also typical. *(Right)* Coronal STIR MR also shows the double line sign ➡. A large effusion is seen, as is extensive edema within the femoral neck ➡. This edema is not always present in AVN; it is hypothesized that it relates to recent collapse or extension of the AVN, and is associated with ↑ in pain.

OSTEONECROSIS, WRIST (SCAPHOID & LUNATE)

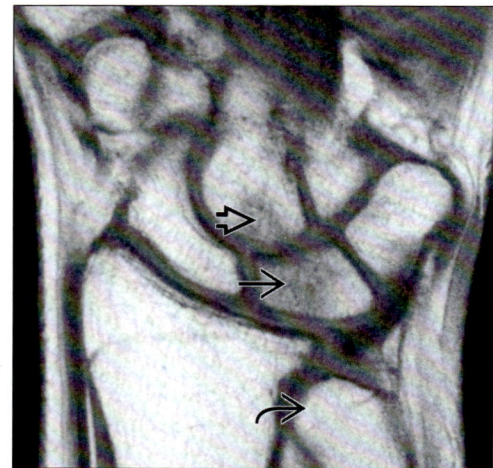

Coronal T1WI MR shows stage I Kienbock disease with diffuse marrow edema in the lunate ➔, and associated negative ulnar variance ➔. There is also mild edema in the proximal aspect of the capitate ➔.

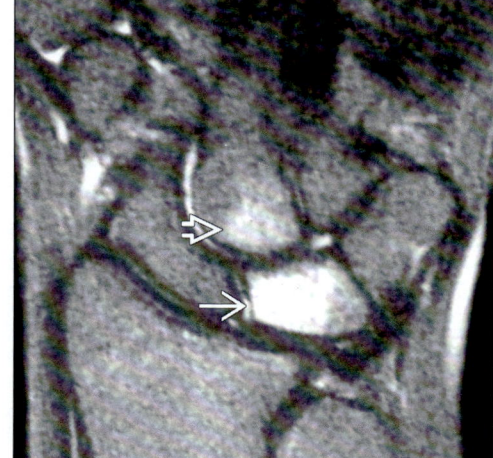

T2WI FS MR confirms diffuse edema in the lunate ➔ & mild edema in the proximal capitate ➔. This finding may be related to altered axial loading mechanics in the wrist due to significant ulnar minus variance.

TERMINOLOGY

Abbreviations and Synonyms
- Preiser disease: AVN of scaphoid without known trauma
- Kienbock disease: AVN of lunate; lunatomalacia, aseptic necrosis

IMAGING FINDINGS

General Features
- Best diagnostic clue: Flattening, fragmentation on radiograph; hypointense on T1 MR
- Size: Ranges from subtle subchondral fx to collapse

Radiographic Findings
- Lunate: Subchondral fx line, sclerosis, → collapse
  - Kienbock's may have associated ulnar negative variance, rarely ulnar positive
  - With collapse, capitate may migrate proximally
- Scaphoid: Usually proximal pole fx & nonunion
  - Rounded, sclerotic fracture edge
  - Sclerosis & fragmentation of proximal pole fragment
  - AVN of scaphoid without prior fracture (Preiser disease) rare: Fragmentation & sclerosis

MR Findings
- T1 MR: Hypointense, centralized to diffuse
  - Early subtle collapse on proximal radial border; later complete collapse & eventual osteoarthritis
- Fluid sensitive sequences
  - Early: Hyperintense marrow, hypointense fx line
  - Late: Hypointense sclerosis, with areas of hyperintensity; osseous collapse
- T1 C+: Viable marrow enhances
- If ulnar negative variance with lunatomalacia, TFCC may be thickened or torn

DIFFERENTIAL DIAGNOSIS

Lunate: Ulnar Impaction Syndrome
- Usually ulnar positive variance
- Chondromalacia, osteophyte & subchondral cysts

Scaphoid: Fx Nonunion without AVN
- Proximal pole or waist of scaphoid fx may develop nonunion, without necessarily having AVN

Other Kienbock Osteonecrosis

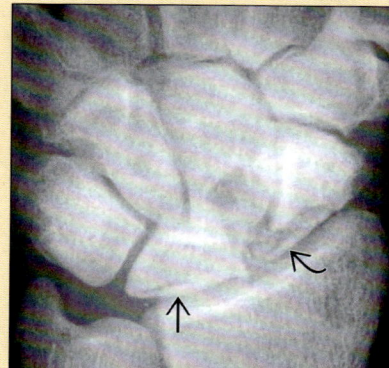
Lunate & Scaphoid AVN: SLE

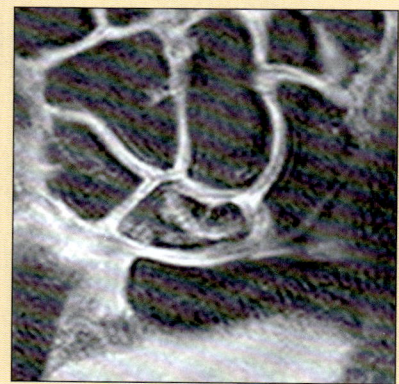
GRE Kienbock

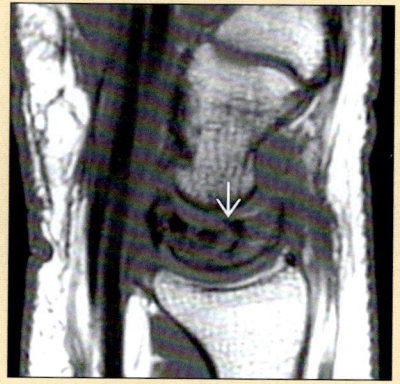
T1: Stage 3 (Flattening)

OSTEONECROSIS, WRIST (SCAPHOID & LUNATE)

Key Facts

Imaging Findings
- Kienbock's may have associated ulnar negative variance, rarely ulnar positive
- Scaphoid: Usually proximal pole fx & nonunion
- AVN of scaphoid without prior fracture (Preiser disease) rare: Fragmentation & sclerosis
- T1 MR: Hypointense, centralized to diffuse
- Early subtle collapse on proximal radial border; later complete collapse & eventual osteoarthritis

- If ulnar negative variance with lunatomalacia, TFCC may be thickened or torn

Top Differential Diagnoses
- Lunate: Ulnar Impaction Syndrome
- Scaphoid: Fx Nonunion without AVN

Diagnostic Checklist
- Contrast-enhanced images may help differentiate viable from non-viable fragments

PATHOLOGY

General Features
- Etiology
  - Lunate: Repeated microtrauma
  - Scaphoid: Usually proximal pole fracture
  - Interrupted blood supply
    - Lunate: 20% have single palmar vessel
    - Scaphoid: Proximal pole fx fragment may have no intact blood supply
  - Risk factors
    - Lunate: Ulnar negative variance
    - Lunate: Susceptible lunate morphology (oblong or square)
    - Scaphoid: Proximal location of fracture
    - Systemic lupus erythematosus (SLE); steroids

Staging, Grading or Classification Criteria
- Lunatomalacia: Lichtman classification
  - Stage I: Normal radiographs ± fracture
  - Stage II: Sclerosis without collapse
  - Stage III: Fragmentation + collapse (IIIA = no instability, IIIB = instability)
  - Stage IV: Sclerosis, collapse + perilunate OA

CLINICAL ISSUES

Presentation
- Most common signs/symptoms: Pain, limited range of motion, grip weakness

Demographics
- Age: 3rd or 4th decades

Natural History & Prognosis
- Chronic pain, arthrosis radiocarpal & midcarpal joints

Treatment
- Conservative
  - Casting: Differentiate transient ischemia from AVN
- Surgical
  - Revascularization
  - Bone graft, osteotomy
  - With arthrosis, may need arthrodesis or proximal row carpectomy for salvage

DIAGNOSTIC CHECKLIST

Image Interpretation Pearls
- Contrast-enhanced images may help differentiate viable from non-viable fragments

SELECTED REFERENCES
1. Zanetti M et al: Role of MR imaging in chronic wrist pain. Eur Radiol. 17(4):927-38, 2007
2. Zafra M et al: Vascularised bone graft and osteotomy of the radius in Kienbock's disease. Acta Orthop Belg. 71(2):163-8, 2005
3. Thienpont E et al: Radiographic analysis of anatomical risk factors for Kienbock's disease. Acta Orthop Belg. 70(5):406-9, 2004

IMAGE GALLERY

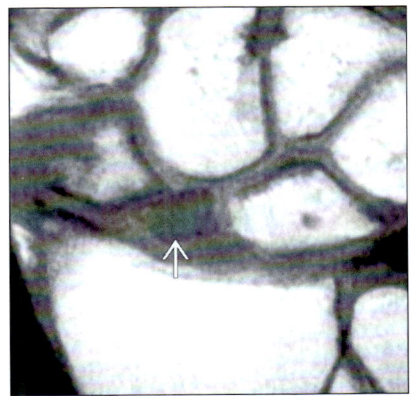 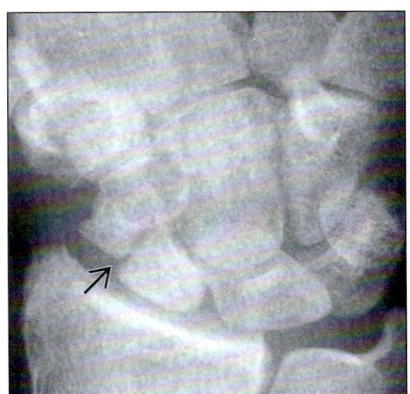 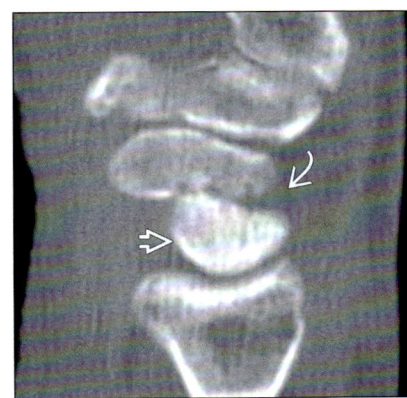

(Left) Coronal T1WI MR shows low signal, displacement, & early fragmentation of a proximal pole waist of scaphoid fracture ➡. There was no enhancement with contrast; this represents AVN as a complication of the fracture. (Center) Anteroposterior radiograph shows a subacute waist of scaphoid fracture ➡, with relative increased density of the proximal pole. (Right) Sagittal bone CT of the same case as previous image confirms increased density of the proximal pole scaphoid ➡, and the typical humpback deformity of the scaphoid fracture ➡.

OSTEOCHONDRITIS DISSECANS

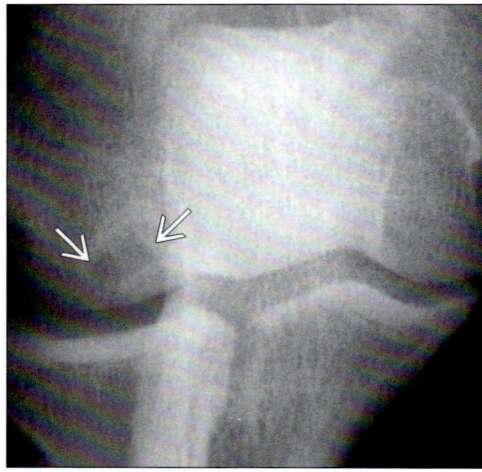

Anteroposterior radiograph shows a lucency within the capitellum ➔. This site is typical for OCD, and is seen in young athletes. It is important to address questions of stability of the fragment with MR.

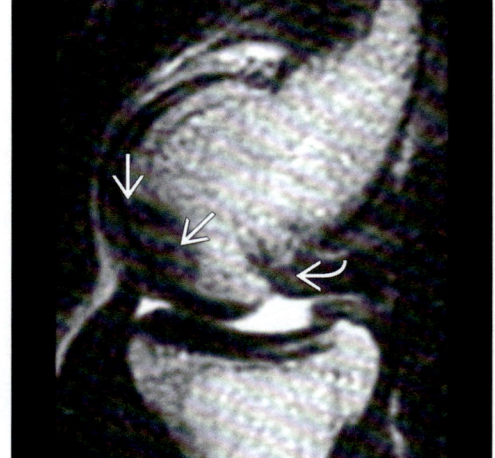

Sagittal T2WI MR confirms low signal within the lesion ➔. There is no peripheral hyperintensity, and the cartilage is intact. These features indicate stability of the fragment. Note the posterior pseudodefect ➔.

TERMINOLOGY

Abbreviations and Synonyms
- Osteochondral defect (OCD), osteochondritis

Definitions
- Lesion of articular surface, usually convex, involving subchondral bone which may extend to articular cartilage

IMAGING FINDINGS

General Features
- Best diagnostic clue: Convex articular surface with concave defect, ± osseous body
- Location
  - Not infrequently bilateral (20%)
  - Knee: Most frequent site
    - Lateral aspect medial femoral condyle
    - Trochlea (femoral sulcus): Usually anterior aspect lateral femoral condyle, close to midline; may occur medially
  - Ankle: Second most frequent site
    - Posteromedial talar dome
    - Anterolateral talar dome
  - Elbow: Anterolateral capitellum
  - Shoulder: Humeral head or glenoid (do not mistake central developmental defect of the glenoid)
  - Wrist: Rare involvement of scaphoid (distal or proximal pole)
- Size: Ranges from small to 3+ cm
- Morphology: Concave bed containing (at some point) osseous bodies

Imaging Recommendations
- Best imaging tool
  - Detection is usually by radiograph
    - May be subtle; MR often demonstrates unsuspected talar dome OCD
  - Evaluation for stability performed by MR

Radiographic Findings
- Radiographic abnormalities occur late in the process
  - Radiograph shows rounded lucency in subarticular region, usually at convex surface of bone
  - If radiograph is profiled properly, a concave defect at the convex osseous surface is seen, often containing an osseous body

DDx: Osteochondritis Dissecans

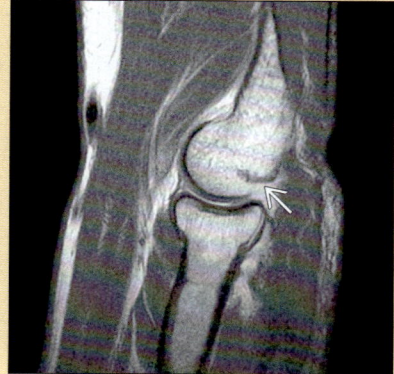

Pseudodefect Capitellum

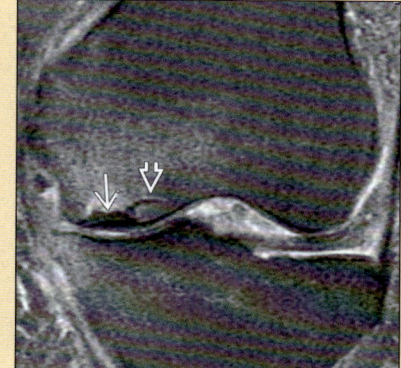

Spontaneous Osteonecrosis

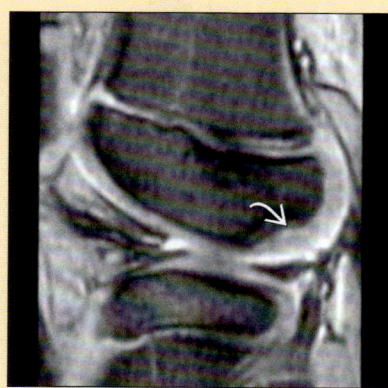

Irregularity Posterior Condyle

OSTEOCHONDRITIS DISSECANS

Key Facts

Imaging Findings
- Radiographic abnormalities occur late in the process
- Radiograph shows rounded lucency in subarticular region, usually at convex surface of bone
- If radiograph is profiled properly, a concave defect at the convex osseous surface is seen, often containing an osseous body
- Loose bodies may be in situ (within the concave "bed" of defect), or may displaced elsewhere within joint
- Earliest MR findings: Subchondral stress reaction
- Enhancement of osseous fragment indicates viability, but does not predict stability
- MR used to determine stability of lesion (92% sensitive, 90% specific for differentiating unstable lesions from stable lesions)
- Fluid sensitive sequences: Hyperintensity at majority of peripheral rim indicates instability
- Fluid entering defect through an articular cartilage defect indicates instability
- Subchondral cysts formed at peripheral rim indicate instability

Diagnostic Checklist
- Main goal for MR is to determine stability of lesion; T2 FS is most important sequence
- Identify loose bodies distant from OCD; these may require removal, even if OCD is stable
- Watch for normal variants at capitellum & posterior femoral condyles
- Enhancement of fragment indicates viability, but not necessarily stability

---

- Oblique view of capitellum or ankle is useful
- For trochlear (femoral sulcus) OCD, axial view of patella is useful
  - Flattening of the normal convexity of the articular surface
  - Loose bodies may be in situ (within the concave "bed" of defect), or may displaced elsewhere within joint

CT Findings
- Requires reformats for full evaluation
- Demonstrates concave defect with sclerotic margin
- Osseous fragments seen within defect; if displaced above articular margin, lesion is unstable
- Loose bodies not adjacent to defect
- Subchondral cysts: Indicate instability of lesion

MR Findings
- Earliest MR findings: Subchondral stress reaction
  - Hypointensity T1, hyperintense on fluid sensitive sequences; enhancement with contrast
  - No fracture line
  - Intact overlying cartilage
- With progression, fracture line forms but articular surface is intact
  - Focal T1 hypointensity may obscure fracture line
  - Focal hyperintensity on fluid sensitive sequences may obscure fracture line
    - Central signal of body variable: Low, high, or mixture of both
- With further progression, articular surface is disrupted; can be directly seen if fluid from effusion surrounds fragment within defect
- Use of contrast
  - Enhancement of osseous fragment indicates viability, but does not predict stability
  - Indirect arthrogram from IV contrast administration may produce enough fluid to demonstrate either intact or disrupted articular cartilage over defect
  - Not routinely required for evaluation of OCD
- MR used to determine stability of lesion (92% sensitive, 90% specific for differentiating unstable lesions from stable lesions)
  - Fluid sensitive sequences: Hyperintensity at majority of peripheral rim indicates instability
    - Etiology of hyperintensity is uncertain: Granulation tissue, edematous fibrous tissue, or fluid
  - Fluid entering defect through an articular cartilage defect indicates instability
  - Subchondral cysts formed at peripheral rim indicate instability
  - Focal osteochondral defect filled with joint fluid

DIFFERENTIAL DIAGNOSIS

Pseudodefect of Capitellum
- Located posteriorly in capitellum, not at the anterior site of OCD
- Normal indentation at junction of cartilage-covered capitellum with non-cartilaginous posterior bone

Panner Disease
- Avascular necrosis of entire capitellum
- Generally in younger patients (5-11 years)

Insufficiency Fracture Femoral Condyle
- Formerly known as SONK, spontaneous osteonecrosis of the knee
- Location generally directly in center of weight-bearing portion of medial femoral condyle
- Occurs in older, osteoporotic age group
- Pain pattern is different; acute, severe pain occurs
- May see depressed fracture fragment, with flattening of cortex, or only marrow edema

Normal Posterior Femoral Cortical Irregularity
- Osseous irregularity & pseudodefect may occur in posterior femoral condyles (not a usual site for OCD)
- Normal overlying cartilage
- Nearly always fills in with normal bone as patient matures
- Younger patient age group (8-12 years)

OSTEOCHONDRITIS DISSECANS

PATHOLOGY

General Features
- Etiology
  - Uncertain; believed to be repetitive microtrauma
    - Likely begins as a chronic shear stress injury within subchondral bone
    - Subchondral trabecular microfractures coalesce into fracture line
    - May extend to overlying cartilage if injury pattern continues without protection
  - OCD capitellum: Sports activities that place repetitive valgus stress on elbow
    - Male baseball pitchers or female gymnasts
    - Increased rotary, compressive, or axial loads: Throwing athletes
- Epidemiology
  - Knee: Most frequent joint
    - Medial femoral condyle: 85%
    - Inferocentral lateral femoral condyle: 13%
    - Trochlea (femoral sulcus): 2%
  - Ankle: Talus far more common than tibial plafond
    - Posteromedial aspect talus: 56%
    - Anterolateral aspect talus: 44%
    - 6.5% of sprained ankles develop OCD (this number is likely an underestimate; MR often shows unsuspected OCD)
  - Elbow (capitellum): About 5% overall

Gross Pathologic & Surgical Features
- Bony defect spectrum
  - May be a true defect
  - May contain osseous bodies
  - May contain fibrous tissue or fibrocartilage
- Osseous fragments spectrum
  - May have intact overlying articular cartilage
  - May be firmly attached by fibrous tissue
  - May be partially or completely detached
- Necrotic bone, granulation tissue, synovitis

Staging, Grading or Classification Criteria
- International Cartilage Repair Society: Classifies OCD at surgery
  - Stage I: Stable lesion in continuity with host bone, covered by intact cartilage
  - Stage II: Partial discontinuity, stable on probing
  - Stage III: Complete discontinuity of the "dead in situ" lesion, but fragment not dislocated
  - Stage IV: Dislocated fragment

CLINICAL ISSUES

Presentation
- Most common signs/symptoms
  - Pain, catching, locking
  - Onset & history usually insidious

Demographics
- Age: 2nd & 3rd decades
- Gender
  - M:F = 6:1 for elbow
  - M:F = 5:3 for knee
  - M:F = 2:1 for ankle

Natural History & Prognosis
- Stable lesions treated appropriately: 50% heal with return to full function
- Instability or loose bodies may result in persistent pain & mechanical symptoms
- Even with treatment, as many as 50% of unstable lesions yield persistent pain in the long term
- Unstable lesion eventually develops osteoarthritis

Treatment
- Major consideration for treatment: Instability of lesion
- What the clinician needs to know
  - Lesion size and location
  - Stability
  - Condition of overlying cartilage
  - Fragment osteonecrosis
  - Loose bodies within joint
- Stable lesions: Non-weight-bearing; muscle strengthening exercises
- Unstable lesions
  - In situ loose body may be pinned, drilled, and/or microfractured if overlying cartilage is mostly intact
  - Removal of loose bodies may be required, with debridement of defect
  - Various transplant techniques may be utilized to address defect

DIAGNOSTIC CHECKLIST

Consider
- Main goal for MR is to determine stability of lesion; T2 FS is most important sequence
- Identify loose bodies distant from OCD; these may require removal, even if OCD is stable

Image Interpretation Pearls
- Watch for normal variants at capitellum & posterior femoral condyles
- Enhancement of fragment indicates viability, but not necessarily stability
- High signal interface between lesion & underlying bone indicates instability

SELECTED REFERENCES

1. Murray JR et al: Osteochondritis dissecans of the knee; long-term clinical outcome following arthroscopic debridement. Knee. 14(2):94-8, 2007
2. Han SH et al: Radiographic changes and clinical results of osteochondral defects of the talus with and without subchondral cysts. Foot Ankle Int. 27(12):1109-14, 2006
3. Kocher MS et al: Management of osteochondritis dissecans of the knee: current concepts review. Am J Sports Med. 34(7):1181-91, 2006
4. Kijowski R et al: MRI findings of osteochondritis dissecans of the capitellum with surgical correlation. AJR Am J Roentgenol. 185(6):1453-9, 2005
5. Boutin RD et al: MR imaging features of osteochondritis dissecans of the femoral sulcus. AJR Am J Roentgenol. 180(3):641-5, 2003
6. De Smet AA et al: Osteochondritis dissecans of the knee: value of MR imaging in determining lesion stability and the presence of articular cartilage defects. AJR Am J Roentgenol. 155(3):549-53, 1990

OSTEOCHONDRITIS DISSECANS

IMAGE GALLERY

Typical

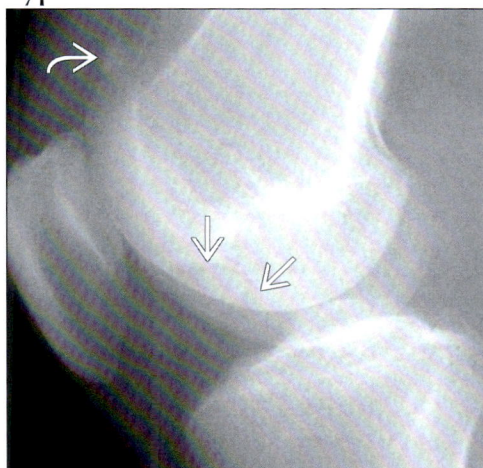
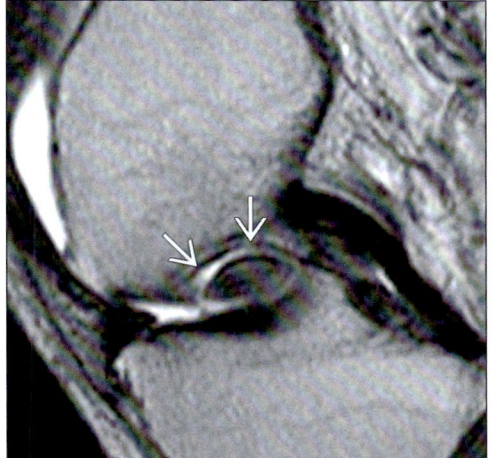

(Left) Lateral radiograph shows a large osteochondral defect in the medial femoral condyle ➔, containing an ossific body. A loose body is also noted within the suprapatellar bursa ➔. *(Right)* Sagittal T2WI MR shows a knee effusion, with fluid surrounding the body ➔. There is a disruption in the cartilage, allowing this fluid to flow around the body; this indicates an in situ loose body, with implied displaceability and instability.

Typical

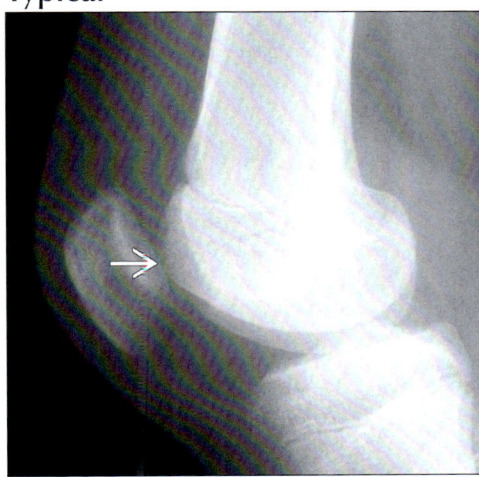
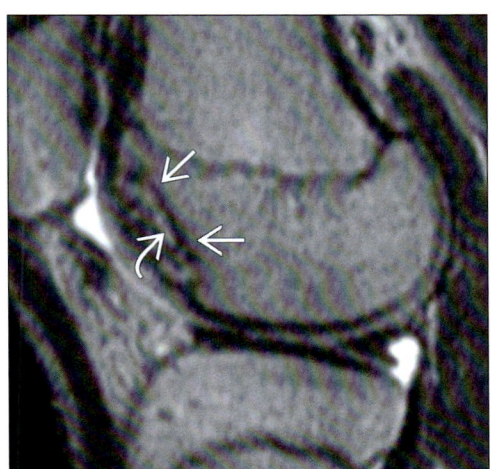

(Left) Lateral radiograph shows a subtle lucency within the lateral trochlea, with flattening of the cortex ➔. This represents an uncommon site of osteochondritis dissecans. *(Right)* Sagittal T2WI MR shows high signal near the lesion periphery ➔, but low signal even more peripheral to that ➔. This knee had been treated with drilling; the subtle hyperintensity represents granulation healing tissue while the surrounding low signal rim suggests healing & stability.

Typical

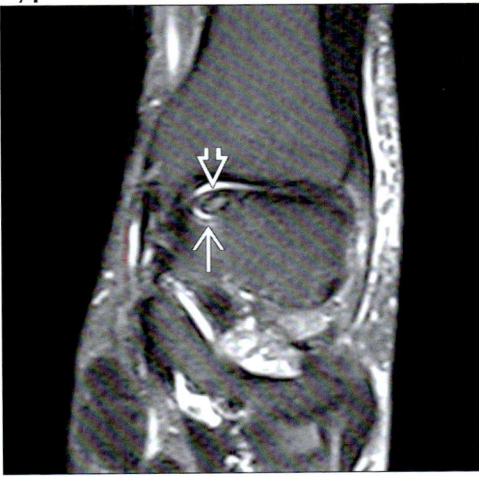
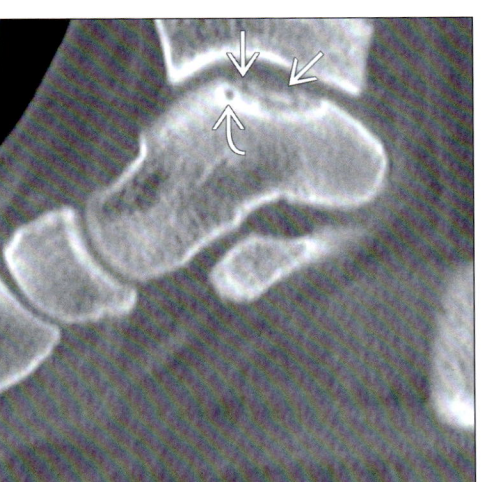

(Left) Coronal T2WI FS MR shows a posteromedial osteochondral defect of the talus, with high signal at the periphery of the lesion ➔, indicating instability. The small amount of fluid overlying the talar cartilage shows that it is thinned ➔. *(Right)* Sagittal bone CT reformat in a different patient shows a large osteochondral defect in the posteromedial talus, with osseous fragmentation & flattening ➔. The presence of a subchondral cyst ➔ confirms lesion instability.

ARTHROPLASTY LOOSENING & DISLOCATION

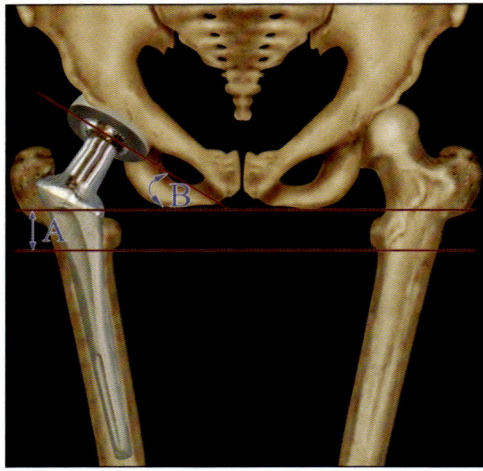

Normal positioning of a THA, with transischial line of reference. The lateral opening of the cup is angle B (nl 40° ± 10°). Limb length (A) is evaluated by a landmark (usually lesser trochanter) relative to transischial line.

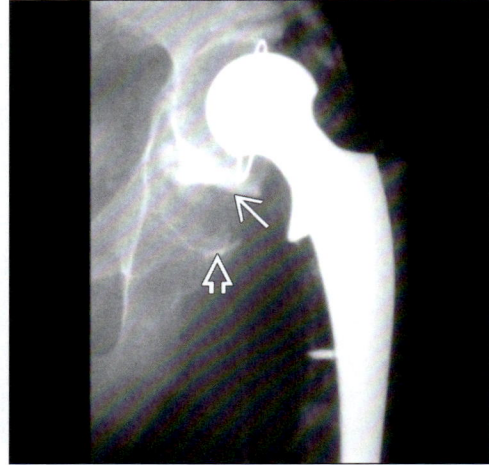

Anteroposterior radiograph shows gross loosening of a cemented acetabular component. There is superior subsidence of the cup by 2 cm ➔ relative to its original position ➔, as well as abnormal lateral opening (tilt).

TERMINOLOGY

Abbreviations and Synonyms
- Total hip arthroplasty (THA)
- Total knee arthroplasty (TKA)

Definitions
- For the purposes of this discussion, hip arthroplasties are discussed in greatest detail
  - THA is the most frequent arthroplasty
  - Most principles of evaluation of THA are generalizable to other prostheses
- Total arthroplasty: Resurfacing of both sides of a joint
- Hemiarthroplasty (endoprosthesis): Replacement of only one side of joint
  - Used in cases of avascular necrosis (collapse with damage on only one side of joint)
  - Used in cases of displaced subcapital fracture of hip where acetabular cup shows no significant arthritis
  - Occasionally used when a single compartment of a knee joint is involved with arthritis
    - Medial or lateral compartment
    - Patellofemoral compartment

IMAGING FINDINGS

General Features
- Best diagnostic clue
  - Loosening of any component
    - Change in component alignment or position
    - Change in angulation of component
    - Change in superior-inferior position (subsidence)
    - Subsidence of cup is in a superior direction
    - Subsidence of femoral component is down the shaft
    - Subsidence of patellar button is usually in a superior direction
    - Subsidence without angulation of TKA femoral or tibial components is rare
    - Progressive change without stabilization is concerning for loosening
    - Component or bone fracture result in loosening
  - Loosening of a cemented component
    - ≥ 2 mm lucency at bone-cement interface, surrounding majority of component
    - ≥ 2 mm lucency at cement-component interface, surrounding majority of component
    - These lucencies often have a sclerotic margin

Cementless Components: Cortical & Endosteal Hypertrophy

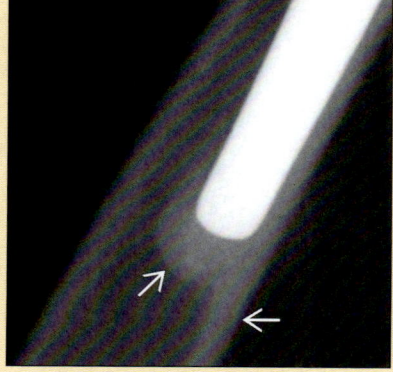

Solid: Nonbridging Hypertrophy

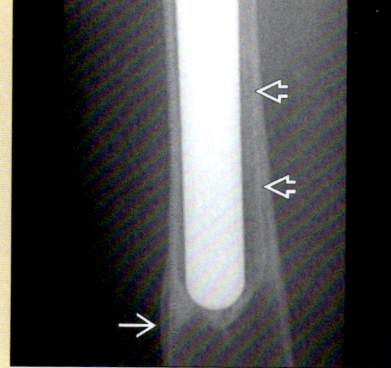

Loose: Hypertrophy & Lucency

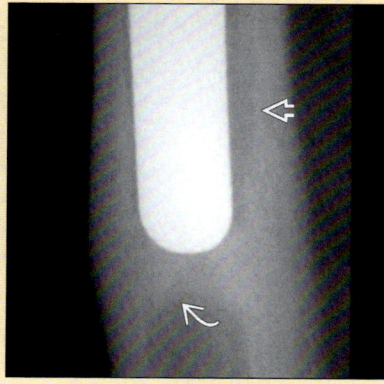

Bridging Hypertrophy & Lucency

ARTHROPLASTY LOOSENING & DISLOCATION

Key Facts

Imaging Findings
- Change in component alignment or position
- Subsidence of cup is in a superior direction
- Subsidence of femoral component is down the shaft
- ≥ 2 mm lucency at bone-cement interface, surrounding majority of component
- ≥ 2 mm lucency at bone-component interface, surrounding majority of component
- Acetabular lateral opening measurement: Angle of cup to transischial line: 40° ± 10°
- Limb length: Choose a landmark (usually lesser trochanter) & measure to transischial line, comparing to contralateral side
- Anteversion: Note that one can observe version of the cup, but CANNOT tell on AP whether is anteverted or retroverted
- Groin lateral: Necessary to determine direction of cup version (ante- or retro-)
- Subsidence or angulation of components may occur without appearance of lucency around component
- Protocol advice: Be certain to include the entire prosthesis stem on image

Diagnostic Checklist
- Watch for subsidence of components without obvious lucency to indicate loosening
- With dislocation, search for malposition of components as a cause
- Do not mistake a femoral hemiarthroplasty for a THA with malpositioned acetabular component
- Compare follow-up image with index radiograph for change in component position

---

- Fracture cement
  - Loosening of a cementless component
    - ≥ 2 mm lucency at bone-component interface, surrounding majority of component
    - Lucency often has a sclerotic margin
    - Normally may resorb calcar, especially with flange at neck of femoral component
    - Normally may have cortical hypertrophy at tip of femoral component
    - Normally may have endosteal hypertrophy at tip of femoral component
    - If the hypertrophy at femoral component tip bridges across marrow space, it is considered evidence of loosening
  - Structural causes of total hip dislocation; these malpositioned components also predispose to component loosening
    - Reconstruction resulting in abnormal limb length
    - Acetabular retroversion or anteversion > 30°
    - Acetabular lateral opening > 50° or < 30°
    - Acetabular component not properly medialized
- Morphology
  - Normal positioning of THA components
    - Length equal to contralateral side
    - Length can be affected by position of cup, femoral stem, or size of neck, head, or polyethylene components
    - Cup open laterally 40° ± 10°
    - Cup anteverted 10-15°
    - Medial-lateral position of cup: horizontal center of rotation should be similar to that of normal head
    - Femoral component in neutral to slight valgus position (prosthesis resting against the lateral cortex proximally & medial cortex distally)
  - Normal positioning of TKA components
    - Femoral component: 5° ± 5° to long axis of femoral shaft on lateral
    - Femoral component: 4-7° valgus on AP
    - Tibial component: 90° ± 5° to long axis of tibial shaft on AP
    - Tibial component: Slight posterior tilt on lateral (normal posterior tilt in native knee is 10°)
    - Patellar button: Center of patella

Radiographic Findings
- AP pelvis
  - Use transischial line as reference for measurements
  - Acetabular lateral opening measurement: Angle of cup to transischial line: 40° ± 10°
    - If > 50°, at risk for dislocation
    - If < 30°, also at risk for dislocation if hip placed in forced abduction
  - Acetabular medial-lateral positioning: Choose a landmark (such as teardrop) to compare position with contralateral hip
    - If over-medialized, excessive thinning of medial wall risks failure
    - If cup is laterally placed, iliopsoas contraction can force dislocation
  - Limb length: Choose a landmark (usually lesser trochanter) & measure to transischial line, comparing to contralateral side
    - Too long: Muscles spasm & result in dislocation
    - Too short: Hip muscles ineffective, leaving hip at risk for dislocation
  - Anteversion: Note that one can observe version of the cup, but CANNOT tell on AP whether is anteverted or retroverted
- Groin lateral: Necessary to determine direction of cup version (ante- or retro-)
  - Note that precise measurement may vary with rotation of pelvis
    - Rotation of pelvis may be controlled by flexing knee over end of table while filming groin lateral

CT Findings
- CT used to evaluate bone stock prior to revision
- Coronal & sagittal reformats minimize metal artifact & allow precision in surgical planning

Imaging Recommendations
- Best imaging tool
  - Radiographs
    - THA: AP & groin lateral
    - TKA: AP, lateral, sunrise

ARTHROPLASTY LOOSENING & DISLOCATION

- Total shoulder: AP & axillary lateral
- Wrist & hand arthroplasties: PA, oblique, lateral
  - Comparison radiographs are essential to evaluate for progressive change
    - Subsidence or angulation of components may occur without appearance of lucency around component
- Protocol advice: Be certain to include the entire prosthesis stem on image

DIFFERENTIAL DIAGNOSIS

Infection
- Rarely, gas may be seen in soft tissues
- Radiographs most frequently show no abnormality if infection is acute
- Subacute infection may show fluffy bone formation about the arthroplasty
- Nuclear medicine studies are often abnormal but nonspecific (abnormal for several months following surgery)
- Diagnosis made by aspiration of joint

Particle Disease (Massive Osteolysis)
- Source of particles may be found
  - Polyethylene wear
  - Osseous debris
  - Metal debris
- Osteolysis tends to be more focal & lytic in particle disease, rather than surrounding the prosthesis

Normal Subsidence in Revision Arthroplasty
- Revisions often are placed in deficient bone related to prior arthroplasty failure
  - Structural or nonstructural bone graft may be placed in osseous defects
    - Either may compress or resorb, resulting in change in position of arthroplasty component
  - Cerclage wires & onlay grafts may help support regions of osseous defects
    - These may not completely secure a long bone component, which then subsides
- Subsidence of several mm or change in angulation may be expected over first 6 months of a revision
- Compare with prior exams & watch for stabilization or continued evidence of component instability

PATHOLOGY

General Features
- Epidemiology
  - Reasons for revision of THA
    - Loose without infection: 52%
    - Instability: 17%
    - Loose with infection: 5.5%
  - Reasons for hip dislocation
    - Positional (hip placed beyond expected range of motion): Most frequent
    - Soft tissue imbalance (reconstruction length either too long or too short)
    - Component malposition (see above): Abnormal acetabular tilt or version

Gross Pathologic & Surgical Features
- Press fit (noncemented) components have a porous surface to allow bone ingrowth for better fixation
  - Surface etched or composed of metal beads
  - Porous surface not always discernible on radiograph
- Ingrowth is mostly fibrous rather than osseous
  - In autopsy series of asymptomatic THA
    - 1/3: No ingrowth
    - 2/3: Ingrowth of only 2-10% of available surface
  - Osseous versus fibrous ingrowth cannot be discerned radiographically

CLINICAL ISSUES

Presentation
- Most common signs/symptoms: Progressive pain

Demographics
- Age
  - Generally older patients have arthroplasties & associated complications
  - Younger patients with arthroplasty due to hip dysplasia have higher rate of complication
    - Related to gracile femoral shaft, limb length discrepancy, & inadequate acetabular bone stock

Natural History & Prognosis
- Loose component generally shows progression to gross loosening
- Dislocated hip without malposition of components likely due to positional mistake
  - Patient may be counseled regarding position and activity
  - If malpositioned components, revision is likely necessary

Treatment
- Revision arthroplasty

DIAGNOSTIC CHECKLIST

Consider
- Watch for subsidence of components without obvious lucency to indicate loosening
- With dislocation, search for malposition of components as a cause

Image Interpretation Pearls
- Do not mistake a femoral hemiarthroplasty for a THA with malpositioned acetabular component
- Compare follow-up image with index radiograph for change in component position

SELECTED REFERENCES
1. Ulrich SD et al: Total hip arthroplasties: What are the reasons for revision? Int Orthop. 2007
2. Taljanovic MS et al: Joint arthroplasties and prostheses. Radiographics. 23(5):1295-314, 2003
3. Manaster BJ: Total hip arthroplasty: radiographic evaluation. Radiographics. 16 (3):645-60, 1996

ARTHROPLASTY LOOSENING & DISLOCATION

IMAGE GALLERY

Typical

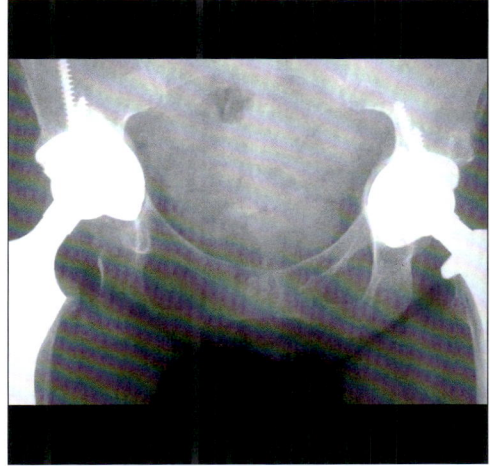
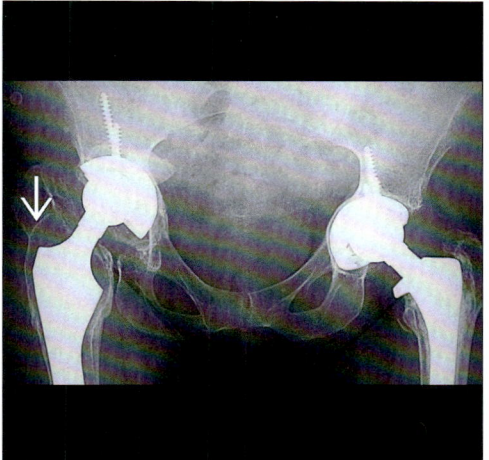

(Left) AP radiograph shows normal placement of the THA. *(Right)* Radiograph obtained 4 years later, shows gross loosening of the femoral component, with inferior subsidence by 1.5 cm ➡. At first glance, the acetabular cup does not appear loose since there is no surrounding lucency. However, compared to the prior image, the cup has subsided superiorly (note its relation to teardrop) & shows an increased lateral tilt. This change in position is diagnostic of loosening.

Typical

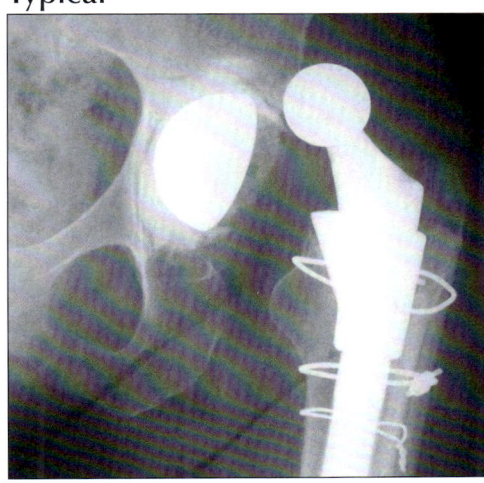
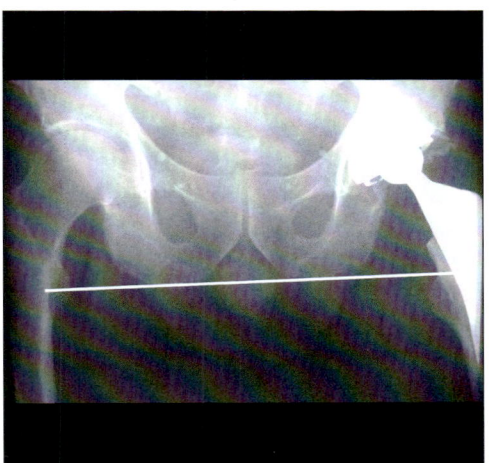

(Left) AP radiograph shows a dislocated THA. The cemented cup is not loose, as the lucency at the bone-cement interface does not exceed 2 mm. However, there is abnormal lateral tilt of the cup (75°), which predisposes the hip to dislocation. *(Right)* This patient had repeated left hip dislocations. Note that the left hip is relatively long compared with the right (distance from transischial line to lesser trochanter: L > R). Increased length puts a THA at risk for dislocation.

Typical

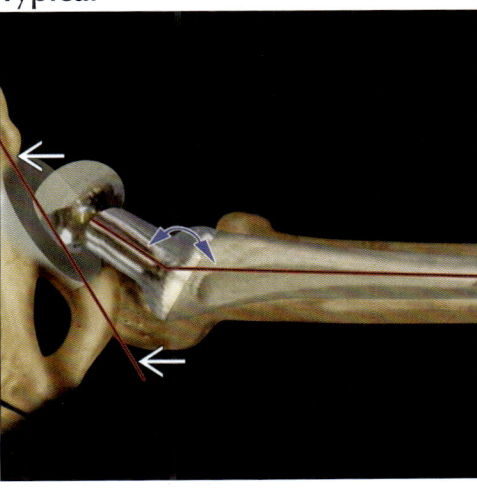
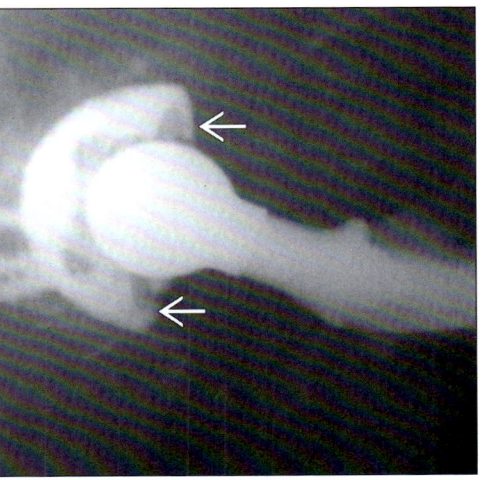

(Left) Groin lateral shows anterior tilt (anteversion) of the acetabular component ➡. The angle describes the neck-shaft angle. *(Right)* Groin lateral view of a THA in a patient with recurrent dislocations shows retroversion of the acetabular component ➡, (compare angulation with that on the prior graphic). One cannot determine retroversion vs. anteversion on AP radiograph; groin lateral is required. Retroversion puts a THA at risk for dislocation.

ARTHROPLASTY HARDWARE/PERIPROSTHETIC FX

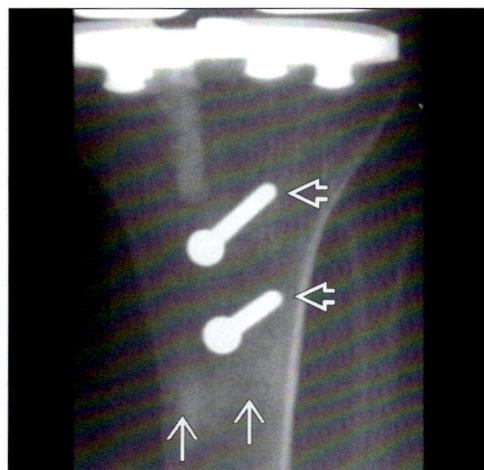 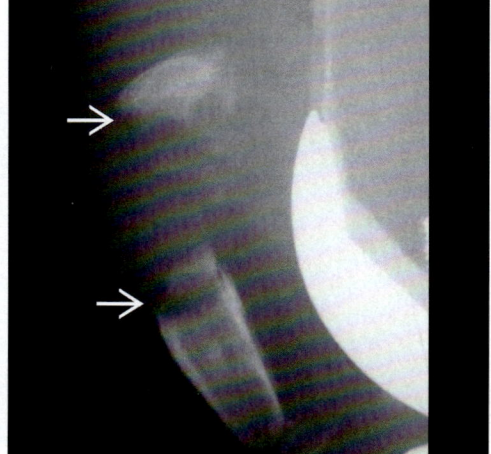

Anteroposterior radiograph shows linear sclerosis, indicating a periprosthetic fx of the tibia ➡. Patients are at risk for periprosthetic fx following TKA, particularly if they have also had a tibial tubercle transfer ➡.

Lateral radiograph shows a displaced patellar fx ➡ following placement of TKA. The patella is at risk due to the osteotomy for placement of the patellar button, which causes devascularization & thinning of the bone.

TERMINOLOGY

Abbreviations and Synonyms
- Total hip arthroplasty (THA)
- Total knee arthroplasty (TKA)

Definitions
- Silastic = silicon for the purposes of this discussion
- Swanson arthroplasty: Silastic arthroplasty utilized for MCP, MTP, or IP joints of hands or feet
  - Rectangular body with triangular flanges extending into phalanges of metacarpal/metacarpals
  - Triangular flanges are not cemented within the long bones & there is no ingrowth potential
  - "Hinge" is just a thinning of the silastic between the body of the prosthesis & its flange

IMAGING FINDINGS

General Features
- Best diagnostic clue
  - Fracture metallic hardware
    - Discontinuity of metal
    - Often nondisplaced & extremely subtle; watch for slight break or angulation
  - Fracture silastic hardware
    - Fracture line in silastic rarely directly seen
    - Secondary sign: Discontinuity, especially between body and flange of implant
    - Secondary sign: Irregularity of the normally smooth edge of the component
    - Abrupt change in alignment of phalanges, such that the flange within the phalanx can no longer be attached to the body of the prosthesis
  - Dislocation metallic hardware
    - Lack of continuity between expected sites of articulation
  - Dislocation polyethylene component
    - Polyethylene is of lower density than the water density of either soft tissue or effusion
    - Because of this lower density, displaced polyethylene components may be seen as a relative lucency in an unexpected position
    - Keep in mind the shape of the polyethylene components; a lucency of the expected shape but in the wrong location is a good hint of the abnormality

Osseous & Hardware Fractures

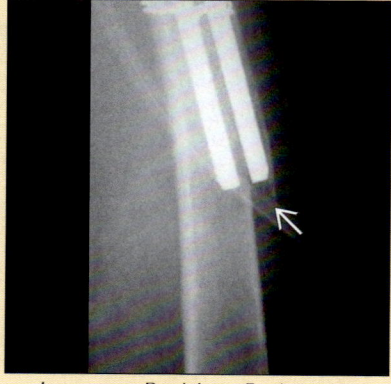 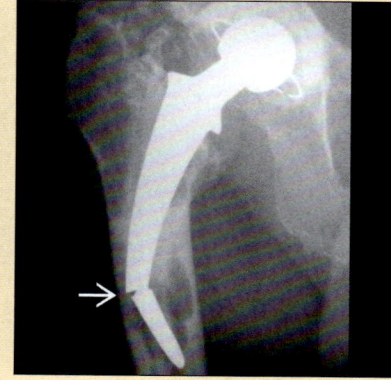 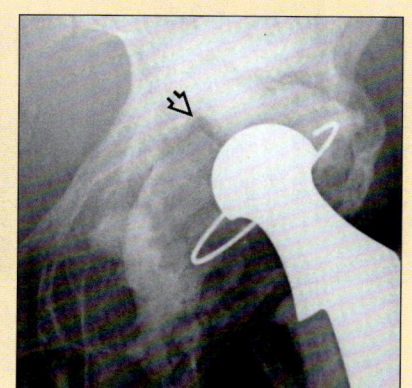

Longstem Revision; Fx Anterior

Fracture Component Shaft

Fracture Polyethylene Cup

ARTHROPLASTY HARDWARE/PERIPROSTHETIC FX

Key Facts

Imaging Findings
- Best chance of seeing subtle hardware or osseous failures is knowing the typical site of failure in each type of arthroplasty

Pathology
- Flange of Swanson arthroplasty within small bones is not cemented (no solid fixation); abnormal repetitive motion is allowed which leads to fragmentation & failure of prosthesis or bone
- TKA in osteoporotic patient: Risk for insufficiency fracture at femoral or tibial metaphyseal sites as patient increases mobility
- TKA in patient with prior tibial apophysis osteotomy & transfer: Increased risk of fracture at tibial metaphysis
- TKA: Patella at greatest risk of fracture: Osteotomy for button placement weakens & devascularizes patella; pegs in button are stress risers
- THA shaft fracture related to cross sectional diameter & length of stem

Diagnostic Checklist
- Watch for relative lucency of a dislocated polyethylene or silastic component
- Watch for malalignment at joint suggesting polyethylene or silastic failure
- Watch for subtle change in alignment or buckle suggesting periprosthetic fracture
- Recognize where the failures occur, and search for subtle signs

---

- THA cup: Polyethylene may become dislodged from metal backing of cup & be seen as a round lucency separate from the cup's backing
- THA cup: With polyethylene dislocation, the small triangular metallic wedges used to secure it may be seen loose in adjacent soft tissues
- TKA patellar button: Convex relative lucency may be seen adjacent to osseous patella
- TKA patellar button: Polyethylene dislocation often takes a "ring" or partial ring of the metallic backing material with it, which makes the dislocation obvious
- Metallosis: Layering of metallic particles along other parts of the joint (polyethylene, synovium); presence demonstrates failure of metal backing & likely polyethylene fracture or dislocation
- Dislocation silastic arthroplasty
  - If there is no flange (as in silastic trapezium at its carpal articulation, or at the MT articulation of an MTP arthroplasty), dislocation seen as complete lack of articulation
  - In Swanson type of arthroplasty, flange may dislocate out of phalanx & extend into adjacent soft tissues
- Periprosthetic osseous fracture
  - Cortical break
  - Buckle/slight change in angulation along cortex
  - Linear sclerosis: Healing in subacute fx
- Location
  - Best chance of seeing subtle hardware or osseous failures is knowing the typical site of failure in each type of arthroplasty
  - THA
    - Cup may fracture anywhere around its convex portion
    - Shaft component tends to fracture near distal tip
    - Periprosthetic fx cup: Generally medial wall
    - Periprosthetic fx shaft: Generally anterior cortex, extending from tip of prosthesis
  - TKA
    - Patellar button dislocates superiorly or medial-laterally
    - Patellar fracture generally transverse; less frequently vertical
    - Femoral fracture through metaphysis
    - Tibial fracture through metaphysis (especially in conjunction with tibial apophysis transfer)
  - Shoulder arthroplasty
    - Humeral shaft at risk for fracture near tip of stem
    - Glenoid component difficult to "seat" in correct position; watch for malalignment or stem extending outside of neck
  - Elbow arthroplasty
    - Humeral stem particularly at risk for abnormal motion & adjacent osseous fracture
  - Silastic implants
    - Swanson arthroplasty particularly at risk for fracture at the thin hinge
    - Thin osteoporotic phalanges are at risk for fracture with abnormal motion of the flange within them

Radiographic Findings
- With correct positioning and exposure, most complications are seen by radiograph

CT Findings
- Used to confirm complications & further define osseous destructive change prior to revision surgery

MR Findings
- Generally not required for evaluation of hardware failure
- Fluid sensitive sequences show silastic-induced synovitis

Imaging Recommendations
- Best imaging tool: Well-positioned radiographs
- Protocol advice
  - Include entire prosthesis in two orthogonal views
  - If MR in presence of metallic hardware, can improve periprosthetic tissue depiction by
    - Thin section imaging
    - Increased frequency-encoding gradient strength
    - Fast spin-echo sequences

ARTHROPLASTY HARDWARE/PERIPROSTHETIC FX

DIFFERENTIAL DIAGNOSIS

Hardware Loosening
- Shift in position or angulation of component
- Lucency surrounding component ≥ 2 mm
- May lead to fracture

Particle Disease & Osteolysis
- Debris of a critical size results in osteolysis
- May lead to fracture

PATHOLOGY

General Features
- Etiology
  - Fracture metallic hardware
    - Instability, abnormal stress
    - Incorrect placement of component
  - Dislocation metallic hardware
    - Positional: Joint placed beyond expected range
    - Example of positional dislocation: THA with hip in forced abduction or adduction
    - Incorrect positioning of components in THA: Abnormal cup lateral open angle or retroversion, incorrect length of components → dislocation
    - Incorrect positioning of components in TKA: External rotation of tibial component leads to dislocation of patella
    - Incorrect positioning of glenoid in total shoulder: Results in subluxation or dislocation of head
  - Fracture or dislocation silastic prostheses
    - Flange of Swanson arthroplasty within small bones is not cemented (no solid fixation); abnormal repetitive motion is allowed which leads to fragmentation & failure of prosthesis or bone
    - Soft tissue imbalance or contractures (as in rheumatoid arthritis) result in abnormal force at the "hinge", putting it at risk for fx/dislocation
    - Carpal soft tissue imbalance (ulnar translocation, instability patterns in rheumatoid arthritis) puts carpal prostheses at risk for dislocation
  - Dislocation polyethylene
    - Instability, abnormal stress
    - Polyethylene wear may add to abnormal stress on component
  - Periprosthetic osseous fracture
    - Acetabular dysplasia or protrusio result in thin medial wall at risk for fracture
    - Long stem femoral revision prostheses increase risk of femoral shaft fracture because the stem is straight but femoral shaft is anteriorly bowed
    - TKA in osteoporotic patient: Risk for insufficiency fracture at femoral or tibial metaphyseal sites as patient increases mobility
    - TKA in patient with prior tibial apophysis osteotomy & transfer: Increased risk of fracture at tibial metaphysis
    - TKA: Patella at greatest risk of fracture: Osteotomy for button placement weakens & devascularizes patella; pegs in button are stress risers
    - Total shoulder (or humeral endoprosthesis) often placed in osteoporotic patient; at risk for fracture at stress riser of stem
- Epidemiology
  - THA shaft fracture related to cross sectional diameter & length of stem
    - Primary cemented THA: 0.4% fracture
    - Primary cementless THA (larger diameter stem): 2.5% fracture
    - Long stem revision THA (larger diameter + long straight stem extending down anteriorly bowed shaft): 7.5% fracture
  - TKA fracture most frequent at patella (1.14%)

CLINICAL ISSUES

Presentation
- Most common signs/symptoms
  - Pain, malalignment
  - Most show sudden onset, though periprosthetic fracture may be incomplete and have more subtle symptoms

Demographics
- Age: Generally older patients, related to age of placement of arthroplasty

Natural History & Prognosis
- Failed arthroplasty generally progresses to worsening disruption
  - Fragmentation of polyethylene, metal, bone, cement
  - Osteolysis & fracture
- Unprotected periprosthetic fracture may complete & displace the fracture

Treatment
- Failed arthroplasty generally needs revision; revision prior to disintegration of bone stock is advisable
- Periprosthetic fracture may respond to rest & protection

DIAGNOSTIC CHECKLIST

Consider
- Watch for relative lucency of a dislocated polyethylene or silastic component
- Watch for malalignment at joint suggesting polyethylene or silastic failure
- Watch for subtle change in alignment or buckle suggesting periprosthetic fracture
- Recognize where the failures occur, and search for subtle signs

SELECTED REFERENCES

1. Furnes O et al: Failure mechanisms after unicompartmental and tricompartmental primary knee replacement with cement. J Bone Joint Surg Am. 89(3):519-25, 2007
2. Chun K et al: Patellar fractures after total knee replacement. AJR. 185:665-0, 2005
3. Van Flandern GJ: Periprosthetic fractures in total hip arthroplasty. Orthopedics. 28(9 Suppl):s1089-95, 2005

ARTHROPLASTY HARDWARE/PERIPROSTHETIC FX

IMAGE GALLERY

Typical

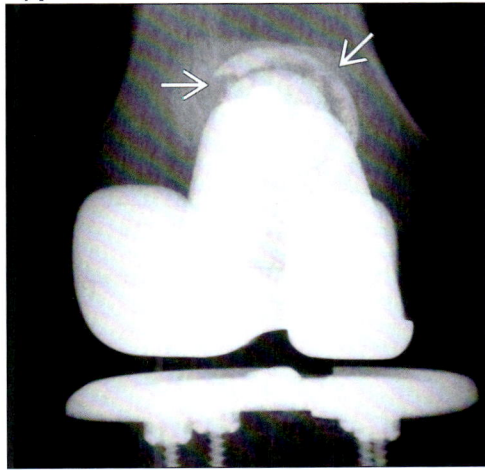
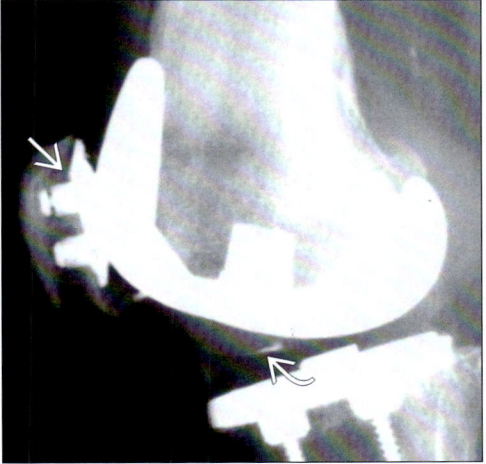

(Left) Anteroposterior radiograph shows fracture of the outer rim of the patellar button, with the metal backing of the button separating ➡. *(Right)* Lateral radiograph of the same knee as previous image confirms the fracture of the metal backing ➡. Some of the separated metal debris is now lining the tibial polyethylene ➡; this appearance is termed metallosis. The patellar button will continue to disintegrate, and the metallosis causes synovitis.

Typical

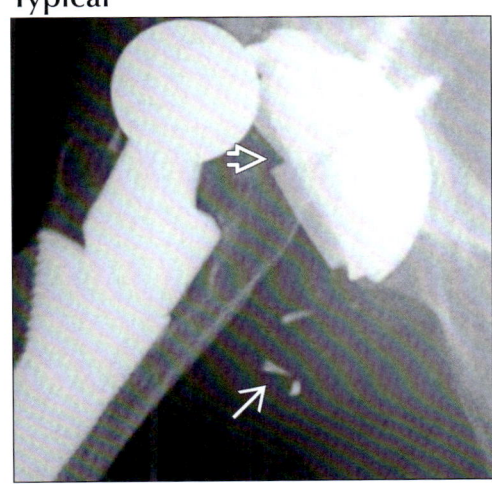
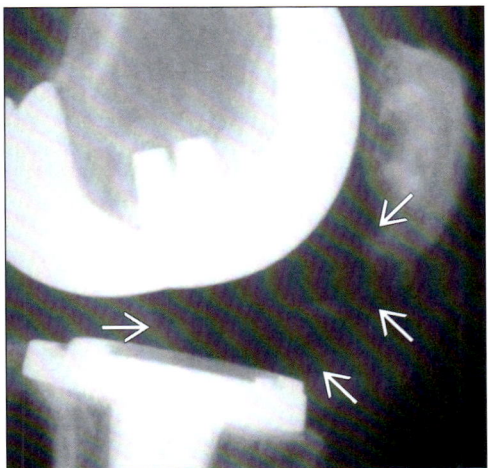

(Left) Frogleg lateral shows a dislocated THA. There are several wedge-shaped metallic densities in the soft tissues ➡. These are used to secure the polyethylene liner in the cup, and their presence in the soft tissues indicates failure. The metallic cup itself is fractured as well ➡. *(Right)* Lateral radiograph shows a lucent structure shaped like the tibial liner, dislocated anteriorly within the joint ➡. It has come loose from the tibial tray & has caused the joint to lock.

Typical

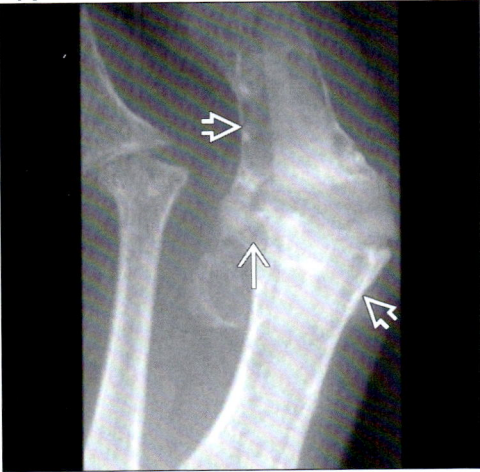
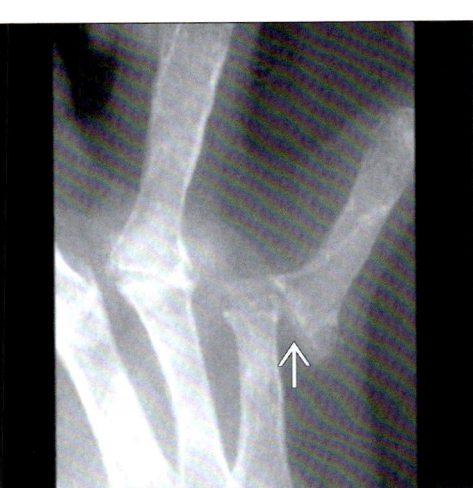

(Left) Anteroposterior radiograph of the great toe shows a silastic MTP arthroplasty. The body of the arthroplasty has fractured ➡. The fx produces particles which in turn result in osteolysis ➡. *(Right)* Anteroposterior radiograph of the MCPs shows silastic arthroplasties placed at MCPs 4 & 5 in a patient with rheumatoid arthritis. The 5th MCP arthroplasty has fractured ➡ at the junction of the body and flange. This is a typical site of prosthesis fracture in patients with RA.

ARTHROPLASTY COMPONENT WEAR/PARTICLE DISEASE

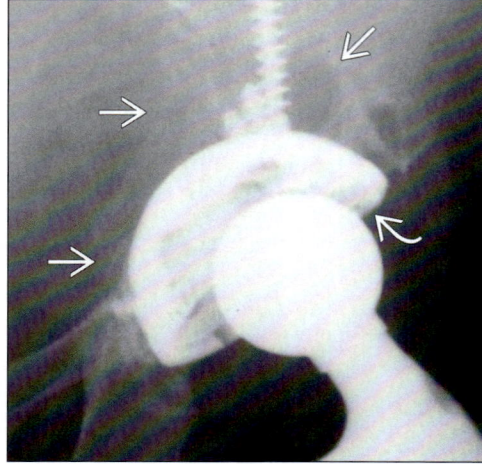

Anteroposterior radiograph shows massive osteolysis ➔ of the acetabulum related to particle disease. The source of particles is wear of the polyethylene acetabular liner, indicated by offset of the head relative to cup ➔.

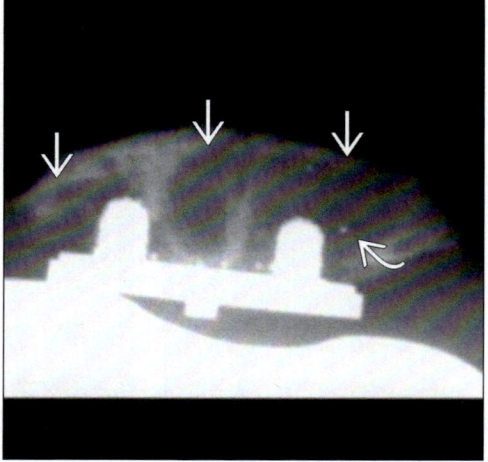

Sunrise radiograph of a patella with TKA shows massive osteolysis ➔. The particles which triggered the inflammatory reaction in this case are metallic beads ➔, shed as the component loosened.

TERMINOLOGY

Abbreviations and Synonyms
- Total hip arthroplasty (THA)
- Total knee arthroplasty (TKA)
- Particle disease = massive osteolysis

Definitions
- Component wear
  - Metal coatings (often microsphere beads) may wear and separate from underlying metal components
  - Polyethylene or silastic components may wear & generate small particles
- Particle disease: Debris of a critical size triggers a cascade in the following manner
  - Debris → inflammatory reaction/synovitis → osteolysis

IMAGING FINDINGS

General Features
- Best diagnostic clue
  - Component wear: May see metallic beads separate from component (bead shedding)
  - Polyethylene wear: Compare regions which are expected to be symmetric
    - Acetabular component of THA: Compare distance between metallic head & acetabulum in the weight-bearing portion (superolateral) with non-weight-bearing portion (inferomedial); wear occurs in the weight-bearing portion, which decreases in size
    - Tibial component: Compare width of lucency at medial & lateral compartments
  - Silastic wear in hand/foot arthroplasties: Abnormal angulation/fracture of component, especially at junction of body & flange of arthroplasty
  - Particle disease: Osteolysis adjacent to evidence of wear or other particle source
- Location
  - THA: Either acetabular or femoral component
  - TKA: Either patellar or tibial component
  - Hands/feet: Silastic components highly prone to wear & debris formation
- Size
  - May be massive (several centimeters)

Polyethylene Wear & Lysis, Confirmed on CT

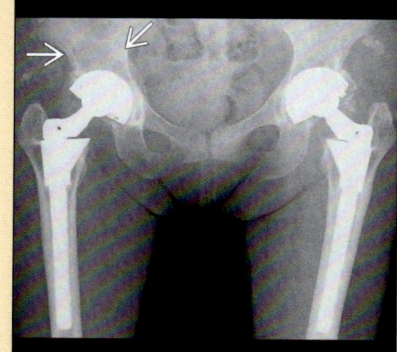

Polyethylene Wear & Lysis

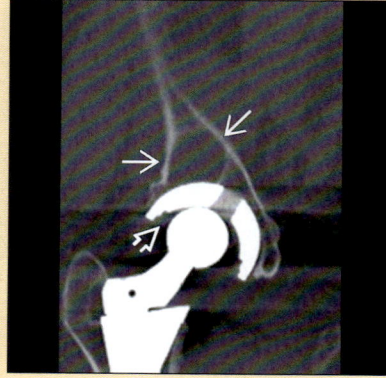

Polyethylene Wear & Lysis

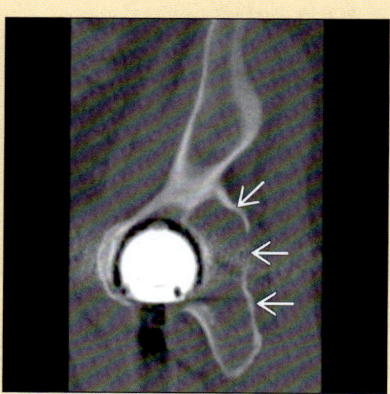

Posterior Column Lysis

ARTHROPLASTY COMPONENT WEAR/PARTICLE DISEASE

Key Facts

Imaging Findings
- Particle disease: Osteolysis adjacent to evidence of wear or other particle source
- It is not the type of particle, but rather the critical size which triggers the lytic response
- Metallic particles: Usually beads (< 1 mm) adjacent to their source
- Polyethylene wear in THA: Offset of polyethylene in acetabular component
- Silastic wear: Abnormal angulation or fx of component with associated osseous lucency
- In wrist, multiple bones in compartment are affected
- Bone CT used for reconstructive planning to evaluate extent & precise location of osseous destruction
- STIR: High signal irregular synovitis & osseous cysts
- CT: If hardware is metallic, artifact is suppressed by ↑ kVp & using coronal & sagittal reformats

Top Differential Diagnoses
- Metastatic Disease or Other Lytic Lesion
- Infected Prosthesis
- Prosthesis Loosening
- Fibrosis at Bone-Metal Interface
- Stress Shielding

Diagnostic Checklist
- Lytic lesion near arthroplasty in elderly patient may not be metastatic, but rather particle disease
- Look carefully for sources of debris, particularly polyethylene wear

---

   - May be quite small, seen as endosteal scalloping
- Morphology
  - It is not the type of particle, but rather the critical size which triggers the lytic response
  - Multiple possible sources of particles
    - Polyethylene/silastic: Due to wear
    - Metal: Due to wear of the particles applied to encourage osseous ingrowth
    - Osseous debris: Mechanical breakdown
    - Fractured cement debris: Mechanical breakdown

Radiographic Findings
- Osteolysis that is not loosening or the normal expected stress shielding
- Metallic particles: Usually beads (< 1 mm) adjacent to their source
  - THA: Acetabulum or proximal femoral component
  - TKA: Patellar or tibial component
- Polyethylene wear in THA: Offset of polyethylene in acetabular component
- Polyethylene wear in TKA: Decrease in "joint space" which may or may not be symmetric
- Osteolysis may have two forms
  - Massive, producing a lytic "lesion"
  - Elongated, due to debris & its reactive tissue tracking along the cement-bone or metal-bone interfaces
- Silastic wear: Abnormal angulation or fx of component with associated osseous lucency
  - In wrist, multiple bones in compartment are affected
    - Prosthesis at trapezium will affect base of thumb, as well as any bone within the middle compartment (trapezoid, capitate, hamate, proximal portions of scaphoid, lunate, trapezium, and bases of metacarpals 2-5)
    - Prosthesis at scaphoid will affect both proximal & distal carpal rows since it bridges these; destruction may be truly massive

CT Findings
- Bone CT used for reconstructive planning to evaluate extent & precise location of osseous destruction

MR Findings
- T1: Low signal regions of synovitis & lysis in bone
- STIR: High signal irregular synovitis & osseous cysts

Imaging Recommendations
- Best imaging tool
  - Radiographs are first line for diagnosis
  - CT used for reconstructive planning
- Protocol advice
  - CT: If hardware is metallic, artifact is suppressed by ↑ kVp & using coronal & sagittal reformats
  - MR: If hardware is metallic, FSE & STIR imaging help suppress metallic artifact

DIFFERENTIAL DIAGNOSIS

Metastatic Disease or Other Lytic Lesion
- Patients with arthroplasties are in the same age group as those who develop metastatic disease

Infected Prosthesis
- Infections are usually suspected clinically prior to radiographic findings developing
- Infections proven by aspiration and culture
- Radiographs most frequently are negative or indistinguishable from prosthetic loosening
- If there are radiographic findings, they include
  - Lytic destructive change
  - Periosteal reaction
  - Occasional fluffy dystrophic bone formation in a periprosthetic location

Prosthesis Loosening
- Lucency at bone-prosthesis or bone-cement interface may be indistinguishable from osteolysis with debris extending along that interface

Fibrosis at Bone-Metal Interface
- Fibrous tissue, rather than bone ingrowth, may occur at bone-prosthesis interface

ARTHROPLASTY COMPONENT WEAR/PARTICLE DISEASE

- Fibrous ingrowth appears as a lucency which may be indistinguishable from either loosening or from osteolysis with debris extending along the interface
- May be asymptomatic

Stress Shielding
- Altered weight-bearing through a prosthesis changes stress on bone
- Bone that has less weight-bearing is resorbed and develops a relative lucency
- Two most typical locations: Lateral metaphysis proximal femur in THA, posterior metaphysis in distal femur in TKA (seen on lateral image)
  - Lateral metaphysis proximal femur in THA (within the greater trochanter, seen on any view)
  - Anterior metaphysis in distal femur in TKA
    - Seen best on lateral view
    - Generally also has thickening of bone along new line of stress, often posterior cortex or extending to one of the femoral prosthesis pegs
- Stress shielding is considered a normal finding; no relation to pain or failure of prosthesis

PATHOLOGY

General Features
- Etiology
  - Polyethylene wear: Multifactorial, with both biological & mechanical factors contributing
    - Theoretically should be so minor and slow in progression that it does not cause problems (0.06 mm/year)
    - In vivo degradation due to oxidation may occur at rim where there is contact with joint fluid
    - Mechanical friction of metal abrades microscopic particles →
    - Incites an inflammatory response in periprosthetic tissues →
    - Secretion of cytokines, growth factors, enzymes →
    - Formation of osteolytic granulomas →
    - Activated macrophages express osteoprotegerin ligands (RANKL)
    - RANKL activates osteoclasts, → lysis
    - Repetitive hydraulic effect of joint fluid brings reactive tissue in contact with susceptible bone
    - Migration of polyethylene debris & its reactive tissue along cement-bone or metal-bone interfaces, or may cause a local lytic "lesion"

Gross Pathologic & Surgical Features
- Lytic lesions, either focal, or along interfaces

Microscopic Features
- Macrophages containing debris, either metal, polyethylene, cement, or osseous

CLINICAL ISSUES

Presentation
- Most common signs/symptoms
  - Pain, slowly progressing over time
  - Occasionally, pathologic fx through region of lysis
  - Occasionally, loosening due to lysis along interface of prosthesis with bone or cement

Demographics
- Age: Older patients, related to presence of arthroplasty
- Gender: No gender preference

Natural History & Prognosis
- Polyethylene wear progresses slowly
- Osteolysis may progress either slowly or rapidly
- If pathologic fx occurs, revision is required
- May control level of pain & treat conservatively

Treatment
- Severe pain, pathologic fracture, or mechanically unsound situation requires revision of arthroplasty
- Revision may be relatively minor
  - Change out the worn polyethylene component
  - Curette & bone graft the site of osteolysis
- Revision may be major, with large defects to fill and little bone to support the arthroplasty
  - May use structural or non-structural bone graft
  - Shaft: may use longstem prostheses, often with onlay graft & modular metaphyseal components
  - Acetabulum: May use oversized cups or cups with reconstructive plates
- Promising therapeutic agents against proinflammatory mediators (such as tumor necrosis factor) and osteoclasts (such as bisphosphonates) shown in animal models; not yet approved

DIAGNOSTIC CHECKLIST

Consider
- Lytic lesion near arthroplasty in elderly patient may not be metastatic, but rather particle disease

Image Interpretation Pearls
- Look carefully for sources of debris, particularly polyethylene wear

SELECTED REFERENCES

1. Purdue PE et al: The cellular and molecular biology of periprosthetic osteolysis. Clin Orthop Relat Res. 454:251-61, 2007
2. Buckwalter KA et al: Multichannel CT Imaging of Orthopedic Hardware and Implants. Semin Musculoskelet Radiol. 10(1):86-97, 2006
3. Kearns SR et al: Factors affecting survival of uncemented total hip arthroplasty in patients 50 years or younger. Clin Orthop Relat Res. 453:103-9, 2006
4. Kurtz SM et al: 2006 Otto Aufranc Award Paper: significance of in vivo degradation for polyethylene in total hip arthroplasty. Clin Orthop Relat Res. 453:47-57, 2006
5. Potter HG et al: Magnetic resonance imaging of joint arthroplasty. Orthop Clin North Am. 37(3):361-73, vi-vii, 2006
6. Parwani AV et al: Particle disease: cytopathologic findings of an unusual case. Diagn Cytopathol. 31(4):259-62, 2004
7. Gallo J et al: Particle disease. A comprehensive theory of periprosthetic osteolysis: a review. Biomed Pap Med Fac Univ Palacky Olomouc Czech Repub. 146(2):21-8, 2002

ARTHROPLASTY COMPONENT WEAR/PARTICLE DISEASE

IMAGE GALLERY

Typical

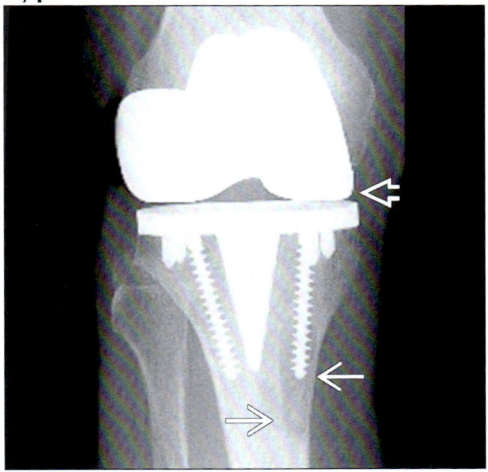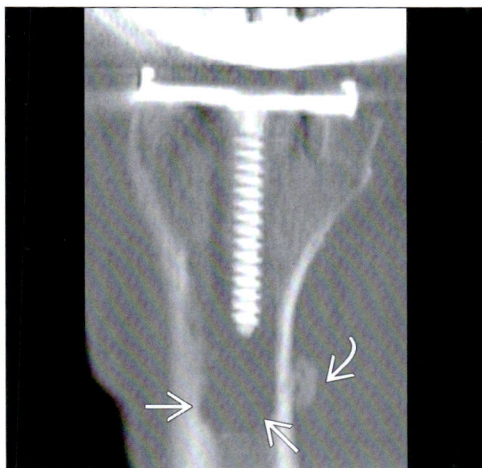

(Left) Anteroposterior radiograph shows osteolysis ⇨ surrounding the medial tibial screw. There is subtle thinning of the polyethylene at the medial side of the joint ⇨. This represents particle disease from polyethylene wear. It is not uncommon for the particles to track along screws due to the hydraulic effect. *(Right)* Sagittal bone CT reformat shows the degree of osteolysis ⇨ as well as callus formation at an incomplete pathologic fracture ⇨.

Typical

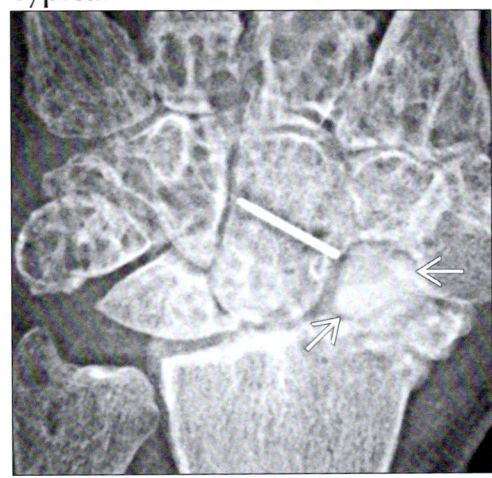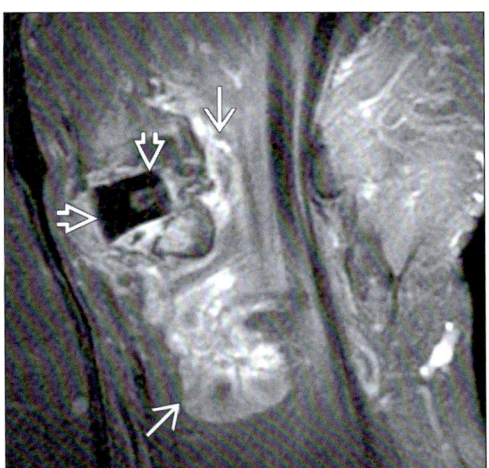

(Left) Anteroposterior radiograph shows osteolysis of all carpal bones as well as the base of metacarpals 2-5. The source of the particles is a silastic scaphoid prosthesis ⇨, which has fractured, rotated and worn down. The fractured K-wire was originally placed to stabilize the prosthesis. *(Right)* Coronal STIR MR near the palmar surface of the wrist shows extensive synovitis ⇨. This is in reaction to a silastic prosthesis, replacing the trapezium ⇨. This patient did not yet have lysis.

Typical

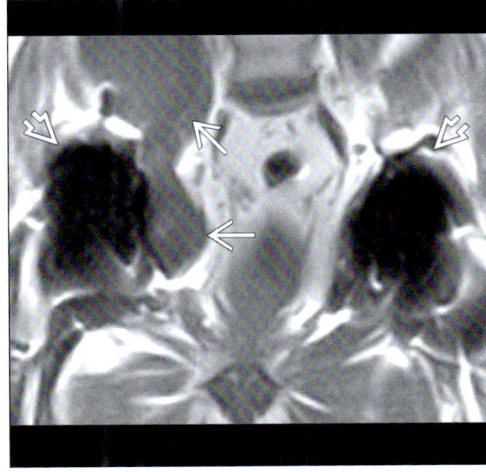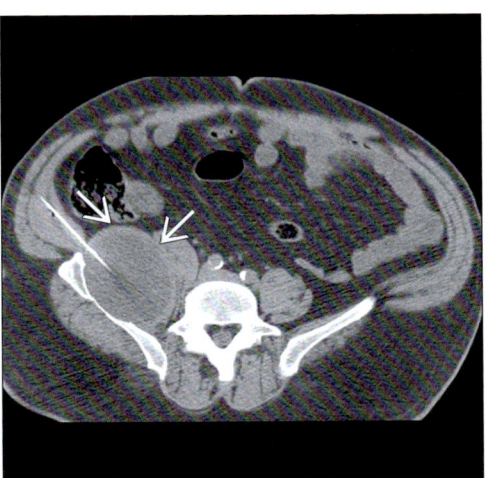

(Left) Coronal T1WI MR shows bilateral THAs ⇨ & large fluid collection in the right iliopsoas bursa ⇨. Concern was for infection vs. synovitis. *(Right)* Axial bone CT confirms large fluid collection in the iliacus bursa ⇨. Needle aspiration yielded thick gelatinous material & debris-laden macrophages. Debris formed from THA polyethylene wear. It thus far has caused a synovitis but not yet osteolysis; the synovitis decompressed into the iliopsoas bursa.

SICKLE CELL ANEMIA: MSK COMPLICATIONS

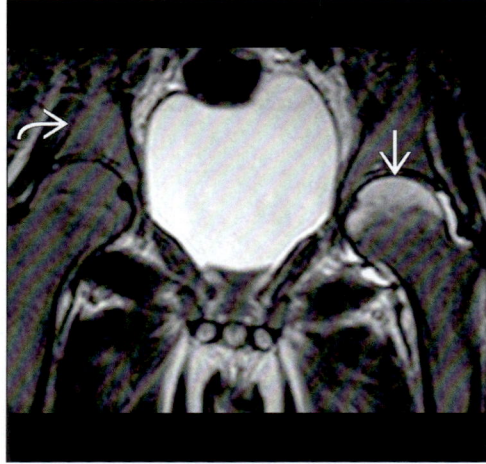

Coronal T2 MR shows diffuse red marrow conversion ➔ in sickle cell patient. Painful left hip shows marrow edema ➔, as well as effusion. This could represent a septic hip; aspirate showed a sterile effusion.

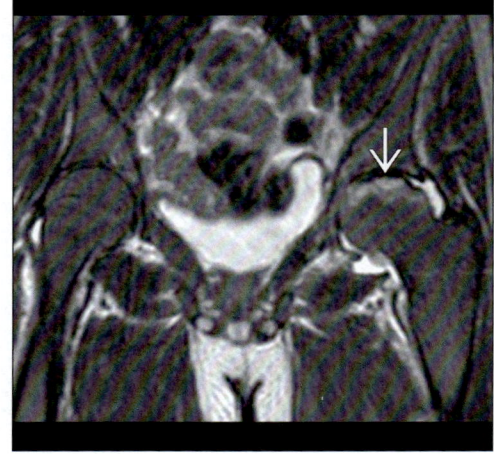

7 months later, the hip shows flattening of the femoral head ➔. This is AVN, with subchondral fracture. This is a common complication of sickle cell anemia; the edema seen earlier was a form fruste of AVN.

TERMINOLOGY

Abbreviations and Synonyms
- Sickle cell disease; HbSS disease

Definitions
- **Autosomal recessive inherited hemoglobinopathy (homozygous, HbSS); radiographic MSK findings reflect one or both of the following processes**
  - Chronic hemolytic anemia
  - Consequences of microvascular occlusion created by sickled cells when exposed to low oxygen tension
- Heterozygous: HbSA (sickle cell trait), HbSC (↓ severe)

IMAGING FINDINGS

General Features
- Best diagnostic clue
  - Generalized patchy bone density, reflecting chronic diffuse bone infarcts
  - Avascular necrosis, especially of femoral head, humeral head, or vertebral bodies
  - May have other associated findings on image
    - Chest: Cardiomegaly, pulmonary infarct
    - Abdomen: Gallstones, absence of spleen (splenic infarct, with eventual autosplenectomy)
- Location
  - Any bone may be involved with infarct
    - Long bones: Femur 96%, humerus 48%
    - Small tubular bones of hands & feet: 20-50%
    - Spine: 43-70%; skull: 25%
  - Avascular necrosis: Femoral head > humeral head > vertebral bodies > other sites

Radiographic Findings
- Bone infarct
  - Long bones
    - Acute: Normal; rare lysis or periosteal reaction
    - Focal (subacute/chronic): Serpiginous calcification
    - Diffuse (chronic): Patchy diffuse sclerosis
    - Occasional associated periosteal reaction
  - Tubular bones of hands & feet (dactylitis)
    - Periosteal reaction initially
    - Patchy sclerosis later
- Avascular necrosis
  - Femoral head: Initially, central increased density
    - Weight-bearing portion: Anterosuperior head

DDx: Thalassemia Major

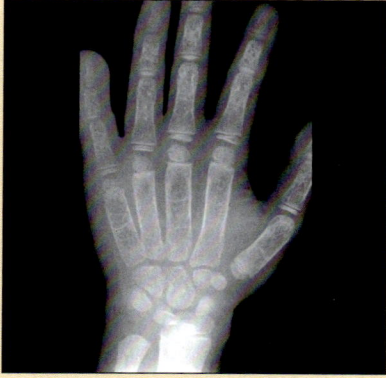

Marrow Hyperplasia: Squaring

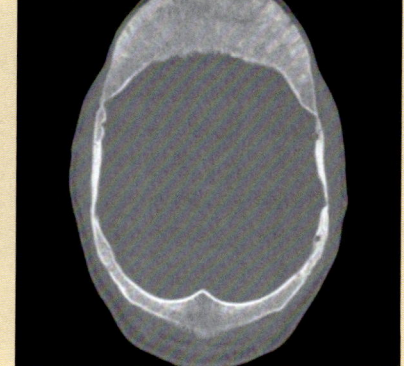

Diploic Space Hyperplasia

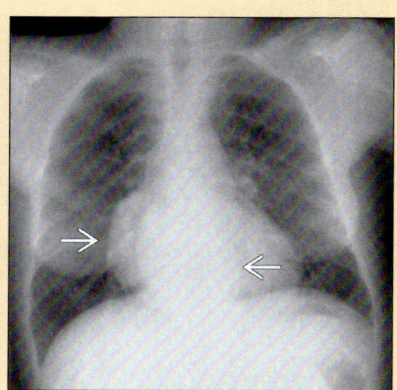

Extramedullary Hematopoiesis

SICKLE CELL ANEMIA: MSK COMPLICATIONS

Key Facts

Terminology
- **Autosomal recessive inherited hemoglobinopathy (homozygous, HbSS); radiographic MSK findings reflect one or both of the following processes**
- Chronic hemolytic anemia
- Consequences of microvascular occlusion created by sickled cells when exposed to low oxygen tension

Imaging Findings
- Generalized patchy bone density, reflecting chronic diffuse bone infarcts
- Avascular necrosis, especially of femoral head, humeral head, or vertebral bodies
- Chest: Cardiomegaly, pulmonary infarct
- Abdomen: Gallstones, absence of spleen (splenic infarct, with eventual autosplenectomy)

Pathology
- Structural defect in hemoglobin HbS: Glutamic acid in position 6 substituted with valine
- **Order of events leading to infarct**: Lowered oxygen tension →
- Altered shape & plasticity of red blood cells →
- Increased blood viscosity, stasis →
- Occlusion of microvasculature by sickled cells → infarct/AVN

Diagnostic Checklist
- Acute infarction & osteomyelitis can be indistinguishable on imaging; pattern of rim-enhancement on MR can be useful
- Red marrow replacement of fatty marrow can be patchy and confusing

---

- Subchondral lucent fracture line, paralleling cortex in weight-bearing region
- Flattening, with mixed lytic & sclerotic density
  - Humeral head: Initial sclerosis
    - Weight-bearing portion: Superomedial head
    - Subchondral lucent fracture line, paralleling cortex in weight-bearing region
    - Flattening, with mixed lytic & sclerotic density
  - Vertebral body: Initial sub-endplate sclerosis
    - Collapse is of the central endplates, either in a biconcave pattern, or a more sharp "H-shape"
- Marrow hyperplasia
  - Uncommon or often so subtle as to not be noted
  - Skull may show mild widening of diploic space, with thinning of calvarium
- Osteomyelitis
  - Periosteal reaction
  - Blurring/obliteration of fat planes
  - Eventual permeative osseous change
- Growth abnormalities: Premature epiphyseal closure (→ growth discrepancy or angulation), coned epiphyses

MR Findings
- Bone infarct
  - Acute: Focal areas of low signal on T1WI and high signal intensity on T2WI MR (edema)
    - T1 C+: Thin linear rim-enhancement
  - Chronic: May be patchy or focal, with classic serpiginous pattern
    - T1WI MR: Serpiginous very low signal pattern outlining red marrow
    - T2WI MR: High signal serpiginous outline; often double line appearance of low and high signal
- Avascular necrosis
  - May present initially as bone marrow edema
  - Later presentation
    - T1WI MR: Low signal in weight-bearing region
    - T2WI MR: Double density (low and high signal) serpiginous rim around region of necrosis in weight-bearing portion of bone
    - Eventual subchondral fracture and flattening
- Marrow hyperplasia
  - T1WI MR: Low signal red marrow replaces fatty marrow; may have focal or patchy retained white marrow
  - T2WI MR: Marrow retains low signal of red marrow
- Osteomyelitis
  - T1WI: Confluent low signal; may not differentiate from low signal of red marrow hyperplasia
  - Fluid sensitive sequences: High signal intensity; adjacent soft tissue edema, cellulitis, or abscess
  - T1 C+: Geographic, thick, irregular rim-enhancement of marrow, adjacent soft tissue reaction or infection
- Myonecrosis: Rare; hyperintensity on fluid sensitive sequences and enhancement of muscle & fascia

Nuclear Medicine Findings
- Bone Scan
  - Marked expansion of hematopoietic marrow
  - Increased uptake in areas of acute infarction
  - Photopenic regions in old infarction
- White cell scan may help differentiate acute infarct from osteomyelitis

Imaging Recommendations
- Best imaging tool
  - Diagnosis generally made on radiograph
  - MR may be required to diagnose early infarct/AVN
  - MR may differentiate acute infarct/osteomyelitis

DIFFERENTIAL DIAGNOSIS

Thalassemia (Cooley Anemia)
- Marrow hyperplasia in long bones
  - Diffuse osteopenia
  - Widening of marrow space, with thinning of endosteal bone
  - Long bones lose morphologic features of diaphysis & metaphysis; "squaring" of bones
- Skull: Severe hyperplasia of marrow, sparing occiput
  - Widened diploic space; "hair on end" appearance
  - Obliteration of paranasal sinuses, with marrow replacing aerated spaces

SICKLE CELL ANEMIA: MSK COMPLICATIONS

- Extramedullary hematopoiesis (usually paravertebral)
- Avascular necrosis & diaphyseal infarcts much less frequent than in sickle cell

Sickle Cell Trait (Heterozygous, HbSA)
- Few musculoskeletal findings
- Rarely will see bone infarcts

Sickle Cell Hemoglobin C (HbSC)
- Marrow hyperplasia of skull
- Avascular necrosis, with few bone infarcts
- Splenomegaly rather than splenic infarction

PATHOLOGY

General Features
- Etiology
  o Structural defect in hemoglobin HbS: Glutamic acid in position 6 substituted with valine
  o **Order of events leading to infarct**: Lowered oxygen tension →
  o Altered shape & plasticity of red blood cells →
  o Increased blood viscosity, stasis →
  o Occlusion of microvasculature by sickled cells → infarct/AVN
    - Small terminal vessels in femoral head and humeral head are particularly at risk
    - In vertebral bodies, terminal vessels loop under the endplates; with focal avascular necrosis at endplates, there is a collapse of the central 75% of the endplates, resulting in "H shape"
  o Dactylitis: Ambient cold temperatures → vasoconstriction in hematopoietic marrow of digits → bone infarct
    - Often first manifestation of disease (6 months to 2 yrs)
    - Periosteal reaction can make infarct impossible to differentiate from osteomyelitis
  o Risk for osteomyelitis is high
    - Majority of cases caused by Staphylococcus
    - Salmonella osteomyelitis more common than in normal population
  o Children are protected for the first 6 months by elevated levels of fetal Hb (HbF)
- Epidemiology
  o 0.2-1% of African-American, 0.1% Hispanic American population; rarely seen in Mediterranean population
  o 8-13% African-Americans carry sickle factor (HbS)
  o 3% of African Americans carry HbC
  o 1:40 with sickle cell trait manifest SC anemia
  o 1:120 with sickle cell trait manifest SC anemia
- Associated abnormalities
  o Thrombosis/infarction
    - Renal papillary necrosis, cholelithiasis, splenic autoinfarction, cardiomegaly, pulmonary infarction, stroke
  o May coexist with thalassemia

Gross Pathologic & Surgical Features
- Dense, hard, sclerotic bone in regions of infarction
- Yellow marrow replaced by red marrow
- Infarcted marrow may contain clotted blood

CLINICAL ISSUES

Presentation
- Most common signs/symptoms
  o Sickle cell crisis
    - Sudden onset severe bone, abdominal, chest pain
    - Often as a result of infection, temperature change (cold), or hypoxia related to altitude or plane flight
    - ± Fever, leukocytosis
    - Time course: Hours to days
  o Hand/foot syndrome
    - Often initial manifestation, in child of 6 months to 2 years of age
    - Swelling, decreased range of motion
    - Occurs with new onset of cold temperatures & resultant vasoconstriction
    - Self limiting, days to weeks

Demographics
- Age: Initial manifestation in first 2 years of life; symptoms persist lifelong
- Gender: No gender difference

Natural History & Prognosis
- Repeated episodes lead to progressive bone infarction
- AVN leads to arthritis and requirement for surgery
- Repeated hospitalizations due to crisis or infection
- Poor prognostic factors: Dactylitis before 1 year of age, Hb levels < 7 gm/dL, leukocytosis without infection
- Early death (average prior to 48 years of age)
  o Pneumonia, meningitis, stroke are leading causes
- Patients with sickle cell trait: Normal life expectancy

Treatment
- Crisis: Oxygen, hydration, pain management
- No prophylactic measure to prevent infarcts
- Avascular necrosis of femoral or humeral head: Osteotomy, core decompression, arthroplasty

DIAGNOSTIC CHECKLIST

Consider
- Acute infarction & osteomyelitis can be indistinguishable on imaging; pattern of rim-enhancement on MR can be useful

Image Interpretation Pearls
- Pay attention to marrow signal
  o Red marrow replacement of fatty marrow can be patchy and confusing
  o Bone marrow edema may be first sign of impending avascular necrosis

SELECTED REFERENCES
1. Sathappan SS et al: Multidisciplinary management of orthopedic patients with sickle cell disease. Orthopedics. 29(12):1094-101; quiz 1102-3, 2006
2. Umans H et al: The diagnostic role of gadolinium enhanced MRI in distinguishing between acute medullary bone infarct and osteomyelitis. Magn Reson Imaging. 18(3):255-62, 2000

SICKLE CELL ANEMIA: MSK COMPLICATIONS

IMAGE GALLERY

Typical

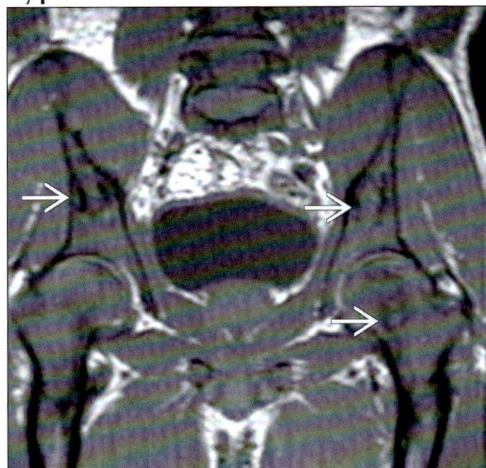 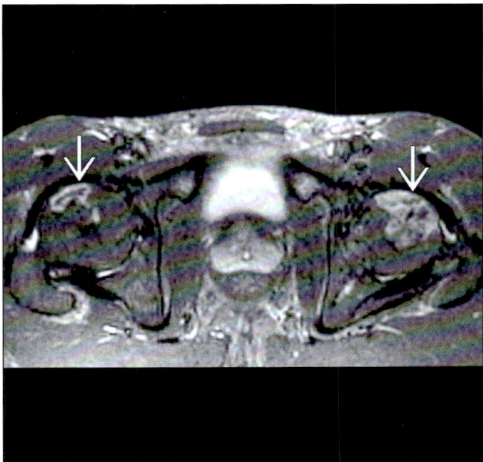

(Left) Coronal T1WI MR shows red marrow conversion of the entire pelvis & proximal femora. Serpiginous low signal bone infarcts are superimposed on this abnormal marrow ➡. *(Right)* Axial STIR MR confirms the serpiginous bone infarcts in the heads & metaphyses of the femora bilaterally ➡. Infarcts are a common complication of sickle cell anemia and may be seen either as discrete serpiginous foci as in this case, or as diffuse patchy bone density changes.

Typical

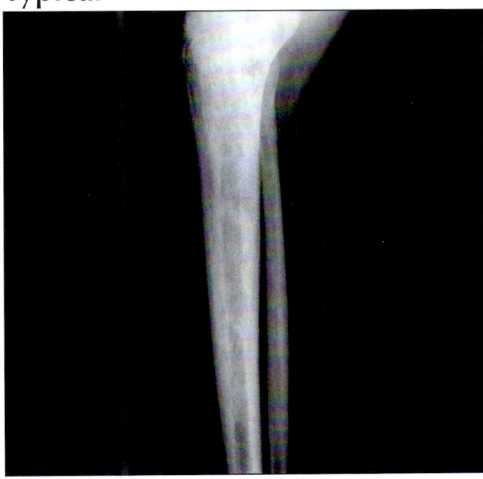 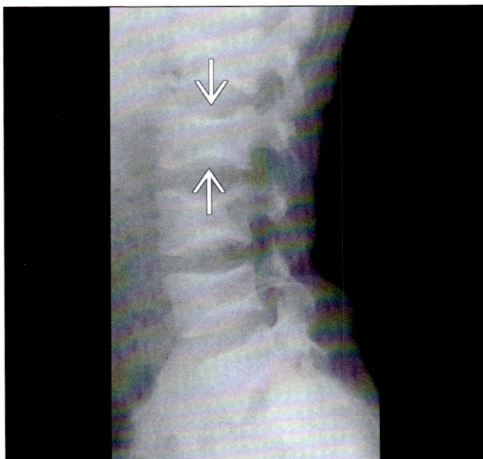

(Left) Lateral radiograph shows diffuse patchy sclerosis throughout the tibia. This appearance is typical of the diffuse bone infarcts that are often seen in sickle cell anemia. *(Right)* Lateral radiograph shows the "H-shaped" vertebral bodies seen in sickle cell anemia ➡. These occur when the sickled cells sludge in the looped vessels beneath the vertebral body endplates. With loss of their vascular supply, the endplates collapse into this configuration.

Typical

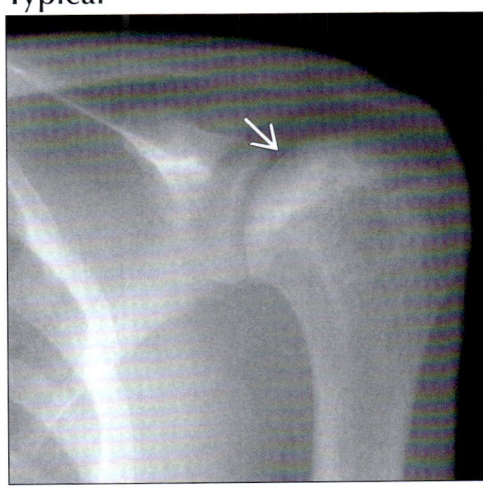 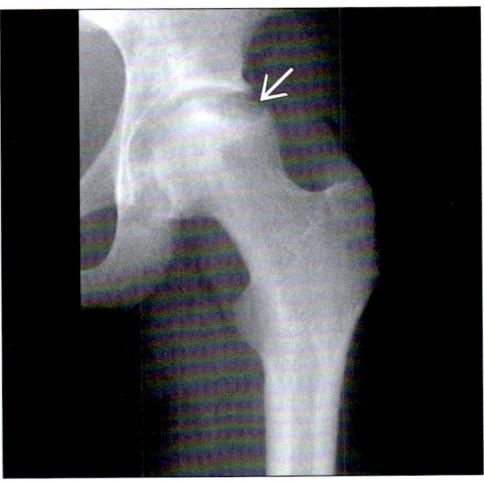

(Left) Anteroposterior radiograph shows abnormal density within the weight-bearing portion of the humeral head ➡. This is avascular necrosis; the humeral head as well as femoral heads are at greatest risk for developing AVN in sickle cell patients. *(Right)* Anteroposterior radiograph shows AVN of the femoral head, with collapse ➡. Note also the diffusely abnormal bone density throughout the visualized pelvic and femoral bones, representing bone infarcts.

HIV-AIDS: MSK COMPLICATIONS

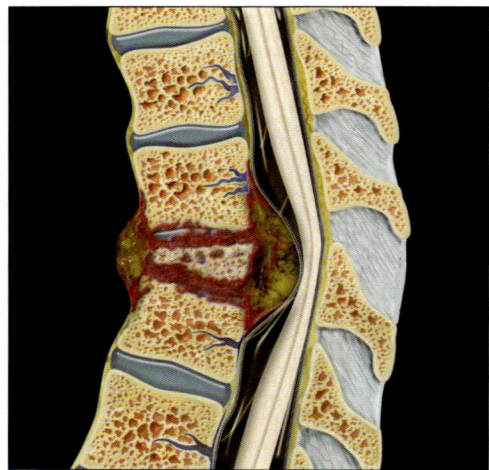

Sagittal graphic shows tuberculous discitis/osteomyelitis of the thoracic spine, with vertebral compression deformity, anterior soft tissue mass, and epidural abscess causing cord compression.

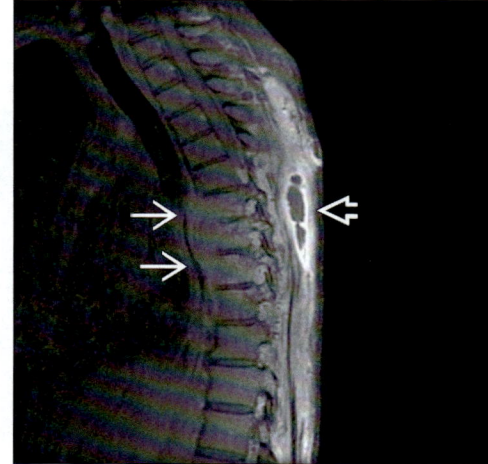

Sagittal T1 C+ FS MR shows subligamentous spread of tuberculous discitis/osteomyelitis of the thoracic spine ➡. Note the large posterior soft tissues abscess ➡.

TERMINOLOGY

Abbreviations and Synonyms
- Acquired immune deficiency syndrome (AIDS), human immunodeficiency virus (HIV), musculoskeletal (MSK)

Definitions
- Severe immunological disorder caused by retrovirus HIV, resulting in defect in cell-mediated immune response → manifested by increased susceptibility to opportunistic infections, neoplasms, inflammatory disorders
- AIDS: CD4 count < 200 cells/mm³

IMAGING FINDINGS

General Features
- Best diagnostic clue
  - Infection most common MSK complication in AIDS
    - Soft tissue infection: Cellulitis, abscess, fasciitis, pyomyositis
    - Osteomyelitis: Bacterial, tuberculosis (TB), bacillary angiomatosis (almost unique to AIDS)
    - Septic arthritis
  - Non Hodgkin lymphoma (NHL) and Kaposi sarcoma most common MSK neoplasms in AIDS
  - Osteonecrosis common in AIDS, most frequently involving femoral head
- Location
  - Soft tissue infection: Superficial and deep soft tissues
  - Osteomyelitis: All long bones, pelvis, spine
  - Neoplasms: Spine, pelvis, long bones
  - Inflammatory disorders: Arthritis (knees, hands, feet), polymyositis (muscles)
- Size: Several cm
- Morphology
  - Infection: Infiltrative soft tissue abnormality, fluid collections
  - Neoplasm: Permeative bone marrow infiltration ± soft tissue mass
  - Arthritis: Erosions, periosteal reaction, soft tissue swelling, joint effusion

Radiographic Findings
- Osteomyelitis: Periosteal reaction, cortical erosions, joint effusion
  - Bacillary angiomatosis: Well-defined lytic lesions

Complications from AIDS, Other Cases

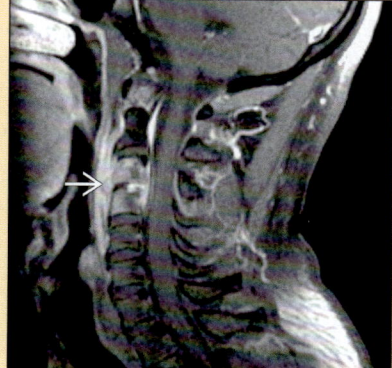

Discitis/Osteomyelitis

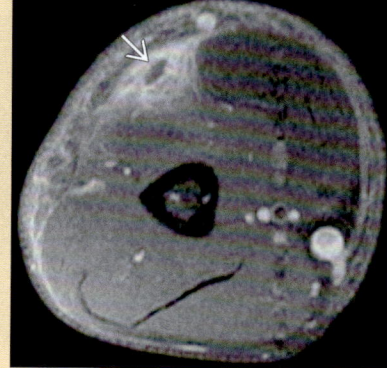

Abscess

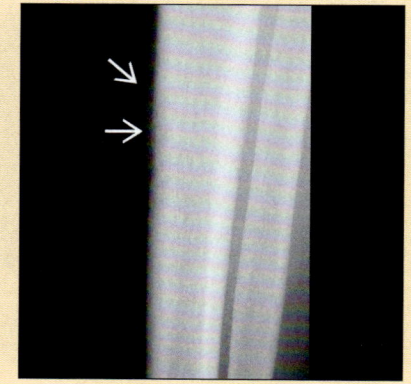

Bacillary Angiomatosis

HIV-AIDS: MSK COMPLICATIONS

Key Facts

Terminology
- Severe immunological disorder caused by retrovirus HIV, resulting in defect in cell-mediated immune response → manifested by increased susceptibility to opportunistic infections, neoplasms, inflammatory disorders

Imaging Findings
- Infection most common MSK complication in AIDS
- Non Hodgkin lymphoma (NHL) and Kaposi sarcoma most common MSK neoplasms in AIDS
- TB: Calcification of paravertebral soft tissues abscesses pathognomonic
- Necrotizing fasciitis: Thickening & fluid collections along deep fascial planes, soft tissue air
- Bacillary angiomatosis: Non-sclerotic lytic lesions, intense enhancement
- Osteomyelitis/discitis: Hyperintense bone marrow, surrounding hyperintense soft tissues
- Pyomyositis: Rim-enhancing intramuscular collection, central hypointensity

Pathology
- MSK complications in late stages of AIDS (CD4 < 200 cells/mm^3)
- 75% of AIDS patients will have MSK complications
- 40 million HIV infections worldwide
- 20 million deaths secondary to AIDS

Clinical Issues
- Fever, weight loss, night sweats
- Treated as chronic disease for many years; eventually almost uniformly lethal due to immune suppression
- HAART (highly active antiretroviral therapy)

- Septic arthritis: Osteoporosis, erosions, joint space narrowing
- Necrotizing fasciitis: Air along fascial planes
- NHL: Lytic lesions, cortical destruction, permeative pattern, soft tissue mass
- Kaposi sarcoma: Cortical lytic lesions, erosions, osseous destruction
  - AIDS defining condition
- AIDS arthritis: Monoarticular, asymmetric, knees and ankles, joint effusion
- Psoriasis/chronic reactive arthritis: Erosions with bone proliferation, asymmetric, hands and feet

CT Findings
- NECT
  - Osteomyelitis/discitis: Periosteal reaction, cortical erosions, medullary changes, joint effusion
    - TB: Calcification of paravertebral soft tissues abscesses pathognomonic
  - Necrotizing fasciitis: Thickening & fluid collections along deep fascial planes, soft tissue air
- CECT
  - Cellulitis: Soft tissue stranding superficial to the superficial fascia, skin thickening
  - Abscess: Rim-enhancing fluid collection, central hypodensity, most common in IV drug abusers
  - Pyomyositis: Muscle enlargement, decreased attenuation, ± central non enhancement (necrosis/abscess)
  - Bacillary angiomatosis: Non-sclerotic lytic lesions, intense enhancement

MR Findings
- T1WI
  - Cellulitis: Hypointense inflammation of the subcutaneous fat
  - Pyomyositis: Low-intermediate signal within muscles, ± hyperintense rim (blood products)
  - Osteomyelitis/discitis: Hypointense bone marrow
  - NHL: Hypointense bone marrow, soft tissue mass
- T2WI
  - Cellulitis: Striated appearance of subcutaneous fat
  - Abscess: Well-defined hyperintense collection with hypointense rim
  - Osteomyelitis/discitis: Hyperintense bone marrow
  - Osteonecrosis: Serpiginous subchondral low and high signal (double line sign)
- PD/Intermediate FS
  - Cellulitis: Hyperintense inflammation of subcutaneous fat, ± septations
  - Abscess: Hyperintense collection with hypointense rim, hyperintense surrounding inflammation
  - Necrotizing fasciitis: Hyperintense signal and fluid collections along deep fascial planes and muscles
  - Pyomyositis: Hyperintense intramuscular collection (abscess) with surrounding hyperintense signal (edema/phlegmon)
  - Osteomyelitis/discitis: Hyperintense bone marrow, surrounding hyperintense soft tissues
  - Septic arthritis: Joint effusion, hyperintense bone marrow and soft tissues, septic bursitis
  - NHL: Hyperintense bone marrow and surrounding soft tissue mass
- STIR: Polymyositis: Symmetric, proximal, increased signal of involved muscles
- T1 C+ FS
  - Cellulitis: Enhancing inflammation of subcutaneous fat
  - Abscess: Hyperintense rim, hypointense center
  - Necrotizing fasciitis: No enhancement
  - Pyomyositis: Rim-enhancing intramuscular collection, central hypointensity
  - Osteomyelitis/discitis: Enhancement ± non-enhancing areas (necrosis)
    - TB: Epidural extension, arachnoiditis (thickened enhancing nerve roots)

Ultrasonographic Findings
- Pyomyositis: Hyperechoic muscles
- Myositis: Hypoechoic muscles

Nuclear Medicine Findings
- In-111 labeled WBC scan most sensitive for detection of early osteomyelitis

HIV-AIDS: MSK COMPLICATIONS

Imaging Recommendations
- Best imaging tool: MR C+
- Protocol advice
  - T1 C+ FS, PD/Intermediate FS
  - CECT

DIFFERENTIAL DIAGNOSIS

None in Presence of HIV/AIDS
- Many of the individual complications can be seen in absence of HIV/AIDS
- Exception is Bacillary angiomatosis, which is virtually pathognomonic

PATHOLOGY

General Features
- General path comments
  - HIV can affect every organ system in the body
    - By direct damage by the virus
    - By rendering host susceptible to opportunistic infections
  - MSK complications in late stages of AIDS (CD4 < 200 cells/mm³)
    - 75% of AIDS patients will have MSK complications
  - Most MSK infections due to Staphylococcus aureus
- Genetics
  - Retrovirus HIV has high affinity to CD4 T lymphocytes and monocytes
  - HIV binds to CD4 cells and replicates itself by generating DNA copy by reverse transcriptase
  - Viral DNA incorporated into host DNA, enabling further replication
- Etiology
  - Transmitted through sexual contact (> 70%)
  - Parenteral transmission among intravenous drug users
  - Transmission by contaminated blood products (rare in US)
  - Transmission from mother to child during pregnancy, birth, breast milk
- Epidemiology
  - 40 million HIV infections worldwide
  - 20 million deaths secondary to AIDS
- Associated abnormalities
  - Pneumocystis carinii pneumonia
  - Tuberculosis

Gross Pathologic & Surgical Features
- Osteomyelitis: Bone destruction with rim of ischemic marrow necrosis
  - TB: Subligamentous spread to intervertebral disc and adjacent anterior vertebral body
- NHL: Pink-tan fleshy lesions with area of necrosis, patchy cortical erosions

Microscopic Features
- Infection: Leukocyte infiltration, vascular compression, necrosis, abscess
- NHL: Bone marrow permeation by round cell tumor
- HIV arthropathy: HIV antigens and DNA can be isolated from synovium

CLINICAL ISSUES

Presentation
- Most common signs/symptoms
  - Fever, weight loss, night sweats
  - Opportunistic infections if CD4 < 200 cells/mm³
- Other signs/symptoms
  - Lymphadenopathy
  - Shortness of breath, cough
  - Diarrhea
  - Oral candidiasis, thrush

Demographics
- Age
  - 25-45 years
  - Children < 15 years: 10% worldwide
- Gender
  - Majority in homosexual men
  - Majority new cases in US: Heterosexual men & women

Natural History & Prognosis
- HIV infection can be latent for many years
- Progression from HIV infection to AIDS: Approximately 11 years after infection
- Treated as chronic disease for many years; eventually almost uniformly lethal due to immune suppression

Treatment
- HAART (highly active antiretroviral therapy)
- Antibiotics
- Antivirals
- Incision and drainage (abscess, pyomyositis)

DIAGNOSTIC CHECKLIST

Consider
- Patients with AIDS have 60x ↑ incidence of NHL

Image Interpretation Pearls
- Always check for presence of necrosis, depth of soft tissue abnormality, and compartmental involvement when evaluating soft tissue infections

SELECTED REFERENCES

1. Restrepo CS et al: Imaging findings in musculoskeletal complications of AIDS. Radiographics. 24(4):1029-49, 2004
2. Tehranzadeh J et al: MRI of large intraosseous lesions in patients with inflammatory arthritis. AJR Am J Roentgenol. 183(5):1453-63, 2004
3. Tehranzadeh J et al: Musculoskeletal disorders associated with HIV infection and AIDS. Part I: infectious musculoskeletal conditions. Skeletal Radiol. 33(5):249-59, 2004
4. Allison GT et al: Osteonecrosis in HIV disease: epidemiology, etiologies, and clinical management. AIDS. 17(1):1-9, 2003
5. Bureau NJ et al: Imaging of musculoskeletal and spinal infections in AIDS. Radiol Clin North Am. 39(2):343-55, 2001

HIV-AIDS: MSK COMPLICATIONS

IMAGE GALLERY

Typical

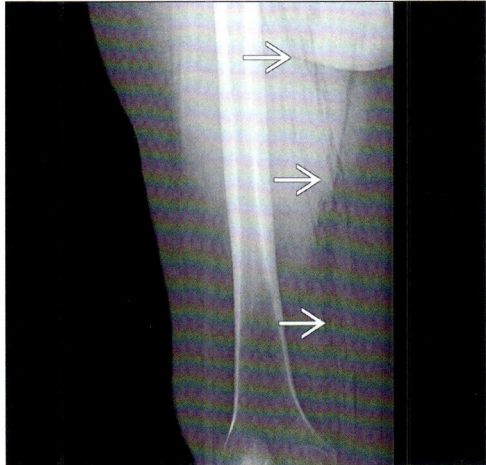
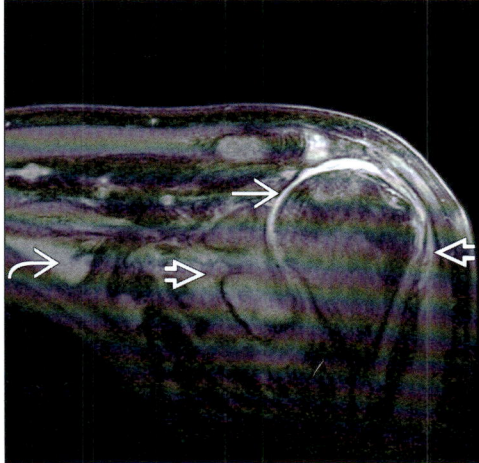

(Left) Anteroposterior radiograph shows gas tracking along fascial planes ➡ in an AIDS patient with necrotizing fasciitis. *(Right)* Coronal PD/Intermediate FS MR shows septic arthritis with destruction of the glenohumeral joint ➡ and inflammatory changes in the surrounding soft tissues ➡ in an HIV infected IV drug abuser. Note the soft tissue abscess in the chest wall ➡.

Typical

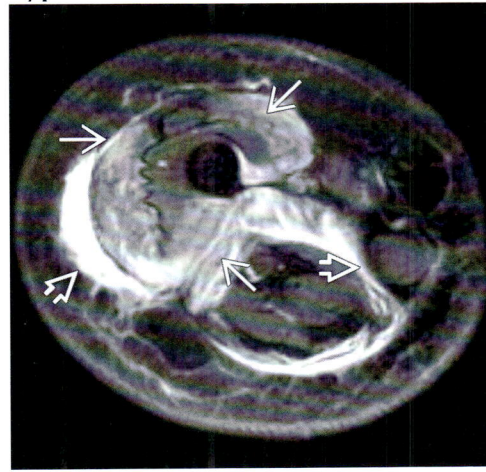
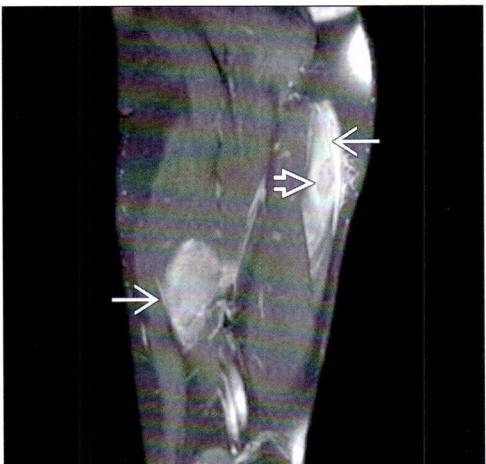

(Left) Axial PD/Intermediate FS MR in a patient with pyomyositis and fasciitis shows enlargement and increased T2 signal in the vastus musculature extending posteriorly ➡. Fluid is tracking along the fascial planes ➡. *(Right)* Coronal T1 C+ FS MR shows abnormal enhancement of the vastus lateralis and semimembranosus ➡. Note the focal non-enhancing area ➡ in this AIDS patient with myositis and myonecrosis.

Typical

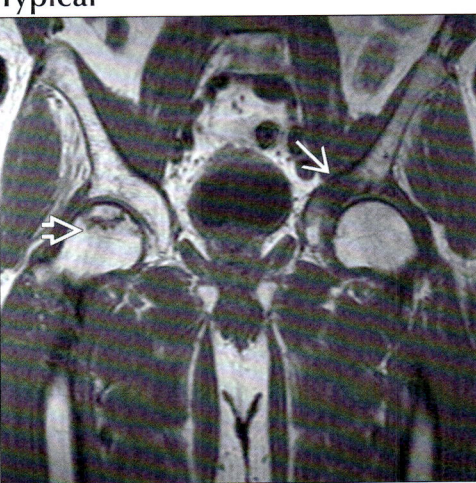
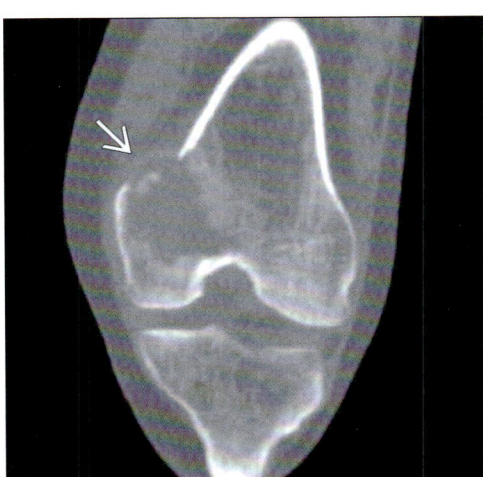

(Left) Coronal T1WI MR shows hypointense marrow replacement of the left acetabulum ➡ in this AIDS patient with lymphoma. Note the avascular necrosis on the right ➡, a common complication from AIDS. *(Right)* Coronal NECT shows a lytic lesion with cortical destruction of the distal femur ➡ in this AIDS patient with lymphoma.

HEMOPHILIA: MSK COMPLICATIONS

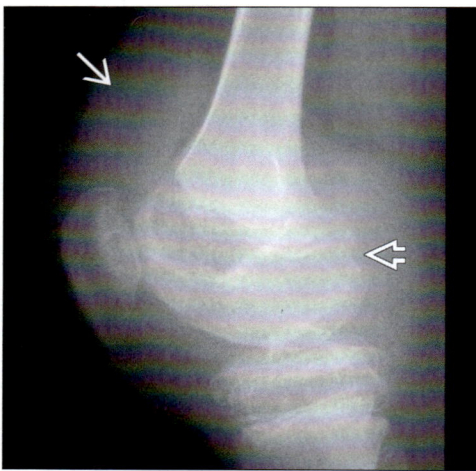 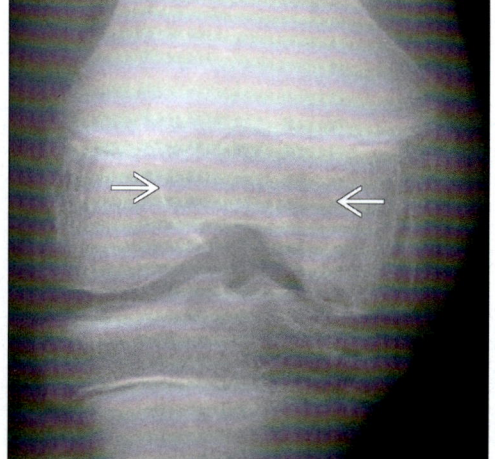

Lateral radiograph of a child's knee shows a large, dense, effusion ➡, along with erosions ⇨ and cartilage narrowing. The metaphyses & epiphyses are significantly overgrown, relative to the gracile diaphysis.

AP shows the widened intercondylar notch ➡, along with erosive changes & overgrowth of the bone. This overgrowth results from chronic hyperemia. Findings are typical of hemophilic arthropathy.

TERMINOLOGY

Abbreviations and Synonyms
- Hemophilia A (factor VIII deficiency), hemophilia B (factor IX deficiency, Christmas disease)

Definitions
- X-linked recessive bleeding disorder resulting from clotting factor deficiencies
- Pseudotumor of hemophilia: Non-neoplastic mass lesion that occurs with repeated focal intraosseous, subperiosteal, or soft tissue bleeding

IMAGING FINDINGS

General Features
- Best diagnostic clue
  - Dense hemarthrosis, arthropathy, growth deformity (balloon-like joints)
  - MR: "Blooming" nodules from hemosiderin deposits
- Location
  - Arthropathy: Knee > elbow > ankle > hip > shoulder
  - May be polyarticular, but usually not symmetric
  - Pseudotumor: Soft tissue > bone > subperiosteal
  - Intraosseous pseudotumor: Femur > pelvis > tibia > small bones of hand > calcaneus
  - Soft tissue pseudotumor: Thigh > gluteal region > iliopsoas muscle
- Size: Pseudotumors may become extremely large, measuring > 20 cm in diameter
- Morphology
  - Chronic hemarthroses & hyperemia → growth deformities
    - Overgrowth of epiphyses/metaphyses
    - Early fusion results in limb length discrepancy

Radiographic Findings
- Hemophilic arthropathy
  - Large effusion
    - Increased density if chronic bleeding results in hemosiderin deposits in synovium
  - Overgrowth pattern
    - Generally, epiphyses & metaphyses show overgrowth (balloon joint) due to hyperemia; diaphyses are gracile
    - In elbow, radial head is particularly enlarged
  - Premature physeal fusion results in limb shortening

Other Cases of Hemophilic Complications

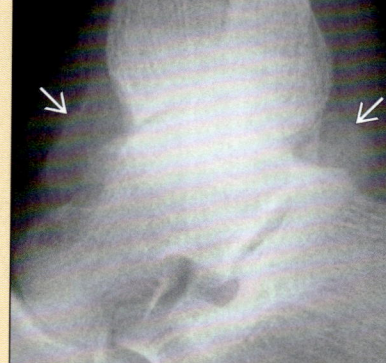 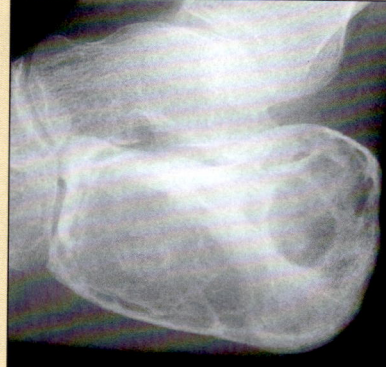 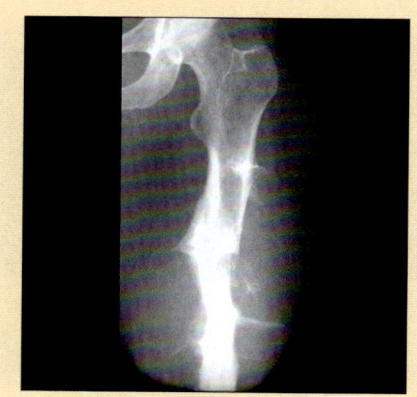

Dense Effusion: Hemosiderin | Intraosseous Pseudotumor | Subperiosteal Pseudotumor

HEMOPHILIA: MSK COMPLICATIONS

Key Facts

Terminology
- X-linked recessive bleeding disorder resulting from clotting factor deficiencies
- Pseudotumor of hemophilia: Non-neoplastic mass lesion that occurs with repeated focal intraosseous, subperiosteal, or soft tissue bleeding

Imaging Findings
- Dense hemarthrosis, arthropathy, growth deformity (balloon-like joints)
- MR: "Blooming" nodules from hemosiderin deposits
- Arthropathy: Knee > elbow > ankle > hip > shoulder
- May be polyarticular, but usually not symmetric
- Pseudotumor: Soft tissue > bone > subperiosteal
- Intraosseous pseudotumor: Femur > pelvis > tibia > small bones of hand > calcaneus
- Soft tissue pseudotumor: Thigh > gluteal region > iliopsoas muscle

Top Differential Diagnoses
- Arthropathy: Juvenile Chronic Arthritis (JCA)
- JCA occurs in skeletally immature patient, so hyperemia results in overgrowth & early fusion
- Arthropathy: Tuberculosis Arthritis (TB)
- If TB arthritis occurs in skeletally immature patient, can get same growth disturbance

Diagnostic Checklist
- Early MR of arthropathy should be obtained; allows early assessment which leads to aggressive prophylaxis & delays joint complications

---

- Osteoporosis
- Pannus causes erosion & widening of intercondylar notch in knee, trochlear notch in elbow
- Inflammatory synovitis causes cartilage destruction, erosions, & subchondral cysts
- Eventual secondary osteoarthritis
- Hemophilic pseudotumor
  - If intraosseous, extremely expanded lytic lesion
    - Appears bizarre due to its size; not permeative
    - May be single lytic lesion, or multilobular
    - Daughter cysts often seen
    - May contain septae
    - Rarely, dystrophic calcification present
    - No predilection for location (epiphyseal, metaphyseal, diaphyseal, central, or eccentric)
    - Endosteal scalloping, cortical thinning
    - Well-marginated; sclerotic rim
    - Adjacent reactive bone formation
  - If subperiosteal or soft tissue in origin
    - Soft tissue density, ± internal calcifications
    - Extrinsic scalloping on bone, with sharp margin
    - Periosteal reaction may be unusual in appearance, with sharp bony excrescences extending perpendicularly from bone

CT Findings
- Valuable in evaluation of septae and thin cortical rim in pseudotumor
- Enhanced CT can define outlines & wall thickness of peripheral capsule
- Central variable attenuation, representing different stages of hemorrhage

MR Findings
- Hemophilic arthropathy
  - Hemosiderin deposits along synovial lining of joint
    - May be nodular
    - Low signal all sequences, bloom on gradient echo
  - Effusion heterogeneous on both T1 & T2: Blood products in various stages
    - Acute: Isointense on T1, hypointense on T2
    - > 1 week: Signal intensity progressively increases on both T1 & T2
    - May contain fluid-fluid levels
  - Cartilage destruction, subchondral erosions & cysts
- Hemophilic pseudotumor
  - Intramedullary cystic lesion
    - Thin low signal rim
    - May have low signal periosteal reaction & adjacent reactive bone formation
    - Low signal hemosiderin deposits within wall
    - Contains fluid components, best seen on T2 & post-contrast T1; may have fluid-fluid levels
    - Complex internal signal (remote & recurrent hemorrhage, clot organization): Mixed high & low signal regions on all sequences
  - Soft tissue/subperiosteal pseudotumor
    - Hemosiderin nodular deposits along capsule of lesion (low signal on all sequences, blooms)
    - Pressure erosions (scalloping) on adjacent bone
    - Low signal bony excrescences extending several centimeters perpendicularly to long bone
    - Pressure may lead to skin necrosis, pain, infection
    - Soft tissue mass heterogeneous on both T1 & T2, representing blood products of various ages
    - May have fluid-fluid levels

Ultrasonographic Findings
- US to follow progression/resolution of pseudotumor

Imaging Recommendations
- Best imaging tool
  - Radiographs make initial diagnosis
  - MR used to confirm presence of hemosiderin & evaluate any "mass lesion" as well as adjacency to peripheral nerves
- Protocol advice: Gradient echo sequences show "blooming" of hemosiderin deposits in synovium

DIFFERENTIAL DIAGNOSIS

Arthropathy: Juvenile Chronic Arthritis (JCA)
- JCA occurs in skeletally immature patient, so hyperemia results in overgrowth & early fusion

HEMOPHILIA: MSK COMPLICATIONS

- Pannus & synovitis causes similar pattern of erosion and cartilage/bone destruction
- Hemophilia may be distinguished from JCA if hemosiderin deposits can be demonstrated either by radiographic density or blooming on MR

Arthropathy: Tuberculosis Arthritis (TB)
- If TB arthritis occurs in skeletally immature patient, can get same growth disturbance
- Cartilage destruction & erosions tend to develop & progress slower in TB than in pyogenic septic joint
- Erosions may have more sclerotic & well-defined rim

Arthropathy: Pigmented Villonodular Synovitis (PVNS)
- Both show low signal intraarticular synovium on all sequences, which "blooms" on gradient echo
- PVNS often has a more focal nodular pattern
- If PVNS occurs in skeletally immature patient, it could result in overgrowth, though typically not to the same extent as hemophilia
- Erosive pattern in PVNS is more focal, related specifically to nodular lesions

Pseudotumor of Bone: May Simulate Multiple Primary or Secondary Tumors
- Giant cell tumor
- Desmoplastic fibroma
- Plasmacytoma
- Metastasis
- Solitary or aneurysmal bone cyst

PATHOLOGY

General Features
- Etiology
  - Hemophilic arthropathy
    - Joints whose stability depends on adjacent soft tissues seem to be most at risk
    - Initial bleed predisposes to recurrent bleed
    - Recurrent bleeding results in hyperemia → osseous overgrowth & early fusion
    - Hypertrophy & inflammation in synovial membrane → cartilage & osseous damage
  - Pseudotumor of hemophilia
    - Recurrent hemorrhage in extraarticular location of musculoskeletal system →
    - Chronic, slowly expanding encapsulated mass →
    - Depending on site, osseous reaction to mass
- Epidemiology
  - Hemophilia A: 1:10,000 males in US
  - Hemophilia B: 1:100,000 males in US
  - Hemarthrosis occurs in 70-90% of hemophiliacs
    - 50% of hemophilic patients develop permanent arthropathy
  - Pseudotumor occurs in 1-2% of patients with severe hemophilia (clotting factor level < 1% of normal)

Gross Pathologic & Surgical Features
- Altered synovial membrane: Inflammatory tissue, pannus, with brownish color
- Discoloration of cartilage, focal areas of fibrillation, erosion, & necrosis

CLINICAL ISSUES

Presentation
- Most common signs/symptoms
  - Acute hemarthrosis: Tense, swollen, red, painful
  - May have leukocytosis & fever
  - Subacute or chronic hemarthrosis: Contractures, severely restricted range of motion
  - Pseudotumor presents with mass
    - Occasional neuropathy
    - Occasional pathologic fracture
    - Occasional compartment syndrome

Demographics
- Age
  - First episode of joint hemorrhage 2-3 years of age
  - Repeated hemarthrosis in adolescents & teenagers
  - Hemarthrosis occurrence decreases in older patients
- Gender
  - Male only (X-linked recessive abnormality)
  - Extremely rare female manifestations seen with various chromosomal abnormalities

Natural History & Prognosis
- Severity varies
  - Least severe: Bleed excessively with surgery or trauma
  - Most severe: Spontaneous bleeding, or minor trauma
- Repeated intraarticular bleeding results in joint contracture & destruction
- Pseudotumor may spontaneously resolve, but usually continues to enlarge

Treatment
- Hemophilic arthropathy
  - Acute: Administer appropriate clotting factor
  - Chronic: Synovectomy; if end-stage, arthroplasty
  - Note: Patients should routinely receive aggressive treatment with synthetic clotting factors
- Hemophilic pseudotumor: Aims at preserving function
  - Conservative: Immobilization
  - Radical resection or radiation

DIAGNOSTIC CHECKLIST

Consider
- Early MR of arthropathy should be obtained; allows early assessment which leads to aggressive prophylaxis & delays joint complications

SELECTED REFERENCES

1. Ng WH et al: Role of imaging in management of hemophilic patients. AJR Am J Roentgenol. 184(5):1619-23, 2005
2. Park JS et al: Hemophilic pseudo tumor involving the musculoskeletal system: spectrum of radiologic findings. AJR 183:55-61; 2004
3. Kilcoyne RF et al: Radiological evaluation of hemophilic arthropathy. Semin Thromb Hemost. 29(1):43-8, 2003

HEMOPHILIA: MSK COMPLICATIONS

IMAGE GALLERY

Typical

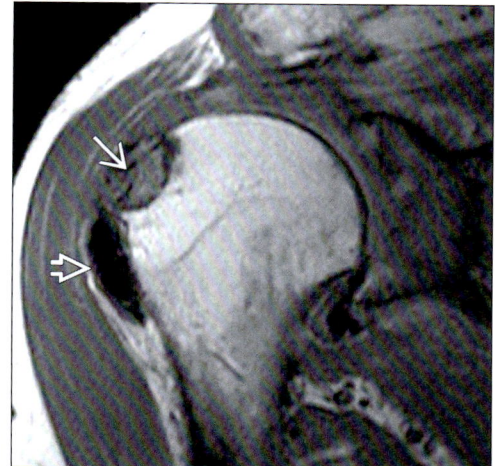 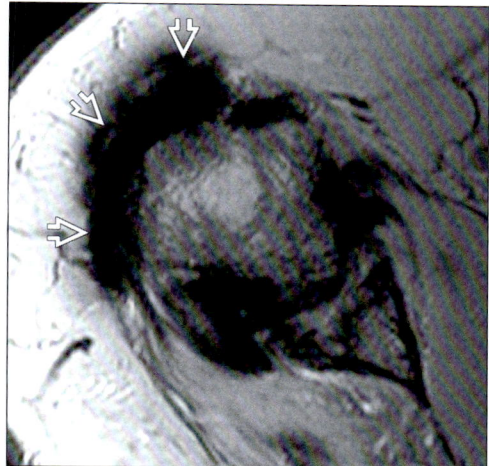

(Left) Coronal T1WI MR shows erosive change in humeral head ➡. Even though this is a T1 image, one can see that there is also a rotator cuff tear. There is, additionally, a low signal mass lining the subdeltoid bursa ➡. *(Right)* Axial gradient echo image at the level of the low signal mass in subdeltoid bursa, shows "blooming" of the mass ➡. This strongly supports the diagnosis of hemophilic arthropathy, with hemosiderin deposition within the synovium.

Typical

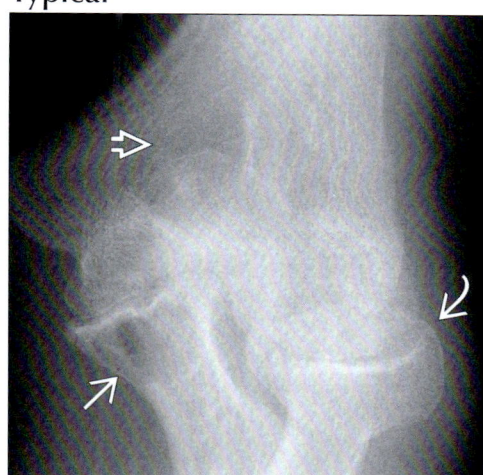 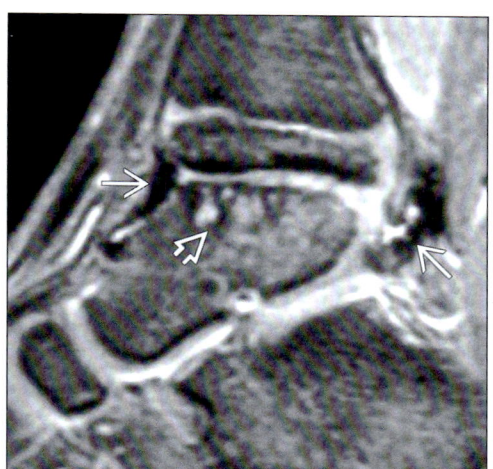

(Left) Anteroposterior radiograph shows typical hemophilic arthropathy of the elbow. There is large subchondral cyst formation ➡, widened trochlear notch ➡, and significant overgrowth of the radial head ➡. *(Right)* Sagittal T2* GRE MR shows hemophilic arthropathy in a 10 year old, with significant erosions & subchondral cyst formation ➡. Note the low signal hemosiderin deposits within the synovium ➡, typical of the disease.

Typical

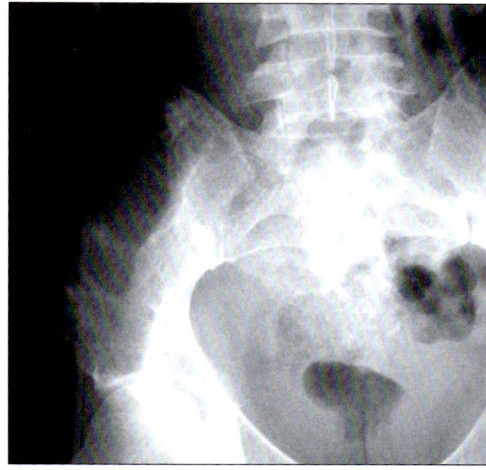 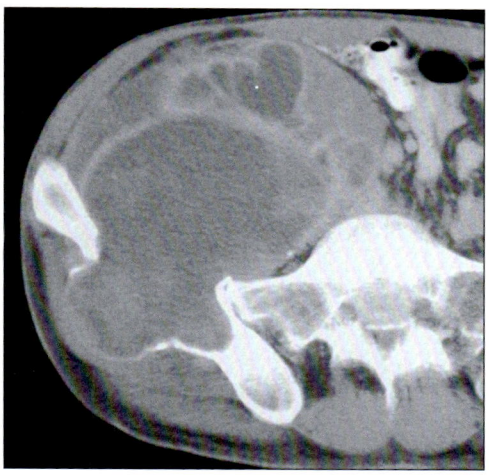

(Left) Anteroposterior radiograph shows a lytic expanded lesion of the iliac wing, with a sclerotic margin. There is pseudotrabeculation within the lesion. *(Right)* Axial CECT shows extent of the expanded lesion and osseous destruction. Multiloculated lesion has a thick enhancing rim. There is varying attenuation and enhancement within the mass, relating to different stages of hemorrhage. Lesion is a classic hemophilic intraosseous pseudotumor.

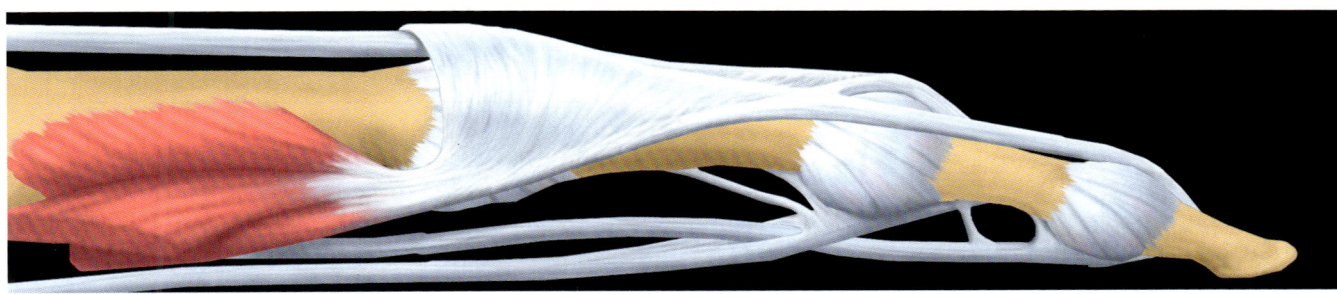

INDEX

A

Abdominal abscess, II:3–4 to II:3–6, **II:3–7i**
  differential diagnosis, **II:3–4i**, II:3–5
Abdominal disorders, II:3–2 to II:3–257. *See also* Abdominal trauma
  abdominal abscess, II:3–4 to II:3–6, **II:3–7i**
  aorto-enteric fistula, II:3–32 to II:3–33
  appendicitis, II:3–76 to II:3–78, **II:3–79i**
  Budd-Chiari syndrome, II:3–134 to II:3–136, **II:3–137i**
  cholangitis
    ascending, II:3–138 to II:3–139
    recurrent pyogenic, II:3–140 to II:3–142, **II:3–143i**
  cholecystitis, II:3–148 to II:3–150, **II:3–151i**
  choledocholithiasis, II:3–144 to II:3–146, **II:3–147i**
  colitis
    infectious, II:3–60 to II:3–62, **II:3–63i**
    ischemic, II:3–92 to II:3–94, **II:3–95i**
    pseudomembranous, II:3–64 to II:3–66, **II:3–67i**
    ulcerative, II:3–70 to II:3–72, **II:3–73i**
  Crohn disease, II:3–34 to II:3–36, **II:3–37i**
  diverticulitis, II:3–80 to II:3–82, **II:3–83i**
  duodenal atresia or stenosis, II:3–190 to II:3–192, **II:3–193i**
  duodenal ulcer, II:3–28 to II:3–30, **II:3–31i**
  ectopic pregnancy, tubal, II:3–254 to II:3–256, **II:3–257i**
  epididymo-orchitis, II:3–178 to II:3–180, **II:3–181i**
  epiploic appendagitis, II:3–84 to II:3–86, **II:3–87i**
  femoral hernia, II:3–16 to II:3–18, **II:3–19i**
  gallstone ileus, II:3–54 to II:3–55
  HELLP syndrome, II:3–122 to II:3–124, **II:3–125i**
  hypertrophic pyloric stenosis, II:3–210 to II:3–212, **II:3–213i**
  ileocolic intussusception, II:3–218 to II:3–220, **II:3–221i**
  imaging issues, II:3–2 to II:3–3
  inguinal hernia, II:3–12 to II:3–14, **II:3–15i**
  intussusception, II:3–56 to II:3–58, **II:3–59i**
  liver
    amebic abscess, II:3–118 to II:3–120, **II:3–121i**
    candidiasis, II:3–110 to II:3–112, **II:3–113i**
    infarction, II:3–126 to II:3–128, **II:3–129i**
    pyogenic abscess, II:3–114 to II:3–116, **II:3–117i**
  Meckel diverticulum, II:3–222 to II:3–224, **II:3–225i**
  meconium ileus, II:3–198 to II:3–200, **II:3–201i**
  meconium peritonitis, II:3–202 to II:3–204, **II:3–205i**
  meconium plug syndrome, II:3–194 to II:3–196, **II:3–197i**
  mesenteric adenitis, II:3–226 to II:3–228, **II:3–229i**
  necrotizing enterocolitis, II:3–206 to II:3–208, **II:3–209i**
  omental infarct, II:3–88 to II:3–90, **II:3–91i**
  ovarian hemorrhage, II:3–246 to II:3–248, **II:3–249i**
  ovarian torsion, II:3–238 to II:3–240, **II:3–241i**
  ovarian vein thrombosis, II:3–242 to II:3–244, **II:3–245i**
  pancreatitis, acute, II:3–152 to II:3–154, **II:3–155i**
  paraduodenal hernia, II:3–20 to II:3–22, **II:3–23i**
  pelvic inflammatory disease, II:3–250 to II:3–252, **II:3–253i**
  peritonitis, II:3–8 to II:3–10, **II:3–11i**
  pneumatosis of intestine, II:3–38 to II:3–40, **II:3–41i**
  portal vein occlusion, II:3–130 to II:3–132, **II:3–133i**
  pyelonephritis, II:3–156 to II:3–158, **II:3–159i**
    emphysematous, II:3–168 to II:3–169
    xanthogranulomatous, II:3–164 to II:3–166, **II:3–167i**
  renal abscess, II:3–160 to II:3–162, **II:3–163i**
  renal infarction, II:3–170 to II:3–172, **II:3–173i**
  renal vein thrombosis, II:3–174 to II:3–176, **II:3–177i**
  small bowel intussusception, pediatric, II:3–230 to II:3–232, **II:3–233i**
  small bowel ischemia, acute, II:3–42 to II:3–44, **II:3–45i**
  small bowel obstruction, II:3–50 to II:3–52, **II:3–53i**
  splenic infarction, II:3–106 to II:3–108, **II:3–109i**

INDEX

splenic infection and abscess, II:3–102 to II:3–104, **II:3–105i**
testicular torsion, II:3–182 to II:3–184, **II:3–185i**
toxic megacolon, II:3–74 to II:3–75
transmesenteric postoperative hernia, II:3–24 to II:3–26, **II:3–27i**
typhlitis, II:3–68 to II:3–69
uterine arteriovenous malformation, II:3–234 to II:3–236, **II:3–237i**
vasculitis, small intestine, II:3–46 to II:3–48, **II:3–49i**
volvulus
    cecal, II:3–100 to II:3–101
    gastric, II:3–214 to II:3–216, **II:3–217i**
    midgut, II:3–186 to II:3–188, **II:3–189i**
    sigmoid, II:3–96 to II:3–98, **II:3–99i**
Abdominal trauma, I:3–2 to I:3–43. *See also* Abdominal disorders
  duodenal trauma/hematoma, I:3–20 to I:3–21
  hepatic trauma, I:3–8 to I:3–10, **I:3–11i**
  hypoperfusion complex, I:3–28 to I:3–30, **I:3–31i**
  imaging issues, I:3–2 to I:3–3
  intestinal trauma, I:3–22 to I:3–24, **I:3–25i**
  pancreatic trauma, I:3–16 to I:3–18, **I:3–19i**
  renal trauma, I:3–12 to I:3–14, **I:3–15i**
  splenic trauma, I:3–4 to I:3–6, **I:3–7i**
  testicular trauma, I:3–26 to I:3–27
Abscess
  abdominal, II:3–4 to II:3–6, **II:3–7i**
  amebic hepatic, II:3–118 to II:3–120, **II:3–121i**
    differential diagnosis, **II:3–118i**, II:3–119
    pyogenic abscess vs., **II:3–114i**, II:3–115
  Brodie
    pediatric stress fracture vs., **I:4–206i**, I:4–208
    stress fracture vs., I:4–11
  cerebral, II:1–48 to II:1–50, **II:1–51i**
  epidural paravertebral, II:1–120 to II:1–122, **II:1–123i**
    differential diagnosis, **II:1–120i**, II:1–121
    traumatic disc herniation vs., **I:1–106i**, I:1–107
  groin, vs. inguinal hernia, **II:3–12i**, II:3–14
  hematoma vs., **I:4–28i**, I:4–29
  lung. *See* Lung abscess
  mediastinal, vs. sternal fracture, **I:2–26i**, I:2–27
  pyogenic. *See* Pyogenic abscess
  renal, II:3–160 to II:3–162, **II:3–163i**
    differential diagnosis, **II:3–160i**, II:3–161
    xanthogranulomatous pyelonephritis vs., **II:3–164i**, II:3–165
  retropharyngeal. *See* Retropharyngeal space, abscess
  soft tissue, II:4–4 to I:4–5
    diabetes complications vs., I:4–20
    differential diagnosis, I:4–5, **II:4–4i**

spinal, vs. fracture., I:2–24
splenic. *See* Splenic infection and abscess
sternoclavicular trauma vs., **I:4–36i**, I:4–37
subperiosteal, of orbit, II:1–92 to II:1–94, **II:1–95i**
subphrenic, vs. diaphragmatic tear, I:2–30
tubo-ovarian. *See* Tubo-ovarian abscess
Acetabular fractures, I:4–126 to I:4–128, **I:4–129i**
  differential diagnosis, **I:4–126i**, I:4–127
Achalasia, vs. pneumomediastinum, **I:2–4i**, I:2–6
Achilles tendon tear/tendinopathy, I:4–162 to I:4–164, **I:4–165i**
  differential diagnosis, **I:4–162i**, I:4–163
Acquired immunodeficiency syndrome. *See* AIDS (acquired immunodeficiency syndrome)
Acromioclavicular dislocation, I:4–42 to I:4–43
  clavicle fracture vs., **I:4–40i**
  differential diagnosis, **I:4–42i**
Acute chest syndrome. *See* Sickle cell disease
Acute disseminated encephalomyelitis, III:1–62
Acute fatty liver of pregnancy, I:3–123
Acute respiratory distress syndrome (ARDS)
  acute interstitial pneumonia vs., II:2–85
  aspiration vs., II:2–109
Adenitis
  mesenteric. *See* Mesenteric adenitis
  retropharyngeal, **II:1–108i**, II:1–109
Adenoma
  hepatic trauma vs., **I:3–8i**, I:3–9
  villous, vs. duodenal trauma, **I:3–20i**, I:3–21
Adhesions, **II:3–54i**
Aerophagia, II:3–51
Agricultural lung diseases, II:2–21
AIDS (acquired immunodeficiency syndrome)
  benign lymphoepithelial disease vs. acute parotitis, **II:1–104i**, II:1–105
  musculoskeletal complications, II:4–74 to I:4–76, **II:4–77i**
    differential diagnosis, I:4–76, **II:4–74i**
  opportunistic infections, II:1–60 to II:1–62, **II:1–63i**
Airway obstruction, II:2–61
Alcoholism, II:2–77
Alveolar hemorrhage, diffuse. *See* Diffuse alveolar hemorrhage
Alveolar proteinosis
  acute interstitial pneumonia vs., II:2–86
  cardiogenic pulmonary edema vs., **II:2–4i**, II:2–6
Amebic abscess, hepatic, II:3–118 to II:3–120, **II:3–121i**
  differential diagnosis, **II:3–118i**, II:3–119
  pyogenic abscess vs., **II:3–114i**, II:3–115
Amiodarone toxicity, II:2–94
Ampullary carcinoma, **II:3–144i**, II:3–145
Amyloid angiopathy, cerebral
  cerebral contusion vs., **I:1–20i**, I:1–21

INDEX

diffuse axonal injury vs., **I:1–24i,** I:1–25
hypertensive intracranial hemorrhage vs., **II:1–24i,** II:1–25
spontaneous intracranial hemorrhage vs., II:1–21
traumatic subarachnoid hemorrhage vs., I:1–17
Amyloidosis
    gout vs., I:4–23
    hematoma vs., I:4–29
    pigmented villonodular synovitis vs., I:4–35
    talcosis vs., II:2–93
Anemia. *See also* Sickle cell disease
    transient tachypnea of newborn vs., II:2–61
Aneurysm
    aortic, **I:2–18i,** I:2–20
    blood blister-like, **II:1–14i,** II:14 to II:1–15
    dissecting vs. fusiform, II:1–13
    fusiform, **II:1–12i,** II:1–12 to II:1–13
    giant serpentine, II:1–12
    mycotic, vs. drug abuse, II:1–65
    saccular, II:1–8 to II:1–10, **II:1–11i**
        blood blister-like aneurysm vs., **II:1–14i**
        differential diagnosis, **II:1–8i,** II:1–9
    thoracic, II:2–129
    traumatic subarachnoid hemorrhage vs., **I:1–16i,** I:1–17
Angiomatosis, bacillary, **II:4–74i,** II:4–76
Angiomyolipoma, **I:3–12i,** I:3–13
Ankle fractures, **I:4–158i,** I:4–158 to I:4–160, **I:4–161i**
Anterior talofibular ligament sprain, I:4–179
Anticoagulation therapy
    spontaneous intracranial hemorrhage vs., II:1–22
    traumatic subarachnoid hemorrhage vs., I:1–17
Aorta
    proximal descending, I:2–20
    spindle, I:2–20
    tortuosity vs. dissection, II:2–129
    ulcer vs. transection, **I:2–18i,** I:2–19 to I:2–20
Aortic aneurysm, **I:2–18i,** I:2–20
Aortic dissection, II:2–128 to II:2–130, **II:2–131i**
    differential diagnosis, **II:2–128i,** II:2–129 to II:2–130
Aortic transection, I:2–18 to I:2–20, **I:2–21i**
    differential diagnosis, **I:2–18i,** I:2–19 to I:2–20
    dissection vs., **II:2–128i,** II:2–130
    spinal fracture vs., **I:2–22i,** I:2–24
Aortic valve stenosis, **II:2–128i,** II:2–130
Aorto-enteric fistula, **II:3–32i,** II:3–32 to II:3–33
Appendicitis, II:3–76 to II:3–78, **II:3–79i**
    differential diagnosis, **II:3–76i,** II:3–77 to II:3–78
    epiploic appendagitis vs., **II:3–84i,** II:3–85
    ileocolic intussusception vs., **II:3–218i,** II:3–219
    Meckel diverticulum vs., **II:3–222i,** II:3–223
    mesenteric adenitis vs., **II:3–226i,** II:3–227
    omental infarct vs., **II:3–88i,** II:3–88 to II:3–89
    ovarian vein thrombosis vs., **II:3–242i,** II:3–243
    pelvic inflammatory disease, **II:3–250i,** II:3–251
    typhlitis vs., **II:3–68i**
Appendicular insufficiency fractures, **I:4–8i,** I:4–8 to I:4–9
Arachnoid granulation, **II:1–36i,** II:1–37
ARDS (acute respiratory distress syndrome)
    acute interstitial pneumonia vs., II:2–85
    aspiration vs., II:2–109
Arterial bleeding, **I:4–122i**
Arterial thrombosis, I:1–41
Arteriovenous fistula, dural
    spinal cord infarction vs., **II:1–124i**
    spinal cord injury vs., **I:1–110i,** I:1–111
    spontaneous low flow vs. carotid-cavernous fistula, **I:1–44i,** I:1–45
Arteriovenous malformation
    hematoma vs., I:4–29
    hemorrhagic, vs. drug abuse, **II:1–64i,** II:1–65
    hypertensive intracranial hemorrhage vs., **II:1–24i,** II:1–25
    spontaneous intracranial hemorrhage vs., II:1–21
    transient tachypnea of newborn vs., II:2–61
    uterine, II:3–234 to II:3–236, **II:3–237i**
Arthritis. *See also* Osteoarthritis; Rheumatoid arthritis
    degenerative, I:4–107
    femoral neck fracture vs., I:4–139
    infectious. *See* Septic joint
    inflammatory
        carpal instabilities vs., I:4–96
        flexor annular pulley tear vs., I:4–107
        gout vs., I:4–23
        neuropathic Charcot vs., I:4–44
        septic joint vs., I:4–16, **II:4–14i**
    juvenile chronic, **II:4–78i,** II:4–79 to I:4–80
    sternoclavicular trauma vs., I:4–37
    tuberculosis, vs. hemophilia, I:4–80
Arthroplasty complications
    component wear/particle disease, II:4–66 to I:4–68, **II:4–69i**
        differential diagnosis, **II:4–66i,** II:4–67 to I:4–68
        hardware/periprosthetic fracture vs., II:1–64
        loosening and dislocation vs., II:1–60
    fibrosis at bone-metal interface, II:4–67
    hardware/periprosthetic fracture, II:4–62 to I:4–64, **II:4–65i**
        differential diagnosis, I:4–64, **II:4–62i**
    loosening and dislocation, II:4–58 to I:4–60, **II:4–61i**

INDEX

differential diagnosis, I:4–60, **II:4–58i**
    hardware/periprosthetic fracture vs., I:4–64
    normal subsidence, I:4–60
    prosthesis infection, II:4–67
    stress shielding, II:4–68
Artifacts. *See also* FLAIR artifact
    chemical shift, vs. subdural hematoma, I:1–9
    magic angle, I:4–152
    post-surgical, vs. subdural hematoma, I:1–9, I:1–13
    streaming, vs. portal vein occlusion., **II:3–130i**, II:3–131
    technical, vs. aortic transection, I:2–20
Ascites
    benign, vs. peritonitis, **II:3–8i**, II:3–9
    loculated, vs. abdominal abscess, **II:3–4i**, II:3–5
Aspiration, II:2–108 to II:2–110, **II:2–111i**. *See also* Meconium aspiration syndrome
    asthma vs., II:2–101
    community acquired pneumonia vs., II:2–26
    differential diagnosis, **II:2–108i**, II:2–109 to II:2–110
    drug abuse vs., II:2–90
    lung contusion vs., **I:2–36i**, I:2–38
    mitral regurgitation pulmonary edema vs., **II:2–8i**, II:2–9
    pulmonary edema vs., I:2–41, I:2–45
    sickle cell disease vs., II:2–77
    silo-filler's disease vs., II:2–22
    smoke inhalation vs., II:2–17
Asthma, II:2–100 to II:2–102, **II:2–103i**
    bronchial foreign body vs., **II:2–116i**, II:2–117
    differential diagnosis, **II:2–100i**, II:2–101
    viral lung infection vs., II:2–37
Astrocytoma, **II:1–32i**, II:1–34
Atelectasis, II:2–27
Atherosclerosis
    aortic dissection vs., **II:2–128i**, II:2–130
    aortic transection vs., **I:2–18i**, I:2–20
    blood blister-like aneurysm vs., II:1–16
    extracranial vascular injury vs., **I:1–40i**, I:1–41
    fusiform aneurysm vs., **II:1–12i**
    intracranial vascular injury vs., **I:1–36i**, I:1–37
Athletic hyperinflation, II:2–97
Atlanto-occipital dislocation, **I:1–60i**, I:1–60 to I:1–61
Atlas
    burst fracture, I:1–62 to I:1–64, **I:1–65i**
        differential diagnosis, **I:1–62i**, I:1–63
    malformations, **I:1–62i**, I:1–63
    pseudospread, **I:1–62i**, I:1–63
Avascular necrosis
    bone marrow edema vs., I:4–47, **II:4–46i**
    femoral head fracture vs., I:4–135
    femoral neck fracture vs., I:4–139

    missed hip dislocation with, **I:4–130i**
    sacral insufficiency fractures vs., I:4–5
Avulsion fractures
    anterior process calcaneal, **I:4–166i**, I:4–168
    extensor digitorum brevis, **I:4–166i**, I:4–168
    finger, I:4–110 to I:4–112, **I:4–113i**
        differential diagnosis, **I:4–110i**, I:4–111
    knee, I:4–142 to I:4–144, **I:4–145i**
        differential diagnosis, **I:4–142i**, I:4–144
    pelvic, I:4–114 to I:4–116, **I:4–117i**
        acetabular fracture vs., I:4–127
        differential diagnosis, **I:4–114i**, I:4–115 to I:4–116
Axonal injury, diffuse, I:1–24 to I:1–26, **I:1–27i**
    differential diagnosis, **I:1–24i**, I:1–25
Autosomal dominant polycystic kidney, 5:42

B

Barton fracture, I:4–75
Benign lymphoepithelial disease, HIV-related, **II:1–104i**, II:1–105
Bezoar, gastric, **II:3–210i**, II:3–211
Bifurcate sprain, I:4–180
Biliary calculi, II:3–144 to II:3–146, **II:3–147i**
    differential diagnosis, **II:3–144i**, II:3–145
Biloma, II:3–5
Bladder rupture, **I:4–122i**
Blood dyscrasia, I:1–17
Bone bruise, I:4–83
Bone cyst, **I:4–14i**
Bone marrow edema, transient, II:4–46 to I:4–47
    differential diagnosis, I:4–47, **II:4–46i**
    osteonecrosis of hip vs., I:4–49
Bone marrow hyperplasia, **II:4–70i**, II:4–71 to II:4–72
Bowel. *See* Intestinal disorders
Brachialis strain, I:4–73
Brain injury, accidental, I:1–29
Brain injury, traumatic, I:1–4 to I:1–45
    carotid-cavernous fistula, I:1–44 to I:1–45
    cerebral contusion, I:1–20 to I:1–22, **I:1–23i**
    child abuse and, I:1–28 to I:1–30, **I:1–31i**
    diffuse axonal injury, I:1–24 to I:1–26, **I:1–27i**
    epidural hematoma, I:1–4 to I:1–6, **I:1–7i**
    imaging issues, anatomic, I:1–2 to I:1–3
    intracranial herniation syndromes, I:1–32 to I:1–34, **I:1–35i**
    neonatal meningitis vs., **II:1–40i**, II:1–41
    subarachnoid hemorrhage, traumatic, I:1–16 to I:1–18, **I:1–19i**
    subdural hematoma
        acute, I:1–8 to I:1–10, **I:1–11i**
        mixed, I:1–12 to I:1–13
        paratentorial, I:1–14 to I:1–15

INDEX

vascular injury
    extracranial, I:1–40 to I:1–42, **I:1–43i**
    intracranial, I:1–36 to I:1–38, **I:1–39i**
Brodie abscess
    pediatric stress fracture vs., **I:4–206i**, I:4–208
    stress fracture vs., I:4–11
Bronchial foreign body, II:2–116 to II:2–118, **II:2–119i**
    croup vs., II:2–53
    differential diagnosis, **II:2–116i**, II:2–117 to II:2–118
    epiglottitis vs., II:2–57
    exudative tracheitis vs., II:2–49
    viral lung infection vs., **II:2–36i**, II:2–37
Bronchial obstruction, II:3–39
Bronchial tear, **I:2–32i**, I:2–33
Bronchiectasis, II:2–110
Bronchiolitis obliterans
    asthma vs., **II:2–100i**, II:2–101
    bronchial foreign body vs., II:2–118
    chronic obstructive pulmonary disease vs., **II:2–96i**, II:2–97
Bronchoalveolar cell carcinoma, II:2–86
Bronchocentric granulomatosis, II:2–101
Bronchogenic carcinoma, **II:2–32i**, II:2–33
Bronchogenic cyst
    bronchial foreign body vs., II:2–118
    round pneumonia vs., **II:2–40i**, II:2–41
Brown tumor of hyperthyroidism, I:4–23, **II:4–22i**
Buckle fractures, I:4–194 to I:4–196, **I:4–197i**
    differential diagnosis, **I:4–194i**, I:4–195 to I:4–196
Budd-Chiari syndrome, II:3–134 to II:3–136, **II:3–137i**
    differential diagnosis, **II:3–134i**, II:3–136
    portal vein occlusion vs., **II:3–130i**, II:3–132
Bulla, infected, II:2–33
Bursitis
    bicipital radial, I:4–72
    olecranon, I:4–65
    patellar tendon tears and tendinosis vs., **I:4–150i**, I:4–151
Burst fracture
    cervical, **I:1–74i**, **I:1–80i**, I:1–81
    chance fracture vs., **I:1–98i**, I:1–99
    compression fracture vs., **I:1–88i**, I:1–89

C

C2-C3 vertebrae, I:1–71
C2 fractures
    hangman's, I:1–70 to I:1–72, **I:1–73i**
        differential diagnosis, **I:1–70i**, I:1–71
    odontoid, I:1–66 to I:1–68, **I:1–69i**
        differential diagnosis, **I:1–66i**, I:1–67
    pathologic, I:1–67

Calcaneal fractures, I:4–166 to I:4–168, **I:4–169i**
    diabetes complications vs., I:4–20, **II:4–18i**
    differential diagnosis, **I:4–166i**, I:4–167
    stress fracture, **I:4–10i**
Calcaneofibular ligament sprain, I:4–179
Calcific periarthritis, II:4–30 to I:4–32, **II:4–33i**
    differential diagnosis, **II:4–30i**, II:4–31 to I:4–32
Campylobacter infections, **II:3–64i**, II:3–65
Cancer. See Carcinoma; Metastasis; Neoplasms
Candidiasis, hepatic, II:3–110 to II:3–112, **II:3–113i**
    differential diagnosis, **II:3–110i**, II:3–111
Capitellar osteochondritis dissecans
    humeral shaft/distal humeral fracture vs., I:4–57
    medial epicondyle avulsion vs., **I:4–210i**, I:4–211
    supracondylar fracture vs., I:4–199
Capitellum pseudodefect, I:4–55, **II:4–54i**
Carbon monoxide poisoning, II:1–78 to II:1–79
    inborn errors of metabolism vs., **II:1–72i**, II:1–73
    near-drowning vs., **II:1–76i**, II:1–77
Carcinoid syndrome, II:2–101
Carcinoma
    ampullary, **II:3–144i**, II:3–145
    bronchoalveolar cell, II:2–86
    bronchogenic, **II:2–32i**, II:2–33
    cecal
        appendicitis vs., **II:3–76i**, II:3–78
        intussusception vs., **II:3–56i**, II:3–57
    colon
        diverticulitis vs., **II:3–80i**, II:3–81
        ischemic colitis vs., **II:3–92i**, II:3–94
        sigmoid volvulus vs., **II:3–96i**, II:3–97
        toxic megacolon vs., **II:3–74i**
    duodenal., **II:3–28i**, II:3–29 to II:3–30
    hepatocellular
        HELLP syndrome vs., **II:3–122i**, II:3–123
        hepatic trauma vs., **I:3–8i**, I:3–9
    pancreatic infiltrating, **II:3–152i**, II:3–153
    renal cell. See Renal cell carcinoma
    squamous cell, **II:1–80i**, II:1–81
    transitional cell
        renal vein thrombosis vs., II:3–175
        xanthogranulomatous pyelonephritis vs., II:3–165
Carcinomatosis
    lymphangitic, II:2–6
    peritoneal, **II:3–8i**, II:3–9
Cardiomyopathy, restrictive, **II:2–136i**, II:2–137
Caroli disease, **II:3–110i**, II:3–111
Carotid-cavernous fistula, **I:1–44i**, I:1–44 to I:1–45
    invasive fungal sinusitis vs., II:1–101
    orbital inflammatory disease vs., II:1–89
Carpal dislocations, I:4–90 to I:4–92, **I:4–93i**
    differential diagnosis, **I:4–90i**, I:4–91

INDEX

fracture dislocation vs., **I:4–86i**, I:4–87
    instabilities vs., I:4–96
Carpal fractures, non-scaphoid, I:4–86 to I:4–88, **I:4–89i**
    differential diagnosis, **I:4–86i**, I:4–87
Carpal instabilities, I:4–94 to I:4–96, **I:4–97i**
    differential diagnosis, **I:4–94i**, I:4–96
    dislocations vs., I:4–91
Carpometacarpal joint
    fifth, fracture/dislocation, **I:4–98i**
    first, dislocation vs. subluxation, I:4–99
Cavernous malformation
    hemorrhagic, vs. drug abuse, II:1–65
    hypertensive intracranial hemorrhage vs., II:1–25
    saccular aneurysm vs., **II:1–8i**, II:1–9
    spinal cord injury vs., I:1–111
CCAM. See Cystic adenomatoid malformation, congenital (CCAM)
Cellulitis
    compartment syndrome vs., I:4–23
    necrotizing fasciitis vs., I:4–27
    orbital
        inflammatory disease vs., **II:1–88i**, II:1–89
        invasive fungal sinusitis vs., **II:1–100i**, II:1–101
    soft tissue abscess vs., I:4–5
Central nervous system disorders, II:1–2 to II:1–125
    See also Central nervous system trauma; Cerebral *terms*
    abnormalities, vs. transient tachypnea of newborn., II:2–62
    abscess, II:1–48 to II:1–50, **II:1–51i**
    blood blister-like aneurysm, II:1–14 to II:1–15
    carbon monoxide poisoning, II:1–78 to II:1–79
    cerebral ischemia-infarction, acute, II:1–32 to II:1–34, **II:1–35i**
    drug abuse, II:1–64 to II:1–66, **II:1–67i**
    dural sinus thrombosis, II:1–36 to II:1–38, **II:1–39i**
    epidural paravertebral abscess, II:1–120 to II:1–122, **II:1–123i**
    extra-axial empyema, II:1–52 to II:1–54, **II:1–55i**
    fungal sinusitis, invasive, II:1–100 to II:1–102, **II:1–103i**
    fusiform aneurysm, II:1–12 to II:1–13
    herpes encephalitis, II:1–56 to II:1–58, **II:1–59i**
    hydrocephalus, II:1–68 to II:1–70, **II:1–71i**
    hypertensive encephalopathy, acute, II:1–28 to II:1–30, **II:1–31i**
    imaging issues, II:1–2 to II:1–3
    inborn errors of metabolism, II:1–72 to II:1–74, **II:1–75i**
    intracerebral hematoma, II:1–16 to II:1–18, **II:1–18i**
    intracranial hemorrhage
        hypertensive, II:1–24 to II:1–26, **II:1–27i**
        spontaneous, II:1–20 to II:1–22, **II:1–23i**
    meningitis, II:1–44 to II:1–46, **II:1–47i**
        neonatal, II:1–40 to II:1–42, **II:1–43i**
    near-drowning, II:1–76 to II:1–77
    opportunistic infection, AIDS-related, II:1–60 to II:1–62, **II:1–63i**
    orbital inflammatory disease, idiopathic, II:1–88 to II:1–90, **II:1–91i**
    osteomyelitis of spine
        granulomatous, II:1–116 to II:1–118, **II:1–119i**
        pyogenic, II:1–112 to II:1–114, **II:1–115i**
    otitis, necrotizing external, II:1–80 to II:1–82, **II:1–83i**
    otitis media, complicated, II:1–84 to II:1–86, **II:1–87i**
    parotitis, acute, II:1–104 to II:1–106, **II:1–107i**
    retropharyngeal space abscess, II:1–108 to II:1–110, **II:1–111i**
    rhinosinusitis, acute, II:1–96 to II:1–98, **II:1–99i**
    saccular aneurysm, II:1–8 to II:1–10, **II:1–11i**
    spinal cord infarction, II:1–124 to II:1–125
    subarachnoid hemorrhage
        aneurysmal, II:1–4 to II:1–5
        nonaneurysmal perimesencephalic, II:1–6 to II:1–7
    subperiosteal abscess of orbit, II:1–92 to II:1–94, **II:1–95i**
Central nervous system trauma, I:1–2 to I:1–113.
    See also Brain injury; Head and neck injury; Spinal *terms*
    imaging issues, I:1–2 to I:1–3
Cephaloceles, **I:1–50i**, I:1–51
Cerebral abscess, II:1–48 to II:1–50, **II:1–51i**
    differential diagnosis, **II:1–48i**, II:1–49
Cerebral contusion, I:1–20 to I:1–22, **I:1–23i**
    cerebral ischemia-infarction vs., **II:1–32i**, II:1–34
    differential diagnosis, **I:1–20i**, I:1–21
Cerebral edema, diffuse, II:1–34
Cerebral ischemia-infarction
    acute, II:1–32 to II:1–34, **II:1–35i**
        differential diagnosis, **II:1–32i**, II:1–33 to II:1–34
        hypertensive encephalopathy vs., **II:1–28i**, II:1–29
        neonatal, vs. meningitis, **II:1–40i**, II:1–41
    hemorrhagic
        cerebral contusion vs., **I:1–20i**, I:1–21
        traumatic subarachnoid hemorrhage vs., I:1–17
    herpes encephalitis vs., **II:1–56i**, II:1–57
    inborn errors of metabolism vs., II:1–73
    subacute, II:1–49
Cerebral palsy, **I:4–150i**, I:4–151

INDEX

Cerebral venous thrombosis. *See* Sinus thrombosis, dural
Cerebritis
    cerebral contusion vs., I:1–21
    cerebral ischemia-infarction vs., II:1–34
Cerebrospinal fluid leak, **I:1–50i**, I:1–50 to I:1–51
Chance fracture, I:1–98 to I:1–100, **I:1–101i**
    compression fracture vs., **I:1–88i**, I:1–89
    differential diagnosis, **I:1–98i**, I:1–99
Charcot
    of hip, I:4–44, **II:4–42i**
    neuropathic, II:4–42 to I:4–44, **II:4–45i**
        diabetes complications vs., I:4–20, **II:4–18i**
        differential diagnosis, I:4–44, **II:4–42i**
        osteomyelitis vs., I:4–8, **II:4–6i**
    of spine, I:4–44, **II:4–42i**
Chauffeur fracture, **I:4–74i**, I:4–75
Chemical shift artifacts, I:1–9
Chest, non-traumatic, II:2–2 to II:2–139
    acute chest syndrome, II:2–76 to II:2–78, **II:2–79i**
    aortic dissection, II:2–128 to II:2–130, **II:2–131i**
    aspiration, II:2–108 to II:2–110, **II:2–111i**
    asthma, II:2–100 to II:2–102, **II:2–103i**
    bronchial foreign body, pediatric, II:2–116 to II:2–118, **II:2–119i**
    chronic obstructive pulmonary disease, II:2–96 to II:2–98, **II:2–99i**
    croup, II:2–52 to II:2–54, **II:2–55i**
    diffuse alveolar hemorrhage, II:2–68 to II:2–70, **II:2–71i**
    drug abuse, pulmonary, II:2–88 to II:2–90, **II:2–91i**
    epiglottitis, II:2–56 to II:2–58, **II:2–59i**
    hypersensitivity pneumonitis, II:2–104 to II:2–106, **II:2–107i**
    imaging issues, II:2–2 to II:2–3
    lung abscess, II:2–32 to II:2–34, **II:2–35i**
    meconium aspiration syndrome, II:2–112 to II:2–114, **II:2–115i**
    pericardial tamponade, II:2–136 to II:2–138, **II:2–139i**
    pneumonia
        acute interstitial, II:2–84 to II:2–86, **II:2–87i**
        community acquired, II:2–24 to II:2–26, **II:2–27i**
        eosinophilic, II:2–80 to II:2–82, **II:2–83i**
        immunocompromised, II:2–28 to II:2–30, **II:2–31i**
        neonatal, II:2–44 to II:2–46, **II:2–47i**
        round pneumonia, pediatric, II:2–40 to II:2–42, **II:2–43i**
    pulmonary edema
        cardiogenic, II:2–4 to II:2–6, **II:2–7i**
        mitral regurgitation, II:2–8 to II:2–10, **II:2–11i**
        noncardiac, II:2–12 to II:2–14, **II:2–15i**
    pulmonary embolism, II:2–120 to II:2–122, **II:2–123i**
    pulmonary interstitial emphysema, pediatric, II:2–64 to II:2–66, **II:2–67i**
    septic emboli, pulmonary, II:2–124 to II:2–126, **II:2–127i**
    sickle cell disease, II:2–76 to II:2–78, **II:2–79i**
    silo-filler's disease, II:2–20 to II:2–22, **II:2–23i**
    smoke inhalation, II:2–16 to II:2–18, **II:2–19i**
    superior vena cava syndrome, II:2–132 to II:2–134, **II:2–135i**
    talcosis, pulmonary, II:2–92 to II:2–94, **II:2–95i**
    tracheitis, exudative, II:2–48 to II:2–50, **II:2–51i**
    transient tachypnea of newborn, II:2–60 to II:2–62, **II:2–63i**
    vasculitis, pulmonary, II:2–72 to II:2–74, **II:2–75i**
    viral lung infection, pediatric, II:2–36 to II:2–38, **II:2–39i**
Chest trauma, I:2–2 to I:2–47
    aortic transection, I:2–18 to I:2–20, **I:2–21i**
    diaphragmatic tear, I:2–28 to I:2–30, **I:2–31i**
    drug abuse vs., II:2–90
    esophageal tear, I:2–32 to I:2–34, **I:2–35i**
    imaging issues, I:2–2 to I:2–3
    lung contusion, I:2–36 to I:2–38, **I:2–39i**
    pneumomediastinum, I:2–4 to I:2–6, **I:2–7i**
    pneumothorax, I:2–8 to I:2–10, **I:2–11i**
    pulmonary edema
        negative pressure, I:2–44 to I:2–46, **I:2–47i**
        neurogenic, I:2–40 to I:2–42, **I:2–43i**
    rib fractures and flail chest, I:2–14 to I:2–16, **I:2–17i**
    spinal fracture, thoracic, I:2–22 to I:2–24, **I:2–25i**
    sternal fracture, I:2–26 to I:2–27
    tracheobronchial tear, I:2–12 to I:2–13
Chiari I malformation, **I:1–32i**, I:1–34
Child abuse
    brain injury, traumatic, I:1–28 to I:1–30, **I:1–31i**
        differential diagnosis, **I:1–28i**, I:1–29 to I:1–30
    inborn errors of metabolism vs., **II:1–72i**, II:1–73
    metaphyseal fracture, I:4–190 to I:4–192, **I:4–193i**
        differential diagnosis, **I:4–190i**, I:4–191 to I:4–192
    neonatal meningitis vs., **II:1–40i**, II:1–41
    toddler's fracture vs., I:4–204
Children. *See also* Pediatric trauma
    bronchial foreign body, II:2–116 to II:2–118, **II:2–119i**
    croup, II:2–52 to II:2–54, **II:2–55i**
    meconium aspiration syndrome, II:2–112 to II:2–114, **II:2–115i**

INDEX

meconium ileus, II:3–198 to II:3–200, **II:3–201i**
meconium peritonitis, II:3–202 to II:3–204, **II:3–205i**
meconium plug syndrome, II:3–194 to II:3–196, **II:3–197i**
meconium pseudocyst vs. Meckel diverticulum, **II:3–222i**, II:3–223
meningitis, neonatal, II:1–40 to II:1–42, **II:1–43i**
osteomyelitis, II:4–10 to I:4–12, **II:4–12i**
pneumonia, neonatal, II:2–44 to II:2–46, **II:2–47i**
pulmonary interstitial emphysema, II:2–64 to II:2–66, **II:2–67i**
round pneumonia, II:2–40 to II:2–42, **II:2–43i**
tracheitis, exudative, II:2–48 to II:2–50, **II:2–51i**
transient tachypnea of newborn, II:2–60 to II:2–62, **II:2–63i**
viral lung infection, II:2–36 to II:2–38, **II:2–39i**
Cholangiocarcinoma
    choledocholithiasis vs., **II:3–144i**, II:3–145
    recurrent pyogenic cholangitis vs., **II:3–140i**, II:3–141
Cholangitis
    AIDS-related, **II:3–138i**, II:3–139
    ascending (bacterial), **II:3–138i**, II:3–138 to II:3–139
    chemotherapy-related, **II:3–138i**, II:3–139
    primary sclerosing
        ascending cholangitis vs., **II:3–138i**, II:3–139
        Budd-Chiari syndrome vs., **II:3–134i**, II:3–136
        choledocholithiasis vs., II:3–145
        recurrent pyogenic cholangitis vs., **II:3–140i**, II:3–141
    recurrent pyogenic, II:3–140 to II:3–142, **II:3–143i**
        ascending cholangitis vs., II:3–139
        differential diagnosis, **II:3–140i**, II:3–141
Cholecystitis, II:3–148 to II:3–150, **II:3–151i**
    differential diagnosis, **II:3–148i**, II:3–149
Choledochocele, II:3–211
Choledocholithiasis, II:3–144 to II:3–146, **II:3–147i**
    differential diagnosis, **II:3–144i**, II:3–145
Cholesteatoma
    complicated otitis media vs., II:1–85
    necrotizing external otitis vs., **II:1–80i**, II:1–81
Chondrodysplasia, metaphyseal, I:4–192
Chondroma, I:4–39, **II:4–38i**
Chondromatosis. See Osteochondromatosis
Chondronecrosis, radiation-induced, I:1–53
Chondrosarcoma
    neuropathic Charcot vs., I:4–44
    pyrophosphate arthropathy vs., II:4–28
    synovial, I:4–39
Choroid plexus papilloma, II:1–70

Chronic obstructive pulmonary disease (COPD), II:2–96 to II:2–98, **II:2–99i**
    differential diagnosis, **II:2–96i**, II:2–97
    pneumatosis of intestine vs., II:3–39
Churg-Strauss vasculitis, II:2–101
Clavicle fracture, **I:4–40i**, I:4–40 to I:4–41
    acromioclavicular dislocation vs., **I:4–42i**
Clay shoveler fracture, **I:1–76i**, I:1–77
Cleft, congenital, I:1–77
Closed loop obstruction. See Small bowel obstruction
Coagulopathies
    HELLP syndrome vs., I:3–123
    hepatic trauma vs., I:3–9
    hypertensive intracranial hemorrhage vs., II:1–25
    intestinal trauma vs., **I:3–22i**, I:3–24
    nonaccidental brain injury vs., **I:1–28i**, I:1–29
Colitis
    granulomatous. See Crohn disease
    infectious, II:3–60 to II:3–62, **II:3–63i**
        differential diagnosis, **II:3–60i**, II:3–61
        pseudomembranous colitis vs., **II:3–64i**, II:3–65
    ischemic, II:3–92 to II:3–94, **II:3–95i**
        differential diagnosis, **II:3–92i**, II:3–93 to II:3–94
        diverticulitis vs., **II:3–80i**, II:3–81
        infectious colitis vs., **II:3–60i**, II:3–61
        pseudomembranous colitis vs., **II:3–64i**, II:3–65
        ulcerative colitis vs., **II:3–70i**, II:3–71
    pseudomembranous, II:3–64 to II:3–66, **II:3–67i**
        differential diagnosis, **II:3–64i**, II:3–65
        diverticulitis vs., **II:3–80i**, II:3–81
        epiploic appendagitis vs., II:3–85
        infectious colitis vs., II:3–61
        ischemic colitis vs., **II:3–92i**, II:3–93
        mesenteric adenitis vs., **II:3–226i**, II:3–227
        typhlitis vs., **II:3–68i**, II:3–69
        ulcerative colitis vs., **II:3–70i**, II:3–71
    radiation-induced, **II:3–80i**, II:3–81
    ulcerative, II:3–70 to II:3–72, **II:3–73i**
        Crohn disease vs., **II:3–34i**, II:3–35
        differential diagnosis, **II:3–70i**, II:3–71
        epiploic appendagitis vs., **II:3–84i**, II:3–85
        infectious colitis vs., **II:3–60i**, II:3–61
        ischemic colitis vs., **II:3–92i**, II:3–93 to II:3–94
        mesenteric adenitis vs., II:3–227
        pseudomembranous colitis vs., **II:3–64i**, II:3–65
Collateral ligament injury, medial, I:4–211
Colles fracture
    die punch fracture vs., I:4–80

INDEX

differential diagnosis, I:4–74i
Colloid cyst
    hydrocephalus vs., **II:1–68i**, II:1–69
    intracerebral hematoma vs., **II:1–16i**, II:1–18
Colon. *See also* Colitis
    atresia, II:3–195
    cathartic, II:3–71
    immature
        meconium ileus vs., **II:3–198i**, II:3–199
        necrotizing enterocolitis vs., II:3–207
    megacolon
        functional, II:3–97
        toxic, **II:3–74i**, II:3–74 to II:3–75
            cecal volvulus vs., **II:3–100i**, II:3–101
            sigmoid volvulus vs., **II:3–96i**, II:3–97
    obstruction
        distal
            cecal volvulus vs., **II:3–100i**
            sigmoid volvulus vs., II:3–97
        small bowel obstruction vs., **II:3–50i**, II:3–52
        toxic megacolon vs., II:3–74
    sigmoid, normal position, II:3–219
Companion shadow, **I:2–8i**, I:2–9
Compartment syndrome, I:4–22 to I:4–24, **I:4–25i**
    differential diagnosis, **I:4–22i**, I:4–23
Compression fractures, spinal, I:1–88 to I:1–90, **I:1–91i**
    burst thoracolumbar fracture vs., **I:1–92i**, I:1–93
    chance fracture vs., **I:1–98i**, I:1–99
    differential diagnosis, **I:1–88i**, I:1–89
    facet-lamina thoracolumbar fracture vs., **I:1–94i**, I:1–95
Condylar fracture, **I:4–198i**, I:4–199
Congenital indifference to pain
    metaphyseal fracture vs., I:4–192
    neuropathic Charcot vs., **II:4–42i**
Congestive heart failure. *See* Pulmonary edema
Connective tissue disease, II:2–86
Cornual ectopic pregnancy, **II:3–254i**, II:3–255
Corpus luteal cyst, II:3–255
Cortical venous thrombosis
    hypertensive intracranial hemorrhage vs., II:1–26
    spontaneous intracranial hemorrhage vs., **II:1–20i**, II:1–21
Craniopharyngioma, II:1–18
Cricoid necrosis, **I:1–52i**, I:1–53
Crohn disease, II:3–34 to II:3–36, **II:3–37i**
    acute small bowel ischemia vs., **II:3–42i**, II:3–43
    differential diagnosis, **II:3–34i**, II:3–35 to II:3–36
    duodenal ulcer vs., II:3–29
    hypoperfusion complex vs., I:3–30
    infectious colitis vs., II:3–61
    ischemic colitis vs., **II:3–92i**, II:3–93 to II:3–94
    mesenteric adenitis vs., II:3–227

    pseudomembranous colitis vs., II:3–65
Croup, II:2–52 to II:2–54, **II:2–55i**
    differential diagnosis, **II:2–52i**, II:2–53
    epiglottitis vs., **II:2–56i**, II:2–57
    exudative tracheitis vs., **II:2–48i**, II:2–49
Cryptosporidiosis, II:3–35
Cuboid fractures
    metatarsal fracture vs., I:4–183
    navicular fracture vs., I:4–175
Cuneiform fractures, I:4–183
Cystadenocarcinoma, biliary
    hepatic amebic abscess vs., II:3–119
    hepatic pyogenic abscess vs., **II:3–114i**, II:3–116
Cystic adenomatoid malformation, congenital (CCAM)
    meconium aspiration syndrome vs., II:2–113
    neonatal pneumonia vs., II:2–45
    pulmonary interstitial emphysema vs., **II:2–64i**, II:2–65
    round pneumonia vs., **II:2–40i**, II:2–41
    transient tachypnea of newborn vs., II:2–61
    viral lung infection vs., **II:2–36i**, II:2–37
Cystic fibrosis
    meconium peritonitis vs., II:3–203
    small bowel intussusception in children vs., II:3–232
    small bowel obstruction vs., **II:3–50i**, II:3–52
Cysts
    bone, **I:4–14i**
    bronchogenic
        bronchial foreign body vs., II:2–118
        round pneumonia vs., **II:2–40i**, II:2–41
    colloid
        hydrocephalus vs., **II:1–68i**, II:1–69
        intracerebral hematoma vs., **II:1–16i**, II:1–18
    corpus luteal, II:3–255
    dermoid. *See* Dermoid cyst
    duplication
        duodenal atresia or stenosis vs., II:3–191
        small bowel intussusception in children vs., II:3–231
    hydatid
        amebic abscess vs., **II:3–118i**, II:3–119
        hepatic, vs. pyogenic abscess, II:3–116
    mucus retention, **II:1–96i**, II:1–97
    paratracheal air, **I:2–4i**, I:2–6
    Rathke cleft, II:1–18
    renal, **II:3–160i**, II:3–161
    splenic
        splenic infarction vs., II:3–107
        trauma vs., **I:3–4i**, I:3–5
Cytomegalovirus infection
    Crohn disease vs., II:3–35
    meconium peritonitis vs., II:3–203

INDEX

D

Dacryocystocele, II:1–93
Deep vein thrombosis
    compartment syndrome vs., I:4–23
    necrotizing fasciitis vs., **I:4–26i**, I:4–27
Degenerative disc disease
    granulomatous osteomyelitis vs., **II:1–116i**, II:1–117
    pyogenic osteomyelitis vs., **II:1–112i**, II:1–113
    traumatic disc herniation vs., **I:1–106i**, I:1–107
Degenerative diseases, **I:1–110i**, I:1–111
Demyelinating disease, **II:1–48i**, II:1–49
Denervation hypertrophy, **I:4–22i**, I:4–23
Dens fracture, I:1–66 to I:1–68, **I:1–69i**
    differential diagnosis, **I:1–66i**, I:1–67
Dermatomyositis, **I:4–26i**, I:4–27
Dermoid cyst
    intracerebral hematoma vs., **II:1–16i**, II:1–17
    ovarian hemorrhage vs., II:3–247
    pelvic inflammatory disease, **II:3–250i**, II:3–251
    subperiosteal abscess of orbit vs., II:1–93
Diabetes
    muscle infarction vs. compartment syndrome in, I:4–23
    musculoskeletal complications, II:4–18 to I:4–20, **II:4–21i**
        differential diagnosis, I:4–20, **II:4–18i**
Diabetic foot, I:4–8, **II:4–6i**
Diaphragm
    eventration vs. tear, **I:2–28i**, I:2–29
    paralysis vs. tear, **I:2–28i**, I:2–29
    rupture. *See* Diaphragmatic tear
Diaphragmatic hernia
    gastric volvulus vs., **II:3–214i**, II:3–215
    pulmonary interstitial emphysema vs., II:2–65
    transient tachypnea of newborn vs., II:2–61
Diaphragmatic tear, I:2–28 to I:2–30, **I:2–31i**
    differential diagnosis, **I:2–28i**, I:2–29 to I:2–30
    esophageal tear vs., **I:2–32i**, I:2–33
Die punch fracture, distal radius, **I:4–80i**, I:4–80 to I:4–81
Differential unilateral acute consolidation, I:2–45 to I:2–46
Diffuse alveolar hemorrhage, II:2–68 to II:2–70, **II:2–71i**
    acute interstitial pneumonia vs., **II:2–84i**, II:2–85
    community acquired pneumonia vs., **II:2–24i**, II:2–25
    differential diagnosis, **II:2–68i**, II:2–69
    eosinophilic pneumonia vs., II:2–82
    immunocompromised pneumonia vs., **II:2–28i**, II:2–29
    noncardiac pulmonary edema vs., **II:2–12i**, II:2–14

Diffuse axonal injury, I:1–24 to I:1–26, **I:1–27i**
    differential diagnosis, **I:1–24i**, I:1–25
Diploic space hyperplasia, **II:4–70i**, II:4–71
Disc herniation
    nontraumatic, I:1–107
    traumatic, I:1–106 to I:1–108, **I:1–109i**
        differential diagnosis, **I:1–106i**, I:1–107
Discitis, AIDS-related, **II:4–74i**
Distraction injury, I:1–99
Diverticulitis, II:3–80 to II:3–82, **II:3–83i**
    cecal
        appendicitis vs., **II:3–76i**, II:3–77
        typhlitis vs., **II:3–68i**, II:3–69
    differential diagnosis, **II:3–80i**, II:3–81
    epiploic appendagitis vs., **II:3–84i**, II:3–85
    hepatic flexure, vs. cholecystitis, **II:3–148i**, II:3–149
    ischemic colitis vs., **II:3–92i**, II:3–93
    sigmoid, **II:3–70i**, II:3–71
    small bowel intussusception in children vs., II:3–231
Dolichoectasia, atherosclerotic, **II:1–12i**
Dorsal hood injury, I:4–104
Dorsal ligament sprain, I:4–175
Down syndrome, **I:1–60i**, I:1–61
Drug abuse, II:1–64 to II:1–66, **II:1–67i**, II:2–88 to II:2–90, **II:2–91i**
    chronic obstructive pulmonary disease vs., **II:2–96i**
    differential diagnosis, **II:1–64i**, II:1–65, **II:2–88i**, II:2–90
    hypertensive intracranial hemorrhage vs., **II:1–24i**, II:1–25
    IV drugs vs. pulmonary edema, I:2–45
    spontaneous intracranial hemorrhage vs., **II:1–20i**, II:1–22
Drug toxicity
    amiodarone, vs. talcosis, II:2–94
    eosinophilic pneumonia vs., **II:2–80i**, II:2–81
    immunocompromised pneumonia vs., II:2–29
Ductus diverticulum, I:2–19
Duodenal atresia or stenosis, II:3–190 to II:3–192, **II:3–193i**
    differential diagnosis, **II:3–190i**, II:3–191
    duodenal ulcer vs., II:3–29
    hypertrophic pyloric stenosis vs., II:3–211
    midgut volvulus vs., **II:3–186i**, II:3–188
Duodenal diverticulum, II:3–29
Duodenal rupture, **I:3–16i**, I:3–17
Duodenal trauma/hematoma, **I:3–20i**, I:3–20 to I:3–21
    pancreatic trauma vs., **I:3–16i**, I:3–17
Duodenal ulcer, II:3–28 to II:3–30, **II:3–31i**
    cholecystitis vs., II:3–149
    differential diagnosis, **II:3–28i**, II:3–29 to II:3–30

INDEX

Silo-filler's disease, II:2–20 to II:2–22, **II:2–23i**
    differential diagnosis, **II:2–20i**, II:2–21 to II:2–22
Sinding-Larsen-Johansson disease, I:4–151
Sinus thrombosis
    cavernous, **II:1–100i**, II:1–101
    dural, II:1–36 to II:1–38, **II:1–39i**
        cerebral ischemia-infarction vs., II:1–34
        differential diagnosis, **II:1–36i**, II:1–37
        hypertensive intracranial hemorrhage vs., II:1–26
        nonaccidental brain injury vs., **I:1–28i**, I:1–29
        with hemorrhagic infarct, vs. drug abuse, II:1–65
    transverse
        drug abuse vs., **II:1–64i**, II:1–65
        paratentorial subdural hematoma vs., **I:1–14i**, I:1–15
    venous, **I:1–20i**, I:1–21
Sjögren syndrome, **II:1–104i**, II:1–105
Skin fold
    pneumomediastinum vs., I:2–6
    pneumothorax vs., I:2–9
SLE (systemic lupus erythematosus). *See* Systemic lupus erythematosus (SLE)
Small bowel ischemia, acute, II:3–42 to II:3–44, **II:3–45i**
    Crohn disease vs., II:3–36
    differential diagnosis, **II:3–42i**, II:3–43
Small bowel obstruction, II:3–50 to II:3–52, **II:3–53i**
    differential diagnosis, **II:3–50i**, II:3–51 to II:3–52
    paraduodenal hernia vs., **II:3–20i**, II:3–21
    transmesenteric postoperative hernia vs., **II:3–24i**, II:3–25
    vasculitis vs., **II:3–46i**, II:3–47
Smash fractures, **I:1–56i**, I:1–57
Smith fracture, I:4–75
Smoke inhalation, II:2–16 to II:2–18, **II:2–19i**
    differential diagnosis, **II:2–16i**, II:2–17
    drug abuse vs., II:2–90
    mitral regurgitation pulmonary edema vs., **II:2–8i**, II:2–9
    pulmonary edema vs., **I:2–40i**, I:2–41, **I:2–44i**, I:2–45
    silo-filler's disease vs., **II:2–20i**, II:2–21
Soft tissue abscess, **II:4–4i**, II:4–4 to I:4–5
    diabetes complications vs. I:4–20
Spinal abscess, I:2–24
Spinal cord infarction, **II:1–124i**, II:1–124 to II:1–125
Spinal cord injury, I:1–110 to I:1–112, **I:1–113i**
    differential diagnosis, **I:1–110i**, I:1–111
    neuropathic arthropathy vs. pyogenic osteomyelitis, II:1–113
Spinal trauma, I:1–60 to I:1–113
    atlanto-occipital dislocation, I:1–60 to I:1–61
    cervical
        hyperextension injury, I:1–76 to I:1–78, **I:1–79i**
        hyperflexion injury, I:1–74 to I:1–75
        hyperflexion-rotation injury, I:1–80 to I:1–82, **I:1–83i**
        lateral flexion injury, I:1–84 to I:1–85
        posterior column injury, I:1–86 to I:1–87
    chance fracture, I:1–98 to I:1–100, **I:1–101i**
    compression fractures, I:1–88 to I:1–90, **I:1–91i**
    disc herniation, traumatic, I:1–106 to I:1–108, **I:1–109i**
    hangman's C2 fracture, I:1–70 to I:1–72, **I:1–73i**
    imaging issues, I:1–3
    Jefferson C1 fracture, I:1–62 to I:1–64, **I:1–65i**
    odontoid C2 fractures, I:1–66 to I:1–68, **I:1–69i**
    sacral traumatic fracture, I:1–102 to I:1–104, **I:1–105i**
    spinal cord injury, I:1–110 to I:1–112, **I:1–113i**
    thoracic fracture, **I:2–22i**, I:2–22 to I:2–24, **I:2–25i**
    thoracolumbar fracture
        burst, I:1–92 to I:1–93
        facet-lamina, I:1–94 to I:1–96, **I:1–97i**
Splenic cysts
    splenic infarction vs., II:3–107
    trauma vs., **I:3–4i**, I:3–5
Splenic infarction, II:3–106 to II:3–108, **II:3–109i**
    differential diagnosis, **II:3–106i**, II:3–107
    splenic infection vs., **II:3–102i**, II:3–103
    trauma vs., **I:3–4i**, I:3–5
Splenic infection and abscess, II:3–102 to II:3–104, **II:3–105i**
    differential diagnosis, **II:3–102i**, II:3–103
    splenic infarction vs., **II:3–106i**, II:3–107
    trauma vs., I:3–5
Splenic trauma, I:3–4 to I:3–6, **I:3–7i**
    differential diagnosis, **I:3–4i**, I:3–5
    infection vs., **II:3–102i**, II:3–103
    laceration vs. splenic infarction, **II:3–106i**, II:3–107
Spondylitis, fungal, II:1–117

INDEX

Respiratory tract infections, **II:2–116i**, II:2–118
Retained products of conception, **II:3–234i**, II:3–235
Retroperitoneal fibrosis, **II:3–32i**
Retropharyngeal space
    abscess, II:1–108 to II:1–110, **II:1–111i**
        croup vs., II:2–53
        differential diagnosis, **II:1–108i**, II:1–109
        epiglottitis vs., **II:2–56i**, II:2–57
        exudative tracheitis vs., **II:2–48i**, II:2–49
    adenitis, **II:1–108i**, II:1–109
    effusion or edema, **II:1–108i**, II:1–109
    hematoma, **II:1–108i**, II:1–109
    suppurative node, **II:1–108i**, II:1–109
Reverse Barton fracture, I:4–75
Rhabdomyolysis, I:4–23
Rhabdomyosarcoma
    complicated otitis media vs., **II:1–84i**, II:1–85
    subperiosteal abscess of orbit vs., II:1–93
Rheumatoid arthritis
    carpal instabilities vs., I:4–96
    flexor annular pulley tear vs., I:4–107
    juvenile, vs. toddler's fracture, I:4–204
    odontoid C2 fracture vs., **I:1–66i**, I:1–67
Rhinorrhea, I:1–51
Rhinosinusitis, acute, II:1–96 to II:1–98, **II:1–99i**
    differential diagnosis, **II:1–96i**, II:1–97
    invasive fungal sinusitis vs., II:1–101
Rib fractures, multiple, I:2–14 to I:2–16, **I:2–17i**
    differential diagnosis, **I:2–14i**, I:2–15
Rib neoplasms, **I:2–14i**, I:2–15
Rickets
    incomplete fracture vs., I:4–196
    metaphyseal fracture vs., I:4–192
    nonaccidental brain injury vs., I:1–29
Rotary extension fracture, **I:1–80i**, I:1–81
Rotational fracture-subluxation, **I:1–76i**, I:1–77
Round pneumonia, II:2–40 to II:2–42, **II:2–43i**
    differential diagnosis, **II:2–40i**, II:2–41

S

Saccular aneurysm, II:1–8 to II:1–10, **II:1–11i**
    blood blister-like aneurysm vs., **II:1–14i**
    differential diagnosis, **II:1–8i**, II:1–9
Sacral fractures
    insufficiency, I:4–4 to I:4–6, **I:4–7i**
        differential diagnosis, **I:4–4i**, I:4–5
    traumatic, I:1–102 to I:1–104, **I:1–105i**
        differential diagnosis, **I:1–102i**, I:1–103
Sacroiliac joint disruption/dislocation, I:1–103
Sacroiliitis, I:4–5
Salter fractures. *See* Physeal fractures
Sarcoid, II:3–103
Sarcoidosis
    asthma vs., II:2–101
    hypersensitivity pneumonitis vs., **II:2–104i**, II:2–106
    orbital inflammatory disease vs., **II:1–88i**, II:1–89
    subdural hematoma vs., **I:1–8i**
    talcosis vs., **II:2–92i**, II:2–93
Scaphoid fractures, I:4–82 to I:4–84, **I:4–85i**
    differential diagnosis, **I:4–82i**, I:4–83
    osteonecrosis of wrist vs., II:4–52
Scaphoid nonunion, **I:4–82i**
Scapula
    fractures, **I:4–44i**, I:4–45
    pneumothorax vs., I:2–9
Scapular trauma, I:4–44 to I:4–46, **I:4–47i**
    differential diagnosis, **I:4–44i**, I:4–45
Scar, vs. hematoma, I:4–29
Scheuermann kyphosis
    burst thoracolumbar fracture vs., **I:1–92i**, I:1–93
    compression fracture vs., I:1–89
Scleroderma, II:3–171
Sclerosis, I:4–107
Scrotum, acute. *See* Epididymo-orchitis
Seat-belt fracture. *See* Chance fracture
Septic emboli, pulmonary. *See* Pulmonary embolism, septic
Septic joint, II:4–14 to I:4–16, **II:4–17i**
    bone marrow edema vs., I:4–47, **II:4–46i**
    diabetes complications vs., I:4–20
    differential diagnosis, I:4–16, **II:4–14i**
    facet-lamina thoracolumbar fracture vs., I:1–95
    neuropathic Charcot vs., I:4–44
    pyrophosphate arthropathy vs., II:4–27
    toddler's fractures vs., I:4–204
Shear injury, I:1–99
Shin splints, I:4–207
Shock abdomen. *See* Hypoperfusion complex
Shock bowel. *See* Hypoperfusion complex
Shock pancreas
    acute pancreatitis vs., II:3–153
    pancreatic trauma vs., I:3–17
Shoulder dislocation, I:4–48 to I:4–50, **I:4–51i**
    differential diagnosis, **I:4–48i**, I:4–49
Sialosis, II:1–105
Sickle cell disease, II:2–76 to II:2–78, **II:2–79i**
    bone marrow edema vs., **II:4–46i**
    differential diagnosis, **II:2–76i**, II:2–77
    musculoskeletal complications, II:4–70 to I:4–72, **II:4–73i**
        differential diagnosis, **II:4–70i**, II:4–71 to I:4–72
    osteonecrosis of hip vs., **II:4–48i**
Sickle cell trait, vs. anemia, II:4–72
Silent sinus syndrome, **II:1–96i**, II:1–97
Silicosis
    hypersensitivity pneumonitis vs., II:2–106
    talcosis vs., **II:2–92i**, II:2–93

INDEX

noncardiac, II:2–12 to II:2–14, **II:2–15i**
   differential diagnosis, **II:2–12i**, II:2–14
   diffuse alveolar hemorrhage vs., **II:2–68i**, II:2–69
   immunocompromised pneumonia vs., II:2–29
   re-expansion vs. mitral regurgitation, II:2–10
   unilateral, II:2–10
Pulmonary embolism, II:2–120 to II:2–122, **II:2–123i**
   aspiration vs., II:2–109
   asthma vs., **II:2–100i**, II:2–101
   chronic, vs. vasculitis, II:2–73
   differential diagnosis, **II:2–120i**, II:2–122
   septic, II:2–124 to II:2–126, **II:2–127i**
      differential diagnosis, **II:2–124i**, II:2–125 to II:2–126
      lung abscess vs., II:2–33
Pulmonary fibrosis
   accelerated idiopathic, II:2–85
   hypersensitivity pneumonitis vs., II:2–105
Pulmonary hemorrhage, **II:2–76i**. *See also* Diffuse alveolar hemorrhage
Pulmonary hypertension, **II:2–100i**, II:2–101
Pulmonary infarction
   community acquired pneumonia vs., II:2–27
   septic pulmonary emboli vs., II:2–125
   vasculitis vs., **II:2–72i**
Pulmonary interstitial emphysema, pediatric, II:2–64 to II:2–66, **II:2–67i**
   differential diagnosis, **II:2–64i**, II:2–65
Pulmonary opacities, migratory, II:2–82
Pulmonary sequestration
   lung abscess vs., II:2–33
   round pneumonia vs., II:2–41
   viral lung infection vs., II:2–37
Pulmonary sling, II:2–118
Pulmonary vein, anomalous left, **II:2–132i**, II:2–133
Pyelitis, emphysematous, **II:3–168i**
Pyelonephritis, II:3–156 to II:3–158, **II:3–159i**
   differential diagnosis, **II:3–156i**, II:3–157
   emphysematous, II:3–168 to II:3–169
      differential diagnosis, **II:3–168i**
   renal infarction vs., **II:3–170i**, II:3–171
   renal vein thrombosis vs., **II:3–174i**, II:3–175
   xanthogranulomatous, II:3–164 to II:3–166, **II:3–167i**
      differential diagnosis, **II:3–164i**, II:3–165
Pyloric stenosis, hypertrophic, **II:3–210i**, II:3–211
Pylorospasm, II:3–211
Pyogenic abscess
   cerebral, **II:1–60i**, III:1–62
   hepatic, II:3–114 to II:3–116, **II:3–117i**
      amebic abscess vs., **II:3–118i**, II:3–119
      differential diagnosis, **II:3–114i**, II:3–115 to II:3–116
Pyomyositis, I:4–20
Pyonephrosis, II:3–165
Pyrophosphate arthropathy, II:4–26 to I:4–28, **II:4–29i**
   carpal instabilities vs., I:4–96
   differential diagnosis, **II:4–26i**, II:4–27 to I:4–28

Q

Quadriceps muscle tear, **I:4–146i**, I:4–147

R

Radial head/neck fracture, I:4–68 to I:4–70, **I:4–71i**
   differential diagnosis, **I:4–68i**, I:4–69
   elbow dislocation vs., I:4–61
   humeral shaft/distal humeral fracture vs., I:4–57
Radial metaphysis osteolysis, I:4–77
Radiation enteritis, II:3–36
Radiation necrosis, **II:4–48i**
Radiation pneumonitis
   eosinophilic pneumonia vs., **II:2–80i**
   immunocompromised pneumonia vs., **II:2–28i**, II:2–29
Radiation therapy, vs. diffuse axonal injury, I:1–25
Radius
   die punch fracture, **I:4–80i**, I:4–80 to I:4–81
   distal, fractures of, **I:4–76i**, I:4–76 to I:4–78, **I:4–79i**
   posterior dislocation, I:4–199
Rathke cleft cyst, II:1–18
Renal abscess, II:3–160 to II:3–162, **II:3–163i**
   differential diagnosis, **II:3–160i**, II:3–161
   xanthogranulomatous pyelonephritis vs., **II:3–164i**, II:3–165
Renal cell carcinoma
   abscess vs., **II:3–160i**, II:3–161
   pyelonephritis vs., II:3–157
   renal vein thrombosis vs., **II:3–174i**, II:3–175
   trauma vs., I:3–13
   xanthogranulomatous pyelonephritis vs., **II:3–164i**, II:3–165
Renal cyst, **II:3–160i**, II:3–161
Renal infarction, II:3–170 to II:3–172, **II:3–173i**
   differential diagnosis, **II:3–170i**, II:3–171
   pyelonephritis vs., **II:3–156i**, II:3–157
Renal scarring, **II:3–156i**, II:3–157
Renal trauma, I:3–12 to I:3–14, **I:3–15i**
   differential diagnosis, **I:3–12i**, I:3–13
   infarction vs., **II:3–170i**, II:3–171
Renal tumors, **I:3–12i**, I:3–13
Renal vein thrombosis, II:3–174 to II:3–176, **II:3–177i**
   differential diagnosis, **II:3–174i**, II:3–175

INDEX

asthma vs., II:2–101
    renal infarction vs., II:3–171
    renal trauma vs., **I:3–12i**, I:3–13
Polychondritis, relapsing, **I:1–52i**, I:1–53
Polycythemia
    cerebral ischemia-infarction vs., II:1–33
    transient tachypnea of newborn vs., II:2–61
Polyps, antral, II:3–211
Portal vein
    extrinsic compression vs. occlusion, **II:3–130i**, II:3–132
    occlusion, II:3–130 to II:3–132, **II:3–133i**
        differential diagnosis, **II:3–130i**, II:3–131 to II:3–132
    preduodenal, vs. duodenal atresia or stenosis, II:3–191
Posterior column injury, cervical, **I:1–86i**, I:1–86 to I:1–87
Posterior communicating artery infundibulum, **II:1–15i**, II:1–16
Posterior reversible encephalopathy syndrome (PRES). *See* Hypertensive encephalopathy, acute
Postoperative complications and artifacts
    aorto-enteric fistula vs., **II:3–32i**
    carotid endarterectomy, II:1–29
    mixed subdural hematoma vs., I:1–13
    post-endoscopic bowel, **II:3–38i**, II:3–39
    postoperative bowel, II:3–39
    subdural hematoma vs., I:1–9
Pregnancy. *See also* Ectopic pregnancy
    didelphys intrauterine, **II:3–254i**, II:3–255
    eclampsia, I:1–17
Pronator muscle injury, I:4–211
Prosthesis infection, II:4–67
Proteinosis, alveolar
    acute interstitial pneumonia vs., II:2–86
    cardiogenic pulmonary edema vs., **II:2–4i**, II:2–6
Pseudo-subarachnoid hemorrhage
    aneurysmal subarachnoid hemorrhage vs., II:1–4
    traumatic subarachnoid hemorrhage vs., I:1–17
Pseudoaneurysm, **II:1–8i**, II:1–9
Pseudocollaterals, **II:2–132i**, II:2–133
Pseudomembranous colitis. *See* Colitis, pseudomembranous
Pseudomyxoma peritonei, **II:3–8i**, II:3–9
Pseudopathologic subcapital fracture, **I:4–14i**, I:4–15
Pseudopneumatosis, II:3–39
Pseudospread of atlas, **I:1–62i**, I:1–63
Pseudosubluxation, I:1–71
Pseudotumor
    of bone, vs. hemophilia, I:4–80
    invasive fungal sinusitis vs., **II:1–100i**, II:1–101
Pterygoid plate avulsion, I:1–57
Pubic ramus
    avulsion, **I:4–114i**, I:4–115
    fracture, **I:4–10i**
Pulmonary artery sarcoma, **II:2–120i**, II:2–122
Pulmonary calcification, metastatic, **II:2–92i**, II:2–93
Pulmonary edema
    cardiogenic, II:2–4 to II:2–6, **II:2–7i**
        acute interstitial pneumonia vs., **II:2–84i**
        aspiration vs., **II:2–108i**, II:2–109
        community acquired pneumonia vs., II:2–26
        differential diagnosis, **II:2–4i**, II:2–6
        diffuse alveolar hemorrhage vs., **II:2–68i**, II:2–69
        drug abuse vs., **II:2–88i**
        immunocompromised pneumonia vs., II:2–29
        negative pressure pulmonary edema vs., I:2–45
        neurogenic pulmonary edema vs., I:2–41
        noncardiac pulmonary edema vs., **II:2–12i**, II:2–14
        pulmonary vasculitis vs., II:2–73
        silo-filler's disease vs., II:2–21
        smoke inhalation vs., II:2–17
    high altitude
        mitral regurgitation vs., II:2–10
        neurogenic pulmonary edema vs., I:2–41
    hydrostatic
        acute interstitial pneumonia vs., II:2–85
        smoke inhalation vs., II:2–17
    mitral regurgitant, II:2–8 to II:2–10, **II:2–11i**
        community acquired pneumonia vs., **II:2–24i**
        differential diagnosis, **II:2–8i**, II:2–9 to II:2–10
        immunocompromised pneumonia vs., **II:2–28i**, II:2–29
        negative pressure pulmonary edema vs., I:2–45
        neurogenic pulmonary edema vs., I:2–41
        sickle cell disease vs., **II:2–76i**, II:2–77
        smoke inhalation vs., **II:2–16i**, II:2–17
    negative pressure, I:2–44 to I:2–46, **I:2–47i**
        differential diagnosis, **I:2–44i**, I:2–45 to I:2–46
        drug abuse vs., II:2–90
        mitral regurgitation vs., II:2–10
        neurogenic pulmonary edema vs., I:2–41
        smoke inhalation vs., **II:2–16i**, II:2–17
    neurogenic, I:2–40 to I:2–42, **I:2–43i**
        differential diagnosis, **I:2–40i**, I:2–41
        drug abuse vs., **II:2–88i**, II:2–90
        mitral regurgitation vs., **II:2–8i**, II:2–9
        negative pressure pulmonary edema vs., **I:2–44i**, I:2–45
        pulmonary vasculitis vs., **II:2–72i**
        smoke inhalation vs., **II:2–16i**, II:2–17

INDEX

partially stable, **I:4–18i**, I:4–119
ring vs. acetabular, I:4–127
stable, I:4–118 to I:4–120, **I:4–121i**
  differential diagnosis, **I:4–118i**, I:4–119
unstable, I:4–122 to I:4–124, **I:4–125i**
  differential diagnosis, **I:4–122i**
Pelvic inflammatory disease, II:3–250 to II:3–252, **II:3–253i**. *See also* Tubo-ovarian abscess
  appendicitis vs., II:3–77
  differential diagnosis, **II:3–250i**, II:3–251
  mesenteric adenitis vs., II:3–228
  ovarian torsion vs., II:3–239
  ovarian vein thrombosis vs., **II:3–242i**, II:3–243
Pelvic varicosities, II:3–235
Peptic ulcer. *See* Duodenal ulcer
Periaortitis, **II:3–32i**
Pericardial tamponade, II:2–136 to II:2–138, **II:2–139i**
  differential diagnosis, **II:2–136i**, II:2–137 to II:2–138
Pericarditis, constrictive, **II:2–136i**, II:2–137
Perimesencephalic venous hemorrhage, I:1–17
Peritonitis, II:3–8 to II:3–10, **II:3–11i**
  differential diagnosis, **II:3–8i**, II:3–9
Petromastoid canal, **I:1–46i**, I:1–47
Petrositis, apical, **II:1–84i**, II:1–85
Phrenic nerve paralysis, **I:2–28i**, I:2–29
Physeal fractures, I:4–186 to I:4–188, **I:4–189i**
  differential diagnosis, **I:4–186i**, I:4–187
  patellar tendon tears and tendinosis vs., **I:4–150i**, I:4–152
  sternoclavicular trauma vs., I:4–37
Pigmented villonodular synovitis, II:4–34 to I:4–36, **II:4–37i**
  differential diagnosis, **I:4–35**, **II:4–34i**
  gout vs., I:4–23, **II:4–22i**
  hematoma vs., I:4–29
  hemophilia vs., I:4–80
  synovial osteochondromatosis vs., I:4–39, **II:4–38i**
Pisiform fracture, **I:4–86i**, I:4–87
Pituitary gland, II:1–9
Plantar calcaneonavicular ligament tear, I:4–175
Plantaris tear, I:4–163
Pleural effusion, I:2–30
Pneumatoceles
  lung abscess vs., **II:2–32i**, II:2–33
  septic pulmonary emboli vs., **II:2–124i**, II:2–125
Pneumatosis of intestine, II:3–38 to II:3–40, **II:3–41i**
  differential diagnosis, **II:3–38i**, II:3–39
  necrotizing enterocolitis vs., **II:3–206i**, II:3–207
Pneumocystitis Jiroveci pneumonia. *See* Pneumonia, immunocompromised
Pneumomediastinum, I:2–4 to I:2–6, **I:2–7i**
  differential diagnosis, **I:2–4i**, I:2–5 to I:2–6

pneumothorax vs., **I:2–8i**, I:2–9
tracheobronchial tear vs., **I:2–12i**
Pneumonia
  acute interstitial, II:2–84 to II:2–86, **II:2–87i**
    differential diagnosis, **II:2–84i**, II:2–85 to II:2–86
  bacterial vs. viral, **II:2–36i**, II:2–37
  community acquired, II:2–24 to II:2–26, **II:2–27i**
    differential diagnosis, **II:2–24i**, II:2–25 to II:2–26
  cryptogenic organizing
    aspiration vs., **II:2–108i**, II:2–110
    community acquired vs., II:2–26
    eosinophilic vs., **II:2–80i**, II:2–81
    pulmonary vasculitis vs., II:2–73
  desquamative interstitial, II:2–86
  diffuse alveolar hemorrhage vs., **II:2–68i**, II:2–69
  drug abuse vs., **II:2–88i**, II:2–90
  eosinophilic, II:2–80 to II:2–82, **II:2–83i**
    acute vs. chronic, II:2–82
    aspiration vs., **II:2–108i**, II:2–110
    asthma vs., II:2–101
    community acquired vs., II:2–26
    differential diagnosis, **II:2–80i**, II:2–81 to II:2–82
    pulmonary vasculitis vs., **II:2–72i**
  immunocompromised, II:2–28 to II:2–30, **II:2–31i**
    acute interstitial vs., **II:2–84i**, II:2–85
    cardiogenic pulmonary edema vs., **II:2–4i**, II:2–6
    differential diagnosis, **II:2–28i**, II:2–29
  lung contusion vs., **I:2–36i**, I:2–38
  mitral regurgitation edema vs., II:2–9
  neonatal, II:2–44 to II:2–46, **II:2–47i**
    differential diagnosis, **II:2–44i**, II:2–45
    meconium aspiration syndrome vs., **II:2–112i**, II:2–113
    transient tachypnea of newborn vs., **II:2–60i**, II:2–61
  noncardiogenic, II:2–73
  nonspecific interstitial, II:2–105
  pulmonary edema vs., I:2–41, **II:2–12i**, II:2–14
  round pneumonia, II:2–40 to II:2–42, **II:2–43i**
  septic pulmonary emboli vs., **II:2–124i**, II:2–125
  sickle cell disease vs., **II:2–76i**, II:2–77
  silo-filler's disease vs., **II:2–20i**, II:2–21
  smoke inhalation vs., II:2–17
Pneumopericardium, I:2–5 to I:2–6
Pneumoperitoneum, II:2–62
Pneumothorax, I:2–8 to I:2–10, **I:2–11i**
  differential diagnosis, **I:2–8i**, I:2–9
  pneumomediastinum vs., **I:2–4i**, I:2–5
  sickle cell disease vs., II:2–77
  tracheobronchial tear vs., I:2–13
Polyarteritis nodosa

INDEX

Otitis, necrotizing external, II:1–80 to II:1–82, **II:1–83i**
   differential diagnosis, **II:1–80i**, II:1–81
Otitis media, complicated, II:1–84 to II:1–86, **II:1–87i**
   differential diagnosis, **II:1–84i**, II:1–85
Otomastoiditis, acute uncomplicated, II:1–85
Otorrhea, I:1–51
Ovarian disorders
   cancer
      hemorrhage vs., **II:3–246i**, II:3–247
      pelvic inflammatory disease vs., **II:3–250i**, II:3–251
   hemorrhage, II:3–246 to II:3–248, **II:3–249i**
      differential diagnosis, **II:3–246i**, II:3–247
      ovarian torsion vs., **II:3–238i**, II:3–239
      tubal ectopic pregnancy vs., **II:3–254i**, II:3–255
   ileocolic intussusception vs., **II:3–218i**, II:3–219
   torsion, II:3–238 to II:3–240, **II:3–241i**
      differential diagnosis, **II:3–238i**, II:3–239
      Meckel diverticulum vs., **II:3–222i**, II:3–223
      ovarian hemorrhage vs., II:3–247
      ovarian vein thrombosis vs., **II:3–242i**, II:3–243
      pelvic inflammatory disease vs., II:3–251
      tubal ectopic pregnancy vs., II:3–255
Ovarian vein thrombosis, II:3–242 to II:3–244, **II:3–245i**
   differential diagnosis, **II:3–242i**, II:3–243
Oxygen therapy
   aneurysmal subarachnoid hemorrhage vs., II:1–5, **II:1–5i**
   meningitis vs., II:1–45
   traumatic subarachnoid hemorrhage vs., **I:1–16i**, I:1–17

P

Pachymeningopathies
   acute subdural hematoma vs., I:1–9
   mixed subdural hematoma vs., I:1–13
Pancreas, annular
   duodenal atresia or stenosis vs., II:3–191
   hypertrophic pyloric stenosis vs., II:3–211
   midgut volvulus vs., II:3–188
Pancreas, shock
   acute pancreatitis vs., II:3–153
   pancreatic trauma vs., I:3–17
Pancreatic disorders
   carcinoma
      choledocholithiasis vs., II:3–145
      infiltrating, **II:3–152i**, II:3–153
   pseudocyst, **II:3–4i**, II:3–5
   trauma, I:3–16 to I:3–18, **I:3–19i**
      differential diagnosis, **I:3–16i**, I:3–17

Pancreatitis
   acute, II:3–152 to II:3–154, **II:3–155i**
      cholecystitis vs., II:3–149
      differential diagnosis, **II:3–152i**, II:3–153
   chronic, vs. choledocholithiasis, **II:3–144i**, II:3–145
   duodenal ulcer vs., II:3–29
   omental infarct vs., II:3–89
   pancreatic trauma vs., **I:3–16i**, I:3–17
   small bowel intussusception vs., **II:3–230i**, II:3–231
Panner disease, I:4–55
Pantothenate kinase associated neurodegeneration (PKAN), II:1–77
Papillomatosis, laryngeal, II:2–126
Paraduodenal hernia, II:3–20 to II:3–22, **II:3–23i**
   differential diagnosis, **II:3–20i**, II:3–21
Paraesophageal hernia
   diaphragmatic tear vs., I:2–30
   esophageal tear vs., **I:2–32i**, I:2–33
Parasitic infections, II:2–81
Paratracheal air cyst, **I:2–4i**, I:2–6
Parotid gland tumors, **II:1–104i**, II:1–105
Parotitis, acute, II:1–104 to II:1–106, **II:1–107i**
   differential diagnosis, **II:1–104i**, II:1–105
Parvovirus infections, II:3–203
Patella
   bipartite, **I:4–146i**, I:4–147
   dislocation., **I:4–146i**, I:4–148
   fracture, I:4–146 to I:4–148, **I:4–149i**
      differential diagnosis, **I:4–146i**, I:4–147 to I:4–148
Patellar tendon tears and tendinosis, I:4–150 to I:4–152, **I:4–153i**
   differential diagnosis, **I:4–150i**, I:4–151 to I:4–152
   patellar fracture vs., I:4–147
Pectus excavatum, **I:2–26i**, I:2–27
Pediatric trauma. *See also* Child abuse; Children
   brain injury, I:1–28 to I:1–30, **I:1–31i**
   incomplete fractures, I:4–194 to I:4–196, **I:4–197i**
   medial epicondyle avulsion, I:4–210 to I:4–212, **I:4–213i**
   metaphyseal fracture, I:4–190 to I:4–192, **I:4–193i**
   physeal fractures, I:4–186 to I:4–188, **I:4–189i**
   stress fractures, I:4–206 to I:4–208, **I:4–209i**
   supracondylar fracture, I:4–198 to I:4–200, **I:4–201i**
   toddler's fractures, I:4–202 to I:4–204, **I:4–205i**
Pellegrini Stieda, **II:4–30i**, II:4–31
Pelvic fractures
   avulsion, I:4–114 to I:4–116, **I:4–117i**
      differential diagnosis, **I:4–114i**, I:4–115 to I:4–116

INDEX

O

Obduratory hernia, II:3–17
Occipital condyle
    congenital variations, I:1–67
    fracture, **I:1–60i**
Ogilvie syndrome, II:3–101
Olecranon
    bursitis vs. triceps tendon rupture, I:4–65
    cortical notch vs. fracture, I:4–65
    fracture
        differential diagnosis, **I:4–64i**, I:4–65
        humeral shaft/distal humeral fracture vs., I:4–57
        supracondylar fracture vs., I:4–199
        stress injury, vs. medial epicondyle avulsion, I:4–211
Omental infarct, II:3–88 to II:3–90, **II:3–91i**
    differential diagnosis, **II:3–88i**, II:3–89
Omental torsion, II:3–89
Ophthalmic vein, superior, I:1–45
Opportunistic infections, AIDS-related, II:1–60 to II:1–62, **II:1–63i**
    differential diagnosis, **II:1–60i**, II:1–61 to II:1–62
Orbit
    infection, II:1–89
    inflammatory disease, idiopathic, II:1–88 to II:1–90, **II:1–91i**
        differential diagnosis, **II:1–88i**, II:1–89
        invasive fungal sinusitis vs., II:1–101
    pseudotumor, II:1–93
    sclerotic inflammation, II:1–89
Orbital vein thrombosis, **II:1–100i**, II:1–101
Orbitopathy, thyroid-associated, **II:1–88i**, II:1–89
Orchitis. *See* Epididymo-orchitis
Orthogonal imaging, I:4–2
Os acromiale, I:4–45
Os hamulus proprius, **I:4–86i**, I:4–87
Os odontoideum, **I:1–66i**, I:1–67
Os trigonum, **I:4–170i**, I:4–171
Osgood Schlatter disease, I:4–151
Ossification accessory centers, I:1–103
Osteoarthritis
    femoral neck fracture vs., I:4–139
    of hip, vs. femoral head fracture, I:4–135
    neuropathic Charcot vs., I:4–44
    radial head/neck fracture vs., I:4–69
    with chondrocalcinosis, **II:4–26i**
Osteochondral injury, I:4–45
Osteochondritis dissecans, II:4–54 to I:4–56, **II:4–57i**
    differential diagnosis, I:4–55, **II:4–54i**
Osteochondroma, **I:4–32i**, I:4–33
Osteochondromatosis
    calcific periarthritis vs., **II:4–30i**, II:4–31
    synovial, II:4–38 to I:4–40, **II:4–41i**
        differential diagnosis, I:4–39, **II:4–38i**
        gout vs., I:4–23
        pigmented villonodular synovitis vs., I:4–35, **II:4–34i**
Osteogenesis imperfecta
    incomplete fracture vs., **I:4–194i**, I:4–195
    metaphyseal fracture vs., **I:4–190i**, I:4–191
    nonaccidental brain injury vs., I:1–29
    transient tachypnea of newborn vs., II:2–62
Osteolysis
    arthroplasty-related particle disease, II:4–66 to I:4–68, **II:4–69i**
    distal clavicle, **I:4–40i**
    radial metaphysis, I:4–77
Osteoma, vs. acute rhinosinusitis, **II:1–96i**, II:1–97
Osteoma, osteoid
    osteomyelitis vs., I:4–8, **II:4–6i**
    pediatric stress fracture vs., **I:4–206i**, I:4–207
    stress fracture vs., I:4–11
    toddler's fractures vs., **I:4–202i**, I:4–204
Osteomyelitis
    adult, II:4–6 to I:4–8, **II:4–9i**
        differential diagnosis, **II:4–6i**, II:4–7 to I:4–8
    chronic, vs. stress fracture, I:4–11
    facet-lamina thoracolumbar fracture vs., **I:1–94i**, I:1–95
    granulomatous, spinal, II:1–116 to II:1–118, **II:1–119i**
        differential diagnosis, **II:1–116i**, II:1–117
        pyogenic osteomyelitis vs., **II:1–112i**, II:1–113
    necrotizing fasciitis vs., **I:4–26i**, I:4–27
    neuropathic Charcot vs., I:4–44
    pedal, I:4–20, **II:4–18i**
    pediatric, II:4–10 to I:4–12, **II:4–12i**
        differential diagnosis, I:4–11, **II:4–10i**
    pyogenic, spinal, II:1–112 to II:1–114, **II:1–115i**
        differential diagnosis, **II:1–112i**, II:1–113
        granulomatous osteomyelitis vs., **II:1–116i**, II:1–117
    sternal fracture vs., **I:2–26i**, I:2–27
    sternoclavicular trauma vs., **I:4–36i**, I:4–37
    toddler's fractures vs., I:4–204
Osteonecrosis
    hip, II:4–48 to I:4–50, **II:4–51i**
        differential diagnosis, I:4–49, **II:4–48i**
    spontaneous, **II:4–54i**
    wrist, **II:4–52i**, II:4–52 to I:4–53
Osteophytosis, I:4–107
Osteoporosis, **I:1–98i**, I:1–99
Osteosarcoma
    myositis ossificans vs., **I:4–32i**, I:4–33
    pediatric stress fracture vs., **I:4–206i**, I:4–207
    surface, vs. stress fracture, I:4–11

INDEX

metacarpal fractures and dislocations, I:4–98 to I:4–100, **I:4–101i**
metatarsal fractures, I:4–182 to I:4–184, **I:4–185i**
myositis ossificans, I:4–32 to I:4–34, **I:4–35i**
navicular fractures, I:4–174 to I:4–176, **I:4–177i**
necrotizing fasciitis, I:4–26 to I:4–27
olecranon fracture/triceps tendon rupture, I:4–64 to I:4–66, **I:4–67i**
patellar fracture, I:4–146 to I:4–148, **I:4–149i**
patellar tendon tears and tendinosis, I:4–150 to I:4–152, **I:4–153i**
pathologic fracture, I:4–14 to I:4–16, **I:4–17i**
pelvic fractures
    stable, I:4–118 to I:4–120, **I:4–121i**
    unstable, I:4–122 to I:4–124, **I:4–125i**
radial head/neck fracture, I:4–68 to I:4–70, **I:4–71i**
scaphoid fractures, I:4–82 to I:4–84, **I:4–85i**
scapular trauma, I:4–44 to I:4–46, **I:4–47i**
shoulder dislocation, I:4–48 to I:4–50, **I:4–51i**
sternoclavicular trauma, I:4–36 to I:4–38, **I:4–39i**
stress fractures
    adult, I:4–10 to I:4–12, **I:4–13i**
    pediatric, I:4–206 to I:4–208, **I:4–209i**
supracondylar fracture, I:4–198 to I:4–200, **I:4–201i**
talus fractures, I:4–170 to I:4–172, **I:4–173i**
tibial plateau fracture, I:4–154 to I:4–156, **I:4–157i**
toddler's fractures, I:4–202 to I:4–204, **I:4–205i**
ulnar collateral ligament tear, thumb, I:4–102 to I:4–104, **I:4–105i**
Mycobacterium avium-intracellulare, II:3–35
Myelitis
    idiopathic transverse, II:1–124
    spinal cord injury vs., I:1–111
Myelomalacia, I:1–111
Myelomeningocele, I:4–192
Myositis
    diabetes complications vs., I:4–20
    orbital, **I:1–44i**, I:1–45
Myositis ossificans, I:4–32 to I:4–34, **I:4–35i**
    compartment syndrome vs., I:4–23
    differential diagnosis, **I:4–32i**, I:4–33 to I:4–34

N

Nasoethmoid fractures, **I:1–56i**, I:1–57
Navicular bone, accessory, **I:4–174i**, I:4–175
Navicular fractures, I:4–174 to I:4–176, **I:4–177i**
    differential diagnosis, **I:4–174i**, I:4–175
    Lisfranc fracture-dislocation vs., I:4–179
    metatarsal fracture vs., I:4–183
Near-drowning, **II:1–76i**, II:1–76 to II:1–77
    inborn errors of metabolism vs., II:1–73

Necrobiotic nodules, II:2–33
Necrotizing fasciitis, **I:4–26i**, I:4–26 to I:4–27
    compartment syndrome vs., **I:4–22i**
    diabetes complications vs., I:4–20
    soft tissue abscess vs., I:4–5, **II:4–4i**
Neonatal diseases. *See* Children
Neoplasms. *See also* Carcinoma; Metastasis; *specific histologic type*
    appendiceal, vs. appendicitis, II:3–78
    bone, vs. pediatric stress fracture, **I:4–206i**, I:4–207
    bowel, vs. intussusception, **II:3–56i**, II:3–57
    calcific periarthritis vs., II:4–32
    compression injury vs. chance fracture, **I:1–98i**, I:1–99
    cranial
        dural sinus thrombosis vs., II:1–37
        spontaneous intracranial hemorrhage vs., II:1–21
    epidural hematoma vs., I:1–5
    extrinsic invasion vs. duodenal ulcer, **II:3–28i**, II:3–29 to II:3–30
    hematoma vs., **I:4–28i**, I:4–29
    hemorrhagic, II:1–26
    low-grade, vs. cerebral contusion, I:1–21
    metatarsal, vs. fracture, I:4–183
    sacral, vs. traumatic fracture, **I:1–102i**, I:1–103
    soft tissue abscess vs., **II:4–4i**
    spinal, compression fracture vs., **I:1–88i**, I:1–89
    spinal cord infarction vs., II:1–124
    splenic
        infarction vs., **II:3–106i**, II:3–107
        infection vs., **II:3–102i**, II:3–103
    sternal, vs. fracture, I:2–26
    sternoclavicular trauma vs., I:4–37
Neuroblastoma
    epidural hematoma vs., **I:1–4i**, I:1–5
    osteomyelitis vs., I:4–11, **II:4–10i**
    round pneumonia vs., **II:2–40i**, II:2–41
    toddler's fractures vs., **I:4–202i**, I:4–204
Neurofibromatosis
    inborn errors of metabolism vs., II:1–73
    incomplete fracture vs., **I:4–194i**, I:4–195
    talcosis vs., II:2–94
Neurosarcoidosis, II:1–45
Neurosyphilis, II:1–57
Non-Hodgkin lymphoma
    Crohn disease vs., II:3–36
    intussusception vs., **II:3–56i**, II:3–57
    orbital inflammatory disease vs., II:1–89
    small bowel intussusception in children vs., II:3–232
    xanthogranulomatous pyelonephritis vs., **II:3–164i**, II:3–165
Nonaccidental trauma. *See* Child abuse

INDEX

epidural paravertebral abscess vs., **II:1–120i**, II:1–121
fracture vs., **I:2–22i**, I:2–24
granulomatous osteomyelitis vs., **II:1–116i**, II:1–117
pyogenic osteomyelitis vs., **II:1–112i**, II:1–113
sternoclavicular trauma vs., I:4–37
Metatarsals
    fractures, I:4–182 to I:4–184, **I:4–185i**
        differential diagnosis, **I:4–182i**, I:4–183
    tumor, I:4–183
Microcalcification, II:1–33
Mitochondrial encephalopathies, II:1–77
Mitral regurgitation. See Pulmonary edema, mitral regurgitant
Mucocele, **II:1–92i**, II:1–93
Mucus retention cyst, **II:1–96i**, II:1–97
Multiple sclerosis
    cerebral abscess vs., **II:1–48i**, II:1–49
    opportunistic infections vs., III:1–62
    spinal cord infarction vs., **II:1–124i**
    spinal cord injury vs., **I:1–110i**, I:1–111
Muscle strain
    compartment syndrome vs., **I:4–22i**, I:4–23
    femoral neck fracture vs., I:4–139
    sacral insufficiency fractures vs., I:4–5
Muscular dystrophy, II:2–62
Musculoskeletal disorders, II:4–2 to I:4–81
    in AIDS/HIV infections, II:4–74 to I:4–76, **II:4–77i**
    arthroplasty complications
        component wear/particle disease, II:4–66 to I:4–68, **II:4–69i**
        hardware/periprosthetic fracture, II:4–62 to I:4–64, **II:4–65i**
        loosening and dislocation, II:4–58 to I:4–60, **II:4–61i**
    bone marrow edema, transient, II:4–46 to I:4–47
    calcific periarthritis, II:4–30 to I:4–32, **II:4–33i**
    Charcot, neuropathic, II:4–42 to I:4–44, **II:4–45i**
    diabetes complications, II:4–18 to I:4–20, **II:4–21i**
    gout, II:4–22 to I:4–24, **II:4–25i**
    hemophilia and, II:4–78 to I:4–80, **II:4–81i**
    imaging issues, II:4–2 to I:4–3
    osteochondritis dissecans, II:4–54 to I:4–56, **II:4–57i**
    osteomyelitis
        adult, II:4–6 to I:4–8, **II:4–9i**
        pediatric, II:4–10 to I:4–12, **II:4–12i**
    osteonecrosis
        of hip, II:4–48 to I:4–50, **II:4–51i**
        of wrist, II:4–52 to I:4–53
    pigmented villonodular synovitis, II:4–34 to I:4–36, **II:4–37i**
    pyrophosphate arthropathy, II:4–26 to I:4–28, **II:4–29i**
    septic joint, II:4–14 to I:4–16, **II:4–17i**
    sickle cell disease, II:4–70 to I:4–72, **II:4–73i**
    soft tissue abscess, II:4–4 to I:4–5
    synovial osteochondromatosis, II:4–38 to I:4–40, **II:4–41i**
Musculoskeletal trauma, I:4–2 to I:4–213
    acetabular fractures, I:4–126 to I:4–128, **I:4–129i**
    Achilles tendon tear and tendinopathy, I:4–162 to I:4–164, **I:4–165i**
    acromioclavicular dislocation, I:4–42 to I:4–43
    ankle fractures, I:4–158 to I:4–160, **I:4–161i**
    avulsion fractures
        finger, I:4–110 to I:4–112, **I:4–113i**
        pelvis, I:4–114 to I:4–116, **I:4–117i**
    biceps tendon rupture, I:4–72 to I:4–73
    calcaneal fractures, I:4–166 to I:4–168, **I:4–169i**
    carpal dislocations, I:4–90 to I:4–92, **I:4–93i**
    carpal fractures, non-scaphoid, I:4–86 to I:4–88, **I:4–89i**
    carpal instabilities, I:4–94 to I:4–96, **I:4–97i**
    child abuse and metaphyseal fracture, I:4–190 to I:4–192, **I:4–193i**
    clavicle fracture, I:4–40 to I:4–41
    compartment syndrome, I:4–22 to I:4–24, **I:4–25i**
    die punch fracture, distal radius, I:4–80 to I:4–81
    distal radius fractures, I:4–76 to I:4–78, **I:4–79i**
    elbow dislocation, I:4–60 to I:4–62, **I:4–63i**
    femoral head fractures, I:4–134 to I:4–136, **I:4–137i**
    femoral neck fractures, I:4–138 to I:4–140, **I:4–141i**
    flexor annular pulley tears, I:4–106 to I:4–108, **I:4–109i**
    forearm fractures, I:4–74 to I:4–75
    foreign body, I:4–18 to I:4–20, **I:4–21i**
    hematoma, I:4–28 to I:4–30, **I:4–31i**
    hip dislocation, I:4–130 to I:4–132, **I:4–133i**
    humeral head/neck fracture, I:4–52 to I:4–54, **I:4–55i**
    humeral shaft/distal humeral fracture, I:4–56 to I:4–58, **I:4–59i**
    imaging issues, I:4–2 to I:4–3
    incomplete fractures, I:4–194 to I:4–196, **I:4–197i**
    insufficiency fractures
        appendicular, I:4–8 to I:4–9
        sacrum, I:4–4 to I:4–6, **I:4–7i**
    knee avulsion fracture, I:4–142 to I:4–144, **I:4–145i**
    Lisfranc fracture-dislocation, I:4–178 to I:4–180, **I:4–181i**
    medial epicondyle avulsion, I:4–210 to I:4–212, **I:4–213i**

INDEX

infection vs., **II:3–102i**, II:3–103
trauma vs., **I:3–4i**, I:3–5

M

Mach band, I:2–6
Macrocrania, benign, II:1–70
Magic angle artifact, I:4–152
Malabsorption syndromes, II:3–232
Marchiafava-Bignami syndrome, I:1–25
Marfan syndrome, **I:1–40i**, I:1–41
Meckel diverticulum, II:3–222 to II:3–224, **II:3–225i**
    differential diagnosis, **II:3–222i**, II:3–223
    ileocolic intussusception vs., **II:3–218i**, II:3–219
    intussusception vs., II:3–57
    small bowel intussusception in children vs., II:3–231
Meconium aspiration syndrome, II:2–112 to II:2–114, **II:2–115i**
    differential diagnosis, **II:2–112i**, II:2–113
    neonatal pneumonia vs., **II:2–44i**, II:2–45
    transient tachypnea of newborn vs., **II:2–60i**, II:2–61
Meconium ileus, II:3–198 to II:3–200, **II:3–201i**
    differential diagnosis, **II:3–198i**, II:3–199
    meconium peritonitis vs., **II:3–202i**, II:3–203
    meconium plug syndrome vs., **II:3–194i**, II:3–195
Meconium peritonitis, II:3–202 to II:3–204, **II:3–205i**
    differential diagnosis, **II:3–202i**, II:3–203
Meconium plug syndrome, II:3–194 to II:3–196, **II:3–197i**
    differential diagnosis, **II:3–194i**, II:3–195
    meconium ileus vs., II:3–199
Meconium pseudocyst, **II:3–222i**, II:3–223
Medial canal fibrosis, post-inflammatory, II:1–81
Medial epicondyle avulsion, I:4–210 to I:4–212, **I:4–213i**
    differential diagnosis, **I:4–210i**, I:4–211 to I:4–212
Medial tibial stress syndrome, I:4–207
Mediastinal abscess, **I:2–26i**, I:2–27
Mediastinal widening
    aortic transection vs., I:2–19
    spinal fracture vs., I:2–24
Medulloblastoma, **II:1–68i**, II:1–69
Megacolon, functional, II:3–97. *See also* Toxic megacolon
Melanoma, malignant, **II:3–56i**, II:3–57
Meningioma
    epidural hematoma vs., I:1–5
    intracerebral hematoma vs., **II:1–16i**, II:1–17
    mixed subdural hematoma vs., I:1–13
    subdural hematoma vs., I:1–9
Meningitis, II:1–44 to II:1–46, **II:1–47i**

    differential diagnosis, **II:1–44i**, II:1–45
    neonatal, II:1–40 to II:1–42, **II:1–43i**
        differential diagnosis, **II:1–40i**, II:1–41 to II:1–42
    opportunistic infections vs., III:1–62
    subdural hematoma vs., I:1–9, I:1–13
    traumatic subarachnoid hemorrhage vs., **I:1–16i**, I:1–17
Menkes syndrome, I:4–192
Mesenteric adenitis, II:3–226 to II:3–228, **II:3–229i**
    appendicitis vs., **II:3–76i**, II:3–77
    Crohn disease vs., II:3–36
    differential diagnosis, **II:3–226i**, II:3–227 to II:3–228
Mesenteritis, fibrosing
    acute small bowel ischemia vs., II:3–43
    omental infarct vs., **II:3–88i**, II:3–89
Metabolic bone disease, I:4–195 to I:4–196
Metacarpal fractures and dislocations, I:4–98 to I:4–100, **I:4–101i**
    differential diagnosis, **I:4–98i**, I:4–99
Metacarpophalangeal joint
    capsular trauma, I:4–103
    dislocations
        flexor annular pulley tears vs., I:4–107
        ulnar collateral ligament tear vs., I:4–103
Metaphyseal fractures, I:4–190 to I:4–192, **I:4–193i**
    differential diagnosis, **I:4–190i**, I:4–191 to I:4–192
Metastasis. *See also* Neoplasms
    calcifications, II:4–31
    cystic
        amebic abscess vs., **II:3–118i**, II:3–119
        pyogenic abscess vs., **II:3–114i**, II:3–115
    dual, II:1–53
    liver, vs. candidiasis, **II:3–110i**, II:3–111
    meningitis vs., **II:1–44i**, II:1–45
    mixed subdural hematoma vs., I:1–13
    pancreatic, **II:3–152i**, II:3–153
    parenchymal, **II:1–48i**, II:1–49
    particle disease vs., II:4–67
    renal
        abscess vs., II:3–161
        renal vein thrombosis vs., II:3–175
        xanthogranulomatous pyelonephritis vs., II:3–165
    retropharyngeal space, II:1–109
    sacrum
        insufficiency fractures vs., I:4–5
        traumatic fracture vs., **I:1–102i**, I:1–103
    septic pulmonary emboli vs., **II:2–124i**, II:2–125
    small bowel
        Crohn disease vs., II:3–36
        intussusception vs., **II:3–56i**, II:3–57
    spinal

INDEX

J

Jefferson C1 fracture, I:1–62 to I:1–64, **I:1–65i**
   differential diagnosis, **I:1–52i**, I:1–63
Joint dislocations, I:4–107
Jones fracture
   Lisfranc fracture-dislocation vs., I:4–179
     progressing to nonunion, **I:4–182i**, I:4–183
Juvenile chronic arthritis, **II:4-78i**, II:4-79 to I:4-80

K

Keratosis obturans, **II:1–80i**, II:1–81
Kidney. *See* Renal *terms*
Knee
   avulsion fracture, I:4–142 to I:4–144, **I:4–145i**
     differential diagnosis, **I:4–142i**, I:4–144
   floating, I:4–155
   impactation fracture, **I:4–142i**, I:4–143
Knee joint malalignment, I:4–143
Köhler disease, I:4–175
Kyphoscoliosis., **I:2–22i**, I:2–24

L

Langerhans cell histiocytosis (LCH)
   complicated otitis media vs., **II:1–84i**, II:1–85
   osteomyelitis vs., I:4–11, II:4–7, **II:4–10i**
Langerhans granulomatosis, **II:2–104i**, II:2–105
Laryngeal papillomatosis, II:2–126
Larynx trauma, I:1–52 to I:1–54, **I:1–55i**
   differential diagnosis, **I:1–52i**, I:1–53
Lateral flexion injury, cervical, **I:1–84i**, I:1–84 to I:1–85
LeFort fractures I-III, I:1–56 to I:1–58, **I:1–59i**
   differential diagnosis, **I:1–56i**, I:1–57
Left heart, hypoplastic, **II:2–60i**, II:2–61
Left heart failure, II:2–9
Left to right shunts, II:2–37
Lesser trochanter avulsion, I:4–115
Leukemia
   metaphyseal fracture vs., **I:4–190i**, I:4–192
   mixed subdural hematoma vs., I:1–13
   nonaccidental brain injury vs., **I:1–28i**, I:1–29
   toddler's fractures vs., **I:4–202i**, I:4–204
Ligaments
   anterior talofibular sprain, I:4–179
   calcaneofibular sprain, I:4–179
   dorsal, sprain vs. navicular fracture, I:4–175
   medial collateral, I:4–211
Lipohemarthrosis, **I:4–154i**
Lipoma
   intracerebral hematoma vs., II:1–17
   saccular aneurysm vs., II:1–9
Lipomatosis, epidural, **II:1–120i**, II:1–121
Liposarcoma, **I:4–28i**, I:4–29

Lisfranc fracture-dislocation, I:4–178 to I:4–180, **I:4–181i**
   differential diagnosis, **I:4–178i**, I:4–179 to I:4–180
   metatarsal fracture vs., I:4–183
Liver disorders. *See* Hepatic disorders
Loose bodies
   calcific periarthritis vs., **II:4–30i**, II:4–31
   medial epicondyle avulsion vs., I:4–212
Lumbar radiculopathy, I:4–5
Lumbosacral dislocation, traumatic, I:1–103
Lunate dislocation, **I:4–90i**, I:4–91
Lunate fracture, I:4–87
Lung abscess, II:2–32 to II:2–34, **II:2–35i**
   contusion vs., **I:2–36i**, I:2–38
   differential diagnosis, **II:2–32i**, II:2–33 to II:2–34
   septic pulmonary emboli vs., **II:2–124i**, II:2–125
Lung contusion, I:2–36 to I:2–38, **I:2–39i**
   differential diagnosis, **I:2–36i**, I:2–38
   pulmonary edema vs., **I:2–40i**, I:2–41, **I:2–44i**, I:2–45
Lung disease, chronic
   bronchopulmonary dysplasia, **II:2–64i**, II:2–65
   hypersensitivity pneumonitis vs., **II:2–104i**, II:2–105
Lung infection, viral, II:2–36 to II:2–38, **II:2–39i**
   differential diagnosis, **II:2–36i**, II:2–37
Lupus. *See* Systemic lupus erythematosus (SLE)
Luxatio erecta, **I:4–48i**, I:4–49
Lymphadenopathy
   bronchial foreign body vs., II:2–118
   femoral hernia vs., **II:3–16i**, II:3–17
   inguinal hernia vs., **II:3–12i**, II:3–14
Lymphangiectasia, congenital, II:2–61
Lymphangioma
   hematoma vs., I:4–29
   subperiosteal abscess of orbit vs., **II:1–92i**, II:1–93
Lymphocele, **II:3–4i**, II:3–5
Lymphoid hyperplasia, II:1–89
Lymphoma. *See also* Non-Hodgkin lymphoma
   CNS., vs. AIDS-related opportunistic infections, **II:1–60i**, II:1–62
   duodenal, **I:3–20i**, I:3–21
   mixed subdural hematoma vs., I:1–13
   osteomyelitis vs., I:4–11
   pancreatic, II:3–153
   renal
     abscess vs., **II:3–160i**, II:3–161
     pyelonephritis vs., **II:3–156i**
     renal vein thrombosis vs., **II:3–174i**, II:3–175
     xanthogranulomatous pyelonephritis vs., II:3–165
   splenic
     infarction vs., **II:3–106i**, II:3–107

INDEX

meconium plug syndrome vs., **II:3–194i**, II:3–195
Ileocolitis, II:3–77
Ileus
    acute, vs. cecal volvulus, II:3–100
    gallstone, II:3–54 to II:3–55
    sigmoid volvulus vs., **II:3–96i**, II:3–97
    small bowel obstruction vs., **II:3–50i**, II:3–51
    toxic megacolon vs., II:3–75
Iliac spine avulsion, **I:4–114i**, I:4–115 to I:4–116
Imaging issues
    abdominal, I:3–2 to I:3–3, II:3–2 to II:3–3
    central nervous system, I:1–2 to I:1–3, II:1–2 to II:1–3
    chest, I:2–2 to I:2–3, II:2–2 to II:2–3
    musculoskeletal, I:4–2 to I:4–3, II:4–2 to II:4–3
Impactation fracture, knee, **I:4–142i**, I:4–143
Inborn errors of metabolism, II:1–72 to II:1–74, **II:1–75i**
    differential diagnosis, **II:1–72i**, II:1–73
    neonatal meningitis vs., II:1–41
Incomplete fractures, I:4–194 to I:4–196, **I:4–197i**
    differential diagnosis, **I:4–194i**, I:4–195 to I:4–196
Incus interposition procedure, **I:1–46i**, I:1–47
Infants. *See* Children
Infections
    arthroplasty loosening and dislocation vs., I:4–60, **II:4–58i**
    congenital, vs. neonatal meningitis, II:1–42
    prosthesis, II:4–67
Inferior vena cava interruption, **II:2–132i**, II:2–133
Inflammation, vs. epidural hematoma, I:1–5
Inflammatory bowel disease, II:3–223
Infraglenoid fracture, **I:4–44i**, I:4–45
Infundibulum, II:1–9
Inguinal hernia, II:3–12 to II:3–14, **II:3–15i**
    differential diagnosis, **II:3–12i**, II:3–13 to II:3–14
    femoral hernia vs., **II:3–16i**, II:3–17
Inguinal node, **II:3–16i**, II:3–17
Insufficiency fractures. *See also* Stress fractures
    acetabular fracture vs., I:4–127
    appendicular, **I:4–8i**, I:4–8 to I:4–9
    femoral head, **I:4–134i**
    sacrum, I:4–4 to I:4–6, **I:4–7i**
        differential diagnosis, **I:4–4i**, I:4–5
        stable pelvic fracture vs., I:4–119
Internal carotid artery dissection, I:1–41
Internal carotid artery stenosis, **I:1–40i**, I:1–41 to I:1–42
Intestinal disorders. *See also* Colon
    atresia, vs. meconium peritonitis, II:3–203
    colitis. *See* Colitis
    Crohn disease. *See* Crohn disease
    diverticulitis. *See* Diverticulitis

duplication, vs. Meckel diverticulum, II:3–223
    inflammatory bowel disease, II:3–223
    ischemia, acute
        Crohn disease vs., II:3–36
        differential diagnosis, **II:3–42i**, II:3–43
    ischemia, vs. gallstone ileus, **II:3–54i**, II:3–55
    necrosis vs. pneumatosis, **II:3–38i**, II:3–39
    obstruction, vs. necrotizing enterocolitis., II:3–207
    perforation, vs. necrotizing enterocolitis, II:3–207
    post-endoscopic bowel, **II:3–38i**, II:3–39
    postoperative bowel, II:3–39
    small bowel. *See also* Duodenal *terms*
        ischemia, acute, II:3–42 to II:3–44, **II:3–45i**
        obstruction. *See* Small bowel obstruction
Intestinal trauma, I:3–22 to I:3–24, **I:3–25i**
    differential diagnosis, **I:3–22i**, I:3–23 to I:3–24
    hypoperfusion complex vs., **I:3–28i**, I:3–29
Intracerebral hematoma, II:1–16 to II:1–18, **II:1–18i**
    cerebral abscess vs., II:1–49
    differential diagnosis, **II:1–16i**, II:1–17 to II:1–18
Intracranial hemorrhage
    drug abuse vs., **II:1–64i**, II:1–65
    hypertensive, II:1–24 to II:1–26, **II:1–27i**
        differential diagnosis, **II:1–24i**, II:1–25 to II:1–26
        spontaneous hemorrhage vs., II:1–21
    spontaneous, II:1–20 to II:1–22, **II:1–23i**
        differential diagnosis, **II:1–20i**, II:1–21 to II:1–22
Intracranial herniation syndromes, I:1–32 to I:1–34, **I:1–35i**
    differential diagnosis, **I:1–32i**, I:1–33 to I:1–34
Intracranial hypotension
    intracranial herniation syndrome vs., **I:1–32i**, I:1–33
    mixed subdural hematoma vs., I:1–13
    subdural hematoma vs., **I:1–8i**, I:1–9
Intracranial shunt malfunction, II:1–69
Intubation, esophageal, **I:2–12i**, I:2–13
Intussusception, II:3–56 to II:3–58, **II:3–59i**
    differential diagnosis, **II:3–56i**, II:3–57
    gallstone ileus vs., II:3–54
    ileocolic, II:3–218 to II:3–220, **II:3–221i**
        differential diagnosis, **II:3–218i**, II:3–219
        small bowel intussusception in children vs., **II:3–230i**, II:3–231
    meconium peritonitis vs., II:3–203
    mesenteric adenitis vs., **II:3–226i**, II:3–227
    small bowel
        in children, II:3–230 to II:3–232, **II:3–233i**
            differential diagnosis, **II:3–230i**, II:3–231 to II:3–232
            hypoperfusion complex vs., **I:3–28i**, I:3–29

INDEX

inguinal, II:3–12 to II:3–14, **II:3–15i**
   differential diagnosis, **II:3–12i**, II:3–13 to II:3–14
   femoral hernia vs., **II:3–16i**, II:3–17
   intracranial, I:1–32 to I:1–34, **I:1–35i**
   obduratory, II:3–17
   paraduodenal, II:3–20 to II:3–22, **II:3–23i**
     differential diagnosis, **II:3–20i**, II:3–21
   paraesophageal
     diaphragmatic tear vs., I:2–30
     esophageal tear vs., **I:2–32i**, I:2–33
   transmesenteric
     internal, **II:3–20i**, II:3–21
     postoperative, II:3–24 to II:3–26, **II:3–27i**
Herpes encephalitis, II:1–56 to II:1–58, **II:1–59i**
   cerebral ischemia-infarction vs., **II:1–32i**, II:1–34
   differential diagnosis, **II:1–56i**, II:1–57
Herpes simplex virus infections, II:1–42
Hiatal hernia
   esophageal tear vs., I:2–33
   gastric volvulus vs., **II:3–214i**, II:3–215
HIE (hypoxic-ischemic encephalopathy). *See* Hypoxic-ischemic encephalopathy (HIE)
Hilar lymph node, **II:2–120i**, II:2–122
Hill Sachs fracture, **I:4–48i**, I:4–50
Hip dislocation, **I:4–130i**, I:4–130 to I:4–132, **I:4–133i**
   acetabular fracture vs., I:4–127
   missed, with avascular necrosis, **I:4–130i**
Hip muscle strain, I:4–119
Hirschsprung disease
   meconium ileus vs., **II:3–198i**, II:3–199
   meconium plug syndrome vs., **II:3–194i**, II:3–195
   necrotizing enterocolitis vs., **II:3–206i**, II:3–207
HIV infections. *See* AIDS (acquired immunodeficiency syndrome)
Humeral head/neck fracture, I:4–52 to I:4–54, **I:4–55i**
   differential diagnosis, **I:4–52i**, I:4–53
   scapular trauma vs., I:4–45
Humeral shaft/distal humeral fracture, I:4–56 to I:4–58, **I:4–59i**
   differential diagnosis, **I:4–56i**, I:4–57
   supracondylar fracture vs., I:4–199
Humpback deformity, **I:4–82i**
Huntington disease, **II:1–76i**, II:1–77
Hydatid cyst
   amebic abscess vs., **II:3–118i**, II:3–119
   hepatic, II:3–116
Hydrocele, **II:3–12i**, II:3–14
Hydrocephalus, II:1–68 to II:1–70, **II:1–71i**
   differential diagnosis, **II:1–68i**, II:1–69 to II:1–70
   nonaccidental brain injury vs., I:1–30
Hydronephrosis, II:3–165

Hydrosalpinx, **II:3–238i**, II:3–239
Hydrothorax, tension, **II:2–136i**, II:2–138
Hydroxyapatite deposition disease, **II:4–26i**
Hygroma
   subdural, **II:1–52i**, II:1–53
   subdural hematoma vs., I:1–9, I:1–13
Hyperextension injury, cervical, I:1–76 to I:1–78, **I:1–79i**
   differential diagnosis, **I:1–76i**, I:1–77
   posterior column injury vs., **I:1–86i**
Hyperflexion injury, cervical, **I:1–74i**, I:1–74 to I:1–75
Hyperflexion-rotation injury, cervical, I:1–80 to I:1–82, **I:1–83i**
   differential diagnosis, **I:1–80i**, I:1–81
   hyperflexion injury vs., **I:1–74i**, I:1–75
   lateral flexion injury vs., **I:1–84i**, I:1–85
   posterior column injury vs., **I:1–86i**
Hyperparathyroidism, I:4–196
Hyperphosphatemia, I:4–196
Hypersensitivity pneumonitis, II:2–104 to II:2–106, **II:2–107i**
   chronic obstructive pulmonary disease vs., **II:2–96i**, II:2–97
   community acquired pneumonia vs., **II:2–24i**, II:2–26
   differential diagnosis, **II:2–104i**, II:2–105 to II:2–106
   drug abuse vs., II:2–90
   silo-filler's disease vs., **II:2–20i**, II:2–21
Hypertension
   diffuse axonal injury vs., **I:1–24i**, I:1–25
   pulmonary, vs. asthma., **II:2–100i**, II:2–101
Hypertensive encephalopathy, acute, II:1–28 to II:1–30, **II:1–31i**
   differential diagnosis, **II:1–28i**, II:1–29
   with hemorrhage, vs. drug abuse, II:1–65
Hyperthyroidism, I:4–23, **II:4–22i**
Hypoglycemia, **II:1–28i**, II:1–29
Hypoperfusion complex, I:3–28 to I:3–30, **I:3–31i**
   acute small bowel ischemia vs., **II:3–42i**, II:3–43
   differential diagnosis, **I:3–28i**, I:3–29 to I:3–30
   intestinal trauma vs., **I:3–22i**, I:3–23
   small intestine vasculitis vs., **II:3–46i**, II:3–47
Hypophosphatemia, I:4–196
Hypoxic-ischemic encephalopathy (HIE)
   near-drowning vs., II:1–77
   neonatal meningitis vs., **II:1–40i**, II:1–41
   perinatal, vs. inborn errors of metabolism, **II:1–72i**, II:1–73

I

Ileal atresia
   meconium ileus vs., **II:3–198i**, II:3–199
   meconium peritonitis vs., **II:3–202i**, II:3–203

INDEX

herpes encephalitis vs., **II:1–56i**, II:1–57
Gout, II:4–22 to I:4–24, **II:4–25i**
   differential diagnosis, I:4–23, **II:4–22i**
   pigmented villonodular synovitis vs., I:4–35, **II:4–34i**
Graft-versus-host disease, I:3–29
Granuloma annulare, I:4–29
Graves disease, **I:1–44i**, I:1–45
Greenstick fractures, I:4–194 to I:4–196, **I:4–197i**
   differential diagnosis, **I:4–194i**, I:4–195 to I:4–196
Groin abscess, **II:3–12i**, II:3–14
Growth plate, unfused, I:4–53

H

Haglund disease, **I:4–162i**, I:4–163
Hair, vs. pneumothorax, I:2–9
Hamartoma, biliary, **II:3–110i**, II:3–111
Hamate fracture, I:4–87
Head and neck injury, I:1–46 to I:1–59
   cerebrospinal fluid leak, I:1–50 to I:1–51
   closed head injury and unstable pelvic fracture, **I:4–122i**
   imaging issues, I:1–2 to I:1–3
   larynx trauma, I:1–52 to I:1–54, **I:1–55i**
   LeFort fractures I-III, I:1–56 to I:1–58, **I:1–59i**
   temporal bone fractures, I:1–46 to I:1–48, **I:1–49i**
Heart disease, congenital
   meconium aspiration syndrome vs., **II:2–112i**, II:2–113
   neonatal pneumonia vs., II:2–45
   transient tachypnea of newborn vs., **II:2–60i**, II:2–61
HELLP syndrome, II:3–122 to II:3–124, **II:3–125i**
   differential diagnosis, **II:3–122i**, II:3–123
   hepatic trauma vs., **I:3–8i**, I:3–9
Hemangioma
   hematoma vs., I:4–29
   Meckel diverticulum vs., II:3–223
Hematoma, I:4–28 to I:4–30, **I:4–31i**
   abdominal abscess vs., II:3–5
   compartment syndrome vs., **I:4–22i**, I:4–23
   differential diagnosis, **I:4–28i**, I:4–29
   duodenal, II:3–30
   epidural. *See* Epidural hematoma
   femoral hernia vs., **II:3–16i**, II:3–17
   inguinal hernia vs., II:3–13 to II:3–14
   parenchymal, **I:1–14i**, I:1–15
   patellar tendon tears and tendinosis vs., **I:4–150i**, I:4–151
   subdural. *See* Subdural hematoma
Hematopoiesis, extramedullary, I:4–72, **II:4–70i**
Hemimegalencephaly, II:1–70
Hemochromatosis, **II:4–26i**, II:4–27

Hemodialysis spondyloarthropathy, II:1–113
Hemodynamically unstable patients, I:3–2 to I:3–3
Hemoglobin C, sickle cell, II:4–72
Hemoglobinuria, paroxysmal nocturnal, II:2–77
Hemoperitoneum, II:3–9
Hemophilia
   arthropathy vs. pigmented villonodular synovitis, I:4–35, **II:4–34i**
   musculoskeletal complications, II:4–78 to I:4–80, **II:4–81i**
   differential diagnosis, **II:4–78i**, II:4–79 to I:4–80
Hemorrhage, spontaneous, I:3–9
Hemosiderin, **II:4–78i**, II:4–79 to I:4–80
Henoch-Schönlein purpura
   hypoperfusion complex vs., **I:3–28i**, I:3–29
   small bowel intussusception vs., **II:3–230i**, II:3–231
Hepatic disorders
   abscess
     amebic, II:3–118 to II:3–120, **II:3–121i**
     cholecystitis vs., **II:3–148i**, II:3–149
     infarction vs., **II:3–126i**, II:3–127
     pyogenic, II:3–114 to II:3–116, **II:3–117i**
   candidiasis, II:3–110 to II:3–112, **II:3–113i**
   cirrhosis, **II:3–134i**, II:3–136
   enlargement, I:2–30
   infarction, II:3–126 to II:3–128, **II:3–129i**
     differential diagnosis, **II:3–126i**, II:3–127
     posttransplant
       amebic abscess vs., II:3–119
       pyogenic abscess vs., II:3–116
   trauma, I:3–8 to I:3–10, **I:3–11i**
     differential diagnosis, **I:3–8i**, I:3–9
     HELLP syndrome vs., **II:3–122i**, II:3–123
     infarction vs., II:3–127
   tumors, bleeding
     HELLP syndrome vs., I:3–123
     trauma vs., I:3–9
   venous outflow obstruction. *See* Budd-Chiari syndrome
Hepatocellular carcinoma
   HELLP syndrome vs., **II:3–122i**, II:3–123
   hepatic trauma vs., **I:3–8i**, I:3–9
Hernia. *See also* Disc herniation
   diaphragmatic
     gastric volvulus vs., **II:3–214i**, II:3–215
     pulmonary interstitial emphysema vs., II:2–65
     transient tachypnea of newborn vs., II:2–61
   femoral, II:3–16 to II:3–18, **II:3–19i**
     differential diagnosis, **II:3–16i**, II:3–17
     inguinal hernia vs., **II:3–12i**, II:3–13
   hiatal
     esophageal tear vs., I:2–33
     gastric volvulus vs., **II:3–214i**, II:3–215

INDEX

F

Farmer's lung, **II:2–20i**, II:2–21
Femoral condyle
    fracture vs. tibial plateau fracture, I:4–155
    insufficiency fracture, I:4–55
    posterior irregularity, I:4–55, **II:4–54i**
Femoral fracture, subcapital, **I:4–138i**, I:4–139
Femoral head fractures, I:4–134 to I:4–136, **I:4–137i**
    acetabular fracture vs., I:4–127
    differential diagnosis, **I:4–134i**, I:4–135
    sacral insufficiency fractures vs., I:4–5
Femoral hernia, II:3–16 to II:3–18, **II:3–19i**
    differential diagnosis, **II:3–16i**, II:3–17
    inguinal hernia vs., **II:3–12i**, II:3–13
Femoral neck fractures, I:4–138 to I:4–140, **I:4–141i**
    acetabular fracture vs., I:4–127
    differential diagnosis, **I:4–138i**, I:4–139
    sacral insufficiency fractures vs., I:4–5
    tibial plateau fracture vs., I:4–155
Fibrodysplasia ossificans progressiva, I:4–33 to I:4–34
Fibromatosis, I:4–29
Fibromuscular dysplasia
    extracranial vascular injury vs., I:1–41
    intracranial vascular injury vs., I:1–37 to I:1–38
Fibrous dysplasia, **I:4–194i**, I:4–195
Fibroxanthoma, I:4–65
Finger
    avulsion fractures, I:4–110 to I:4–112, **I:4–113i**
        differential diagnosis, **I:4–110i**, I:4–111
    dislocation, I:4–111
Flail chest, **I:2–14i**, I:2–14 to I:2–16, **I:2–17i**
FLAIR artifact
    aneurysmal subarachnoid hemorrhage vs., II:1–5
    meningitis vs., **II:1–44i**, II:1–45
    nonaneurysmal perimesencephalic subarachnoid hemorrhage vs., **II:1–6i**, II:1–7
Flexor annular pulley tears, I:4–106 to I:4–108, **I:4–109i**
    differential diagnosis, **I:4–106i**, I:4–107
Flexor digitorum profundus tear, **I:4–106i**, I:4–107
Flexor muscle injury, I:4–211
Flexor pollicis longus tear, **I:4–102i**, I:4–104
Floating knee, I:4–155
Forearm fractures, **I:4–74i**, I:4–74 to I:4–75
Foreign body. See also Bronchial foreign body
    airway, vs. asthma, II:2–101
    musculoskeletal, I:4–18 to I:4–20, **I:4–21i**
        differential diagnosis, **I:4–18i**, I:4–20
    soft tissue abscess vs., **II:4–4i**
Fractures. See also specific bone or region fracture
    avulsion. See Avulsion fractures
    Barton, I:4–75
    burst. See Burst fracture
    clay shoveler fracture, **I:1–76i**, I:1–77
    Garden IV, non-pathologic, **I:4–14i**, I:4–15
    incomplete, I:4–194 to I:4–196, **I:4–197i**
        differential diagnosis, **I:4–194i**, I:4–195 to I:4–196
    insufficiency. See Insufficiency fractures
    pathologic, I:4–14 to I:4–16, **I:4–17i**
        differential diagnosis, **I:4–14i**, I:4–15 to I:4–16
    periprosthetic, II:4–62 to I:4–64, **II:4–65i**
    stress. See Stress fractures
    whiplash. See Whiplash fracture
Fungal sinusitis, invasive, II:1–100 to II:1–102, **II:1–103i**
    differential diagnosis, **II:1–100i**, II:1–101
Fusiform aneurysm, **II:1–12i**, II:1–12 to II:1–13

G

Gadolinium administration, I:1–17
Gallstone erosion, II:3–29
Gallstone ileus, **II:3–54i**, II:3–54 to II:3–55
Gallstones, dropped, **II:3–54i**
Gastric perforation, **II:3–206i**
Gastrocnemius muscle, **I:4–162i**, I:4–163
Gastroenteritis
    ileocolic intussusception vs., II:3–219
    small bowel intussusception in children vs., II:3–231
Gastroesophageal reflux
    hypertrophic pyloric stenosis vs., **II:3–210i**, II:3–211
    midgut volvulus vs., **II:3–186i**, II:3–187
Gaucher disease
    osteonecrosis of hip vs., **II:4–48i**
    sickle cell disease vs., II:2–77
    splenic infection vs., II:3–103
Germ cell tumors, mediastinal, II:2–129
Gestational trophoblastic disease, **II:3–234i**, II:3–235
Giant cell tumor
    pyrophosphate arthropathy vs., II:4–28
    of tendon sheath, vs. gout, I:4–23, **II:4–22i**
Giant serpentine aneurysm, II:1–12
Glenohumeral dislocation
    humeral head/neck fracture vs., I:4–53
    scapular trauma vs., I:4–45
Glenoid fracture, I:4–53
Glioblastoma multiforme, **II:1–48i**, II:1–49
Glioma
    hemorrhagic, **I:1–24i**, I:1–25
    herpes encephalitis vs., II:1–57
    tectal, **II:1–68i**, II:1–69
Gliomatosis cerebri
    acute hypertensive encephalopathy vs., II:1–29

INDEX

perforated
- acute pancreatitis vs., **II:3–152i**, II:3–153
- emphysematous pyelonephritis vs., **II:3–168i**
- trauma vs., **I:3–20i**

Duodenal web
- duodenal atresia or stenosis vs., **II:3–190i**, II:3–191
- midgut volvulus vs., **II:3–186i**, II:3–188

Duodenitis, II:3–29

Duplication cyst
- duodenal atresia or stenosis vs., II:3–191
- small bowel intussusception in children vs., II:3–231

Dural sinuses
- hypoplasia-aplasia, **II:1–36i**, II:1–37
- normal infant, **II:1–36i**, II:1–37

Dystrophic calcifications
- calcific periarthritis vs., II:4–31
- knee avulsion fracture vs., **I:4–142i**, I:4–144

E

Eclampsia, I:1–17

Ectopic pregnancy
- cornual, **II:3–254i**, II:3–255
- tubal, II:3–254 to II:3–256, **II:3–257i**
  - differential diagnosis, **II:3–254i**, II:3–255
  - ovarian torsion vs., II:3–239

Ehlers-Danlos IV, **II:1–12i**

Elbow dislocation, I:4–60 to I:4–62, **I:4–63i**
- differential diagnosis, **I:4–60i**, I:4–61
- humeral shaft/distal humeral fracture vs., **I:4–56i**, I:4–57

Emphysema. See also Pneumomediastinum
- bullous, I:2–9
- lobar
  - bronchial foreign body vs., **II:2–116i**, II:2–118
  - pulmonary interstitial emphysema vs., **II:2–64i**, II:2–65
  - transient tachypnea of newborn vs., II:2–61
- pulmonary interstitial, pediatric, II:2–64 to II:2–66, **II:2–67i**
  - differential diagnosis, **II:2–64i**, II:2–65

Empyema
- epidural, **I:1–4i**, I:1–5
- extra-axial, II:1–52 to II:1–54, **II:1–55i**
  - differential diagnosis, **II:1–52i**, II:1–53
- subdural, **I:1–12i**, I:1–13
- subdural hematoma vs., I:1–9

Encephalitis. See also Herpes encephalitis
- AIDS-related opportunistic infections vs., **II:1–60i**, II:1–61
- inborn errors of metabolism vs., II:1–73
- limbic., II:1–57
- near-drowning vs., **II:1–76i**, II:1–77

Encephalomalacia, II:1–34
Encephalomyelitis, acute disseminated, III:1–62
Endobronchial obstruction, II:2–110
Endometrial implants, II:3–57
Endometrioma, **II:3–246i**, II:3–247

Enteritis
- infectious, II:3–227
- ischemic
  - intestinal trauma vs., **I:3–22i**, I:3–24
  - small intestine vasculitis vs., II:3–47

Enterocolitis
- infectious, I:3–30
- necrotizing, II:3–206 to II:3–208, **II:3–209i**
  - differential diagnosis, **II:3–206i**, II:3–207
- neutropenic. See Typhlitis

Ependymoma, II:1–69

Epididymo-orchitis, II:3–178 to II:3–180, **II:3–181i**
- differential diagnosis, **II:3–178i**, II:3–179
- testicular torsion vs., **II:3–182i**, II:3–183

Epidural hematoma, I:1–4 to I:1–6, **I:1–7i**
- differential diagnosis, **I:1–4i**, I:1–5
- epidural paravertebral abscess vs., II:1–121
- mixed subdural hematoma vs., I:1–13
- subdural hematoma vs., **I:1–8i**, I:1–9

Epidural paravertebral abscess, II:1–120 to II:1–122, **II:1–123i**
- differential diagnosis, **II:1–120i**, II:1–121
- traumatic disc herniation vs., **I:1–106i**, I:1–107

Epidural tumors
- epidural paravertebral abscess vs., **II:1–120i**, II:1–121
- traumatic disc herniation vs., **I:1–106i**, I:1–107

Epiglottitis, II:2–56 to II:2–58, **II:2–59i**
- croup vs., **II:2–52i**, II:2–53
- differential diagnosis, **II:2–56i**, II:2–57
- exudative tracheitis vs., **II:2–48i**, II:2–49

Epiphrenic diverticulum
- esophageal tear vs., I:2–33
- gastric volvulus vs., **II:3–214i**, II:3–215

Epiploic appendagitis, II:3–84 to II:3–86, **II:3–87i**
- differential diagnosis, **II:3–84i**, II:3–85
- mesenteric adenitis vs., II:3–228
- omental infarct vs., **II:3–88i**, II:3–89

Erdheim-Chester disease, II:2–6
Esophageal fistula, I:2–33
Esophageal tear, I:2–32 to I:2–34, **I:2–35i**
- diaphragmatic tear vs., **I:2–28i**, I:2–30
- differential diagnosis, **I:2–32i**, I:2–33
- tracheobronchial tear vs., **I:2–12i**, I:2–13

Esophagectomy, II:3–215
Essex-Lopresti fracture, I:4–68 to I:4–70, **I:4–71i**
Ewing sarcoma, I:4–11, **II:4–10i**
Extraocular muscle, **I:1–44i**, I:1–45

INDEX

Spondylolysis, primary, I:1–71
Spondylometaphyseal dysplasia, **I:4–190i**, I:4–192
Squamous cell carcinoma, **II:1–80i**, II:1–81
Status epilepticus
    acute hypertensive encephalopathy vs., **II:1–28i**, II:1–29
    herpes encephalitis vs., **II:1–56i**, II:1–57
Steatosis, focal, **II:3–126i**, II:3–127
Sternal fracture, **I:2–26i**, I:2–26 to I:2–27
Sternal neoplasms, I:2–26
Sternoclavicular trauma, I:4–36 to I:4–38, **I:4–39i**
    differential diagnosis, **I:4–36i**, I:4–37
Streaming artifact, **II:3–130i**, II:3–131
Stress fractures. *See also* Insufficiency fractures
    adult, I:4–10 to I:4–12, **I:4–13i**
        differential diagnosis, **I:4–10i**, I:4–11
    calcaneal, **I:4–166i**
    compartment syndrome vs., I:4–23
    pathologic fracture vs., I:4–15 to I:4–16
    pediatric, I:4–206 to I:4–208, **I:4–209i**
        differential diagnosis, **I:4–206i**, I:4–207 to I:4–208
    pelvic avulsion fracture vs., I:4–115
    pubic ramus, I:4–119
    sacral, **I:1–102i**, I:1–103
Stress injury
    olecranon, I:4–211
    physeal fractures vs., I:4–187
Stroke. *See* Cerebral ischemia-infarction, acute
Subarachnoid hemorrhage
    aneurysmal, II:1–4 to II:1–5
        differential diagnosis, **II:1–4i**, II:1–5
        meningitis vs., **II:1–44i**, II:1–45
        nonaneurysmal perimesencephalic hemorrhage vs., **II:1–6i**, II:1–7
    nonaneurysmal perimesencephalic, **II:1–6i**, II:1–6 to II:1–7
        aneurysmal hemorrhage vs., **II:1–4i**
    nontraumatic vs. traumatic, **I:1–16i**, I:1–17
    rapid decompression, II:1–29
    spontaneous, **I:1–36i**, I:1–38
    traumatic, I:1–16 to I:1–18, **I:1–19i**
        aneurysmal vs., **II:1–4i**
        differential diagnosis, **I:1–16i**, I:1–17
        perimesencephalic hemorrhage vs., **II:1–6i**, II:1–7
Subcapital femoral fracture, **I:4–138i**, I:4–139
Subdural effusion, **II:1–52i**, II:1–53
Subdural hematoma
    acute, I:1–8 to I:1–10, **I:1–11i**
        differential diagnosis, **I:1–8i**, I:1–9
        dural sinus thrombosis vs., II:1–37
        epidural hematoma vs., **I:1–4i**, I:1–5
        extra-axial empyema vs., **II:1–52i**, II:1–53
        interhemispheric vs. paratentorial, **I:1–14i**, I:1–15
        mixed, **I:1–12i**, I:1–12 to I:1–13
        paratentorial, **I:1–14i**, I:1–14 to I:1–15
Subperiosteal abscess of orbit, II:1–92 to II:1–94, **II:1–95i**
    differential diagnosis, **II:1–92i**, II:1–93
Subperiosteal hematoma, **II:1–92i**, II:1–93
Subphrenic abscess, I:2–30
Substance abuse. *See* Drug abuse
Subtalar dislocation, **I:4–170i**
Subtalar sprain, I:4–180
Superior vena cava (SVC) syndrome, II:2–132 to II:2–134, **II:2–135i**
    differential diagnosis, **II:2–132i**, II:2–133
Superolateral major fissure, **I:2–8i**, I:2–9
Supracondylar fracture, I:4–198 to I:4–200, **I:4–201i**
    differential diagnosis, **I:4–198i**, I:4–199
    elbow dislocation vs., I:4–61
    humeral shaft/distal humeral fracture vs., **I:4–56i**
Surfactant deficiency disease
    neonatal pneumonia vs., **II:2–44i**, II:2–45
    pulmonary interstitial emphysema vs., II:2–65
Swyer-James syndrome, II:2–118
Synovitis
    of hip, toddler's fractures vs., I:4–204
    viral, vs. septic joint, I:4–16, **II:4–14i**
Syphilis
    neurosyphilis, II:1–57
    nonaccidental brain injury vs., I:1–29
Systemic lupus erythematosus (SLE)
    acute interstitial pneumonia vs., II:2–86
    chondritis vs. larynx trauma, **I:1–52i**, I:1–53
    enteritis vs. acute small bowel ischemia, **II:3–42i**, II:3–43
    pneumatosis of intestine vs., **II:3–38i**, II:3–39
    renal infarction vs., II:3–171

T

Talcosis, pulmonary, II:2–92 to II:2–94, **II:2–95i**
    differential diagnosis, **II:2–92i**, II:2–93 to II:2–94
Talofibular ligament, anterior, I:4–179
Talus
    fractures, I:4–170 to I:4–172, **I:4–173i**
        differential diagnosis, **I:4–170i**, I:4–171
        unfused posterior process, **I:4–170i**, I:4–171

INDEX

Temporal bone fractures, I:1–46 to I:1–48, **I:1–49i**
    differential diagnosis, **I:1–46i**, I:1–47
Tendinosis, I:4–115
Tendon tear
    Achilles tendon, I:4–162 to I:4–164, **I:4–165i**
    patellar, I:4–150 to I:4–152, **I:4–153i**
    pelvic avulsion fracture vs., I:4–115
    tibial posterior, **I:4–174i**, I:4–175
Tenosynovitis, **I:4–106i**, I:4–107
Tension hydrothorax, **II:2–136i**, II:2–138
Testicular disorders
    infarct
        epididymo-orchitis vs., **II:3–178i**, II:3–179
        trauma vs., I:3–27
    torsion, II:3–182 to II:3–184, **II:3–185i**
        differential diagnosis, **II:3–182i**, II:3–183
        epididymo-orchitis vs., **II:3–178i**, II:3–179
        trauma vs., **I:3–26i**, I:3–27
    torsion appendix testis
        epididymo-orchitis vs., II:3–179
        testicular torsion vs., II:3–183
    trauma, I:3–26 to I:3–27
        differential diagnosis, **I:3–26i**, I:3–27
        epididymo-orchitis vs., II:3–179
        testicular torsion vs., **II:3–182i**, II:3–183
    tumors
        epididymo-orchitis vs., **II:3–178i**, II:3–179
        testicular torsion vs., **II:3–182i**, II:3–183
        testicular trauma vs., **I:3–26i**
Thalassemia, II:4–71
Thenar muscle injury, **I:4–102i**, I:4–104
Thoracic abnormalities, II:2–62
Thoracic aneurysm, II:2–129
Thoracolumbar fractures
    burst, **I:1–92i**, I:1–92 to I:1–93
    facet-lamina, **I:1–94i**, I:1–94 to I:1–96, **I:1–97i**
Thoracoplasty, **I:2–14i**, I:2–15
Thoracostomy, **I:2–14i**, I:2–15
Thumb, **I:4–102i**, I:4–102 to I:4–104, **I:4–105i**
Tibial fractures
    distal, vs. physeal fractures, **I:4–186i**, I:4–187
    plateau, **I:4–154i**, I:4–154 to I:4–156, **I:4–157i**
Tibial tendon tear, posterior, **I:4–174i**, I:4–175
Toddler's fractures, **I:4–202i**, I:4–202 to I:4–204, **I:4–205i**
TORCH infections, II:1–41
Torsion appendix testis
    epididymo-orchitis vs., II:3–179
    testicular torsion vs., II:3–183
Toxic megacolon, **II:3–74i**, II:3–74 to II:3–75
    cecal volvulus vs., **II:3–100i**, II:3–101
    sigmoid volvulus vs., **II:3–96i**, II:3–97
Tracheitis, exudative, II:2–48 to II:2–50, **II:2–51i**
    croup vs., **II:2–52i**, II:2–53
    differential diagnosis, **II:2–48i**, II:2–49
    epiglottitis vs., **II:2–56i**, II:2–57
Tracheobronchial tear, **I:2–12i**, I:2–12 to I:2–13
Tracheoesophageal fistula, II:2–61
Transient interruption of contrast, II:2–122
Transient post-ictal changes, I:1–21
Transient tachypnea of newborn, II:2–60 to II:2–62, **II:2–63i**
    differential diagnosis, **II:2–60i**, II:2–61 to II:2–62
    meconium aspiration syndrome vs., **II:2–112i**, II:2–113
    neonatal pneumonia vs., **II:2–44i**, II:2–45
Transitional cell carcinoma
    renal vein thrombosis vs., II:3–175
    xanthogranulomatous pyelonephritis vs., II:3–165
Transmesenteric hernia
    internal, **II:3–20i**, II:3–21
    postoperative, **II:3–24i**, II:3–24 to II:3–26, **II:3–27i**
Transscaphoid lunate fracture/dislocation, **I:4–90i**
Trapezium fracture, I:4–87
Trapezoid fracture, I:4–87
Traumatic effusion, **I:1–12i**, I:1–13
Triceps muscle, contusion or hematoma, I:4–65
Triceps tendon rupture, **I:4–64i**, I:4–64 to I:4–66, **I:4–67i**
Triquetrum fracture, I:4–86 to I:4–87
Tuberculosis
    arthritis vs. hemophilia in, I:4–80
    Crohn disease vs., **II:3–34i**, II:3–35
    duodenal ulcer vs., II:3–29
    epidural hematoma vs., I:1–5
    lung abscess vs., II:2–33
    renal, vs. infarction, **II:3–170i**, II:3–171
Tuberculous spondylitis. *See* Osteomyelitis, granulomatous, spinal
Tubo-ovarian abscess. *See also* Pelvic inflammatory disease
    ovarian hemorrhage vs., **II:3–246i**, II:3–247
    ovarian torsion vs., **II:3–238i**, II:3–239
    ovarian vein thrombosis vs., **II:3–242i**, II:3–243
Tumor emboli, **II:2–120i**, II:2–122
Tumoral calcinosis, **I:4–32i**, I:4–33
Typhlitis, **II:3–68i**, II:3–68 to II:3–69
    pseudomembranous colitis vs., II:3–65
    ulcerative colitis vs., II:3–71

U

Ulna
    neuritis vs. medial epicondyle avulsion, I:4–211

INDEX

posterior dislocation vs. supracondylar fracture, I:4–199
stress fracture, I:4–65
Ulnar collateral ligament tear
    elbow dislocation vs., I:4–61
    supracondylar fracture vs., I:4–199
    thumb, I:4–102 to I:4–104, **I:4–105i**
        differential diagnosis, **I:4–102i**, I:4–103 to I:4–104
Ulnar impaction syndrome, II:4–52
Uremia, **II:2–4i**, II:2–6
Ureteral obstruction, II:3–175
Uterine arteriovenous malformation, II:3–234 to II:3–236, **II:3–237i**
    differential diagnosis, **II:3–234i**, II:3–235

V

Valgus trauma, I:4–199
Vascular injury
    extracranial, I:1–40 to I:1–42, **I:1–43i**
        differential diagnosis, **I:1–40i**, I:1–41 to I:1–42
    intracranial, I:1–36 to I:1–38, **I:1–39i**
        differential diagnosis, **I:1–36i**, I:1–37 to I:1–38
Vascular loop, **II:1–8i**, II:1–9
Vascular malformation, hemorrhagic, **II:1–64i**, II:1–65
Vasculitis
    intestinal trauma vs., **I:3–22i**, I:3–24
    intracranial vascular injury vs., **I:1–36i**, I:1–37
    pulmonary, II:2–72 to II:2–74, **II:2–75i**
        differential diagnosis, **II:2–72i**, II:2–73
    renal infarction vs., II:3–171
    renal trauma vs., **I:3–12i**, I:3–13
    small intestine, II:3–46 to II:3–48, **II:3–49i**
        differential diagnosis, **II:3–46i**, II:3–47
    spontaneous intracranial hemorrhage vs., **II:1–20i**, II:1–22
Vasculopathies, fusiform, II:1–13
Vasospasm
    blood blister-like aneurysm vs., **II:1–15i**, II:1–16
    extracranial vascular injury vs., I:1–42
    intracranial vascular injury vs., I:1–37
Venous infarction, **II:1–40i**, II:1–41
Venous malformation
    spinal, I:1–17
    superior vena cava syndrome vs., **II:2–132i**, II:2–133
Ventriculomegaly, II:1–70
Vertebral disc extrusion, **II:1–120i**, II:1–121
Vertebral wedging, I:1–89
Vestibular aqueduct, enlarged, **I:1–46i**, I:1–47
Visceral imaging grading systems, I:3–3
Vocal cord dysfunction
    asthma vs., II:2–101
    paralysis treatment vs.. larynx trauma, I:1–53
Volvulus
    cecal, **II:3–100i**, II:3–100 to II:3–101
    gastric, **II:3–214i**, II:3–214 to II:3–216, **II:3–217i**
    midgut, II:3–186 to II:3–188, **II:3–189i**
        differential diagnosis, **II:3–186i**, II:3–187 to II:3–188
        duodenal atresia or stenosis vs., **II:3–190i**, II:3–191
        hypertrophic pyloric stenosis vs., **II:3–210i**, II:3–211
        meconium peritonitis vs., **II:3–202i**, II:3–203
        meconium plug syndrome vs., II:3–195
    sigmoid, II:3–96 to II:3–98, **II:3–99i**
        cecal volvulus vs., **II:3–100i**
        differential diagnosis, **II:3–96i**, II:3–97
        toxic megacolon vs., **II:3–74i**

W

Wegener granulomatosis
    lung abscess vs., **II:2–32i**, II:2–33
    orbital inflammatory disease vs., II:1–89
Werdnig Hoffman disease, II:2–62
West Nile virus infections, II:1–57
Wet lung disease. *See* Transient tachypnea of newborn
Whiplash fracture
    cervical hyperextension injury vs., **I:1–76i**, I:1–77
    cervical hyperflexion injury vs., I:1–75
    hyperflexion-rotation injury vs., I:1–81
Wilm tumor, II:3–157

X

Xanthofibroma, I:4–23, **II:4–22i**
Xanthofibromatosis, **I:4–162i**, I:4–163

Y

Yersiniosis, **II:3–34i**, II:3–35

Z

Zygomaticomaxillary complex fractures, **I:1–56i**, I:1–57